1973

MSU and Nebraska College of Technical Agriculture are the first programs accredited by the AVMA.

The Association of Animal Technician Educators (AATE) is formed at the Third Symposium on Animal Technician Training.

AVMA House of Delegates passes a resolution proposing "registration" but not "licensing" of animal technicians.

The Committee on Accreditation for Training of Animal Technicians changes its name to the Committee on Animal Technician Activities and Training.

1975

Washington State Association of Veterinary Technicians (WSAVT) is established.

The AATE constitution is adopted, and the first officers are elected. The name of the organization is later changed to the Association of Veterinary Technician Educators (AVTE).

1976

CATAT is recognized by the U.S. Office of Education as the accrediting body for animal technician training programs.

The first professional journal for veterinary technicians is published in the U.S. and is titled *Methods: The Journal for Animal Health Technicians.*

The Veterinary Technicians and Assistants Association of Pennsylvania (VTAAP) is created.

1977

New York offers the first written state examination for animal health technicians.

1978

The Virginia Association of Licensed Veterinary Technicians is established.

AVMA's annual conference includes continuing education classes for animal health technicians for the first time.

The Alberta Association of Animal Health Technologists is formed.

1980

At the AVMA's annual conference in Washington, an ad hoc committee of Canadian and U.S. veterinary technicians and members of the AATE agree to develop an international veterinary technicians association. Plans are made to continue the discussion at the 1981 Western States Veterinary Conference and 1981 AATE Symposium (JAVMA Vol 177 #7 p. 596).

The Compendium on Continuing Education for the Animal Health Technician (later called Veterinary Technician) is first published.

Association Technician Sante Animal du Quebec (ATSAQ) begins, with 25 members.

1981

At the AATE Symposium at Michigan State University, groundwork for the establishment of the North American Veterinary Technician Association (NAVTA) occurs. A name for the new organization, a constitution, and pro tem officers are established this year.

The Association of Zoo Veterinary Technicians is formed.

1982

NAVTA publishes *The Compendium on Continuing Education for the Animal Health Technician.* The title of this publication is changed in 1984 to include the term "veterinary technician."

NAVTA proposes a professional oath.

1984

NAVTA adopts a national code of ethics for veterinary technicians.

First student chapter of NAVTA is formed at Michigan State University.

1985

The AVMA Executive Board establishes the Animal Technician Testing Committee, which generates the Animal Technician National Examination (ATNE) in conjunction with Professional Education Services (PES).

The Association of Animal Technician Educators (AATE) changes its name to the Association of Veterinary Technician Educators (AVTE).

1986

The first ATNE is given in Maine.

The NAVTA Newsletter is developed and distributed.

1988

In Canada, the Eastern Veterinary Technician Association (EVTA) is established.

The AVMA votes no to a resolution that would change terminology from "animal technician" to "veterinary technician."

1989

The Canadian Association of Animal Health Technologists and Technicians (CAAHTT) is formed.

The AVMA House of Delegates approves use of the term "veterinary technician," which replaces the term "animal health technician."

Consequently: CATAT name is changed to CVTEA, ATTC is changed to VTTC, and ATNE is changed to VTNE.

1990

NAVTA adopts its official mission statement and begins a strategic planning process.

NAVTA produces *The World of the Veterinary Technician* videotape and other promotional materials.

The Ontario Association of Animal Health Technicians (OAAHT) establishes a registry.

First annual liaison meeting of NAVTA and AVMA representatives is held at AVMA headquarters in Schaumberg, IL.

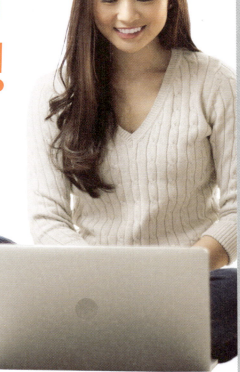

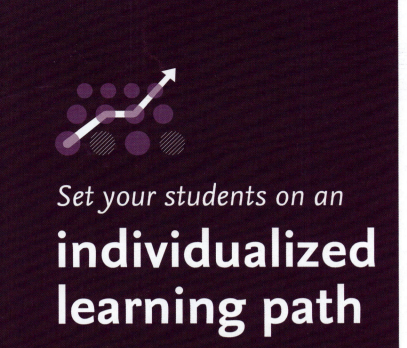

Set your students on an
individualized learning path

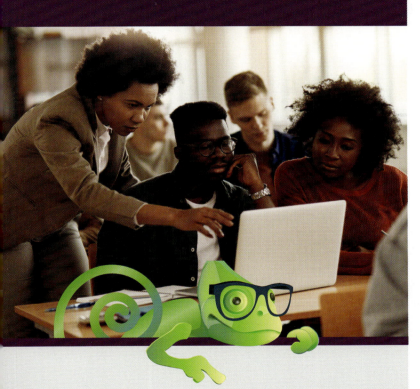

Elsevier's trusted, market-leading content serves as the foundation for all questions, which are written, reviewed, and leveled by experienced educators, item writers, and authors.

Detailed rationales for each question and essential test-taking tips and strategies help students learn how to successfully dissect and tackle different question types and improve test-taking skills for both course exams and summative exams.

A robust educator dashboard highlights usage and performance summaries; areas of strength and weakness tied to topics for each student and class; and data that you can use to modify lectures according to content misconceptions and intervene with struggling students, where necessary.

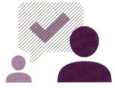

STUDENTS — **Ask your instructor** about enhancing your course experience with EAQ!

INSTRUCTORS — Visit **myevolve.us/EAQ** to learn more!

Elsevier Adaptive Quizzing (EAQ) offers a bank of high-quality practice questions that allow students to advance at their own pace — based on their performance — through multiple mastery levels for each chapter, topic, or concept. EAQ integrates seamlessly into your course to help students of all skill levels focus their study time and effectively prepare for class, course exams, and summative exams.

23-0687 TM/AF

ELSEVIER

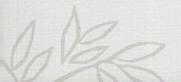

McCURNIN'S
Clinical Textbook for Veterinary Technicians and Nurses

ELEVENTH EDITION

Oreta M. Samples, DHSc, MPH, BS, AAS, RVT

Assistant Professor
Department of Veterinary Science and Public Health,
Program Coordinator, MPH Program
Department of Veterinary Science
Fort Valley State University
Fort Valley, Georgia;
AVA Sub-Review Committee,
Editorial Board - AVTA Journal
National Association of Veterinary Technicians of America
Bridgewater, New Jersey

Paige A. Allen, MS, RVT

Assistant Director for Academic Advising (Retired)
Department of Veterinary Nursing
Purdue University
West Lafayette, Indiana

ELSEVIER

Elsevier
3251 Riverport Lane
St. Louis, Missouri 63043

MCCURNIN'S CLINICAL TEXTBOOK FOR VETERINARY TECHNICIANS
AND NURSES, ELEVENTH EDITION

ISBN: 978-0-323-93651-4

Notice

Previous editions copyrighted 2022, 2014, 2010, 2006, 2002, 1998, 1994, 1990, and 1985.

Content Strategist: Melissa Rawe/Samantha Hart
Senior Content Development Specialist: Kristen Helm
Publishing Services Manager: Deepthi Unni
Senior Project Manager: Beula Christopher
Senior Book Designer: Amy Buxton

Printed in India

Last digit is the print number: 9 8 7 6 5 4 3 2 1

Working together
to grow libraries in
developing countries

www.elsevier.com • www.bookaid.org

To our students, who inspire us, and to the many veterinary technicians, who have taught us the true meaning of dedication.

To three major influences in my life, Kathy Holston, who encourages me constantly to reach for my dreams and never give up, Dr. S. Mobini, who encouraged me in my pursuit to be a writer and never stopped believing in me, and my sister, Lisa Robin Harris, who has shown me what it means to survive ... I hold you all close to my heart.

Oreta M. Samples

To my parents, who believed in me and showed me the importance of always being true to myself. To my mentors, who guided me and challenged me to be better. To my husband, who loves me no matter what, and to my kids and grandkids, who are the future of this world.

Paige A. Allen

Contributors

Beth Overley Adamson, VMD, DACVIM (Oncology)
Veterinary Oncologist
Department of Oncology
Metropolitan Veterinary Associates
Norristown, Pennsylvania

Darcy Adin, DVM, DACVIM
Clinical Professor
Department of Small Animal Clinical Sciences
University of Florida
Gainesville, Florida

Paige A. Allen, MS, RVT
Assistant Director for Academic Advising (Retired)
Department of Veterinary Nursing
Purdue University
West Lafayette, Indiana

Leilani Alvarez, DVM, DACVSMR, CVA, CCRT
Director
Department of Integrative and Rehabilitative Medicine
Schwarzman Animal Medical Center
New York, New York

Courtney Beiter, RVT, VTS (Anesthesia and Analgesia)
Technician
Department of Small Animal Emergency and
    Critical Care
The Ohio State University Veterinary Medical Center
Columbus, Ohio

Mary Lynn Berg, BS, LATG, RVT, VTS (Dentistry)
President and Founder, Consulting
Beyond the Crown Veterinary Education;
Treasurer
Academy of Veterinary Dental Technicians
Lawrence, Kansas;
Adjunct Professor
Department of Veterinary Technology
St. Petersburg College
St. Petersburg, Florida;
Adjunct Professor
Department of Veterinary Nursing
Colby Community College
Colby, Kansas

Leiah Brooks, AAS (Veterinary Technology), RVT
Registered Veterinary Technician
Department of Veterinary Science and Public Health
Fort Valley State University
Fort Valley, Georgia

Kara M. Burns, MS, MEd, LVT, VTS (Nutrition)
Founder
Academy of Veterinary Nutrition Technicians;
Independent Consultant of Nutrition
Lafayette, Indiana

Michelle Campoli, AS, CVT, CVPM
Business Analyst
Veterinary Software and Services
IDEXX Laboratories
Westbrook, Maine

Karen Capps-McMullan, MBA, CPA, RVT
Animal Care Technical Paraprofessional
Department of Veterinary Technology
Fort Valley State University
Fort Valley, Georgia

**Deana Cappucci, BS, LVT, CCRVN, CCMT, VTS (Physical
    Rehabilitation)**
Physical Rehabilitation Nurse
Department of Physical Rehabilitation
West Delray Veterinary
Delray Beach, Florida

Ellen M. Carozza, AAS, LVT, VTS (CP-Feline)
Licensed Veterinary Technician
Private Consulting
The CAT LVT LLC
Herndon, Virginia

Heather Carter, RVT, VTS (Anesthesia and Analgesia)
Animal Health Technician
Department of Small Animal Anesthesia
The Ohio State University Veterinary Medical Center;
Lead Anesthesia Technician
Veterinary Dentistry and Oral Surgery of Ohio
Ohio, Columbus

Michele D. Coarsey, MS, ASCP(SV), RVT
Laboratory Manager II
Department of Serology/Virology
Veterinary Diagnostic and Investigational Laboratory; College of
    Veterinary Medicine; University of Georgia
Tifton, Georgia

Edward Cooper, VMD, MS, DACVECC
Professor - Clinical
Department of Veterinary Clinical Sciences
The Ohio State University
Columbus, Ohio

Danielle DeCormier, AAS Veterinary Technology, LVT, VTS (Oncology), CFE
Director
Clinical Services Education
MedVet
Columbus, Ohio

Lorelei D'Avolio, BS, LVT, CVT, VTS (Clinical Practice- Exotics), CVPM
Assistant Director of Nursing
Department of Emergency and Critical Care, Exotics
Cape Cod Veterinary Specialists
Dennis, Massachusetts

Monique Feyrecilde, BA, LVT, VTS (Behavior)
Owner
Teaching Animals
Maple Valley, Washington

Amy A. Geeding, BS, MS, CVT
Director of Nursing
Veterinary Teaching Hospital
School of Veterinary Medicine - Louisiana State University
Baton Rouge, Louisiana

Mary Ellen Goldberg, BS, LVVN, CVT, SRA (Retired), CCRVN, CVPP, VTS (Physical Rehabilitation and Laboratory Animal Medicine (Research Anesthesia)- Retired)
Certified Veterinary Pain Practitioner,
Independent Contractor,
Faculty/Instructor
Clinical Courses
VetMedTeam, LLC
Boynton Beach, Florida;
Examination Coordinator
Faculty
Canine Rehabilitation Institute
Wellington, Florida

Maxon M. Graham, BS, RVT
Veterinary Technician 3
Large Animal Hospital
LSU School of Veterinary Medicine
Baton Rouge, Louisiana

Temple Grandin, BS, MS, PhD
Professor
Department of Animal Sciences
Colorado State University
Fort Collins, Colorado

Jamie Guiberson, AS, BS, CVT, VTS-EVN
Emergency and Critical Care Nurse
Department of Nursing
New Bolton Center, University of Pennsylvania
Kennett Square, Pennsylvania;
Adjunct Instructor
Veterinary Nursing Program
Harcum College
Bryn Mawr, Pennsylvania

Justin T. Hayna, DVM, Dipl. ACT
Clinical Assistant Professor
Department of Veterinary Clinical Sciences
Purdue University
West Lafayette, Indiana

Holly LeBeau, BS, RVT, AS (Veterinary Technology)
Large Animal Veterinary Technician
Large Animal Hospital,
LSU Veterinary Teaching Hospital
Baton Rouge, Louisiana

Phillip Lerche, BVSc, PhD, DipACVAA
Professor - Clinical
Department of Veterinary Clinical Sciences
The Ohio State University
Columbus, Ohio

Joseph Lozier, DVM, MS, DACVS-LA
Associate Professor- Clinical
Department of Veterinary Clinical Sciences
The Ohio State University
Columbus, Ohio

George W. McCommon, BSA, DVM
Professor
Department of Veterinary Science and Public Health
Fort Valley State University
Fort Valley, Georgia

Rachel McGinty, AAS, RVT
Medical Health Physics Technician
Department of Environmental Health and Safety - Radiation Safety
The Ohio State University
Columbus, Ohio

Tasha McNerney, BS, CVT, CVPP, VTS (Anesthesia)
CEO
Veterinary Anesthesia Nerds
Glenside, Pennsylvania

Samantha Moraux, CVT, VTS (Oncology), AS
Nursing Manager
Department of Emergency
Veterinary Emergency Group
Philadelphia, Pennsylvania;
Oncology Veterinary Technician Specialist
Department of Oncology
Eclipse Specialty and Emergency Pet Care
Wippany, New Jersey

Margaret Mudge, VMD, DACVS, DACVECC
Clinical Professor of Equine Emergency and Critical Care and Surgery
Department of Veterinary Clinical Sciences
The Ohio State University
Columbus, Ohio

Amy Newfield, MS, CVT, VTS (ECC)
Professional Unicorn,
Owner
Veterinary Team Training
Boston, Massachusetts

Carl O'Brien, AAS (Veterinary Technology), RVT, VTS (Anesthesia and Analgesia)
Supervisor
Department of Large Animal Anesthesia
The Ohio State University Veterinary Medical Center
Columbus, Ohio

Heather Prendergast, BS, AS, RVT, CVPM, SPHR
President
Synergie Consulting
Las Cruces, New Mexico

Kara Richmond, CVT
Certified Veterinary Technician
Animal Poison Control Center
American Society for the Prevention of Cruelty to Animals (ASPCA)
Champaign, Illinois

Kristina L. Rothers, BS, CVT, VTS-EVN
Technician
Department of Equine Medicine
Colorado State University, Johnson Family Equine Hospital
Fort Collins, Colorado

Oreta M. Samples, DHSc, MPH, BS, AAS, RVT
Assistant Professor
Department of Veterinary Science and Public Health,
Program Coordinator, MPH Program
Department of Veterinary Science
Fort Valley State University
Fort Valley, Georgia;
AVA Sub-Review Committee,
Editorial Board - AVTA Journal
National Association of Veterinary Technicians of America
Bridgewater, New Jersey

Erin Scott, AAS (Veterinary Technology), LVT, VTS (ECC)
Vet Tech III
Department of Cardiology and Cardiac Surgery
Colorado State Veterinary Teaching Hospital
Fort Collins, Colorado

Philip J. Seibert Jr., CVT
Consultant
SafetyVet
Calhoun, Tennessee

David L. Shuey, LMSW, DMA
Veterinary Social Worker
Department of Veterinary Wellness
Indevets
Philadelphia, Pennsylvania

Nanette Walker Smith, MEd, RVT, CVT, LVT
Licensed Veterinary Technician,
Practice Consultant (Veterinary) and Coach,
Fear Free Independent Consultant,
Teacher
Secondary - Substitute
Lewis-Palmer School District 38
Monument, Colorado
Events Coordinator
Happy Cats Haven
Manitou Springs, Colorado;
Advisory Committee
Colorado Academy of Veterinary Technicians
Colorado Springs, Colorado

Andrea M. Steele, MSc, RVT, VTS(ECC)
Chair
Animal Care Programs
Conestoga College
Kitchener, Ontario, Canada

Lori L. Stose, DVM, BA
Assistant Professor
Department of Veterinary Science and Public Health
Fort Valley State University
Fort Valley, Georgia

Margaret L. Trenta, BA, LVT
Surgery Suite Supervisor
Veterinary Teaching Hospital
Louisiana State University
Baton Rouge, Louisiana

Ann B. Weil, DVM, DACVAA
Clinical Professor
Department of Veterinary Clinical Sciences
Purdue University
West Lafayette, Indiana

Jarred Williams, MS, DVM, PhD, DACVS-LA, DACVECC-LA
Clinical Professor
Department of Large Animal Medicine
University of Georgia
Athens, Georgia

Olivia M. Holt Williams, RVT
Licensed Veterinary Technician,
Director of Nursing
Veterinary Teaching Hospital
University of Georgia
Athens, Georgia

Tina Wismer, DVM, MS, DABVT, DABT
Senior Director
ASPCA Animal Poison Control Center
Champaign, Illinois

Anni Wojcieszko, DVM, JD, LLM
Relief Veterinarian, Self-Employed
Attorney, Self-Employed
Cleveland, Ohio

Moges Woldemeskel, DVM, MVSc, PhD, DACVP
Professor
Department of Veterinary Pathology
Tifton Veterinary Diagnostic and Investigational Laboratory
University of Georgia, College of Veterinary Medicine
Tifton, Georgia

Ann Wortinger, BIS, LVT, VTS (ECC)(SAIM)(Nutrition), Elite FFCP
Content Development Coordinator
Department of Education
Appalachian State University
Belleville, Michigan

Liza Wysong Rudolph, BAS, RVT, VTS
Program Director
Department of Veterinary Technology
Rowan College of South Jersey
Sewell, New Jersey

Preface

Dear Reader,

Paige Allen and I proudly present the 11th edition of *McCurnin's Clinical Textbook for Veterinary Technicians and Nurses*. This textbook represents a longstanding tradition of academic excellence in veterinary technology. We hope this latest version will be a treasured resource for educating veterinary technicians. As a labor of love directed toward animals and a reflection of our dedication to advancing the profession of veterinary nursing, we continue to select topics that are relevant to the needs of the 21st century veterinary technician student, particularly those enrolled in programs accredited by the American Veterinary Medical Association (AVMA).

We hope that this textbook will serve as the foundation for study, not only in college but also later when new graduates prepare for the Veterinary Technician National Examination and beyond—when they face questions and when decisions are to be made regarding the immediate care of their patient. No textbook can cover the full spectrum of knowledge required by today's veterinary technicians to succeed. Our goal is to focus on key topics aligned with the directions of AVMA requirements for accredited programs, to build a foundation of veterinary nursing supportive of both general and specialty practices.

Key Features

This edition is generously illustrated with beautifully curated and updated photographs, line drawings in full color, and numerous tables and boxes. Each chapter begins with a **Chapter Outline**, a list of **Key Terms**, and a series of **Learning Objectives**. **Technician Notes** continue to be a helpful study tool for students. An updated and comprehensive **Glossary** reflective of the key terms in each chapter appears at the end of the text.

Organization

The book is divided into eight sections that are delineated by different-colored pages:
- Part 1 introduces the profession; it focuses on practice management, computer applications, medical records, and health and safety.
- Part 2 transitions into topics related to essential patient management and nutrition. This section begins with animal behavior, restraint, handling, and physical examination. Subsequently, it offers an overview of preventive health medical nursing, small and large animal nutrition, and reproduction.
- Part 3 covers the four major disciplines in laboratory clinical sciences and concludes with chapters on diagnostic imaging and basic necropsy procedures.
- Part 4, Medical Nursing, includes diagnostic sampling and therapeutic techniques for both small and large animals,

including a series of illustrations that emphasize the veterinary technician's role in collecting specimens. This section also provides information on small and large animal medical nursing, veterinary oncology, alternative medicine and rehabilitation techniques, and physical therapy. This part of the textbook also includes a chapter covering the care of birds, reptiles, and small mammals.
- Part 5, Emergency and Critical Care, begins with fluid therapy and transfusion medicine. Subsequent chapters address the emergency and critical care patient, toxicology, wound management, and bandaging.
- Part 6, Anesthesia, Analgesia, and Pharmacology, is a critical part of the textbook for veterinary nurses and covers the fundamentals of these three disciplines.
- Part 7 covers surgical instrumentation, aseptic technique, operating room conduct, assisting, and suture materials. Surgical nursing topics specific to small and large animals are subsequently covered, followed by a chapter on veterinary dental technology.
- Part 8 concludes the textbook by focusing on end-of-life issues, including geriatric and hospice care, the importance of the human-animal bond, and euthanasia.

The Learning Package

The 11th edition of *McCurnin's Clinical Textbook for Veterinary Technicians and Nurses* is designed as a comprehensive learning package.

The student package includes:
- Textbook
- Student Workbook
- Evolve website

The faculty package includes:
- Textbook
- TEACH Instructor Resources
- Student Workbook
- Evolve website

The entire package has been designed with the student and the educator in mind. The ease of reading each comprehensive chapter, along with the additional materials, provides students with the maximum opportunity to learn. The driving force in developing this package was to provide an educational structure to accredited veterinary technology programs to help them produce knowledgeable and clinically proficient veterinary technicians.

Student Workbook

The Student Workbook is designed to be a supplement to the learning process. The content of the Workbook matches the book chapter by chapter to help students master and apply key concepts and procedures in a clinical situation. Multiple choice questions, matching exercises, photo quizzes, labeling exercises, crossword puzzles, and other activities to guide the learning process are included.

TEACH Instructor Resources

Available on Evolve, TEACH Instructor Resources are designed to save the instructor time and to take the guesswork out of classroom planning and preparation. The resources include Lesson Plans, PowerPoint Slides, Student Handouts, an updated Test Bank, and answers to the Workbook Exercises.

Evolve Website

Elsevier has created a website dedicated solely to supporting this learning package: http://evolve.elsevier.com/Samples/McCurnin/. The website includes a student site and an instructor site.

Student site resources include:

- Medical Record Forms: 25 medical records that correlate directly with the medical records chapter in the book. These full-size forms can be printed and used. They are listed alphabetically.
- Chapter Review Questions.
- Expanded Glossary.
  Faculty site resources include:
- TEACH Instructor Resources
- Lesson Plans
- PowerPoint Lecture Presentations
- Student Handouts
- Test Bank, consisting of 1500 questions
- Answer Key, containing answers to the questions included in the Workbook
- Image collection
- Access to all student resources

Oreta M. Samples
Paige A. Allen

Acknowledgments

We would like to acknowledge those who held this role before us—Dennis McCurnin, Joanna Bassert, John Thomas, and Angela Beal. Their dedication to this book provided us with an amazing foundation and we hope that we have made you proud.

Thank you to all the contributors for their time, knowledge, and dedication to making the content accurate and useful. Their love of this profession and their belief in the future veterinary nursing profession shines in each word.

We also want to thank the team at Elsevier, for without them the development of the 11th edition of *McCurnin's Clinical Textbook for Veterinary Technicians and Nurses* would not have been possible.

Oreta M. Samples
Paige A. Allen

Contents

Part 2   Patient Management and Nutrition

Part 7 Surgical Nursing

How to Use This Learning Package

McCurnin's Clinical Textbook for Veterinary Technicians and Nurses, 11th edition, is the ultimate learning package for preparing students to become veterinary technicians. It provides a solid foundation for the basic and advanced clinical skills that students must master to achieve competence, and its student-friendly style clarifies even the most complex concepts and procedures to help prepare for the Veterinary Technician National Examination (VTNE) and certification.

Textbook Features

- **Chapter Outlines** introduce you to the chapter material, allowing you to see at a glance how the subject material is organized. It also helps you focus on one topic at a time by showing you relationships to other topics in the chapter.
- **Learning Objectives** help you focus on key concepts and procedures.
- **Key Terms** listed at the beginning of the chapter reinforce new terminology.
- **Introduction** gives an overview of the chapter that distills the key points and focuses your study.
- **Case Presentations** challenge you to apply your knowledge of chapter content to realistic clinical scenarios to solve problems and make appropriate decisions.
- **Technician Notes** are interspersed throughout each chapter to help you retain key information related to the technician's role.
- **Procedure boxes** present clear, step-by-step guidelines for performing important tasks.
- **Put Into Practice boxes** demonstrate and suggest ways that the technician can utilize the knowledge they are studying into hands-on clinical practice with their patients.
- **Glossary** with definitions of the key terms from each chapter reinforces new terminology and helps you comprehend the reading material.

Student Workbook

The Student Workbook, sold separately, includes review exercises for all chapters, including definitions of key terms; matching, fill-in-the-blank, true-false, and review questions; and photo quizzes, word searches, and crossword puzzles.

Evolve Website

The Evolve website includes learning resources available to instructors and students using *McCurnin's Clinical Textbook for Veterinary Technicians and Nurses,* 11th edition. At the beginning of this textbook is a page introducing the Evolve site. All you need to get started is a computer and an Internet connection. To register as a Student or an Instructor, enter the following URL: http://evolve.elsevier.com/Samples/McCurnin/. Follow the directions for "Instructors" or "Students" to create an Evolve account. You will have to do this only one time.

Student resources include the following:
- Medical Record Forms: 25 medical records that correlate directly with the medical records chapter in the book. These are full-size forms that can be printed and used.
- Chapter review questions that are mapped to VTNE.
- Expanded Glossary.

Faculty resources include the following:
- TEACH Instructor Resources
- Lesson Plans
- PowerPoint Lecture Presentations
- Student Handouts
- Test Bank
- Answer Key, containing answers to the questions provided in the Workbook
- Image Collection, containing all the images from within the book, plus some additional images
- Access to all student resources

Additional Resources

Coville & Bassert
Clinical Anatomy and Physiology for Veterinary Technicians, 3e
Combining expert clinical coverage with engaging writing and vivid illustrations, this popular text is key to understanding the anatomic and physiologic principles that will carry you throughout your career.

Brown & Brown
Lavin's Radiography for Veterinary Technicians, 7e
This concise, step-by-step text gives you the knowledge and skills you need to produce excellent radiographic images. It covers the physics of radiography, the origin of film artifacts, and positioning and restraint of small, large, avian, and exotic animals.

Christenson
Veterinary Medical Terminology, 3e
Reader-friendly and organized by body system, this textbook helps you quickly gain a solid understanding of veterinary terminology. Essential word parts and terms are presented in the context of basic anatomy physiology and disease conditions giving you the tools to immediately apply new terminology to practical clinical situations.

Hendrix & Robinson
Diagnostic Parasitology for Veterinary Technicians, 6e
This book features clear and concise discussions of the most commonly encountered internal and external parasites.

Holmstrom

Veterinary Dentistry: A Team Approach, 4e

From radiology to anesthesia to patient needs and client education, this handy, full-color guide covers everything you need to know about veterinary dentistry!

Prendergast

Front Office Management for the Veterinary Team, 3e

Focusing on the day-to-day duties of the veterinary team, this book offers a complete guide to scheduling appointments, billing and accounting, communicating effectively and compassionately with clients, managing medical records, budgeting, marketing your practice, managing inventory, and using outside diagnostic laboratory services.

Sirois

Laboratory Procedures for Veterinary Technicians, 7e

This book covers the broad spectrum of laboratory procedures that veterinary technicians need to perform effectively in the private setting.

Studdert, Gay, & Blood

Saunders Comprehensive Veterinary Dictionary, 5e

This is the most comprehensive dictionary in the field, offering a wide range of full-color illustrations and over 60,000 main entries and subentries, including information on large animals, small animals, and exotics, in an all-new, user-friendly format.

Taylor

Small Animal Clinical Techniques, 3e

With step-by-step instructions for more than 60 procedures, this must-have textbook includes everything you need to learn the techniques you need for everyday practice.

Martini-Johnson

Applied Pharmacology for Veterinary Technicians, 6e

This book helps you learn how to administer prescribed drugs to animals, calculate drug dosages accurately, and instruct clients about side effects and precautions. Coverage of drug information includes pharmacokinetics, pharmacodynamics, clinical uses, dosage forms, and adverse effects.

1

Introduction to Veterinary Nursing and Technology: Its Laws and Ethics

ANNI WOJCIESZKO

CHAPTER OUTLINE

LEARNING OBJECTIVES

When you have completed this chapter, you will be able to:

1. Pronounce, define, and spell all the key terms in this chapter.
2. Describe the events from 1963 to 2019 that led to the development of modern veterinary technology in the United States and Canada.
3. Describe the educational and credentialing requirements established in most states and provinces for entry into the profession of veterinary technology.
4. Explain the structure, format, and scheduling of the Veterinary Technician National Examination (VTNE).
5. List the six features that characterize a profession.
6. Describe the five steps of the veterinary technician practice model.
7. Describe the scope of practice for veterinary technicians and list five duties performed only by veterinarians.

1

8. Describe areas of responsibility for veterinary technicians in clinical practice.
9. List the members of the veterinary health care team and describe their respective roles; include a list of the veterinary technician academies recognized by the National Association of Veterinary Technicians of America (NAVTA) in your definition of veterinary technician specialist.
10. Describe professional appearance, conduct, and communication.
11. Name the organizations represented by the acronyms AVMA, CVMA, CVTEA, NAVTA, AAVSB, and RVTTC and describe their roles in the education and credentialing of veterinary technicians.
12. Describe professional ethics.
13. Differentiate between statutes (laws) and regulations.
14. Describe the role of state boards in the credentialing of veterinary professionals.
15. List possible grounds for disciplinary action by state or provincial boards, list three levels of supervision defined in the NAVTA Model Rules and Regulations and describe how these levels affect the veterinary technician's scope of practice.
16. Describe steps and possible sanctions carried out during disciplinary action against a licensee.
17. Describe how laws related to labor, contracts, medical waste, controlled substances, and animals relate to the profession of veterinary technology.
18. Name and describe animal laws.

KEY TERMS

American Animal Hospital Association (AAHA)
American Association for Laboratory Animal Science (AALAS)
American Association of Veterinary State Boards (AAVSB)
American Veterinary Medical Association (AVMA)
Analgesia
Anger
Animal Care Committee (ACC)
Animal Welfare Act (AWA)
Assistant laboratory animal technician (ALAT)
Association of Veterinary Technician Educators (AVTE)
Canadian Association of Laboratory Animal Science (CALAS)
Canadian Veterinary Medical Association (CVMA)
Committee on Veterinary Technician Education and Activities (CVTEA)
Committee on Veterinary Technician Specialties
Drug Enforcement Agency
Horse Protection Act (HPA)
Institutional Animal Care and Use Committee (IACUC)
Laboratory animal technician (LAT)
Laboratory animal technologist (LATG)
National Association of Veterinary Technicians of America (NAVTA)
Practice acts
Professional Examination Service (PES)

Registered master laboratory animal technician (RMLAT)
Registered Veterinary Technologists and Technicians of Canada (RVTTC)
Registered Veterinary Technologists and Technicians of Canada/ Technologues et Techniciens Vétérinaires en Registrés du Canada
Registry of Continuing Education (RACE)
Resolution
Rules and regulations
Societies
Technician evaluation
Technician intervention
U.S. Fish and Wildlife Service (US FWS)
Validation
Veterinarian
Veterinary assistant
Veterinary nurse
Veterinary practice
Veterinary technician
Veterinary Technician National Examination (VTNE)
Veterinary technician practice model
Veterinary technician specialist (VTS)
Veterinary technologist
Veterinary technology

Introduction

The care and treatment of injured and sick animals is an important, challenging job that requires intelligence, excellent observational skills, and the ability to work efficiently within a collaborative clinical team. It also requires patience, compassion, and tenacity. These talents are embodied within the profession commonly known as *veterinary technology* or *veterinary nursing*. The term *veterinary technician* is commonly used in the United States and Canada, while *veterinary nurse* is uniformly used in countries throughout Europe. As the terms *technician* and *technology* are increasingly associated with the use and maintenance of technical equipment, such as computers, use of the term *veterinary nurse* is becoming more popular in the United States, because it is believed to more accurately reflect the job at hand and the level of education and skill required in modern veterinary practices today. A movement to increase use of the term *veterinary nurse* in the

United States and Canada is known as the *Veterinary Nurse Initiative*. In this edition, the terms *veterinary technician* and *veterinary nurse* are both used throughout the text.

Veterinary technicians and veterinary nurses are essential members of the veterinary health care team, because they perform all animal care duties except those that by law may *only* be performed by veterinarians. Like the registered nurse in the human health care field, the veterinary nurse assesses hospitalized patients, gathers clinical information, and uses critical thinking to generate nursing care plans that help alleviate a hospitalized patient's reaction to disease and improve patient comfort and recovery. As part of the veterinary health care team, the veterinary nurse carries out the medical orders of the *veterinarian* and is aided by *veterinary assistants*. In addition, veterinary technicians and nurses, particularly those working in general small- and large-animal practices, are expected to perform the duties of radiology and laboratory technicians and those of medical, surgical, and anesthesia nurses (Fig. 1.1). Finally, veterinary

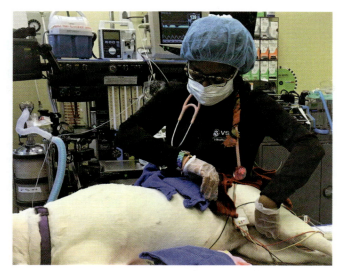

• **Fig. 1.1** The veterinary nurse has emerged as a critical component of the veterinary health care team. This nurse-anesthetist monitors pulse rate and pulse intensity immediately after a surgical procedure. (Courtesy Dr. Joanna Bassert.)

nurses and technicians must be prepared to work with multiple species and ready to address a broad range of clinical responsibilities.

Over the past 60 years, veterinary medicine has become highly sophisticated, giving rise to the expanded role and critical importance of veterinary nurses and technicians. It is no longer possible to provide high levels of medical care while attaining acceptable profit margins without the support of veterinary nurses and technicians. A skilled practitioner of patient assessment and critical thinking, the veterinary nurse or technician regularly evaluates the status of hospitalized patients and independently carries out nursing interventions to improve patient comfort and morale. Monitoring patient progress and pain level and providing wound care as ordered by the veterinarian are some of the essential services veterinary nurses and veterinary technicians provide. Also, these important professionals carry out the treatment orders of the supervising veterinarian, keeping doctors apprised of patient status such as pain level, wound status, and patient mentation. In outpatient clinics and many general veterinary practices, veterinary nurses and technicians assist veterinarians with daily appointments, including routine health care. In our televised modern world, veterinary-centered television programs have heightened the awareness of modern **veterinary practice** and have led to heightened public expectations that animal patients will receive excellent care from the veterinary nurse and veterinarian.

PUT INTO PRACTICE

Finding your place in veterinary medicine is about investigating the opportunities for you as a technician to practice at your highest skill level. Explore employment options such as specialization as well as nontraditional career options.

This chapter presents an overview of the profession of veterinary nursing, including the profession's history, educational requirements, range of duties, salaries, specialties, professional organizations, and expectations for professional conduct. It introduces the veterinary technician practice model in the United States and the steps that define the veterinary nursing process. The laws and ethics that define the profession of veterinary technology in the United States and Canada, govern its credentialing process, and support animal welfare are also discussed.

Veterinary Technician Oath

"I solemnly dedicate myself to aiding animals and society by providing excellent care and services for animals by alleviating animal suffering and by promoting public health.

I accept my obligations to practice my profession conscientiously and with sensitivity, adhering to the profession's code of ethics and furthering my knowledge and competence through a commitment to lifelong learning."

History of Veterinary Technology

Historically, many veterinarians practiced independently and performed many of the laboratory and nursing duties themselves. Often, spouses, family members, and other laypersons served as assistants, receptionists, and office managers. Today, corporations or teams of veterinarians own many practices. Modern practices often employ many veterinarians and require a staff of credentialed veterinary technicians, assistants, receptionists, and kennel workers to carry out the many duties required in running a successful veterinary hospital. This team approach is a fundamental part of veterinary practice management today, and the veterinary technician often serves as an important link between the veterinarian, support personnel, and pet owner.

The profession of veterinary nursing and technology in the United States began to take form in the early 1960s with the establishment of the first formal university-level program for the education of animal health technicians. The period since then has been rich with the accomplishments of dedicated veterinary technicians and veterinarians who committed themselves to the advancement of patient care by defining, developing, and advancing the profession of veterinary technology (refer to the Timeline on the inside covers of this textbook).

Veterinary technicians were first called *animal health technicians* in the United States and Canada. The adjective "veterinary" referred exclusively to veterinarians until 1989, when the term *veterinary technician* was formally approved by the House of Delegates of the American Veterinary Medical Association (AVMA). Now, hundreds of accredited programs of veterinary technology are available in Canada and in the United States, and this number is steadily increasing. Current listings of the programs accredited by the AVMA can be found at the AVMA website (www.avma.org). Programs in Canada that are accredited by the Canadian Veterinary Medical Association (CVMA) and by the **Registered Veterinary Technologists and Technicians of Canada/Technologues et Techniciens Vétérinaires en Registrés du Canada (RVTTC)** can be found at their website (www.rvttcanada.ca). Thousands of individuals have graduated from these programs, and the number of veterinary technology programs continues to grow as demand for educated, skilled veterinary personnel increases.

The Veterinary Nurse and Technician Today

The veterinary technicians and nurses in North America and the veterinary nurses in Europe work in a wide range of facilities, perform many kinds of tasks, and may work with diverse types of animal species. Veterinary nurses and technicians may work in private or corporate veterinary practices, such as companion-animal, large-animal, or mixed-animal practices. (A *mixed-animal practice* is one that treats both farm and companion animals.) They also may work in zoos, aquariums, wildlife rehabilitation centers, and research facilities, and in industry as sales representatives of veterinary products. They may become entrepreneurs by establishing their own kennel facility or pet-sitting business. Veterinary nurses and veterinary technicians who earn advanced degrees may become instructors in veterinary nursing and technology programs or in other related academic programs. The range of job opportunities for veterinary nurses and technicians today is broader than ever before.

Within this diverse array of opportunities, veterinary nurses and technicians may narrow their field of work and concentrate on specific areas. For example, a technician or nurse working in a practice that treats exotic species, such as birds and reptiles, will develop skills and knowledge particular to that aspect of veterinary nursing. In addition, some veterinary practices are specialty or *referral practices*, because they employ veterinarians who have completed specialized advanced training in a particular aspect of veterinary medicine or surgery. Pet owners may be referred to a veterinary specialist for advanced care of their pets. Specialty areas may include dermatology, surgery, internal medicine, cardiology, etc.

Veterinary nurses and technicians who work in specialty practices see unusual cases and become skilled in addressing the needs of these often critically ill patients. Specialty practices often share facilities with an emergency, critical care, or trauma practice that is open all day and all night. Some veterinary nurses and technicians prefer the challenge, excitement, and unpredictability of emergency practice and have dedicated their careers to this aspect of veterinary nursing, and some others prefer the relative predictability of working in specialty areas, such as dermatology, cardiology, or internal medicine.

As interest in veterinary technician specialties grew in the United States, the **National Association of Veterinary Technicians of America (NAVTA)** developed the **Committee on Veterinary Technician Specialties (CVTS)** to help guide and structure the development of specialties for veterinary technicians. The CVTS provides a standardized list of criteria and assistance for societies interested in attaining academy status. Each academy establishes the standards and requirements for the **Veterinary Technician Specialist (VTS)** designation in its discipline. Therefore each veterinary technician awarded a VTS designation has completed requirements for formal education, clinical training, and standardized testing. **Societies** may be formed by veterinary technicians who share a common interest in a particular aspect of veterinary technology. The formation of a society by veterinary technicians often precedes the formation of a NAVTA-approved specialty in that same field. Further information about societies and specialties can be found at https://navta.net/.

Employment Prospects, Salaries, and Attrition

Widespread shortages of veterinary technicians continue to be reported throughout the United States and Canada, providing graduates of veterinary technology programs with ample job opportunities. According to the US Bureau of Labor Statistics website, employment of veterinary technologists and technicians is projected to continue to grow at a rate of 20% from 2014 to 2031, much faster than the average for all occupations. Although job opportunities are plentiful, salaries vary, depending on the field of interest, the location of employment, and the level of experience of the veterinary technician. It also depends on the level of respect and recognition the employer has for the education and training of the credentialed veterinary technician. It is recommended that veterinary technicians avoid working at practices that do not appropriately distinguish between veterinary technicians (or

veterinary nurses) and veterinary assistants. This may be evident on the "meet our staff" section of a practice's website.

In May 2021, the US Bureau of Labor Statistics reported that the median wage for veterinary technicians and technologists nationwide was $36,850 per year. In addition, the level of experience, location of work, and field of interest may also have a significant impact on income potential. For example, veterinary technicians working for the federal executive branch of government, such as the US Department of Agriculture (USDA), and veterinary technologists working in colleges and universities, earn on average more than technicians working in social advocacy organizations, such as community animal shelters or in veterinary practices. Veterinary technicians living in states where there is a higher density of veterinary practices earn more than technicians living in less populated states. Texas, California, Florida, Pennsylvania, and New York, in this order, employ the greatest number of veterinary technicians at the highest average salary in the United States. Because demand for credentialed veterinary technicians and technologists is particularly high in these states, the median salaries in these areas reflect this demand.

The sector in which a veterinary technician works also affects income. Veterinary technicians in general practice may earn $33,000 to $50,000, depending on the levels of experience and responsibility. VTSs and veterinary technicians who work in education earn salaries significantly higher than those of technicians working in other areas. An experienced VTS in emergency and critical care nursing who oversees an intensive care facility may earn $50,000 to $75,000 per year in the greater Philadelphia area, while in New York City, the salary for the same work may be significantly higher. Technicians who assume practice management duties may be paid a higher salary. The range of salaries for veterinary technicians can be surprisingly broad, depending on the technician's level of experience, credentials, work sector, and geographic location.

Before beginning a job search, veterinary technicians are encouraged to determine their living expenses, student loan payments, transportation, and insurance costs. This provides a clear assessment of financial needs and enables the veterinary technician to move into a job search with the knowledge of their own salary requirements. Veterinary technicians who make this calculation are better able to judge job offers, to ask for 100% of what they want with confidence (based on what they need), and to establish sound financial goals for themselves moving forward.

In addition to salary compensation, many employers offer a range of benefits, including health insurance, retirement plans, and allowances for continuing education (CE) and professional membership fees. Large corporations are generally better equipped to provide benefit packages compared with small private businesses. However, veterinary practices that are owned by for-profit corporations have obligations to stockholders. To pay dividends or meet income benchmarks, they may offer lower salaries and fewer benefits to employees compared with privately owned veterinary hospitals and may also expedite the handling of clients and patients to maximize profits. As veterinary technicians evaluate employment sites, it is important to read and understand the mission and the vision statement of each practice. These drive the veterinary hospital's culture and the relative value placed on patients and the medical professionals who care for them.

The profession of veterinary technology has a high rate of attrition. Graduate technicians report leaving the profession because of lack of appreciation, underutilization, low pay, and lack of advancement opportunities. Attrition from the profession is a critical part of the current technician shortage problem. Many states have shortages of many sectors, including veterinarians, veterinary assistants, and veterinary technicians and technologists.

Because employee attrition is extremely costly to practices, both fiscally and in terms of the morale and efficiency of the veterinary health care team, improved staff management and retention of veterinary technicians is particularly important to the fiscal health of veterinary practices. Statistics gathered by the AVMA indicate that the most financially sound practices are those that make full use of their veterinary nursing and assistant staff, delegating to them all the patient care duties except those tasks that, by law, may only be performed by veterinarians.

In most states, only veterinarians may perform surgery, prognose, diagnose, prescribe, and attest to the health status of a patient. All other tasks may be delegated to the veterinary technician and the assistant. Those veterinary practices that make maximal use of veterinary technicians/nurses while acknowledging and respecting the difference between veterinary technicians/nurses and veterinary assistants generally have higher staff retention rates and revenues compared with practices that do not distinguish between these two different cohorts.

> **TECHNICIAN NOTE**
>
> Veterinarians in well-managed veterinary practices complete only the tasks that, by law, they alone are permitted to do. All other animal care tasks should be delegated to veterinary technicians or veterinary nurses and, where applicable, to veterinary assistants.

Education

Programs of Veterinary Technology

Like nursing schools in the human health care field, programs of veterinary technology may include undergraduate courses and bestow an associate degree or a baccalaureate degree. Programs in the United States are accredited by the Committee on Veterinary Technician Education and Activities (CVTEA), which is under the auspices of the AVMA. Programs in Canada are accredited by the Animal Health Technology/Veterinary Technician Program Accreditation Committee (AHT/VTPAC), which is under the auspices of the CVMA. When a program is accredited, it must meet 11 essential criteria for curricula, faculty, facility, and admissions requirements. Each program must submit reports to the accrediting body for review semiannually, annually, or biannually, depending on the age and stability of the program. In addition, the accrediting body carries out on-site visits of each program. Based on on-site evaluation and preassessment documentation, recommendations by the accrediting body are classified into three categories: critical, major, and minor deficiencies. Programs must report to the accrediting body any progress made in addressing the deficits cited by the on-site review committee.

The curriculum of veterinary technology programs includes general college-level courses, such as biology and chemistry, and courses specific to clinical practice, such as veterinary parasitology, medicine, medical terminology, and clinical chemistry. In addition, more than 350 "essential" and "recommended" tasks are listed in the *Accreditation Policies and Procedures Handbook* of the CVTEA, which constitutes the foundation of the hands-on curriculum for laboratory and practical training (Fig. 1.2). Some baccalaureate degree programs include advanced veterinary technology courses in the junior and senior years in addition to the

standard curriculum required by the associate AVMA-accredited programs. As the profession continues to grow, greater numbers of baccalaureate programs are expected to be established, and a few of these programs will offer increasing numbers of advanced veterinary technology courses. Refer to Box 1.1 for a list of courses typically offered in veterinary technology programs.

Standard Criteria

Through the development of standard criteria for each required task, AVMA-accredited programs ensure consistency of standards among various faculty members and classroom sections, and between distance education and traditional on-campus courses. In addition, programs are required to document that every student has successfully completed each of the required tasks before graduation.

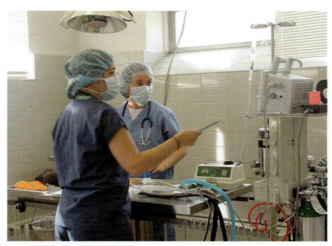

• **Fig. 1.2** An instructor *(left)* in an accredited veterinary technician program draws a student's attention to a patient monitor in a small-animal clinical laboratory.

• **BOX 1.1**   **Types of Courses Required in Veterinary Technology Programs**

Basic Math and Science Courses
Technical Math
Biology
Chemistry
Microbiology
Comparative Mammalian Anatomy and Physiology
Medical Terminology
Computer Science

Veterinary Technology Courses
Introduction to Veterinary Technology
Veterinary Practice Management
Animal Management and Nutrition
Farm Animal Clinical Procedures
Companion Animal Clinical Procedures
Laboratory Animal Science
Animal Medicine
Veterinary Radiology
Animal Parasitology
Veterinary Hematology
Veterinary Clinical Chemistry and Urinalysis
Veterinary Surgical Assisting
Veterinary Pharmacology and Anesthesiology

Distance Education

Although most veterinary technology programs are offered to students in the traditional on-campus fashion, programs are available via web-based distance education. Distance education programs provide educational opportunities to students around the world. The courses are rigorous and require a high degree of self-discipline from students, who often must work independently. Communication with teachers and classmates is encouraged and sometimes required by the courses. The flexibility of distance education programs makes them particularly well suited for mature students who are already working in veterinary practices and who may not live near a college or university.

Many distance education programs require that students work in veterinary practices while completing online course work. This enables students to be supervised by an employer or another mentor as they develop the required hands-on skills. In addition, it offers ready access to many of the materials and animals needed to complete required clinical tasks. For documentation, distance learning students are often asked to videotape themselves successfully completing tasks in keeping with the program's standard criteria and the AVMA requirements. They may be asked to complete projects such as blood films, radiographs, laboratory tests, written assignments, and examinations.

Continuing Education (CE)

Most states and provinces require veterinary technicians to attend CE lectures and workshops to maintain credentials (licensure, certification, or registration). These lectures are available at various national, regional, and local professional conferences and workshops throughout the United States and Canada, and through AVMA- and CVMA-accredited programs of veterinary technology. CE is also available online via webinars or web-based lectures and through the websites of many professional associations and veterinary information centers. See Table 1.3 (later in the chapter) for a list of professional associations and veterinary information links. As veterinary medicine rapidly progresses and changes, it is particularly important for veterinary technicians to commit themselves to a career of lifelong learning.

The Veterinary Technician National Examination (VTNE)

After completing the requirements to graduate from a program of veterinary technology, students prepare to take the **Veterinary Technician National Examination (VTNE)**, which is required in the vast majority of states and provinces in the United States and Canada, respectively. The VTNE is designed to evaluate the competency of entry-level veterinary technicians. Most states and Canadian provinces require that applicants are graduates of an AVMA-accredited or CVMA- accredited program of veterinary technology to be eligible to take the VTNE.

The VTNE was first developed under an agreement between the American Association of Veterinary State Boards (AAVSB) and the Professional Examination Service (PES). The AAVSB is represented by the Veterinary Technician National Examination Committee (VTNEC), which is composed of veterinarians and veterinary technicians engaged in clinical practice, national professional associations, AVMA-affiliated specialty boards, and academia. Members of the committee are recommended by the executive boards of the AVMA, NAVTA, Association of Veterinary Technician Educators (AVTE), RVTTC, and AAVSB. Once recommended, these representatives are then formally appointed by the Board of Directors of the AAVSB.

The VTNE is a computer-based examination that is available in English and French. Only 150 of the 170 questions count toward the final score. The additional 20 questions are piloted for possible use in the future. The PES provides the committee with three draft examinations for their review and **validation**. These drafts are developed from a computerized bank of questions, originally written by veterinarians and veterinary technicians from all aspects of the veterinary medical profession. The questions are reviewed independently for accuracy, relevance to the field of veterinary technology, and level of difficulty. In addition, the questions are screened for grammar, style, and conformity to psychometric principles.

The VTNE is offered at testing centers throughout North America. Three 30-day windows are available for candidates to complete the VTNE: March 15 to April 15, July 15 to August 15, and November 15 to December 15.

Candidates may apply to take the VTNE on the AAVSB website (www.aavsb.org) and can list their preferences for the testing center location and the date and time when they would like to take the examination. In addition, the candidates must send to the AAVSB proof of having graduated from an AVMA- or CVMA-accredited veterinary technician program.

Immediately after the candidate completes the examination, a provisional pass or fail is given. Scaled scores are subsequently tallied by the PES, and the AAVSB dispatches these scores electronically to both the candidate and the school from which the candidate graduated.

The examination is composed of 150 multiple-choice questions that cover the following 10 primary areas or domains within the profession of veterinary technology:

1. Pharmacy and pharmacology, 13%
2. Surgical nursing, 13%
3. Dentistry, 7%
4. Laboratory procedures, 9%
5. Animal care and nursing, 20%
6. Diagnostic imaging, 6%
7. Anesthesia, 13%
8. Emergency medicine/critical care, 7%
9. Pain management/**analgesia**, 7%
10. Communication and veterinary professional support services, 5%

Twenty new questions are added to each examination. These additional questions do not count toward the final score of the candidate but are inserted to determine how well the candidates answer them and whether the questions qualify as repeatable questions. Candidates are not aware of which questions are confirmed and which are untested.

Candidates who wish to have their VTNE scores sent to multiple state boards must register with the Veterinary Information Verifying Agency (VIVA) through the AAVSB. A fee is required for registration with the VIVA, along with an additional fee for each transfer. It is important to note that requirements for the credentialing of veterinary technicians vary among the states and the provinces. Therefore to obtain information regarding credentialing requirements specific to a jurisdiction, veterinary technicians who relocate to other states or provinces are encouraged to consult the respective AAVSB and state or provincial boards.

The Profession of Veterinary Technology and Veterinary Nursing

The roles of the veterinary technician and the veterinary nurse are varied. The type of facility, the location of the practice, and the range of species that are treated all dramatically affect the spectrum of responsibilities. Some veterinary technicians and nurses are also leaders within the practice and have management and clinical responsibilities. Veterinary technicians and nurses who work in large urban specialty hospitals, for example, may have enormous responsibilities such as caring for critically ill patients, maintaining inventory, and hiring and scheduling support staff. Veterinary technicians and nurses who work in modest, small rural communities with one or two attending veterinarians may have fewer responsibilities. In this way, the range of responsibilities for veterinary technicians and nurses can be quite broad.

In general, practicing veterinary technicians administer nursing care to hospitalized animals in a conscientious and knowledgeable manner. They regularly assess each hospitalized patient's status and report significant findings and status changes to the supervising veterinarian. Veterinary technicians may develop and implement their own care plans to address the hospitalized patient's changing reaction to the following:

1. A procedure or illness
2. A patient's risk for future problems
3. An owner's knowledge deficits and limitations in coping with pet care at home

What Defines a Profession?

Professions such as veterinary technology are characterized by six features:

1. The profession comprises individuals who have completed specific undergraduate or graduate education programs within the framework of a higher learning institution and successfully passed national and/or state qualifying examinations.
2. The profession is based on a specific body of knowledge that leads to defined skills, abilities, and conduct.
3. The profession provides a specific service.
4. The profession comprises individuals who act independently and make decisions based on observation, knowledge, critical thinking, and independent analysis.
5. The profession has a code of ethics and conduct.
6. In the United States, the profession is structured by **practice acts** and corresponding **rules and regulations** in each state. These laws and regulations are enforced and upheld by an overseeing committee, which is typically the state licensing board or board of governors.

What Structure Is in Place to Define and Guide the Clinical Responsibilities of Veterinary Technicians?

The Veterinary Technician Practice Model

Veterinary technicians are responsible for the independent assessment and care of hospitalized patients and for carrying out the medical orders of the veterinarian. Patient assessment, critical thinking, the analysis of patient data, and the development of nursing care plans tailored to each patient are all part of the veterinary technician's responsibilities. The **veterinary technician practice model** provides a structured approach to patient care and ensures that consistent excellent care is provided to each patient. In this way, the practice model is the foundational discipline of veterinary technology. For the veterinary technician student, it offers a systematic approach to critical thinking and problem solving.

The veterinary technician practice model consists of five steps that are performed cyclically throughout a patient's hospitalization period. Routinely hospitalized patients, such as healthy postoperative (spayed and neutered) patients and emergency and critical care patients, should both be evaluated by using this same systematic approach:

1. Gather data about the patient.
2. Identify and prioritize patient evaluations.
3. Develop and implement a plan for patient care by establishing a series of veterinary nursing interventions.
4. Evaluate the patient's response to the plan of care.
5. Gather additional data (go back to Step 1 and re-evaluate the patient).

Step 1: Gather Data

When patients are admitted for hospitalization, veterinary technicians assist veterinarians in gathering data to establish an initial database. The database is composed of subjective and objective information. The subjective information includes observable information, such as the patient's history and nonmeasurable physical examination findings. Examples of subjective data include observations about the patient's mentation, hydration status, and appetite level.

Objective data includes measurable patient information, such as vital signs (heart rate, respiratory rate, blood pressure, and body temperature) and laboratory results (complete blood count [CBC] and serum chemistry analysis).

Step 2: Identify and Prioritize Patient Evaluations

Once the database is collected, the veterinary technician uses reasoning to develop a list of patient evaluations. These evaluations are analogous to those leading to a nursing diagnosis in the human nursing profession. They reflect the animal's response to physiologic and psychological changes caused by a particular disease process, trauma, treatment, change in diet, owner neglect, etc. **Technician evaluations** are not made exclusively in emergency and critical care practices. Rather, they are made as a routine part of all levels of veterinary nursing.

A veterinarian is responsible for diagnosing and curing the patient, whereas a veterinary technician assesses and alleviates the patient's reaction to disease, surgery, or trauma; assesses the patient's risk for future problems; and educates the pet owner. Patient evaluations therefore fall into one of three categories:

1. Evaluations that relate to actual physical and psychological problems of the patient, such as "hypovolemia," "abnormal eating behavior," and "fear."
2. Evaluations that relate to the risk of or potential for problems in the future, such as "risk for infection" and "risk of aspiration."
3. Evaluations that relate to the owner (also called the *client*), such as "client knowledge deficit" and "noncompliant owner."

Next, the veterinary technician prioritizes the evaluations so that the most life-threatening problems are addressed first (Table 1.1). The most critical problems are considered foundation issues because, if they are not addressed first, the animal may not live. For this reason, the foundation evaluations are listed at the bottom of Table 1.1 in the same way that the foundation of a house, which is closest to the ground, is the most important component of a healthy, well-built building. Evaluations are divided into nine categories; the *most important* issues at the bottom relate to oxygenation, and the least important issue at the top pertains to utility. All evaluations that are related to oxygenation, such as "obstructed airway," "altered ventilation," and "altered gas diffusion," would be addressed early in the technician's plan of care.

Step 3: Develop a Plan of Care and Implement Interventions

After the evaluations have been prioritized, the veterinary technician develops a written plan of care. The veterinary technician uses

TABLE 1.1 Identification and Prioritization of Patient Evaluations in the Veterinary Technician Practice Model

Priority	Category	Evaluation
9 *Lowest priority* Address these evaluations last	Utility	Aggression Anxiety Client coping deficit Client knowledge deficit Fear Inappropriate elimination Reproductive dysfunction
8	Activity	Exercise intolerance Reduced mobility Sleep disturbance
7	Chronic pain/ acute pain (mild to moderate)	Mild to moderate pain Acute pain Chronic pain
6	Noncritical safety	Altered mentation Altered sensory perception Noncompliant owner Hyperthermia Hypothermia Impaired tissue integrity Owner knowledge deficit Risk of infection Risk of infection transmission Self-inflicted injury Status within appropriate limits
5 *Middle priority*	Nutrition	Altered oral health Abnormal eating behavior Ineffective nursing Overweight Self-care deficit Underweight Vomiting/diarrhea
4	Elimination	Altered urinary production Bowel incontinence Constipation Diarrhea Inappropriate elimination Self-care deficit Urinary incontinence
3	Hydration	Hypervolemia Hypovolemia
2	Critical safety/ acute pain (severe)	Acute pain Electrolyte imbalance Hyperthermia (severe) Hypothermia (severe) Postoperative compliance Preoperative compliance
1 *Highest priority* Address these evaluations first!	Oxygenation	Altered gas diffusion Altered ventilation Cardiac insufficiency Decreased perfusion Obstructed airway Risk of aspiration

critical thinking and creativity to develop a unique series of **technician interventions** for the patient. These interventions should address the technician evaluations of the patient listed in Step 2. For example, if a technician evaluation indicates that the patient is hypothermic, the veterinary technician can include the intervention "Place and monitor warming devices and blankets" as part of the technician plan of care. Similarly, if the patient is experiencing pain, the technician can list the intervention "Notify the veterinarian about pain" as part of the technician nursing plan so that pain medication is ordered.

Step 4: Evaluate Patient Response

Re-evaluation of the patient and adjustment of the technician's plan of care ensure that the patient's condition is monitored as it improves or worsens with treatment. The technician may examine and re-evaluate the patient several times throughout the day.

Step 5: Add Data

As the patient's condition changes with treatment and hospitalization, additional tests, laboratory studies, and physical examinations may be needed. These processes yield additional data for the technician to analyze and evaluate. In this way, this step is similar to Step 1, because it includes the continued collection of new or additional data that could influence the patient's recovery.

TECHNICIAN NOTE

The veterinary technician practice model consists of five steps that are performed cyclically throughout a patient's evaluation period. Routinely hospitalized patients, such as healthy postoperative spayed and neutered patients, and emergency and critical care patients should all be evaluated using this same systematic approach. The veterinary technician practice model therefore is not exclusive to emergency and critical care practice; it is the foundation of veterinary nursing of all patients. Independently evaluating your patients is what it means to practice veterinary nursing.

Scope of Practice

As the sophistication of veterinary medicine has increased, the responsibilities of the veterinary technician in clinical practice have also broadened. However, much variability has been noted among veterinary practices in the ways in which veterinary technicians are employed and used. In well-managed practices, veterinary technicians perform all duties associated with the care and treatment of animal patients except those tasks that can only be legally performed by a veterinarian. In addition, veterinary technicians are empowered to delegate appropriate tasks to veterinary assistants. Although state laws differ, it is widely accepted and has been proposed by both the AVMA and the AAVSB that *only* veterinarians may do the following:

1. Prescribe
2. Diagnose
3. Prognose
4. Perform surgery

In other words, veterinary technicians cannot diagnose or prognose; prescribe any treatments, drugs, medications, or appliances; or perform surgery or attest to the health status of an animal. However, they are allowed to carry out all other patient care duties, including placement of catheters by all routes. Therefore it is important that the veterinary technician, when completing veterinary medical records, enter the notation, "as ordered," after administering each treatment, drug, medication, or appliance ordered by the veterinarian.

In addition to patient care and client education, the veterinary technician may be involved in nonclinical tasks, such as personnel management, management of facilities and equipment, and inventory control. Modern veterinary practices are organized into distinct working areas. Depending on their job description and the size of the practice, a veterinary technician may work in all, a few, or only one of the areas discussed in the sections below.

Responsibilities of the Veterinary Technician in Practice

Reception Area

Although many practices hire receptionists, not veterinary technicians, to work in the reception area, it is important for the clinical staff to be cross trained in this aspect of the practice so that important information gathered by the receptionist can be accessed easily when they are not available. The veterinary technician should be familiar with the computer system and the practice management software used by the practice. This will facilitate obtaining existing records, creating new patient records, and accessing medical histories and billing information during emergencies that may occur after hours.

Outpatients and Examination Rooms

The veterinary technician helps ensure that office visits are handled efficiently and professionally. This involves directing clients to the examination room or treatment area, obtaining a history and physical exam, weighing the patient, and acquiring vaccines, instruments, and materials needed for the visit. The veterinary technician may also collect blood at this time and may obtain skin scrapings and fecal, urine, and cytology samples for laboratory testing. In addition, the veterinary technician provides information to clients about preventive care, diet, behavior modification, medication, discharge instructions, and surgical procedures.

Because pet owners are often more at ease talking to the veterinary technician than to the veterinarian, the technician can be a valuable support person for bereaved or worried pet owners. The veterinary technician answers clients' questions both in person and over the telephone, and occasionally must address difficult or angry pet owners.

Laboratory and Pharmacy

The veterinary technician has the skills to perform laboratory tests used in practice (Fig. 1.3). The number of laboratory tests performed on site varies. In veterinary hospitals that make full use of these skills, veterinary technicians perform CBCs, differential counts, and morphologic examinations of blood. They perform urinalysis, including examination of urine sediment, and fecal analysis for evidence of parasites. Veterinary technicians are skilled in the use of enzyme-linked immunosorbent assay (ELISA) test kits, glucose meters, refractometers, and dry chemistry analyzers. In addition, veterinary technicians are familiar with the interpretation of common cytologic preparations, such as ear swabs and vaginal smears.

Once a diagnosis is made, the veterinarian prescribes, in writing or orally, a treatment for the animal patient. The veterinary technician interprets the prescription language and then fills and dispenses the medication to the pet owner, along with instructions for its use. In addition, veterinary technicians are often responsible for ensuring that the pharmacy is well stocked, that expired drugs are discarded, and that controlled substances are handled appropriately.

Radiology and Special Imaging

The veterinary x-ray examination (also known as *radiography*) is an important diagnostic tool. Veterinary technicians are skilled in radiographic techniques, including patient positioning, selecting the proper settings, and taking exposures at appropriate times. In addition, technicians ensure that hospital staff members protect themselves from harmful radiation by wearing appropriate protective clothing (lead aprons, gloves, and thyroid shields) and that dosimeters are used routinely to monitor x-ray exposure. Technicians may be responsible for managing the ordering and mailing of dosimeters as well.

Modern veterinary technology programs teach students to use digital radiographic equipment and software, which allows for adjustment of the image to maximize accurate image detail (Fig. 1.4). Digital imaging has many advantages over standard radiographic techniques. It is faster to produce, easier to adjust, and convenient to store. Digital images can be sent electronically to specialists for evaluation or to referring veterinary hospitals. Similarly, special imaging techniques, such as computed tomography (CT), and magnetic resonance imaging (MRI), are being used

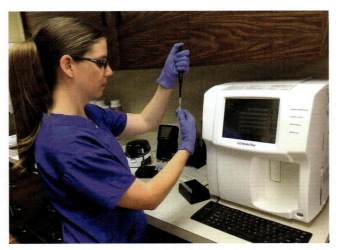

• **Fig. 1.3** A certified veterinary technician in Pennsylvania completes laboratory tests using automated analyzers. (Courtesy Joanna Bassert.)

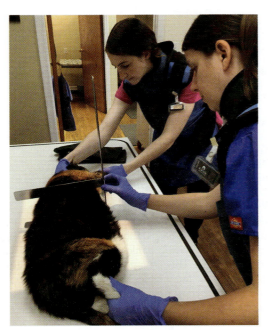

• **Fig. 1.4** Veterinary technicians are skilled in the use of radiographic equipment. (Courtesy Dr. Joanna Bassert.)

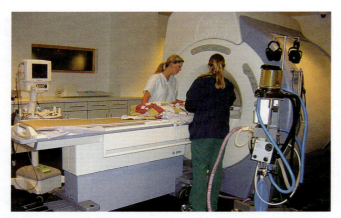

• **Fig. 1.5** Advanced imaging techniques, such as the use of magnetic resonance imaging (MRI), as shown, are becoming an important diagnostic tool in veterinary medicine today. (Courtesy Dr. Joanna Bassert.)

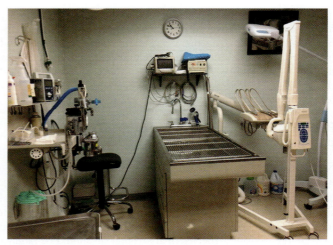

• **Fig. 1.7** This dental suite is used by veterinary technicians who perform oral examinations, dental charting, and prophylactic teeth cleaning. (Courtesy Dr. Joanna Bassert.)

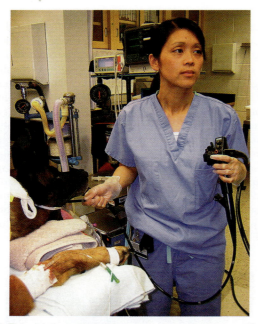

• **Fig. 1.6** This veterinary technician works in a specialty practice where she has become proficient in using fiberoptic endoscopes. (Courtesy Dr. Joanna Bassert.)

with increasing frequency in veterinary medicine (Fig. 1.5), particularly in specialty practices and veterinary teaching hospitals. Veterinary technicians are also playing a greater role in collecting images using ultrasonography and endoscopy (Fig. 1.6), which are subsequently interpreted by a radiologist.

Treatment Room

Most veterinary hospitals have a treatment room for various procedures and surgical preparation. The treatment area may be a large central room with a bank of cages for postoperative and critical care patients. This arrangement facilitates monitoring of hospitalized patients and enables the technical staff to be efficient in completing important treatment duties. Dental units and procedure sinks may be used in the main treatment room, where dentistry and minor surgical procedures are performed.

Veterinary technicians and veterinary nurses are responsible for carrying out orders for the administration of medication. This involves giving medications by all routes (i.e., orally,

intramuscularly, and intravenously). It may also involve placing catheters, setting up, and monitoring intravenous (IV) fluid administration. Blood may be collected, and the animal may be routinely checked for alertness, temperature, pulse, respiration, urination, and defecation. For critical cases, treatment may include changing bandages, lavaging open wounds, placing and monitoring nasal oxygen, and maintaining chest, tracheal, urethral, or abdominal tubes. Veterinary technicians are responsible for documenting all treatments, data, and physical findings in the patient's record. The patient record is an important legal document and serves as a means of ensuring that errors in treatment are not made.

The veterinary technician or nurse prepares the patient before entry into the operating room (OR). This involves ensuring that the animal has been appropriately fasted and has urinated before surgery. The technician is responsible for weighing the animal and for calculating and administering preoperative anesthetic agents. In many veterinary practices, the veterinary technician is also responsible for induction and maintenance of anesthesia. Although an animal can be anesthetized in many ways, this procedure usually involves placing an IV catheter, setting up fluids, placing an endotracheal tube, and administering IV and/or gas anesthetic agents. Monitoring equipment, such as the pulse oximeter, capnograph, esophageal stethoscope, Dinamap monitor, Doppler ultrasonography machine, or blood pressure monitor, may be used by the technician to monitor the anesthetized patient. Before moving the patient to the OR, the technician clips hair and performs an initial skin preparation of the surgical area. Often, a technician is responsible for carrying out routine dental procedures that must be performed while the animal is anesthetized (Fig. 1.7). In this situation, the technician must perform two important jobs at once, namely, monitor the patient under anesthesia and complete oral examinations and dental health procedures, such as scaling and polishing the patient's teeth. The veterinary technician must be prepared for anesthetic emergencies and should be familiar with emergency drugs and procedures needed to resuscitate animals in crisis.

Operating Room

The OR nurse positions the animal patient on the operating table and completes the final surgical scrub. Necessary instruments, equipment, and materials are made available (Fig. 1.8). The OR nurse retrieves any additional materials requested during

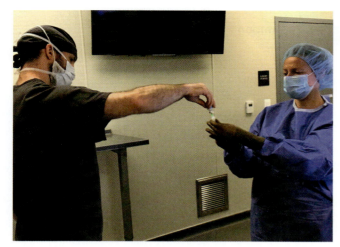

• **Fig. 1.8** An operating room technician *(left)* offers a vial of medication to the surgeon *(right)*, who uses a sterile syringe to draw up the medication without touching the vial. (Courtesy Dr. Joanna Bassert.)

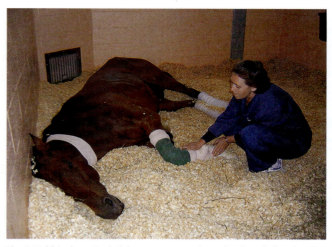

• **Fig. 1.10** Veterinary technicians assess and monitor hospitalized patients and are often the first to notice an animal in pain or distress. Technicians are responsible for alerting the attending veterinarian and ensuring that ward patients receive effective pain management, as ordered. (Courtesy Dr. Joanna Bassert.)

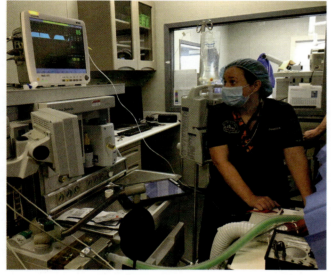

• **Fig. 1.9** Administering anesthetics and monitoring anesthetized patients constitute some of the most challenging aspects of veterinary technology and are associated with a high level of responsibility for the life of the patient. This technician is monitoring a patient undergoing an orthopedic procedure. The head of the patient *(not visible)* is to the right, under the blue drape. (Courtesy Dr. Joanna Bassert.)

the patient, and intraoperative monitoring of blood pressure and heart and respiratory rates. A negative change in vital signs might require the veterinary nurse to give compensational and resuscitative drugs. Although modern anesthetic agents are considered safe to use, risk exists whenever an anesthetic is administered. Unexpected reactions to anesthetic agents, surgical complications, and human error can be fatal. The nurse-anesthetist must be meticulous about checking and rechecking the functionality of the anesthesia machine. The valves, tubing, vaporizer, oxygen delivery systems, and rebreathing bags must all be in good working condition. The nurse-anesthetist is also responsible for checking and rechecking the equipment before anesthetizing the patient.

Wards

Veterinary nurses also play an important role on the wards, not only in ensuring that treatments are given correctly and in a timely manner but also in providing compassion and a gentle touch to animals. The nurturing that animals receive when they are sick is an important part of their recovery. Even healthy animals that are being boarded benefit from special care and reassurance from technical staff members.

The veterinary nurse is often the first to observe changes in a patient's status (Fig. 1.10). Difficulties with IV lines, infusion pumps, or monitoring equipment are also first noticed by the veterinary nurse. Immediate patient assessment and interventions are carried out by the ward nurse, documented in the medical record, and communicated to the veterinarian. Throughout the patient's hospitalization, the veterinary nurse assesses and reassesses patient status, develops new evaluations, and adjusts the nursing care plan. During these periodic patient assessments, the veterinary nurse looks for signs of pain in the patient and ensures that appropriate pain management is provided as ordered by the veterinarian.

Hospital Management and Communications

Veterinary technicians and nurses, particularly those with an interest in business, may pursue additional education in hospital management and become employed as hospital managers. They may oversee the veterinary staff and assist with scheduling, hiring, personnel and client management, bookkeeping, and inventory

the procedure, adjusts the surgery lights, tilts the surgery table, and, in general, does whatever is necessary to support the surgeon. In some practices, the veterinary nurse acts as both anesthetist and circulating nurse. Technicians may be asked to assist during a particularly challenging operation and must be skilled in proper sterile techniques, including gloving and gowning. After the procedure has been completed, the technician cleans the surgical instruments and reorganizes them into surgical packs for sterilization. The technician may also perform the duties of the postoperative care nurse for the recovering patient.

Being an anesthetist is one of the most important duties of the veterinary nurse (Fig. 1.9). In some practices, veterinary nurses are responsible for completing dosage calculations for preoperative, postoperative, and intraoperative drugs. The veterinary nurse is also responsible for the induction of anesthesia, intubation of control. Increasingly, veterinary technicians and nurses, particularly those in large practices, are drawn into management duties, such as management of technical staff and ordering of supplies. In states or provinces where it is legal for nonveterinarians to own veterinary practices, veterinary technicians have become practice owners and managers.

Terminology and the Veterinary Health Care Team

Productive and efficiently managed veterinary practices depend on the dedication of a team of veterinary professionals and support personnel (Table 1.2). As described in the following sections, each member of the team plays a collaborative role in providing quality health care to the animal patient (Fig. 1.11).

Veterinarian

A veterinarian typically completes 4 years of study at an AVMA- or CVMA-accredited college of veterinary medicine after completing 4 years of undergraduate study. Graduates of veterinary medical schools are distinguished by the initials DVM after their names unless they have graduated from the University of Pennsylvania, in which case they will have the initials VMD after their names. To practice, veterinarians must be licensed by the state or province in which they work. Typically, this requires successful completion of national and state/provincial examinations and payment of a licensing fee. For a current listing of accredited colleges of veterinary medicine in the United States and Canada, go to the AVMA website (www.avma.org). In some states, exceptions for licensure are made for veterinarians who are employed in university veterinary teaching hospitals.

Veterinarians who have completed an educational program and examination in a particular medical or veterinary medical specialty are "board certified." In veterinary medicine, the specialty boards are associated with the AVMA. For example a veterinarian may become board certified in surgery by the specialty organization known as the *American College of Veterinary Surgeons* (ACVS). A board-certified veterinary surgeon may use the initials "ACVS" after their name and advertise as a "specialist" in surgery. To *maintain* the specialty certification, the veterinarian must complete CE in the chosen specialty as mandated by the specialty board. Board-certified veterinarians often practice in groups as "referral" hospitals and primarily see patients referred by other practicing veterinarians for a second opinion or for the performance of complex diagnostic, surgical, and therapeutic procedures.

Veterinary Technician Specialist

In February 1994, NAVTA formed the CVTS to address the growing interest among veterinary technicians in attaining higher levels of skill and knowledge in a particular aspect of veterinary technology. For this reason, the CVTS established a process and a list of criteria for the formation of academies in specialized fields of veterinary technology.

To form a specialty, a group of veterinary technicians with an interest in a particular field of veterinary technology would first establish a professional society. After the society has grown, it may then petition the CVTS for recognition as an academy. The

TABLE 1.2	Common Professional Terminology
Acronym	**Name**
Veterinary Health Care Team	
ACT	Animal care technician
AHT	Animal health technician
CVPM	Certified veterinary practice manager
CVT	Certified veterinary technician
DVM	Doctor of veterinary medicine
LVN	Licensed veterinary nurse
LVT	Licensed veterinary technician
OJT	On-the-job–trained (veterinary assistant)
RAHT	Registered animal health technician
RVN	Registered veterinary nurse
RVT	Registered veterinary technician
VA	Veterinary assistant
VHM	Veterinary hospital manager
VMD	Veterinary medical doctor (University of Pennsylvania)
American Laboratory Animal Technology	
AALAS	American Association of Laboratory Animal Science
ALAT	Assistant laboratory animal technician
LAT	Laboratory animal technician
LATG	Laboratory animal technologist
Canadian Laboratory Animal Technology	
CALAS	Canadian Association of Laboratory Animal Science
ARLAT	Associate registered laboratory animal technician
RLAT	Registered laboratory animal technician
RMLAT	Registered master laboratory animal technician

organizing committee of the proposed academy, together with the CVTS, establishes the advanced requirements and the examination process for becoming a VTS in the field of interest. As of this printing, NAVTA (www.navta.net) has recognized 16 areas of specialty in veterinary technology (Box 1.2).

Thus the VTS is a veterinary technician who has reached a higher level of skill and understanding in a particular field of veterinary technology (Box 1.3). The VTS must meet the criteria set by each academy. The most common criteria are:

- Must be a graduate of an AVMA-accredited program of veterinary technology and/or be legally credentialed to practice veterinary technology in their respective state, province, or country.
- Must have successfully completed the education, training, and experience requirements established by the respective academy of specialists.
- Must be reviewed and approved for specialist status by the academy.

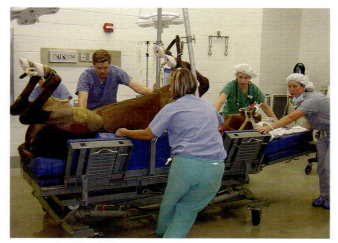

• **Fig. 1.11** The veterinary health care team must work collaboratively to provide the best possible veterinary medical care. Here, a veterinary team moves an anesthetized horse to the recovery stall. (Courtesy Dr. Joanna Bassert.)

• BOX 1.2 NAVTA-Recognized Areas of Specialty for Veterinary Technicians

The Academy of Veterinary Emergency and Critical Care Technicians
The Academy of Veterinary Dental Technicians
The Academy of Internal Medicine Veterinary Technicians
The Academy of Veterinary Technicians in Anesthesia and Analgesia
The Academy of Laboratory Animal Veterinary Technicians and Nurses
The Academy of Veterinary Behavior Technicians
The Academy of Veterinary Clinical Pathology Technicians
The Academy of Veterinary Technicians in Clinical Practice
The Academy of Dermatology Veterinary Technicians
The Academy of Equine Veterinary Nursing Technicians
The Academy of Physical Rehabilitation Veterinary Technicians
The Academy of Veterinary Nutrition Technicians
The Academy of Veterinary Ophthalmic Technicians
The Academy of Veterinary Surgical Technicians
The Academy of Veterinary Zoological Medicine Technicians
The Academy of Veterinary Technicians in Diagnostic Imaging

To learn more about a particular specialty, search for the academy name to find the website.

It is also recommended that applicants maintain membership in national, state/province, and local veterinary technician associations, and join the specialty society.

As mentioned earlier, veterinary technicians who have achieved specialty status are signified by the initials VTS (with their field of specialty in parentheses) after their names. For example, the technician Mary Jones, CVT, VTS (dentistry), is a specialist in veterinary dentistry.

The VTS often works in specialty and referral veterinary hospitals and in teaching hospitals associated with universities. In these environments, the VTS can concentrate on their field of interest and can share knowledge with veterinary medical and veterinary technology students.

Veterinary Technologist

In the United States, the **veterinary technologist** holds a bachelor of science (BS) degree in veterinary technology from an AVMA-accredited program. The veterinary technologist works in such positions as project leader, practice supervisor, or teacher in a veterinary technology program and may require a greater level of education than is required for the veterinary technician position. Some veterinary technologists, particularly those employed in teaching hospitals of veterinary medical schools, become highly skilled in a particular aspect of veterinary technology. Some institutions and practices use the term *veterinary technologist* to refer to a veterinary technician who holds a bachelor's degree in any field.

In Canada, the term *veterinary technologist* is synonymous with the term *veterinary technician* or a graduate of a college program in Ontario.

Veterinary Technician

A **veterinary technician** is a person who has earned an associate of science (AS) degree in veterinary technology or veterinary nursing. After graduating, veterinary technicians are required to complete national and state examinations before they can be credentialed (licensed, registered, or certified).

Frequently, veterinary technicians pay a fee to the state veterinary association to receive a license, certification, or registration. The term *veterinary nurse*, rather than *veterinary technician*, is used in European countries.

Veterinary Assistant

The term *veterinary assistant* is used to describe a person who is involved in the care of animals and is not a veterinary technician, laboratory animal technician, or veterinarian. Typically, veterinary assistants are responsible for assisting the veterinary technician and the veterinarian by restraining animals, setting up equipment and supplies, cleaning and maintaining practice and laboratory facilities, and feeding and exercising patients. Most veterinary assistants are trained on the job by a supervising veterinary technician or veterinarian, but some assistants complete 4 to 6 months of training in a formal course of study.

The profession of veterinary technology started to take form in the early 1960s. Before this time, the position of a veterinary technician, as defined today, did not exist, and veterinary practices depended exclusively on the skill of on-the-job–trained veterinary assistants. Today, veterinary assistants continue to constitute a large and important portion of the workforce in veterinary practices nationwide. Veterinary technicians and veterinary assistants work together in many veterinary practices, and although the AVMA and NAVTA make clear distinctions between the two groups, some states do not have such distinctions between these roles.

The growing number of traditional and distance AVMA- and CVMA-accredited programs make education in the field of veterinary technology more accessible to veterinary support staff members who wish to become veterinary technicians.

Laboratory Animal Technicians and Technologists

The American Association for Laboratory Animal Science (AALAS) and the Canadian Association of Laboratory Animal Science (CALAS) have established a certification program that

Each veterinary technician academy has its own requirements for becoming a technician specialist. Specific requirements can be found on each of the academy websites. The Academy of Emergency and Critical Care Technicians (AVECCT) was the first technician academy to be recognized by the National Association of Veterinary Technicians in America (NAVTA).

Requirements for sitting the AVECCT examination[1]:

Section 1. Credential requirements dictate that each applicant, before they are declared eligible for examination, must:

A. Be a graduate of an American Veterinary Medical Association (AVMA)–approved veterinary technician school and/or legally credentialed to practice as a veterinary technician in some state or province of the United States, Canada, or another country.

B. It is strongly encouraged that the candidate be a member of a local, state, provincial, or North American veterinary technician association and a member of the Veterinary Emergency Critical Care Society.

C. After graduating from a recognized school of veterinary technology and/or becoming credentialed to practice as a veterinary technician and meet training requirements, as specified:

1. Three years' full-time work experience or its equivalent (5760 hours) in the field of veterinary emergency and critical care medicine. All experience must be completed within 5 years before the application.

   a) For the purpose of this eligibility requirement, the definitions of emergency care and critical care as established by the Veterinary Emergency Critical Care Society will be used.

   (1) Emergency care: action taken in response to an emergency. The term implies emergency action directed toward assessment, treatment, and stabilization of a patient with an urgent medical problem.

   (2) Critical care: care taken or required in response to a crisis; in medicine, treatment of a patient with a life-threatening or a potentially life-threatening illness or injury whose condition is likely to change on a moment-to-moment or hour-to-hour basis. Such patients require intense and often constant monitoring, reassessment, and treatment.

2. A minimum of 25 hours' continuing education related to veterinary emergency and critical care.

   a) Continuing education must be completed within the last 5 years before the application is submitted.

   b) Continuing education must be received from a nationally recognized program. Proof of attendance is required.

D. Provide documentary evidence of advanced competency in veterinary emergency and critical care nursing through clinical experience.

1. Completion of the Advanced Veterinary Emergency Critical Care Nursing Skills Form. The skills form documents those nursing skills that have been mastered by the candidate and are necessary to practice veterinary emergency critical care nursing at an advanced level. The list will be provided by the Credentials Approval Committee. The skills form is subject to change based upon the current state of the art in veterinary emergency critical care nursing.

2. A case record log is maintained from January 1 to December 31 of the year immediately preceding submission of the application. A minimum of 50 cases should be recorded. These cases should reflect management of the emergent or critically ill patient and mastery of advanced nursing skills. The log should include the following: date, patient identification (name or number), species/breed, age, sex, weight, diagnosis, length of care, outcome, and summary of nursing care techniques and procedures performed by the applicant on the patient.

3. Four case reports of no more than five pages each, double spaced. Case reports must demonstrate expertise in the nursing management of a variety of veterinary patients requiring emergency and critical care. Case reports should be selected from the case record log. Case reports must be the original work of the applicant.

4. Two letters of recommendation from an AVECCT member—a Veterinary Emergency Critical Care Society (VECCS) veterinarian or a diplomate of the American College of Veterinary Emergency and Critical Care.

   a) Until sufficient numbers of the aforementioned are provided, letters of recommendations will be accepted from the following: non-VECCS emergency clinic veterinarians and board-certified specialists in anesthesia, internal medicine, and surgery.

[1]Requirements are subject to change.

Additional information on specialties can be found at: navta.net/veterinary-technician-specialties and at http://www.avecct.org.

---

certifies laboratory animal technicians. In the United States, there are three designations: assistant laboratory animal technician (ALAT), laboratory animal technician (LAT), and laboratory animal technologist (LATG). In Canada, there are four designations: associate registered laboratory animal technician administrative (ARLATA), associate registered laboratory animal technician (ARLAT), registered laboratory animal technician (RLAT), and registered master laboratory animal technician (RMLAT).

AALAS- and CALAS-certified animal technicians care for the laboratory animals used in research facilities and teaching institutions. These facilities are registered by the USDA and may be in pharmaceutical companies, universities, and colleges. A technician does not need to be a graduate of an AVMA- or CVMA-accredited program of veterinary technology to be eligible for AALAS or CALAS certification. Graduates of AVMA- and CVMA-accredited programs must complete 6 months of additional training in a registered facility before they are eligible for the Level 1 ALAT examination.

Similar to the VTNE, AALAS/CALAS certification examinations are developed and administered by the PES, but they fall under the auspices of the AALAS, rather than those of the AAVSB. After passing the examination, the candidate may use the designation of registered laboratory animal technician (RLAT), for example. Candidates must complete a specified length of on-the-job experience to qualify for the next level of AALAS or CALAS certification.

Professionalism

As with all professions, veterinary technology is best represented by the excellent skill, ethical conduct, and passion of its members. Veterinary technicians are bound by a code of ethics and ideals established by NAVTA (Box 1.4), and by societal expectations of what constitutes professionalism. Although the ethics and ideals of veterinary technology may be clearly defined in writing, the nuances of professional conduct may be less clear, much like the subtleties of social interpersonal conduct. Therefore it is challenging for programs of veterinary technology to instill a common understanding of professional manners in a diverse student body. To this end, programs may have mandatory dress codes and rules about comportment on campus, particularly in the classroom. A portion of a laboratory grade, for example, may assess the professional conduct of the student. Did they come to class on time, in uniform, and with a positive attitude?

• BOX 1.4   NAVTA Veterinary Technician Code of Ethics

Each member of the veterinary technology profession has the obligation to uphold the trust invested in the profession by adhering to the profession's code of ethics. No code can provide the answer to every ethical question faced by members of the profession. They shall continue to bear their responsibility for reasoned and conscientious interpretation and application of the basic ethical principles embodied in the code to individual cases.

A veterinary technician shall uphold the laws/regulations of their state or province that apply to the technician's responsibilities as a member of the veterinary medical health care team.

The code of ethics shall be subject to review and timely revision by the Association.

Preamble

The code of ethics is based on the supposition that the honor and dignity of the professional of veterinary technology lies in the just and reasonable code of ethics. Veterinary technology includes the promotion and maintenance of good health in animals, the care of diseased and injured animals, and the control of diseases transmissible from animals to humans. The purpose of the code of ethics is to provide guidance to the veterinary technician for carrying out professional responsibilities to meet the ethical obligations of the profession.

Code of Ethics

- Veterinary technicians shall aid society and animals through providing excellent care and services for animals.
- Veterinary technicians shall prevent and relieve the suffering of animals.

- Veterinary technicians shall promote public health by assisting with the control of zoonotic diseases and informing the public about these diseases.
- Veterinary technicians shall assume accountability for individual professional actions and judgments.
- Veterinary technicians shall protect confidential information provided by clients.
- Veterinary technicians shall safeguard the public and the professional against individuals deficient in professional competence or ethics.
- Veterinary technicians shall assist with efforts to ensure conditions of employment consistent with the excellent care for animals.
- Veterinary technicians shall remain competent in veterinary technology through commitment to lifelong learning.
- Veterinary technicians shall collaborate with members of the veterinary medical profession in efforts to ensure quality health care services for all animals.

Ideals

- In addition to adhering to the standards listed in the code of ethics, veterinary technicians may also strive to attain a number of ideals. Some of these are:
- Veterinary technicians shall strive to participate in defining, upholding, and improving standards of professional practice, legislation, and education.
- Veterinary technicians shall strive to contribute to the profession's body of knowledge.
- Veterinary technicians shall strive to understand and support the attachment between a person and their companion animal.

National Association of Veterinary Technicians in America (NAVTA). https://navta.net/policies

---

CASE PRESENTATION 1.1

Larry, a veterinary technician, learned that he had passed the Veterinary Technician National Examination (VTNE), and 2 weeks later, he received his state credentials. The very next day, Larry received a call from Pleasant Veterinary Practice (PVP), where he had had an interview a week before. The person who called congratulated Larry and told him that PVP had decided to hire him as a "tech," beginning the next day.

On his first day Larry, is prohibited from drawing blood from a patient by the "head tech," because Larry has not yet been authorized to do so. He is told that he must "work his way up the ladder" before he is allowed to perform that level of task. Larry recalls learning to draw blood during the first semester of his freshman year, and he is now proficient in performing phlebotomy and a wide range of other tasks, such as inducing and monitoring anesthesia. Larry learns that there is a three-tier hierarchy of "techs" at the practice and that he must advance through all three tiers before he can draw blood. It will take about a year to advance to the top level.

Larry also learns that the "head tech" has been employed at the practice for many years but was not credentialed in the state and did not graduate from an accredited program of veterinary technology. As the day goes on, Larry finds himself being prevented from performing many technician duties and is merely asked to hold and restrain animals. He also learns that half the "techs" on staff are veterinary assistants, not veterinary technicians. On his second day, Larry notices that the veterinarians place catheters, intubate, and administer anesthesia themselves. He also notices one of the senior "techs" extracting two premolars by using a root elevator after performing dental prophylactic cleaning and oral examination of an animal patient.

Case Assessment:

List the concerns that you may have about PVP. What roles in the veterinary health care team are being confused, if any? It turns out that there is a high level of turnover among credentialed veterinary technicians on staff at PVP.

How would you account for this? List the changes you would make in staff management if you were the practice manager.

Student Assessment:

Did the student work well with classmates and teachers? These assessments help guide and prepare the student for work in a clinical environment, where pet owners and the employer will judge their conduct.

Professional Appearance

The first impression a veterinary technician makes is usually based simply on their appearance. Neat, clean, well-fitting, and ironed uniforms are essential. Long hair should be pulled back, and fingernails are best kept short and free of polish. Minimal jewelry, makeup, or perfume should be worn.

Uniform

Veterinary technicians wear a variety of "uniforms," depending on the field in which they work. In equine practice, for example, many technicians wear collared shirts, khaki pants, and solid protective footwear that is durable, warm, and practical in the rugged and often unheated setting of hospital barns (Fig. 1.12A). Sturdy shoes are important to protect the feet from injury if trampled by a hoof. Sneakers, sandals, and other open-toed shoes would be inappropriate in a barn. Technicians who work in bovine practices are likely to wear insulated coveralls and weatherproof boots to stay warm while working in muddy cattle pens.

Veterinary technicians who work indoors as in laboratory animal facilities (see Fig. 1.12B) and in companion-animal practices often wear scrubs and clean white sneakers or orthopedic clogs. Some companion-animal or mixed-animal practices prefer that

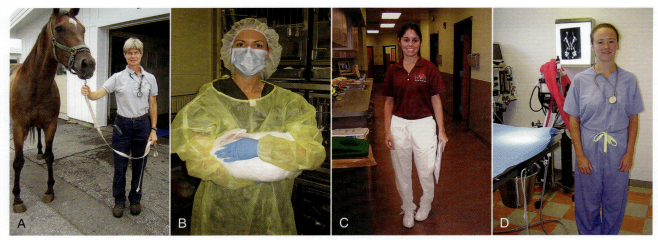

• **Fig. 1.12** (A) Many veterinary technicians who work in equine practice wear collared shirts, pants, and solid protective boots, which have proved to be practical in the rugged setting of hospital barns. (B) A technician who works in a laboratory animal facility must wear gloves and protective gowns to ensure that contagions are not transmitted to the animals in the vivarium. (C) Some veterinary technicians working in companion-animal practice wear collared shirts that carry the practice name and logo. (D) An operating room nurse wears clean scrubs and is equipped with a watch and a stethoscope to evaluate the status of anesthetized and recovering patients. (Courtesy Dr. Joanna Bassert.)

the staff wear collared shirts (or scrub shirts) with the practice name and khaki pants (see Fig. 1.12C).

In a working environment where one can become quickly soiled by animal hair and bodily fluids, such as saliva, blood, or urine, a clean, neat uniform may be challenging. It is helpful to have garment brushes and adhesive rollers on hand to remove hair from the uniform, particularly before entering an examination room with a client. Having an extra uniform available is essential when handling animals with suspected contagious diseases, such as parvovirus enteritis and panleukopenia, because the pathogens can be transmitted to other animals via contaminated clothing.

Uniforms should be clean and fit appropriately. Cleavage or the backside should never be revealed. Maintaining a professional appearance for many technicians therefore includes wearing white crew-neck T-shirts under a V-neck scrub shirt, for example, and scrub pants with elastic waistbands rather than drawstrings. The pants should be the correct length and hemmed to avoid the risk of tripping (see Fig. 1.12D).

Veterinary technicians are encouraged to wear professional pins on their shirts with their name or practice logo. Many programs of veterinary technology award college or university pins bearing the veterinary asclepius and college name to graduating students. NAVTA awards pins to its longtime members, as do several state or provincial veterinary technician associations. Although college rings and other jewelry are not acceptable because they are prohibited in the OR, wearing pins as symbols of the profession is encouraged.

Finally, the uniform of all veterinary technicians, regardless of field of interest, must include a watch with a second hand. Vital signs cannot be measured without a watch. Other items, such as a functional pen, digital thermometer, and a stethoscope, are also critical tools for veterinary technicians.

Hands and Nails

Contagions on the hands, especially under the nails, of health care workers can be spread from one patient to another. For this reason, it is important to make a habit of washing hands often, particularly between contacts with different animals. In addition, fingernails should be kept as short as possible and free of nail lacquer, which can chip off into sterile surgical fields. Not only can long nails harbor infectious agents, but they also interfere with daily nursing tasks, such as restraining animals, putting on surgical gloves, and placing IV catheters.

Jewelry, Face, and Hair

Veterinary technicians must be proficient in restraining animals and must be prepared to do so. The risk of injury to the technician and other staff members is increased if jewelry and long hair can be caught up in claws and flailing limbs. Necklaces, dangling earrings, and loose bracelets are particularly dangerous and should be discouraged for the safety of staff and patients. Finally, because of the close working conditions of most operating rooms and ward facilities, veterinary technicians should avoid wearing strong cologne, as there may be coworkers and pet owners who are allergic.

Professional Conduct

The way in which a veterinary technician behaves represents the most important aspect of their professionalism. Like many health care professionals, technicians are held to a high standard of conduct. For this reason NAVTA developed a list of professional ideals, as listed in Box 1.5. Specific guidelines for professional conduct both in and outside the workplace are given below.

In the Workplace

1. Be honest and forthright in communications with coworkers and clients. Take responsibility for making a mistake and, if possible, take immediate action to correct the error.
2. Maintain a positive attitude and an even, controlled disposition. Be respectful of coworkers and pet owners. Avoid expressing **anger**, sarcasm, and cynicism, because this has a

• BOX 1.5 Questions That Help Determine a Course of Good Conduct

1. Do the practice act and the regulations of the state board require that the technician act in a certain manner or prohibit the technician from acting in a certain manner?
2. Are there any other laws that require that the technician act in a certain manner or prohibit the technician from acting in a certain manner?
3. Do the ethics of the profession of veterinary medicine or veterinary technology require that the technician act in a certain manner or prohibit the technician from acting in a certain manner?
4. Do the individual technician's personal ethics require that the technician act in a certain manner or prohibit the technician from acting in a certain manner?

demotivating effect on the veterinary health care team and often worsens the situation.

3. Be tactful and careful in both verbal and written communications. Be considerate of the time, place, and quality of a query when asking questions.
4. Be a collaborative team player. Provide ideas and positive energy to help improve the efficiency of the health care team and the quality of the medical services.
5. Be attentive to the concerns and needs of both coworkers and pet owners. Avoid tuning out mentally. Take the initiative to pitch in and help where needed.
6. Respect the veterinarian-client-patient relationship. Keep in mind that some communications are most appropriately delivered to clients by the veterinarian.
7. Be aware of the clinical and professional competence of others. When concerned about incompetence in the workplace, address the issue promptly and tactfully to protect the integrity of the practice. Do not turn a blind eye.
8. When a conflict arises, address it promptly, privately, and calmly with those directly involved. Avoid drawing in those who are not directly involved in the conflict. Doing this undermines trust and is a poor substitute for direct communication.
9. Maintain the confidentiality of professional and personal information about clients and coworkers that was learned directly or indirectly. Do not gossip.
10. Be committed to being competent and skilled. Be receptive to innovative ideas and suggestions for improvement. Be enthusiastic about teaching others.
11. Be aware of and abide by the laws and regulations that define the scope of practice in your state.

Outside the Workplace

1. Join and participate in national, state/provincial, and local professional organizations.
2. Participate in high school career days and give presentations about the profession when the opportunity arises.
3. Attending national, state/provincial, and local veterinary conferences. Stay current on issues affecting the profession.
4. Support legislation in your state/province that better defines and strengthens veterinary technology.
5. Maintain state/provincial licensure, certification, or registration.
6. Seek healthy ways to manage stress, such as exercise, meditation, and taking time for personal interests.

Professional Communication

Verbal Communication

Clear and frequent communication with coworkers and clients is an important part of an efficient health care team. Veterinary technicians should ensure that they use correct grammar and well-articulated speech. Confirming with clients their understanding of medical terminology and avoiding medical jargon is paramount to good communication.

Written Communication

Medical Records

The medical record is a legal document owned by the veterinary practice or the supervising institution. The medical record must completely and accurately document all care provided to a patient and all relevant observations made pertaining to a patient. For example, if a patient is hospitalized overnight, the record must include notations of care provided, including feeding, and of monitoring performed, such as vital signs. If care is not documented, it may be presumed that care was not provided.

The medical record may be subpoenaed by a court of law. In most states, the practice must provide medical records upon demand by the profession's regulatory authority. Both courts and regulatory authorities closely scrutinize medical records in evaluating the care that was provided to a patient. Errors in the document can render the medical record invalid; this could have adverse legal ramifications for the practice. In addition, medical records of animals used for teaching in veterinary technology programs and in colleges of veterinary medicine are examined by a USDA inspector, who could cite deficiencies during an inspection if the written record contains errors. Using correct spelling and grammar in these legal documents is important. Refer to Chapter 3 for additional information about addressing errors in medical records.

Email

Email is a common form of written communication today, and although emails are often considered less formal than letters, use of correct spelling and grammar in emails to clients and colleagues is important. Moreover, from a legal perspective, emails could be introduced as evidence in civil and administrative proceedings against veterinarians and veterinary technicians. Although email "feels" less formal, it is important to remember that all written communication should be carefully drafted and reviewed for accuracy and appropriateness before it is sent. It is helpful to get into the habit of doing the following when sending emails to professional contacts:

1. Begin with a salutation that includes the name of the person you are writing to (e.g., "Hi, Mary," or "Good evening, Dr. Brown"). Email accounts can be shared, and it is important to be clear when identifying the intended recipient of the email. Salutations may not be necessary during frequent exchanges but should be included when first making contact.
2. Compose a concise email that is grammatically correct. Use a spell checker.
3. Keep in mind that email can be forwarded to others and tone can be misinterpreted. *Never* write an angry email or one that is critical of a colleague or coworker. Be careful with the use of humor to avoid it being misinterpreted.
4. Always end with a closing and your name. Many professionals program their computers to automatically end each email with a preset closing. Typically, this includes the person's full name, title, address, and telephone number.

5. Ensure that your email address does not leave a bad impression. Silly, cutesy, and animal-related email addresses, such as bunnyluvr@comcast.net or pintaday@msn.com, may not represent a professional image. A simple email address that includes your first initial and last name works well. Similarly, make sure that recorded answering machine greetings are appropriate for professional colleagues, particularly if you are actively searching for a new position and expect potential employers to call.

6. If possible, avoid using email to communicate difficult news to a client. It is better to speak directly with the client on the telephone.

> **TECHNICIAN NOTE**
>
> Keep in mind that email and text messages can be forwarded, and tone can be misinterpreted. Always assume that email and text messages are *not* private, and *never* write an angry email (or text message) or one that is critical of a colleague or coworker.

Text Messaging

In some practices, texting is now used to send reminders or to let a pet owner know that a pet has come out of surgery. Accurate and professional communication may be more difficult with text messaging than with email or written letters. Text messages should be sent only to clients who wish to receive information that way and should be used only to send information that can be accurately and professionally conveyed in a few words. Tips for text messaging include the following:

- Do not use acronyms or emoticons that you are not sure the recipient will understand—the message needs to be unambiguous and clear.
- Communicate briefly and succinctly.
- Do not use text messaging for serious topics or to communicate difficult news. These conversations would optimally occur over the phone or in person.

Professional Organizations and Acronyms

As the profession of veterinary technology matures, increasing numbers of professional organizations are being formed at the national, state, or provincial, and local levels. These organizations support the education, professional interests, and activities of veterinary technicians. NAVTA and the RVTTC, for example, represent the professional foundation of veterinary technology in the United States and Canada, respectively. However, many organizations are now being formed based on the special interests of their members. Examples include the Association of Zoo Veterinary Technicians, the Society of Veterinary Behavior Technicians, and the American Association of Equine Veterinary Technicians. The continued growth of veterinary technology depends heavily on the efforts of individuals within these and other professionally related organizations (Tables 1.3 and 1.4). Graduate veterinary technicians can aid in advancing their profession by joining and being active members.

National Association of Veterinary Technicians in America

NAVTA has been the leader in shaping and supporting the profession of veterinary technology in the United States. It has written the code of ethics, the veterinary technician oath, and the

veterinary technician model practice act and has brought about significant changes in the profession. In addition, NAVTA is an important source of support and information for veterinary technicians. Its mission is simple and elegant—to advance veterinary technology and veterinary nursing through advocacy, awareness, and professional development.

There are three classifications of membership in NAVTA: active, associate, and student members. To be an active member, one must live in the United States, be a graduate of an AVMA-accredited program of veterinary technology, and/or must be licensed, certified, or registered as a veterinary technician. Associate members of NAVTA typically include veterinarians, veterinary assistants, and veterinary personnel living outside the United States. Associate members may serve on NAVTA committees but may not vote or hold an elected office. Student members must be enrolled in an AVMA-accredited program of veterinary technology and are given the same membership privileges as associate members.

Registered Veterinary Technologists and Technicians of Canada/Technologues et Techniciens Vétérinaires en Registrés du Canada

The RVTTC, formally CAAHTT (Canadian Association of Animal Health Technologists and Technicians), was founded in 1989 and represents the joining together of seven provincial associations. Each association maintains its own membership base and submits funding (proportionate to the size of its membership) to the RVTTC. In this way, individuals who are members of a provincial association are automatically given membership in the RVTTC.

The RVTTC's mission is "to unite, advance, and strengthen the RVT profession across Canada through leadership and advocacy to promote excellence in animal healthcare." By uniting the various provincial veterinary technician and technologist associations, they enable a united, collaborative effort to support and advance the profession of veterinary technology in Canada. The interconnectedness of the RVTTC helps streamline communication among provinces, facilitates collaboration on projects, and brings nationwide awareness to the importance of animal health care.

> **TECHNICIAN NOTE**
>
> The National Association of Veterinary Technicians of America (NAVTA) and the Registered Veterinary Technologists and Technicians of Canada/ Technologues et Techniciens Vétérinaires en Registrés du Canada (RVTTC) have designated the third week of October as National Veterinary Technician Week. Mark your calendars! For more information, check the NAVTA website (www.navta.net) or the RVTTC website (www.rvttcanada.ca).

Professional Ethics

"Rules or principles that govern right conduct. Each practitioner, upon entering a profession, is invested with the responsibility to adhere to the standards of ethical practice and conduct set by the profession."

– SAUNDERS COMPREHENSIVE VETERINARY DICTIONARY, 5TH ED. ST. LOUIS, MO: SAUNDERS; 2020.

How does one discern good from bad and right from wrong? Is the technician's primary concern the animal, the owner, or the employer? In the practice of the healing arts, practitioners often

TABLE 1.3   Professional Associations

Organization	Acronym	Website
American Association of Equine Practitioners	AAEP	www.aaep.org
American Association of Feline Practitioners	AAFP	www.catvets.com
American Animal Hospital Association	AAHA	www.aahanet.org or www.healthypet.com
American Association for Laboratory Animal Science	AALAS	www.aalas.org
American Association of Veterinary Laboratory Diagnosticians	AAVLD	www.aavld.org
American Association of Veterinary Medical Colleges	AAVMC	www.aavmc.org
American Association of Veterinary State Boards	AAVSB	www.aavsb.org
American College of Laboratory Animal Medicine	ACLAM	www.aclam.org
American College of Veterinary Emergency and Critical Care	ACVECC	www.acvecc.org
American College of Veterinary Internal Medicine	ACVIM	www.acvim.org
American College of Veterinary Surgeons	ACVS	www.acvs.org
Animal Medical Center of New York	AMCNY	www.amcny.org
American Society of Laboratory Animal Practitioners	ASLAP	www.aslap.org
American Society for Veterinary Clinical Pathology	ASVCP	www.asvcp.org
American Veterinary Dental College	AVDS	https://avdc.org/
American Veterinary Medical Association	AVMA	www.avma.org
Association of Veterinary Technician Educators	AVTE	www.avte.net
British Small Animal Veterinary Association	BSAVA	www.bsava.com
British Veterinary Nurses Association	BVNA	www.bvna.org.uk
Canadian Association for Laboratory Animal Medicine	CALAM	www.calam-acmal.org
Canadian Association for Laboratory Animal Science	CALAS	www.calas-acsal.org
Canadian Council on Animal Care	CCAC	www.ccac.ca
Centers for Disease Control and Prevention	CDC	www.cdc.gov
Canadian Food Inspection Agency	CFIA	www.inspection.gc.ca
Canadian Veterinary Medical Association	CVMA	www.canadianveterinarians.net
Committee on Veterinary Technician Education and Activities	CVTEA	www.avma.org
Food and Drug Administration	FDA	www.fda.gov
Federation of European Companion Animal Veterinary Association	FECAVA	www.fecava.org
International Veterinary Emergency and Critical Care Symposium	IVECCS	www.veccs.org
National Animal Health Laboratory Network	NAHLN	www.aphis.usda.gov
International Council for Veterinary Assessment	ICVA	www.icva.net
Occupational Safety and Health Administration	OSHA	www.osha.gov
Professional Examination Service	PES	www.professionalexamservices.com
Veterinary European Transnational Network for Nursing Education and Training	VETNNET	www.vetnnet.com
Veterinary Hospital Managers Association, Inc.	VHMA	www.vhma.org
Veterinary Information Network	VIN	www.vin.com
Veterinary Support Personnel Network	VSPN	https://www.vin.com/vspn/default.aspx
Workplace Hazardous Materials Information System	WHMIS	https://www.canada.ca/en/health-canada/services/environmental-workplace-health/occupational-health-safety/workplace-hazardous-materials-information-system.html
The World Small Animal Veterinary Association	WSAVA	www.wsava.org

TABLE 1.4	**Veterinary Nurses and Technician Associations**	
Country	**Organization**	**Website**
International	The International Veterinary Nurses and Technicians Association (IVNTA)—an association of member countries that seeks to foster and promote links with veterinary nursing/ veterinary technician staff worldwide by communication and cooperation	www.ivnta.org
Australia	Veterinary Nurses Council of Australia	www.vnca.asn.au
Canada	Registered Veterinary Technologist and Technicians of Canada	www.rvttcanada.ca
Finland	Klinikkaeläinhoitajatry (native language site)	www.klinikkaelainhoitajat.fi
Ireland	Irish Veterinary Nursing Association	www.ivna.ie
Japan	Japan Veterinary Nurses and Technicians Association (native language site)	www.jvna.or.jp
New Zealand	New Zealand Veterinary Nursing Association	www.nzvna.org.nz
United Kingdom	British Veterinary Nurses Association	www.bvna.org.uk
United States	National Association of Veterinary Technicians of America	www.navta.net

face situations where the right course of conduct is not immediately apparent. This is magnified in veterinary medicine, because not only are veterinarians and technicians responsible for the care of a patient, but they also have responsibilities to the animal's owner and, in some cases, to the public. For this reason, when considering the question of "right conduct," one must first ask, "Right for whom?"

In addition to having an ethical dimension, many of the issues that a veterinary technician may encounter also have a legal dimension. The state or province in which a veterinary technician practices may place specific responsibilities on veterinarians and veterinary technicians. Many other laws, including pharmacy laws, laws on the use of controlled substances and other drugs, and food safety laws, may affect how a member of the veterinary medical team addresses the issue.

Ethical questions are often complicated in veterinary medicine, because veterinarians and technicians serve not only the patient, but also the client. Conflicts may arise when the client does not adopt the recommendations of the veterinary medical team. The veterinary medical team must work within the limits set by the client, who is often balancing the desire to provide the best care for the animal within the constraints of financial, work, and familial commitments. In such circumstances, it is important to remember that the client is often the owner of the animal and, as such, has the ultimate decision-making authority regarding the care provided to the animal.

However, there are exceptions to the general rule that the client has ultimate decision-making authority regarding the care provided. The veterinary medical team is not required to "do things the client's way" if the team determines that the client's choices would cause harm to the patient or if doing so would violate the practice act or other law. Consider the following examples:

1. A client presents his young, healthy dog to be spayed and informs the practice that he has lost his job and therefore cannot pay for any "extras," such as pain medication, but that he will keep the dog quiet and in a confined space after the surgery. Should the team provide this surgical service without providing postoperative analgesic medication for the dog? Why, or why not?

2. A person who is not a known client brings a dog to be neutered. On the initial intake examination, the technician discovers that the dog is microchipped, but the information on the microchip does not match the information provided by the new client. What are the responsibilities of the technician? What are the responsibilities of the veterinarian?

3. While a technician is on a farm call with her employing veterinarian to attend to a client's cattle, the technician notices an emaciated dog tied outside the client's house that has a swollen face and pus oozing from one of its eyes, which is crusted shut. The technician brings the dog's condition to the attention of the veterinarian, who asks the client about the dog. The client replies that he invited the veterinarian and technician to the property to only work on the *cattle, not the dog*. The veterinarian assents to the client's request and does nothing further with regard to the dog. What options does the technician have in this situation, and what should the technician do?

In discussing these questions, from a legal perspective, consider the following:

1. What is the legally mandated minimum standard of care in your state or province? Would doing what the client asks violate the minimum standard of care?

2. Who is permitted to request that services be provided to an animal? What must a veterinary practice do to determine whether the person requesting the services is legally authorized to make the request?

3. Do members of the veterinary team have a *legal* responsibility to report suspected animal abuse or neglect to any authority? Do members of the veterinary team have an *ethical* responsibility to report suspected animal abuse or neglect to any authority? Do members of the veterinary team have a legal or ethical responsibility to intervene when they believe they have seen animal abuse or neglect?

Finally, the technician will need to determine whether acting or not acting in a certain manner will conflict with their own personal ethics. Meaningful discussions regarding professional ethics can arise when examples of situations frequently encountered by technicians in practice are considered and when ethical queries are applied to help resolve dilemmas (see Box 1.5). The three scenarios presented above depict various legal and ethical issues.

CASE PRESENTATION 1.2

You have an employment interview scheduled with a veterinarian who has been in practice for 30 years. The veterinarian had told you that she has no veterinary technicians and is looking for someone to be her "right hand." On entering the practice, you notice a strong odor of urine, and the floor feels sticky as you walk through the facility. The veterinarian does not have modern equipment (e.g., the facility does not have digital radiography, but only film radiography, and there is no monitoring equipment for surgical patients). When you ask about the existing outdated equipment and lack of monitoring equipment, the veterinarian tells you that she has been using the same x-ray machine for 30 years and that it works just fine. Furthermore, she says her fingers are experienced at assessing pulses. What should you do?

Profession-related Laws and Regulations

The practices of professions and occupations are governed by each state or province. A veterinary technician does not need to be an expert in all the laws and regulations that affect the profession; however a technician should have a strong grasp of the state law that governs the licensing, professional conduct, and discipline of veterinary technicians and veterinarians. In addition, a veterinary technician should be familiar with some of the areas governed by other state and federal laws so that if a question arises, the technician will know where to look for the right information.

TECHNICIAN NOTE

Most laws and regulations that govern the practice of veterinary technology are state based. However, many federal laws govern services provided to farm animals and the handling of veterinary drugs.

Laws (Statutes)

In the United States, each state has a practice act, which is the primary law that governs the practice of veterinary medicine and veterinary technology. The practice act and any changes to it must be "enacted" by the state legislature. In other words, the original act and any amendments to the act must be approved by both the state house of representatives and the state senate and signed into law by the governor. A proposed amendment or change to the practice act is called a *bill*.

The practice act is enacted to promote public health, safety, and welfare by ensuring the delivery of competent veterinary medical care and to protect the public from incompetent, unethical, or unauthorized practice. A practice act mandates that only licensed veterinarians practice veterinary medicine in that specific jurisdiction (state). It may also include the function and powers of the state board of veterinary medicine, licensing requirements, examinations, and possible disciplinary actions.

The veterinary practice acts of some states include jurisdiction over veterinary technicians; in other states, there are separate veterinarian and veterinary technician practice acts. If a veterinary technician violates the state's practice act or the regulations of the profession's governing body, the penalty can include loss of licensure, monetary penalties (fines), or other disciplinary requirements. Because practice acts vary from one jurisdiction to another, every veterinary technician must be sure to understand the laws that govern the practice of veterinary technology in the state in which the technician plans to practice.

The AVMA and the AAVSB have proposed model practice acts as templates for states that are preparing to revise their practice acts. Refer to Box 1.6 for the AAVSB model practice act. Refer to the Evolve site for the complete AVMA model practice act.

The practice act in most states includes a definition of the practice of veterinary medicine and veterinary technology, although in some states, it has been left to the state board to define the practice of veterinary technology. The definition of the practice is important, because it informs veterinarians and technicians of the practices they may engage in and lists the specific clinical activities that unlicensed persons should not perform.

Rules that attempt to define the scope of practice for veterinary technicians are often vague. A common provision prohibits veterinary technicians from performing surgery. Would the prohibition against performing surgery preclude a technician from suturing a small laceration? Would this preclude a technician from suturing skin to close an incision made by the veterinarian in performing surgery?

In addition, the definition of "practice" is important, because it prohibits unlicensed individuals from performing activities that are defined as part of the practice of the profession. Unlicensed individuals who practice veterinary medicine or veterinary technology may be subject to monetary penalties (fines) imposed by

---

• BOX 1.6   American Association of Veterinary State Boards (AAVSB) Veterinary Technology State Practice Act Model

Veterinary Technician Means:
A person who is duly licensed to practice veterinary technology under the provisions of this Act.

The Practice of Veterinary Technology Means:
Any person practices veterinary technology with respect to animals when such person performs any one or more of the following:
1. Provides professional medical care and monitors and treats animals under supervision of a licensed veterinarian.
2. Represents oneself directly or indirectly as engaging in the practice of veterinary technology.
3. Uses any words, letters, or titles under such circumstance to induce the belief that the person using them is qualified to engage in the practice of veterinary technology, as defined; such use shall be prima facie evidence of the intention to represent oneself as engaged in the practice of veterinary technology.

Nothing in this section shall be construed to permit a veterinary technician to do the following:
1. Surgery
2. Diagnosis and prognosis of animal diseases
3. Prescribing of drugs, medicine, and appliances

Regulations Defining Tasks of Veterinary Technicians
The board shall adopt regulations establishing animal health care tasks and the appropriate degree of supervision required for those tasks that may be performed only by a veterinary technician or a veterinarian.

the board. In most states, it is also a crime and may subject an unlicensed individual to criminal penalties, including imprisonment. Often, "practice" by an unlicensed individual could also constitute animal cruelty, for which that individual may be subject to criminal prosecution. Criminal violations must be investigated and charged by the appropriate authorities. An unlicensed individual purporting to practice veterinary medicine could be charged criminally with animal cruelty *and* charged (before the state or provincial licensing authority) for practicing without proper licensure.

> ### TECHNICIAN NOTE
> Violation of the state practice act or of a board's regulations may subject the violator to loss of licensure or practice restrictions, monetary penalties, and possibly imprisonment.

Rules and Regulations

Rules and regulations are often written by each state's board of veterinary medicine, which is known simply as "the board." The review process of regulations varies from state to state, but, in general, regulations do not have to be approved by the legislature or the governor. They are therefore usually easier and less costly to change and update than the practice act [amendments]. The [rules and] regulations, together with the state practice act, are posted on the state board's website. It is important for veterinary technicians to be familiar with these documents and to understand that both the practice act and the [rules and] regulations must be followed.

The overriding purpose of the board is to protect the public by enforcing the practice act and the rules and regulations. To do this, it ensures that those seeking professional licensure have completed all the requirements set forth in the law to be licensed and that the requirements for maintaining a license, such as completion of CE and payment of a renewal fee, have been completed.

Regulations are said to have the "force and effect" of law, because they must be followed or the violator will be subjected to sanction by the board. Because regulations have the force and effect of law, violating a regulation written by an agency, such as the board, will subject the violator to the possibility of the same sanctions as those for violating the practice act itself. These sanctions include the imposition of a reprimand or a monetary penalty, restrictions placed on a license, suspension of a license, or revocation of a license. In other words, the license that the board "giveth," the board may "taketh away." Most state boards also have the authority to impose sanctions designed to remediate the conduct of the violator. Remedial sanctions may require that an individual complete additional CE or be monitored while practicing.

The public may have input into the formulation of both the practice act and the regulations. The public may influence laws by providing information and opinions to legislators. The public may affect regulations by providing information and opinions to the state board members who are rewriting the regulation. Veterinary technicians may influence regulations that affect their scope of practice by providing information and opinions to the state board of veterinary medicine.

The practice act and the regulations sometimes do not address certain questions faced by technicians. Technicians may write to their state board to ask for clarification and guidance; however, some state boards are prohibited from providing such guidance. In such a case, a technician seeking advice may wish to contact the state veterinary technician association or a former professor in the technician's educational program for guidance. The board

may be able to inform the technician if other laws or regulations (e.g., regulations of the state department of agriculture related to rabies disclosure) affect the particular question facing the technician. The technician may consult model acts and regulations of organizations for additional guidance while keeping in mind that model acts and regulations are not mandatory. In addition, the technician may consult codes of professional ethics set forth by NAVTA and the AVMA for guidance.

Entry Into Practice

Licenses, Certificates, and Registrations

Because the practice of veterinary technology is regulated by each state or province, some variety is noted in the terminology used to designate an individual authorized by the board to practice. This variety can be confusing, because one state may issue a license, whereas another may issue a certificate. Granting of a license by a state board implies that the board has reviewed and approved the qualifications of the individual to practice (Fig. 1.13). Granting of a certificate implies that some other entity has reviewed and approved the qualifications of the individual to practice and has certified that the person is competent to practice. Some states issue a license but call the person a "certified" technician (e.g., in Pennsylvania, technicians' qualifications are reviewed by the board, and the board issues a license bestowing the title *certified veterinary technician*). Some jurisdictions "register" rather than license technicians. The term *registered* implies that neither the board nor an independent entity has reviewed and approved the qualifications of the technician to practice; however, to lawfully practice veterinary technology, the individual must register and provide information to the board. Some boards that provide registration do review and approve the qualifications of technicians. A technician should check with the state's board before beginning practice to ensure that they have obtained the proper authorization to practice, as almost all jurisdictions in the United States have implemented some form of regulation of the profession. The AAVSB website provides updated information on jurisdictional regulations of the profession.

In Canada, the practices of veterinary medicine and veterinary technology are legislated on a province-by-province basis. Registration is mandatory in six provinces: Alberta, British Columbia, Manitoba, Ontario, and Saskatchewan. In provinces where registration is voluntary, a licensed veterinarian may delegate tasks

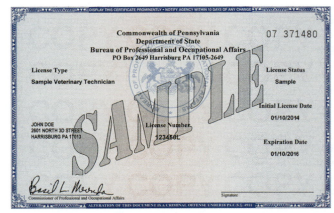

• **Fig. 1.13** Sample of a license to practice veterinary technology from the state of Pennsylvania.

to both *registered veterinary technicians* (the term used in Eastern Canada) and *registered veterinary technologists* (the term used in Western Canada) and to unregistered individuals. Registration in Canada requires successful completion of an approved educational program, passing of the VTNE, and membership in the province's professional association. Completion of CE is required to maintain current registration. RVTs seeking to move from one province to another should contact the provincial licensing authority for information and to obtain a valid registration to practice in the province to which the RVT plans to relocate.

In April 2019, officials at the RVTTC identified the most common grounds for disciplinary sanctions imposed on RVTs. These included theft from the practice, issues related to unlawful diversion of veterinary drugs, and misrepresentation/unlicensed practice. As with the licensing boards in the United States, the provincial governing bodies may impose fines, suspend, or revoke an RVT's registration, or require an RVT to complete additional education in an area specified by the licensing authority.

The terminology used in the state or province in which you plan to practice is not as important as the distinction made between those authorized to practice and those *not* authorized to practice. In most states, only a person who has been issued some credential by a state may perform the functions defined as the practice of veterinary technology.

In Europe, the European Union Recognition of Professional Qualifications Regulations of 2015 set minimum qualifications for licensure as a veterinary nurse or veterinary nurse assistant. Some European schools are accredited by the Accreditation Committee for Veterinary Nurse Education (ACOVENE), which accredits veterinary nurse educational programs in Belgium, Italy, Norway, Portugal, The Netherlands, the United Kingdom, and Ireland. Entry into the profession requires a Level 3 diploma in veterinary nursing, foundations of science, or a BS degree. The European Union also recognizes veterinary nursing specialties, including anesthesia and analgesia, emergency and critical care veterinary nursing, advanced practice veterinary nursing, diagnostic imaging, cardiology, emergency medicine, and oncology. Additional information may be obtained from the European Board of Veterinary Specialization (EBVS) or the Academy of Internal Medicine for Veterinary Technicians.

Demonstrating Good Moral Character

State and provincial laws vary widely in how the board determines whether an applicant possesses the good moral character required for licensure. In some jurisdictions, the applicant merely verifies (signs a statement under legal penalty of prosecution for perjury or for making a false statement) that they have good moral character. Other requirements can include submitting letters of recommendation attesting to the applicant's good moral character, a criminal history record check from the jurisdiction where the applicant has lived in the last 5 years, a federal criminal history record check, or a signed document verifying that the applicant has never been convicted of a crime.

Background Checks

The nationwide trend across all professions is to require applicants for licensure to submit criminal history record checks. Citations for "underage drinking," "disorderly conduct," "driving while under the influence of alcohol" (DUI), and "driving while intoxicated" (DWI) are crimes that must be reported on the application for licensure. Generally, traffic offenses, such as "speeding" or "failure to yield" do not need to be reported. The applicant should

read the application carefully and err on the side of reporting any criminal convictions the person may have. If the board does not have the authority to refuse to issue a license based on the crime committed, the board will disregard the information.

How does a board view an applicant with a criminal record? The answer to this question varies from state to state. Some states have absolute bars to licensure; that is, if a person has been convicted of certain crimes, they may not be issued a license. It is rare to find a state that has an absolute lifetime bar to licensure regardless of the crime that the applicant has committed; to do so would be contrary to the theory that a person who has committed a crime can be rehabilitated. It is not unusual, however, to see a 5- or 10-year bar to licensure. For example, in some states, a person who has been convicted of a felony-level criminal offense involving drugs may be barred from licensure for 10 years. In other states, a person who has been convicted of any violent crime may be barred from licensure for 5 years.

Refusal of Licensure

State boards may use an applicant's criminal convictions to support the board's finding that the applicant does not have good moral character and may then refuse to bestow licensure. The most common criminal convictions that lead boards to refuse to license an applicant are convictions involving crimes of moral turpitude. A *crime of moral turpitude* is one that involves dishonesty or deception, immorality or depravity, or interference with justice. All theft offenses, such as shoplifting, theft by unlawful taking, theft by deception, embezzlement, false swearing, forgery, and writing bad checks, are considered crimes of moral turpitude, because they involve dishonesty. *Crimes of depravity* include murder, rape, distribution of drugs, and misdemeanor offenses, such as stalking, harassment, and assault. Crimes that involve *interference with justice* include eluding a police officer and interfering with the conduct of a criminal investigation.

> **TECHNICIAN NOTE**
> The most common criminal conviction that lead boards to refuse to license an applicant are convictions involving crimes of moral turpitude.

If the applicant has a criminal conviction in their background, the individual should review the practice act and the regulations of the board in the jurisdiction in which they plan to practice to determine whether the conviction will bar the applicant from being licensed in that jurisdiction. When a licensing board is faced with a decision on whether to license a person who has a background that includes a criminal conviction, it will seek to determine whether the person is rehabilitated (unlikely to commit further criminal offenses). Positive indications of rehabilitation include no additional criminal convictions, a steady work history, admission of responsibility for the crime, and a positive outlook toward the future.

Other information commonly required on an application for licensure includes whether the applicant has held any other professional license in any state, whether the applicant has ever had a license disciplined by a state, and whether the applicant is now or has ever been addicted to alcohol or drugs. In most states, the simple fact that a person has held a professional license that has been subject to discipline is a legal ground to deny the application for licensure. A veterinary technician in one state who has had their license revoked for stealing drugs from the practice will not likely be granted a veterinary technician license in another state.

License Renewal and Continuing Education

Every state that issues a license to practice veterinary technology requires that the license be renewed. The length of time that a license is valid varies from state to state. In most states, the applicant will be able to renew the license online.

To renew the license, the applicant will be required to fill out a renewal application and pay a renewal fee. Although renewal applications vary from state to state, the common theme of renewal applications is to determine whether the licensee remains fit to hold the license. Some states (e.g., New Mexico) require veterinary technicians to register with the state board annually and inform the board of their employment. In addition, a technician may be required to inform the board whenever they change employment.

Most jurisdictions require professional licensees, including veterinary technicians, to complete CE to renew their licenses. The number of hours and the types of CE required for licensure renewal vary from state to state. Be sure to check with the board in the jurisdiction in which the applicant intends to practice for detailed information about its CE requirements.

A common scheme used by many states is to have a list of approved CE providers. For example, in the United States, many states accept CE credits offered by the state's schools of veterinary technology, the AVMA or the state veterinary medical association, NAVTA or the state technician association, programs approved by the Registry of Continuing Education (RACE) of the AAVSB, and most of the large national veterinary medical conferences. Some states limit the number of CE hours that may be earned from "distance learning" sources, which usually include Internet-based courses, teleconferences, and journal articles with test questions that are mailed to the journal's publisher.

Many states permit technicians to obtain CE credits for other educational activities, but technicians must seek board approval in advance for a nontraditional educational activity. A state board will approve an educational program for credit when it appears that the program will enhance the technician's knowledge and skills and will advance the practice of veterinary technology.

Grounds for Disciplinary Action

Technical Violations

The grounds for which a board may discipline a licensee (or refuse to grant an application to an applicant for licensure) are set forth in the state practice act. Additional grounds for discipline may be set forth in the state board's regulations. Some violations of the practice act are spoken of as *technical violations*. These technical violations include practicing on a lapsed license, failing to complete mandatory CE, having a record of a criminal conviction that is not related to the practice of the profession, and being disciplined by the licensing board of another state. These violations are considered technical violations, because there is no direct link between the licensee's misconduct and harm to an animal. It is important to note that in virtually every state, a licensee may be prosecuted and disciplined for misconduct, even if the licensee's misconduct did not cause any harm to an animal.

Substantive Violations

The so-called substantive violations of the practice act and regulations are violations that bear directly on the licensee's conduct in practicing the profession. Common grounds for discipline include unprofessional conduct, malpractice, incompetence, deviation from the standards of acceptable and prevailing practice, practicing beyond the scope of practice authorized in the state, or violating any rules of the board or any rules set forth in the practice act. Other examples include engaging in acts of moral turpitude, fraud, or deceit in the practice of the profession or during entry into the practice of the profession; misrepresentation; animal abuse; animal neglect or animal cruelty; engaging in any act that is illegal and is related to the profession; aiding another person to violate the practice act; impairment by reason of addiction to drugs or alcohol or by mental disease that prevents safe practice; and a criminal conviction.

Fraud and Deceit

A licensee may be prosecuted and disciplined for violating any rule of the board or any rule set forth in the practice act, even if it is not specifically mentioned as grounds for discipline. A licensee may be prosecuted and disciplined, or an applicant may be prevented entry into the practice of the profession, for committing fraud or deceit in the practice of the profession. This includes falsifying information submitted on an application for licensure, omitting requested information on an application, and cheating on the licensure examination. It also includes such conduct as falsifying a health certificate or other document and signing a form for the veterinarian that the veterinarian is required to sign. Finally, violations under this section may include fraudulent or deceitful conduct related to the client, such as charging for services not performed, and may include fraudulent or deceitful conduct related to the technician's employer, for example, stealing from the practice.

Crimes of Moral Turpitude

In some states, a licensee may be prosecuted and disciplined for engaging in acts of moral turpitude and engaging in immoral conduct. Because *moral turpitude* is a well-defined term in criminal law, a licensing board will usually look to the criminal law in its state to determine what conduct by a licensee involves moral turpitude. In addition to being authorized to discipline a licensee who has been convicted of a crime of moral turpitude, a licensing board may have the authority to discipline a licensee for engaging in acts of moral turpitude, even if the licensee was not convicted of a crime related to the conduct. Some state practice acts include a definition of immoral conduct, some refer to the criminal statutes for the definition of immoral conduct, and some do not specify what kind of conduct is considered immoral conduct.

Misrepresentation

A licensee may be prosecuted and disciplined for misrepresentation. Misrepresentation is saying something that is not accurate. Telling a client that a certain treatment will cure a patient is a misrepresentation, because virtually nothing in medicine is an absolute certainty, and a technician may not give a prognosis. However, it is not a violation to say, "Your pet is in good hands. We are doing everything we can for your pet."

Animal Abuse

A licensee may be prosecuted and disciplined for animal abuse, animal neglect, or animal cruelty. States and provinces vary on whether the abuse, neglect, or cruelty applies to any animal or only to animals that are under the care of the technician. In the United States, some state boards consider abuse, neglect, or cruelty to be a deviation from the standards of acceptable and prevailing practice, rather than a separate offense.

Committing or Aiding Illegal Professional Acts

A licensee may be prosecuted and disciplined for engaging in an illegal act that is related to the profession. For example, a licensee who provides a performance-enhancing drug to the owner of a competition animal could be prosecuted for engaging in an illegal act related to the profession.

A licensee may be prosecuted and disciplined for aiding another person to violate the practice act. If you were to give unauthorized assistance to another person in taking the licensing examination, you would be guilty of aiding another person to violate the practice act. The most common example of this misconduct occurs when a noncredentialed person is working in a veterinary practice and the credentialed persons in the practice know, or even instruct, the noncredentialed person to perform tasks that only those with credentials are allowed to perform. This situation occurs fairly often when veterinarians who are licensed to practice in another country come to the United States and become employed as noncredentialed veterinary assistants. It may take a year or longer for them to become licensed veterinarians in the United States. However, because they may have been practicing veterinary medicine outside the United States for a number of years, they may appear to be competent to perform a wide variety of tasks within a hospital. It is important to remember that noncredentialed individuals are limited to performing only those tasks that the statute and board regulations authorize, regardless of the knowledge or skill level of the individual. Any credentialed person who assists a noncredentialed person in performing tasks that the statute includes as the practice of the profession may be aiding unlicensed practice of veterinary medicine.

TECHNICIAN NOTE

The most common example of misconduct occurs when a noncredentialed person is working in a veterinary practice and credentialed persons in the practice know, or even instruct, the noncredentialed person to perform tasks that only those with credentials are allowed to perform.

Working Impaired

Licensees may be prosecuted and disciplined for working while impaired by addiction to drugs or alcohol, or by an untreated mental disease. Disciplinary action may require that the licensee practice only under supervision and that the licensee must actively participate in a treatment program. In addition, the licensee must submit random urine samples that are tested for misuse of drugs, including alcohol.

TECHNICIAN NOTE

The most common reason a technician is disciplined by a licensing board is that they have exceeded the scope of practice authorized by law.

CASE PRESENTATION 1.3

Tina works with animal rights groups and helped start the first no-kill shelter in her community. To further her knowledge and be able to better help animals, Tina attended an American Veterinary Medical Association (AVMA)–accredited program, passed the VTNE and state board, and became a credentialed veterinary technician.

Tina now works for Dr. Jones. George has just become a client of the practice and brings his new puppy in for examination. The puppy is sickly; Dr. Jones diagnoses parvovirus enteritis. George does not want to pay for the treatment, even though Dr. Jones advises George that the puppy would make a full recovery with treatment. George instructs Dr. Jones to put the puppy to sleep and pays for the procedure and cremation. After George leaves, Tina tells Dr. Jones that she is involved in the local shelter and that the shelter will pay for the puppy's treatment and then place the puppy for adoption. Can Dr. Jones begin the treatment and let Tina take the puppy? What should Dr. Jones do? What should Tina do?

CASE PRESENTATION 1.4

A few weeks have passed since Tina started work at Dr. Jones's hospital. Barbara comes in for an appointment with her elderly cat. The cat has terminal cancer and has been crying for the past five hours. Barbara elects euthanasia and then leaves the hospital. Dr. Jones directs Tina to administer the euthanasia solution. Tina is vehemently opposed to euthanasia and believes that animals should be permitted to die naturally when it is their time. Can Tina refuse to follow Dr. Jones's instructions?

Practicing Beyond the Scope of Practice

As previously noted, a licensee may be prosecuted and disciplined for practicing beyond the scope of practice authorized in the state. This violation is considered one of the most serious examples of misconduct that may be committed by a licensee, because it demonstrates a fundamental misunderstanding of the role of the licensee or deliberate disregard for the role of the licensee.

Most states prohibit veterinary technicians from performing surgery, diagnosing an animal's ailment, attesting to an animal's health status, offering a prognosis for the animal, and prescribing treatments or drugs for an animal. In addition, states often require a level of supervision by a veterinarian for a veterinary technician to perform any particular task, such as administration of anesthetic. These items usually are set forth in the regulations of the state board.

TECHNICIAN NOTE

If a veterinary technician is found to have deliberately practiced beyond the scope of practice authorized by the state, it is likely that the sanction imposed will be severe.

Unprofessional Conduct

A licensee may be prosecuted and disciplined for unprofessional conduct. *Unprofessional conduct* usually refers to conduct that disparages the profession in the eyes of the public.

Malpractice (Negligence)

A licensee may be prosecuted and disciplined for malpractice (also called *negligence*). *Malpractice* refers to deviation from or failure to conform to acceptable standards of practice. Licensing law borrows the concept of a "tort" from civil law; in civil law, a tort is a wrong or injury for which a court will provide a remedy. The usual remedy in a tort action is the award of monetary damages. For a person to recover damages for infliction of a negligent tort, the person must prove the existence of a legal duty owed to the person by another, the other's breach of the duty, a causal relationship between the breach and the person's injury, and damages suffered by the person. However, in laws governing professionals (unlike in civil lawsuits), the state's prosecuting attorney need only establish a duty to the patient and a breach of that duty by the licensed practitioner. The patient does not have to suffer any injury for the professional to be disciplined for malpractice. An additional difference is that a state board does not award monetary damages to the animal's owner; the state board's authority is limited to imposing disciplinary sanctions on the professional. Veterinarians can carry professional liability insurance, which is similar to malpractice insurance. The veterinarian's professional liability insurance covers acts, errors, and omissions performed while legally responsible to render professional services as a veterinarian or a veterinary technician.

Veterinarians can also be found negligent or guilty of malpractice as a result of the actions of a staff member. Veterinary technician–committed errors, such as purchase errors, record omissions, and medication errors, are examples whereby the veterinarian can be found guilty, even though it was the staff working on them who committed the error.

The ultimate safeguard to ensure that there is proof of standard veterinary practice is a complete and thorough patient record that accurately documents all therapeutic actions conducted. Communications and discussions with clients regarding the patient should be documented by staff members who speak with the client. Refer to Chapter 3 for more information about documentation and completion of veterinary medical records.

TECHNICIAN NOTE

In the laws governing professionals (unlike in civil lawsuits), the state's prosecuting attorney needs only to establish a duty to the patient and a breach of that duty by the licensed practitioner. The patient does *not* have to suffer any injury for the professional to be disciplined for malpractice.

Incompetence. Finally, a licensee may be prosecuted and disciplined for incompetence. *Incompetence* is conduct that increases the risk of negligence, even if negligence has not yet actually occurred. For example, sloppy laboratory practices, incomplete record keeping, and improper sanitation may demonstrate incompetence, because these practices increase the risk of something going wrong. Sloppy laboratory practices increase the risk of tainted samples and misdiagnoses; incomplete record keeping increases the risk of an animal being given the wrong medication; and improper sanitation increases the risk of animals (or humans) being infected by a pathogen.

Responsibility for Actions

As a credentialed professional, a veterinary technician is responsible for their conduct. Because a technician is employed by and acts under the supervision and direction of a veterinarian, the veterinarian is also responsible for the conduct of the technician. For this reason, as a general rule, whenever a veterinary technician is disciplined by a licensing board for exceeding the technician's authorized scope of practice, incompetence, or negligence or malpractice, the veterinarian responsible for supervising the technician may also be disciplined by the board.

CASE PRESENTATION 1.5

Two weeks ago, Tom learned that he had passed the Veterinary Technician National Examination (VTNE), and he received his state license yesterday. Today, Tom received a call from a busy four-veterinarian practice, where he had an interview last week. Tom was informed that a decision has been made to hire him as a veterinary technician, beginning tomorrow.

On his first day at work, Tom is assigned to shadow Annette during his orientation. Annette is introduced to Tom as the "head technician"; he is told that she has been working at the practice for 9 years and that she will show him how things are done in the "real world." Annette's nametag identifies her as "technician" and "behavior specialist." Tom notices that Annette does not have a technician license displayed on the facility wall where the other licenses are displayed.

Annette takes Tom to the back and introduces him to Bassie, a young Basset Hound that was dropped off that morning to be spayed. Annette takes the dog's vitals and listens to her heart. Annette then tells Tom that everything is normal and that there is no need to do preoperative blood work, because that will make the owner happy when she gets her bill. Annette directs Tom to administer preanesthetic medications to Bassie and then carry the dog into the surgical room. Annette then administers intravenous medication to Bassie; scrubs, clips, and drapes her; and instructs Tom to call Dr. White on his cell phone and let him know that Bassie is ready for surgery. Dr. White is just pulling up to the hospital when he takes Tom's call and tells Tom that he will be right in. When Dr. White arrives, he asks Annette how everything is; Annette says everything is okay. Dr. White begins the surgery, but Bassie's heart fails, and she cannot be revived. Necropsy reveals that Bassie had a serious heart condition that should have been identified on auscultation. Does Tom have any legal or ethical responsibilities in this situation?

Process of Disciplinary Action

Notice

The board must notify the licensee in writing of the specific allegations for which disciplinary action has been initiated. For example, a state may allege that a technician is subject to discipline under the practice act because they have been convicted of a crime, and a particular section of the practice act gives the board the authority to take disciplinary action against licensees who have been convicted of certain crimes. The notice is usually sent by certified mail, return receipt requested, but may also be sent by first-class mail. In some cases, a board will have the notice delivered to the accused licensee by personal service (i.e., hand delivery). If the board cannot locate the licensee because the licensee has moved and has not provided the board with a forwarding address, notice may be accomplished by publishing an announcement in a publication of legal record within the state. This publication is generally the same publication in which a board publishes notice of new regulations governing the practice of the profession.

Right to a Hearing

In addition to setting forth the factual allegations that give rise to the action against the licensee, the notice will inform the licensee that they have a right to a hearing to defend against the allegations and tell their side of the story. The hearing may be held before an administrative law judge or hearing officer, or may be held before one or more members of the licensing board.

The licensee is not required to be represented by an attorney at a disciplinary hearing before a licensing authority. There is no "right" to an attorney in disciplinary matters, as there is in criminal matters; therefore the state will not appoint (and pay for) an attorney to represent the licensee if the individual cannot afford legal representation. However, an attorney is likely to recommend legal representation by an attorney, because the disciplinary action before the board is a legal proceeding, and attorneys have expertise in the law. The administrative law judge or hearing officer will often assist an unrepresented licensee in the technical aspects of presenting the evidence. Although it is not necessary to retain legal counsel, it is advisable to do so.

Hearings Procedures

The opportunity to be heard requires that a licensing authority hold a hearing so that the licensee can present evidence and provide responses to the allegations. Hearings are matters of public record, which means that the public may come to a hearing or may obtain a transcript of the hearing. In lieu of a hearing on alleged violations of the practice act, the state's attorney may offer the licensee a settlement (or consent) agreement. Settlement agreements are documents wherein the licensee admits that they violated the practice act and agrees to a sanction set forth in the agreement. In some cases, more lenient sanctions are offered if the licensee will agree to settle the matter through agreement, because this **resolution** of a case saves the state time and money by not requiring the formal presentation of evidence at a hearing. The state board must approve the agreement before it is considered final.

A hearing generally begins with an announcement of the time and location that the hearing is being held and an introduction of officials present. Generally, a presiding officer, usually an administrative law judge or hearing officer, will be present. A prosecuting attorney who works for the state will represent the state (the state's attorney). The licensee may have legal counsel or may proceed without legal counsel. The state's attorney will proceed first, because the state bears the responsibility for demonstrating that the licensee has committed a violation of the law or regulations. The state's attorney may call witnesses, including the licensee, and may present documents. In turn, the licensee may question the state's witnesses. After the state's case has been presented, the licensee will have an opportunity to call witnesses and produce documents. The state's attorney may question the licensee's witnesses. The hearing officer or any board member may also question any witness. The hearing usually concludes with closing arguments. Each side makes a statement about what it believes the evidence introduced at the hearing has shown and whether it believes the licensee has violated the licensing law or regulations. The state's attorney and the licensee may also make recommendations regarding the disciplinary sanction, if any, that they believe should be imposed. After the hearing, the parties are generally given an opportunity to file a written argument regarding what they believe the evidence has shown. The board will issue a written opinion later, generally anywhere from 2 months to 1 year after the hearing. The written opinion issued by the board will set forth what the board believes happened and whether the licensee is subject to discipline. If the board finds that the licensee is subject to discipline, the written opinion will include an order setting forth the disciplinary sanction imposed by the board.

In some states, a licensing board may offer to resolve a matter through an "informal conference" rather than a formal hearing. You may work in a state that uses formal hearings or in one that uses informal conferences to resolve disciplinary matters against licensees; however, the licensee should learn as much as possible about the process that is followed in that jurisdiction and how the outcome can be disputed if it is not favorable.

Disciplinary Sanctions

Revocation of a License

Revocation of a license is considered the most severe sanction that a board may impose. In some states, revocation is the permanent preclusion of an individual from the practice of a profession. In other states, an individual may apply for relicensure after 5 or 10 years. To be relicensed, the individual must demonstrate all qualifications for licensure, including good moral character, and/or must retake the licensure examination.

Suspension of a License

Suspension is also considered a severe sanction that may be imposed by a board, as a suspension prohibits the sanctioned individual from practicing the profession. A suspension may be imposed for either a set period or an indefinite period, in which case the suspension is lifted after the licensee has completed specific tasks assigned by the board. For example, in a disciplinary case where the board found that the technician exceeded the scope of practice of the profession, the board might require the technician to cease practice until the technician has completed CE in the role of a veterinary technician and a CE course on the state's law governing veterinary technicians. When the sanctioned technician is permitted to return to practice, the board may further limit the technician by means of the terms of probation.

> **TECHNICIAN NOTE**
>
> Suspension of a license is considered a severe sanction, because a suspension prohibits the sanctioned individual from practicing the profession for a set period or an indefinite period.

Probation of Licensee

A licensing board may place a licensee on probation. A licensee who is on probationary status with the board is permitted to practice the profession; however, boards generally place limits on the practice of an individual who is on probation. Limits may include ongoing CE, practicing under a higher level of supervision, or restriction from performing specific tasks. For example, a technician who made an error in administering an anesthetic may be required to observe the administration of anesthetics during 10 surgical procedures and then may be directly monitored by another technician for 10 surgical procedures before being able to resume normal practice.

Reprimand

A *reprimand* is a public censure of a licensee without suspension or probation. This sanction is generally reserved for violations or repeat violations that warrant more than a civil penalty.

Civil Penalty

A *civil penalty* is a fine paid to the licensing board. In the United States, virtually every state has statutory limits on the amount of the civil penalty that may be imposed for a violation of the state's licensing laws. Although this varies from state to state, caps are commonly set at $1000 (Pennsylvania, Tennessee), $5000 (Illinois), and $10,000 (Connecticut) per violation. Some boards permit licensees who have been sanctioned with a civil penalty to make installment payments on the penalty.

Additional Laws Governing Veterinary Practice

Labor Laws

Labor laws define the rights and obligations of both employees and employers. They specify the requirements for employment standards, such as annual vacation pay, minimum wage, layoff procedures, and severance pay. Every jurisdiction has some type of labor law. Employees and employers should be aware of the labor legislation that governs employment in their state or province and should be familiar with the government agency that regulates these types of laws.

Hostile Work Environment

A *hostile work environment* can be defined as any workplace where:
1. The actions, including remarks of workers or employers, are overtly discriminatory regarding age, race, gender, sexual orientation, or disability. The actions may or may not also include inappropriate physical contact, sexual harassment, physical abuse, or intimidation.
2. An employee is unable to perform their work reasonably well because of certain behaviors by management or coworkers.
3. In retaliation for the previous actions of a worker, a manager engages in behavior designed to make the worker quit.
4. A worker feels physically threatened. Violence is a criminal offense and should be reported to the police. A police report will document the actions of the hostile person.

Many jurisdictions have few, if any, laws prohibiting hostile work environments. However, civil rights acts, discrimination in employment acts, and disabilities acts play a role in how a complaint is addressed, prosecuted, and resolved.

Safety in the Workplace

The Occupational Safety and Health Administration (OSHA), which resides in the US Department of Labor, was created by Congress to enforce federal employment laws that help to ensure safe working environments for US workers. The primary goal of OSHA is to prevent employment-related accidents and illnesses. It confirms that all workers have a fundamental right to a safe workplace. Safety is also supported by working with stakeholders to establish, promote, and enforce safe work practices, standards, and procedures. Stiff penalties or fines may be imposed on businesses that fail to comply with OSHA.

Most jurisdictions also have a Radiation Health and Safety Act, which imposes certain minimum mandatory conditions for the protection of persons exposed to radiation and engaged in the operation and use of radiation equipment. Refer to Chapter 4 for additional information about OSHA compliance and safety in veterinary practices.

Medical Waste Management Laws

Health care facilities, such as hospitals, physicians' offices, dental practices, and veterinary hospitals, generate a plethora of medical waste. Disposal of this waste is regulated by the municipalities, the states and provinces, and the federal government. Although the states and provinces impose regulations for office, municipal, and medical waste, including potentially infectious waste, the federal government imposes regulations for hazardous waste, such as mercury and radioactive wastes. Medical waste includes cultures and stocks of infectious agents, body tissues, blood wastes and blood byproducts, sharps, contaminated carcasses and stall/cage beddings, surgery or autopsy waste that was once in contact with infectious agents, laboratory waste, medical equipment that has encountered infectious agents, and other contaminated biological materials.

In the United States, the Environmental Protection Agency (EPA) enforces the Medical Waste Tracking Act. This act defines medical waste, regulates its management and transport, and outlines enforcement processes. Most jurisdictions have a government agency that regulates the disposal of medical waste.

Controlled Substances

A *controlled substance* is a drug or chemical whose manufacture, possession, or use is regulated by the government. In veterinary medicine, controlled substances are used on a daily basis. Federal and state legislation, such as the federal or state controlled substance acts, establish limitations and guidelines for the possession, use, storage, exportation, and production of specific drugs. Controlled drugs are categorized into specific classes or schedules based on risk of addiction. In the United States, Congress has empowered the **Drug Enforcement Agency (DEA)** to enforce federal regulation of controlled substances. Controlled substance logbooks, used in many veterinary practices, are required by government regulatory agencies and legislation to document the distribution and use of controlled substances. State controlled substance acts frequently apply to all drugs and devices, not just those drugs that are on the state or federal controlled substances lists. Veterinarians may only prescribe drugs for their animal patients within the veterinarian-client-patient relationship. They may not prescribe (or dispense from their own pharmacy) drugs for themselves or others. No state permits veterinary technicians to prescribe drugs.

Emerging Issues

With the increasing prevalence of state laws that authorize the use of medical cannabis products by authorized patients and of laws legalizing the sale of cannabis products to the public, technicians may encounter veterinary clients with questions about using cannabis products on their animals. Despite legalization of most cannabis products at the state level, some are considered controlled Schedule I substances at the federal level. By definition in federal law, 'hemp' cannot contain more than 0.3% THC (tetrahydrocannabinol). Products with more THC are classified as 'marijuana' and are considered 'Schedule I' drugs. However, many states have independently legalized the sale and use of marijuana, even though it has NOT been legalized nationally. All hemp-based CBD products should be regarded as drugs.

The nonpsychoactive CBD, believed to be one of 100 active ingredients in cannabis, has received the most attention as a potential treatment for pain management, anxiety, and seizures. A study published in *Frontiers in Veterinary Science* on January 10, 2019 used data created from an anonymous online survey in collaboration with the Veterinary Information Network (VIN) to report on veterinarians' knowledge of and comfort with discussing or recommending CBD products for pet animals. Funding for research on the use of cannabis and CBD products has increased in recent years, and the report "The Health Effects of Cannabis and Cannabinoids: The Current State of Evidence and Recommendations for Research" was published by the National Academy of Sciences in January 2017. In the animal world, the American Kennel Club's (AKC) Canine Health Foundation awarded funding to researchers at the Colorado State University College of Veterinary Medicine and Biological Sciences to conduct a clinical trial to test the effects of CBD on 60 dogs that had responded poorly to standard treatments. The results of this study were promising, and the use of cannabinoids in dogs will continue to be of interest as an alternative to traditional pharmaceuticals. Awards have also been made by other organizations to researchers at the Auburn University College of Veterinary Medicine in Alabama for study.

Because veterinary technicians are prohibited from prescribing drugs under the practice acts that govern the profession in the United States and because the legal status of all cannabis-derived products is a matter of great uncertainty, technicians should refer questions from clients to their supervising veterinarian. Veterinarians may find more information to guide their discussions with clients in the guide provided by the AVMA Council on Biologic and Therapeutic Agents, "Cannabis: What Veterinarians Need to Know." Although two states—California and New York—have pending legislation to address the use of cannabis products in animals, no state has yet given veterinarians explicit authority to discuss the use of cannabis products as medicine in animals or to recommend or use these products.

Intellectual Property and Contract Law

Intellectual property (IP) law protects the rights of owners of intangible creations, such as inventions, writings, trademarks, and trade secrets. Such creations may not be used without the owner's permission. Anything an employee develops or writes in the course of employment is covered under IP law. The employer generally owns the created work unless otherwise agreed.

When hiring new employees, most companies now present the employee with an employment contract. The contract spells out the basic employment terms, such as salary and benefits. Noncompete (NCA) and nondisclosure (NDA) agreements are now often included in employment contracts.

Noncompete agreements are worded to protect the employer from unfair competition. Terms may include limitations on working within a certain distance of the employer's location for a specified time after employment is terminated. Most states still recognize these agreements, as long as the distance and time periods of employment restrictions are "reasonable." The NCA also prohibits an employee from soliciting the employer's clients and staff after termination of employment. Nondisclosure agreements create a confidential relationship between a person in possession of sensitive information and another person who will have access to the same information. This information could include client account information or other protected information related to the business.

These types of agreements are usually between the veterinarian and the employer, but a technician may be asked to sign such an agreement, especially if the technician performs management duties.

One should carefully read and have an attorney review any employment contract before signing, as the contract terms may limit their ability to work in an area after leaving the employer. If the contract terms are enforceable in your jurisdiction, breaking the terms of the contract may subject you to a civil lawsuit.

Animal-Related Laws

Anticruelty Laws

In the United States, state and federal criminal code prohibits animal cruelty. However, variations exist in state laws prohibiting animal cruelty regarding the animals that are protected under the laws and the specific acts that are prohibited. Every state prohibits dogfights and cockfights and other intentional acts that injure or kill certain animals in a cruel manner. In addition, state anticruelty laws rarely provide the same protection to farm animals. In the United States, most states also prohibit neglect of animals. In Canada regional ordinances often include cruelty laws. Humane investigators and police officers may investigate complaints of animal cruelty.

Unfortunately, it may be common for veterinary technicians to encounter in professional practice an animal that they suspect might be a victim of cruelty. In some states, technicians and veterinarians have a legal duty, imposed in the practice act or the anticruelty law, to report suspected cruelty to an animal. Other states do not mandate reporting but leave the decision to report the matter to criminal authorities up to the individual.

Extensive research has established a link between cruelty to animals and violence against children, spouses, older adults, or others in the home and has demonstrated that violence against animals in a household is a reliable indicator of a higher level of violence against humans in the same household. Because of this link, some states have considered or enacted laws that require government to establish an animal abuse registry in addition to the state's existing child abuse registry, and, importantly, to require cross reporting of abuse among databases. Technicians should be familiar with the reporting requirements in the jurisdiction in which they practice.

Animals Used in Research and Education

In the United States, the Animal Welfare Act (AWA) requires that minimum standards of care and treatment be provided for some warm-blooded animals bred for commercial sale, used in research and higher education, transported commercially, and exhibited to the public. The AWA does not apply to mice and rats bred for research, farm animals used for food or fiber, amphibians and reptiles, horses not used for research, invertebrates, or birds, which represent approximately 90% of animals used in research and higher education. Animals regulated under this law include those exhibited in zoos, circuses, and marine mammal facilities; pets transported on commercial airlines; and animals used in research and for teaching purposes. The AWA prohibits staged dogfights and bear and raccoon baiting.

The AWA was passed in 1966 and was amended in 1970, 1976, 1985, 1990, 2002, 2007, 2008, 2013, and 2019. Inspectors from Animal Care (a subsidiary of the USDA) conduct randomly scheduled, unannounced inspections to ensure that all regulated facilities are compliant with the AWA. If an inspection reveals deficiencies in meeting AWA standards and regulations, the inspector instructs the facility to correct the problems within a specific time frame. If follow-up inspections show that the deficiencies have not been corrected, the inspector documents repeat violations and may pursue more forceful legal action.

USDA-registered research facilities are required to have Institutional Animal Care and Use Committees (IACUCs) that help enforce the AWA through the actions of employees within and near the institution. This form of self-assessment helps the institution stay on course with AWA compliance. Enforcing standards regarding animal housing, feeding, handling, and veterinary care and review of animal use protocols are included among the responsibilities of the IACUC. In Canada, the Animals in Research Act governs the use of animals in research and education. This act is enforced by the Canadian Council on Animal Care (CCAC), and registered research and educational institutions in Canada are required to have Animal Care Committees (ACCs) to help institutions oversee the care of institution-owned animals. AVMA-accredited programs of veterinary technology are required to have IACUCs or ACCs if the school owns regulated species. Each program must create protocols for clinical procedures that use animals. These protocols are subsequently reviewed by the IACUC or the ACC for discussion, amendment, and approval.

Horse Protection Act

The US Horse Protection Act (HPA) is a federal law enacted in 1970 (PL 91-540, as amended, 15 USC § 1821 et seq.) to prohibit horses that are subjected to practices known as *soring* from participating in shows, sales, exhibitions, or auctions. Soring has been a widespread problem in the Tennessee Walking Horse show community and includes such horrific practices as the external application of caustic chemicals to the pasterns of horses, coupled with exercising the horse with heavy chains ("action devices") fastened around its pasterns to create pain, and various methods of "pressure shoeing" to cause pain to the horse every time the horse places its front feet on the ground. The HPA is enforced by the USDA's Animal and Plant Health Inspection Service (APHIS), but the enforcement program has always been underfunded, and only a very small number of violators have been prosecuted. In early 2011, the USDA announced new minimum civil penalties for violations of the HPA and its regulations. The HPA also prohibits drivers from transporting sored horses to or from any of these events. Several states have specifically addressed soring as part of the state's criminal statutes related to prosecutions for animal cruelty. On June 14, 2012, the AVMA and the American Association of Equine Professionals (AAEP) called for a USDA ban on all "action devices" and "performance packages" (a type of elevated shoeing) in both the training and showing of the Tennessee Walking Horses. Technicians working in an equine practice should consider their legal and ethical responsibilities should they encounter horses that they believe have been abused by soring.

Endangered Species Act

The primary goals of the Endangered Species Act are to prevent the extinction of imperiled plant and animal life, and to recover and maintain those populations by removing or lessening threats to their survival. This act is administered by two federal agencies—the US Fish and Wildlife Service (FWS) and the National Oceanic and Atmospheric Administration (NOAA).

Laws Specific to Canada

Criminal Code of Canada

The Criminal Code sections 444 to 447 contain laws specific to the injury or endangerment of cattle and other animals, such as dogs and birds, and which cause unnecessary suffering or failure to exercise reasonable care of animals. It also has references to the illegality of cockfights.

Canada Wildlife Act

This act allows for the creation, management, and protection of conserved lands for the purpose of supporting wildlife, wildlife research, and conservation. The purpose of conserving land is to preserve habitats that are critical to migratory birds and other wildlife species, particularly those with critically diminished populations.

Canadian Food Inspection Agency

The Canadian Food Inspection Agency (CFIA) enforces the criminal code through routine inspections, unannounced site inspections, and response to reports of noncompliance.

Provincial Legislation on Animal Welfare

Each province has legislation concerning animal welfare. Provincial legislation and regulations tend to be general in scope, covering a wide range of animal welfare interests. Some provinces have regulations pertaining to specific species.

Nongovernment Animal Welfare Organizations

A number of Canadian nongovernment organizations have animal welfare mandates and assume responsibility for various aspects of animal welfare. The National Farm Animal Care Council (NFACC), for example, facilitates collaboration among all its members with respect to the care and management of farm animals. The NFACC also facilitates sharing of information and monitors the trends and initiatives in domestic and international marketplaces.

Humane Transportation of Animals

The CFIA ensures humane transport of food animal species. Regulations prohibit overcrowding, transport of incompatible animals in the same stall, and transport of animals unfit for travel. These regulations specify appropriate conditions for loading and unloading animals, adequate feeding and watering regimes, maximum transit times, minimum rest periods, and bedding requirements. Regulations also require animal handlers to take animals to the nearest veterinary medical facility for care if they are compromised in transit.

Canadian Meat Inspection Act

The Meat Inspection Act established standards for the humane handling and slaughter of food animals in federally inspected slaughter facilities. The CFIA places inspectors at federally registered slaughter establishments to monitor the handling and slaughter of food animals.

Acknowledgment

The authors wish to acknowledge Joanna M. Bassert and Teresa Lazo for their work on the previous edition version of this chapter.

Recommended Readings

Bureau of Labor Statistics, Occupational Employment Statistics, Occupational Employment and Wages, May 2015, 29-2056 Veterinary Technologists and Technicians. Available at: http://www.bls.gov/oes/current/oes292056.htm#nat (Accessed on June 4, 2016).

Canadian Vet Tech (a newsmagazine for veterinary technologists and technicians). It features in-depth articles and continuing education for veterinary technicians. International Institute for Animal Law: Available at: www.animallaw.com (Accessed on June 27, 2011).

Rockett J, Lattanzio C, Anderson K. *Patient Assessment, Intervention and Documentation for the Veterinary Technician: A Guide to Developing Care Plans and SOAP's*. Florence, KY: Delmar Cengage Learning; 2008.

Benson GJ, Rollin BE. *The Well-Being of Farm Animals: Challenges And Solutions*. 1st ed. Ames, IA: Wiley-Blackwell; 2004.

Rollin BE. *Animal Rights & Human Morality*. 3rd ed. Amherst, NY: Prometheus Books; 2006.

Shapiro LS. *Applied Animal Ethics*. Albany, NY: Delmar Thomson Learning; 2000.

The *NAVTA Journal* is the official publication of the National Association of Veterinary Technicians in America (NAVTA) and is exclusive to NAVTA members (www.navta.net).

The *RVT Journal* is published by RVTs, for RVTs, and distributed to more than 3000 RVTs across Canada (www.oavt.org).

The *Trends Magazine* provides perspectives on the art and business of companion animal veterinary practice to all members of the practice team (https://www.aaha.org/publications/trends-magazine/).

US Department of Agriculture; National Agriculture Library. Animal Welfare Act. Available at: https://www.nal.usda.gov/animal-health-and-welfare/animal-welfare-act.

2
Veterinary Practice Management

HEATHER PRENDERGAST

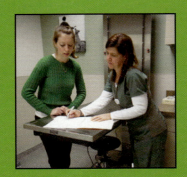

CHAPTER OUTLINE

LEARNING OBJECTIVES

When you have completed this chapter, you will be able to:

1. Pronounce, spell, and define each of the key terms in this chapter.
2. List the terms used to describe various types of veterinary facilities.
3. List the roles and responsibilities of each member of the veterinary health care team.
4. Describe the basic flow of clients, patients, and employees through a typical veterinary hospital.
5. Outline the key elements of effectively working with clients, including the importance of communication skills, myths about communication skills, and how to diffuse the anger of difficult clients.
6. Describe the major job management functions needed to run a veterinary hospital efficiently.
7. Describe the primary components of excellent practice management.

8. List examples of stressors in the veterinary workplace and describe ways to ameliorate the effects of those stressors on veterinary personnel.
9. Describe the major areas in which veterinary practices employ internal and external marketing techniques.
10. List some of the major tasks associated with good financial management.
11. List reasons why management and financial analysis are important to the business of veterinary medicine.
12. Discuss the importance of efficient operations for practice revenue.
13. Discuss key areas in which computerization adds to the efficiency and productivity of veterinary practice.

KEY TERMS

Accounts receivable
American Animal Hospital Association (AAHA)
Appointment system
Basic animal husbandry
Bereavement
Cash flow
Center
Certified Veterinary Practice Manager (CVPM)
Clinic
Contamination
Emergency facility
Frustration
Gross revenue
Haul-in facility

Hospital
Mixed animal practice
Mobile facility
Net income
Office
Outpatient
Practice inventory management system (PIMS)
Profits
Referral facility
Specialty facility
Strategic planning
Technician supervisor
Veterinary teaching hospital
Walk-in system

Introduction

Veterinary technicians today have diverse employment opportunities available to them. Some of these include working in laboratory animal medicine and in the pharmaceutical industry; however, most veterinary technicians work in clinical practice. Although there are many corporately owned veterinary practices, most practices are operated as independently owned, for-profit businesses, and many offer a full complement of veterinary services, including care for sick and injured animals and preventive and wellness care. A growing number of nonprofit animal shelters and rescue groups offer veterinary services both to their own pets and to the public. The services offered by these practices are sometimes, but not always, more limited compared with those offered by for-profit veterinary practices.

The revenue and **profits** generated by a practice make it possible for the veterinary health care team members to provide good quality medical care to patients. In the long run, it is not possible for a practice to offer excellent veterinary care if it is not economically successful. The revenue and profits earned by practices are reinvested in equipment, drugs, and supplies; in hiring staff; and in updating and maintaining the hospital building. In addition, revenue is used to pay all employees of the practice, including the practice owner. Only if the practice does well economically can the people who work in the practice thrive economically.

PUT INTO PRACTICE

Becoming an integral part of the team will require you to do some work. It is important to demonstrate your knowledge, show humility, and support others. You can be a leader in your practice without a title. Showing you care for your patients and others is vital to building trust with each other.

It is not easy to operate a veterinary practice successfully. Much time and money must be invested in the activities necessary to make the practice a success. Effective management of a veterinary practice as a business has become a complex task because of increased competition; growing malpractice threats; new technology; the availability of information on the Internet; shifting client expectations; and continued inflation of the costs of medical equipment, supplies, and personnel.

Not all practices are structured in the same way. Some are focused solely on companion animal care, others treat horses exclusively, and still others offer veterinary care for a variety of species, large and small. Some practices are located in their own

facilities, others offer only ambulatory care, and some provide both ambulatory and nonambulatory services. Most practices focus on general medicine, but a growing number offer emergency or specialty care. No matter the type of practice, most team members will have some role in management activities that allow the practice to thrive. Therefore students need to develop a working knowledge of the principles of practice management to be effective technicians, to contribute to the financial success of the practice, and to prepare for future advancement in the veterinary technology profession. This understanding is critical for assessing practice differences when searching for the best employment opportunity.

TECHNICIAN NOTE

In the long run, it is not possible for a practice to offer excellent veterinary care if the practice is not economically successful. Only if the practice does well financially can the people who work in the practice thrive financially.

Types of Veterinary Practices

Most practices have two to three full-time–equivalent veterinarians who work 30 hours or more each week, while some practices have a solo veterinarian who is also the owner. Many practices are still privately owned, but a large number are corporately owned, especially emergency and specialty.

Most veterinary hospitals have limited their practice to the treatment of some species but not others. For example, they may offer care exclusively to cats or horses, to companion animals (dogs, cats, exotic pets), or to large animals (livestock and/or horses). Some practices, known as *mixed animal practices*, see a variety of species, including companion animals, livestock, and horses. A few practices may be limited to exotic animals, such as reptiles, birds, and small mammals.

Most practicing veterinarians are general practitioners who offer primary care services. Complex cases are often referred to veterinarians who are specialists working in **referral facilities** or veterinary schools. These veterinary specialists are generally board certified in surgery, internal medicine, dermatology, ophthalmology, or other areas. Veterinary technician specialists (VTSs) also work in referral practices and in hospitals affiliated with veterinary medical schools.

Veterinary **emergency facilities** can be found in all major cities and also in many smaller communities. Some are part of a referral and **specialty facility** or a veterinary teaching hospital, but most often, they are standalone businesses. These facilities are usually open at times when general practices are not, such as at night and on weekends and holidays. This network of referring practitioners provides access to the best quality of care possible while also serving as the foundation of clinical research at both specialty centers and veterinary medical schools.

Most general practices open between 7:00 a.m. and 8:00 a.m. and close around 6:00 p.m. during the week, and also have some Saturday hours. An increasing number of practices are open in the evening to serve clients who cannot make appointments during the day. Specialty hospitals generally open around 8:00 a.m. and close between 5:00 p.m. and 6:00 p.m. and usually do not offer Saturday or Sunday hours. Emergency practices are open nights, weekends, and holidays—the times general practices are closed. Teaching hospitals at veterinary colleges tend to have similar hours for their general and specialty practices but accept emergencies 24 hours a day, 365 days of the year. Veterinary practice *names* can be described in various ways, such as a **clinic**, a **hospital**, or a **veterinary teaching hospital** (Box 2.1).

Typical Employee Positions

Regardless of the size and type of the practice, overall types of staff positions tend to be similar. Most practices have the following types of employees: management personnel; veterinarians; veterinary technicians and technologists; veterinary assistants; receptionists; and kennel, ward, or barn attendants. Veterinary technicians are graduates of an American Veterinary Medical Association (AVMA)-accredited program of veterinary technology; veterinary technologists have graduated from an accredited 4-year program. In large practices, the roles may be further subdivided; for example, the practice may have **outpatient** technicians and surgery technicians, or the management staff may consist of a hospital administrator, a practice manager, and an accounting staff member.

In smaller practices, staff members may have dual roles. For example, a veterinary technician may also handle some management duties, or a veterinary assistant may also work in the kennel. In these practices, staff members are often cross trained in several positions so that the practice can continue to function when sickness, vacation, or emergencies arise and a key individual is out for the day.

In most practices, everyone is expected to perform certain activities; for example, it may be the receptionist's job to answer the telephone, but if the receptionist is busy and the phone keeps ringing, any of the staff members should be willing to answer it. Entering charges into a client's invoice may be the primary responsibility of the technician, but veterinarians and receptionists will also sometimes need to do this. In all practices, everyone is expected to communicate well and contribute to outstanding client service.

To be effective, the veterinarian-owner must act as the chief executive officer for the clinic overall and must delegate appropriate areas of responsibility to veterinary technicians and other members of the team. In the best-run practices, job duties are delegated to the lowest-level person who can do the job well within the legal scope of practice (Fig. 2.1).

• BOX 2.1 Guidelines for Classifying Veterinary Facilities

Veterinary teaching hospital: A veterinary teaching hospital is a facility in which consultative, clinical, and hospital services are rendered and in which a large staff of basic and applied veterinary scientists perform significant research and teach professional veterinary students (DVM [Doctor of Veterinary Medicine] or equivalent degree) and house officers.

Hospital/Clinic: A veterinary or animal hospital is a facility in which the practice is conducted typically or may include inpatient and outpatient diagnostics and treatment.

Outpatient clinic: A veterinary or animal outpatient clinic is a facility in which the practice conducted may include short-term admission of patients but where all patients are discharged at the end of the workday.

Mobile practice: A mobile practice is conducted from a vehicle with special medical or surgical facilities or from a vehicle suitable for making house or farm calls. Regardless of mode of transportation, such practice shall have a permanent base of operations with a published address and telecommunication capabilities for making appointments or responding to emergency situations.

Emergency facility: A veterinary emergency facility is one with the primary function of receiving, treating, and monitoring of emergency patients during its specified hours of operation. A veterinarian is in attendance at all hours of operation, and sufficient staff is available to provide timely and appropriate care. Veterinarians, support staff, instrumentation, medications, and supplies must be sufficient to provide an appropriate level of emergency care. A veterinary emergency service may be an independent, after-hours service; an independent 24-hour service; or part of a full-service hospital.

Specialty facility: A specialty facility is a veterinary or animal facility that provides services by board-certified veterinarian(s)/specialists.

Referral facility: A referral facility provides services by those veterinarians with a special interest in certain species or a particular area of veterinary medicine.

Center: The word "center" in the name of a veterinary or animal facility strongly implies advanced depth or scope of practice (e.g., Animal Medical Center, Veterinary Imaging Center, Canine Sports Medicine Center).

TECHNICIAN NOTE

In the best-run practices, job duties are delegated to the lowest-level person who can do the job well within the legal scope of practice. This is why successful practices delegate all clinical care duties to veterinary technicians and other members of the veterinary health care team, except those tasks that, by law, must be performed exclusively by veterinarians.

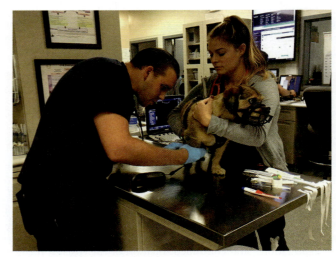

• Fig. 2.1 Members of the veterinary health care team work collaboratively to provide excellent health care to animals. Financially successful practices delegate duties to the lowest-level person who can do the job well within the legal scope of practice. (Courtesy Dr. Joanna Bassert.)

This kind of delegation is a key component of good management. Unfortunately, it is not uncommon to see veterinarians doing tasks that a well-educated technician is legally allowed to do. Many practices hire veterinary technicians but have them perform the duties of veterinary assistants and caretakers. Consequently, the practice spends more money than necessary on personnel, causing **frustration** among veterinarians and among veterinary technicians who are not given the opportunity to fully exercise the skills they were educated to perform. It is important to remember, however, that most veterinary practices are small and have a limited number of employees; except in the largest practices, it is difficult to fully limit duties to just one individual or one staff position.

Regardless of position in the hospital setting, all personnel should have detailed job descriptions. A job description will allow both the employee and management to maintain a clear understanding of areas of responsibility. Job descriptions are also useful when new employees are hired or employees are replaced. Common duties of each employee are discussed in the sections below. However, it is important to remember that some variation may occur depending on the way in which an individual practice is structured.

Although each position in the hospital has its own specific responsibilities, it is essential that all employees work together as a team to maximize the veterinarians' effectiveness and productivity and the pet owners' service experience. Team members must be selected on the basis of their ability to work together efficiently, rather than just on their ability to perform isolated duties. Last but not least, each employee should take it upon themselves to continue developing their technical competencies and professionalism through educational opportunities. Continuous development allows for greater networking within the veterinary technician profession and more opportunities for advancement.

Management Personnel

Veterinary practices are small businesses that must be efficiently operated and financially successful if they are to offer high-quality patient care. To survive as a veterinary *hospital,* the practice must survive as a *business.* Ensuring survival is the job of practice owners and management staff.

Historically, veterinarians who owned a veterinary practice often performed the management tasks necessary to keep the practice economically viable and running smoothly. As practices have gotten bigger and the challenges of management have become greater, increasing numbers of veterinarians are delegating business management responsibilities to managers. The quality of management among veterinary practices varies widely; some practices are managed well and others poorly.

The organization of management staff varies according to practice size and management philosophy. Three commonly seen management positions are office manager, practice manager, and hospital administrator. Job descriptions for these can be obtained from the Veterinary Hospital Managers Association (VHMA); however, the duties assigned to each of these positions and the quality of work performed in them can vary widely. The scope of work for each position is provided here.

- *Office manager:* Office managers generally report to the practice owner or the practice manager. Their duties include hiring and training office and reception staff, scheduling shifts and supervising receptionists, acting as a client liaison when problems or complaints arise, preparing bank deposits, collecting **accounts receivable**, and performing clerical work.
- *Practice manager:* Practice managers generally report to the practice owner or to the hospital administrator. They often have more extensive management training and experience than office managers and have a wider range of management responsibilities. Typically, duties include hiring, training, scheduling, and supervising staff; carrying out marketing activities; and preparing or supervising the preparation of accounting and financial documents, such as accounts receivable, accounts payable, budgets, and financial analyses. Establishing budgets and fees; purchasing supplies and equipment, including maintaining inventory control; serving as a client liaison; managing the computer network; and supervising and organizing workflow are added responsibilities of the practice manager. Practice managers generally are not involved in medical management duties, although they may oversee the nonmedical aspects of veterinarians' work.
- *Hospital administrators:* These individuals are generally responsible for all activities of the hospital, both medical and administrative, and run the hospital in conjunction with practice owners. Hospital administrators are also responsible for the tasks commonly performed by office managers and practice managers, in addition to hiring and supervising veterinarians and veterinary technicians.

In some hospitals, head receptionists and head technicians may perform some management duties in their area, in addition to their regular responsibilities. Large hospitals may have management personnel solely responsible for human resources, finance, or marketing.

The size of the practice generally influences the management structure. In small practices, management tasks may be shared among several individuals. Practice owners, for example, may delegate some tasks, such as inventory control and staff scheduling, to receptionists, technicians, or office managers but may do the planning-, finance-, and employee-related work themselves. Team members handling management tasks may report directly to the practice owner or to the office manager. Office managers report to practice owners.

Some particularly large practices have technician supervisors who recruit, hire, and train the technician staff. This position may include writing job descriptions, performing annual reviews, and determining staff advancement and raises. Technician supervisors might also arrange in-house continuing education for the nursing staff.

Medium-sized practices often have a full-time practice manager, whose responsibility is to handle most management duties. Some duties may still be delegated to other team members, and the practice may also have employees in head technician and head receptionist positions. Practice owners generally remain involved in some high-level tasks, such as hiring veterinarians, **strategic planning**, and managing financial issues. Most often, the head technician, the head receptionist, and others doing management tasks report to the practice manager, and the practice manager, in turn, reports to the practice owner.

Large to very large practices often have both a practice manager and a hospital administrator on staff and, in addition, may have a human resources (HR) manager, a finance manager, a bookkeeper or accounting department, and clerical staff. Usually, the HR manager, the finance manager, the accounting staff, and other low-level management personnel report to the practice manager. The practice manager reports to the hospital administrator and the administrator to the practice owner.

Many nonowner-veterinarians working in clinical practice do not have formal management duties assigned to them. It would be expected, however, that they would demonstrate the traits of good managers and leaders in client service, communication, teamwork, and other areas.

It is not uncommon to see veterinary technicians who have an interest in management moving into the role of practice manager. The obvious advantage to this is that the technician generally has worked at the practice for a long time and knows how the practice operates. The disadvantage is that the technician may not have the management or leadership skills necessary to run the practice well and may have too many friendships among the staff to be able to effectively deal with personnel issues. Not all practice owners, many of whom are veterinarians, offer the training and support necessary for veterinary technicians to be successful in new management roles. Technicians who are interested in management can learn more about what management work entails by attending management-related continuing education classes before moving into these new roles.

> ### TECHNICIAN NOTE
>
> It is not uncommon to see veterinary technicians who have an interest in management moving into the role of practice manager.

The VHMA is the only organization that can certify veterinary practice managers. Managers who complete the program become Certified Veterinary Practice Managers (CVPMs). Candidates must document veterinary management work experience and completion of continuing education in management, submit letters of recommendation, and pass an examination administered by the CVPM board. The CVPM program is accredited by the Institute for Credentialing Excellence.

> ### TECHNICIAN NOTE
>
> The Veterinary Hospital Managers Association is the only organization that can certify veterinary practice managers. Managers who complete the program become Certified Veterinary Practice Managers (CVPMs).

Veterinarians

The primary activities of veterinarians in clinical practice include diagnosing and treating ill or injured animals and providing preventive or wellness care to animals to reduce the likelihood of disease or accident in the future. Generally, a full physical examination is performed on each animal presented for care, or an assessment of herd health is completed, and findings from these assessments, along with results from various laboratory and imaging and other diagnostic tests, are used by the veterinarian to generate a diagnosis. Treatment can consist of a broad range of activities, including surgery, dental cleaning and extractions, oral or parenteral medication, hospitalization, acupuncture, and many others.

Preventive care or "wellness care" activities for companion animals include an annual physical examination, vaccinations, and administration and/or prescription of parasiticides. Pet owners, even those who have owned pets before, often do not understand what care is needed for their pets or why it is important. A critical component of veterinary care is communication about these issues with pet owners.

Large animal practitioners and those who work in shelter medicine focus on the care of the animal group as a whole and on the care of individual animals.

Ideally, the veterinarian delegates most animal care tasks (as allowed by the state practice act) to veterinary technicians and technologists; examples of these tasks include providing anesthesia, dental prophylaxes, imaging, laboratory procedures, and client communications. Delegation of these duties to the veterinary technician allows the veterinarian to increase their own efficiency and allows the veterinary technician to carry out the job that they were educated to do and, in this way, to have a meaningful role in the hospital.

Veterinary Technicians and Technologists

As discussed in Chapter 1, a veterinary technician has an associate degree from an AVMA-accredited program in veterinary technology, and a veterinary technologist has a baccalaureate degree in veterinary technology. Unlike the veterinarian, who is responsible for making the diagnosis and treating the patient, the veterinary technician and veterinary technologist evaluate the patients' responses to disease. Assessing and reassessing the patient, making technician evaluations, and using independent critical thinking to develop and implement a technician plan of care are the primary steps in the veterinary technician practice model. Veterinary technicians and veterinary technologists are responsible for carrying out the medical treatment plans of the veterinarian, alerting the veterinarian to changes in patient status, educating the client about disease processes and home treatment protocols, and completing medical record entries (see Fig. 2.2). Recognizing and addressing patient discomfort and anticipating potential complications are additional important responsibilities of the veterinary technician.

> ### TECHNICIAN NOTE
>
> Assessing and reassessing the patient, making technician evaluations, and using independent critical thinking to develop and implement a patient plan of care are the primary steps in the veterinary technician practice model.

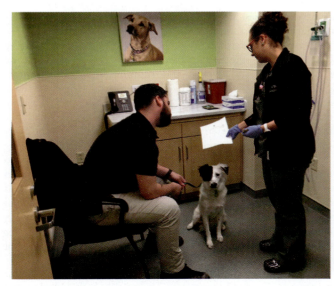

• **Fig. 2.2** Veterinary technicians and technologists are responsible for educating the client about their pet's condition and how to carry out take-home instructions. (Courtesy Dr. Joanna Bassert.)

The role of veterinary technicians and assistants can vary greatly among veterinary hospitals, depending on the size of the hospital and the organization of workflow. Many hospitals do not have credentialed veterinary technicians; therefore veterinarians and veterinary assistants perform all animal care duties. Other hospitals have a mixture of technicians and assistants.

The term *technician*, or *tech*, is often used erroneously in veterinary practices to describe any or all animal care personnel, regardless of their educational background, credential level, or skill set. It is important for veterinary practices to use proper terminology so that clients are clear about the qualifications of each member of the veterinary health care team.

Staff members who wear name tags that use unapproved terminology and practices that make no distinction between veterinary assistants and veterinary technicians or technologists cause confusion in pet owners, and the practice is doing a disservice to its employees in not recognizing those with true credentials. Indeed, the Internet-informed client of today may construe this as an intentional effort on the part of the practice to deceive the client by inflating the image of noncredentialed personnel. The establishment of terminology approved by the National Association of Veterinary Technicians in America (NAVTA) and the AVMA decades ago, together with official terminology as outlined in state practice acts, offers the pet owner and the veterinary practice owner clear terminology to distinguish credentialed from noncredentialed staff.

> **TECHNICIAN NOTE**
>
> The term *technician*, or *tech*, is too often used erroneously in veterinary practices to describe any or all animal care personnel regardless of their educational background, credential level, or skill set. It is important for veterinary practices to use proper terminology so that clients are clear about the qualifications of each member of the veterinary health care team.

Large private practices, such as specialty and referral practices, and veterinary teaching hospitals often have large caseloads that allow veterinary technicians to work exclusively in one area of a hospital, such as in the operating room (OR), the intensive care unit (ICU), and the departments of anesthesiology, cardiology, internal medicine, ophthalmology, dermatology, radiology, and clinical pathology. This may lead to technicians working toward a VTS specialty designation.

Veterinary Assistants

Veterinary assistants generally perform animal care and ward maintenance duties under the supervision of a veterinarian or a veterinary technician. These duties may include using animal restraint; performing laboratory work; filling prescriptions; preparing patients for surgery; administering and monitoring treatments; bathing animals; cleaning cages; feeding, watering, and walking hospitalized patients and boarders; and performing other duties as needed to create a smooth patient flow in the hospital.

Assistants may be responsible for cleaning and maintaining the building, wards, and barn (in large animal practices). However, in some practices, kennel or barn attendants perform these tasks. The role of the assistant is generally determined by the size and type of practice and the number of staff members.

Receptionists

Receptionists fill a key position in any hospital operation. They are the first and last person a client sees and are often instrumental in leaving the pet owner with a good impression. Typical receptionist duties include making appointments, answering questions in person or on the phone, greeting clients, updating client and patient information, setting up the medical record for the current visit, checking clients in and out, quoting fees, maintaining appointment schedules for veterinarians and veterinary technicians, handling money and bank deposits, and managing accounts receivable.

Movement of patients and their medical records from the receptionist in the front to the veterinary technician in the back is critical for an efficiently functioning hospital. Both receptionists and technicians should have some understanding of the other's duties and how their tasks affect those of others. They should regularly work together to resolve issues that are impeding the ability of each group to do its job well.

> **TECHNICIAN NOTE**
>
> Movement of patients and their medical records from the receptionist in the front to the veterinary technician in the back is critical for an efficiently functioning hospital. Both receptionists and technicians should have some understanding of each other's duties and how their tasks affect those of others.

Kennel, Ward, and Barn Attendants

Attendants perform the basic husbandry required to keep patients clean, groomed, fed, watered, and exercised, with the safety and comfort of each patient taken into consideration. Ward staff should observe and record the patient's appetite, attitude, bowel movements, and urinary output, and must alert the staff about observed abnormal behavior. They also move patients from the ward to the treatment area, to the reception area for discharge, or to surgery. Ward staff can double as veterinary assistants through cross training. Attendants are usually responsible for ongoing cleaning and maintenance of all areas of the hospital. Cleaning and sanitation are critical in a hospital environment to prevent nosocomial infections—those inadvertently acquired by patients from the hospital environment (Box 2.2).

> **TECHNICIAN NOTE**
>
> Although each position in the hospital has its own specific responsibilities, it is essential that all employees work together as a team to maximize the veterinarians' effectiveness and productivity and the pet owners' service experience.

Practice Facilities and Workflow

The facilities of veterinary practices vary greatly depending on the needs of clients and the species of animals seen by the practice. Facility design must accommodate the needs of patients, the number of clients served, the interests of the veterinarians, the level of care to be provided, and the level of financing available for investing in the facility.

As discussed previously, the practice may limit veterinary service to a single species (feline, equine, swine, cattle), to small animals (dogs, cats, exotic pets), to large animals (livestock and horses), or to exotic animals, or it may serve as a mixed practice (many species). Each type of practice has unique requirements for facility design and construction. Large animal and mixed practices may provide all veterinary services on the animal owner's premises, may have haul-in facilities for these species, or may provide both options as a convenience to the client. Some companion animal practices provide house calls in addition to work done at the practice facility, and a few veterinarians operate house call–only practices.

Many state practice acts and other regulations that apply to veterinary practices have not only been updated to specify standards of practice and professional competency for both veterinarians and technicians, but they also have adopted facility and equipment requirements. Some states require facility registration and have inspectors to ensure that standards established by the state are being met.

The American Animal Hospital Association (AAHA) offers voluntary accreditation programs for veterinary hospitals. The AAHA is the only organization in North America that has nearly 50 mandatory standards (and several applicable standards) to drive high-quality patient care. The process is designed to help practices refine and improve their services in five areas:

1. Quality of care
2. Management
3. Medical records
4. Facility
5. Diagnostics and pharmacy

The most common type of veterinary facility is a small animal practice devoted to general care that employs two to three veterinarians; this will be used as the model for discussing facility design and client, patient, and employee workflow. Issues unique to larger general practices, referral hospitals, emergency clinics, veterinary teaching hospitals, large animal or mixed animal practices, and ambulatory practices will be discussed at the end of this section.

Hospital facilities are generally designed to include sufficient examination rooms for outpatient services, overnight hospitalization, and complete surgical facilities. They must have ancillary support areas, such as a reception area, a laboratory, a pharmacy, and space for imaging, diagnostic procedures, and treatment. Some hospitals also offer boarding and grooming services. The appropriate size and location of each area in the hospital are related to the types of services offered by the hospital, the number of veterinarians and support staff in the practice, and the number of clients and patients served.

General maintenance within the building is an ongoing challenge. Floors, flat surfaces, walls, cages, runs, and stalls must be kept clean and odor-free. Counters, magazine racks, and pictures need to be organized and dusted frequently. The reception area, examination rooms, and public bathrooms must be inspected and cleaned regularly throughout each day. Everyone in the practice must assume some of the cleaning responsibility. One of the reasons cleanup in a veterinary practice is challenging is the large quantity of hair shed by animals. Clients notice hospital cleanliness. Only one client may complain, but many others may also be forming a negative impression of the practice. If the veterinary hospital is to be considered a modern and progressive medical facility, all personnel must strictly monitor odors and sanitation. Whenever a pet soils an area or a cage, it must be cleaned thoroughly as soon as possible. Appropriate disinfectants must be used to prevent odor buildup. Deodorizers may be of benefit to help clean the area but should not be used to cover up a sanitation problem. Appropriate ventilation systems should be in place throughout the building, with frequent filter changes.

Equipment cleaning must be an ongoing activity. Each major piece of equipment should be assigned to a specific member of the hospital team to keep it well maintained. It is recommended that the person most familiar with each piece of equipment be assigned to maintain it. If this is done, all equipment will last longer and will always be ready for use when needed for quality patient care. Regular maintenance of nonmedical equipment, such as calculators, computers, air conditioning and heating units, lawn mowers, and related equipment, should also be performed. Important medical equipment, such as anesthesia machines, endoscopes, and ultrasound machines, should have a documented, regular maintenance schedule to ensure proper servicing and consistent functioning of the equipment. The responsibility to maintain this equipment is most commonly assigned to those who use it most often.

Small Animal General Practices

Facility Exterior

Pet owners generally choose a practice that is conveniently close to their homes; therefore, most companion animal practices are located in or near populous residential areas. The practice facility, both inside and out, should convey an attractive and professional image and should meet the needs of patients, clients, and employees (Fig. 2.3). In most communities, pet owners have many choices when it comes to selecting a veterinary practice. Practices that will be most successful are those that best meet the needs and expectations of the pet owner. Ideally, veterinary practices are located in areas of high visibility and easy access. Not only is well-placed, well-lit professional signage a marketing tool, but it also allows clients to find the practice easily at night and during an emergency.

A client's initial impression of a practice is based on the appearance of the building and grounds. Regular maintenance, including

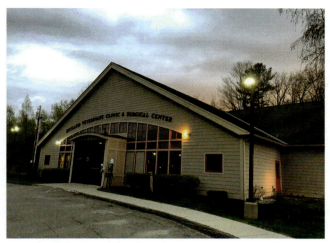

• **Fig. 2.3** The exterior appearance of the hospital should provide a positive image, and client parking should be clearly designated and clean. Pictured is the façade of Rutland Veterinary Clinic and Surgical Center, Rutland. (Courtesy Rutland Veterinary Clinic and Surgical Center, Rutland, VT.)

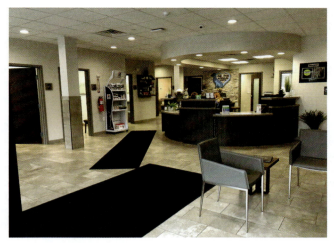

• **Fig. 2.4** The reception area should be welcoming, clean, and spacious enough to accommodate dogs and cats comfortably. (Courtesy Park Ridge Animal Hospital, Park Ridge, NJ.)

painting and repair, is therefore very important. Landscaping should be regularly attended to, as dead plants and weeds do not send the right message. The parking lot should be clean, neat, and well lit, and should offer easy access to the hospital entrance. The parking lot entrance and exit should be clearly marked by signs. Parking spaces should be reserved for clients only, with employee parking located behind the building or in a remote area away from the building entrance.

The entrance to the veterinary facility should be in full view and clearly marked to allow easy access. If more than one entrance is available, as is occasionally done to separate small and large animals or canines and felines, each entry should be well marked. To prevent client congestion, the entrance and the exit should be separated. Practice employees should not use the public entrance of the building. Furthermore, those providing routine deliveries and service activities should enter and exit the building away from client areas when possible.

Professional activities within a veterinary hospital can be grouped into four areas: outpatient, inpatient, surgical, and support.

Outpatient Areas

Most patients visit a veterinary hospital as outpatients. This means that the pet will not be admitted to the hospital and will not be staying overnight. Outpatient areas are composed primarily of the reception area and the examination rooms, but the laboratory, pharmacy, and treatment areas are used for outpatients and for hospitalized patients. Clients generally cannot judge the quality of medicine in a veterinary practice; much of their evaluation of the quality of the practice is based on their impressions of the facility and the level of client service. A disorganized, dirty, smelly, noisy hospital will not inspire confidence in clients regarding the level of patient care, nor will it convey value for the fees charged. It is important for employees to impress clients by wearing clean, neat uniforms and by maintaining a well-groomed appearance at all times.

TECHNICIAN NOTE

Most patients visit a veterinary hospital as outpatients. This means that pets will not be admitted to the hospital and will not be staying overnight.

Clients and their pets typically first enter the reception area, where the admission process begins. Most reception areas have a large counter behind which the receptionist sits. If the practice uses hard copy medical records, an area for filing them often adjoins the receptionist's work area. The receptionist checks the client in, locates the client record, and coordinates the business and medical records needed for the visit. Some practices have a separate telephone area where additional receptionists take telephone calls and schedule appointments.

The waiting area for clients and their pets often dominates the reception space, while some space may be devoted to the sale of pet food and other products. Clients often spend time waiting in the reception area, so it is important that this area be neatly organized, attractive, and clean (Fig. 2.4). Seating should be comfortable, and tables or other raised areas on which pet owners can set carriers should be available. The waiting area should be scrupulously cleaned, and it should be ensured that there are no unpleasant smells. It is helpful to provide separate areas for dog owners and cat owners, as cats are very sensitive to the presence of dogs. The reception area should be reasonably quiet; interesting magazines and pet information can be provided; a client restroom should also be available. Any reading material provided should be complete and should not have torn or missing pages; pictures should be neatly framed and matted. A coffee or soft drink station is a welcome touch. In addition, a children's play area, television, and access to wireless Internet can also help clients feel more comfortable during their wait.

Receptionists should be mindful of how their conversations and actions are perceived by clients. Personal phone conversations, arguments among staff members in view of clients, and staff members who do not appear to be working while clients are waiting to be served do not create a good impression.

Clients do not like to be kept waiting. They should spend only a short amount of time in the reception room before they are escorted to one of the examination rooms. This requires effective appointment scheduling and dedication to timely service. As a general rule, two examination rooms should be available in the outpatient area for each veterinarian working on a given day. Therefore in the typical two-veterinarian practice, four examination rooms should be available, with the staff and veterinarians moving between them and facilitating timely service.

A patient presenting in an emergency always receives priority. If any question exists as to whether the case is truly an emergency, the pet should be placed in an examination room or taken back to the treatment area for an immediate triage examination by a veterinary technician or veterinarian. If the case is not an emergency, it can be worked back into the normal scheduling.

Examination rooms generally include an examination table, seating for the client, and a counter and cabinets to hold equipment and supplies needed by the veterinarian and other staff members. Computers and monitors are often present in each room. Examination areas should be clean, well organized, and attractive; the same guidelines described for reception areas apply to examination rooms as well (Fig. 2.5). Medications are generally not kept in examination rooms where clients may have unsupervised access to them. Examination equipment and supplies should be secured or kept out of sight so that neither clients nor their children will be tempted to look at or handle them. In addition, cats should ideally be placed in cats only examination rooms, and cat carriers should be placed on the examination table and not on the floor, where the patient would feel more insecure.

After the client is escorted into one of the examination rooms, a veterinary technician will obtain a brief history and gather all the materials needed for the visit. The veterinary technician will also obtain the pet's weight and temperature, pulse rate, and respiratory rate (TPR). All materials needed for the visit will also be gathered at this time by the veterinary technician.

When all the initial patient information has been gathered, the veterinarian typically performs a thorough physical examination on the pet and further discusses the pet's history with the client. A veterinary assistant should assist the veterinarian during the physical examination by restraining the patient as necessary. This frees the technician to move on to the next appointment and/or to gather additional materials that may be anticipated for the current patient. For example, if blood, urine, or skin specimens are needed, a technician should obtain these samples in the examination room or, if necessary, move the pet to a treatment area and obtain the samples out of sight of the owners. Clients should not be allowed to restrain their own pets because of the risk of being bitten; however, they may be allowed to see the process, because this adds to the client's value, as discussed later in the chapter.

After the examination is completed, the results of the examination and of the diagnostic procedures will be discussed with the client. Recommendations for additional diagnostics and for treatment or preventive care are made if necessary. The veterinary technician will often administer some treatments, such as immunizations, and will fill prescriptions according to the order by the veterinarian. In addition, the veterinary technician will educate the owner regarding the administration of home medications and treatments.

After the examination with the veterinarian, some patients may be admitted to the hospital for further diagnostics and treatment. In this case, the patient will be taken to the treatment areas, and the client will be escorted to the reception area to leave contact information for further follow-up with the veterinarian and the team. If the patient is going home, both the client and the patient will be escorted back to the reception area to settle the account and schedule any necessary future appointments.

The laboratory (Fig. 2.6) and pharmacy areas are usually located near the examination rooms. They often separate the "front" of the hospital, which includes the reception area and examination rooms, from the "back," which includes the treatment area, the surgical area, hospital runs, wards, and the boarding area. This high-functioning area is critical, because every team member uses it, regardless of working with inpatient or outpatient pets (Fig. 2.7A). Both areas should be well organized, and shelves should be clearly labeled. Signs prohibiting the use of refrigerators for human food storage should be posted clearly (see discussion of Occupational Safety and Health Administration [OSHA] in Chapter 4). In some practices, the laboratory and the pharmacy are combined for more efficient use of floor space. The pharmacy may also house the safety data sheets required by OSHA. Refer to Chapter 4 for more information about safety in a veterinary practice.

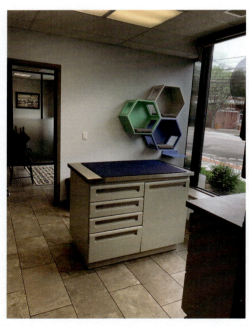

• **Fig. 2.5** Examination rooms should be warmly decorated, clean, and in excellent condition. (Courtesy Park Ridge Animal Hospital, Park Ridge, NJ.)

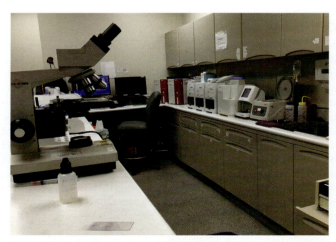

• **Fig. 2.6** The laboratory is located just beyond the examination and treatment rooms. A well-equipped clinical laboratory has microscopes, automated analyzers, a desktop computer, and a chair. (Courtesy Dr. Joanna Bassert.)

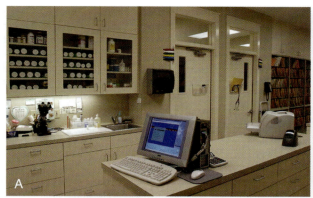
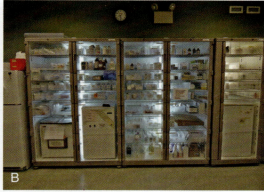
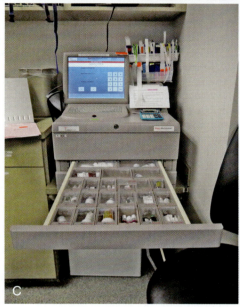
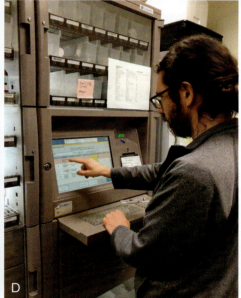

• **Fig. 2.7** (A) The pharmacy is located near examination rooms and inpatient treatment area. (B) Cardinal Health glass refrigerators. (C) Pyxis MedStation units provide environmentally appropriate storage for biologicals and pharmaceuticals. (D) Electronic door and drawer monitoring helps keep track of staff use of pharmacy products. (Courtesy Dr. Joanna Bassert.)

CASE PRESENTATION 2.1

Veterinary Technician Licensing

Scenario: Alisha Smith is a "veterinary technician" who has worked at the ABC Animal Hospital for over 10 years. She is a great "technician" and knows how to do a lot of technical tasks. ABC also has several "veterinary assistants," who have all been employed for less than 2 years. Within the last year, ABC Animal Hospital hired Michelle, who is a recent graduate of a Veterinary Technology program and has passed the Veterinary Technician National Exam (VTNE) and is fully credentialed.

Because Alisha is the head technician, she is responsible for training and onboarding new team members. As Michelle is going through the training process, she begins to realize some of the training and information provided are inaccurate and are unsafe for patients. She asks Alisha when and where she went to school because she tries to understand the misinformation. She learns that Alisha never went to school, and in fact, Alisha stated directly to Michelle that "one does not need to go to school to be a veterinary technician."

Query: What should Michelle do?

Response: Michelle should first research the information presented during training and obtain accurate documentation of the appropriate procedures. Second, she should research the state practice act to determine whether

title protection for the term "veterinary technician" exists in the state's law. In addition, she should find out if there is a scope of practice, listing specific duties in the law that define what tasks veterinary technicians (versus noncredentialed employees) can and cannot perform. Last, she should present her findings and concerns to the practice manager and owner. Some issues and questions that need to be discussed include the following:
- Does title protection exist in the state, and if so, what are the potential ramifications for *incorrectly* using the term *veterinary technician*?
- If a scope of duties exists, what are the potential ramifications if noncredentialed veterinary assistants perform the duties of veterinary technicians?
- What are the risks associated with the existing training program, and how can it be updated to better protect the patient?

Tips:
- Always seek to understand first, before asking for change. There may be a reason the training protocols are in place.
- Use empathy and compassion when addressing this topic. It may be a sensitive one to all those involved.

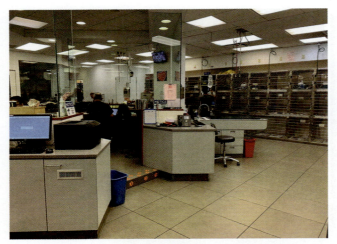

• **Fig. 2.8** Centralized treatment areas are convenient for both the veterinarian and the veterinary technician and offer easy access to both outpatient and inpatient treatment. (Courtesy West Chelsea Veterinary Hospital, Manhattan NY.)

Inpatient Areas

Inpatients are those pets that have been admitted to the hospital for various kinds of diagnostics or treatments, including laboratory work, radiography, dental care, and surgery. The pet may be admitted for an hour or two or for many days. This second work area in the hospital is devoted to these types of procedures and generally consists of a treatment area; special procedure rooms for radiography, ultrasonography, and endoscopy; patient wards; an isolation ward; an exercise area; a kitchen; boarding cages and runs; and a bathing and grooming area.

The treatment area is the central hub of the hospital. Patients from the wards (inpatients) and from examination rooms (outpatients) will be moved to this area for diagnostic procedures, medication administration, and recheck procedures, such as cast, bandage, or splint changes. In some specialty, emergency, and critical care hospitals, the centralized treatment area may be subdivided by workstations that create designated space for each of the specialty departments (Fig. 2.8). The treatment room may also be used for the preparation of surgical patients.

> **TECHNICIAN NOTE**
>
> The treatment area is the central hub of the hospital. Patients from the wards (inpatients) and from examination rooms (outpatients) will be moved to this area for diagnostic procedures, medication administration, and recheck procedures, such as cast, bandage, or splint changes.

In most hospitals, the radiology suite is near or connected to the treatment room and provides easy access to the surgery area as well (Fig. 2.9A). The radiology suite includes areas for taking, viewing, enhancing, and interpreting radiographs (x-ray films). Clients should not visit the radiology section when the x-ray machine is in use because of the risk of exposure to radiation. All personnel in radiology should wear personal protective equipment (PPE), such as leaded aprons, gloves, and thyroid shields (see Fig. 2.9B). In addition, veterinary technicians should wear their own dosimeters to monitor their level of exposure to radiation (see Fig. 2.9C). The level of exposure varies from person to person, depending on their caseload and the type of cases seen;

therefore, staff should not share dosimeters. Lead goggles are also helpful PPE that technicians should ask for and wear every time they are exposed to radiation. Ultrasonographic, dental, or other procedures may occur in rooms adjacent to the radiology suite.

Cages and runs for hospitalized patients are generally included in the treatment area, although some hospitals have small rooms off the treatment area for less seriously ill hospitalized patients. Critical patients are generally kept directly in the treatment area, where they can be easily monitored. This area is often referred to as the *ICU*. To reduce their anxiety, cats are kept in quiet areas away from dogs and preferably in a space located well above floor height.

The veterinarian will establish a medical treatment regimen for each hospitalized patient. The veterinary technician assesses the hospitalized patient frequently and generates a list of technician evaluations relevant to the patient. These evaluations are subsequently prioritized, and a patient care plan is developed; specific interventions are developed and implemented by the veterinary technician. The veterinarian writes SOAP (subjective, objective, assessment, and plan) notes to assist in the diagnostic process; the veterinary technician prepares SOAP notes to support the technician process and to ensure that all technician evaluations are addressed. Many practices, particularly those that use electronic medical records (EMRs), employ a truncated method of making medical notations in the patient record. For purposes of instruction and for teaching critical thinking skills, veterinary medical schools and veterinary technology programs instruct students in the formal method of writing SOAP notes. Refer to Chapters 1 and 7 for additional information about patient assessment and to Chapter 3 regarding medical record keeping.

During hospitalization, the veterinary technician makes repeated assessments of the patient; carries out medical treatments and diagnostic tests as ordered by the veterinarian; and delegates exercising, feeding, restraining, and grooming of the patient to veterinary assistants and animal caretakers. Often, daily communication with the client is carried out by the veterinary technician. A large whiteboard or computer screen in the treatment areas may be used to summarize the diagnostic, treatment, and surgery schedules for hospitalized patients. Computerized schedules may be generated with the same information. All patients should be assessed several times each day by the attending veterinary technician, and these assessments should be documented with appropriate entries into the medical record. Daily ward rounds can be helpful in keeping each member of the veterinary health care team up to date on the status of hospitalized patients.

When animals with infectious and contagious diseases are hospitalized, they are placed in an isolation ward. The isolation area should have one entrance and exit, preferably with access to the outside so that infectious patients do not walk through the common areas of the hospital. Isolation areas are designed to restrict the shedding of infectious microbes to a single region that can be easily sanitized. Disinfectants and protective disposable gloves, booties, and gowns should be available at the entrance to the isolation ward. The air handling system for the isolation area must be separate from that used in other parts of the building to prevent aerosol transmission of contagions. If adequate isolation facilities are not available on the premises, the case should be referred to a practice that has the proper facility. All treatment and handling of the infectious patient should be done by just one or two people. The patient should be treated and housed in the isolation facility and should never be taken to any other part of the hospital, including the main treatment room. Staff must be trained to

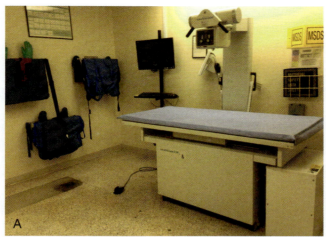

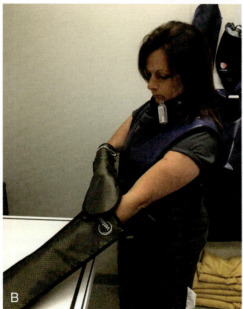

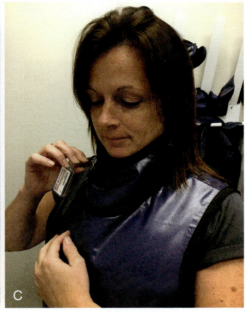

• **Fig. 2.9** A radiology room with an x-ray machine. Note the lead aprons, thyroid shields, gloves, and personal protective equipment (PPE) hanging on wall-mounted racks. (Courtesy Dr. Joanna Bassert.)

follow stringent isolation protocols to prevent the transmission of nosocomial infections to other patients.

When hospitalized pets are ready for discharge, the client is given written instructions for home care. The veterinary technician reviews discharge instructions with the owner and ensures that the owner is clear about home care. Copies of all client communication documents that are sent home with the client should be kept in the medical record; this allows team members to easily refer to the printed documents and provides proof of communication at discharge. Surgical incisions, bandages, splints, and casts must be clean and dry before the patient is discharged. Clients should be asked to settle their account before their pet is brought to them.

TECHNICIAN NOTE

When hospitalized pets are ready to be discharged, the veterinary technician reviews the discharge instructions and home care with the client.

Clients often wish to visit their pets when they are hospitalized. In this event, the client usually makes an appointment with the receptionist to visit the animal at a specific time that is convenient for both the client and the hospital operation. During the owner's visit with the pet, a technician or veterinarian should be present to answer questions concerning the status of the patient. Client visits are generally beneficial for both the hospitalized patient and the client. The mental states of the client and the patient can be strengthened, and communication between veterinarian and the client can be improved.

Most hospitals have an inside or outside exercise area for dogs. Outside areas are enclosed in escape-proof fencing or walls and generally are positioned directly outside boarding kennels to decrease the risk of a kenneled animal escaping (Fig. 2.10). The hospital and practice owners assume legal responsibility when hospitalized or boarded animals escape.

The room used for food preparation and storage is sometimes referred to as the *kitchen* (Fig. 2.11). This room is used to store a variety of canned and dry foods kept in dry, rodent-proof

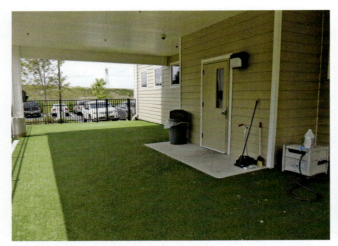

• **Fig. 2.10** For the security and safety of the patients, outside exercise should always occur in fenced enclosures.

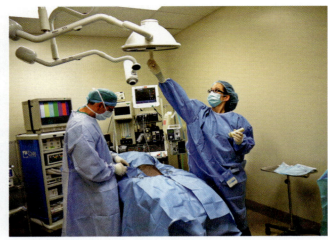

• **Fig. 2.12** A surgical room, with one door for entrance and exit, ceiling-mounted lights, and minimal countertops.

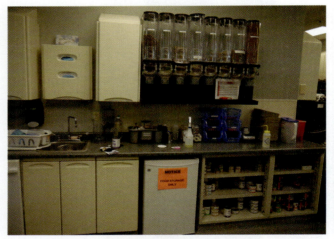

• **Fig. 2.11** Food preparation for hospitalized patients occurs in the hospital's kitchen, which is outfitted with ample counter space, a refrigerator, and a dishwasher.

containers. Automatic dishwashers are frequently used to sanitize food and water bowls. It is helpful to acquire quiet dishwashers if they are close to the wards, as well as ones that heat water to high temperatures. A sink with hot and cold running water, ample countertop space, and a refrigerator should be available in the kitchen. OSHA regulations dictate that human food and drink must *not* be stored in the same refrigerator with pet food, biological samples, and/or pharmaceuticals.

Apart from hospitalized patients, regional zoning laws may preclude practices from boarding animals. Most hospitals, however, do include kennels if zoning permits. Boarding facilities are typically located in the back of the hospital and often include separate areas for dogs and cats. If the hospital offers grooming services, they are often located in this area as well. Although some veterinary hospitals board only pets who are regular clients of the practice, others offer boarding services for both clients and nonclients. Some practices have extensive and elaborate boarding, grooming, and pet spa areas; others offer a simpler array of services.

Not all practice owners find boarding and grooming to be profitable services. These services are often more labor intensive (and

thus more expensive) than others offered by practices. However, many practices have found that if done well, boarding kennels complement the medical side of the business. Practices that offer luxury boarding with attractive dog suites and cat condos, extra playtimes, swimming, and socialization with other pets or people can charge more for these services and make this a very profitable enterprise.

The second way of capitalizing on boarding and grooming is by generating as many spin-off medical services as possible. In hospitals that do this, technicians or veterinarians will give each boarding or grooming pet a mini-examination to identify obvious eye, ear, nose, teeth, skin, and other easily recognizable problems. Groomers and all those involved in working with the boarders will be trained to identify these issues and report them to a doctor for follow-up.

Even if a hospital does not offer grooming services, most practices have a small area for bathing pets. This usually consists of a raised bathtub, a combing table, and a dryer cage. It is important that all patients be clean and dry before they are discharged. Some hospitals have a separate entrance and reception area for pets that are solely for boarding or grooming; others check in and discharge animals to be groomed via the main hospital entrance and exit.

Surgical Area

The third work area in the hospital, the surgical area, consists of the surgical preparation room, ORs, and a recovery room. All three areas in the surgical section are typically located close to each other.

As stated earlier, surgical preparation may be done in the treatment room in some hospitals. All preoperative preparation of the patient, surgeon, and technician should take place outside the OR to keep the OR as clean as possible. These preoperative activities include instrument preparation and sterilization, clipping and scrubbing of the patient, and hand scrubbing, gowning, and gloving of the surgical team.

The OR itself should be a "dead-end" room with only one entrance and exit (Fig. 2.12). Dust-carrying bacteria are easily stirred into the air when people walk through the room and will settle into an open surgical incision. No one should enter the OR without proper clothing, shoes, cap, and mask. Clients will not be permitted in this area except in unusual circumstances.

The OR should be used only for surgical procedures and must not double as a treatment or examination room. Storage cabinets should be kept to a minimum and should contain only items that are used in surgery. Items used elsewhere in the hospital should not be stored in the OR. Countertops should be kept to a minimum, because flat surfaces collect dust and must be wiped down daily. Surgery lights, oxygen outlets, and patient monitors should be ceiling or wall mounted, when possible. Floors, walls, and ceiling should be washable, smooth, and seam-free to allow complete and easy cleaning. Cleaning the underside of the surgery table base, the tops of surgical lights, and the floor and other flat surfaces (window ledges, countertops, etc.) should be done daily. The air handling system for the OR should be separate and should create slight positive pressure to prevent dust and other debris from entering the room from other areas when the door is opened. All cleaning materials and utensils used in the OR should be restricted to use in this room. Mops and sponges that are used elsewhere in the building and then used in the OR will bring additional **contamination** into the room. The cleanliness of the OR should be everyone's concern to prevent nosocomial infection of the surgical patient.

Some practices have a separate surgical recovery room; others place recovering pets in areas of the hospital ward where they can be carefully monitored. Whenever surgical recovery occurs, the patient should be closely monitored by the technical staff. Under no circumstances should any patient recovering from anesthesia be left unattended in the ward, in a stall, or elsewhere with an endotracheal tube in place.

Support Area

The fourth work area of the hospital is the hospital support area. This area contains, somewhat by default, the "leftover spaces," but it also contains the critical planning and management areas of the hospital. The support area includes the veterinarians' **offices**, the business management office, the library, the employee lounge, and storage areas. In smaller practices, the professional office, the business management office, and the library may all be in one room.

From a management viewpoint, hospital storage space is the most expensive floor space in the building, because this space generates the least income. Therefore storage areas must be given close attention so that this valuable space is used as efficiently as possible. Supplies and equipment that are no longer used or usable should be removed to make room for essential items. Inventory control (avoiding overstocking or understocking) and space organization will ensure maximal use. Items that can be hung on the wall or ceiling should be removed from the floor. Metal or wooden shelving will organize space for bulk drugs, food, and cleaning supplies. Flammable or toxic materials should be safely marked and stored away from food or drugs (refer to Chapter 4 for additional information about safety).

The smaller the practice, the less distinct the four areas in the practice (outpatient, inpatient, surgery, and support). Furthermore, the smaller the practice, the fewer technical staff members and assistants are needed, resulting in less opportunity for the veterinary technician to focus on one work area. This is not to imply that the smaller practice is less ideal. The small practice sometimes can provide greater personal satisfaction because of closer contact with the entire operation and increased diversification of job roles.

CASE PRESENTATION 2.2

Pet Sitting

Scenario: Ben Johnson is a veterinary technician employed by the Fairview Veterinary Hospital. The hospital offers a wide variety of boarding services and has a spacious, attractive, and comfortable boarding facility for both dogs and cats. Pets are appropriately cared for when boarded.

A client of the practice is reluctant to board her anxious cat and asks Ben if he would do some in-house pet sitting. She wants Ben to come over twice a day, check on Fluffy, change the litter box, feed her, and make sure the water bowl is full. The amount she offers in payment seems fair, and Ben is enthusiastic about taking on the job.

Queries: Should Ben take the position? Does he have any obligation to the practice to say no to the client?

Response: Many small businesses have policies in place regarding employee work that is done outside the primary job at the practice. Ben should check to see if such a policy exists at his practice and, if it does, whether pet sitting would violate the policy. Ben should also discuss the new job offer with an appropriate person at the practice, such as his immediate supervisor, the practice manager, or the practice owner. Ben should be careful not to engage in work that could be in competition with the practice. In this way, Ben can avoid creating any unintended ill will in his full-time position at the veterinary hospital. Some important queries for Ben to consider before accepting additional work are as follows:

- Has Ben informed his employer about the offer, and did the practice approve of Ben doing the outside work?
- How will the client's regard of the practice change if the practice discourages Ben from taking on the outside work?
- Does the practice have a legal right to dictate Ben's actions in this scenario?
- Would the practice approve of Ben marketing his pet-sitting services?
- Would the practice approve if Ben lists his employment at the Fairview Veterinary Hospital in his marketing materials?
- Will the practice give out Ben's name to clients who request in-home pet-sitting services?

Small Animal House-Call Practices

A few small animal practices do not have a permanent hospital facility but instead offer house-call services and operate from a mobile veterinary vehicle that is specially equipped for treating pets at home. Veterinarians can perform basic surgical and diagnostic procedures in a **mobile facility**. In addition, ambulatory veterinarians frequently establish a relationship with a nearby veterinary hospital that allows the use of the facility for the treatment of more complex cases.

Specialty and Emergency Practices

These practices are usually larger and offer more advanced care compared with most general practices. Although their facilities include the same types of areas as are found in general practice (reception area, examination rooms, surgical area, etc.), more space is allocated to each area, and the hospital may be divided by department. For example, internal medicine has its own examination rooms, treatment area, and hospitalization ward, as do the other services (surgery, dermatology, ophthalmology, etc.). Services often share an ICU, some hospitalization space, and pharmacy and laboratory areas.

Large Animal Mobile Units

Veterinary diagnostic and preventive medicine services for a herd of animals require the veterinarian to visit the owner's farm or

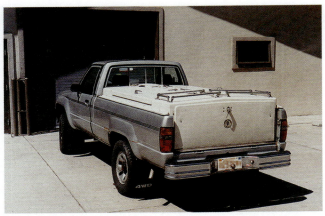

• **Fig. 2.13** A veterinary mobile unit is equipped with hot water, a refrigerator, and many compartments for equipment and supplies.

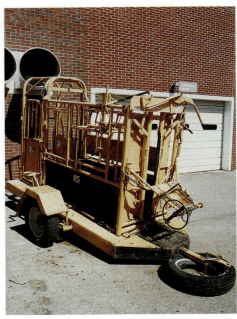

• **Fig. 2.14** A portable cattle chute on wheels is pulled behind the ambulatory truck to the farm.

stable. The large animal practice often makes use of a specially designed mobile vehicle for conducting farm visits (Fig. 2.13). These visits require stringent sanitary precautions to prevent transmission of disease from one client facility to another. Washing hands, changing to clean coveralls, chemically disinfecting boots, and cleaning equipment between farm calls are paramount to prevent disease transmission among farms, and to gain and keep the confidence of the livestock or equine owner. Some large animal practices offer only mobile services, whereas some others also have a permanent facility to which animals can be brought.

> **TECHNICIAN NOTE**
>
> Mobile large animal practices employ stringent sanitary precautions to prevent transmission of disease from one farm to another. Washing hands, changing to clean coveralls, chemically disinfecting boots, and cleaning equipment between farm calls are paramount to prevent disease transmission from farm to farm.

Mobile facilities used to serve large animal patients and clients may range from a car with a few portable "grips" in the trunk, to a van with a set of drawers and containers, to a specially designed mobile truck unit. Truck units usually are fully equipped with refrigeration for biologicals plus hot water and a supply of disinfectants, drugs, vaccines, medical supplies, restraints, diagnostic and treatment equipment, and sometimes even mobile x-ray units. Everything needed for a series of planned visits plus unexpected emergencies must be on board. The water supply and disinfectants are used to clean and disinfect hands, boots, and equipment after every farm call. A portable cattle chute may be pulled behind the mobile unit to the farm to process herds of cattle (Fig. 2.14).

A veterinary technician or assistant may be responsible for stocking, organizing, and maintaining the large animal mobile unit. The mobile unit inventory will vary, depending on the nature of the practice, the preferences of the veterinarian, and the species served. Preparing inventory lists and patient appointment lists for the day's activity ensures that the veterinarian will have what is needed on every call. Obviously, a wide range of specific supplies is necessary for the routine practice of large animal veterinary medicine. This inventory must be replenished frequently, organized for easy and quick access, and cleaned and disinfected daily and after every farm call. Technicians often assist veterinarians on

farm calls and become efficient at maintaining and organizing the mobile unit.

Large Animal Haul-in Facilities

Some veterinarians with mixed and large animal practices provide haul-in facilities for individual patients to be trucked or brought by trailer into the practice. Unloading chutes and gates for cattle trucks and stock trailers are provided at the large animal outpatient entrance. A few even provide holding corrals and squeeze chutes for processing a truckload of cattle or sheep. Unloading chutes for cattle, sheep, and swine must adjust to different heights to accommodate the trucks, pickups, and trailers used for transporting animals. It is paramount that fencing and panel arrangements be constructed to prevent escape from the premises if the animal escapes from the head catch or alleyway or when unloading.

When haul-in facilities for large animals are provided, each of the areas previously discussed for a small animal facility will be present for serving large animal patients. Frequently, some areas (e.g., reception area, laboratory, conference rooms, pharmacy, etc.) will be used for both small animal and large animal services. Large mixed animal hospitals may have a separate pharmacy for large animal supplies, separate public restrooms, and possibly a separate reception area. The nature of the large animal facilities of each practice varies, depending on the needs of the livestock and equine population and owners served by the practice.

The large animal inpatient treatment area may be the same as the outpatient examination area for large animal patients. An alleyway with a head catch or a squeeze chute is used for bovine patients, a stock is used for equine patients, and pigs, goats, or sheep may be treated in their stalls. Patient wards are available in large animal veterinary hospitals. Some equine hospital barns have large ward areas with ceiling-mounted tracks that allow recumbent horses to be harnessed and hoisted into a standing position or transported to another stall or region of the barn (Fig. 2.15). An equine hospital may also include separate barns for surgery and

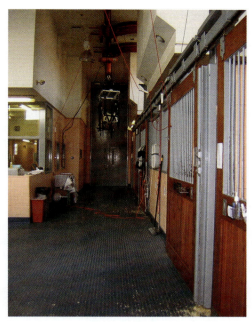

• **Fig. 2.15** Some equine veterinary hospitals are equipped with a ceiling-mounted rail and harness system that supports nonweight-bearing horses and is used to move patients from one location to another within the hospital.

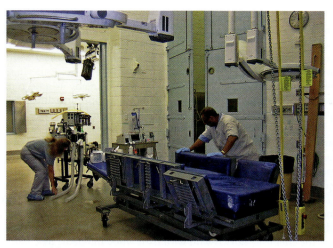

• **Fig. 2.16** After surgery, a large animal operating room, with anesthesia machine *(right)* and mobile operating table *(foreground)*, is being prepared for the next surgical procedure. The blue doors to the adjacent recovery stall are visible to the right behind the movable operating table. (Courtesy Dr. Joanna Bassert.)

for medical patients. In addition, many equine hospitals include an isolation barn to limit the spread of contagious microbes such as *Salmonella.* Outdoor pens and turn-out paddocks may be available for recovering patients and used in good weather.

Examination rooms in equine hospitals include stocks that restrain horses for examination and standing procedures. Because of the large size of both horses and cattle, all veterinary staff should be well trained in restraint and safety procedures; this ensures protection for large animal patients, owners, and staff. A variety of restraint procedures may be followed (see Chapter 6).

Most large animal practices also use the treatment area as a nonsterile surgical room for minor procedures. Because of the large size of patients and the extensive amount of hair and excrement left in these areas by large animals, high-pressure hoses and disinfectant systems are used frequently, along with removable floor drain traps.

The surgical room in the equine practice facility is organized to provide the same stringent asepsis as is provided in a small animal surgical area. However, because these patients are much larger, mechanical or hydraulic equipment designed to lift the animal is necessary, particularly to move anesthetized animals from the presurgical area to the OR and from the OR to the recovery room. The surgical area is equipped with a padded mechanical or hydraulic surgical table on which the horse is placed after induction of general anesthesia (Fig. 2.16). Equine practices may include an induction room and a padded recovery stall. (Fig. 2.17A and B). Anesthesia is maintained with an equine gas anesthesia machine.

An area must be available for the proper performance of large animal necropsy (see Chapter 16). Necropsies are performed more frequently on large animals than on small animals. Because of the economic value of large herds or flocks, necropsies are often done when animals die to determine whether the rest of the herd or flock is threatened. Confirmation of the diagnosis will often require the submission of specimens to a state or university diagnostic laboratory for testing and review by a board-certified pathologist. Necropsy of several animals may be performed (more commonly on sheep, pigs, and poultry) to determine which of several concurrent diseases is the probable cause of death. Necropsies are valuable as a preventive measure to stop the spread of disease and to prevent it in the future. They also serve as a great learning tool for veterinary staff to be better prepared to recognize similar cases in the future.

Clients and Client Services

The most important person in any practice is the client; no animal visits a veterinary practice without an accompanying human. The practice of veterinary medicine, particularly in general practice, is truly a people business. Clients generally judge a practice based on client service, not on the quality of medicine. Although the availability of the Internet allows clients to be more informed about medical matters, it is still difficult for most clients to know whether they received good care or not until an obvious mistake has been made. Clients tend to assume that all practices offer a similar level of medical care; therefore they use nonmedical factors to evaluate the quality of care. For example, to a client, dog urine in the reception room indicates a dirty hospital and thus poor care, because everyone knows that sanitation and sterility are essential parts of good medicine. A technician's view of this same scenario demonstrates an opportunity to collect a sample from an animal before immediate clean-up begins.

TECHNICIAN NOTE

Because of the large size of equine patients, mechanical or hydraulic equipment is necessary to move anesthetized horses from one area to another within the surgical suite.

TECHNICIAN NOTE

The most important person in any practice is the client; no animal visits a veterinary practice without an accompanying human. The practice of veterinary medicine is truly a people business.

It is important to realize that clients judge a practice based on *perceived* value rather than *true* value, and the perceived value comes from the customer service experience. Clients did not go to veterinary school and often do not understand medical words; however, they are customer service experts. For example, if the receptionist tells the client that Fluffy will be ready at 3:00 p.m., but the client has to wait around the reception area until 3:25 p.m., the client *knows* that a client service error has occurred.

The availability of veterinary services in the United States is at an all-time high and the net result of the increased number of practices is competition for clients among established and new practices. Practices that will financially survive must offer outstanding client service experience in addition to outstanding care. The practice will collapse unless existing clients are retained, and new clients are continually coming into the practice. Clients are the lifeblood of the practice, and everyone in the practice works for the client. Loyalty is won with hard work and dedicated, caring service to each client. If the staff attitude becomes negative toward clients, the practice clientele will dwindle. A practice's facilities, equipment, and techniques may be the finest available, but they will remain unused unless enough clients willingly authorize or request that practice's services.

How does a client select a veterinary practice? Historically, most clients will select the practice with the most convenient location or one that is recommended by friends and colleagues. With increasing use of social media, pet owners also make use of online reviews.

Once a practice has been selected, it is judged on the following client service attributes:
- Professional, friendly, and caring personnel
- Attention to the client's needs and desires
- Consistency in care and service
- Availability of a wide range of services
- Convenience—hours, location, respect for clients' time, online appointment booking, online pharmacy
- Reliability
- Clean, attractive, and updated facility
- Clear and understandable communication of recommendations and benefits to client and pet

In large animal practices, retention and satisfaction issues are the same for clients as those encountered by small animal owners, with the addition of economic return. In food animal practices, the veterinarian must become an economic asset to overall farm profitability or the client cannot afford to seek and use veterinary services. The sentimental and emotional attachment (human-animal bond) of the client to the animal extends that economic limit in companion animal and some equine practices but is not a factor in food animal practices.

Importance of Client Communication

In study after study, the importance of good communication skills in well-run veterinary practices has been demonstrated. Clear communication must occur not only among members of the veterinary staff but also between staff members and clients.

TECHNICIAN NOTE

Most complaints against veterinary practices are the result of ineffective communication between the practice and the pet owner.

PUT INTO PRACTICE

While your clinical skills are important, communication is vital at all levels. Listening to understand instead of listening to respond can go a long way in building relationships and defusing challenging situations.

Communication Myths

Myths regarding communication skills abound. The first is that communication is a personality trait, and you either have it or do not have it. The truth is that communication consists of a series of

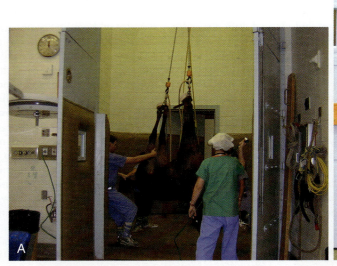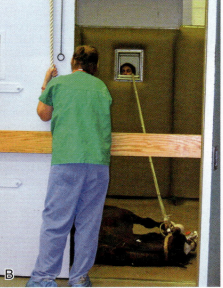

• **Fig. 2.17** (A) An anesthetized horse is moved to a recovery stall via rails mounted to the ceiling. (B) The walls and floor of the recovery stall are lined with thick pads. Small windows in stall doors allow veterinary personnel to visually monitor and control the patient, using ropes when it attempts to stand. (Courtesy Dr. Joanna Bassert.)

learned skills, and anyone who wants to *can* learn them. Another common myth is that it takes too much time for veterinary health care team members to communicate well with clients. Practices are busy, and good communication is not possible when the veterinary health care team is under time pressure. In reality, good communication is more efficient in the long run, because it results in fewer errors, greater client satisfaction, and better medical care for patients.

A message has three main components: (1) 55% of the message is provided nonverbally, (2) 38% of the message is delivered paraverbally, and (3) only 7% of the message is communicated through the words chosen. It is then that much more important to apply the six aspects of excellent communication as discussed below.

Six Aspects of Excellent Communication

Clear and frequent verbal communication with coworkers and clients is an important part of effective veterinary health care. The components of what makes good communication are as follows:
1. *Clarity:* Be clear in speech by using correct grammar and articulation.
2. *Courtesy:* Always be courteous and respectful. Avoid using words that might offend, such as curse words and unprofessional slang.
3. *Positive nonverbal communication:* Be aware of your own nonverbal communication and use open body postures and direct eye contact to build trust.
4. *Open-ended inquiry:* Obtain important information from the client using open-ended inquiries.
5. *Reflective listening:* Employ active and reflective listening to let clients know that you understand what they are saying.
6. *Empathy:* Show sincere empathy by putting yourself in the position of others. Let them know that you understand how they must be feeling.

Clarity

Clarity is particularly important in medical communication. Only 57% of veterinary clients surveyed in the 2011 Bayer Veterinary Care Usage Study[1] fully agreed with the following statement: "My veterinarian communicates with me using language I understand." Only 44% agreed with the statement, "My veterinarian clearly explains when I need to bring my pet in for various procedures or tests." It is clear from this study's findings that improvement is needed in the communication that veterinarians and other staff members have with clients.

It is easy for veterinarians and veterinary technicians to use medically precise words that mean nothing to a pet owner. The veterinary staff should use terminology that the client will understand and not overwhelm the client with too much information. They should ensure that the client understands exactly what needs to be done, why, and when. Simply *saying* all this to a client is often not enough. Verbal communication needs to be reinforced by providing printed take-home information and by making a reminder phone call or other communication subsequently. Last, clients should be specifically asked if they understand or have any questions.

Courtesy

Common courtesy, genuine concern, and respect are important parts of communication in all professions and businesses, as in personal relationships. When a veterinary practice loses sight of the individual client, the feeling of getting personal service is lost for both the client and the patient. Courtesy begins with acknowledging clients as soon as they enter the reception room, addressing them by name, and asking after their families—in short, treating clients as important guests in the practice. Courtesy also extends to telephone manners. All calls should be answered promptly; the caller should be welcomed with a greeting, such as, "Good morning, this is ABC Animal Hospital; my name is Kathy. How may I help you?" In this way, the caller immediately knows that they have reached the correct hospital and that someone is there to help. Telephone courtesy is just as important as face-to-face courtesy, because most clients make their first contact with the hospital through the telephone.

Nothing is more important for the veterinary professional than talking to a client; one should not rush through information just because one is feeling hurried or because the information asked for appears to be "common knowledge." It is important to remember that what is common knowledge to a veterinarian, veterinary technician, or other practice staff person is very likely new information to the client; one should not assume a superior manner or tone that makes the client feel "put down."

Positive Nonverbal Communication

In all communication, 55% is nonverbal communication, which includes all the behavioral signals that pass between interacting individuals exclusive of verbal content. For example, when a client is asked whether all medication was given to the dog, they may say "Yes" but with a tentativeness that indicates either "No" or "Not sure." Practicing open, nonverbal communication (uncrossing legs and arms and maintaining good eye contact) builds greater levels of trust. Nonverbal signals are generally involuntary and are interpreted as reflecting a person's true feelings. When mixed messages are sent, the nonverbal message is instinctively perceived as being more accurate than the verbal message.

Open-Ended Inquiry

Open-ended questions are particularly important when taking history; they encourage the client to elaborate or to tell a story freely, with no shaping or focusing of content by the person asking the questions. The goal is to find the meaning of the communication, not just the facts. Simple examples include questions that start with "Tell me…" or "Describe for me…"; "What" and "How" questions are also effective. "Why" questions are less effective; they tend to provoke defensiveness. Open-ended questions are part of a "funnel approach" to gathering information—the inquiry should start with broad questions and end with more specific ones. For example, the first broad, open-ended question might be, "How does Fluffy behave in the morning when you see him acting strangely?" After the full story has been elicited, the time is right to focus on specifics. Closed-ended questions are used to clarify details, such as "Which leg do you think he is favoring?"

Reflective Listening

Listening is extremely important because it represents half the communication process. The skill of active and reflective listening must be practiced on a regular basis. Many people prefer to talk rather than listen; when other individuals are speaking, they may be preoccupied with formulating their responses rather than truly listening to what is being said. Veterinary staff should keep in mind that clients have much to contribute to the diagnostic process by providing important clues in the patient's history.

Active and reflective listening first involves offering encouragement to the speaker by nodding and making direct eye contact.

After the speaker has finished talking, the listener reflects to the speaker what was said and asks the speaker if the reflection is correct. This helps ensure that the listener has an accurate understanding of the information communicated and helps the speaker feel heard and understood. One example of reflective listening is verifying the information provided: "So, Fluffy threw up twice last night. Is that correct, Mrs. Jones?"

Empathy

Empathy is the ability to understand the position of another person and to communicate that understanding to the person. Examples include the following: "I can see how hard it is to make this decision about Fluffy," or "It seems you did all that you could for Fluffy."

Dealing With Difficult Clients

Dealing with an angry client is not easy and requires skill. There should be a clear understanding within the practice about how difficult clients are to be dealt with and whose role this is. Although there is no way to completely prepare for a client's outburst, it does help to role play such situations during staff training.

The following guidelines may help defuse the situation:

- "Invite" an angry client immediately to a private area, such as an examination room or an office away from other clients, or to a place without distraction or interruption.
- Create a friendlier environment by sitting down side by side, without a desk or an examination table between you and the client.
- Start the conversation immediately by thanking the client, in a friendly fashion, for allowing the practice to find out what is wrong.
- Sometimes the client will burst out complaining, in detail, about everything that is wrong. Although this may be unpleasant, it is essential to listen to the client's perspective to achieve eventual resolution. If the client does not initiate a discussion, you must speak first: "Could you explain to me what is wrong?"
- Employ active and reflective types of listening. Being empathic will help understand the client's point of view.
- Try to find points of agreement. Any part of the client's experience during which the pet owner confirms that something went well or that they are satisfied with a particular aspect of service is beneficial to the process of resolving problems.
- Be careful not to justify a clinical action that the client is criticizing. If the client is right about a mistake that has been made or about the poor quality of service delivered, accept it and correct the situation immediately.
- When it does become appropriate to explain hospital procedures, try to put them in a positive light; for example, clients hate to hear that their pet needs rabies vaccination because it is your "policy." Talk to clients in terms of what constitutes the best health care for their pet: "Did you know that Texas has the highest incidence of rabies in the nation?"
- Try to find a solution to create a "win-win" situation. Asking the client what they would recommend to help resolve the problem would be helpful.
- Allow the client to save face whenever possible.
- Do not take problems and problematic people personally—be professional and see this as part of the job.

The staff member should keep in mind that clients may have other "major" issues going on in their personal lives. The difficult client may be going through a divorce or have recently lost a loved one. This added stress prevents them from being able to understand and communicate clearly with veterinary personnel. This is one more reason to not take angry clients personally; one may never understand what the other person is currently experiencing.

Even if it is ultimately the role of the practice manager to deal with an angry client, some of the tips already presented should be used by all staff members to help control the situation while the veterinarian or the practice manager is being contacted. It is always important to review the client's complaint after the situation has been resolved to determine whether the practice should do some things differently in the future to avoid a repeat situation.

The most difficult people to reason with are those who are under the influence of alcohol or drugs. Staff members should be careful about how they interact with these individuals. They should not argue with them or confront them, because persons under the influence could become violent and uncontrollable, and law enforcement officials should be contacted to handle the situation.

Management of the Veterinary Practice

Effective management of the people, facilities, and processes in a veterinary hospital makes it possible for veterinarians, technicians, and other staff members to practice high-quality medicine and serve clients in a way that makes them want to return to the hospital. What would happen if no one was available to order medicines and medical supplies; to hire competent veterinarians, technicians, and receptionists; to make sure the facility was clean and equipment in good working order; and promote the hospital while making sure the workflow was efficient? First, no clients would show up; second, even if they did, no appropriately trained people or medicines and supplies would allow for the practice of high-quality medicine.

Management is essential for efficient operation. Management roles are commonly divided into the following categories:

- *Planning*—strategic and operational
- *Human resources*—hiring, managing, and training employees who work in the practice and fulfilling related legal and regulatory requirements
- *Marketing*—all activities necessary to obtain and retain clients and to enhance awareness and standing of the hospital in the community
- *Financial*—accounting, bookkeeping, financial analysis, capital acquisition, budgeting, pricing strategies, risk management, and related compliance with legal and regulatory requirements
- *Operations*—a broad category that has to do with all systems, policies, and procedures that make the hospital operate smoothly on a day-to-day basis, including inventory control, patient and staff scheduling, purchasing, patient flow, management of the front desk, and many other activities
- *Facility and equipment*—acquisition and maintenance

Technicians have an ever-increasing role in practice management. In most practice situations, technicians are involved in management of patients, clients, equipment, and inventory. They may also be involved in hiring and supervising employees and in conducting training and marketing activities. To develop management skills, one must be willing to assume increasing levels of responsibility. As the practice changes in terms of staffing, numbers of cases, the facility, types of clients, new technologies, and so forth, veterinary technicians must adapt their management skills to these changes.

The role of the veterinary technician in management will vary depending on the type of practice and the previous experiences of the technician and the veterinarian. The technician who can (1) conceptualize the vision and goals set by the veterinarian for the practice, (2) efficiently organize each area in which they are given responsibility, (3) become a productive team player and a good communicator, and (4) develop the ability to solve problems constructively to enhance patient care and the veterinary team usually will be given a greater role in practice management, greater responsibility overall, and greater financial rewards.

CASE PRESENTATION 2.3

Inventory

Scenario: Tiffany Smith is a veterinary technician who has worked at an animal hospital for several years and has recently been asked to manage the practice's inventory. This new responsibility includes ordering drugs and supplies, entering received items into the practice inventory management system (PIMS), and regularly counting the products on the shelves and comparing with the counts in the PIMS. Previously, these tasks were completed by several receptionists and other technicians in the hospital. Tiffany was told by the practice owner that the "inventory system was in great shape" and this would be an easy task.

When Tiffany takes on the new responsibility, she quickly realizes that the inventory system is disorganized and that the records of what is ordered, received, and put on the shelves are inconsistent with the data in the PIMS. In addition, Tiffany has observed other employees order drugs and supplies for their own pets without reimbursing the practice.

Query: How should Tiffany address the inventory discrepancies and her concerns?

Response: Tiffany needs to schedule a time with the practice owner to discuss her findings in private. During this time, it is important that Tiffany presents only what she knows to be true. For example, she knows that there are discrepancies between the inventory list and the amounts of products that are on the shelves. It is important that Tiffany does not speculate about the cause of these irregularities or share suspicions with colleagues, because this can lead to damaging gossip and speculation. Instead, Tiffany should speak exclusively with the practice owner who, once informed, can decide what, if any, actions should be taken. The practice owner may then lead further investigations. In addition, Tiffany should not speculate about the reasons for the discrepancies. Instead, she should confine her role to putting a stronger inventory system in place. If Tiffany feels she does not have either the knowledge or the training to develop an inventory system, she needs to communicate this knowledge deficit directly and immediately to the practice owner. The practice owner can then either provide appropriate training or reassign the responsibility to another employee.

Planning

Businesses that are most successful in the long run are those that can grow and adapt to changing circumstances. Medical and surgical standards necessary to provide high-quality care, the expectations of clients and employees, and the business skills necessary to run a financially successful practice are not the same now as they were 5 years ago and will not be the same when 5 more years have passed. Practices that do not engage in formal planning activities will ultimately deteriorate and close. Some changes are forced upon a practice, such as changes in medical standards or business regulations; other changes occur internally and are obvious to an owner or manager as something that must be dealt with, for example, deterioration in the quality of the facility or equipment and poorly trained staff.

> ### TECHNICIAN NOTE
> Businesses that are most successful in the long run are those that can grow and adapt to changing circumstances.

Other changes may not be as apparent to a hospital owner or manager as those mentioned above, but they are identified through ongoing monitoring of practice metrics. Examples include lack of transaction growth, decreased client compliance with medical recommendations, and lack of profitability. In addition to appropriately reacting to the types of negative changes mentioned, practices should be proactive and engage in activities that will grow the practice, such as adding new services or adopting new forms of technology that improves client communication and medical standards. All practices need to have systems in place to identify problems and plan for all contingencies. Some of these activities will be performed on a monthly or quarterly basis; others may be done annually or on an as-needed basis.

One of the most important times for business planning is before a practice is started or purchased or when a significant change is being made to the practice, for example, the addition of specialty services to a general practice or the opening of a satellite clinic. The document prepared most frequently during this planning process is known as a *business plan*. A business plan is a written document that describes the current nature of the business and plans, both short term and long term. The business plan should cover all key areas of the business.

> ### TECHNICIAN NOTE
> One of the most important times for business planning is before a practice is started or purchased or when a significant change is being made to the practice, for example, the addition of specialty services to a general practice or the opening of a satellite clinic.

As noted previously, strategic planning activities should be engaged in and take place monthly, quarterly, and yearly once the practice has begun operating. Monitoring activities that should take place monthly and quarterly include comparing the budget against actual revenue and expense numbers, the number of active clients and patients, accounts receivable, and other key performance metrics. Tracking metrics often allows the practice to pivot and adapt as needed to ensure strategic goals are achieved.

Yearly strategic planning involves a retreat away from the practice and may need to be moderated by an outside party. The retreat should last two or three days and include all key employees of the practice. All areas of the practice should be analyzed, including medical and surgical services, client services, staffing, marketing, finance, operations, facilities, and general management. Practices that do the most effective job at planning will ask technicians and other staff members to contribute their thoughts about how the practice could function better, the kind of feedback they receive from clients, and other matters related to the management of the hospital. Additionally, the practice's long-term vision should be reviewed, along with the mission/purpose statement and core values of the practice. Planning must be in accordance with the vision and ensure that all plans fall in alignment with the mission/purpose and under the guidance of the core values.

Human Resources

The term *human resources* is used to describe the department or activities related to hiring, training, managing, and terminating the people who work in a business. Finding and keeping good employees is arguably one of the most difficult tasks facing the veterinary profession today. Without these employees, veterinarians will not be able to offer the high levels of medical and surgical care that they wish to, nor will they be able to provide the type of client service that keeps clients returning to a practice, which would lead to the business prospering financially.

Hiring

The way hiring duties are handled varies among practices, depending on the size of the practice, management personnel being on the staff, and the management philosophy of the individuals involved. If the hospital has a practice manager, this person generally will oversee hiring lower-level management personnel, technicians, receptionists, veterinary assistants, and kennel/ward/barn personnel. Practice owners usually will be significantly involved in the hiring of veterinarians and upper-level management personnel. Other staff members may also participate in the process of formal and/or working interviews.

Before effective hiring can take place, the practice must have a full understanding of the position it wishes to fill. Preparation or updating of two key documents will help with this task: the organizational chart and the job description.

An *organizational chart* (also referred to as the "org chart") is a visual representation of how departments and employee positions in a business are aligned. It shows how authority and responsibility flow between departments and individuals. All key individuals in the practice should be included in the org chart, along with clear indications of who reports to whom. Both direct and indirect reporting relationships may be noted. For example, technicians may formally report to the practice manager but on a day-to-day basis may work regularly for and informally report to the veterinarians in the practice.

TECHNICIAN NOTE

Before effective hiring can take place, the practice must have a full understanding of the position it wishes to fill. Preparation or updating of two key documents will help with this task: the organizational chart and the job description.

A *job description* outlines the duties and other attributes of someone who fills a particular position and should be prepared for all positions in the practice. These documents allow both the employee and management to maintain a clear understanding of current and new areas of responsibility and must be reviewed and updated annually. Technicians are often involved in updating these descriptions for their positions. Components of a well-written job description include the following:

- Position title
- Reporting relationship
- Basic purpose or mission of the job
- Principal job duties and responsibilities (both technical and interpersonal)
- Minimum education, experience, and skill and personal characteristic requirements
- The Americans with Disabilities Act requirements

Once the practice has a clear idea of the educational, experiential, technical, and interpersonal skills needed for the job, the recruiting process can begin. Applicants can be attracted to the practice in several ways, with the highest opportunity through Indeed, veterinary technician programs, vendor representatives, or personal contacts. Recruiting for a veterinarian or practice manager may also utilize recruiters or placement services.

Once suitable applicants have been identified, the practice must obtain more detailed information about their skills and experience. This is usually done through the job application, resume, interview, and references.

The best way to gather this information and determine whether a candidate is a good fit for the practice is by conducting an interview. Current interviewing theory states that past behavior is the best predictor of future behavior. Therefore the hiring manager's goal is to identify situations in the candidate's past that are similar to circumstances that they will encounter in this job position and to find out how they reacted to them. Questions should also be asked that clarify or expand on information provided in the candidate's resume. Once all candidates have been interviewed and their references checked, a decision will be made about which one to hire. Attitude and interpersonal skills are generally considered to be as important as, if not more important than, technical skills. All candidates should be notified of the practice's decision as soon as possible.

It is not uncommon for practices to ask a candidate to participate in several interviews and to include technicians and other staff in these sessions. Some interview questions are unlawful or discriminatory and must not be asked (e.g., questions on race, religion, national origin, gender, disabilities, marital status); it is important to ensure that no one in the practice asks them.

One of the most important techniques that anyone involved in an interview should remember is to listen. It is more important to find out all one can about someone who may be coming to work in the practice than to talk about oneself or the hospital. It is important not only to ask a lot of questions but also to listen to the answers.

Compensation

Another key task performed by the HR department is the determination of compensation for veterinarians, technicians, and other staff members. Total compensation is composed of both salaries/wages and benefits.

Objectives of a compensation system include the following:
- Attract, retain, and motivate high performers
- Maintain internal consistency and external competitiveness
- Recognize and reward performance

The first step in creating an equitable and effective wage and compensation system is to develop a consistent procedure for setting pay levels for each position. It is essential to know not only the pay ranges for veterinary practices in the area but also the going rates for positions in other businesses where current staff members or job candidates might apply for equivalent positions. To find and keep better-than-average people, it is necessary to pay better-than-average salaries.

Pay should be based on performance. A good correlation is generally found between the productivity of employees and their level of education, skill sets, and work experiences, although more experience and more education do not always translate into better work performance. In salary determination, the key is to make sure that the education, skills, and experiences being rewarded are specific requirements of the position that will contribute to better job performance. Seniority by itself is not a reason for higher pay. Those who do not perform well should not be paid in the same manner as those who do perform well.

The Fair Labor and Standards Act (FLSA) governs how the practice can pay people (salary vs. hourly rate) and when overtime must be paid. Some states have stricter guidelines to follow and, when that is the case, the stricter guidelines are enforced. FLSA does state that only employees that serve in an executive, professional, or upper management level can be paid a salary; other employees receive hourly rates. To clarify, only veterinarians and practice managers/administrators should receive salary wages; veterinary technicians (and all other support personnel) are hourly employees.

> **TECHNICIAN NOTE**
>
> A good correlation is generally noted between the productivity of employees and their education level, skill set, and work experience.

Benefits vary among staff positions and between full-time and part-time employees. However, those often seen in veterinary practices include health insurance, vacation pay, sick pay, paid holidays, and reimbursement for dues, licenses, continuing education, and retirement plan contributions.

Training and Orientation

In an ideal world, all employees would come to the practice knowing everything they need to know to be productive team members. Unfortunately, this is not the case. Even if a veterinarian, a technician, or a receptionist has worked in another practice, they will not know the policies and procedures in their new hospital. The quality of educational programs can vary greatly among schools. The most successful hospitals are those with good-quality, formalized onboarding programs.

Employee orientation is usually the first training experience a new employee encounters. The goal of the orientation is to introduce the employee to colleagues, give the employee an overview of how the practice operates, instruct the employee in the policies and procedures necessary for the efficient operation of the practice, supply OSHA training, and provide the employee the basic, practical information needed for a successful start—work hours, pay dates, and so on.

Employees should then receive a longer, more detailed training program dedicated to their role in the hospital. Some components of the training will be the same across positions; for example, everyone needs to know how to use the PIMS. Other components of training will be specific to the position.

The best hospitals offer ongoing education and training in both medical and client service matters. Technology and medical standards change rapidly, and ongoing training of all employees is essential if good quality medicine and client services are to be offered. Education and training lead to improved efficiency, better work quality, and improved client service and makes the job more interesting for the employee.

Continuing education should be done internally, often as a part of staff meetings held on a weekly or monthly basis or at other intervals. Another important aspect of ongoing education is the opportunity to attend outside veterinary meetings or conferences as they relate to the goals of the veterinary practice. In addition to attending sessions given by recognized experts in their field, these meetings give all staff members a chance to meet and talk with people from other hospitals. Information learned in these conversations can be as helpful as that learned in formal sessions.

Employee Management and Retention

Another formal task of HR is the ongoing management/relations of employees in the practice. Leading, coaching, and growing team members is 80% of a practice manager's role. With that being said, the process is a two-way street between the employer/manager and the employee. The employer/manager needs to communicate expectations to the employee and to work with the employee to set mutually agreed-upon performance goals and contributions needed from the employee for practice success. The employer/manager also needs to provide guidance and feedback to the employee as needed and the tools and resources needed by the employee to be successful. The employee has a role in this as well through goal setting and achievement, communicating concerns, and asking for help when needed to seek out training opportunities, guidance, and direction.

An important management task that is generally performed or coordinated by the practice manager is that of performance appraisals. One of the most common mistakes in personnel management is putting off regular employee evaluations. Personnel problems resulting from poor work performance do not just go away; they only become worse. Employees cannot improve their performance unless they are given an opportunity to identify shortcomings. Employers also need to identify and reward employees for work done well.

Good managers do not wait for the annual performance review to let their employees know which areas they excel in and where they need help and guidance. However, it is important that this feedback be conveyed formally and documented at least annually. Written performance appraisals are a formalization of the day-to-day appraisal process. They often help reduce misunderstandings, can be more convincing than words, and create a permanent record. However, nothing in the formal evaluation should be a surprise to the employee, unless it has to do with an incident that occurred five minutes before the performance appraisal meeting. All positive and negative feedback should have been communicated to the employee at the time the behavior occurred. Ideally, the performance review process is a positive one wherein management and employees work together to help the employee perform better and reach personal work goals.

> **TECHNICIAN NOTE**
>
> Good managers do not wait for annual performance reviews to let their employees know which areas they excel in and those in which they need help and guidance. However, it is important that this feedback be conveyed formally and documented at least annually.

Formal reviews are typically given after 3 months for a new employee and, after that, once a year. The review should cover technical skills (e.g., is the employee able/unable to do specific tasks?) and the employee's willingness, motivation, and general attitude toward their work.

Employees are sometimes asked to complete self-evaluation forms before the time of the review. Employees frequently know more about their performance than any other single person does, and they often set higher standards for their own performance than others do.

Even if the person performing the review has not asked the employee to do a self-assessment, this is a good exercise for the employee to go through in preparation for the meeting.

Addressing Employee Stress

Veterinary medicine, like other healthcare professions, involves a fair amount of stress. Veterinary personnel who work in clinical practices are on their feet for most of the day. Many technicians feel that they have little time for lunch or other breaks and are challenged to keep up with the pace of a busy practice. Animals can be uncooperative and owners, who may be stressed themselves (particularly if their pet is ill), can be difficult at times. In addition, the close-knit staff that constitutes many veterinary health care teams can be particularly susceptible to stress if conflict arises within the team. Finally, pet loss resulting from euthanasia or illness, particularly unexpected death, can cause sadness and lower morale which, in turn, exacerbate an already stressful working environment. With time, experienced technicians learn to pace themselves and to recognize and address potentially stressful situations as they arise. Nevertheless, stress is an all-too-common aspect of working in veterinary medicine.

Physical signs of stress include gastric reflux, ulcers, nausea, and muscle tension leading to muscular aches and pains. As stress gets worse or goes on for a long period, anxiety, depression, anger, and a reduced ability to cope are commonly seen.

Not everyone experiences stress in the same way. Whether or not a person can adapt to stress depends on the situation, the level and duration of the stress, and the personality of the individual. Some personality types are susceptible to stress; others are stress resistant. People who tend to be competitive, perfectionistic, and often angry are more susceptible to stress. They are called "type A personalities." In contrast, "type B personalities" are more stress resilient. They tend to have realistic expectations of what they can accomplish and are less worried about failure.

Stressors

The extent to which a person is self-confident and possesses self-esteem is important in the level of stress experienced by the person. For example, an individual who is confident in their abilities, intelligence, and organizational skills may be relatively calm while planning a wedding, working full time, and volunteering to run the community fundraiser. In contrast, a less-confident individual might feel tremendously stressed when performing the simplest tasks.

Previous experiences, personal backgrounds, and the circumstances of one's living situation can affect an individual's susceptibility to the stress of clinical practice. Life events play a key role in the performance of workers and in the level of stress they experience. A person who feels supported by family and friends, for example, is more stress resilient in the workplace than someone who does not have support. Stress can come both from positive events, such as getting married, and from negative events, such as the death of a loved one. Both events are stressful. Employees who have overextended themselves in their activities outside of the workplace may feel tired and short-tempered, even though such activities are designed to be fun. Thus moderation is an important part of a balanced and happy life.

Reducing Stress in the Workplace

Veterinary technicians who are leaders within the veterinary health care team can help create a positive working environment for the team by minimizing stress and by building a culture of collaboration (Box 2.3). Enforcing a no-gossip policy, for example, and removing staff members who incite conflict can eliminate a huge source of stress in the veterinary health care team. Technicians can help create an environment in which staff members feel free to admit mistakes and where individuals are not singled out and shamed. Finally, veterinary technician leaders can decrease stress by arranging regular meetings where open and clear communication with team members takes place.

• BOX 2.3   **Five Steps for Reducing Stress**

1. Plan for the unexpected.
   - Keep time slots free for emergencies and delays.
   - Arrange for emergency backup personnel in the event that a team member unexpectedly cannot work and when more emergencies than expected arrive for treatment.
   - Cross train staff.
   - Have backup generators that keep the practice (and the computer system) functional during power failures.
   - Prepare written standard operating procedures and review them with staff.
2. Create reasonable work schedules.
   - Avoid scheduling excessively long hours.
   - Insist that each member of the health care team take at least one break per 8-hour period.
   - Schedule and take vacation time.
3. Create a culture of collaboration, trust, and mutual support (rather than of gossip, blame, and finger pointing).
   - Model professional behavior and respect for coworkers.
   - Never reprimand a staff member in front of others.
4. Recognize and counsel staff members who are particularly stressed.
5. Provide clear communication with staff members.
   - Have regular staff meetings.
   - Support open communication but at the same time, limit complaining.

Employee Substance Use Disorder and Stress: Important and Not to Be Ignored

The combination of a stressful workplace and the availability of drugs in both veterinary and human medical practices put personnel at risk of engaging in illegal drug use. Although there has been much study of addiction issues among health care workers in human medicine, far less is known about addiction among veterinary personnel. Empirical reports from recovery workers indicate that veterinarians are more advanced in their addiction and mental illness before they are reported. It is thought that this may be attributed to greater levels of isolation among veterinarians who tend to work in small private practices, making them less likely to investigate prevention education. As a result of working long hours, high levels of stress, easy access to drugs, decreased levels of reporting, and the lack of established support programs specific to veterinary professionals, addiction is a significant but generally ignored problem in veterinary practice, particularly relative to professionals in human medicine. Because of a lack of concrete data on addiction among veterinary personnel, it is unclear how many animals are harmed by veterinary health care workers with addiction problems. One survey reported that 14% of veterinary practice managers left their positions because of drug misuse. This compares poorly with the addiction rate in the general population in the United States.

The central nervous system, including the brain, and emotions are dependent on the normal action of neurotransmitters. Alcohol and drugs can enhance, distort, or even eliminate information normally exchanged by nerve cells. Some individuals may turn to drugs and alcohol as a form of self-medication to cope with stress. The evidence seems to indicate that genetic susceptibility to substance use disorder may be present as well. Some cultural groups have established patterns of drug use, and some age groups seem to be more susceptible. When the individual has knowledge about drugs and has access to them, that individual is at risk. In general, a veterinarian or a veterinary staff member with a substance use problem will exhibit a change in behavior. They may neglect duties in the clinic, appear disorganized, or exhibit poor judgment in the practice of veterinary medicine. Other signs may include prescriptions written for themselves, friends, or family, and drugs going missing from the clinic during the hours in which they were on duty. Financial or legal problems may arise. Unexplained absences, conflicts with others, and career instability may result.

Some type of intervention and action is needed any time that substance misuse interferes with work activities. Client, patient, and coworker safety is of primary importance. The entire practice may be at risk of malpractice suits because of the substance misuse by an employee. In every state, a board of veterinary medicine awards, reviews, and can suspend licenses of veterinarians (and veterinary technicians, if licensed) in that state. Most governing boards for health care professionals have stipulations by which the professional found impaired is denied renewal of license. Generally, the impaired professional should be counseled, preferably by a peer or a superior, to seek treatment.

All 50 states offer resources and guidance for impaired veterinarians through the governing board or through the state professional association. However, there is little support for veterinary staff, including veterinary technicians. Because many states do not credential veterinary technicians, fewer rehabilitation opportunities are available for them via state licensing boards or state technician associations. Most states have a list of qualified counselors and treatment centers that work with impaired doctors, dentists, and veterinarians. For these medical professionals, counselors will do an evaluation to determine what type of treatment is recommended.

Marketing

The term *marketing* often gets confused with the term *advertising;* however, marketing is composed of much more than advertising. Marketing includes all activities necessary to obtain and retain clients and enhance the awareness and standing of the hospital in the community. To obtain and retain clients, the practice must offer services/products that are of value to the pet owner at a price consistent with that value and in a way that is appealing to the client. Therefore marketing is not only about the service/product itself but also about client service. And, of course, part of marketing involves communicating the offerings of the hospital to clients and potential clients. Some professionals feel uncomfortable with the idea of marketing, because the concept gets confused with the idea of sales or trying to get pet owners to buy something they do not really need. Another way to think of marketing is as client education, that is, helping pet owners understand the care needed for their pets to live a long and healthy life. The veterinary technician must understand marketing principles to be an effective communicator of professional services and goods offered by the practice.

TECHNICIAN NOTE
Marketing includes all activities necessary to obtain and retain clients and enhance the awareness and standing of the hospital in the community.

Animals are totally dependent on their owners' awareness of their health care needs and the willingness of the owners to meet those needs. Some practitioners believe that as long as high-quality medical and surgical skills are delivered, the client will continue to use their services based on this alone. However, the average client lacks the professional background to accurately judge the quality of medical or surgical services performed. Instead, clients judge the quality of services and caring communication that they receive, which influences their perception of the value of medical and surgical services received. A client's perceived value of services is their reality of the quality of the practice.

Veterinary medicine is a people-service business. Veterinary professionals care for animals but ultimately, they provide services and products to the owners of the animals. As discussed in an earlier section, patients cannot come to the practice without their owners. This is a key concept that should underpin everything a practice does. When clients call on the telephone, for example, this should not be regarded as an interruption of the team member's time; those clients are the only reason the practice continues to exist. Only satisfied clients return and refer others to the practice.

Every activity the hospital engages in is part of marketing. The professional appearance of the hospital, clinic, or ambulatory vehicle is suggestive of the quality of care it provides. Verbal and nonverbal communication between doctors or technicians and pet owners does not just convey information; it also conveys interest in the pet and the pet owner, warmth and concern, and a desire to help the pet owner. Technicians are actively involved in marketing the practice through everything they do.

Marketing activities are often categorized into two types: internal and external. Internal marketing is generally aimed at the existing client base, and much of this is focused on day-to-day client service and communication, and other activities that occur within each practice. External marketing is focused more outwardly, but current clients are also reached through external marketing. Much of the goal of these activities is to attract new clients. The line between the internal and the external techniques is fuzzy; however, the purpose of both is to increase the number of clients served by the practice and the frequency of their visit.

Internal Marketing

Internal marketing targets the existing client base and includes client relationships, the practice's appearance, services offered, reminders, client-oriented materials, and digital marketing (including social media and target marketing). Internal marketing techniques attempt to educate current clients about the health needs of their pets and the various veterinary services and service programs available to meet those needs. Much of the internal marketing carried out within a practice is handled by veterinary team members, including technicians.

TECHNICIAN NOTE
Internal marketing is aimed primarily at the existing client base. Internal marketing techniques attempt to educate current clients about the health needs of their pets and about various veterinary services and service programs that are available to meet those needs.

The veterinarian and the support staff must work together as a service team, all delivering the same high-quality educational messages, care, and service.

Client Relationships

The most important technique that can be used in any marketing program is personalized, sincere care of the client. Many clients require as much attention and care as patients do. Personalized service that emphasizes each individual client is critical. This concern and caring cannot be faked; people who work in veterinary practices need to be genuinely concerned about the clients they serve.

Practice Appearance

The importance of the appearance of the clinic, hospital, or ambulatory vehicle was discussed previously. A practice facility does not have to be new or have the latest equipment to project a positive professional image, but it must be attractive and clean, and it must be given proper care and maintenance to send the desired marketing messages of warmth, caring, and professional competence. Weeds and pet feces in and around the parking lot area, urine stains on exterior walls, and a poorly maintained, filthy examination room will all convey a poor impression to clients. The practice does not need to smell like a veterinary facility. The odor of anal glands and urine can permeate the facility when not immediately cleaned up; therefore every team member must be engaged in maintaining the practice's appearance and be committed to correcting odors as they arise.

The client's perception is the reality to them; what can they see, smell, and hear when they enter the practice? Team members are encouraged to walk through the front door at least weekly with a client "hat" on, and see, smell, and hear what clients do.

Full-Service Care

Part of the marketing process involves identifying what clients want and providing it to them. In general, pet owners, like all other consumers in today's busy world, want convenience. In a small animal practice, full-service care includes pediatric care, preventive medicine, nutritional management, behavior counseling, veterinary-supervised boarding, geriatric care, dentistry, surgical options, in-house emergency care, **bereavement** counseling, and cremation services. Many clients also want their veterinary practice to offer online product purchases and delivery of medications and food purchases, nonmedical boarding, grooming, and pet daycare. Anything that makes it simpler and faster for pet owners to take care of their pets is important to them. Full-service care sends a strong marketing message regarding convenience and respect for the client's time and needs.

Providing a Low-Stress Practice Experience

A veterinary visit is very stressful for many pets and consequently for their owners. Many pet owners do not obtain veterinary care on a regular basis, because the experience is stressful and difficult for both the pet and the owner. Therefore practice owners and managers have become increasingly interested in creating a welcoming and comfortable environment for both pets and their owners. The importance of feeling welcomed and comfortable in a veterinary practice helps ensure continued veterinary medical care. Several initiatives in the veterinary profession are aimed at giving practice team members the tools and resources they need to reduce fear, anxiety, and stress in both pets and their owners when visiting veterinary practices. This is done by making thoughtful changes to the clinical environment, including changes to the facility layout and to the workflow. Reducing pet stress also makes for a less anxious owner. By employing low-stress handling and restraint techniques, such as using pheromones to reduce anxiety in pets and providing positive food enticements at the same time help make a potentially awful experience more pleasant. This is true for both the pet and its owner. In particularly fearful animals, pharmacologic intervention can also be employed.

In addition, instructing cat owners to acclimate their cats to carriers in advance of veterinary appointments can make it easier for cats to get the care they need. In addition, providing a separate reception area and hospital ward for cats helps to ease both feline and owner anxiety.

Additional information about creating a low-stress environment for pets can be found at the following websites:
- Fear Free initiative: www.fearfreepets.com
- Low Stress Handling University: https://lowstresshandling.com
- American Association of Feline Practitioners Cat Friendly Practice initiative: www.catvets.com

Client Reminders

Most practices have a system in place in which reminders are sent to clients when it is time for various services to be performed, such as annual examinations, vaccinations, and medication refills. As noted previously, clients are increasingly busy and want to be reminded when care is due. All the most used practice management computer software packages have the capability of capturing information regarding reminders.

The most successful reminder protocols in practices have the following characteristics:
- Multiple reminders (usually up to three) will be sent if the client does not respond to the first or second one.
- Reminders are sent using the format preferred by the client—some may choose mail, others email or text, or a phone call.
- Reminders are sent not just for vaccinations but for a wide variety of services, including dental care, follow-up laboratory testing, food refills, ovariohysterectomy or castration, and refills for heartworm, flea, tick, or other preventive medications.
- The language used in the reminder does not just name the recommended service; "FVRCP" (which stands for feline viral rhinotracheitis [herpes], calici, panleukopenia) vaccine means nothing to a client. Instead, the reminder should briefly describe the service offered and should emphasize the benefits for both the pet and the client.

Personal Appearance

The personal appearance and hygiene of each staff member reflect the quality of the practice. Many clients relate personal appearance to sanitation and the level of medicine practiced. For clients to build trust and respect for the veterinary technician, technicians must always appear professional. A positive appearance includes wearing a clean, well-fitting uniform with neatly maintained hair. Personal appearance is very similar to building appearance; it serves as an outward signal of internal quality and impacts the perception the client has of the practice.

Client Materials

Client handouts can range from a practice brochure outlining hours and services to educational materials discussing preventive care and specific diseases (Fig. 2.18). The use of handouts is important for several reasons. Not only do they reinforce the information that was provided at the practice, but they also make it possible for others involved in the pet's care to understand the medical condition of the pet and the recommendations made by the practice.

Not everyone learns best by listening to oral information; many people take in information better by reading it and others when seeing pictures or models or through direct observation of the pet's problem. Handouts are particularly useful to clients if after returning home they forget some of the details of what was discussed with the veterinary technician or veterinarian. Written handouts provide critically important information and instructions to the pet owner that can be referenced frequently as needed.

Dental Report Card

Last name_____ Pet _____ Date _____

Stage 1 – Gingivitis

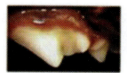

Plaque and tartar buildup can lead to an infection causing inflammation of the gums around the dog's teeth. Gum tissue around the teeth can become inflamed and swollen.

Stage 2 – Mild Periodontitis

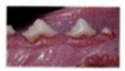

Inflammation progresses to an infection that starts to destroy gum and bone tissue around the teeth. This can lead to discomfort for the dog. and bad breath may be noticeabie.

Stage 3 – Moderate Periodontitis

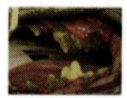

The continuing infection destroys more tissue around the teeth, often causing bleeding of gums and loosening of teeth. The discomfort and pain can affect eating habits.

Stage 4 – Severe Periodontitis

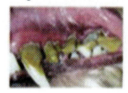

Extensive infection is tearing down even more of the attach-ment tissues (gum and bone). Teeth are at risk of being lost.

Just like human beings, dogs are susceptible to plaque and tartar buildup that can lead to gingivitis and periodontitis, a chronic form of the disease that can be painful.

Periodontal disease, which includes gingivitis and periodontitis, is an inflammation and/or infection of the gums and bone around a dog's teeth. It is caused by bacteria that accumulate in the mouth. forming soft plaque that later hardens into tartar. If untreated, periodontal disease can eventually lead to tooth loss.

Over time, plaque and tartar buildup can lead to inflammation of the gums around the dog's teeth: **gingivitis.**

Periodontitis is a potentially irreversible infection that, if left untreated, can result in the destruction of gum and bone and other tissues around the teeth. In most severe cases, periodontitis can ultimately lead to loss of teeth, fracture of the jawbones, and other serious consequences that can dramatically affect quality of life and overall health. When-ever possible, preventing disease is preferable to treating it!

Dental disease can also lead to cardiac and/or kidney disease.The bacteria that collect in your pet's mouth also circulate throughout the body, contributing to a variety of other diseases.

The good news is that periodental disease can be prevented with a good dental care program, including:

- Daily home oral care: brushing your pet's teeth can be fun!
- Dental toys: rope toys, rawhides that are dissolvable, and Denta-Bones. Remember, hard toys can fracture teeth. Any chew toy should be slightly pliable.
- NEVER give you pet beef, chicken, or pork bones!
- Veterinary dental cleaning as advised.

• **Fig. 2.18** Client information handout. Dental report card shows photographs of stage 1 gingivitis, stage 2 mild periodontitis, stage 3 moderate periodontitis, stage 4 severe periodontitis in dog, followed by the causes of periodontal disease and prevention tips. (Courtesy Jornada Veterinary Clinic, Las Cruces, NM.)

Although some practices create their own handouts, others use commercially available versions. The quantity and quality of handouts received from veterinary professional organizations, such as the AVMA, the AAHA, or the American Association of Equine Practitioners (AAEP), or from companies in the animal health industry are often excellent; however, these pieces should be carefully reviewed by the practice to make sure they conform to the philosophy and recommendations of the practice. Preprinted labels with the practice name, address, telephone number, website, and email address can be affixed to any commercial brochure to personalize the material.

Like reminders, client education materials should be available in multiple formats, including videos, models, and PDFs that can be printed, emailed, or placed on the practice website. All client materials should have a consistent look and feel (logo, font, colors) and should not have any spelling or grammatical mistakes.

A vital role of the veterinary technician in the practice is cli-ent education. Veterinary technicians should be familiar with all educational materials and should have them available for clients at each appointment. In addition, the veterinary technician is responsible for explaining printed home care instructions to the pet owner. Pets will improve more quickly if the home treatments are carried out correctly and consistently (Fig. 2.19).

Condolence and Thank-You Communications

A condolence/sympathy card and personalized note sent to a client when a pet dies demonstrates concern for the feelings of the client during the time of bereavement. This expres-sion helps the client deal with the loss and allows the client to understand the "I care" attitude of the practice for both clients and their pets.

Thank-you notes to clients for referring another client, to new clients, or to those who bring cookies or other gifts to the practice are not only common courtesy but reflect good marketing. The practice may choose to use commercially prepared cards or may develop a letter format on the computer that can be personalized. Regardless of the format used, the sentiments expressed should be sincere and professional.

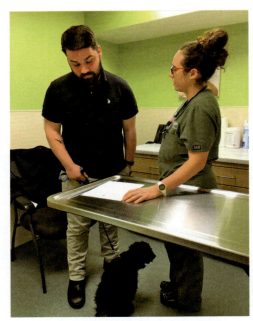

• **Fig. 2.19** Technician reviewing take-home instructions with a client. (Courtesy Dr. Joanna Bassert.)

Digital Marketing

Many practices reach out to their clients through e-newsletters, blogs, and social media. Human interest stories that help educate clients about husbandry items related to their animals, things the owners can do to keep their pets healthy, and necessary veterinary services get the most attention. News about the practice and its team members is also popular. Photos, graphics, and an easy-to-read style all increase the likelihood that the material will be read. Topics included can range from information about seasonal illnesses/accidents to signs and symptoms noticed by an owner that should be discussed with a veterinarian to ensure the health of the pet. Digital marketing material should always refer the reader to the practice's website for further information on a specific subject found in the electronic library of the website.

Most veterinary teams do not have the experience or the time to compose blogs and develop engaging social media posts, and owners should consider engaging with a veterinary-specific marketing company to produce relevant materials that help the practice achieve its strategic goals.

Targeted Mail

Another way of educating clients is through targeted emails. These are specific notifications that focus on one topic, for example, spring allergies. These mailings can be sent to specific segments of clients or to all clients, depending on the applicability of the information, and should focus not only on why this is important for the pet, but what the practice recommends to keep the pet more comfortable, safe, etc. In companion animal practices, targeted emails must be personalized with the pet's name and sex and should be graphically pleasing. When using marketing techniques such as this, the receptionist team must ensure that email addresses are collected and verified each time the client visits the practice.

TECHNICIAN NOTE

Findings from the Bayer Veterinary Care Usage Study[1] indicate that a large number of pet owners do not have a complete understanding of the care their pet needs to live a long and healthy life.

A Practice App

With the increased use of smartphones and tablets among clients, having a veterinary-specific practice app allows the client easy access to the practice. The app can be loaded onto most electronic devices and provides the client the opportunity to make appointments, refill medications, see their pet's reminders, review client education materials, and even receive loyalty rewards for money spent in the practice. The practice can send messages to the client (push notifications), send alerts for lost pets, and let them know that their medication refill is ready to be picked up. In these ways, practice apps make it easy for the client to do business with the veterinary practice.

External Marketing

As noted previously, the line between internal and external marketing is not a clear one; however, external marketing efforts are directed more outwardly to attract new clients, but some will reach current clients too.

External marketing activities are implemented by individual practices, veterinary professional organizations, and commercial companies in the animal health arena. Marketing done by professional organizations and the animal health industry focuses on general messages, such as "Visit your veterinarian twice a year" or on specific product-related messages. External marketing efforts initiated by the practice generally include educational content but also focus on the benefits of visiting that particular practice.

Commonly seen types of external marketing efforts used by veterinary practices include advertising through digital marketing and participating in community activities. All practices should have clear signage—not only does this help clients locate the practice, but it is also a marketing tool. Signs should be large and well lit and should be placed in a highly visible area. They should be professionally created with messaging that can be changed or that will stand the test of time. Signage should be well maintained, along with the rest of the building exterior.

Digital Marketing

Digital marketing represents the most common form of advertising for veterinary practices and organizations. Websites are the most common attractor for new clients and provide a resource for existing clients. They should be professionally designed, with professional photos of the team. A web page should provide practice clientele with the ability to make an appointment online, order medications, and access their pets' health records through the practice app. The practice web page should be updated frequently and must be attractive and easy to use. Search engine optimization and mobile phone applications are critical in maximizing the usefulness of these communication tools.

Digital marketing also includes the use of social media, using Facebook, Instagram, and occasionally TikTok. Posts need to be interesting, timely and done frequently. Facebook readers expect new information to be provided much more frequently than on a website. Social media should be used to market the practice's blogs.

Community Activities

Veterinary practices that engage in community activities have found them to be personally rewarding and a way to increase their client base. Many opportunities arise for veterinarians and technicians to become involved in community service through

Girl Scouts, Boy Scouts, 4-H programs, school boards, rescue organizations and shelters, country clubs, Rotary clubs, Lions clubs, and church activities. Potential contacts with clients are made in the course of being involved in and contributing to these organizations. Practices will often sponsor local activities, such as sports teams or animal fairs; this is another good way to increase awareness of the practice.

Financial

Managing the finances of a practice well is critical. If the practice is not financially successful, it will not be able to offer high-quality medicine and surgery, invest in its employees, or ultimately survive. Some of the tasks associated with good fiscal management include the following:

- Bookkeeping and accounting, including payment of bills and collection of fees
- Management analysis
- Budgeting
- Price setting
- Capital equipment acquisition
- Risk management
- Compliance with legal and regulatory requirements

Bookkeeping and Accounting

All small businesses, including veterinary practices, must perform the following bookkeeping tasks: collect payments for services performed or products sold, make payments for products purchased and services received, run payroll, and prepare financial statements. Most practices do not prepare their own tax returns, but they must keep the financial records in such a way as to make it easy for their accountant to do it.

All client financial information, including invoices for services performed or products purchased, returns, credits, and payments, is initially entered into the PIMS. Each evening, the daily transactions entered into this system are reconciled with the payments collected during the day, and a bank deposit is made. This information is then entered into the practice's accounting software. The most commonly used software in small businesses is QuickBooks®. Bills are generally paid on a regular schedule, often weekly, and this information is also captured in the accounting software. Payroll is most often handled by an outside payroll service, with the information entered into the practice accounting software.

The practice accounting software is used to generate regular reports for use in preparing the tax return and managing the practice's finances and operations. The most commonly used reports are the balance sheet, the income statement, and the statement of **cash flows**. The balance sheet summarizes the financial *position* of the practice at a point in time and shows all assets and liabilities of the practice. The income statement reflects the financial *performance* of a business between two points in time. It includes the total **gross revenue** generated by the practice for a specified period (typically monthly, quarterly, or yearly) and expenses incurred to generate that revenue during the same period. The income statement is often called by other names, including *profit and loss statement (P&L)*, *statement of operations*, and *statement of revenue and expenses*. The amount left over after the expenses are subtracted from the revenue is **net income**, which is hoped to be a positive number. The statement of cash flows reflects the sources and uses of cash during a particular period (monthly, quarterly, or yearly).

The accounting system must be set up to capture all financial data simply and accurately. Various checks and balances must be included in the system to identify inadvertent mistakes or deliberate fraud or theft. The people involved in all aspects of the accounting process must have the training to do this job properly; these are not generally tasks that employees can pick up intuitively. Technicians are not usually involved in the actual preparation of the accounting reports unless they have moved into a management role; however, they are often involved in some of the activities that feed into the accounting system, such as the preparation of client invoices and inventory control. Performing these tasks properly is very important to the accuracy of financial reports.

Management Analysis

The accounting system is also used to generate information for management analysis (i.e., to gain a better understanding of how well the practice is doing operationally and financially and which areas could be improved). The financial statements discussed previously are used in this type of analysis; however, it is also important to review other metrics that provide information about practice operational performance.

Key Performance Indicators

Key performance indicators (KPI) are metrics used by the practice to evaluate performance. The term is used loosely and can include a wide range of figures, many of which come from the PIMS. In addition to the items already discussed, some of the most used include the following:

- *Revenue and transactions per full-time-equivalent (FTE) doctor:* An FTE doctor is usually considered to be one who works 40 hours per week, 52 weeks per year. FTE doctor figures are used instead of absolute numbers of doctors, because doctors do not always work the same number of hours per week. Transactions are equivalent to client invoices; invoices are generated for all services provided and may range from a small dollar amount for a bag of food or a prescription refill to a much greater amount for a complicated surgical or medical case. These metrics are used to measure the productivity of doctors. Technicians are instrumental in helping doctors to be productive.
- *Patient visits:* Patient visits are different from transactions. Transactions (invoices) include all services or products purchased by a client, whereas patient visit figures include only times that a patient actually visited the hospital and had some kind of procedure performed, such as an examination, surgery, or dental work.
- *Average transaction charge:* This figure is calculated by dividing the total revenue of a practice by the total number of transactions; it represents the average amount a client spends during a visit to the practice.
- *Revenue by category* (dentistry, surgery, product sales, etc.): These metrics are used to analyze the types of services clients are choosing to receive.
- *Numbers of new clients and active clients:* A new client is considered to be one who has never visited the practice before; an

active client is one who has visited the practice within the past 12 months.

- *Accounts receivable aging:* Accounts receivable represents amounts owed to the practice by clients who are allowed to charge at the practice (i.e., they do not pay for their services at the time of purchase but are billed later). The aging report shows the dollar amount owed by these clients and how long the money has been owed.
- *Overtime hours:* It is often difficult to schedule employee hours to exactly meet the needs of the practice because of emergencies and last-minute additions to the appointment schedule; therefore overtime is sometimes incurred by staff members. Overtime pay is a higher amount than regular time pay, so practice owners and managers strive to keep it to a minimum.
- *Work hours per transaction:* This metric is calculated by dividing the total number of hours worked by doctors and staff by the total number of transactions. The resulting figure serves as a measure of staff and veterinarian efficiency.

TECHNICIAN NOTE

Key performance indicators (KPI) are metrics used by the practice to evaluate practice performance.

Clinical signs of poor business management that can be identified through the types of review described previously include increasing accounts receivable, reduced amounts of cash, increased debt, a decline in gross revenue and/or profitability, increasing personnel costs, declining productivity, declining client numbers, and a declining average transaction charge. These are all fixable problems, but they must first be identified.

Technicians often are not involved in the management analysis itself, but they are instrumental in improving the operational and financial success of the practice through their client service, communication, and medical roles.

Budgeting

Budgeting, however dull or intimidating, is an essential tool for managing the finances of a veterinary hospital. A budget is generally prepared at the end of one fiscal year for the following year; it includes estimated amounts for revenue and expenses.

Besides providing specific financial data, a budget forces the practice to plan, and planning helps identify problems early, determine why circumstances might be expected to change in the future, and decide what can be done about this.

Budgeting is also an excellent way to communicate the goals of the practice to the entire hospital staff, to ensure that these goals are coordinated, and to monitor actual performance against expectations.

Price Setting

All practices do not charge the same amounts for services or products. This type of price setting among competing practices would, in fact, be illegal. Each practice determines its own fees based on what has been charged in the past, how much it costs to provide the service, what value the practice believes the service brings to the client, and other factors. Setting fees is as much art as it is science.

For a long time, the cost of veterinary medicine was very low. Over the past 15 years or so, it has risen significantly, and client displeasure regarding the cost of veterinary care has been observed.

This increase in cost is not just a result of increases in fees charged to clients; it has also occurred because of the expanded range of care now available for pets and because pets live longer than they used to and require care for aging-related issues.

Practices will have to use more sophisticated fee strategies in the future and will need to focus on increasing profitability through ways other than fee increases. Owners and managers need to understand the drivers of profitability. In addition to the fees charged to clients, key drivers include the number of clients in the practice, the frequency of their visits to the practice, the quantity of services they choose to accept each time they visit, the amounts of discounts or missed charges, and whether the amounts charged to clients are collected. All else being equal, fee increases will increase profitability, but those same fee increases may also cause declines in some of the other profitability drivers (e.g., number of new clients, the frequency of pet owners' visits to the practice). The expected impact of all changes must be understood before the level of fee increases that are beneficial to the practice can be determined.

Whether or not a pet owner is willing to pay for a service or a product is not always about the absolute price charged for the item. Willingness to pay also has to do with whether an owner finds value in the item and thinks it is important to the pet's health. Findings from the Bayer Veterinary Care Usage Study[1] indicate that many pet owners do not understand the need for veterinary care. Technicians play a vital role in educating pet owners about veterinary care and in explaining why it can help their pets live happier, healthier lives.

Even if the price and the value are acceptable to the client, if they do not have the money, they are not going to be able to afford the services. Therefore the availability of payment options is critical. Even clients who are fully committed to providing quality care are looking for payment alternatives. Payment options for clients generally fall into four categories: in-house delayed billing of various types, third-party payment plans, pay-by-the-month preventive care plans, and pet insurance. This is another area in which technicians have a critical role; they need to understand the various payment options offered by the practice and must be able to communicate this clearly to clients.

TECHNICIAN NOTE

Even if the price and the value of pet services are acceptable to clients, they cannot afford the services if they do not have the money. Therefore the availability of payment options is critical.

It is also critical that everyone in the practice actually charges the stated fee for services and products sold. All charges related to the pet's care should be included on the invoice. Many practices offer care at a reduced cost to some deserving clients or to charitable organizations; any discounts included on an invoice by technicians should be approved by the practice owner/manager in advance.

The goal of the practice is to charge fair and equitable fees to cover the practice's cost of providing high-quality care and service to clients. The fees should support investment in equipment, competitive salaries and benefits for veterinarians and staff, and a fair return on the investment to practice owners for the business risks involved.

TECHNICIAN NOTE

It is also critical that everyone in the practice charges the stated fee for services and products sold. All charges related to the pet's care should be included on the invoice.

Operations

As discussed earlier in the chapter, this is a broad category that has to do with all the systems, policies, and procedures that make the hospital operate smoothly on a day-to-day basis, including patient scheduling, client check-in and check-out, inventory control, patient flow, and many other activities. Additionally, the efficient flow of operations depends on the proper use and implementation of technology, allowing the team to work smarter, not harder. Third-party integration platforms can integrate with the PIMs to allow clients to make appointments online, order medications and request refills, and text back and forth with the veterinary team, allowing their questions to be asked in their time. This can also be considered "being easy to do business with," resulting in happier, less frustrated clients.

Front Desk Management

Appointment Scheduling

Companion animal practices may use an **appointment system** or a **walk-in system**. Each system has advantages and disadvantages. Most practices employ an appointment system. Appointments allow the practice to channel the flow of clients and patients into specific periods, because this helps improve the efficiency of the work schedule. On the one hand, when more clients are scheduled, more staff can be made available during the busier periods; on the other hand, when no appointments are scheduled, staff numbers can be reduced.

Practices using the appointment system generally schedule client/patient visits in 15-, 20-, or 30-minute blocks. When 15-minute blocks are used, four appointments per hour can be scheduled. Some practices book all appointments for the same length of time; others adjust appointment length depending on the reason for the animal being brought to the practice. Time for surgeries, dental treatments, and other procedures is also scheduled.

Because of clients' work schedules, practices are now also scheduling appointments in the evening to meet the needs of animal owners. Saturdays are also popular for the same reason. In many practices, Saturday is the busiest day of the week. Some practices may be open even on Sundays.

Practices that do not schedule appointments simply let clients "walk in," and they are seen on a "first come, first served" basis, except, of course, for emergencies (Fig. 2.20). Advantages for the

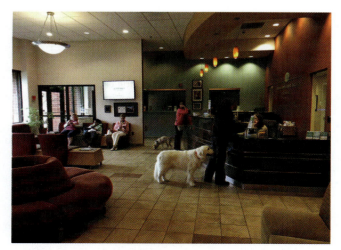

• **Fig. 2.20** Practices that do not schedule appointments simply let clients "walk in," and they are seen on a first come, first served basis.

client include not having to make an appointment and having the ability to drop in at the practice whenever it is convenient. Disadvantages include the length of wait time and the congestion that may occur when several clients come in at the same time. For the practice, the major disadvantage is not having the ability to plan proper staffing and control the workload.

Many practices also take "drop-offs" (i.e., the client brings the pet and leaves it to be seen when a veterinarian is available). Examination of these pets is worked into the schedule when veterinarians become free. Some clients will just show up in practices that generally operate by appointment, and most practices try to accommodate them.

The receptionist generally makes appointments either by phone or when the client is in the practice. Forward booking is defined as booking the patient's next appointment before the client leaves the practice. Next appointments may include a vaccination booster, medical progress examination, a spay or neuter procedure, a dental prophylaxis, a semiannual or annual examination.

Studies show that when appointments are booked before the client leaves, compliance is greater than when waiting for a client to call and schedule the appointment. The technician's role is to help ensure that clients and patients are seen at their scheduled times and that all the various activities that need to occur during the appointment (physical examination, diagnostics, client communication) happen in a timely fashion. Veterinarians, technicians, receptionists, and other staff members must work as a team to make this happen. It is very frustrating for both clients and practice staff members when appointments run late.

Estimates and Client Payments

Once the pet has been examined and the veterinarian has discussed the recommendations with the pet owner, a written treatment plan/estimate should be prepared and agreed to by the client before care is provided. One clear exception to this is true life-threatening emergencies; the pet should be stabilized before the treatment plan/estimate is prepared.

The treatment plan estimate should be verbally reviewed with the client after it is prepared. A credentialed veterinary technician or a well-experienced veterinary assistant should be able to detail the estimate. It is important that the person talking to the client can answer questions not only about the proposed charges but also about the need for care and why the recommended services are important. Client concerns about money often reflect a lack of understanding of the need for care than concern about the absolute cost. At this time, the practice's payment options can also be discussed.

Most practices require clients to pay in full at the time the service is provided. Traditionally, practices accepted the same payment options seen at most retail businesses—cash, checks, and bank credit cards (MasterCard, Visa, Discover, American Express, etc.). The demand for payment options continues to increase as clients deal with the increasing costs of veterinary care resulting from the availability of more sophisticated medical options, the extended life span of pets, and fee increases. Because some hospitals have found it challenging to collect fees using in-house billing options, the preferred trend has been toward using third-party payment plans and educating clients about pet insurance. Large animal ambulatory practices are an exception, because livestock owners often are not available during farm calls and therefore are billed later. However, many ambulatory practitioners now require credit card payments.

These payment options make a difference in the care that clients provide for their animals. Multiple studies have shown that pet owners with pet insurance, those who have a third-party payment option, and those enrolled in a practice's pay-by-the-month preventive care plan spend significantly more on their pet's care.

Not all third-party medical payment plans are the same but, in general, their financing arrangements require the pet owner to make monthly payments against the cost of the care financed. Clients can apply for the financing while at the veterinary practice and receive immediate approval. The practice receives its money soon after it provides the care and is not responsible for collecting from the client.

Another financial option for clients is pet health insurance. As with all insurance, this is a form of risk management. The transaction involves the pet owner (the insured) assuming a guaranteed and known relatively small loss in the form of a premium payment to the insurer in exchange for the insurer's promise to compensate the insured in case of a large, possibly devastating expense. Pet insurance is classified as indemnity insurance and is similar to other forms of indemnity insurance, such as automobile insurance. Pet health insurance is vastly different from human health insurance.

As with third-party payment plans, an understanding of plan options and the companies providing them will help practice team members make intelligent and useful recommendations to clients. Generally, the reason for veterinarians, their staff, or their clients becoming unhappy with pet insurance is lack of understanding of what can be reasonably expected from pet insurance.

Once pet owners decide that pet insurance is for them, they need to pick a company and a plan. Many options are available, and it can be quite daunting for the client to sort through them all. Therefore practices can be helpful by prescreening and recommending a few (two to three) policies for the client's consideration.

Pay-by-the month wellness plans are essentially annual preventive care plans that include the specific services the practice feels a pet owner should provide to each pet during a year to keep it healthy. These are wellness or preventive services, such as vaccines, physical examinations, heartworm testing and other diagnostic blood work, and deworming. The plans are not generally meant to provide care for sick pets although, of course, there is a little overlap. The total cost of the plan is generally billed to the client in equal monthly installments, although they can use the services whenever desired during the year. These plans are popular with pet owners, because they spread the annual cost over 12 months and are easier to manage from a cash flow perspective.

Technicians can play a significant role in helping clients understand not only why the recommended care is so important but also what financial options are available. Effective communication related to the cost of care begins with confident receptionists, technicians, and veterinarians who understand how the fee is computed and represents the quality of service provided. Clients will be more willing to accept the fees charged if they perceive value not only in the care recommendations but in the client service experience as well. Technicians can contribute significantly to increasing the value that clients receive.

OSHA and Safety Management

OSHA is a federal agency that ensures employee safety. There are many hazards that are present in veterinary practice, and part of the management duties must include the development and overseeing of a safety program. Yearly hazard and chemical inspections are required, along with the development of safety plans, training of staff members, and annual OSHA reporting. Chapter 4 provides more information on OSHA requirements and the technician's role in keeping a hospital safe.

Inventory Management

One of the most significant expense categories in veterinary practices is the one that includes inventory items, such as pharmaceuticals, vaccines, pet food, surgical supplies, laboratory reagents and test kits, and drugs and supplies necessary to provide medical and surgical care. Effective inventory management is important for keeping these costs under control and making sure that necessary items are on hand when needed. Inventory control is sometimes seen as a boring and tedious task, but it can have a huge impact on practice efficiency and profitability and is, in fact, one of the easier things that can be done well in practice.

A significant amount of money can be lost through inadequate inventory control procedures. This loss may occur because the business was billed for materials that were never shipped or never received at the practice or was double billed for a single shipment, billed for damaged goods, or billed for more or different items than were received. Back orders that are not canceled when the product is reordered elsewhere double the inventory. Losses also occur when products expire and are no longer effective or legally safe to use. Oversupply also crowds the shelf space and the storage space, leading to misplacement and overordering.

Technicians are frequently involved in inventory management and can do much to keep this part of the hospital operation running smoothly.

> **TECHNICIAN NOTE**
>
> A significant amount of money can be lost through inadequate inventory control procedures. This loss may occur because the business was billed for materials that were never shipped or never received at the practice, or double billed for a single shipment, billed for damaged goods, or billed for more or different items than were received.

Goals of an effective inventory system include the following:

- The smallest quantities of drugs and supplies needed by the practice are maintained and procured at the lowest overall cost while ensuring that the practice has everything needed to provide the highest quality care without running out of drugs and supplies.
- Systems and controls are in place to keep theft and other shrinkage to a minimum, to make sure that accurate records are kept, and that drugs and supplies are available when needed. Shrinkage may result from product expiration, broken bottles, and torn bags.
- Accurate records are readily available to evaluate the efficiency of the system and to improve on it.
- The system is simple for all to use.
- The inventory is well organized within the facility, is easy to find, and is not susceptible to theft or misplacement.
- Vendor numbers are kept to a minimum.
- Vendors selected are reputable, are interested in the success of the practice and of the profession, and supply products necessary for the practice, good service, and fair prices.
- All medications and products sold to clients are included on the invoice and are charged appropriately.
- Inventory is sold to clients before payment to the vendor has to be made (there will be some exceptions to this when good deals

present themselves); generally, this means that inventory needs to turn over once a month.

- Controlled drug storage and record keeping is done in accordance with legal requirements. A reasonable profit is realized from sales.

Generally, one person should be put in charge of the inventory system, although in some hospitals, one person oversees the drugs and supplies inventory and another oversees food inventory. The person in charge of the inventory system may perform all or most of the tasks related to inventory or may delegate some activities while supervising the overall system. All tasks should be assigned to specific individuals to maintain accountability.

The inventory should be ordered on a regular basis, often weekly. The practice must have a system in place for determining what items need to be ordered. This can be done in many ways. Sometimes a list is kept; at other times, reorder reports from the PIMS are used; and in other hospitals, the person doing the ordering goes through each cabinet to see what needs to be replenished.

Practices generally have a group of distributors and manufacturers (vendors) from which they order; ideally, this list is kept relatively small. Many practices have found that picking one distributor from whom they order most of their items works best; they get good service, and average prices tend to be reasonable and competitive.

A list of items ordered or actual purchase orders should be maintained for the items ordered. When the order is received, the list of items ordered should be compared with the items received, and the order list initialed by the person doing the comparison. Procedures should be in place to follow up on discrepancies and track backorders.

When supplies are delivered to the practice, the packing slip or invoice included in the box should be checked against the items received and discrepancies investigated. Quantities received and item prices should be entered into the computer after the order is received. The packing slip and invoices should then be given to the accounting department. If the practice receives both an invoice and a packing slip, items should be compared from one to the other and missing items investigated. Procedures should be in place to identify, use, and/or return short-dated and out-of-date products.

One of the most important inventory management procedures involves regular counting of products on the shelves. Most practices do not count their inventory on a regular basis. At best, they do it once a year for tax purposes. The count done for tax purposes is not sufficient to make sure that an inventory system is working effectively. All items need to be counted on a more regular basis.

Items most susceptible to theft include food, heartworm preventive medication, and flea/tick medications; these should be counted monthly to make sure they are not being stolen or given to clients without charge. In the beginning, these items may need to be counted more frequently if the practice is having problems keeping track of inventory. A list of all these items should be made (with each size listed individually) and then divided by four so that each item is counted once a month. The product on hand is counted and the balance for this product, as indicated in the computerized tracking program, is immediately checked. To ensure accuracy, it is important to do these two steps in close succession. If discrepancies in the counts are noted, follow-up will be necessary:

- Are there any product purchase invoices that have not been entered into the inventory module?

- Was any product used in-house that has not been recorded in the inventory module (e.g., through a dummy client account)?
- Was any product sent home with clients or with employees that has not yet been recorded on an invoice? This is a problem more often with hospitalized or boarding patients than with outpatients.
- Was any product that was returned to the manufacturer still included in the inventory module?
- Was the product used for any other reason and not deleted from the inventory module?
- Is the product stored in some other location that may not have been counted?
- Do staff members have any other ideas as to why the discrepancies exist?

TECHNICIAN NOTE

Items most susceptible to theft include food, heartworm preventive medication, and flea/tick medications; these should be counted monthly to make sure they are not being stolen or given to clients without charge.

Depending on the extent of the discrepancies and whether reasonable explanations can be found for them, it may be necessary to institute more stringent inventory control procedures until the problem can be identified.

Unless the practice is experiencing a problem, counts on the other products usually do not need to be done as frequently. The frequency will be determined by the dollar value of the item, its likelihood of being stolen or given away, and experience with the use of this product in the clinic.

Good physical control of the inventory is important for several reasons:

- Good physical control helps ensure that the inventory is properly stored based on its physical requirements (e.g., temperature, light).
- An inventory that is well organized and easy to find makes it easier to assess how much is on hand, facilitates keeping track of short-dated products, and allows for quicker and more accurate physical counts.
- Proper organization and storage serve as a deterrent against theft and makes it easier to keep track of in-house usage.
- Sensible organization facilitates good record keeping.

In general, good physical control of the inventory requires the following:

- A locked central storage area with limited access—even here, only small quantities of product should be kept
- Small quantities of products kept in examination rooms, pharmacy and laboratory areas, and other areas easily accessible to employees
- Empty boxes displayed in public areas

Ideally, drugs would be used and replaced every 30 days (i.e., a turnover rate of 12 times per year). Unfortunately, the turnover rate is much lower in many practices.

It is also important to set up an inventory master list of all items stocked in the hospital; keep a pharmacy library of all company product inserts, catalogs, and ordering procedures; and keep a file of safety data sheets for all products as required by OSHA.

All practice information management systems have inventory modules, although practices frequently do not use them to their full capacity. It is almost impossible to have accurate inventory information without a computerized system.

A "controlled" drug is a one that is tightly controlled by government regulation because of its potential for misuse. Some controlled drugs are substances with known medical use and are available only by prescription from a licensed medical professional; others have no medical use and are illegal in the United States. Regulations cover how the drug is made, used, handled, stored, and distributed. Storage and record-keeping requirements for controlled drugs used in a veterinary practice are much more stringent than for other inventory items.

Computerization of the Veterinary Practice

Today, many veterinary practices use computers to perform practice management duties, including maintaining patient medical records, invoicing, and performing inventory and operational analyses. A wide range of management options are available in software products, providing practices with an indispensable tool for increasing efficiency and productivity.

Currently, at least 25 PIMS are available for veterinary practices. Most of these systems are currently server based, but cloud versions are becoming increasingly popular and available. A wide range of available features is seen in these systems and, although some activities are common to almost all systems (e.g., invoicing and inventory modules), other features, such as the ability to interface with diagnostic equipment or the ability to enter all medical information about a pet, may be available only on more sophisticated systems.

CASE PRESENTATION 2.4

Medical Records

Scenario: Angie, a recently hired veterinary technician, reviews a medical record before checking in a surgical patient. She notes that the medical record is incomplete and missing several important notes needed for the surgery check-in. On the previous visit, taking of the patient's vital signs and assessment and planning were not completed. To check the patient in, Angie must find the veterinarian to obtain information to complete the check-in process. The incomplete medical record made Angie "feel" incompetent and unable to deliver excellent customer service to the client, because the client's waiting time was longer than expected. At the end of the day, the client wrote a poor online review outlining her experience.

Query: Angie finds that this is a common experience in this veterinary practice, resulting in low self-confidence, reduced job satisfaction, and decreased sense of well-being. What should Angie do?

Response: Angie has two options. She can leave the practice without saying anything, or she can bring the issue to the attention of the practice manager or owner. Approaching the leadership should be the first choice, with the following points of consideration:

- Complete, legible medical records result in improved patient care.
- Complete medical records are required to be kept for each patient seen by the veterinary practice.
- Complete medical records allow everyone on the team to deliver a consistent message to the client and improve client satisfaction rates, which ultimately drive improved revenue and new client retention.
- Complete medical records prevent missed charges.

Angie could help ensure that medical records are completed thoroughly by volunteering to develop a medical record standard for all team members to follow. In addition, the development of a medical record audit process and an audit form would help the practice identify missed charges, missed recommendations, and any incomplete medical records. This would prevent the recurrence of experiences such as the one described above.

Each client and pet combination has a central electronic patient record created during the first visit to the practice. Information is added with each client or patient visit or during communication between the pet owner and the veterinary health care team. During a visit, veterinary personnel enter information as procedures are performed on a particular patient. All this data is stored in a database and becomes part of the patient's EMR. At the conclusion of an office visit or hospitalization, the receptionist prints out an invoice that itemizes procedures performed on the pet. The PIMS is also used to record payments made by the client to the hospital.

Electronic Medical Records

Historically, a paper medical record would be maintained for each patient in veterinary practice. This record would include the history, physical examination and diagnostic testing results, and SOAP assessments. The patient's computerized record would include a list of all procedures done for the patient and the amounts charged. Most practices have moved toward a complete EMR for each pet in which the information traditionally kept on paper is kept as part of the EMR. The use of EMRs improves communication and efficiency within the veterinary healthcare team. Refer to Chapter 3 for more information about EMRs.

Patient Scheduling

An important feature in a PIMS is the appointment scheduler (Fig. 2.21). When the appointment scheduling is not computerized, only one staff member at a time can record or change appointments. Computers make it possible for multiple staff members to be able to add or delete appointments concurrently, and this feature alone decreases the chaos created at the front desk when all client contacts require the services of the receptionist.

Different software systems have different capabilities in the scheduling module. An important feature is appointment time customization. Different types of appointments can be assigned specific lengths of time. Instead of a standard 15- or 30-minute appointment scheduled for all clients, appointment length can be customized to an appropriate length for the service to be provided. For example, suture removal may be set up as a 5-minute appointment, but a new client examination may require a 30-minute appointment.

Another related feature is the ability of the PIMS to show where patients are physically within the hospital. For example, all pets visiting the hospital for grooming are shown in the grooming section, all surgery patients are shown in surgery, and so on. This facilitates locating the patient if questions arise or if the client calls for a progress update (Fig. 2.22).

Reminders

The reminder module includes information about services that each pet needs in the future. For example, at the time that vaccinations are provided, the pet's record will be updated with the date the next vaccinations are due. The reminder module can also be used for heartworm preventive medication and other medications, blood work related to drug monitoring, therapeutic diets, and other needed services or product refills. Reminders can then be mailed, emailed, or sent through a text message—whichever communication method the client prefers.

Billing

An electronic invoice is created for each patient upon entry into the practice facility. As staff members perform medical tasks or

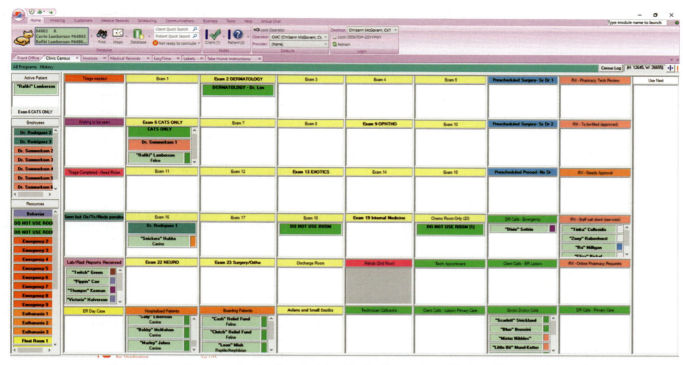

• **Fig. 2.21** Computer screen showing the schedule of the health care team. (Courtesy Dr. Joanna Bassert.)

dispense products to clients, they enter those services directly into the computer. The veterinary software updates the invoice for each item entered. When the client is ready to check out, the receptionist prints a fully itemized invoice for the client. The receptionist enters into the computer the payment made by the client.

When the software system is installed, one of the first tasks is to enter all services and products offered by the practice and the amount charged to the client for each. Not only does automation of this task reduce the number of billing errors, but it also allows practices to easily provide estimates to clients before diagnostics or treatment are initiated.

> **TECHNICIAN NOTE**
>
> An invoice is created for each patient upon entry into the practice facility. As staff members perform medical tasks or dispense products to clients, they enter those services directly into the computer.

Inventory

Inventory management is a critical module included in most PIMS. Inventory items are entered into the system, along with information about the price to be charged to clients when items are received; as items are sold, the quantity on hand is reduced. Inventory reports from the PIMS can be used to compare quantities on hand in the practice with what the PIMS says should be on hand. This process may help in identifying potential theft, shrinkage, or distribution of products to clients without charge. Other reports can be used to analyze the usage of products or reorder points.

Many practices do not use the PIMS inventory to its full advantage. Because expenses for drugs, medical supplies, and food are one of the largest in all practices, this is an area on which practices should focus more attention.

Client Communication

As discussed previously, many clients do not fully understand the care needed by their pet. Information entered into the pet's

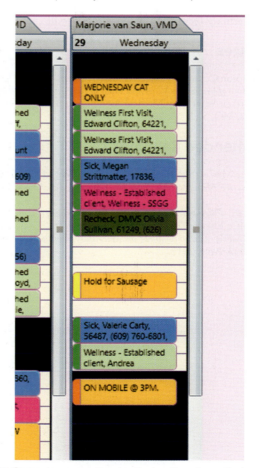

• **Fig. 2.22** Computer screen showing the location of a particular veterinarian and patient. A quiet, "cats only" examination room offers a low-stress environment for cats sensitive to noise and to lingering odors from dogs. (Courtesy Dr. Joanna Bassert.)

medical record can be retrieved later for educational and marketing purposes. For example, information about the benefits of blood work for senior pets could be sent electronically to all owners of pets that are over 7 years of age. The computer could also be asked to produce a list of all patients that received recommendations for dental work. Phone calls then can be made to those clients who have not yet booked appointments. Many other similar educational and marketing activities can now be done much more easily with the advent of computerization in veterinary practices.

Accounts Receivable

As noted previously, when medical services are added to the medical record, charges are added to the invoice. Payment by the client is recorded on the invoicing/payment screen. Most clients pay the full balance at the time of service, but some are allowed to pay off their invoices over time. The veterinary software keeps track of these accounts receivable—that is, amounts owed to the practice.

Accounts are generally considered overdue if left unpaid for 30 days. Monthly bills can be sent out to all "past due" accounts. The software is capable of adding a late fee, depending on the length of delinquency. Today's software also makes it possible to block clients from charging fees in the event that they are habitually negligent in paying their bills.

Although the PIMS is an essential part of most practices, other software is needed for a few activities. None of the currently available PIMSs have a good quality accounting or general ledger program integrated within their software. Practices therefore need separate accounting software to produce the necessary financial statements for tax and management purposes. Bookkeepers input revenue information from the billing and invoicing features of the PIMS to the accounting software, and this financial software manages accounts payable, prints checks, and tracks expenses.

Summary

Practices that flourish now and will continue to thrive in the future are those that empower veterinary health care staff to perform all patient care except those tasks that, by law, should be performed only by veterinarians. In particular, credentialed veterinary technicians who are educated in AVMA-accredited programs of veterinary technology and have passed the VTNE and state requirement are educated to deliver excellent care. Following the veterinary technician practice model will enable practices to provide high-quality medical and surgical services. They will be able to maintain excellent client-practice contact and internal communications, maintain thorough written and digital medical records, and assist in the management of attractive, efficient veterinary facilities. These flourishing practices will be exciting and rewarding enterprises for all who are affiliated with them, including clients, their animals, and the entire veterinary health care team.

References

1. Von Simpson C, Volk J, Felsted KE. *Bayer Veterinary Care Usage Study: The Decline of Veterinary Visits and How to Reverse the Trend.* Presented at: American Veterinary Medical Association Annual Convention. St. Louis, MO: Slide 68; 2011.

Recommended Readings

Heinke ML, McCarthy JB. *Practice Made Perfect: A Guide to Veterinary Practice Management.* 2nd ed. Lakewood, CO: AAHA Press; 2012.

Prendergast H. *Practice Management for the Veterinary Team.* 4th ed. St. Louis, MO: Elsevier; 2023.

Smith C, Rose R. *Career Choices for Veterinary Technicians.* Lakewood, CO: AAHA Press; 2013.

Journals

DVM 360, Cleveland, OH, MJH Associates, Inc. Monthly.

The NAVTA Journal, Schaumburg, IL. Bi-Monthly.

Today's Veterinary Nurse; NAVC Publications; Gainesville, FL. Quarterly.

Trends, Denver, CO, American Animal Hospital Association. Monthly.

Veterinary Practice News, BowTie, Mission Viejo, CA. Monthly.

Management Short Courses

American Animal Hospital Association Veterinary Management Institute. Purdue University Veterinary Practice Management Program.

Patterson Veterinary University. www.PattersonVetUniversity.com.

Internet Sites

www.avma.org.

www.vhma.org.

www.dvm360.com.

www.aaha.org.

3

Veterinary Medical Records

MICHELLE CAMPOLI AND PAIGE A. ALLEN

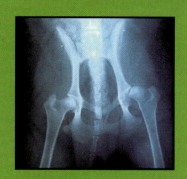

CHAPTER OUTLINE

LEARNING OBJECTIVES

When you have completed this chapter, you will be able to:

1. Pronounce, define, and spell all key terms within this chapter.
2. Describe the key principles of the medical record's function.
3. List and describe the primary and secondary purposes of the medical record.
4. Explain the legal issues related to ownership of medical records, release of medical information, and maintenance of medical records.
5. Describe methods for formatting medical records and explain their respective advantages and disadvantages.
6. List and describe each problem-oriented veterinary medical record (POVMR) component.
7. Explain each portion of the veterinary technician subjective, objective, assessment, plan (SOAP) note and the types of information included in each portion, and describe how each portion correlates to the steps in the veterinary technician practice model (presented in Chapter 1).
8. Describe the importance of cage cards, discharge instructions, discharge summary, and medication administration/order record (MAOR) forms and why they are valuable in organizing the care of hospitalized veterinary patients.
9. Explain the advantages and disadvantages of electronic medical record keeping.
10. Compare and contrast the types of filing systems commonly used for paper medical records.
11. List and describe the types of forms and logs commonly used in veterinary practice.
12. Describe methods for collecting and storing medical information in ambulatory veterinary medical practices.
13. Locate your state's record keeping and retention requirements.

KEY TERMS

Consultations
Electronic medical records (EMRs)
Master problem list
Medication administration/order record (MAOR)
Previous history
Problem-oriented veterinary medical record (POVMR)
Progress notes
Recent history

Signalment
Subjective, objective, assessment and plan (SOAP)
Source-oriented veterinary medical record (SOVMR)
Veterinarian-client-patient relationship (VCPR)
Veterinary technician evaluations
Veterinary medical databases
Working problem list

Introduction

This chapter offers an overview of the veterinary patient record's organization, components, and functions by using illustrations from both electronic and paper-based platforms. In addition, it discusses the ethical and legal issues that accompany the record-keeping process and introduces the importance of consistently maintaining neat, thorough accounts of patient care. It also introduces the reader to **SOAP** (subjective, objective, assessment, plan) notes and the technician's care plan, and describes their importance in helping support excellent patient care.

Patient Medical Record

The patient medical record is one of the core tenets of veterinary practice. Regardless of the practice type (general, emergency, referral, equine, etc.) or record-keeping methodology (electronic, paper chart, or a hybrid of the two), the most important functions of the medical record are accurately identifying the patient and the client/owner and providing continuity of care of the patient. In addition, the medical record serves as a legal record of the specific veterinary care provided to every patient.

Veterinary technicians play a critical role in fostering the development of complete and accurate patient records and often are responsible for assisting the veterinarian with the documentation of both outpatient and inpatient cases. The saying "If it is not documented, then it did not happen" is important regarding the legal aspects of care and should be always on the minds of clinicians and practice owners. With the litigious nature of our society, keeping accurate, detailed, and complete medical records is paramount to the success of any veterinary practice.

PUT INTO PRACTICE

Medical records are legal documents, so it is important that as a veterinary technician, you are comfortable with writing clearly and accurately. It is a great idea to ask others to review what you have written until you are confident in writing medical records.

The term *medical record* refers to the total body of information regarding a patient, including client information, patient identification and handling notes, patient exam findings, laboratory and imaging results, surgical and anesthetic records, hospitalization treatment sheets, prescribed medication, supplement and diet information, outcomes from special studies, referral recommendations, communications, authorization, and consent agreements, and even billing and payment information. Keeping this ever-increasing expanse of patient documentation organized and accessible is often managed primarily with a veterinary practice management software system, and secondarily with hard copy files.

Fortunately, a plethora of veterinary practice management software products are available to help practices efficiently organize and access the increasingly complex and amount of patient data. Refer to Table 3.1 for a list of some of the more prevalent computer systems used in veterinary practices today. Given the large volume of information gathered for each patient and the many clients and patients each practice serves, computerization is an industry standard for storing veterinary client and patient information. Although there are some practices that continue to use only written medical records, most practices today use computers and applications to support the management of medical record keeping. In addition, managing patient data, client and staff scheduling, billing, inventory management, payroll, marketing, data collection, accounting, and client communications can all be managed using various technologies.

Principles and Functions of the Medical Record

The importance of the medical record cannot be overstated for veterinary practices that maintain the health of and treat sick and injured animals. A thorough, accurate medical record is a critical component of excellent veterinary care and a prudent responsibility of well-managed and successful veterinary practices. The breadth of information that makes up the veterinary medical record has increased over the years due to more advanced diagnostics; client communication platforms have become more accessible; and practice specializations and state medical board and accreditation requirements have expanded. In addition, state regulations and client expectations have grown.

The pandemic (2020) induced changes to practice workflow and shifted some patient care models to a more remote format to expand already stretched-thin veterinary teams. Telemedicine, emerging artificial intelligence (AI) technologies, and accessibility to care pushes the sharing of records to tie into continuity of care. In addition, client expectations to access patient records and information on their pets have shifted to a more technology-driven expectation with generational shifts in both clients and veterinary team members. Multiple sources of patient data now exist and must be integrated into the patient's record.

Although the approach to and the format of the record itself have remained essentially the same, the methodology for recording and storing of medical records has changed dramatically from paper records to **electronic medical records (EMRs)**. A variety of

TABLE 3.1   Examples of Veterinary Practice Management Software

Name of Software	Company Name	Description
Animal Intelligence	Animal Intelligence Software	Meets the specialized needs of innovative general, specialty, and emergency and critical care veterinary practice.
AVImark	Covetrus	Manages all practices and scalable enough to grow with any clinic.
Cornerstone Practice Management	IDEXX Laboratories	Comprehensive software package, including appointment scheduler, time clock for employees, electronic medical record (EMR), inventory, reporting and more. An American Animal Hospital Association (AAHA)-endorsed PIMS (Practice Information Management Software) for electronic records.
DVMax	IDEXX Laboratories	Practice management solution with records management, laboratory support, inventory management, treatment plans, medical record entry (MREs), and diagnoses.
eVet Practice	Covetrus	Cloud-based practice management system in the United States; supports clinics of all sizes.
ezyVet	ezyVet Software	Cloud-based; includes accounting, hospital regimes, and electronic whiteboard; used in all practice types.
Impromed Infinity	Covetrus	Helps increase profits, reduce expenses, and recover missed charges.
IntraVet	Patterson Veterinary	Estimates, laboratory results, medical history, patient images, invoices, and client communications are integrated with patient records.
NaVetor	Patterson Veterinary	Built from the cloud up, NaVetor veterinary software is a modern, efficient, remarkably easy way to streamline the workday and navigate the business. Because it is cloud based, it can be used anywhere without the need for installation or new hardware investments.
Neo	IDEXX Laboratories	IDEXX Neo is brilliantly simple and completely ready to go. Cloud-based veterinary software is designed for ease of use and ability to access practice information on any Internet-connected device, anywhere.
Smart Flow Sheet	IDEXX Laboratories	A cloud-based veterinary software module for patient treatment and workflow tracking.
VetBlue Clinic	VetBlue	For veterinary offices of all sizes and types, including mobile veterinary and equine veterinary practices. Cloud based.
Vetter	Vetter Software	Cloud practice management software for veterinarians.

software tools are available and continue to be developed to meet the growing electronic record needs of the veterinary community. Although the way in which veterinary medical data are recorded and stored has changed dramatically, the format of the medical record is remarkably the same and includes the same key elements as those of paper-based records. Therefore the key tenets of excellent medical record keeping remain true today, as discussed below:

1. A medical record should be maintained in such a manner that another veterinary professional could, by reading the record, easily understand the case and proceed with proper care of the patient.
2. Medical records should include all clinical information to support the diagnosis and the treatment given.
3. Entries should:
   i. Be entered in chronologic order by date and time so that the patient's history can be readily traced.
   ii. Be accurate and concise, yet thorough and objective. It should avoid emotional or editorial language, such as derogatory or negative comments about the client, patient, or other professionals. Comments about a pet owner may be relevant but should be added to the record only when interactions and/or observations affect the health and treatment of the pet. For example, making an entry that the client was rude is inappropriate; however, a client's refusal to sign discharge instructions would be important to document. Keep in mind that clients may obtain copies of the medical record, making the practice vulnerable to the consequences of any unprofessional or casual entries.

   iii. Use only standard abbreviations (refer to the American Animal Hospital Association [AAHA] standard abbreviations publication—Recommended Reading and Resources).
   iv. Be written as if the client or a lawyer were reviewing it.
4. Entries indicating future care (e.g., "Recheck in five days") should be documented, whether the client follows through or not.
5. In paper medical records, corrections should be made overtly. For example, if an error was made, a single dark line should be drawn through the error and the change initialed and dated. Avoid writing in the margins or between entries. This can be mistaken as an alteration of the record, which would compromise the validity of the entry and could also bring into question the integrity of the entire medical record.
6. Clients have the right to see or have a copy of their pets' medical records upon request. In the current ethos of social media, when anything can be shared with the world with a few taps on a phone, it is important to always act in an ethical and professional manner when recording medical findings about patients.
7. Although there are no definitive rules regarding the time frame for completing a patient's record (most states define this as "in a contemporaneous manner"), record keeping should be done as much in real time as possible so that important information is not forgotten. Details about a patient can be overlooked or forgotten if they are not written down during or soon after a particular appointment or treatment. In other words, make notations in the medical record immediately after each treatment, assessment, or interaction with a patient. Mistakes are most likely to happen when written entries are made after working

with several other patients and when record write-ups are left for a later time. Another cause of potential problems occurs when a patient transfers to another veterinary hospital or emergency clinic before their records have been updated with examination findings, latest diagnostic test results, and treatments provided. These data would be vital to future veterinary services to avoid complications from overdosing or adverse drug interactions and unnecessary repetition of diagnostic tests.

The Institute of Medicine has organized the functions of the medical record into two broad categories: primary purposes and secondary purposes. Primary purposes support the patient's medical care and include documentation of diagnostic procedures, diagnoses, prognoses, and treatment. Secondary purposes are not clinically based; they include evaluations of medical information for business, legal, and research purposes (Box 3.1).

Primary Purposes

Supports Excellent Medical Care

The medical record is a critical tool that in many ways enables and supports effective treatment and care of animals. First, it assists the veterinary health care team in correctly identifying the patient and the owner. After all, many black Labrador Retrievers look alike, may have the same name, and may have owners with the same last name. The medical record helps prevent confusion among the identities of patients and their owners. Second, it aids in the generation of effective diagnostic and treatment plans. It documents physical examination findings of the veterinarian and the veterinary technician, lists diagnostic procedures and tests to be performed, and records the veterinarian's ideas regarding differential diagnoses. The medical record also enables the veterinary health care team to document the patient's responses to treatment so that plans may be adjusted as needed. As time passes and members of the health care team change, the medical record supports continuity of care. It helps those who are not familiar with the case to understand the medical history and conditions of the patient. In this way, it provides an avenue for communication among all members of the veterinary health care team so that treatment can be accurately and effectively administered. This is especially important in multidoctor practices where veterinary care can be delivered by more than one veterinarian. It may also be relevant when a case is shared with another general practice or specialist.

• BOX 3.1   Summary Chart: Functions of the Medical Record

Primary (medical care based)
- Identifies the correct patient and client
- Documents and supports diagnostic procedures, diagnoses, prognoses, and treatment plans
- Supports continuity of care
- Supports communication between health care team members and the client
- Personalizes the veterinarian-client-patient relationship (VCPR)

Secondary (business & legal based)
- Billing verification
- Supports business analysis (income, budgeting, staffing)
- Supports inventory maintenance marketing strategy
- Supports hospital and individual accreditation
- Serves as a legal document
- Supports research (case studies, registries and databases, education)

Documents Communications

The medical record also documents communications with the client; this is particularly important when many members of the veterinary health care team are communicating with the same pet owner. A copy of take-home instructions, for example, will be included in the medical record so that any confusion about home care provided by the client (owner) can be quickly clarified. In addition, the medical record assists in the generation of reminders that help pet owners stay current with their pet's preventive medical care plan or maintenance of chronic health issues, such as diabetes or renal insufficiency. Expansion of third-party applications enhance communications between practice and client and should be considered for inclusion into record. Point of exam (POE) apps and services share records; in these ways, good communication is critical for providing a logical, continued plan of patient care for both health care providers and pet owners.

Interactions with clients and their pets are also aided using medical records. Financial limitations, for example, and the behavioral idiosyncrasies of the pet may be recorded. In addition, the veterinarian-client-patient relationship (VCPR) can be further enhanced when the names of other family members and important family activities are noted in the record as reminders for future topics of informal discussion.

Secondary Purposes

Supports Business and Legal Activities

The medical record lists all services rendered to the pet owner, whether they involve boarding a dog or spaying a cat. This documentation verifies billing and serves as legal evidence of services received by the owner. It can be used to assess staff members' workloads, formulate income analyses, make budgetary plans, perform actuarial calculations, maintain inventory, and generate a marketing strategy. In addition, it plays an important role during hospital and team member accreditations or during the evaluation of team members. It also helps assess compliance with standards of care.

The medical record is used as a legal document in the event of an examining board hearing or in a court of law and is valuable during litigation. It serves as evidence of procedures performed and treatments administered, and it provides specific dates and times of events. In this way, the medical record is critical in defending against malpractice suits. Special care must be taken to ensure that the record is complete and accurate. One must be kept in mind that in a court of law, the prevailing view is "If it is not recorded, it was not done." In addition, insurance companies may require the medical record to assess whether a claim is to be paid.

Supports Research

The medical record is a key element in the preparation of case studies, and presentations for conferences. Information from medical records is collected to develop registries and veterinary medical databases, which assist in the conduct of retrospective studies and in predicting clinical outcomes. It is used to teach veterinary medical and veterinary technician students. To maintain confidentiality, all patient markers are removed from the record before they are used for any purpose other than patient care.

TECHNICIAN NOTE

A comprehensive medical record supports excellent medical care, communication, research, and good business practices. It helps defend practices during malpractice litigation and when complaints are filed against a practice with the state boards of veterinary medicine.

Medical and Legal Requirements

Not surprisingly, the most common deficit cited by state veterinary examining boards in investigations of complaints is incomplete medical records. It is particularly critical that veterinary personnel understand and carry out state mandates for medical record keeping. Other requirements may be imposed by certifying or accrediting organizations, such as the AAHA, the American Association of Feline Practitioners (AAFP), Fear Free–certified practitioners and hospitals, and others.

Veterinarian-Client-Patient Relationship

The VCPR serves as the foundation of the interactions among veterinarians, their clients, and their patients. Medical records must be maintained for all patients with whom a VCPR exists. VCPR can be applied to individual animals and to a group of animals within an operation (production system). According to the American Veterinary Medical Association (AVMA), a VCPR occurs when the following conditions have been met:

- The veterinarian has assumed responsibility for making clinical judgments regarding the health of the animal(s) and the need for medical treatment, and the client has agreed to follow the veterinarian's instructions.
- The veterinarian has sufficient knowledge of the animal(s) to initiate at least a general or preliminary diagnosis of the animal(s)' medical condition. This means that the veterinarian has recently seen and is personally acquainted with the keeping and care of the animal(s) by virtue of an examination of the animal(s), or through medically appropriate and timely visits* to the operation where the animal(s) are kept.[†]
- The veterinarian is readily available or has arranged for emergency coverage for follow-up evaluation in the event of adverse reactions or failure of the treatment regimen.
- The veterinarian provides oversight of treatment, compliance, and outcome.
- Patient records are maintained.

> **PUT INTO PRACTICE**
>
> While you are not technically a part of the VCPR, it is important that you make sure a VCPR is in effect prior to dispensing any medication to a client. Make sure you are up to date on the requirements for your state regarding the establishment of a VCPR.

It is important to note that the AVMA's position regarding the practice of telemedicine, at the time of this chapter's writing, is articulated in the following section of the Veterinary Medical Model Practice Act: "…a veterinarian-client-patient relationship (VCPR) cannot be established solely by telephonic or other electronic means." Therefore with current technologic capabilities and considering existing state and federal regulatory laws, veterinary telemedicine should only be conducted within an existing VCPR. Further information is located at the AVMA website.

---

*Some state regulatory boards include a specific period to clearly define the term *timely* relating to examinations and visits.
[†]When establishing a VCPR in the case of large operations, "sufficient knowledge" can be further specified by some state boards by means of: examination of health, laboratory, or production records; or consultation with owners, caretakers, or supervisory staff regarding a health management program for the patient; or information regarding the local epidemiology of diseases for the appropriate species.

However, the COVID-19 pandemic brought about state-mandated changes to delivery of care methods which, in some cases, modified the definition of the VCPR or the loosening of telemedicine use to establish and maintain the VCPR. The pandemic also brought about a drastic increase in veterinary telehealth platforms, many of which integrate with a practice's software. As technologies advance and evidence-based research on the impact of telemedicine on access to care and patient safety becomes available, methods for establishment of VCPR may change. Ultimately, a state's board rules should be a technician's reference point on how telehealth can dovetail with the VCPR and health care delivery.

Importance of Informed Consent

A common complaint of pet owners is delivery of veterinary care to a pet without request or authorization from the owner. Clients may also dispute services that were authorized but without complete understanding of the full cost, or other implications of the services such as euthanasia, expensive diagnostics, and high-risk procedures. It is very important for veterinary practices to ensure that *informed* client consent is obtained in all cases to minimize potential disputes. *Informed consent* is defined as a person's agreement to allow something to happen, such as a medical, diagnostic, or surgical procedure, based on full disclosure of facts necessary to make an intelligent decision. In other words, the client or the representative must be educated by using language that they can understand. This includes all facts regarding the pet's medical condition, diagnosis, prognosis, risks, and treatment options, and justification for the cost of treatment. The prognosis and the risk to the animal if the owner refuses treatment should also be included in the disclosure. In addition, in-clinic and home care, monitoring, follow-up, emergency procedures, and preventive health care plans should all be discussed with the client and documented in writing. Informed consent should include both verbal and written descriptions of treatments and procedures under consideration. This is important, because consent forms are often not read thoroughly by clients and even a signed consent form can be contested if the client is not made fully aware of *all* the ramifications of a particular procedure or action.

Informed consent is generally determined and applied based on three standards:

1. Reasonable practitioner standard—requires disclosure of all facts the doctor believes relevant to the client.
2. Reasonable client/patient standard—requires disclosure of all risks to a reasonable, prudent person in the client's position.
3. Individual client/patient standard—requires determination of what risks are material to the client being addressed and disclosure of those risks.

Giving the client a written handout describing the treatment or procedure and asking if there are any questions is insufficient in obtaining informed consent. Because the veterinarian is best able to explain a particular procedure to a pet owner and answer questions, they are in the best position to obtain the owner's consent for the procedure. However, it may be permissible for a veterinary technician to obtain consent from an owner if the technician is familiar with the procedure or treatment. In this case, it is prudent for the veterinary technician to ask the pet owner if they would prefer to discuss the procedure with the veterinarian. It is also important for the veterinary technician to answer any questions that the owner may have until it is confirmed that the client has no more questions.

In documenting informed consent, communications with clients should be recorded in the medical record, including the content of face-to-face consultations, email or text communications, and conversations on the phone. If an animal is co-owned, it may be helpful to note the specific party involved in the conversation, because co-owning clients do not always communicate effectively with each other. Written communication with clients via email or text should be maintained, because it offers a dated and timed record. When consent is offered over the phone, it is preferable for the conversation to be witnessed by another staff member on speakerphone or on another line. This discussion should later be summarized in the medical record and signed by both the veterinarian and the staff/witness.

Consent and Authorization Forms

Consent and authorization forms document in writing the understanding between the veterinary practice and the pet owner. Forms should outline specific conditions, risks of procedures, and responsibilities of both parties. In keeping with the doctrine of informed consent, completed authorization forms provide veterinary practices with legal evidence that the owner was informed of important information and that the owner agreed to pursue a particular course of action based on the circumstances and information given to them. One should be aware that consent must be given by legal adults 18 years of age or older. In addition, the competency of the owner at the time of consent is observed and noted. Consent by a minor may not be considered legal consent, even if they are the established caregiver of the patient. One must be aware that even considering a signed consent form, a client can claim that they were not duly informed.

In most practices, client education followed by obtaining a signed consent form is standard operating procedure to proactively address potential client concerns and ensure that excellent communication was carried out. Surgery, euthanasia, and necropsy are a few examples of situations in which written owner permission and verbal communication are critical. During emergencies, for example, owners can be particularly emotional and may have difficulty making clear decisions. Owners who decide to euthanize their sick or injured pet may regret their decision later. They may blame the veterinary staff for "being pressured into it" or may believe that they were not given all the information needed to make a sound choice. Authorization forms verify the identity of the owner and reduce the practice's liability in performing euthanasia. Because complications and complaints can arise months later, it is important to make consent forms a permanent part of the medical record.

A common source of consternation in veterinary practices is miscommunication regarding the cost of services. Many veterinary hospitals have developed forms for fee estimation and for treatment consent. These forms give owners a written estimate of the costs of procedures, verify ownership, document any declined services, and establish an agreement if the animal is abandoned by the owner. This empowers the practice to act if the owner cannot meet their responsibility to pay for services and/or retrieve the pet.

Obtaining consent from the owner is recommended whenever there are indications that a problem could arise with a client. Legal difficulties can often be prevented by identifying potentially difficult clients in advance. Having the owner's written consent to restrain their pet during an examination, for example, may protect the practice later if the client is bitten. Sometimes an owner who normally insists on holding their pet during an office visit may decide not to do so after reading and signing a consent form that lists the risks of restraining an animal. Consents can be maintained in either electronic or paper form by means of electronic signatures and/or by scanning printed and signed forms into the medical record.

Documentation: Protection Against Complaints and Litigation

In some cases, it is state law to provide drug information handouts and document prescription consultations when medications are dispensed to a veterinary patient, like a human pharmacy consult. For example, in California, Lizzie's Law requires a doctor, a duly authorized registered veterinary technician, or a veterinary assistant to counsel clients on the administration, proper use and storage, potential risks, side effects, and drug interactions of a prescribed drug and document that the consult occurred or was declined in the patient's medical record.

When a lawsuit or a complaint is filed against a veterinarian, a veterinary technician, or a practice, a complete, accurate, and legible (and unalterable) medical record is one of the most convincing pieces of evidence used to refute allegations. An incomplete, inaccurate, or illegible record may be construed as evidence of professional incompetence and substandard care, which may lead to stiff fines or worse imposed by the state board of veterinary medicine.

Disgruntled pet owners often present at hearings with a plethora of evidence against the practice, including transcripts of phone and/or email and text conversations and office visits, retrieved foreign objects, copies of medical records, itemized receipts, pill vials, sworn witness testimony, and before and after photographs of their pet. Maintaining a discipline of generating consistently complete and accurate medical records is essential to ensure protection from legal action.

The following rules of thumb must be kept in mind:

1. If it was not entered into the patient's medical record, either written down or electronically, it did not happen. Refer to Box 3.2, Clinical Application 1.
2. If the writing is illegible, the information was not written down.
3. If one part of the electronic or written medical record shows signs of tampering or is inaccurate, the integrity of the *entire* medical record becomes questionable. Electronic records should have a locking or closing record functionality and/or a clear audit trail of changes or additions made to the record. Although rare, veterinary technicians are sued for malpractice. Therefore veterinary technicians, like veterinarians, must ensure that they have protected themselves from potential litigation by recording all treatments and interactions with patients and clients. In addition, veterinary technicians should avoid employment with veterinary practices that preclude them from making independent assessments of their patients and from recording those findings in the medical record.

Scribe, ChatGPT, or other AI powered tools can be used; however, it is ultimately the doctor's responsibility for accuracy of record entries (align with other references to record ownership/responsibilities). Some guidelines for generating clear, complete, and accurate records are as follows:

1. Entries should be typed or written neatly in black ink. This improves clarity of images during copying or faxing.
2. In a court of law, handwriting alone is not an adequate way to identify the author of a notation. All written entries should be signed or initialed by the author and include the author's credentials (e.g., CVT, DVM), the date, and the time. The

• BOX 3.2 | Clinical Application 1

Take a look at the following written records for Fenway, a 6-year-old Golden Retriever. His owners noted a soft mass on his left side and asked their veterinarian about it at the dog's annual examination. According to the owners, they were told it was a lipoma. Fenway was examined at a different practice the next year for limping. The mass had grown, and it was now affecting Fenway's left forelimb. The mass was identified as a mast cell tumor. Luckily, it was localized and excised successfully.

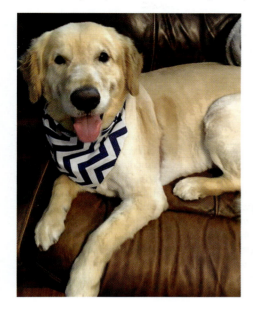

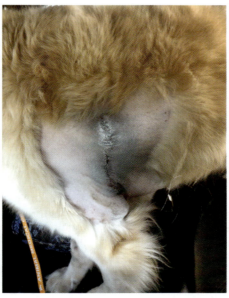

Discussion points:
Can you locate the lipoma diagnosis in the annual examination entry?
Do you think the client can file a complaint?

practice should also maintain a log that associates each person's full name, which is typically typed into the log, with signatures and initials listed in separate columns. In this way, initials and signatures are accurately and clearly linked to specific veterinarians or veterinary technicians. Entries into electronic patient records similarly must verify the employee's identity and include the date and time the entry is made.

3. In hard copy medical records, errors should *not* be scratched out, erased, or blotted out with marker or correction fluid. Instead, a single line should be drawn through the mistake and the word *error* written in the margin, along with the correct information. The change is also signed and dated by the person who made the error, with a brief explanation for the correction entered.

Progress Notes

Date/Time	Initials	Progress Notes
7/7/xx 6 pm	JS	Notation: "Fluffy" exhibits moderate pain in the cranioventral abdomen. ~~Small~~ Firm oval mass palpable approx. 2 cm x 2.5 cm.

Error, Jane Smith 7/7/13 6:03pm

Any erasure or blotting out may suggest tampering with the record and could render the document inadmissible in a court of law. Computerized medical records must be able to track input, changes, addendums, and deletions and ideally lock the records to ensure an unalterable state. If the history of electronic entries, deletions, addendums, and changes cannot be tracked, the medical record is not credible as evidence.

1. Entries to written records may be initialed rather than signed if the form includes a signature box in which an individual's signature is listed with their initials or if the practice maintains a logbook of employee names, signatures, and initials.
2. Only approved standard abbreviations should be used in veterinary medical records.

The medical record is considered legal evidence of services and procedures performed by the veterinary health care team. In the event of litigation, as during a malpractice or insurance suit, a subpoena for the record is often issued and the record admitted as evidence.

Legal guidelines for medical records vary among the states or provinces and may dictate the type of information that should be included, how long the record should be kept, and restrictions on the release of medical information. It is highly recommended that all members of the veterinary health care team be familiar with the laws of the state or province in which they work. The "Recommended Readings and Resources" section at the end of this chapter provides links to the requirements for each state or province.

TECHNICIAN NOTE

In hard copy records, errors should *not* be scratched out, erased, or blotted out. Instead, a single line should be drawn through the mistake and the word "error" written in the margin, along with the correct information. This change should be signed and dated by the person who made the error. Any erasure or blotting out may suggest tampering with the record and could render the document inadmissible in a court of law.

Ownership and Release of Medical Information

In general, veterinary medical records are the property of the veterinary practice and its owners. Although the client purchased the veterinary services that generated the medical information, the client is not, by law, the owner of the medical record. However, the client may make a written request at any time for a copy of a pet's medical record. It is customary for clients to request copies of their pet's medical record when they are moving and changing veterinary practices. This facilitates continued care of the patient and prevents repetition of immunizations or diagnostic tests. It is recommended that copies of medical records be sent directly to the successive veterinarian by either electronic or other means and not hand delivered by the owner, who may be apt to misinterpret entries in the medical record. A cover letter or email should be included with the attached copy of the record so that the original veterinary hospital and veterinarian can be easily contacted, if necessary. A fee may be charged for sending a copy of the record, based on the state board's rules.

It is considered best practice to obtain a signed authorization form or a written letter of request for record copies from the animal's owner before any information is released to the owner, another veterinarian, or another third party. Although the Health Insurance Portability and Accountability Act (HIPAA) does not cover pet medical records, some states have laws that mimic HIPAA regulations. The AVMA maintains a list of each state's privacy laws (See "Recommended Reading and Resources").

The practice owner should be the only person to authorize the release of information contained in the record. One should keep in mind that the patient record is a confidential document and that confidentiality must always be protected. Therefore in most states/provinces, the patient record may be released to a third party only with permission from the client. The following circumstances are exceptions to this rule, when information in the medical record must be given to the appropriate authority without client permission.

- The veterinarian has diagnosed a reportable disease and must alert local, state/provincial, and federal agencies as required by law. *Reportable diseases* may be dangerous to the public and to the health of animals in general and include a wide variety of diseases, such as rabies, brucellosis, and equine encephalitis. Additional regulations regarding reportable diseases can be found in the *US National List of Reportable Animal Diseases (NLRAD) System Standards,* which is published by the US Department of Agriculture (USDA).
- A court of law subpoenas the medical record.

Clients give permission for their pet's medical record to be copied and sent to a third party for a variety of reasons. Some examples are given below:

- The patient is moving to another veterinary practice, and the client would like the new practice to have a copy of the medical record.
- The pet has bitten a person, and the client would like to give proof of the animal's immunization against rabies.
- The animal's health, life, or ability to perform was insured. The client cannot collect from an insurance company until official proof indicates that the animal did indeed die or become injured.
- Scientists studying epidemiology, zoonoses, and medical trends examine patient records for data that are relevant to their research. The client agrees to release patient information if the confidentiality of the owner is maintained (Box 3.3).

American Veterinary Medical Association (AVMA) Ethics and Medical Records (excerpt from the Principles of Veterinary Medical Ethics)

1. Veterinary medical records are an integral part of veterinary care. These records must comply with standards established by state and federal laws.
2. Medical records are the property of the practice and the practice owner. The original records must be retained by the practice for the period required by law.
3. The information within veterinary medical records is considered confidential. It must not be released except as required or allowed by law or by consent of the owner of the patient.
4. Veterinarians are obligated to provide copies or summaries of medical records when requested by the client. Veterinarians should secure a written consent to document that provision.
5. Without the express permission of the practice owner, it is unethical for a veterinarian (or a veterinary technician) to remove, copy, or use the medical records or any part of any record for personal or professional gain.

American Veterinary Medical Association. *Principles of Veterinary Medical Ethics of the AVMA.* https://www.avma.org/KB/Policies/Pages/Principles-of-Veterinary-Medical-Ethics-of-the-AVMA.aspx. *Accessed October 1, 2016.*

Format of Veterinary Medical Records

The medical record is very important in securing a strong legal defense, but the most important reason for maintaining excellence in medical record keeping is to provide optimal patient care. Incomplete or lost medical information leads to incomplete and suboptimal patient care. Because it is impossible to remember all clinical details associated with each case, a thorough, well-written medical record often contains extensive information. Medical information must therefore be organized in such a way that veterinary personnel can locate pertinent details quickly and easily. Computers and veterinary practice management software have dramatically improved the organization, storage, and accessibility of patient information.

Historically, medical record information was stored in hard copy and could be organized in several ways. Most methods fall into one of three categories:

1. Source-oriented veterinary medical record (SOVMR)
2. Problem-oriented veterinary medical record (POVMR)
3. A combination of SOVMR and POVMR

Today, veterinary medical record keeping is maintained partly or fully via computerized practice management software, which has transformed the way in which veterinary medical records are maintained. Computers can effortlessly maintain records by using the aspects of both the SOVMR and POVMR approaches.

Source-Oriented Veterinary Medical Record

In a **source-oriented veterinary medical record (SOVMR)**, patient information is organized by subject matter. Laboratory reports, for example, may be kept separate from **progress notes**, which are written in chronologic order. Clinical observations are entered as they become evident. In this way, the most recent information is located last, and the oldest information is found first. In a hard copy (paper) record and many electronic systems, chronologic history is displayed with the most recent entries first.

The source-oriented method is easy to learn and takes little time to complete; however, it can lack detailed documentation, which may prove vital during litigation. Remember, if it is not recorded, it did not happen. In addition, and perhaps most important, individual medical problems may be difficult to monitor. A veterinary technician, for example, may have to search several different sections of a SOVMR to follow the progress of a cat with diabetes, because blood work results, physical examination findings, and diagnostic imaging details may be in three different areas of the medical record. The organization of medical information in a SOVMR format may be further complicated in practices that include different departments and specialty groups.

Problem-Oriented Veterinary Medical Record

The **problem-oriented veterinary medical record (POVMR)** provides an organized approach to clinical veterinary care in that information in the medical record is grouped by problem, and each problem is addressed separately. Notes are entered on progress forms using the SOAP format. A SOAP note is written for each visit or examination performed during a patient's hospital stay. Both veterinarians and veterinary technicians may write SOAP notes in the POVMR, although the focus of each is different. The veterinarian focuses on identifying the cause of illness and subsequently a cure, whereas the veterinary technician focuses on the patient's psychological and physiologic reactions to the medical condition. The POVMR fosters excellent communication and team-oriented medical care and encourages ongoing assessment and revision of the health care plan by all members of the health care team. The AAHA endorses the use of problem-oriented veterinary medical record keeping and insists on its use in practices seeking AAHA certification.

Components of the Problem-Oriented Veterinary Medical Record

Although POVMR medical records vary somewhat, they most commonly include the following:

1. Database
   i. Client and patient information
   ii. History (current history, chief presenting complaint, and **previous history**)
   iii. Physical examination findings
   iv. Pertinent test results (radiography, special imaging, and laboratory reports)
2. Master problem list and working problem lists
3. Initial plan and progress notes
   i. Progress forms that include SOAP notes for each visit.
   ii. Treatment-related forms, medication administration/order record (MAOR) forms, surgical reports, and anesthesia forms
4. Case summary and discharge instructions

These components can be further subdivided into more specific units of information (Box 3.4).

The Database

A database is a collection of all available information that would contribute to the diagnostic process of a patient when originally seen for a particular problem. Initial data may include the following: client and patient information, details gleaned through

• BOX 3.4   Standard Information for Veterinary Medical Records

Client Information

Name of owner
Address (mailing and email)
All applicable phone numbers (home, cell, and work phone numbers) and
  fax numbers
Additional information if co-owned:
  Other adult family members or responsible parties/authorized agents
  Alternative emergency contact information
  If applicable, referring person

Patient Information

Name of animal
Signalment: species, breed, age, sex, and spayed/neutered
Color and markings
Tattoo, microchip number, and identification (ID) number

Pertinent History

Presenting complaint
Last normal (last time patient was known to be normal)
Frequency of episodes
Client observations and/or concerns
Current medications
Allergies
Current diet
Transfusion history
Recent travel history

Previous History

Previous problems
Previous treatments and responses
Previous surgeries
Previous medications
Previous diagnostic tests
Immunization history
Patient's weight history
Previous diet
Geographic region of origin/birth and travel history
Previous reactions to drugs, anesthesia, and transfusions

Physical Examination

Initial physical examination findings
Progress notes and SOAP (subjective, objective, assessment, planning) notes
Master problem list
Working problem list

Diagnosis

Tentative diagnoses
Definitive diagnoses

Prognoses

Diagnostic results
Laboratory reports
Reports and assessments of diagnostic procedures (endoscopy, radiography,
  ultrasonography, and special imaging)
Description of surgical and dental procedures, including duration of
  procedure and name of surgeon
Anesthetic record
Consultation reports with specialists or other referring veterinarians
  (dermatology, oncology, cardiology, ophthalmology, surgery, internal
  medicine, dentistry, and neurology)
Necropsy report

Therapeutic Plans

Changes in therapy
Medication administration and order record (MAOR)
Name of medication
Time
Date
Dosage and directions
Fluid rate
Route of administration
Frequency
Duration of treatment
Identification of individuals administering treatments

Cautionary Notes

Slaughter withdrawal and/or milk withholding dates (food animal)
Client communications
Signed consent forms
Client waivers or deferrals of recommendations
Client phone communication log
Discharge instructions
Financial records

Derived from Peden AH. Comparative Records for Health Information Management. *2nd ed. Florence, KY: Delmar; 2004;* The American Veterinary Medical Association (AVMA) guidelines on basic information for records; and The American Animal Hospital Association (AAHA) standards of accreditation.

interviews with the owner regarding the pet's recent and prior histories, findings of health assessment or physical examination of the animal, photograph of the animal, (Fig. 3.1), and results of various laboratory and radiologic tests.

It is recommended that the database be as complete as possible, restricted only by potential risk to the patient, including pain, and by limitations of the owner's financial resources.

Client and Patient Information

Typically, the receptionist takes the name and contact information of the client (and/or agent of the client) when the first appointment is made. Contact information includes the client's mailing address; home, cell, and office phone numbers; and email address. This information will be confirmed later when the owner arrives

for the appointment. It is particularly important to record the correct spelling of the owner's first and last names. Even seemingly simple names, such as Megan Brown, may be spelled differently, for example, Meaghan Brown or Meghan Browne. One should not presume to know the correct spelling of the client's name; it should always be confirmed with the client to prevent subsequent confusion and the risk of errors in client or patient identity.

In addition, the receptionist may want to have a general idea of the client's schedule for the day and how they can best be reached; the use of cell phones has made quick location somewhat easier. This is particularly critical if the pet is being admitted and is undergoing surgery or a procedure that requires anesthesia. Unexpected events or findings can occur during clinical procedures, and the veterinarian may need to consult the owner immediately.

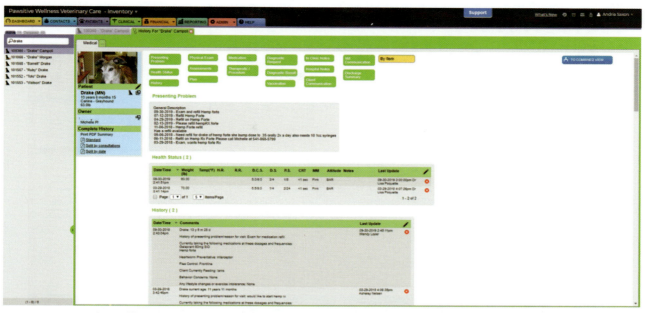

• **Fig. 3.1** The initial physical examination is an important part of a patient's database. (Courtesy ezyVet Software.)

Sometimes the owner must make important decisions over the telephone, such as the extent of treatment to be performed, while the animal is on the surgery table and/or under anesthesia. In this situation, good communication and care provided for the patient are maximized if the client can be contacted immediately. In addition to client information, the receptionist records co-owner information and the name of the referring individual.

Patient identification (ID) is also recorded at the time of admission and includes the name of the animal; any electronic ID, such as a microchip or tattoo number; species; breed; gender; reproductive status (e.g., intact, spayed, neutered, pregnant); age; color; and any distinctive markings, such as ear notches or cropping, scars, and tail docking. Collectively, this information identifies the individual patient and is known as *signalment*. Hospitals that employ computer-based patient records include this information automatically in each electronic view of the patient record. For practices that use handwritten medical records, they should employ a wide range of forms for various diagnostic tests and different departments. In these hospitals, it is important to stamp every form with the client information and the patient's signalment, including the back of the form if it is two-sided. The identity of the patient and client is automatically recorded in the EMR. Fig. 3.2A and B are examples of electronic and hard copy client-patient information forms. It should be noted that computer-based records separate data into windows that can be opened individually and edited. In the patient information window, many practice management software programs issue alerts to veterinary personnel regarding special handling of the patient, drug allergies, and other important reminders (Fig. 3.3).

Before the patient is examined, valuable information about the patient is obtained from the patient's signalment. Physiologic changes related to age, breed, and gender, for example, can influence a patient's rate of healing, its resolve when stressed, and its behavior toward other animals. In this way, signalment assists the veterinary technician to assess the patient more accurately and to anticipate potential risks during hospitalization.

History

A comprehensive history includes both previous and recent historical information. Previous historical information is typically taken during each new patient visit. Some practices have two history forms: one on which the previous history information is recorded and the other for **recent history** information.

Previous history information may include the following:
1. *Origin:* Animal's birthplace and date
2. *Preventive medicine program:* Immunizations, parasite control, dental care program, ear care program, spay/neutering, and exercise program
3. *Behavior:* Usual disposition and temperament, unusual behavioral events
4. *Environment:* Kept indoors or outdoors, presence of other pets and humans in the home, level of exposure to non–family-owned pets, travel history
5. *Nutritional history:* Current weight, daily diet, and weight changes
6. *Known allergies and reactions:* Atopy, food, contact with substances, medications, blood transfusions
7. *Reproduction:* Neutered, estrus cycles, when bred, number of litters
8. *Previous conditions:* Medical illness, trauma, or surgical operations
9. Medications, treatments, and responses
10. *Prior referral history*

Recent history information may include these items:
1. Presenting complaint and circumstances
2. Date when last normal
3. Location and character of problem, such as quality, severity, onset, duration, time of day, frequency, triggers, associated problems, and progression
4. Current medications
5. Treatment efforts (if any)
6. Comments and concerns of the owner
7. Current diet

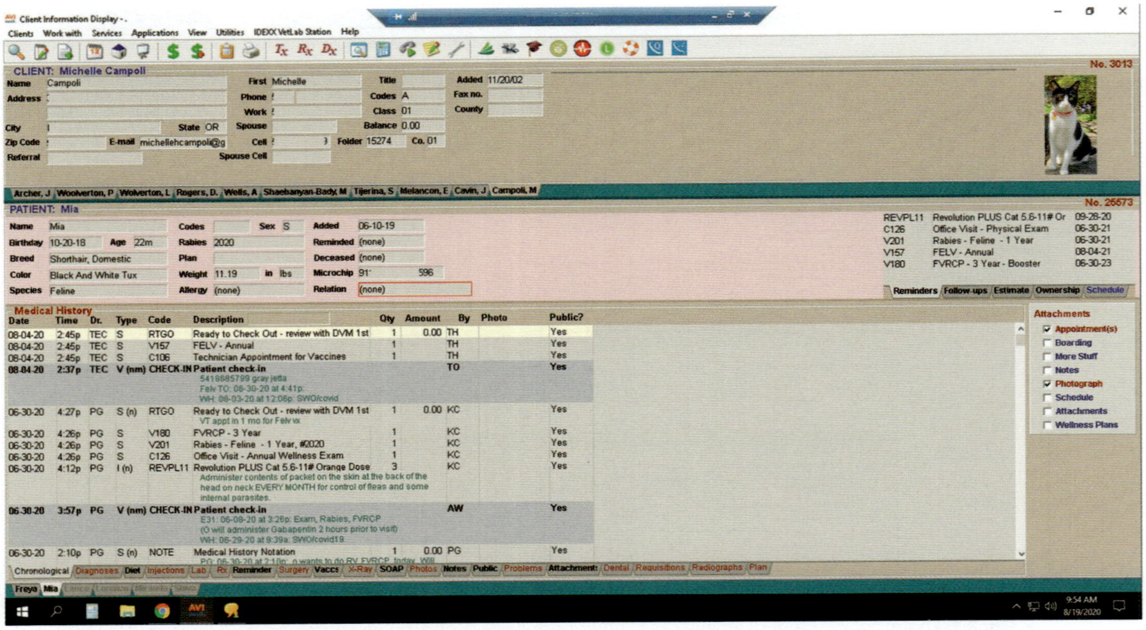

A

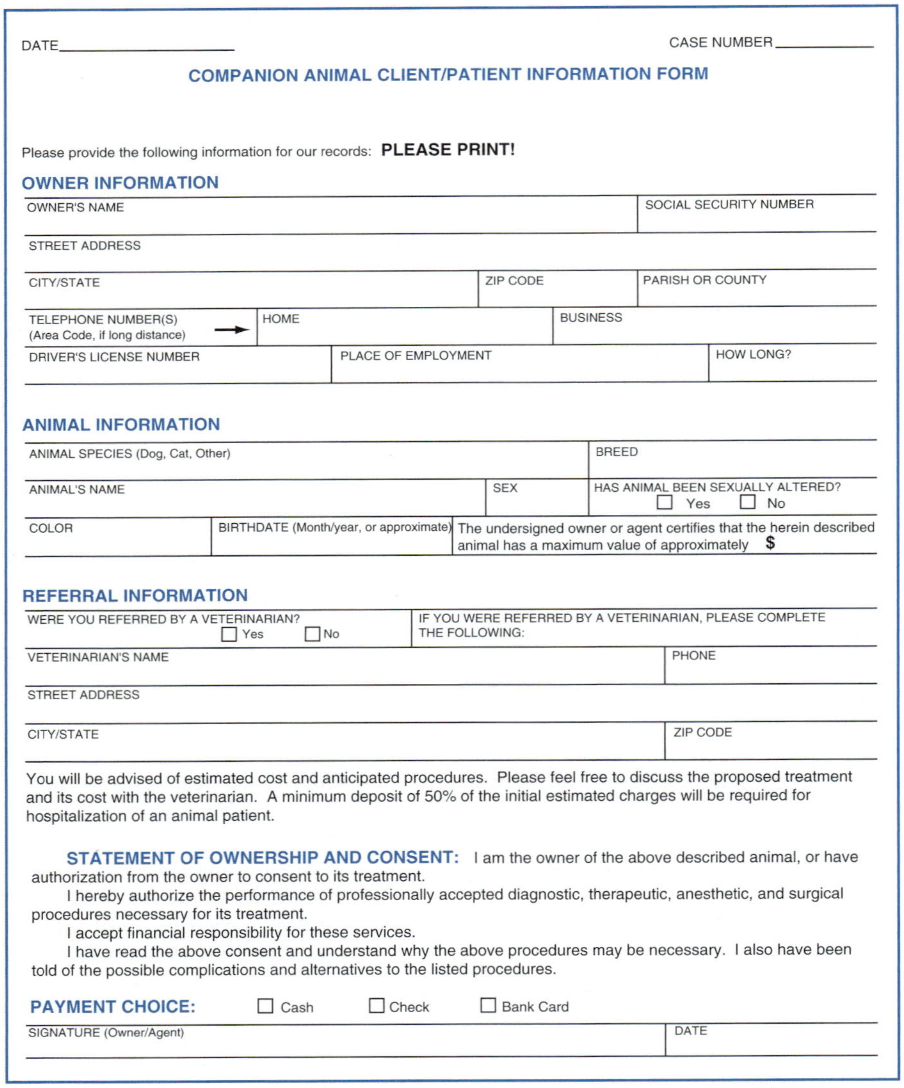

DATE__________ CASE NUMBER__________

COMPANION ANIMAL CLIENT/PATIENT INFORMATION FORM

Please provide the following information for our records: **PLEASE PRINT!**

OWNER INFORMATION

OWNER'S NAME	SOCIAL SECURITY NUMBER

STREET ADDRESS

CITY/STATE	ZIP CODE	PARISH OR COUNTY
TELEPHONE NUMBER(S) (Area Code, if long distance) →	HOME	BUSINESS
DRIVER'S LICENSE NUMBER	PLACE OF EMPLOYMENT	HOW LONG?

ANIMAL INFORMATION

ANIMAL SPECIES (Dog, Cat, Other)		BREED
ANIMAL'S NAME	SEX	HAS ANIMAL BEEN SEXUALLY ALTERED? ☐ Yes ☐ No
COLOR	BIRTHDATE (Month/year, or approximate)	The undersigned owner or agent certifies that the herein described animal has a maximum value of approximately $

REFERRAL INFORMATION

WERE YOU REFERRED BY A VETERINARIAN? ☐ Yes ☐ No	IF YOU WERE REFERRED BY A VETERINARIAN, PLEASE COMPLETE THE FOLLOWING:
VETERINARIAN'S NAME	PHONE
STREET ADDRESS	
CITY/STATE	ZIP CODE

You will be advised of estimated cost and anticipated procedures. Please feel free to discuss the proposed treatment and its cost with the veterinarian. A minimum deposit of 50% of the initial estimated charges will be required for hospitalization of an animal patient.

STATEMENT OF OWNERSHIP AND CONSENT: I am the owner of the above described animal, or have authorization from the owner to consent to its treatment.

I hereby authorize the performance of professionally accepted diagnostic, therapeutic, anesthetic, and surgical procedures necessary for its treatment.

I accept financial responsibility for these services.

I have read the above consent and understand why the above procedures may be necessary. I also have been told of the possible complications and alternatives to the listed procedures.

PAYMENT CHOICE: ☐ Cash ☐ Check ☐ Bank Card

SIGNATURE (Owner/Agent)	DATE

B

• **Fig. 3.2** (A) Within veterinary practice management software, client and patient information is stored in specified windows. AVImark software (Covetrus) combines client and patient information windows on the same screen. (B) An example of a client and patient information form for hard copy medical records.

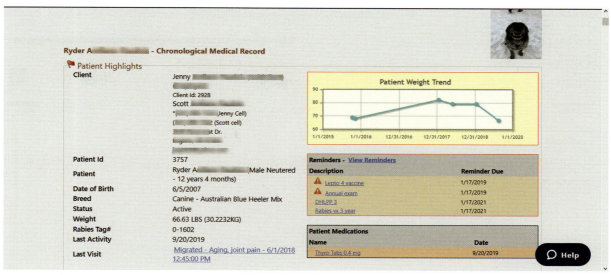

- **Fig. 3.3** Patient information window from eVet Practice (Covetrus), displaying reminders and other important patient information. (Courtesy Michelle Campoli, CVT, CVPM.)

8. Recent changes in environment, household schedule, or pets/humans in household
9. FAS (fear, aggression, stress) score (required by Fear Free–accredited practices)
10. Information from previous or referring veterinarian

Physical Examination Findings

The physical examination is one of the most important diagnostic procedures. Although the physical examination of the veterinarian and that of the veterinary technician differ regarding focus, both are important components of the patient's database. If performed carefully and systematically, the physical examination can provide veterinary technicians with valuable information to accurately assess hospitalized patients under their care. Typically, data entry is organized by anatomic system, and prompts are available to the examiner as they move through the examination. Notes are made directly on the physical examination form or are entered into the computer at the time of the examination. In some veterinary hospitals, voice recognition software allows members of the veterinary health care team to dictate findings while performing the examination. Refer to Chapter 7 for more information on physical examination forms and instructions for performing a thorough examination.

Each anatomic system is examined, and abnormalities are typically recorded in detail; normal systems are noted with the notation "WNL" (within normal limits) or as "NSF" (no significant findings). This confirms that the system was indeed examined and was found to be normal. Electronic forms can include a "shorthand" box to click if the system is WNL. Absence of WNL or NSF would imply that the system was not examined. Another common shorthand notation is "BAR" (bright, alert, and responsive). As previously stated, use of standard abbreviations supports efficient and accurate medical record keeping and creates a common language for all referring and collaborating health care providers.

Laboratory, Diagnostic Imaging, and Other Pertinent Forms

Animals may have a variety of diagnostic tests performed, such as complete blood count (CBC), chemistry profile, urine and fecal analysis, radiology, ultrasonography, electrocardiography (ECG), electroencephalography (EEG), endoscopy, scintigraphy, computed tomography (CT), and magnetic resonance imaging (MRI). This part of the database can vary, depending on the needs of the patient and the specific orders of the veterinarian. Depending on the size and caseload of the veterinary practice, separate forms or windows in the practice management software may be used for recording data from various diagnostic procedures (Fig. 3.4, A and B). Anesthesia, surgery, recovery, and pain management records may also be pertinent to a patient that has undergone a surgical procedure.

Laboratory Diagnostic Summary and Flow Sheet

The laboratory diagnostic flow sheet is a compilation of laboratory data collected for an individual animal. It can be used for outpatients or inpatients. It shows, briefly, the different laboratory values for tests that have been performed on the patient (Fig. 3.5). Specific values on different dates can be compared for blood counts, chemistry panels, blood gases, urinalyses, and coagulation rates. This sheet is of value when internal medicine cases are evaluated, such as animals with diabetes or any of the following disorders: anemia, chronic renal failure, hepatic failure, Addison disease, and Cushing disease. This information is created manually in the event of a paper chart practice or can be a function of the practice's software or by means of an integrated third-party laboratory application.

Consultants

Referral and specialty hospitals have specialty departments, such as behavior, dermatology, internal medicine, neurology, nutrition, oncology, ophthalmology, orthopedics, and surgery. As cases are worked up, specialists may be consulted to address specific problems that the patient is experiencing. A consultation form would be completed, and the consulting veterinarian's findings, diagnosis, and recommendations would be recorded. These findings, together with results of special imaging or other diagnostic tests, would be emailed to the referring practice or practitioner.

Master Problem List and Working Problem List

A defining part of the POVMR is the **master problem list** (also referred to as the *diagnosis list*). The master problem list includes

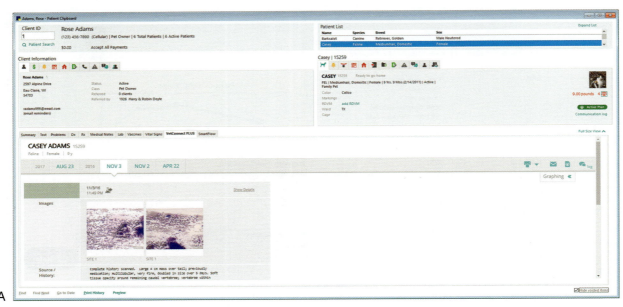

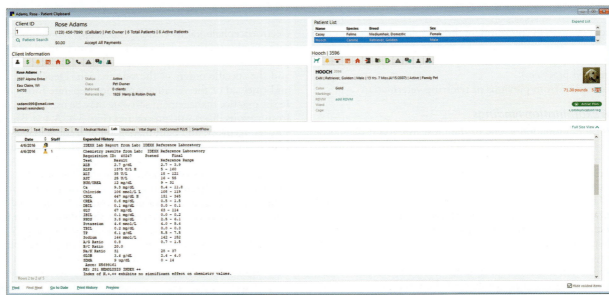

• **Fig. 3.4** (A) Histopathology report and image. (B) Clinical chemistry results. (Courtesy IDEXX Cornerstone, IDEXX Laboratories.)

the major medical disorders experienced during a patient's lifetime. Each problem represents a conclusion or a decision resulting from examination, investigation, and analysis of the database. The master problem list is typically arranged in five columns: a chronologic list of each problem, the date of onset, the action taken, the outcome or resolution, and the date of the outcome or resolution. In this way, the master problem list serves as an index to the patient's medical history. Problems may be added, and intervention or plans for intervention may be changed. Briefly, the veterinary technician can determine what happened, when it happened, and how long it lasted. A summary of the preventive medical history may accompany the master problem list, which includes the dates when immunizations were administered and the results of fecal analysis and routine screenings for heartworm and contagious viral diseases.

The **working problem list** is often used in veterinary practices to assist the veterinary health care team in working through current problems. For example, if the patient is hospitalized and is subsequently diagnosed with autoimmune hemolytic anemia, the initial working problem list may include symptomatic and reactive problems until the final diagnosis is made by the veterinarian.

The master problem list is essentially a list of final diagnoses generated by the veterinarian, whereas the working problem list is a dynamic tabulation of clinical problems and symptoms generated by the veterinary technician and the veterinarian. The veterinary technician may list exercise intolerance and the veterinarian might list nonregenerative anemia. In this way, the working problem list helps the veterinary health care team prioritize problems, think critically, and formulate interventions as problems become apparent, without offering a specific diagnosis. When a final diagnosis, for example, autoimmune hemolytic anemia, is reached by the veterinarian, it is added to the master problem list.

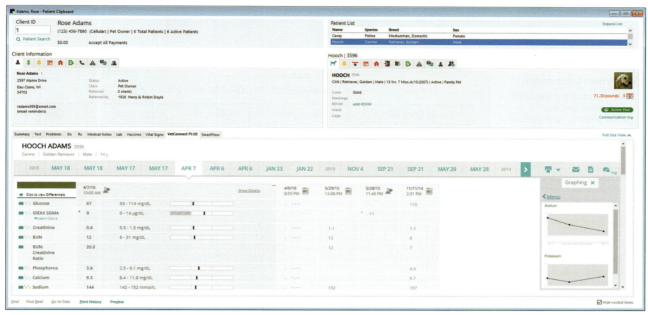

• **Fig. 3.5** Example of compiled laboratory data in an electronic record. (Courtesy IDEXX Cornerstone and VetConnect PLUS, IDEXX Laboratories.)

Hospitalized Patient Records

Overview

Each separate problem is named and described in the initial plan in progress notes by using the SOAP format (Fig. 3.6). If an animal is hospitalized, ongoing daily management of the patient is also documented as a medical record note or progress note (Fig. 3.7). Therapeutic interventions and plans are evaluated and adjusted according to the progress of the patient; evaluations are made, and the working problem list is modified as needed. If diagnostic procedures are performed, findings relevant to the current problem may be entered in the SOAP notes or added later as a notation independent of the SOAP notes. Test results, either printed on separate hardcopy forms or downloaded into the EMR, are included elsewhere in the medical record and can be referenced in the SOAP notes or medical record notes without the need to restate the results. If laboratory test results, such as the results of an in-house CBC, are printed on a small slip of paper, the slip can be taped directly to the progress sheet in a hard copy medical record, or a copy may be made, as some machine-printed results will fade over time. Placing a signature and a date across both the progress sheet and the piece of paper helps to authenticate the information. If a definitive diagnosis is made by the veterinarian, it is added to the medical record, together with the patient's prognosis and therapeutic plans. Communications with the client and any changes in therapy are also noted on the progress sheets.

When the patient is ready to be discharged, a summary is written, relating the overall assessment of the animal and its progress during treatment, with plans for follow-up or referral. The summary includes a review of all problems initially identified and encourages continuity of care for the patient at home and via subsequent follow-up visits or referral appointments. One should keep in mind that any entries made indicating future care (e.g., "Recheck in 5 days") should be documented accordingly, whether it was performed or not. If not performed and not documented, it will give the appearance of a gap in care.

Medications and take-home instructions are dispensed and reviewed with the owner. Each subsequent time a patient visits the veterinary hospital, SOAP notes and other notations are made to summarize the visit and address new problems.

Veterinary Technician SOAP Notes

Patient evaluation and assessment are documented in the progress notes by using a structured SOAP format. Although SOAP notes may be written by both veterinarians and veterinary technicians, the focus of their notes differs significantly. The veterinarian seeks to find a primary cause and a cure for illness, whereas the veterinary technician assesses the patient's physiologic and psychosocial responses to illness and strives to ameliorate those responses as a technician. In this way, the technician's evaluation of the patient is distinctly different from that of the veterinarian, much like the nurse's veterinary technician SOAP notes are decidedly different from those of the doctor in human medicine. The motivation of the veterinary technician is to put the patient's comfort first. In addition to assessing the patient, the veterinary technician anticipates future changes, complications, and sequelae to current problems. This forward thinking is noted in the SOAP notes as risks, such as "risk for infection" or "risk for transmission of infection." Because veterinary technicians may not prescribe medication, the notation "as per order" would be made in the patient's medical record to indicate the role the veterinarian plays in prescribing medical treatment. Refer to Table 1.1 in Chapter 1 for a complete listing of patient evaluations.

Anatomy of In-Patient Progress Notes

1 Patient Information

This includes the patient's signalment and the owner's name and mailing address, which together help confirm the correct identity of the patient. The signalment guides veterinary personnel towards a list of possible diagnoses relevant to the sex, age and breed of the patient.

2 Signature and Credentials Verification

Veterinary personnel complete this section to correlate staff signatures with their respective initials. The "title" column identifies the role on the veterinary health care team member as either a veterinarian or veterinary technician.

3 Date, Time, and Author of Entry

Because the medical record is a legal document, every entry must be dated and timed. In addition, the signature or initials of the author should be noted to indicate who made the entry and when.

4 Subjective Patient Information

Assessment of the patient begins from a distance before the cage or stall door is opened and may include:
a. A brief summary of presenting complaint and recent historical information from the owner.
b. Subjective observations such as the patient's posture, behavior, mentation, and the appearance and frequency of defecation, urination and vomition.
c. Observations about food and water consumption are also noted.

A physical examination of the patient follows and all relevant, non-quantifiable findings are recorded.

IN-PATIENT PROGRESS NOTES

Patient ID	Allergies	Initials	Signature	Title
"Freddy" Henderson 3/18/XX Chow Mix, FS 14 Briar Cliff Road Misty, KY 23564	Clavamox	SP	Sarah Pace	CVT
	Weight: 54 lb			

Date	Time, Signature	SO AP	Progress Notes
9/3/XX	4:45 PM Sarah Pace, CVT	S	Owner reports patient is lethargic with poor appetite and licking flanks. PE: geriatric patient, slow stiff gate, multi-focal, ulcerative skin lesions with sl. serous exudate on R and L flanks, dull brittle coat, matting in perianal region and flanks. Flea dirt evident. PE othrwise WNL
		O	T=103.5F, P=80, RR=panting, MMC=blue (chow), MMM=tacky, BCS: 2/5, CRT=2.5 sec, Skin turgor= 2 sec., PCV=49%, TP=7.9 g/dl
		A	Hypovolemia, hyperthermia, impaired tissue integrity, risk of infection, pain/pruritis, self-inflicted injury, altered appetite, underweight, self-care deficit, client knowledge deficit, decreased mobility.
		P	1. Place IV catheter and administer 0.9% NaCl IV as per order of Dr. Fox 2. Collect culture and sensitivity of affected dermal areas as per order 3. Clip and lavage affected regions, remove mats 4. Administer trimethoprim sulfa, Rymadil, Frontline as per order 5. Install cage mat and soft bedding in cage 6. Apply E-collar 7. Client education re: flea control, import. of regular grooming and mod. exercise in geriatric animals. 8. Dispense prescription diet as per order

5 Objective Patient Information

All quantifiable information such as vital signs, test results, capillary refill time, and dehydration indicators are recorded.

6 Assessment

The veterinary technician identifies pertinent patient evaluations and prioritizes them in order of importance according to the physical and psychological needs of the patient. Risks for complications and client knowledge deficits are also noted and prioritized.

7 Plan

Using logic and independent critical thinking, a technician intervention is formulated to address each of the technician evaluations listed in the Assessment section. In this way, a nursing care plan is formulated. The interventions are carried out in order of importance.

• **Fig. 3.6** Anatomy of the veterinary technician's SOAP (subjective, objective, assessment, and plan) notes.

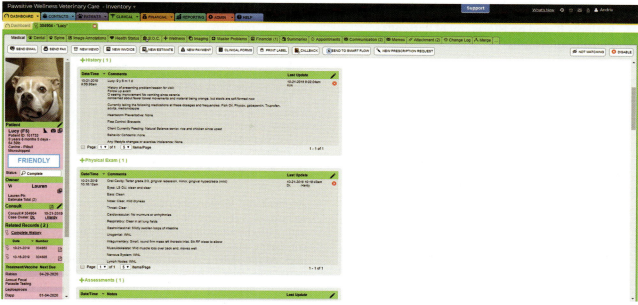

• **Fig. 3.7** An example of a progress note medical record. (Courtesy eZyVet Software.)

Subjective/Objective

Although it is widely agreed that information from the database constitutes the "S" and "O" portions of the SOAP notes, there are differences of opinion regarding what constitutes subjective or objective information. Different schools teach different approaches. In this chapter, all *nonmeasurable* information will be categorized as "subjective" and all *measurable* information as "objective." Relevant historical information, such as the presenting complaint, and most of the physical examination findings would therefore be entered in the subjective section. This can also include the FAS level (fear, anxiety, stress spectrum, an assessment used by Fear Free–certified practices). Observations of the patient's posture, attitude, and appetite may also be included, such as "standing, panting, and wagging tail," or "awake, in left lateral recumbency." Pain level scoring can also be considered objective if the pain scoring system is uniformly employed within the veterinary practice. Other measurable data, such as laboratory results, temperature, heart and respiratory rates, weight, skin retraction time, capillary refill time, numbers of bowel movements, and measured urine output, would also be noted in the objective information section.

Assessment

Completion of the *assessment* portion of the SOAP notes requires analysis of all subjective and objective data that have been gathered by the veterinary technician thus far. Based on this data, the veterinary technician uses critical thinking to generate a list of technician evaluations of the patient that reflect the patient's physical, psychological, social, and environmental conditions. In this way, the veterinary technician assessment of the patient is holistic, considering all aspects of the individual's experience and generating a custom-tailored nursing care plan to address each of the patient's needs. One should keep in mind that in a true veterinary technician's SOAP, the assessment portion includes veterinary technician evaluations and is *not* delegated to the veterinarian to fill in a list of medical or surgical differential diagnoses. (Refer to Table 1.1 in Chapter 1 for a list of veterinary technician evaluations.)

In 1943, the famous psychiatrist Abraham Maslow developed a hierarchal pyramid of needs to account for motivating forces observed in the human psyche. This concept was later applied to the nursing profession to help guide prioritization of clinical problems and to improve understanding in addressing the needs of patients. Veterinary technicians similarly can make use of Maslow's concept by prioritizing patient evaluations to generate an effective nursing care plan that addresses the most important issues first. Table 3.2 illustrates a hierarchy of animal health needs and offers examples of corresponding **veterinary technician evaluations**. Note that the most important needs of the patient are listed first and that the less critical ones are listed next, in decreasing order of importance. In the SOAP notes, each patient evaluation is assigned a number such that the most important evaluation in the hierarchy of physiologic needs is in the number one position. This organization supports the veterinary technician's practice model of addressing the most important health problems first. Refer to Chapter 1 for a discussion of the veterinary technician practice model. Examples of veterinary technician evaluations include hypothermia, altered mentation, inappropriate elimination, and risk of infection. Evaluations that require urgent attention, such as those related to inappropriate oxygenation, are first in the hierarchy of patient needs. As part of the veterinary technician practice model, veterinary technicians re-evaluate their patients and reassess and adjust the plan. Patient progress and adjustments to the list of evaluations are noted in the assessment portion of the veterinary technician SOAP notes.

Plan

In the last portion of the SOAP notes, the veterinary technician methodically develops an intervention for each of the evaluations listed in the assessment portion. The compilation of these interventions constitutes the technician *care plan* for patient care, and it is hoped that carrying out the plan will restore patient comfort and well-being. Plans may include, for example, client education, administration of medications as ordered by the attending veterinarian, moderate daily exercise, daily cold compresses, and follow-up appointments. Perhaps the patient will be discharged from the veterinary hospital, or perhaps the patient will require additional diagnostic testing and evaluation. The nursing care plan should

TABLE 3.2	Prioritization of Technician Evaluations of Patients Based on Hierarchy of Patient's Physiologic Needs	
Priority	**Physiologic Need**	**Technician Evaluation of Patient**
1	Oxygenation	Altered gas diffusion Altered ventilation Cardiac insufficiency Decreased perfusion Obstructed airway Risk of aspiration
2	Critical safety and/or severe pain	Acute pain Electrolyte imbalance Hyperthermia (severe) Hypothermia (severe) Postoperative compliance Preoperative compliance
3	Hydration	Hypervolemia Hypovolemia
4	Elimination	Altered urinary production Bowel incontinence Constipation Diarrhea Inappropriate elimination Self-care deficit Urinary incontinence
5	Nutrition	Altered oral health Abnormal eating behavior Ineffective nursing Overweight Self-care deficit Underweight Vomiting and/or diarrhea
6	Noncritical safety	Altered mentation Altered sensory perception Noncompliant owner Hyperthermia Hypothermia Impaired tissue integrity Owner knowledge deficit Risk of infection Risk of infection transmission Self-inflicted injury Status within appropriate limits
7	Chronic pain or mild-to-moderate acute pain	Acute pain Chronic pain
8	Activity	Exercise intolerance Reduced mobility Sleep disturbance
9	Utility	Aggression Anxiety Client coping deficit Client knowledge deficit Fear Inappropriate elimination Reproductive dysfunction

Modified from Rockett J, Lattanzio C, Anderson K. *Patient Assessment and Interventions and Documentation for the Veterinary Technician.* Clifton Park, NY: Delmar Cengage Learning; 2009.

• BOX 3.5　Clinical Application 2

Discuss which of the following client communications should be included in a patient medical record:

A client's email to the practice's general inbox providing a rave review of a boarding kennel the practice recommended

A phone call from the owners with a status update regarding their hospitalized pet

A text message from the clients requesting a refill of their pet's prescription diet

A chance encounter at a restaurant in which the clients mention that they are not giving the prescribed medication to their chronically ill dog as instructed

---

augment and support the medical treatment plan. The veterinary technician is responsible for discussing the suggested nursing care plan with the attending veterinarian in advance to ensure that it is consistent with and supportive of the medical/surgical treatment plan. As the patient is evaluated and re-evaluated by the veterinary technician, their plan of care is adjusted to address any new developments and changes in the status of the patient. It is important that the veterinary technician keeps the attending veterinarian abreast of any changes in patient status.

Notations

Any incoming information that is entered in the progress notes but is independent of the SOAP notes is entered as a *notation*. Additional information from a referring veterinarian, for example, or any relevant communication with an animal's owner in person, or by telephone, text, or email, may be recorded in the progress notes as a notation. Refer to Box 3.5.

If additional results are not downloaded into the electronic record, small sheets of paper with laboratory results or physiologic test results may be taped directly onto the progress sheet near to the notation that references the test result in hard copy medical records. To further verify the authenticity of the addition, the veterinary technician should sign across the junction of the progress sheet and attached piece of paper. The entry should be dated and timed, and the date on the laboratory paper should be circled or underlined.

Medication Administration/Order Record

The **medication administration/order record (MAOR)**, also known as a *ward treatment sheet*, is used to ensure that hospitalized patients are given treatments, diagnostic tests, and diet as requested by the attending veterinarian. Management of hospitalized patients can be complex, particularly in busy practices with heavy caseloads and in those that treat emergency and critical care patients. To assist the veterinary health care team in carrying out treatment orders efficiently, grids are used to record which treatments were delivered, when, and by whom (Fig. 3.8, A and B). Although MAORs are often used in hard copy, they can be generated and used electronically as well by means of a practice management software "electronic whiteboard" or as an integrated third-party program, such as SmartFlow or Instinct. The advantages to an electronic MAOR include legibility, retrievability from any computer, visibility to multiple patients simultaneously, and, in some platforms, dual functionality by not only indicating a treatment is completed as a date- and time-stamped patient record entry but also capturing the billing information (Fig. 3.9, A and B).

In addition, the MAOR offers an at-a-glance summary of the patient's management during hospitalization. Treatments to be given and the dates and specific times throughout the day when

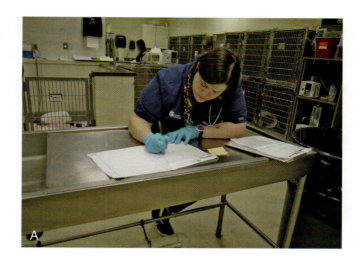

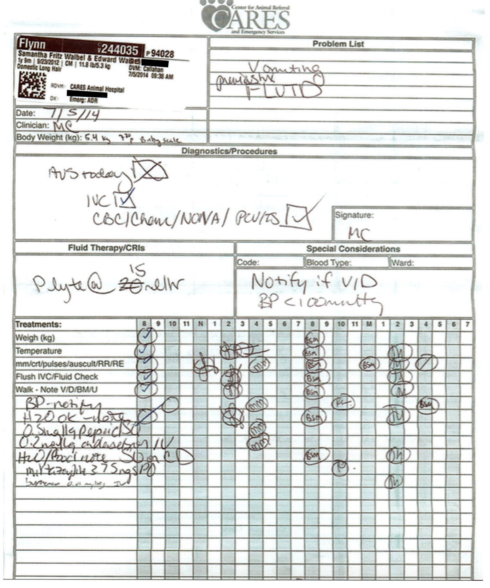

• **Fig. 3.8** (A) A veterinary technician enters notations in a patient's medical record regarding patient assessment findings and treatments that were completed. (B) An example of a completed ward treatment sheet. Hard copies are later scanned and added to the patient's electronic medical record.

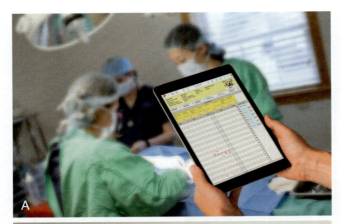

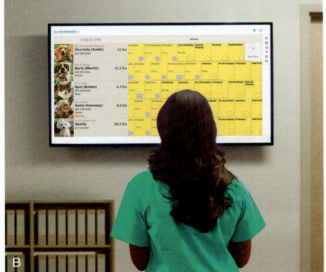

• **Fig. 3.9** (A) SmartFlow System. (B) Example of an electronic whiteboard. (Courtesy SmartFlow, IDEXX Laboratories.)

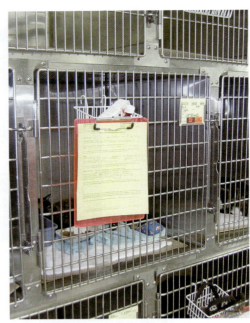

• **Fig. 3.10** Some practices store patient medications in wire baskets that can be attached directly to the door of the patient's cage. Medical records can also be attached to the cage. Both the record and the medications must be labeled clearly.

each of the treatments should be completed are listed. Doses, methods of administration, and cautionary notes should be written for each medication. In addition, MAORs should always include the patient's full name, patient ID number, and/or signalment, and any known allergies that the patient may have. For hard copy sheets, if a signature logbook is not kept in the wards, MAORs should also include a signature chart that lists the full name of each member of the health care team with corresponding initials. This allows team members to use the shorthand approach of initialing boxes in the chart without having to sign their full names.

When paper MAORs are completed, the following guidelines apply:

1. Each order entered in the MAOR should be written exactly as the veterinarian wrote it. The full name of the medication and its dose and route of administration should be listed. It is important for the veterinary technician to ask for clarification if instructions are not clear. Medications given during surgery or anesthesia are entered on surgical or anesthesia forms and are *not* entered on the MAOR.

2. When a treatment is given, the person giving the treatment writes their initials in the column that indicates the time of administration. A treatment that is given one hour before or after the ordered time is typically considered "on time." However, when the time of administration is significantly different from the requested time, the veterinary technician enters the actual time that the treatment was administered.

3. When a treatment is not given, this should be clearly noted in the patient's medical record. In addition, the veterinary technician must notify the attending veterinarian if a treatment was not administered and notate this also.

4. When a dose is ordered for a specific period, an "X" should be placed in the boxes representing the dates when the medication is *not* to be given.

5. When a medication is discontinued, the veterinary technician should make an entry in the medical record that the medication was discontinued. Erasing, crossing out, or blotting out the record of a discontinued medication should never be done.

6. If the patient was discharged and the full recommended duration of medication was not given by hospital personnel, the remaining boxes of dates and times should be left blank.

In most practices, medications and supplies needed to complete treatments are kept near the patient for convenience. Some practices store a patient's medications and treatment supplies in bins on a table or shelf, along with the patient's medical record. Other practices prefer to use baskets that can be suspended from the patient's cage, together with the MAOR, (Fig. 3.10). Hospitals for equine and food-animal patients often maintain medications and supplies in treatment carts that can be wheeled easily in barn aisles from stall to stall. Regardless of the approach used, it is important to clearly label medications and supplies with the patient's name, signalment, and owner information.

Cage Cards and Patient Identification

Cage and stall cards are used to identify the patient and the reason for the hospitalization. Cards are either produced manually or through the practice management system. The owner and patient information are entered or printed on the card. Many practices apply identifying collars to each patient so the cage card can be matched to the identification on the patient. In equine practices, the identification strip is applied to the horse's halter. In some practices that do not use separate ward treatment sheets or MAORs, the treatment grid is also stamped on the cage and the stall card and lists the procedures to be performed. In some specialty and referral practices, the color of the cage card may be used to indicate the hospital division that is treating the patient. A red card, for example, might indicate surgery, whereas a blue card might indicate internal medicine or cardiology.

> **TECHNICIAN NOTE**
>
> Veterinary technicians need to be sure that owners have the necessary information and resources to continue any prescribed home care and home monitoring of their pets.

Discharge and Summary Forms

It is important to discharge patients in a fashion that ensures a desirable outcome for the patient and the owner. To this end, veterinary technicians need to ensure that owners have the necessary information and resources to continue any prescribed home care and home monitoring of their pet. A clear, concise summary of the pet's illness, prognosis, and treatment during hospitalization and specific discharge instructions are written in simple language that the client can understand. Either a printed copy of the form is given to the owner, or it is brought up on the computer and the veterinary technician reviews it with the owner before the animal leaves the hospital. It is advisable to have the client sign the form to acknowledge the information and for a copy of the signed form remain in either the hard copy or the EMR. In this way, the veterinary technician directly educates the pet owner about the pet's disease process and the clinical signs and symptoms of potential complications. Take-home instructions regarding administration of medications or special diet or feeding instructions, use of Elizabethan collars, and recommended follow-up examinations or tests, for example, are also discussed directly with the client. Pre-printed instructional brochures or handouts may be attached to the instructions or all forms and informational content emailed for further edification of the client. This one-on-one communication offers an opportunity for the pet owner to ask questions and allows the veterinary technician to ensure that appropriate care of the pet will be continued at home. The veterinary technician's name and the clinic's contact information are often included on the form so that the owner can call if questions or problems arise.

Management of Electronic Medical Records

Overview

With the rapidly changing rate of technology, growing, cloud-based platforms, information applications, operating systems, etc., the daily use and maintenance of medical records is a constantly evolving landscape. Although a background in Information Technology (IT) is not required, general comfort with technology, including various applications and software, and with hardware, such as laptops, tablets, and smartphones, is an essential skill in today's practice.

Advantages of Electronic Medical Records

There is no shortage of currently available veterinary practice management software products. Each program uses its own approach to management and organization of patient medical records. However, most, if not all, offer improved legibility, increased speed of access to data, and ease of use by multiple users at the same time. Consistency and complete records are achieved when using standardized examination notes, promoting consistent capture of history, presenting problems, SOAP notes, and diagnosis. Integration with diagnostics and monitors also simplify record keeping and having all patient information in a single information source, and this can also include trending of vitals and laboratory results to further assist the team in making medical decisions for the patient.

In addition, if appropriate precautions are employed, digital medical record keeping decreases the risk of loss. Finally, EMRs can include all patient information, including digital radiographs, laboratory results, endoscopic examination findings, surgical images, and ECG tracings. Even the frequency of pharmaceutical use, the storage of controlled substances, and the restriction of access to certain drugs by certain personnel can all be managed and recorded electronically (Fig. 3.11, A and B). In these ways, the EMR offers numerous advantages over paper-based records.

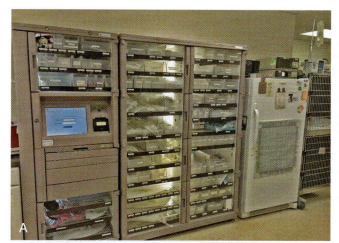

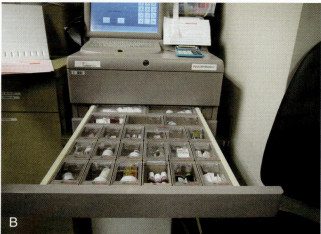

• **Fig. 3.11** (A) Storage and restricted access to medical supplies can be managed electronically. (B) Inventory management systems such as Cubex record activity and track inventory with detailed records, and communicates with a hospital's Practice Information Management System (PIMS).

EMRs are easily retrievable and can be viewed by multiple people at the same time from different workstations. This level of accessibility allows practices to run more efficiently and faster, and with fewer errors compared with the traditional system using hard copy medical records.

Computerization has also improved the quality and completeness of patient information; this is especially evident in multiple doctor practices where medical record entries are consistent across providers. Entries into EMRs are consistently legible and organized. When notable findings are made, veterinary personnel can type or dictate information directly into the medical record, use macros, or choose from a drop-down menu of common findings (Fig. 3.12, A and B).

Templates for physical examinations list all anatomic systems, and thus the veterinarian and the veterinary technician are prompted to assess each aspect of the patient. Some software systems allow the examiner to click on "WNL" or "normal" to verify that a system was examined (Fig. 3.13).

To speed up data entry or for those who do not type well, voice recognition software can be employed in the examination room, doctor's office, or operating room with use of a connected headset or computer microphone. With this setup, using either a specific dictation software, such as Dragon, or integrated operating system (OS) speech-to-text applications, such as Windows speech recognition, veterinary personnel can dictate physical examination findings or can describe the appearance of organs during an exploratory laparotomy, for example. Voice recognition software transcribes the spoken word into text, which is either directly entered or cut and pasted into the patient's medical record, according to the practice management system's ability to interface with speech to text.

Veterinary practice management software permits direct entry of digital radiographs, laboratory results, intraoperative photographs, ECG tracings, microscopic images, and referral reports, just to name a few, into the patient's medical record (Fig. 3.14, A and B). This reduces staff time spent searching for reports (e.g., "pulling radiographs") and enables images and other findings to be conveniently emailed to referral specialists for further evaluation.

Validating the Electronic Record

As with all veterinary hospitals, it is important for paperless practices (e.g., EMR) to be able to show an accurate, neat, and complete medical record. The practice must also be able to demonstrate that the record is void of tampering and that it gives an accurate representation of patient care. Because digital records are easy to change, it is important that a historical account of the EMR be automatically collected and stored in the data management system. For example, some practice management software programs allow the veterinary health care team to make entries and changes to entries in a patient record within the first 24 to 48 hours of patient care. Entries made within this time frame are regarded as the primary document. After this period, however, either the record is locked or finalized with no further changes allowed other than a date/time-stamped addendum, or the system records the date and time of all subsequent changes in the form of an audit trail and/or maintains a copy of the primary document. For this reason, it is best for veterinarians and veterinary technicians to make prompt, accurate entries. To ensure confidentiality and integrity, AAHA standards include the EMR system automatically closing record notations after a user-specified period (maximum of 24 hours). Amendments/addenda are clearly recorded in an audit trail. During a hearing in a court of law, it can be argued that information entered after the fact is more prone to inaccuracy owing to lapses in memory of the veterinary professional. Some practices make use of off-site services that store their electronic information in heavily secured servers. Companies that specialize in housing medical databases can also act as third-party agents to verify the originality of the records and the absence of tampering. Many of the current software systems make use of cloud storage.

Risk of Loss

The risk of loss of digital information is a concern during lightning storms and unexpected power surges that can destroy hard drives in servers and take out printers, monitors, televisions, and most electrical instrumentation and monitoring devices. Using surge suppressors and unplugging computers during storms is important and can save practices from unnecessary loss of equipment and valuable patient information. In addition, practices can guard against data loss by incorporating backup servers into their practice network and by using backup generators or battery power in the event of a regional brownout or blackout (Fig. 3.15).

Logs

Historically, logbooks have been kept as hard copy documents, but increasingly, electronic logs are becoming the norm. The information in logs may include specific data for a particular hospital department, piece of equipment, or procedure. Many practices have logs for radiology and special imaging, surgery, anesthesia, controlled substances, ultrasonography, clinical laboratory, and euthanasia. In addition, some practices have unexpected death, drug reaction, and medical waste logs. Any division of the veterinary hospital or any specific activity could conceivably have a log that records daily activity in that aspect of the hospital. Some large practices may have 8 to 12 different types of logs, whereas smaller practices may have two to four logs. Take note that a particular state may require specific details for logs, and accrediting bodies, such as AAHA, Fear Free, specialty boards, and others may have other log standards to maintain.

Logs serve two purposes:
1. They provide additional documentation for legal support.
2. They provide data for quick analysis and retrospective studies.

A practice that is interested in examining the average length of surgery, for example, can quickly calculate that figure based on data in the surgery log. In radiology, techniques could be evaluated by examining the recorded settings in the radiography log.

Management of Paper Medical Records

In contrast to electronic records, handwritten medical records represent the original record-keeping method before computers were readily available and are still found in some practices today. The advantages of one are often the disadvantages of the other and vice versa. Paper charts do not require a power source, are not subject to OS updates, and will not break if dropped, but they can be readily misplaced, can only be accessed by one person at a time, and may contain inconsistently formatted or illegible entries.

Consistency with paper records can be improved with the use of examination forms, labels, or stamps. Legibility is paramount, because illegible writing can impede patient care and can lead to errors in both health care delivery and client communications.

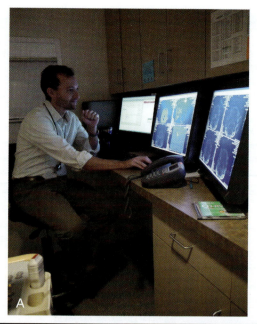

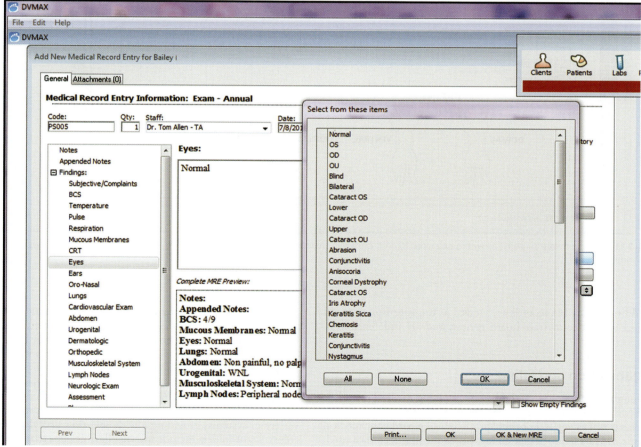

• **Fig. 3.12** Veterinary personnel can type or dictate patient information directly into the medical record. (A) Electronic medical records are easily retrievable and can be viewed by multiple people at the same time from different workstations throughout the veterinary hospital. Veterinarians can dictate or type findings into the patient's medical record as they are discovered. This creates greater efficiency and improved organization and communication, which can lead to improved patient care. (B) An electronic record example using macros to insert common findings into the patient's exam note. (A, Courtesy Dr. Joanna Bassert. B, Courtesy IDEXX DVMax, IDEXX Laboratories.)

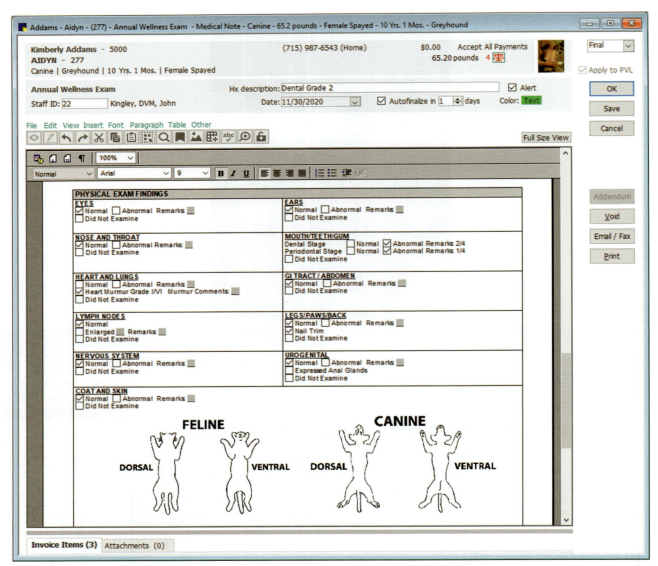

• **Fig. 3.13** Some software systems allow the examiner to click on "WNL" (within normal limits) or "normal" to confirm that a physiologic system has been examined.

In addition, illegible records are viewed as unprofessional, could subject a practice to state board review, and are indefensible in court.

Organization and Filing

Although the dominant method of maintaining medical records is via EMR systems, familiarity with paper medical records and filing systems is still essential. For those practices using hard copy medical records, AAHA requires that an individual medical record, if used, be maintained for each patient and that hard copy records be stored in standard letter-sized folders (Fig. 3.16). Tabs are located at the edge of one end of the folder to facilitate the placement of color-coded decals. Some folders have grids printed on the outside of the cover on which critical information, such as the animal's immunization history, can be written. In this way, the staff can quickly locate key pieces of information. More commonly, however, veterinary practices use folders with a plain manila cover.

The folders are stored vertically on shelves, which are kept behind or near the receptionist's desk for easy retrieval. Some practices may have record rooms, where a mobile shelving system may be employed. These systems have large shelves mounted on tracks which can be moved easily from one location to another and may be positioned up against one another when access to the records is not needed.

Many veterinary hospitals use a folder system that is developed specifically for veterinary medicine. Several companies make a variety of systems, providing a wide selection of styles, sizes, and colors. Most folders include internal flexible clips that hold forms, printed diagnostic results and reports, and medical notes in the correct order (Fig. 3.17). Medical note pages can also be color coded (pink and blue) to quickly identify the patient's gender to avoid use of the wrong pronoun when talking with the client. In addition, the folders are designed to accommodate color-coded tabs or stickers (known as *signaling devices*) that are applied to the outer edge of the folder, making filing more efficient and filing errors easier to identify.

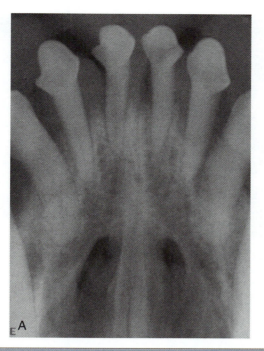

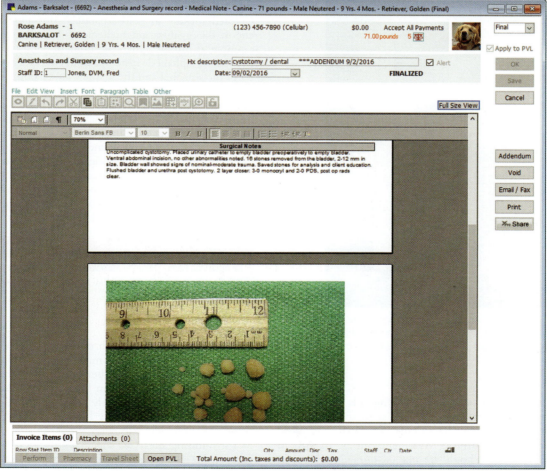

• **Fig. 3.14** (A) An example of a digital dental radiograph from a dog. The photo is stored as a permanent part of the patient's electronic medical record. (B) A postcystotomy image entered as part of the surgical record. (A, Courtesy Dr. Joanna Bassert, IDEXX Laboratories. B, Courtesy IDEXX Cornerstone, IDEXX Laboratories.)

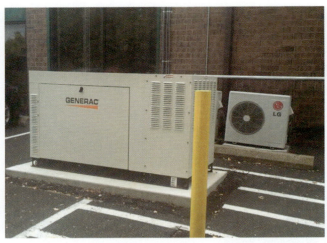

• **Fig. 3.15** A natural gas–powered electric generator that automatically turns on during power outages. This ensures the continuation of patient care and is particularly vital for the most vulnerable patients, such as intra-operative patients and those on ventilators and constant rate infusions in critical care wards. (Courtesy Dr. Joanna Bassert.)

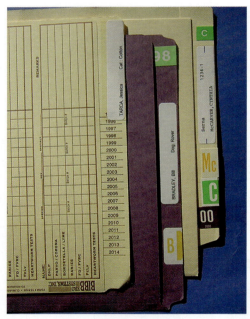

• **Fig. 3.16** Shown are a variety of letter-size folders. The color and the style of the folders can vary, as can use of stamping charting notes on the cover. Color-coded decals are placed on the edges of the folders to facilitate filing.

Colored tabs can not only serve as filing aids but can also be applied to files to alert the receptionist to specific client-patient issues. For example, the records of animals that need immunizations and deworming treatment can be flagged to indicate that reminders should be mailed out. Colored flags may indicate those clients that have an outstanding bill or that have not returned to the practice in a long time by means of year tab from date of last visit. In this way, colored signaling devices can be added to identify groups of files that need attention.

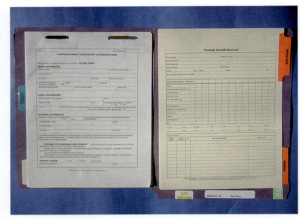

• **Fig. 3.17** Letter-size folders contain flexible metal clips that hold forms in their correct order. Dividers allow for rapid retrieval of laboratory reports, operative notes, and progress notes.

Use of "file out" place holders are also used to indicate a record folder is in use, and the place holder itself may be color coded or labeled to indicate the chart's location, such as pending laboratory results, prescription request, or in-progress appointment.

Alphabetic Filing

Colored stickers are sold separately; this allows the practice to choose the organizational scheme of the color-coding system. For example, it can be alphabetic, numeric, or a combination of the two. In the alphabetic system, a different color is given to each letter of the alphabet and the first few letters of the client's last name are used to label the patient's chart. The system is easy to learn and does not require cross referencing with a master list of clients. The primary challenge in using the alphabetic system, however, is that the employee doing the filing must be careful to correctly apply the alphabetic order and spell clients' names correctly in all instances. Unfortunately, errors in spelling and filing do occur from time to time, so misfiled records tend to be more common with the alphabetic system than with the numeric system, although misfiles can be visualized to a degree if the color coding of nearby files does not correspond to the incorrectly placed file.

> **TECHNICIAN NOTE**
>
> The American Animal Hospital Association (AAHA) requires that each patient have its own medical record and that paper records, if used, be stored in standard letter-sized folders.

Numeric Filing

In the numeric system, each client is assigned a number. The number assigned to the file may be a hospital-generated number. Each digit in the number has a different color, and files are shelved numerically from lowest to highest (Fig. 3.18). In this way, it is easy to correctly sequence the files, and any misfiled records are more easily identified than in an alphabetic system, because the file color sequence does not match that of surrounding files (see Fig. 3.19 for example of a misfiled record). To retrieve a particular file, the receptionist first must check a cross reference that lists the client's name and the corresponding file number. The list is commonly computerized, allowing for a search by client or patient name, phone number, and other parameters, although paper-based systems, such as a Rolodex, can still be employed.

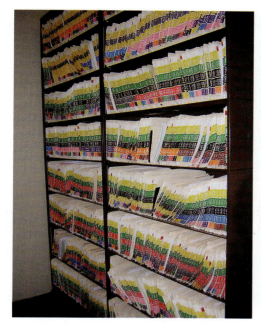

• **Fig. 3.18** Numeric color-coding systems allow for rapid retrieval and filing.

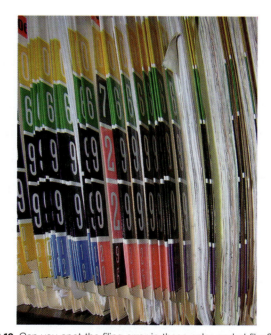

• **Fig. 3.19** Can you spot the filing error in these color-coded files? (Courtesy Dr. Joanna Bassert.)

One of the advantages of the numeric filing system is that fewer filing errors occur, because numbers are easier to read and interpret compared with letters, and spelling is not a factor. In addition, numeric filing systems are practical for large-volume practices, because no file duplication occurs, whereas in the alphabetic system, many clients may have the same surname. An added benefit is also the protection of client identification not being readily visible from the external record folder. The disadvantage of the numeric system, however, is that a cross-reference list must be generated and maintained.

File Purging

Periodically, the collection of hard copy medical records should be reviewed and purged of files that are not in current use. Each veterinary hospital has its own review and purging schedule. The following guidelines and suggested timeframes can serve as a helpful starting point, but the practice should follow the state's file retention requirements.

1. The collection of medical records is reviewed at least once per year. (If using hard copy charts, use the previous year's label on the record.)
2. Active records (those with a visit/transaction) covering a 3-year period (or other period established by your practice) are maintained in the primary medical records collection. This may be further restricted because of space limitations, and immediate active records may need to be kept in the primary area for 1 to 2 years, based on the hospital's policy and determining factor as immediate active (visit/transaction in last XX months) and the remaining "recent active" (visit/transaction in prior XX months after immediate actives) files are moved to a readily accessible secondary area.
3. Records that have been inactive for 4 years or longer (or other period established by your practice and/or state requirement) are moved to a storage location, which should be easily accessible.
4. Inactive records 8 years old or older may be removed from storage and shredded. (Refer to your state's requirements.)

Use of color-coded tabs with the year can be of value when the annual review of medical records is completed. They enable the receptionist to quickly identify older records by their specific colors.

Lost Records

Loss of records is problematic, and records may be lost through misfiling, incorrect spelling of names, or misplacement. At times, even after an exhaustive search, the record remains untraceable, and the loss may not be discovered until the animal comes to the practice for a return visit.

In this case, it is best to explain to the client that the record has been misplaced. A new record should be started, and information requested from the client and the veterinarian. In addition, copies of laboratory data, pathology reports, and radiologic information, any computer records from billing to establish examination and other service dates, prescription history, or reminders should be obtained to re-establish the file.

Although the problem of lost records is embarrassing for the practice and inconvenient for the client, it could happen even with the most elaborate record keeping system; however, every effort should be made to file each record quickly and accurately after each visit. Clients feel more at ease and reassured if the record is complete and is easily accessible.

Management of Ambulatory Practice Records

Ambulatory food-animal and equine practitioners work long hours and put many miles on their trucks as they travel from farm to farm (Fig. 3.20A), although small-animal mobile practices in urban areas are also a reality. Transporting lengthy medical record files is impractical in a situation where there is limited storage space (in the vehicle) and risk of physical record loss or damage. Although some ambulatory practitioners may continue

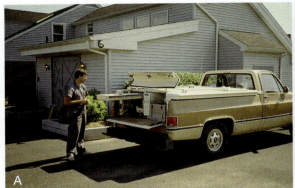
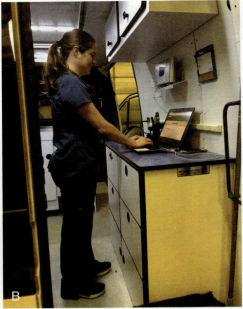

• **Fig. 3.20** (A) An ambulatory large-animal veterinarian has little room in his truck for large, cumbersome medical records. (B) Many practitioners now travel with laptop computers or tablets. Digital entries are subsequently transferred to the practice's main server if not connected to the practice's Practice Information Management System (PIMS) via Wi-Fi.

to make handwritten notes or use other methodology to be transcribed into the actual record upon return to the office, many carry a mobile device, such as a laptop or tablet, in their vehicles to assist with record keeping. The practitioner enters information about diagnosis, treatment, and billing with the mobile device (Fig. 3.20B). Depending on the practitioner's practice management system, access may be in real time through a wireless Internet connection or mobile hotspot using either a mobile phone or the vehicle's system. Alternatively and in the absence of Internet connection, a "checked out" copy of the practice database is used and is later synchronized back into the main database upon return to the office. Some ambulatory practitioners use an index of bar codes (similar to retail outlets), each one representing a different diagnosis, procedure, or medication. The veterinarian scans the appropriate bar codes to create an invoice and to document the diagnosis and treatments rendered. Instructions to the owner might also be generated. This information can be either emailed while on site or upon return to the office, or it can be printed out and given to the owner on site via a small portable printer carried in the vehicle.

It is impractical for food-animal veterinarians who are responsible for the health of entire herds of livestock to maintain an individual record for every animal treated. In this situation, the veterinarians keep records for the herd. Immunizations and reproductive histories are maintained for the group, although individual records may be generated for animals that have undergone special surgical or treatment procedures.

Large-animal teaching hospitals and full-service large-animal private practices commonly have hospitalized surgical, medical, and neonatal patients. In this context, each large-animal patient has its own medical record. In-house treatments and procedures are recorded in the medical record by hospital staff members on hard copy or electronically. Computer terminals and keyboards are prone to be affected by the dust commonly found in barns, but they work well in enclosed technicians' stations or treatment

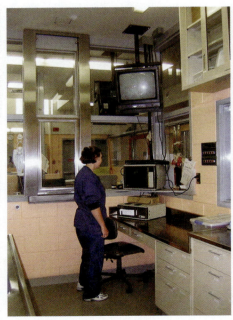

• **Fig. 3.21** Computers and telemetry monitoring equipment can be housed in glass-enclosed nursing stations, such as the one shown, to protect the delicate circuitry from exposure to dust and water. (Courtesy Dr. Joanna Bassert.)

closets, which are commonly constructed in a central area of the wards (Fig. 3.21). In particularly dusty areas, patient-side medical record keeping can be accomplished by using tablets that are enclosed in protective cases (Fig 3.22). Dust covers can also help protect computer hardware when not in use. Computer terminals are also found in the treatment, radiology, and surgical facilities in large-animal practices for easy entry and retrieval of veterinary medical information.

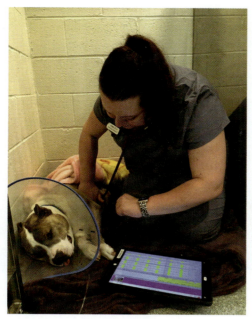

• **Fig. 3.22** The use of tablet computers in patient wards is a common practice in veterinary hospitals today. (Courtesy Dr. Joanna Bassert.)

Conclusion

The organization, components, and functions of the veterinary patient medical record are important for the entire team to understand and utilize properly. There are many parts to the record, including the **SOAP** notes and the technician's care plan, diagnostic test results, hospitalization information, diagnosis and treatment plans, and important client information. The most important aspect to remember is that the medical record serves as a legal record of the specific veterinary care provided to every patient. While taking care of the patient is an important aspect of the veterinary technician, it is also important to keep accurate medical records.

Recommended Readings and Resources

AAHA Resources

AAHA. *Standard Abbreviations for Veterinary Medical Records*. 3rd ed. Lakewood, CO: American Animal Hospital Association; 2010.

AVMA Resources

AVMA: Veterinary State Board websites: https://www.avma.org/KB/Resources/Reference/Pages/Veterinary-State-Board-Web-sites.aspx.

AVMA. Confidentiality of veterinary patient records: avmajournals.avma.org/view/journals/javma/255/3/javma.255.3.282.xml.

For access to all of the medical record forms discussed in this chapter, see the Evolve site associated with this textbook.

Publications

Heinke ML, McCarthy JB. In: Lakewood CO, ed. *Practice Made Perfect: A Complete Guide to Veterinary Practice Management*. 2nd ed. American Animal Hospital Association; 2012.

Potter PA, Perry AG. *Fundamentals of Nursing*. 7th ed. St. Louis, MO: Mosby; 2009.

Rockett J, Christianson C. *Case Studies in Veterinary Technology: A Scenario-Based Critical Thinking Approach*. Heyburn, ID: Rockett House Publishing, LLC; 2010.

Rockett J, Lattanzio C, Anderson K. *Patient Assessment and Interventions and Documentation for the Veterinary Nurse*. Clifton Park, NY: Delmar Cengage Learning; 2009.

Related Associations

American Animal Hospital Association, 14142 Denver West Pkwy., Ste 245, Lakewood, CO 80401www.aaha.org.

American Health Information Management Association, 233 North Michigan Avenue, 21st floor, Chicago, IL 60601-65809, www.ahima.org.

American Veterinary Medical Association, 1931 N. Meacham Road, Suite 100, Schaumburg, IL 60173-4360. www.avma.org.

National Association of Veterinary Technicians in America, 750 Route 202 Suite 200 Bridgewater, NJ 08807. www.navta.net.

4

Occupational Health and Safety in Veterinary Hospitals

PHILIP J. SEIBERT JR.

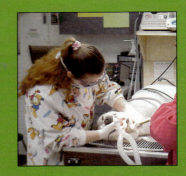

CHAPTER OUTLINE

LEARNING OBJECTIVES

When you have completed this chapter, you will be able to:

1. Pronounce, spell, and define all key terms in the chapter.
2. Do the following regarding safety in the veterinary hospital:
   - Explain the acronym OSHA and describe the role it plays in the development of safety programs in veterinary hospitals.
   - List the safety rights and responsibilities of veterinary hospital staff members.
   - List the safety rights and responsibilities of veterinary hospital owners and leaders.
3. List common workplace hazards in a veterinary facility, describe precautions that can be taken to reduce the risk of these hazards, and do the following:
   - Explain proper methods for lifting objects and animals.
   - List the hazards associated with the use of ethylene oxide, formalin, glutaraldehyde, anesthetic gases, and compressed gases.

- Describe the requirements of the OSHA "right to know" law.
- Explain the acronym SDS and describe the components of an SDS.
4. Do the following regarding medical and animal-related hazards:
   - List the hazards related to the capture and restraint of small and large animals.
   - Explain risks associated with excessive noise and methods taken to minimize these risks.
   - Describe hazards related to bathing and dipping animals and explain methods to minimize these risks.
   - Define the term *zoonotic disease* and list zoonotic and nonzoonotic diseases commonly encountered in veterinary practices.
5. Explain the importance of wearing goggles, gloves, and a surgical mask when performing dental procedures on animals.

6. List methods to minimize the risks associated with exposure to radiation, anesthetic gases, and medical waste.
7. List the equipment and supplies needed to protect veterinary personnel when handling hazardous pharmaceuticals, such

as chemotherapeutic drugs, and describe methods for safely handling contaminated bedding and waste from oncology patients.

KEY TERMS

Bone marrow disorders
Coccidia
Cutaneous larval migrans
Cytotoxic drugs (CDs)
Diarrhea and cramping
Ergonomic principles
Giardia
Ground-fault circuit interrupter
Hazardous chemical
Hazardous materials plan
Hospital Safety Manual
Lyme disease
Occupational Safety and Health Act

Occupational Safety and Health Administration (OSHA)
Panleukopenia
Parvoviral enteritis
Personal protective equipment (PPE)
Rabies
"Right to know" law
Ringworm
Safety data sheet (SDS)
Sarcoptic mange
Toxoplasmosis
Visceral larval migrans
Waste anesthetic gas (WAG)
Zoonotic disease

Introduction

Working as a veterinary technician and as part of the veterinary health care team can be deeply rewarding. However, with every reward comes responsibility. One of the responsibilities as a veterinary technician is to help ensure the safety of coworkers, patients, and clients, as well as one's own safety. If someone is hurt on the job, the damage extends beyond the physical pain and disability suffered. The hospital is also affected, both financially and operationally, because the veterinary health care team loses an important member—you. Other staff members of the practice must work harder to cover the personnel shortage. In addition, the quality of health care delivered to patients may be adversely affected by having less than a full team of caregivers.

As a staff member in a veterinary hospital, you are exposed to hazards in the day-to-day routine of clinical practice. These hazards include exposure to infectious diseases, harmful chemicals, and radiation, and the risks of being scratched, bitten, shoved, stepped on, and kicked. That is the bad news. The good news is that when properly identified, these hazards can be managed and the risk of injury minimized or even eliminated. To that end, it is important to educate yourself about all hazards, particularly those listed in this chapter, and integrate safety procedures into the everyday habits of your job.

Safety

Objectives of a Safety Program

The **Occupational Safety and Health Administration (OSHA)** enforces federal laws that help ensure a safe workplace for US workers. These laws require all businesses to have a safety program. The primary purpose of a safety program is to reduce or eliminate the possibility of injury or illness to staff members. The three main methods for achieving that goal are (1) training that enables you to develop your skills, (2) focusing on the task at hand and minimizing distractions, and (3) adhering to the proper procedures for a given task.

Remember, we can never totally avoid every hazard, but we can minimize our exposure to them by understanding the job that needs to be done, paying attention to the task at hand, and following established procedures.

Your Safety Rights

One can never eliminate every hazard completely, but each of us can minimize our exposure to hazards in most cases.

> **TECHNICIAN NOTE**
>
> You have the right to expect your workplace to be reasonably free from unnecessary hazards, but no one can guarantee that a workplace is completely free of *all* risk.

The ability to participate in a safety program at work is an important part of your rights. It is often assumed that the owner or manager of a business knows all there is to know about the business, but too often, it is the staff member who first becomes aware of potential safety problems. As a veterinary hospital staff member, you have the right and a responsibility to bring those concerns to the attention of the hospital leadership without fear of reprisal. In most instances, the complaint is first presented to the immediate supervisor, but be aware that not all complaints will bring about changes to the operation of the practice. Some complaints stem from a lack of familiarity with standard safety procedures, and in these cases, instruction by a supervisor is all that is needed to resolve the issue. However, if a complaint is not taken seriously by the hospital leadership or if a dangerous situation is not adequately addressed, you have the right to bring the issue to the attention of the regional OSHA office.

> **PUT INTO PRACTICE**
>
> When presenting potential safety issues to your supervisor, bring one to two solutions to the issue. This will show your supervisor that you care and are willing to work on solutions.

When medical evaluations, radiation exposure reports, and other such reports are collected by the hospital leadership, they must be made available to the staff member for review. This does not mean that you are entitled to see private or sensitive information about other staff members, but it does mean that you are entitled to see data that is relevant to your safety. You are also entitled to know about the nature and type of accidents that have occurred in your hospital. If your practice employs more than 10 staff members, you have the right to view the summary of work-related injuries and illnesses (OSHA Form 300A), which should be posted on the employee bulletin board at certain times of the year.

Your Safety Responsibilities

It is your responsibility to learn and follow the safety rules and practices that have been established for your position in the hospital. Even though OSHA will not cite or fine a staff member directly for violations of these responsibilities, they are required under the **Occupational Safety and Health Act** (hereafter referred to as "the Act") to "comply with all occupational safety and health standards and all rules, regulations, and orders issued under the Act." Not only does this include specific OSHA standards, but it also applies to workplace-specific rules established by the leadership at your hospital.

TECHNICIAN NOTE

It is your responsibility to learn and follow the safety rules and practices that have been established for your position in the veterinary hospital.

Although you cannot be disciplined by your employer for exercising your rights under the Act, you can be disciplined for willful or repeated violations of any safety rule or standard. In some cases, this discipline can be as simple as a verbal reprimand, but in severe or chronic situations, it can include termination. In most states, if you are terminated for the willful violation of safety rules, you will likely be denied unemployment benefits.

In addition to the responsibility to follow the rules, the Act requires you to do the following:
- Read the OSHA poster (Fig. 4.1).
- Comply with all applicable standards.
- Wear or use prescribed **personal protective equipment (PPE)** while working (Fig. 4.2).
- Report hazardous conditions to your supervisor.
- Report any job-related injury or illness to the proper person and seek treatment promptly.

The Leadership's Rights

Although the Act and OSHA require the leadership of a business to maintain safety standards, this is not meant to restrict the right of the business to set rules of conduct or operation for its staff. The hospital owner, for example, has the right to set and enforce rules for their own business if those rules are consistent with federal and state safety laws. Practice owners must have ample time to correct any safety-related problems. In other words, a staff member should not rush off to file a grievance with the regional OSHA office without first giving the hospital leadership ample time to correct the deficiency.

If a hospital is inspected, the hospital owner has the right to be present, because the business is considered their personal property. A staff member is not authorized to admit an OSHA inspector into the practice in the absence of the hospital owner (unless, of course, the hospital owner specifically gives that staff member the authority

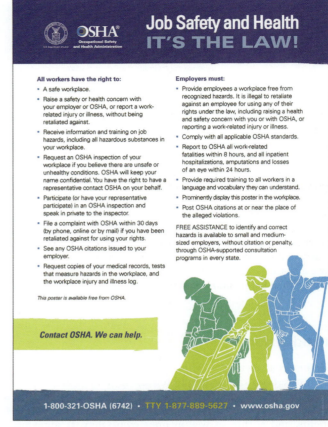

• **Fig. 4.1** Locate and read all safety notices where you work. (From www.osha.gov.)

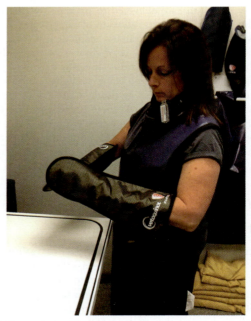

• **Fig. 4.2** Preventive protective equipment (PPE) is essential for safely working in veterinary facilities. Use of lead aprons, gloves, and a thyroid shield is required when working with radiologic equipment. (Courtesy Dr. Joanna Bassert.)

to act on their behalf). However, OSHA inspectors may enter a practice without the presence of the owner and without permission by a staff member if the inspectors have a court order to do so.

The Leadership's Responsibilities

The leadership of a veterinary hospital is responsible for providing a safe work environment for all staff members. This does not mean providing a facility with zero hazards—that would be impossible. It means that the leadership must make a reasonable effort to identify the hazards present, correct those that can be eliminated, and control the hazards that cannot be eliminated. The hospital leadership must establish safety procedures for the hospital, including emergency procedures for preventing workplace accidents. The leadership must enforce these rules as diligently as it would be expected to enforce any other rule in the practice.

The hospital leadership is also responsible for providing practice-specific safety training to staff members. Even if a veterinary technician has years of prior experience, the practice is required to make sure that the technician can do their job safely. This training can be provided in a formal setting, as in staff meetings or a continuing education course, or it can be given within the hospital in a one-on-one manner. A great deal of learning takes place in many practices every day. On-the-job training can be an effective way to obtain knowledge about safety, but be sure you know your limits and abilities. Ultimately, you are the best person to determine whether you are competent to do a job safely. If you think you need extra safety training in a particular area, do not hesitate to ask for it. Tell your supervisor immediately so that arrangements can be made for proper instruction.

Working While Pregnant

Sometimes, it is difficult to reconcile one's need for privacy with the need to keep a supervisor informed. Most hospitals take this notification seriously and will keep the news confidential until you are ready for others to know. With a little common sense, a little planning, and a little adaptation, a pregnant woman can work in a veterinary hospital right up to delivery.

- If you become pregnant, be honest and forthcoming about what is going on. Notify the hospital leadership as soon as you have confirmed your pregnancy. Hospitals can become lax in their safety measures from time to time and, because studies show that hazards introduced during the first trimester can be most damaging to the developing fetus, telling the leadership early will initiate a hazard assessment to get procedures back on track.
- Know your rights and responsibilities. Employers are prohibited by law from removing you from a hazardous job simply because you are or may become pregnant and the fetus may be affected. However, you must be capable of performing the essential elements of the job to be protected by the law.
- Follow the safety rules. Although there are numerous hazards pregnant women face in everyday life as well as on the job, following the safety requirements will minimize risk.
- Be flexible. No matter what your intentions are today, no one can predict the future. The progress of your pregnancy may change what you can—or are willing—to do.

General Workplace Hazards

Every practice should have a collection of written safety-related policies, known as the **Hospital Safety Manual**. You should know

where the *Hospital Safety Manual* is in your hospital and should take time to become familiar with it. Memorize the "dos and don'ts" for your particular hospital, and always follow the safety rules. No one can protect you from an injury or illness better than you can.

Safety Starts With Healthy

Staying safe at work starts with taking care of yourself in life. Your body needs adequate rest for physical and mental health, increased concentration and memory, a healthier immune system, and even reduced stress. Most adult bodies crave about 8 hours of sleep a night. Try to achieve that by giving yourself a bedtime and sticking to it! Improve the quality of your sleep by turning off your cell phone or at least leaving it and other electronics in another room so that you are not disturbed by texts and alerts. If you use your cell phone as an alarm, try turning off the alerts so your sleep is not disturbed.

Your body is an engine, and engines need fuel. Your fuel is your diet, and the best way to keep your body healthy is to eat a balanced diet. Junk food, caffeine, and sugar are all fine in moderation, but your body's engine cannot perform when it is fueled by the wrong stuff!

A factor in many workplace accidents is fatigue. Our bodies and minds need regular "respites" from the task at hand. Although most hospitals do not have formal "break times," it is important to periodically give yourself a break from the grind of the daily chores to simply do things like get some water or go to the bathroom. And take that lunch break! There is an abundance of information to show that people who work all day but skip a lunch break are less productive in the afternoon, are more prone to making mistakes, and suffer a higher rate of injuries from accidents!

Most of us are in the veterinary profession because of our love for animals. But just like everything else, that love can become unhealthy. Let's face it, we care, but we cannot solve all the problems of every animal we see. And when we become too emotionally involved with the outcome of every single animal, we eventually burn out. And no one wants that! We need you, your family needs you, and your patients certainly need you. So it is important to live a balanced life.

One of the best ways to find that balance in life is to find a hobby. People with hobbies are less likely to suffer from stress, low energy, and depression. Activities that get you out and about can make you feel happier and more relaxed. By engaging in a "non-animal—related" hobby, you are going to be better able to deal with the emotional side of caring for animals.

Don't skip vacations! The tradition of people taking vacation time away from work is rooted in centuries of evolution in the workplace. Many years ago we realized that people are happier AND PERFORM BETTER at work when they take regular vacations from work. You don't have to travel for a vacation; you can do whatever you want, but it is important for the quality of your work and for your health to occasionally take some time to recharge.

Dressing Appropriately for the Job

One of the most basic rules of safety is to dress appropriately for the job at hand. In the veterinary hospital, this includes protective footwear and minimal or no jewelry. You can reduce the chances of getting injured by wearing sturdy shoes that cover your entire foot (not sandals or slip-on or open-toed shoes) and that have nonslip soles. Be especially cautious when walking on uneven or wet floors. Never run inside the hospital or on uneven footing. Excessive jewelry can present a hazard in many clinical situations but particularly when an animal struggles during restraint and can inadvertently snag a piercing, an earring, or a necklace with a claw. If your hospital's dress code allows visible piercings and jewelry, it is best to choose a post style instead of one that dangles or is loose.

Save Your Back!

According to insurance statistics, back injuries account for one in every five workplace injuries among US and Canadian workers. To minimize your chances of suffering one of these painful injuries, remember the rules for lifting: keep your back straight and lift with your legs (Fig. 4.3). Never bend over at the waist to lift an object or animal. If your hospital does not have a motorized lift table, get help when lifting patients weighing more than about 40 lb. Remember to follow sound ergonomic principles when positioning or restraining patients, especially when working with horses or food animals (Case Presentation 1).

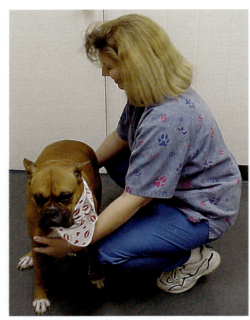

• **Fig. 4.3** Remember to keep your back straight and to lift with your legs.

CASE PRESENTATION 4.1

A 22-year-old male has been a veterinary technician for 2 years. He worked at a companion animal practice in the past but has recently started working in an equine-only hospital. During his first week on the job, he suffered a debilitating back injury while trying to capture and restrain a fractious patient. Because he has a background in companion animals, the technician viewed restraint as primarily a physical overpowering of the patient. Had he received proper training when he first started the job, he would have known that tranquilization and sedation are the primary methods of restraint used for horses that become fractious when physical restraint (e.g., placement in a stock) is not practical.

The technician was confined to bed for 3 days by the physician and was restricted in his physical activities for 2 weeks to recover from the muscle strain.

Clean Up After Yourself

Some injuries are caused by cluttered or dirty work areas. In addition, clutter is known to contribute to the severity of accidents that otherwise would be minor. Cleanliness and organization are good business standards, especially in a health care facility. Always clean up spills as soon as they happen. You should always clean and return equipment to the proper storage place immediately after use. Remove all trash from your work area at least daily.

Everything in Its Place

Supplies and equipment should always be stored properly. Organize drawers, cabinets, and counters so that items can be found easily and clutter is reduced. Heavy supplies or equipment should be kept on lower shelves to prevent unnecessary strain in trying to lift them overhead and to reduce the risk of material falling on your head. Never use stairways or exit hallways as storage areas. Do not overload shelves or cabinets (Fig. 4.4). Store liquids in containers with tight-fitting lids and always replace the lids when finished using the product. Whenever possible, store chemicals on

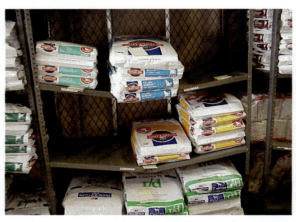

• **Fig. 4.4** Improper storage of materials can lead to serious injury. Do not overload shelves.

shelves at or below eye level; this will minimize the possibility of accidental spilling of the chemical on you when you are getting or replacing a container. Never climb into or on cabinets, shelves, chairs, buckets, or similar items. Use an appropriate ladder or step to reach high locations.

Beware of Break Times

Accidental ingestion of pathogenic organisms or harmful chemicals while eating on the job is a real possibility in veterinary hospitals. Therefore it is important to eat and drink (including simple snacks, sodas, and even water) only in areas that are free of toxic and biologically harmful substances. Examination and treatment areas, the laboratory, animal housing areas, and even the reception area are all potential sources of contamination and are not appropriate locations for the consumption of food or beverages. These rules also apply to the preparation of foods and beverages. Make sure that coffee makers and utensils are away from sources that could contaminate food, such as laboratories and treatment and bathing areas. Check the cabinets or shelves above the food preparation areas to ensure that there is no risk of any hazardous material spilling onto the area. Always store food, drinks, condiments, and snacks in a refrigerator separate from the one used to store biological or chemical hazardous materials, such as vaccines, drugs, and laboratory samples.

> **TECHNICIAN NOTE**
>
> Always store food, drinks, condiments, and snacks in a refrigerator separate from the one used to store biological or chemical hazardous materials, such as vaccines, drugs, and laboratory samples.

Machinery and Equipment

Never operate machinery or equipment without all proper guards in place. Equipment such as fans and cage dryers have moving parts that can severely hurt or even sever a finger. Long hair should be tied back or pinned up to prevent it from getting caught in fans or other moving parts.

When using such equipment as autoclaves, microwave ovens, cautery irons, or other heating devices, be sure to understand the proper rules for safe operation. Burns, especially from steam, are painful and serious, and almost always can be prevented. Autoclaves also present a danger from the pressure that is used for proper sterilization. Before opening an autoclave, be sure to first release the pressure by activating the vent device and at the same time, keeping your hands and face away from the steam. Let the steam dissipate completely before opening the door fully and be careful when removing the packs, because they may still be hot. Always assume that cautery devices and branding irons are hot and use the insulated handle whenever you touch them. Never place heated irons on any surface where they could overheat and start a fire or where someone might accidentally touch them.

Electrical

Many commonly performed procedures require the use of electricity. Although new equipment and buildings have safety features built into their design, you must be conscious of preventing a situation that could cause a fire or physical harm to yourself, another person, or a patient.

Do not remove or tamper with light switch or electrical outlet covers. Always keep circuit breaker boxes closed and never block access by stacking supplies or equipment in front of them. Only persons trained to perform maintenance duties should repair electrical appliances, outlets, switches, fixtures, or breakers.

If you must use a portable dryer or other electrical equipment in a wet area, make sure it is properly grounded and is plugged into only a ground fault circuit interrupter outlet. Extension cords should be used only for temporary applications and should always be of the three-conductor, grounded type. Never run extension cords through windows or doors that may close and damage the wires or across aisles or floors where a tripping hazard may be created.

Surge suppressors should only be used to protect sensitive electronic equipment and should never be overloaded (Fig. 4.5). Surge suppressors should never be used with portable heaters, autoclaves, coffee makers, or other heat-generating appliances, because they may overheat and cause a fire.

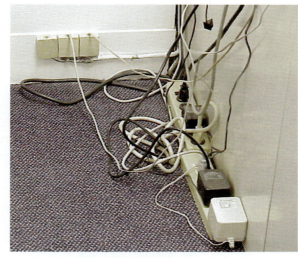

• **Fig. 4.5** Overloaded surge suppressors or extension cords can start a fire.

Equipment with grounded plugs must never be used with adaptors or with nongrounded extension cords. Never alter or remove the ground terminals on plugs. Appliances or equipment with defective ground terminals or plugs should not be used until repaired.

Fire and Evacuation

The potential for dramatic loss of life (both human and animal) and destruction of property makes a fire one of the most feared accidents imaginable. Fortunately, the danger of such an event can be significantly reduced by taking a few simple precautions:

- Never use power adaptors or surge suppressors as a substitute for permanent wiring. Overloaded or faulty electrical cords can overheat or short out and start a fire, even when the equipment is turned off.
- Always store flammable liquids properly; many fluids, such as gasoline, paint thinner, and ether, should never be stored inside the hospital except in an approved flammable storage cabinet. Some components of specialty dental and large animal acrylic repair kits are also flammable. Very small amounts of these components usually are not a problem, but always ensure that they are stored and used in an area with good ventilation and that the containers have tight-fitting lids that are replaced immediately after use.
- Flammable materials, such as newspapers, boxes, and cleaning chemicals, must always be stored at least 3 feet away from an ignition source, such as a water heater, furnace, or stove.
- Always take extra care when using portable heaters. Never leave them unattended and always make sure that they are placed no closer than 3 feet from any wall, furniture, or other flammable material.

You should learn about the emergency warning system in your hospital. If the facility is equipped with an electronic alarm system (Fig. 4.6A), be sure you know how to activate it manually. In the absence of an electronic alarm system, a verbal alarm is effective. You can use the telephone intercom feature to alert everyone that there is a fire in the building (in small buildings, simply yell in a loud, clear voice to get the message out).

You should become familiar with the locations of emergency exits in your facility (see Fig. 4.6B and C). Never store materials,

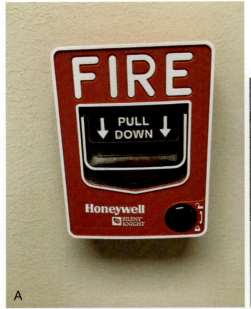

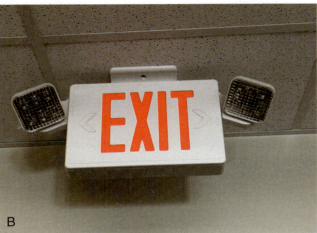

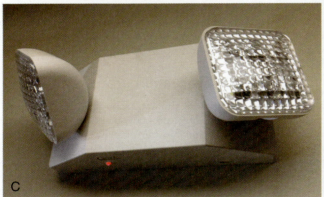

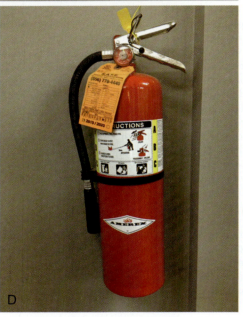

• **Fig. 4.6** Learning the emergency warning system and safety measures in your hospital is vital in the event of an emergency. Safety measures may include: (A) an electric fire alarm system, (B) illuminated emergency exit signs, (C) emergency lights, and (D) a fire extinguisher.

equipment, garbage, or recycling in a way that would impede the emergency exit, even if it's "temporary." Security doors can be locked from the outside, but make sure the emergency exits are always able to be opened from the inside without a special key or device when you are in the building.

Know your duties in the event of a fire. Although you will feel the need to rescue animals during an evacuation, it is imperative that you FIRST report to the designated assembly area for accountability, to formulate a plan for rescue, and to establish a triage area where rescued animals can be evaluated, treated, and housed during the crisis. If you do not know your designated assembly area, ask your supervisor.

Know where the fire extinguishers are located (see Fig. 4.6D) and how to use them (Procedure 4.1). Most veterinary hospitals are equipped with dry chemical fire extinguishers. Before you decide to use a fire extinguisher, make sure the alarm has been sounded, everyone has left the building (or is in the process of leaving), and the fire department has been called.

> **TECHNICIAN NOTE**
>
> Become familiar with the locations of emergency exits in your facility. Make sure that emergency exits are always left unlocked from the inside and free from obstruction when you are in the building.

The National Fire Protection Association recommends that you never attempt to fight a fire if any of these conditions are true:
- The fire is spreading beyond the immediate area where it started or involves any part of the building or structure.
- The fire could block your escape route.

PROCEDURE 4.1

Using a Fire Extinguisher

- If you must use a portable fire extinguisher, remember the mnemonic PASS:
  - **P**ull the pin: Some extinguishers require releasing a lock latch, pressing a puncture lever, or another motion. (Check your extinguishers to be sure.)
  - **A**im low: Point the extinguisher (or its horn or hose) at the base of the fire.
  - **S**queeze the handle: This releases the extinguishing agent.
  - **S**weep from side to side at the base of the fire until it appears to be out.
- Watch the fire area. If fire breaks out again, repeat use of the extinguisher.
- Most portable extinguishers work according to these directions, but read and follow the directions on your specific extinguisher.

- You are unsure of the proper operation of the extinguisher.
- You are in doubt that the extinguisher you are holding is designed for the type of fire at hand or is large enough to suppress the fire.

Natural Disasters

Natural disasters such as lightning, tornados, and earthquakes will strike with little or no warning. Your practice should have a plan to respond to those events, and you should be familiar with that plan. Other natural disasters, such as hurricanes and blizzards, are usually predictable, so plans can be made to accommodate the safety needs of patients and staff. Ask your supervisor for the details of your practice's natural disaster plan.

Do Not Become a Victim of Violence

Just as in any occupation, you are at risk of injury from accidents not directly related to your job. Vehicle accidents, personal assault, and robbery have resulted in injury to veterinary technicians while on duty. Although no one can prevent every possible scenario, preparation can certainly help and sometimes will minimize injury. When outside the hospital building, be aware of your environment and do your best to avoid placing yourself in a situation that could go bad.

Do not make it easy for the wrong people to get in and surprise you! Always keep "nonclient" doors locked from the outside to prevent anyone from gaining unauthorized or undetected entry into the building (Fig. 4.7). Do not keep them open for any reason. Do not share your pass code or key to the hospital with others.

When leaving the hospital building, especially after dark, always be aware of your environment and try to avoid risky situations. Avoid leaving alone—it is best to leave in pairs or in a group. Have your keys in hand before you leave the building so you won't be distracted in the parking lot. Lock the doors immediately after you get into your vehicle and, if someone approaches you, do not roll down the window to speak to them, even if they ask for assistance. Offer to call the police for them from your cell phone.

If you are working alone, you should have a plan for getting help if you are attacked, injured, or become "trapped" in a run with an animal and cannot get to the phone. Use the following tips every time you go into work alone, and safety will become part of your normal routine:

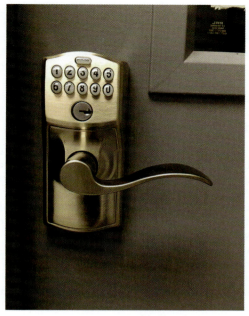

• **Fig. 4.7** Personal safety includes the diligent use of locks and barriers to deter unauthorized persons from entering the facility. Keep all nonclient doors locked from the outside to prevent access by unauthorized personnel.

- Let someone you trust (spouse, friend, or relative) know where you are going and that you will be working alone. Arrange to call them at a specific time to let them know that you are okay. Then, if you do not call at the arranged time, they can check on you.
- When you arrive at work, take note of your surroundings. If possible, drive all the way around the building once before parking. Pay attention to any cars or people that do not belong there.
- Once you are inside, lock the door behind you. If the business is open and you are alone, make sure all the doors except the client entrance are locked and there is a visual or audible notice when the client door is opened. If other staff members or deliveries must come and go throughout the day, they should use the front door or have a key or the combination to the back door.
- Although it may not be allowed during regular operations, carry a cell phone on your person when you are working alone to be able to summon help if you are incapacitated or trapped.
- Before leaving, look for people loitering in the parking lot or near the building. If there are cars in the parking lot that do not belong there, be cautious and do not leave the building until you have assistance.

If you work in critical care or a 24-hour practice, you should use the "barriers" that are usually available. Such things as buzzers to control access through the front door and one-way locks on the remaining doors (to let you out in case of an emergency while keeping the door locked from the outside) are essential in these environments, so do not prop doors open, disassemble the locking system, or turn the system off.

In any business that keeps money or stores valuable items, there is a risk of robbery. If you ever find yourself in a situation where someone demands money, drugs, or other material items while threatening your personal safety, do *not* withhold the things they demand. Cooperate with the person's demands and hand over what is demanded but do not go with the person. Resist physical assault or battery to the best of your abilities; preferably, go outside the building so that passersby can see what is happening and can render assistance or call the police. As soon as it is safe, let everyone else know of the situation. You should attempt to contact the police if this can be safely done without the person's knowledge; otherwise, do it immediately after the person has left.

Hazardous Chemicals: Right to Know

You may not think about it, but many products that you use every day can be **hazardous chemicals**. Every chemical, even common ones, such as cleaning supplies, has the potential to cause you harm. Most chemicals are dangerous, because they are a health hazard or because of a physical property that can cause injury. The most common chemicals in use in the veterinary practice include the following:

- Cleaning and disinfecting agents
- Insecticides and pesticides
- Drugs and medications (including anesthetic gases)
- Sterilization agents (including lab chemicals, formaldehyde, and ethylene oxide)
- Radiology processing fluids

Planning and training are the keys to safely handling any chemical, so every business, including your hospital, must follow the requirements of OSHA's **"right to know" law**. This law requires that you be informed of all chemicals you may be exposed to while doing your job. The "right to know" law also requires that you wear all safety equipment prescribed by the manufacturer and the hospital when using any product containing a hazardous chemical. Safety equipment must be provided to you at no cost, but it is not optional—you must wear what is required.

PUT INTO PRACTICE

Offering to create standard operating procedures (SOPs) for the handling of hazardous materials or other safety aspects in your practice can help make everyone safer and offer an invaluable service to your employer.

When a product is used in a work setting, such as your hospital, you may be exposed to that product to a greater extent than you would as an average consumer, so your risk may be different. When you receive a product from the manufacturer or distributor, every bottle will be identified with a label containing directions for use and the appropriate warnings. The warnings will include the following:

- *A product identifier:* The product identifier can simply be the product's name, but it will often include the name of the hazardous chemical as an ingredient of the product.
- *A signal word:* Signal words are used to indicate the relative level of severity of the hazard and alert the reader to a potential hazard on the label. There are only two words used as signal words: "Danger" and "Warning." "Danger" is used for the more severe hazards, and "Warning" is used for the less severe hazards.
- *Hazard statements:* Hazard statements describe the nature of the hazards of a chemical, including the degree of the hazard. An example of a hazard statement could be "Causes damage to kidneys through prolonged or repeated exposure when absorbed through the skin."
- *Precautionary statement(s):* Precautionary statements describe recommended measures that should be taken to minimize or

• **Fig. 4.8** Examples of hazard pictograms on product labels.

prevent adverse effects resulting from exposure to the hazardous chemical or improper storage or handling. There are four types of precautionary statements:
Prevention (to minimize exposure)
Response (in case of accidental spillage or exposure, emergency response, and first aid)
Storage
Disposal
- *Pictogram(s):* Pictograms are graphic symbols used to communicate specific information about the hazards of a chemical. There are a total of nine pictograms that can be used to convey hazards on labels (Fig. 4.8).
- *Name, address, and telephone number* of the chemical manufacturer, importer, or other responsible party.

You should always read, understand, and follow all the directions and warnings printed on the label.

Chemicals that are used in significant quantities may be obtained in large containers and subsequently transferred to smaller containers or spray bottles for ease of use in the hospital. It is important to remember to apply a hazard warning label (Fig. 4.9) to those "working" containers to ensure that the product is used safely. In addition, the manufacturer of a product that contains a hazardous chemical will prepare a **safety data sheet (SDS)** (formerly known as *Material Safety Data Sheets* [MSDSs]) that gives you additional precautions, instructions, and advice for handling that product in the workplace (Fig. 4.10). Your hospital is required to keep an SDS library for the chemicals that you use. Ask your supervisor where your hospital's SDS library is located and take the time to review the SDSs for the products you use frequently. Although SDSs may look complex at first glance, the information that is important to you is easy to find. Section II contains hazards identification, Section IV contains the first aid measures, Section VII gives safe handling and storage instructions, and Section VIII explains the controls you should employ when using that product, including any protective equipment recommended by the manufacturer (Box 4.1).

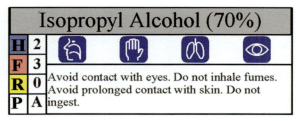

Isopropyl Alcohol (70%)

H	2
F	3
R	0
P	A

Avoid contact with eyes. Do not inhale fumes. Avoid prolonged contact with skin. Do not ingest.

• **Fig. 4.9** Example of a secondary container hazard warning label.

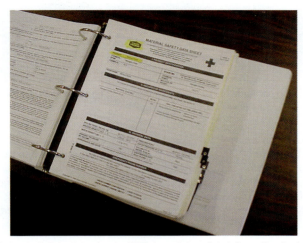

• **Fig. 4.10** Safety data sheets (SDSs) contain safety information that may not be indicated on the product label.

TECHNICIAN NOTE

Your practice is required to keep a safety data sheet (SDS) library for the chemicals that you use. Ask your supervisor where your hospital's SDS library is located.

Working bottles of hazardous products should always have tight-fitting, screw-on lids. Always remember to place the cap back on the bottle after using any chemical product. You should endeavor to store chemical bottles in a closed cabinet; this will help prevent injury to animals if they escape. Ideally, the cabinet or shelf should be at or below eye level. This will minimize the chance of the product spilling on to your face if the cap is not secure. Never store or use hazardous products near food, beverages, or food preparation areas.

When two chemicals are combined, the result is seldom a simple mixture. It is often a new, sometimes different, and possibly dangerous chemical, so never mix any chemicals unless you are directed to do so by the label or an SDS. When it is necessary to dilute a concentrated product with water, be careful to keep the material from splashing on to your hands, clothes, or face. If it is likely that the product will splash on you, wear PPE, such as a pair of protective latex or nitrile gloves and protective goggles or glasses. When making solutions from a concentrated chemical, you should always start with the correct quantity of water and *then* add the concentrate.

Minor spills of most chemicals can be cleaned up with paper towels or absorbent material (e.g., cat litter) and disposed of in the trash; however, dangerous chemicals, such as chemotherapy drugs, radiographic fixer solution, mercury, or ethylene oxide, require special procedures, so before you use a new chemical, review the SDS and learn the procedures you must follow for cleaning up a

• BOX 4.1   Safety Data Sheets (SDSs)

Safety data sheets (SDSs) are formatted to conform to the Globally Harmonized System (GHS), which includes 16 standard sections that are arranged in the order given below. Like the former materials safety data sheets (MSDSs), SDSs are prepared by a manufacturer to relay detailed information about a product.

Section 1: Identification—includes product identifier; manufacturer or distributor name, address, and phone number; emergency phone number; recommended use; restrictions on use

Section 2: Hazard(s) identification—includes all hazards regarding the chemical; required label elements

Section 3: Composition/information on ingredients—includes information on chemical ingredients; trade secret claims

Section 4: First aid measures—includes important symptoms/effects, acute, delayed; required treatment

Section 5: Firefighting measures—lists suitable extinguishing techniques, equipment; chemical hazards from fire

Section 6: Accidental release measures—lists emergency procedures; protective equipment; proper methods of containment and clean-up

Section 7: Handling and storage—lists precautions for safe handling and storage, including incompatibilities

Section 8: Exposure controls/personal protection—lists OSHA's permissible exposure limits (PELs); threshold limit values (TLVs); appropriate engineering controls; personal protective equipment (PPE)

Section 9: Physical and chemical properties—lists the chemical's characteristics

Section 10: Stability and reactivity—lists chemical stability and possibility of hazardous reactions

Section 11: Toxicologic information—includes routes of exposure; related symptoms, acute and chronic effects; numerical measures of toxicity

Section 12: Ecologic information

Section 13: Disposal considerations

Section 14: Transport information

Section 15: Regulatory information

Section 16: Other information—includes the date of preparation or last revision

---

spill. When cleaning up any spill, remember to wear gloves and any other special PPE mandated on the SDS. Keep other people and animals away from the spill until it is safe. Unless prohibited by instructions on the SDS, wash the spill site and any contaminated equipment with a detergent soap and water—avoid the use of disinfectant chemicals (Procedure 4.2).

Familiarize yourself with the locations of the eyewash stations in your hospital. Test them regularly and know how to use them before you are in a position to need them. Do not use the spray attachments on sinks or tubs as a substitute for an eyewash station, because the unregulated spray may injure your cornea.

Special Chemicals

Some chemicals pose more or different threats than everyday products; therefore additional precautions apply for these chemicals.

Mercury Thermometers

Although digital thermometers have largely replaced glass and mercury thermometers in medicine, there are some still in use. The bad news is that exposure to mercury can cause serious health problems. The good news is that the amount of mercury in a clinical glass thermometer is usually less than 0.5 mL and is not likely to create a serious health hazard. Because mercury can be a problem in the environment, special precautions are necessary when cleaning up broken mercury thermometers. The best protection

PROCEDURE 4.2

Chemical Spill Cleanup

Step 1. Keep unnecessary people and pets out of the area to prevent the spread of spilled material.

Step 2. If the area is small or if the fumes are extremely strong, increase ventilation by opening a window or turning on an exhaust fan. Do not use an electrical exhaust fan or electrical equipment. Avoid turning switches on or off when cleaning up spilled flammable materials.

Step 3. Put on a pair of protective latex or nitrile gloves. If it is likely that your clothing will become contaminated during the cleanup, put on a protective apron and protective eyewear.

Step 4. As soon as possible, cover the spill with absorbent materials, such as paper towels or cat litter. Allow the absorbent material to fully collect the liquid.

Step 5. Using a broom, gently sweep the saturated absorbent into a dustpan and deposit it into a plastic trash bag.

Step 6. When all material has been picked up, seal the trash bag and dispose of it as regular waste unless your institution, city, or county requires you to do otherwise.

Step 7. Wash the contaminated area thoroughly with plain water or detergent soap (not with a disinfectant) if permissible by instructions in the safety data sheets (SDSs). Allow the area to air dry.

Step 8. Remove any protective equipment used during the cleanup. Dispose of single-use items as regular trash unless your institution, city, or county requires you to do otherwise.

Step 9. Wash your hands thoroughly and change any clothing that has become contaminated during the cleanup process.

Step 10. Replace used materials in the spill kit.

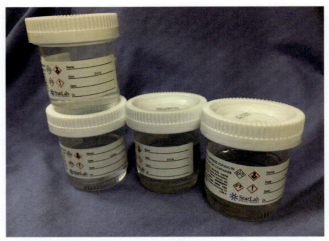

• **Fig. 4.11** When possible, use only biopsy jars prefilled with formalin to prevent excessive exposure.

may be to switch to digital thermometers. The clean-up procedure for a broken mercury thermometer is listed here:

- Read the SDS carefully and follow all instructions.
- Clean up the spill promptly so the mercury does not vaporize and get inhaled.
- Remove animals and other people from the area.
- Put on a pair of latex or nitrile gloves. Do not touch the liquid mercury with your hand.
- Use a mercury absorption sponge to collect the mercury "beads" that form, then dispose of the sponge into household garbage. Do not use a broom or vacuum to clean it up and do not flush mercury down the drain.
- Be careful of broken glass fragments. After all the mercury is collected, use a broom and dustpan to clean up the broken glass. Dispose of the glass in an appropriate trash container.
- Wash the affected area with a detergent soap and allow the area to air dry before using it.
- Throw the protective gloves in the trash.
- Thoroughly wash your hands with detergent soap.

Ethylene Oxide

Many hospitals use gas sterilization for items that would be damaged by other procedures. Electrical drills, rubber products, and sharps are commonly exposed to ethylene oxide (EtO) as a sterilization agent in human and veterinary medicine. This method has distinct advantages, but because EtO is thought to be a human carcinogen, special precautions must be maintained:

- Read the SDS carefully and follow all instructions.
- Store the ampules of EtO in a closed cabinet away from sources of heat, ideally in the same room where the sterilizer is located, to avoid the risk of breakage during transport and handling.

- Use only approved devices for the procedure.
- Read, understand, and follow all written procedures and safety precautions relevant to your hospital.
- Complete the machine manufacturer's Certified Operator Training program.
- Know the emergency procedures that should be performed in case of accidental release of EtO.

Formalin

Historically, formalin has been used in the veterinary profession for tissue preservation, diagnostic tests, and even sterilization. Because formaldehyde is also a suspected human carcinogen, OSHA takes its use seriously. Standards for the use of formaldehyde are like those put forth for the use of EtO:

- Read the SDS carefully and follow all instructions to minimize your exposure.
- Store supplies safely (including jars containing specimens).
- Use only with good ventilation in the room and avoid breathing vapors.
- Wear gloves and goggles when handling the chemical or tissues prepared with the chemical.

Whenever possible, you should obtain formalin in small, premeasured containers (also called *biopsy jars*) so that serious risk is minimized (Fig. 4.11). The diagnostic laboratory will often supply prefilled biopsy jars at no charge, so be sure to ask.

Glutaraldehyde

Glutaraldehyde is a potent chemical used to sterilize hard instruments without the use of an autoclave. Because it is so effective at killing germs, glutaraldehyde can be harmful to other living organisms, including you (Fig. 4.12). Be sure to follow the manufacturer's rules for safe handling when using this "cold sterilization" solution. Wear gloves when handling the liquid or instruments wet with the liquid, wash your hands after handling instruments exposed to glutaraldehyde, and keep sterilization trays covered to minimize evaporation.

Cryogenic Materials

Liquid nitrogen and solidified carbon dioxide (also known as "dry ice") are common chemicals used in veterinary reproductive, dermatologic, and laboratory procedures. The hazards of these materials include frostbite on contact with skin, asphyxiation, pressure

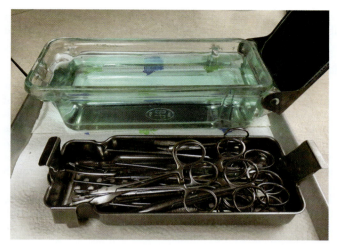

• **Fig. 4.12** Chemicals used to disinfect instruments and to clean surfaces, such as glutaraldehyde, are designed to kill living organisms, so they must be handled safely.

buildup, and explosions when improperly contained. When using cryogenic materials, always wear protective eyewear and thermally protective gloves and a thermally protective apron if there is the possibility that the chemical could splash on you. Liquid nitrogen and carbon dioxide displace oxygen readily; therefore it is important to store and use these products only in well-ventilated areas. Because the liquid-to-gas expansion ratio of nitrogen is 1:694 at 20°C (68°F), it quickly generates a tremendous amount of pressure, so liquid nitrogen storage containers must be fitted with special lids that control spills but also allow decompression of internal pressure.

Medical and Animal-Related Hazards

The purpose of our work is the care and treatment of animals, but sometimes handling our patients can itself be a hazard. Just about anyone who has worked with animals under stress or pain can tell stories of being injured by a patient. Insurance statistics show that animal-related accidents are the most common type of injury among workers in veterinary-related jobs, including that of veterinary technicians.

> **TECHNICIAN NOTE**
>
> Insurance statistics show that animal-related accidents are the most common type of injury among workers in veterinary-related jobs. This is particularly pertinent to veterinary technicians who work directly with animals for long periods.

Unfortunately, this hazard cannot be eliminated, so we must do the next best thing—minimize and control it. The best way to protect yourself from this hazard is to obtain training and practice in reading animal body language and by anticipating and pre-emptively lowering animal stress. Learning and mastering effective restraint techniques and knowing when to employ them is also critically important in decreasing the likelihood of an animal-related injury.

The most basic safety rule when working around animals is to stay alert. Animals sometimes react to situations unexpectedly. Sudden noises, movements, or even light can be the stimulus that would cause an animal to react, so if you are the person responsible for restraining the animal, keep your attention focused on the animal's reactions, not on the procedure. You must learn the proper restraint positions for each of the species of animals with which you work. Refer to Chapter 6 for additional information about the restraint and handling of animals and to Chapter 5, "Animal Behavior," for methods of pre-emptively lowering stress in veterinary patients.

Remember that capture–restraint equipment is available if the animal is fractious or is not cooperating; sometimes, just a piece of rope to hobble a leg or a piece of gauze for a hasty muzzle will make all the difference. Do not forget that the use of chemical restraint rather than physical restraint is often better for both you and the animal but be sure to ask the veterinarian for approval before administering any medication to a patient.

Large animals, such as horses and cattle, are dangerous simply because of their size and may severely injure or even kill a person when trying to escape restraint. Never put your hand or leg or any other part of your body between the animal and the side of the enclosure or chute; use a hook or a pole to pass ropes or belts through the chute. If you must enter a stall, paddock, or trailer with a large animal, stay on the side of the animal nearest the door so that you can escape if the situation becomes hazardous. If you must capture a fractious animal from a cage or a pen, make sure that another person is nearby to assist you if you run into trouble.

If your job entails handling exotic or nondomestic animals, remember that they all have their own unique methods of defense. You should know and understand their possible reactions before you attempt to restrain or treat them.

Although animal bites from otherwise healthy animals present a very low risk for rabies transmission, there is always a risk of infection and subsequent problems from these types of puncture wounds. If you are bitten, be sure to wash the area thoroughly with disinfectant soap and plenty of water and cover the wound. Always report the bite to your supervisor and see a physician for evaluation or care.

Noise

Dogs in cages will inevitably bark, and constantly barking dogs can adversely affect your hearing, especially if you work in an indoor kennel. Noise levels in dog wards can reach as high as 110 decibels (dB). Relatively short-duration exposure to these noise levels, as when going into the kennel only to retrieve a patient, poses no serious damage to your hearing. However, chronic and long-term exposure can contribute to hearing loss. When working in noisy areas for extended periods (e.g., while cleaning cages), you must wear personal hearing protectors. It does not matter what styles or types of hearing protector you use (earplugs or muffs), provided they are rated to filter the noise at levels of 20 dB or more (the package label will indicate the sound reduction rating).

> **TECHNICIAN NOTE**
>
> Noise levels in dog wards can reach as high as 110 decibels, making hearing protection an important necessity when working in those areas for more than a few minutes a day. Kennel workers are therefore particularly at risk for hearing loss without proper protection.

Bathing, Dipping, and Spraying Areas

Probably no area of an animal hospital is associated with greater risk for injury than the bathing or insecticide application area.

Although newer parasite control products significantly reduce exposure to pesticides and insecticides, shampoos and medical dips are still a big concern.

Products used for bathing and dipping animals can be harmful to your health and the environment. Even "all-natural" shampoos can cause eye irritation, and you can develop sensitivities to even the mildest products if you are exposed often enough. Because it is impossible to prevent animals from splashing and shaking, it is important to always wear protective glasses or goggles when bathing or dipping animals. In most cases, it is also important to wear gloves and an apron to prevent the product from getting on your skin or clothing; this minimizes the amount absorbed through the skin.

Bottles of dips, shampoos, and insecticides should be stored in a cabinet at or below eye level. Bottles should be properly labeled with the contents and any hazard warning that is appropriate (refer to the discussion on chemicals in this chapter for additional details). To prevent accidental spillage, always replace the cap or lid on the container after each use.

Always use a ventilation fan to keep the fumes from shampoos and dips at a safe level. When exhaust fans are too large, they waste heating or air conditioning, so you may be hesitant to use them in some situations. Ideally, a smaller fan installed directly over the tub will exhaust fumes without sacrificing environmental comfort in the room.

If you ever splash a chemical in your eyes, do not rub your eyes with your hands. Immediately call out for help; someone is usually nearby. With a coworker's assistance, go to the eyewash station and flush both eyes (even if only one eye is affected). Avoid using spray attachments for tubs and sinks, because the water pressure is unregulated, and streams of water from these devices can be fine enough to lacerate your cornea.

Zoonotic Diseases

Infectious diseases that can be passed between animals and humans are known as *zoonotic diseases*. You can be exposed to the organisms that cause disease by several means: inhalation, contact with broken skin, ingestion, contact with eyes and mucous membranes, and accidental inoculation by a needle. A veterinary technician may be exposed to a wide variety of zoonotic agents—certainly more than can be discussed in this chapter. However, some important ones are discussed in the sections below.

Viral Infections

Rabies is a serious (almost always fatal) viral disease that can affect any warm-blooded animal (including humans). The virus is spread by contact with an infected animal's saliva. Usually, the virus is transmitted through a bite, but it has also been transmitted when open wounds or mucous membranes encounter virus-rich saliva.

Although the disease is ever present in wild animal populations (primarily bats, raccoons, and skunks in the United States and Canada), in recent years, many states have confirmed record high numbers of rabies cases in domestic species, such as cats, dogs, horses, and cattle. Although rare, it is possible that you will encounter a rabid animal at the hospital where you work.

It is important that you are aware of the prevalence of rabies and its incidence among wild species in your area, because it varies among different regions of the country. There is a very safe and effective human rabies vaccine that can be administered to people who work in high-risk animal environments, such as a shelter or wild animal rehabilitation center. Ask your hospital administrator about the availability of pre-exposure vaccines at your hospital or workplace.

Bacterial Infections

You may be exposed to a wide variety of pathogenic and non-pathogenic bacteria during your professional life. Examples of pathogenic bacteria include *Salmonella* spp., *Pasteurella* spp., *Escherichia coli*, *Pseudomonas* spp., or resistant *Staphylococcus* spp. The evolution of methicillin-resistant *Staphylococcus pseudointermedius* (MRSP) is causing great concern among public health authorities and health care facilities alike. Bacteria can be transferred through direct contact with animals and their exudates. This is particularly likely if you have any cuts or open sores. Some bacteria may be aerosolized and inhaled or absorbed through mucous membranes. The best protection against exposure to bacteria is simply good personal hygiene. Always follow the personal hygiene rules as discussed later in this chapter.

Lyme disease is a serious concern for animals and people. When an infected deer tick bites a host (an animal or person) to feed, the bacterium *Borrelia burgdorferi* is transferred to the host. Lyme disease in humans is characterized by aches in the joints, fever, and a host of other flulike symptoms. The best defense against this disease is to check oneself daily for ticks and remove them promptly. If you work in a food animal or mixed animal hospital, it is a good idea to use an insect repellent when you go out into fields or woods to work.

Fungal Infections

Contrary to its name, **ringworm** is not a parasite or a worm. It is an infection of the skin caused by a fungus known as *Microsporum* spp. and is easily passed between animals and humans. Cats and horses are particularly susceptible to ringworm infection. The most effective protection from ringworm infection is to wear gloves when handling or treating animals diagnosed with the condition and to practice good personal hygiene. Be especially careful about preventing contamination of your clothing when treating patients with *Microsporum* spp. because it is believed that fungal spores can be carried to other locations (e.g., your home) on clothing and can infect other animals or other people.

Internal Parasites

When the eggs of common internal parasites, such as canine or feline roundworms, infect humans, they usually do not mature into adult parasites, but they do cause other problems. Roundworm larvae can migrate to virtually any organ in the body and develop into a cystlike growth known as *visceral larval migrans*. These "cysts" usually are not clinically noticeable unless they develop in a vital organ; for example, in the eye, they can do permanent damage to the retina and cause blindness. Puppies almost always have some level of roundworm infestation, because passage of worms from the adult female to the fetus occurs through the placenta and via lactation. When the infected puppy defecates in soil, roundworm eggs can survive for long periods until they are picked up and ingested by another mammal.

Another common internal parasite, hookworms, can also cause problems in humans by a condition known as *cutaneous larval migrans*. This condition is particularly prevalent in the southern areas of the United States, where winters are warm and humid. Unlike the visceral cysts from roundworms, *cutaneous larval migrans* is relatively easy to spot. This appears as small red lines in the regions where the parasite from the soil has burrowed into the skin. These marks are often itchy and lengthen as the parasite moves subcutaneously from one part of the body to another.

Protozoal Infections

Infestation with a protozoan known as *Toxoplasma gondii* is called *toxoplasmosis*. Although it is usually not harmful to most adults, this event can have devastating effects on the development of a human fetus by causing hydrocephalus and intellectual disability. Immature *Toxoplasma* eggs are shed in the feces of infected cats and sporulate approximately 2 to 4 days later. Three-day-old sporulated oocysts—if ingested by a pregnant woman—are particularly dangerous to her fetus. Pregnant women working in a veterinary hospital can reduce potential exposure to *Toxoplasma* by avoiding cat litter pans when possible, particularly those that contain feces older than 2 days. If cleaning litter pans is unavoidable, wear gloves when handling the litter box and wash your hands when you are finished. Women working in the veterinary professions are encouraged to discuss *Toxoplasma* titers with their physician before and during pregnancy.

Other zoonotic protozoal agents, such as **Giardia** and **coccidia**, may cause diarrhea and gastrointestinal cramping in humans. They are typically spread to humans through contact with infected animals (particularly puppies and kittens), but they can also be acquired by drinking contaminated water. Good personal hygiene is the best defense against these infections.

External Parasites

The irritating and itchy mite that causes **sarcoptic mange** can spread easily to humans from animals. Typically, this occurs in regions where clothing is tight, such as along bra lines and waistbands. When treating animal patients for mange, always wear gloves and a gown and wash your hands thoroughly with disinfecting soap immediately after the procedure.

Nonzoonotic Diseases

Some infectious diseases, such as **parvoviral enteritis** in dogs and **panleukopenia** in cats, are not a serious concern for human health, but these conditions are so highly contagious that you can carry the live virus home to your pets on your clothes and shoes. For this reason, some technicians who have worked with animals with parvoviral infection leave their shoes outside the front door and change their clothes immediately upon entering the home; some even change clothes before they leave the hospital. When treating patients with contagious diseases, be sure to:

- Wear PPE, such as an apron, a surgical mask, examination gloves and, when appropriate, eye protection.
- Thoroughly wash your hands with a disinfecting agent, such as chlorhexidine or povidone-iodine scrub, at completion of treatment.
- Change your clothes before handling your own animals.

Because you are likely to encounter infectious disease agents in your duties, particular attention to personal hygiene and sanitary work practices is especially important. Good personal hygiene includes making sure clothing is not soiled by chemicals or biological material and, of course, performing regular hand washing. In general, you should wash your hands at the following times:
1. After handling medications, laboratory samples or chemicals
2. After treating patients or cleaning cages
3. Before and after you use the restroom
4. Before eating
5. Before you leave work at the end of your shift

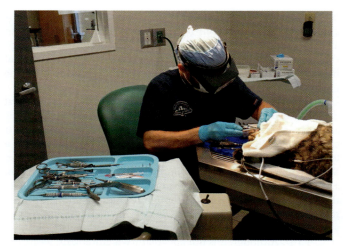

• **Fig. 4.13** Always wear eye protection, a mask, and gloves when performing dental prophylactic procedures.

A Dirty Mouth? Precautions for Dentistry Operations

Dental procedures that include use of high-speed or ultrasonic scalers aerosolize oral microbes, making personal protection a necessity. One of the most common pathogens in the mouths of animals is *Pasteurella multocida*, an organism that has been linked to cardiac and pulmonary problems in humans and animals alike.

When performing any procedures in the mouth of an animal, always do the following:
- Wear goggles, protective glasses, or a face shield to reduce the amount of splatter or spray that gets on your face and in your eyes (Fig. 4.13).
- Wear gloves to prevent opportunistic pathogens from gaining entry to your body through cuts or scrapes on your hands.
- Wear a tightly woven surgical mask that covers both your nose and mouth to prevent inhaling the spatter and aerosols.
- Wear a cap and a long-sleeved smock or gown that you can remove after the procedure to reduce the amount of spatter that winds up on your clothing.
- Stay an arm's length away from the animal's mouth. Avoid getting your face too close.
- Clean all instruments and wipe the tables and machines with a disinfecting detergent at the conclusion of the procedure before removing your protective gloves.
- Be sure to wash your hands, forearms, and even your face after the procedure.

Radiology

The ability to "see inside the body" is a great tool in medicine. In most cases, the method of choice is diagnostic radiography. Short-duration, infrequent exposure to x-ray radiation, such as having a radiograph taken of yourself, is considered an acceptable level of exposure (the benefits outweigh the risks). However, long-term exposure to low doses of radiation has been linked to many medical disorders. High-dose exposure can cause skin changes, cell damage, and gastrointestinal and bone marrow disorders that can be fatal. Fortunately, you can protect yourself while using this tool in your duties. By following simple safety precautions and adhering to the ALARA (As Low

As Reasonably Achievable) principle, you can safely use radiographic equipment in your hospital. These precautions apply to all radiographic operations—even digital procedures. Although the image is "captured" by a receptor plate instead of chemical film in a digital operation, the x-rays that are produced by the machine are the same!

Although modern radiographic machines, including digital devices, have many safeguards integrated into their design, they all emit x-ray radiation, so it is essential to protect yourself against exposure. When you are performing radiography, *always* wear a lead apron if you must be in the room when the exposure is made. When you must be near the primary beam to restrain or position a patient for a radiograph, you must also wear protective gloves that cover your entire hand. Although restraint of animals during radiographic studies can be challenging, never place any part of your body, even a gloved hand, in the path of the primary beam (Fig. 4.14). Although it is not a regulatory requirement, wearing a thyroid shield is also recommended.

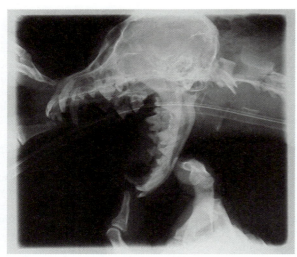

• **Fig. 4.14** Never place your hand or any other part of your body in the primary beam when taking radiographs.

CASE PRESENTATION 4.2

A 40-year-old veterinary technician noticed dark-colored spots that were not typical aging spots on her hands. Her dermatologist diagnosed her with skin cancer. It was later determined that the cancer was a type that is typically associated with exposure to radiation.

An investigation into the case revealed that the technician had worked at various veterinary hospitals and even in a research facility throughout her career. In most of these positions, her duties included exposing and processing radiographs. Because the technician was "small in size," she found the protective gloves used for the procedure bulky and cumbersome. Therefore she most often chose to restrain patients without using gloves. At one job in a mixed animal hospital, she even held the cassette for lameness evaluation with her bare hand. Her desire to help patients without regard for her own safety was compounded by the perpetual "hurry up and get it done" attitude, which unfortunately is prevalent in veterinary practice.

In this case, the damage was not evident and no physical pain had been experienced at the time of exposure; the technician therefore assumed that the practice of taking radiographs without gloves was safe. Her failure to follow the instructions given when she was a technician student and during the continual safety training throughout her career was the primary cause of her incurable condition.

Before you operate an x-ray machine, make sure you know the purpose of every knob and button. Always use the collimator to restrict the primary beam to a size smaller than the size of the cassette—in other words, "cone down" to the area to be radiographed so that scatter radiation is minimized. A properly collimated radiograph shows a well-defined border around the image inside of the cassette or receptor plate's maximum size.

To eliminate unnecessary exposure to radiation, do it right the first time! Always follow the written operational and safety procedures provided by the hospital or the machine manufacturer. If you have not already done so, create an exposure chart specific to your machine so that you can replicate the best techniques for various studies. By following a proven technique chart and positioning the patient correctly the first time, the number of "retakes" and thus unnecessary exposure can be reduced.

Portable machines, such as those used in dental procedures and large animal or mobile operations, can be particularly dangerous because of their multipurpose uses. These machines can be aimed in any direction and, because of their limited power, they must use longer exposure times to produce diagnostic images. When using a portable machine, always make sure no one is in the path of the primary beam (even at a distance). Always use a cassette-holding pole and never hold a cassette or receptor plate with your hands—even with gloves—while the exposure is being made. Remember to wear a lead apron and gloves when near the machine during exposure.

If you are involved in the exposure portion of radiography, you must have and use an individual dosimetry badge. This badge is worn on your collar outside your protective apron during any radiographic procedures. It is important to return the badge to the designated storage location (outside the radiography area) when it is not being used. Unless you are taking radiographs "in the field," do not wear your badge outside, because exposure to sunlight will result in false readings. As a result of the relatively low numbers of radiographs taken in most practices, the availability of safer machines, and the use of good protective equipment, most technicians receive little, if any, occupational exposure to radiation.

Although digital radiology is fast becoming the standard in veterinary hospitals, procedures that use films and chemicals (developer and fixer) are still common enough that you may encounter them in your career. Those chemicals can be corrosive to materials and organic tissues, so use PPE, such as gloves and goggles, when mixing and pouring the chemicals. When using manual processing, stir the chemicals with care and avoid splashing. After handling radiographic developing chemicals, always wash your hands. It is important to avoid breathing in the fumes from processing chemicals, so make sure that there is adequate ventilation in the darkroom; an exhaust fan is usually necessary.

Radiographic developing solutions can react dangerously with other chemicals. For this reason, never pour chemicals down the drain used for developing solution. When mixed with developer solutions, some liquid drain openers can produce toxic gases. Others can produce extreme heat from exothermic reactions and can damage pipes.

Anesthesia

Anesthesia is as common to veterinary medicine as antiseptic wound care, so we sometimes become overly comfortable with the procedure. Although modern inhalation aesthetics are much safer for our patients, long-term exposure to **waste anesthetic gases (WAGs)**, as is possible when one works with the machines on a regular basis, has been linked to congenital abnormalities, spontaneous abortions, and even liver and kidney damage. The National Institute of Occupational Safety and Health (NIOSH) estimates that more than 250,000 workers in the United States may be at risk for exposure to WAGs, primarily from unmetabolized gas exhaled by recovering patients, poor work practices such as disconnecting the patient from the machine without first turning off the flow of gas, and from leaks in the anesthetic circuit during the procedure.

Using a proper scavenging system is the single most effective means of reducing exposure to WAGs in the operating room. There are three general types of scavenging systems available: active scavenging, passive exhaust, and absorption. Each has a place but rarely does one method fit all circumstances, so it is common to have several styles available for different anesthetic scenarios. Regardless of the system used, make sure it is properly connected and fully operational before turning on the anesthesia machine. If you use absorption canisters, be sure to check them (by weighing with a gram scale) before each procedure, because once the canister becomes saturated with gas, it is ineffective. Replace adsorber canisters before they gain the maximum amount of weight designated by the manufacturer (typically 50 g).

According to some research findings, as much as 90% of the anesthetic gas levels found in the room during a procedure can be attributed to leaks in the anesthesia machine, so be sure to perform a leak check before use. Refer to Chapter 30 for instructions on checking the anesthesia machine for leaks. Also, make sure that correctly sized hoses and rebreathing bags are used. Intubation tubes should be placed and the cuff inflated before the animal is connected to the anesthesia machine. Start the flow of the anesthetic gases only after the patient is connected to the machine. When the surgical procedure is finished, turn off the vaporizer and increase the flow of oxygen to the patient. Be sure to use the "flush" feature to purge the circuit before disconnecting the machine.

Before filling the vaporizer, move the anesthesia machine to a well-ventilated area. Use a pouring funnel or adapter and be careful to avoid overfilling the vaporizer or spilling the liquid anesthetic. If you accidentally break a bottle of anesthetic or spill more than a few milliliters of liquid, immediately evacuate all nonessential people from the area. Any windows in the area should be opened, and exhaust fans should be turned on to evacuate the room air as efficiently as possible. Quickly control the spread of any liquid by pouring a generous amount of cat litter on the spill and placing a plastic bag over it to reduce evaporation. Pick up the cat litter that has absorbed the liquid by using a dustpan and place the cat litter inside a plastic garbage bag. Seal the bag tightly and dispose of it in an outside trash can. Leave the exhaust fans on and the windows open until you are sure the gas level has been reduced to a safe level.

Protocols that deliver the anesthetic agent to the patient via a mask or tank for induction are more likely to generate a larger quantity of WAGs. Since they are difficult to scavenge properly, they are not recommended as a primary or frequent method to induce anesthesia. When these protocols must be used, be sure to use an appropriate flow rate and a proper reservoir bag for the size of the patient—do *not* turn up the oxygen flowmeter to maximum when masking a patient. Induction chambers should always be connected to an active or passive scavenging system; adsorption canisters are not a good choice for tank inductions, because the flow rates will not allow adequate contact time in the canister to absorb the gas. For both processes, make sure that general ventilation in the room is adequate and use exhaust fans when available.

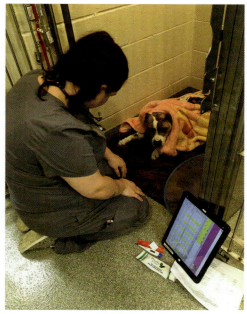

• **Fig. 4.15** Monitor recovering anesthesia patients "at arm's length" to minimize exposure to gases emitted during respiration.

> **TECHNICIAN NOTE**
> The OSHA-recognized safe exposure limit for all halogenated anesthetic agents, including isoflurane and sevoflurane, is less than 2 parts per million (ppm).

Anesthetized animals do not metabolize all the anesthetic gas that they have inhaled. They exhale some of it into the room after they have been extubated and while they are recovering. When monitoring patients during their recovery, you should avoid putting your face close to the animal's face (Fig. 4.15). In addition, keep the number of recovering patients at an acceptable number, based on the size of the area and the capability of the ventilation system. For as long as possible, delay extubating and allow the patient to partially recover while still connected to the anesthesia machine (oxygen only) and the scavenging system.

When changing the soda lime (carbon dioxide absorbent) in anesthesia machines, wear rubber or latex gloves. When the soda lime is wet, as is often the case from humidity in the system, it can be caustic to tissues and some metals. Dispose of used soda lime granules in a plastic trash bag as regular trash.

You can also test your exposure level to waste gases during procedures using a badge similar to the one used in radiology. Testing exposure levels on a regular basis is expected in workplace safety regulations.

> **TECHNICIAN NOTE**
> In anesthetized animals, not all of the inhaled anesthetic gas is metabolized. The animals exhale some of it into the room after they have been extubated and while they are recovering.

Compressed Gases

Every year, hundreds of workers are injured while working with compressed gas cylinders, such as those we use for oxygen and medical gases, usually because of improper storage or handling of the cylinders. Regardless of the size of the cylinder or whether the

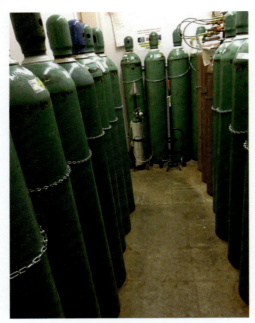

• **Fig. 4.16** All compressed gas cylinders, including small-sized tanks, must be secured to prevent them from falling over.

cylinder is empty, full, or in use, store cylinders in a dry, cool place away from potential heat sources, such as furnaces, water heaters, and direct sunlight. Always secure the tanks, even small ones, in an upright position by means of a chain, strap, or holder to prevent them from falling and causing physical injury (Fig. 4.16). Cylinders that are stored inside a closet should also be secured, because they can fall against the door, causing injury when the door is opened. If cylinders are equipped with a protective cap, it must be firmly screwed in place when the cylinder is not in use. If you must move a large cylinder, do not roll or drag it; always use a hand truck or a handcart and remember to strap the tank to the cart to prevent it from falling.

Sharps and Medical Waste

The most obvious hazards from needles or sharp objects are from punctures and lacerations and the associated bacterial infections, but the most serious danger is from exposure to the drug or chemical in the needle. To prevent these types of accidents, follow these tips:

- Always keep sharps, needles, scalpel blades, and other sharp instruments capped or sheathed until ready for use.
- Do not attempt to recap the needle after use unless the physical danger from sticks or lacerations cannot be prevented by any other means.
- When possible, place the entire needle/syringe unit in a sharps container immediately after use.
- Never throw needles or sharps directly into regular trash containers, regardless of whether they are capped.
- When it is necessary to recap a needle, you should use the "one-handed" method (Procedure 4.3). Although some practice is needed before the one-handed method becomes second nature, it is the safest and most practical approach for most veterinary situations.
- Do not remove the needle from the syringe for disposal, because this unnecessary handling often results in injury.

- Do not overfill a sharps container—when it is full, it is full! When the sharps container is full, seal it and replace it with a new one. Likewise, you should not collect sharps in a smaller container and transfer them to a larger container for disposal.
- Never open a sharps container that has already been sealed or stick your fingers into one for any reason.
- Do not destroy the needle by bending, cutting, or grinding before disposal, because that may aerosolize the contents of the needle, increasing your exposure.

"Medical waste" refers to waste materials generated in the treatment or testing of animals or humans that may be contaminated with a pathogen that can still infect humans.

Table 4.1 explains which materials are usually considered medical waste and which are not. Although this chart is essentially accurate, some states have special rules for discarding medical waste, so be sure to follow the rules prescribed by your state or province.

Hazardous Drugs and Pharmacy Operations

Medicines are designed to cure diseases and make patients better, but it is important to remember that nearly all medicines are chemicals, and chemicals can be dangerous. In the veterinary pharmacy, you can be exposed to all kinds of drugs just by handling them. Liquids can splash in your eyes when you pour them, or they can release vapors that you may inhale. Handling, crushing, or breaking tablets can leave powder residue on your hands that will be ingested the next time you put your hands near your mouth or mucous membranes.

No matter what the drug is, the biggest rule to remember when handling any medication is to practice good personal hygiene, especially thorough hand washing. Avoid counting pills by pouring them in your hand. Cleaning the tray between uses will also help prevent cross contamination of medications.

Some animal medications can be very toxic to humans. When you are handling drugs like chloramphenicol, misoprostol, strong hormones, and others designated by the safety officer, you should always wear disposable examination gloves and wipe the outside of the drug vial after using it to remove residue. The labels of bottles containing hazardous medications should also be clearly identified and the products segregated in a designated place in the pharmacy.

Some drugs, such as cytotoxic drugs (CDs) used to treat patients with cancer, are so potent that even very small exposures can cause harm. Always store CDs in a closed cabinet or container so that cross contamination is minimized. Never eat food or snacks; drink water, soda or coffee; chew gum; smoke cigarettes; or apply cosmetics or personal care products (such as lip balm) in areas where CDs are used or stored.

When preparing CDs for patient administration, always wear powder-free chemotherapy gloves, a disposable apron or gown that is not used for any other purpose, a tightly woven surgical mask, and eye protection. The use of a closed-system transfer device (CSTD) to draw up CDs has become the expectation in both veterinary and human medical situations. Even with the use of a CSTD, OSHA requires the use of a biological safety cabinet (BSC) for the preparation of CDs (Fig. 4.17).

When handling or cleaning up after patients that have received chemotherapeutic treatments, remember that some drugs are excreted in bodily fluids, so it is important to always wear powder-free chemotherapy gloves and dispose of them into yellow chemo waste containers when finished. Be sure to follow all instructions on the SDS, on the package insert, and in your practice's chemotherapy safety plan. Refer to Chapter 20, "Veterinary Oncology," for additional information regarding the safe use and handling of chemotherapeutic drugs.

PROCEDURE 4.3

One-Handed Needle Recapping

Step 1. Place the cap on a flat surface, such as a countertop, and carefully slide the needle into the cap.

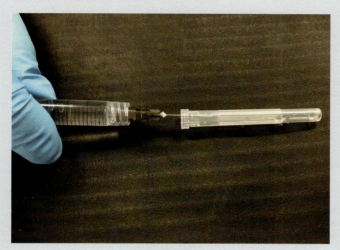

• Fig. 4.18

Step 2. Slowly raise the tip of the syringe, allowing the cap to cover the full length of the needle.

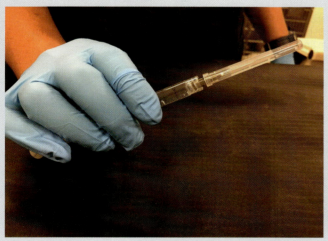

• Fig. 4.19

Step 3. Raise the tip of the syringe until the cap falls and fully covers the needle.

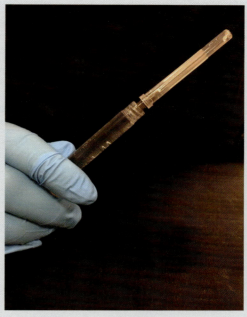

• Fig. 4.20

Step 4. Finally, use your other hand to securely "seat" the cap.

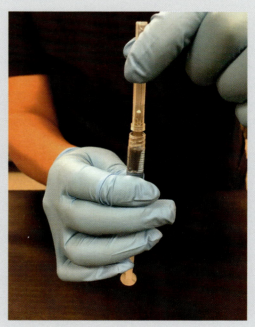

• Fig. 4.21

TABLE 4.1   **Typical Medical Waste Definitions**

Material	Medical Waste	Normal Trash
Sharps (any device with characteristics that make it possible to puncture, lacerate, or penetrate the skin)	Any used needles and scalpel blades Glass or hard plastic that is contaminated with a *human disease*–causing agent	Glass or hard plastic that is not contaminated with *human disease*–causing agents can be disposed of as normal waste
Medical devices, such as blood tubes, vials, catheters, intravenous tubes, etc.	Considered biomedical waste only when they contain *human* pathogens or they have been used for chemotherapy	Devices that simply contain or are contaminated with animal blood (except from primates); normally not considered biomedical waste
Animal blood or tissues	Only dead animals or animal parts that are infected with zoonotic diseases; include but are not limited to rabies, brucellosis, systemic fungal diseases, tuberculosis, and atypical mycobacteriosis	Tissues from routine surgical procedures (castration, ovariohysterectomy, etc.); should be considered regular waste
Laboratory cultures	Microbiological cultures (bacterial, fungal, or viral) of *human* pathogens; considered biomedical waste	In some cases, culture media from negative tests; may be considered regular trash but probably wise to just classify all laboratory cultures as biomedical waste for simplicity
Bandages/sponges	Used absorbent materials, such as bandages, gauze, or sponges that are saturated with blood or body fluids that contain *human* pathogens that may splash or drip	Sponges or bandages used on animals not infected with a disease transmissible to humans
Primate materials		Normal waste generated from work on primates; considered regular waste *unless it fits into another category* (e.g., from research studies using human pathogens)
Animal waste	Waste from animals with an infection that is contagious to *humans* and can be transmitted by means of the waste; waste from chemotherapy patients for up to 48 hours after the last treatment	Normal waste from animals not infected with *human disease*–causing agents; should be disposed of as regular trash

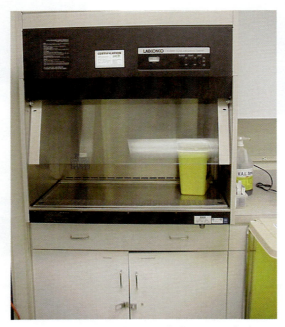

• **Fig. 4.17** A biological safety cabinet is required when cytotoxic drugs are prepared.

Summary

In this chapter, we have discussed the hazards associated with your career and the actions you should take to protect yourself. We all face dangers in life, but that does not mean we have to place ourselves in unnecessary danger to get our job done. Strive to find the balance between getting the job done, being productive, and staying safe. Safety is not something that will keep you from doing your job—it should be the reason you can stay in your career for a long time.

Internet Resources/Recommended Reading

Canadian Centre for Occupational Health & Safety: www.ccohs.ca
Centers for Disease Control and Prevention: www.cdc.gov
Department of Labor: www.dol.gov
Environmental Protection Agency: www.epa.gov
Infection Control Today: www.infectioncontroltoday.com

National Institute of Occupational Safety and Health (NIOSH): www.cdc.gov/niosh
OSHA: www.osha.gov
SafetyVet: www.safetyvet.com
The Veterinary Information Network (VIN): www.vin.com/vin
The Veterinary Support Personnel Network (VSPN): www.vn.com/vspn/default.aspx
The Virtual Anesthesia Machine: http://vam.anest.ufl.edu/

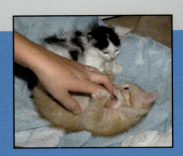

5

Animal Behavior

MONIQUE FEYRECILDE

LEARNING OBJECTIVES

When you have completed this chapter, you will be able to:

1. Pronounce, spell, and define all key terms in the chapter.
2. Explain why behavior problems can be life threatening to pets.
3. Summarize the veterinary technician's role in supporting behavioral health.
4. Describe how and when learning occurs in animals.
5. Understand the mechanisms and possible applications for:
   - Classical conditioning and counterconditioning
   - Desensitization
   - Operant conditioning
   - Applied behavior analysis
6. Recognize and protect against common problems with the use of punishment.
7. Understand the role of animal development in animal behavior.
8. Describe, identify, and respond to body language signals of canine, feline, equine, bovine, and small ruminant patients.
9. Understand and counsel clients and fellow professionals in meeting the behavioral and social needs of animals in their care.
10. Recognize how to prevent and screen for the three most common unwanted behaviors in dogs and cats.
11. Recognize common behavior concerns in equine, bovine, and small ruminant patients.
12. Identify and immediately triage behavior emergencies in canine, feline, equine, and ruminant patients.
13. Describe how patients learn in the veterinary setting, and what technicians can do to influence the learning experience.
14. Define the fundamentals of Fear Free veterinary care for canine and feline patients.
    - Determine a numeric fear, anxiety, and stress (FAS) score.
    - Apply considerate approach before and during patient interactions and handling.
    - Use Touch Gradient to create a more relaxed and safer handling experience.
    - Describe the use of gentle control to stabilize and restrain patients.
    - Describe what information should be included in Emotional Medical Records.

KEY TERMS

Aggression
Allogrooming
Antecedent
Anthropomorphism
Anxiety
Backward conditioning
Behavior
Body language
Buller steer syndrome
Classical conditioning
Compassion
Consequence
Considerate approach
Conspecific
Counterconditioning
Diplomate of the American College of Veterinary Behaviorists
Displacement behaviors
Delay conditioning
Desensitization
Diagnosis
Emotional Medical Record
FAS
Fear
Fear, anxiety, and stress (FAS)
Fear-related aggression
Fear Free

Gentle control
Gregarious
Habituation
Negative punishment
Negative reinforcement
Nostrils
Operant conditioning
Play-related aggression
Pheromone
Phobia
Positive punishment
Positive reinforcement
Punishment
Reinforcement
Repetitive behavior
Sensitization
Simultaneous conditioning
Socialization
Stress
Touch Gradient
Trace conditioning
Unconditioned response
Unwanted behaviors
Unwanted elimination
Veterinary technician specialists
Zoonosis

Introduction to Behavior and Motivation

Understanding the behavior of animals, including humans, is crucial to the success of every veterinary professional. Animals exhibit behaviors for a reason, and every behavior has a "function," from the perspective of the individual. In other words, animals "do what works for them." The function of a behavior may be improving social ties, remaining safe, decreasing stress, increasing access to food or reproductive opportunities, increasing or decreasing distance from a social interaction, experiencing feelings of enjoyment, tactile pleasure, etc. Individual behaviors can also have more than one function. Recognizing the difference between normal and abnormal behaviors, being familiar with how animals learn, understanding basic prevention strategies, and knowing how to apply common behavior modification methods for animal learning are key skills needed by the veterinary technician.

Every animal should be allowed to display and engage in species-normal behavior. However, some clients find normal behaviors objectionable. This chapter serves as an introduction to animal behavior, behavioral wellness, and the role of the veterinary team in recognizing and changing adverse animal behavior in the veterinary environment and in the home. Animal behavior is relevant to veterinary medicine in general. More than half the pet owners surveyed reported unwanted behaviors as the cause for surrendering their pet to a shelter. In this way, unwanted behaviors can damage and even sever the human-animal bond. In addition, without veterinary care, animals may suffer and/or be considered unsuitable and euthanized. By practicing behaviorally aware medicine, veterinary professionals can steward and nurture the human-animal bond, improving overall wellness in pets and their owners. Many unwanted behaviors are normal for the species but may be objectionable to humans. Some behaviors, such as human-directed **aggression** or interanimal aggression, present a particular risk to the life of the animal. In addition, many pet owners report concern that their pet will experience undue stress during veterinary appointments. This concern sometimes prevents owners, particularly cat owners, from seeking veterinary care for their pets. Being aware of potential animal stressors, helping families prevent and respond appropriately to unwanted animal behaviors, and helping animals adjust to the challenges of their home life will help keep families and their pets together. In this way, providing low-stress veterinary care is critically important and will ensure that pets and their owners keep coming back.

Animals do not use speech to communicate with humans. Therefore veterinary professionals must rely on their understanding of animal development, nonverbal communication, prevention and intervention strategies, motivation of behavior, and learning theory to help promote and maintain a positive human-animal bond between clients and their pets. In this way, veterinary professionals can help keep animals safe. Anthropomorphism (attributing human characteristics to nonhuman animals or objects) presents a significant risk to animal welfare. When people label animal personality or motivation with such terms as *mean, fractious, angry,* or *difficult,* these labels may preclude accurate interpretation of an animal's behavior. Working with animals requires keen observation skills. Veterinary technicians need to watch for behaviors that can be both observed and quantified so that such behaviors may be addressed. Attempting to determine what the animal is thinking and define its behavior by using human labels (i.e., anthropomorphizing) can lead to errors in the understanding and management of cases of problematic veterinary behaviors. Some material in this chapter is devoted to changing adverse emotional responses in animals. Interpreting these emotional responses relies on the use of clearly defined, well-developed tools for observing, correctly interpreting, and effectively responding to animal body language.

Animal experiences, particularly those associated with **fear**, **anxiety**, and **stress**, affect both the animals' behavior and clients' future decision making. Fear and stress are adaptive. These feelings keep animals safe by helping them avoid dangerous situations. Fear and stress can also enhance memory consolidation; that is, when the animal is stressed, detailed and long-lasting memories will be formed. Stress also decreases memory retrieval: during times of stress, it is difficult for animals to think clearly and make rational decisions, much as it is for people. Diminishing stress, fear, and anxiety should be the primary objective for anyone who works with and handles animals, both for the welfare of the animals and for the safety of those who work with them.

Every animal is an individual entity, with a unique combination of genetics and experience contributing to how it responds to stimuli, makes decisions, takes action, and engages with or avoids situations. Genetics play an important role in animal behavior and personality. Each animal has certain genetic predispositions, including innate behavioral tendencies. **Socialization**, training, and behavior modification will never cause an animal to "out-run" or exceed what is possible based on its best genetic potential. However, lack of proper socialization, training, and behavior modification can prevent any animal from achieving its own personal best. When working with animals, it may be impossible for the veterinary workers to differentiate between qualities intrinsic to the animal and those that are the result of environmental influences. One must always assume that clients are doing their best and resist the urge to pass judgment on a client's efforts. All animals learn by the same methods, and consistent use of positive reinforcement works with humans and animals. All involved in the care of animals are on the same team dedicated to improving animal welfare by protecting and strengthening the human-animal bond. Supporting colleagues and clients is crucial to fulfilling this important mission.

> **TECHNICIAN NOTE**
>
> Diminishing patient fear and stress is an important primary objective for every veterinary professional.

The Roles of Professionals in Behavior

Veterinarians and Behavior

Veterinarians are responsible for diagnosing medical conditions that may affect an animal's behavior. They are also responsible for diagnosing, prescribing medications, generating and delineating treatment plans, and performing all surgical procedures. Many veterinarians who work in general practice have taken advanced continuing education classes in the field of animal behavior and therefore are qualified to diagnose and treat behavior disorders. Veterinary behavior is a recognized specialty for both veterinarians and veterinary technicians. Veterinarians with the designation **Diplomate of the American College of Veterinary Behaviorists** (DACVB) have completed a formal residency and passed a rigorous examination process. **Veterinary technician specialists** (VTSs) in Behavior have also completed advanced continuing education and have demonstrated extensive knowledge and skill by passing a stringent professional examination that is administered by the Academy of Veterinary Behavior Technicians. Veterinarians in general practice are responsible for assessing their own competence in treating a particular case. Patients requiring care beyond the level of skill offered by a practitioner should be referred to a DACVB. Because veterinarians who specialize in behavior are still relatively uncommon, the behavior specialists often provide veterinarian-to-veterinarian remote consultations to assist with patient management and treatment. Table 5.1 provides helpful resources for veterinarians and veterinary technicians seeking to advance their training in animal behavior management.

Veterinary Technicians and Behavior

Veterinary technicians cannot make diagnoses. By law, only veterinarians can establish a **diagnosis**. Therefore determining whether a cat that is urinating outside the litter box has a urinary tract

TABLE 5.1 Additional Resources for Veterinary Teams

AVBT: The Academy of Veterinary Behavior Technicians—www.avbt.net
SVBT: The Society of Veterinary Behavior Technicians—www.svbt.org
ACVB: American College of Veterinary Behaviorists—www.dacvb.org
AVSAB: American Veterinary Society of Animal Behavior—www.avsab.org

disorder or a behavioral elimination disorder is the exclusive responsibility of the veterinarian. However, diagnosis, prescribing, and surgical intervention represent only a small part of what patients need when they are ill.

Veterinary technicians are not only skilled in caring for patients, but they also serve as patient and owner advocates. Indeed, medical and surgical tasks other than surgery, diagnosis, prognosis, and attesting to health status for veterinary patients are best completed by veterinary technicians.

Tasks completed by veterinary technicians in behavior are as follows:

- Consulting with families regarding preacquisition guidelines
- Triaging incoming patients and assessing emergencies and high-risk cases
- Collecting detailed behavior histories from pet owners who report unwanted or abnormal behaviors
- Reviewing behavior histories with the veterinarian
- Providing client education to improve patient outcomes and to meet the basic needs of animals by ensuring that:
  - pets receive appropriate preventive medicine
  - medication and home-care instructions are carried out as prescribed
- Screening pets and situations for risk factors for unwanted behaviors
- Collecting all laboratory samples and analyzing them, when appropriate, and reporting the results to the veterinarian
- Educating clients about the diagnosis and prescribed treatment plan
- Discussing prescribed medications and relevant drug interactions with the client
- Determining the best way to administer medications and educating clients on proper administration
- Demonstrating behavior modification protocols and coaching clients on proper implementation
- Demonstrating training protocols and coaching clients on appropriate techniques for success
- Assisting clients with implementing management strategies
- Acting as a "case manager" or client liaison among the client, the veterinarian, and all other professionals involved in the case
- Assisting in the evaluation of nonveterinary referral professionals (trainers, etc.)
- Providing emotional support for families before, during, and after treatment
- Providing grief support in cases where the human-animal bond has been severed

On occasion, there is overlap between roles. For instance, many technicians and veterinarians are also skilled and certified in training or consultation regarding animal behavior. However, nurses, trainers, consultants, and animal behaviorists must all be stringent in maintaining their integrity by staying within their own scopes of practice.

TECHNICIAN NOTE

Advocate for every one of your patients while staying within the scope of practice for veterinary technicians.

Behavior Consultants and Trainers and Behavior

There is little regulation in the training and consulting business for animals. Although there are multiple certifications, such as Certified Applied Animal Behaviorist (CAAB) for those with a PhD in Applied Animal Behavior and Applied Animal Behaviorist (AAB) for those with a master's degree, there is no external regulation regarding what consultants and trainers may or may not do (aside from those tasks restricted to veterinarians by law). The term *behaviorist* is used by many professionals with varying skill sets, but the term *veterinary behaviorist* is restricted to veterinarians who are DACVBs. Behavior consultants may coach clients in implementing behavior modification and training plans. Trainers assist families by teaching clients how to train animals to perform behaviors consistent with what the family requires and what the animal deserves and needs. Trainers often offer both group classes and individual coaching sessions, whereas consultants and behaviorists usually work on a one-on-one basis with a family.

Every veterinary team needs a "referral village," including behavior consultants and trainers. The veterinarian, the veterinary technician, the consultant, and the trainer all fulfill different roles to assist animals and their owners in working together. A veterinarian may make a diagnosis and prescribe a behavior modification plan and medications. The veterinary technicians may work out the details of the plan, educate the client on administering medications, and establish a specific strategy for implementing the plan. The veterinary technician frequently provides ongoing support and instruction. The consultant may provide in-home, hands-on coaching to further the client's understanding of the modification plan, whereas a trainer works to give the client and the animal specific skills. The veterinary team is obligated to verify that the referred professionals use methods that are safe, appropriate, and effective, and have low risk of fallout for both the client and the animal. When assessing trainers and consultants, it is important to directly observe the individual's skills, aptitude, understanding, and values. In addition, veterinary team members should investigate the education, certification, and experience of consultants and trainers and observe them at their workplace. Table 5.2 provides guidelines that will help veterinary professionals evaluate consultants, behaviorists, and trainers prior to referral.

How Animals Learn

All animals, including humans, learn via the same basic principles. The effectiveness of animal learning is dictated by what they feel, what they experience, their decision-making ability, and their specific behavior patterns. Because behavior is such a critical factor in the success of the human-animal relationship, every technician should understand the basics of the science of learning to help create the best possible outcomes both during veterinary visits and during family life at home. The success of behavior modification and training is the result of aligning the animal's behavior and the human's expectation. This process often requires modifying both factors: human expectations *and* an animal's behaviors. Both expectation and behavior are fluid and subject to both intentional and accidental change. The animal's emotional state, the environment, the context or situation, and individual learning history will

TABLE 5.2	Factors to Consider When Evaluating Behavior Professionals Prior to Referring Clients

Education and evidence of continuing education

Certifications advertised (if any) are accurate, current, and in good standing

Carries appropriate insurance

No prior charges or convictions for animal-related crimes

Allows and welcomes observation of a class or consultation

Does not guarantee or warrant results

Emphasizes the use of humane methods without causing pain, fear, and distress

Uses primarily positive reinforcement for both animal and human learners

Makes baseline measurements to quantify behavior and refers to these to assess results

Understands and articulates the possible adverse effects of punishment

Does not recommend devices causing pain (prong and choke collars, electric shock devices, etc.)

Sets animals and people up for success (environment, knowledge, planning)

Has excellent client communication skills

Shows good awareness of the emotional state and needs of all animals and responds immediately and appropriately

Provides effective feedback to clients in a way that builds both skills and trust

impact and inform behaviors. The basic concepts discussed in this chapter will encompass classical conditioning, counterconditioning, desensitization, sensitization, habituation, operant conditioning, and the advantages and possible disadvantages of specific methods. These terms are used to **describe** what we observe about animal behavior. None of the techniques or concepts exists in a vacuum: they are all in action at all times. Dividing up concepts for the purpose of discussion allows a better and deeper understanding of the factors in action, but these applied principles overlap and occur simultaneously.

TECHNICIAN NOTE

Learning theory applies to all animals, including humans—we all learn the same way!

Classical Conditioning

Classical conditioning occurs when a learner associates a previously meaningless stimulus with one that already evokes a response. When the meaningless and meaningful stimuli are *paired* over time, the previously meaningless stimulus will evoke the same meaningful response. For example, a leash (previously meaningless) shown to the dog before a walk (exciting stimulus) enough times will often result in the dog showing excitement at the sight of the leash, even before a walk has begun. Box 5.1 provides another example of a classically conditioned response (CR). Classical conditioning results in responses the animal does not

• BOX 5.1	Example of Classical Conditioning to a Pill Bottle

Before Conditioning
Bottle of pills rattles → no response
Bitter pill placed in animal's mouth → Salivation and head shaking

During Conditioning
Bottle of pills rattles → Bitter pill placed in animal's mouth → Salivation and head shaking

Result of Conditioning
Bottle of pills rattles → Salivation and head shaking *without* administration of pill

consciously control, such as emotions, reflexes, and secretions. Classical conditioning is extremely common in veterinary environments and can be either beneficial or detrimental to the patient and the veterinary team. Classical conditioning has a number of deeper complexities not discussed in this chapter, which is intended to provide an introduction to the concept rather than a comprehensive discussion. To learn more about the intricacies of learning theory, refer to the Recommended Readings at the end of this chapter.

Classical conditioning is an excellent technique for conditioning animals to have a positive emotional response to husbandry and veterinary care. Individual animals experience pleasure in their own ways—what is pleasurable is determined by, and only by, the individual animal.

To ensure that the CR is the desired one, it is important to first determine ways to elicit the *desired* CR. How can we prompt the feeling we want the animal to have? Does the animal have a preferred food treat that causes salivation and food seeking, a favorite way to be scratched, a stroke or touch that results in blissful relaxation and soft ears? In these examples, salivation, pleasure, bliss, and relaxation would be the *unconditioned responses* (UR). No training is needed to cause UR—it is intrinsic to the animal. The animal learner is observed carefully to ensure that it is showing the desired response before the trainer moves forward with the conditioning plan. If a piece of chicken is completely uninteresting to a cat, but she purrs and bunts a brush, the learner is communicating that the brush, rather than the chicken, is the more effective conditioning tool at that moment. Once it is determined how the desired UR can be elicited, it can be paired with the goal of a *conditioned stimulus* (CS), such as the sight of nail clippers for grooming. Through this pairing process, the sight of the nail clippers will predict food, tactile stimulus, and so on and eventually the sight of nail clippers alone will elicit the purring and bunting behavior. Purring and bunting in response to the sight of the nail clippers would now be a *CR*.

Injections are a good example of using classical conditioning for the benefit of the patient in the veterinary environment on a daily basis. For patients that have not previously received injections, preparation of the syringe and injection will be meaningless stimuli at first. However, all injections cause at least a small amount of discomfort because of the use of a needle. Patients can quickly be conditioned to show a fear or pain response at the sight of a syringe because of this pairing. By planning a proactive pairing sequence, veterinary technicians can minimize unwanted conditioning and maximize desired conditioning.

Present syringe and touch injection site → Provide pleasurable experience (food, preferred touching, such as pat or a scratch) → Animal experiences pleasure
Repeat
Present syringe and touch injection site, inject → Provide pleasurable experience (food, preferred touching, such as pat or a scratch) during injection → Animal experiences pleasure
Future response
Present syringe, and touch injection site → Animal shows anticipation of pleasurable food, scratching, etc.

In some situations, proactive pairing in a rapid sequence is insufficient, or the animal may have a preexisting fear of injections.

Desensitization and Counterconditioning

Counterconditioning is an interventional technique to *replace* an existing CR. For example, if a dog sees the nail clippers and runs away to hide behind the sofa, counterconditioning would be used to *replace* the conditioned fear response with a different response, such as anticipating food treats. However, patients that are undergoing counterconditioning, by definition, already have an unwanted CR to the stimulus, such as the dog that runs away in fear at the sight of the nail clippers. The nail clippers would need to be introduced gradually during the retraining process to allow the response to be changed more efficiently and effectively. Gradually introducing a stimulus to a learner such that the learner does not respond to it is a form of classical conditioning called desensitization.

Desensitization involves identifying a nonstressful starting point, providing gradual planned exposures that do not elicit a visible response from the learner, and very gradually increasing the stimulus intensity over repeated exposures. If the learner shows a response, even a subtle one, the process is stopped temporarily, and the most recent successful exposure is repeated. Desensitization is often best implemented simultaneously with classical conditioning or counterconditioning for fastest results, as discussed later in this chapter.

One helpful mental image which may help illustrate desensitization is that of climbing the rungs of a ladder. The ladder must be placed on stable ground—the nonstressful starting point. Each rung of the ladder represents a gradual increase in stimulus intensity. If the rungs are too far apart, the ladder may feel scary or unsafe, and the learner may respond by showing fear or anxiety. If the learner is asked to climb the ladder too quickly, a fear response may occur. By controlling the rate of ascent up the ladder and making sure that there are plenty of "rungs" (exposures) placed closely together, the animal can be helped to learn that there is no need for stress. If the rungs are close enough together, a ladder can even become a ramp—easier to ascend than any ladder! Fig. 5.1 shows an example of a possible desensitization hierarchy, or exposure ladder, to gradually present injections.

Controlling the stimulus intensity requires some creativity. Keeping a training log or a series of training plan worksheets can help track progress during this process. Depending on the nature of the stimulus and the logistics of planning exposures, one can determine how best to control the stimulus intensity. For a tactile stimulus, the length of time the animal is touched, the location the animal is touched, and how firm a touch will be part of controlling the intensity. For something the learner sees, such aspects as size of the object, distance from the learner, and realism of the object can all be used to control the intensity. For example, if we are conducting a desensitization protocol for a person who is afraid of spiders, we may have to start with a photo from an ad

Administer injection
Sham injection with capped syringe and sharp pinch
Sham injection with capped syringe
Move syringe while repeating gentle tent, firm tent, pinch
Move syringe toward patient while touching injection area
Hold syringe while touching patient
Hold syringe
Increase pressure and add firm pinch
Increase pressure and duration, tent firmly
Lightly pinch/make a tent gently
Stroke injection area
Glide to injection area
Touch nonsensitive area
Handle syringe and medication vial
Open syringe wrapper
Approaches handler, indicating a nonstressful starting point

• **Fig. 5.1** Example of desensitization ladder for injections.

of a stuffed spider toy presented 6 feet away for 3 seconds, or even asking a person to think about what a picture of a stuffed spider might look like. In this example, we control three factors: time exposed, distance from the learner, and realism (photo of a toy—two layers of protection). For a cat that will be receiving injections, we may start with showing our hand to the cat, or reaching 1 inch toward the probable injection location. The learner dictates where this process needs to start and how quickly we may progress through the plan.

TECHNICIAN NOTE

Monitor animals closely for subtle signs of stress during desensitization. If the animal is stressed, stop the process and go back to the most recent successful exposure. You may need to stop the process for a few seconds or even for a few days. The animal always sets the pace. Refer to the section "Communication" and the discussion on body language for help with interpreting possible stress-related signals.

Desensitization and Counterconditioning: Combinations

The goal of desensitization is to develop a nonresponse or a favorable response in an animal to a particular stimulus. Desensitization occurs over time to a particular stimulus. By gradually exposing the learner to the stimulus and carefully controlling the intensity of the stimulus (from the learner's perspective), the learner can learn that the stimulus is not a concern. However, desensitization alone is a very slow process. The goal of desensitization is to prevent or eliminate an undesirable response and to develop a desired response, which may be a nonresponse. The end goal of most conditioning and behavior modification plans is to elicit a *desired* response. By combining desensitization with classical conditioning and/or counterconditioning, effective and efficient behavioral change can be elicited in a pet.

TECHNICIAN NOTE

Desensitization alone is a very slow process. The goal of desensitization is to prevent or eliminate an undesirable response and to develop a desirable response, which may be a nonresponse. The end goal of most conditioning and behavior modification plans is to elicit a *desired* response. By combining desensitization with classical conditioning and/or counterconditioning, effective and efficient behavioral change can be elicited in a pet.

To combine desensitization and classical conditioning or counterconditioning, a plan needs to be generated, not only for desensitization but also for creating a desired emotional response. To do this, it is important to get to know the learner's preferences. Does a particular cat like whipped cream? Consider using a dog's favorite tennis ball or a piece of steak. A horse might enjoy sweet cob, peppermints, or alfalfa pellets. Perhaps a pig would like being scratched, tapped, or lightly poked with a back scratcher or fork (called "forking"), or perhaps the pig would prefer food, such as tiny bits of apple. Take time to explore what each patient finds pleasurable.

Once a detailed plan for desensitization has been made and a happy anticipation or pleasure response is predictably elicited, then one is in a position to generate an effective protocol of desensitization with classical conditioning (DS-CC) or desensitization with counterconditioning (DS-CCC). In DS-CC, each step of desensitization is paired with something the animal finds wonderful. For example, every rung on the injection desensitization ladder (see Fig. 5.1) might be paired with a bit of steak for a particular dog.

> ### TECHNICIAN NOTE
> Make a desensitization ladder and determine how to elicit the desired pleasure response in an animal before starting a desensitization with classical conditioning (DS-CC) or desensitization with counterconditioning (DS-CCC) protocol.

Timing is important when pairing stimuli during classical conditioning or counterconditioning. Four different timing options exist, and each has its benefits and drawbacks. Fig. 5.2 shows the timing options for classical conditioning: **backward conditioning** (distraction), **simultaneous conditioning**, **delay conditioning**, and **trace conditioning**. For examples, we will use the idea of providing delicious food to condition a response to touching the ear. The goal is for the animal to have a pleasure response when the ear

is touched. Table 5.3 illustrates the timing options for this example, with the benefits and possible drawbacks of each method. Use of tools (Fig. 5.3), such as lickable mats or pads, remote treat delivery systems, food dispensing toys, or food bowls, can help with creative food delivery if food needs to be given while using hands to touch the animal during the conditioning protocol.

Sensitization

Sensitization occurs when the animal develops a stronger response over time to the same stimulus. Consider, for example, a cat that needs daily ear drops. On day 1, the cat crouches and shakes her head during the drops; on day 2, the cat crouches and growls; on day 3, the cat crouches, growls, and runs away to hide; on day 4, the cat crouches and growls and then strikes with a front paw before running away; on day 5, the cat runs and hides at the sight of the owner coming; and on day 6, the cat growls when the owner pets it on the head even when ear drops are not present. The stimulus, ear drops, did not change the intensity, but the cat's response changed, becoming much stronger over time.

Sensitization is a very common result of veterinary handling and treatments. The use of proactive preventive desensitization and classical conditioning plans when introducing new stimuli can reduce the risk of sensitization. Closely monitoring how animals respond to touching, treatments, and environmental experiences (sounds, odors, sights, etc.); watching for body language signals of stress; and then stopping and making a new plan, when necessary, all help prevent sensitization. Refer to the section "Communication" for a discussion on body language signals of stress in a variety of species.

Habituation

Habituation is a type of conditioning in which the learner's response to the same stimulus decreases in intensity over time. A good human example of habituation is moving to a home

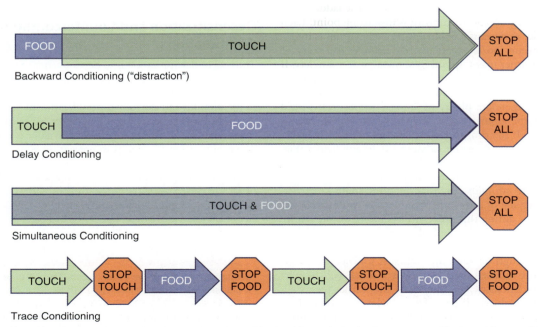

• **Fig. 5.2** Timing procedures for classical conditioning: backward conditioning (distraction), simultaneous conditioning, delay conditioning, and trace conditioning.

TABLE 5.3	Timing Options for Classical Conditioning/Counterconditioning Pairing Food With Touching an Animal		
Type of Conditioning	**Timing Example**	**Benefits**	**Challenges**
Backward	1. Begin food	Easy to perform, intuitive	Food *predicts* touch: this may teach the animal to fear the food rather than liking the touch
	2. Start touch	Fast to perform for short procedures	Food can "mask" fear—a very-high-value treat may make it difficult for the person to observe changes in body language, even though the animal is uncomfortable
	3. End both food and touch		
Simultaneous	1. Begin food and begin touch	Easy to perform, intuitive	Can be difficult for one person to perform (touching and delivering food at the same time)
	2. End both food and touch	Good for short procedures	May result in fear of food, as with backward conditioning
		Creates strong responses	
Delay	1. Begin touch	Creates very strong responses	Can be difficult for one person to perform
	2. Begin food after touch starts	Good for longer or repeat procedures	
	3. End both food and touch	Easy to implement	
Trace	1. Begin touch	Creates very strong responses over multiple short trials	Requires higher-order brain processing—sometimes inhibited by medications
	2. End touch	Easy for one person	Distractions may inhibit acquisition of response
	3. Begin food	Easy for one person to observe animal responses—food less likely to "mask" effects	
	4. End food	Excellent for long-term conditioning for procedures	

near the airport. At first, each time a plane takes off or flies low overhead, its noise is heard and the residents tend to look up, orienting toward the plane. After a few weeks, most will not even hear the planes anymore. The stimulus of the plane noise does not change in intensity, but the brain determines that this stimulus is unimportant and does not require attention, so the people stop noting it. Box 5.2 summarizes the key differences among the several types of conditioning.

TECHNICIAN NOTE

Sensitization and habituation share a common factor—exposing the animal to a stimulus without controlling or modulating the stimulus intensity. Attempts at habituation can result in a potentially harmful sensitization response.

Operant Conditioning

Operant conditioning, also known as *instrumental conditioning,* is a form of learning in which consequences drive future behavior. For the purposes of operant conditioning, the term *consequence* simply means what comes after a behavior. It does not have a negative connotation.

Operant conditioning differs from classical conditioning, which deals in unconscious responses; operant conditioning focuses on voluntary behavior, where the animal makes choices

and these choices lead to consequences. The learner is exposed to situations, stimuli, cues, environments, and events. Each exposure will lead to a given consequence from the animal's point of view. The nature of that consequence will influence the animal's future choices. Essentially, operant conditioning can be used to better understand how animals "do what works," and operant conditioning can be employed to create a picture of "what works" from the trainer's perspective. Operant conditioning describes four kinds of consequences (Fig. 5.4), which are described below.

The term *operant conditioning* describes two basic categories of consequences for any behavior: reinforcement and punishment. **Reinforcement** is anything that increases the *future* frequency, intensity, or duration of the behavior. **Punishment** is anything that decreases the *future* frequency, intensity, or duration of the behavior. Consequences, whether reinforcement or punishment, drive future behavior. It is not possible to know in a given moment whether a consequence is reinforcement or punishment. Tracking the intensity, duration, and frequency of the behavior over time will show whether reinforcement or punishment was occurring. It is possible to predict whether a consequence is likely to be punishing or reinforcing, such as a delicious treat being reinforcing and a painful shock from a collar being punishing, but the only true way to tell is to keep a log of the animal's behavior over time.

Within the categories of punishment and reinforcement, there are two types: positive and negative. When discussing operant conditioning, *positive* means adding something to the situation,

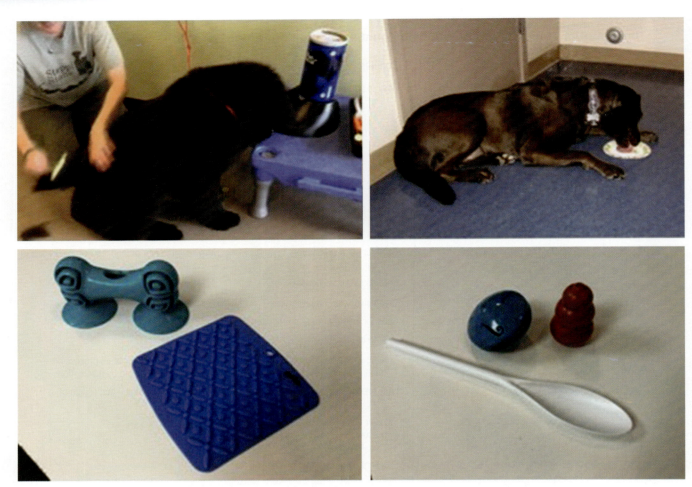

• **Fig. 5.3** Hands-free food delivery items are helpful for some conditioning plans.

• BOX 5.2	Summary of the Differences Among Several Types of Conditioning	
Conditioning Type	**Stimulus Factors**	**Responses**
Habituation	Stimulus is the same all the time	Decreases over time
Desensitization	Stimulus is carefully controlled and intensity gradually increased	Does not develop (prevention) Decreases after conditioning (intervention)
Sensitization	Stimulus is the same all the time	Increases in intensity over time

and *negative* means removing something from the situation. This can be thought of as the math of training. *Positive* and *negative* do not refer to how a consequence feels or is perceived; these terms simply indicate whether something is added or subtracted from the situation after a behavior occurs. The combinations of the two categories and the two types result in positive reinforcement, negative reinforcement, negative punishment, and positive punishment. The quadrants do not apply only to training situations. Reinforcement and punishment can happen in the environment completely separate from animal interactions with humans and also occur during interactions between animals. For the purposes of this chapter, we will focus mainly on training scenarios, because this is where this information is most likely to be used by veterinary technicians.

> **TECHNICIAN NOTE**
>
> Learning happens all the time, and operant conditioning does not happen only during training sessions.

Positive Reinforcement

As mentioned, with operant conditioning, *positive* and *negative* do not mean "good" and "bad"; instead, these terms should be thought of as mathematical terms. *Positive* means adding something to a situation, and *reinforcement* means the behavior strengthens over time. If something is added to the situation after a behavior and the behavior strengthens over time, **positive reinforcement** is happening. Positive reinforcement training is popular with many trainers of various species around the world because it is designed to help the animal understand how to succeed without causing stress or fear in the animal. This method teaches the learner exactly what the desired behavior is and allows the trainer and the learner to have a relationship based on predictability, pleasant interactions, and trust.

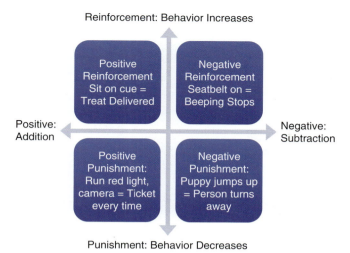

Reinforcement: Behavior Increases

| Positive Reinforcement Sit on cue = Treat Delivered | Negative Reinforcement Seatbelt on = Beeping Stops |
| Positive Punishment: Run red light, camera = Ticket every time | Negative Punishment: Puppy jumps up = Person turns away |

Positive: Addition — Negative: Subtraction

Punishment: Behavior Decreases

• **Fig. 5.4** The quadrants of operant conditioning.

| TABLE 5.4 | **Examples of Treats Commonly Used for Dogs and Cats** |

Cats	Dogs
Kibble	Kibble
Canned cat food	Canned dog food
Canned cat food, pureed	Canned dog food, pureed
Commercially produced cat treats, soft and crunchy	Commercially produced dog treats, soft and crunchy
Squeeze cheese/canned cheese	Squeeze cheese/canned cheese
Cream cheese packets	Cream cheese packets
Butter pats	String cheese
Bonito Flakes/Kitty Kaviar	Flavored pastes, commercially prepared (e.g., KONG)
Flavored pastes, commercially prepared (e.g., KONG)	Nut butters (*Caution:* Some humans are allergic)
Freeze dried meats/organ meats/fish	Freeze dried meats/organ meats/fish
Baby food	Baby food
Liver paste/pate/braunschweiger	Liver paste/pate/braunschweiger
Deli meat slices or cubes	Deli meat slices or cubes
Canned whipped cream	Canned whipped cream
Anchovy paste	Pretzel rods to administer soft foods
Green olives (diced tiny)	Canned meats (SPAM, tuna, chicken, etc.)
	Greenies Pill Pockets
	Popcorn
	Goldfish crackers
	Cheerios or similar small cereals

When positive reinforcement is used in training, the animal will perform certain behaviors, and the trainer will respond by delivering something the animal enjoys during or immediately after performance of the desired behavior. The animal performs a desired behavior, and the trainer immediately delivers a probable reinforcer, such as a treat, toy, praise, attention, or touch. How can the trainer tell if what is delivered is truly reinforcing? One has to simply wait to see if the animal repeats that same behavior in the future more frequently, with greater intensity, or with longer duration. Some of the most common tools used for positive reinforcement training in the veterinary hospital are food treats. Table 5.4 shows examples of a variety of food treats frequently used for training in the clinic.

Example: Teaching a dog to walk onto a weighing scale. A handler stands next to the head of a dog that is on leash and together they face the direction of a walk-on scale. Using her voice, the handler encourages the dog to move toward the scale. Each time the dog takes a step toward the scale, the handler offers the dog a treat by tossing the treat to the floor directly under the dog's nose and in the direction of the scale. Behavior: Step forward. Consequence: A treat is added.

TECHNICIAN NOTE

Positive reinforcement training is the preferred method to decrease learner stress and improve the relationship between the trainer and the learner.

Clicker training or marker-based training is a common technique when using positive reinforcement. A training clicker can be used to "mark" desired behaviors and predict a piece of food is on the way. Using a word such as "good" or "nice," a whistle, a tongue-click, a hand signal, or specific touch can all be markers—as long as they predict a desired reward is on the way. Marker-based training relies on the classically CR to the click, word, or signal. By pairing the marker with something the learner enjoys and desires, the marker can be used to precisely communicate which behavior is the target of reinforcement. Example: Handler presents their palm to a dog. When the dog reaches to sniff the palm, the handler clicks, then delivers a treat. The click marks the instant the dog touched the palm with its nose, and the treat is then delivered. It is not possible for the dog to simultaneously touch the palm with their nose and also be eating a treat, so the marker allows some additional communication about the desired

behavior. Marker-based training is not a requirement, but understanding the use of markers is a useful tool for anyone engaging in training.

Negative Reinforcement

Negative reinforcement is the removal of something to increase the likelihood that a particular behavior will happen again. Remember, *negative* does not mean "bad"; it means "subtract." Sometimes, with negative reinforcement, we are adding something that the learner will work to avoid. This means potentially something the animal finds unpleasant has been added, or the animal is put in a situation that is causing aversion. Intentionally causing unpleasant feelings or experiences presents an ethical dilemma, so negative reinforcement should be used with caution. In general, when working with animals, the least invasive, minimally aversive, and maximally comfortable method should be chosen for each individual animal. Refer to Fig. 5.5 for Dr. Susan Friedman's hierarchy for behavioral change. The graphic illustrates the road to behavioral change. Note that each exit is in order of what will be the least likely to cause emotional or physical harm to both the animal and its relationship with the trainer.

Hierarchy of Behavior-Change Procedures

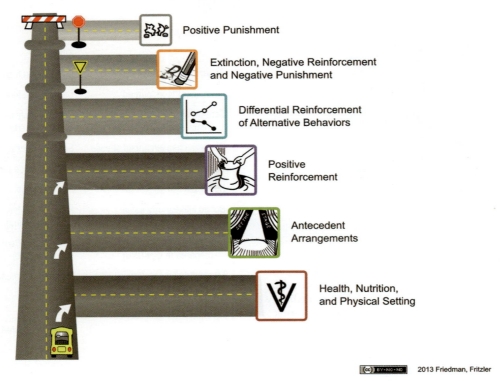

Positive Punishment

Extinction, Negative Reinforcement and Negative Punishment

Differential Reinforcement of Alternative Behaviors

Positive Reinforcement

Antecedent Arrangements

Health, Nutrition, and Physical Setting

(cc) BY-NC-ND 2013 Friedman, Fritzler

• **Fig. 5.5** Dr. Susan Friedman's hierarchy for selecting procedures to change behavior.

Example: Fastening a safety belt. The driver climbs into the car and turns on the engine. An obnoxious beeping noise occurs. As the driver fastens the seatbelt, the annoying beep stops. In the future, the driver fastens the seatbelt before starting the engine (increase in belt-buckling behavior), and the beeping is removed (negative). Negative reinforcement is used to increase the rapid seatbelt-fastening behavior. Because the stimulus removed is a relatively benign beep and the learner is able to comprehend immediately the effect of their actions, this is a low-risk use of negative reinforcement.

Example: Teaching an animal to stand still when restrained. A dog is standing and the trainer has placed their arms around the dog to restrain it. The dog begins to struggle against the pressure of the trainer's arms. As soon as the struggling ceases, the trainer reduces the arm pressure applied to the animal. The trainer removed something (pressure), and the animal stands more quietly in the future (increase in behavior), so negative reinforcement for the behavior (i.e., standing still) occurred. The risk with this technique is that the trainer held the animal while it was exhibiting likely signs of fear and stress. Struggling is an attempt by the animal to communicate discomfort with restraint, and this method could damage the trust between the trainer and the learner, because fear or stress is an unpleasant feeling. Negative reinforcement requires the learner to avoid something and the trainer to remove it in a timely fashion. The appropriateness of causing intentional avoidance and the possible fallout from doing so should be carefully considered.

When animals struggle during handling, Howell and Feyrecilde's 2-2-3 rule should be kept in mind.[1] This is a modified version of the guideline set forth in Yin's *Low Stress Handling*.[2] If it requires more than two tries, two arms to stabilize, or the animal struggles for more than 3 seconds, a different handling plan is recommended (refer to Chapter 6).

Negative Punishment

Decreasing a behavior over time by removing something from the situation is called *negative punishment*. In general, negative punishment removes something the learner wants, so through trial and error, the learner realizes that its behavior does not achieve any pleasing result. When something the learner wants is removed after an undesired behavior, the undesired behavior should decrease over time. Because this method only teaches what *not* to do rather than what to do, it can cause frustration and confusion and diminish the trust relationship between the learner and the trainer. Training will, by necessity, involve stopping some unsafe or unwanted behaviors at times, but the use of punishment should always be undertaken with caution.

Example: Teaching a cat not to bite during play. When the owner is playing with the cat, the cat bites the owner's hand. The owner immediately removes their hands and walks away (negative—removal of attention and access to play). Over time, the cat's biting behavior during play decreases (punishment—decrease in behavior). This approach may result in decreased biting, but it might also result in frustration and confusion, because all behavior serves a function in the mind of the learner, and this scenario does not instruct the cat about appropriate or acceptable play.

Positive Punishment

Positive punishment means adding something to the situation to decrease a behavior in the future. Positive punishment should be reserved as the last resort, if it is used at all in training, and is not appropriate for use in the veterinary setting.

Positive punishment raises welfare concerns. Whatever is added as the consequence must be sufficiently unpleasant so that the learner will actively try to avoid it. Furthermore, the animal needs to understand precisely how the behavior and the punishment are connected. Often, the animal may connect the punishment with the person or item delivering it, developing a fear of the person, object, or experience, rather than simply decreasing the unwanted behavior. Additionally, the punishment must happen promptly and every single time the unwanted behavior occurs; otherwise the behavior will not decrease as anticipated.

Example: Stopping drivers from speeding. Speed limits are considered "guidelines" by many drivers, and many people speed every single day. On occasion, the speeding driver is pulled over and given a ticket. Imagine that a speeding ticket is given perhaps once every 2 years, but the speeding behavior occurs daily. Everyone hates receiving speeding tickets, so why do people still speed every day, even if they have received one or more tickets in the past? The reason is that issuing speeding tickets does not meet the criteria for punishment. The behavior of speeding is not decreasing. Rather, the behavior of slowing down only when the police are visible or when passing through a known "speed trap" is reinforced by the lack of being ticketed. For speeding tickets to be effective, they would need to be given every single time a driver speeds, and the dollar amount would need to be high enough for every driver to be willing to work to avoid having to pay the fine. Speeding tickets are a great example of a failed attempt at positive punishment.

Example: Stopping drivers from running red lights. Many neighborhoods have started installing red light cameras. The camera takes a photo of the license plate of any car passing through the intersection while the light is red, and the driver is mailed a ticket. Intersections have signs indicating that the red light camera is present, so drivers can choose whether to run the red light or not. The behavior of running red lights with installed cameras has been documented to have reduced considerably after cameras were installed (positive punishment—adding the ticket reduces running red lights). However, not every intersection has cameras. Some drivers may take a different route to avoid cameras. The real behavior being reduced is running red lights only when cameras are present.

The above examples illustrate the complexity of applying punishment, even when the learner has every opportunity to understand the complete picture of both the behavior and its possible outcomes in advance.

Possible Problems With Punishment

The use of punishment is challenging. For punishment to be effective:

- The punishment must be consistent and constant: it must happen every time the behavior occurs. Often, when the attempted punishment protocol ends, the behavior returns.
- Punishment must occur promptly, preferably within 1 second of the behavior.
- Punishment must be so unpleasant that it stops the behavior and the learner will work to avoid it.

In general, the most effective training strategies focus on teaching a learner what to do, as opposed to teaching the learner what *not* to do—for example, teaching a puppy *to* sit for greeting, instead of teaching a puppy *not* to jump up; teaching a cat *to* play with a toy instead of teaching it *not* to bite at hands; or teaching a horse *to* place its nose into a halter, instead of teaching it *not* to toss or raise its head.

Punishment teaches learners what *not* to do but does not, in any fashion, teach them the desired behavior. The learner may learn not to give "wrong" answers, but the animal may not determine the correct behavior on its own. When animals are working to avoid wrong responses, they will offer fewer behaviors overall and may learn to fear the trainer, the location where training is performed, and the idea or the setup of training. Fear suppresses acquisition of new behaviors, and training relies on learners acquiring new behaviors. Punishment can significantly slow down the training process and compromise animal welfare by causing signification stress and anxiety. Positive punishment can harm the human-animal bond.

When animals are fearful, they have a limited number of ways to communicate their fear (refer to the section "Communication"). Most animals will try to leave or flee (avoid); fidget or move around randomly (displacement); or fight (defensive aggression). The use of positive punishment, such as prong collars, choke chains, shock collars, shocking mats, striking the animal, intentionally scaring the animal (e.g., with booby traps, yelling), or physically manipulating the animal (by using "alpha roll," "scruff and shake"), have been documented in dogs to cause the animal to avoid the situation or show aggressive behaviors. Using pain or force to train and handle large animals can easily put the handler or the trainer in physical danger. Any training protocol that elicits aggression from the animal should be stopped immediately and a new plan designed before resuming training.

> **TECHNICIAN NOTE**
>
> The use of punishment, particularly positive punishment, can slow down learning and present emotional and physical risks both to the trainer and to the animal.

Behavior Modification

Modification of animal behavior is a valuable tool for every veterinary technician. In fact, the behavior of animals is modified both intentionally and passively or by accident every time an interaction takes place. As discussed earlier in this chapter, a veterinarian's diagnosis is often needed prior to initiating a behavior modification plan. An understanding of basic behavior modification protocols will empower the technician to handle animals more successfully in the clinical environment and to provide better stewardship of the human-animal bond by helping clients and their animals.

Management

Behavior modification generally involves a combination of management and active behavioral change. Management means controlling the animal's environment and experiences to prevent an unwanted behavior. Behavior modification takes time, and the way any animal becomes more proficient in a behavior is through repetition and rehearsal. Until the animal has the skills and experience to perform the desired behavior, and the trainer, client, or handler has the skills to elicit the desired behavior, management can be used to prevent repetitions of unwanted behaviors. In some cases, management alone can result in an acceptable outcome.

Relying entirely on management for unwanted or concerning behaviors carries some risk. Any management plan will eventually break down from time to time. For example, a family trying to teach a dog to stay on the floor, rather than jumping onto the counters, might employ a management plan of never leaving food out on the countertops. At some point, someone will forget and leave a bit of food within the dog's reach. The dog may jump on the counter and reach the food, thus receiving accidental positive reinforcement for jumping onto the counter. For this reason, everyone working with the dog needs to be completely familiar with any management protocol. Management is only one part of a behavior modification plan.

Management can require some creativity but is a helpful part of every behavior modification plan. A few examples of management are as follows:

- Having a dog wear a harness and a long line while learning the recall cue. The long line prevents accidental errors until the dog has learned to come when called, and is a safety net.
- A cat growls and runs away when seeing a neighbor's cat outside the living room window. Placing frosted cling film on the window provides a visual barrier, preventing the cats from seeing each other.

The ABC of Behavior

One way to understand behavior and how to modify it is to use the applied behavior analysis (ABC) model. The ABC model first determines the animal's motivation for performing a particular behavior. In the clinical setting, veterinary professionals will most commonly be presented with scenarios where an unwanted behavior is present and a different behavior is preferred. What positive outcome does the unwanted behavior provide the animal? The second step is to provide the animal with a desirable alternative behavior that also achieves a positive outcome for the pet. By studying what happens immediately before and after an animal demonstrates a particular behavior, veterinary technicians are better able to understand the factors that trigger a particular behavior. Technicians can then design a plan to teach and reinforce a *different* behavior that is more desirable to the owners and that will also (most importantly) be rewarding to the animal. The retraining plan includes motivators and specific outcomes that teach the animal a desirable alternative behavior.

A stands for **Antecedent**. Antecedents are stimuli that precede the unwanted behavior. Antecedents can be contextual, location based, visual, tactile, olfactory, auditory, taste related, and anything in the environment that is distinctive and predictive. For example, the presence of the carrier predicts a cat running away to hide, and the sound of the doorbell happens before a dog begins barking and a stranger then enters the home.

B stands for **Behavior**. Behavior is what the animal actually does. There may be many behaviors happening close together and in rapid succession. The trainer needs to focus on individual behaviors to best understand the options for modifying the unwanted behaviors.

C stands for **Consequence**. Consequences, as discussed earlier in this chapter, follow behavior and drive future decision making by the learner.

By observing the behavior of interest and then analyzing what happens both before and after the behavior, the veterinary technician can map out the ABC of any given behavior. Sometimes, multiple antecedents will be present, and multiple possible consequences occur. Careful observation will help the trainer respond appropriately in the training context to achieve the desired behaviors.

When setting up an ABC analysis, follow these steps:
1. Identify the **B**ehavior of interest.
2. Identify the **C**onsequences that are likely maintaining the behavior.
3. Identify the **A**ntecedents that predict the occurrence of the behavior.

Changing the antecedent, the consequence, or both will generally result in a change in the animal's behavior. Although examples can be extremely complex, simple examples are used in this text for the purpose of teaching.

Example: A cat runs away when it sees the carrier.

B = Running away
C = Negative reinforcement—distance from the carrier is increased
A = Presence of the carrier—likely past history of being captured and pushed into the carrier, a likely past unpleasant experience

Antecedent arrangement is always a place to start when attempting to modify behavior—in this case, arranging antecedents differently. If the goal behavior is for the cat to walk into the carrier, the arrangement would look something like this:

B = Cat is present while the carrier is visible.
C = Treats and toys are placed in the room where the carrier is kept.
A = The color and shape of the carrier are changed to begin the training process. All chasing and capturing attempts cease.

The ABCs will change throughout a behavior modification plan. The arrangement above is only the first step in the plan. As the cat becomes comfortable eating treats and playing with toys in the presence of the carrier, the behavior of the cat and the consequences of the behavior can be changed to teach the cat to walk into the carrier, which is the ultimate goal.

B = Cat glances at carrier
C = Click and treat
A = Presence of new carrier, trainer, clicker, and treats

    Possible next step:

B = Cat takes one step at a time toward carrier
C = Click and treat after every step
A = Presence of new carrier, trainer, clicker, and treats

    Possible next step:

B = Cat walks to carrier and sniffs door
C = Click and treat after every two to three steps and the sniff
A = Presence of new carrier, trainer, clicker, and treats

Gradually, the behavior required to earn a click and treat can be changed or increased. This is called ***changing criteria***. By slowly increasing the criteria over time, the trainer can guide the learner to understand the new behavior. If the criteria are increased too quickly or if the time elapsed between clicks and treats becomes long, the learner may stop making progress. The art of increasing and decreasing criteria to maintain sufficiently frequent treat delivery requires time and practice to master. When the veterinary technician is taking history, there is great opportunity to record target behaviors, examine possible antecedents and consequences, and become part of the team modifying both antecedents and consequences to illustrate the desired behavior to a learner.

Example: Using descriptors in a scenario.

We have introduced numerous terms in this chapter which can be applied to our understanding of how animals learn, and ways we can change their feelings, experiences, and behaviors over time. No one method is happening alone at any given moment: the full suite of learning concepts are always at work. Here is an example to consider, with some of the concepts labeled.

Scenario: Injection training for a cat

The cat does not have a preexisting fear of injections but has been prescribed a medication to be injected twice weekly.

Question: What does the cat like and enjoy?
Answer: Churu paste is the cat's favorite treat.
Question: Does the cat have any known fear of handling or sensitive body areas?
Answer: No.
Possible training scenario:

Identify a nonstressful starting point: injection is already drawn up, Churu is available, cat is on its favorite perch.

Consider an exposure ladder (Figure 5.1).

Steps:

Cat is sitting on perch, offer two licks of Churu, cat licks Churu, and remains sitting on perch
Exposure 1, offer two licks of Churu, cat licks Churu, and remains sitting on perch
Exposure 2, offer two licks of Churu, cat licks Churu, and remains sitting on perch

Continue through exposure ladder until injection is administered. Cat showed no signs of moving away, stress-related body language, or avoidance.

What happened?

A desensitization-type classical conditioning protocol using an exposure ladder to help the cat accept and allow the injection procedure while on a station or perch. Operant conditioning terms can be used to describe positive reinforcement for the behaviors of coming to the perch, stillness, remaining on the perch, allowing touching, and injection. Positive emotions around the person, the syringe, the injection protocol, the perch, and the entire training picture occur. In this example, both emotions and specific behaviors are being examined. No single technique is occurring but rather, an entire training session is described, using several different terms and definitions to give a more complete understanding of what is happening from the learner's perspective.

Animal Development

Canine and Feline Development

Puppies and kittens are born without the ability to control their own body temperatures and with both their eyes and ears closed. Once the eyes and ears are open, the first socialization period begins. Kittens have a primary socialization period approximately at age 2–7 weeks. Puppies have a primary socialization period at age 3–16 weeks. For kittens, the primary socialization period ends prior to the typical age of adoption or acquisition into a family. This presents unique challenges, because the family has fewer opportunities to provide positive socialization during the first socialization period. For puppies, the primary socialization period extends into the first weeks usually spent with a new family, providing the family valuable opportunities to help the puppy become a well-adapted pet for the family's projected lifestyle.

What is the socialization period? It is a time of mental flexibility when animals learn who their primary social partners are (same species, other species), how to navigate social interaction, what is pleasurable or dangerous in the environment, and how to respond to potential threats. Animals can and do continually add to their database of social knowledge throughout their lifetimes, but the brain is most elastic regarding these experiences during the primary socialization periods.

Clients should be advised to strategically arrange pleasurable exposures to as many features of their pet's planned adult life as possible. These strategic exposures should give the puppies and kittens opportunities to interact with a great variety of people, objects, sounds, sights, odors, textures, surfaces, and events. Because during the socialization period, puppies and kittens more easily learn both what is safe and what should be feared, these exposures must be planned well to be both pleasurable and safe in the mind of the puppy or the kitten. The socialization period is an opportunity to create important positive associations (garbage truck sound = chicken treats!) that can last a lifetime. By providing proper socialization for puppies and kittens, clients can provide a form of behavioral vaccination, protecting these animals against the common causes of fear and stress as they mature.

Every animal has a certain genetic potential with regard to behavior. Sociability, interactions with animals of the same species and other species, interactions with people, and responses to environmental stimuli all have some genetic potential. Temperament, preference, sociability, and responses to environmental stimuli can be highly heritable. The goal of socialization is to allow the animal to reach its best genetic potential. However, no amount of socialization and training will allow an animal to "outrun" its genetics. A puppy from two very shy parents is likely to be on the end of the shy-bold spectrum. A kitten born to and raised by parents who display fear aggression toward humans is likely to grow into a fearful adult.

Kittens and puppies visiting the veterinary hospital around age 7–8 weeks should be prosocial. Young animals should be willing to interact with team members and explore the environment. Kittens and puppies that are shy, fearful, "slow to warm up," or not prosocial during these first visits may need immediate effective intervention. These young animals require rapid treatment to reach their full potential. General practices with advanced knowledge of behavior, DACVBs, and CAABs should be able to help these patients. If there are no local referral options available, many DACVBs offer long-distance veterinarian-to-veterinarian consultations to provide support and guidance.

After the socialization period comes the juvenile period. For dogs and cats, this period is the time from the end of the socialization period until sexual maturity. Most dogs reach sexual maturity at age 5–18 months, with larger breeds maturing later. Most cats reach sexual maturity at age 4–10 months.

During the primary socialization period and the juvenile period, some dogs will experience what have been referred to as "fear periods." Fear periods have not been extensively researched and are not well understood. During these times, the dog may become more easily frightened or startled, often by previously familiar objects or events. The dog may also have prolonged recovery times from fear-provoking experiences. If a client suspects that their dog is experiencing a fear period, efforts should be made to temporarily protect the dog from probable fear-provoking experiences, for example, fireworks displays or a high-powered dryer used for grooming. Fear periods are by definition brief and temporary. If the animal is showing fear responses with regularity and for longer than 1–2 weeks, a referral for a behavior modification and support plan should be considered, as this behavior pattern is not a part of normal development.

Cats in the juvenile period may show new avoidance of humans around age 8–10 weeks, but this generally resolves on its own in well-socialized kittens.

Adolescence begins for both dogs and cats at the onset of puberty and continues through social maturity. Most dogs reach social maturity at age 2 to 3 years and cats between age 2 to 4 years. Adolescent animals often have an increased need for both physical and mental activity. Enhanced management during this life stage is recommended to prevent unwanted behaviors. As dogs and cats mature, they may begin to show signs of fears, **phobias**, territorial behavior, decreased social flexibility, and increased independence from the owners. It is extremely common for clients to surrender adolescent pets to animal shelters. Compared with the socialization period and the juvenile period, the adolescent age group also has less frequent contact with the veterinary team. Contacting clients with adolescent pets to ensure things are going well is a valuable service the veterinary technician can offer between wellness visits.

The adult period for both dogs and cats begin at social maturity (age 2–4 years) and continues until the senior period. Cats are generally considered to be at the senior stage at age 10–11 years, with giant dogs entering their senior years around age 6 years, large dogs around age 7–8 years, and small breed dogs around age 10–11 years. Adult dogs and cats require plenty of physical and mental stimulation and will need maintenance of their training (see the section "Meeting Animal Needs"). Senior dogs and cats often develop changes in their sensory acuity, mobility, and muscle mass. They may display decreases in their cognitive ability, disturbances of the sleep-wake cycle, and changes in their social awareness of owners or other animals. Changes in the daily routine, expectations, and management strategies may be appropriate for senior dogs and cats. Senior pets should visit the veterinarian regularly, and technicians should question the owners carefully about any changes in the animal's activity, social acuity, sensory acuity, mobility, and sleep-wake cycle.

Equine Development

Horses from birth until weaning are referred to as *foals*. Immediately after birth, mares and foals begin the bonding process, with the mare licking and nuzzling her foal and licking amniotic fluid from the foal and the bedding. Nuzzling, licking, and close contact generally continue for at least 30 to 60 minutes and are presumed to be crucial to the bonding of the mare and the foal. Mares bond to foals rapidly, but foals will follow any larger object for the first week of life until they are able to distinguish their individual dam.

Foals should begin to nurse within 2–3 hours. It is normal for mares to protect the foal from other horses and even from familiar humans while the foal is young. Caution should be used when entering enclosures, and threatening of new mothers should be avoided (Fig. 5.6). A technique for improving adult equine behavior through early handling of foals, often called *imprint training*, is a matter of disagreement among experts. This technique suggests a series of handling exercises that begin within 48 hours of birth. Studies looking to confirm the efficacy of this technique have been equivocal, and much concern has been expressed about this approach interfering with mare-foal bonding and with the foal's early nursing attempts (potentially preventing timely transfer of immunoglobulins). Some studies have looked at the effects of similar habituation and desensitization techniques on older

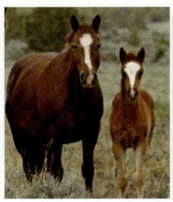 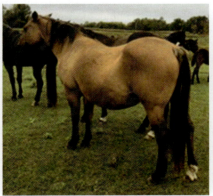 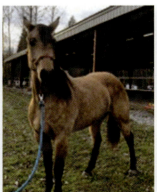 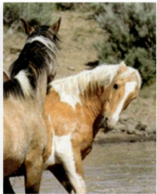

• **Fig. 5.6** Quick reference for equine body language. Relaxed *(left)* progressing to most stressed *(right)*.

foals and have found them to be similarly effective without any potential negative side effects. Much remains to be learned about the sensitive period of the foal and the ideal time at which early handling and socialization will be most beneficial. Nevertheless, foals learn faster compared with adult horses, and early habituation to humans can be achieved without interfering with the mare-foal bonding. One should make an effort to ensure that all interactions with foals are positive ones to avoid creating a learned fear of human approach or handling. Gentle, regular handling of the mare in the foal's presence may be equally important.

Horses are highly social animals and in free-living situations, they would always stay in groups. Until about a month of age, most foals play by spending time running and jumping near their mothers. Turning out mares and foals together with other mares and foals can improve social behavior among horses, because the foals can rehearse adult behavior through safe play. Foals raised in group living conditions with other socially appropriate horses tend to grow into more socially well-adjusted adults, in addition to other health benefits. Foals housed singly with only their dams may show a limited variety of social behavior because of lack of experience.

The developmental stages of foals vary considerably between free-living animals and animals living with humans. Free-ranging mares do not wean their foals until age 5–15 weeks before the birth of their next foal. Before this time, as the foal begins to graze more, the mare's aggression toward the foal will peak to prevent nursing. Horses weaned by humans rather than by their dams are generally weaned considerably earlier, at age 4–6 months. Significant stress during weaning can correlate with unwanted behaviors in the adult horse. Abrupt separation of mares from foals to induce weaning results in the highest stress levels. Foals separated from the dam and kept alone may panic, resulting in injury. Gradual weaning, where the mare and foal are allowed to see one another and interact through a fence, but the foal cannot nurse, is less stressful. Group weaning, where mares and foals are together at pasture for a period before the mares are removed, also appears to be less stressful, because the foals are left with other foals for companionship and remain in a familiar location.

After weaning until the age of one year, horses are referred to as *weanlings*. Weanlings are often learning about humans and about interactions with equipment, such as halters and handling systems, and forming social bonds with their herd mates. Weanlings have increased social receptivity; because their primary point of attachment has always been the dam until the point of weaning, forming additional social bonds at this time is useful for health and safety. When interacting with weanlings, handlers may want to teach the young horse to wear a halter, pick up its feet for grooming, tolerate the sound of clippers, and so on. This early training helps prepare the young horse for adult life. Handling experiences should be kept short and positive. Attention should be paid to the horse's body language. If the horse is fearful, the process should be slowed down. Pairing handling and training experiences with things the horse enjoys, such as special treats and specific kinds of scratching or touching, help the horse develop a positive CR to handling. Desensitization procedures, antecedent arrangement, and the use of positive reinforcement as discussed earlier in this chapter apply to all animals, and these techniques are recommended.

Horses older than 1 year of age but younger than 3 years of age are referred to as *yearlings* and *2-year-olds*. Females will achieve sexual maturity at age 9–18 months, whereas males reach sexual maturity, on average, at age 12–15 months. Adolescence is the period between puberty and adulthood. Adolescent horses will have a strong desire to explore the environment, and many trainers start introducing adolescent horses to equipment and ground training. Some horses are ridden prior to physical maturity during the late adolescent period at age 2 to 3 years.

Horses are not full grown and mature adults until age 4 to 5 years. Although younger horses have gone through puberty and are theoretically capable of reproduction, social opportunities for reproduction are rarely available to subadult horses. Adult horses are ready to be trained and to learn to carry a load or a rider. During the adult period, horses need plenty of attention, exercise, and ongoing maintenance of positive experiences, training, and husbandry to preserve ease of handling.

The average life span of horses is 25–30 years. Most horses are in the senior life stage during their late teens. Senior horses may show decrease in muscle mass, changes in mobility associated with arthritis, and changes in their vision. Hearing changes and cognitive changes are less common in horses than in dogs and cats. Senior horses require additional vigilance from owners, because they may need special considerations in their environment, feed type, frequency of veterinary care, and social interactions compared with horses in the young adult period. Some changes in behavior described as "reluctance to load," "not standing well for the farrier," or "becoming face shy during halter placement" can be traced back to physical changes in the senior horse and should be addressed accordingly by the veterinarian.

> **TECHNICIAN NOTE**
> Horses have a long maturation period, and this should be considered during any training and behavior modification.

Cattle and Small Ruminant Development

Like horses, range cattle and dairy or beef cattle have significantly different natal and juvenile periods, depending on their housing and living situations. Dairy calves may be separated from their mothers within 24 hours of birth to facilitate commercial milk production. The calves may be housed singly or in groups and will be fed milk replacer, often via a mechanical feeder. Beef cattle and particularly, range-raised calves, will generally wean at age 8 to 11 months.

Less has been studied about the social interactions and milestones of cattle compared with those of dogs, cats, and horses. Dairy calves housed in groups rather than singly show increased social contact and closeness with other cows as they mature. In studies evaluating response to handling for veterinary procedures, calves raised with their dams took the longest to approach a person, whereas calves raised singly approached most quickly. Calves raised with their dams and in groups with other calves showed significantly less struggling during veterinary handing compared with singly housed calves.

Bulls and cows both reach sexual maturity around age 12 months, but most cattle producers do not breed cows until they are approximately 18 months of age to allow them to become more physically mature prior to parturition.

The small ruminant species most often kept are sheep and goats.

Communication Body Language

Body language is the primary language our animal patients use to communicate with one another and with us. Body language cues have meaning and function. The signal may be asking to increase distance from a person, object, or situation, decrease the distance, interact, stop an interaction, communicate reproductive status, provide food-finding information, and more. Although animals do use vocalizations to communicate, they do not use speech or language like humans do. By studying body language and continuously monitoring patients for signs of fear, anxiety, and stress, the veterinary staff can respond to their needs promptly, creating a better experience for the animal and a safer experience for the veterinary team. There will always be individual variations among animals, even within a single species or breed; however, this chapter is designed to provide a basic guide to common body language signals associated with a relaxed state, mild stress, moderate stress, and severe stress.

Most clients are not fully aware of the body language of animals. While they may notice overt signs such as growling or escape behavior, subtle communication signs are not always clear to clients. The veterinary team must be skilled not only in observing and interpreting body language but also in communicating with clients about signs of body language. Interacting with animals in a respectful way while decreasing stress as much as possible means pausing interactions when the animal shows signs of stress. By being sensitive to these cues in a variety of species and communicating effectively with owners about body language cues, the veterinary technician can be an effective and valuable part of the behavioral health care team for a variety of species.

When interpreting body language, it is important to observe the whole animal rather than just individual body parts. Each of the sections that follows will describe individual body parts to observe, but the overall effect of the entire animal, including whether the animal chooses to approach or stay at a distance, how the animal responds to movement or touch, if the animal can accept food or tactile interactions, and where the interaction takes place all factor into interpreting body language.

Metacommunication is part of context. A dog that growls or shows its teeth while crouching with its elbows touching the floor, rump in the air, and a high, softly wagging tail is likely inviting play. The "play bow" posture gives special meaning to the growl, indicating it is nonthreatening. A growling dog that is crouching with a tucked tail and moving away is giving a distance-increasing signal and should be left alone. Animals will often give multiple signals at once while trying to communicate clearly or even to communicate mixed feelings or internal indecision. Familiarity with a variety of signs will improve the quality of the technician's interpretation of body language cues. Table 5.5 gives a summary of the body language signals of dogs and cats.

TECHNICIAN NOTE

Animals must use body language to communicate with each other and with humans. Developing the skill of rapid, complete observation of body language cues will improve the technician's ability to handle and interact with patients safely with reduced patient stress.

Canine Body Language

The body language cues discussed in this chapter are generalities. Certain breed characteristics, such as the eyes of Pugs and Chow Chows, the muzzle and lips of Shar-Pei, lack of tails, and so on may diminish the animal's signaling capacity with individual body parts. Context is key! Also, breed variation matters in body posture. A tucked tail in a Labrador Retriever has a different significance from the same tail carriage in a Greyhound or a Border Collie, breeds in which holding the tail down is normal. Showing the whites of the eyes by a Boston Terrier may be normal all the time, but for a Pointer, the whites of the eyes are rarely visible when the animal is relaxed.

In this chapter, we will describe the body language in four conditions: relaxed, mild stress, moderate stress, and severe stress. This scale is adapted from *Cooperative Veterinary Care*.[1] Fig. 5.7 provides a quick reference for canine body language cues.

Relaxed Dog

The body language of a relaxed dog includes soft muscles; a soft facial expression; normal pupil size; ears oriented forward or relaxing low for drop-ear breeds; whiskers held in a neutral position; tail held in the natural carriage or lower and softly wagging or hanging soft; mouth closed and soft or panting with a relaxed jaw; and the tongue soft, sometimes with a curled tip. Relaxed dogs will normally solicit social interaction and will accept food. When touched, the dog's body will feel soft and will bend readily when moving.

Mildly Stressed Dog

Mildly stressed dogs will show signs of stress, particularly during handling but will rapidly return to their baseline body language when the interaction is stopped. Mildly stressed dogs will often show **displacement behaviors** or behaviors that are out of context. These might include licking the lips when not hungry, turning away and sniffing when no compelling odor is present, leaning on the owner, soliciting attention by pawing at or climbing on the owner or the veterinary technician, yawning when not tired, shaking off when not wet, and licking or nosing at the client's or veterinary technician's chin or cheeks. For example, if treats are tossed on the ground and the dog goes to sniff them, this is contextually appropriate. If someone reaches out to pet the dog and it turns away and begins sniffing, this is out of context and may indicate that the dog is mildly stressed when the person reaches toward it.

Mildly stressed dogs will generally approach and accept treats but may stop accepting treats when touched. The dog will have soft muscles; a soft facial expression, sometimes with mild pinching between the eyes; normal to mildly increased pupil size; ears oriented forward or slightly to the side or back; whiskers held in a neutral position; tail held in the natural carriage or lower and softly wagging or hanging soft; mouth closed and soft or panting with a relaxed jaw; and the tongue soft, sometimes with a curled tip.

Moderately Stressed Dog

Moderate stress can encompass any and all of the mild stress signs plus the following: intermittently refusing food previously accepted or taking food with a rough grab when previously gentle. The moderately stressed dog may take treats with mixed feelings, reaching out with its weight shifted backward and stretching out the neck to reach the treats. The dog may also approach only when treats are visible and then rapidly move away. The dog may respond by averting its gaze or looking away, choosing not to interact and moving away; it may exhibit a furrowed brow, moderately dilated pupils, ears held back or down, tense lips held back and little tongue visible, tense muscles, inability to settle/sit still, attention seeking from the owner, and general fidgeting. Signs of stress increase with handling, and it becomes difficult for the animal to return to baseline.

High-value treats can sometimes mask mild and moderate stress. If the food offered is delicious enough, the dog may follow

TABLE 5.5	Body Language Reference Table for Dogs and Cats			
Individual Physical Characteristics	**Relaxed**	**Mild Stress**	**Moderate Stress**	**Severe Stress**
Pupils	Normal for ambient light	Normal to mild dilation	Mild to moderate dilation	Fully dilated
Muscles	Soft	Soft	Some tension	Tense Some will be frozen
Haircoat	Flat	Flat	Flat	Some piloerection Cats may puff tail
Tail	*Dog:* Midline or lower, soft *Cat:* Midline or higher, crook tip	Midline or lower, soft	*Dog:* Above or below midline, tense *Cat:* Tucked, tense, tip may flick	*Dog:* High or tucked tight, tense *Cat:* Tucked or lashing, tense
Gaze	Freely moves, chooses to look at and interact with people	Freely moves but looks away	Gaze will fix on threat or fix away from threat	Looking directly at or completely away from threat Direct staring
Mouth	Soft lips, closed mouth	Mouth may open, lips relaxed Dogs may pant lightly	Mouth tense, commissure of lips tight Dogs may pant, with lips pulled back	Mouth tense, lips may be retracted to show teeth Dogs may pant heavily with lips pulled back, or close mouth with tight tense lips
Paws	All paws on the ground, freely moving	Dogs may lift a front paw, may place paws on humans	*Cats:* Conceal one or several paws *Dogs:* Lifting a front paw, pawing at humans	*Cats:* All paws tightly tucked, may strike with front paws *Dogs:* Standing or crouching with weight forward or backward

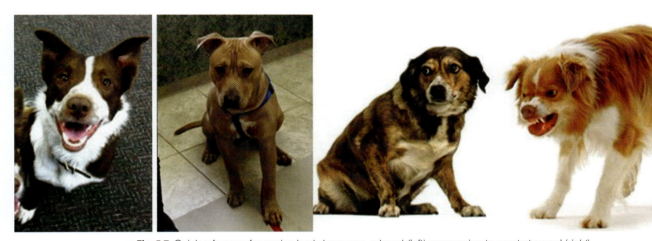

• **Fig. 5.7** Quick reference for canine body language, relaxed *(left)* progressing to most stressed *(right)*.

the food and do something it would otherwise be unable to do. Veterinary team members must use caution in such situations; fear can be intensified during future visits. Imagine this scenario: I have a friend who is afraid of snakes. I bring out my very friendly pet snake and ask my friend to touch the snake, explaining it is friendly. My friend declines. I pull a $100 bill out of my pocket, and tape it to the snake. I then tell my friend she can keep the $100 if she touches the snake to pick up the bill. My friend stretches her hand out, and then she pulls off the $100 bill with the minimum contact necessary and as fast as possible. If I ask my friend after the fact if she still fears snakes, she is likely to say, "Snakes are scary, but thanks for the $100." Because of the high-value item on offer, my friend did something she ordinarily would never do. Consider this example when working with animals that tentatively reach for treats and then rapidly move away.

Moderate stress compromises welfare. Any treatments that are not immediately needed should be stopped and a new plan made.

Severely Stressed Dog

Dogs experiencing severe stress are in a state of significant emotional distress. These dogs may show defensive aggression and threatening postures, but this is uncommon. Usually, dogs in severe stress caused by fear will use hiding and avoidance, rather than overt aggression. In most cases, dogs experiencing severe stress should be given stress-relieving medications prior to attempting handling.

Dogs in severe stress may show any and all signs of mild and moderate stress combined with any of the following signs: moving away from the veterinary team and not approaching, inability to accept food, or accepting food only from the owner. The dog may have a furrowed brow; dilated pupils; ears held tightly back or down; panting, with tense lips held back and little tongue visible; tense muscles; and very slow or very frantic movements. The dog may urinate, defecate, or express its anal sacs. The dog may also enter a state called *learned helplessness,* in which the dog no longer tries to escape but, rather, looks statue like and stoic, because it has learned there is no escape. Dogs displaying learned helplessness may appear cooperative on the surface but are in extreme emotional distress.

Dogs in severe stress may show defensive aggression if approached. This may include becoming stiff or freezing; showing the whites of the eyes; giving direct eye contact or staring; and lunging, growling, snarling, snapping, or biting. A dog displaying these signs needs immediate stress relief. This degree of stress is harmful to the patient and compromises the safety of the veterinary health care team.

> **TECHNICIAN NOTE**
>
> Severely stressed animals can present significant safety risks for veterinary technicians attempting to handle them.

Feline Body Language

As with dogs, there is considerable variation among individual preferences and signals shown by cats. Some cats are very social and comfortable in a variety of environments, including the veterinary hospital. Socially confident cats will often explore, rub on people and furniture, and pursue interactions with the veterinary team members. Often, these cats also feel more confident about showing how they feel and, when they are fearful, this is often misunderstood as resistance or fractious behavior. Fear and stress inhibit behavioral expression in many animals. When the baseline fear level of cats is slightly lower, they will sometimes more readily express defensive aggression. Careful monitoring of every patient, throughout every visit, for changes in stress levels is crucial. A patient's stress level can change rapidly, and the veterinary team needs to be able to adapt just as quickly. Fig. 5.8 provides a quick reference for feline body language cues.

Relaxed Cat

The body language of a relaxed cat includes soft muscles, a soft facial expression, normal pupil size, ears erect and soft, relaxed brow, whiskers held neutral or slightly back, mouth closed, and tail held up, with a soft curve in the tip. Relaxed cats will readily exit the carrier on arrival and show willingness to explore the environment, sometimes rubbing their cheeks or top of the head on people or objects. They will walk around the room with a horizontal topline. Relaxed cats will sometimes jump onto a shelf or table and sprawl out.

Relaxed cats will often accept food treats, and many like tactile interactions, such as cheek and chin rubbing or gentle brushing with a soft-bristled brush.

Mildly Stressed Cat

Mildly stressed cats will often approach and retreat or show interest with gazing and sniffing but choose not to approach. They may choose or prefer to remain in the carrier. Mildly stressed cats will show some or all of these signs but with low frequency: looking away without moving away; mildly dilated pupils; ears held slightly to the side; legs, tail, and whiskers held closer to the body.

Moderately Stressed Cat

Cats in moderate stress may show any of the signs listed under mild stress plus any or all of these signs: reluctance to leave carrier/preferring to hide when the top of the carrier is removed; generally choosing to stay in the carrier rather than coming out; refusing food previously accepted; not exploring the environment; holding the tail tight to the body; choosing a sternal instead of sprawling position and pulling the legs under the body if lying down; holding ears to the side or slightly back; alternating the gaze between looking toward possible threats and looking away; and twitching of the tip of the tail.

Moderate stress represents changes in the animal's welfare. Often, cats displaying signs of moderate stress will rapidly escalate to severe stress when handled or if the handling period is prolonged. Medication to reduce stress should be considered for moderately stressed cats prior to any procedures beyond very brief handling.

Severely Stressed Cat

Cats experiencing severe stress are experiencing decreased welfare. For the safety of the animal and the veterinary team, severely stressed cats should receive medications to relieve stress before initiating treatments.

Severely stressed cats will generally show either some level of defensive aggression or learned helplessness. These cats generally

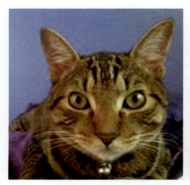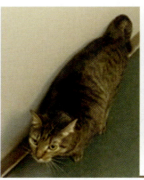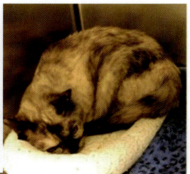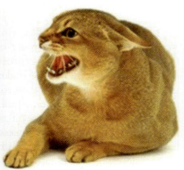

• **Fig. 5.8** Quick reference for feline body language, relaxed (*left*) progressing to most stressed (*right*).

have no interest in exploring the environment and will prefer to hide or escape. The cat will try to appear small initially, but if handled, may puff up and try to appear larger in self-defense. If the cat does move around the room, the back will be hunched, haircoat may be standing up, and the tail may be bushy. The cat may lower its head and initially look away, but then stare directly at a perceived threat. Severely stressed cats will show any or all of the signs of mild to moderate stress in addition to the following: pupil dilation, ears held flat against the head and back, whiskers held completely flat or forward, body flattened, tail tucked tightly against the body or held out low from the base, vocalization with hisses or growls, show of the teeth, striking with the front paws, and biting.

Equine Body Language and Communication

Dogs and cats certainly present dangers to the veterinary team when experiencing significant stress, but large animal medicine can come with increased risk of team injuries when animals try to avoid or object to handling and treatments. It should be kept in mind that animals that cannot flee when fearful (confined to a halter, crossties, stall, small pen, tether, etc.) and have limited options to communicate their feelings of fear and stress. Chapter 6 discusses specific handling strategies to keep both the animals and the veterinary team members safe.

Horses use a variety of means to communicate with each other and with humans. Their unique senses and herd life as prey animals rather than potential predators influences the motivation behind communication and the nature of long-distance or long-range communication.

Communication and the Senses

Typical of most prey animals, horses' eyes are set laterally, allowing them to have a wide field of monocular vision on either side of their body and a narrow binocular field of view directly in front of their noses. This leaves the horse with two blind spots: one directly behind them and one directly below its nose. It is necessary for the horse to raise or lower its head to change its field of vision and its depth perception. Horses can see color, but their vision is dichromatic; that is, they mostly see shades of pale blue, green, gray, and yellow.

Horses, unlike dogs and cats, use a wide variety of auditory signals to communicate. Foot stomping and pawing can communicate stress or fear of a threat, whereas pawing can be linked to frustration. Foals will engage in snapping (sometimes called *champing* or *teeth clapping*). The foal will pull back its lips and snap its teeth rapidly. This behavior is sometimes paired with sucking and tongue-clicking sounds. Snapping is shown when foals approach adult horses, when adults direct aggression toward foals, when the foal's dam is copulating with a stallion, and when approached by cattle, humans, or mounted riders. Snapping is sometimes displayed with no apparent provocation, and the meaning of the behavior is not well understood.

Horses also use a variety of vocalizations to communicate. Refer to Box 5.3 for a key to horse vocalizations and their meanings.

Olfaction is another important means of communication among horses. In addition to the conventional olfactory system, horses have a well-developed accessory olfactory system, the vomeronasal organ (also referred to as the *Jacobson organ*). When investigating other horses' urine or feces, and sometimes in response to novel smells or flavors, the horse may exhibit the *flehmen response* (Fig. 5.9). Horses recognize foods by their odor and investigate

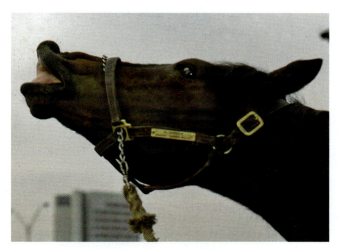

• **Fig. 5.9** Flehmen response in a horse.

most foreign objects by smelling them. They also greet **conspecifics** nose to nose, smelling the "breath" from their **nostrils**. One method by which horses recognize individuals is by their odor, and odor plays an important role in a mare's recognition of her own foal. Stallions use odor cues and a variety of other cues to determine when a mare is in estrus.

The sensitivity of the horse's skin varies depending on the location, and tactile communication is important among horses and between the horse and the rider. The density of the skin receptors and the thickness of the skin contribute to the differences in sensitivity. The vibrissae (Fig. 5.10) around the eye and muzzle are well innervated and help the horse determine the distance from its muzzle to a surface. The withers, flank, and elbow regions are other sensitive areas. Some horses may be sensitive to having their ears, groin, area under the tail, or bulbs of the heels touched. When horses perform **allogrooming**, they tend to stand shoulder to shoulder and nibble at the areas over each other's withers, neck, and back (Fig. 5.11). The withers are a good place to begin stroking a horse after greeting it, because grooming of this area has been shown to reduce the heart rate in the horse.

TECHNICIAN NOTE

Horses have specialized senses and communication strategies as a result of their lifestyle.

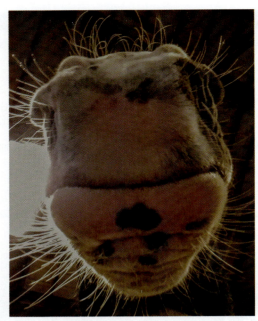

• **Fig. 5.10** Vibrissae, specialized sensory hairs in the horse.

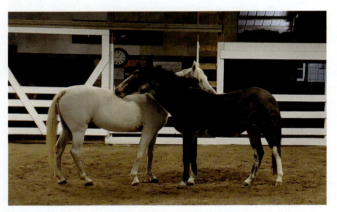

• **Fig. 5.11** Allogrooming in horses is an important communication and bonding behavior.

Relaxed Horse

A relaxed horse's ears will usually be relaxed and held to the side, but the horse will rotate its ears toward objects, individuals, or sounds of interest. The head may be held low or may be raised when the horse is looking at something of interest. The horse may graze or nap. The horse's muscles will feel and appear soft, and the tail will usually be hanging down or lightly swishing in response to flies on its skin. Eyes will appear soft, with relaxed eyelids, and the blinking will be slow, with pupils being the appropriate size for ambient light. The horse may stand on all four hooves with one foot "cocked," the toe touching the ground while bearing most of its weight on the opposite rear foot. The nostrils are relaxed and the breathing calm.

Mildly Stressed Horse

The mildly stressed horse shows concern about something, deciding whether to investigate. It will have an alert expression. The ears may be fixed, facing a specific direction, and the head raised or lowered. The nostrils may widen intermittently. Pupils may mildly

dilated but are difficult to appreciate in low-light conditions (e.g., inside a barn or stall) and in dark-eyed horses. The horse may move slowly toward or away from an object or individual causing concern or may approach after initial hesitation.

Moderately Stressed Horse

Moderately stressed horses are experiencing fear and distress. The horse will often raise its head high, and the ears will swivel, be fixed toward a specific direction, or begin to lie back or be "pinned." The horse may trot away with the tail held high or held low against the rear legs. Some stressed horses will drop the head and stand with splayed legs. The nostrils will flare and the eyes will widen, with wrinkles above or behind the eye. The eyes may dart around rapidly, assessing for possible escape routes. The horse may pinch its lips, holding them closed with the corners pulled forward. Some moderately stressed horses will paw the ground.

Severely Stressed Horse

Severely stressed horses are experiencing significant impacts on welfare and can present serious danger to anyone attempting to handle them. They may show any of the mild or moderate stress signs, plus some signs of severe stress. The horse may pin its ears back and may raise its head high and toss it or "snake" its head low from side to side. The horse's muscles will appear tense and may even tremble. The eyes will be wide, often with the whites showing and the pupils dilated. Nostrils will flare, the lips may be pulled tight, and the horse may show teeth or bite. The tail may be held very high, wringing, or slashing rapidly from side to side. Some horses will stamp their front hooves and may strike out or rear and strike. The horse may sway back and forth on its hindquarters, preparing to kick.

Cattle Body Language

Cattle, like horses, are herd animals and prey species. They have a blind spot behind them near each hip and have dichromatic vision. They also use vocalizations to call to companions or family members or to express alarm. Cows and other ruminants have less developed facial musculature, so facial expression plays a less crucial role in communication. Cows can present danger during handling with kicking, pushing or pressing, charging, butting, or, in the case of horned animals, even goring with their horns. Keeping the stress and fear levels low for cattle will diminish danger to the handler. Furthermore, stress has a negative impact on the production of meat and milk. Calmer animals experiencing less stress will be more profitable for producers. Fig. 5.12 provides a quick reference for cattle body language.

Relaxed Cattle

Relaxed cattle will be standing or walking quietly and often grazing or lying down ruminating. The tail will hang down in a neutral position. If curious, the cow may calmly approach, with its head raised and the tail raised in an inverted "U" shape. Cows will orient their ears toward noises or objects of interest or particular threat, but there is limited detailed research on ear position and arousal. When feeling calm, cows will groom their companions to cement bonds and may nuzzle each other or people by using their noses or lips.

Mildly Stressed Cattle

Mildly stressed cattle may widen the eyes slightly, close the mouth, raise the head slightly and turn it to the side, and then move away.

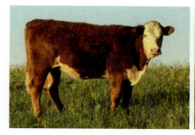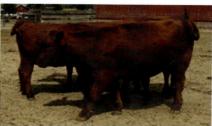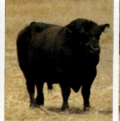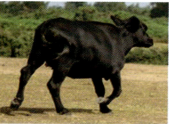

• **Fig. 5.12** Quick reference for cattle body language. Relaxed (*left*) progressing to most stressed (*right*).

If grazing or lying down, the cow will stop eating and stand, observe potential threats, and generally move closer to herd mates and away from fear-provoking stimuli. The tail may sway slowly or remain hanging in a relaxed position.

Moderately Stressed Cattle

Moderately stressed cattle will show wide eyes, often with the sclera visible. The eyes may dart around. The cattle may actively try to escape by lowering the head and galloping away or balk and freeze, unable to move forward. The tail is clamped low next to the body or tucked between the rear legs when the animal is fearful, or held up in an inverted "U" shape if it is alert and considering approaching the threat. Stressed cattle will startle easily, exhibiting large twitches or jumps. When galloping in flight, a cow's tail will be held straight out, with the tip drooping.

Severely Stressed Cattle

Severely stressed cattle experience significant welfare concerns and can present serious danger to handlers. The eyes may be wide open and rolling, with the sclera visible. Bulls considering a charge will stand with their front legs wide, head lowered, and chin tucked. They will sometimes paw the ground and orient the top of their head and horns toward the threat. Cows will stand facing the threat, with their heads low and swinging from side to side. Cattle may rapidly wag their tails if experiencing pain and when preparing to kick. Severely stressed cattle may kick rapidly and accurately to the front, sides, and back with the hind hooves.

> **TECHNICIAN NOTE**
>
> Stress in large animals leads to a decrease in the animals' quality of life and fitness and in income for agricultural businesses. Decreasing stress is good for both the animals and the industry.

Small Ruminant Body Language

Small ruminants have two primary defense mechanisms when stressed and fearful: flocking closely with other animals and fleeing. Sheep will flock, whereas goats will scatter. All will run rapidly away from threats, when possible. Sheep and goats can recognize the faces of many different humans and identify them from a great distance. Although rams and goats may charge or head butt threats, this is often done during times of reproductive competition or territorial pressure rather than out of fear caused by a specific event or procedure. Both sheep and goats prefer to be with others of their own species and use vocalizations to call to the young and to companions and to alert others to possible danger. Chapter 6 provides tips for moving sheep and goats in a nonstressful way. As with cattle, with less stress, all commercial livestock produce better, have higher conception rates, and

provide improved meat and milk yield. Sheep raised for wool also have less wool breakage and yield higher-quality fleece when they experience less stress.

Relaxed Sheep and Goats

Relaxed sheep and goats will often be grazing or lying down near companions. The ears will be relaxed and held to the side. Eyes will show slow movements, and the animals may blink slowly. The nostrils will be relaxed and respiratory rate even. When interested by something, the animals may raise their heads, sniff intently with the lips pulled forward, and orient the ears toward the object of interest. Tails, if present, will generally be relaxed and down or swaying gently.

Mild to Moderate Stress in Small Ruminants

Mild stress will lead sheep to seek out companions and flock together. Goats may flock under mild stress. Sheep and goats will raise their heads, and scan the environment for an escape route by using rapid eye, ear, and head movements. Ears may be oriented toward the threat, toward companion animals, or toward potential escape routes. Sheep and goats will hold their heads high when they are preparing to bound away.

Severe Stress in Small Ruminants

Severe stress almost always provokes a flight response in small ruminants. Panicked small ruminants attempting to flee may run into barriers, fences, humans, and young animals. Animals may sustain serious injury and even die from running in a state of panic. When animals show signs of mild or moderate stress, the stressor should be reduced for the safety of the animals.

Prior to flight, sheep will band together, whereas goats will scatter. Ears may be held back and down. If the threat is smaller than the animal (e.g., a sheep or a goat being threatened by a dog), the animal may stand tall to appear larger; stamp its feet; lower its head toward the threat, with ears held far forward; and make small charges toward the threat. This behavior is uncommon toward humans by females and the young but may be displayed by bucks and rams.

Meeting the Needs of Animals

The five freedoms, which every animal is entitled to, were developed by Roger Brambell in response to requests for improving the welfare of livestock. These five freedoms are:
1. Freedom from hunger and thirst
2. Freedom from discomfort
3. Freedom from pain, injury, and disease
4. Freedom to express normal behaviors
5. Freedom from fear and distress

Every species has species-specific behaviors which they must be allowed to express and specific needs with respect to housing, exercise, mental stimulation, and social contact to remain physically and behaviorally healthy. Every animal deserves safety and access to adequate feed, shelter, water, veterinary care, and species-appropriate husbandry. Animals need opportunities for physical and mental exercise and stimulation on a daily basis, and their social needs should be met so that they can enjoy good physical and mental health. Refer to Table 5.6 for a quick reference guide for meeting the needs of dogs, cats, horses, cattle, sheep, and goats.

Special Considerations for Horses

In free-ranging conditions, the horse is virtually never alone. Horses live in small groups, called *bands,* consisting of several mares, their offspring under 3 years of age, and, in most cases, a single stallion. When young horses reach sexual maturity, they leave their natal band but quickly join up with other bands of horses. The mares in the herd form a relatively stable dominance hierarchy among themselves, and the oldest mare in the band is likely to be the highest-ranking mare. Free-ranging horses spend most of their day grazing.

Within any group, horses usually have preferred associates. Preferred associates will allogroom and conduct most of their daily activities in proximity with one another. If they are at some distance from each other when a threat is perceived, they will often move closer together. When possible, group housing of horses provides the animals opportunities to engage in these species-normal behaviors. When bonded pairs are separated, for whatever reason, varying degrees of distress may be seen in both parties.

Free-ranging equids dedicate most of their time budget to walking and feeding. Horses rarely stand in one place longer than required to take a few mouthfuls of grass before moving a few steps. Horses naturally eat many small meals in a 24-hour period. In captivity, the average horse is not allowed to do any of these things. Its locomotion is frequently limited to moving around a stall or a paddock, and meals are provided at the convenience of its owner or caretaker.

When horses are frequently moved from place to place for training, for competition, or after being purchased by new owners, and often housed singly, they are prevented from establishing normal stable relationships with conspecifics. The general lack of stable social relationships may serve as one of several predisposing factors to the variety of behavior problems that afflict the domestic horse.

Meeting the Needs of Gregarious Animals

Gregarious animals live in groups with others of their own species. One of the advantages of social living is the improved ability, merely because of numbers, to recognize danger more efficiently. Numbers provide each individual with a statistically better chance of not being the one caught by the predator. When a group of horses, cattle, or sheep is alarmed, the response of those first seeing the alarming stimulus will be to alert their companions through body language cues and vocalizations regarding the possible threat. After the initial alert response, the animals may investigate or take flight.

A solitary animal without conspecifics will be even more cautious, and one should be prepared for it to take flight more quickly, without taking time to investigate the perceived threat. A frightened animal may attempt escape regardless of the harm it may cause to itself or to individuals nearby. Fleeing horses and cattle can cause serious and even fatal injury to handlers and serious harm to themselves. Fleeing smaller animals are likely to cause self-injury during panic. It is important to discuss with clients about the nature and preferences of individual animals and to monitor the body language of animals continuously and closely when working with them to avoid injury.

TABLE 5.6	Meeting the Basic Needs of Animals: Species-Specific Animal Care
Canine	Safety, nutrition, regular veterinary care and husbandry
	Adequate clean spaces to reside, explore, and rest
	Environment of plenty, freedom from competition for resources
	Daily aerobic and mental exercise
	Each animal reaches its own personal maximum speed daily
	Mental stimulation
	Foraging opportunities (feeding strategies)
	Olfactory variety
	Intellectual pursuits such as training, sports, instinctive work
	Social contact with preferred associates (human and animal)
Feline	Safety, nutrition, regular veterinary care and husbandry
	Adequate clean spaces to reside, explore, and rest
	Environment of plenty, freedom from competition for resources
	High perching areas, secluded hiding spots
	Scratching posts/areas in socially important locations
	Social contact with preferred associates (human and animal)
	Daily physical and mental exercise
	Feeding strategies consistent with the feeding needs of cats
	Numerous small meals through the day
	Seek, hunt, play, consume, groom, and sleep
Equine	Safety, nutrition, regular veterinary care and husbandry
Bovine	Adequate clean spaces to reside, explore, and rest
Small Ruminant	Environment of plenty, freedom from competition for resources
	Social contact with preferred associates
	Group housing when possible
	Opportunity for grazing, allogrooming, feelings of safety and security
	Protection from conspecific aggression, especially during breeding/rut
	Sufficient daily physical and mental exercise
	Time budget is spent largely on walking and grazing
	Access to outdoor grazing and exploration
	Protection from predation and harassment

Common Unwanted Behaviors, Active Prevention, and Intervention

Pet Selection Counseling

Pet selection counseling is one way technicians can help match clients and pets for a successful lifelong relationship. Many conflicts between people and pets stem from mismatched expectations, desires, or abilities. By helping clients determine which pets are most suitable for them prior to acquisition, technicians can prevent, in a timely manner, any conflict and damage to the human-animal bond.

Clients should be questioned about how much time they would like to devote to different aspects of pet care, their level of experience, their training and the willingness to spend time training, and the desired lifestyle of the pet and whether everyone in the household is on the same page with these ideas. Box 5.4 provides examples of questions intended to guide the recommendations for a family considering acquiring a pet.

Whenever possible, clients should meet an animal pet prior to acquisition. Although sometimes this is not possible, every effort should be made to do so. In the case of purchasing animals from a breeder, the client should also try to meet the parent animals; inquire about the temperament, personality, and health of the parent animals; and ensure that the pet can be returned to the breeder if necessary. Breeders or animal producers who forbid visits from potential adopters or buyers should be avoided, because there may be some animal welfare concerns. Purchasing or adopting animals sight unseen carries a much greater risk compared with meeting the animal prior to bringing it home.

After the client has adopted or purchased a new pet, the veterinary team has a valuable opportunity to educate the client about strategies for preventing unwanted behaviors and how to meet the needs of the pets. Table 5.7 provides an example checklist of topics to discuss with each owner throughout their preventive health visits during the juvenile years of the animals.

Common Unwanted Behaviors of Dogs and Cats

The most common **unwanted behaviors** described by cat and dog owners who surrender their pets to shelters are **unwanted elimination**, destructive behavior, and aggression. In many cases, these three indications require a veterinarian's diagnosis and treatment planning. The strategies discussed below may help prevent these common problems before they begin, thus better protecting the human-animal bond.

The veterinarian should screen the animals for any elimination disorders. In some cases, these patients will be prescribed medications in addition to a treatment plan involving management, supervision, and behavior modification.

Unwanted Elimination: Dogs

Housetraining

Housetraining can be done at any age; it is not restricted to puppies. Incomplete housetraining is a common cause of unwanted elimination in dogs. Adult dogs, convalescing dogs, and dogs

---

• BOX 5.4   Example of a Pet Selection Questionnaire and the Insight it May Provide to the Veterinary Technician

Question

Does everyone in the family want to adopt or purchase this animal?
What kind of animal do you want most?

Have you had this animal, breed, etc. before?
What was the outcome?

How much time would you like to devote for
    grooming
    exercise
    training
    feeding
    walking?

What is the composition of your family? Adults, children, frequent visitors?
High-energy or low-energy household?

What is the family budget for pet care?
Have you considered pet insurance or a pet care savings account?
Are you familiar with the costs for training classes and any sports you might wish to try?

Are there any deal-breakers for you regarding a new pet?

Insight for Technician's Recommendation

"No" answers point to possible conflict, which may complicate acquisition.
Discuss pros/cons of this specific pet.
Screen for dissent among family members.
No history with animal or breed points to opportunities for education.
Prior rehoming, surrender, or early age euthanasia requires further investigation before recommendations.
Social interactions and attention, training, grooming, exercise, and veterinary care all take time.
Higher energy pets and breeds will require more exercise, and young pets will require more supervision and training.
Some animals described as highly intelligent, such as Bengal cats or Malinois dogs, require more extensive time commitments to training and exercise than a client may anticipate.
Long-coated animals and those with continuously growing hair will need daily grooming and often professional grooming.
Recommend an animal usually good with children for families with children. Some animals are very stressed by busy households or city life, whereas others thrive in a buzzing household.
Younger animals have less predictability about future personality and temperament, but they are also more adaptable to change.
Training, grooming, vetting, feeding, walking, boarding for vacations, and more all require varying degrees of financial commitment, depending on the needs of the individual pet.
For example, brachycephalic breeds and senior pets generally have higher veterinary costs, and giant dog breeds will cost more to feed and house.
Animals with long hair will likely need a budget for professional grooming.
Size? Slobber? Incompatible with children or other specific pets?
Prepare in advance so that the client is better ready to screen pets, breeds, and individual animals for possible deal-breakers.

TABLE 5.7	Example New Puppy and New Kitten Checklists for Important Discussion Topics During Juvenile Wellness Visits

Example Puppy Visit Topic Checklist	Example Kitten Visit Topic Checklist
• Choosing a puppy class • Housetraining • Crate training, travel training • Appropriate play, including bite inhibition during play • Introductions between the puppy and other pets • Family lifestyle meeting: socialization to people, places, surfaces, sounds, odors, experiences • How to choose food and treats • Making a vaccine schedule and understanding exposure risks • Antipulling devices, such as harnesses for walking • Teething and chewing—selecting appropriate chew items • Internal and external parasite control and zoonosis • Learning to accept handling and restraint for grooming and health care • Tooth brushing • Nail trimming • Ear cleaning • Skin and coat care • Breed-specific health concerns and behavior tendencies • Neutering: what, why, and when?	• Housetraining, including common litter issues • The health benefits of keeping cats indoors • Crate training to make trips outside the house easy • Appropriate play, including bite and claw inhibition during play • Introductions between the kitten and other pets • How to choose food and treats • Making a vaccine schedule and understanding exposure risks • Appropriate toy choices and avoiding foreign object ingestion • Teething and clawing—selecting appropriate items and developing good scratching habits • Internal and external parasite control and zoonosis • Learning to accept handling and restraint for grooming and health care • Tooth brushing • Nail trimming • Ear cleaning • Skin and coat care • Breed-specific problems and tendencies • Neutering: what, why, and when?

experiencing physical or cognitive changes may require housetraining plans.

Any adult dog that had been housetrained well but shows new elimination behaviors inside the home should be thoroughly screened by the veterinarian for any health-related causes. Any disease leading to polyuria or polydipsia, gastrointestinal (GI) upset, pain on elimination, pain or discomfort in assuming the position to eliminate, or change in the odor or appearance of eliminations can be associated with changes in elimination patterns.

When educating clients about housetraining of dogs of any age, it is important to stress the following four factors: realistic expectations; management, supervision, and training; forming good habits; and being consistent.

Realistic Expectations

Housetraining a dog requires investment of time. Puppies are not fully housetrained until they have gone 12 consecutive weeks without eliminating in unwanted locations. Most puppies are not physically capable of meeting this benchmark until the age of 6 months. Preparing clients for the time investment in advance sets everyone up for success.

Management, Supervision, and Training

Clients should be ready for puppies or dogs to be under constant supervision and management until they have met the benchmark of 12 weeks clean in the house. While in training, the client should keep the dog:

1. Safely confined in a place where it will not eliminate, such as a playpen or a crate
2. On a leash, even in the house, with the owner closely supervising
3. Safely confined or leashed in a place where elimination is allowed, such as a fenced yard, a dog walk, or a park

To teach dogs to eliminate in designated locations, the client will first need to carefully choose the areas. It must be kept in mind that physiologically, puppies have immature bodies that require practice to fully empty both bladder and colon, and that

they may have little biological warning before elimination takes place.

To encourage correct elimination patterns, the dog should be taken out after sleeping, eating, drinking, and high-energy activity periods, such as play sessions. The dog should also be taken out anytime it displays sniffing, circling, or revisiting of areas where it has previously eliminated. For elimination trips, the client should take the dog outside on leash at first, even if the area is fenced. This allows for monitoring the quantity and quality of eliminations and for detecting any possible health problems early. As soon as the pet finishes eliminating, the owner should offer quiet, happy praise and a delicious treat in an effort to provide positive reinforcement of the desired elimination behavior. Being allowed off leash to investigate safely fenced yards, play sessions, and training sessions are also excellent rewards.

Mistakes are inevitable. If the client finds the dog eliminating in an inappropriate area, the dog should be calmly interrupted and guided to the designated elimination area to finish eliminating. Being startled will sometimes stop the elimination, and it may take some time for the dog to finish, so the owner needs to be patient. Feces found after the fact should be removed and the area cleaned up with a quality product, and efforts to supervise should be redoubled. Punishment will likely cause stress and confusion, and it is not effective unless it occurs within one second of the behavior, which is not possible. Mistakes found after the fact indicate a breakdown in management or supervision. In addition, scolding a dog for eliminating in front of a human can lead to covert elimination, difficulty collecting samples for the laboratory should they be needed later, and stress associated with elimination when a person is present.

Forming Good Habits

Following these guidelines will result in a dog that reliably eliminates quickly when taken to the elimination area and in few or no mistakes after the training period is complete. Habits are formed through repetition: clients should be reminded to ensure that the dog is performing the desired behavior repeatedly. Every mistake is a rehearsal of the unwanted behavior. For best results, the client should do everything possible to ensure that all repetition is only that of the desired behavior.

Being Consistent

Providing food, water, sleep, and exercise on a predictable schedule will help dogs eliminate on a more predictable schedule. Predictability of elimination will help clients successfully housetrain their pets, because the clues to when and how much the pet will eliminate are easier to anticipate.

Unwanted Elimination: Cats

Unwanted elimination is the single most commonly described objectionable behavior. Early diagnosis, treatment, and behavior modification help improve the prognosis for unwanted elimination. The longer the unwanted elimination persists, the more difficult it can be to change. Every client presenting a cat of any age should be questioned during the visit about litter use. "Are there any eliminations outside the litter box or in any unwanted locations?" By screening cats during every single visit for this common problem, the chances that a veterinary technician can assist with early detection improve. In addition, hearing this screening question during every visit alerts clients to call the veterinary hospital if they see a change in their pets' elimination habits at home.

Housetraining

Many clients assume that cats self-train for elimination and, to some extent, this is true. Cats provided with a litter area that meets their personal preferences and needs, is readily and easily accessible, and is kept clean and tidy will often require little additional training. Young cats eliminating outside the litter box should be assessed right away, as discussed in the next section.

Litter Box Preferences

Research has demonstrated that most cats prefer fine-textured, unscented, clumping litter placed in a box with a large surface area and without a cover. Fig. 5.13 shows examples of converting storage containers into litter boxes matching this description. Most pet store suppliers and litter manufacturers cater to the preferences of humans rather than those of cats. Clients should be educated about proper litter selection and maintenance as early as possible.

Litter box size and cleanliness should facilitate cats to enter the box, turn in a circle, eliminate, bury the elimination, circle again, and exit without touching the sides of the litter box or any clumps of previously soiled litter. To achieve this goal, clients should provide a large box and scoop all soiled litter from the box at least once a day. Once weekly, all the litter should be removed, and the container scrubbed with soap and water before being refilled with clean litter. Annually, clients should consider replacing the litter box itself as plastic will inevitably start to develop residual odor, no matter how well the client has kept the box clean.

Although most cats prefer fine-clumping litter, some have a different substrate preference. Providing exposure to many types of litter early on in the training process can help identify individual preferences for substrate. During this process, the client will provide several litter types in separate boxes placed in one location. The litter type that is used most often by the cat should point to its substrate preference. If the cat uses all litter types with equal frequency, the cat may have flexibility with regard to substrates.

Meeting the needs of indoor cats, as discussed earlier in this chapter, will go a long way toward maintaining desired elimination

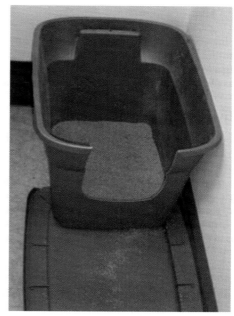

• **Fig. 5.13** Litter boxes that are custom made from storage containers are affordable and ideal for many cats.

patterns and preventing other common unwanted behaviors. The Ohio State University Indoor Pets Initiative provides a great deal of information regarding meeting the needs of indoor cats.

In rare situations, cats that have undergone diagnosis and treatment for unwanted elimination will not respond, and the behavior will continue. For these cats, allowing safe and controlled outdoor access may reduce unwanted elimination and is preferable over euthanasia. The use of cat enclosures ("Catios"); use of fencing products, such as deer fencing or Purr-fect fence; and training of cats to walk with a leash and harness all allow safe exposure while protecting cats from harm from cat fights, dog attacks, and vehicular accidents. These measures also prevent cats from negatively impacting local wildlife through predation.

Urine Marking

Urine marking is a normal behavior of dogs and cats. Depositing urine, feces, and anal sac secretions is unpalatable to humans but normal for animals. Prevention strategies against urine marking by both dogs and cats include adequate supervision; reduction of stressors, such as competition for resources among animals; providing adequate physical and mental exercise and enrichment; and allowing opportunities for acceptable marking, such as outdoor walks for dogs and scratching posts for cats.

Some suggestions for decreasing unwanted urine marking by dogs are as follows:
- Veterinarian consultation to diagnose and treat underlying medical concerns
- Ceasing all physical punishment or training based on fear or intimidation
- Screening the pet for stress and reducing stressors as much as possible, including conflicts between pets in the household or between the pet and the owner
- Providing an opportunity for urine marking in acceptable locations (e.g., on walks)
- Direct supervision and management to reduce opportunity to mark in unwanted areas

Aggression During Play

Aggression in the form of chasing, barking, biting, scratching, and physical contact is a normal part of play for both puppies and kittens and is called *play-related aggression*. Puppies and kittens use play fighting to gain coordination and learn social communication with conspecifics during their youth. Clients need to be prepared to direct the play behavior of their pets starting at a young age and to foster appropriate play to avoid unwanted aggressive behavior.

Rough play is often accidentally reinforced by clients. When puppies or kittens bite during play, they are overly excited and are showing an interest in continuing with escalating levels of rough play. Physical punishment, loud voices or shouting, and high-pitched voices or squeaking can send the wrong message to the animal, which will interpret it as the client's desire for escalation of rough play. Attempts to punish rough play can also damage the human-animal bond if the client scares the animal or causes pain. Fear and pain harm the trust between the pet and the owner and can result in the animal avoiding interactions with its owner or in display of defensive aggression when fearful of the owner.

When playing with puppies and kittens, clients should use toys rather than hands. For puppies, using plush toys that are small enough for the puppy to bite but have a large surface area available is helpful. The client should be instructed to hold onto a small part of the toy, giving the puppy access to the majority of the toy. If the puppy bites the client during play, the client should calmly stop play, take a brief break (a few seconds to a few minutes) so that the excited puppy can calm down, and then redirect play to an appropriate toy. Some kittens also enjoy biting or kicking a large stuffed toy, but most prefer to chase and capture smaller items instead. Clients should play with kittens by using fishing-pole type toys or small toys that can be tossed and chased. If kittens begin to bite at the client's hands or feet, the client should stop play immediately and take a brief break so that the kitten can calm down before starting play again. Any client who sustains repeated bites or scratches from a puppy or kitten should seek the advice of the veterinary team.

Fear and Aggression

Socialization, which has been discussed elsewhere in this chapter, plays an important role in protecting dogs and cats from future fears of common events, interactions, and objects. When kittens and puppies have a variety of positive, nonfrightening exposures to different stimuli in their youth, they have the opportunity to learn that these items and experiences are not a threat and thus do not warrant a fear response. The goals of these early learning experiences are to teach the animal that the stimulus is not dangerous, that it leads to good things happening, and that the client will support and protect the animal. Pairing potentially concerning experiences with pleasurable ones can be done during every veterinary visit. Veterinary technicians can pair greeting of the animal with treats, touching, and praise. Further pairing can happen with each step of collecting vital signs, each part of the physical examination, any necessary treatments such as vaccinations or sample collection, and grooming such as nail care. When performing these pairing exercises, the veterinary technician can and should educate the client about the body language of dogs and cats and the reason for pairing these experiences. Veterinary technicians can lead by example, showing clients in the examination room how to watch for signs of stress, stop if the animal feels worried, and

how to provide positive, safe, and pleasurable experiences with new places, people, and handling.

If puppies and kittens show fear of the veterinary team or of handling, the veterinarian should be alerted. Early intervention with the use of desensitization and counterconditioning can reverse mild fear when the pet is still young.

Educating clients about the body language of fear and stress helps clients provide effective and save socialization and social interactions. For example, many clients do not know about out-of-context behaviors, such as panting when not hot, shaking off when not wet, sniffing when there is no appealing odor, or licking the lips when not hungry. Clients may not understand that when a cat rolls on its side or back, it is relaxed but most likely is not inviting touching of its abdomen. Alerting clients to subtle signs of fear and asking them to monitor for these signs in response to people, places, odors, sounds, surfaces, experiences at home and in any context may provide a protective effect against **fear-related aggression** or disorders in the future. At a minimum, educating clients that fearful body language indicates that pets need space and to be removed from a stressor, and a visit to the veterinarian will improve the quality of life for fearful animals in the home and contribute to early detection of behavior concerns.

Medical Treatment of Fear and Anxiety in Dogs and Cats

In some cases, the veterinarian may prescribe medications to prevent or treat fear and anxiety in animals and as part of a comprehensive behavior treatment plan. Behavior medications for animals fall into two basic categories: (1) baseline or mainstay medications, which are administered every day during a long-term behavior treatment, and (2) event-based or short-term medications, which are effective for only a few hours at a time and can be given prior to anticipated stressful events or exposure to known triggers.

Baseline or mainstay medications work to gradually change the animal's brain chemistry. The medications upregulate or downregulate the production, use, and turnover of neurotransmitter chemicals, which are the messengers of the central nervous system. Changing the activity of neurotransmitters can influence the way animals experience stress, fear, or arousal and help them succeed during behavior modification protocols. As with any medication, psychoactive medications generally have the best effect when they are begun at the time of diagnosis rather than late in the process. Much like a patient with a urinary tract infection, who will be provided antibiotics rather than sent home with advice to drink plenty of water and cranberry juice, patients experiencing emotional or psychological distress should, in many cases, also receive medical treatment as a first line of care. Stigma surrounding the use of psychoactive medications and concerns about side effects or unwanted personality changes may cause reluctance to use them. The veterinary team should be nonjudgmental and supportive and provide support and education for clients throughout the treatment period. Table 5.8 provides a list of commonly used behavior-modifying medications used in veterinary medicine.

Event-based medications or short-acting medications may be used before veterinary visits, travel, storms or fireworks, or any event the patient may find temporarily stressful. Event-based medications are extremely useful to many patients before veterinary visits and should be considered for any patient displaying moderate or severe stress in the veterinary environment. Providing medical relief of fear, anxiety, and stress gives the pet a better

TABLE 5.8 Mainstay or Baseline Medications Commonly Used During Behavior Treatment

Drug Class Generic(Brand)	Common Uses	What to Expect	Contraindications	Time to Effect	Notes
Selective serotonin reuptake inhibitor (SSRI)	Off-label use for dogs and cats Chronic fear, anxiety, and/or stress, compulsive disorders, aggression				
Fluoxetine (Reconcile, Prozac)		Most common side effects are mild and include transient sedation (calmness, lethargy, or depression) or reduced appetite; other gastrointestinal (GI) signs may include (nausea, diarrhea, or constipation) May produce paradoxical agitation, anxiety, or aggression when first starting or adjusting dose	Caution with combining with other serotonergic medications because of risk of serotonin syndrome Caution in patients with a known history of seizures or platelet abnormalities Unregulated diabetes mellitus	3–6 weeks	Reconcile is approved by the US Food and Drug Administration (FDA) for use in dogs for the treatment of separation anxiety
Paroxetine (Paxil)		Same as fluoxetine plus increased urinary sphincter tone and constipation	Same as fluoxetine plus history of urinary blockage, glaucoma	3–6 weeks	
Sertraline (Zoloft)		Same as fluoxetine	Same as fluoxetine	3–6 weeks	
Citalopram (Celexa)		Same as fluoxetine	Same as fluoxetine plus caution in patients with cardiac conduction abnormalities	3–6 weeks	
Tricyclic antidepressants (TCAs)	Off-label use in dogs and cats Chronic fear, anxiety, and/or stress				
Clomipramine (Clomicalm)	Possibly for compulsive disorders as more serotonin selective	Anticholinergic effects Sedation, ataxia, dry mouth, dry eye, mydriasis, increased intraocular pressure, cardiac arrhythmia (tachycardia), constipation, urine retention Common are sedation, wobbliness, GI (taste aversion, transient vomiting, constipation or diarrhea), appetite changes (usually reduction), and urinary retention (cats) May produce paradoxical agitation, anxiety, or aggression when first starting or adjusting dose	Seizure predisposition Ocular abnormalities (keratoconjunctivitis sicca, glaucoma) Unregulated diabetes Hepatic disease Cardiac conduction abnormalities (arrhythmia) Thyroid disorders and concurrent thyroid or sympathomimetic medication Concurrent MAOI Prostate disease or history of urinary outflow obstruction	3–6 weeks	Clomicalm is FDA approved for use in dogs for the treatment of separation anxiety

Continued

TABLE 5.8	Mainstay or Baseline Medications Commonly Used During Behavior Treatment—cont'd				
Drug Class Generic(Brand)	Common Uses	What to Expect	Contraindications	Time to Effect	Notes
Amitriptyline (Elavil)		Same as clomipramine	Same as clomipramine	3–6 weeks	
Monoamine oxidase inhibitor (MAOI)	Cognitive dysfunction syndrome Off label • For chronic or unavoidable fear, social anxiety, panic disorder, and aggression • Use in cats				
Selegeline (Anipryl, L-deprenyl)		Common in dogs are gastrointestinal (vomiting and diarrhea), may see restlessness, repetitive movements, lethargy, salivation, and anorexia	Do not use with any other serotonergic drug, herbal, or supplements because of serotonin syndrome	4–6 weeks	Anipryl is FDA approved for use in dogs for the treatment of canine cognitive dysfunction syndrome (and pituitary-dependent hyperadrenocorticism)
		CNS stimulant because of amphetamine content metabolites	Seizure predisposition		This medication seems to be more likely to result in serotonin syndrome when combined with other serotonergic products
		May produce paradoxical agitation, anxiety, or aggression	Unregulated diabetes		Concurrent use of α^2 agonists or opioids could result in risky blood pressure fluctuations

experience, reduces the risk of the pet developing a worsening fear of the veterinary environment over time, and improves the safety of the veterinary team. Patients who show avoidance and aggression in the veterinary hospital are not "bad," "mean," or "spoiled." They are simply fearful and are using the only form of communication available to them (their behavior) to communicate. Table 5.9 provides a list of commonly used event-based medications for dogs and cats.

Sedatives should never be used alone to treat fear. Fearful animals receiving only sedatives (e.g., acepromazine) will experience physical sedation. Their movements will be slower, and they may show fewer outward signs of stress. In some cases, these animals are experiencing no reduction in their fear level, and it may even increase because they are physically less able move away from perceived threats. Studies have demonstrated that dogs administered acepromazine repeatedly for noise-related fear displayed an *increased* fear response over time. Sedatives are an extremely useful tool when animals are experiencing anxiety. However, instead of administering sedatives as sole agents, they should be used in combination with medications that relieve fear and stress when the animals are experiencing anxiety.

For hospitalized patients experiencing stress, treatment for stress should be included in the hospitalization protocol. Veterinary technicians who observe stress and fear in hospitalized patients should alert the veterinarian and advocate for the patient's needs. Stress

and fear delay healing and have a harmful effect on overall wellness. Providing medical relief of stress and fear while a patient is in the hospital may speed healing, improve the patient experience, facilitate treatments, and improve the safety of the veterinary team.

TECHNICIAN NOTE

Veterinary technicians who observe stress and fear in hospitalized patients should alert the veterinarian and advocate for the patient's needs. Stress and fear delay healing and have a harmful effect on overall wellness.

Common Equine Behavior Concerns

Training Techniques

Historically, training techniques for horses have relied predominantly on negative reinforcement, the release of pressure when a desired behavior occurs. As with all species, the use of negative reinforcement requires astute observation of body language and behaviors, deft application, and the immediate removal of pressure when a desired behavior or approximation occurs. As more is learned about animal welfare and training practices, more information is becoming readily available for the safe use of positive reinforcement–based training for horses and other large animals. Choosing a welfare-forward approach to training that minimizes stress, maximizes sensitivity to communication from the animal,

TABLE 5.9 Short-Acting or Event-Based Medications Used During Times of Predictable Stressors or Triggers

Drug Class (Brand)	Common Uses	What to Expect	Contraindications	Time to Effect	Notes
α² agonist	Acute fear, anxiety, panic, phobia Noise aversion, Hyperactivity/excitability or arousal Impulse control/situations of social aggression Sedation (dose related) with analgesic/antinociceptive effects				
Dexmedetomidine oromucosal gel (Sileo)		Adverse reactions include transient pale mucous membranes at the site of application; uncommonly emesis, drowsiness, or sedation	Severe cardiovascular, respiratory, liver, or kidney diseases or otherwise compromised or debilitated dogs	30–60 minutes	Sileo is approved by the US Food and Drug Administration (FDA) for treating noise aversion in dogs; coaching owners on use of the dosing syringe is important to prevent accidental overdosing
Clonidine (Catapres)		Possible sedation (usually dose dependent), vomiting, dry mouth, constipation, transient hyperglycemia, hypotension, and bradycardia	Same as dexmedetomidine	1–2 hours	Treatment of fear, anxiety, and stress and hyperexcitability Its use has not been studied in cats
Antiepileptics					
Gabapentin	Anticonvulsant, acute or chronic fear, anxiety, panic, phobic conditions, Fear Free veterinary visits for dogs and cats; generalized, separation, and social anxiety; chronic neuropathic pain	Extremely well tolerated in dogs and cats with mild appetite stimulatory effects and memory impairment Common are dose-dependent sedation and/or ataxia; less common are gastrointestinal (GI) (vomiting, diarrhea) Rare, urinary incontinence	Few as primarily secreted renally unchanged and not metabolized; known hypersensitivity	Rapid, 2 hours with as-needed administration Delayed, 1–3 weeks for reduction in neuropathic pain and anxiety, and control of seizures	Wide dosage range Higher doses are often used for preventing or treating acute fears, such as veterinary visits
Imepitoin (Pexion)	Anticonvulsant, noise aversions in dogs	Ataxia, increased appetite, lethargy, vomiting, and possibly aggression	Unknown	Recommended dosing is to give twice daily starting 2 days before the noise event	Pexion is FDA approved for treating noise aversion in dogs At the time of completion of the chart, the medication was not yet available in the United States Use with caution in dogs that have a history of aggression
Benzodiazepines	Acute fear, anxiety, panic, phobia Increased social behavior and "friendliness" Anxiety-related urine marking in cats (diazepam) Submissive- (fear-) related urination in dogs Reduced appetite because of anxiety Muscle relaxation Hypnosis, sedation, insomnia Anticonvulsant for status epilepticus				

Continued

TABLE 5.9   Short-Acting or Event-Based Medications Used During Times of Predictable Stressors or Triggers—cont'd

Drug Class (Brand)	Common Uses	What to Expect	Contraindications	Time to Effect	Notes
Diazepam (Valium)		Sedation or lethargy, polyphagia, muscle relaxation, ataxia inhibits learning, amnesia, hepatic necrosis (cats), increased affection or possible paradoxical reactions: increased excitability, disinhibited aggression	Narrow angle glaucoma; use with caution in cases of aggression resulting from the possibility of disinhibited aggression	1–2 hours	Increased appetite can result in food-searching behavior and restlessness
Alprazolam (Xanax)		Same as diazepam; thought to be less sedating	Same as diazepam	1–2 hours	Same as diazepam
Lorazepam (Ativan)		Same as diazepam; possibly safer on the liver in cats	Same as diazepam	1–2 hours	Same as diazepam
Clonazepam (Klonopin)		Same as diazepam; thought to be less sedating and cause less polyphagia	Same as diazepam	1–2 hours	Same as diazepam
Serotonin antagonist and reuptake inhibitor (SARI)					
Trazodone	Acute or chronic fear, anxiety, panic disorders, generalized anxiety disorder, separation anxiety disorder, aggression and/or agitation, compulsive disorder, postoperative confinement of dogs, sedation/anxiolytic prior to travel and with veterinary visits	GI effects (vomiting and diarrhea), sedation, yet may produce ataxia, hypotension, excitement or agitation, and panting	Seizure predisposition Priapism Conjunction with monoamine oxidase inhibitors (MAOIs)	*Rapid:* 1–2-hour sedation effects when used as needed *Delayed:* 2–4 weeks for SARI when used every 8–12 hours as mainstay or adjunct	Administration without food speeds absorption, whereas with food slows absorption and reduces GI side effects Although less likely to produce agitation and aggression than other behavior drugs, use with caution in patients with aggression as agitation may occur in some individuals Caution with layering other serotonin agonists, such as tramadol as there is an increased risk of seizure or serotonin syndrome; priapism is a rare side effect that may be seen in dogs Caution with use in patients with a history of priapism
Tranquilizer/ neuroleptic/ antipsychotic					

TABLE 5.9 Short-Acting or Event-Based Medications Used During Times of Predictable Stressors or Triggers—cont'd

Drug Class (Brand)	Common Uses	What to Expect	Contraindications	Time to Effect	Notes
Acepromazine	Acepromazine is approved for dogs and cats as aid in controlling intractable animals, to alleviate itching, as an antiemetic for vomiting associated with motion sickness, and as a preanesthetic agent; A neuroleptic tranquilizer	Sedation, weakness, central nervous system (CNS) depression with suppression of the sympathetic nervous system (SNS) and without significant respiratory depression. Hypotension. Changes in cardiac rate (bradycardia with reflex tachycardia) and function (cardiovascular collapse). Impaired thermoregulation (hypothermia/hyperthermia). Paradoxical reactions. CNS stimulation with anxiety, agitation, and idiosyncratic aggression	Known hypersensitivity (breed sensitivities). Cardiac disease. Hypovolemia or shock. Patients with organophosphate toxicity	Rapid sedation, 30 minutes to 1 hour in most patients after oral administration	Not recommended as a monotherapy for treating behavioral issues because while immobilized, patients may experience anxiety, being more sound sensitive and reactive to other sensory inputs. When used, must be combined with medications to treat fear, anxiety, and stress. Effects can last for 24 hours, which can be disturbing for pet owners. Cautionary statements—Use cautiously as a restraining agent in aggressive dogs as it may make the animal more prone to startle and react to noises or other sensory inputs. Phenothiazine use in seizure-prone patients or those with epilepsy is controversial, with cautionary statement that it lowers the seizure threshold; yet evidence suggests that it does not precipitate seizures. Reduce dose in debilitated or geriatric animals, those with hepatic or cardiac disease, or when combined with other agents. Giant breeds, sight hounds, dogs with *MDR1* mutations (Collies, Australian Shepherds, etc.) may be more sensitive to effects; Terriers may be more resistant to effects

and selects positive reinforcement–based approaches is best for the animal and safest for the people working around the animal. It is not the goal of this chapter to provide a comprehensive guide to training but to prompt the reader to consider welfare and safety as the primary factors of importance when selecting training methods. Refer to the Recommended Readings at the end of this chapter for resources detailing newer approaches to training large animals.

Aggression Among Horses

Aggressive threats are common among groups of horses. These displays are generally ritualized and alleviate conflict through communication, reducing the actual incidence of harmful encounters between animals. Generally, offensive aggression arises from the fore end and commonly includes head threats, in addition to bite threats, bites, threats to strike, and actual strikes. Kicking and kick threats are believed by some to be limited to defensive behavior but may, in fact, be used whenever danger or an opponent is closer to the hindquarters than to the forequarters. When a head threat does not result in the offending party moving away or otherwise deferring, teeth may be bared as a threat or an actual bite may occur. Horses may also threaten to strike with their forelegs by simply moving one foreleg forward and pinning their ears. A kick threat may involve simply shifting weight or cocking or lifting a leg, but a thrashing tail may also be a threat to kick as discussed earlier in this chapter (refer to the section "Body Language"). Sometimes a slight hop on the hind legs is performed before the horse kicks out with one or both legs. Horses can be very fast and accurate in the placement of strikes and kicks, so it should always be assumed that when the legs do *not* make contact, the intent was only to threaten.

Horses can cause serious injury to conspecifics in the process of establishing a social group. Injuries may be more likely if horses that have been confined in isolation are subsequently reintroduced to other horses within confined quarters. In preparing to house two horses together, using management to separate the horses physically but still allowing olfactory, visual, and limited tactile contacts is recommended. Using protected contact allows owners to screen the interaction between horses and possibly prevent injuries caused by surprise aggression between unfamiliar horses.

Competition for resources or perceived scarcity can be a common cause of aggression among horses housed together. Providing an environment with multiple feeding stations placed a distance apart, attractive resting areas with plenty of distance between them, and multiple watering areas can help decrease conflict over resources. In addition, the area holding multiple horses must be large enough that horses can use their normal visual cues for deference or appeasement and have sufficient space to escape aggressors. Moving away is a primary communication mechanism horses use to de-escalate encounters. Sufficient space must be provided to allow horses to move away from one another.

Human-Directed Aggression

As with dogs and cats, some unwanted behavior that is normal for horses may be objectionable to humans. Some common causes of human-directed aggression include flight responses associated with fear, frustration, confusion or conflict about responding to signals, high arousal states, and pain or discomfort. Equine aggression directed toward humans is unfortunately common and is more often seen in stalled horses compared with pastured horses. When horses feel threatened or fearful, they will demonstrate this initially via subtle changes in their body language. When these signals fail to communicate their discomfort, the horse will then escalate their body signals. If the stronger signals result in the retreating of the perceived threat or a stop to the painful or fear-inducing stimulus, the horse learns that the more overt signals but not the subtle ones are effective. The horse may subsequently abandon lower-level signals in favor of more overt threats. It is important to keep in mind that these behaviors are based on fear and that the handler can control the behavior by reducing the animal's fear in response to subtle changes in the horse's body language immediately, and by using welfare-forward training plans to recondition fear-based behavior in the future.

Fear of husbandry and veterinary care is common among horses. When a particular person, equipment setup, or context predicts pain or discomfort, the horse may become conditioned to repel these stimuli. Horses can develop fears of being caught, clipped, saddled, or ridden. In many cases, chronic pain and the fear of pain may be the cause of aggression. If a horse has subclinical orthopedic pain, for example, it may learn to be aggressive toward people who carry tack and attempt to saddle them. Underlying pain in a horse must always be ruled out as a cause of aggression, irritability, and reluctance to work. Once pain has been identified and treated, the behavior modification techniques described earlier in this chapter can be used to implement training plans.

Veterinarians should be consulted when horses display unwanted behaviors or a change in behavior. Changes in behavior may result from illness, injury, or pain and will require a thorough physical examination by a veterinarian. Conditioned behavioral disorders should be identified and treatment and behavior modification plans should be established to change the unwanted behavior. Treatment for horses is available through DACVBs, as with dogs and cats.

Repetitive Behaviors

Unwanted **repetitive behaviors,** such as wind sucking, cribbing, wood sucking, wood chewing, stall walking and weaving, kicking stalls, and frequent pawing are often called "stable vices." A more accurate description, in some cases, may be "displacement" or "redirection": the animal is performing this behavior because it is unable to engage in its true target behavior. Some of these behaviors are true stereotypies, repetitive behaviors with no discernible, immediate function. Stereotypies are not observed in free-ranging horses but are observed in wild equids held in captivity. This suggests that stereotypies may be a stress response to captivity and husbandry. In any case, the label "stable vice" suggests that the animal is somehow "deficient," "damaged," or "defective." Such pejorative labels should no longer be used. Instead, the specific behaviors observed should be identified and described while considering possible antecedents and consequences. Horses displaying repetitive behaviors should be examined by a veterinarian, and the veterinary technician should take a thorough history and assist in educating the horse owner about the prescribed behavior modification plan.

Repetitive pawing behavior can be a displacement behavior in horses. Pawing is a normal part of accessing food and water by horses. Particularly around feeding time, horses may paw the stall floor as a result of not engaging in pawing as part of normal foraging. Kicking the inside of the stall may be a redirected behavior when a horse is unable to communicate with another horse via body language or when horses are restricted from responding to visual cues by the barriers of stall walls or by large distances from one another.

Free-ranging horses chew on and eat bark as a normal part of their diet, so wood chewing and wood eating may be a normal behavior in many cases. In some situations, however, the horse may exhibit the redirected behavior of wood ingestion when insufficient fiber is present in its. Correcting deficiencies in horse husbandry will often decrease wood ingestion.

Wood eating should not be confused with cribbing or crib biting. Cribbing is usually considered a stereotypy. When cribbing, or crib biting, the horse grasps a fixed object with its incisors, arches its neck, and leans backward, sometimes but not always gulping air, and making a distinctive grunting noise. Cribbing is not observed in free-ranging horses. Cribbing has been linked to management factors, such as diets that are low in forage and housing that limits normal social behavior among horses. However, many horses are kept stalled, with limited access to forage, and are fed concentrates twice daily, and they do not all become cribbers. This fact suggests that the origin of cribbing is complex and multifactorial, and research continues to provide fascinating information about this problem. Cribbing may be associated with the stress of coping with an abnormal environment in the adult horse and with the stress of weaning in foals. The likelihood of cribbing is greater in weanling foals given concentrate feeds. Treatment for cribbing should be guided by the veterinarian and, when possible, a DACVB. Some remedies commonly chosen by clients such as cribbing collars and cribbing rings cause intentional pain to the horse when it tries to crib. These devices compromise welfare, can cause harm, and should not be used. Further, their efficacy is not proven.

Common Cattle Behavior Concerns

Human-Directed Aggression

Most of the species of domestic livestock used by humans today were selected because they possessed a certain amount of tolerance for human proximity and handling. Nevertheless, some individual animals may display aggression toward humans. This is more common among hand-raised animals because they are more likely to direct their normal species-typical behaviors toward humans as though the humans are conspecifics. Therefore whenever possible, orphaned animals should be raised with conspecifics or fostered in such a way as to prevent this problem.

Cattle that spend much of their life on an open range may also be more difficult to handle and more aggressive than other cattle. These animals do not have the learning history to understand that humans do not pose a threat and have lived in an environment where they had to protect themselves from threats to remain safe. In contrast to hand-raised orphans, the fear of free-range cattle stems from the *lack* of exposure to human handling. Exposure can make considerable difference in the ease with which cattle can be worked. Whenever possible, simply moving cattle through a chute without performing any procedures can help familiarize cattle with the process, reduce stress, and ultimately save time. A positive effect on herd behavior may be achieved after only two or three practice runs through a chute.

Dairy cows are selected for ease of handling, but all bulls should be handled with caution, especially by people unfamiliar to them or those associated with a history of unpleasant experiences. The veterinary technician should remain aware that all livestock species can recognize individual humans by their appearance. These animals remember people, and such memories of specific handling events and/or humans will influence the behavior of livestock in the future. Raised voices and slapping and hitting have been shown to be aversive to cattle. Whistling; gentle, consistent touch; and scratching are generally considered less aversive. Setting up handling facilities with an understanding of animal perceptions of the environment and moving and treating animals with patience and tolerance will pay off if the animals do not learn to associate your approach with fearful stimuli.

Buller Steer Syndrome

Buller steer syndrome has a considerable negative economic impact on feedlot production, representing a sizable loss second only to respiratory diseases. It is also a welfare concern for the buller steer, sometimes resulting in direct injury and death. Buller steer syndrome occurs when one steer repeatedly stands and tolerates mounting by other steers. A normal steer would not allow mounting but would exhibit avoidance behaviors or turn and threaten the animal attempting to mount. Instead, "buller" steers allow it and may be injured by the persistent mounting, often becoming debilitated. Buller steers are more common in large groups of cattle in crowded conditions. The metabolism of hormones commonly administered to feedlot steers may influence the development of buller steers, but this effect requires more research. Why or how steers develop this syndrome is unknown, and treatment generally involves removing buller steers from the group. Maintaining a separate pen of only bullers can be helpful as bulling is not generally observed in these pens.

Milking Avoidance

Milking results in oxytocin release during let-down, which should provide a natural, positive, classically CR to milking. Animals that previously willingly entered the milking parlor can exhibit a change in milking tolerance for a variety of reasons. Changes in the handling practice, changing the location of entry or the side the cow presents for milking, traction problems in the handling system, changes in the appearance or shape of the handling system, changes in sounds of the milking or handling system, or changes in feeding patterns during milking can all influence the cow's willingness to enter the milking parlor. Pain during milking may also result in parlor avoidance. Monitoring for pain in general, lameness, and particularly pain of the teat or bag should be performed for any cow newly avoiding the parlor.

Cows exhibiting changes in milking behavior should be examined by the veterinarian to ensure that they do not have any decline in visual acuity, orthopedic pain, ulcers, or mastitis. A review of husbandry and handling practices should be conducted, with pain-related and fear-related handling practices being replaced with welfare-improving handling methods (refer to Chapter 6, "Restraint and Handling").

Small Ruminant Behavior Concerns

Small ruminants can display aggression toward other members of the flock or toward humans, as discussed for cattle. Fear, territorial behavior, sexual behavior, and competition for resources can all contribute to aggressive displays directed toward herd- or flockmates, as well as humans. Rams and bucks should be monitored for aggression toward other rams and bucks and toward humans, particularly during breeding season. Welfare-centered handling should be used for all animals, and a history of forceful handling can contribute to fear-related aggression in small ruminants.

Rejection of Young

Small ruminants may sometimes reject their lambs or kids. Ewes and does generally spend time bonding with their young immediately after birth. They clean the young, consuming amniotic material and vocalizing so that the lamb or the kid will be able to recognize and follow the dam. Stress during birth, competition between animals for birthing space and food, inexperience (first-time mothers), or multiple births of more than two offspring all may result in rejection of the young. Rejecting lambs or kids presents a significant production challenge. Hand rearing or bucket rearing the young is costly and time intensive. When possible, bonding of the lamb or the kid and the mother should be attempted.

To encourage bonding, mother and young can be housed together in a small pen or "jug." If the mother is striking at the lamb or kid, the mother may need to be placed temporarily in a halter or stanchion to ensure the safety of the young. To encourage a lamb or a kid to nurse, it should be helped to stand facing the teats, with its rear toward the mother's shoulder. Rubbing or bumping the rear of the youngster will encourage it toward the teat and stimulate nursing. Forcibly placing the animal's mouth on the teat will almost always create resistance, may decrease the urge to nurse out of fear of handling, and should not be done.

When mothers reject their young and other new mothers are readily available, the young can sometimes be "grafted" onto another mother to be fostered. This is best done when the young are within 1–2 days of the same age, during or immediately after the birth of the foster mother's young. The lamb or the kid to be grafted should be rubbed all over with the amniotic fluid and placenta of the foster mother's newly delivered lamb or kid. Feces or urine of the foster mother's own young may be rubbed near the genital area of the fosterling as well. The grouping must be monitored to ensure that the new mother is not showing aggression toward the fosterling. In cases where neonatal death has occurred, mothers may be willing to accept fosterlings dressed with the skin of the deceased young. This practice requires direct supervision to ensure the dressed skin does not cause health or welfare problems. Because of the behavioral, emotional, and financial benefits of young being reared by mothers rather than by hand, fostering is a worthwhile attempt, though not all fosters will be accepted by the new mother, or there may be a shortage of mothers, necessitating hand rearing.

Behavior Emergencies

TECHNICIAN NOTE

There are few true behavior emergencies, but it is crucial for veterinary technicians to immediately recognize and triage behavior emergencies for immediate care when they occur. Animal lives depend on rapid recognition and action by the entire veterinary team.

Canine and Feline

There are few true behavioral emergencies in dogs and cats. By its nature, behavior evolves over time. It takes time for clients to notice changes in animal behavior. Clients often seek out trainers in an attempt to adapt to the animal's behavior and to solve the problem on their own. Some clients may not be aware they should discuss concerning behaviors and changes in behavior with the veterinary team. Taking a short behavior history during every appointment will help catch problems early before they become emergencies.

What constitutes a behavior emergency in dogs and cats?
1. *The human-animal bond compromised:* If the client is considering severing the human-animal bond and taking the pet to a shelter or rescue, finding a new home, or considering euthanasia, this is an emergency, even if the behavior is a longstanding one. Clients who seem to be at risk for severing the human-animal bond should be seen immediately, whenever possible. The most common emergent situation in cats is elimination outside the litter box. Although this condition is seldom medically urgent, if the client is ready to give up, these cases should be triaged appropriately (not only on the basis of the patient's condition, but also on the basis of the condition of the human-animal bond, the owner's level of frustration, and their intention to euthanize or give up the pet).
2. *Human-directed aggression with sustained injuries:* As discussed earlier in this chapter, the vast majority of aggression shown by dogs and cats is defensive and related to fear. If a client describes injuries sustained or fear of being injured by the animal, this is an emergency and they should be seen as soon as possible. *A full behavior history and safety risk assessment should be performed prior to interacting with any patient with human-directed aggression.* The practitioner should have clear guidelines about what level of human-directed aggression they are comfortable with and skilled enough to treat, and a list of referral options for cases beyond the scope or comfort of the current practitioner. Veterinary technicians can and should triage and urgently schedule or refer these cases as appropriate based on their veterinarian's triage guidelines.
3. *Any situation in which the animal is harming itself:* For example, a dog breaking teeth or toenails during escape attempts, or any animal the client describes as panicked.
4. *Aggression toward other animals:* The behavior causes injuries to other animals.

Equine and Large Animals

Situations involving self-injury by the animal, interactions where humans are injured, and interactions where other animals are injured should all be triaged as urgent. If the human-animal bond is at risk, this is also an urgent situation.

Foal rejection is one of the few recognized true behavior emergencies in horses. It is critical to the foal's survival that it receives colostrum within several hours of birth. Foal rejection can result in failure of passive transfer of immunity, or FPT. After 36 hours, the foal's digestive tract is incapable of absorbing the important macromolecules found in the colostrum. Many mares, particularly **primiparous** mares, resent manipulation of the inguinal fold and the udder. These mares may avoid the foal's approach and may kick, squeal, and even bite when the foal attempts to nurse. Pain associated with mastitis, passage of the placenta, or uterine contractions that occur because of oxytocin released when the foal suckles may contribute to this problem.

A more serious form of foal rejection occurs when the mare acts as if she is afraid of the foal itself and actively attacks it. In these situations, the mare may attempt to escape the foal and may injure it in the process and/or kick the foal whenever it approaches. Other mares may attack the foal by biting it and throwing it across the stall. These mares often have a history of not having licked the fetal membranes or the foal in the minutes after birth and generally behave in a less protective manner toward the foal. These mares have been shown to have lower concentrations of serum progesterone compared with mares that accept their foals. Because foal rejection occurs more frequently in Arabian mares, the behavior likely has a heritable component. Mares with a history of rejecting a foal should be carefully evaluated if rebreeding is considered. However, the likelihood of foal rejection does appear to decrease with parity.

A variety of methods have been used to manage and treat foal rejection. A combination of tranquilization and restraint can be used to allow the foal to nurse and to teach the mare that suckling relieves tension and pressure on the udder, resulting in improvement in physical comfort. A combination of gradual desensitization of the flank/udder region and counterconditioning to change the mare's emotional response to the foal has also been used successfully to treat this problem. If the mare does not accept the foal, a nurse mare can sometimes be located to accept the foal. Foals should be raised by mares rather than by hand whenever possible.

Learning in the Veterinary Setting

Learning happens all the time. Animals are constantly taking in information and developing conscious and unconscious responses. When the veterinary setting involves pheromone signals of stress and fear or social signals from other animals, the animals easily develop an aversion to the environment. Animals that are injured or ill may associate pain or feeling unwell with the veterinary environment. Veterinary technicians need to approach these animals with compassion for their feelings of pain, illness, fear, and stress while maintaining their own safety as the highest priority.

Safety Considerations

As discussed earlier in the chapter, patients experiencing fear, anxiety, and stress will usually first try to avoid the fear-inducing stimulus or event. Ultimately, fear is adaptive under certain circumstances; it keeps animals safe by allowing them to avoid potential harm. If they are unable to escape from perceived threats, animals may defend themselves in fear. Veterinary technicians must understand the body language of fear in multiple species, recognize early warning signs of patient discomfort, and respond appropriately.

Reducing Patient Stress and Anxiety in Veterinary Practices

In the past two decades, the importance of reducing stress and anxiety during veterinary appointments has been well documented. Compared with calm patients, those that experience anxiety are more likely to resist treatment and may exhibit more aggression toward veterinary personnel. In addition, fear in patients may prevent veterinary technicians from carrying out important treatments and diagnostic studies. Fear can also raise cortisol levels, which in turn can delay healing. Finally, veterinary patients are more cooperative when the clinical environment has calming, rather than excitatory, stimuli.

Leaders, such as veterinarians Dr. Sophia Yin, Dr. Marty Becker, and Dr. Karen Overall, have dedicated much of their careers to understanding and improving the experience of animals in veterinary hospitals. To this end, Low Stress Handling University and Fear Free Pets are education programs developed to teach veterinary personnel a kinder and more effective approach to patient handling. Lowering the stress of veterinary patients also helps create a more pleasurable experience for pet owners and veterinary personnel and for the patient. Over the past two decades, new awareness of the significance of stress on animal patients and the adverse role it plays on patients during routine office visits and overnight hospitalizations has been well documented and discussed.

Implementing low-stress approaches to veterinary practice requires veterinary technicians to carefully monitor the behavior and responses of each patient and balance the need for a particular treatment against the potential stress it may cause the patient. Some procedures may be paused briefly or postponed indefinitely until a new plan that is better suited to the individual needs of the patient can be implemented.

Fear Free Fundamentals

Fear Free is a certification program for members of the veterinary profession and other pet care professionals (trainers, groomers, walkers, shelter teams, etc.). Certification is available for canine/feline, equine, avian, and small exotics, with more courses underway at the time of this publishing. The certification programs provide in-depth instruction on how to interact with animals. Fear Free strives to provide the highest quality veterinary medical care by protecting the emotional welfare of the patient.

According to studies conducted by Bayer and the American Association of Feline Practitioners (AAFP), 34% of cat owners avoid making veterinary care appointments because they feel that the visit would be too stressful. Greater than 50% of pet owners describe their pets as very stressed in the veterinary setting. Providing care with attention to the emotional welfare of pets is less stressful for owners and their animals. Owners who are less stressed are more likely to bring their pets to the veterinarian earlier, more frequently, and with less reluctance, which in turn maximizes the potential health of the animal.

Experiencing fear, anxiety, and stress can lead to physiological changes that alter both the short- and long-term health of the animal. Increased heart rate, respiratory rate, blood pressure, temperature, blood glucose, and cortisol levels are immediate physiologic responses to stress. The body prepares for fight or flight as the hypothalamic-pituitary-adrenal (HPA) axis and the sympathetic nervous system (SNS) launch physiologic protective measures by increasing sensory alertness and masking pain. Stress-related diarrhea, stress leukograms, and stress-related urinary tract disease are all examples of physiologic changes attributed to stress. Long-term stress can result in immunosuppression, influence GI health, increase dermatologic permeability, delay wound healing, and, in severe cases, may shorten the animal's life span. Decreasing avoidable activations of the stress response therefore improves the animal's health and welfare.

The FAS Score

Fear Free uses the abbreviation FAS for fear, anxiety, and stress. The FAS score is a numeric value assigned to the patient's level of fear, anxiety, and stress. FAS scores can change rapidly, can be specific to certain procedures or experiences, and can vary by individual patient. The FAS score is determined by observing the animal's body language indicators as described in the body language sections of this chapter. The FAS score ranges between 0 and 5, with 0 being completely relaxed and 5 often involving defensive aggression. Fig. 5.14 shows an example of FAS scores and the actions associated with them. Animals displaying FAS scores of 0 and 1 are responding well to treatment: green light = proceed. These animals are relaxed or have mild stress as described earlier in the chapter. FAS scores of 2 to 3 may mean that the animal would benefit from a different plan, especially for longer procedures or for procedures that will need to be done repeatedly: yellow light = proceed but with caution. FAS scores of 2 to 3 correspond to the descriptions of moderate stress as described earlier in this chapter. FAS scores of 4 to 5 mean that the animal is experiencing active distress: red light = pause the treatment and make a new plan before proceeding. FAS scores of 4 to 5 correspond to severe stress and represent a significant threat to patient welfare.

Tracking, recording, and referring to FAS scores is a way to quantify and communicate about patient emotional welfare and behavior while in the veterinary setting.

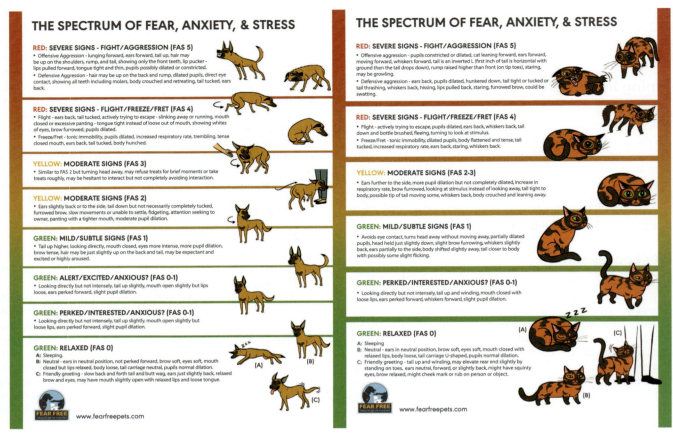

• **Fig. 5.14** Fear Free spectrum of fear, anxiety, and stress (FAS).

Considerate Approach

The **considerate approach** concept encompasses "the interaction between the veterinary team and the patients and inputs from the environment while veterinary care is being administered." This approach means setting up the environment and each interaction to be sensitive to the needs of patients. Table 5.10 lists the common strategies used to implement the considerate approach.

Touch Gradient

Touch Gradient is a method of touching animals in a systematic and sensitive way to decrease fear, anxiety, and stress during handling. The Touch Gradient has two main components:

1. Maintaining **continuous hands-on contact** with the patient throughout the entire procedure or examination
2. Acclimating the patient to **increasing levels of touch intensity** while continuously measuring the patient's acceptance and comfort

When initiating tactile contact with a pet, the animal's touch receptors receive the touch information and send it to the brain. The animal then responds to that stimulus. After the first touch, many pets respond favorably if some level of tactile contact is maintained. Repeatedly removing and replacing the hands on the patient's body can amplify the sensitivity of the touch receptors (known as "wind-up") and can cause the patient to startle when touched.

Touch varies in several ways. Location on the body, duration of contact, pressure applied, and sharpness of sensation are all aspects

of touch that can be altered to accommodate the sensitivities of the patient and thus improve patient trust, comfort, and cooperation.

Animals have an uneven distribution of touch receptors over their bodies. In general, the most sensitive areas, with the highest density of touch receptors, include the face (nose, lips, ear tips, eyelids, tongue), the legs (increasing distally with paws and toes being most sensitive), the anal and genital areas, and the tail. One way to employ the Touch Gradient is to initiate touch in the less sensitive areas, such as the sides of the shoulders or lateral midthorax, and then glide to more sensitive areas, as needed. This allows the animal to become accustomed to touch and adjust gradually to increasing intensities of sensations. For example, rather than reaching directly for the paw when starting a nail trim, one should begin by touching the shoulder and *then* move to the paw. A sudden contact with a sensitive area, such as the paw, may startle the animal and cause a negative response.

Use of the Touch Gradient concept may help change the way in which physical examination is performed. For example, if the animal is known to have a sensitive area that triggers a fear response or defensive aggression, that area should be examined last. With each physical examination, it would be wise to start with less invasive touching and gradually work up to more invasive touching. The face, lips, nose, and ears are highly sensitive body parts, whereas the thorax and trunk are generally less sensitive. The assessment should begin with a skin examination, body condition score and muscle condition score, lymph node evaluation, and auscultation. Next, the head is examined, followed by gliding the hand down the limbs to the paws, and deep palpation of the abdomen is done last. During this process, the most sensitive areas are examined

TABLE 5.10 Implementing Considerate Approach as Part of Fear Free Care

Environment	Patient Interaction	Client Interaction
Synthetic calming pheromones	Work where pet is comfortable	Previsit questions:
Clean away odors without strong perfumes	Mat on floor, table, couch, carrier bottom, car, house call	- Location
Remove urine and feces promptly from entrance areas	Provide what pet likes	- Provider
Nonslip surfaces for pets	Treats (lots!), toys, tactile, catnip, etc.	- Favorite treats
Scale, floor, table, kennel	Approach calmly and from side	- Known fear triggers
Prevent social interaction between patients	Avoid direct eye contact	- Motion sickness
Prevent interactions between pets and strangers/other clients	Calm, confident voices	Safe travel plan
Calming music	Allow pet to approach team	Encourage family presence
No sounds of distressed animals	Gently reposition: no dragging	Explain all measures taken for patient comfort
Water bowl and litter box		Verbalize FAS (fear, anxiety, stress) scores
Hiding areas and high spots for cats		Explain body language cues—many clients do not recognize them
Kennel without facing other pets		Explain welfare
Visual barriers/partial cage covers		Discussing medications
Separate dog/cat examination rooms and housing whenever possible		

last. This approach helps the animal become better conditioned to handling and improves patient responses to handling in the future.

Thoughtful Control of the Patient

The veterinary team comfortably and safely positions the patient to allow for the administration of veterinary care. This involves using distractions and gentle handling to stabilize patients for procedures, and recognizes that use of the "less is more" concept is often the best strategy. If animals cannot be stabilized and treated easily without using forceful restraint techniques, medication may be warranted to decrease the FAS score, and veterinary technicians should consult the veterinarian. It may also be prudent for the veterinarian to consider a house call so that the pet can be treated in a familiar, safe environment. Additional information regarding restraint and handling techniques is provided in Chapter 6.

Factors of Gentle Control

The following are the components of the **gentle control** concept.
- Use of distractions when possible
- Stabilization rather than forcible restraint to encourage stillness
- Animal made to feel secure—no slipping, gently supported
- Animal gently kept in place with attention paid to all six directions of possible movement (up, down, right, left, forward, back)
- Safely preventing harm to the pet and the veterinary team
- A plan for ways to stop the procedure and safely move away if the FAS score increases rapidly

> **TECHNICIAN NOTE**
>
> Providing optimal care for animal patients involves using animal-aware handling strategies combined with medications when appropriate to provide the lowest stress and safest experience for the animal and the veterinary team.

Happy Visits and Victory Visits

Patients benefit from positive emotional responses to the veterinary environment. One way to achieve these positive responses, especially for dogs, is the use of the Happy Visits concept. Happy visits involve visiting the hospital; receiving treats or other preferred interaction (toys, tactile) in the parking lot, lobby, and examination room; and leaving. No medical care nor simulated medical care is administered during happy visits. If a pet appears stressed during a visit, the visit should be stopped and a new plan made. Stressed pets are experiencing repeated unpleasant events rather than happy ones, and this will have the opposite of the desired effect.

The Victory Visits concept involves scheduling time for the patient to visit the hospital for specific training to accustom the animal to veterinary and husbandry procedures. Skilled team members can conduct victory visits, or an outside trainer or behavior consultant may need to conduct these visits. During victory visits, the techniques of desensitization, classical counterconditioning, and operant conditioning, as discussed earlier in this chapter, are all used to teach patients how to receive care with less fear, anxiety, and stress.

Behavior and the Emotional Medical Record

It is crucial for the veterinary team to keep accurate records about how animals respond to veterinary care and how best to successfully provide care for specific animals.

When recording behavior and treatment notes in the medical record, choose language that accurately reflects the body language and behavior of the patient without labels. For example, "Standing lateral saphenous blood draw with cheese distraction" is a more helpful note than "fractious for blood draw." The first note tells a team member how to try to succeed in animal handling. The second note can lead to the veterinary technician approaching the animal with some apprehension and a plan for assertive restraint. The Emotional Medical Record should include what the animal prefers for distractions, the best location to work with this animal, whether there is a provider preference, and specific handling notes and responses for each visit. The Emotional Medical Record requires a small investment of time during each appointment. This time investment pays off by team members being able to refer to the emotional record prior to animal handling. This saves a great deal of time in trial-and-error handling attempts during future visits while also alerting the veterinary team member to safety concerns and protecting the patient from handling events and techniques known to potentially compromise the welfare of that specific patient.

References

1. Howell A, Feyrecilde M. *Cooperative Veterinary Care*. Newark: John Wiley & Sons; 2018.
2. Yin SA. *Low Stress Handling. Restraint and Behavior Modification of Dogs & Cats: Techniques for Developing Patients Who Love Their Visits*. Davis, CA: CattleDog Pub; 2009.

Recommended Readings

Becker M, Radosta L, Becker M. *From Fearful to Fear Free: A Positive Program to Free Your Dog From Anxiety*. Health Communications Inc; 2018.

Ellis SLH, Rodan I, Carney HC, et al. AAFP and ISFM feline environmental needs guidelines. *J Feline Med Surg*. 2013;15(3):219–230.

Erber R, Wulf M, Rose-Meierhöfer S, et al. Behavioral and physiological responses of young horses to different weaning protocols: A pilot study. *Stress*. 2012;15(2):184–194.

Grandin T. *Temple Grandin's Guide to Working with Farm Animals: Safe, Humane Livestock Handling Practices for the Small Farm*. North Adams, MA: Storey Publishing; 2017.

Grandin T. *Improving Animal Welfare: A Practical Approach*. 3rd ed. Wallingford, UK: CABI; 2020.

Hartmann E, Søndergaard E, Keeling LJ. Keeping horses in groups: A review. *Appl Anim Behav Sci*. 2012;136(2-4):77–87.

Herron ME, Shofer FS, Reisner IR. Survey of the use and outcome of confrontational and non-confrontational training methods in client-owned dogs showing undesired behaviors. *Appl Anim Behav Sci*. 2009;117(1-2):47–54.

Hout MVD, Merckelbach H. Classical conditioning: still going strong. *Behav Psychol*. 1991;19(1):59.

Kurland A. *Modern Horse Training: A Constructional Guide to Becoming Your Horse's Best Friend*. Delmar, NY: The Clicker Center; 2023.

Landsberg G, Hunthausen W, Ackerman L. *Behavior Problems of the Dog & Cat*. 4th ed. Elsevier; 2023.

Loryman B, Davies F, Chavada G, Coats T. Consigning "brutacaine" to history: a survey of pharmacological techniques to facilitate painful procedures in children in emergency departments in the UK. *Emerg Med J*. 2006;23(11):838–840.

Martin D. *Canine and Feline Behavior for Veterinary Technicians and Nurses*. 2nd ed. Ames, IA: John Wiley & Sons; 2023.

Miklósi A. *Dog Behaviour, Evolution, and Cognition*. Oxford: Oxford University Press; 2016.

Neilson JC. House soiling by cats. In: Horwitz DF, Mills DS, eds. *BSAVA Manual of Canine and Feline Behavioural Medicine*. Gloucester, UK: BSAVA; 2009:117–126.

Nellis J. The developmental behaviour of foals and its relevance to husbandry. Part 1: The first 3 months. *UK-Vet Equine*. 2022;6(2):80–84.

Ohio State University Indoor Pet Initiative: https://indoorpet.osu.edu/home.

Overall KL. Pharmacologic treatments for behavior problems. *Vet Clin North Am Small Anim Pract*. 1997;27(3):637–665.

Salman M. Behavioral reasons for relinquishment of dogs and cats to 12 shelters. *J Appl Anim Welf Sci*. 2000;3(2):93–106.

Seibert L. Diagnosis and management of patients presenting with behavior problems. *Vet Clin North Am Small Anim Pract*. 2008;38(5):937–950.

Starling M, McLean A, McGreevy P. The contribution of equitation science to minimising horse-related risks to humans. *Animals*. 2016;6(3):15.

6

Restraint and Handling of Animals

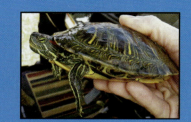

MONIQUE FEYRECILDE, JAMIE GUIBERSON, AND TEMPLE GRANDIN

CHAPTER OUTLINE

LEARNING OBJECTIVES

When you have completed this chapter, you will be able to:

1. Pronounce, spell, and define all the key terms in this chapter.
2. List three indications for animal restraint and describe methods for approaching dogs and cats before attempting restraint.
3. Do the following regarding canine and feline capture and restraint:

- List the actions taken to diminish stress in dogs and cats during physical examinations and hospitalization.
- List some of the equipment and methods used in capturing and restraining both cooperative and uncooperative dogs and cats.

- List the advantages and disadvantages of chemical restraint in dogs and cats.
- Describe various positions for restraining cats and dogs, specifically for nail trimming and venipuncture of the cephalic vein.
4. Do the following regarding equine capture and restraint:
   - Explain the principles that affect equine perception and behavior.
   - Describe the physical abilities of horses and how these affect the ways in which horses are handled.
   - Describe methods for approaching and capturing adult and juvenile equine patients, including using restraint equipment, diversions, and pharmaceutical products, and identify special restraint techniques for horses and the circumstances in which they are used.
5. Do the following regarding capture and restraint of cattle:
   - Describe the principles that affect cattle behavior, and list principles used to move cattle in an effective and low-stress manner.
   - Explain the differences in housing between dairy and beef cattle, and describe how these differences affect methods to handle and restrain them.

- List the types of bulls known to be particularly dangerous to handle.
- List the equipment used to restrain cattle in general and to restrain specific parts of their body. Also, describe the circumstances of their use.
6. Describe methods for observing and approaching swine of each gender and age group, and discuss methods used to capture and restrain adult and young pigs.
7. Do the following regarding small-ruminant capture and restraint:
   - Describe the behavioral tendencies of small ruminants and explain how this influences the approach and capture of herds.
   - List the factors that affect levels of aggression in camelids and describe how aggression presents in these species.
   - Describe the approach, capture, and restraint of individual sheep, goats, and camelids.
   - List additional restraint techniques used in camelids but not in sheep or goats.
8. Describe restraint and handling techniques used with birds, small mammals, and reptiles.

KEY TERMS

Binocular vision	Manual twitch
Blind spot	Near side
Cat bag	Pig board
Chemical restraint	Point of balance
Cow kick	Primiparous
Cross-ties	Passerine
Defensive aggression	Physical restraint
Diversionary restraint	Rabies pole
Double barrel kick	Raptorial species
Emergency muzzle	Rule of Twos
Fear, anxiety, stress (FAS)	Stocks
Fight-or-flight response	Tail tie
Freeze	Tortoise
Flight zone	Turtle
Hobbles	Twitch
Humane twitch	

Introduction

Most people entering the field of veterinary technology have had prior experience working with animals, but few have had the experience necessary to safely handle *all* types of animals that are encountered in veterinary practice today. Animals are diverse, not only across species, but also as individuals. Each animal possesses its own unique behaviors and idiosyncrasies, and therefore reacts to the world in its own way. For this reason, veterinary technicians must be prepared to address the unique behavioral tendencies of the individual animal and those of a species. It does not take long to realize that each animal is unique. Therefore stabilization and restraint techniques will need to be tailored to each patient, and the veterinary technician must be attentive to the changing needs of veterinary patients. To do this veterinary personnel must develop a solid understanding of both species-specific behaviors and the unique behavioral patterns of individual patients. Armed with this information, veterinary technicians will be prepared to carry out optimal animal handling, stabilization, and restraint

techniques. In addition, knowledgeable veterinary technicians will provide a safer clinical environment for both the patient and the veterinary health care team.

This chapter provides a fundamental introduction to the handling and restraint of animals commonly encountered in veterinary practice. It is not, however, a comprehensive guide to the restraint and handling of *all* animals. Rather, it provides a foundation for effective handling of a few species in commonly encountered clinical circumstances. Several complete guides and certification programs exist for animal handling. Refer to the "Recommended Reading" section at the end of this chapter for additional information and resources.

Minimizing Stress

The mission of the veterinary health care team is to prevent and relieve animal suffering and promote wellness. Therefore it is important to be aware of the changing emotional state of each patient while medical care is being provided.

Receiving medical care in either the home or the veterinary hospital frequently sparks fear, anxiety, stress (FAS) in animal patients. However, veterinary patients are usually confined to a carrier or restrained by a leash and are therefore prevented from running away. Restrained veterinary patients may therefore demonstrate signs of distress, including defensive aggression toward veterinary personnel. Closely monitoring the behavioral signals of FAS in patients (refer to Chapter 5) helps veterinary professionals avoid the fear-induced defensive aggression of their patients. In this way, knowing the signs of FAS helps veterinary personnel avoid injury caused by defensive aggression. Refer to Chapter 5 for specific signs of animal distress. Handling animals in a way that reduces fear improves the safety and welfare of both the patient and the veterinary team. Thoughtful handling improves the patient's overall experience and the quality of veterinary care that can be provided.

Animal Stabilization and Restraint

Stabilizing veterinary patients so that they can receive medical care includes working with the animal to help it stay calm, unafraid, and cooperative. This approach helps keep both the patient and the veterinary team safe. When strong restraint is considered, such as manually holding an animal immobile, the situation should be thoughtfully evaluated and considered. Is the proposed procedure a medical need or a want? Is the procedure needed immediately or can it wait until the animal is calmer and better acclimated?

"Less is more" is an important approach to the restraint and handling of veterinary patients, because it helps reduce patient stress and ensure successful interaction between the patient and veterinary personnel. It is not uncommon for veterinary patients to express more, not less, FAS when aggressive restraint and handling techniques are used. In contrast, medical treatment of FAS does not have this escalating effect.

Animals are flexible, strong, and coordinated. They can respond suddenly and with great strength, especially when they are in pain or experiencing FAS. Many injuries to veterinary team members, and sometimes to the patient, occur during attempts to physically control fearful and defensively aggressive animals. To maintain the safety of both the patients and veterinary personnel, strong physical restraint should be minimized and used only at times when the treatment provided is a true, immediate medical necessity. Many animals that are urgently in need of medical care are often sick or injured. They are often weakened by their condition and therefore require little stabilization or restraint during treatment. Examples of exceptional times when there is an urgent medical need that may warrant strong restraint include the following:

- The animal is in critical danger if intervention is not swift and immediate.
- The animal is having a seizure and needs immediate anticonvulsant treatment.
- The animal is in extreme pain and needs the immediate administration of analgesic and sedative medications.
- The animal is choking and will asphyxiate without immediate airway intervention.
- The animal is actively injuring itself or a team member. (Refer to Chapter 29 for more information.)

In all other situations, veterinary personnel can wait for a moment, an hour, a day, or even months while the animal is given time to calm down and a plan to safely and compassionately handle the patient can be implemented. This may involve delaying treatment to allow for a cool-down period and/or rescheduling the appointment altogether.

Providing a supportive and low-stress environment for veterinary patients is an important part of excellent veterinary medicine. The responsibility of the veterinary medical team to provide excellent care to animal patients must include an awareness of and compassion for the fear that many patients experience in veterinary facilities. Prophylactic care, diagnostic testing, routine treatments, and medical orders, in many cases, can be delayed until the patient has calmed down. It is well known that many fearful animals with elevated FAS can become defensively aggressive, endanger the safety of veterinary personnel, and exacerbate their own condition. However, when the patient's condition requires immediate attention, the "needs" of the veterinary team to examine the patient, collect samples, run diagnostic imaging, and provide treatment must be pursued immediately to prevent serious harm to the veterinary patient. In general practices, where preventive medicine plays a large role, the *immediate* medical needs of most patients are relatively small compared with those of patients in an emergency or critical care practice. This allows the veterinary health care team in many small-animal practices greater flexibility in the way it approaches frightened and stressed veterinary patients.

The veterinary patient communicates, via its behavior, whether it perceives a particular treatment to be aversive, frightening, or uncomfortable. Although the veterinary team may perceive a routine nail trim or a vaccination as a nonpainful or nonfrightening procedure, it is the animal's perspective that determines how the animal responds, not the human perspective. An analogy to this is the diverse feelings humans have about snakes. A person who is afraid of snakes may scream and run away from one, even though it is, for example, a harmless garter snake sunning itself on the sidewalk. The fact that the snake is harmless does not diminish the person's fear of it. Explaining why a snake is harmless does not help calm the person, diminish the adrenaline release, or help the individual relax. During a procedure, if an animal's body language communicates that it is stressed, a new plan is needed, regardless of how noninvasive or nonpainful the treatment may seem from the human perspective. Animals do their best to communicate with humans during office visits. Taking the time to observe the animal's signals and responding in a compassionate and sensitive way will improve the quality of care the animal receives.

Safe and appropriate stabilization and physical restraint of animals is critical in veterinary practice for the following reasons:

1. *To safely position a patient so that it can receive medical care.* Some animals may experience fear during parts of, or during the entirety of, a physical examination or diagnostic and therapeutic procedure. Fear of handling and treatment may cause the animal to physically resist the interaction. Keeping the patient and veterinary technician safe during this time will facilitate the administration of life-saving medical care.
2. *To prevent the animal from harming itself while it is receiving medical care.* During an attempt to escape frightening treatments, animals may injure themselves and/or may harm members of the veterinary health care team. These assertive attempts to flee are displays of *defensive aggression.* For their own benefit, veterinary patients must be protected from acts of defensive aggression, such as jumping off or falling off an examination table, or from injuring themselves by chewing the bars of their kennels while attempting to escape. With rising FAS in

veterinary patients, arousal and the **fight-or-flight response** also increases and may cause catastrophic results and injury to the frightened patient. Maintaining a safe environment, including well-constructed stalls, cages, and fencing, is therefore a crucial part of protecting the patient from injury.

3. *To protect personnel.* The safety of veterinary technicians, clients, and handlers is a priority when working with animals. Veterinary team members can sustain serious and even fatal injuries when working with animals. Injuries can lead to loss of income, expensive litigation, anxiety, decreased morale, and loss of livelihood. Increased costs of insurance, liability coverage, and workers' compensation are also a financial burden to hospitals but are secondary to team member injuries. Practice owners are responsible for the safety of all veterinary personnel during the performance of veterinary procedures. For this reason, many practitioners believe that the ability to perform safe and appropriate animal stabilization and restraint is one of the most important skills in veterinary technicians.

TECHNICIAN NOTE

Safe and appropriate stabilization and restraint of the patient is vital to ensure that prompt and efficient medical care is provided to the patient. It is also essential to ensure the safety of the veterinary medical team.

Preparing for the Visit

The interaction between veterinary technicians and their patients begins long before the animal is approached or touched. As discussed in Chapter 5, many veterinary patients may have a conditioned fear response based on previous frightening experiences in veterinary medical settings. Preparing the environment in advance may help reduce the fear response of these previously conditioned patients. The following are helpful strategies to lower animal stress during visits to veterinary facilities:

- Maintain the exterior of the hospital such that it is free of urine and feces; these may contain pheromones, which send messages of fear and anxiety.
- Minimize patient contact with other patients and strangers in the parking lot and reception area, and when moving through the hospital.
- Use calming music and calming pheromones inside the veterinary facility (Feliway, Adaptil: Ceva Animal Health).
- Provide comfortable nonslip surfaces and create spaces where patients can hide.
- Have a wide variety of treats available.
- Provide access to water.
- Provide frequent opportunities for the patient to eliminate.
- Clients should be questioned by the customer service team prior to the visit to screen for any potential known triggers of fearful behavior and to help ensure the smoothest and least fearful arrival possible for the patient.

Every patient has a certain "emotional account balance" available on a given day and in each situation. Each time the animal experiences stressors, a small withdrawal is made from the emotional account. Positive experiences make deposits into the emotional account. Maintaining an adequate balance in the emotional account will help patients tolerate and participate in treatment in a more positive way.

Ideally, the waiting area should be set up in such a way that animals have private areas separate from other animals while waiting and when moving through various parts of the veterinary hospital. The use of visual barriers to form individual seating areas, strategically placed food or retail displays, or a pheromone-treated towel placed over a carrier can all help reduce patient stress. Decreasing

wait times, offering alternate entry locations, scheduling appointments for fearful animals during quiet times of the day, and ensuring that the client care team is skilled in reading and interacting with animals are all strategies for helping to create a positive emotional environment for patients.

Greetings and First Impressions

Chapter 5 describes methods for evaluating the emotional status of patients based on changes in body language and level of interaction with—or avoidance of—staff members. When first entering a space where a patient is present, whether it is an examination room, a treatment ward, or a boarding area, the patient's behavior should be observed before attempting to handle the patient. When the technician is speaking to the patient, does it approach the technician or move away? Does the pet show any interest in treats or social interaction? (Refer to the table in Chapter 5 for signs of relaxation and of mild, moderate, and severe stress.) Animals experiencing moderate or severe stress are likely to respond by displaying "distance-increasing signals" and may show "fear-based, defensive aggression" when approached. Some animals show out-of-context displacement behaviors or mixed signals. Patients that manifest mixed signals are likely to be fearful and should be treated with caution.

TECHNICIAN NOTE

No single behavior can convey the full complexity of an animal's state of mind. Ear position, vocalization, tail movement, and other behaviors are all open to interpretation and must be evaluated collectively to determine whether a patient is exhibiting threatening behavior.

PUT INTO PRACTICE

Your ability as a veterinary nurse/technician to recognize each patient's need when preparing to restrain them is one of your greatest strengths. Strive to learn the animal behavior for all of the species you will work with in your job.

Veterinary patients should be observed from afar before any interaction whenever possible. These observations can reveal valuable information about the animal's emotional state. For example, a dog that freely walks onto the scale, greets staff members, and calmly enters the examination room is likely to be more comfortable with care compared with a dog that hides under the client's chair or scrambles to avoid the scale. Cats looking out the carrier door with interest and rubbing their cheeks or the top of their head on the carrier door are likely to be relaxed when handled. In contrast, cats with dilated pupils that stay in the rear of the carrier and vocalize frequently are likely stressed and may resist handling. How well the pet obeys the owner's commands in an unfamiliar setting, such as in the waiting room, may also reflect the level of stress the patient is experiencing. If the pet ignores commands while in the waiting area, it may continue to do so in the examination room.

TECHNICIAN NOTE

Cat owners should be advised to acclimate their cat to the carrier before veterinary office visits. Leaving the carrier door open on the floor at home and placing catnip or treats inside can make the carrier more pleasant for the cat. Cat owners can also place pheromone-sprayed familiar towels, catnip, and treats in the carrier to help reduce the animal's anxiety during transport.

Patients that are hospitalized should be observed for a few moments before an attempt is made to approach them or to access their cages. Consider gently speaking to sleeping or resting pets initially or softly calling an animal by name to wake it up *before* approaching or opening the cage door. If the pet is awake in the cage, its posture and activities and its reaction to people and other animals that pass by it should be observed. Consolidating medical treatments so the patient is handled with less frequency and allowing improved opportunities to rest between handling events help to reduce stress and can improve responses to treatment. Using the Touch Gradient introduced in Chapter 5 before, during, and after treatments will improve the patient experience.

First Interactions

Before interacting with patients, veterinary technicians should review the medical record for any information about the patient's behavior in the veterinary clinic during prior visits and consult with the customer service team about the client's answers to questions during scheduling. The technician should also double-check with the client before interacting with the patient. The technician should ask specifically how the pet responds to being touched; whether there are any specific sensitive areas; behavior during veterinary examinations in the past; procedures at home, such as nail care or toothbrushing; whether medications or devices, such as muzzles, have been used in the past; and prior behavior during any medical treatments. While taking the medical history, the pet should be allowed to become accustomed to the surroundings, and assessment of their body language and comfort level occur without direct interaction. Fearful pets are often easier to handle if they are given time to adjust before any attempt at greeting or approaching them.

Pets observe their surroundings just as veterinary team members observe their patients. Pets rely heavily on scents to interpret their environment, so a lingering aroma of anal gland secretions, urine, or feces can affect the behavior of the next pet that enters the area. It is therefore important for veterinary personnel to wash their hands between patient examinations and try to keep the examination room, table, and waiting area as clean and odor-free as possible between appointments. If possible, establishing a cat-only examination room at the quiet end of a hallway is helpful in establishing a fear-free environment for cats, minimizing the perception of dogs. Feline facial pheromone spray is also helpful for improving the perception of aromas for cats. A dog-appeasing pheromone spray (e.g., Adaptil; Ceva Animal Health, Inc., Libourne, France) can be sprayed on towels, muzzles, veterinary team members, and all other equipment used by dogs. Many pheromone products are available as plug-in diffusers that can be used in strategic areas around the practice. Both feline and canine pheromones may be used on scrubs several times a day to help create a calming effect in patients.

When possible, the technician should allow the patient to come to them, rather than approaching the patient directly. When approaching a patient, the technician should approach at an angle from the side, gazing indirectly at the patient. Hands should be kept at the sides or in a relaxed posture, and a calm, quiet voice and gestures should be used. Movements should be smooth, obvious, and predictable. Loud noises such as clapping hands; large, rapid movements; and appearing tall or imposing should be avoided. The technician should speak softly and use the pet's name. Sitting in a chair, squatting, or bending the knees to touch the patient is preferable; reaching over or looming over the patient should be avoided.

The technician should assess the pet's interest in treats, toys, and other forms of interaction, such as play, especially in kittens. However, if the patient is presenting for immediate anesthesia or for gastrointestinal illness, the veterinarian should be consulted before offering food or water to the patient. If allowed,

the technician can offer treats by dropping them on the ground or rolling them gently toward the pet. When the pet approaches, treats can be offered on the end of a pretzel rod, on a treat mat, or on a flat hand, though never the fingers, as some pets may take treats aggressively, harming the technician's fingers. Some fearful pets may approach the treat with interest but may also exhibit conflicted body language, because they are moving closer than they want toward the veterinary team member. If pets are leaning backward while taking treats, reaching out with a long, extended neck to snatch treats quickly, or taking the treat and then moving far away to eat it, FAS is present in the patient. It should be remembered that animals' behaviors can change rapidly, and even an apparently relaxed pet can respond unexpectedly if it is suddenly frightened or in pain. Continuous observation is necessary for safe animal handling.

In rare situations, some dogs may display territorial behavior when the client is approached by a stranger. The technician should closely monitor the dog while greeting its owner, avoid moving between the client and their pet, and if reaching out for a handshake or making other contact with the owner, making sure to monitor the dog's response at the same time.

A fearful patient should be allowed to back away temporarily and should *not* be pursued or cornered, because this may increase the animal's fear and potentially prompt a defensive action. Reaching toward a fearful dog, even with the intent of encouraging the dog to sniff, can appear intimidating or threatening from the dog's perspective. Therefore the technician should let the dog approach them. Some dogs can be coaxed forward by speaking softly to them by using gentle words of encouragement while assuming a less threatening posture and/or backing away so that the animal does not feel pursued. Asking the client to walk calmly around the examination room while encouraging the pet to explore can help dogs feel more comfortable to move around and explore. Offering a small treat (by gently rolling it on the floor near the dog) may encourage the dog to move. However, a dog that is extremely stressed may have no interest in treats.

Patient-Handling Fundamentals

All handling of patients, from placing a leash to picking up a small dog or cat or removing a pet from a carrier, should always be done with caution. Veterinary team members are often close enough to the patient for potential bites or scratches to occur. Even frequent and familiar patients should be monitored continuously during interactions for potential changes in fear, anxiety, and stress levels. Anxious patients may display the fight-or-flight response when the veterinary team member attempts handling. Stimulation of the sympathetic nervous system increases heart rate and blood pressure; increases blood flow to the skeletal muscles, lungs, and brain; and causes other changes in the body that prepare the animal to increase distance from a threat by escaping ("flight") or by showing defensive aggression ("fight"). When interaction with a patient progresses from observation and approach to direct interaction, the veterinary technician is shown that the patient is likely in a state of physiologic excitement. If a pet is not permitted to escape (flee) and the stress level continues to escalate, the next logical step is for the animal to defend itself (fight). By responding to changes in the patient's stress level promptly, defensive aggression can generally be avoided. As discussed in Chapter 5, some patients that are experiencing extreme stress may appear unusually still or even stoic but may have entered a state of learned helplessness. Learned helplessness may give the appearance that the animal is comfortable with the interaction because it is still, but the animal is, in fact, in a state of significant emotional distress. Some behaviorists have included a third term— "freeze"—along with "fight" and "flight." Many pets (especially cats) become very still when they are nervous. This allows easier handling but does not necessarily mean that the pet is relaxed, so continued cautiousness on the part of the handler is warranted.

Minimizing fear, anxiety, and stress in patients improves the patients' acceptance of handling and of various procedures. However, it is important to use time efficiently so that the length of stressful activity is kept to a minimum. To this end, veterinary technicians should be sure to have all needed instruments and equipment ready so that the appointment time and, consequently, the duration of patient stress are kept to a minimum. Thus the technician should be sure to prepare the environment in advance:

- All equipment is ready and in the room before handling begins and has been cleaned thoroughly between every patient to remove residual odors.
- Comfortable, nonslip surfaces are provided on the floor and any examination surfaces.
- When possible, a designated room is reserved for cats, minimizing the odors and sounds of dogs.
- Many cats and small dogs appreciate warm towels and small, round, soft beds.
- Synthetic pheromone products are used.
- Calming music is played.
- Frequent entrance and exit of the examination room are avoided.
- Client educational materials, such as posters explaining animal body language and handouts about reducing fear and anxiety during visits, are placed in each room.

Cat carriers are placed on the floor of the examination room or on an elevated surface where the cat can see the exit point and safely walk out of the carrier without falling. Cats should be allowed to choose to exit or stay inside the carrier until handling and other examination procedures are ready to begin. Some cats respond best if allowed to remain in their carriers for the majority of the visit. Coach clients to choose carriers that open from the front and top or that can be disassembled so that the top can be removed entirely to facilitate removal of the pet. This allows the cat to remain in its preferred space and, at the same time, allows the veterinarian or veterinary technician to perform clinical tasks. Many animals find being on the examination table much more stressful than being in the carrier or on the floor, so the amount of time spent on the table should be minimized.

Once the examination has begun, the technician should proceed at the pet's pace, quietly and with calm assurance, until the examination is completed. After the examination, the pet should be allowed to return to its carrier or to explore the room freely. No attempt should be made to restrain the animal while speaking with the client.

TECHNICIAN NOTE

If pet owners perceive that coming to the veterinarian's office is too stressful for their pets, they are more likely to forgo regular visits. This means that patients will not receive the medical care they deserve.

Moving and Transferring Dogs

Moving or transferring dogs is part of daily practice in the veterinary setting. Whenever moving dogs into and out of kennels, dogs should be on a leash for safety and ease of movement. Dogs should always be walked by using a double leash system to prevent escapes. Owners of small dogs sometimes prefer to hold their dogs in their arms or on their laps without a leash. The technician should encourage the client to place a leash on the pet by politely offering the loan of a hospital leash. Retractable leashes are not appropriate for use in the hospital.

Slip leashes help prevent escapes, but some dogs will respond to the unfamiliar tightening of a slip leash around the neck by backing up or panicking. Thicker and wider leashes are more comfortable and cause less pressure compared with narrow leashes. Long slip leads can be fashioned into an escape-proof harness. A harness-leash or similar product can be used in combination with a collar to provide better control without causing increased pressure on the animal's airway or neck. Fig. 6.1 shows an array of leashes with different diameter slip leads, a slip leash harness, and a commercially available harness-leash product.

If the client is present, the technician should ask the client to apply the leash. Before picking up any animal, the client should be asked how the animal normally responds to being lifted and whether the pet has any sensitive or painful areas that should be avoided. If the client is not present, the technician should begin by speaking to the dog quietly and gently, apply the leash by opening the neck loop very wide, and move alongside the dog, rather than face to face (Fig. 6.2). Using the other hand, a treat is offered at nose level through the open loop, and the large loop is gently lowered over the animal's head and shoulders and the loop then carefully closed. If the animal is in a cage or kennel, the leash loop is opened and prepared in advance before opening the cage or run. Then the technician stands sideways or with their back toward the kennel door and opens the door while holding the leash at the door opening. Many dogs will voluntarily place their heads at the door opening and subsequently into the leash loop. If the dog does not do this voluntarily, the technician should carefully reach into the cage and place the loop over the dog's head. When entering kennels, the technician should move with their side toward the dog to maintain a small body profile. Nonthreatening body language should be used, as described earlier in this chapter, and a soft, comforting voice while approaching the dog. If the dog is showing signs of increased FAS, the technician should be extremely careful, because reaching into a small space and looming over the dog can elicit defensive aggression in the patient.

Once the leash is placed, large dogs can be led to the next desired location. However, small- to medium-sized dogs may need to be picked up. To do this, first, a leash is placed on the dog while speaking quietly and calmly. Then the technician stands next to the dog and squats beside it in a side-by-side position (Fig. 6.3). The leash is shortened, and the arm placed over the back of the dog. The technician then runs the hand under the dog's chest with the palm facing up and positions it on the sternum between the forelimbs. The dog is secured against the side of the technician's thigh or hip, and the technician then raises the dog into their arm and stabilizes the dog before standing. Treats are offered with the free hand when possible. When transferring dogs from one person to another (client to team member or between team members), one must be sure that the dog is oriented such that its head is facing away from both handlers and that the handlers approach the dog's *side* and not the *front*. Medium and large dogs often require two handlers to be picked up—one to stabilize the head and thorax and the other to support the abdomen and hind limbs (Fig. 6.4).

When moving a dog through the hospital, the technician should be sure to check the route in advance to ensure that it is

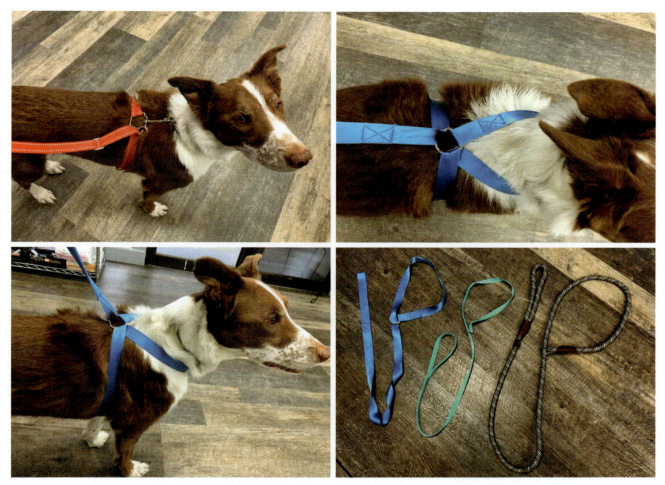

• **Fig. 6.1** An array of different diameter slip leads, a slip lead harness, and a commercially available harness-leash product.

clear. It is best to move a dog through an area without encountering other animals. The leash is kept short, and the technician faces the direction the dog is expected to go. The technician then walks calmly and encourages the dog to come along by using treats and soft verbal encouragement (Fig. 6.5). A dog should never be dragged by the neck, because this can result in injury and might induce rapid defensive aggression if the animal panics. If the patient becomes uncooperative, it is important to ask for help rather than use physical force. Pre-emptive sedation may be an appropriate intervention for some patients, particularly for dogs that cannot be safely approached and handled. Refer to latter sections in this chapter regarding emergency sedation.

Moving and Transferring Cats

Before removing a cat from a pet carrier or kennel, close all accessible doors and windows and the secure examination or treatment room. If the cat is in a carrier, the methods previously described to disassemble the carrier are used or the cat is invited to walk out of the carrier on its own. If the cat is in a kennel, a towel or blanket is kept available. The technician then walks to the kennel and speaks softly, opening the door of the kennel with their side or back facing the cat. Many cats will come to the front of the kennel to investigate and can be gently picked up. For cats that are fearful and remain in the back of the cage, a pheromone-infused *thick* towel or small blanket (thicker than the length of a cat's canine

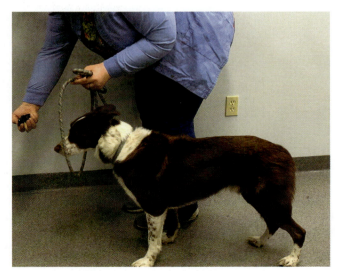

• **Fig. 6.2** Placing a leash onto a dog speaking gently from the side-by-side position. Offer a treat through the open loop and then gently lower the loop over the animal's head and shoulders.

tooth) can be gently placed over the cat and used to pick up the cat and carry it. This method helps protect the handler from potential scratches and bites. Some cats prefer to be moved in a carrier.

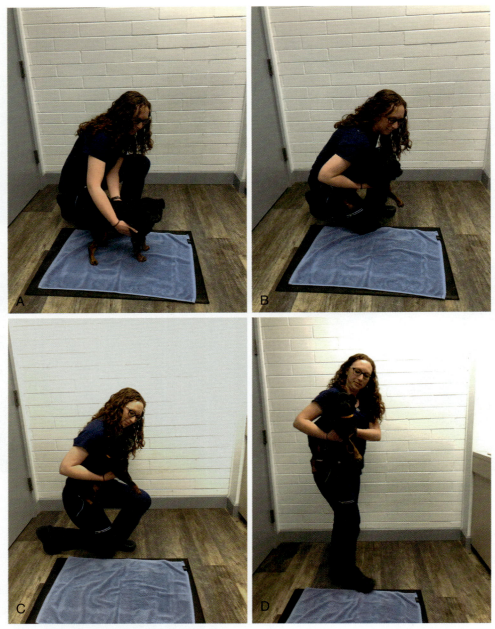

• **Fig. 6.3** (A) When picking up a small- to medium-sized dog, speak quietly and calmly while placing a leash on the dog. (B) Squat next to the dog, shorten the leash, place your arm over the dog's back, run your hand under the dog's chest with your palm facing up. (C) Position palm on the sternum between the forelimbs. (D) Secure the dog against the side of your thigh and stand.

For these cats, an open cat carrier is placed in the cage, the cat is allowed to move into the carrier on its own, and then the carrier door is closed and used to transport the cat.

If it is necessary to reach into a carrier to remove a cat, it must be done with extreme caution. If the cat is growling, hissing, refusing to make eye contact, or has the ears pulled back, another technique should be tried. If the cat seems calm but simply does not want to come out, the cat's cheek and chin should be stroked for a few moments. If the cat remains calm after being touched, the technician can reach underneath the cat's chest and remove the cat from the carrier. Using the scruff of the neck to pull or otherwise move a cat is not recommended.

Escaped Animals

Sometimes animals escape from their handlers. When this happens, it is important to first secure the area to ensure that the animal cannot leave the immediate area and that it cannot leave the building. One should resist the desire to immediately chase the animal. Escaped animals are generally fearful and in a state of panic. Pursuing these animals increases their fear and causes them to try even more to escape. If cornered, these fearful animals may demonstrate defensive aggression. Whenever possible, the escaped animal should be observed from a safe distance to see if it settles in one location. Often, it does. However, it may not be safe to wait

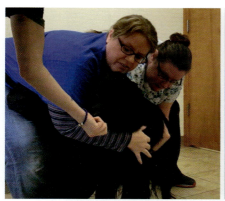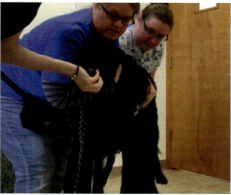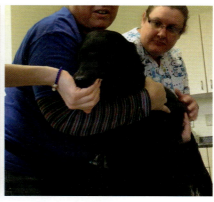

• **Fig. 6.4** Medium- and large-sized dogs often require two handlers to be picked up—one to stabilize the head and thorax, and the other to support the abdomen and hind limbs.

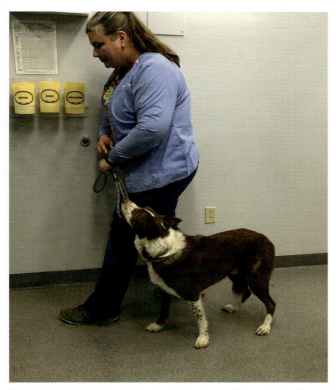

• **Fig. 6.5** Proper body positioning to help a dog walk through the hospital. Keep the leash short and face in the direction you want the dog to go. Walk calmly and encourage the dog to accompany you by using treats and soft verbal encouragement.

and observe the animal. In some situations, the immediate environment is not safe, and quick attempts at capturing an escaped animal are necessary for its safety.

However, most veterinary facilities are designed to discourage escaped animals from moving. Once an escaped animal has settled, dogs can often be leashed using the above technique. Very small dogs may be covered with a thick towel or small blanket and then wrapped securely and picked up.

In contrast, cats are agile and flexible and move very quickly. They are effective biters and jumpers, and can scratch with all four feet. Even small kittens can injure a team member. With their subtle body language, cats sometimes rise emotionally through the ladder of stress responses more quickly than a veterinary team may anticipate. Therefore it is important to carefully monitor cats and to respect their unique physical attributes when handling them.

Escaped cats can climb cabinets and walls. They can fit into remarkably small spaces, such as under cages and behind appliances, and have been known to displace acoustic ceiling tiles and disappear into the dark area above a clinic's dropped ceiling. Commonly, feline patients retreat into their pet carriers and require both encouragement and assertive prodding to get them out for an appointment or examination. However, once they escape, they can be formidable animals to capture.

Escaped cats can be captured in a variety of ways. In many circumstances, it is possible to throw a thick towel or blanket over the cat as soon as it becomes stationary. Once covered, it can then be wrapped in the material before being picked up. If the cat displays considerable defensive aggression, the handler can use long, thick gloves in combination with a towel or a blanket. Using gloves alone to capture a cat may put both the cat and the handler at risk of injury. Gloves dull tactile sensations and dexterity, and protect only the lower part of the arm. In addition, cats have been known to bite through some gauntlets (stout gloves with long loose wrists). Other equipment, such as a clamshell cat capture device or a large, soft net with a long handle, may prove to be more useful to safely capture escaped cats than cumbersome leather gloves. Refer to Fig. 6.6 for equipment associated with the emergency handling of cats. It is widely felt that these latter items minimize the risk of injury to both veterinary team members and to the escaped veterinary patients.

The use of emergency devices, such as a rabies pole, animal control pole, or come-along, should be undertaken with extreme care and caution. If an animal is so aggressive that it must be captured with a rabies pole, it should be ensured that the most experienced team members are available to assist, and the capture process should be as brief as possible. Animals can easily harm the handlers if the capture does not go smoothly; worse, animals can harm themselves when desperate. Fearful animals have been known to sustain injuries, such as tooth and jaw fractures, neck injuries, self-inflicted bites and scratches, or, rarely, fatal injuries when these devices have been used.

TECHNICIAN NOTE

Even the most experienced technician may need help when handling a patient. It is better to ask for help than to risk injury of either the patient or a veterinary team member.

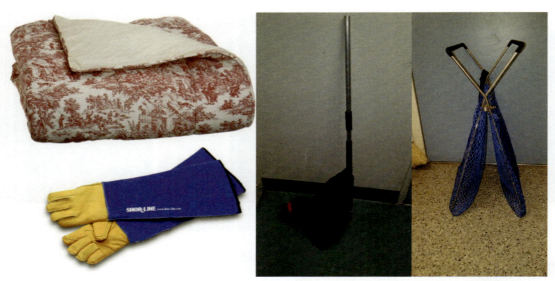

• **Fig. 6.6** Equipment for emergency handling of cats, including a soft, long-handled net; a thick blanket; gloves; and a clamshell-type handling device.

Stabilization and Restraint for Common Procedures

Many procedures in veterinary hospitals today are performed with animals in a variety of positions. Animals are moved into a variety of positions appropriate for each patient and circumstance. Table 6.1 shows a list of procedures and common body positions and locations for these procedures. When handling animals, the technician should consider what position will be most comfortable for the animal while maintaining the safety of the veterinary team. It is important to always have a plan for ways to support the animal, making sure the animal feels safe and secure, and to know how to rapidly stop the handling by having a planned handling-cessation routine.

Communication between veterinary team members is important during the handling and positioning of veterinary patients. In most cases, one person may be performing a procedure while another person(s) stabilizes the patient. When performing a procedure, the technician should communicate with the animal handler about what position(s) will facilitate the procedure when beginning to touch the animal and before administering any potentially painful stimulus, such as a needle stick, or a startling one, such as turning on hair clippers or pressing an x-ray pedal. The handler should, in turn, communicate with the technician. The animal is monitored for decreased interest in food if treats are being used, body tension, expression, attempts to move away, or risk of scratches or bites. When handling an animal, the technician should maintain the body in a position where they can move away if needed. If positions need to be changed or an animal must be let go for any reason, this should be communicated verbally before acting, whenever possible. For example, sitting on a rolling stool or squatting with one knee on the floor rather than kneeling on both knees allows the handler to rapidly move away from the patient if needed. Sitting completely on the floor may diminish handler response time.

One should remember to incorporate the "Considerate Approach" factors described in Chapter 5 and earlier in this chapter to ensure that the environment and the techniques used help promote success and comfort. When handling animals, it is important to use the Touch Gradient and the "less is more" concepts. If

very firm physical restraint appears necessary, the handlers should consider pausing and making an alternative plan rather than causing increased pressure in the animal. Severe restraint of stressed patients compromises the welfare of the patient and the safety of the veterinary team.

TECHNICIAN NOTE

Many procedures can be performed with the animals placed in a variety of positions. Some animals find restraint extremely stressful. Therefore it is particularly important to find a position that works well for both the animal and the veterinary technician. Avoid causing injury to the patient and *never* leave an animal unsupervised on an elevated surface, such as an examination table.

Family Presence During Veterinary Care

The presence of family can be calming for many pets. Hearing the owner's voice, seeing the owner, receiving treats and attention from the owner, and being able to seek comfort will all help patients relax in many situations. It is imperative that the veterinary team keep the client safe. Family presence does *not* mean expecting clients to be properly trained to safely restrain their animals. It means considering the potentially positive effects of family presence on both the patient and on the client's perception of veterinary care. In human medicine, healing times are hastened, overall hospital stays are decreased in length, and the patient's perception of time spent in the hospital is more favorable if their family is encouraged to be present during visits.

Sometimes clients will speak to, touch, or attempt to restrain a pet in a way that increases patient anxiety rather than decreasing it. When this happens, the technician should be prepared to offer the client useful instructions to follow. This benefits the client by demonstrating appropriate methods while protecting the patient and the veterinary team. For example, when a client is petting roughly and speaking in a high or nervous voice, a bowl may be placed in front of the dog, and the client is handed 20 very tiny treats and asked to offer them to their pet every 2 seconds while speaking kindly to the animal (Fig. 6.7). Another option is to ask the client to distract the patient by using a large pretzel rod with

TABLE 6.1 Positioning Options for Common Procedures

Procedure	Possible Positions and Locations
Physical examination	Floor, table, or other elevated surface Inside cat carrier Inside hospital housing Standing Sternal recumbency Partial towel wrap
Subcutaneous or intramuscular injection	Floor, table, or other elevated surface Inside cat carrier Inside hospital housing Standing Walking Sitting Sternal, lateral, or voluntary dorsal recumbency Partial towel wrap
Jugular venipuncture	Standing Sitting Lateral recumbency Sternal recumbency Partial towel wrap
Cephalic venipuncture	Standing Sitting Sternal recumbency Partial towel wrap
Lateral saphenous venipuncture	Standing Sternal recumbency on a hip with hind limbs extended Lateral recumbency Neck towel
Medial saphenous venipuncture	Sternal recumbency on a hip with hind limbs extended Lateral recumbency Partial towel wrap
Cystocentesis	Standing Sternal recumbency (cats) Lateral recumbency Dorsal recumbency Partial towel wrap
Nail care	Standing Sitting (forelimbs) Sternal recumbency on a hip with hind limbs extended Lateral recumbency Voluntary dorsal recumbency Partial towel wrap

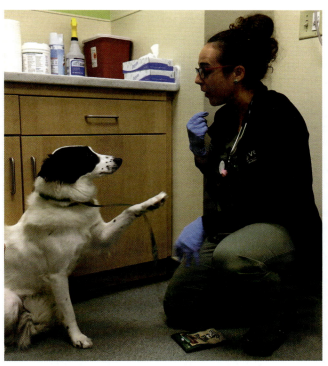

• **Fig. 6.7** Keep the client and the patient occupied by giving the client instructions and treats to feed the patient.

soft, sticky treats on one end to be licked by the patient. This is a particularly helpful and positive distraction for a pet. The following beneficial outcomes often result from including the client in creating a low-stress experience for their pet:
- The client is kept away from harm by moving the client further from the patient.
- The clients' hands are kept occupied so that they are unlikely to try to touch the patient.
- Both the client and the dog have a common focus that keeps the head of the patient facing one direction.

The client speaks to the patient in a soothing voice, which reduces anxiety. The client sees that the veterinary team is committed to the welfare of the patient. Often, veterinary team members perceive pets as "better behaved" without the owner present. Most patients who appear "better behaved" or "more cooperative" without the client are often displaying the freezing behavior described in Chapter 5 in the section "Learned Helplessness." When the comfort of family presence is removed, the patient's behavior becomes suppressed, and fear inhibits the animal from showing normal responses. Clients do not need to touch or be within reach of a pet to create a beneficial presence. Technicians should keep clients safely out of harm's way while allowing them to participate when appropriate.

In the past, animals were frequently separated from their owners and treated in a separate, large treatment area where they were forcibly restrained and clients would not be made uncomfortable seeing the distress of their animal. Under these circumstances, patients experienced high levels of FAS and were more likely to display defensive aggression toward staff members, increasing the likelihood that veterinary technicians and assistants would be injured. This used to be the standard of care.

Client trust in the veterinary health care team can be undermined when animal FAS is high. High FAS causes emotional distress, and patient emotional distress can undermine client trust in the veterinary team. For this reason, procedures were sometimes performed away from the client. Providing care with clients present can be helpful to both clients and patients. A client's presence can help calm the patient and, at the same time, allow the client to see the true value of the care provided and the compassion with which it is delivered. In this way, a stronger bond between the client and the veterinary team is forged. This trust will help improve both the quality and the quantity of veterinary care that a patient receives during its lifetime.

The presence of a family member is not always feasible, particularly when caring for hospitalized patients. During specialized imaging, anesthesia, chemotherapy, radiography, and emergency stabilization, the client and the pet will be separated out of necessity. During these times, when family is not present, it is important to preserve low FAS levels by consistently employing thoughtful methods of restraint and handling. A method of restraint that one would not use in the presence of the client should never be used. If heavy physical restraint is necessary, alternative techniques should be considered.

When providing stabilization or restraint to a resistant patient, consider the following questions:

- If I am using a distraction, is the distraction stationary? If the distraction is moving, the pet will follow its movements.
- Is the patient experiencing discomfort or pain? If so, is the pain or discomfort caused by the procedure or secondarily because of positioning?
- Is the patient's FAS level increasing? Does the patient's resistance represent attempts to escape?
- Is the patient's body position comfortable and within the normal range of motion?
- Is the patient distracted by something, such as the client moving around the room or noises coming from outside the room?
- Can the Touch Gradient be improved or another technique, such as rapid desensitization and counterconditioning, be used? (Refer to Chapter 5.)

Relaxed or Mildly Stressed Dogs and Cats (FAS 0–3)

Many relaxed patients are easily treated with the use of distractions. Proper positioning of the patient and keeping distractions within view and at nose level are important skills for veterinary technicians to master. While the patient is engaged by a distraction, another veterinary technician can position the patient and provide stabilization techniques by using gentle control of the head, body, and limbs as needed.

Standing or Sitting Positions

The procedure for the standing and sitting positions is as follows. Face the direction you want the patient to face, with your side to the patient. Place the distraction at nose level in the location you want the animal's head. Once the patient is interested in the distraction, gently place one arm or hand under the cranial aspect of the patient's neck. Place the other hand over or under the animal's trunk (over for most animals, under for those requiring assistance standing or balancing). Support the head and neck against your body, using the "seatbelt" technique. Position one arm to prevent sudden movement of the head toward the operator and the other arm to hold the patient's trunk against your body. Use only the amount of support needed to keep the patient in the correct position. At the same time, be ready to provide more support and protection to the operator if the animal moves unexpectedly. While the patient is engaged with a distraction, communicate clearly and frequently with team members. Perform the procedure by using the Touch Gradient approach. If the procedure involves lifting the limbs, be sure to keep the limbs within the pet's normal range of motion rather than twisting or lifting them out to the side. This helps ensure the comfort of the patient.

When presenting a limb for venipuncture, first support and, if necessary, extend the limb from the joint proximal to the vessel. Avoid pulling on the animal's paw. Apply pressure gradually, rather than abruptly, to distend and position the vein. If clippers, disinfectants, or topical anesthetics are used, introduce them gradually to avoid startling the patient. Fig. 6.8 shows a dog in a standing position for common procedures, such as immunizations, blood collection, cystocentesis, and nail care. Note the "seatbelt" position of the arms.

Sternal, Lateral, and Dorsal Recumbency

Before handling the patient, it is helpful to inform the client what position is desired of the animal. Some veterinary patients can follow cues from the client, such as to lie down, for example, or to lie on the side or back. Relaxed or mildly stressed patients can be coaxed into the desired position by using distractions, such as a long-lasting lickable food item. In this way, the patient assumes the desired position on its own. Many pets are sufficiently motivated by food to voluntarily follow a treat lure to a position, such as on a scale, an examination table, or into and out of a hospital kennel.

To coax animals into a particular position, the technician should first allow the animal to be drawn to a treat. The treat is like a magnet that is attached to the pet's nose and that follows the nose as the animal moves. If the pet's nose disconnects from the treat or the pet loses interest and moves away from the treat, the technician should stop and assess the situation:

- The patient's interest in the food magnet may not be strong enough to hold the patient's attention. In this case, using a different type of food should be considered.
- The magnet may be moving too quickly, making it overly challenging for the patient to follow.
- The patient may be inexperienced in following a lure.
- The patient may feel uncomfortable about entering the requested position and therefore resist following the lure.

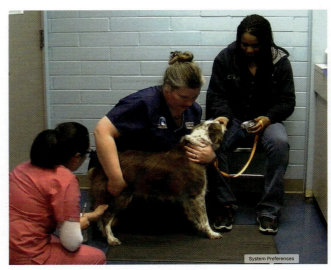

• Fig. 6.8 Standing and sitting positions for common procedures, such as immunizations, blood collection, cystocentesis, and nail care. Note the "seatbelt" position of the arms.

For animals that willingly follow lures, the following actions should be used to encourage body position changes.

Desired movement—standing or sitting to sternal recumbency:

- Hold the treat (lure) on the patient's nose, then move the treat slowly downward between the animal's front paws.
- Draw the treat slightly forward and away from the animal's nose. Maintain this position.
- With the other hand, stroke the animal along its back with gentle scratching to encourage the patient to stay in position.

Desired movement—sternal to lateral recumbency:

- Hold a treat to the nose of the patient, then draw the letter "C" with the treat, gently moving it laterally and then caudally toward the animal's tail.
- When the animal rolls onto a hip, pause in that position and let the patient settle. This position (sternal recumbency on one hip, with hind limbs laterally extended) is commonly used for a variety of procedures (see Table 6.1).
- Move a hand-held treat up the animal's back from the tail toward the shoulders. This encourages the animal to lean onto its dependent elbow and look caudally toward the treat.
- Move the treat toward the animal's nose and encourage the head to lower. Calmly support or assist the animal using the Touch Gradient approach to place the animal on its side.
- Place one arm lightly over the animal's neck with your hand positioned near the dog's dependent (down) thoracic limb.
- To maintain the animal in position, place the other arm lightly over the animal's flank and rest your hand on the dependent pelvic limb. Continue to offer treats in this position throughout the procedure.

Desired movement—lateral to dorsal recumbency:

- With the animal starting in lateral recumbency, encourage the animal to roll onto its back by using a treat. To do this, place the treat on the ground near the animal's nose.
- Move the treat slowly upward from the ground, toward the ceiling, forming the letter "C" in this movement.
- Gently guide the animal's body to follow the head movement and support the animal when it achieves dorsal recumbency.

Mildly and Moderately Stressed Patients (FAS 2–3)

Many mildly and moderately stressed patients will respond well to the same techniques used on relaxed patients, but some will need more help. For these patients, the technician should begin by reviewing the list of orders; work with the veterinarian to prioritize the requested treatments; and develop a plan of care that will help keep patient stress low. Some treatments, for example, may be given at another time, less frequently, or only as needed. Using the *Rule of Twos* can also help keep patients calm. If a procedure requires more than two attempts, causes more than two seconds of intense struggling, or requires more than two arms on the animal to stabilize it, a different plan is likely to be both beneficial to the animal and safer for the veterinary team.

Standing or Sitting Positions

The procedure for the standing and sitting positions is as follows. Encourage the dog to stand and walk to a particular location by walking next to the dog or by asking the client to walk with the dog. Position yourself beside the dog. Using the Touch Gradient approach, introduce first one hand and then two hands to the dog's body. Glide one hand and then the other hand to the trunk-support position as described previously.

Provide only the amount of support required to keep the animal stationary. This support can be "disguised" as petting or massage while simultaneously keeping the animal stationary. Keep the animal from turning its head toward the operator and be ready to provide additional support if the animal moves unexpectedly.

Canine: Standing to Lateral Recumbency

When establishing recumbency from the standing position, it is best to have at least two people reposition the dog (Fig. 6.9). After the dog is recumbent, the number of handlers needed to maintain recumbency may be decreased. The animal's *torso* should always be moved *toward* the handlers, while the limbs are moved *away* from the handlers. This helps protect veterinary personnel from being bitten and scratched. It also allows for slow, controlled movement of the patient. Grasping animals by their limbs and "tipping" them away from the handler put animals at risk for injury, particularly if the handlers lose control and cause the patient to fall on its side. This can lead to broken teeth, for example, if the patient's face hits the floor.

Moving into Lateral Recumbency: Step by Step

1. Two team members squat or kneel side by side on the floor and next to the standing dog. One person is positioned at the dog's neck and shoulders, while the other is positioned at the animal's flank and hip. A third technician may be at the patient's head with a lure, such as food treats, to distract the dog.
2. Before positioning the patient, the first veterinary technician strokes the standing dog by using the Touch Gradient approach, then glides the hands over the dog, reaching under the dog's chest to control what will become the dependent (down) thoracic limb.
3. Using the Touch Gradient approach, the second handler strokes the dog, then glides the hands over the flank and under the abdomen to control what will become the down side of the pelvic limb.
4. The team members communicate with one another, working together and, at the same time, gently hugging the dog against the front of their own bodies.
5. Working in collaboration, the team members gradually lift both the fore- and hind limbs away from the floor, supporting the animal's body with their bodies so no part of the animal is unsupported or hanging "in mid air."
6. The animal's body gently slides down the fronts and thighs of the technicians until the dog is placed into lateral recumbency. One technician holds the patient's dependent (down) thoracic limb and uses the other arm to control the dog's head and neck. A second veterinary technician holds the dependent pelvic limb and controls the rump with the upper arm and elbow. Both veterinary technicians support the spine of the dog, allowing the dog to rest on its side with its dorsum pressed against the technicians' knees and thighs. This is the final position when restraining large dogs.
7. Small- and medium-sized dogs may be lifted onto an examination table by one veterinary technician, using one arm to support the hind end while the other arm controls the front end.
8. The dog can then be moved into lateral recumbency and stabilized in place. To do this, the veterinary technician places one arm across the dog's neck and grasps the dependent (down) thoracic limb. The technician's other arm is placed across the dog's flank, where the dependent pelvic limb (down hind limb) is grasped. The grip should be relaxed as much as possible whenever the animal is still and relaxed.

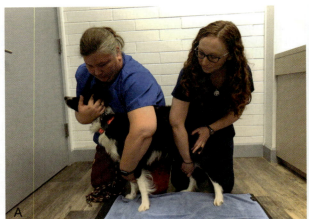
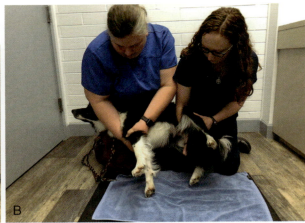
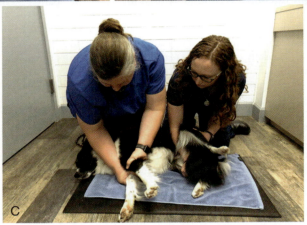

• **Fig. 6.9** (A) Placing a dog in lateral recumbent position using two people to gently cradle the dog before (B) lowering dog onto its side with feet facing outward. (C) Finally, the dog is gently but firmly restrained by controlling the forelimbs and hind limbs.

Canine: Standing to Dorsal Position

This is very similar to the lateral positioning technique mentioned previously, but with the use of a soft V-shaped positioner.
1. Place a V-shaped padded patient positioner in the desired handling location.
2. Move the dog next to the V-positioner. Avoid moving the V-positioner toward the dog, as many dogs would find this movement startling.
3. Two veterinary team technicians position themselves, squatting or kneeling, side by side, next to the dog. One person is at the neck and shoulders, while the other is positioned at the animal's flank and hip. For small dogs, being positioned side by side at a table may work better. The V-positioner should be placed between the dog's feet and the handlers' knees.

As the animal slides down the handler's thighs, the dog's dorsum can be directed to land in the trough of the V-positioner. One veterinary technician stabilizes the thorax, taking care to minimize handling of the paws and to avoid placing the face next to the animal's up-turned mouth. The second technician stabilizes the animal's hips while minimizing the handling of paws and taking care not to crush the tail. (See Fig. 6.10, which shows positioning in dorsal recumbency by using the Gentle Control approach.)

Feline: Standing or Sitting Positions

The procedure for the standing and sitting positions is as follows. Work in a location where the cat is comfortable. Gently place the cat in the desired position or invite it into the desired position by using treats, toys, and help from the client. Position yourself beside the cat. As with dogs, using the Touch Gradient approach, first introduce one hand and then two hands. Glide one hand to the back of the neck, stroking the top of the head, behind the ears, and the sides of the cheeks. Use the other hand to stroke the cat's flank or rump. Stroke gently but firmly. Avoid reaching under the cat to manipulate the abdomen, because most cats respond negatively to abdominal stroking. Provide only the amount of support required to keep the animal stationary. Often, this support can be perceived as "disguised" petting or massage by the animal. The hand used to scratch and stroke the cat's head can be used if needed to redirect the head safely. Simply make a "C" with the hand and place it behind the cat's ears, turning the head as needed until the procedure can be paused.

Feline: Standing to Lateral Recumbency

Cats rarely need to be placed into lateral recumbency for examination but are often placed in this position for imaging and procedures. When establishing recumbencies, cats can be moved by one or two people. The animal's torso should always be positioned

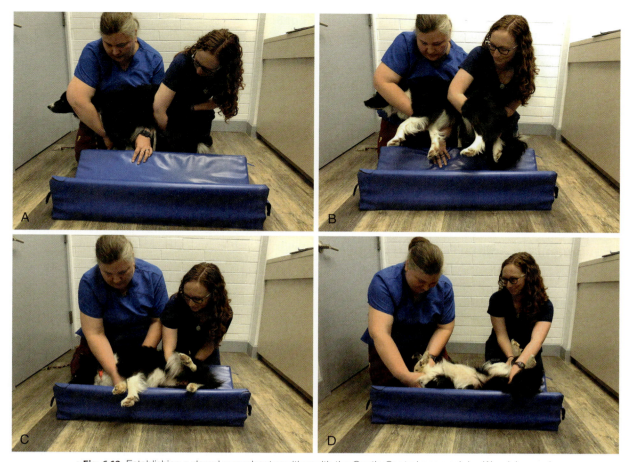

• **Fig. 6.10** Establishing a dorsal recumbent position with the Gentle Control approach by (A) gaining positive control over the animal before (B) lowering it into the padded sling. (C) Animal should then be firmly but comfortably restrained in the device on its side before (D) rolling on its back with positive control.

toward the handlers and the limbs positioned *away from* the handlers. This helps protect the handlers from being bitten or scratched and allows for slow, controlled repositioning of the patient. Grasping animals by their limbs and "tipping" them away from the handler puts the animal at risk of injury when it falls into lateral recumbency. Animals can fracture teeth and sustain other trauma if their faces hit the floor or tabletop when being restrained in this way. Handlers may also be at risk as the cat is positioned in such a way that its teeth are close to the handler's hands, making a bite more likely.

The steps for positioning of cats are as follows:

1. Position the cat on an elevated surface, such as an examination table, and stand beside the cat. The examiner typically stands on the opposite side of the table from the veterinary technician.
2. Using the Touch Gradient approach, stroke the cat's body and gently move the animal's torso against your abdomen.
3. Use one hand to stroke the cat's head and cheek, and then glide the hand down the cat's chest and between the forelimbs. Gently encircle the forelimbs above each elbow. Apply only enough pressure so that the elbows do not easily slip out of your grasp. Do not squeeze the *distal* limbs.
4. Use the opposite hand to stroke the cat's rump, then glide the hand down along the hip and between the hind limbs. Using this hand, gently encircle both hind limbs above the hocks. Encircle the tibial/fibula area just tight enough that the hocks will not easily slip out of grasp. Do not squeeze the distal limb.

5. Gently roll the cat's body onto its side, with the cat's dorsum against the handler's abdomen and the limbs extended.

Feline: Standing to Dorsal Position

1. Place a V-shaped padded positioner in the desired handling location with the cat between the handler and the positioner.
2. Follow steps 1 to 5 in "Feline: Standing to Lateral Recumbency."
3. Once the body and limbs are supported, lift the cat. The cat's body is supported by the handler's abdomen. The handler then leans forward and gently slides the cat into the trough of the V-positioner.
4. Two handlers are recommended to maintain the cat's position in the V-positioner. One handler stabilizes the head and thorax, taking care to minimize handling of the paws and avoid placing their face next to the animal's upward-pointing mouth. The second handler stabilizes the hips, again minimizing the handling of paws and taking care not to crush the tail.

Severely Stressed Patients (FAS 4–5)

As previously discussed, severely stressed patients are in a state of significantly diminished welfare and can represent serious risk of harm to the veterinary team and any clients who may be present. Severely stressed patients often benefit from the administration of medications to mitigate their fear, stress, and anxiety prior to handling. In emergent situations where the animal's need for medical care precludes administration of medications to decrease FAS, emergency tools, such as basket muzzles, towels, blankets, and gloves, may be necessary to keep team members safe.

Once the animal has received treatment for FAS or the situation has been deemed too dire to wait, the instructions for the basic maneuvers to establish recumbency are the same. These handling maneuvers must be undertaken with the utmost care to keep all veterinary personnel and the patient safe.

> **TECHNICIAN NOTE**
>
> When restraining a dog or a cat, use the minimal amount of restraint necessary to prevent injury and facilitate examination. Remember, "less is more."

Special Equipment for Animal Handling

Muzzles

For examinations and short procedures, muzzles can be used to improve the safety of personnel during required animal handling. Some patients may have a negative conditioned emotional response to the muzzle, particularly if one was used before a painful procedure. When planning to use muzzles, the technician should first discuss with the client whether one has been previously used on the patient. It is important to positively acclimate young animals to the use of muzzles so that their handling and restraint during future veterinary visits is facilitated.

A wide variety of muzzles for dogs and cats are available on the market. Dogs may be fitted with basket muzzles, air muzzles, or nylon fabric or mesh muzzles (Fig. 6.11). A plastic Elizabethan collar or, in an emergency, a gauze or tape muzzle may be used (even a necktie can serve as a muzzle during an emergency). For cats, hard plastic or soft nylon fabric muzzles can be used. Air muzzles and plastic Elizabethan collars may also be helpful. The risks and benefits of each of these types of muzzles are listed in Table 6.2.

All restraint equipment and positioning must be safe for both the patient and the handler, and should be appropriate for the type of procedure and its duration. As successful restraint methods are developed for each patient, a notation should be entered into the patient's record so that the effective restraint technique can be repeated during future appointments.

Cat Bags

Cat bags are nylon restraining sacks that typically include a Velcro-closure collar and side zippers that give access to the cat's limbs. The bag restricts the patient's movements and theoretically helps protect veterinary personnel from scratches and bites. However, it is important to note that stressed, fearful patients tend to become *more* stressed and fearful when put into a cat bag. In other words, if a cat has a high enough FAS level that a cat bag is being considered, applying the bag to the cat may present significant safety issues for the team. The bag also restricts access to the cat's body, often making physical examination more challenging.

Towels and Blankets

Towels and blankets are incredibly versatile tools for handling both dogs and cats. Many dogs and cats will become calmer when gently covered with a pheromone-infused blanket or towel. In general, towels and blankets used for handling patients with high FAS should be selected to be tightly woven (no loose knits) and thicker than the length of the animal's longest tooth. This helps prevent accidental bites and scratches through the fabric. Many animals are fearful of having their faces and heads restrained or of having human hands on or around their necks. Towels can be rolled lengthwise and placed around an animal's neck as an alternative to the use of the hands, making a thick scarf, almost like a cervical collar. The scarf can then be held to direct the animal's head from behind if needed, and the support around the neck makes it more difficult for the animal to turn its head toward the handlers working on the animal's body. The towel must be snug enough to control the animal's movement but loose enough to allow free flow of air and blood. The animal should be monitored at all times when a towel scarf is used.

The use of a thick towel or blanket draped over an animal and then gathered around its body can be a useful temporary tool to safely stabilize the patient. By covering the patient's head, sensory input is reduced, and a barrier between the animal's teeth and the handler's body is created. A beach towel can be used both as a scarf, as described above, and as a wrap. Using this combination (wrap and scarf) is particularly helpful during short procedures in cats. When wrapping cats, the key is for the towel to fit snugly around the cat without being

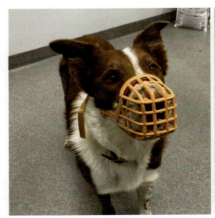
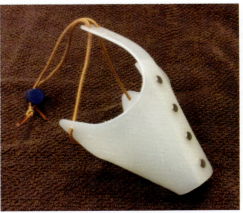

• **Fig. 6.11** An array of muzzles: Making a notation in a patient's medical record regarding the specific size and type of muzzle used saves time during appointments.

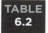

TABLE 6.2   Additional Resources for Detailed Small-Animal Handling Techniques and Protocols

Equipment Type	Benefits	Risks
Nylon dog muzzle	Quick to apply Inexpensive	Restricts panting: risk of patient harm Must be used very briefly only Low-strength materials Diminishes ability for patient monitoring Easy for patient to remove Many animals are already fearful of these
Nylon cat muzzle	Quick to apply Inexpensive	Presses on whiskers—may overstimulate Easily covers nares/can restrict breathing Can restrict airway if cat tries to remove and tightens around neck
Basket dog muzzle: Plastic Vinyl Custom biothane Custom leather	Preferred equipment Available in many sizes Allows panting Dog can eat treats and drink Can be used for long time periods (supervised) Many custom brands and materials available Easy to train acceptance Clients can train acceptance at home	Fingers can be inserted into the basket Moderate cost compared with nylon Patients can remove if no forehead strap
Plastic cat muzzle: "WonderMuzzle"	Easy to apply If well tolerated, cats become calm Prevents bites effectively	For brief use only If poorly tolerated, may make further handling impossible until patient is calm Restricts airway if improperly applied Patient can easily remove Difficult to safely remove if patient panics when applied
Air muzzle	Allows panting Easy patient observation Better fit for brachycephalics and felines Can be worn for longer periods (supervised)	Heavy Hands can be inserted into ball Sometimes poorly tolerated Costly compared with other options
Elizabethan collar	Can be worn throughout hospitalization Allows panting and easy patient observation Better tolerated if patient is already fearful of muzzles	Less protection to handlers Difficult to apply in fearful patients
Emergency muzzle: Gauze Shoe string Necktie	Fast to apply Can be used in the field in an emergency if other muzzles are not available	Can break during application Emergency use only Restricts panting Restricts patient monitoring Can cause edema and pain Dog can easily remove

uncomfortably tight (Fig. 6.12). It is also important to swaddle the cat in a way that restricts the cat's movement in all six directions (up, down, left, right, forward, back).

Gloves

A variety of animal handling gloves are commercially available. When combined with towels and blankets, gloves can facilitate the restraint and handling of fractious patients and the rapid sedation of patients that display aggression. Gloves may also be helpful when moving items, such as food and bedding, into and out of the cages of aggressive animals. However, gloves do not completely protect the handler. Most cats can bite through gloves with their narrow, sharp, cone-shaped canine teeth. And although gloves are scratch resistant, many adult cats can reach beyond the glove-covered portion of the arm when feeling sufficiently defensive. Gloves also diminish the tactile feedback

and dexterity of the wearer. For example, gloves make it more difficult to make fine adjustments to hand positions, such as increasing pressure in tiny increments during patient handling. They also make routine procedures, such as giving injections or drawing blood, difficult to perform. Additionally, patients handled with gloves may develop a significant fear of the approaching hands and of hand-shaped objects in the veterinary setting. As with any handling tool, gloves should be used judiciously rather than routinely.

TECHNICIAN NOTE

Adopting safe, effective, and low-stress handling techniques protects everyone—the veterinary technician, the veterinarian, the pet, and the owner. It also strengthens the relationship between the client and the practice.

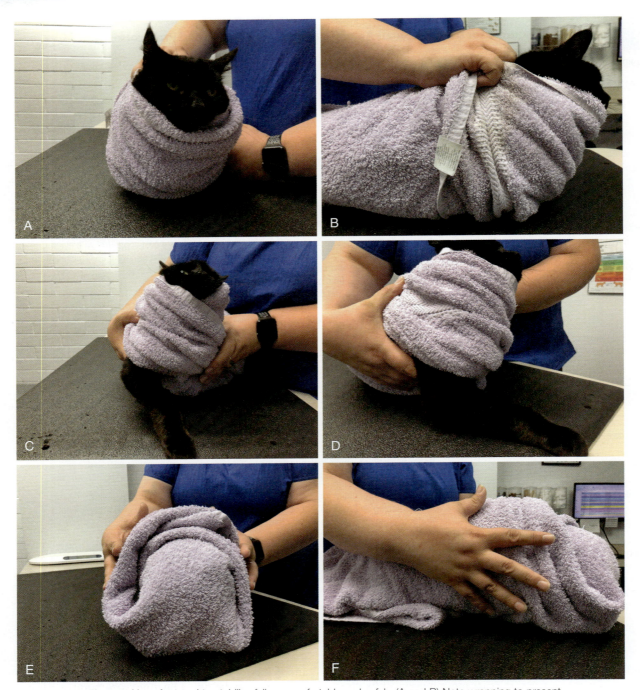

• **Fig. 6.12** Use of a towel to stabilize felines comfortably and safely. (A and B) Note wrapping to present head for treatment, (C and D) cephalic veins, and (E and F) to restrain entirely for the purpose of moving safely and securely.

Scruffing Feline Patients

Grasping the skin over the back of the neck and shoulders of a cat is referred to as "scruffing." Grasping the scruff of the neck was a routinely practiced and accepted form of restraining cats but is used less routinely today. Adult cats grasp one another by the scruff during breeding and fighting. Queens grasp their kittens by the scruff if they must relocate the kittens in an urgent situation. The queen may also put its mouth on the scruff of a kitten, seemingly to stop the kitten's behavior.

Veterinary patients that are trying to escape or that are showing defensive aggression are in a state of significant emotional distress. Although the use of scruffing may subdue a cat long enough to perform a short procedure, it also raises FAS in the patient. Focusing on handling methods that prevent cats from reaching FAS levels of 4 or 5 is a preferred course of action than routinely raising stress levels by scruffing them. To this end, some veterinary hospitals have designated their clinics "scruff-free zones." With the goal of maintaining low FAS levels in patients and by using towels, blankets, gloves, and appropriate medical treatment (as needed), scruffing can be avoided.

Using scruffing to routinely control cats also carries risk. Some points to consider regarding scruffing cats are as follows:

- Few cats become calm when scruffed, although they may freeze and stop moving.
- If the cat responds negatively or becomes highly aroused or defensive when scruffed, it is unlikely to return to its baseline emotional state for the remainder of the handling session.
- Cats are extremely flexible and can deliver serious scratch wounds with both the front and hind paws while the scruff is held. Those cats that are placed in a stretch position and are restrained by the hind limbs while being scruffed can scratch with the front paws.
- Scruffing can result in injury to the cat's skin and neck.
- If the team member attempts to grasp the scruff and is unsuccessful, the unprotected hand is at risk of being bitten, and the cat may escape.

Scruffing should be reserved for immediate emergencies, such as when there is imminent danger to a person or pet. As soon as possible, an alternative handling method should be used, and the animal should be safely confined. An updated treatment plan should be prepared. Cats should never be lifted or suspended by the scruff of the neck, because this can cause discomfort, pain, and physical injury, especially in elderly, fragile, sick, or obese animals.

Medical Treatment of Fear, Anxiety, and Stress

There are many commercially available oral medications that can be used alone or in combination to diminish the stress and fear a patient may experience during veterinary visits. The use of these medications, combined with a plan for behavior modification and training, is a good long-term solution for patients that display fear in the veterinary setting. For patients with FAS levels 1 and 2, natural supplements and nutraceuticals are available to help diminish mild fear.

The technician should remember that whenever the patient experiences significant fear during a visit, a permanent memory is formed. Enough negative experiences teach the patient that veterinary care is unpleasant or dangerous and trains the animal to display defensive aggression to protect itself.

A wide variety of safe and effective agents are available for medical management of FAS before and during veterinary visits. Sedation or chemical restraint carries risk, as does the use of traditional physical restraint. Choosing when sedation is appropriate and what agents to use is the responsibility of the veterinarian. However, every member of the veterinary team should be empowered to pause in their handling of patients and assess their effectiveness as caregivers. Giving stressed and fearful animals a break from handling may provide a better opportunity later. Delaying treatment or diagnostic testing to give patients time to acclimate can make a difference in the experience of both the veterinary technician and the patient. In addition, regular review of handling and medication plans can lead to patient-specific variations that improve the experience of the individual animal. Like humans, each veterinary patient is unique and responds to restraint and handling techniques in its own fashion. Sedating a pet or requesting sedation for a pet does not represent a failure to effectively perform restraint or treatment. Rather, it represents an awareness of and compassion for a fearful veterinary patient. Sound veterinary nursing requires compassion and patience. In this way, veterinary technicians set an example for others and help preserve both the physical and emotional welfare of their patients and the people who care for them.

Talking About Medical Treatment of FAS With Clients

When providing treatment for FAS in animals, the veterinary team may choose from a variety of medical interventions, such as nutraceuticals, oral medications, sedation, and (very rarely) general anesthesia. Maintaining communication with the client is crucial to patient success. As the veterinary health care team becomes increasingly aware of animal body language and of the risk of causing emotional harm to animal patients, the importance of providing consistently thoughtful and positive patient care increases. Clients are more likely to return to a practice that provides a positive experience for their pets. In other words, veterinary case volume increases when both clients and animals feel comfortable coming to a veterinary practice.

When talking with clients about the use of medications, they should be described as medicines to reduce fear and stress, relieve any pain the animal may be experiencing, and allow safe handling for both the patient and the team. Veterinary professionals would do well to eliminate deprecatory labels for fearful patients. Terms such as *mean, fractious, unruly, poorly behaved, evil,* and *spoiled* do little to describe specifically observed behaviors and even less to advance the conversation with clients to steward the patient's care. A few example scripts for discussing the use of medications before treatment are given below.

Example 1: "Mr. Jones, Rex is not bearing any weight on this leg at all. The veterinarian has recommended that we take x-rays of Rex's leg. See how he leans away, looks away, and moves away when I try to touch him? These signs tell us he is in pain and a bit anxious about what we are going to do. The veterinarian has ordered some medicine for Rex prior to his x-rays that will decrease the pain he is feeling and help him relax. With your permission, I would like to give that medicine now."

Example 2: "Mrs. Stone, Fluffy is a senior-aged cat and needs to have important blood work performed. However, the test does not have to be performed today. See how Fluffy pulls her legs tightly under her and flicks the tip of her tail when I approach her? She is telling me she is worried about my approach and may act defensively. The stress of forcing Fluffy to give a blood sample today can change the results, and it may also make it more difficult for us to collect lab samples next year. Dr. Smith has arranged to send you home with some medication to give Fluffy tonight and again tomorrow morning. Then, tomorrow afternoon, you can return with Fluffy so that we can collect a blood sample when she is feeling calmer. Giving her a better experience this year will make the process easier next year. It will also ensure that the test results are as accurate as possible."

Mastering client communication regarding animal handling and stabilization is an important key to providing the best care for every patient, every time.

TECHNICIAN NOTE

Pet owners expect their pets to be handled in a respectful, compassionate manner. Wrestling with a pet or using what may be perceived as excessive force can damage a client's perception of the practice and its staff.

An Introduction to Herd Animals

Introduction

Herd animals, such as cattle and horses, are grazing prey species. When they enter a new place they may react to stimuli in their environment that people may not notice. Some examples are refusing to walk over a drain on the floor or becoming agitated when a loud intercom makes sharp intermittent sounds. Distractions in the environment, such as changes in the flooring, a reflection off a vehicle, a coat on a fence, or a hose on the floor, may cause large animals to refuse to move through a chute. The coat and the hose should be removed. When a distraction such as a floor drain cannot be moved, the animal should be given the opportunity to put its head down and look at the drain. After it has looked at it, smelled it, and raised its head back up, it can then be urged to move forward.

Flight Zone and Point of Balance

A tame horse that can be led with a halter and that allows people to touch and handle it without anxiety has no **flight zone**. Dairy cows may have a small flight zone of 0.5 meters to 1.5 meters (2–4 feet). These animals are often milked twice daily and are accustomed to being handled, particularly from the rear end. Extensively raised beef cattle may have a large flight zone of 2 to 6 meters (6–20 feet). *The flight zone is the animal's personal space.* The size of a flight zone is determined by both previous experiences and genetics. When an animal is held in either a single-file chute or a restraining chute, a common mistake made by many is to remain standing inside the flight zone. This may cause the animal to become agitated, because the person is inside the flight zone and the animal is not able to move away. Signs of agitation in cattle and horses is tail swishing and defecation. Handlers should back up and move away from the flight zone. During a medical procedure, tail swishing is often an early warning signal that a horse may kick or bite.

When moving a single bovine forward, the handler works on the edge of the flight zone and is located behind the **point of balance** at the shoulders. A common mistake that many people make is standing at the animal's head and poking its hindquarters with a driving aid. This gives the animal confusing signals. An effective method for moving a *group* of cattle forward, particularly in a single-file chute, is for the handler to briskly walk in the opposite direction of the desired movement. When the point of balance at the shoulder of the first animal is crossed, the animal will usually move forward, and the other cattle will follow. The handler breaks away and circles back to repeat the process.

Keeping Animals Calm

If a horse or cow becomes severely agitated, 20 to 30 minutes will be required to allow it to calm down. Often it is best practice to allow an animal to calm down before additional attempts are made to perform a medical procedure. Yelling at animals is extremely stressful to them. Calm talking or a little "shhhh shhhh" sound is all that is needed. Nonslip flooring is essential to help keep animals calm, because slipping causes animals to panic. Often, a cow or a horse will experience numerous small slips and become increasingly agitated. Slipping can be prevented by using a rubber mat, grooved concrete floor, or rods welded to a metal floor.

Cattle and horses are herd animals, and they often become fearful and agitated when they are separated from their herd mates or stable companions. Animals that are isolated from others have caused many injuries to both animals and people. Some cattle and horses will remain calmer if a companion is brought into the veterinary facility along with it.

Effects of Novelty

New things can be both attractive and scary. A horse or a cow may voluntarily approach a novel object that is left in a pasture. Animals will often walk up to a coat that is left on a fence. However, new things may be frightening when they are introduced suddenly. This explains why a horse that is calm at home may become highly agitated at a show. Flags, bikes, and balloons that may be present at a show are scary, because they move rapidly and are unfamiliar. Horses and show cattle need to be carefully acclimated to these objects *before* they are taken to a show.

Making a New Experience Positive

It is important for an animal's first experience with something new, such as a horse trailer or a new corral, to be a *good* first experience. If the first experience is painful or scary, it may be more difficult to get the animal to go through a subsequent experience, such as re-entering a trailer or corral, in a positive manner. A good approach is to give it positive associations with the new place. Feeding it in the new place is one way of giving the animal a positive experience. Painful procedures must be performed sometimes, but ensuring that such procedures are not the animal's first experience with a new person, a new place, or a new piece of equipment is highly recommended. Sometimes, an animal will associate a person dressed in a white coat or other distinctive clothing with someone to be feared. This may result from a previously painful or scary experience that is now associated with a white coat. If a veterinary technician determines, for example, that a certain piece of clothing they are wearing is aversive to a particular animal, then the technician should stop wearing it.

Introduction to Equine Restraint

Before working with horses, it is important to have a general understanding of their behavior, their innate instincts, how they perceive the world around them, and how they might react when handled by humans. Horses are a prey species and are therefore "flight animals." When frightened or startled, it is instinctual for them to flee. When fleeing, they will search for the easiest escape route, and you should be prepared that this may be in your direction. Consequently, when approaching a horse in the field, it is important to speak from a distance so that the animal hears and then sees you approaching. The technician should use a soothing tone of voice while approaching the horse. This is an effective way to avoid startling the animal. One should also keep in mind that horses are far-sighted. They see best looking far into the distance but have poor vision close. In addition, they have blind spots, such as the areas directly in front of them or directly behind them, in their vision. Therefore while approaching a horse, the technician should talk to the animal from a distance to let the horse know about the approach. The technician should approach from the left side of the horse and stand at the shoulder, not directly in front or behind, so that they can be optimally seen by the horse. The technician then places their hands on the animal and always stays close to its torso.

Within herds, there is a hierarchy. Horses may fight to establish their places within the herd; however, horses are not typically aggressive. Certain factors can make horses aggressive. The most antagonistic horses seem to be protecting something; mares with foals can become unpredictable as they defend their foals, stallions will guard their herd of mares, and even racehorses can become extremely protective of the stall. These horses can be very quick to bite, strike, or wheel around and kick at a perceived threat. More commonly, what veterinary professionals encounter when dealing with horses is fear or anxiety. Horses that are isolated from the herd because of illness or injury can become anxious; being transported to a new environment full of strange people only increases equine stress levels. It should be remembered that horses are prey animals and that humans can be perceived (by the horse) as predators. The horse's instinct in this situation is to evade human contact and capture; this is similar to the flight-or-fight response seen in nature. Fearful horses will try anything to escape capture; this can result in injury to humans or animals. Both aggressive and fearful horses can quickly turn away from the person attempting to restrain them, leaving the handlers in a potentially dangerous situation.

Safely Working with Horses

The safest place to stand when working with a horse is at its left shoulder (Fig. 6.13). Horses have monocular vision; that is, they have separate vision in each eye. Therefore their peripheral vision is excellent, and their field of view is extremely broad. In addition, they have strong binocular vision for spotting potential predators from a remarkably far distance. In fact, they can see things in the distance that humans cannot. Some things they see may startle them unexpectedly and trigger the flight response. This could be surprising and a little scary to the veterinary technician who, for example, is trying to lead a frightened horse into a clinic barn. The veterinary technician may have been surprised and left wondering later about what had frightened the horse. In addition, horses do not see well directly behind them. In general, it is important for all personnel handling horses to expect the unexpected when leading horses and, whenever possible, to avoid stimuli that might trigger the flight response.

The equine field of vision is almost 360 degrees. Horses have 60- to 70-degree **binocular vision**, that is, vision in which both eyes are used synchronously to produce a single image. This makes judging distances directly in front of them difficult without moving their head. Horses have three areas where their vision is extremely limited: directly behind them, directly in front of their nose, and between their eyes on the forehead. These locations are known as ***blind spots***. To compensate for these blind spots, horses will turn their head quickly toward objects in these areas to determine whether they are a threat. Blind spots are one reason people should not approach a horse if it is not aware of their presence or if the horse's hind end is facing them.

Veterinary personnel need to be cautious when moving into and around equine blind spots, where they are more vulnerable to being injured. Horses generally give a warning before kicking. Typical warning signs include but are not limited to lifting a limb quickly, stomping a foot, and pawing. However, a frightened horse can be unpredictable and can kick without warning. Horses can kick with both fore- and hind limbs. When horses use their forelimbs to kick, it is known as *striking*. A single limb strike is the most common way a person can be injured when in front of a horse. Strikes occur if the horse is prone to this behavior or is agitated. A single forelimb strike usually is not fatal but can cause bruising, hematoma, or even a fractured limb. However, some horses, especially young horses, will rear up and strike out with both forefeet, usually causing damage to the handler's upper body and head. This reaction has the potential to cause serious and

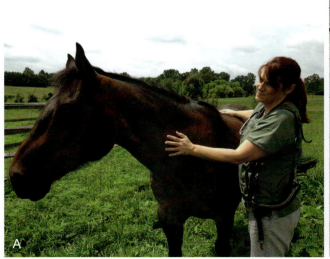

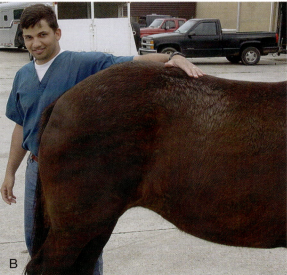

• **Fig. 6.13** (A) When approaching a horse from a distance, use a soothing tone of voice to let it know you are coming. Extend a hand to the horse, particularly if the horse extends its neck to you. Place a hand on the horse's shoulder and back to communicate your presence in a nonthreatening manner. Always stand at the horse's left shoulder. (B) Because their vision is limited regarding that which is directly behind them, be sure to place your hand on the croup or loin when circling behind them to let the horse know your location.

sometimes fatal injury to the handler. The handler should always stand on the side of the horse at the shoulder and never directly in front of or behind the horse.

It is important for the technician to let the horse know where they are standing at all times. An effective way to do this is to keep the torso close to the horse's body and place a hand on its back so it can *feel* where the technician is standing. The technician can also use their voice and gently speak to the horse so that it can *hear* where the person is standing. When moving around horses, it is safer to move in front of them than behind them. Standing in blind spot areas, such as directly in front or behind them, could put the technician at risk of being kicked by the hind limbs, or struck by the forelimbs.

Horses can kick in several ways, some of which can be fatal to both humans and other animals. Horses are able to kick straight back with one or both hind limbs ("double-barrel kick"), to the side ("cow kick"), and as far forward as their ears. Fatal kicks usually occur with a straight back kick or a double-barrel kick, when the limb/limbs are at full extension. These kicks can reach the chest and head of a person easily and have the most power behind them. When working with horses (particularly near the hind end), it is important to use one's voice, stay close to the animal's torso, and maintain a hand on the animal as much as possible to let the horse know where one is. Staying close to the horse does not prevent it from kicking, but it does shorten the distance of a kick and therefore reduces the force of the impact (Fig. 6.14).

> **TECHNICIAN NOTE**
>
> When working with horses, it is important to stay close to the torso of the horse and to always stand to the side, *not* directly in front or behind the animal.

To ensure the safety of both humans and horses, proper restraint is very important, particularly when working with horses outside. The type of procedure that needs to be done should be considered when selecting the type of restraint to use. Many procedures can be performed with a basic lead, either attached to the bottom ring of the halter or with a chain placed over the horse's muzzle. Physical examinations, venipuncture, and intravenous (IV) catheter placement are all typically performed with minimal restraint, but some horses may need additional restraint, depending on their temperament and sensitivity.

It is also important to keep in mind that horses will react to the comfort level of the handler, so if you are not comfortable handling a horse on your own, you should ask for assistance. For example, if you are nervous or jumpy around a horse's normal movements, the horse may be more likely to feed off that energy and become more nervous in its actions. If you are relaxed and comfortable with the horse's natural movements, it will relax in your presence.

Approach

Domesticated horses are curious creatures and will typically approach a person or will allow a person to approach them if they do not perceive a threat. This understanding can be helpful when attempting to catch horses in a pasture or in a stall. Patience is important, especially when working in the field environment. In this latter scenario, horses may begin by appearing curious but may not allow themselves to be caught. As the game of cat and mouse continues, endorphin levels rise in the bloodstream of the free horse,

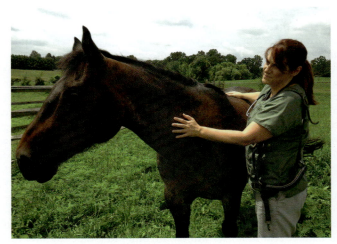

• **Fig. 6.14** Staying close to the horse does not prevent it from kicking, but it does shorten the distance of a kick and therefore reduces the force of the impact.

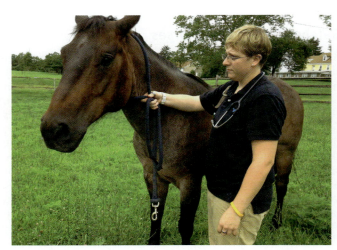

• **Fig. 6.15** Stand at the horse's left shoulder and place the lead rope around the horse's neck to secure the horse before placing the halter.

giving it a pleasurable experience. For this reason, the game continues indefinitely to the dismay, frustration, and ultimate failure of the human. Using a lead rope to initially capture the horse is sometimes necessary, and a halter can be placed later in a controlled and nonthreatening manner. In many cases, the horse will get close enough for the technician to drape the lead rope over its neck (Fig. 6.15). This is a safe way to make initial contact because if the animal bolts, the technician can quickly release the rope and not have a dangling lead attached to the horse. The halter is subsequently placed and the lead rope attached to the bottom ring of the halter. Both the halter and lead provide sufficient restraint for the performance of many procedures (Fig. 6.16).

It is important to keep in mind that if a horse does not want to be caught, one cannot catch it. Horses that have had a negative experience with their handlers, for example, may fear being caught. Additionally, if the only time a horse is brought into the barn is to undergo procedures such as floating their teeth or trimming their hooves, the horse may develop an aversion to being caught under any circumstance, especially if the procedure is uncomfortable for them. Educating clients to add some positive experiences, for instance, coming into the barn for just feeding or

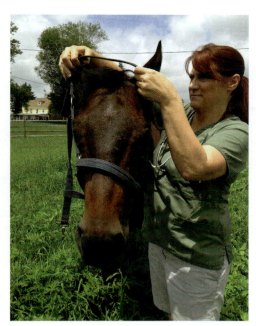

• **Fig. 6.16** Restraint of the horse should begin with a well-fitting halter and lead rope.

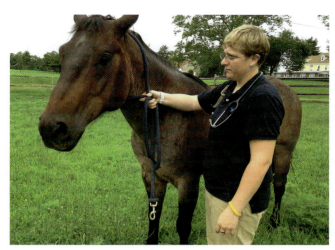

• **Fig. 6.17** Once bonding and acceptance have occurred, a lead rope can be placed around the neck. The lead rope provides minimal restraint but usually enough that a halter can be placed.

grooming, is an enjoyable way to balance out the experience of being caught and coming into the barn.

When working around horses, it is important to be calm and avoid making abrupt movements or loud noises. Applying equine restraint can be an intimidating procedure, even for those with horse experience. A horse's stature alone can be menacing, making restraint appear to be a daunting task. Learning proper and safe handling techniques may ease personal fears and lead to greater respect for horses. The technicians should observe and assess a horse before entering its enclosure and watch closely for signs of fear or aggression. A handler can observe subtle cues before capture that can help suggest how the horse is going to react. Signs of aggression in horses include but are not limited to pinning the ears, pawing at the ground, snorting, lunging forward, and turning the head quickly and biting. Signs of fear are much more subtle and include tension; tightening of muscles around the mouth, eyes, and neck; widening of eyes with show of the sclera (the whites of the eyes); and an increased respiratory rate. Nostrils are flared, and the horse takes deep breaths. Although the ears are forward and alert, the head is high, and the horse has a heightened awareness of everything around it. (For further information on equine behavior, refer to Chapter 5.)

Adult equine patients who have been properly handled and trained seem familiar with common restraint techniques. Horses typically and traditionally are handled on the left side, probably because people lead horses with their right hands. The left side of the horse is known as the *near side*. Horses handled this way tend to be more accepting of capture; this does not mean that they cannot and will not lash out. Any horse that has teeth or feet can bite, strike, or kick. The handler should try to remain calm when around a horse; horses can sense when a person is nervous. It is important to move gradually; keep the hands low; talk in a light, calm tone; and avoid quick, jerking motions or loud noises. Patience is key; the horse should be allowed to get used to the handler's presence in the stall. The handler should reach out slowly and attempt to touch the horse near its withers. The horse should be rubbed in this area and along the neck. These techniques are

like the bonding and grooming rituals of horses in a herd. Once bonding and acceptance have occurred, a lead rope can be placed around the neck (Fig. 6.17). The lead rope provides minimal restraint but usually enough that a halter can be placed if it is not already on the horse. Once the halter is placed, the lead rope can be attached to the tie ring on the halter, and head control can be obtained. It should be kept in mind that slow, gentle movements and talking are still necessary so as not to "spook" the horse and minimize stress and unacceptable behaviors.

Hospitalized horses in a stall are somewhat more agreeable to being captured compared with horses in the field. Field service personnel can be faced with a bigger challenge during capture of a horse for examination as horses typically have a large flight zone. The normal flight distance of most horses is approximately 10 to 30 feet; once inside this area, it is most important to remain calm and to never move quickly. Startling a horse or a herd of horses in the flight zone will cause the herd to run and can create a dangerous situation for all involved. Horses that evade capture may be enticed with some grain; often, food is all that is needed to catch the horse. Veterinary personnel can request that the horse needing examination be caught or placed in a stall before their arrival. Sometimes, using the buddy system works well too by capturing a herd mate, making the capturing of the patient easier.

> **TECHNICIAN NOTE**
>
> Horses that evade capture may be enticed with some grain. Often, food is all that is needed to catch the horse.

Juvenile horses (weanlings and yearlings)—that is, horses approximately 6 months to 2 years of age—present a unique challenge for veterinary personnel. Certain breeds will be introduced to handling only when veterinary care is needed, and these young horses often are just being introduced to halters and restraint. Young horses typically are more anxious compared with their adult counterparts; however, they often are more curious, which can be used to one's advantage. Squatting down, avoiding eye contact, and making the handler appear small will often make a nervous but inquisitive young horse come close enough to touch on the shoulder and scratch. The handler can try scratching the withers at the caudal aspect of the neck and work cranially without touching the halter. Grabbing the horse by the halter at this point or at any time is ill advised and dangerous. Juvenile horses most likely will pull back hard to escape and, when they realize that this maneuver is not working, they may try to rear up or flip over backward. To avoid injury, it is advisable to use slow movements and a soothing voice while attempting to apply the lead rope to the tie ring under the chin *without* touching the young horse (Fig. 6.18). While scratching with one hand, the handler reaches under with the other to clip the lead to the tie ring on the halter. One should never put a chain over a juvenile horse's nose; the horse does not know what it is and will not react favorably to the application, making future attempts to handle the young horse very difficult. It is necessary at times to use enticements, such as grass or grain, to gain the juvenile horse's trust.

Foals require a lot of patience and understanding. Ideally, three people should be charged with capturing a foal: one to restrain the mare and two to catch the foal, although often this is not the reality. The key to capturing a foal is using the mare, as it will run behind the mare when threatened. The foal's head will be directly behind the mare, with the foal's hind end facing the person who is attempting capture; be careful to avoid being kicked. The handler needs to approach from the side of the foal *farthest* from the mare. Moving in between the mare and the foal can be detrimental to capturing the foal; instead, this could stress out the mare, especially if she cannot see the foal. She will most likely move, allowing the foal to escape. Foals, just like adult horses, will be more difficult to catch the second time around. The same techniques (i.e., slow, steady movement; calm voice) used for adults apply to restraint of the foal, including scratching or rubbing the foal's neck or withers when first contact is made, then using only the arms and the body to restrain the foal (Fig. 6.19).

Regardless, once it is captured, it is important to allow the animal time to adjust before starting any examination or procedure. Rewarding the horse with a neck scratch and soothing words will help it to relax. One should not assume that high levels of restraint are necessary; restraint can begin with calm, pleasant interactions. If greater levels of restraint are needed, the horse will give behavioral signals. The handler should wait until the animal gives these signals before increasing the level of restraint to avoid an uncooperative patient.

Before physical contact with the horse, the veterinary team should develop a plan to include how to approach the horse, how much restraint will be required, and what escape route should be used if things should go wrong. The veterinary technician should prepare necessary supplies ahead of time to reduce the animal's stress. It is wise to always have a backup plan to allow for a horse that dodges initial approach and capture. Horses learn quickly; if they evade capture once, it will be harder to catch them the second time around. Having a plan ensures that an examination will occur, even if the initial attempt to restrain the animal goes awry. Horses generally are housed in boarding facilities and may be transported to clinics by hauling companies. Often, an owner is not present during veterinary visits, but a farm manager may be. If an owner or a farm manager are present, they should be questioned about the horse for invaluable input. They should be asked the about the horse's normal behavior and attitude, previous contact with veterinary personnel and procedures, and restraint techniques used by the owner/farm manager and by veterinary personnel during previous veterinary care visits. It is important to listen to the owner, but ultimately, the veterinary personnel should decide the best course of action regarding restraint. Even the best-behaved horses can be unpredictable when sick or injured.

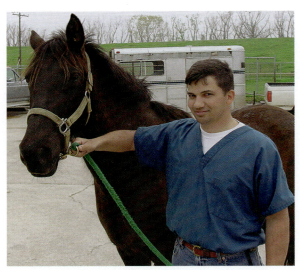

• **Fig. 6.18** Attempt to apply the lead rope to the tie ring under the chin without touching the young horse.

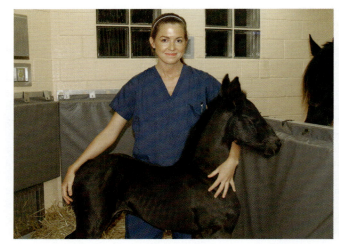

• **Fig. 6.19** Scratch or rub the foal's neck or withers when first contact is made, then use only your arms and body to restrain it.

It is also important to note that behaviors may change throughout the hospitalized experience. Horses who come in nervous and fractious may settle when feeling better, whereas some horses may start to become more averse to treatments and may become more difficult to work with.

> **TECHNICIAN NOTE**
> The key to successful restraint is reducing the animal's stress.

When performing procedures at the rear of the horse, it is important for the technician to alert the horse to their presence before jumping into the work. Greeting them using one's voice from a distance, holding the hand out to be smelled, and placing the hand on the horse's neck and back are all effective ways of communicating one's presence in a nonthreatening manner. When working directly with horses, it is important to stand to the side and as close to them as possible to lessen the force of any potential kick. This is especially true when taking the horse's rectal temperature.

You should run your hand down their back, scratch at the base of their tail head to relax them, and then stand up against their hip while reaching around to insert the thermometer. If the horse tries to kick, you will feel the movement and can move away to safety, whereas if you were standing an arm's length away, the horse could put enough force behind a kick to cause significant injury. The technician should be mindful of the horse's feet, however, to avoid being inadvertently stepped on if the horse takes a step to the side. When horses feel an aversion to something in front of them, they may lift a forelimb and bring it up and out to strike whatever it is. Therefore when performing procedures such as nasogastric intubation, it is important to stand at the animal's side.

In stalls, horses may have similar fears or anxieties. For example, a horse may become defensive of its feed and hay and may demonstrate signs of aggression when people enter its stall. In these cases, veterinary technicians must be strategic and have a plan for working around these fears and consequent defensiveness. In such instances, it is best to feed animals hay in their stall close to the doorway, making it easier to catch them. Procedures or treatments may need to be performed before the animal is offered a grain meal; however, some animals do better with the diversion of feed.

When entering the horse's stall or field, personal safety comes first. A person capturing a horse should never enter an area if the horse is not aware of the person's presence. As a general rule, a stall should not be entered if the horse has its hind end facing the handler. A clicking noise made with the tongue or talking to the horse is usually enough to get its attention. The handler should not enter a stall without having the horse's attention; doing so can startle ("spook") the horse. A startled horse can wheel around quickly, pinning the handler into a corner or pressing them against the wall. A handler trapped in a stall with a nervous, stressed, and startled horse would result in a disaster. It is important to make sure there is room for escape, if necessary. Once the horse is aware of the presence of the person, it is safe to approach and capture it. Once the horse is restrained, the handler and the examiner should always work on the same side of the horse.

TECHNICIAN NOTE

Patience is imperative when working with horses; it will go a long way toward easing the horse's fears and keeping everyone safe.

Horses do not typically act aggressively without provocation and mostly exhibit behavioral signals when they are becoming defensive. It is important for veterinary technicians and handlers to heed these behavioral signals and proceed with caution. Some animals are protective of their herd mates and will try to lead fellow horses away from being caught, a behavior often seen in stallions and in geldings that adopt a harem of sorts. In a stall, it is important to have control of the animal before fully entering the stall so that the technician does not get stuck in a corner without an avenue for easy escape. It is of utmost importance to have control of horses that exhibit defensive or threatening behavior *before* entering the stall. The technician may be able to coax the horse to the front of the stall with feed. After gaining control of the horse, the technician can start building a positive experience. Developing a positive relationship with these animals means that sometimes the technician needs to work on providing positive experiences a few times before the actual procedure. For horses that are very averse to being caught, a catch rope can be left in place on the halter to make it easier to catch them in the future. A catch rope is about 12 inches of a lead or braided twine that stays attached

to the halter, even when the horse is not being held. It must be ensured that the rope is not long enough to cause harm as the horse moves about. Positive behavior during this process should always be rewarded. Sometimes, positive interactions, such as grooming the patient or just giving them some attention, should be made without treatments or procedures to build trust.

Positive reinforcement along with frequent treatments is also recommended. For instance, some eye conditions will need to be treated with medication every 2 to 4 hours. These treatments will cause some mild and temporary discomfort to the eye, and some horses will become averse to seeing you enter the stall every few hours. If you provide a small handful of grain or a treat with every treatment, they should start to associate the treatment with a treat instead of the discomfort of the medication. Placing grain or a treat in a small bag that will make a sound when crinkled is also a good auditory stimulus that the horse should associate with a treat.

When performing procedures on horses, it is important to have one person restrain the patient while another performs the procedure. Having a designated handler frees veterinary personnel to complete important clinical tasks and helps ensure a high level of safety when performing the procedures. The handler must stand on the same side of the horse as the person performing the procedure. This way, if the horse has an averse reaction, the handler can quickly direct the horse's hind end *away* from the clinician when a handler is not available. A rope or nylon lead can be used to tie the horse to a fixed area in the stall, barn, or field.

When tying a horse, it is important to use a quick-release knot (Fig. 6.20) and to never tie a horse with a chain over its nose or on its gums. Veterinarians may request that horses be placed in **cross-ties** to prevent further injury from lying down. Cross-ties are another form of restraint that may be used to restrain horses when working alone (Fig. 6.21). They are a way to control the horse's head and restrict the horse to a small area, typically in a barn aisle or stall. However, horses can still move a little on cross-ties, but their range is limited by the length and flexibility of the ties. Horses accustomed to cross-ties typically do well on them, particularly for physical examination, minor procedures, and grooming. However, horses should never be left unattended on cross-ties, because they may panic, rear up, slip, or flip over backward.

Cross-ties require a quick-release or breakaway option in case the animal becomes stressed.

Restraint Techniques and Devices

Restraint is defined as the control of an animal for the purpose of examination or treatment. There are three major methods for achieving adequate restraint, which can be divided into the following categories: physical restraint, diversionary restraint, and chemical restraint. When working with large-animal species, this involves the following:

Physical restraint—the use of stocks, halters, and lead ropes, etc.

Diversionary restraint—the use of various techniques or devices designed to distract the patient; this may include manual (e.g., light tapping on the horse's head) or mechanical (use of a **twitch** or other instrument) methods, or providing grain to distract the animal.

Chemical restraint—the use of specific drugs to achieve an appropriate level of patient compliance for successful completion of specific veterinary procedures and ensuring the safety of both the veterinary medical team and the patient.

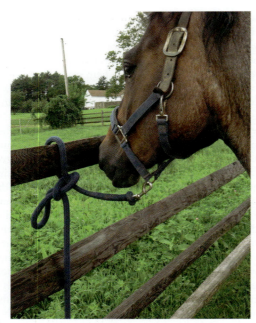

• **Fig. 6.20** A quick-release knot. Horses can be trained to be ground-tied, cross-tied, or tied to a ring in the stall or to some other sturdy structure, such as a fence post.

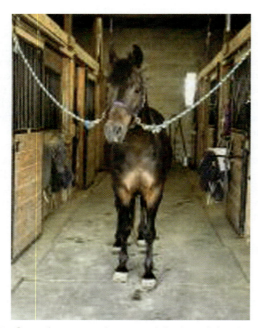

• **Fig. 6.21** Cross-ties are used to control the horse's head and restrict movement when working alone.

Physical restraint of the adult equine begins with the halter. A halter is placed around the horse's head. Halters can be made of leather, nylon, or rope. The halter consists of the noseband (which consists of the nose piece and the chin piece), the connecting strap, the throat latch, a cheek piece that runs up either side of the face, the crown piece, a buckle, and/or a snap. Other pieces of the halter include the metal tie ring, the square metal nose pieces, and the metal cheek rings. Specialty halters are used for medical procedures, such as anesthesia or laryngotomy. These halters are usually composed of burlap or nylon; they lack the connecting strap and the throat latch piece and are temporary. Anesthesia and laryngotomy halters provide little restraint. Veterinary technicians should know the different types of halters and should be able to list their parts for proper use and application.

Lead ropes can have a single snap or chain at one end and are made from leather, rope, or nylon. The lead rope provides some head control, and the rope end can be placed around the horse's neck for control while haltering. Once attached to the halter, the lead rope should be held close to the snap end with the right hand, and the extra length should be folded and grasped in the left hand. The lead rope, although like a dog leash, is *not* a dog leash and should never be wrapped around hands or arms. Mistaking the lead rope for the leash and wrapping it around an arm could lead to the handler getting dragged by a horse that "spooks" and decides to take off running. The rope end of the lead should not be allowed to drag on the ground; the handler or the horse could step on the end. Stepping on the end of a lead rope by a horse or person can cause a horse to panic and potentially get injured.

Placing a knot at the end of the lead is useful in case the horse tries to pull the lead out of your hand, as it will provide a larger area to grab. Also, when holding the lead, it is important to always keep two hands on it. One hand should be close to the snap or chain, whereas the other should be further down the lead. Horses need to be able to move the head as they are led, so you should not hold them too tightly.

Chain shanks have a chain and a single snap on one end. Like other lead shanks, the lead portion of the shank is made of rope, nylon, or leather. Depending on how they are used, chain shanks can provide greater restraint than shanks that lack chains. For example, when managing excitable horses, the chain can be placed through the square metal nose pieces and over or under the nose (Fig 6.22). This creates a distraction to the horse and improves handling. A fractious horse, however, may benefit by placing the chain over the nose, or in extreme cases, under the upper lip on the gums. This is known as a *gum chain* or a *lip chain* and is a severe form of restraint. The chain needs to be slowly and carefully tightened over the gums when it is placed (see Fig. 6.23). Only experienced handlers should attempt to apply and use a gum chain. Damage to the horse's gums, stress, and handling aversions may ensue if this technique is employed improperly. The gum chain is used often with young athletes that do not respond to traditional restraint practices. When used correctly, a gum chain can also trigger a small endorphin release. When this restraint is applied, there should be only gentle and steady pressure. One should never put extreme pressure on the horse's gums or make aggressive movements with the chain. The gum chain should only remain in place for a few minutes.

You should also never loop a chain through the ring under the chin and clip it to itself. This will make a dangerous loop such that if a horse is allowed to move freely, for example, when grazing, it could accidentally bring a foot up and step through the loop made in the chain.

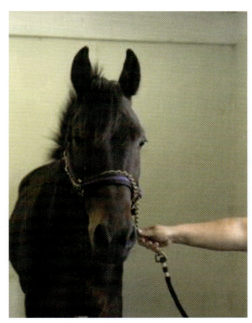

• **Fig. 6.22** A chain shank.

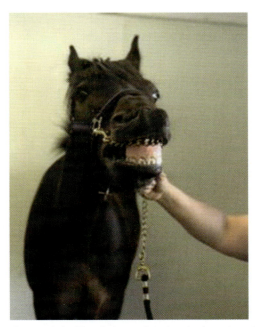

• **Fig. 6.23** A gum chain. The chain needs to be slowly and carefully tightened over the gums when it is placed.

Diversionary restraint techniques help reduce unwanted behaviors when performing short, relatively nonpainful procedures. When selecting a method, it is important to keep in mind the safety of both the horse and the veterinary staff. Manual diversions use the handler's hand to assist in providing a distraction; this can include diversions such as tapping on the forehead or under the eye of the patient. Manual twitches may also include applying pressure to the upper lip or rolling the skin on the neck or shoulder (Fig. 6.24A) by using one's hand. These diversions distract the horse and divert its attention away from the procedure being performed. The use of diversions works well for short, relatively nonpainful procedures, such as venipuncture and physical examination, but can lose effectiveness over time and should be used for only a few minutes when short procedures are performed.

Starting with a slight neck twitch may be enough of a distraction, and it is done by rolling the skin at the area of the scapula. The manual twitch can be used for horses that are not averse to having their faces touched, because they do not know what is coming. When applied properly to the horse's muzzle, the twitch puts pressure on acupressure points that stimulate endorphin release (Fig. 6.25). The technician must wait for the endorphin release for this procedure to fully work. Most horses will lower the head and appear almost sedate when the acupressure is working fully. This twitch should be in place for no longer than five minutes or the endorphin release will have subsided, creating an unpleasant situation.

A few different types of mechanical twitches are used as diversions. A common one consists of a wooden handle with a chain or rope loop attached to a wooden handle. The loop is typically placed around the upper portion of a horse's muzzle and then twisted. The muzzle contains pressure points that when pressed stimulate the release of endorphins. These endorphins are powerful hormones that relax the horse and block pain perception. The endorphin release, however, is not immediate. Like the use of chemical sedation, it takes about 3 minutes for the release of endorphins, and it provides pain modulation for approximately 15 to 20 minutes. It is therefore counterproductive to attempt a procedure when the twitch is initially applied.

Typically, the use of a rope or a chain twitch requires two people, the restrainer and the examiner. Several different types of twitches are available, but the most commonly used ones are the hand or ones that have a wooden handle and a rope loop (Fig. 6.24B). In contrast, the **humane twitch** (Fig. 6.26) is a mechanical restraint device composed of a metal hinge that is placed over the upper lip of the horse, squeezed, and clipped to the halter. It is designed for personnel who must perform procedures or examinations alone.

Another option for physical restraint when it is important for the horse to stand still is to simply pick up and hold one of the its feet (Fig. 6.27). When any quadruped does not stand still for a procedure, this simple approach works well and should be considered. If clinical work is being done on a particular limb, the opposing limb should be picked up and held off the ground by a handler, forcing the horse to shift its weight to the other three limbs and making it stand still.

Diversionary restraint is a well-received approach, especially if the animal has no feed restrictions and is food motivated. For horses that need a diversion for a quick procedure, such as an injection or eye medication using a subpalpebral lavage system, a small handful of grain may provide just the right amount of diversion needed to complete the task. Other ways of diversion include massaging certain areas, such as the base of the ears or the area near the withers, or scratching the area near the withers. This mimics the communal grooming that occurs within herds and may be comforting.

Performing an ear twitch is not acceptable under any circumstances, and for a good reason. Ears are sensitive areas of the

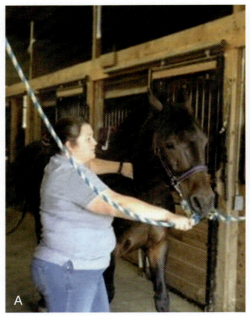 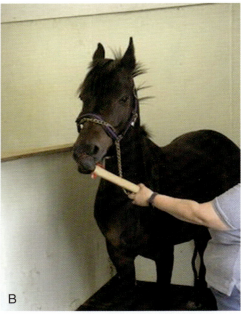

• **Fig. 6.24** (A) Rolling the skin on the neck or shoulder are examples of manual twitching. (B) A person twitches the upper lip of horse using a rope loop attached to a wooden handle.

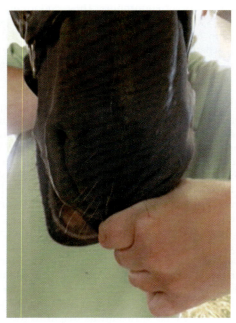

• **Fig. 6.25** Manual twitch—applying pressure to the upper lip. When applied properly to the horse's muzzle, the twitch puts pressure on acupressure points that stimulate endorphin release.

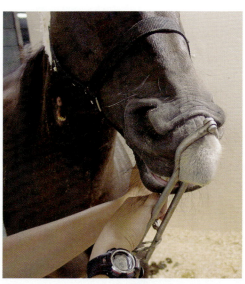

• **Fig. 6.26** The humane twitch is designed for personnel who have to perform procedures or examinations alone.

Foal and Young Horse Handling and Restraint

Before working with a foal that is still with its dam, it is imperative to be mindful of one's position in relation to the mare and the foal. Some mares are protective of their foals and may not tolerate anyone standing between them. In situations where the foal needs to be restrained on the ground, it is a good idea to have someone restraining the mare. The best plan is to hold the mare in an area from which she can see the foal but cannot step on the people performing the procedure.

Foal restraint requires a lot of patience. Once caught and restrained, the foal will still fight and try to get away. Using the following guidelines for foal restraint will make foal management less

horse's body and, if too much pressure is placed while twisting and squeezing the ear, damage can be done to the auricular cartilage. The more an ear twitch is used, the greater the likelihood that it is creating a new aversion which, in turn, could affect the owner's relationship with the horse. Horses need to be comfortable with people moving around their heads and ears, especially when a halter or a bridle is being placed. A much nicer and sometimes equally effective technique is rubbing the base of the horse's ear. It has been shown to have a calming effect.

stressful for the foal, the mare, and the handler. First, to prevent the foal from startling and running, the handler should approach the foal slowly and gradually and remain calm. Once the foal is within reach, an arm should be placed around the foal's chest and hind end. The foal will struggle to escape; the handler should just hold on until it settles down.

A particularly good distraction for foals is scratching them. Scratching foals up near their withers or caudal dorsum simulates

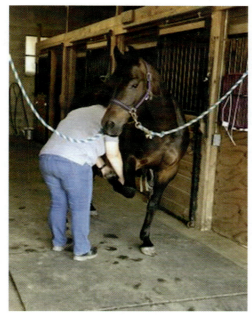

• **Fig. 6.27** Another option for physical restraint when it is important that the horse stands still is to simply pick up and hold one of the horse's feet.

grooming by their dams. Many foals will try to reciprocate the efforts of scratching and may turn to groom the technician. Typically, the technician can redirect the foal's mouth, but this is something to be mindful of. Another acceptable spot is the area around the base of the ears, where gentle massage is usually well received. It is very important to not grab a foal's ear as a handle for restraint, because this will likely cause future aversion or could do damage to the fragile cartilage.

When working with foals, it is important to remember that even though they are up and walking within hours of birth, it does not mean that they are similar to an adult. Foals that are imprinted early in life may provide the veterinary staff with an advantage, but all young equines need to be taught the basics of wearing a halter and being led. Foals are easily moved with their dams and follow them closely (Fig. 6.28A). If actual restraint is necessary to walk a foal, the technician should use a rope lead and a figure-of-eight rope around the foal's chest and behind its hindquarters (see Fig. 6.28B). This type of rope will allow the technician to coax the foal forward by gently pulling on the rear and slow it down by gently holding or pulling the rope at its chest. The figure-of-eight rope works well for moving foals to and from a stall or field and can also be used to teach them how to enter a trailer.

A halter may be used in foals from a very early age, even when only a few days old, and may merely be ornamental fixtures at this time. Although it is appropriate to acclimate foals to wearing halters early in their lives, it is *not* appropriate to restrain or handle foals by their halters until they become used to them. Grabbing a foal's halter may startle it and cause it to flip over backward or to rear up and strike out, putting both the foal and the technician at risk. The best approach is to place an arm around the foal's neck or in front of the chest. This way there is a bit of a barrier, but the technician can easily release the foal if necessary.

Diversionary restraint, such as gently lifting up the tail, using a skin twitch, or rubbing the base of an ear, can help veterinary

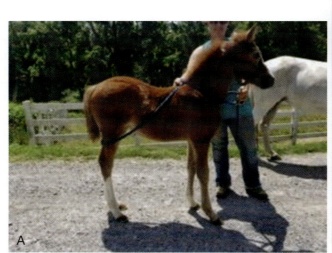 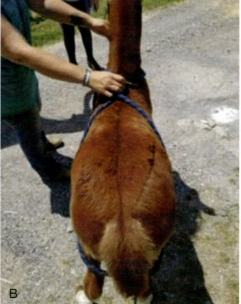

• **Fig. 6.28** (A) Foals are easily moved with mares and follow their dam closely. (B) If actual restraint is necessary to walk a foal, you should use a rope lead to make a figure of eight with the rope around the foal's chest and behind its hindquarters.

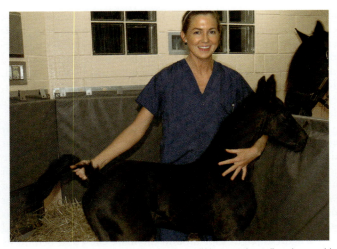

• **Fig. 6.29** Diversionary restraint, such as lifting up the tail, using a skin twitch, or squeezing an ear, can help veterinary personnel perform examinations and procedures.

personnel perform examinations and procedures (Fig. 6.29). Mechanical restraint such as twitches or chains should not be used on foals. Grabbing a foal's ear to use as a twitch is unacceptable, as damage can be done to the cartilage.

When performing a procedure on a foal, mainly a neonate, you should first identify if this procedure will be safer to do with the foal standing or on the ground. If the foal is standing, it may be beneficial to position the hind end towards a corner of the stall while continuing the restraint around the chest. Keep in mind to keep your head out of the way of theirs, especially in the case of jugular venipuncture. When stuck, the foal may toss its head up and thrust into the handler, causing injury.

If the foal is small enough to safely restrain on the ground, it is first key to have someone helping with the mare, or at least position the foal in an area near a doorway. If the foal is not already on the ground, two people can easily pick the foal up and lay it down by grasping it at bony points (sternum and stifles usually) and picking the foal up while directing the limbs towards them to gently lay the foal down. Care should also be used to protect the foal's head. Use caution to only pick foals up by bony structures such as the sternum and stifles, and never pick a foal up with pressure on the abdomen. When the foal is down, someone should straddle the hind limb and hug them tightly with their legs, and someone should do the same with the forelimbs while also restraining their head, if possible.

Weanling and yearling foals are generally unfamiliar with being haltered and led. They also tend to be nervous, especially when away from familiar surroundings. A short catch rope is sometimes attached to the tie ring of their halter when they present. It is advisable not to grab the catch rope. Young horses tend to resist their halter being grabbed and can rear up, flip over, or slip on the stall floor while trying to escape. The best method for catching a juvenile horse is to use a calm, quiet approach. Treats can be used as enticement and, once the handler is close enough, a lead rope is quietly clipped to the halter, if possible. If not, the handler can stroke the horse's neck and withers, and wait to gain its trust before attaching the lead rope. Once the juvenile is on the lead, the handler should move with it as it moves without pulling on the lead rope, because this could cause the young horse to pull back and rear up. It is important to understand that a weanling or yearling may panic

and try to rear up or escape. Sticking with the young horse as it moves, keeping calm, and having patience are very important. The handler should never try to lead a juvenile horse with a chain over its nose.

A key principle to remember with these young animals is that pressure can work with or against you. When young horses comply with the pressure of leading with you, their reward should be a small release in pressure. Learning about the amount of pressure to apply will take patience but is a very useful tool to accomplish your goal. It is important to not use excessive pressure and know when to relax it to avoid injury.

TECHNICIAN NOTE

For their own and the animal's safety the handler should never try to lead a juvenile horse with a chain over its nose.

Chemical Restraint

For some procedures, physical restraint may not be enough to ensure the safety of everyone involved. Evaluate the procedure and the animal *before* starting a procedure. If the animal is already showing aversions or acting in an unsafe manner, chemical restraint may be indicated.

Chemical restraint is the use of medications (tranquilizers, sedatives, and anesthetics) to achieve a desired level of patient relaxation that permits patient care as ordered. Chemical restraint is often used immediately in colicky horses that are violently painful on presentation. Chemical restraint can also be used in horses that are generally uncooperative and/or are resistant to certain procedures such as nasogastric intubation. Drugs commonly used for chemical restraint include acepromazine, butorphanol, detomidine, and xylazine. For further information on pharmacology and the management of equine pain, refer to Chapter 29.

Acepromazine at a dose of 0.01 to 0.03 mg/kg is commonly used for minor procedures and can be given via the intravenous (IV), intramuscular (IM), or both routes for a combination of short-acting and longer durations. If the animal's behavior has already escalated, then an α^2-agonist may be a better choice. Xylazine at a dose of 0.2 to 0.4 mg/kg IV provides a desirable plane of sedation and is quick acting and quickly metabolized. Detomidine may be used at a dose of 5 to 8 µg/mL IV or IM, especially if the animal needs to stay very still for the procedure. The onset of drug action is quick, but the effect lasts a little longer. If the procedure is expected to be painful, butorphanol may be combined with these sedatives to add analgesia. The common dose range is 0.01 to 0.02 mg/kg. For animals that have an aversion to the needle, detomidine is also available in a gel form and is administered sublingually.

Other Forms of Restraint

In some cases, veterinary technicians may be part of a procedure that requires more control of the animal than is possible with traditional restraining devices. In veterinary hospitals or at large farm operations, stocks may be available (Fig. 6.30). Stocks can contain entire animals in a very small space, preventing them from moving sideways or stepping forward or backward and providing personnel extra protection from being kicked. However, some large animals have been witnessed kicking above the top rail of stocks to injure nearby handlers, although this is rare. YouTube is a good place to find film clips of these unusual events. Stocks

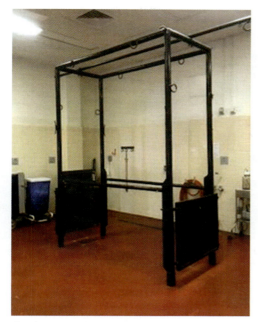

• **Fig. 6.30** Stocks contain the entire animal in a very small space, preventing them from moving sideways or stepping forward or backward. They also provide protection from injury for veterinary personnel and handlers.

offer optimal restraint for many procedures, including rectal, uterine, and endoscopic examinations. Restraining the head of a horse in stocks with a lead is important, particularly during endoscopic examination and other procedures that involve contact with the head.

Distraction can be used for minor procedures or working with younger animals and those that are food motivated. Placing a small amount of food in a bucket held at the mouth may distract horses enough for an injection or blood draw. Horses respond well to positive reinforcement, and the technician may find that the horse looks forward to these treats and associates veterinary technician visits with the treat and not the injection.

Trailering

Caution should be used when loading a distressed animal; if possible, such animals should be loaded as they normally are. Horses may be used to a type of trailer, for example, a slant-load stock trailer or a straight-load trailer with a ramp. It is best not to add a new element at a crucial time. Most horses load well, whereas some need to be coaxed onto the trailer, typically starting with grain. Other methods include gentle pressure and release as the horse makes a forward movement. Pulling or tugging on the horse forcefully should be avoided, as this is ineffective. If the horse is close, one can try picking up a front foot and placing it on the trailer or ramp. Other acceptable methods include blindfolding the horse, sedation, and using a rear strap. Putting on the rear strap is achieved when a person stands on either side of the horse's shoulder, each holding the end of a long rope. As the person leading the horse moves forward, the person at the rear should give a pull. Light taps with a lunge whip may be used, but lashing the animal or smacking at it with a broom is unacceptable behavior, which usually only makes the situation worse.

When unloading a horse, the trailer is accessed first. Can the horse be turned around and walk off the trailer or will it need to be backed off? This may depend on any injury that the horse has.

If the horse needs to back off a straight-load trailer, it may be necessary to have someone on the side of the ramp to help guide the horse safely backward.

Equine Restraint: Special Circumstances for Specific Procedures

Tying a horse is generally done for noninvasive procedures, such as grooming. Horses can be trained to be ground-tied, cross-tied, or tied to a ring in the stall or to some other sturdy structure, such as a fence post. Another reason to tie a horse is to prevent further injury. For example, preventing a horse that has undergone orthopedic repair of a severe fracture from lying down could be crucial for its recovery, and the veterinarian may decide that this horse should be cross-tied. Any horse that is tied needs to be monitored closely and never left alone. A horse should never be tied with the chain over the nose or under the chin, because if the horse becomes anxious or tries to escape, it will be injured. A quick-release knot or breakaway snaps should always be used to set the horse free if it panics. Tying a horse should be done only when necessary, and invasive procedures should not be completed while the horse is tied.

> **TECHNICIAN NOTE**
> Tying a horse is generally done for noninvasive procedures, such as grooming. Any horse that is tied needs to be monitored closely and never left alone.

Lifting a forelimb or hind limb is done to keep other limbs on the ground and reduce the risk of a practitioner being kicked. Lifting a limb is easy, but keeping the limb up can sometimes be difficult, particularly if the horse falls asleep standing and uses the handler who is holding the limb up as a crutch. It is important for the handler to prompt the horse to shift its weight evenly to the other three limbs. Hobbles are used rarely on horses. The general purpose of hobbles is to connect two limbs together, such as the hind limbs, to prevent kicking. Breeding hobbles, for example, can be used to prevent a mare from kicking and injuring the stallion during live cover. *Nurse mares*—mares that nurse rejected or orphaned foals—might be hobbled on the hind limbs to prevent the mare from kicking and injuring the foal, particularly during introduction and until bonding between mare and foal has occurred.

Stocks are vertical metal or wooden pillars arranged in a rectangular shape and connected by horizontal bars and designed to restrain horses or cattle. Stocks are commonly found in most large-animal hospitals. They can be used during many procedures but are most used during abdominal palpations per rectum, reproductive examinations, or endoscopic procedures. Stocks serve as a safe alternative to handler restraint for these procedures; however, it must be noted that horses have been known to spook and jump over or out of stocks, causing serious injury. Also, horses are still able to cow kick and strike out when in stocks. The handler should always be present and holding the horse's lead when a horse is in stocks to ensure the safety of the animal and other barn personnel (Fig. 6.31).

A tail tie can be applied with rope or brown gauze and tied around the horse's neck and chest to prevent movement of the tail during abdominal palpation per rectum or reproductive examination. A brown gauze tail tie is more commonly used; it is applied at the base of the tail and is wrapped around the tail to the end

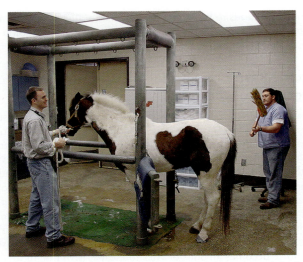

• **Fig. 6.31** The handler should always be present when a horse is in stocks to ensure the safety of the animal and other barn personnel.

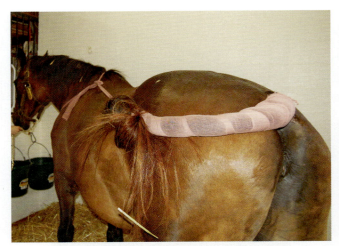

• **Fig. 6.32** Brown gauze is put through a loop and stretched over the back of the horse and around its neck. It is then secured with a quick-release knot.

of the tailbone. The hairs that hang from the end of the tail are then folded over and the brown gauze is wrapped around, creating a loop in the tail. The brown gauze is put through this loop and is stretched over the back and around the neck; it is then secured with a quick-release knot (Fig. 6.32). The purpose of the brown gauze wrap is to cover the bulk of the small hairs at the base of the tail and prevent them from getting into a clean field. A tail tie is applied to the hairs at the end of the tail and is secured in a similar fashion; however, small hair coverage will not be attained.

In conclusion, many methods of restraint are known; however, no one way is the correct way. Every horse is different and should be treated as an individual. The entire situation should be assessed before restraint. Regarding equine restraint, the safety of personnel should always be a priority. Learning and understanding proper and safe restraint techniques will minimize stress on the animal and will keep all those working with the animal safe. Ask for assistance if you are not comfortable, as horses will feed off your energy. If you are nervous, they may appear the same, whereas if you are comfortable and confident, they will be more trustworthy of your intentions. Building rapport with equine patients in the clinic is an important part of the treatment strategy. This will take more time up front but could have great benefits in the long run.

Capture and Restraint of Cattle

The Approach

The fundamental difference between working with livestock species and working with companion animals is the predator-prey interaction that serves as the foundation of human-livestock interactions. This relationship causes cattle to alter their behavior when they observe a predator to avoid being chosen as prey. Therefore it is important to complete as much of the physical examination as possible before the cow notices that you are evaluating it or are moving to restrain it. General conditions, such as attitude, lameness, rumination/cud chewing, appetite, and respiratory rate, can be included in an initial observation. Much like evaluating dogs and cats in the waiting room, the reaction of the cow or the herd when they observe you can provide information about how to proceed. Cattle that startle at your presence and begin to flee need to be handled more carefully and quietly compared with cattle

that approach you with curiosity. Be particularly cautious when separating sick or injured animals from the larger herd. Elevated anxiety levels caused by separation can lead both the patient and other members of the herd to be defensive and aggressive.

Low-stress Handling

The predator-prey relationship, as mentioned above, can be dangerous if cattle are stressed and feel threatened; however, it also serves as the basis of the way veterinary professionals work with cattle. Cows have an inherent fear of humans and will try to maintain a distance at which they feel safe. This distance is called the *flight zone*, and it varies from 0 to 25 feet, depending on the tameness of the animal (Fig. 6.33A). Because of their daily contact with the farmer during milking time, adult dairy cattle tend to have relatively small flight zones (5–10 feet) compared with beef cattle. Beef cattle that typically graze on open grasslands have a larger flight zone of 15 to 25 feet.

> **TECHNICIAN NOTE**
>
> Pet cattle have no flight zone. The best method of moving these animals usually involves placing a rope halter on their heads and leading them.

When humans or other predators enter the flight zone of cattle, the cattle tend to bunch together and move away as a group from the perceived threat. As they relocate to a more comfortable distance, they turn back and look at the perceived threat. This is an indication that the flight zone has been re-established.

Behavioral cues, such as those mentioned above, underscore the importance of the "pressure and release" system that influences the management of herd animals, such as cattle and sheep. Handlers move cattle by invading their flight zone and then allowing the animals to re-establish this distance (release). Repetition of this pressure and release system uses the species' innate flight distance to move both single animals and groups of animals in a particular direction. It is important that the "release" portion of herding lasts for the duration of time when the cattle are moving in the desired direction. Only when the herd stops or needs to be redirected should a corrective pressure be used. However, handlers should be careful not to invade the flight zone of the cattle too

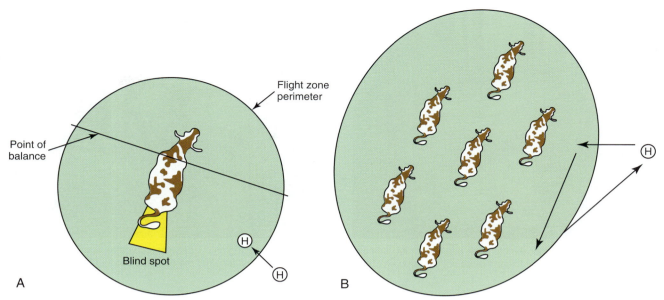

• **Fig. 6.33** (A) Correct position for moving a single bovine. As the handler moves into the flight zone from behind the point of balance, the bovid will move forward and to the left. (B) A handler walking briskly in the opposite direction of the desired movement of a herd is an effective method for moving cattle or horses forward. After passing the cattle and initiating their movement, the handler must step out of the flight zone and move to the head of the herd before repeating the process. (Redrawn from JC Fisher, IAN Image Library website. ian.umces.edu/imagelibrary.)

aggressively or they may generate a fear response that could cause panic within the herd. A frightened animal is a dangerous one; this is especially true of cattle, because they are large, strong, and able to push through or jump over fences, potentially injuring themselves and the handlers.

The flight zone of cows may also be affected by the way in which the herd is handled. Cows should be worked by using calm and deliberate movements. Quick or sudden movement and loud noises, such as yelling, can cause cows to panic and attempt to flee. Cows do not understand vocal commands, but they do understand body language. Calm and quiet handlers are often more successful in handling cows and herd animals in general compared with aggressive, frustrated, and loud handlers.

The point of balance in most herd animals is at the shoulder. This means that when standing at the shoulder, a step in either direction (toward the head or toward the tail) will prompt the animal to move in the *opposite* direction. To move a single cow forward, for example, one would enter its flight zone from *behind* the shoulder and wait for the cow to re-establish a comfort distance. It should be remembered that as long as the cow continues to move in the desired direction, no further pressure is needed. When the cow stops or begins to move in an undesired direction, the handler would then have to re-enter its flight zone to redirect it. Cattle prefer to stay in a group and follow the herd's leader. When groups of cattle are moved in a working chute system or in a pasture, pressure is placed on the point of balance of the leader or on cattle in the middle of the leading group. Fig. 6.33B shows the handler entering the flight zone near the front of the group, walking toward the rear of the group, and then exiting the flight zone. This triangular movement pattern moves the herd forward as the point of balance is crossed. The handler then releases pressure by exiting the flight zone. The pattern can be repeated as often as necessary.

As cattle approach a holding area, handlers should initially move outside the flight zone, releasing pressure. If cattle balk at the entrance and turn back, a small amount of pressure should be added. However, continuous pressure can make a cow feel trapped and can make the animal begin to panic. Cattle will run over and through obstacles, including humans, if they are pressured to the point of panic. Like horses, cattle have very poor vertical vision and cannot focus at close range. These traits result in cattle balking at things that do not cause much concern for humans (Fig. 6.34). Common causes of balking include shadows, changes in floor or wall color, flapping clothes or bags, extension cords, discarded cups or cans, and changes in flooring texture. Removal of the offending item is the easiest solution, although some items require more long-term planning. The use of electric prods to push cattle into or through a poorly designed system is unacceptable and, in this author's opinion, inhumane. Electric prods should be used in less than 5% of cattle working through a chute system.

Capture

Handling facilities for beef and dairy cattle differ significantly from one another. In the United States, most dairy cows are housed in a barn for some portion of the day, particularly during milking times. Those that are turned out to pasture will willingly come to the barn for milking when their udders are full and causing discomfort. This eliminates the need to aggressively herd them. If better control is necessary, especially of the head, a rope halter can be placed on the cow's head (Fig. 6.35). A cow halter is often made of braided rope and has two loops and a tail. The loop that is reduced in size when you pull on the tail goes over the nose and under the jaw. The other loop is changed in size by adjusting a portion of the nose loop; it is placed over the poll and around the ears and horns, if present. Some find it easier to adjust the poll and ear loop and place it first and then place the nose and jaw loop

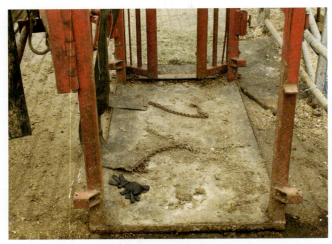

• **Fig. 6.34** Cattle have very poor vertical vision and cannot focus at close range, resulting in cattle balking at things that do not cause much concern in humans.

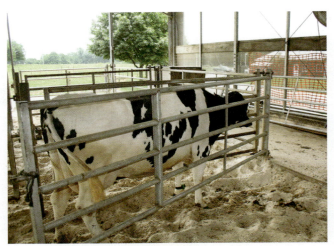

• **Fig. 6.36** Trapping a cow between two gates is an effective way to limit its movement and allow for medical care and for placing a halter.

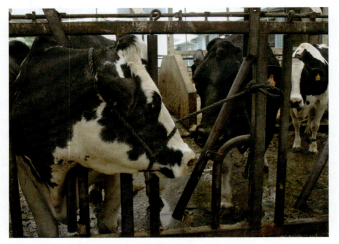

• **Fig. 6.35** A cow halter is often made of braided rope and has two loops and a tail. The loop that is reduced in size when you pull on the tail goes over the nose and under the jaw.

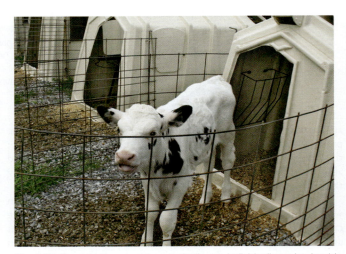

• **Fig. 6.37** On dairy farms, calves typically are individually maintained in their own hutches.

or vice versa, but either order is acceptable. The halter is secured by pulling on the tail of the halter after both loops are placed. Technically, the tail of the halter should exit from the left side of the cow's mandible, but head restraint will be more secure if the tail exits to the side of the cow where it will be tied.

TECHNICIAN NOTE

Place a halter *upside down* on a cow so that the part that tightens when the tail is pulled is around the ears and *not* the mouth. This provides additional head control and, at the same time, maintains the ability to open the cow's mouth for an oral examination or speculum placement.

When placing a halter over the poll, the technician should be very careful to keep their own head from being directly over the cow's head. Cattle will occasionally lift their heads straight up, colliding with the restrainer's head, chin, and/or nose. To avoid injury, the cow should be kept at arm's length or approached from the side instead of directly from the front. Cows are sometimes in individual "box stalls" for additional treatment and care. In these situations, the cow may be more nervous, because it is separated

from the herd. In this situation, successful placement of a halter may be aided by trapping the cow between two gates to limit its movement (Fig. 6.36).

A smaller halter of identical design is used for calves. Adult halters may work on calves, but often, the nose piece is too large. On dairy farms, calves are typically individually maintained in their own hutches (Fig. 6.37). A halter provides sufficient restraint for most procedures. However, much like working with a foal in a stall with her dam, extreme caution should be exercised while attempting to restrain a calf in the same pen as the calf's dam. It is safest to work with a calf in a separate pen or close to the stall's exit gate so that a quick exit is possible if needed.

When working with cows, the halter should be tied with a quick-release knot that maintains the desired lead length and allows the handler to release the cow with one pull of the rope. This is critically important, because some cows will react negatively to being handled or treated and will lie down while tied. Depending on the type of restraint used, this can be potentially harmful to the cow, and a quick-release knot allows the animal to be freed quickly as needed.

Beef cattle are typically handled less often compared with dairy cattle, so additional handling facilities are required for working with them. This may be composed of a holding pen, a crowding pen, an alley, and a chute. Cattle are moved into holding and crowding pens by using the principles of pressure and release. Movement into the holding pen can be safely and effectively conducted by using a simple flag attached to a stick. The same principles of pressure release and point of balance apply but, in this case, the stick serves as an extension of the handler, allowing the handler to safely work from the outside of the pen. The crowding pen is often round, allowing a large, swinging gate, like the minute hand on a clock, to follow the cows into the alley. Cows enter the alley in single file and follow the cow ahead. Alleys should have solid sides to avoid distractions, should be slightly wider than the cow, but not wide enough to allow it to turn around, and may be curved to take advantage of the cow's preference to return to where it came from. Handlers should never enter the alley unless necessary and never without identifying a method of escape. A frightened or injured cow is very dangerous and will seek an exit by moving forward or backward and through the handler if needed.

Extreme caution should be used when working with bulls. Beef and dairy bulls may be commingled with female cattle and can easily be overlooked. When handling cattle, it is important to always ask if a bull is present. Beef bulls tend to be less aggressive toward humans compared with their dairy counterparts, but both can be deadly to handlers. If a bull is present, the handler should watch for signs that the bull is showcasing its size and is becoming aggressive. Such signs include the bull showing its side, pawing the ground, or lowering its head. If a bull is exhibiting these signs, the handler should slowly back away out of the bull's flight zone; without running, they should exit the pen or pasture as soon as possible. Bulls may have nose rings as additional aids in handling and restraint, similar to a halter. The nose of a cow or a bull is very sensitive, and a ring placed in the nasal septum provides additional but not total control of the bull.

Restraint Techniques and Devices

When working animals through handling facilities, a chute with a head gate or head catch is the final destination (Fig. 6.38). This piece of equipment has two doors that close horizontally with a vertical opening in between. Initially, the doors are opened slightly to allow the animal to see a path for escape. When the animal's head enters the opening, the gate is quickly closed and tightened around the neck. This restrains the cow and limits forward movement to the length between head and shoulder. The head gate can also be self-locking, but this type is less common in a chute system because of the need to adjust the head gate for animals of different sizes to prevent frequent escapes. If a cow gets part of its shoulder through, it will escape; it should then be released to prevent injury to the handler. On some chutes, additional restraint is provided via a collapsing side that squeezes the cow and prevents additional movement. These chutes can be run manually or operated hydraulically. Each chute operates slightly differently, with multiple handles and moving parts; time should be taken to become familiar with the handling equipment to avoid injury. For dairy cattle, a simpler, automatic head-catch system may be used at the feed bunk and in a box stall. This head-restraint system is called a *head lock* (Fig. 6.39). This system automatically secures a cow's head between two vertical bars when the cow puts her head down to eat. A head-lock system provides an opportunity to restrain an entire pen of cows for routine management practices while ensuring that they stay with the herd and have access to feed. However, cows should not be locked up for longer than an hour, because this impinges on a cow's time budget and prevents lying down and rumination.

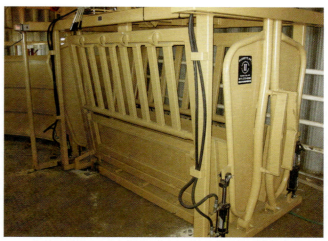

• **Fig. 6.38** When working animals through handling facilities, a chute with a head gate or head catch is the final destination.

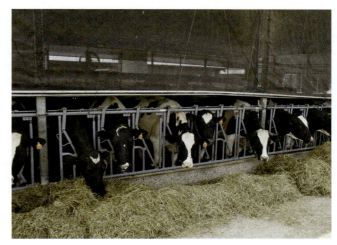

• **Fig. 6.39** A simple automatic head-catch system may be used at the feed bunk and in a box stall of dairy cattle. This head-restraint system is called a head lock.

A physical examination in cattle can often be completed with simple head restraint. In dairy cattle, head locks are commonly used for routine postpartum health monitoring. In beef cattle, many chutes provide drop-down sides or windows in the side of the chute for access to the bovine. An oral examination can often be accomplished without further restraint, and the use of a halter is contraindicated (unless placed upside down), because the halter tightens over the nose and under the jaw, effectively closing the mouth. A towel can be used to grasp and move the tongue to allow examination of the oral cavity and detection of tongue paresis, common in cases of botulism.

TECHNICIAN NOTE

Protective gloves and sleeves should always be worn for examination of the oral cavity of a cow that is exhibiting neurologic signs, because rabies is a differential diagnosis and, if contracted, may cause potentially fatal complications in the examiner.

Oral medication or fluids can often be administered to cows by using only a head lock or a head gate. Oral administration of a bolus, a magnet, or fluid is often easier without a halter. To administer a bolus using a pill gun or a balling gun, the procedure is as follows. Stand on the cow's left side, facing the same direction the cow is facing (i.e., with your back to the cow). Reach over the nose with your right hand and brace the cow's head against your hip. Maintaining the cow's head and neck as straight as possible will facilitate administration of oral medications. Next, place your first two fingers into the mouth at the oral commissure. Recall that cows do not have upper incisors, so the risk of being bitten is very low, especially if you keep your fingers in the space between the lower incisors and the molars, termed the *dental pad*. Once your fingers are in the cow's mouth, the cow will open it slightly. The cow will then open further as you move your fingers to the hard palate (Fig. 6.40). When the cow's mouth opens, insert the pill gun with your free hand.

A similar approach can be used when administering oral fluids. For pumps that have soft rubber hosing, a speculum is required to prevent a potential rumen foreign body if the cow chews through the hose and swallows the distal portion. A Frick speculum can be placed in a similar manner to the pill gun and held in place by hand. Often, a Frick speculum comes with a set of nose tongs attached that maintain placement of the speculum when an oro-gastric tube is placed and fluids are administered. Some pumps are made with protective metal encircling the esophageal tube, allowing the tube to be passed directly into the mouth without the need for a speculum. When passing an esophageal tube, care should be taken to keep the head level such that the nose stays below the poll to avoid accidental introduction of the tube into the trachea.

Additional Head Restraint

To access the jugular vein or for invasive procedures of the head, a halter should be used in combination with a head lock or a head gate to restrain the bovine patient. The cow should be pulled straight ahead to get the shoulder as close to the head lock as possible before turning the cow's head and tying the halter. This procedure minimizes the ability of the cow to move in a cranial–caudal direction and exposes the maximum length of the jugular vein for venipuncture or catheter placement. In fractious bovine patients, applying pressure to the nasal septum with one's fingers can provide better control over the head.

> **TECHNICIAN NOTE**
>
> Temporarily grasping the nasal septum between the thumb and the index finger provides additional control of fractious patients while a second handler provides treatment.

Pressure can be applied by inserting metal nose tongs that squeeze the nasal septum. The tongs are connected to a rope, which can be tied off and allows the examiner to maintain use of both hands for procedures. Although useful when necessary, nose tongs occasionally elicit an escalation of fractious behavior, and some behavior experts have indicated that nose tongs may cause increased adverse reactions with repeated use.

Tail Restraint

During obstetric procedures, the cow's tail can be restrained with a simple tail tie. Like the tail tie described in the previous equine restraint section, a rope is tied into the hair at the end of the tail (the cow's switch) by placing a rope horizontally across the switch and folding the hair upward. The rope is then tied into a quick-release knot incorporating all the switch tail, with the other end of

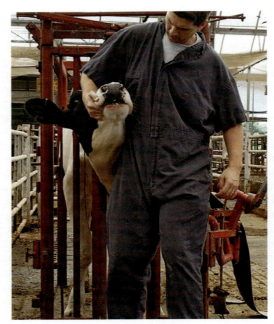

• **Fig. 6.40** Using a pill gun or administering oral fluids may require opening the cow's mouth manually.

the rope encircling the cow's neck. To prevent injury, the remainder of the rope should be tied to the cow, not to the surrounding structure.

Another tail restraint method is the TailJack. This simple method of restraint is thought to provide nerve stimulation like that of the twitch in horses. It is a useful method for restraint of nervous patients when a minor procedure, such as the administration of local analgesia, infusion of intramammary mastitis treatment, or rectal palpation, is being conducted. The TailJack is accomplished by grasping the tail 6 to 10 inches from the tail head. The tail is pushed straight up and over the dorsum of the cow until it forms a 60-degree angle with the spine of the cow (Fig. 6.41). This method of restraint is also useful for venipuncture, because it provides access to the coccygeal vein and artery of the cow. For small quantities of blood (<20 mL), coccygeal venipuncture using a Vacutainer (BD, Franklin Lakes, NJ) and collection tube is the easiest, safest, and most efficient method.

Foot Control and Restraint

Lameness is a common disease of dairy cows, often requiring corrective trimming as treatment. Cattle are much more reluctant than horses to raise their feet for examination and treatment. Professional hoof trimmers will often use a tilt table or standing chute to access one or more feet as needed. When these restraint systems are not available, a pulley system can be constructed by using a rope, alone or with block and tackle.

Lifting and restraining a cow's forefoot is typically the most difficult step, perhaps because cows bear most of their weight on their forelimbs. The best approach (which has been effective for this author) is to place a slip knot or use a rope with a quick-release honda to encircle the forelimb to be examined as close to the pastern as possible. Then the rope is placed over a bar or beam, and the examiner comes back to the foot and loops back around the foot and over the same bar or beam. Now a double-pulley system has been constructed and will allow the examiner to lift the foot with relative ease. Once the forelimb is lifted, it is secured to

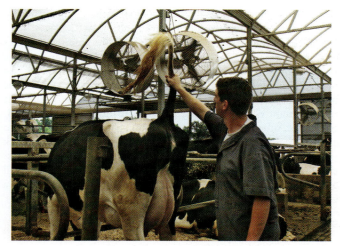

• **Fig. 6.41** The "TailJack" is accomplished by pushing the tail straight up and over the dorsum of the cow until it forms a 60-degree angle with the spine of the cow.

an adjacent bar or pole for further restraint if needed. One should always be cautious when lifting a cow's foot, because this requires a shift in balance that may cause the cow to fall over, occasionally onto the person lifting the foot. Fortunately, approximately 90% of lameness occurs in the hind feet, which are relatively easier to handle.

In practice, this author has successfully used a 2-inch-wide leather strap fitted with a belt buckle and a semicircular metal fitting. This strap is applied tightly, proximal to the hock, to apply pressure to the calcaneus tendon and thus limit movement. A block-and-tackle device is attached to the metal fitting and to a bar or beam above the cow, and the cow's foot is raised to the desired level. Alternatively, a rope can be tied with a slip knot or by placing a honda proximal to the hock. The rope is passed over a bar or beam, and the cow's hind limb is raised for examination. With both methods, the cow retains some ability to extend its limb, so the examiner must be cautious when trimming or applying treatment. Hoof knives and other lameness equipment can be dangerous to examiners when it is not under their control.

For lameness procedures causing moderate pain and distress to cattle or for cattle unwilling to submit to the restraint required to deliver an appropriate treatment, regional analgesia is often very effective. In this case, a rubber IV hose is applied as a tourniquet just distal to the hock. The lateral branch of the saphenous vein is located, and 20 to 30 mL of 2% lidocaine is infused by using a butterfly catheter. Analgesia develops in 10 to 15 minutes and persists for as long as the tourniquet remains in place. This technique provides a safer environment for the cow and for the veterinarian or veterinary technician treating the lameness.

Casting Cows

Occasionally, it becomes necessary to place a cow in lateral or dorsal recumbency for a treatment procedure. This straightforward procedure can usually be accomplished by one or two individuals without the need for exerting great force. First, the cow must be haltered and tied to a post or other bar that will withstand some force. The length of the rope should be such that the cow is able to lie down comfortably with its head and neck extended in a normal position. Then one of two rope patterns is applied to the cow. The author's preference is the half-hitch pattern, which starts with a slip knot or honda around the neck, followed by two half-hitch

knots, one at the withers and one just proximal to the hips. The tail of the rope comes off the cow's spine, with all three knots positioned dorsally. A strong pull of the free end should result in the cow's lying down.

The rope should be placed such that it can be easily removed from the recumbent cow without entangling the rope under the patient's abdomen. Entangled rope can potentially cause damage to recent surgical sites and is often very difficult to retrieve from under the weight of the cow. The udder or the prepuce should not be included in the knot, because pressure can cause inflammation and injury.

> **TECHNICIAN NOTE**
>
> When the half-hitch method is used to cast a cow, a large loop can be made on one side to facilitate removal of the rope after the procedure is completed.

The other method is the Burley or "running W" method. Again, after the patient is securely tied with a halter of sufficient length, the rope is placed over its back with the center at the point of the shoulder. The ends are carried between the forelimbs and are crossed at the sternum. One end is carried up each side of the animal's body, and two are crossed again over the back. Each end passes downward between the hind limbs, going between the inner or medial surface of the limbs and the udder or the scrotum. Pulling on both ends of the rope applies pressure on the cow, causing it to lie down, with the cow favoring the side on which the greatest pressure is applied. Application of hobbles to the fore- and hind limbs at the level of the pastern before pulling on the rope limits the bovine patient's ability to balance, resulting in quicker and easier progression to recumbency with both casting methods.

After the cow has been cast, kneeling on the head at the angle of the mandible or just caudal to the head on the neck of the cow prevents the cow from rising while additional positioning is completed. This procedure can also be used to maintain lateral recumbency after the casting rope has been removed. Hobbles can be used to place the cow in dorsal recumbency. A small, square bale of hay or straw can further aid in positioning and support of the cow. When cows are cast, they should be carefully observed for signs of bloat or regurgitation. The use of xylazine, an α^2-agonist often used for sedation of cattle, may exacerbate these issues.

Cows that are already in recumbency and are unable to rise because of hypocalcemia, endotoxemia, or other disease can be tied to maintain recumbency during treatment. The bovine patient should be placed in sternal recumbency and can be braced with a straw bale if necessary. After a halter is placed on the cow's head, the head is turned to the side where its feet are visible. The free end of end of the halter is then tied to the most lateral (outside) limb above the hock, bringing the cow's nose as close as possible to the hock. A quick-release knot is used to secure the halter. This enables exposure of the jugular vein for IV fluid administration while effectively restraining the cow.

Capture and Restraint of Swine

Observation

Observation of pigs before handling and restraint is a critical part of the physical examination. This is especially true when the examiner is evaluating the entire herd, not just an individual pig. When and where pigs are lying, their interactions with each other, and their gait and dunging patterns are important parts of a thorough barn evaluation.

Approach

When the examiner enters the pen, adult pigs are often curious and may seek out the examiner by using their excellent sense of smell to investigate. Adult pigs may also attempt to chew on the examiner's boots, coveralls, or limbs if given the opportunity. This is normal behavior and does not indicate that pigs are not being fed appropriately. When an examiner enters a farrowing room or nursery, nursing and weaned piglets may demonstrate avoidance behaviors. Often, they will be startled when the examiner is first observed and may run into a corner to escape (Fig. 6.42). As with other livestock species, lactating females with offspring, injured animals, and adult males should be considered dangerous and handled with extreme caution. Lactating sows may be confined to a lactating crate to prevent them from crushing their offspring (Fig. 6.43). Caution should be exercised, because sows can reach through bars to bite handlers. Intact male pigs, called *boars*, are kept on farms to elicit estrous behavior from gilts and sows during artificial insemination. When boars are exposed to a female in standing heat, they often become aggressive and present a danger to the handler. A solid board should always be used when handling boars and should be kept between the handler and the boar to prevent injury from the boar's tusks.

Pigs have the least herding instinct of all food animal species but do become nervous when separated from herd mates. Swine have a flight zone like that of ruminants, with a blind spot directly behind them. Compared with other livestock species, pigs can be more stubborn and difficult to move, perhaps because of their poor eyesight or their reliance on scent to investigate new environments. When pigs are moved within a barn or are loaded onto a ramp, the same principles of minimizing stress among livestock should be followed. The path should be cleared of obstacles or distractions to facilitate the movement of pigs. Moving pigs in small groups of five or six allows them to remain together and move as a group without becoming uncontrollable.

> **TECHNICIAN NOTE**
>
> If you attempt to move a large group of pigs, the leaders often will turn back before entering the intended pen, making the remainder of the group difficult to move successfully.

A pig board can be placed transversely in the direction of movement and used to apply gentle forward pressure to the back of the group of pigs as they explore their new surroundings. This prevents the group from turning around (Fig. 6.44). Exertion of extra pressure, loud noises, and rough or aggressive treatment can cause pigs to panic and make any directed movement difficult. Handling equipment for pigs should adhere to the same principles that are followed for other livestock: solid walls of a bright and similar color and a well-lit area facilitate positive pig movement. If a pig does turn to face the handler and the board, it must be ensured that the board is flush with the floor. Pigs have a natural rooting instinct and will pick the board up with their nose if given the opportunity. The board should be angled such that the end closest to the pig is slightly ahead of the other end. This provides leverage for the handler and prevents the pig from pushing through the board and past the handler.

When in open pens, adult pigs can often be approached while resting and given injections with little need for capture or restraint (Fig. 6.45). If this approach is not successful, they can be captured individually or worked in small groups. The handler should wear ear protection to protect hearing when working with pigs, because they signal agitation and distress through loud squeals of up to 130 decibels (85 decibels may cause hearing loss).

Capture and Restraint Techniques

In many commercial operations adult pigs are often housed in stalls or crates, reducing or eliminating the need for capture. In open-pen systems or when new gilts are introduced into a barn, pigs can be crowded into a small pen to facilitate vaccination, ear tag placement/removal, or other necessary procedures. Handlers should bring as many pigs into the pen as can be accommodated to limit movement and minimize the length of time for capture and restraint; pigs can become hyperthermic if stressed or crowded for an extended period, and the stress can be exacerbated by a genetic predisposition (porcine stress syndrome). This author has had little problem with groups of 10 to 12 commercial gilts restrained in a 10-by-10-foot pen.

To capture individual pigs, a pig board can be also used as a third wall to trap the pig in a corner. The handler should move the pig into a corner by using the solid board and the pig's point

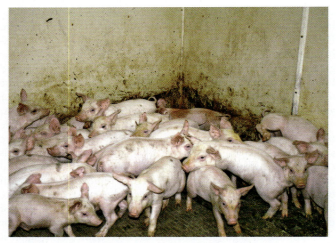

• **Fig. 6.42** Weaned piglets may avoid handlers by running into a corner in an effort to escape.

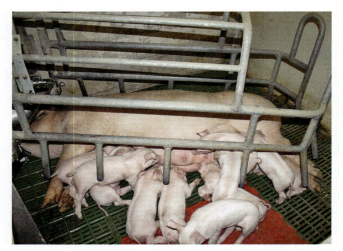

• **Fig. 6.43** Lactating sows may be confined to a lactating crate to prevent them from crushing their offspring.

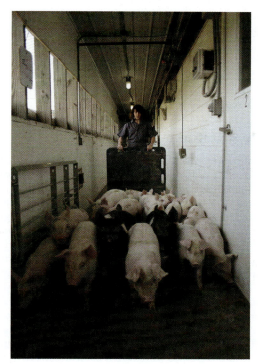

• **Fig. 6.44** A pig board can be placed transversely to the direction of movement and used to move a group of piglets forward, preventing them from turning around.

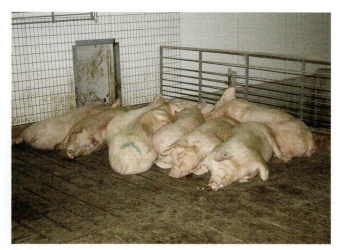

• **Fig. 6.45** When in open pens, adult pigs often can be approached while they are resting and given injections with little need for capture or restraint.

of balance. When the pig is facing the corner, the board is placed parallel with the pig, and pressure is applied to the board, squeezing the pig between the wall and the board. As soon as treatment is completed, the pig should be released.

If greater control of the pig is needed or if a more invasive procedure is required, a snare can be used. The loop of the snare is adjusted for the size of the pig and is offered to the pig. Pigs are curious and like to chew; many will readily accept the wire loop into their mouths and over the snout and the maxilla. The snare handle is held vertically while the loop is positioned caudally on the pig's snout as much as possible and then is tightened carefully. The handler then secures the pig by keeping pressure on the handle

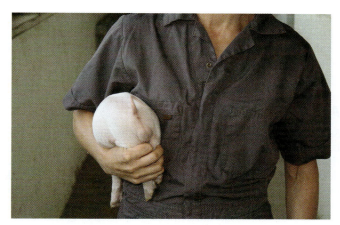

• **Fig. 6.46** Male piglets can be positioned in a football-type hold for castration.

while the procedure is completed by a second person. Two people are required to treat a pig by using this technique. The snare should *never* be tied or used to move the pig, because this can cause injury to the palate and the oral cavity of the pig. Once the procedure is completed, the snare is released, and the pig is returned to its pen.

For smaller pigs, lifting and manual restraint are preferred. Piglets are often weighed and given injections, and boars are castrated in the first few days of life. As with other species, care should be taken when capturing piglets in a pen with a nursing dam. Piglets younger than 1 week old often weigh 3 to 5 pounds and can be grasped dorsally by the thorax, then restrained. For larger piglets, grasping a hind limb provides an initial hold, then the other hand should slip under the chest to provide support while lifting the piglet in a horizontal position. The piglet can be held in a football-type hold, with the piglet resting on the forearm with the rump toward the elbow and the head in the hand. The opposite hand is free to conduct an examination or administer treatment. Restraint for castration of male piglets can be done in a similar manner, with the piglet's head toward the handler's elbow (Fig. 6.46). The head is restrained between the handler's elbow and chest while the hand of the same arm grasps the hind feet.

Pet Pigs

Pet pigs, pot-bellied or other types, are raised more as companion animals and should be handled and restrained accordingly when possible. These pigs are often trained to walk on a leash with a harness like that of a dog, with the restraint of these pet pigs similar to that of a dog. These pigs can also be suspended in a mesh or canvas that allows all four limbs to protrude through the ventral aspect of the sling. More invasive procedures are best accomplished with the animal under sedation or general anesthesia for the benefit of the animal and the owner.

TECHNICIAN NOTE

Pet pigs are pets first and pigs second. Treat them (and their owners) as if they were companion animals.

Capture and Restraint of Small Ruminants

Observation

Shifting population demographics and a growing interest in alternative livestock enterprises have resulted in increasing numbers of small-ruminant producers in the United States. When confronted by humans, sheep, goats, and camelids (primarily llamas and alpacas) exhibit predator-prey interactions like cattle. Observation of these animals from beyond their flight zone is therefore an important step in identifying animals in need of medical intervention.

Approach

Small ruminants flock together when confronted by a threat. This behavior can be used to the handler's advantage by first bunching the herd tightly and then moving them as a group. Sheep flocks demonstrate this behavioral trait most consistently. Some flock owners will employ dogs to bring flocks into holding facilities, although the owner should have complete control over the dog. Dogs are less commonly used in handling herds of goats, because some goats will challenge the dogs or become agitated and act unpredictably.

> **TECHNICIAN NOTE**
>
> Guardian dogs are sometimes used to protect small-ruminant flocks against predators; these dogs should not be confused with herding dogs.

Small ruminants have flight zones inversely proportional to their domestication level. The flight zone and the point of balance are used to move small ruminants into smaller pens for treatment. Handling facilities are like those used for cattle: solid walls with alleyways that are wide enough for one animal to pass through but not to turn around. If an individual animal requires attention, it can be examined as part of a smaller group or separated from the flock or herd within the handling facilities.

Small ruminants are the safest of the livestock species to work with. Sheep and goats rarely kick or bite, and only aggressive males will challenge handlers. Working around camelids, however, requires greater caution, because they are known to spit fermented stomach contents to up to 6 feet when agitated. A gurgling sound emits from a llama or an alpaca before expulsion of stomach contents. Camelids may also kick and bite when very agitated. Like horses, the ear and tail positions of the camelid can indicate the animal's attitude. Ears that are flattened caudally against the head and a vertical tail indicate a high level of aggression in the camelid patient. Conversely, a lowered head and a tail that is curled forward demonstrate submissive behavior, as most seen in imprinted camelids. Imprinted llamas and alpacas, especially males, can also be dangerous, because they view humans as competitors instead of predators and will attack to defend their territory.

Capture

When possible, small ruminants should be worked in small groups (three to four animals) to mitigate the panic associated with being separated from their peers. Sheep and goats can be confined in alleyways and small pens that allow handlers to conduct a variety of management procedures. Caution should be taken when crowding the animals or when working heavily fleeced sheep during hot weather, because they can develop life-threatening hyperthermia.

> **TECHNICIAN NOTE**
>
> The normal temperature of sheep (101°F–103°F) makes development of hyperthermia a greater risk. Be careful when working heavily fleeced sheep in hot weather.

Goats can also be crowded into small pens but often exhibit such reactions as jumping over gates, pushing through weak spots in a fence, or lying down. Camelids can be crowded together into a corner or pen by having two handlers stretch a rope approximately 35 feet in length 3 to 4 feet off the ground. If the camelid challenges the rope, it may be worked through individual squeeze chutes like those used for cattle.

Individual Restraint

After the animal has been moved into a smaller pen, the first step of restraint for all small-ruminant species is to control the head. This can be accomplished by grasping the neck just under the jaw. This is also the first step in flipping a sheep into a sitting position. After the neck and head are controlled with the left hand, the right hand is moved to the sheep's right hind limb. By flexing the neck and turning the nose back and toward the handler and by lifting the right hind limb, the handler can push the sheep into a sitting position. A second method of setting sheep up is to use the right hand to apply firm pressure over the pelvis; the left hand can turn the sheep's nose back and away from the handler. The sheep's weight is shifted onto the handler's legs and, with continued flexion of the head, the sheep is made to sit down, with its back leaning against the handler's legs. With both methods, once the sheep is sitting up, the left forelimb is grasped with the left hand and the right forelimb with the right hand, and the weight of the sheep rests against the handler's legs (Fig. 6.47). In this position, the sheep can be sheared, administered medication, held for hoof trimming or, in the case of lambs, castrated and have the tail docked.

Goats can be initially restrained by positioning a hand under the jaw. However, they are more athletic than sheep and resist being tipped onto their rump as sheep can be. Instead, a goat can be held by placing the neck in the crook of the elbow and the head against the restrainer's chest while using the other hand to grab the tail. Caution should be exercised because in this position, horned goats may be able to injure the handler by head butting. A safer alternative for restraining a goat is backing it into a corner with a hand on its jaw and then straddling the goat with its rump against the wall and squeezing with the handler's knees. Handlers can use the horns of *mature* goats as an additional method of restraint in this position (Fig. 6.48). Immature goats should *not* be restrained by their horns, because they can fracture and break off. Dairy goats and those that are accustomed to routine handling may be restrained by using a halter, their neck collar (if present), or a milking or trimming stand.

> **TECHNICIAN NOTE**
>
> Never grab the wool or hair of a small ruminant for restraint. In addition to being painful, this can cause damage to the fiber and the underlying meat, decreasing the value of both. In addition, never restrain an immature goat by its horns, because they can fracture and break off, causing pain and hemorrhage.

Camelids can also be restrained by initially placing a hand under the jaw and then squeezing the neck in a flexed elbow against the handler's chest. The other hand can be used to grasp the tail or press down at the shoulders.

Restraint Techniques for Camelids

Some restraint techniques that can be used in sheep or goats should not be used in camelids. If additional restraint is needed,

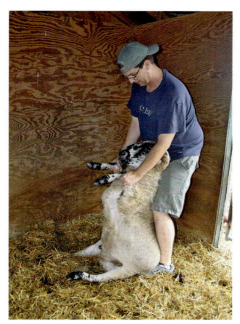

• **Fig. 6.47** Once the sheep is sitting up, grasp the left forelimb with the left hand and the right forelimb with the right hand, and rest the weight of the sheep against your legs.

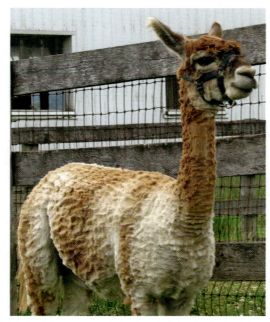

• **Fig. 6.49** A miniature pony halter is often used effectively in camelids. However, to ensure that the nose strap does not pinch the soft tissue of the nasal passages, the nose strap should be positioned just rostral to the eyes.

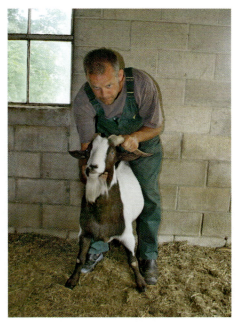

• **Fig. 6.48** Handlers can use the horns of mature goats as an additional method of restraint in this position. Immature goats should not be restrained by their horns, because they can fracture and break off.

pressure can be applied at the base of the ear. The right hand is moved up the neck to the base of the ear, and pressure is applied. Twisting or other manipulation is not necessary and does not increase the restraint available to the handler. When pressure is initially applied, the llama or the alpaca will retreat from the hold, so a firm grip should be employed and caution exercised to avoid sudden jerks of the animal's head, which may collide with the handler's face. As in horses, halters and lead ropes can also be applied to camelids as methods of control and restraint. A miniature pony halter is often used effectively in camelids. To ensure that the nose strap does not pinch the soft tissue of the nasal passages (Fig. 6.49), the nose strap should be positioned just rostral to the eyes. Camelids that are accustomed to halters can also be cross-tied like a horse for examination and for minor procedures. When working with and restraining camelids, they may "kush," or lie down. Maintaining pressure over the back and shoulders with the hands can keep them in this position, enabling completion of treatment, examinations, and minor procedures.

Capture and Restraint of Avian and Exotic Species

As the popularity of avian and exotic species increases, so will the presence of these species in veterinary hospitals. Veterinary medical care is as important for birds and exotic animals as it is for domestic species. Veterinary technicians who work with exotic species must therefore have a solid understanding of the natural history, husbandry needs, and safe restraint techniques needed to provide competent medical care to these species. Typically, exotic pet practices see a variety of avian and exotic animals that can be categorized as predators or prey species. As with all animals, the hospital visit should be as stress-free as possible, because it is well known that convalescence is hindered by stress. One important rule of thumb for reducing stress in hospitalized animals is to house predator and prey species separately.

PUT INTO PRACTICE

If you are working in a general practice, you may not see many exotics or birds, but this is a niche where you can build expertise. When those patients do come into your practice, you will be able to assist your veterinarian and provide proper restraint and care for those patients.

Restraint of Avian Species

Psittacines

The initial reaction of most avian species to an unfamiliar environment is fear; this may lead to the flight-or-fight response. As you can imagine, prey species, such as psittacines (parrot species), become guarded when sensing a predator species, such as a cat, dog, or ferret, nearby. Fleeing birds tend to head for windows and can crash into glass panes or walls when they panic.

> **TECHNICIAN NOTE**
> Make sure all windows in examination and treatment rooms are closed and shaded with curtains or blinds. Fleeing birds will go straight for a clear glass pane during an escape and can critically injure themselves.

In addition, a psittacine can smell the scent of a predator on the hands of veterinary personnel during an examination and while being restrained. This can cause the animal to startle and try to flee without warning. Care must be taken to wash hands between patients. Practicing good hygiene not only reduces the risk of spreading communicable diseases, but it also decreases previous patients' scent and the possibility of the handler being bitten or the patient being injured when attempting to flee what it perceives to be a dangerous environment.

Observation and Approach

Psittacines should be observed and evaluated from a distance before being handled. Subtle behaviors may provide information about the pet's stress level, attitude, and overall health. Psittacines that are stressed may emit an alarm call during most of the visit, whereas a comfortable parrot might readily step out of its carrier and onto the owner's hand. Transferring a calm bird to a veterinary technician to restrain during the visit goes more smoothly.

> **TECHNICIAN NOTE**
> To ensure the safety of all animals visiting a veterinary practice, exotic animals should be transported in enclosed carriers or cages.

Even when a bird is comfortable on the hand of its owner, the pet may not be willing to go to a new person. Parrots that lean backward when approached by a veterinary handler are expressing their resistance to being handled by a stranger. In addition, parrots will contract and dilate their pupils in rapid succession when they are focusing to strike at an object. This behavior is called *pinning* and is another warning sign to handlers. Ideally, stressed parrots are given time to acclimate to the new environment of the examination room before any attempt is made to handle it. Offering parrots a favorite snack can also help diminish anxiety in the patient before the animal is restrained. As with any veterinary visit, all supplies needed to carry out the examination and veterinary care should be gathered and made available *before* the patient is restrained.

Restraint Techniques

A calm bird can be examined by using hand restraint, but a stressed bird that makes repeated alarm calls and displays defensive body posture will have to be captured and restrained by using a towel. With crushing beaks, sharp, penetrating nails, and strong wings, psittacines, particularly large parrots, can injure veterinary personnel if not restrained properly and safely. Handling parrot species with leather gloves is fruitless, because their beaks can cause crushing, not tearing, trauma, as with raptors. In addition, when working with multiple larger parrot species within a short period, ear protection should be worn by veterinary personnel. The alarm cry of the hyacinth macaw, for example, rivals in decibels the screams of swine.

> **TECHNICIAN NOTE**
> A macaw can crack a Brazil nut with minimal effort, which indicates that leather gloves are a useless defense against its powerful beak.

Most parrot species, regardless of size, can be trained to accept hand restraint for grooming and medical examinations. To restrain small birds with one hand, the handler should gently control the head at the base of the mandible with the thumb and index finger while allowing the bird to grip on the lower digits (ring or pinky finger). The pet's dorsum lies against the palm of the handler's hand so the wings can be controlled, but the keel is not restricted. Typically, this is adequate for examinations, but not for procedures, because the other hand will be needed to restrain the feet (Fig. 6.50).

To restrain small- to medium-sized parrots with two hands, the head and wings are restrained as described earlier, but the opposite hand is used to restrain the limbs. The limbs are restrained at the level of the tibiotarsus, with the thumb and the index finger holding one limb and the index finger and the middle finger holding the other (Fig. 6.51). This technique has a few benefits. First, movement of the keel is not restricted, so the risk of compromising the bird's ability to breathe is reduced; second, the position of the bird affords both the handler and the veterinarian excellent visualization of the pet's respiratory effort and rate. Last, with this technique, the patient is less likely to overheat, as sometimes happens with prolonged use of towels. The owner is the best person to train the pet to voluntarily accept gentle restraint for claw and wing feather trims, and physical examinations (Fig. 6.52). During training, owners should be sure to desensitize the pet to every aspect of the physical examination process. If any question about the temperament of a bird arises, the handler should always err on the side of caution during office visits and use the restraint technique that is safest for both patient and veterinary personnel.

Many avian patients may be too big or too resistant to be restrained with hands alone. For these patients, using a towel is necessary. When the wings and the torso are wrapped in a towel, the handler can concentrate on restraining the head and the feet. For small- to medium-sized patients, the capture technique is typically performed while the bird is perched on the handler's hand. While the owner grips the toes of the bird, a towel is slowly raised in front of the bird and draped over it. The back of the head is then restrained, and the remainder of the bird is wrapped in the towel, being careful not to cover the face. This enables the bird to breathe without obstruction.

For particularly resistant birds, capture should be done with a towel while the patient is still in the carrier. The towel is used to gently cover the patient from the back and simultaneously restrain the bird's head and beak. Once the head and the beak are adequately restrained, the towel can be wrapped around the patient, with the opening along the keel. This opening enables direct observation of the keel and associated respirations. It also provides easy access to the wings and the feet, but at the same time, restricts wing motion until the wings are needed and are gently pulled

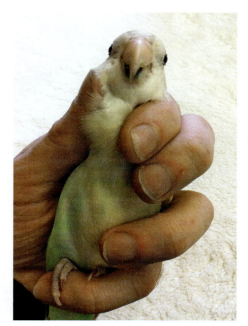

• **Fig. 6.50** Many birds, such as this lovebird, can be trained to accept hand restraint for grooming and medical examinations.

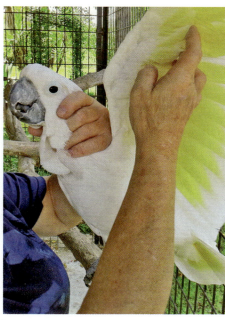

• **Fig. 6.52** Owners of this cockatoo trained their pet to voluntarily accept gentle restraint for claw and wing feather trims and physical examinations.

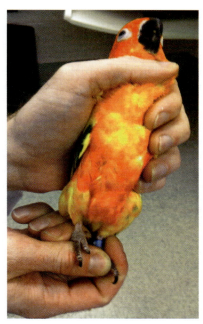

• **Fig. 6.51** When using two hands to restrain small- to medium-sized birds, such as this sun conure, the head and wings are restrained with one hand, while the limbs are restrained with the other hand.

> **TECHNICIAN NOTE**
>
> When wrapping a bird in a towel, care must be taken not to restrict normal movement of the thoracic wall and cause inadvertent suffocation.

If the animal appears to be overheating, the physical examination should stop and the patient should be allowed to recover. With repeated towel-restraint sessions for grooming or clinical procedures, the bird will grow to become fearful of towels and will react violently at even the sight of them. Desensitization techniques can be employed by owners to prevent the bird from developing a fear of towels.

Chemical Restraint

For those avian patients that are too anxious or need prolonged restraint for clinical procedures, a dose of an anxiolytic medication, such as midazolam, given intramuscularly or intranasally can aid in decreasing anxiety. If the animal is so stressed that it is refractory to the administration of medication, a brief "chill period" may be necessary. This should be followed by use of the inhalant isoflurane delivered via face mask to the point of twilight anesthesia or immobilization. Once immobilized, a physical examination and any nonpainful clinical procedures, such as grooming, blood sampling, and positioning for radiographs, can be performed with relative ease. If the animal is in need of a procedure that includes noxious stimuli, injectable analgesics and greater depths of inhalant anesthesia are needed for pain management.

Passerines

Small **passerines**, such as finches and canaries, are restrained very gently, as described in the section on small psittacines, using the single-handed method. Dimming the overhead lighting can facilitate the capture of the animal with minimal chasing.

from underneath the towel. Once the towel is in place and the head and beak are restrained, the feet are secured with the remaining hand (Fig. 6.53). With towel restraint, one must pay special attention to respiratory rate and effort and to body temperature, ensuring that the animal does not inadvertently suffocate or overheat. Because birds do not have diaphragms, respiration is dependent on expansion of the thoracic wall. Holding a bird too tightly across the chest can therefore hinder respiration.

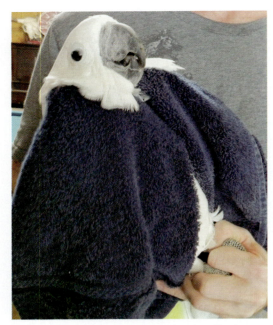

• **Fig. 6.53** Once the towel is in place and the head and beak are restrained, the feet are secured with the remaining hand. Make sure the keel is unrestricted, but the wings are well restrained.

Birds of Prey

Because most birds of prey (**raptorial species**), such as falcons, vultures, hawks, owls, and eagles, have dangerously sharp beaks and talons, leather gloves must be worn by handlers when restraining these species. Once the animal has been captured, a gloved hand restraint technique is used, as described for parrots. The aid of a towel may be helpful, depending on the demeanor and size of the animal and the procedure to be performed. Raptors used as falconry animals and those that reside in wildlife sanctuaries or zoos are often handled by people and are calmed by the application of a leather hood over the head and eyes. In addition, leather jesses are applied around the lower limbs, enabling control via a string while the animal is perched on the handler's gloved hand.

Restraint of Small Mammals

Rabbits

The rabbit can be a highly stressed patient, especially when placed in an environment where predators may be detected. Questioning the client about the home environment and the presence or absence of other pets in the home can be helpful in predicting the level of stress experienced by a particular patient when it is removed from its carrier, as individuals not normally exposed to natural predators in the home environment will be much more stressed in the hospital environment, where these predators are likely to be present.

The posture and respiratory rate of rabbits may offer clues about stress levels and the type of restraint that would be appropriate for the patient. For example, if the animal is at the front of the carrier, sniffing and trying to explore the world outside the carrier, it is likely that the rabbit is comfortable in the presence of humans and will require minimal restraint. A fearful rabbit, on the other hand, often hides in the back of the carrier, grunts, and has rapid breathing, with flared nares. Some rabbits slap a hind limb on the carrier floor, known as *thumping*, as an offensive warning. When threatened, they can charge

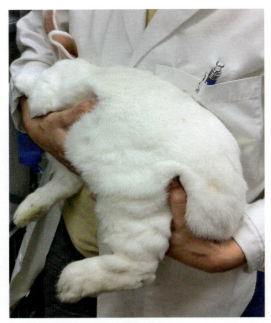

• **Fig. 6.54** A secure way to carry a rabbit is holding it like a football, giving the handler complete control of the head and hind limbs. Never carry a rabbit by the scruff alone.

veterinary personnel, with their forelimbs outstretched in a lurching motion.

Restraint

Removal of the animal from the carrier or hospital cage is accomplished by using a football hold. The handler places one arm under the ventral portion of the rabbit, supporting both the chest and the hindquarters from underneath. While the supporting hand controls the hind limbs, the rabbit's face is buried into the crook of the handler's forearm, and the opposite hand is placed on the dorsum of the animal. In essence, the rabbit is carried like a football, giving the handler complete control of the head and hind limbs (Fig. 6.54). A rabbit should never be carried by the scruff alone.

> **TECHNICIAN NOTE**
>
> An improperly restrained rabbit can kick forcefully with its hind limbs and subluxate or fracture its thoracolumbar vertebrae, resulting in paralysis. Therefore it is important that the hind limbs are always under the handler's control.

Using a towel is the safest way to restrain an uncooperative rabbit for examinations, nail trims, and nonpainful clinical procedures. The rabbit is placed on a towel, and both sides of the towel are lifted and wrapped around the patient, leaving the head exposed for examination and subsequent procedures (Fig. 6.55).

> **TECHNICIAN NOTE**
>
> Rabbits are obligate nasal breathers; that is, they do not breathe through the oral cavity but only through the nose. Therefore care must be taken to ensure that the nares are not obstructed during restraint.

For those patients that are calm and acclimated to human handling, a towel may not be needed during most of the examination. To examine the perianal area, the rabbit can be rotated into a dorsal position (either toweled or untoweled), with the hind

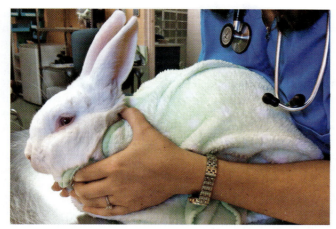

• **Fig. 6.55** Using a towel is the safest way to restrain an uncooperative rabbit for examinations and nonpainful clinical procedures.

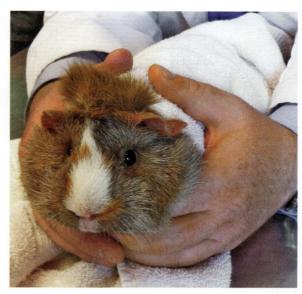

• **Fig. 6.56** Towel restraint, as previously described for rabbits, is ideal for restraining the uncooperative guinea pig.

limbs restrained by the handler. However, most rabbits object to manual manipulation of the oral cavity, making toweling a common requirement for the dental portion of the examination.

Chemical Restraint

Anxiolytic medications, such as midazolam, can be beneficial for most rabbits during short, nonpainful clinical procedures, such as blood sampling or positioning for radiographs. If further sedation is needed, a drug combination that consists of midazolam and other analgesics, tranquilizers, or dissociative drugs can be given. Care must be taken when giving rabbits drug combinations that could potentially cause respiratory depression, because they can be *extremely difficult* to intubate without a great deal of practice. However, experienced veterinarians and veterinary technicians who have become skilled in the procedure can intubate rabbits without the use of a laryngoscope.

Guinea Pigs and Chinchillas

As prey species, guinea pigs and chinchillas may be on high alert if not well socialized to the presence of and handling by humans. Guinea pigs tend to emit high-pitched alarm calls and can defend themselves by biting. Chinchillas often struggle and thrash during restraint to flee.

Well-socialized guinea pigs typically need little restraint for grooming and examinations, whereas even the best-behaved chinchillas are still a bit too restless for minimal restraint to be effective. Towel restraint as previously described for rabbits is ideal for both the uncooperative guinea pig and the squirmy chinchilla (Fig. 6.56).

> **TECHNICIAN NOTE**
>
> Handling guinea pigs with intensely pruritic (itchy) dermatologic disorders, such as sarcoptic mange, can elicit a grand mal seizure of short duration. Always forewarn the owner of this potential complication before handling an extremely itchy guinea pig.

Ferrets

Ferrets are generally mild-tempered predators that eat and play for most of their waking hours. Be cautious in approaching ferrets, particularly females, because they can nip and tend to be more independent and aggressive than males. Ferrets explore the world using their exquisite sense of smell, making distraction with the use of treats (Hills A/D Recovery Diet for Cats [Hill's Pet Nutrition Co., Topeka, KS]) an effective form of light restraint during physical examinations, minor clinical procedures, and grooming. Ferrets may react strongly to noxious smells, such as isopropyl alcohol, when used during venipuncture and ultrasonography. Using a skin sanitation substance such as chlorhexidine surgical scrub instead of alcohol is helpful in reducing stress when ferret skin is prepared for IV catheter placement or phlebotomy. Warmed, unscented ultrasound gel used judiciously for ultrasound procedures is acceptable; however, some ferrets will groom the affected area for hours if it is not completely washed off at the end of the procedure.

Restraint

A gentle scruffing technique is effective in restraining ferrets. The handler scruffs the dorsum of the neck and holds the animal in the vertical position with one hand while the other hand is used to stabilize the hind limbs (Fig. 6.57A). Ferrets held in this position often make a yawn reflex, which facilitates an examination of the oral cavity. If the patient is uncooperative despite treat distractions, the ferret can be scruffed and positioned in lateral recumbency in the same way that aggressive cats are restrained. Care must be taken when scruffing very active ferrets with generalized alopecia, because skin bruising will be quite noticeable after the restraint.

Chemical Restraint

Chemical restraint can be an effective form of restraint and is used as a last resort (see Fig. 6.57B). In this author's experience, a low dose of butorphanol adequately tranquilizes most ferrets for noninvasive diagnostic procedures, such as blood collection and positioning for radiography and ultrasonography.

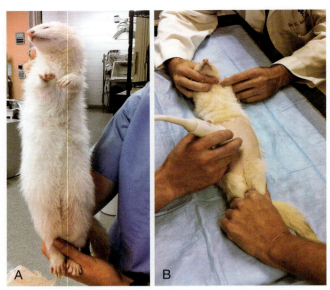

• **Fig. 6.57** (A) Scruffing a ferret induces a physically relaxed state. (B) With low-dose butorphanol, this ferret is easily positioned during an ultrasound examination.

Hamsters, Mice, Hedgehogs, Sugar Gliders, and Gerbils

Caution should be taken when capturing and handling hamsters. Most hamsters are aggressive and will bite when threatened. Scruffing has been used in the past for restraint, but it is not optimal, because there is risk that the eyes will proptose bilaterally if the scruffing is too taut around the eyes and face. However, if the animal is scruffed along the neck to avoid the face, the animal can readily turn and bite the handler. A small hand towel is often successful in the safe restraint of hamsters. Inhalant isoflurane for immobilization is sometimes warranted after a small fasting period until the animal has emptied out its cheek pouches of foodstuffs. If seeds or food are present in the cheek pouches during gas sedation, the patient is at high risk of aspiration, causing tracheal obstruction and suffocation.

Mice are more easily handled than hamsters, but their small size makes them difficult to control during clinical procedures. Mice can be gently restrained by scruffing the available skin along the neck and dorsum with the thumb and index finger while restraining the tail with the pinky finger. Chemical or gas immobilization may be needed for certain clinical procedures, such as blood collection and radiography.

Hedgehog quills are a defensive feature worth respecting. The quills are modified hairs and are very stiff and sharp—like those found on porcupines. When threatened, hedgehogs quickly curl up, protecting their vulnerable abdomen and head. Contrary to common belief, hedgehogs cannot actively shoot their quills; rather, when threatened, the quills become easily epilated, allowing them to stay in the predator's mouth, tongue, and face, for example, when attacked. In addition, hedgehogs generate frothy sputum, which they apply to the tips of their dorsal quills. No one knows the precise reason for this behavior, but it is thought to help conceal the scent of the hedgehog as the sticky froth readily absorbs odors from the surrounding environment. When handling hedgehogs, the technician should be sure to use leather gloves to prevent accidental injury from the quills. Use of inhalant anesthesia may be needed to facilitate a thorough physical examination

and any clinical procedures. Because hedgehogs can vomit, a short fasting period and cotton-tipped applicators kept on hand to clean out the oral cavity when needed are advisable. Sugar gliders are challenging to handle during a physical examination. They are agile animals and excellent at jumping out of the hand and gliding a good distance through the air. Sugar gliders have sharp nails used for climbing and have sharp incisors designed to extract gum from trees in their native habitat, making their bites and scratches very painful for the handler. Control of the head is carried out with the thumb and the index finger, with care taken not to damage their very large eyes, which are designed for seeing at night. Most clinicians elect to use isoflurane immobilization to facilitate completion of the physical examination and clinical procedures. A short fasting period is needed, because gas anesthesia commonly induces vomiting in this species. Cotton-tipped applicators should be immediately available to clean out the oral cavity if vomiting occurs.

Gerbils may be restrained manually or with the use of gas anesthesia as described in the previous section on hamsters. When using manual restraint, the technician should never grab gerbils by their tails, because the connective tissue under the skin loosens during stressful events, causing the skin and the fur of the tail to deglove, called *fur slip*. Needless to say, witnessing fur slip is upsetting to gerbil owners, because only the raw, exposed flesh of their pet's tail is left behind.

Restraint of Reptiles

Lizards

Knowing the species of lizard and its temperament enables the handler to quickly select a safe form of restraint for each patient. The green iguana is probably the most challenging species of lizard to restrain, because it is territorial and naturally aggressive, particularly during breeding season. These large lizards can reach 5 feet in length in captivity. An iguana has remarkably sharp teeth and nails and a muscular tail, which the animal uses to defend itself by whipping it back and forth. These are the weapons that the handler must guard against when planning to restrain these lizards. Some green iguanas that have been well socialized to humans may be complacent during an examination, but the handler should be careful not to confuse a well-behaved animal with an ill one, because many reptiles that present to veterinary hospitals are sick.

Care should be taken when approaching a patient for the first time to read its body language (Fig. 6.58). A defensive lizard has a hunched back, and it may whip its tail back and forth. In addition, some iguanas bob their heads up and down in a threatening gesture. The easiest and safest capture technique for most medium- to large-sized lizards is the towel-restraint method. To reduce stress, capture should be attempted while the animal is still in its transport carrier. When attempting to capture a small lizard, the handler should keep in mind that these animals are particularly quick movers, making their escape relatively easy when the carrier door is opened or the top of the carrier is removed.

Towel restraint is usually the preferred method for medium- to large-sized lizards; however, the handler should be careful to watch for signs of overstressing the patient, or worse, inadvertently restricting respiration. It must be kept in mind that like birds, lizards lack diaphragms and therefore rely on movement of the thoracic wall to draw air into and out of the lungs. The towel must not be wrapped too tightly around the animal, because restricting the movement of the thorax will suffocate a lizard.

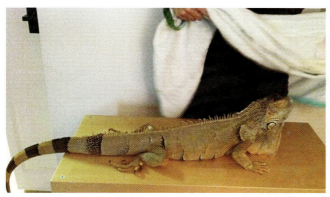

• **Fig. 6.58** A green iguana with a relaxed body posture has been preconditioned for handling. This relaxed posture demonstrates that reptile training and desensitization are beneficial for decreasing stress during physical examination.

Slipping a towel over the animal as the top of the carrier is being removed usually works well. However, carrying out this approach successfully requires at least two people. The person performing the restraint should be prepared with a towel and possibly leather gloves, depending on the size, previous conditioning, and temperament of the lizard, and the skill of the handler (Fig. 6.59). The towel should be slipped over the patient's head and back. The handler should quickly gain control of the head at the base of the neck while at the same time, wrapping the animal's trunk with a towel that also restrains the limbs and feet. When picking the animal up, one hand should always maintain control of the head. The opposite hand and forearm are slipped under the animal's trunk to support the body, and the tail is restrained between the handler's arm and body.

TECHNICIAN NOTE

As much as possible, use gentle restraint when capturing and examining reptiles. Many reptiles are presented to veterinary hospitals with calcium and vitamin D deficiencies, making them prone to iatrogenic bone fracture with rough handling.

For blood collection, once the animal is properly restrained by using the towel method, the tail can be exposed to allow access to the tail veins for venipuncture. This can be accomplished with the patient in a dorsal or ventral position (Fig. 6.60). In some cases of very calm or ill lizards, wrapping the head and covering the eyes with gauze while being careful not to obstruct the nose will relax the patient enough for some procedures, such as radiographic studies, to be performed (Fig. 6.61).

If the lizard is displaying defensive or threatening gestures, such as head bobbing and tail flicking, the overhead lights should be dimmed to allow the patient to calm down. Then, with the aid of another staff member, the pet is slowly covered and wrapped with a towel. It is important to keep in mind that this technique works well with diurnal species but may not be as effective with nocturnal species, such as geckos.

For smaller, more docile lizards, such as bearded dragons, uromastyx, and geckos, minimal hand restraint is typically all that is needed (Fig. 6.62). However, these smaller creatures may inflict bite wounds, especially during minor procedures such as blood sampling, so the handler must always have control of the head.

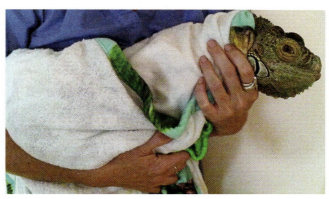

• **Fig. 6.59** Careful use of a towel during restraint of a green iguana ensures that its respiration is not compromised.

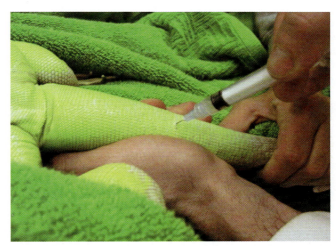

• **Fig. 6.60** For blood collection of this green iguana, once the animal is properly restrained in dorsal recumbency, the tail can be exposed to allow access to the tail veins for venipuncture.

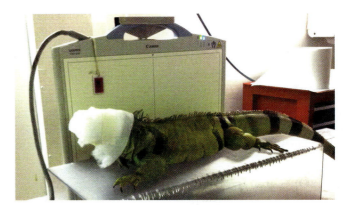

• **Fig. 6.61** In some cases of very calm or ill lizards, such as this green iguana, wrapping the head and covering the eyes with gauze while being careful not to obstruct the nose will relax the patient enough for some procedures, such as radiographic studies, to be performed.

Snakes

Because both venomous and nonvenomous snakes can be purchased by pet owners, the handler should be sure to know the species of snake that is being presented for examination. A quick

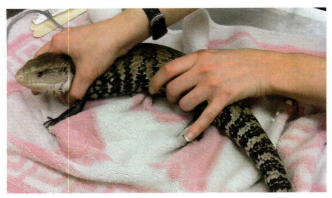

• **Fig. 6.62** For small- to medium-sized lizards, such as bearded dragons, uromastyx, and geckos, minimal hand restraint is typically all that is needed.

Internet search may be required to be sure of the species; however, it is better to know in advance for the protection of all veterinary personnel. The handler should never reach into a transport device without visually identifying the species beforehand, because several venomous species are available on the market.

Smaller species, such as corn snakes, king snakes, and legless lizards (discussed here because the restraint is the same as for snakes), are docile and are easily handled. Large constrictors, such as pythons and boas, may not be as complacent, and large snakes, such as Burmese pythons, may require multiple handlers—one to control the head and several others to control and support the immense body. The safest way to restrain any nonvenomous snake is to control the head, with the thumb and middle finger just behind the animal's mandible and with an index finger on top of the animal's head. The rest of the hand gently encompasses the neck. The opposite hand is then available to support the remainder of the snake's body (Fig. 6.63).

Snakes may show defensive and threatening behavior by raising their heads and hissing. This behavior should not be confused with signs that a snake is ill with a respiratory infection. Snakes in respiratory distress will extend the head and neck to facilitate breathing. They may also hiss and make gurgling sounds as they blow bubbles from the nares and mouth.

Turtles and Tortoises

Turtles and tortoises are easily captured and held. During restraint, caution should be used around the head, because the beaks of these animals, especially those of snapping turtles, can inflict a serious wound. The nails of turtles, especially those on the forelimbs, can inflict deep scratch wounds if the animal is improperly restrained. Restraint can be accomplished in small- to medium-sized animals by grasping behind the plastron (bottom shell) and carapace (top shell) with a one-handed "sandwich" grip. The other hand is then free to grasp the head just behind the mandibles when and if the animal relaxes and extrudes its head (Fig. 6.64). This technique

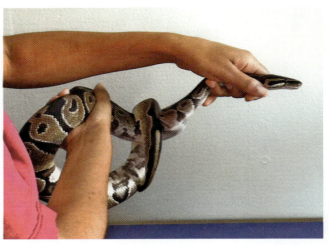

• **Fig. 6.63** The safest way to restrain any nonvenomous snake is to control its head. Place the thumb and middle finger just behind the animal's mandible, with the index finger on top of the animal's head. The rest of the hand gently encompasses the neck. The opposite hand is then available to support the remainder of the snake's body. (Photo courtesy R La Toya Latney, 2011.)

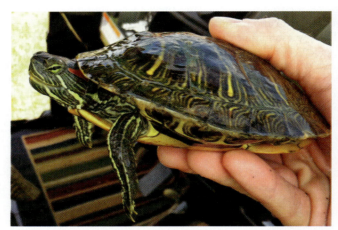

• **Fig. 6.64** Restraint can be accomplished in small- to medium-sized animals by grasping behind the plastron (bottom shell) and carapace (top shell) with a one-handed "sandwich" grip.

may be advantageous in restraining small snapping turtles, because they have remarkably long necks and can bite a hand that is not well out of the way. Box turtles have hinged plastrons and are able to close the cranial and caudal hinged portions over the front and back openings, respectively, creating a kind of box. The handler should be careful to ensure that their fingers are not injured by being closed into the box. Medium-sized turtles can be restrained using a two-handed sandwich method by grasping both sides of the shell (top and bottom) at the same time. A veterinary technician or a veterinarian will need to control the head subsequently.

Acknowledgments

The authors and publisher wish to acknowledge Karen Todd-Jenkins, Barbara Dugan, Darren W. Remsburg, and Chris Montgomery for their previous contributions to this chapter.

Recommended Readings

Canine and Feline Restraint and Handling
Textbooks

Howell A, Feyrecilde M. *Cooperative Veterinary Care*. Hoboken: John Wiley & Sons, Inc.; 2018.

Moffat K. Addressing canine and feline aggression in the veterinary clinic. *Vet Clin North Am Small Anim Pract*. 2008;38:983.

Yin S. *Low Stress Handling, Restraint, and Behavior Modification of Dogs and Cats*. Davis: CattleDog Publishing; 2009.

Articles

Rodan I. Understanding feline behavior and application for appropriate handling and management. *Topics Comp Anim Med*. 2010;25:178.

Rodan I, Sundahl E, Carney H, et al. AAFP and ISFM feline-friendly handling guidelines. *J Feline Med Surg*. 2011;13(5):364–375.

Shaw JK, Martin D. *Canine and Feline Behavior for Veterinary Technicians and Nurses*. Hoboken: John Wiley & Sons, Inc.; 2014.

Equine Restraint and Handling

Hanie EA. Physical restraint of horses. In: *Large Animal Clinical Procedures for Veterinary Technicians*. St Louis: Elsevier Mosby; 2006:47.

Higgins AJ, Snyder JR. *The Equine Manual*. 2nd ed. Edinburgh: Elsevier Saunders; 2005.

Marlborough LC, Knottenbelt DC. Basic management. In: Coumbe K, ed. *Equine Veterinary Nursing Manual*. London: Blackwell Science Ltd; 2001:1.

Reeder D, Miller S, Wilfong DA, et al. *AAEVT's Equine Manual for Veterinary Technicians*. Ames, IA: Wiley-Blackwell; 2009.

Restraint and Handling of Cattle, Swine, Small Ruminants, Camelids, and Cervids

Fowler M. *Medicine and Surgery of South American Camelids. Llama, Alpaca, Vicuña, Guanaco*. 2nd ed. Ames, IA: Blackwell Publishing Professional; 1998.

Fowler M. *Restraint and Handling of Wild and Domestic Animals*. 3rd ed. Ames, IA: Wiley-Blackwell; 2008.

Grandin T. Behavioral principles of livestock handling. *Prof Anim Sci*. 1989;5(2):1–11.

Grandin T. Teaching principles of behavior and equipment design for handling livestock. *J Anim Sci*. 1993;71:1065.

Restraint and Handling of Exotic Species

Fowler M. *Restraint and Handling of Wild and Domestic Animals*. 3rd ed. Ames IA: Wiley-Blackwell; 2008.

Mader D. *Reptile Medicine and Surgery*. 2nd ed. Philadelphia: Saunders; 2006.

Mitchell MA, Tully TN. *Manual of Exotic Pet Practice*. Philadelphia: Saunders; 2009.

Tully TN, Mitchell MA. *A Technician Guide to Exotic Animal Care*. Denver: American Animal Hospital Association; 2001.

Wilson L. Considerations on companion parrot behavior and avian veterinarians. *J Avian Med Surg*. 2000;14:273.

7

History and Physical Examination

GEORGE W. McCOMMON

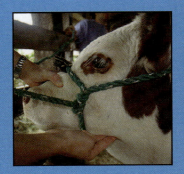

CHAPTER OUTLINE

LEARNING OBJECTIVES

When you have completed this chapter, you will be able to:

1. Pronounce, spell, and define all the key terms in this chapter.
2. Obtain an accurate and complete medical history in small animals by:
   - Explaining the role of the veterinary technician in obtaining the patient's medical history.
   - Listing questions commonly used to obtain a dog's or a cat's medical history.
   - Differentiating between an open-ended question and a leading question and why they are important.
   - Describing the type of information contained in each section of the patient's medical history for dogs and cats.
   - Explaining what a patient's signalment and mentation are and how they relate to patient assessment.
   - Listing the aspects of an animal's origin, background, and past medical history that may be relevant to a presenting complaint.
3. Describe the general procedures used to perform and document a physical examination in dogs and cats, including a subjective assessment of the patient in its surroundings and the measurement of temperature, pulse, and respiration.
4. Discuss methods for performing a comprehensive evaluation of each of the body systems in small animal species.
5. Obtain an accurate and complete medical history in large animals by:
   - Explaining the importance of determining owner/agent information.
   - Describing how the signalment and mentation of a large animal relates to patient assessment.
   - Discussing the individual history and chief complaint of the large animal.
   - Discussing the medication and treatment history.
   - Describing why the process of gathering historical information on herd health differs from taking an individual patient's history.
6. List and describe unique procedures used in the physical examination of horses and ruminants.

KEY TERMS

Abdominal pinging
Abscess
Alopecia
Anisocoria
Aortic stenosis
Ataxia
Aural
Axillary
Barbering
Body condition score
Borborygmus
Colitis

Excoriation
Fever
Glycosuria
Halitosis
Hyperthermia
Hypothermia
Hypovolemia
Icterus
Mentation
Nares
Patent ductus arteriosus
Perineal

Perineal hernia
Petechiation
Pleural effusion
Pneumothorax
Polydipsia
Pruritic
Pulmonary edema
Pulse deficit
Pulse pressure

Pyometra
Renomegaly
Shock
Signalment
Stenotic nares
Stertor
Stridor
Thrombocytopenia

Introduction

The history and physical examination is the first step in the technician's observation of any patient or group of patients. Information obtained during a physical exam serves as the basis for subsequent assessment and intervention. It is essential that veterinary technicians can obtain complete and accurate historical information in both individual patients and herd populations. Similarly, good physical examination skills enable rapid identification of significant problems and provision of appropriate therapeutic measures by the veterinarian. This can be lifesaving in emergency situations. This chapter will stress the importance of a systematic approach to both obtaining historical information (i.e., health history) and performing a physical examination. Veterinary technicians are often the first to observe changes in patient status, and the level of skilled observation and ability to correctly interpret physical examination findings has a significant impact on patient outcomes.

History and Physical Examination of Small Animals

History

Obtaining a complete history is the first step toward creating a diagnostic and therapeutic plan for veterinary patients. Pertinent historical information is an important part of the assessment of the patient by the technician. The veterinary technician should ask questions that clarify the nature of current and previous clinical problems and confirm the accuracy of all information. This may require asking the same question more than once in a different way and repeating responses back to the owner while following up with: "Do I have this correct?"

Obtaining a health history in a clear and organized manner is the foundation of a comprehensive patient evaluation, but it can be challenging. For example, it is difficult to extract information from some owners, because they may say too little or may talk incessantly about unrelated issues. When faced with the former, the veterinary technician must stress the importance of the information, explaining to the owner that the more information they can provide, the more likely it is that the veterinary team will be able to help the pet. In the latter situation, the veterinary technician should refocus the owner's attention on the matter at hand. This may require interrupting the owner and suggesting, "We can talk about that later, but for now, let's focus on this problem." In some cases, the person presenting the patient to the practice may not be the patient's owner and may not know the answers to the questions that the technician is asking. Finally, certain problems or disease states may require specifically tailored questions. The goal of this chapter is to present an organized approach to

obtaining a complete and accurate history for every patient. This method serves as a foundation on which questions based on the owner's knowledge and the patient's specific complaints and pre-existing diseases can be added.

The Role of the Veterinary Technician

The veterinary technician who can obtain a complete and accurate history plays a critical role in the practice. Obtaining information from clients is often time consuming, and veterinary technicians who do this well can free the veterinarians to complete other work. By using historical information in conjunction with new information, the veterinary technician should be able to generate technician evaluations helpful to the veterinarian in formulating appropriate interventions to support the patient. The historical information obtained, however, is useful only if it is complete and accurate. Acquiring inaccurate information could be worse than obtaining no historical information at all. Faulty information might result in unnecessary diagnostic tests, treatments, and loss of client trust. Use of excellent interpersonal skills and careful questioning will aid in gaining the trust and confidence of the pet owner while providing much needed information.

Developing Rapport With the Client

Before obtaining a medical history, it is important for the technician to introduce themselves to the client and explain what is being done so that the client feels comfortable and is willing to share information. The technician must be sure they know the client's name and the pet's name and sex before entering the room to prevent embarrassing mistakes during the conversation. In situations where the pet has been taken away from the client before the history is obtained (e.g., emergency stabilization after trauma), it is essential that the technician come to the client armed with information on pet's status. A comfortable rapport must be established before beginning to gather information via questions.

Asking the Questions

Some owners have medical training, and medical jargon can be used with them; however, most owners do not understand medical terminology, so the technician must be careful to use simple language without making the client feel talked down to. For example, if the technician is doing a follow-up examination of a diabetic cat whose owner is checking the cat's urine daily for glucose, it would be inappropriate to ask, "Have you noted glycosuria since your previous visit?" It would be equally inappropriate to ask, "Is the little square pad on your dipstick changing color when you dip it in Fluffy's pee-pee?" Finding words that are appropriate for the client is important so that they do not feel confused or insulted. It is safest when the technician asks, "Has the urine strip been positive for sugar since your previous visit?" It is important to strike an appropriate balance and tailor the questions to the individual client to avoid losing the client's trust. Clients will often ask for clarification if they are unsure of what the technician is asking, either verbally or through body language.

It is also important to ask open-ended questions rather than leading questions. An open-ended question is one that requires clients to fill in the information themselves, whereas a leading question is one that potentially guides them to a specific answer. For example, if you are trying to determine whether a pet has polydipsia, it is best to ask the open-ended question, "Have you noticed any changes in his water intake during this illness?" rather than "Has he been drinking more water than usual?" When leading questions are asked, clients sense which response the interviewer prefers and are likely to give it. Leading questions can generate inaccurate historical information and should be avoided.

When questioning clients, the technician must avoid appearing judgmental regarding care and management of the pet, because this may make clients feel uncomfortable with providing truthful answers. The questions asked should not reflect the technician's biases or personal beliefs. For example, when questioning an owner about their dog that has acute vomiting and diarrhea, it would be unhelpful to ask, "You don't feed her table scraps, do you?" Faced with that question, the owner is likely to say, "No, of course not," even if they do. It would be better to ask, "What is her normal diet?" or "Did she eat anything outside of her normal diet recently?" or "What human food does she typically eat?" Making clients feel comfortable with talking about their actions, as opposed to defending them, will generate more accurate information.

> **TECHNICIAN NOTE**
>
> Explaining your position and role to clients and tailoring your questions to their level of understanding will allow you to gain the client's trust and obtain more detailed information.

Documenting the Information

Historical information is useless if it cannot be read and therefore should be written carefully, neatly, and accurately on a structured medical record form. All veterinary hospitals should have a standardized history form as part of the medical record; this allows efficient recording of the information presented. The form also provides prompts to remind the technician to obtain certain pieces of information. Information should be recorded in the medical record as it is obtained to prevent any subsequent misunderstanding. Practices that use medical practice management software enter historical data digitally into prescribed fields. If using a hard copy form, it must be remembered that entries must be written legibly or typed using appropriate medical terminology and that the medical record is a legal document and must therefore be written with the utmost care and precision. The medical history will provide a reference for the veterinary health care team as it implements and revises treatment plans for the patient. Please refer to Chapter 3, which provides an appropriate outline of necessary information.

The Information

The following sections provide a general listing of important information that should be obtained in most medical histories. This is meant to serve as a guideline to ensure that complete and accurate historical information is obtained in an efficient manner. Some additions or deletions may be appropriate in specific cases.

> **TECHNICIAN NOTE**
>
> The major focus of any medical history is the presenting complaint; however, it is equally important to obtain general background information.

Signalment

Every patient record should contain the pet's signalment, which includes age, breed (or dominant breed if mixed), sex, and reproductive status (spayed or neutered). It is important to confirm the signalment during the first meeting with the client, because this information often provides important clues about the case. Certain diseases appear more commonly in animals of certain signalments, such as congenital diseases, which are more likely to be diagnosed in very young patients than in very old patients.

Background Information

Background information should begin with documentation of how long the pet has been owned and where and when it was obtained. If it was obtained from a breeder, it may be useful to note whether the client still has contact with the breeder, and if the client knows of any diseases diagnosed in related dogs. Any previous medical problems should be recorded. When discussing the pet's origins, the technician should ask whether there has been any recent travel away from the pet's normal living areas. This information is most important when there is suspicion of a disease that is endemic to a region where the pet has visited in the past 6 months.

This is also a good time to find out where the pet is kept during the day and what its normal routine is. If it is kept indoors, is it in a crate or is it restricted to a certain part of the home? If it is kept outdoors, is it in a fenced yard or is it allowed to run free? At this time, the technician should always get a thorough nutritional history, including the type of food eaten, the amount, and the frequency. It is also important to note whether any recent changes have been made to the diet or whether the animal was fed anything unusual (or if it got into something it should not have) just before the onset of illness.

Preventive Medicine. Complete information regarding vaccination history should be obtained if the pet is a new patient. The technician should note which vaccines were given, when they were given, and the expiration date of the vaccine (i.e., date for boosters). This is also the time to ask about other preventive medications, such as heartworm and flea and tick prevention medications, and how consistently these medications are given; whether they are given year-round or only during warmer months is important. When discussing flea and tick medications, it is a good idea to ask whether the owner has seen fleas or ticks on the pet or in its environment. In new patients, an effort should be made to secure medical records from previous veterinary care providers.

Behavioral Information. The technician should ascertain what the pet's normal behavior is on a day-to-day basis and note any changes in behavior relative to the illness (i.e., mentation). This helps determine if the pet is aggressive toward people or other animals, which may affect how the animal is handled during physical examination or hospitalization. Second, it helps determine whether any behavior changes, such as increased aggression, disorientation, unusual elimination habits, and so on, may explain the underlying illness.

Household Information. The health status of other members of the patient's household can be important in determining the cause of the pet's illness, especially in cases of infectious diseases. The technician should determine to what extent the pet is exposed to other animals: what species, how many, and for what duration. The technician should also determine whether any of these animals are ill, regardless of whether symptoms are like those of the presenting patient. Illnesses among humans in the family should be explored to establish the possibility of zoonotic disease transfer. This is especially important in some cases of infectious dermatologic diseases, such as sarcoptic mange, and may also provide information regarding the patient's exposure to toxins, such as medications taken by family members.

Allergy History. Before beginning medical therapy, it is important to note any known allergies or other adverse reactions to medications or food that the pet may have experienced. Even if these reactions have not been confirmed to be related to the exposure in question, they are important to note. At this time, the technician should also ask whether the pet has ever received a blood product transfusion. If it has, attempt to determine what product, when it was administered, whether any adverse reaction occurred, and if the pet's blood type is known. This information will help guide any subsequent blood product therapy.

Reproductive History. Although the current reproductive status of the patient will be noted in the signalment, as discussed earlier, it is important to ask for historical information regarding the patient's prior reproductive history. If an animal is neutered, it is important to note at what age this occurred, because this information may pertain to disease prevalence. For example, mammary tumors are much more common in female dogs after they have gone through a single heat than in those spayed before their first heat. If an animal is not neutered, the technician should ask whether it is currently being bred and if it has previously been bred. The timing of the most recent heat cycle should be noted for all intact female dogs, because pyometra occurs most commonly 2 weeks to 2 months after a heat cycle.

Pertinent Past Medical History

It is important to identify any prior medical problems that the pet has experienced. Recurrent bouts of similar problems may be an indication of chronic disease. Some previous historical problems may be of no significance to the current presentation and can be ignored. However, if a previous problem sounds as though it may be relevant to the current complaint, this is an opportunity to question the owner more thoroughly about it.

Presenting Complaint

The presenting or chief complaint is the most important information to be addressed in the current medical history. Every patient will have a presenting complaint, and owners are often anxious to discuss this. During emergencies, it is important to quickly obtain information regarding the presenting complaint before obtaining any background information, because time is of the essence in treating life-threatening problems. The presenting complaint can be obtained simply by asking, "What brings you to the practice today?" A patient may have more than one presenting complaint. In this case, it is best to record, triage, and discuss each complaint separately. It must not be assumed that all symptoms can be tied to a single medical disorder; there may be several mitigating factors contributing to the reason for the current visit.

> **TECHNICIAN NOTE**
>
> In emergency situations where rapid patient stabilization is necessary, information regarding the presenting complaint should always be obtained first to assist in generating an immediate response and treatment plan for the patient.

Last Normal

A good way to get a sense of the duration of a problem is to ask the client, "When would you say your pet was last normal?" This often helps the client recall a pleasant time when the pet was acting normally, which is easier than trying to remember how long the pet has been sick. The duration of each presenting complaint varies. A clear timeline of clinical events offers diagnostic clues to the veterinary team, assisting in formulating evaluations and interventions in the event the patient is hospitalized.

Progression

Once a problem list is established, each problem is prioritized (triaged) according to the order in which it appeared and how long it lasted. How each problem progressed is also ascertained. In other words, is the problem getting better, getting worse, or unchanged? A problem that is rapidly worsening may warrant a more immediate course of therapy than a problem that is stable or improving.

Systems Review

A review of body systems through questioning of the client may provide information that otherwise may be overlooked by owners, because they only focus on the presenting complaint. All clients should be asked about the presence of coughing, sneezing, vomiting, diarrhea, polyuria, and polydipsia (remember, use language that the owner can understand). Current appetite, energy level, and any perceived weight loss or weight gain should be noted.

Medications

Reviewing the patient's current medication protocols is important, with the goal being identification of the following: type of medication, dose and frequency of medication, duration for which it has been given, reason it has been given, and whether it has provided benefit to the pet. This includes over-the-counter preparations that may be purchased at the local pet store (i.e., vitamins, supplements). If not immediately known, the client should be asked to call back the information after returning home. The technician should ask about the use of topical eye and ear preparations and medicated shampoos or dips, because some owners do not regard these as "medications." Finally, any preventive medications that are being given, such as heartworm and flea and tick products, should be reviewed.

CASE PRESENTATION 7.1

Signalment: 6-year-old intact male Boston Terrier
Past pertinent history: None
Presenting complaint: Vomiting
Last normal: Three days prior
Progression: The dog was normal when the owners left for work 3 days ago but was vomiting when the owners returned home. They took him to another veterinary hospital, where abdominal radiographs were taken. Based on normal results from radiography and lack of abdominal pain, the dog was given subcutaneous fluids and was discharged with instructions to withhold food and water for 24 hours before beginning a bland diet. Since discharge, he has continued to vomit and has become progressively more lethargic.
Systems: No coughing, sneezing, diarrhea, polyuria, polydipsia, or weight loss noted. No recent weight loss. (As the admitting technician, you are responsible for obtaining the patient's history.) As you discuss the case with the owners, they recall that the dog was chewing a "cow trachea" when they left for work the day that he was last normal. Upon further questioning, it becomes clear that the dog is bringing up white foamy material in the absence of abdominal retching. These specific questions allow you to determine whether the dog is truly vomiting or is displaying regurgitation (Table 7A). You suspect that regurgitation is the actual presenting complaint.

Table 7A Historical Differentiation Between Regurgitation and Vomiting

	Regurgitation	Vomiting
Bile	Rarely to never	Often
Digested food	Sometimes	Often
Active abdominal retch	Rarely to never	Always
Hypersalivation	Sometimes	Sometimes
Gagging	Sometimes	Rarely
Odynophagia	Often	Never

The most useful pieces of information are the presence or absence of bile in the expelled material and the presence or absence of active abdominal retching during expulsion.

Agreeing with your assessment that regurgitation may be the problem, the veterinarian orders cervical and thoracic radiographs (Fig. 7.A). These reveal a radiopaque foreign body in the cervical esophagus, with esophageal dilation proximal to the foreign body. An emergency endoscopy is performed, and the presence of the foreign body is confirmed (Fig. 7.B). The foreign body (a "cow trachea") is removed with endoscopic guidance (Fig. 7.C), and the dog proceeds to make a full recovery.

The owners are grateful that you took the time to obtain an accurate and complete history.

Summary: This is an example of how important good history-taking skills are. At the dog's initial visit, the individual obtaining the history did not discern that the dog was regurgitating (as opposed to vomiting). The erroneous historical diagnosis of vomiting resulted in the ordering of abdominal radiographs, which resulted in a missed diagnosis, inappropriate treatment, and unnecessary costs. By taking the time to obtain a complete and accurate history, you ensured that diagnostic and therapeutic plans were appropriate.

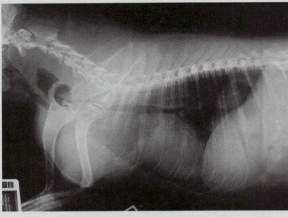

• **Fig. 7.A** Lateral cervical and thoracic radiograph showing a circular radiopaque foreign body in the cervical esophagus with the dilated esophagus proximal to it.

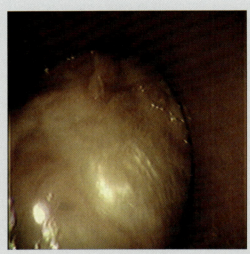

• **Fig. 7.B** Endoscopic image of the cervical esophagus obstructed by foreign body.

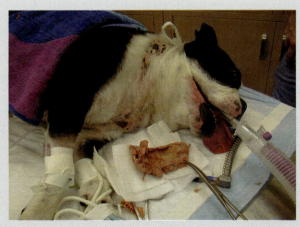

• **Fig. 7.C** Cow trachea foreign body immediately after endoscopic removal from the patient.

Physical Examination

A thorough physical examination should be the first and most important diagnostic test performed on a patient. Because technicians must rely on an owner's interpretation of the pet's illness and the symptoms that pets show are often vague, the physical examination is more important than the past medical history in determining the source of illness. The physical examination serves as the technician's initial observation of a patient, both during the initial presentation and when monitoring changes in a hospitalized patient. An efficient physical examination and recognition of changes will help guide the veterinary nursing process through identifying pertinent issues and subsequently formulating a list of interventions.

The key to performing a good physical examination is careful completion of all parts of the examination every time it is performed. The technician should perform all aspects of the physical examination in the same order in every patient. Developing this sort of routine will help avoid forgetting to evaluate one area because of overly focusing on another. The routine may have to vary slightly from patient to patient, and the technician will find that certain areas of the examination will be covered more carefully in some patients than in others. For example, a complete neurologic examination may be unnecessary on a patient that is seen for coughing and is ambulating normally, with no historical complaints regarding the nervous system. Similarly, in a patient that has hindlimb paralysis, the technician may limit the respiratory examination to a brief auscultation and spend more time performing a complete neurologic examination, including reflex testing. The key is to perform some evaluation of every system during every examination. The guidelines given below are one example of the method by which physical examination could be performed, but with growing experience, the technician can develop their own routine. If the same routine is followed every time a physical examination is performed, the technician can be sure that the examination will be thorough. It must be kept in mind that it is important to examine the patient frequently throughout the period of hospitalization and to maintain a dynamic nursing plan that effectively addresses changes in patient status.

> **TECHNICIAN NOTE**
>
> As with the patient's history, following a consistent routine for every physical examination will prevent overlooking any important findings. A consistent routine also aids in developing continued proficiency in recognizing the normal from the abnormal.

Documenting the Information

It is important that the physical examination must be documented appropriately. All veterinary hospitals should have a standardized physical examination form as part of the medical record. This form should include areas for recording body weight, temperature, pulse rate, and respiratory rate (RR). It should also provide prompts reminding the technician to examine each of the body systems and specific areas in the form where that information should be recorded. For an in-depth look at medical records, please see Chapter 3. As with any part of a medical record, recorded information should be typed or legibly written, medical terminology should be used, and content should always remain professional. Information should be documented in as much detail as possible so that findings can be compared with those from future physical

examinations. The medical record is a legal document and should be treated as such. Mistakes should be crossed out (not scribbled over) and initialed before corrections are made.

> **TECHNICIAN NOTE**
>
> Historical and physical examination findings should be recorded thoroughly, professionally, and legibly in every patient's medical record; they are legal documents.

The SOAP Documentation

The acronym SOAP stands for Subjective, Objective, Assessment and Plan and is used to formulate the plan for treatment as well as documentation of the physical exam. Every physical examination should begin with a subjective assessment of the patient in its surroundings. Several pieces of useful information can be obtained with just a quick visual inspection of the animal from a distance as it behaves in the waiting room, the examination room, or the kennel. The technician can obtain a general sense for the animal's **mentation**. Is the patient bright, alert, and responsive? Is the patient quiet but alert and responsive? Such observations may suggest a less emergent condition. Is the patient dull, depressed, or even unresponsive? This could indicate a more serious disease or neurologic dysfunction. In addition to mentation, the technician can visually inspect the animal as it rests for increases in RR or effort. While the animal walks, quickly look for evidence of lameness, **ataxia**, or visual deficits which may allow you to identify asymmetry or swelling of the patient. This is a good time to evaluate the body condition of the patient and to assign a **body condition score**.

> **TECHNICIAN NOTE**
>
> Taking a moment to observe the patient in its surroundings before performing a physical examination can provide important information.

Temperature, Pulse, and Respiration

Measurement of body temperature, pulse rate, and RR (TPR) will be a part of every physical examination and will be obtained and noted in records by the technician before the veterinarian's examination is performed. For the veterinarian and the veterinary technician, these values provide a quick reference to a substantial amount of information regarding the status of the patient. As mentioned previously, these values should be recorded in a dedicated area on the standard physical examination form or in designated fields in digital records for quick reference.

The body temperature is optimally measured rectally by using a rectal probe thermometer. The probe should always be lubricated to make insertion easier. Most rectal thermometers in current use report the temperature through a digital display window. These thermometers work quickly and are safe and accurate. Although less commonly used, glass liquid capillary thermometers, which rely on a column of liquid (usually alcohol or mercury) rising inside the thermometer may be seen in older practices. When using the liquid capillary type of thermometer, one must remember to shake the thermometer with the insertion tip down so that the liquid level falls from where it was left after its most recent use. Forgetting this step could result in an inaccurate measurement. A protective cover should always be used with all thermometers to minimize disease transmission, and instruments should be sanitized between uses. An **axillary** or **aural** temperature measurement may be used in cases where the rectum or nearby anatomy is swollen or painful, as in severe **colitis** or with a **perineal hernia**. These measurements are less accurate compared with a rectal measurement and should be used only when necessary and noted within the record.

Variations from normal body temperature are helpful in determining the nature or severity of a patient's illness. An elevated body temperature (**fever** or **hyperthermia**) may signify the presence of infection, inflammation, or neoplasia. However, mild elevations may be noted secondary to the anxiety associated with a visit to the practice. Significant true hyperthermia may be present when heat-dissipating mechanisms cannot overcome excessive ambient temperatures (heatstroke) or secondary to certain drugs. Severe elevations (>107°F) can lead to organ dysfunction and can warrant initiation of gradual cooling mechanisms. Decreased body temperature (**hypothermia**) is seen less commonly and usually results from impaired thermoregulation in any sick animal, especially cats. Inability to maintain body temperature is more common in patients that are young, old, or thin. Conditions that commonly result in impaired thermoregulation include chronic renal failure, hypothyroidism, and central nervous system disease. Severe hypothermia (<90°F) can be life-threatening and requires immediate attention. Normal body temperature ranges, pulse, and RRs for dogs and cats are noted in Table 7.1.

Peripheral arterial pulses should be palpated to determine pulse rate and pulse quality in every patient. Pulses generally are palpated by way of the femoral artery, which is located high on the medial thigh of the animal. Digital pressure should be applied over the femoral artery by using the tips of the fingers. Some degree of pressure will be required to feel the pulse, but excessive pressure could compress the vessel, making the pulse difficult to feel. The degree of pressure needed will vary from patient to patient. The pulse rate (per minute) is calculated by counting the number of pulses palpated for 15 seconds and multiplying by 4. It is essential to auscultate the heart while palpating pulses. Heart rate (HR) and pulse rate should be identical, and a pulse of approximately equal quality should be produced by each heartbeat. Absence or a significant change in pulse quality in the presence of an audible heartbeat is called a *pulse deficit*. Pulse deficits usually indicate an abnormal heart rhythm and warrant further evaluation, such as with electrocardiography (ECG).

It is important to determine the pulse quality when palpating peripheral arterial pulses. The pressure felt when palpating a pulse is called the *pulse pressure* and represents the difference between systolic and diastolic arterial pressures. The intensity of the palpated pulse will vary, depending on the body condition of the animal, appearing stronger in thin animals and weaker in obese or heavily muscled animals. Pulse quality is a subjective measurement that is likely to vary among technicians, according

to the level of experience attained in palpating peripheral pulses. An attempt should be made to describe the intensity of the pulse by using such terms as *weak, moderate,* or *strong.* In general, a weak peripheral pulse is indicative of poor perfusion and may be caused by decreased cardiac output (i.e., congestive heart failure or **hypovolemia**) or increased peripheral resistance (i.e., **shock**). Pulses may be described as "slow to rise" if the peak of intensity comes late in the pulse wave, a condition that is seen with obstruction to cardiac output, as occurs with **aortic stenosis**. A pulse that feels stronger than normal may also indicate a problem and is described as *bounding, tall,* or *hyperkinetic.* Bounding pulses may be palpated in hyperdynamic states (early septic shock, anemia) or when a rapid drop-off in diastolic pressure occurs (i.e., **patent ductus arteriosus**). Whenever pulse quality is abnormal, evaluation of blood pressure using direct or indirect means is warranted, and all readings should be documented.

RR and effort should be noted in all patients. An initial notation of RR and effort should be made before any stressful manipulation of the patient is performed as stress will commonly cause an increase in those parameters. RR is generally obtained visually first and then by auscultation to hear lung sounds. To calculate RR (per minute), the number of breaths is counted for 15 seconds and multiplied by 4. Determination of respiratory effort is more subjective. Animals breathing with normal effort should appear comfortable and lack any abdominal effort. If abnormal effort is detected, the technician should attempt to determine the phase of respiration when effort is increased. Increased inspiratory effort may indicate an upper airway problem, especially if an associated noise is noted, as with laryngeal paralysis. Increased expiratory effort may indicate small airway obstructive disease, such as asthma.

Systems Review

After visual inspection of the animal in its surroundings and notation of temperature, pulse, and respiration, a more thorough examination of individual body systems should be performed. Each system is described below, including what should be assessed and recorded as part of the physical examination process.

> **TECHNICIAN NOTE**
> Every major body system should be examined briefly in every patient. Special attention may be paid to specific systems, depending on the individual patient.

Oropharyngeal System

Diseases of the oral cavity may cause loss of appetite, difficulty chewing, or **halitosis**. Dental disease (e.g., periodontal disease) is common in small animal patients. Oropharyngeal examination

TABLE 7.1	Normal TPR Values for Adult Small Animals		
	Rectal Temperature, °F	Heart Rate	Respiratory Rate
Dog	100.0–102.2	60–160/minute (smaller breeds may have higher rates; puppies can have rates up to 200)	16–32/minute
Cat	100.0–102.2	140–220/minute	20–42/minute

TPR, Body temperature, pulse rate, and respiration rate.

is an important part of the physical examination that can be easily performed in most patients by lifting the animal's lips with its mouth in the closed and open positions. Caution should be exercised during an oral examination, especially in uncooperative patients, to avoid being bitten. Teeth should be examined visually for any evidence of discoloration, fracture, or excessive tartar formation. Abnormal teeth should be gently palpated to assess for pain and to determine whether a tooth is loose (suggesting periodontal disease). Any missing teeth should be noted and recorded in the medical record. The gums should be examined for redness, a sign of gingivitis, the precursor to periodontal disease. Any gingival swelling that may represent neoplastic masses or tooth root abscesses should be noted. More diffuse swelling can be seen with gingival hyperplasia. Gingival ulcers may be seen with renal disease, feline viral upper respiratory disease (herpesvirus, calicivirus), or ingestion of caustic substances. Examination of the animal with its mouth open allows inspection of the lingual surfaces of teeth and gums and examination of the tongue for swelling, discoloration, or ulceration. To inspect the tongue, the technician should push upward from the jaw between the two rami of the mandible. Inspection under the tongue may reveal abnormalities, such as masses (i.e., sublingual squamous cell carcinoma [see Fig. 7.1]), swelling (a ranula or a salivary mucocele), or foreign material (string around the base of a cat's tongue). An open-mouth examination also allows inspection of the roof of the oral cavity (soft and hard palate) and the back of the oral cavity (pharynx, larynx). These areas should be visually inspected for any swelling or mass, discoloration, or foreign material. Some pharyngeal masses may be large enough that they can be palpated externally by feeling the area just caudal to the mandible and cranial to the tracheal cartilage. Greater detail regarding an oropharyngeal examination and dental disease can be found in Chapter 35.

> **TECHNICIAN NOTE**
>
> A thorough oropharyngeal examination should include both open-mouth and closed-mouth examinations.

Eyes

An ocular examination can be performed with no specialized equipment and should include examination of the eyelids and of the external and internal structures of the eyes. It should also include an assessment of the patient's visual status. An examination of the eyelids should aim to identify any redness or swelling. Eyelid margins should be evaluated for evidence of masses or abnormal hairs (especially if they appear to be growing in toward the eye, causing irritation). Finally, the position of the lower eyelid should be examined to see whether the lower lid is rolling in toward the eye (entropion) or out away from the eye (ectropion) as both conditions can lead to ocular problems. Any ocular discharge should be noted and described regarding symmetry (unilateral, bilateral) and character (serous, mucoid, purulent, hemorrhagic). Sampling by use of a sterile swab may be microbiologically useful to diagnose and treat. Excessive tearing or squinting of the eye may indicate irritation and should be noted. A general visual inspection of the globes should be performed to determine whether they are symmetric and whether they are enlarged and/or protruding (as can be seen with glaucoma or lesions behind the eye) or sunken. The globes can be gently pressed with the thumbs over the eyelids. They may feel extremely firm when intraocular pressure is high (as with glaucoma) or soft when intraocular pressure is low (as with uveitis). If the eyes cannot be pushed backward (retro pulsed) slightly, a lesion (e.g., a mass) may be present behind one or both eyes.

> **TECHNICIAN NOTE**
>
> Although a complete ocular examination requires specialized ophthalmologic equipment, a significant amount of information can be obtained without the use of any equipment.

The external parts of the eye that can be evaluated include the conjunctiva, sclera, nictitating membrane, and cornea. The conjunctiva is the pink membrane that can be seen by pulling back the upper or lower eyelids; it covers the outer part of the eye up to where the cornea begins. Redness of the conjunctiva (conjunctival hyperemia) is seen with many diseases of the external part of the eye, such as conjunctivitis. The sclera is the normally white part of the eye; yellow discoloration indicates icterus (Fig. 7.2). Redness noted in the sclera may be caused by conjunctival hyperemia (usually diffuse, with small, movable blood vessels), episcleral injection (large, straight blood vessels, often indicative of internal ocular disease), or subconjunctival hemorrhage (usually large, round to irregular blotches). Any eye redness should be recorded and reported to the veterinarian for further evaluation. The nictitating membrane ("third eyelid") rests beneath the lower eyelid on the medial aspect of the orbit and is either not visible or partially visible. If the nictitating membranes are visible, this is an abnormality

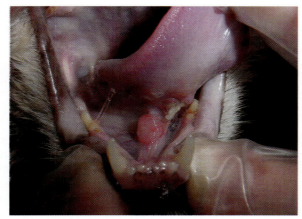

• **Fig. 7.1** Sublingual squamous cell carcinoma visualized during examination of the underside of the tongue of a cat.

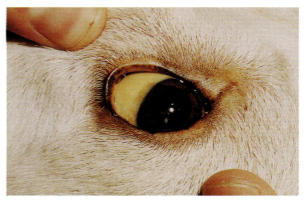

• **Fig. 7.2** Yellow discoloration of the sclera seen with icterus.

and should be noted. If not visible, they can be briefly examined by pressing inward on the eye, causing the nictitating membrane to rise so that it can be evaluated for swelling, redness, masses, or foreign material. The cornea is the transparent covering of the front of the eye, and it should be clear. It should be examined for cloudiness or other precipitates (e.g., pigment). Corneal ulcers are common and, although fluorescein staining is usually required for recognition of a corneal ulcer, deeper ulcers may be identifiable with only visual inspection. A diseased cornea may have blood vessels growing into it (especially toward an area of ulceration to help with healing); these should be noted.

The internal structures of the eye that can be evaluated without specialized equipment include the iris, lens, and anterior chamber. The iris is the colored part of the eye. It should be evaluated for swelling, discoloration, irregularity, or masses. The pupil is the opening of the iris which should always be evaluated for degree of constriction or dilation, and for symmetry of size. If the pupils are of differing sizes, this is referred to as *anisocoria*. The pupillary light response should be examined in all patients. When a light of sufficient strength shines into one pupil, both pupils should constrict. Anisocoria and abnormal pupillary light responses can indicate various ocular and neurologic diseases. The lens is located inside the pupillary opening and is the part of the eye responsible for focusing images onto the retina. In a normal patient, the lens cannot be seen without specialized equipment. However, increased lens opacity may be seen with nuclear sclerosis (a normal aging change seen commonly in dogs) or cataract formation. The anterior chamber is the part of the eye behind the cornea but in front of the iris and should normally be clear; there should be no difficulty seeing the structures behind it. Cloudiness, pus, or blood may be present in the anterior chamber in association with severe ocular inflammation. Rarely, masses may be seen in the anterior chamber.

A simple evaluation of the patient's visual ability can be made as it is walking into or around the examination room. Most blind patients have difficulty getting around in the unfamiliar setting of the veterinary hospital, even if they have accommodated well for their blindness at home. Another way to assess a patient's ability to see is to test its menace reflex by covering one eye (so that only one eye is tested at a time) and making a menacing gesture toward the other eye with your hand (making sure not to touch the patient or create excessive air movement that it could feel). A patient with sight will close the eye in response to this gesture (assuming it is old enough to recognize that your gesture is menacing, has an intact facial nerve, and is capable of blinking). Vision may also be assessed by dropping cotton balls in front of the patient from above its head and noting whether it visually follows the cotton balls as they pass in front of the eyes.

Ears

Examination of the ears should begin with visualization and palpation of the pinnae. During visualization, the pinnae should be evaluated for symmetry (although in some patients, asymmetry may be normal) and inspected inside and outside for swelling, redness, **alopecia**, crusting, or evidence of **excoriation**. The interior part of the pinnae is a common place to recognize **petechiation**, which is indicative of a primary hemostatic defect (e.g., **thrombocytopenia**) (Fig. 7.3). Palpation of the pinnae will allow for recognition of focal swelling (as seen with aural hematoma) or diffuse thickening (as might be seen with chronic otitis). Lifting and/or pulling back the pinnae will allow visual inspection of the external ear canal. Canine and feline ear canals consist of a vertical

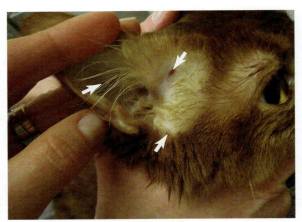

• **Fig. 7.3** Petechiae (*arrows*) inside and in front of the pinna in a cat.

canal, which opens to the external environment and runs inward parallel to the skull, and a horizontal canal, which is a short section between the vertical canal and the eardrum and runs more perpendicular to the skull. Only the vertical canal may be visualized without specialized equipment. This area should be evaluated for discharge, thickening and/or swelling, or masses. Aural discharge should be described in terms of amount (mild, moderate, severe) and appearance (waxy, black, hemorrhagic, purulent). Sampling with sterile swabs is encouraged and labeled R and/or L ear. Evaluation of the horizontal canal and eardrum requires the use of an otoscope.

Most otoscopes found in veterinary practice are wall mounted or portable. They typically consist of a handle, which allows the examiner to hold the instrument; a head, through which the examiner visualizes the structures; and detachable cones. The cone is a gradually tapering tube that fits nicely into the ear canal, through which the otoscope light shines to allow visualization. Most otoscopes can also be used as ophthalmoscopes by changing the head. Wall-mounted otoscopes usually have a base that plugs into an electrical outlet and hangs on the wall. The handle is attached to the base via a cord that supplies the power to light the otoscope. The handle is permanently attached to the base, and the cones may be changed to match the size of the patient undergoing an examination. The cone should be large enough to allow clear visualization of structures inside the ear canal but small enough so as not to cause the patient discomfort. Wall-mounted otoscopes offer the advantage of always being ready for use and requiring little assembly, but they lack the flexibility of the portable units in terms of where the patient is positioned. Cones are generally washed and cold sterilized for reuse.

TECHNICIAN NOTE

An otoscopic examination must consist of a thorough ear examination performed by visualizing the vertical and horizontal canals.

With wall-mounted units, the patient must be fairly close to the wall-mounted base, but portable units allow for examination of the patient anywhere. The portable unit consists of a handle that contains a rechargeable battery to power the light source, a connecting piece that attaches the handle to the head, and the head (Fig. 7.4). As with the wall-mounted unit, a cone must be attached to the head for an examination. Disadvantages of the portable otoscope are that the battery requires recharging and may

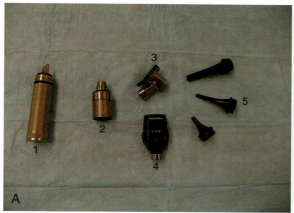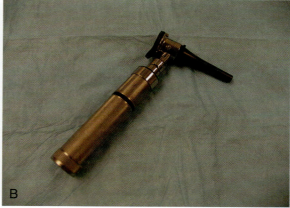

• **Fig. 7.4** (A) Components of a portable otoscope/ophthalmoscope. *1,* Handle. *2,* Connecting piece. *3,* Otoscope head. *4,* Ophthalmoscope head. *5,* Otoscope cones of varying sizes. (B) Assembled portable otoscope.

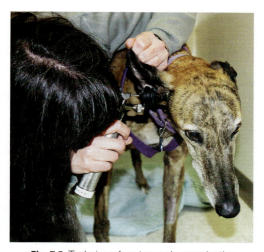

• **Fig. 7.5** Technique for otoscopic examination.

not always be ready when needed and that the otoscope needs to be assembled before use.

To examine the horizontal canal and eardrum using an otoscope, the pinnae are first gently pulled upward (opposite the direction of the patient's legs) to lessen the angle between vertical and horizontal canals. At this point, the otoscope cone is gently passed into the vertical canal while the examiner is looking through the otoscope's head. The cone is gently advanced into the horizontal canal until the eardrum is visualized or until the patient shows evidence of discomfort (Fig. 7.5). During passage of the otoscope through the vertical and horizontal canals, those areas should be examined for evidence of redness, swelling, masses, discharge, excess hair, or foreign material. The eardrum should appear as a gray-to-white, slightly transparent, round membrane separating the inner ear from the external ear canal. Abnormalities of the eardrum that should be noted include tears or perforation of the eardrum, increased thickness (or decreased transparency), and evidence of discharge behind the eardrum. It should be noted that otoscopy is technically challenging and is resisted by many patients. Visualization of the eardrum may be difficult for the novice technician; only through frequent practice and the help of a dedicated restrainer will the technique become comfortable.

Respiratory System

The initial examination of a patient's respiratory status involves visual determination of RR and effort, as discussed previously. Patients in significant respiratory distress should be provided with supplemental oxygen and should be minimally stressed. The remainder of the physical examination should be brief or may be postponed until the patient is in a more stable condition.

TECHNICIAN NOTE

Patients in significant respiratory distress should be placed on oxygen and stabilized before a complete respiratory examination is performed.

In a stable patient, examination of the respiratory system should begin with evaluation of the upper respiratory tract. The **nares** should be visually inspected to ensure symmetry and patency. Patency can be evaluated by holding a glass slide in front of the nares and looking for condensation to form from each nostril as the animal exhales. The nares should also be evaluated for normal opening size, especially in brachycephalic breeds of dogs, in which **stenotic nares** are common. Nasal discharge should be described in terms of symmetry (unilateral, bilateral), severity (mild, moderate, severe), and character (serous, mucoid, purulent, hemorrhagic). Sampling should be done utilizing sterile swabs and labeled R or L naris. Opening the patient's mouth and briefly visualizing the hard and soft palates at the roof of the mouth will allow a basic inspection of the nasopharynx for masses, which may appear as a downward bulging of the palate. Any clinical signs of upper airway disease noted during an examination should be recorded, such as sneezing, **stertor**, or **stridor**.

Auscultation with the use of a stethoscope completes the respiratory examination (Fig. 7.6).

A stethoscope should be used such that the earpieces are pointing toward the examiner's nose when they are placed into the ears. The chest-piece on most stethoscopes consists of two sides: a flat side, called the *diaphragm*, and a cup-shaped side, called the *bell*. The diaphragm, which transmits high-frequency sounds, is used most and is appropriate for lung auscultation. The bell, which transmits low-frequency sounds, is used less frequently and may enhance the ability to hear certain cardiac sounds, such as those associated with a galloping rhythm. Twisting the chest-piece

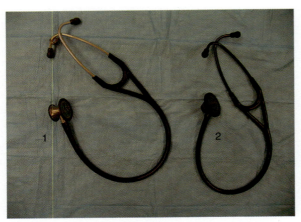

• **Fig. 7.6** Stethoscopes. *1.* Chest-piece with separate bell and diaphragm. *2,* Chest-piece with integrated bell and diaphragm.

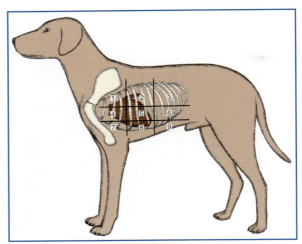

• **Fig. 7.7** Division of the lungs into nine quadrants for auscultation and description of location of abnormal lung sounds. (From McCurnin DM, Poffenbarger EM. *Small Animal Physical Diagnosis and Clinical Procedures.* St. Louis, MO: Saunders; 1991.)

180 degrees within the tubing will change whether the bell or the diaphragm is active. Some stethoscopes do not have a separate bell and diaphragm but can function as both if the pressure with which the chest-piece is applied to the patient is varied.

When respiratory auscultation is performed, the patient should be in a quiet room. Many things can hamper the ability to effectively auscultate a patient, including ambient noise, patient movement (causing hair rubbing to be heard through the earpieces), panting, and purring. In a panting dog, the mouth should be held gently closed to improve auscultation. Attempts should be made to quiet a cat's purring, such as temporarily covering the nares, running water near the cat, holding alcohol-soaked cotton to the nares, or tapping the nose. Once conditions are optimal, respiratory auscultation should begin with the chest-piece over the trachea. Normal tracheal airflow is turbulent, and respiratory sounds should be loud and harsh. Abnormal sounds heard over the trachea suggest a problem in the upper airway (trachea or more cranial). For example, a high-pitched inspiratory sound may indicate partial upper airway obstruction, as can be seen with laryngeal paralysis. Although these abnormal upper airway sounds will likely be transmitted to the lungs and audible during lung auscultation, they do not indicate lung disease. The lungs should be auscultated on both sides of the patient, generally dividing the lung fields into nine quadrants on each side (Fig. 7.7). Each quadrant should be auscultated through at least two to three respiratory cycles of inspiration and expiration. In a normal patient, air movement will be audible during both inspiration and expiration but should be of minimal intensity. The intensity of normal lung sounds will vary, depending on the body condition of the patient; sounds are more intense in thin patients and less intense in obese or well-muscled patients. The most identified abnormal lung sounds are crackles and wheezes. Inspiratory crackles usually indicate the presence of fluid within the alveoli, as can be seen in **pulmonary edema.** Wheezes may occur during inspiration and/or expiration when air is moving through a narrowed airway, as seen with feline asthma. Failure to hear any air movement is a sign of a different problem. Absence of lung sounds in the ventral lung fields in the standing animal usually indicates **pleural effusion,** because fluid tends to settle in the ventral areas. Conversely, absence of sounds in the dorsal lung fields often indicates a **pneumothorax,** because air will rise to the dorsal areas. Space-occupying masses and lung consolidation can also result in the absence of lung sounds. When abnormal lung sounds are auscultated (or lung sounds are absent),

the technician should note whether they occur during inspiration or expiration and in which lung fields they were identified.

Cardiovascular System

Examination of the cardiovascular system begins with a look into the mouth to assess the perfusion status. The gingival mucous membranes should be pink and moist, although some animals will have normally pigmented gingivae. Pallor of the mucous membranes usually indicates anemia, parasitism, or poor perfusion. Hyperemia of the mucous membranes can occur in stressed animals or can be seen in hyperdynamic states, such as the early phase of septic shock. If the mucous membranes are dry or tacky, this is usually an early sign of dehydration, although in a patient that is panting excessively, the mucous membranes may be dried by air movement associated with panting and therefore will not be a good indicator of hydration status. The gingival mucous membranes are also used for measuring capillary refill time (CRT), which serves as another indicator of perfusion. With the patient's lip raised, the gingival surface is gently pressed with a finger to occlude blood flow until the color fades from the mucous membrane beneath the finger. The finger is removed, and the time it takes for the mucous membrane color to return to normal is measured (Fig. 7.8). In a normal animal, this CRT will be less than 2 seconds. Refill times longer than 2 seconds are indicative of poor perfusion, as can be seen in hypotensive states. Extremely rapid refill (<1 second) may be seen in stressed patients or in hyperdynamic states, such as the early phase of septic shock. Peripheral arterial pulse quality will also provide information regarding perfusion, as was discussed previously.

TECHNICIAN NOTE

A complete cardiac examination includes assessment of perfusion status, heart rate (HR), heart rhythm, and heart sounds.

Cardiac auscultation allows evaluation for abnormal HR, rhythm, and sounds. In dogs, the heart should be auscultated on each side of the chest around the level of the costochondral junction (just behind the level of the elbow in a standing patient). By moving the chest-piece around slightly, the technician will

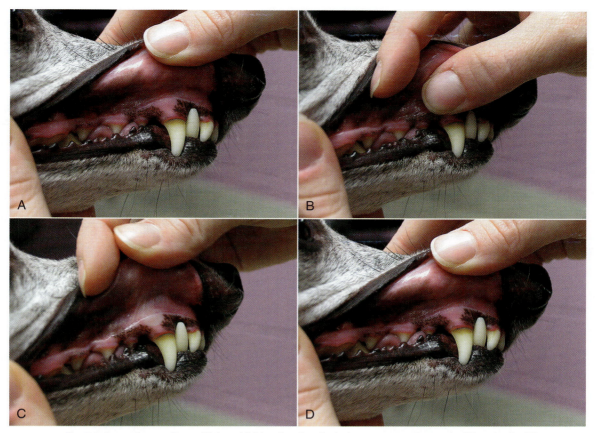

• **Fig. 7.8** Assessing capillary refill time. (A) Visualize the gingival mucous membranes by lifting the lip. (B) Apply gentle pressure with the thumb onto the mucous membranes. (C) Resultant area of pallor when the thumb is removed. (D) Note time to return of normal mucous membrane color.

be able to auscultate in the vicinity of each heart valve. The pulmonic, aortic, and mitral valves can be best auscultated on the left side, whereas the tricuspid valve is best auscultated on the right side. In cats, it is best to auscultate directly over the sternum initially before moving the chest-piece gradually up to the left side and back over to the right side. Valve positions are like those in the dog, but in cats, abnormal heart sounds are more commonly auscultated in the sternal area. The heart rhythm should be regular—that is, each heartbeat is separated from the next one by an identical time interval. Dogs may normally have a slight variation in heart rhythm such that HR increases slightly during inspiration and decreases slightly during expiration. This is called *respiratory sinus arrhythmia,* and it is a sign that a dog has normal cardiac function. To best evaluate cardiac rhythm, the pulses must be palpated during auscultation. As discussed previously, a pulse of approximately equal intensity should be generated with each heartbeat. In a patient with an abnormal heart rhythm or with pulse deficits, ECG should be performed to determine the exact nature of the abnormality.

The heart sounds typically audible during auscultation in a normal patient are S_1 (the first heart sound), which is created by closure of the mitral and tricuspid valves at the start of systole, and S_2 (the second heart sound), which is created by closure of the aortic and pulmonic valves at the end of systole. These two short heart sounds result in the typical "lub-dub" sound of the normal heartbeat. The presence of a third heart sound is termed a *gallop rhythm* because the resulting heart rhythm sounds like the galloping of a horse. A gallop rhythm is not actually an abnormal

rhythm in the sense of electrical activity but is caused by an extra heart sound termed S_3 or S_4. S_3 is usually associated with ventricular dilation, as with dilated cardiomyopathy, whereas S_4 is usually associated with decreased ventricular compliance and hypertrophy (hypertrophic cardiomyopathy). S_3 and S_4 cannot be differentiated via auscultation. Rarely, the second heart sound (S_2) may be split and may sound like a third heart sound; this is uncommon.

A heart murmur is an abnormal sound caused by turbulent blood flow, which typically sounds like a "swishing" noise. Identification of heart murmurs can indicate cardiac disease, although they can occur with noncardiac disease (e.g., anemia) or can be normal in some young animals. Heart murmurs should be described by their intensity, when they occur in the cardiac cycle, and where they are heard loudest. The intensity of a heart murmur is typically graded on a scale from I to VI, as shown in Table 7.2. Systolic murmurs occur between S_1 and S_2 (i.e., during systole) or may mask those two sounds. Diastolic murmurs occur after S_2 and before the next S_1 (i.e., during diastole). A continuous murmur occurs throughout the cardiac cycle. The area on the chest where a murmur is loudest is termed the *point of maximal intensity.* For dogs, this point is usually identified in relation to the location of heart valves, as shown in Fig. 7.9. For cats, this point may more easily be described in relation to the sternum (e.g., midsternum or left parasternum), where many feline murmurs are best auscultated.

The final part of a thorough cardiovascular examination consists of evaluation of jugular veins. In a short-haired patient, the

TABLE 7.2	Grading of Heart Murmurs in Small Animals	
Grade	**Description**	
I	Very low intensity murmur that can be heard only in a quiet area	
II	Murmur of soft intensity that can be heard immediately	
III	Murmur of moderate intensity	
IV	Loud murmur	
V	Loud murmur with a palpable thrill on the body wall	
VI	Loud murmur that can be heard with the stethoscope held some distance from the thoracic wall	

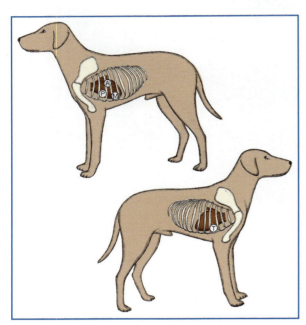

• **Fig. 7.9** Point of maximum intensity of heartbeat. Aortic Valve (A): Controls flow of blood from left ventricle to aorta. Pulmonic Valve (P): Controls blood flow from the right heart to the pulmonary artery which supplies blood to lungs. Mitral Valve (M): The valve that controls blood flow from the left atrium to the left ventricle. Tricuspid Valve (T): Regulates flow of blood from right atrium to right ventricle.

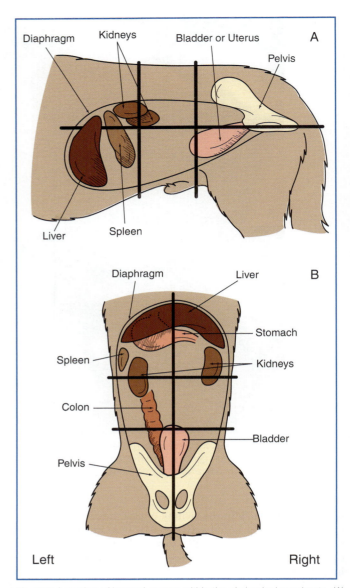

• **Fig. 7.10** Location of internal organs within the abdominal quadrants. (A) Lateral projection. (B) Dorsoventral projection.

jugular veins can be visualized on either side of the trachea when the patient's muzzle is lifted dorsally with the patient in the standing or sitting position. In animals with thicker or longer coats, the hair may need to be clipped or moistened to allow evaluation. Normal patients should have jugular pulsations that do not extend beyond one-third up the neck. The jugular veins drain blood into the right atrium, and their pulsations and distention give a direct indication of right atrial pressure. Distended jugular veins extending farther up the neck can be seen in any disease causing elevated central venous pressure, especially those causing increased right atrial pressure, such as pericardial effusion or pulmonic stenosis.

Gastrointestinal System

Abdominal palpation involves assessment of more than just the gastrointestinal (GI) tract. During abdominal palpation, other abdominal organs, including liver, spleen, kidneys, and urinary bladder, will be examined. The technique of abdominal palpation can be difficult for the novice technician, but with practice, they

can become proficient. As with the physical examination, following a consistent routine every time abdominal palpation is performed will ensure that nothing is missed. A thorough understanding of the anatomic location of abdominal organs within the abdominal cavity is essential for effective palpation. Fig. 7.10 shows the location of abdominal organs within the abdomen. The abdomen can be divided into six sections: cranial-dorsal, cranial-ventral, middorsal, midventral, caudal-dorsal, and caudal-ventral. For most dogs, the two-handed technique is the best method (Fig. 7.11). For small dogs and cats, the one-handed technique (Fig. 7.12) may be easier, with use of the general principles discussed later for the two-handed technique. With the patient in the standing position, the examiner should stand just behind the patient or should stand straddling the caudal end of the patient. This will allow the placement of one hand on either side of the abdomen. The hands should be in a flat, relaxed position. Palpation should begin in one section (e.g., cranial-dorsal), with the hands moving gently toward each other in a smooth, fluid motion. The hands and fingers should remain relaxed, and

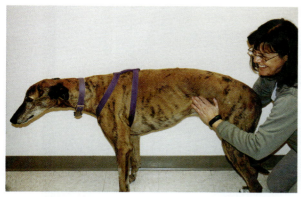

• **Fig. 7.11** Two-handed abdominal palpation in the dog.

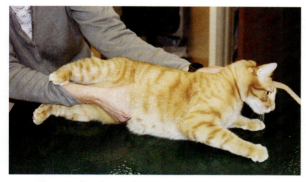

• **Fig. 7.12** One-handed abdominal palpation in the cat.

excessive pressure should not be exerted. If the patient tenses its abdominal muscles, delineation of organs by touch becomes difficult. The palpation should move slowly and methodically through all other sections of the abdomen, and the progression should be the same each time a patient is palpated. Within each section, the technician should be noting any pain, swelling, firmness, or fluid. These findings should be recorded as to their severity and location (which section, left or right side).

> **TECHNICIAN NOTE**
>
> Abdominal palpation should be performed using a consistent routine in every patient to avoid omitting evaluation of any area.

Specific organs should be palpated in their respective regions. The liver should not be palpable in the normal animal, but if it is enlarged or contains a mass, it may be palpated in the cranial-ventral abdomen just caudal to the rib margin. The spleen is usually palpable in the cranial-ventral or midventral abdomen on the left side and should be gently palpated for enlargement or masses. The kidneys reside in the cranial-dorsal or middorsal abdomen and cannot be palpated in most dogs, because they are encased in quite a bit of fat and are not movable. However, they may be palpated in thin dogs or when **renomegaly** is present. Indications of pain in those sections of the abdomen may represent renal pain. In cats, the kidneys are much more movable and much more easily palpable. They usually are just caudal to the ribs in the dorsal abdomen and can be freely moved in most cats. They should be palpated for irregularities in size or shape and for evidence of pain. The urinary bladder can be easily palpated in the caudal-ventral abdomen,

assuming it is not empty and that the patient is cooperative. Identification of the urinary bladder facilitates performance of cystocentesis. The urinary bladder should also be gently palpated for distention or thickness. Care should be taken in bladder palpation as this may encourage the animal to urinate spontaneously. On rare occasions, bladder stones may be palpable on physical examination. In male dogs, the prostate gland may be palpable in the caudal-dorsal abdomen, especially if it is significantly enlarged, though it is best examined via a rectal examination.

The GI tract can be examined to some extent during abdominal palpation. The stomach usually is not palpable if it is empty, but if gastric distention or a mass is present, it may be palpable in the cranial-dorsal abdomen (or farther caudal with severe distention). The small intestines are generally palpable as loops passing through the fingers in much of the midabdomen. It is not possible to delineate the different sections of small intestine by palpation. Small intestinal masses should be easily palpable, but other intestinal changes, such as wall thickening, are usually subtle and difficult to appreciate. The large intestine usually can be palpated in the middorsal and caudal-dorsal abdomen as it courses toward the rectum, if it contains formed feces. If it is empty, it may not be as easily palpated. Good palpation may allow for identification of large intestinal masses or constipation or obstipation. It is important to remember that a complete GI examination includes examination of the oral cavity, pharynx, rectum, and anus.

Rectal Examination

A rectal examination should be considered in every canine patient and will be performed by the veterinarian. In cats and small dogs, a rectal examination may be prohibitively painful and should be performed only in patients with a presenting complaint related to that area. In preparation for the veterinarian's exam, the technician may inspect the rectum, the **perineal** area, and anus for redness, swelling, masses, discharge, or other abnormalities. Dorsal to the rectum, the medial iliac lymph nodes are present on either side of the midline and may be palpated if they are enlarged. The character of any stool presented should be noted and sampled for testing for parasites, blood, etc. The anal sacs should be palpated where they lie just behind the anal mucosa one on either side, located at approximately the 5 o'clock and 7 o'clock positions (Fig. 7.13A). Palpation may be done through moving the finger within the rectum laterally and caudally while gently pressing with the thumb on the outside of the anus. Normal anal sacs should be small (<1 cm) and firm but slightly fluctuant. Distended anal sacs likely contain normal anal sac fluid but could contain a mass. Both sacs must be fully expressed to confirm whether a mass is present. This should be done in any patient with a palpably distended anal sac. Each sac opens at the rectal-anal junction adjacent to the location of the sac. The anal sacs are expressed by gently applying pressure with the thumb and finger during palpation until one feels a slight "pop" (see Fig. 7.13B). Anal sac fluid can vary in appearance and consistency from whitish to dark brown and from watery to thick, and it can have a noxious odor. Evidence of blood or pus may indicate anal sac infection and should be noted. Thick material can result in an anal sac impaction, which can be uncomfortable for the patient and can lead to "scooting" of the rear end. Anal sac expression can be difficult in patients with an impaction and may require sedation.

> **TECHNICIAN NOTE**
>
> The rectal examination provides an impressive amount of useful information and should be performed on every patient except those that will experience significant discomfort from the examination.

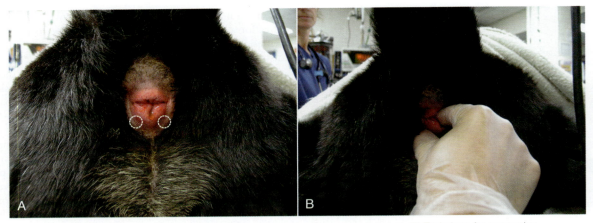

• **Fig. 7.13** (A) Approximate location of the anal sacs in a dog *(dotted circles)*. (B) Technique for expression of the left anal sac in a dog.

Urogenital

Much of the urinary system is evaluated during abdominal palpation and a rectal examination, as discussed previously. The kidneys, urinary bladder, and proximal urethra have already been examined. The only part of the urinary system left to be evaluated is the distal urethra, which opens at the tip of the penis in the male and into the vestibule in the female. In male dogs, the penis should be gently extruded by pulling back the skin of the prepuce. Any discharge within the prepuce should be noted and possibly sampled. The penis should be evaluated to ensure that the urethral opening is normal and appears patent. Any masses or wounds on the penis should be noted. Penile examination is not typically performed in the male cat except when the patient is sedated, such as in the case of urethral obstruction.

Examination of the vagina and vestibule is not routinely performed in dogs and cats. In cases with a presenting complaint referable to the lower urinary tract, a vaginal examination may be indicated. A digital vaginal examination may be performed by the veterinarian on the nonsedated dog, but often, sedation will be necessary. Sedation will always be required in the cat. In either case, the examiner should wear sterile gloves and should use copious lubrication to avoid causing trauma and discomfort to the patient.

In the United States, a vast majority of dogs and cats are sterilized. Therefore an examination of reproductive organs is not commonly performed. In the intact male dog or cat, the testicles should be examined gently with palpation of the scrotum to ensure that both testicles are present. Testicles should descend into the scrotum by 8 weeks of age in most patients and by 6 months in all patients. The testicles should be gently palpated to assess for asymmetry in size, masses, heat, or pain. The penis should be extruded and examined, as described earlier. In the intact female dog or cat, the reproductive organs are not as easily examined. A vaginal examination may be performed if pathology is suspected but is not part of a routine examination. The uterus cannot be palpated during abdominal palpation unless it is enlarged, as with pregnancy or pyometra. The ovaries cannot be palpated. It is good practice to palpate the mammary chains in all female dogs and cats, but it is especially important in sexually intact patients, because they have a much higher risk of mammary cancer. Most dogs and cats will have five mammary glands on each side of the ventral abdomen. They should be gently palpated for heat, swelling, masses, or discharge. In lactating animals, milk should be expressed and examined for blood or pus.

> **TECHNICIAN NOTE**
>
> A urogenital examination and mammary palpation are most important in patients that are sexually intact and are generally performed by the veterinarian.

Integument

A complete evaluation of the integumentary system will include examination of the hair, skin (including footpads and nails), and subcutaneous tissues. The character of the normal hair coat can vary greatly among breeds and among individual patients, but in general, it should be thick and shiny. Abnormal hair coats may be dull, greasy, or "rough" looking and may contain scale (flakes of shed epidermis). The coat should be visually evaluated for areas of thinning or *alopecia* (Fig. 7.14). If alopecia is noted, it should be described in terms of location (focal versus diffuse versus patchy, unilateral versus bilateral, symmetric versus asymmetric) and degree (partial versus complete). The coat should be inspected closely in alopecic areas to detect evidence of broken hairs, which may indicate that the alopecia is caused by scratching or **barbering,** excoriation, or underlying disease. The hair should be gently parted in several areas to look for evidence of ectoparasites, such as fleas. In extremely **pruritic** (itchy) animals, a flea comb can be used to improve the chances of identifying live fleas or their excrement.

> **TECHNICIAN NOTE**
>
> Dermatologic diseases are common in small animal patients. Familiarity with skin pathologies and the terminology for skin lesions will be useful.

The extent to which the skin is directly examined depends on the presenting complaint of the patient. A patient with no complaints referable to the skin (e.g., pruritus, flaking, or odor) need only have a cursory skin examination. Patients with complaints referable to the skin warrant a more thorough evaluation. In any patient lacking alopecia, the hair must be parted for evaluation of the skin. The ventral-caudal abdomen has a light covering of hair in many patients and is a good place to visualize the skin. Common abnormalities that can be identified on the skin include papules and pustules, which are seen commonly with bacterial skin infections. A papule is a pink or red elevated skin lesion smaller than 0.5 cm in diameter. A pustule is similar in size to a papule but is a raised area containing pus; it usually has a pink or red base with a white tip. Scales and crusts are caused by any inflammatory process affecting the outer layers of skin. Both appear as flakes and contain shed epidermal cells with crusts also containing inflammatory cells. They can be difficult to differentiate based on visual inspection alone and may require laboratory analysis. Excoriations are areas of self-trauma caused by scratching in a pruritic animal. The skin is a good area in which to see petechiae and ecchymoses, which usually indicate a primary hemostatic defect. Erythema (redness) of the skin may be noted focally or diffusely. Nail beds and footpads should be examined, especially in patients with diseased skin, to evaluate for redness, discharge, or ulceration.

Masses are commonly found on the skin and within the subcutaneous tissues in veterinary patients. Most masses will be caused by benign neoplastic processes, although palpable masses may represent malignancy, vaccine reactions, abscesses, or swelling caused by trauma. It is important that any masses be noted in the medical record in detail so that any changes in their size or appearance can be noted. Masses should be described based on their location, including whether they are on the surface of the skin (cutaneous) or under the skin (subcutaneous). Their exact location can be recorded in the medical record by using a body map, which allows for the precise marking of the location of the mass and is much more effective than written descriptions for comparison in future examinations. The size and shape of the mass should be noted. The size is most precisely recorded by using measuring calipers, although an estimation can be made if calipers are not available. The mass should be described as soft, fluctuant, or firm, and adherence to underlying structures should be noted by recording whether it is movable or fixed. Careful monitoring of cutaneous and subcutaneous masses is important in determining a diagnostic and therapeutic plan.

Lymph Nodes

In the normal patient, peripheral lymph nodes that can be palpated are the mandibular, prescapular, and popliteal lymph nodes. The axillary and inguinal lymph nodes typically are palpable only when they are significantly enlarged. Similarly, enlarged medial iliac lymph nodes may be palpable via a rectal examination, as discussed earlier. The mandibular lymph nodes are located on either side of the neck just caudal-dorsal to the ramus of the mandible and cranial-ventral to the mandibular salivary glands. They can be differentiated from the salivary gland because they tend to be more movable, slightly firmer, and smaller (in the normal patient). The prescapular lymph nodes are in the subcutaneous tissue just medial to the scapular-humeral joint on either side of the patient. These nodes often are encased in fat and may feel slightly softer than other normal nodes (Fig. 7.15A). The popliteal lymph nodes are located on the caudal aspect of each hindlimb at the level of the stifle joint (Fig. 7.15B). The axillary lymph nodes, if palpable,

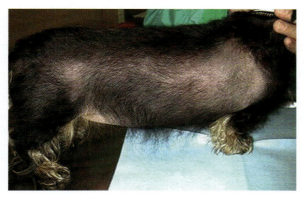

• **Fig. 7.14** Bilaterally symmetric truncal alopecia in a dog with hyperadrenocorticism.

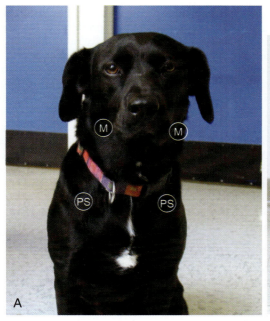
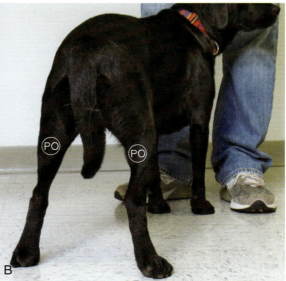

• **Fig. 7.15** (A) Dog showing the location of mandibular lymph nodes *(M)*. (B) Dog showing the location of popliteal lymph nodes *(PO)*.

will be in the subcutaneous space on the lateral aspect of the ventral thorax under the arm. The inguinal lymph nodes are in the most caudal part of the ventral abdomen just medial to the thighs on either side of the midline.

Lymph nodes should be palpated by gently isolating them between thumb and index finger. Ideally, the left and right lymph nodes are palpated simultaneously at each location to determine whether they are identical in size and shape. Normal lymph nodes are round to oval, slightly movable, and firm but slightly compressible. Abnormal lymph nodes may be enlarged, firm, warm, or painful. The most common abnormality palpated is an enlarged lymph node. It should be noted that lymph nodes in young animals (younger than 6 months of age) are normally mildly enlarged compared with the size they will be during adulthood. Lymph node enlargement may indicate that the node is infected, is reacting to local inflammation, or is neoplastic. Enlargement should be noted as focal (single node or single region) or generalized (all palpable nodes enlarged). The specific enlarged nodes should be noted, and their size measured with calipers or estimated.

TECHNICIAN NOTE

The peripheral lymph nodes that should be palpable in every patient are the mandibular, prescapular, and popliteal lymph nodes.

Musculoskeletal System

Examination of the musculoskeletal system will vary greatly depending on the patient's presenting complaint. In a patient without symptoms referable to the musculoskeletal system (e.g., lameness, swelling, difficulty rising, or pain), the examination will be cursory. All patients should be observed as they walk around the examination room or waiting area for signs of lameness that the owner may not have perceived. In patients without lameness, the musculoskeletal examination should include a visual inspection of the standing animal for asymmetry of the limbs. This is followed by gentle palpation of each limb and the vertebral column over the neck and back. Initial palpation of limbs should be performed such that opposite sides (i.e., left and right forelimbs, left and right hindlimbs) are examined simultaneously. This will allow for comparison with the opposite leg when swelling or pain is evaluated.

In a patient that is seen with a complaint related to the musculoskeletal system such as lameness or one in which the examination revealed an abnormality, a more thorough examination is indicated. This should start with observation of the animal walking or jogging on a lead for identification of lameness. Animals will put less weight on a painful limb when walking or shift the weight to the good limb. This results in the patient putting the head down when stepping on the good limb and pulling the head up when stepping on the painful limb. Once the affected limb has been identified, the veterinarian may place the patient in lateral recumbency, and each limb thoroughly examined one at a time. The soft tissues and long bones of the limb should be palpated with gradually increasing levels of pressure to identify swelling or pain. Then, starting at the toes, every joint should be put through a range of flexion and extension to isolate the examined joint and not move any other joints. It is important to examine all limbs so that the limb with perceived discomfort can be compared with the opposite limb. If the practitioner identifies pain in one limb and the patient does not show a similar response in the other limbs, it is likely that a problem has been identified. Similarly, the

technician should restrain the animal for the veterinarian to palpate the vertebral column one bone at a time by pressing down on their dorsal surface on the animal's back. The neck should be put through a full range of motion and any pain noted. These manipulations should only be performed by a veterinarian; the technician should act only as a dedicated restrainer during the process.

TECHNICIAN NOTE

In a patient with lameness, all limbs should be thoroughly examined to allow comparisons to be made and to isolate the affected area. Technicians should never attempt manipulation of the musculoskeletal system as unintentional patient injury may occur.

Nervous System

Like the musculoskeletal examination, the time allotted for the neurologic examination will vary greatly depending on the individual patient. The examination of every patient will include a subjective visual evaluation of mentation, visual acuity, and gait as it enters the examination room, as described in the section on observing patients in their surroundings. Most patients will have menace reflex and pupillary light reflex testing performed as part of the eye examination. If these parameters are considered normal and the patient does not have any complaints that could be related to the nervous system, the neurologic examination need not be any more extensive.

A patient with an abnormality noted on the cursory examination or one with a complaint that could be related to the nervous system should have a more complete neurologic examination carried out by the veterinarian. Presenting complaints that could be related to the nervous system include but are not limited to behavior changes, depression, lethargy, blindness, head tilt, circling, lameness, weakness, or paralysis. A complete neurologic examination includes an evaluation of mentation, gait and posture, muscle tone, cranial nerves, postural reactions, and reflexes. Mentation is noted by the technician during patient intake and is assessed subjectively during visual observation of the patient. It may be described as bright and alert, quiet, dull, obtunded (not interested in surroundings), stuporous (responsive only to noxious stimuli), or comatose (unresponsive to stimuli). Gait and posture are also observed at this time. The patient should be walked or jogged on a lead and made to turn when gait is assessed. Although animals with neurologic disease can have normal gait and posture, ataxia is a common gait abnormality in these patients. *Ataxia* refers to uncoordinated muscle movements when walking. When a patient's gait is evaluated, ataxia is identified when you are unable to predict where the foot will fall on the patient's next step. Ataxia can vary in type and severity, and it is often confused with lameness by owners. Muscle tone is subjectively assessed by visual inspection and palpation by the practitioner and involves determination of the anal sphincter tone. During a rectal examination, the anal sphincter muscles should tighten around the finger. Muscle atrophy or decreased tone may be noted in denervated muscle.

A cranial nerve examination is an essential part of every complete neurologic examination and is also completed by the veterinarian, with the technician serving as dedicated restrainer. Cranial nerve reflex tests are summarized in Table 7.3. The olfactory nerve (cranial nerve [CN] I) is not routinely tested, because a patient's response to scent is difficult to evaluate. The spinal accessory nerve (CN XI) is not evaluated. Lesions in this nerve cause atrophy of the trapezius muscle, which can be difficult to identify. The

TABLE 7.3 Examination of the Cranial Nerves

Nerve	Test	Normal	Abnormal
I. Olfactory	Volatile substance	Sniff, recoil, nose lick	No response
		Blink	No blink
II. Optic	Menace Pupillary light reflex	Direct, consensual responses present	No direct or consensual responses
III. Oculomotor	Pupillary light reflex Observe eye following an object	Direct, consensual responses present Normal eye movement	No direct response, consensual intact Impaired ocular movement in ventral, dorsal, and medial directions Dorsomedial strabismus
IV. Trochlear	Observe	Normal eye position	Muscle atrophy
	Palpate temporalis	Normal muscle tone	No blink
	Corneal reflex	Eye blink	No blink
	Palpebral reflex	Eye blink	
V. Trigeminal	Observe ability to chew	Normal jaw movement	Inability to chew
	Palpate masseter muscle	Normal muscle tone	Muscle atrophy
	Pupillary light reflex	Direct, consensual responses present	No direct or consensual response present
VI. Abducens	Observe	Normal eye position	Medial strabismus
VII. Facial	Observe	Facial symmetry	Lip droop
	Corneal reflex	Eye blink	No blink
	Palpebral reflex	Eye blink	No blink
	Menace	Eye blink	No blink
VIII. Acoustic	Hand clap	Startle response	No response
	Move head horizontally, vertically	Normal nystagmus	No response, resting or positional nystagmus
IX. Glossopharyngeal	Gag reflex	Swallow	No response
X. Vagus	Gag reflex	Swallow	No response
	Oculocardiac reflex	Bradycardia	No response
	Laryngeal reflex	Cough	No response
XI. Accessory	Palpate neck muscles	Normal muscle tone	Muscle atrophy
XII. Hypoglossal	Tongue stretch	Retraction of tongue	No response

From McCurnin DM, Poffenbarger EM. *Small Animal and Physical Diagnosis and Clinical Procedures.* Philadelphia, PA: Saunders; 1991

position of the eyes at rest and the doll's eye reflex (physiologic nystagmus) will evaluate CN III, the trochlear nerve (CN IV), and the abducens nerve (CN VI). The doll's eye reflex is performed by turning the patient's muzzle and head from left to right. As the head moves in one direction, the eyes should initially move to the opposite direction and then snap back to the center. The palpebral reflex is tested by tapping the medial and lateral canthus of the eye to induce a blink. The corneal reflex is tested by holding the eyelids open and gently touching the cornea with a wet cotton swab. Gently pinching the lips with a hemostat or placing the hemostat inside either nostril should cause the patient to move away and

will evaluate the sensory portion of the trigeminal nerve (CN V). Facial symmetry should be assessed because a droop to one side compared with the other can indicate a lesion of the facial nerve (CN VII). The eyes should be examined for nystagmus, which can indicate a lesion in the vestibulocochlear nerve (CN VIII). The gag reflex is performed by pressing with a finger on the back of the patient's tongue; this should elicit contraction of the pharyngeal muscles, which can be used to evaluate the glossopharyngeal nerve (CN IX) and branches of the vagus nerve (CN X). A visual examination of the tongue to identify deviation to one side or another can identify lesions of the hypoglossal nerve (CN XII).

A neurologic examination of the limbs involves assessment of postural reactions, reflexes, and sensation. Conscious proprioception is tested in the standing patient by picking up one paw and placing its dorsal surface onto the floor. The normal patient will quickly lift and turn the foot so that the palmar or plantar surface is touching the floor. This test should be performed on each leg. Note that patients with significant muscle weakness may not have the strength to lift the limb to turn it, so you should help support the patient's weight. Limb strength can be assessed by forcing the patient to hop on one limb at a time and comparing their strength to do so between limbs. In small patients, this can be done easily by supporting the weight of the other three limbs while the patient is moved from side to side on one limb. In larger dogs, it may be necessary to hold up only one forelimb and move the patient from side to side on the opposite forelimb while keeping the hindlimbs still. A similar technique can be used to evaluate the hindlimbs. Reflex testing should be performed with the patient in lateral recumbency and relaxed. Forelimb reflexes to be tested include the withdrawal reflex, the biceps reflex, and the triceps reflex. Forelimb reflexes can be difficult to obtain, and the withdrawal reflex is the most reliable. It is performed by pinching the patient's toe, which should result in strong flexion of the limb. Hindlimb reflexes are more reliable and include the withdrawal reflex, the patellar reflex, and the cranial tibial reflex. Reflex responses should be scored from 0 to 4, as described in Table 7.4. Although not a limb reflex, the cutaneous trunci reflex can provide information regarding the integrity of spinal segments. It is performed by gently pinching the skin on either side of the lateral thorax, which should cause twitching of superficial muscles. Pinching the anal mucosa should result in a reflex contraction of the anal sphincter muscles (the perineal reflex). Sensation should be tested in paralyzed limbs by aggressively pinching the bones of the toes with a hemostat. The animal with intact sensation will vocalize or will try to bite. Note that pulling the leg back into flexion does not indicate normal sensation, but rather, indicates an intact withdrawal reflex. Absence of sensation suggests a more severe lesion. Results of the complete neurologic examination should allow for anatomic localization of the source of neurologic symptoms.

TABLE 7.4	Grading of Reflex Responses
Grade	**Description**
0	No response
1	Hyporeflexia (less than normal response)
2	Normal response
3	Hyperreflexia (greater than normal response)
4	Clonus (repetitive response)

History and Physical Examination of Large Animals

When a large animal patient is presented for an evaluation, the medical record is generated. The history and physical examination are the most important parts of the medical record and serve as the starting point for identifying the patient's problems. Once this initial information is collected, the record may be expanded to include laboratory tests, diagnostic imaging, and special examinations of body systems, according to the purpose of the examination and the condition of the patient.

History

Husbandry practices, animal environments, and economic factors affecting large animals differ significantly from those of small animals; however, the basic approach to effective history taking is the same for both large and small animal patients. Experienced clients can provide an excellent history with little coaching, but most clients do not know how to give a concise, useful summary of their animal's condition. The technician will need to ask specific, open-ended questions to obtain relevant information, keeping the information on an organized timeline. Once the history is obtained, the accuracy of the information must be evaluated as owners may unknowingly give inaccurate information, believing it to be true. Occasionally, owners provide false information to avoid embarrassment, not wanting to appear ignorant or to admit that they may have made a mistake in management of their animal.

Even though the history will focus on the chief clinical problem of an animal or group of animals, the technician must keep the bigger picture of herd health and husbandry in mind when taking a history on large animal patients.

Owner/Agent Information

It is common for large animals to be attended by a person (or persons) other than the owner, such as a trainer, groomer, farm hand, stable owner, or lessee (animal lease agreements are not uncommon). It is important to determine the identity of the person presenting the animal and to establish their relationship to the animal. If the owner is not present, it is necessary to obtain appropriate contact information so that the veterinarian can communicate directly with the owner and to determine who has the decision-making responsibility for the animal, because some owners may entrust the trainer or agent to make decisions about the animal's treatment and care.

The economic value of certain large animals created a need many years ago for an insurance industry to protect owners' investments. Equine insurance coverage is common in the United States, and valuable ruminant breeding animals are often insured; therefore the insurance status of the animal should be determined. *Mortality insurance* covers the value of the animal in case of death. *Surgical insurance* covers specific costs of surgery and hospitalization with some limitations—like human health insurance policies. *Loss of use insurance* states specifically the intended use of the animal (breeding, racing, etc.) and, if the animal cannot perform its intended function because of illness or injury, the owner may

TABLE 7.5 Age/Sex Terminology for the Horse

Term	Description
Foal	Young horse, from birth to weaning (weaning usually at 4–7 months old)
Weanling	Young horse, from weaning to first birthday
Yearling	1–1½ years
Long yearling	1½ years to second birthday
Colt	Intact male 2–3 years old
Filly	Female 2–3 years old
Stallion	Intact male after third birthday
Mare	Female after third birthday
Gelding	Castrated male of any age

TABLE 7.6 Age/Sex Terminology for Ruminants

Age	Cattle	Sheep	Goat
Parturition (freshening)	Calving	Lambing	Kidding
Neonate	Calf	Lamb	Kid
Male (<1 year)	Bull calf	Ram lamb	Buck kid
Female (<1 year)	Heifer calf	Ewe lamb	Doe kid
Immature female (has not given birth)	Heifer	Yearling ewe	Yearling doe
Mature female	Cow	Ewe	Doe (nanny)
Mature male	Bull	Ram	Buck (billy)
Castrated male	Steer	Wether	Wether

be reimbursed for lost potential income. Contact information for the insurance company and insurance agent should be noted in the medical record as they may be involved in the decision-making process for the affected animal. The type of insurance policy and the estimated economic value of the animal should also be recorded, because these factors often play an important role in the diagnostic and treatment options provided for the animal.

Signalment of the Animal
The signalment of the animal typically includes age, sex, breed, color, and reproductive status. This information helps in formulating the patient's rule-out list of potential diagnoses, because certain disease conditions have known predilections for subsets of the population according to signalment. For example, gray coat color in horses is associated with a higher incidence of melanoma than other coat colors; obstructive urolithiasis in ruminants is almost always associated with males; and β-mannosidase deficiency has been reported only in the Nubian breed of goats.

Another important part of large animal signalment is the intended use of the animal. Most large animals are kept for specific purposes, such as breeding, athletic performance, and commercial production of meat, milk, hair, or other products. The animal's occupation may predispose it to certain diseases or injuries, such as the increased occurrence of osteochondral "chip" fractures in racehorses versus pleasure horses, and the higher incidence of mastitis in dairy cattle than in beef cattle.

The terminology used by clients with large animals to describe their animals is species specific, and the technician should be familiar with commonly used terms for the sex, age, and reproductive status of various large animal species (Tables 7.5 and 7.6).

Individual History and Chief Complaint
The history is usually obtained before the physical examination is begun, because it may contain helpful information for the examiner. However, in emergency situations, it may be necessary to evaluate and stabilize the animal before proceeding with obtaining details about the animal's history. For example, an animal's vaccination and deworming history has little immediate value for an animal in need of treatment for severe shock and can be determined after the animal is stabilized.

TECHNICIAN NOTE
In an emergency, it may be necessary to perform the physical examination before taking a detailed history.

The individual history includes two major components: the history of the current problem and the general history of the animal. The history of the current problem is usually taken first and includes the client's chief complaint, also known as the *primary reason* for requesting an examination, although it is not always the animal's primary problem. It is important to listen to the client and to avoid any perception of discounting or disregarding their concerns. Once the chief complaint has been determined, the technician can begin a more directed line of questioning to accurately characterize the problem in terms of duration, progression, severity, frequency, and response to any previous therapy. Further questioning will focus on specific body systems affected by the current problem; in an animal with respiratory disease, the presence and character of a cough, nasal discharge, or respiratory noise are important. Information on appetite, dental care, abdominal pain, and fecal volume and consistency are important in assessing an animal with GI disease.

The general history includes information on the animal before the current problem developed and may include information on diet, exercise, preventive health maintenance, reproductive status, and previous medical problems and surgical procedures.

Medication and Treatment History
Most large animal facilities keep first aid kits and pharmaceuticals on the premises, and animals are often treated before the veterinarian is called. This situation is common in large animal practices, especially with production animals, where economics often dictates whether the owner calls the veterinarian immediately or attempts to solve the problem themselves. Owners may be reluctant to report this and may need to be asked specifically whether they have treated the animal and how.

Herd Health History
Large animals are seldom kept as isolated individuals and therefore commonly share resources with other large animals. Similarly, animals often receive care for preventive health maintenance, such as vaccination, deworming, and external parasite control as a group.

After the individual history is obtained, it may be important to gather information on the size and nature of the group or herd and the resources that they share, such as food and water, shelter facilities, and common land areas (i.e., pastures and pens). Animals may be grouped randomly, but more commonly, large animals are grouped by age, sex, reproductive status, and other common attributes. If other animals are affected, the signalment of those animals can hold vital clues to the nature of the problem. Shared food, water, and grazing sources allow ready transmission of infectious agents and widespread distribution of parasites and toxins. Even horses that are housed in individual stalls are usually placed in common turnout areas for daily exercise, encountering other animals and/or their fecal material and possible parasites. Herd conditions may also create competition for food and water, preventing some individuals from getting adequate nutrition.

TECHNICIAN NOTE

Large animals often share resources, such as food, water, shelter, and turnout areas, with other animals. This should be noted on health forms.

The source of feed, hay, bedding, and water may not always be the farm on which the animals are kept. Under pasture conditions, stream, creek, or pond water may provide water for the animals' use. The purity of such water sources may be affected by "upstream" agricultural activities and runoff or even the local wildlife population. Feed, hay, and bedding are often purchased and shipped to the farm by outside vendors; their quality and content may not be guaranteed. For example, poisonous plants may be inadvertently harvested when hay is cut and baled, proving toxic if animals consume it. In certain areas of the country, black walnut trees may be included in the production of wood shavings, but no labeling requirements for packaging have been put forth; black walnut shavings may cause severe laminitis in horses when used for bedding. Also, the potential for wildlife or rodents sharing large animal habitats may lead to disease spread. For instance, the Virginia opossum has been implicated in the spread of equine protozoal myelitis.

A summary of basic large animal history information is presented in Box 7.1.

Physical Examination of Large Animals

Combined with a thorough history, the physical examination forms the basis for identifying a patient's actual problems. Most clinicians use a problem-oriented approach to diagnosis and treatment. History and physical examination also serve as the basis for the technician evaluation, to be prioritized according to the urgency of the situation.

A consistent and systematic approach to physical examination will increase the proficiency of the examiner and will decrease the likelihood of overlooking important findings regardless of animal size or species.

Physical Examination of the Equine

The diagnostic physical examination may range from a basic TPR examination to a thorough multisystem or system-specific evaluation, depending on the patient's problems. In addition to the diagnostic type of physical examination, horse owners may request other types of "routine" physical examinations for their horses. The *insurance examination* may be required by the insurance company before a horse can receive insurance coverage. It

• BOX 7.1   Large Animal History

The following information should be obtained and recorded in the medical record:

Person Providing Information
   Owner, agent, trainer, or farm employee
Insurance Information
   Company name, contact information
   Policy number
   Type of insurance
Patient Signalment
   Age, sex, breed, color, and identifying markings
Diet
   Feed schedule
   Forage/hay
   Type
   Source
   Grain
      Type
      Source
   Supplements
   Dietary changes
      Intake: increased or decreased
      Change in appetite for certain foodstuffs
      Change in source of foodstuffs
   Water
   Sources
   Availability
Housing Type
Reproductive Status
Vaccination History
Deworming History
Production History: any Increase or Decrease in Production
Previous Illnesses/Surgical Procedures
Presenting (Chief) Complaint
   Time of onset
   Speed of onset: peracute, acute, or chronic
   Duration
   Progression of severity: improving, worsening, or static
   Previous treatments/medications
Herd Information
   Number of animals in herd
   Number affected
   Number of deaths

may range from a basic physical examination to a thorough, in-depth examination of all body systems; the type of insurance and the value of the animal will dictate the depth of examination required by the insurance company. The *prepurchase examination* is conducted before the sale of an animal is completed and is a common procedure in equine practice. A seller and a buyer are identified, and the veterinarian performing the examination is presumed to be working in the buyer's best interests (the veterinarian is paid by the buyer). The scope of the prepurchase examination is dictated by the intended use of the horse and its estimated value; it may be a simple physical examination or an in-depth examination, including biopsy, blood work, endoscopy, ECG and/or echocardiography, and diagnostic imaging. Prepurchase examinations are a potential source of lawsuits against the veterinarian; therefore veterinarians go to great lengths to document the findings of prepurchase examinations without overstating their findings as predictions or guarantees of future performance.

The technician should understand the potentially sensitive nature of insurance and prepurchase examinations and should help ensure the accuracy and privacy of the results.

Getting Started

The basic physical examination always begins with observation of the animal from a distance. Good examiners will take advantage of this opportunity to observe the animal before and during interaction, considering the total picture of the horse and its environment. The attitude, alertness, and general body condition of the horse are noted. Movements of the horse provide an opportunity to observe lameness. If food and water are available, appetite, mastication, and swallowing reflexes can be observed. Interactions with other animals can also provide useful information.

After the horse is observed and its temperament, presence or absence of pain, and possible body systems that will need to be evaluated are gauged, the most appropriate method of physical restraint can be selected. All physical examinations begin with appropriate physical restraint. Physical restraint is necessary for the safety of the personnel and of the horse. Depending on the body system (or systems) to be evaluated, the method of physical restraint may change during the examination. Chemical restraint may need to be applied to supplement physical restraint of painful or uncooperative patients (see Chapter 6, "Restraint and Handling of Animals").

After proper restraint has been applied, the hands-on physical examination can begin. It includes TPR measurements, heart and lung auscultation, abdominal auscultation, determination of hydration status, examination of mucous membranes, and height and weight measurement.

Body Temperature

Temperature is almost always taken rectally, using a standard mercury or digital thermometer. Although any thermometer may be used on large animals, thermometers designed strictly for large animals are commercially available and are typically 5 inches long with a thicker glass casing than a regular thermometer and a "ring top," which allows the user to attach a short (<12 inches) string. This allows for managing two commonly encountered situations: aspiration of the thermometer into the rectum and unexpected expelling of the thermometer out of the rectum. Some horses may pull the anus inward while the thermometer is in place, resulting in the entire thermometer being pulled into the rectum. This is potentially serious if the thermometer breaks inside the rectum or if the horse strains to defecate, at which point life-threatening perforation of the rectum by the thermometer may occur. The presence of the thermometer in the anus may also stimulate defecation, causing the thermometer to be passed out of the rectum, fall to the ground, and break. Broken thermometer glass can puncture hooves or skin or may be eaten as the horse browses for food. A firm grip should be maintained on the thermometer through the entire procedure, or a string tied at one end to the ring top and the other end to an alligator clip which may be secured to the horse's tail hairs or hair coat (not the skin). If the horse pulls the thermometer into the rectum, the string can be used to gently retrieve it or to digitally follow the string into the rectum for retrieval. If the horse pushes the thermometer out of the rectum, the secured string prevents it from falling on the ground.

The string should be no more than 12 inches long, because longer strings result in the thermometer dangling against the legs, causing some horses to kick.

Inserting the rectal thermometer requires some skill. The thermometer should be lubricated with petroleum jelly, mineral oil, or water; however, dipping the thermometer in the horse's water bucket should be avoided, because it will be viewed as unsanitary by onlookers. To insert the thermometer, the technician should stand next to the horse's hindquarters (never behind the horse), facing in the caudal direction (Fig. 7.16). If the horse is likely to resist by kicking or appears agitated by the manipulations of the tail and hindquarters, the technician can stand behind a stall door or a stack of hay bales for protection. The tail is grasped near the base and elevated or gently pushed to the opposite side. The tail should be moved only enough to get clear entrance to the anus (Fig. 7.17). Some horses respond best to gentle rubbing of

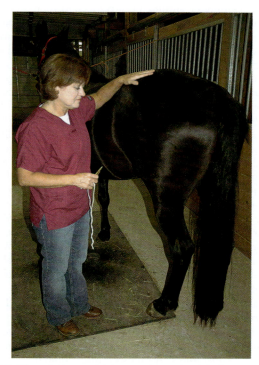

• **Fig. 7.16** When taking rectal temperature, stand facing caudally and maintain contact with the horse.

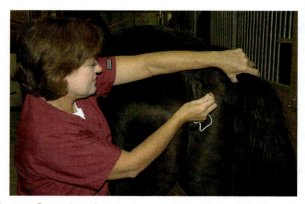

• **Fig. 7.17** Grasp the tail at the base and move it gently to the side; the thermometer can then be inserted through the anus into the rectum.

the perianal area before the anus is touched with the thermometer, rather than thrusting the thermometer into the anus with no warning. The anal opening may be identified visually or by feel and the thermometer gently inserted with a twisting motion. If the thermometer does not advance easily, it should never be forced, because the rectal wall can be easily perforated. If the horse strains in resistance, the technician should stop and try distracting the animal by offering feed or having the handler tap on the horse's forehead while the thermometer is being inserted. The thermometer usually enters horizontally, but some horses require tipping of the thermometer slightly upward (dorsally) to enter the rectum.

> **TECHNICIAN NOTE**
> Rectal thermometers should be inserted and advanced into the rectum without use of force to avoid perforation.

The thermometer should be advanced several inches into the rectum and then either held in the hand or clipped to the tail or coat hairs and left in place for at least 60 seconds (mercury type) or until the audible or visual signal is heard or seen (digital type).

Normal rectal temperature varies, depending on the age, breed, and environment of the animal. Body temperature is typically lowest in the morning. Normal rectal temperature of the adult horse at rest is 99.0°F to 101.5°F. Temperatures from 101.5°F to 102.0°F indicate a "gray zone" that may be normal for some individuals, especially in hot weather or after workout. A temperature greater than 102.0°F is always suspicious except after physical exercise, which can temporarily elevate temperature to 102°F and greater. As the animal cools down, the temperature should decrease. All elevated temperatures should be retaken 15–20 minutes later to allow for this. Normal values for TPR are given in Table 7.7.

Other factors may influence temperature. Large breeds and draft horses tend to have rectal temperatures at the lower end of the temperature range. Neonatal foals may lack the ability to generate body heat and often have low body temperatures immediately after birth. As the heat-generating mechanisms develop, older foals may have, on average, an approximately 1°F higher temperature compared with adults for the first few days to weeks after birth. Rectal procedures, such as a manual or endoscopic rectal examination, may allow air to enter the rectum, causing falsely lower rectal temperatures. The temperature should be taken before any rectal procedure is performed.

If the rectum contains feces, the thermometer tip sometimes may be inadvertently inserted into a fecal ball. This is the most common cause of unusually low readings and necessitates repeating the procedure. If the temperature reading is suspicious, it should be taken again at the end of the examination after the horse has rested.

Pulse Rate and Heart Rate

HR and pulse rate are not the same; *heart rate* refers to the number of heart beats per minute (beats/min [bpm]); *pulse rate* refers to the number of palpable arterial pulse waves per minute. In normal animals, HR and pulse rate are equal.

Pulse rate is taken by palpation of arteries. As blood passes from arteries through capillary beds, a dampening effect on arterial blood pressure fluctuations (waves) is noted; therefore veins do not have palpable pulses.

Auscultation of the heart allows for taking HR, not pulse rate, and is done because some heart abnormalities may produce audible heart sounds that are not necessarily accompanied by an arterial pulse. For accuracy, when the heart is auscultated, the arterial pulse should be simultaneously palpated to ensure that every audible heartbeat is accompanied by a palpable pulse wave (Fig. 7.18). If each audible heartbeat is not accompanied by a pulse wave—a condition called *pulse deficit*—the clinician should be notified.

Arterial pulses may be palpated at several locations. The most convenient location is the facial artery, where it crosses the ventral aspect of the mandible, rostral to the origin of the masseter muscle (Fig. 7.19). Two or three fingers are lightly rolled back and forth across the ventromedial aspect of the mandible just rostral to the masseter muscle to identify the facial artery and facial vein; these vessels lie side by side and form a tubular, compressible type of structure. Once identified, the vascular bundle is firmly pressed against the mandible to feel the arterial pulse (Fig. 7.20). Care should be taken not to press too tightly as the artery may be occluded and pulse not easily felt. Large animal HR is much lower than that of their small animal counterparts, often requiring more patience to identify a palpable pulse.

> **TECHNICIAN NOTE**
> The point where the facial artery crosses the ventromedial aspect of the mandible is the most convenient location for obtaining pulse rate.

TABLE 7.7	Normal TPR Values for Adult Large Animals		
	Rectal Temperature, °F	Heart Rate	Respiratory Rate
Horse	99.0–101.5	28–44/minute	6–16/minute
Cattle	101.5 (range, 100.4–103.1)	40–80/minute	10–30/minute
Sheep	102.5 (range, 102.0–104.0)	70–90/minute	12–25/minute
Goat	102.0 (range, 101.5–104.0)	70–90/minute	15–30/minute

TPR, Body temperature, pulse rate, and respiration rate.

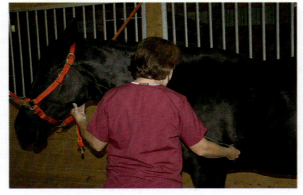

• **Fig. 7.18** Simultaneous palpation of arterial pulse on the facial artery and auscultation of the heart for possible pulse deficit.

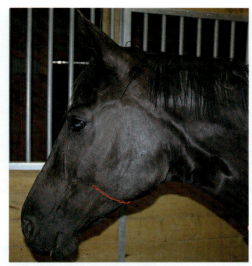

• **Fig. 7.19** The facial artery *(red highlight)* courses along the rostral aspect of the masseter muscle and crosses the ventromedial aspect of the mandible.

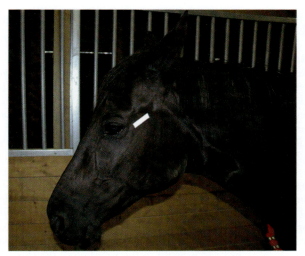

• **Fig. 7.21** Location of the transverse facial artery *(white mark)*.

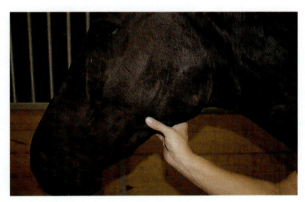

• **Fig. 7.20** Press the vascular bundle firmly against the medial aspect of the mandible.

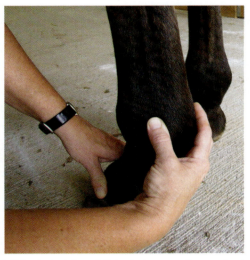

• **Fig. 7.22** Palpation of the digital arteries over the proximal sesamoid bones.

Other arteries are available for obtaining pulse rates. The transverse facial artery is in a horizontal depression about 1 inch caudal to the lateral canthus of the eye, just below the zygomatic arch (Fig. 7.21). The coccygeal artery is located along the ventral midline of the tail, supplying blood to the tail. The dorsal metatarsal artery is located between metatarsals 3 and 4 (cannon bone and lateral splint bone) on the hindlimbs. The lateral and medial digital arteries can be palpated where they cross over the abaxial aspect of the proximal sesamoid bones of each leg or just proximal to the collateral cartilages of each hoof (Fig. 7.22). The carotid artery has a pulse wave but is difficult to accurately palpate in large animals because of its deep position and therefore is seldom useful for palpation.

The main features of the pulse are rate and rhythm. The rate is recorded as the number of beats per minute (bpm); 28 to 48 bpm is normal in adult horses at rest. Foals have a rate of 60 to 80 bpm immediately after birth: this climbs to 75 to 100 bpm during the first week or two of life before gradually decreasing toward the adult rate over the next several weeks to months. Athletic horses may normally have rates less than 28 bpm; 24 bpm is not uncommon in racehorses.

The pulse rhythm is recorded as regular or irregular. Irregular rhythm likely indicates arrhythmia of the heart. The most common cause of pulse irregularity in horses is second-degree atrioventricular (AV) block, a type of heart arrhythmia caused by failure of the electric current generated by the atria to reach the ventricles. Intermittent blockage of current occurs at the AV node, resulting in "dropped" pulse beats, which usually occur in *a regular pattern* every third or fourth heartbeat. Second-degree AV block is readily identified by palpating the pulse. The regular rhythm is interrupted by a single "lost" (dropped) beat, with "lost" beats occurring at regular intervals (beat-beat-beat-no beat-beat-beat-beat-no beat, etc.). Even though second-degree AV block is usually considered a normal finding in horses, its presence should be noted in the medical record. Horses with this arrhythmia may have low resting HR—less than 28 bpm. Second-degree AV block is more common in athletically fit horses. It should disappear in any horse after exercise and is believed to be caused by increased tone from the vagus nerve, part of the parasympathetic nervous system.

Pulse quality is often described subjectively in nonspecific terms, such as *strong*, *bounding*, *weak*, or *thready*. The usefulness of such results depends on the technician's experience in assessing the pulse and should not be overinterpreted.

Respiratory Rate

The number of respirations per minute can be counted in several ways: (1) by using the stethoscope, listening to air movements in and out of the trachea or chest; (2) by touch, feeling the movement of air in and out of a nostril; and (3) by visually observing/counting chest movements per minute.

Respirations should be characterized by effort and depth and may be described as "shallow," "deep," "labored," or "gasping." Horses normally use a combination of thoracic and abdominal muscles to breathe; this is called *costoabdominal breathing*. Some painful conditions of the chest may lead to increased use of abdominal muscles to breathe, referred to as an *increased abdominal effort*. Normal horses cannot breathe through the mouth; mouth breathing is considered abnormal and, if observed, should be noted in the medical record and brought to the attention of the clinician.

Respiratory noises are not uncommon in horses and are often significant findings. Noises may be characterized as "wheezing," "whistling," "honking," "snoring," or "fluttering" and may be heard only when the horse is at rest or only during exercise. It is important to note the horse's activity when the noise is heard and whether the noise occurs during inspiration, expiration, or both.

The normal RR of an adult horse at rest is 6–16 breaths per minute and is higher during hot weather or after physical activity. Foals have a high RR at birth because of residual fluid in the lower airways with newborn foals. The birth RR of 80 to 90 will slow to 60 to 80 in the first 5 to 10 minutes after birth before gradually decreasing to 20–40 for the first week or two of life.

> **TECHNICIAN NOTE**
>
> Open-mouth breathing in horses is never normal and should be reported to the clinician immediately.

Heart Auscultation

Auscultation may be done on the left or right side of the chest, although most of the heart valves and sounds are heard best from the left side. However, the right side should not be overlooked; some murmurs are audible only on the right side and will be missed if the horse is auscultated only from the left.

Horses are athletes; the heart of the average horse may be as large as a basketball. The landmarks for basic auscultation of the heart are the same on either side of the chest. Dorsoventrally, the landmarks of the heart are the level of the shoulder joint for the heart base and the point of the elbow (olecranon) for the heart apex (Fig. 7.23). Craniocaudally, the landmark is defined by the caudal border of the triceps muscle, which roughly divides the heart into cranial and caudal halves.

Heart sounds are easier to hear when performing auscultation cranial to the caudal border of the triceps muscle. Because the triceps muscle is too thick to allow any heart sounds to be heard through it, the head of the stethoscope must be placed directly against the chest wall. To expose the chest wall at this location, the triceps muscle can be gently elevated away from the chest wall before the stethoscope is positioned (Fig. 7.24). Another approach is to advance the forelimb to a more forward position, as if the horse were taking a step forward, moving the triceps cranially. Many horses are reluctant to hold this position for any length of time.

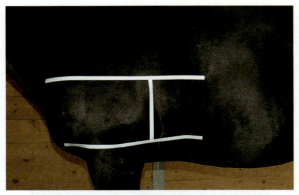

• **Fig. 7.23**

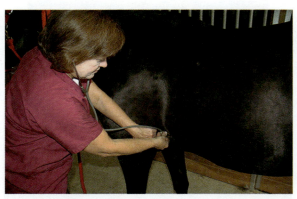

• **Fig. 7.24** The triceps muscle is gently lifted away from the chest wall to provide access for the stethoscope.

HR is counted as beats per minute. The cardiac sounds S_1 (lub) and S_2 (dub) are components of one heartbeat. A common error, especially for those accustomed to small animal auscultation, is to count S_1 and S_2 as separate beats, essentially doubling the actual HR. HR in large animals is slow with loud, distinct heart sounds, which may lead to possible confusion.

Auscultation is also used to detect abnormal heart sounds. Murmurs are not uncommon in horses, although most equine murmurs are normal heart sounds that are simply the result of large volumes of blood moving at high speeds through the heart valves. Because of the large heart size, these sounds are amplified and are referred to as *ejection murmurs*, which are commonly heard in horses and should disappear when the horse is exercised. True cardiac disease is unusual in horses but usually will be accompanied by murmurs or other abnormal sounds.

Heart murmurs are assessed for loudness, character, and the timing of the murmur in the cardiac cycle (systolic, diastolic, or continuous). The horse may be exercised to see if the abnormal sound disappears, stays the same, or gets louder with exercise. Using these initial criteria, the veterinarian decides whether further evaluation of the cardiovascular system is warranted.

> **TECHNICIAN NOTE**
>
> Ejection murmurs are commonly auscultated in the horse and regarded as normal findings.

Lung Auscultation

Despite the large size of equine lungs, breath sounds may be difficult to hear. A quiet environment is important for an accurate evaluation, with lung auscultation *always* being performed on *both* sides of the chest. Respiratory diseases do not necessarily affect both lungs and pleural cavities, resulting in markedly different auscultation findings over both the right and left lung fields of a single individual. Because of the large size of the lungs and possible uneven distribution of disease, auscultation findings may vary, even over different areas of the same lung.

The borders of the lung fields are the same for the right and left sides of the chest and are outlined in Fig. 7.25. The lung field basically consists of a cranioventral area and a caudal-dorsal area; a part of the cranial-ventral field is obscured by the shoulder musculature and cannot be heard. The stethoscope is placed in several locations within the lung field, and several breaths are listened to at each location (Fig. 7.26). Normally, air movement in and out of the airways should be heard with each chest excursion; sounds may be amplified in foals, thin animals, and any animal after exercise. Occasionally, it is desirable to induce deep breathing to accentuate the lung sounds. This is easily accomplished by occluding the nostrils temporarily until the horse begins to object to the lack of air; at the first sign of discomfort, the examiner releases the nostrils and immediately moves to auscultate the chest. Abnormal respiratory sounds include wheezes, crackles, and moist gurgling sounds; the absence of breath sounds may also be significant. The veterinarian should be alerted when abnormal sounds are detected.

Abdominal Auscultation

A stethoscope is used to listen to abdominal sounds, which are created by movements of the intestines. This is commonly referred to as *gastrointestinal motility,* a term that is somewhat misleading, because some sounds are generated by the passive movement of gas and liquids within the intestines without being propelled by the intestinal musculature. It is not completely accurate to assume that all intestinal sounds are from functional intestines; patients with GI disease or diseased portions of intestine may have little or no purposeful motility, yet passive fluid and gas sounds may be heard. Experience is required to distinguish active motility from passive sounds.

Abdominal auscultation should be performed on both sides of the horse. Although auscultation can be performed at any location on the abdominal wall, common sites for auscultation are in the areas known as the *right* and *left flanks,* which are slightly depressed areas between the pelvis and the caudal margin of the rib cage. The point of the hip (tuber coxae) identifies the dorsal extent of the flank area (Fig. 7.27), an area where horses often display sensitivity to being touched; these areas should be approached slowly and gently. A good approach is to place the hand with the stethoscope on the horse's back and slowly slide it to the flank or lower abdominal area.

A standard four-point auscultation is sufficient for most patients. A stethoscope is used to auscultate the upper and lower flanks on both sides of the abdomen. The four points of auscultation are referred to as *upper left, upper right, lower left,* and *lower right abdominal quadrants* (Fig. 7.28). Intestinal motility sounds, also called *borborygmi,* have been described as sounding like thunder rumbling or an approaching freight train and are associated with coordinated, normal

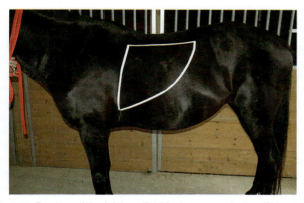

• **Fig. 7.25** Borders of the left lung field for lung auscultation. Side view of horse shows a cone-shaped mark on the periphery of the lung.

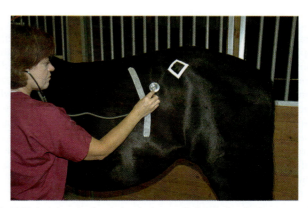

• **Fig. 7.27** Landmarks for abdominal auscultation in the flank area are the point of the hip (tuber coxae) and the last rib. The hip point of the horse is marked.

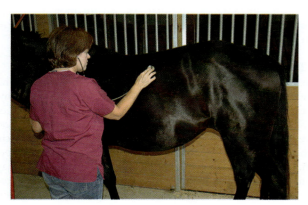

• **Fig. 7.26** Auscultation of the left caudal-dorsal lung field.

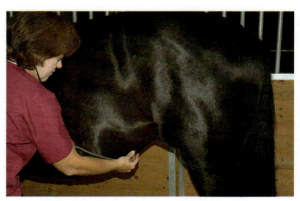

• **Fig. 7.28** Auscultation of the lower left abdominal quadrant.

• BOX 7.2 | Four-Point Abdominal Auscultation

Findings from the four-point auscultation are recorded in the medical record by using a grid that identifies each abdominal quadrant.

Upper Left Quadrant	Upper Right Quadrant
Lower Left Quadrant	Lower Right Quadrant

Results of auscultation at each location are recorded as follows:
0 = no motility heard
+ 1 = hypomotility (<1 borborygmus/minute)
+ 2 = normal motility (1–3 borborygmi/minute)
+ 3 = hypermotility (>3 borborygmi/minute)

For example, a horse with hypomotility in the lower right quadrant and a normal number of borborygmi in all other quadrants would be recorded as follows:

+2	+2
+2	+1

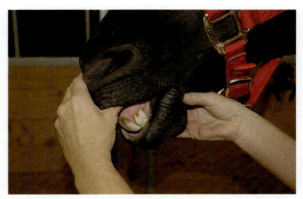

• **Fig. 7.29** Examination of the gums. The upper lip is gently elevated to the extent necessary for the gum tissue to be seen.

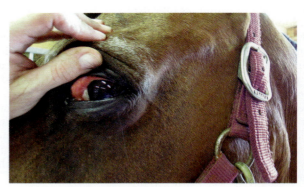

• **Fig. 7.30** Examination of the conjunctiva. The upper lid is gently elevated upward, without pinching or pressing.

patterns of large intestinal motility. The number of borborygmi per minute is counted in each abdominal quadrant, leaving the stethoscope in place for *at least 1 minute* at *each* of the four auscultation points to get an accurate count. "Normal" motility is considered to be one to three borborygmi per minute in each abdominal quadrant. More than this is hypermotility, whereas a lesser rate is regarded as hypomotility. The complete absence of **borborygmus** is equated with "intestinal standstill," properly termed *ileus*, a condition indicative of serious intestinal disease associated with increased morbidity and mortality seen in colic patients. Auscultation in colic patients may be confusing, because gas and fluid "tinkling" sounds may still be heard in horses with complete ileus. These are passive sounds and are not to be confused with the motility of normally functioning intestines.

Findings of four-point abdominal auscultation are recorded in the medical record by using the grid system, as shown in Box 7.2.

TECHNICIAN NOTE

The presence of intestinal sounds does not always indicate the presence of intestinal motility.

Mucous Membranes

Mucous membranes are tissues that can produce and secrete mucus; their color is helpful in the diagnosis of disease. Several mucous membranes are readily visible to the examiner: the gums (gingiva), conjunctiva of the eye, lining of the nostrils, and inner surfaces of the vulva (Figs. 7.29 and 7.30). The inner surface of the ear pinna is not a mucous membrane, although it may be useful for detecting icterus and clotting disorders.

Mucous membrane color is usually light to dark pink. The color may change with abnormalities of blood perfusion, the oxygen content of blood, and certain diseases. Cyanosis imparts a bluish tint, usually indicating extremely low oxygen content in tissues. Brick-red coloration indicates bacterial septicemia and/or septic shock. Endotoxemia in the horse exhibits the unique characteristic of producing a purple gum color that appears along the margin of teeth and gums; this is commonly referred to as a *toxic line*. Yellowish coloring of gums indicates icterus, associated with liver dysfunction or abnormal hemolysis of red blood cells. Pale mucous membranes may indicate anemia or poor perfusion, although many normal horses have naturally pale pink gums. Clotting disorders may produce visible hemorrhage in mucous membranes. Small pinpoint hemorrhages less than 1 mm in diameter are called *petechial hemorrhages* or *petechiae*; ecchymotic hemorrhage produces slightly larger hemorrhages 1 mm to 1 cm in diameter.

Mucous membranes are often assessed for moisture and are commonly described as "moist," "dry," or "tacky"; this information is considered less useful than the membrane color.

Hydration Status

The hydration status of an animal is important information which may be measured with laboratory tests or estimated from the physical examination by using the skin turgor test or CRT measurement.

Skin turgor is assessed by the *skin pinch* or *skin snap* test. Loose skin over the lateral aspect of the neck is briefly and firmly pinched with the fingers and is allowed to retract back to its original position. In normally hydrated animals, the skin should return ("snap") promptly back to its original position in approximately 1 second or less. Dehydration (>5% dehydration) prolongs the response to greater than 1 second. Severely dehydrated animals may take

8 seconds or longer for the skin to retract. This test is less reliable in obese animals, because the fat in the cervical area may falsely improve the skin snap; thin horses and horses older than 15 years may also have delayed skin snap response, regardless of hydration status.

CRT reflects cardiac output, which is directly affected by hydration status. Prolonged CRT is usually associated with low cardiac output, likely caused by inadequate hydration of the animal or from decreased heart function. CRT is assessed by pressing briefly but firmly on the gums with a fingertip to produce a "blanched" white spot before releasing; the time for the original gum color to return to the blanched spot is counted in seconds. The original color should return in less than 2.5 seconds. A CRT greater than 2.5 seconds is considered abnormally delayed, whereas severe dehydration and severe shock may produce a greatly prolonged CRT—5 to 8 seconds. Dehydration and shock are the most common causes of prolonged CRT in the horse.

TECHNICIAN NOTE

Measurement of capillary refill time (CRT) is more accurate than that of skin turgor in determining an animal's hydration status.

Height and Weight Measurement

Height and weight measurements are needed for a variety of purposes, for example, for insurance or prepurchase examination, breed registration, or entry into certain horse show classes. The weight measurement is usually obtained for calculating the proper dose of drugs and therapeutic substances and for dietary formulation.

Height may be estimated or measured precisely. Rough estimates may be made with the height-weight tape. This instrument is essentially a tape measure, marked on one side for height measurement in hands (1 hand = 4 inches) and on the other side for weight measurement. Ideally, the horse should stand on a firm, level surface, with its weight distributed evenly on all four legs. The horse's head should not be elevated or lowered but should be in a horizontal position, with the neck parallel to the ground. One end of the measuring tape is held on the ground just behind the horse's forelimb. The tape is then stretched vertically to the withers, and the height is read at the level of the highest point of the withers. For precise determination of height, commercially made rigid measuring rulers are available. These rulers are made of metal and include bubble-style levels to ensure that the ruler is not tilted when the measurement is taken. The animal should stand squarely on a firm, level surface, with the head and neck held parallel to the ground. The measurement is taken at the last mane hair or the highest point of the withers, depending on the breed registry or rules of competition.

Weight may be roughly estimated with the height-weight tape or taken more precisely with a livestock scale. The height-weight tape has one side that is calibrated for weight measurement; weight tick marks are based on measurements around the girth of the horse. The tape is applied to encircle the horse at its girth, the area caudal to the withers and just behind the forelimb (Fig. 7.31). The weight tape is formulated from logarithms of "normal" animals and may be inaccurate for excessively thin or obese animals. The build of an animal may also affect the results. Height-weight tapes designed for cattle are not accurate for horses.

Precise weights for large animals may be obtained with livestock scales. Digital livestock scales have a walk-over design and are popular at many hospitals and practices. Traditional livestock scales are somewhat cumbersome to use and have largely been replaced by digital walk-over scales.

CASE PRESENTATION 7.2

Signalment: 9-year-old Standardbred gelding
Presenting complaint: Colic
History: A nine-year-old Standardbred gelding was admitted to the equine hospital with a history of abdominal pain of 3 days' duration. The referring veterinarian treated this horse on the farm with mineral oil and water administered via nasogastric intubation and provided medication as needed for pain control. All grain and hay had been withheld since treatment began, but free access to water had been allowed. The horse had not defecated in 3 days, and its discomfort was increasing. The horse was referred to the hospital for further assessment and treatment, including surgery, if necessary.

Subjective:

Mentation: Alert but slightly depressed
Behavior: Paws occasionally; frequently assumes urination stance but does not urinate
Mucous membrane color: Pale pink with mild yellowish discoloration
Eyes: Mild yellowish discoloration of sclerae
GI motility: Hypomotility, all abdominal quadrants

Objective:

Temperature (T) 100.8°F; **pulse (P)** 52 beats per minute; **respirations (R)** 12 breaths per minute
Capillary refill time (CRT) = 3 seconds
Lies down and rolls 2 to 3×/hour
Defecated three hard, dry fecal balls during examination

Assessment (prioritized technician evaluations, with rationale):

1. Abdominal pain (patient displays clinical signs consistent with abdominal pain: pawing; stretching as if to urinate; rolling; elevated pulse rate)
2. Dehydration (increased CRT, increased pulse rate)
3. Icterus (yellowish cast to mucous membranes and sclerae)

Plan (prioritized technician evaluations, with interventions):

1. *Abdominal pain:* Closely monitor for signs of increasing pain and notify veterinarian immediately if pain increases. Risk for self-trauma and injury to veterinary staff.
2. *Dehydration:* Anticipate need for IV catheterization and IV fluid therapy. Monitor vital signs.
3. *Icterus:* Anticipate need for blood work (complete blood count [CBC] and chemistry panel).

TECHNICIAN CASE NOTES

- The most accurate indicator of the need for exploratory abdominal surgery in a case of colic is the horse's level of pain. Pain is more accurate than any other physical examination finding or laboratory result. Close monitoring of the patient's pain level is crucial in case management; signs of increasing pain constitute a true emergency.
- Although the passing of three fecal balls may seem insignificant compared with normal fecal volume, when observing a colic patient, this finding can be highly significant to the clinician. Not only small fecal volumes but the character of feces should be noted on the patient's chart. If mineral oil has been administered via nasogastric intubation, its appearance on feces or around the anal/perineal area is highly significant and should be noted.
- Horses may develop icterus when food is withheld for 24 hours or longer. This type of icterus is properly referred to as *fasting hyperbilirubinemia* and usually occurs with no clinical signs of liver dysfunction. Serum chemistry will show an increase in total bilirubin (unconjugated), but all other liver parameters are typically normal. The icterus requires no special treatment and will resolve rapidly when the patient is allowed to eat.

solid pellets. The color of the feces depends on the diet and ranges from green to dark brown. Undigested roughage fibers in the fecal material are an abnormal finding that may indicate dysfunction of the rumen and/or the reticulum.

Recommended Readings

Fubini SL, Ducharme NG. *Farm Animal Surgery*. St. Louis, MO: Saunders; 2004.

Hanie EA. *Large Animal Clinical Procedures for Veterinary Technicians*. St. Louis, MO: Mosby; 2006.

McCurnin DM, Poffenbarger EM. *Small Animal Physical Diagnosis and Clinical Procedures*. Philadelphia, PA: Saunders; 1991.

Pugh DG. *Sheep and Goat Medicine*. 2nd ed. St. Louis, MO: Saunders; 2012.

Smith MC, Sherman DM. *Goat Medicine*. 2nd ed. Hoboken, NJ: Wiley-Blackwell; 2009.

Speirs VC. *Clinical Examination of Horses*. Philadelphia, PA: Saunders; 1997.

8

Preventive Health Programs

GEORGE W. McCOMMON

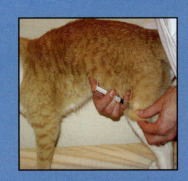

CHAPTER OUTLINE

LEARNING OBJECTIVES

When you have completed this chapter, you will be able to:

1. Pronounce, define, and spell all of the key terms in this chapter.
2. Compare and contrast the issues and information discussed during wellness visits at various life stages of a dog or a cat (puppy/kitten, adult, and senior/geriatric), and discuss the importance of grooming.
3. Do the following regarding immunity in cats and dogs:
   - Differentiate between active and passive immunity and discuss why it is necessary to administer a series of vaccinations to young puppies and kittens.
   - Differentiate between noninfectious and infectious types of vaccines and explain the purpose of adjuvants.
   - Describe the storage, handling, reconstitution, and dosing of animal vaccines.
   - List the recommended administration locations for various canine and feline vaccinations.

- Distinguish between core and noncore vaccines and explain what is meant by duration of immunity.
- Identify the core and noncore vaccines that are used for dogs and cats.
- Describe potential adverse vaccine events and how to deal with various adverse events should they occur.
4. Explain the importance of discussing potential canine and feline parasitic infections with owners and describe general preventive measures that can be taken.
5. Describe a routine preventive health program for horses, including physical examination, vaccinations, parasitic infection prevention, dental and hoof care, and nutrition.
6. Describe vaccines and other preventive measures that can be used during various life stages of pigs, cattle, sheep, and goats.

KEY TERMS

Active immunity
Adjuvant
Anaphylaxis
Antitoxin
Biosecurity
Canine adenovirus type 2 (CAV-2)
Canine parainfluenza vaccine (CPiV)
Canine parvovirus type 2 (CPV-2)
Colostrum
Congenital
Distemper, adenovirus 2, parainfluenza, parvovirus (DA2PP)
Feline calicivirus (FCV)

Feline herpesvirus type 1 (FHV-1)
Feline immunodeficiency virus (FIV)
Feline leukemia virus (FeLV)
Feline panleukopenia virus (FPV)
Feline viral rhinotracheitis, calicivirus, panleukopenia (FVRCP)
Fomite
Needle teeth
Passive immunity
Thrush
Thyroxine (T4)
Toxoid

Introduction

Preventive health programs are an important part of veterinary practice and encompass a wide range of issues. Through these programs, veterinary health care team members can anticipate the risks of disease for each patient and tailor recommendations to the owner based on information specific to the animal, such as its age and the environment in which it lives. Routine examinations, screening tests, and client education are key components of responsible health care. In this way, many diseases and disorders that once were common can be entirely avoided or detected early on to facilitate successful, early treatment and prevention.

Preventive health programs are especially important in situations where animals are housed in group situations, including animal shelters or animal-centered farming enterprises. In these situations, preventive health care may decrease the likelihood of large populations of animals contracting contagious diseases, which could have catastrophic consequences for the health of the animals and the economic viability of the business.

This chapter offers a general overview of preventive health measures for dogs, cats, horses, and common livestock species. For information about preventive health care specific to the neonate, refer to Chapter 21. Preventive health care information for geriatric patients can be found in Chapter 36. Finally, information about training and behavior modification of young animals can be found in Chapter 5.

Preventive Health Programs for Dogs and Cats

Lifelong Wellness

Regular wellness visits are important for maintaining health in dogs and cats throughout their lives. The American Association of Feline Practitioners (AAFP) has identified six life stages in cats: kitten (0–6 months); junior (7 months–2 years); adult (3–6 years); mature (7–10 years); senior (11–14 years); and geriatric. Refer to the AAFP's online Feline Life Stages Guidelines (www.catvets.com) for specific recommendations regarding preventive health care in cats.

In the past, regular visits to a veterinary practice were predominantly driven by the need for annual immunizations for pets. As vaccination recommendations have changed in more recent years, other important themes that were addressed during these visits are being emphasized more. A thorough physical examination should be performed during each appointment. Routine examinations establish what is normal for healthy animals and help detect abnormalities that the owner may not be aware of. When a problem is detected early in the disease process, a favorable outcome of treatment for the condition becomes more likely. Routine wellness visits also give the veterinary health care team an opportunity to update subjective patient data, such as changes in the animal's life, and to make recommendations accordingly. They provide an important opportunity to educate the client on the various physical and psychological needs of the patient as the animal matures and to ensure client compliance when the pet becomes ill.

Wellness in Puppies and Kittens

The initial visit to a veterinary practice for a healthy puppy or kitten typically occurs at age 6 to 8 weeks. In many practices, extra time is designated for a pet's first visit, because many topics may be discussed with the owner. The pet is examined, with emphasis on identifying any congenital defects that may be present. Depending on the contractual agreement of sale and on the laws of the state where the animal was purchased, the first appointment may identify a serious condition, deeming the animal unfit for purchase, and the owner may be entitled to reimbursement or may be allowed to exchange or return the animal to the dealer. For kittens, the initial visit often involves performing a blood test to check for feline leukemia virus (FeLV) and feline immunodeficiency virus (FIV). Other blood tests that address specific genetic diseases are available and may be discussed with and offered to owners of breeds predisposed to specific diseases. Both internal and external parasite control is addressed, and owners may be instructed to bring their pet's fecal specimen for analysis during the visit and subsequent treatment of parasitism. This is an important opportunity to educate clients about the need for routine parasite control and the zoonotic risks of certain parasites to humans. Depending on the results of the fecal flotation test and any previous history of deworming, antiparasitic medications may be prescribed. During initial visits, clients are also educated about the risks of heartworm disease and flea infestation in both cats and dogs.

The initial visit is a good time for the veterinary health care team to educate the client on basic husbandry practices and the normal progression of a pet's development. This is especially important for new pet owners, who may not be aware of what is involved in properly caring for a pet. Topics that are typically addressed include the following:

1. Instruction on house breaking for puppies and litter box training for kittens
2. Nutritional information, including appropriate diet, amounts, and frequency of feeding and use of "treats"
3. Basic socialization and animal training techniques
4. Housing requirements for the pet, including appropriate outdoor shelters
5. Tooth development, eruption times, and the importance of dental care throughout the animal's life
6. Techniques on animal-proofing the house, including recognizing and removing potential foreign bodies from the pet's environment and informing owners about foods, plants, and common household products that are toxic to animals
7. Exercise requirements
8. Grooming requirements
9. The importance of spaying and neutering and the ideal ages at which these procedures should be performed on pets

Details about spaying or neutering should be discussed with owners if they do not intend to breed their pet. The client must be informed about both the medical benefits and the surgical and anesthetic risks in spaying and neutering. Spaying eliminates unwanted pregnancies, heat-related behaviors, ovarian cancer, and pyometra. It also decreases the likelihood of mammary carcinoma if spaying is performed before the second heat. Neutering may eliminate roaming, intermale aggression, enlargement of the prostate gland, and testicular cancer. Surgical risk to the animal has been minimized with the use of state-of-the-art anesthetics and sterile techniques; nevertheless, certain risks, such as adverse reactions to medications, unexpected hemorrhage, and postoperative complications, do exist. Informed consent forms should be signed by the owner before all surgical procedures are performed.

After the initial visit, puppies and kittens are examined at 3- to 4-week intervals until they are approximately 16 weeks of age.

During these visits, the pet receives booster vaccinations and anti-parasitic medications, if needed. At this time, the veterinary staff can get updates on how the pet is doing at home and answer any questions that the owner may have.

Initial puppy and kitten wellness visits are extremely important in setting a client on a path toward responsible pet ownership. In addition, these appointments give the veterinary health care team an opportunity to provide excellent service and to create a positive experience for first-time clients in the hope that it will give rise to a lasting relationship through the life of the pet.

TECHNICIAN NOTE

Initial wellness visits for puppies and kittens typically occur every 3 to 4 weeks until the animal is approximately 16 weeks of age and usually coincide with the animal's vaccination schedule.

Wellness in Adult Dogs and in Adult and Mature Cats

As young dogs and cats develop into adults, their physical and psychological needs change. New recommendations regarding the pet's nutrition must be made as the animal transitions from food required for growth to maintenance and finally geriatric diets. Immunization protocols also change. After 1-year boosters have been administered, many of the core vaccines are recommended to be administered every 3 years. This does not mean, however, that adult dogs and cats do not need to continue to visit the veterinary practice regularly. According to current American Animal Hospital Association (AAHA)-American Veterinary Medical Association (AVMA) Canine and Feline Preventive Health Guidelines, dogs and cats should be examined annually, with some animals requiring more frequent examinations. This allows the veterinarian to detect potential changes that may have gone unnoticed by the owner and to address any current problems that the animal may be experiencing.

Dental health should be assessed regularly. As dogs and cats age, dental diseases and the amount of tartar tend to increase, and the veterinary health care team can make recommendations on dental care. Testing for various regional infectious diseases, such as heartworm disease in dogs and cats, are conducted at this time. Currently, owners will also acquire medications for parasite control, such as heartworm prevention and flea and tick control. As the pet ages, routine blood and urine tests (complete blood count [CBC], chemistry panel, and urinalysis) are recommended to establish baseline levels and to screen for underlying disease.

Finally, these visits offer veterinary technicians' important opportunities to educate clients about the changing requirements of their pets as they age and to make recommendations based on the risks and needs of the patient. It is especially important to impress on clients the importance of regular preventive health care to ensure the long-term health of their pets (Case Presentation 8.1).

TECHNICIAN NOTE

The American Animal Hospital Association (AAHA)-American Veterinary Medical Association (AVMA) Canine and Feline Preventive Health Guidelines recommend that adult dogs and cats be examined annually, with some animals requiring more frequent visits.

CASE PRESENTATION 8.1

Bailey, a gray-and-white 4-year-old spayed female domestic shorthair cat, is presented for the annual preventive health appointment. The veterinary technician escorts the client and the patient back to an examination room and obtains the following information about Bailey:
- Weight: 17 lb
- Heart rate (HR): 170 beats per minute (beats/min)
- Respiratory rate (RR): 24 breaths per minute
- Temperature (T): 101.5° F

Information from owner: Bailey's appetite is good, and she has no problems that the owner has noticed. The cat is not on any medications. Bailey is an indoor-only cat but occasionally goes out onto a patio area that is enclosed by a fence. Bailey is the only pet in the house.

Physical Examination Findings

A moderate amount of tartar is present on the cat's teeth. When the cat is combed, a few small black flecks of material, mixed in with hair, are visible in the comb. All other examination findings are unremarkable. The client is asked if she has noticed the cat scratching herself lately, and the client confirms that Bailey has been scratching herself occasionally but by no means regularly. The technician prepares vaccines and other materials for the veterinarian and enters the following information into the medical record, using the SOAP (subjective, objective, assessment, and plan) format:

Date: 8/18/XX, Barb Smith, CVT

S: Good appetite; not on any medications; owner reports "indoor only," but cat has access to enclosed patio; sole pet in household; no problems according to owner; moderate tartar on teeth, evidence of flea dirt; occasionally scratches; all other physical examination findings WNL (within normal limits)

O: Weight = 17 lb; HR = 170 beats/min; RR = 24 breaths per minute; T = 101.5°F

A:
1. Altered oral health
2. Overweight
3. Flea infestation and risk of transmission
4. Client knowledge deficit

P:
1. If ordered, dispense:
   - Dental and oral care products
   - House treatment products and flea medications
   - Prescription weight-reduction diet
2. Educate client:
   - Treatment for fleas in house, in yard, and on pet
   - Home dental health care
   - Importance of regular professional dental cleaning
   - Weight loss program

Senior and Geriatric Animal Wellness

According to the AAFP Senior Care Guidelines, cats are classified as "senior" when they are 11 to 14 years of age. At 15 years and beyond, cats are considered geriatric. For dogs, exact age ranges are not as well defined, because wide variations have been noted in the life spans of large-breed dogs versus small-breed dogs. The AAHA Senior Care Guidelines for Dogs and Cats define as "*senior*" animals that are in the last 25% of their predicted life span. As animals reach this stage of their lives, it becomes more likely that some sort of illness will develop. Because one of the goals of preventive health programs is to detect disease early in its onset, it is recommended that animals in this age group visit the veterinary practice every 6 months. Specific attention is paid to weight, mobility, dental health, hearing, vision, and psychological needs. A thorough history is necessary to determine how the owner feels the pet is doing. It is also common for animals to

TABLE 8.1	Recommended Sites of Administration of Feline Vaccines[a]			
Vaccination	Route	Body Region	Location on Limb
FVRCP	SQ	Right front leg	Lateral side, distal to elbow
FeLV or FIV	SQ	Left hind leg	Lateral side, distal to stifle
Rabies	SQ	Right hind leg	Lateral side, distal to stifle
Giardia	SQ	Left front leg	Lateral side, distal to elbow

[a]Based on recommendations made in the 2013 American Association of Feline Practitioners Feline Vaccine Advisory Panel Report.

FeLV, Feline leukemia virus; *FIV*, feline immunodeficiency virus; *FVRCP*, feline viral rhinotracheitis (herpesvirus), calicivirus, and panleukopenia virus; *SQ*, subcutaneous.

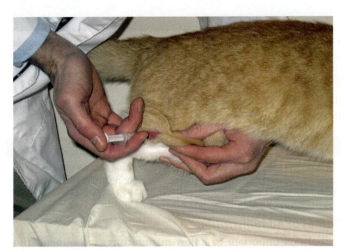

• **Fig. 8.2** The American Association of Feline Practitioners (AAFP) recommends that the feline rabies vaccine be administered subcutaneously in the right hind leg, distal to the stifle.

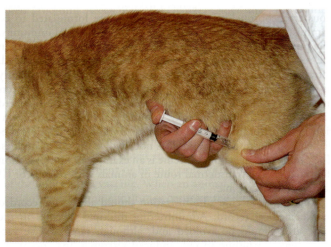

• **Fig. 8.3** The American Association of Feline Practitioners (AAFP) recommends that the feline leukemia virus (FeLV) vaccine be administered subcutaneously in the left hind leg, distal to the stifle.

for veterinary health care teams to follow a similar protocol, with rabies vaccines administered subcutaneously into the right hindlimb, DA2PP (distemper, adenovirus 2, parainfluenza, parvovirus) vaccines administered subcutaneously into the right front

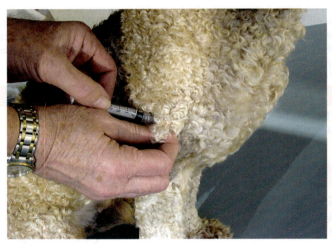

• **Fig. 8.4** The right front limb is a common site of administration of the DA2PP (distemper, adenovirus 2, parainfluenza, parvovirus) vaccine in dogs.

limb (Fig. 8.4), and noncore vaccines, such as leptospirosis or *Borrelia burgdorferi* (Lyme disease) vaccines, administered subcutaneously into the left hindlimb. These administration sites may vary by veterinary practice and by veterinarian. Because of the invasive nature of vaccine-induced sarcomas, it is now recommended that immunizations be administered on the distal limb. In the event of a local vaccine-induced sarcoma, the leg could be amputated to completely remove the mass.

TECHNICIAN NOTE

Always be aware of the appropriate route of administration of a vaccine. Intranasal vaccines should never be administered subcutaneously or intramuscularly.

Core Versus Noncore Vaccines

Vaccines have had a profound effect on preventing diseases in both humans and animals. Despite all the good that can come from immunization, there are potential risks. For this reason, it may not be advisable to immunize every animal with every vaccine that exists for that species. Both the AAFP and the AAHA have published guidelines for vaccines that they consider core and those that they consider noncore (Tables 8.2 and 8.3). Core vaccines are those that are recommended for all animals of a species. These vaccinations stimulate immunity against diseases that are highly contagious and prevalent in the environment. In

TABLE 8.2   Recommended Feline Vaccination Protocol[a]

Vaccine Type	Category	Route	Initial Vaccination Age (≥6 weeks and ≤16 weeks) Protocol	Initial Vaccination Age (>16 weeks) Protocol	Booster Interval Following Initial Vaccination Series	Subsequent Revaccination Interval	Comments
Rabies							
Canarypox virus–vectored recombinant, nonadjuvanted	Core	Injection	1 dose when ≥8 weeks of age	Same as (≥6 weeks and ≤16 weeks) protocol	1 year later	Every year	Must follow state/local regulations regarding interval, route, initial age, etc.
1-year killed virus, adjuvanted	Core	Injection	1 dose when ≥12 weeks of age	Same as (≥6 weeks and ≤16 weeks) protocol	1 year later	Every year	Must follow state/local regulations regarding interval, route, initial age, etc.
3-year killed virus, adjuvanted	Core	Injection	1 dose when ≥12 weeks of age	Same as (≥6 weeks and ≤16 weeks) protocol	1 year later	Every 3 years	Must follow state/local regulations regarding interval, route, initial age, etc.
Feline Herpesvirus-1 and Feline Calicivirus							
MLV, nonadjuvanted	Core	Injection	Every 3–4 weeks until 16–20 weeks of age	2 doses 3–4 weeks apart	1 year later	Every 3 years	
Killed virus, adjuvanted	Core	Injection	Every 3–4 weeks until 16–20 weeks of age	2 doses 3–4 weeks apart	1 year later	Every 3 years	
MLV, nonadjuvanted	Core	Intranasal	Every 3–4 weeks until 16–20 weeks of age	2 doses 3–4 weeks apart	1 year later	Every 3 years	
Feline Panleukopenia Virus							
MLV, nonadjuvanted	Core	Injection	Every 3–4 weeks until 16–20 weeks of age	2 doses 3–4 weeks apart	1 year later	≥Every 3 years	
Killed virus, adjuvanted or nonadjuvanted	Core	Injection	Every 3–4 weeks until 16–20 weeks of age	2 doses 3–4 weeks apart	1 year later	≥Every 3 years	
MLV, nonadjuvanted	Core	Intranasal	Every 3–4 weeks until 16–20 weeks of age	2 doses 3–4 weeks apart	1 year later	≥Every 3 years	
Feline Leukemia Virus							
Canarypox virus–vectored recombinant, nonadjuvanted	Noncore	Transdermal	2 doses 3–4 weeks apart when ≥8 weeks of age	Same as (≥6 weeks and ≤16 weeks) protocol	1 year later	As determined by risk factors	AAFP highly recommends for all kittens
Killed virus, adjuvanted	Noncore	Injection	2 doses 3–4 weeks apart when ≥8 weeks of age	Same as (≥6 weeks and ≤16 weeks) protocol	1 year later	As determined by risk factors	AAFP highly recommends for all kittens
Feline Immunodeficiency Virus (FIV)							
Killed virus, adjuvanted	Noncore	Injection	3 doses 2–3 weeks apart when ≥8 weeks of age	Same as (≥6 weeks and ≤16 weeks) protocol	1 year later	Every year	Vaccinates will test positive with antibody-based FIV test

Continued

TABLE 8.2 Recommended Feline Vaccination Protocol[a]—cont'd

Vaccine Type	Category	Route	Initial Vaccination Age (≥6 weeks and ≤16 weeks) Protocol	Initial Vaccination Age (>16 weeks) Protocol	Booster Interval Following Initial Vaccination Series	Subsequent Revaccination Interval	Comments
Chlamydophila felis							
Avirulent live organism, nonadjuvanted	Noncore	Injection	2 doses 3–4 weeks apart when ≥9 weeks of age	Same as (≥6 weeks and ≤16 weeks) protocol	1 year later	Every year	
Killed organism, adjuvanted	Noncore	Injection	2 doses 3–4 weeks apart when ≥9 weeks of age	Same as (≥6 weeks and ≤16 weeks) protocol	1 year later	Every year	
Bordetella bronchiseptica							
Avirulent live organism, nonadjuvanted	Noncore	Intranasal	1 dose when ≥8 weeks of age	Same as (≥6 weeks and ≤16 weeks) protocol	1 year later	Every year	
Feline Coronavirus							
MLV, nonadjuvanted	Noncore	Intranasal	2 doses 3–4 weeks apart when 16 weeks of age	Same as (≥6 weeks and ≤16 weeks) protocol	1 year later	Every year	AAFP generally does not recommend
Giardia lamblia							
Killed organism, adjuvanted	Noncore	Injection	2 doses 2–4 weeks apart when ≥8 weeks of age	Same as (≥6 weeks and ≤16 weeks) protocol	1 year later	Every year	AAFP generally does not recommend

[a]Based on recommendations made in the 2013 American Association of Feline Practitioners Feline Vaccine Advisory Panel Report.

AAFP, American Association of Feline Practitioners; *MLV*, modified live virus.

TABLE 8.3 Recommended Canine Vaccination Protocol[a]

Vaccine Type	Category	Route	Initial Vaccination Age (≤16 weeks) Protocol	Initial Vaccination Age (>16 weeks) Protocol	Booster Interval Following Initial Vaccination Series	Subsequent Revaccination Interval	Comments
Rabies							
1-year killed virus	Core	Injection	1 dose when ≥12 weeks of age	Same as (≤16 weeks) protocol	1 year later	Every year	Must follow state/local regulations regarding interval, route, initial age, etc.
3-year killed virus	Core	Injection	1 dose when ≥12 weeks of age	Same as (≤16 weeks) protocol	1 year later	Every 3 years	Must follow state/local regulations regarding interval, route, initial age, etc.
Canine Distemper Virus							
MLV or recombinant	Core	Injection	Every 3–4 weeks when ≥6 weeks until 14–16 weeks of age	1 dose	1 year later for (≤16 weeks) protocol	≥Every 3 years	

TABLE 8.3   Recommended Canine Vaccination Protocol[a]—cont'd

Vaccine Type	Category	Route	Initial Vaccination Age (≤16 weeks) Protocol	Initial Vaccination Age (>16 weeks) Protocol	Booster Interval Following Initial Vaccination Series	Subsequent Revaccination Interval	Comments
					≥3 years later for (>16 weeks) protocol	≥Every 3 years	
Measles Virus							
MLV	Noncore	Injection (IM only)	1 dose when >6 weeks and <12 weeks of age	Not recommended	Not recommended	Not recommended	
Canine Adenovirus, Type 2 (CAV-2)							
MLV	Core	Injection	Every 3–4 weeks when ≥6 weeks until 14–16 weeks of age	1 dose	1 year later for (≤16 weeks) protocol	≥Every 3 years	
					≥3 years later for (>16 weeks) protocol	≥Every 3 years	
MLV	Noncore	Intranasal	1 dose when ≥3–4 weeks of age	Same as (≤16 weeks) protocol	≤1 year later	≤Every year	May not provide protection against CAV-1 and should not replace MLV injectable vaccine. Recommended for dogs at risk for infectious tracheobronchitis. Available only as a combination vaccine.
Canine Parvovirus							
MLV	Core	Injection	Every 3–4 weeks when ≥6 weeks until 14–16 weeks of age	1 dose	1 year later for (≤16 weeks) protocol	≥Every 3 years	
					≥3 years later for (>16 weeks) protocol	≥Every 3 years	
Canine Parainfluenza Virus							
MLV	Noncore	Injection	Every 3–4 weeks when ≥6 weeks until 14–16 weeks of age	1 dose	1 year later for (≤16 weeks) protocol ≥3 years later for (>16 weeks) protocol	≥Every 3 years	Available only in combination with canine distemper virus, CAV-2, and canine parvovirus
MLV	Noncore	Intranasal	1 dose when ≥3–4 weeks of age	Same as (≤16 weeks) protocol	≤1 year later	≤Every year	May be administered more often than annually for high-risk animals. Available only as a combination vaccine.
Leptospira interrogans							
Four-way killed whole-cell or subunit bacteria	Noncore	Injection	2 doses 2–4 weeks apart when ≥12 weeks of age	Same as (≤16 weeks) protocol	1 year later	Every year	

Continued

| TABLE 8.3 | Recommended Canine Vaccination Protocol[a]—cont'd | | | | | | |

Vaccine Type	Category	Route	Initial Vaccination Age (≤16 weeks) Protocol	Initial Vaccination Age (>16 weeks) Protocol	Booster Interval Following Initial Vaccination Series	Subsequent Revaccination Interval	Comments
Two-way killed bacteria	Noncore	Injection					AAHA does not recommend
Bordetella bronchiseptica							
Inactivated cellular antigen extract	Noncore	Injection	Doses administered at 8 and 12 weeks of age	2 doses 2–4 weeks apart	1 year later	Every year	Second dose in initial vaccine series should be given ≥1 week before exposure
Bordetella bronchiseptica							
Live avirulent bacteria	Noncore	Intranasal	1 dose when ≥3–4 weeks of age	Same as (≤16 weeks) protocol	≤1 year later	≤Every year	May be administered more often than annually for high-risk animals
Borrelia burgdorferi							
Killed whole-cell bacteria or recombinant subunit OspA	Noncore	Injection	2 doses 2–4 weeks apart when ≥12 weeks of age	Same as (≤16 weeks) protocol	1 year later	Every year	
Canine Influenza							
Killed virus	Noncore	Injection	2 doses 2–4 weeks apart when ≥6 weeks of age	Same as (≤16 weeks) protocol	1 year later	Every year	

[a]Based on recommendations made in the 2011 American Animal Hospital Association Canine Vaccination Guidelines.

AAHA, American Animal Hospital Association; *CAV*, canine adenovirus; *IM*, intramuscular; *MLV*, modified live virus.

most cases, all animals, regardless of their lifestyle, have at least the potential to be exposed to these diseases. According to the 2022 AAHA Canine Vaccination Guidelines, core vaccines for dogs include rabies, parainfluenza, distemper, hepatitis (adenovirus 2), and canine parvovirus (CPV) vaccines. According to the 2020 AAFP Feline Vaccine Advisory Panel, core vaccines for cats include rabies vaccine, FeLV, FHV-1 + FCV, and FPV + FHV-1 + FCV. Noncore vaccines for felines include *Bordetella* and chlamydia.

Noncore vaccines are not recommended for every animal. These vaccines are recommended for animals at risk for contracting specific diseases. Therefore veterinary health care team members must discuss with the owner the lifestyle of the animal and must weigh the risks of the animal contracting the disease versus the risks of potential adverse effects of the vaccine.

Both the AAFP and the AAHA have classified a few vaccines as "not recommended." In these cases, it is the opinion of the advisory committee that these vaccines have little to no indication for use, either because the vaccines have been associated with adverse events or because they have failed to induce adequate protection against the disease.

> **TECHNICIAN NOTE**
>
> Core vaccinations are recommended for all animals of a particular species, because they provide protection against highly contagious common pathogens.

Onset and Duration of Immunity

The onset of immunity varies between infectious-type and noninfectious-type vaccines; it generally takes longer for immunity to develop after administration of a noninfectious type of vaccine than after administration of an infectious type of vaccine.

Duration of immunity is the length of time that an animal retains an adequate level of immunity to protect itself from disease or infection if it were naturally exposed to the pathogenic organism. In many cases, infectious vaccines provide a longer duration of immunity compared with noninfectious vaccines. However, this is not an absolute rule because certain rabies vaccines (noninfectious type) can provide immunity for 3 years in animals that have received 2 vaccines 1 year apart, but annual boosters are recommended for intranasal *Bordetella bronchiseptica* vaccines (infectious type). After the initial puppy or kitten series and a 1-year booster, 3-year revaccination intervals are recommended for both the canine combination (DA2PP) and the feline combination (FVRCP) core vaccines. Many boarding facilities will require proof of immunizations (especially *B. bronchiseptica*) before accepting animals for boarding.

Feline Immunizations

The recommendations discussed below are based on the 2013 AAFP Feline Advisory Panel Report. A summary of these recommendations can be found in Table 8.2.

Rabies Vaccine (Noncore Vaccine). Rabies, a zoonotic disease caused by a rhabdovirus, affects the central nervous system (CNS) and is a reportable disease. It is spread through saliva and CNS tissue and is most commonly transmitted through bite wounds. Rabies is an endemic disease in the United States, where skunks, bats, foxes, raccoons, and coyotes act as natural reservoirs of the disease-causing organism. Clinical signs in animals vary widely but typically involve neurologic signs, such as increased aggression, agitation, solitude seeking, incoordination, and/or paralysis. No treatment for the disease is available, and it is almost always fatal after the onset of clinical signs. Injectable adjuvanted, killed virus vaccines and nonadjuvanted, recombinant virus, canarypox-vectored vaccines are available. In many regions, pets are required by law to receive rabies vaccinations, and the law may even dictate the route of administration (intramuscular vs. subcutaneous) and/or the frequency of administration (annually vs. triennially).

> **TECHNICIAN NOTE**
>
> Veterinary health care team members must be aware of local or regional rabies immunization laws before administering the vaccination.

Feline Herpesvirus Type 1 and Feline Calicivirus Vaccines (Core Vaccines). Feline herpesvirus type 1 (FHV-1), which frequently causes feline viral tracheitis, is an upper respiratory disease in cats. Common clinical signs include sneezing, ocular and nasal discharge, and fever. Feline calicivirus (FCV), of which there are many strains, is also a frequent cause of upper respiratory disease in cats. FCV causes similar signs as FHV-1 but also may cause oral ulceration. In both cases, viruses are shed via oropharyngeal, conjunctival, and nasal secretions for up to 3 weeks. In addition, FCV can be shed in urine and feces. FCV can survive in the environment for a longer period (up to 1 week); FHV-1 can survive in the environment for only 24 hours. Direct contact between cats is the most common means of viral spread, although indirect contact with infective secretions is also possible. Latent infections are normal with FHV-1 infection and involve the virus lying dormant within the cat for a certain period. After episodes that are stressful for the cat, clinical signs of upper respiratory disease and/or viral shedding typically recur. A carrier state is also possible in cats infected by FCV; however, these cats tend to shed virus continuously.

Both FHV-1 and FCV are commonly found in cat populations, making exposure to these organisms likely. Cats of any age are susceptible to upper respiratory disease, although kittens tend to be most severely affected. Both modified live and inactivated vaccines are available, and both types have relatively good efficacy in protecting against disease. These vaccines do not, however, protect against infection or carrier state. In the case of FCV, the vaccine does not cover against all strains. Vaccines are available in an injectable form, which is administered subcutaneously, and in an intranasal form. It is possible for vaccinates to develop mild signs of upper respiratory disease, especially after receiving the

intranasal vaccine, and lameness may develop secondary to the calicivirus component of the vaccine. FHV-1 and FCV vaccines are commonly combined with the feline panleukopenia vaccine to form the combination vaccine FVRCP.

> **TECHNICIAN NOTE**
>
> Feline herpesvirus type 1 (FHV-1) and feline calicivirus (FCV) are common causes of upper respiratory disease in cats.

Feline Panleukopenia Virus Vaccine (Core Vaccine). Feline panleukopenia is caused by a parvovirus, the feline panleukopenia virus (FPV), and is highly contagious; it is commonly found in the environment, and cats of all ages are susceptible. Clinical signs include fever, lethargy, anorexia, dehydration, vomiting, and diarrhea. Sudden death is also possible, especially in younger cats. As the name implies, a low white blood cell (WBC) count (leukopenia) is typical. Neurologic signs are possible, because infection during late gestation or the first few weeks of life can lead to cerebellar hypoplasia. The virus is shed in all body secretions but is most commonly found in feces and urine, and the virus can survive in the environment for up to 1 year. Direct contact with an infected cat or with infectious secretions is the most common means of viral spread. Both modified live and inactivated vaccines are available in injectable forms and provide excellent immunity. An intranasal modified live vaccine is also available. It is possible for modified live vaccines to cause cerebellar disease in fetuses and neonates, so this vaccine type should not be administered to kittens younger than 4 weeks of age or to pregnant queens. FPV vaccine is commonly combined with FHV-1 and FCV vaccines to create the combination vaccine FVRCP.

Feline Leukemia Virus Vaccine (Noncore Vaccine). FeLV is a retrovirus of the subfamily Oncornavirus. It is shed in saliva and nasal secretions and is typically spread through mutual grooming, sharing of food and water dishes, and biting. The disease can also be spread in utero, through nursing, and via blood transfusions. The virus can survive in the environment for up to 48 hours. Cats of all ages can be infected; however, kittens and young cats seem to be most susceptible. Cats infected with FeLV experience clinical signs secondary to immunosuppression, anemia, and/or lymphoma. Inactivated injectable, nonadjuvanted recombinant injectable, and nonadjuvanted recombinant transdermal vaccines are available. This immunization is recommended for cats that are at risk of contracting the disease, such as cats that have access to the outdoors or cats that have contact with those of unknown FeLV status. It is also recommended that cats test negative for FeLV before vaccination. The AAFP Feline Vaccine Advisory Panel highly recommends vaccination of all kittens because of the potential for change in their risk status.

Feline Immunodeficiency Virus Vaccine (Noncore Vaccine). FIV is a lentivirus that causes immunosuppression in cats. It is spread primarily through saliva and blood via bites, wounds, and other fighting-related injuries. Adult male cats that have access to the outdoors are considered most susceptible because of their predisposition for fighting. An inactivated injectable vaccine is available. Cats receiving the vaccine should test negative for FIV before their first injection. After vaccination cats will test positive on the antibody-based FIV screening test. This is because the screening test is incapable of differentiating between antibodies formed secondary to the vaccine and antibodies formed secondary to the actual disease. Therefore it is important to educate owners on the implications of the test results. It is recommended that a cat receiving this vaccine also receives a microchip for identification to increase the likelihood that if it ever goes missing, it will be returned to the owner and will not be euthanized because of its false-positive FIV test result. The FIV vaccine is recommended for cats at risk of contracting the disease, such as cats that have access to the outdoors and have a predisposition to fighting, and FIV-negative cats that live in a household with an FIV-positive cat.

> **TECHNICIAN NOTE**
>
> Feline immunodeficiency virus (FIV)–negative cats that receive the FIV vaccine will test positive on the antibody-based FIV screening test.

***Chlamydophila felis* Vaccine (Noncore Vaccine).** *C. felis* causes a bacterial disease that infects the conjunctiva and respiratory tract of cats. It primarily causes signs of conjunctivitis, including unilateral or bilateral serous ocular discharge, which may progress to mucopurulent discharge. Signs of upper respiratory tract disease, such as mild nasal discharge and sneezing, occur less commonly. The pathogen is spread by direct contact between cats and may be shed for months beyond clinical resolution of the disease. Infections are treatable. Some evidence suggests that zoonotic transmission of this organism is possible. Injectable inactivated, adjuvant, and modified live vaccines are available and stimulate some protection against the disease. Like other vaccines that protect against feline upper respiratory disease, this immunization does not prevent infection or shedding. The vaccine is recommended for cats that live in multicat environments and have a previous history of *C. felis* infection.

***Bordetella bronchiseptica* Vaccine (Noncore Vaccine).** *B. bronchiseptica* causes a bacterial infection in which clinical signs of upper respiratory disease include sneezing, submandibular lymphadenopathy, oculonasal discharge, and sometimes coughing. Cases most frequently occur in animal shelters and multicat households. The disease is often most severe in young kittens, but cats of all ages may be affected. *B. bronchiseptica* is shed in oropharyngeal and nasal secretions, and transmission occurs via direct contact with other cats or with secretions. The bacteria can be shed for up to 19 weeks after infection. It is possible for this organism to be transmitted between cats and dogs. A modified live intranasal vaccine is available and is recommended for cats at risk of contracting the disease, such as those entering boarding facilities, animal shelters, or catteries that have had confirmed cases of the disease. The vaccine should be administered at least 72 hours before the cat enters the facility.

Feline Coronavirus Vaccine (Noncore Vaccine). Feline coronavirus (FCoV) is the causative agent of feline infectious peritonitis (FIP); however, only certain strains of the virus actually cause the disease. It is not uncommon for cats to be exposed to FCoV, but only a small percentage of cats develop FIP. Two forms of the disease have been identified. Clinical signs of the "dry" form include fever, decreased appetite, and weight loss. The main clinical sign of the "wet" form is effusion, which occurs in the abdomen and/or the thoracic cavity. FCoV is shed in feces, respiratory secretions, saliva, and urine. Transmission of the virus occurs through direct contact with secretions or excretions or via mutual grooming. Cats of all ages are susceptible, although kittens seem to be most at risk of developing the disease. An intranasal modified live vaccine is available, but its efficacy is controversial in that studies have shown varying results. It may be helpful in preventing the disease in cats that have never been exposed to FCoV. Therefore testing for FCoV is recommended before vaccination. According to the AAFP Feline Vaccine Advisory report, this vaccine is generally not recommended.

***Giardia lamblia* Vaccine (Noncore Vaccine).** *Giardia lamblia* is a protozoan parasite that causes gastrointestinal disease in many animals, including cats. If clinical signs occur, the most common sign is diarrhea. Weight loss is also reported. The organism is transmitted via the fecal–oral route, and infection commonly occurs secondary to ingestion of contaminated water or infected prey, sharing of litter boxes with an infected animal, and mutual grooming. The organism can survive in wet, cold environments for several months. An injectable adjuvanted inactivated vaccine is available. Because of the insufficient numbers of research studies, its efficacy is controversial. Therefore it is not generally recommended by the AAFP Feline Vaccine Advisory Panel.

Canine Immunizations

The recommendations discussed below are based on the 2011 AAHA Canine Vaccination Guidelines. A summary of these recommendations can be found in Table 8.3.

Rabies Vaccine (Core Vaccine). Rabies vaccination is required by law in many regions. State, local, and/or provincial laws may dictate the frequency of administration of the vaccine—either annually or triennially. The route of administration, which may be subcutaneous or intramuscular, is also specified by some laws. Injectable killed virus vaccines are available for use in dogs. For further information on the disease, refer to the "Rabies" section under "Feline Immunization."

Canine Distemper Virus Vaccine (Core Vaccine). Canine distemper is caused by a paramyxovirus. Many different clinical signs, including decreased appetite, fever, lethargy, and signs of respiratory disease, can be associated with the disease. In more severe cases, vomiting, diarrhea, anorexia, and dehydration may occur. The disease has been associated with neurologic signs, such as seizures, ataxia, paresis, and/or hyperesthesia. Hyperkeratosis of the planum nasale and foot pads may also be observed later in the disease process (hence the nickname "hardpad disease"). Dogs of any age may be affected; however, young dogs are most at risk. This disease can also affect many other species, including foxes, raccoons, skunks, wolves, and ferrets. The virus is shed in all secretions but is mostly transmitted through respiratory exudates. The virus does not survive in the environment very long under normal conditions. Injectable recombinant and modified live vaccines are available and are considered core vaccines. Canine distemper virus is often combined with vaccines for other canine diseases to create the DA2PP vaccine or the DHPP (distemper, hepatitis, parainfluenza, parvovirus) vaccine. In addition, a measles virus vaccine is available for use in puppies younger than 16 weeks of age. The use of measles vaccine in young puppies can provide some temporary protection against canine distemper disease, because the measles virus shares some similarities with the distemper virus. It is also able to stimulate an immune response in the presence of lower levels of acquired maternal antibodies. Thus the advantage of using this vaccine is that it can cross protect young dogs against canine distemper potentially at an earlier age than distemper vaccine alone. Measles vaccine must be administered intramuscularly and is considered a noncore vaccine by the AAHA Canine Vaccination Task Force.

> **TECHNICIAN NOTE**
>
> Measles vaccine can provide some temporary cross protection against canine distemper virus in young puppies.

Canine Adenovirus Type 2 Vaccine (Core Vaccine). Canine adenovirus type 2 (CAV-2) is one of the causes of canine infectious tracheobronchitis ("kennel cough"), while canine adenovirus type 1 (CAV-1) causes infectious canine hepatitis. Signs of the latter disease include vomiting, diarrhea, abdominal pain, clotting disorders, and fever. Ocular signs, such as anterior uveitis and corneal edema, may occur as the dog recovers from the infection. Acute death may also occur, especially in young puppies. Dogs of all ages may be infected, although young dogs are most affected. CAV-1–modified live vaccines were found to cause renal and ocular disease in some animals. The injectable modified live vaccine using CAV-2, however, rarely causes any side effects and induces protection against CAV-1 and CAV-2. This core vaccine is often combined with canine distemper, CPV, and canine parainfluenza (CPiV) vaccines to create the DA2PP or DHPP vaccine. The "A2" and "H" in these vaccine names are used interchangeably, depending on the brand, and stand for adenovirus type 2 and hepatitis respectively. An intranasal vaccine for CAV-2 is also available and is used in combination with *B. bronchiseptica* and CPV vaccines to provide protection against canine infectious tracheobronchitis. This form does not protect against CAV-1 and should not be used as a substitution for the injectable vaccine. The intranasal CAV-2 combination vaccine is classified as a noncore vaccine by the AAHA Canine Vaccination Task Force.

Canine Parvovirus Vaccine (Core Vaccine). Canine parvoviral enteritis is a serious, highly contagious disease. Canine parvovirus type 2 (CPV-2) is shed in feces, and the disease is spread by fecal–oral transmission. The virus is resistant to many disinfectants and is able to survive in the environment for weeks to months. Parvocidal disinfectants and 1:30 solutions of dilute bleach are effective in killing the pathogen. Clinical signs of the disease include diarrhea, vomiting, dehydration, leukopenia, and fever. Dogs of all ages are susceptible to illness, but young dogs are at highest risk. An increased incidence of the disease is found in certain breeds, such as Doberman Pinschers and Rottweilers. Injectable modified live vaccines are available and are often combined with vaccines against canine distemper virus, CAV-2, and CPiV vaccines to create the DA2PP combination vaccine. Modified live vaccines are expected to provide immunity to all variants of CPV.

TECHNICIAN NOTE

Canine parvoviral enteritis is a highly contagious disease; infected patients must be housed in designated isolation areas during hospitalization.

Canine Parainfluenza Virus Vaccine (Noncore Vaccine). CPiV is a paramyxovirus that is one of the causes of canine infectious tracheobronchitis ("kennel cough"). The main clinical sign of the disease is a self-limiting cough, which is typically nonproductive. Both injectable and intranasal modified live vaccines are available. The injectable CPiV vaccine is available only in combination with canine distemper, CPV, and CAV-2 vaccines (DA2PP). The injectable form only protects against clinical signs and does not prevent infection or viral shedding. The intranasal CPiV vaccine is available only in combination with *B. bronchiseptica* and CAV-2 vaccines. The intranasal form is considered superior in protection against parainfluenza virus because, in addition to protecting against clinical signs, it prevents infection and viral shedding.

Leptospirosis (Noncore Vaccine). Leptospirosis is caused by the bacterium *Leptospira*, of which there are many serovars. Leptospirosis is transmitted through exposure to contaminated water, food, soil, or bedding and through bite wounds, by placental and venereal transfer, and through direct contact with infected urine. The bacterium can survive for weeks in warm, moist environments. It is uncommon in dry, arid regions. Clinical signs in infected dogs depend, in part, on the infecting serovar and may include fever, anorexia, polyuria, polydipsia, vomiting, and diarrhea. Renal failure, with or without liver disease, is possible. Some of the most implicated serovars in canine leptospirosis infection include *L. icterohemorrhagiae*, *L. grippotyphosa*, *L. pomona*, and *L. canicola*. Leptospirosis is a zoonotic disease, and precautions must be taken when treating animals that have or are suspected of having this disease. Four-way, injectable killed virus, whole-cell, and subunit *L. interrogans* vaccines are available. Each type provides protection against *L. canicola*, *L. pomona*, *L. grippotyphosa*, and *L. icterohemorrhagiae*. The leptospirosis vaccine is considered a noncore vaccine and is recommended for animals at risk of contracting the disease, depending on the prevalence of the disease in the area in which the animal lives and its risk of exposure to the pathogen. It should be kept in mind that several other serovars can cause leptospirosis, and existing vaccines do not protect against these other serovars. An older, injectable, two-way killed bacteria vaccine that contains serovars for *L. icterohemorrhagiae* and *L. canicola* is currently not recommended by the AAHA Canine Vaccination Task Force. The four-way *L. interrogans* vaccine can be administered as an individual immunization or is sometimes combined with canine distemper, CAV-2, CPiV, and CPV combination vaccine (DA2PPL).

TECHNICIAN NOTE

Many serovars can cause leptospirosis. The vaccine provides protection against four of the most common ones.

Bordetella bronchiseptica (Noncore Vaccine). *B. bronchiseptica* is one of the primary causes of canine infectious tracheobronchitis ("kennel cough"). Clinical signs include a dry, honking cough and possible nasal discharge. Bacteria are shed in respiratory secretions and are transmitted via airborne contact with secretions or through direct dog-to-dog contact. The infection is easily spread in highly populated closed environments, such as boarding kennels, animal shelters, and pet shops. An injectable inactivated cellular antigen extract and an intranasal live avirulent bacterial vaccine are available. These vaccines are considered noncore and should be administered to animals at risk for contracting infectious tracheobronchitis. It is not uncommon for boarding facilities to require this immunization before admission. *B. bronchiseptica* vaccines may be administered individually or may be combined with CPiV and CAV-2 vaccines.

TECHNICIAN NOTE

B. bronchiseptica intranasal vaccines are often preferred over the injectable forms of the vaccine, because they stimulate both local immunity and systemic immunity.

B. burgdorferi Vaccine (Noncore Vaccine). Canine Lyme disease is caused by the bacterium *B. burgdorferi*. The disease is spread by ticks (*Ixodes* species). Although only a small percentage of infected dogs show evidence of clinical disease, signs may include fever and polyarthritis. A small portion of infected dogs may also develop a protein-losing glomerulopathy and experience signs associated with renal failure. Injectable killed whole-cell bacteria and recombinant subunit OspA vaccines are available. OspA is an outer surface lipoprotein of *B. burgdorferi*. The vaccine is recommended for use in dogs with an increased risk of exposure, such as those living in or visiting areas where the risk of *Ixodes* tick exposure is high or where the disease is endemic. Tick control plays an important role in the prevention of Lyme disease.

Canine Influenza Vaccine (Noncore Vaccine). Canine influenza virus causes upper respiratory disease in dogs. Clinical signs include cough, fever, and possible nasal discharge. A small percentage of dogs may develop pneumonia secondary to the infection. Currently, an injectable killed virus vaccine is available. Although the AAHA Canine Vaccination Task Force does not make any specific recommendations regarding the vaccine, the same principles as those for other noncore vaccines against upper respiratory disease would apply. Dogs that are at risk of contracting the disease are those that live in, are traveling to, or may encounter dogs coming from endemic areas.

Canine Coronavirus Vaccine (Noncore Vaccine). Canine coronavirus causes an infectious form of enteritis that infrequently affects dogs. It is a highly contagious disease that spreads rapidly via fecal–oral transmission. Clinical signs include diarrhea, decreased appetite, lethargy, and possibly vomiting. Young animals tend to be most severely affected by the disease. Injectable killed virus and modified live virus (MLV) vaccines are available. The vaccine provides incomplete protection by decreasing but not eliminating canine coronavirus replication. This vaccine is not recommended by the AAHA Canine Vaccination Task Force.

Adverse Vaccine Events

Adverse vaccine events are side effects that may sometimes occur secondary to vaccination. Most of these events are transient, typically lasting a few days, and are not life threatening. Examples of side effects that typically do not require treatment include lethargy, mild fever, soreness at the injection site, and/or decreased appetite. Before their pet receives vaccination, owners should be warned that these side effects may occur and should be instructed to contact a veterinary health care team member if signs last longer than 2 to 3 days or are otherwise progressive. With many intranasal vaccines, it is not uncommon for a small percentage of animals to develop mild signs of transient upper respiratory disease, such as sneezing, nasal discharge, and coughing. With any immunization, the client must also be instructed to monitor the pet for any signs of an allergic reaction. A veterinary health care team member should be contacted immediately if the client observes the pet displaying signs such as facial swelling, difficulty breathing, vomiting, diarrhea, urticaria (hives), and/or seizures. In the most severe cases, systemic anaphylaxis can occur; this is a severe allergic or hypersensitivity response to a foreign substance. In these cases, cardiovascular collapse, respiratory arrest, and death may result if treatment is not immediately instituted. Treatment for allergic reactions may involve administration of an injectable antihistamine and/or administration of an injectable steroid. For more severe cases, the animal may also require administration of epinephrine and intravenous fluids.

Other types of adverse events may occur days to weeks (or more) after vaccination, and additional factors could play a role. Examples include immune-mediated hemolytic anemia, immune-mediated thrombocytopenia, immunosuppression, hypertrophic osteodystrophy, and thyroiditis.

Another potential adverse event related to vaccination is the development of a mass at the injection site, which is especially problematic in cats. Although this is considered rare, it is possible for a sarcoma to develop in the location of a vaccination. It is recommended that immunizations be given in a limb instead of the shoulder blade region, where tumor removal would be more difficult. Not all masses that develop at the injection site are cancerous. Sometimes benign inflammatory masses (granulomas) may develop and typically resolve within several weeks of administration. According to the Vaccine-Associated Feline Sarcoma Task Force, any mass that appears at an injection site should be documented. It is important to note the size, shape, and location of the mass and when it was first observed, and the owner should be instructed to monitor the mass for any changes. It is recommended by the task force that a biopsy should be performed on any mass that is greater than 2 cm in diameter, is still present months after vaccination, and/or continues to enlarge beyond 1 month after injection to determine whether the mass is cancerous.

All adverse vaccine events should be reported to the manufacturer of the vaccine. If multiple vaccines were administered to an animal during the same appointment, all vaccine manufacturers involved should be contacted. In addition, adverse vaccine events should be reported to the US Department of Agriculture Animal and Plant Health Inspection Service (USDA-APHIS) Center for Veterinary Biologics (CVB). Reports may be submitted online, via telephone (1-800-752-6255), or by fax or mail. Links to online submission forms and a printable pdf form that can be used to submit the report by mail or fax can be found at the USDA-APHIS CVB website (https://www.aphis.usda.gov/veterinary-biologics/adverse-event).

In most cases, the protection afforded by immunization outweighs the potential risk of an adverse event occurring in an immunologically naïve animal. For animals with suspected or known reactions to vaccines, the veterinary health care team must discuss with the owner the risks and benefits of administering the vaccine. Depending on the previous reaction, an antihistamine injection may be recommended up to 30 minutes before vaccine administration. Another option may be to administer a different brand of vaccine. In other cases, the owner and the veterinarian may elect to forgo vaccinating the pet given adequate antibody titer levels, which can be measured to determine whether protective immunity against the disease is present. Other potential actions that can be taken to decrease the likelihood of an adverse event occurring include selecting vaccine types that are less likely to cause local inflammation (nonadjuvanted) and/or spreading out the immunization process by administering core vaccinations first and noncore vaccinations later.

TECHNICIAN NOTE

The "1-2-3" recommendations for biopsy or removal of a postvaccination mass are as follows:
1. The mass is still growing after **1** month.
2. The mass is greater than **2** cm in diameter.
3. The mass persists for longer than **3** months.

Parasite Prevention

Parasite control is an important aspect of preventive health programs as parasites not only cause diseases but can also be carriers of other diseases that they transmit to pets. Fleas, for example, can cause flea-allergy dermatitis, but if they are ingested by a cat or a dog, they can also transmit tapeworms. A primary concern of ticks is the transmission of tick-borne diseases, which include

TABLE 8.4	Examples of Commonly Used Heartworm Preventive Products That Also Aid in the Treatment and Control of Other Parasites							
Product	**Heartworms**	**Hookworms**	**Roundworms**	**Whipworms**	**Fleas**	**Ear Mites**	**Sarcoptic Mange**	**Ticks**
Heartgard Plus Chewable (ivermectin and pyrantel pamoate)								
Canine	+	+	+	–	–	–	–	–
Heartgard Chewable (ivermectin)								
Feline	+	+	–	–	–	–	–	–
Revolution (Selectin)								
Canine	+	–	–	–	Adults and eggs	+	+	*Dermacentor variabilis*
Feline	+	+	+	–	Adults and eggs	+	–	–
Interceptor (milbemycin oxime)								
Canine	+	+	+	+	–	–	–	–
Feline	+	+	+	–	–	–	–	–
Sentinel (milbemycin oxime and lufenuron)								
Canine	+	+	+	+	Eggs and larvae	–	–	–
Trifexis (spinosad and milbemycin oxime)								
Canine	+	+	+	+	Adults	–	–	–

ehrlichiosis, Rocky Mountain spotted fever, and Lyme disease. There are many safe and effective products currently available to treat and prevent flea and tick infestations. These include oral medications that sterilize flea eggs or kill fleas in contact with the animal and monthly topical spot-on treatments that kill and/or repel fleas and ticks. It is important to note that some tick products that are safe and effective for use in dogs are not safe for use in cats; canine parasiticides should never be used on cats. It is especially important that owners are aware of this information if they have both dogs and cats in their household. The veterinary health care team should make recommendations to clients regarding the products that are best indicated for all their pets based on the animals' lifestyle.

Internal parasites also pose a risk for dogs and cats. All puppies and kittens should receive deworming medication. Annual fecal examinations to check for intestinal parasites are also recommended. Heartworms as an internal parasite may infect dogs, cats, and ferrets. According to the American Heartworm Society, the dog is the natural host for this parasite. The cat is an atypical host in which heartworm larvae do not typically mature into adults. The ferret is susceptible to infection, and one to two worms may be damaging to the heart because of its small size. Canine heartworm-preventive medications should not be used in cats or ferrets. An added advantage of many canine heartworm preventives available now is that they also treat for common intestinal parasites (Table 8.4).

Wellness examinations are a good time to educate owners on the dangers that parasites pose to their pets and about the benefits and ease of administering these products. For further information regarding diagnosis and treatment of parasites, refer to Chapters 13 and 28.

Preventive Health Program for Horses

A preventive health program for horses should be designed to meet the specific needs of the individual animal or herd. Such programs may vary from one stable to another and from one veterinary practice to another, depending on expected exposures, management styles, and personal preferences of attending veterinarians and horse owners. An example of one preventive health program for horses is outlined in Box 8.1.

Physical Examination

All new additions to a stable or an established herd should have a negative Coggins test result for equine infectious anemia (EIA) before arrival. Ideally, upon arrival, the horse(s) should immediately be placed in quarantine for 1 month before entering the general population. During this time, the first physical examination of the preventive health program can be performed. If quarantine facilities are not available, a thorough physical examination should be performed, and any signs of illness or parasite infection should be addressed before the horse is allowed to meet any animals in the resident population.

Vaccinations

Vaccination schedules are based on the age of the horse, anticipated exposure to infectious organisms, and the duration of immunity provided by the vaccine. Tables 8.5 and 8.6 list the vaccination guidelines provided by the American Association of Equine Practitioners. A variety of commercially available vaccines are approved for use in healthy horses, and the choice of product often depends on geographic location and personal experience and familiarity.

Young horses that are immunologically naïve or any horse that has an unknown immunization history should receive an initial immunization followed by a second booster immunization. The time between initial and booster vaccinations can vary based on the type of vaccine and the manufacturer but is generally 4 weeks.

TECHNICIAN NOTE

Young horses and those with an unknown vaccination history should receive an initial immunization followed by a booster in 4 weeks.

In rare instances, anaphylactoid reactions can occur with the use of any vaccine. These life-threatening crises must be handled quickly. Other complications, such as fever, lameness, and swelling or abscess formation at the injection site, may occur with routine use of the vaccines. The horse owner should always be informed of these possibilities before any vaccine is administered and be advised to notify their veterinarian if any signs are observed.

Tetanus Vaccines

Tetanus or lockjaw is a disease characterized by muscular rigidity that may culminate in death from respiratory arrest or convulsions. Tetanus is caused by toxins produced by the anaerobic bacterium *Clostridium tetani*. Active immunity to tetanus is produced by administration of a tetanus **toxoid**, which is a purified, inactivated toxin of *C. tetani*.

C. tetani is routinely found in the environment, and yearly vaccinations are recommended for all horses. Tetanus toxoid booster vaccinations are routinely given by many veterinarians when treating horses with penetrating injuries or at surgery.

Tetanus **antitoxin** is produced by hyperimmunization of donor horses with tetanus toxoid. Tetanus antitoxin provides protection by binding to the *C. tetani* toxin and can be used locally at the site of infection or given parenterally. Administration of tetanus

• BOX 8.1   General Outline of a Preventive Health Program for Horses

Spring
- Perform annual physical examination.
- Vaccinate all horses; vaccinate broodmares approximately 30 days before foaling.
- Obtain fecal egg count; deworm those with egg counts greater than 150 eggs/g.
- Perform annual dentistry examination; remove wolf teeth in 2-year-olds.
- Trim feet every 6–8 weeks.

Summer
- Give booster vaccinations for herpesvirus and influenza in high-risk animals.
- Vaccinate foals beginning at 3–4 months of age (can delay until age 6 months for foals born to vaccinated dams).
- Trim feet every 6–8 weeks.
- Obtain fecal egg count; deworm those with egg counts greater than 150 eggs/g.

Fall
- Give booster vaccinations for herpesvirus and influenza in high-risk animals.
- Give booster vaccinations for equine encephalitis viruses (WEE, EEE, VEE) and WNV in endemic areas.
- Trim feet every 6–8 weeks.
- Obtain fecal egg count; deworm those with egg counts greater than 150 eggs/g.
- Perform dentistry examination on horses younger than 5 years of age and on horses with known dental problems.

Winter
- Trim feet every 6–8 weeks.
- Deworm all horses with ivermectin–praziquantel or moxidectin–praziquantel to treat tapeworms and bots acquired over the summer and fall.

antitoxin to unvaccinated horses induces immediate protection, which lasts approximately 2 weeks, but its use should be restricted to high-risk cases because it can cause acute hepatitis.

Tetanus antitoxin and tetanus toxoid should never be mixed in the same syringe and should be injected at distant sites if administered at the same time.

TECHNICIAN NOTE

Tetanus antitoxin and tetanus toxoid should never be mixed in the same syringe.

Western, Eastern, and Venezuelan Encephalitis Vaccines

Equine encephalomyelitis is a viral neurologic disease of horses caused by Eastern, Western, and Venezuelan virus strains. These viruses are maintained in nature by bird and animal reservoirs and are transmitted to horses via biting insects. Venezuelan equine encephalomyelitis occurs primarily in South and Central America and has not been found in the United States for many years. The trivalent vaccine is commonly used for horses in states bordering Mexico to create a buffer zone, which may prevent the spread of Venezuelan equine encephalomyelitis into the United States.

The equine encephalomyelitis vaccines currently used for active immunization are inactivated virus vaccines and should be administered annually before the biting insect season. Vaccine protection

TABLE 8.5 Vaccinations for Foals[a,b]

Disease	Foals and Weanlings (<12 months of age) of Mares Vaccinated in the Prepartum Period for the Disease	Foals and Weanlings (<12 months of age) of Unvaccinated Mares	Comments
CORE VACCINATIONS: Protect against diseases that are endemic to a region, those with potential health significance, required by law, virulent/highly infectious infections, and/or those posing a risk of severe disease. Core vaccines have clearly demonstrated efficacy and safety and thus exhibit a high enough level of patient benefit and low enough level risk to justify their use in all equids.			
Tetanus	Three-dose series: First dose at 4–6 months of age Second dose 4–6 weeks after first dose Third dose at 10–12 months of age	Three-dose series: First dose at 1–4 months of age Second dose 4 weeks after first dose Third dose 4 weeks after second dose	
Eastern/Western equine encephalomyelitis (EEE/WEE)	Three-dose series: First dose at 4–6 months of age[c] Second dose 4–6 weeks after first dose Third dose at 10–12 months of age, before onset of next vector season	Three-dose series: First dose at 3–4 months of age[d] Second dose 4 weeks after first dose Third dose at 10–12 months of age, before onset of next vector season	Note: Primary vaccination series scheduling may be amended with vaccinations administered earlier to younger foals that are at increased disease risk owing to the presence of vectors. A foal born during the vector season may warrant beginning vaccination at an earlier age than a foal born before the vector season.
Rabies	Three-dose series: First dose at 6 months of age Second dose 4–6 weeks after first dose Third dose at 10–12 months of age	Three-dose series: First dose at 3–4 months of age Second dose 4 weeks after first dose Third dose at 10–12 months of age	
West Nile virus (WNV)	Inactivated vaccine[e] Three-dose series: First dose at 4–6 months of age Second dose 4–6 weeks after first dose Third dose at 10–12 months of age, before onset of next vector season	Inactivated vaccine[f] Three-dose series: First dose at 3–4 months of age Second dose 4 weeks after first dose Third dose at 10–12 months of age, before onset of next vector season	Note: Primary vaccination series scheduling may be amended with vaccinations administered earlier to younger foals that are at increased disease risk owing to the presence of vectors. A foal born during the vector season may warrant beginning vaccination at an earlier age than a foal born before the vector season.
	Recombinant canarypox vaccine Three-dose series: First dose at 5–6 months of age Second dose 4 weeks after first dose Third dose at 10–12 months of age, before onset of next vector season	*Recombinant canarypox vaccine* Three-dose series: First dose at 5–6 months of age Second dose 4 weeks after first dose Third dose at 10–12 months of age, before onset of next vector season	No data are available for use of the recombinant or chimera product in foals <5 months of age. If either product is administered to foals at <5 months of age, the recommended primary schedule should still be completed.
	Flavivirus chimera vaccine Two-dose series: First dose at 5–6 months of age Second dose at 10–12 months of age, before onset of next vector season	*Flavivirus chimera vaccine* Two-dose series: First dose at 5–6 months of age Second dose at 10–12 months of age, before onset of next vector season	
RISK-BASED VACCINATIONS: These have applications that may vary among individuals, populations, and geographic regions. Risk assessment should be performed by, or in consultation with, a license veterinarian to identify which vaccines are appropriate for a given horse or equid population (i.e., herd). The listing of a vaccine here is *not* a recommendation for its inclusion in a vaccination program. Vaccine scheduling is provided for use after it has been determined which, if any, risk-based vaccines are indicated.			

Continued

TABLE 8.5   Vaccinations for Foals[a,b]—cont'd

Disease	Foals and Weanlings (<12 months of age) of Mares Vaccinated in the Prepartum Period for the Disease	Foals and Weanlings (<12 months of age) of Unvaccinated Mares	Comments
Anthrax	Not applicable. Because it is not recommended to vaccinate mares during pregnancy, no foals of mares will be vaccinated prepartum	No age-specific guidelines are available for this vaccine. Manufacturer's recommendation is for primary series of 2 doses administered subcutaneously at 2–3-week intervals	Antimicrobial drugs must *not* be given concurrently with this vaccine. Caution should be used during storage, handling, and administration of this live bacterial product. Consult a physician immediately should accidental human exposure (via mucous membranes, conjunctiva, or broken skin) occur.
Botulism	Three-dose series: First dose 2–3 months of age Second dose 4 weeks after first dose Third dose 4 weeks after second dose	Three-dose series: First dose 1–3 months of age Second dose 4 weeks after first dose Third dose 4 weeks after second dose	Maternal antibody does not interfere with vaccination; foals at high risk may be vaccinated as early as 2 weeks of age.
Equine herpes virus (EHV)	*Inactivated or modified live vaccine* Three-dose series: First dose 4–6 months of age Second dose 4–6 weeks after first dose Third dose at 10–12 months of age Revaccinate at 6-month intervals	*Inactivated or modified live vaccine* Three-dose series: First dose 4–6 months of age Second dose 4–6 weeks after first dose Third dose at 10–12 months of age Revaccinate at 6-month intervals	
Equine viral arteritis (EVA)	Colt (male) foals Single dose at 6–12 months of age (see comments)	Colt (male) foals Single dose at 6–12 months of age (see comments)	*Before initial vaccination, colt (male) foals should undergo serologic testing* and be confirmed negative for antibodies to EVA. Testing should be performed shortly before or preferably at the time of vaccination. Because foals can carry colostrum-derived antibodies to EVA for up to 6 months, testing and vaccination should *not* be performed before 6 months of age.
Equine influenza	*Inactivated vaccine* Three-dose series: First dose at 6 months of age Second dose 3–4 weeks after first dose Third dose at 10–12 months of age *Modified live vaccine* Two-dose series administered intranasally: First dose at 6–7 months of age Second dose at 11–12 months of age Revaccinate at 6-month intervals	*Inactivated vaccine* Three-dose series: First dose at 6 months of age Second dose 3–4 weeks after first dose Third dose at 10–12 months of age *Modified live vaccine* Two-dose series administered intranasally: First dose at 6–7 months of age Second dose at 11–12 months of age Revaccinate at 6-month intervals	Increased risk of disease may warrant vaccinations of younger foals. Because some maternal anti-influenza antibody is likely to be present, a complete series of primary vaccinations should still be given after 6 months of age.
Potomac horse fever (PHF)	Two-dose series: First dose at 5 months of age Second dose 3–4 weeks after first dose	Two-dose series: First dose at 5 months of age Second dose 3–4 weeks after first dose	If risk warrants, vaccine may be administered to younger foals. Subsequent doses are to be administered at 4-week intervals until 6 months of age.
Rotavirus	Not recommended in foals	Not recommended in foals	

Continued

TABLE 8.5 Vaccinations for Foals[a,b]—cont'd

Disease	Foals and Weanlings (<12 months of age) of Mares Vaccinated in the Prepartum Period for the Disease	Foals and Weanlings (<12 months of age) of Unvaccinated Mares	Comments
Strangles (*Streptococcus equi*)	*Killed vaccine* Three-dose series: First dose at 4–6 months of age Second dose 4–6 weeks after first dose Third dose 4–6 weeks after second dose	*Killed vaccine* Three-dose series: First dose at 4–6 months of age Second dose 4–6 weeks after first dose Third dose 4–6 weeks after second dose	Vaccination is *not* recommended as a strategy in outbreak mitigation. If risk warrants, the MLV may be safely administered to foals as young as 6 weeks of age. However, vaccine efficacy in this age group has not been adequately studied. If MLV is administered to younger foals, a third dose of vaccine should then be administered 2–4 weeks before weaning.
	Modified live vaccine Three-dose series, administered intranasally: First dose at 6–9 months of age Second dose 3–4 weeks after first dose Third dose at 11–12 months of age	*Modified live vaccine* Three-dose series, administered intranasally: First dose at 6–9 months of age Second dose 3–4 weeks after first dose Third dose at 11–12 months of age	

[a]ALL vaccination programs should be developed in consultation with a licensed veterinarian.

[b]The two categories (core and risk-based vaccinations) reflect differences in the foal's susceptibility to disease and ability to mount an appropriate immune response to vaccination based on the presence (or absence) of maternal antibodies derived from colostrum. The phenomenon of maternal antibody interference is discussed in the text portion of these guidelines.

[c]*Foals in the Southeastern United States:* The primary vaccination series should be initiated with an additional dose at 3 months of age because of early seasonal vector presence.

[d]*Foals in the Southeastern United States:* The primary vaccination series should be initiated at 3 months of age because of early seasonal vector presence.

[e]*Foals in the Southeastern United States:* Owing to early seasonal vector presence, the primary vaccination series should be initiated earlier with the addition of a dose at 3 months of age.

[f]*Foals in the Southeastern United States:* The primary vaccination series should be initiated at 3 months of age because of early seasonal vector presence.

MLV, Modified live virus.

TABLE 8.6 Vaccinations for Adult Horses[a]

CORE VACCINATIONS: Protect against diseases that are endemic to a region, are virulent/highly contagious, pose a risk of severe disease, have potential public health significance, and/or require vaccination by law. Core vaccines have clearly demonstrated efficacy and safety with a high enough level of patient benefit and low enough level of risk to justify their use in all equids.

Disease	Broodmares	Other Adult Horses (>1 year of age) Previously Vaccinated for the Disease	Other Adult Horses (>1 year of age) Unvaccinated or Lacking Vaccination History	Comments
Tetanus	*Previously vaccinated* Annual: 4–6 weeks prepartum *Previously unvaccinated or having unknown vaccination history* Two-dose series: Second dose 4–6 weeks after first dose Revaccinate 4–6 weeks prepartum	Annual	Two-dose series: Second dose 4–6 weeks after first dose Annual revaccination	Booster at time of penetrating injury or before surgery if last dose was administered more than 6 months previously
Eastern/Western equine encephalomyelitis (EEE/WEE)	*Previously vaccinated* Annual: 4–6 weeks prepartum *Previously unvaccinated or having unknown vaccination history* Two-dose series: Second dose 4 weeks after first dose Revaccinate 4–6 weeks prepartum	Annual: spring, before onset of vector season	Two-dose series: Second dose 4–6 weeks after first dose Revaccinate before onset of next vector season	*Consider 6-month revaccination interval for* 1. Horses residing in endemic areas 2. Immunocompromised horses

Continued

TABLE 8.6	Vaccinations for Adult Horses[a]—cont'd			
Rabies	Annual: 4–6 weeks prepartum or before breeding (see comments)	Annual	Single dose: annual revaccination	*Note on vaccination before breeding:* Because of the relatively long duration of immunity, this vaccine may be given after foaling but before breeding and thus may reduce the number of vaccines given to a mare prepartum
West Nile virus (WNV)	*Previously vaccinated* Annual: 4–6 weeks prepartum	Annual: spring, before onset of vector season	*Inactivated vaccine* Two-dose series: Second dose 4–6 weeks after first dose Revaccinate before onset of next vector season	When using inactivated or recombinant product, consider 6-month revaccination interval for: 1. Horses residing in endemic areas 2. Juvenile (<5 years of age) 3. Geriatric horses (>15 years of age) 4. Immunocompromised horses
	Unvaccinated or lacking vaccination history • It is preferable to vaccinate immunologically naive mares when open • In areas of high risk, initiate primary series as described for unvaccinated adult horses		*Recombinant canarypox vaccine* Two-dose series: Second dose 4–6 weeks after first dose Revaccinate before onset of next vector season	

RISK-BASED VACCINES: Are selected for use based on risk assessment performed by/or in consultation with a licensed veterinarian. Use of these vaccines may vary between individuals, populations, and/or geographic regions.
NOTE: Vaccines are listed in this table in alphabetical order, not in order of priority of use.

			Flavivirus chimera vaccine Single dose Revaccinate before onset of next vector season	
Anthrax	Not recommended during gestation	Annual	Two-dose series: Second dose 3–4 weeks after first dose Annual revaccination	Do not administer concurrently with antibiotics. Use caution during storage, handling, and administration. Consult a physician immediately if exposure occurs by accidental injection, ingestion, or otherwise through the conjunctiva or broken skin.
Botulism	*Previously vaccinated* Annual: 4–6 weeks prepartum *Previously unvaccinated or having unknown vaccination history* Three-dose series: First dose at 8 months of gestation Second dose 4 weeks after first dose Third dose 4 weeks after second dose	Annual	Three-dose series: Second dose 4 weeks after first dose Third dose 4 weeks after second dose Annual revaccination	

TABLE 8.6 **Vaccinations for Adult Horses[a]—cont'd**

Equine herpes virus (EHV)	Three-dose series with product labeled for protection against EHV abortion: Give at 5, 7, 9 months of gestation	Annual (see comments)	Three-dose series: Second dose 4–6 weeks after first dose Third dose 4–6 weeks after second dose	Consider 6-month revaccination interval for: 1. Horses younger than 5 years of age 2. Horses on breeding farms or in contact with pregnant mares 3. Performance or show horses at high risk
Equine viral arteritis (EVA)	Not recommended unless high risk	Annual: Stallions, teasers: vaccinate 2–4 weeks before breeding season Mares: vaccinate when open	Single dose (see comments)	Before initial vaccination, intact males and any horses potentially intended for export should undergo serologic testing and be confirmed negative for antibodies to EVA. Testing should be performed shortly before or preferably at the time of vaccination.
Influenza	*Previously vaccinated* *Inactivated vaccine* Semiannual with one dose administered 4–6 weeks prepartum *Canarypox vector vaccine* Semiannual with one dose administered 4–6 weeks prepartum *Previously unvaccinated or having unknown vaccination history* *Inactivated vaccine* Three-dose series: Second dose 4–6 weeks after first dose Third dose 4–6 weeks prepartum *Canarypox vector vaccine* Two-dose series: Second dose 4–6 weeks after first dose but no later than 4 weeks prepartum	*Horses with ongoing risk of exposure* Semiannual *Horses at low risk of exposure* Annual	*Modified live vaccine* Single dose administered intranasally; Revaccinate semiannually to annually *Inactivated vaccine* Three-dose series: Second dose 4–6 weeks after first dose Third dose 3–6 months after second dose; Revaccinate semiannually to annually *Canarypox vector vaccine* Two-dose series: Second dose 4–6 weeks after first dose; Revaccinate semiannually	
Potomac horse fever (PHF)	*Previously vaccinated* Semiannual, with one dose given 4–6 weeks prepartum *Previously unvaccinated or having unknown vaccination history* Two-dose series: First dose 7–9 weeks prepartum Second dose 4–6 weeks prepartum	Semiannual to annual	Two-dose series: Second dose 3–4 weeks after first dose Semiannual or annual booster	A revaccination interval of 3–4 months may be considered in endemic areas when disease risk is high.
Rotavirus	Three-dose series: First dose at 8 months of gestation Second and third doses at 4-week intervals thereafter	Not applicable	Not applicable	

Continued

TABLE 8.6	Vaccinations for Adult Horses[a]—cont'd			
Strangles (*Streptococcus equi*)	*Previously vaccinated* *Killed virus vaccine containing M-protein* Semiannual with one dose given 4–6 weeks prepartum *Previously unvaccinated or having unknown vaccination history* *Killed virus vaccine containing M-protein* Three-dose series: Second dose 2–4 weeks after first dose Third dose 4–6 weeks prepartum	Semiannual to annual	*Killed virus vaccine containing M-protein* Two- to three-dose series: Second dose 2–4 weeks after first dose Third dose (where recommended by manufacturer) 2–4 weeks after second dose Revaccinate semiannually *Modified live vaccine* Two-dose series: administered intranasally Second dose 3 weeks after first dose Revaccinate semiannually to annually	Vaccination is not recommended as a strategy in outbreak mitigation

[a]All vaccination programs should be developed in consultation with a licensed veterinarian.

lasts approximately 6 to 8 months; in areas where winter freezes are uncommon or in endemic areas, semiannual vaccinations are advisable.

Equine Herpesvirus Vaccines

Equine herpesvirus (EHV), also known as *rhinopneumonitis*, frequently causes respiratory disease but can also cause abortion, neurologic disease, and neonatal illness. Although multiple herpesviruses have been identified, current vaccines offer protection against EHV-1 and EHV-4. These viruses cause respiratory disease; however, EHV-1 is also associated with infections of the CNS and the reproductive tract. EHV-4 is most frequently associated with upper respiratory tract disease in young horses and is rarely a cause of abortion.

Both inactivated and MLV vaccines are available for protection against the respiratory form of EHV; no currently available vaccine is licensed for protection against neurologic disease. Because immunity is short-lived, high-risk animals should be vaccinated every 6 months. Pregnant mares should be vaccinated during the fifth, seventh, and ninth months of gestation with an approved vaccine to aid in control of abortion.

Equine Influenza Vaccines

Equine influenza is a highly contagious viral disease with worldwide distribution. Influenza is contracted through inhalation and infects the upper and lower airways. Influenza is frequently seen in mobile populations of horses, and disease outbreaks usually occur in horses 1 to 3 years of age after mixing with infected horses at racetracks, training barns, or show grounds.

Both inactivated and MLV vaccines are available. MLV vaccines for influenza are administered intranasally and provide a greater duration of immunity. Booster vaccines are recommended every 6 months in high-risk animals.

Strangles Vaccines

Strangles is a respiratory disease caused by infection with the bacterium *Streptococcus equi*. Strangles is easily transmitted through direct contact with mucopurulent discharge from infected horses or from contaminated **fomites**, such as feeding utensils, buckets,

or other equipment. Strangles is characterized by sudden onset of fever and nasal discharge followed by acute swelling and abscess formation in submaxillary, submandibular, and retropharyngeal lymph nodes.

Several inactivated injectable vaccines and one low-virulence live strain intranasal vaccine are available to aid in the control and prevention of strangles. Intramuscular strangles vaccinations may cause postinjection reactions or abscesses at the site of administration. Because of these adverse effects, vaccination against strangles is recommended only for horses with a high likelihood of exposure to the pathogen. Vaccination is not 100% effective for preventing disease but does often reduce the severity and incidence of disease. Purpura hemorrhagica (immune-mediated vasculitis) is a possible adverse effect of all strangles vaccines.

TECHNICIAN NOTE

Administration of intranasal vaccines often results in contamination of hands and clothing by the modified live virus (MLV). Intranasal vaccines should be given last if a series of injections is being given, and hands should be washed thoroughly after administration.

Equine Viral Arteritis Vaccine

EVA is a contagious viral disease. Although infection is rarely serious in healthy adult horses, it is a matter of concern to horse breeders, because it can lead to abortion or neonatal death and can cause stallions to become permanent carriers of the virus.

Only one MLV vaccine against EVA is commercially available. Vaccination is recommended for colts intended to be breeding stallions and broodmares with no evidence of previous exposure to the virus before being used with carrier stallions for breeding. Vaccination is tightly controlled in some states, and there may be problems importing or exporting seropositive horses to certain countries.

Potomac Horse Fever Vaccines

Potomac horse fever (PHF) is caused by *Neorickettsia risticii* (formerly known as *Ehrlichia risticii*). It is most prevalent in the eastern

United States, particularly near large waterways, but has been identified throughout the United States and in other countries.

Approved vaccines are available for use in the control and prevention of PHF, and their use should be considered in areas where the disease is known to occur. The antibody response to vaccination is reportedly poor; however, vaccinated animals may exhibit reduced severity of clinical signs.

Botulism Vaccine

Botulism is caused by toxins produced by the bacterium *Clostridium botulinum* and results in gradual progressive muscular weakness. Multiple types of *C. botulinum* exist, although type B is most common in horses and is associated with the consumption of decaying forage.

The currently available equine botulism vaccine is a *C. botulinum* type B toxoid and is recommended for use in endemic areas. This vaccine requires an initial three-dose series followed by annual vaccination. Foals from unvaccinated mares may benefit from vaccination beginning as early as 2 weeks of age.

Anthrax Vaccine

Anthrax is caused by the bacterium *Bacillus anthracis*. Infection results from ingestion of soil, forage, or water contaminated by spores of the bacterium.

The currently available vaccine is an avirulent live-spore vaccine. Because swelling and abscesses have been associated with vaccination, its use is generally limited to animals in high-risk areas.

Rabies Vaccines

Rabies is a viral disease affecting the CNS and resulting in death. Approved killed virus vaccines are available for use in horses and should be used annually. Rabies vaccines induce a strong immunologic response; therefore only a single dose is required annually in adult horses.

West Nile Virus Vaccines

West Nile virus (WNV) was a foreign animal disease before 1999, when the disease was detected in humans and horses on the East Coast of the United States; however, WNV is currently prevalent throughout the United States. The disease is caused by a flavivirus that infects numerous species of birds and mosquitoes; humans and horses are dead-end hosts.

Several vaccines are available for protection against WNV. They should be administered annually ahead of the biting insect season. Vaccine protection lasts approximately 6 months; in areas where winter freezes are uncommon, semiannual vaccinations are advisable.

Parasites

A good preventive health program should account for control of internal and external parasites. Heavy parasite burdens decrease athletic and reproductive performance and can cause weight loss and colic. A good deworming program should target ascarids, small and large strongyles, bots, and tapeworms. See Chapter 13 for more information on parasite recognition, treatment, and prevention in small and large animal species.

Dental Care

Routine examination and care of the teeth is an important part of any horse's preventive health program. Signs of a dental problem can vary and include weight loss, bad breath, drooling, swelling of the face or jaw, dropping feed while eating, head tossing, excessive chewing of the bit, and problems while being ridden (bucking, tail ringing, fighting against the bit). Proper and thorough examination of the oral cavity usually requires sedation, a light source (e.g., a headlamp or a flashlight), and a mouth speculum.

In the horse, teeth are continually erupting, and the lower jaw is narrower than the upper jaw. As the horse grinds its food from side to side, the teeth are worn down unevenly. The inside (near the tongue) of the upper teeth is worn, as is the outside (near the cheek) of the lower teeth. Thus sharp points develop on the outside of the upper teeth and the inside of the lower teeth. These sharp enamel points can become severe, resulting in lacerations of the tongue and cheek. The cheek teeth of the upper jaw are often positioned slightly forward of the teeth in the lower jaw and, because of the offset positioning, hooks and ramps can form. *Hooks* are sharp points found on the first upper cheek teeth. *Ramps* are sharp points found on the last lower cheek teeth. Most enamel points, hooks, and ramps can be removed by regularly scheduled floating (rasping).

Wolf teeth are the small, pointed, rudimentary first premolars located just in front of the first cheek teeth. Wolf teeth do not appear in all horses, are more common in the upper jaw than in the lower jaw, and vary in size. In some horses, the position of these teeth causes interference with the position and function of the bit. For this reason, wolf teeth are often removed before a horse enters training (around age 12–18 months). Wolf teeth are generally removed while the horse is sedated, yet still standing.

Normally, the deciduous premolars are replaced by the permanent premolars without a problem between 2 and 4 years of age. Occasionally a deciduous premolar fails to fall out—a condition known as a *retained cap*. This can result in discomfort, leading to decreased feed consumption and lowered performance. Caps are easily removed in standing sedated horses.

Routine dental maintenance can prevent or minimize many of the dental problems observed in horses. Annual examinations are recommended for mature horses. Young horses lose deciduous teeth and gain their permanent teeth between the ages of 2 and 5 years of age. During this time, 24 teeth are lost and replaced, providing ample opportunity for dental problems to occur. Young horses should undergo a thorough dental examination before starting training and then twice yearly until all permanent teeth are in. Finally, horses with a history of dental problems should have their teeth examined biannually or even more frequently if required.

> **TECHNICIAN NOTE**
>
> Young horses (younger than 5 years of age) and those with a history of dental problems should have their teeth examined biannually.

Hoof Care

The roles of the veterinarian and the veterinary technician in hoof care are largely advisory, because most routine hoof care is provided by farriers. However, education of the client on the importance of proper and frequent hoof care is important.

Horse hooves grow an average of one-quarter inch per month, depending on ground surface, exercise frequency, nutrition, and individual growth rates. Based on the average growth rate, hooves should be trimmed every 6 to 8 weeks to maintain proper shape, balance, and movement. Keeping the hooves trimmed short and maintaining the correct hoof–pastern axis helps prevent excess stress on tendons and ligaments of the limb. In foals, some minor conformation problems, such as splayfoot or pigeon toe, can be corrected or minimized with frequent hoof trimming.

Hoof cleaning not only removes rocks and debris from the foot, but it also helps in the prevention of thrush. Thrush is caused by anaerobic bacteria that grow in moist and dark conditions, such as in the sulci of the frog and under dirt that has accumulated and packed into the sole. Thrush appears as a moist, malodorous accumulation in the sulci of the frog and sometimes over the sole. Frequent cleaning removes dirt and exposes these bacteria to drying, aerobic conditions. Copper- or iodine-based solutions can be applied to the sulci of the frog to treat thrush.

Nutrition

Proper nutrition is the foundation for any preventive health program as many health issues, such as laminitis, colic, and ulcers, can be directly related to nutritional problems. Owners should be encouraged to feed a balanced diet and to work closely with their veterinarian or equine nutritionist to develop proper diets for their animals. Equine nutrition is discussed in greater detail in Chapter 9.

Preventive Health Programs for Livestock Species

Preventive medicine is especially important in livestock species to maintain the productivity of the herd. Management, nutrition, and vaccination all play a role in minimizing the incidence of disease. This section is not intended to provide a comprehensive review of all of the vaccines available for livestock; the goal is to describe typical preventive management procedures and commonly used vaccination programs.

Swine

Birth to Weaning

Preventive medicine in swine herds begins with piglets, which must be kept in a warm, draft-free environment. When young pigs are cold, they lie on top of each other, increasing the risk of rectal prolapse. Within the first week of life, piglets have their needle (canine) teeth trimmed and tails docked to prevent them chewing on each other. Within the first few days, the piglets are commonly given iron supplement injections to prevent anemia, and male piglets that will not be used for breeding are castrated.

Growing Pigs

At weaning, when piglets are removed from the sow, they are vaccinated against erysipelas. Erysipelas (nicknamed "diamond skin disease"), which is caused by the bacterium *Erysipelothrix rhusiopathiae*, is characterized by fever, skin lesions, and sudden death in infected piglets. Animals that survive the acute infection may develop chronic arthritis or endocarditis and consequently experience poor growth. Pens into which weaned piglets are moved must be cleaned, disinfected, and well ventilated, without being cold or drafty. Newly grouped weaned piglets should not be mixed with older pigs, because this could increase stress, competition for food, and risk of disease exposure. Overcrowding must also be avoided. Weaning is a stressful time for piglets, and some farms will add antibiotics to the feed for a few weeks after weaning to help counteract the increased risk of infectious disease because of stress-induced suppression of the immune system during the post-weaning period. Piglets may be dewormed at weaning, if necessary, and vaccinated against pathogens that may cause pneumonia, such as *Mycoplasma* bacteria.

Biosecurity (protocols preventing introduction of disease organisms on the farm) should be strictly practiced in swine production. On some farms, all visitors, including veterinarians and their staff, are asked to shower and change into clothing provided by the farm before meeting any animals. The risk of spreading disease may also be minimized by working with the youngest pigs first and then proceeding progressively through older groups of pigs.

Breeding Animals

Pigs are commonly vaccinated for leptospirosis, parvovirus, and again for erysipelas before entering the breeding herd. Leptospirosis, an infection with *L. pomona*, *L. bratislava*, or other members of the genus *Leptospira*, may cause infertility, abortion, stillbirth, or the birth of weak piglets. Animals purchased for breeding should be tested for brucellosis and for pseudorabies if the animals are not from a pseudorabies-free area. Commercial pigs in the United States are considered pseudorabies-free, but feral pigs in some southern states and California may still carry the disease. Brucellosis may cause abortion or infertility, and it is zoonotic. Pseudorabies causes infertility, death in young pigs, and respiratory disease, with the possibility of chronic infection in older animals. Animals entering a herd free of porcine reproductive and respiratory syndrome (PRRS) should also be tested for the PRRS virus, which causes reproductive failure, respiratory disease, and chronic infections. Depending on their origin, animals may need to be treated for internal and external parasites. New additions to the herd should always be quarantined away from the herd for 30 days or longer before they are introduced to the rest of the herd. Quarantine prevents new animals from spreading diseases that they may have been carrying asymptomatically when they were purchased or some diseases, such as pneumonia, that they may have developed during transport to the farm.

Sows in the breeding herd should have booster vaccinations against erysipelas and leptospirosis when their litters are weaned; boars may be given the same vaccines every 6 months. Sows and gilts (young sows) may also be vaccinated against the bacterium *Escherichia coli* to prevent diarrhea in their offspring and against parvovirus, which may cause infertility and abortion.

> **TECHNICIAN NOTE**
>
> Because swine in modern production systems may never be outdoors, many pigs do not require deworming at any time.

Cattle

Although beef and dairy production systems have many differences, they are discussed together here, because many of the principles of disease control and diseases of concern are the same in both systems.

Birth to Weaning

In cattle, preventive medicine often starts before birth because many pregnant cows are vaccinated against *E. coli*, rotavirus, and coronavirus to protect their calves from diarrhea. Colostrum from vaccinated cows provides extra protection to calves from diseases against which the cow has been vaccinated. Calves should be born into a dry, draft-free environment. It is essential that calves receive an adequate amount of good-quality colostrum soon after birth. In beef herds, this is ensured by frequent monitoring of cows during calving season, whereas dairy herds typically hand-feed colostrum to newborn calves. Dairy farms will keep frozen colostrum or colostrum replacer on hand to feed orphan calves or calves from dams that fail to produce adequate colostrum or leak colostrum before calving.

TECHNICIAN NOTE

The first step in keeping calves healthy is ensuring that they receive an adequate amount of good-quality colostrum shortly after birth.

Weaning is the discontinuation of milk consumption by the calf. Dairy calves are raised away from their dams, so weaning is primarily a dietary adjustment. In beef calves, weaning is usually achieved by separating the calves from their dams. Vaccination in beef calves should begin before weaning, because weaning is a stressful time and stress may suppress the immune system, increasing the risk of contracting infectious diseases. Refer to Table 8.7 for a list of vaccines used in cattle. Dairy calves are weaned when they are younger compared with beef calves (younger than 2 months of age vs. about 6 months of age), so vaccination in dairy calves is commonly delayed until after weaning. For any young cattle, vaccination at less than 3 months of age is likely to be

somewhat ineffective because of interference from maternal antibodies obtained through colostrum; maternal antibodies against the antigen in a vaccine may bind the antigen and prevent it from stimulating a good response from the calf's own immune system. Calfhood vaccination programs usually include a clostridial vaccine, a combination vaccine against respiratory and reproductive viruses, and brucellosis vaccination (often called "Bangs" vaccination). Clostridial diseases, such as tetanus, blackleg, and malignant edema, are caused by bacteria from the genus *Clostridium*, occur primarily in young animals, and often are rapidly fatal. Respiratory and reproductive viral diseases are commonly included in one "five-way" or "six-way" product, usually with the brand name indicating the strength of the vaccine rather than what it is designed to protect against. The viral reproductive and respiratory pathogens commonly included in combination vaccines are bovine viral diarrhea virus (BVDV), which may cause diarrhea, mucosal ulcers, abortion, and immunosuppression, plus infectious bovine rhinotracheitis (IBR), parainfluenza 3 (PI3) virus, and bovine respiratory syncytial virus (BRSV), which are primarily respiratory pathogens. These combination vaccines also frequently include the bacterial pathogens *Histophilus somnus*, which may cause sudden death, fever, and depression, and/or *Leptospira* species, which cause infertility and abortion. Bangs vaccination protects against brucellosis (i.e., Bangs disease), an infection with *Brucella abortus* that is associated with abortion and infertility. Brucellosis vaccination is reported to the USDA and vaccinates are marked with an orange ear tag and a tattoo in the right ear. Only heifers younger

TABLE 8.7	Vaccines Used in Cattle		
Disease	**Typical Schedule**	**Comments**	
Viral diseases[a] (IBR-BVDV-PI3-BRSV)	Two doses in calfhood, annually thereafter	IBR, BVDV, PI3, and BRSV are respiratory pathogens. BVDV can cause a variety of disease syndromes and depressed immune function.	
Leptospirosis[a]	Two doses in calfhood, every 3–12 months in adulthood	Leptospirosis is commonly included in viral combination vaccines. Leptospirosis decreases reproductive performance.	
Brucellosis[a]	One dose in calfhood, females only	Commonly called Bangs vaccine. Vaccination of heifers makes interstate shipment and sale easier. Brucellosis decreases reproductive performance.	
Clostridial diseases[a]	Two doses in calfhood, optional in adults	Most vaccines include several clostridial components, often referred to as 7-way or blackleg vaccine.	
Campylobacteriosis	Annually before breeding season in beef herds	Also called vibriosis or "vibrio"; decreases reproductive performance.	
Bacterial respiratory diseases	Before weaning or upon entrance to the feedlot	These vaccines are often multivalent, including antigens from *Pasteurella*, *Mannheimia*, and *Haemophilus* bacteria.	
Gram-negative mastitis	Follow label directions	Commonly used in dairy cows.	
Rotavirus and coronavirus	Administered to pregnant cows	Designed to protect calves from diarrhea via antibodies in the cow's colostrum.	

Vaccines may be used in other situations such as anaplasmosis, anthrax, Johne disease, pinkeye (*Moraxella bovis*), foot rot, and trichomoniasis.

[a]Core vaccines.

This table is not intended to be comprehensive.

BRSV, Bovine respiratory syncytial virus; *BVDV*, bovine viral diarrhea virus; *IBR*, infectious bovine rhinotracheitis; *PI3*, parainfluenza 3.

than 1 year of age may be legally vaccinated against brucellosis and, in some states, the maximum age for vaccination is less than 1 year. Vaccination against brucellosis is especially important for animals that may be sold as breeding stock. Special care is taken in the handling and administration of RB51, the brucellosis vaccine, because the vaccine contains live organisms and the disease is zoonotic. Unlike clostridial and viral vaccines, the brucellosis vaccine is given only once; there is no "booster" vaccination.

Beef and dairy cattle that naturally have horns are commonly dehorned to protect other animals and farm personnel from injury. In dairy calves, this is usually done within the first few weeks of life, whereas in beef animals, dehorning may be done at the time of weaning.

> **TECHNICIAN NOTE**
>
> Cattle vaccines should be administered as labeled (intramuscularly or subcutaneously) only in the neck region to maintain meat quality. In addition, most vaccines for food animals have withdrawal or withholding periods, at which time the animal and its products (e.g., milk) may not be sold for human consumption.

Growing Cattle

Disease in growing cattle is best prevented by appropriate nutrition and clean, well-ventilated housing (or good pasture), in addition to vaccination. Growing cattle that are at risk will need to be treated for external and internal parasites as necessary. Adequate fly control will help prevent infectious bovine keratoconjunctivitis (pinkeye), an infection of the eye caused by *Branhamella ovis* and *Moraxella bovis*, which are carried between animals on flies. Heifers commonly receive another dose of viral respiratory and reproductive vaccine before being bred for the first time. Beef cattle are typically given a repeat vaccination against viral respiratory pathogens upon entering the feedlot; in addition, such animals are commonly vaccinated against the bacterial respiratory pathogens *Histophilus somnus*, *Mannheimia hemolytica*, and *Pasteurella multocida*.

Breeding Animals

To protect the health of the herd, care must be taken when breeding bulls are obtained. Beef herds are more likely to purchase bulls, because they generally employ natural breeding throughout the herd, whereas dairy herds use artificial insemination extensively. In addition to a breeding soundness examination for fertility, purchased bulls should at least have a negative test result for BVDV, which may cause infertility, abortion, diarrhea, death, or chronic poor condition. It is also advisable to test bulls for the venereal disease trichomoniasis, which is passed to cows during breeding and causes fertility problems. It is preferable to purchase the bull from a herd that is free of Johne disease, which is caused by *Mycobacterium paratuberculosis* and manifests as chronic diarrhea and weight loss, and bovine leukosis virus (BLV), which may cause cancer. Bulls should be vaccinated before the breeding season against respiratory and reproductive viral pathogens; campylobacteriosis, which is caused by *Campylobacter fetus* and may be passed to cows when breeding and cause infertility; and leptospirosis. Cows also should be revaccinated against these diseases before the breeding season.

> **TECHNICIAN NOTE**
>
> Nearly all adult cattle receive vaccinations against viral respiratory and reproductive pathogens (infectious bovine rhinotracheitis [IBR], parainfluenza 3 [PI3] virus, and bovine respiratory syncytial virus [BRSV]), frequently combined with antigens for one or more bacterial pathogens, at least once a year.

In dairy cows, mastitis (an infection of the mammary gland) is an important disease and a key focus of preventive efforts. Dairy cows are commonly vaccinated against mastitis, which is caused by *E. coli* and can be severe and life threatening. The vaccine does not prevent *E. coli* mastitis, but it does reduce the frequency and severity of the disease on the farm. Most cases of mastitis cannot be prevented by vaccination; prevention also relies on management steps. These include keeping the housing and milking areas clean, cleaning the teats well before milking, dipping the teats into disinfectant before and after milking (called *predipping* and *postdipping*), and providing proper nutrition.

Only the most commonly used vaccines have been mentioned here, but many more are available. Not all available vaccines are considered effective. Vaccine protocols should be tailored to each herd, specifically based on the needs and risks of the herd. However, even an excellent vaccination protocol cannot compensate for poor management and nutrition. Additional information about common infectious diseases in cattle can be found in Chapter 19. Hoof trimming is especially important in dairy animals. The hooves in cattle may not wear down as quickly as they grow, and in animals that have suffered an episode of lameness, the hooves may not wear down evenly. Dairy cows should have their feet trimmed at least once a year or more often if problems develop. Because they walk more, beef animals do not usually need routine hoof trimming, but this measure may be necessary for animals with abnormal hoof growth patterns, such as "corkscrew claws," in which the wall of the hoof spirals under the sole. This is thought to be a hereditary problem, so cows that display corkscrew claws should be removed from a breeding program.

As with bulls, purchased cows should be tested and quarantined before being introduced into a herd. It is preferable to buy cows from a herd that is free of Johne disease and BLV infection, and all animals should have a negative test result for BVDV. In addition, the milk of purchased dairy cows should test negative for the presence of mastitis infection.

Small Ruminants: Sheep and Goats

Newborn and Growing Animals

As with cattle, preventive health programs for sheep and goats begin before birth, when pregnant ewes and does are vaccinated against *Clostridium perfringens* types C and D and *Clostridium tetani*, which cause usually fatal diseases such as lamb dysentery, overeating disease, and tetanus. Protection for lambs and kids is provided through colostrum from their vaccinated dams. Previously vaccinated ewes and does should be vaccinated against these clostridial diseases again at least 4 weeks before their due date; if they have not previously been vaccinated, they should be vaccinated twice during pregnancy. Refer to Table 8.8 for a list of vaccines used in sheep and goats. The offspring of vaccinated dams should be vaccinated twice at 6 to 10 weeks of age. If ewes and does do not get vaccinated during pregnancy, kids or lambs should be vaccinated just after birth and again at age 2 to 3 weeks. In selenium-deficient areas, ewes should be supplemented with selenium orally or by injection to prevent weakness caused by selenium deficiency ("white muscle disease") in their lambs.

During the first 2 weeks of life, most sheep in the United States have their tails docked, or shortened. This is believed to decrease feces collecting on the tail and the risk of infestation of the tail by fly larvae (maggots). In addition, sheep with docked tails may be

TABLE 8.8 Vaccines Used in Sheep and Goats

Disease	Typical Schedule	Comments
Clostridial diseases[a]	Two doses during growth, periodically thereafter	Commonly called "CD-T"; includes protection against *Clostridium perfringens* types C and D (bloody scours and pulpy kidney disease) and *Clostridium tetani* (tetanus).
Sore mouth	Annually	Also called *contagious ecthyma* or *orf*. Caused by a poxvirus and is zoonotic. Vaccine is live and should not be used on farms that do not already have sore mouth on the premises. Care in handling vaccine should be taken.
Rabies	Annually	Not practical or necessary in commercial flocks but recommended for pets.

Vaccines may be used in other situations, such as foot rot, chlamydia, vibriosis, and caseous lymphadenitis.

[a]Core vaccine.
This table is not intended to be comprehensive.

easier to shear and fetch a higher price when sold for meat. Tail docking is usually performed by using a hot metal instrument that cuts off the tail and cauterizes the blood vessels at the same time or by applying a very tight elastic band to the tail, which causes a part of the tail to undergo necrosis (tissue death) and to fall off after a few weeks. It is recommended that the tail be left long enough to cover the animal's anus; if the tail is docked too short, it may damage local nerves and increase the risk of rectal prolapse. Male animals that will not be sold young or used for breeding are usually castrated, either by surgically removing the testicles or by applying a tight elastic band to the scrotum (i.e., banding), as in docking of the tail.

Most goats will grow horns if they do not have their horn buds removed; this removal is best done in the first week of life and is usually performed by using a hot iron instrument that destroys the horn-growing cells of the horn bud. If the horn bud was not removed when the goat was young and an animal without horns is desired, the goat will have to be dehorned, which is a more complex procedure. Horns are removed to protect people and other animals from injury.

At the time of castration, horn bud removal, dehorning, and/or tail docking, tetanus antitoxin should be administered to the offspring of ewes and does that were not vaccinated against clostridial diseases during pregnancy.

> **TECHNICIAN NOTE**
>
> Diseases caused by *Clostridium* species are especially dangerous to sheep and goats. Pregnant ewes and does should be vaccinated against clostridial diseases to protect their offspring.

Small ruminants may also be vaccinated against contagious ecthyma, also called *orf* or *sore mouth*. It is a viral disease that causes painful skin lesions on the mouths of young animals and the mouths and teats of ewes and does, resulting in decreased nursing by young animals. Sore mouth vaccination is performed by scratching the skin in an area without wool (inner ear or under the tail in older animals, inner thigh in young animals) and introducing a live virus into the scratch. This must be done well before lambing or kidding so that newborn animals will not be affected. In addition, great care must be taken by the person administering the vaccine, because it contains a live virus that can cause zoonotic

disease. The vaccine should not be used in herds that have not had problems with the disease.

Coccidia are present in all sheep and goats and may cause diarrhea, weight loss, and illness in young animals under stress. Coccidia are controlled by effective management steps, such as preventing overcrowding, providing good sanitation, and not placing feed on the ground. A coccidiostat drug, such as lasalocid or decoquinate, may be added to the feed to prevent outbreaks of coccidiosis at times of stress.

The Breeding Herd

For small ruminants kept as pets, rabies vaccination is probably worthwhile, although it is not used in commercial flocks. As in other species, many other vaccines are available for use in sheep and goats; decisions about whether to use them in particular animals or herds should be made in consultation with a veterinarian and in consideration of specific needs and risks.

> **TECHNICIAN NOTE**
>
> Rabies vaccination is not administered to all animals in commercial sheep and goat flocks, but it should be considered for pet sheep and goats.

Parasitism is a serious problem in sheep and goats, particularly infestations by *Haemonchus contortus*, also called the *barber pole worm*. *H. contortus* attaches to the wall of the abomasum and consumes the animal's blood. If left untreated, the infestation may lead to severe anemia and death. No strategy eliminates internal parasites in sheep and goats, but the parasite burden can be reduced in several ways. One approach is good nutrition; well-nourished animals are less susceptible to parasitic infestations. To reduce contamination of feed by feces, the feed should be kept elevated from the ground in a trough that young animals cannot climb into. Goats that can browse above-ground plants, instead of just grazing as sheep do, will have reduced parasite burdens. Parasitism in sheep may be reduced by rotating them through pastures that have been kept empty or have been used by cattle or horses (not goats) or for growing crops in the previous 3 to 6 months. Culling of animals with chronic severe parasitism is recommended, because such animals have low parasite resistance—a trait that may be passed on to offspring. Oral deworming agents, such as those of the benzimidazole (e.g., thiabendazole) and aver-mectin (e.g., ivermectin) families, are used in small ruminants, but these drugs must be used strategically, because overuse promotes resistance. Some experts have recommended deworming only ani-mals that show signs of disease. Sheep may develop external para-sites, such as ticks and lice, which should be treated as necessary with sprays, dips, or ivermectin-type drugs.

> **TECHNICIAN NOTE**
>
> Sheep may be evaluated for anemia caused by parasitism with *Haemonchus contortus* by examining the conjunctiva of the eyes. If it is white, not pink, the animal is likely to be anemic and heavily parasitized. The FAMACHA (FAffa MAlan CHArt) technique is useful in determining whether an animal is suffering from parasitism.

Summary

Many aspects of preventive medicine must be applied in live-stock species. Vaccination is important, but it is not a substitute for proper management. Disease is prevented through proper nutrition, good hygiene, appropriate housing, parasite control, and vaccination. To prevent diseases, new animals must be tested and quarantined before they are introduced into a herd.

Acknowledgments

The authors and publisher wish to acknowledge the contributions of Carolyn J. Hammer, Stacey M. Ostby, Christopher T. Reetz, and Sarah A. Wagner to previous editions of this chapter.

Recommended Readings

Dogs and Cats

American Association of Feline Practitioners. *American Association of Feline Practitioners 2020 Feline Vaccination Guidelines.* Available at: https://www.catvets.com/guidelines/practice-guidelines/aafp-aaha-feline-vacciantion.

Vaccine-Associated Feline Sarcoma Task Force: Vaccine-Associated Feline Sarcoma Task Force guidelines: diagnosis and management of sus-pected sarcomas, American Veterinary Medical Association website. Available at: http://www.avma.org/vaccine-associated-feline-sarcoma-task-force-guidelines-diagnosis-and-managment-suspected-sarcoma.

Vogt AH, Rodan I, Brown M, et al. AAFP-AAHA feline life stage guide-lines. *J Am Anim Hosp Assoc.* 2020. Available at: https://www.aaha.org/aaha-guidelines/life-stage-feline-2021/feline-life-stage-home/.

Welborn LV, DeVries JG, Ford R, et al. 2019 AAHA canine vaccination guidelines. *J Am Anim Hosp Assoc.* 2011;47:1. Available at: https://www.aaha.org/aaha-guidelines/life-stage-canine-2019/life-stage-canine-2019.

Horses

American Association of Bovine Practitioners, AABP Vaccination Guidelines. Available at: aabp.org/committees/resources/VaccGuide-lines2021.pdf.

9

Animal Nutrition

KARA M. BURNS

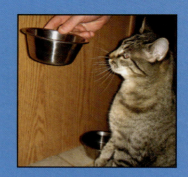

CHAPTER OUTLINE

LEARNING OBJECTIVES

When you have completed this chapter, you will be able to:

1. Pronounce, spell, and define the key terms in this chapter.
2. Compare and contrast the concepts of energy units, energy partitioning, metabolizable energy measurement, Atwater factors, energy density, and measurements of energy expenditure.
3. List the macronutrients and micronutrients found in pet food. Do the following regarding nutrients:
   - List the building-block molecules that make up proteins, fats, and carbohydrates.
   - Discuss the requirements for protein, fat, carbohydrates, fiber, vitamins, and minerals in the diet of dogs and cats.
   - List the energy-producing and nonenergy-producing components of food.

- Differentiate between microminerals and macrominerals and give examples of each.
4. Explain the rationale for and steps of the nutritional assessment of small animals.
   - Calculate the resting energy requirement (RER) for a cat and dog.
   - Determine the body condition score of a cat and dog.
5. Describe the unique feline physiology and the impact on nutrition.
   Explain various aspects regarding commercial pet food, including the following:

a. Explain how pet food manufacturing is regulated in the United States and identify the government agencies and organizations involved in the regulation of pet food.

b. Describe which marketing language bears little nutritional significance and explain how veterinary therapeutic diets may be used appropriately and inappropriately.

c. List the components of pet food labels and explain how the information provided in each component should be interpreted.

6. Explain the myths that are associated with small animal nutrition.

7. Describe feeding protocols for healthy dogs and cats at each stage of life, including pregnant and lactating females.

8. Describe the rationale and indications for assisted feeding in cats and dogs.

9. Regarding the nutrition of horses:
   - Explain the importance of grass and hay in the equine diet.
   - Describe how pregnancy and lactation alter a mare's nutritional requirements.

- List steps taken to provide appropriate nutrition to foals and young, growing horses.
- Describe general guidelines for feeding sick horses.

10. Describe the rationale and method for performing an assessment of nutrition status in large animals.
    - List the variables affecting energy requirements of livestock.
    - Describe how nutrient excesses and deficiencies lead to toxicity in large animals.
    - Describe how the nutritional requirements of each of these species are affected by the animal's stage of life and by its energy expenditure (maintenance, growth, lactation, etc.).
    - List advantages and disadvantages of pasture feeding livestock.

11. Discuss the requirements for protein, fat, carbohydrates, fiber, vitamins, and minerals in the diets of birds, small mammals, and reptiles.

KEY TERMS

Amino acid
Assisted feeding
Atwater factors
Average daily gain
Biological value (BV)
Body condition score (BCS)
Calorie
Complete feeds
Concentrates
Daily energy requirement (DER)
Digestible energy (DE)
Digestion
Energy density
Enteropathy
Esophagostomy tube
Fatty acid

Forage
Gastrostomy
Gross energy (GE)
Kilocalorie (kcal)
Kilojoule
Lipid
Metabolizable energy (ME)
Metabolizable (maintenance) energy requirement
Net energy (NE)
Nonprotein nitrogen
Nutrient
Palatability
pH
Resting energy requirement (RER)
Roughage
Total digestible nutrients

Introduction

Nutrition is one area of veterinary medicine that affects all animals, large and small. Of the three components that affect an animal's life—genetics, environment, and nutrition—nutrition is the only factor that the veterinary health care team can positively impact. Health and healing depend on proper nutrition and feeding management. As a member of the veterinary health care team, it is important for veterinary technicians to understand nutrition and how it relates to the animals that they care for each day.

Basics of Nutrition

Proper nutrition and feeding management are fundamental to good health in both small and large animals. When discussing nutrition, we will begin with a review of nutrients. Many pet and livestock owners want to discuss the ingredients of feeds and pet foods. However, it is important to keep in mind that there are many different types of ingredients that can provide the same vital nutrients. For this reason, nutrients are the fundamental

part of nutrition not the source of those nutrients. A nutrient is any food component that helps support life. These have been divided into six major groups. Three of these groups supply energy, and three do not provide energy. Energy-producing nutrients include proteins, fats, and carbohydrates. Nonenergy-producing nutrients include vitamins, minerals, and water. In the wild, animals eat to satisfy their energy needs. However, companion animals, such as dogs and cats, rely on their owners to feed them, and livestock rely on farmers to ensure proper feeding practices. Consequently, many pet foods and livestock feeds are nutritionally balanced preparations. A complete and balanced diet for a particular species is one that provides the correct balance of proteins, fats, carbohydrates, vitamins, minerals, and water in the proper proportions and, at the same time, meets the animal's energy needs.

> **TECHNICIAN NOTE**
>
> Proper nutrition and proper feeding management are fundamental to good health in both small and large animals.

Energy

Energy is not merely one of the major nutrients, but it is the most critical component of the diet (after water). Energy needs are always the first requirement that needs to be met in an animal's diet. After energy needs have been met, nutrients become available for other metabolic functions. Approximately 50% to 80% of the dry matter (DM) in a dog's or a cat's diet, for example, is used for energy. The body obtains energy from nutrients by oxidation of the chemical bonds found in the fundamental nutrient molecules: proteins, carbohydrates, and fats.

> **TECHNICIAN NOTE**
>
> Approximately 50% to 80% of the DM in a dog's or a cat's diet is used for energy. The body obtains energy from nutrients by oxidation of the chemical bonds found in the fundamental nutrient molecules: proteins, carbohydrates, and fats.

The process of a substance combining with oxygen and resulting in the loss of electrons is known as *oxidation* and occurs during **digestion**, absorption, and transport of nutrients into the body's cells. The most important energy-containing compound produced during this oxidative process is adenosine triphosphate (ATP), a common high-energy compound composed of a purine (adenosine), a sugar (ribose), and three phosphate groups.

The biochemical reactions that occur within the body either use energy or release energy. Anabolic reactions require energy for completion, and catabolic reactions release energy upon completion. ATP and other energy-trapping compounds pick up part of the energy released from one process and transfer it to other processes. This energy is used in a variety of ways, such as for pumping ions, molecular synthesis, and activating contractile proteins. These processes principally describe the total use of energy by the animal. Without the energy supplied through the diet, these reactions would not occur, and death would follow.

When discussing energy, the veterinary profession uses the term *kilocalorie*. A kilocalorie (kcal) is the amount of heat required to raise the temperature of one kilogram of water by 1° Celsius (°C). Kilocalories are also referred to as "**Calories**" (with a capital "C") when discussing food or exercise. The term **digestible energy** refers to the food's **gross energy** minus the energy that is nonabsorbable and lost in feces.

"**Metabolizable energy**" (ME) is the food's gross energy minus the energy lost in feces and urine. It is the amount of energy that is available to the pet's body for metabolism after digestion and absorption. "**Net energy**" (NE) is calculated from the measurement of energy used for digesting, absorbing, and using food. Because the acts of eating and digesting use energy, the subtraction of this amount from the ME provides an estimate of how much is left over for metabolism.

> **TECHNICIAN NOTE**
>
> The food's gross energy minus the energy lost in feces and urine is known as *metabolizable energy* (ME).

Energy Terms

1. Digestible energy (DE) = gross energy (GE) from food – energy lost in feces.
2. Metabolizable energy (ME) = digestible energy (DE) – energy lost in urine and gas. ME is the most common estimate of how much energy (kcal) is supplied from pet food.
3. Net energy (NE) = metabolizable energy (ME) – energy used in digesting, absorbing, and using food.

When GE values are readjusted for digestibility and urinary losses, ME values of 3.5 kcal/g are assigned to proteins and carbohydrates and 8.5 kcal/g to fats; these values are called *modified* **Atwater factors**. These were developed by the Association of American Feed Control Officials (AAFCO) to produce an equation that would more accurately reflect the digestibility of commercial pet foods, which tend to have lower digestibility compared with typical human foods.

Proteins

Proteins serve as a dietary nitrogen source for animals and are the primary part of many body tissues, enzymes, and hormones. Proteins are also essential components of deoxyribonucleic acid (DNA), ribonucleic acid (RNA), hemoglobin, and antibodies; in addition, in blood vessels, plasma proteins maintain an important oncotic force that prevents fluid from leaking out of the vessels and into the surrounding tissues. They also serve as transport molecules in the blood. Proteins supply approximately 4 kcal of energy per gram when consumed in the diet and are composed of combinations of building-block molecules called **amino acids**. Amino acids that are called "essential" are those that cannot be synthesized by the body and must be supplied in the diet. Dogs require 10 essential amino acids, whereas cats require 11. One of the essential amino acids required by cats is taurine. The amount of dietary protein required varies by species, age of the animal, and quality of the protein being used.

The *quality* of protein used is not identifiable on the labels on pet food packaging. Rather, protein quality is assessed by its digestibility and amino acid profile. Measuring a protein's biological value (BV) is one way of determining quality. The higher the quantities of essential amino acids found in a particular protein, the higher its BV and quality. The higher the BV of a particular protein, the more likely it is to be absorbed and metabolized by the body. Thus the higher the quality of a particular protein, the less it is required in the diet to meet the protein needs of the animal. Protein supplied that is more than the animals' nutritional needs is *not* stored as protein. The liver converts excess protein into energy, and the nitrogenous waste product (urea) from this process is excreted by the kidneys in urine. Subsequently, too much dietary protein cannot be stored in adult cats and dogs, and it has the potential to increase the workload of the kidneys.

> **TECHNICIAN NOTE**
>
> The quality of a protein is not identifiable on a pet food label. Protein quality is assessed by its digestibility and amino acid profile.

Proteins from animal sources, such as meats and by-products, contain more essential amino acids than proteins from plants. However, proteins from the two types of sources, meats and plants, are often complementary. Proteins enhance the overall BV of the diet when combined with other nutrients in the correct proportions. Cats have a higher protein need and therefore require at least twice as much protein as dogs. Young animals require more protein than adults. Cats have a high protein requirement, because they must metabolize some protein for energy. Cats also have a greater need for meat-based proteins than plant-based proteins. Thus cats do not have metabolic flexibility where protein is concerned. This is one major reason that cat food is higher in protein than dog food. This is also the reason dogs should not be allowed to eat cat food and vice versa.

In ruminants, digestion is supported by microbes in the rumen, where protein from feed is converted into their subunits of short peptide chains and amino acids. Subsequently, these smaller molecules are further broken down into ammonia, organic acids, and carbon dioxide (CO_2). The ammonia released by microbial degradation of feed-based protein is removed from the rumen by absorption through the rumen wall, or it is used by rumen microorganisms for the synthesis of protein. The microbial flora in the rumen generates a consistently excellent quality of protein that is subsequently passed on to the lower digestive tract. For this reason, protein in moderate- to poor-quality feeds is typically improved through rumen metabolism. However, the opposite can occur if high-quality protein is fed to ruminants. Common nonprotein nitrogen (NPN) sources include urea, ammonium salts, ammoniated by-products, or free amino acids. These NPN sources should be used cautiously in ruminants to prevent potential excess or deficiency, which may result in toxicity.

Carbohydrates

Cats and dogs have no minimum requirement for carbohydrates. However, carbohydrates are added to commercial pet foods as an energy source to supply calories and to add variety, fiber, and palatability to the diet. Carbohydrates are also typically less expensive ingredients in pet foods. Dietary carbohydrates provide approximately 4 kcal of energy per gram, and cereal grains are the most common source in pet foods. Carbohydrates are classified into two segments, based on their digestibility: soluble and insoluble. Raw carbohydrates are not digested well by carnivores (e.g., cats) and omnivores (e.g., humans, bears, and dogs). However, simply grinding or cooking raw ingredients can increase their digestibility.

TECHNICIAN NOTE

Grinding or cooking raw sources of carbohydrates increases their digestibility in cats and dogs.

Soluble carbohydrates are also referred to as *nitrogen-free extract* (NFE). Carbohydrates can consist of simple sugars, or monosaccharides; complex sugars, or disaccharides; and polysaccharides. Carbohydrates aid in digestion with the help of enzymes, such as maltase, sucrase, and lactase. These are found in the intestinal tract lining and break down disaccharides. Therefore any impairment of the intestinal tract may affect the pet's ability to digest some forms of carbohydrates—specifically disaccharides (complex sugars). Soluble carbohydrates over the amount needed to meet the animal's energy requirements are stored in the body as glycogen or fat and may lead to obesity.

Insoluble carbohydrates, sometimes referred to as *dietary fiber*, include cellulose, hemicellulose, and lignin, among others. Monogastric animals lack the intestinal enzymes to completely digest insoluble carbohydrate sources and rely on key bacterial flora to break down these fibers and permit partial assimilation. Various fiber sources have different degrees of digestibility or solubility. Dietary fiber, especially cellulose, has been shown to normalize the gastrointestinal (GI) tract. Components of dietary fiber have

also been shown to alter fat and glucose metabolism and decrease the absorption of other nutrients. Diets high in insoluble carbohydrates are inappropriate for dogs and cats with high energy requirements (e.g., puppies and kittens); pregnant and lactating females; and stressed or working animals. However, insoluble carbohydrates are helpful in overweight animals, because they aid in weight control and weight reduction by promoting a sense of fullness without adding calories.

Carbohydrates often used in livestock feeds are as follows:
- Fiber-forage: structural carbohydrates, cellulose, hemicellulose
- Sugars (molasses, growing plants): glucose, sucrose, fructose
- Starches: stored carbohydrates, grains

Fats

Fats serve as a more concentrated source of energy in a diet, providing 9 kcal of energy per gram. Fats are the primary energy source of most commercial pet foods. In addition:
1. Fats enhance palatability.
2. They are necessary for the absorption, storage, and transport of the fat-soluble vitamins A, D, E, and K.
3. They are the source of the essential fatty acids (EFAs) required by dogs and cats, including linoleic acid, linolenic acid, and arachidonic acid (AA).

EFAs are necessary components of cell membranes. They are also responsible for the synthesis of prostaglandins and related compounds and for the control of epidermal water loss. Cats require dietary sources of AA, which is found only in animal fats; this is another indication that cats are true carnivores and that to survive, they require meat tissue sources in their diet. Dogs can synthesize AA from linoleic acid. EFA deficiencies occur in dogs when they are fed low-fat dog food containing beef tallow as the sole source of fat in the diet or when the diet has been improperly stored for an extended period. Dietary fat needs to be stabilized with an antioxidant or preservative to preserve the quality of the dry food to which it has been added and to prevent the fat from becoming rancid. The same does not apply to canned foods, because canned foods are pasteurized and sealed. Signs of fat deficiencies in cats and dogs include delayed wound healing, dry hair coat, scaly skin, and *pyodermas* (skin infections).

Vitamins

Vitamins are important for the chemical reactions of metabolism, functioning as enzyme precursors or coenzymes. Vitamins are divided into the following two basic categories:
1. Fat-soluble vitamins
   a. Vitamin A
   b. Vitamin D
   c. Vitamin E
   d. Vitamin K
2. Water-soluble vitamins
   a. Vitamin B complex
   b. Vitamin C

Fat-soluble vitamins can be stored in body fat and in the liver. Therefore dietary excesses of fat-soluble vitamins may result in toxicities. The water-soluble vitamins are not stored to any great extent in the body. Owners and health care teams must be careful of excessive water loss in animals (i.e., excessive urination, diarrhea, etc.), because vitamins may be decreased through the loss of water, necessitating vitamin supplementation. Cats have additional vitamin requirements compared with dogs. Cats are unable to convert beta-carotene, present in plants, into vitamin A. Therefore they require a dietary source of preformed vitamin A found only in animal tissues. In addition, niacin must be added to a cat's diet, because cats cannot convert the amino acid tryptophan into the B vitamin niacin.

Minerals

Minerals are categorized into two major groups: (1) macrominerals, which include calcium, phosphorus, potassium, sodium, and magnesium; and (2) microminerals or trace minerals, which include iron, zinc, copper, manganese, iodine, cobalt, and selenium. It is the balance of the *amount* of minerals in the diet that is important. Excess intake of any one mineral may be harmful. In addition, any unabsorbed portion may bind with other minerals, adversely affecting their availability and resulting in a deficiency or imbalance within the pet. The best approach is to feed a diet known to contain the proper amount and balance of minerals for each species and for the animal's particular life stage or activity level.

Calcium is required in the largest amount in the diet, but it is also important that calcium is present in the diet in the proper proportion in relation to phosphorus. Too much calcium in livestock feed and in pet food will result in a decrease in the absorption of phosphorus, iron, zinc, and copper. This will cause delayed bone growth and maturation in puppies and kittens. Dietary supplements, such as calcium carbonate, dicalcium phosphate, bone meal, or vitamin D, are not recommended and should not be given with high-calcium diets and free-choice feeding. Supplements are most often the cause of calcium excess. Calcium deficiency is primarily associated with phosphorus excess, such as when dogs are fed high levels of meat and organ tissue in their diet. The correct calcium-to-phosphorus ratio is approximately 1.1 and 1.4 to 1.

TECHNICIAN NOTE

Calcium is the mineral required in the largest amount in the diet, but it is important to have calcium in the proper proportion and amount in relation to phosphorus.

Phosphorus has an important role in cell metabolism and bone and teeth composition. Too much dietary phosphorus, however, increases the glomerular filtration rate and results in greater work for the kidneys. High phosphorus levels in conjunction with calcium may result in soft tissue calcification, which may lead to kidney damage. Sodium is the main cation of extracellular body fluids, whereas potassium is the main intracellular one. Sodium chloride, or salt, is a main taste factor in many pet and human foods. Too much salt in the diet, however, can lead to high blood pressure and fluid buildup and may worsen heart and kidney diseases. Although 4 to 8 mg/kg of sodium is adequate to maintain homeostasis, many commercial pet foods contain 10 to 40 times the amount needed, that is, 80 to 150 mg/kg! In both small and large animal species, the excess intake of any one mineral may be harmful.

The term *ash* is used a lot in small animal feeds, particularly cats. High ash content in some cat foods has been linked to urinary tract disease. It is important to know that the term *ash* refers to *all the minerals* in a food product. It is the mineral magnesium that seems to be the main contributor in the appearance of struvite urolith–related lower urinary tract disease (LUTD). Low-ash foods could still contain excess levels of magnesium, making

them harmful to urinary tract health. It is important to look at the specific minerals in a particular food as opposed to its ash content. Additionally, promoting production of urine with mean **pH** (acidity) of 6.2 to 6.4 can inhibit the production of struvite crystals and urinary stones.

Water

Water is the most critical nutrient for life. Therefore all animals, large and small, should always have access to fresh, clean water. Water is vital to all species and is required to sustain life. Water is necessary to complete body functions, such as digestion, transport of nutrients, and excretion, and for all metabolic reactions to occur normally in the body. It is therefore important to remind owners to always provide fresh, clean water for their pets. Water loss of 5% will result in sluggishness and an overall unwell feeling in pets. A 10% loss in total body water causes serious illness, and a 15% loss may result in death. The water requirement of a dog or a cat, expressed in milliliters per day (mL/day) is roughly equivalent to the animal's energy requirement in kilocalories per day (kcal/day).

TECHNICIAN NOTE

A rule of thumb for water requirement for a dog or a cat, expressed in milliliters per day (mL/day), is roughly equivalent to the animal's energy requirement in kilocalories per day (kcal/day).

Palatability

Palatability is *not* a nutrient, nor does it relate to the nutritional value of the food. Palatability is a measure of how well overall an animal *likes* a food. *Acceptability* of food by a pet indicates whether the amount of food eaten will be enough to meet the animal's caloric requirements. A *balanced* food only needs to be palatable enough to ensure acceptability along with adequate nutrient intake, and a food's performance does not improve by higher consumption of it. In fact, higher consumption may predispose the animal to obesity. Pet owners, however, often judge the quality of a food by how quickly their pets consume it. Some palatability factors include odor, temperature, texture or feel of the food in the pet's mouth, fat content, water content, and salt content. When a pet owner needs to improve the palatability of the diet without altering the nutritional profile of the food, simple things, such as moistening dry food, warming a food to body temperature, hand feeding, or simply adding the canned version of the selected diet to the dry food in the bowl, can be helpful.

PUT INTO PRACTICE

Communication with clients regarding the importance of nutrition is imperative to the health of your patients. Helping clients to understand nutrition labels and what their pets need to thrive is a way you can increase patient care and revenue for your practice.

Digestibility

Digestibility can be defined as the amount of nutrients in a food that are available for absorption by an animal's body. It is those nutrients that are "used" by the body. Factors that can negatively affect a food's digestibility include inclusion of poorquality ingredients and high levels of fiber, ash, and phytate. Inadequate processing and extreme heat treatment of foods will also have a harmful effect on digestibility. In contrast, pet food digestibility is increased by inclusion of high-quality ingredients and the use of proper processing techniques. Therefore in less digestible foods, the body will not be able to use the nutrients and thus create more waste. Although lower quality, less digestible food may cost less money up front, given the poor digestibility, the pet will need to eat a larger quantity of food to truly gain the nutrients the body needs.

Supplements

Several other compounds found in foods also play a role in nutrition. Antioxidants are substances that delay or prevent oxidation (breakdown) of other compounds or structures, such as cell membranes. Although certain vitamins and minerals serve as antioxidants (e.g., vitamin E, selenium), nonnutrients, such as flavonoids and polyphenols, can be found in certain plants used in pet foods or may be added separately. Carotenoids act both as provitamins (partially converted to vitamin A in the body) and as antioxidants. Carotenoids are typically found in colorful vegetables. Choline is a compound that acts like a B vitamin, although choline is most often synthesized in the liver as opposed to being a dietary requirement. In certain instances, choline can be an essential nutrient. Another vitamin-like compound is L-carnitine, which can be found in animal tissue (meat) and synthesized in the body. L-carnitine is often added to pet food for its beneficial effects on health—especially in weight management.

Many clients themselves take supplements and want to give supplements to their pets as well. If a vitamin/mineral supplement is given to a pet whose diet contains adequate minerals, the owner may create a vitamin or mineral imbalance in that pet. It is important to understand the dangers of supplementing minerals. Oversupplementation of calcium in a growing puppy will have dramatic negative effects on the skeletal system and may result in several developmental orthopedic diseases. Feeding high levels of calcium will not cause that puppy to grow taller. Genetics determine the size of the dog. As discussed earlier, macrominerals and microminerals affect the absorption of other minerals. Therefore if a client supplements one mineral, it undoubtedly will affect many others. Malnutrition due to nutrient excess is more common than malnutrition resulting from nutrient deficiencies. However, both can exist simultaneously. Microminerals, also called *trace minerals*, include iron, manganese, copper, and selenium. Companion animals can experience trace mineral deficiencies. These deficiencies can occur either by consuming a food too low in microminerals or by consuming a food that has been supplemented with another mineral that might interfere with the absorption of microminerals.

> **TECHNICIAN NOTE**
>
> Clients who often take supplements themselves may also want to give supplements to their pets. However, owners must be educated that if a vitamin/mineral supplement is given to a pet whose diet contains adequate minerals, a vitamin or mineral imbalance may be created in that pet.

Nutritional Evaluation of Small Animals

Health care teams know that proper nutrition is a critical component for maintaining the health of pets. Every patient, healthy or ill, that enters the veterinary hospital should have an evaluation of its nutritional status, and health care team members should make a nutritional recommendation based on this evaluation. However,

in some practices, it may be difficult for health care team members to get involved in helping clients make nutritional decisions for their pet. Therefore the role of the veterinary health care team in nutrition needs to be reviewed and practical guidelines and tips applied.

The positive impact of proper nutrition on health and disease is well established in all animals. Appropriate feeding throughout all life stages can help prevent diet-associated diseases and assist in the management of other diseases. Because good nutrition is integral to optimal pet care, it is important to incorporate nutritional assessment and specific nutritional recommendations into each annual visit. To help health care teams integrate nutrition into their practice routines, the American Animal Hospital Association (AAHA) offers the Nutrition and Weight Management Guidelines which may be found at: https://www.aaha.org/aaha-guidelines/2021-aaha-nutrition-and-weight-management-guidelines/home/. The World Small Animal Veterinary Association (WSAVA) launched its publication, the *V5 Global Nutrition Guidelines*, to be found at: https://wsava.org/global-guidelines/global-nutrition-guidelines/. Evaluation of nutritional status, which is considered the "fifth vital sign," should be performed during each patient visit. Nutritional screening during the standard physical examination and history taking requires little to no additional time or cost. However, incorporating nutritional assessment and recommendations into the care of small animals helps develop a partnership between the practice management and the veterinary health care team, resulting in healthier pet patients.

Nutritional Assessment

Nutritional assessment considers several factors, including the animal, its diet, feeding management, and environmental factors. It is critical to remember that nutritional assessment is an iterative process in which each factor affecting the animal's nutritional status is assessed and reassessed as often as required. Although the impact of nutrition on health is a complex area of study, the AAHA and the WSAVA nutritional guidelines can be summarized into three easy-to-implement steps:

1. Incorporate a nutritional assessment and specific dietary recommendation for every pet at every visit.
2. For every patient, perform a screening evaluation (nutritional history/activity level, body weight (BW) and body/muscle condition score).
3. Perform an extended evaluation for a patient with abnormal physical examination findings or nutritional risk factors, such as life stage issues, abnormal body condition score (BCS) or muscle condition score, poor skin or hair coat, systemic or dental disease, diet history of snacks or table food that is greater than 10% of total calories, unconventional diet, GI upset, or inadequate or inappropriate housing.

Every animal that presents to the hospital should be assessed to establish its nutritional needs and feeding goals, which depend on the pet's physiology and/or disease condition. The role of the veterinary technician is to ascertain patient history, determine the patient's BCS, work with the veterinarian to determine the proper nutritional recommendation for the patient, and communicate this information to the pet owner.

> **TECHNICIAN NOTE**
>
> Incorporate a nutritional assessment and specific dietary recommendation for every pet at every visit.

The first step in evaluating a pet and determining its nutritional status is to obtain a complete history, including signalment (i.e., species, breed, age, gender, reproductive status, activity level, and environment). Next, a nutritional history should be taken to determine the quality and adequacy of the food being fed to the pet, the feeding protocol (e.g., whether the pet is fed at designated meals or has free choice, the amount of food given, the family member responsible for feeding the pet), and the type or types of food given to the pet. Refer to Fig. 9.1 for an example of a nutritional history form. When evaluating a pet, the technician should ask the owner the following questions:

- What brand and type of food do you feed your pet?
- What brand and type of snacks or treats do you give your pet?
- Tell me about any supplements you give to your pet.
- Tell me what medications your pet has been prescribed or recommended to take.
- What type of chew toys does your pet play with?
- What human foods does your pet consume?

Nutritional History Questionnaire

Date_____ Pet's name_____ Species_____

Breed_____ Date of Birth_____ Weight_____

Gender_____ Neutered/Spayed - No___ Yes___ BCS_____ MCS_____

1. Tell me about your pet's living environment - Indoors ☐ Outdoors ☐ Both ☐
2. Tell me about your pet's activity level.
   a. Plays/walks **3 times/day**_____ **1-2 times/day**_____ **Never**_____
3. Do you have other pets? **No**_____ **Yes**_____
   a. If yes, list here_____
4. Tell me the arrangements for feeding your pets._____
5. Does your pet have access to other, unmonitored food sources? No ☐ Yes ☐
   a. If yes, please describe_____
6. Tell me about your pet's appetite. _____
7. Who feeds your pet? _____
8. What changes have been made to your pet's diet in the past 30 days? _____
9. Please list the brands and product names (if applicable) and amounts of ALL foods, treats, snacks, dental hygiene products, rawhides, and any other foods that your pet is currently eating.

Food/Treat	Form	Amount	How Often	Date Started

10. Tell me what supplements your pet receives._____
11. What medications is your pet taking and how is each administered? _____
12. Tell me about the toys your pet enjoys. _____
13. Tell me about food or treats not formulated for pets that your pet receives._____
14. Tell me what foods/treats are NOT tolerated by your pet._____
15. If you are going on vacation and I am your pet sitter, tell me everything I need to do for your pet while you are gone._____
_____

©Kara M. Burns

• **Fig. 9.1** Nutritional history form. (Copyright Kara M. Burns.)

- Tell me about any other sources of food to which your pet may have access.

Asking open-ended questions requiring more than a one-word answer is the best way to get information. The above questions are common, but to truly find what is going into the pet, it is beneficial to ask questions such as the following:

- Tell me what types of things your pet eats in a 24-hour period.
- If you have a pet sitter watch your pet, tell me what directions you leave for the pet sitter.

Answers to these open-ended questions will help the health care team determine what the patient is truly receiving from the owner. Closed-ended questions may put owners on the defensive or imply that they are giving something to their pets that they should not be giving.

Owners should also be asked about their pets' access to foods, supplements, and medications and how much of each substance the pets consume each day. Pets also may be fed by more than one family member or receive numerous treats throughout the day. All these factors play a role in the proper nutrition of pets.

All members of the health care team should be familiar with taking a nutritional history. Through this mechanism, the team can pinpoint a breakdown in owner compliance (e.g., more than one person in the household is feeding the pet, the pet is getting more calories than are recommended, etc.) and begin to establish a feeding protocol to ensure proper calorie consumption by the pet.

Feeding Methods

There are three different ways to feed a companion animal. The client should understand these three feeding methods, and the health care team should make a recommendation based on the pet, the client, and the type of food. The three methods include portion-controlled feeding (meal feeding), time-restricted feeding, and ad lib (free) feeding.

Portion-Controlled (Meal) Feeding

Portion-controlled (or meal) feeding requires the owner to measure out a specific amount of food and give it to the pet in a "meal" or a portion at a specific time of day. The pet should consume the food within a few minutes but is not required to finish it. The food amount is typically divided into morning and evening feedings. This method is recommended, because it is aimed at preventing the pet from overeating. This method is also preferred, because the client always knows how well the pet is eating each day.

Time-Restricted Feeding

Time-restricted feeding allows the client to feed as much food as the pet will eat in 5 minutes. How well the pet eats is critical to the pet's eating enough food to meet its needs. This method keeps clients informed on how well their pet is eating. However, it is also possible for the pet to overconsume with the use of this method. Small-breed dogs may not eat enough in the time provided, and large-breed dogs may eat too much. This method is quite variable and is not typically the best recommendation for pets.

Ad Lib (Free) Feeding

Ad lib (or free) feeding is common, because little effort is required and owners prefer this to accommodate busy schedules. This method allows the client to place unlimited food in front of the animal, allowing it to eat at its leisure. The pet owner is much less aware of how much their pet consumes. Frequently, large bowls of food are offered to the animal, enabling the pet to eat during the entire day. When this method is used, many pets will often consume 15% to 20% more calories than they should and subsequently, their weight management becomes difficult. Owners of cats are known for using this method—more so than owners of dogs. Ad lib feeding makes it difficult to know if and how much the pet is eating. And if the client is feeding multiple cats, then monitoring food intake is even more difficult. This method is often not recommended—but is used too often.

> **TECHNICIAN NOTE**
>
> Although the ad lib feeding method may be more convenient for pet owners, it results in higher calorie consumption and may lead to obesity in the pet.

Nutritional Calculations

The amount of food that is fed to an animal is established on a calculation of the animal's daily energy requirement (DER). The formula demonstrates how many calories an animal should be fed to maintain its weight in a controlled environment, known as the **resting energy requirement** (RER). If the animal faces additional factors, such as working, lactation, or growth, a further calculation is required. This constitutes the DER. Once the calculation is complete, the client will understand how many calories must be provided. It is important to realize that this calculation is a starting point. Every pet is unique and should be evaluated individually; some pets may require more calories, and some may require fewer. The health care team can educate clients on how to monitor the pet's weight and body condition by incorporating body condition scoring and BW assessment.

Veterinary health care teams should be comfortable with calculating the amount of food or the appropriate energy intake of the patient. The pet's DER reflects the pet's activity level and is a calculation based on the pet's RER.

There are some basic formulas that all veterinary health care team members should memorize or have on laminated note cards in every examination room (along with a calculator!). The most accurate formula to determine the RER for a cat or a dog, regardless of the breed, is:

$$\text{RER kcal / day} = 70 \, (\text{Ideal BW in kg})^{0.75}$$

The second equation is

$$(BW_{kg} \times BW_{kg} \times BW_{kg}, \sqrt{}, \sqrt{}) \times 70$$

Once the RER is determined, the DER may be calculated by multiplying the RER by "standard" factors related to energy needs.

Body Condition Scoring

The health care team should document the pet's **body condition score** (BCS) and weight at every visit as part of the physical examination. BCS is a subjective assessment that is important when determining whether a dog or a cat is at a healthy weight and when substantiating a diagnosis of obesity in a pet. It allows health care team members to assess a patient's fat stores and muscle mass, helps in evaluating weight changes, and provides a value that can be used in team communication. The two most common body condition scoring systems are the five-point scale and the nine-point scale. Both rating scales use nine points, but the five-point scale is scored to the nearest half-point, whereas the nine-point scale is scored to the whole point. It is important for all members of the health care team to use the same scoring system from the outset to avoid confusing or miscalculating the patient's weight. Body condition is assessed beginning at the head of the pet and working toward the tail. Fat cover is evaluated over the ribs, down the topline, around the tail base, and ventrally along the abdomen. On the five-point scale, a score of 1 represents "too thin" and 5 represents "obese"; a score of 3 means "ideal." According to body composition studies in cats and dogs, a body condition of 15% to 25% fat is optimal; therefore a pet with an ideal BCS has 15% to 25% body fat. A pet with a BCS indicating overweight has 26% to 35% body fat, and a pet with a BCS indicating obesity has greater than 40% body fat. Refer to Figs. 9.2 and 9.3 for the body condition scoring scales from the 2021 AAHA Nutrition and Weight Management Guidelines for dogs and cats.

Muscle Condition Scoring

Muscle condition scoring is the evaluation of muscle mass independent from body fat content assessed by BCS. Muscle condition scoring includes visual examination and palpation over temporal bones, scapulae, lumbar vertebrae, and pelvic bones. The loss of muscle unfavorably affects the strength, immune function, and wound healing of pets. After all the information is collected and analyzed in the assessment phase a treatment plan is implemented. This is followed by repeated assessment and adjustment of the plan, remembering that nutrition is an iterative process. Figures of feline and canine muscle condition scoring from the 2021 AAHA Nutrition and Weight Management Guidelines are given in Figs. 9.4 and 9.5.

Establishing a written protocol to ensure that every patient receives a nutritional assessment and specific dietary recommendation at every visit is simple. Each practice should develop a customized protocol.

Pet owners want and expect the very best for their pets. Even pets that are not "sick" may still not have ideal health. Pet owners who understand that preventive care preserves and lengthens the lives of their pets are much more likely to become regular users of veterinary medical services, regardless of their economic conditions. All members of the veterinary health care team should focus on proper nutrition for every pet that presents to their hospital. To do this, the health care team must perform a complete nutritional history and patient assessment and be knowledgeable about the wide variety of foods that are available on the market today. The health care team members must familiarize themselves with the nutritional requirements of pets, assess

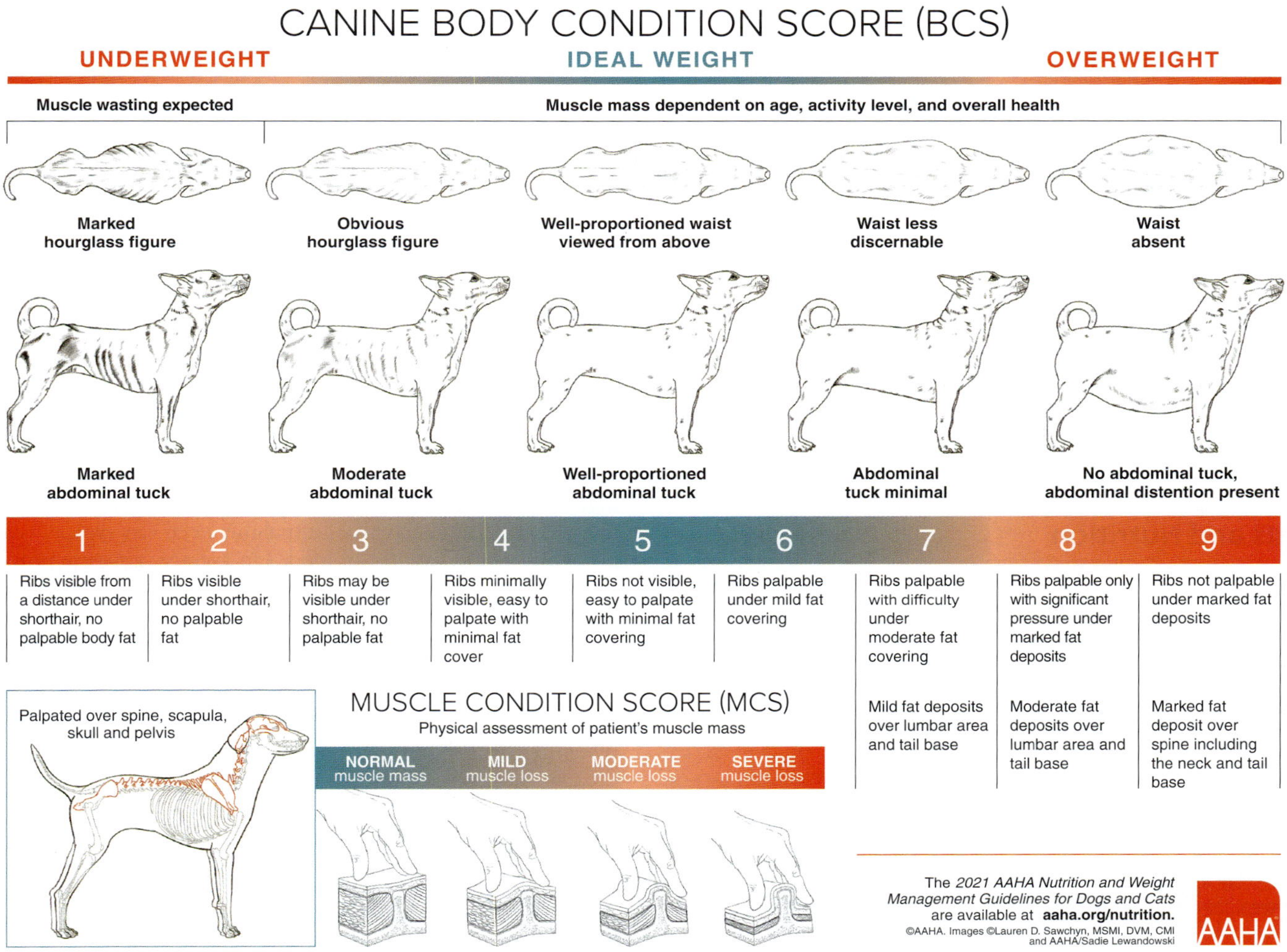

CANINE BODY CONDITION SCORE (BCS)

UNDERWEIGHT		IDEAL WEIGHT				OVERWEIGHT		
Muscle wasting expected		Muscle mass dependent on age, activity level, and overall health						
Marked hourglass figure	Obvious hourglass figure	Well-proportioned waist viewed from above		Waist less discernable		Waist absent		
Marked abdominal tuck	Moderate abdominal tuck	Well-proportioned abdominal tuck		Abdominal tuck minimal		No abdominal tuck, abdominal distention present		
1	2	3	4	5	6	7	8	9
Ribs visible from a distance under shorthair, no palpable body fat	Ribs visible under shorthair, no palpable fat	Ribs may be visible under shorthair, no palpable fat	Ribs minimally visible, easy to palpate with minimal fat cover	Ribs not visible, easy to palpate with minimal fat covering	Ribs palpable under mild fat covering	Ribs palpable with difficulty under moderate fat covering	Ribs palpable only with significant pressure under marked fat deposits	Ribs not palpable under marked fat deposits
						Mild fat deposits over lumbar area and tail base	Moderate fat deposits over lumbar area and tail base	Marked fat deposit over spine including the neck and tail base

Palpated over spine, scapula, skull and pelvis

MUSCLE CONDITION SCORE (MCS)
Physical assessment of patient's muscle mass

NORMAL muscle mass	MILD muscle loss	MODERATE muscle loss	SEVERE muscle loss

The *2021 AAHA Nutrition and Weight Management Guidelines for Dogs and Cats* are available at **aaha.org/nutrition.**
©AAHA. Images ©Lauren D. Sawchyn, MSMI, DVM, CMI and AAHA/Sadie Lewandowski

AAHA

• **Fig. 9.2** 2021 AAHA Guidelines body condition scoring of dogs. (From the 2021 AAHA Nutrition and Weight Management Guidelines for Dogs and Cats, aaha.org/nutrition. Copyright AAHA. Images copyright Lauren D. Sawchyn, MSMI, DVM, CMI and AAHA/Sadie Lewandowski. Used with permission.)

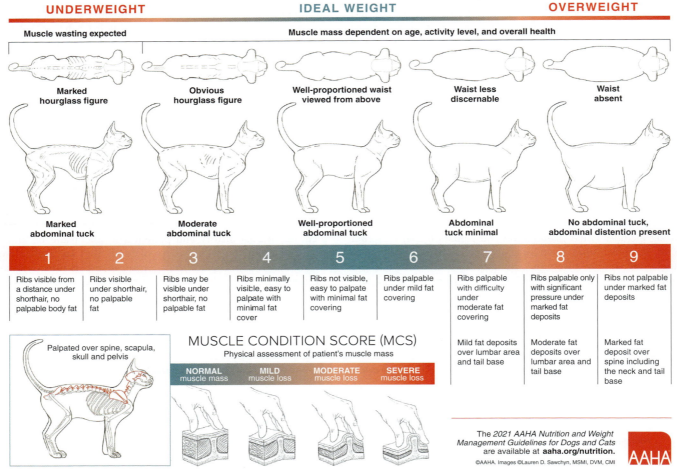

FELINE BODY CONDITION SCORE (BCS)

UNDERWEIGHT   **IDEAL WEIGHT**   **OVERWEIGHT**

Muscle wasting expected   Muscle mass dependent on age, activity level, and overall health

Marked hourglass figure	Obvious hourglass figure	Well-proportioned waist viewed from above	Waist less discernable	Waist absent
Marked abdominal tuck	Moderate abdominal tuck	Well-proportioned abdominal tuck	Abdominal tuck minimal	No abdominal tuck, abdominal distention present

1	2	3	4	5	6	7	8	9
Ribs visible from a distance under shorthair, no palpable body fat	Ribs visible under shorthair, no palpable fat	Ribs may be visible under shorthair, no palpable fat	Ribs minimally visible, easy to palpate with minimal fat cover	Ribs not visible, easy to palpate with minimal fat covering	Ribs palpable under mild fat covering	Ribs palpable with difficulty under moderate fat covering / Mild fat deposits over lumbar area and tail base	Ribs palpable only with significant pressure under marked fat deposits / Moderate fat deposits over lumbar area and tail base	Ribs not palpable under marked fat deposits / Marked fat deposit over spine including the neck and tail base

Palpated over spine, scapula, skull and pelvis

MUSCLE CONDITION SCORE (MCS)
Physical assessment of patient's muscle mass

NORMAL muscle mass	MILD muscle loss	MODERATE muscle loss	SEVERE muscle loss

The *2021 AAHA Nutrition and Weight Management Guidelines for Dogs and Cats* are available at **aaha.org/nutrition**.
©AAHA. Images ©Lauren D. Sawchyn, MSMI, DVM, CMI

AAHA

• **Fig. 9.3** 2021 AAHA Guidelines body condition scoring of cats. (From the 2021 AAHA Nutrition and Weight Management Guidelines for Dogs and Cats, aaha.org/nutrition. Copyright AAHA. Images copyright Lauren D. Sawchyn, MSMI, DVM, CMI/Sadie Lewandowski. Used with permission.)

patients, and educate clients regarding nutrition and the health of their pets.

Cats and Nutrition

Cats and dogs are members of the order Carnivora and are therefore classified as carnivores. However, when considering cats and dogs from a dietary perspective, dogs are considered omnivores, and domestic cats are strict or obligate carnivores. This difference between cats and dogs is supported by specific behavioral, anatomic, physiologic, and metabolic adaptations of cats to a strictly carnivorous diet.

TECHNICIAN NOTE

From a dietary perspective, dogs are considered omnivores, and domestic cats are strict or obligate carnivores. Veterinary technicians should be aware of the characteristics of cats that make their nutritional needs distinctly different from those of dogs.

Feline Feeding Behaviors

Cats display certain feeding behaviors that are like felids in the wild. Cats typically do not display a regular daily rhythmic sleep-wake cycle or regular cycles of activity, feeding, and drinking. Cats are known to eat 10 to 20 small meals throughout the day and the night. This reflects the relationship between cats and their prey in the wild. Cats are known to hunt alone. Feral cats typically catch prey/mice as their source of food. On average, a mouse provides approximately 30 kcal of ME. This amount is about 12% to 13% of a feral cat's DER. As one can see, hunting throughout the day and the night is necessary to obtain sufficient food by an average cat. Therefore meal feeding—especially once per day—conflicts with the natural feeding behaviors of cats. But it has also been seen that free feeding has contributed to the obesity epidemic that is seen in cats and in other species; thus it is important to feed to the cats' natural instincts, but not overfeed.

Feline Metabolism

Feline metabolism is unique. Feline nutrition must be closely monitored to meet the specific nutritional requirements of a true carnivore. Some of these unique attributes include:
1. Strict requirement for the amino acid arginine
2. Lack of arginine in the diet for longer than 24 hours may have life-threatening consequences
3. Inability to synthesize taurine from cysteine

CANINE MUSCLE CONDITION SCORE (MCS)

MCS is the physical assessment of patient's muscle mass.

MCS is scored by visual examination and palpation of musculature over the spine, scapulae, skull, and pelvis:

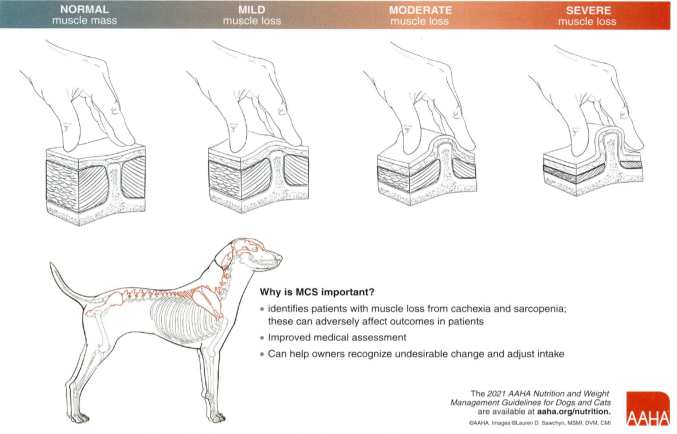

| NORMAL muscle mass | MILD muscle loss | MODERATE muscle loss | SEVERE muscle loss |

Why is MCS important?

- identifies patients with muscle loss from cachexia and sarcopenia; these can adversely affect outcomes in patients
- Improved medical assessment
- Can help owners recognize undesirable change and adjust intake

The *2021 AAHA Nutrition and Weight Management Guidelines for Dogs and Cats* are available at **aaha.org/nutrition.**
©AAHA. Images ©Lauren D. Sawchyn, MSMI, DVM, CMI

AAHA

• **Fig. 9.4** 2021 AAHA Guidelines Muscle Condition Score (MCS) canine. Muscle condition scoring in dogs. (From the 2021 AAHA Nutrition and Weight Management Guidelines for Dogs and Cats, aaha.org/nutrition. Copyright AAHA. Images copyright Lauren D. Sawchyn, MSMI, DVM, CMI/Sadie Lewandowski. Used with permission.)

4. Inability to synthesize vitamin A from beta-carotenes
5. Inability to synthesize niacin from the amino acid tryptophan

Cats are very sensitive to the form, odor, and taste of foods. The flavor and texture preferences of individual cats are often influenced by early experience that can affect preferences throughout life. Cats familiar with a certain texture or type of food (i.e., moist, dry, semi-moist) may refuse foods of different texture or type. Cats do prefer certain "flavors," such as animal fat, protein hydrolysates (digests), meat extracts, and certain free amino acids found in animal muscle (i.e., alanine, proline, lysine, histidine, and leucine). The temperature of food plays a role in the cat's acceptance and consumption of the food. When feeding canned/moist foods, the preference is for the moist food to be at or near body temperature (38.5°C [101.5°F]). These factors are important to ensure proper nutrition of a cat.

TECHNICIAN NOTE

Cats are highly sensitive to the form, odor, and taste of food.

As we have discussed, cats are carnivores, with unique anatomic, physiologic, metabolic, and behavioral adaptations that support eating foods higher in protein and lower in carbohydrates compared with dogs. Cats are well-adapted hunters, with increased visual acuity, upright ears, sensitive facial whiskers, tactile hairs, retractable claws, and conical, sharply pointed teeth. Cats have low liver glucokinase activity, which means that they have limited ability to metabolize large amounts of simple carbohydrates. Cats also demonstrate decreased activity in the enzymes responsible for the digestion and uptake of starches and sugars. These adaptations support consumption of natural prey such as small rodents, which are estimated to contain around 55% protein, 45% fat and 1% to 2% carbohydrate on a DM basis (DMB). It is important to note that despite these specific adaptations, cats can and do use carbohydrates, and carbohydrates provide a good source of energy. Dry foods containing 40% or greater dietary carbohydrates with an average digestibility of 85% are well tolerated by healthy cats.

FELINE MUSCLE CONDITION SCORE (MCS)

MCS is the physical assessment of patient's muscle mass.

MCS is scored by visual examination and palpation of musculature over the spine, scapulae, skull, and pelvis:

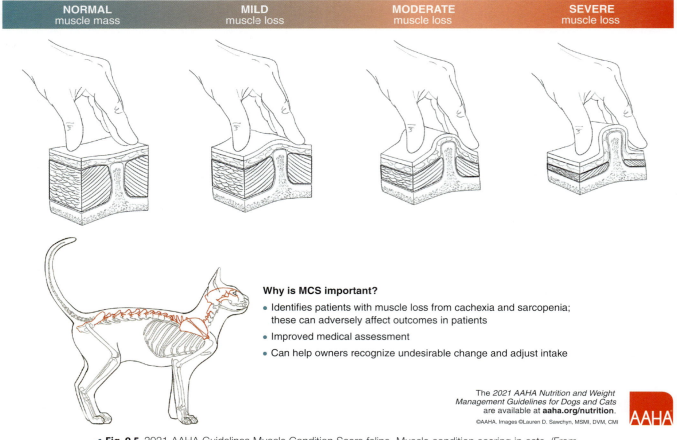

| NORMAL muscle mass | MILD muscle loss | MODERATE muscle loss | SEVERE muscle loss |

Why is MCS important?

- Identifies patients with muscle loss from cachexia and sarcopenia; these can adversely affect outcomes in patients
- Improved medical assessment
- Can help owners recognize undesirable change and adjust intake

The *2021 AAHA Nutrition and Weight Management Guidelines for Dogs and Cats* are available at **aaha.org/nutrition**.

©AAHA. Images ©Lauren D. Sawchyn, MSMI, DVM, CMI

AAHA

• **Fig. 9.5** 2021 AAHA Guidelines Muscle Condition Score feline. Muscle condition scoring in cats. (From the 2021 AAHA Nutrition and Weight Management Guidelines for Dogs and Cats, aaha.org/nutrition. Copyright AAHA. Images copyright Lauren D. Sawchyn, MSMI, DVM, CMI/Sadie Lewandowski. Used with permission.)

Unique Anatomic and Physiologic Features in the Cat

The eyes of the cat are well adapted for hunting. Their visual acuity is greater than that of dogs because of their larger optic cortex. Cats' ears are upright, face forward, and have 20 associated muscles to provide the fine control needed to locate sound precisely. Cats also respond to high-pitched sounds, which represent the range of sound frequencies emitted by typical prey. Facial whiskers and tactile hairs, as can be seen in Fig. 9.6, are very sensitive and are responsible for helping cats to hunt in dim light and to protect their eyes.

Cats and dogs have the same number of incisor, canine, and carnassial teeth, but cats have fewer premolar and molar teeth. Also, cats' teeth do not possess fissured crowns, which are a hallmark of omnivorous animals. The jaws of cats have limited grinding ability. The scissorslike action of the carnassial teeth is ideal for delivering the cervical bite used to transect the spinal cord and immobilize or kill prey. It is important to note that cats lack salivary amylase, which is used to initiate digestion of dietary starches.

Cats have evolved to eat small, frequent meals; thus the stomach is less important for storage compared with that in dogs. The stomach of domestic cats is relatively smaller, with a smaller glandular fundus. Likewise, the length of the intestine is shorter in felines compared with that in omnivores and herbivores. A greater villus height in cats increases the absorptive surface area. The intestinal villi are small, fingerlike projections that protrude from the epithelial lining of the intestinal wall. Villi increase the internal surface area of the intestinal walls, thus providing a greater surface area for absorption. The absorptive capacity of felines is estimated to be 10% less than that of canines. The sugar transport system of the small intestine is not adaptive to varying levels of dietary carbohydrate. Also, cats have low activities of intestinal disaccharidases (i.e., sucrase, maltase, and isomaltase). Pancreatic amylase production is also reduced compared with dogs. Pancreatic amylase production is relatively nonadaptive in cats, as would be expected in a species unaccustomed to significant changes in dietary carbohydrate levels. Cats, unlike omnivores, have been found to harbor higher concentrations of bacteria in the small intestine. Remarkably, the numbers typical for cats would be diagnostic for small

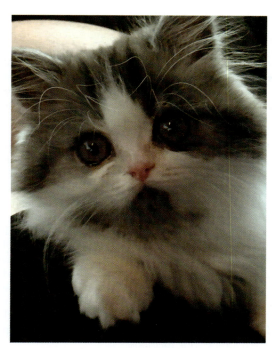

• **Fig. 9.6** Feline facial whiskers and tactile hairs. (Copyright Kara M. Burns.)

constantly active. Consequently, specific amounts of dietary protein are always catabolized for energy.

Arginine

Arginine deficiency results in a dramatic response in cats, more so than any other nutrient deficiency. Cats cannot synthesize adequate ornithine or citrulline to convert to arginine, which is needed for the urea cycle. With deficiency of arginine, the urea cycle cannot convert ammonia to urea, resulting in ammonia toxicity. Even eating one meal devoid of arginine may result in hyperammonemia in less than 1 hour. Affected cats exhibit severe signs of ammonia toxicity (i.e., vocalization, emesis, ptyalism, hyperactivity, hyperesthesia, ataxia, tetanic spasms, apnea, cyanosis) and may die within 2 to 5 hours.

Taurine

Taurine (a β-amino sulfonic acid) is abundant as a free amino acid in the natural foods of cats, such as the meats of small rodents, birds, and fish. Dietary taurine is essential in cats, and clinical disease results if insufficient amounts are present. Many species can use either glycine or taurine to conjugate bile acids into bile salts before they are secreted into bile. Cats need taurine to conjugate bile acids. The loss of taurine in bile coupled with a low rate of taurine synthesis contributes to the obligatory taurine requirement in cats.

> **TECHNICIAN NOTE**
>
> Dietary taurine is essential in cats, and clinical disease results if insufficient amounts are present.

Methionine and Cysteine

Methionine and cysteine are sulfur-containing amino acids that are required in higher amounts by cats, especially during growth. Methionine and cysteine are considered together, because cysteine can replace up to half of the methionine requirement in cats. Methionine serves as a precursor to cysteine; therefore cysteine is not an essential amino acid. Cysteine cannot be converted to methionine; however, a minimal requirement for methionine must be met with dietary methionine. The potential for nutritional deficiencies exists, especially in cats fed home-prepared or vegetable-based foods. Clinical signs of methionine deficiency include poor growth and a crusting dermatitis at the mucocutaneous junctions of the mouth and nose. To meet the requirement in kittens, approximately 19% of a food must be composed of animal protein. Foods that are higher in plant proteins will require additional methionine. Supplementation can be supplied as DL-methionine, a crystalline form of the amino acid.

Fat Metabolism

Cats can digest and use high levels of dietary fat. Being true carnivores, cats have a special need for AA (20:4n6) because of their limited ability to synthesize AA from linoleic acid (18:2n6). An exogenous source of AA is especially important for more demanding life stages (e.g., gestation, lactation, growth). The basis for this additional requirement is the low hepatic delta-6 desaturase activity in cats. Cats are also better able to digest higher-fat foods compared with dogs.

Vitamin Metabolism

The vitamin needs of cats are different from those of dogs in several ways. It is known that cats do not convert enough tryptophan

intestinal bacterial overgrowth in dogs. Certain amino acid transporters in the small intestines of cats are highly adaptable, particularly the transporter responsible for arginine uptake. This finding underscores the importance of the amounts of protein and specific amino acids in foods for cats. Cats are unable to synthesize significant quantities of ornithine or citrulline within the intestine. Both are precursors to arginine synthesis. It is because of this inability that cats have an absolute requirement for arginine in their foods.

Key Nutritional Factors for Felines

Most animal's livers have two enzyme systems—hexokinase and glucokinase—for converting glucose to glucose-6-phosphate. This conversion must take place before the liver can use glucose. Adult cats have very low hepatic glucokinase activity and a limited ability to metabolize large amounts of simple carbohydrates. Kittens ingest digestible carbohydrates (i.e., lactose or milk sugar) before weaning. Adult cats must rely primarily on gluconeogenesis from glucogenic amino acids, lactic acid, and glycerol for maintenance of blood glucose concentration. Immediately after a meal and during the absorptive phase, gluconeogenesis is maximal in cats.

Protein

Protein metabolism is unique in cats, which have a higher maintenance requirement for protein versus dogs. Cats also are known for having a special need for four amino acids: arginine, taurine, methionine, and cysteine. The protein requirement for growth in kittens is only 50% higher than that in puppies, whereas the protein requirement for feline maintenance is twice that of adult dogs. The higher protein requirement of cats is a result of high activity of hepatic enzymes (i.e., transaminases and deaminases) that remove amino groups from amino acids so that the resulting ketoacids can be used for energy or glucose production. Felines have a limited ability to decrease the activity of these enzymes when fed low-protein foods. In cats, hepatic enzyme systems are to niacin. An animal tissue–based diet is well supplied with niacin from nicotinamide adenine dinucleotide (NAD) and nicotinamide adenine dinucleotide phosphate (NADP) coenzymes; therefore cats do not need to produce niacin from tryptophan. The niacin requirement in cats is 2.4 times higher than that in dogs. Cats have high transaminase activities, which is consistent with consuming a diet high in energy derived from dietary protein. Thus it is logical to expect that their pyridoxine turnover and requirement would be higher than those of omnivores. Pyridoxine requirement in cats is estimated to be 1.7 times higher than that in dogs. Vitamin A occurs naturally only in animal tissue. Plants synthesize vitamin A precursors (e.g., β-carotene). Omnivorous and herbivorous animals can convert β-carotene to vitamin A; cats cannot, because they lack intestinal dioxygenase that cleaves β-carotene to retinol. In addition, cats have insufficient 7-dehydrocholesterol in the skin to meet the metabolic need for vitamin D photosynthesis, thus resulting in a requirement for a dietary source of vitamin D. Vitamin D is relatively abundant in animal liver; therefore the need for dermal production is minimal, and alternative pathways rapidly metabolize 7-dehydrocholesterol. Both niacin and pyridoxine are needed at four times the level required by dogs. Consequently, feeding *dog food to a cat or vice versa is never advised.*

Water

It is well established that water is the most important nutrient. The water needs of cats differ from those of dogs because of the adaptation of the ancestors of cats to environmental extremes. Domestic cats are believed to have descended from the African wildcat *(Felis silvestris libyca)*, known to be a desert dweller. Adaptation to a dry environment may explain a few special features of water balance in cats. Cats can survive on less water compared with dogs and may fail to increase water intake at minor levels of dehydration, up to 4% of BW. Highly concentrated urine is formed in cats to compensate for reduced water intake. However, this strong concentrating ability, in addition to a weak thirst drive, may result in highly saturated urine. Highly saturated urine increases the risk of crystalluria or urolithiasis. Cats consume 1.5 to 2 mL of water per gram of DM. This 2:1 ratio of water to DM is similar to that of typical prey. This ratio represents approximately 0.5 mL water/kcal ME intake. Practical recommendations for water provision are higher at 1 mL water/kcal ME. Water ingested from moist foods containing 78% to 82% moisture will result in diuresis.

> **TECHNICIAN NOTE**
>
> Cats can survive on less water compared with dogs and may fail to increase water intake at minor levels of dehydration, up to 4% of body weight (BW).

Cats have unique requirements when it comes to nutrition. This is based on many factors, most importantly the fact that cats are obligate carnivores. Proper nutrition and care throughout a cat's life maximize health, longevity, and quality of life. Veterinary technicians should have a thorough understanding of the nutritional needs of cats to maximize the care of their feline patients.

Feeding Pets

Pet Food Labeling

The pet food label is more than a package for the pets' food—it is a legal document. The pet food label is the primary way in which product information is communicated from the manufacturer or distributor to pet owners, veterinarians, health care team members, and regulatory officials. Reading and interpreting pet food labels is one method for finding information about pet foods. However, the pet food label does not necessarily provide information about food quality (e.g., digestibility and **biological value**). One of the best recommendations for learning more about pet foods is to contact individual pet food manufacturers or nutrition experts for additional information that can be used to evaluate the quality of various pet foods.

Pet food labels communicate information about the product and serve as a legal document. Several agencies and organizations regulate the production, marketing, and sales of pet foods in different countries. Each agency has different responsibilities, with varying degrees of authority. Some of these agencies are responsible for regulating information provided on pet food labels, whereas others influence the regulatory process. Pet foods are regulated at the point of sale. For example, pet foods manufactured in the United States but sold outside the United States must meet labeling requirements of the country in which the food is sold. Pet foods sold in the United States must comply with Food and Drug Administration (FDA), AAFCO, and state pet food labeling requirements.

The AAFCO is an elected body of officials who are the recognized source for pet food labeling, ingredient definitions, and standardized food testing methods.

The AAFCO defines what can be placed on the label and what is prohibited. AAFCO guidelines help ensure that manufactured pet foods are formulated, or test fed to be complete and balanced, and that they meet the animal's needs during growth, lactation, gestation, and maintenance.

> **TECHNICIAN NOTE**
>
> The Association of American Feed Control Officials (AAFCO) is an elected body of officials who are the recognized source for pet food labeling, ingredient definitions, and standardized food testing methods.

The FDA is responsible for certain pet food labeling regulations. It also specifies certain ingredients, drugs, or additives and enforces regulations on pet food contamination (chemical or microbiological). If a pet food manufacturer makes a health claim for a product, the FDA will investigate and could require the manufacturer to alter the label if the claim cannot be proven.

The United States Department of Agriculture (USDA) is responsible for making sure that pet food packages are labeled correctly and are not mistaken for human foods. All pet food labels must specify the intended species, such as "cat food" or "dog food." The USDA also inspects the animal ingredients used in pet foods. The pet food label is the primary way in which product information is communicated from the manufacturer or distributor to pet owners, veterinarians, health care team members, and regulatory officials. Reading and interpreting pet food labels is one method for finding information about pet foods. However, as mentioned, pet food labels do not provide information about food quality (e.g., digestibility and biological value). One of the best recommendations to learning more about pet foods is to contact individual pet food manufacturers or nutrition experts for additional information that can be used to evaluate the quality of various pet foods.

Pet Food Assessment

There are literally thousands of pet foods that come in various types, shapes, flavors, and sizes. How does one choose the ideal pet food? By looking down the pet food aisle for an appealing label or advertisement? By asking friends what they feed their pets? By asking the veterinary care team for their recommendations? After deciding what food to feed, is the decision based on data or emotion? Time and again, a client will see an advertisement for a pet food that might create interest in that brand. That might cause them to ask you for the veterinary technician's opinion. This chapter will discuss different types of foods, labeling requirements, and methods for evaluating pet foods. Also addressed are homemade foods. However, the focus will be on commercially prepared pet foods. It should be remembered that thousands of pet food brands are available. The veterinary technician's goal is to educate the client on the best food for their specific pet. But how does the technician ensure that the food recommended is the right food? There are some basic labeling guidelines and definitions that will help determine this. First, a food should be "complete and balanced," which means that the food will meet the nutritional requirements of the specific animal. There are two other types of foods: all-purpose and special-purpose foods. All-purpose foods are formulated to meet pets' nutritional needs from birth through the senior years. Generally, these foods are sold as off-brand or generic foods. The concept of all-purpose feeding is based on the premise that one product meets all nutritional requirements during all stages of the pet's life. Therefore these products must contain adequate nutrients to support the most demanding life stages—growth, gestation, and lactation. All-purpose foods or all life stage foods provide nutrients excessive of the allowances for adult maintenance and geriatric diets. Special-purpose foods are formulated for animals with special needs or to meet the requirements at a specific life stage. The obesity-prone pet and the working dog are examples of animals that might need special-purpose foods. The obesity-prone pet requires fewer calories, whereas the working dog requires additional calories.

A pet food product is following and ensures nutritional adequacy if it either has been formulated to meet the nutritional needs of a pet or has been test fed. However, the feeding trial method is much more effective than the formulation method in determining whether a food product will provide adequate nutrition. Foods formulated to meet nutritional standards based on a computer program are never test fed to ensure that they maintain adequate nutrition. The AAFCO's feeding trials are performed for the growing puppy, the gestating and lactating dog, and the adult dog. There is no AAFCO feeding trial protocol for the senior animal.

Types of Pet Foods

There are three types of pet foods generally fed to client-owned animals: canned foods, dry foods, and semimoist foods. Each type of food has its advantages and disadvantages. Canned food is very palatable but is more expensive than dry food. Water, protein, and fat all contribute to a more palatable product. Canned food contains approximately 78% to 82% moisture, which increases the food's palatability and its cost. Canned foods are more profitable for the manufacturer because of the water content. The canned food may appear as a loaf, an "all-meat" product, or a combination of meats and flours bound together with gums and guars. If a client wants to feed a preservative-free food, a canned food product would be recommended. The food is sterilized during the canning process and does not require additional preservatives. The can seals out bacteria and contaminants. Once

the can is opened, it must be refrigerated and can be safely fed for only 3 to 5 days—at most. Semimoist foods also are very palatable and may appeal to the picky eater or to a pet owner trying to provide variety. The food contains approximately 25% to 30% moisture. The popularity of semimoist foods was much higher in the past; however, because of the level of preservatives and development of other product choices, the current demand for this product type is much lower. Semimoist foods have higher levels of preservatives to maintain shelf life. They are also formulated to be higher in soluble sugars and simple carbohydrates, which may not be beneficial for diabetic animals. The most common food type is dry food, which has approximately 7% to 12% moisture. Dry foods are not found to be as palatable as canned foods overall, but they are much more affordable. Dry foods are also the most convenient food type to feed. Dry foods can be made through an extrusion process or a baking process. During the extrusion process, the dry ingredients are mixed together, moisture is added, and the dough is pushed through an extruder. The extruder uses pressure and heat to cook the dough. The product emerges from the extruder and is sliced off to make the kibbles. Palatability enhancers are then applied to the outside of the kibble. In the baking process, which is less common, the dry ingredients are combined with moisture, and the dough is rolled flat onto a large cooking surface. Once the dough has been cooked, the product is broken into small pieces.

> **TECHNICIAN NOTE**
> If a client wants to feed preservative-free food, a canned food product would be recommended.

Homemade foods are also quite popular with some pet owners. There are numerous good-quality recipes that are believed to ensure adequate nutrition. However, many homemade foods are not balanced, or may become unbalanced if the directions are not understood and followed exactly. It is very important to understand that formal testing has not occurred with foods made at home. Also, the pet owner must follow the recipe exactly and completely. No ingredient substitutions can be made. With homemade diets, there is a high risk of the pet receiving food that is nutritionally inadequate.

There are a few factors that may affect the pet's desire to eat. Canned food is generally more palatable than dry food. Adding warm water to dry food or warming the food to slightly above room temperature will increase its palatability. Adding a small amount of chicken broth to canned or dry food also may increase its appeal. Adding garlic powder, onion powder, or salt to the diet is not recommended, because this can be dangerous to the pet.

Giving a pet a treat is commonplace in many households. Treats may be a snack from the kitchen or a product purchased by the pet owner. Treats do not fall under the same regulations as pet foods. There are no AAFCO guidelines regarding treats. Many treats have higher than recommended levels of sodium, phosphorus, protein, and fat. Feeding greater than 10% of the diet in treats could alter the pet's nutritional intake.

> **TECHNICIAN NOTE**
> Advise pet owners to feed no greater than 10% of the daily energy requirement (DER) in treats and subtract this number of calories from the overall DER.

Understanding Feeding Costs

Most pet owners do not understand how to calculate the cost of feeding their pet. The perceived cost of food is the price paid at the grocery store, pet store, or veterinary clinic. It is important for the client to understand that pet foods are not alike, that they are not created equally, and that the cost of the purchased food is thus not the "real" cost. The pet owner should be advised to write down the date the product was purchased and the purchase price. The feeding guidelines or amount to be fed should also be written on the bag. The cost of feeding daily can now be calculated more accurately.

Regulation of Pet Foods

Pet food labels communicate information about the product and serve as a legal document. Several agencies and organizations regulate the production, marketing, and sales of pet foods in different countries. Each agency has different responsibilities, with varying degrees of authority. Some of these agencies are responsible for regulating the information provided on pet food labels, whereas others influence the regulatory process. Pet foods are regulated at the point of sale. For example, pet foods manufactured in the United States but sold outside the United States must meet labeling requirements of the country in which the food is sold. Pet foods sold in the United States must comply with FDA, AAFCO, and state pet food labeling requirements.

Interpreting Pet Food Labels

Pet food labels include two main parts:
1. The principal display panels
2. The information panels

Principal Display Panel

The principal display panel is defined by the FDA as "the part of a label that is most likely to be displayed, presented, shown, or examined under customary conditions of display for retail sale." Certain pieces of information are required on each part of the label, whereas others are optional.

The principal display panel is the main way to attract the customer's attention and should immediately communicate the product identity. The product identity must include a designator or the species for which the food is intended, such as "dog food," "cat food," "for puppies," or "for dogs and puppies." The brand name is the name by which pet food products of a given company are identified. The product name is not essential and may be the same as the brand name. However, most often, it gives a description of the food and is subject to regulations dealing with the composition of ingredients. The product vignette is a visual representation of the product and must accurately show the contents of the package (e.g., the food pictured on the label cannot appear better than the actual product).

The amounts of ingredients that must be present to use a certain product name are determined by percentage rules. For example, the term "chicken" requires that at least 70% of the product contains chicken; "chicken dinner/entrée, etc." must contain 10% chicken if moist and 25% chicken if dry; "with chicken" means that the product contains at least 3% chicken; "chicken flavor" means that chicken is recognizable by the pet (<3% chicken). A nutrition statement may be provided on the display panel; it is usually brief and may include such terms as "complete and nutritious," "100% nutritious," or "100% complete nutrition." The use of these terms suggests that the product contains ingredients

in amounts sufficient to provide the estimated nutrient requirements of a dog or a cat, or the product contains a combination of ingredients that when fed to a normal animal as the only source of nourishment will provide satisfactory results.

Information Panel

The information panel is adjacent to the principal display panel and includes product information. The ingredient statement must be shown on the label and includes a list of ingredients (which must conform to the AAFCO terms) in descending order by weight. Ingredients are listed on an "as-is" basis, which makes interpretation of ingredient lists difficult, because many key ingredients are added with different moisture contents. Because meats contain more moisture, they may be listed first on the ingredient list, although the primary component of the food may be a mixture of grains. This is often misleading to pet owners. We know many pet owners think they want a meat-first food product for their pet. The perception is that the product is made up mostly of meat. A pet food that lists several related ingredients or different forms of the same ingredient separately (e.g., brown rice, rice bran, rice gluten, etc.) could make rice-based ingredients appear to be a lower portion of the food than is the fact. However, as discussed above, this is misleading, because the product is portrayed as a "meat-heavy" food. Also, the ingredient statement does not provide information about the quality of ingredients. Likewise, because an ingredient's position on the list includes its water content, this allows dry ingredients to appear lower on the list compared with ingredients that are naturally high in moisture.

> **TECHNICIAN NOTE**
>
> The ingredient statement must be shown on the label and include a list of ingredients in descending order by weight. Ingredients are listed on an "as-is" basis, which makes interpretation of ingredient lists difficult, because many key ingredients are added with different moisture contents.

One limitation of the ingredient statement is that such terms as "meat by-products" are difficult to evaluate. Many owners are under the impression that "by-products" are not healthy and may even be harmful to their pets. However, the nutritive values of various meat by-products vary widely. It is often misinterpreted that foods containing meat by-products are inferior to foods containing whole meat. The AAFCO defines meat, as listed on an ingredient label, as any combination of skeletal muscle, striated muscle, or muscle found in the tongue, diaphragm, heart, and esophagus, with or without the overlying fat and the portions of the skin, sinew, nerves, and blood vessels that normally accompany muscle. Meat must be suitable for use in animal foods and therefore excludes feathers, head, feet, and entrails.

Meat by-products do not include hair, horns, teeth, or hooves. Nutritive values in meat by-products also vary greatly. Meat by-products such as liver, kidney, and lungs have excellent nutritive value. By-products are simply secondary products added to the principal product. Many human foods contain by-products, and most pet foods contain by-products. For example, by-products of milk for human consumption would be ice cream, cheese, and butter. Many by-products are excellent sources of nutrients for pets and for people.

Guaranteed Analysis

The guaranteed analysis includes crude protein (minimum), crude fat (minimum), crude fiber (maximum), and moisture (maximum).

Additional guarantees are optional and may be included by the manufacturer. The guaranteed analysis is a general idea of the nutrient content of a food but is of little value in comparing foods, because specific nutrient contents are not given and values are listed on an "as is" basis. Although crude protein is an accurate index of protein quantity, it does not indicate protein quality. Crude fat may be used to estimate the energy density of a food product. Crude fiber is an estimate of the indigestible portion of a food product; it usually underestimates the true level of fiber in the product. Food products that contain higher levels of fiber are generally lower in calories. The moisture content represents the water content in the product; in the United States, it cannot exceed a maximum of 78%. Foods that have greater than 78% moisture content must use a different name, such as "in gravy," "in sauce," or "in aspic." Dry matter contains all nutrients (except water), and subtle changes in moisture content may result in marked differences in DM, which subsequently affects amounts of nutrients in a food product.

Nutrient Content of Pet Foods

Pet food manufacturers in the United States are required to include minimum percentages for crude protein and crude fat and maximum percentages for crude fiber and moisture. Guarantees for other nutrients may follow moisture but do not need to be listed unless their presence is highlighted elsewhere on the label (e.g., "contains taurine," "calcium enriched"). Guarantees for substances not listed in the AAFCO dog or cat nutrient profiles (e.g., vitamin C, L-carnitine, glucosamine, chondroitin sulfate) should immediately follow the listing of recognized nutrients and be accompanied by an asterisk referring to the disclaimer "Not recognized as an essential nutrient by the AAFCO Dog (or Cat) Food Nutrient Profiles." It is important to recognize that these percentages generally indicate the "worst-case" levels for these nutrients in a food product. They do not reveal the exact or typical amounts of these nutrients."

Crude Protein

Crude protein refers to a specific analytical procedure that estimates protein content by measuring nitrogen. Crude protein is an index of protein quantity but does not indicate protein quality (amino acid profile) or digestibility.

Crude Fat

Crude fat refers to a specific analytical procedure that estimates the lipid content of food obtained through either ether extraction or acid hydrolysis. It should be kept in mind that fats have more than twice the energy density of proteins and carbohydrates and can be used to estimate the energy density of a food product. If the moisture and crude fiber content of two products are somewhat similar, the one with the higher crude fat guarantee will usually have the higher energy density.

Crude Fiber

Crude fiber represents the organic residue that remains after plant material has been treated with dilute acid and alkali solutions. Crude fiber is used to report the fiber content of commercial pet foods but typically underestimates the true level of fiber in the product. Crude fiber is an estimate of the indigestible portion of the food for dogs and cats. The crude fiber method typically recovers a large percentage of cellulose and lignin in a sample, a variable percentage of hemicellulose, and even ash.

Moisture

Moisture is determined by drying a sample of the product to a constant weight. The drying procedure measures water in the product as a whole. Subtle differences in moisture content of moist products can result in marked differences in DM content and therefore the financial side of feeding a given pet food. It should be remembered that the DM content of the food contains all nutrients except water.

Example: Compare the DM content of three different moist cat foods:
1. Food A contains 72% moisture.
2. Food B contains 78% moisture.
3. Food C contains 82% moisture.

Food A 100 – 72% water = 28% DM
   Food B* 100 – 78% water = 22% DM
   Food C† 100 – 82% water = 18% DM

As can be seen above, a small difference in the water content of a food makes a large difference in its DM content. Guarantees are expressed on an "as-is" or "as-fed" basis. To ensure that pet foods are looked at equally, it is important to remember to convert these guarantees to a DM basis when comparing foods with differing moisture contents (e.g., moist vs. dry foods).

> **TECHNICIAN NOTE**
>
> To ensure that pet foods are looked at equally, it is important to remember to convert the guaranteed analysis to a dry matter (DM) basis when comparing foods with differing moisture contents.

Ash

Although not "required," many pet food manufacturers in the United States will include the maximum ash content on their food labels. "Low ash" claims are not allowed because the term *ash* per se does not truly mean anything. What is of more significance is the level of certain minerals. Ash has historically been tied to the urinary tract health of cats, whereas it is the specific minerals in "ash" that should be reviewed by the pet owner. "Low magnesium" claims on cat food labels are allowed if the product meets certain FDA criteria. In such cases, a maximum magnesium guarantee is required. To be labeled as a "low magnesium" food, the product must contain less than 0.12% magnesium on a DM basis and less than 25 mg per 100 kcal ME. The estimation of magnesium content based on calculation from the guaranteed analyses must meet these criteria as well. The only exception occurs when the label bears an AAFCO calorie content statement that is higher than would be estimated from the guaranteed analysis. Ash consists of all noncombustible materials in the food, usually salt and other minerals. "High ash content" in dry and soft-moist foods generally indicates high magnesium content. However, the ash content of moist cat foods usually correlates poorly with the magnesium content. Excessive magnesium intake may be one risk factor for feline struvite urolithiasis.

Nutritional Adequacy Statement

The nutritional adequacy statement on the information panel is often more detailed than the brief statements found on the principal display. Examples include "Complete and balanced nutrition for growth of kittens" and "meets … requirements for the entire life cycle of all dogs." The nutrition statement will help determine whether the manufacturer is making claims for a specific-purpose

*28 – 22 ÷ 22 × 100 = 27% more DM in Food A (72% moisture) vs. Food B (78% moisture)
†28 – 18 ÷ 18 × 100 = 55% more DM in Food A (72% moisture) vs. Food C (82% moisture)

food versus an all-purpose food. Pet foods with no statement of adequacy include snacks, treats, and some therapeutic foods.

The basis of the nutrition claim is documented on the pet food label by one of two methods: the formulation method or the feeding trial method. The formulation method is simply a laboratory nutrient profile analysis and does not require any feeding or digestibility trials to prove availability of the nutrients in the profile analysis. This method is recognized on a label by such statements as "Meets or exceeds the minimal nutritional levels established by AAFCO" or "Formulated to meet the AAFCO dog nutrient profile for … ." AAFCO nutrient profiles are published for two categories or life stages: (1) growth and reproduction and (2) adult maintenance.

The feeding trial method is the preferred method for substantiating a claim. Feeding trials can result in adequacy claims for four categories:

1. Gestation and lactation
2. Growth
3. Maintenance
4. Complete for all life stages

A food product that has successfully passed a sequential growth and gestation/lactation trial can make the claim "complete for all life stages." The required wording for labels that have passed these tests is "Animal feeding tests using AAFCO procedures substantiate that (brand) provides complete and balanced nutrition for (life stage)." Pet foods that do not meet AAFCO requirements by either of the standard methods will have a nutritional statement as follows: "This product is intended for intermittent or supplemental feeding only."

TECHNICIAN NOTE

The feeding trial method is the preferred method for substantiating a nutrition claim.

An important point to make to owners is that those foods that make a claim for "all life stages" have met the growth, gestation, and lactation nutritional profile. These life stages are higher in nutrient requirements. If these are met and the claim is "complete for all life stages," the food being fed is, in essence, a "puppy/kitten" formula. Care must be taken when discussing nutrition with owners of adult or older pets, because some of the nutrients in an all life stage formulation may be too high in certain nutrients to suit adult or older pets.

Dog and cat foods labeled as "complete" and "balanced" for any or all life stages must list feeding directions on the product label. At a minimum, feeding directions should include the instructions "feed (weight/unit) per (weight) of dog or cat" and frequency of feeding. These feeding directions are general guidelines and should serve as a starting point; adjustments may be needed to maintain optimal body condition. It is important to talk with owners about how much to feed their pets and to ensure that owners know that these are only guidelines. The exact amounts to feed should be discussed with the veterinary health care team. If a Pug weighs 40 lb, this does not necessarily mean it should be fed the amount on the bag for a 40-lb dog. Also, an important point to discuss with owners is the size of the cup. A cup is intended to be an 8-ounce measuring cup—not a 56-ounce convenience store beverage container!

Pet Food Myths

There are a number of myths and misperceptions surrounding pet foods today. Many of these have been perpetuated by word

of mouth and through unreliable sources of information, such as those found on the Internet. Some will be reviewed here. The technician should remember to use credible veterinary resources when researching questions and communicating and educating pet owners.

By-products

There is rampant misinformation about a common ingredient—by-products. A by-product is something that is just that—a side product resulting from the making of another product. By-products are not, by definition, of poor quality. The term refers only to the anatomic parts included, not to the nutritional quality of the parts. The AAFCO defines a meat by-product as "the non-rendered, clean parts, other than meat, derived from slaughtered mammals. It includes, but is not limited to, lungs, spleen, kidneys, brain, livers, blood, bone, stomachs and intestines freed of their contents. It does not include hair, horns, teeth, and hooves … ."

Many of the items included in "by-product" (e.g., organ meats) may be higher in essential nutrients—amino acids, minerals, and vitamins—and may be more palatable to the pet. Interestingly, many items that would be appropriately classified under the label "by-product" (e.g., bully sticks [bull penis], lung, liver, pig ears, tendons, etc.) are popular dog treats. Many pet owners who would not consider feeding a diet containing any animal "by-product" will feed the same ingredients as treats without any concern. Ironically, the quality control of these treat items is much less stringent than that of pet foods that include by-products offered by reputable pet food manufacturers.

Corn

Although corn has been commonly included in pet foods for years, some consumers now perceive corn as an undesirable ingredient. Many pet owner concerns about corn are scientifically invalid. The misperception and misinformation surrounding corn is so widespread that many pet food manufacturers have gone to great lengths and great cost to remove corn from their products and ingredient panels. The chapter will address the misperception of corn because, in the veterinary profession, we are still getting many questions about corn.

Corn is believed to be a common allergen; however, true food allergies are not as prevalent as many pet owners believe. In fact, food allergies are rare in dogs and cats and are rarely the causes of GI (e.g., chronic vomiting or diarrhea) and dermatologic problems (e.g., pruritus, otitis, pyoderma) in dogs and cats. Only 1% of all skin diseases can be attributed to food allergies! Flea allergy and atopy account for the vast majority of dermatologic signs. Some dogs and cats experience a food-sensitive disease with the introduction of a new diet. This is not food allergy but rather, a response to a change in the properties of foods, such as differences in digestibility, fat, fiber content, or other properties. In the very small number of animals with true food allergies, documented allergies to corn are quite rare and are much less common than allergies to other ingredients, such as beef, dairy, and chicken.

TECHNICIAN NOTE

Only 1% of all skin diseases can be attributed to food allergies.

The digestibility of corn and other carbohydrate sources (oats, potato, barley, wheat, etc.) increases with processing and with cooking. Whole corn that is ground and cooked via extrusion (the way that most dry foods are made) has been shown to have digestibility of 97% or greater in both dogs and cats. Misinformation regarding corn's digestibility may be the result of pet owners' experience of feeding whole corn and seeing undigested kernels in feces. Properly prepared corn is highly digestible by both dogs and cats and provides several essential nutrients to a pet's diet. Corn is a source of essential nutrients, including protein, fiber, and fatty acids, specifically linoleic acid. Corn is not a "filler." The true definition of "filler" is an ingredient that does not contribute any nutrients or beneficial properties to a food and is rarely used in pet foods. We see now that corn does the opposite and provides valuable nutrients.

Grain-free

Many pet owners believe that grain-free pet foods are easier to digest, provide pets with better nutrition, and are less likely to cause allergies compared with pet foods containing grain. Properly processed grains are highly digestible. Although uncooked grains are poorly digested by dogs and cats, those that are properly cooked are highly digestible. In fact, dogs and cats can digest carbohydrates from grains with greater than 90% efficiency.

Foods that contain grains provide exceptional nutrition. It should be remembered that grains are carbohydrates, which are an important source of energy. Another misperception is that "grain-free" means carbohydrate-free. This is certainly not the case. Grains also contain fiber, which promotes GI health. EFAs and other nutrients in grains contribute to a healthy skin and coat.

Protein sources from grains, such as corn gluten meal, can be highly digestible sources of many essential amino acids for dogs and cats. Also, grains are unlikely to cause allergies. It should be remembered that less than 1% of dogs are sensitive to grains. Food allergies are caused by immune reactions to proteins in the diet. Properly processed grains provide necessary nutrients as part of a nutritionally complete and balanced diet.

Feeding Trials Are Not Necessary

The feeding trial protocol, as established by the AAFCO for adult maintenance, lasts a minimum of 6 months and requires only eight animals per group. Many parameters are monitored in these animals. These parameters are set at the minimum nutrient requirements as defined by the National Research Council. Typically, these levels tend to be lower than the recommended daily intake (RDI). Requirements are minimum levels of nutrients which over time are sufficient to maintain the desired physiologic functions of the animals in the population. The RDI of a nutrient is the level of intake that appears to be adequate to meet the known nutritional needs of practically all healthy individuals. The National Research Council recommendations provide a guide to diet formulations, but they do not account for digestibility or nutrient availability. It is the AAFCO feeding trials that provide a reasonable guarantee of nutrient availability and sufficient palatability to ensure acceptability of a food product by the pet. The feeding trial also provides some assurance that the product will support certain functions, such as gestation, lactation, and growth.

The feeding trial is also the only way to accurately assess the quality of the protein in a diet, because this is the only valid way to determine the digestibility of a protein and thus its quality. Passing the feeding trial does not ensure that the food will be effective in preventing long-term nutritional/health problems or in detecting problems that have a low prevalence in the general population. The feeding trial is also not designed to ensure optimal growth or maximize physical activity. If a product has not gone through a feeding trial conducted by the manufacturer, pet owners should perform the feeding trial for them using their own pets. Although feeding trials (especially those involving therapeutic diets) cannot be expected to detect all deficiencies or excesses (which may also result from malabsorption or maldigestion), they do give veterinary professionals the added advantage of having someone evaluate a product before recommending it to clients. Feeding trials are conducted on healthy dogs and cats with controls that are the same breed and gender. During the trials, the animals must receive the test food as their only source of nutrition. The same formula must be fed throughout the entire trial. The trials are conducted to measure the following:

- Daily food consumption
- Weekly BW measurement
- Stated laboratory parameters measured at the end of the trial
- Complete physical examination by a veterinarian at the beginning and the end of the trial

A few animals, not greater than 25%, may be removed from the trial for nonnutritional reasons or poor food intake. At the end of the feeding trial, the results obtained from the test animals are compared with those from the control group, a historical group average, or reference values published by the AAFCO.

TECHNICIAN NOTE

The feeding trial is the most accurate way to assess the quality of the protein in a diet, because this is the only valid way to determine the digestibility of a protein and thus its quality.

To verify if a feeding trial has been conducted on a food product, the product label should be checked to find the source of the AAFCO certification; if a feeding trial has been done, it will be stated on the label as such.

Pet Food Preservatives Are Bad

A *preservative* is defined as any substance that is capable of inhibiting or retarding the growth of microorganisms or of masking the evidence of such deterioration. The primary nutrient needing protection from preservatives during storage is dietary fat, which can be in the form of vegetable oils, animal fats, or the fat-soluble vitamins A, D, E, and K. These nutrients have the potential to undergo oxidative destruction, called *lipid peroxidation*, during storage. Antioxidants are included in foods to prevent this lipid peroxidation. Oxidation of fats in pet foods also results in loss of calorie content and formation of toxic forms of peroxides that can be harmful to the health of pets. The FDA defines an *antioxidant* as any substance that aids in the preservation of foods by retarding deterioration, rancidity, or discoloration as the result of oxidation processes. Various types of antioxidants have been accepted for use in human and animal foods since 1947. Antioxidants do not reverse the oxidation of foods once it has started but rather, delay the oxidative process and prevent the destruction of fats in foods. Because of this, for antioxidants to be fully effective, they must be included in the product when it is initially prepared and processed. This inclusion helps prevent rancidity, maintaining the food's flavor, odor, and texture, and preventing the accumulation of the toxic end products of lipid degradation.

Antioxidants can be divided into two basic types: naturally derived products and synthetic products. Naturally derived products are commonly found in certain grains, vegetable oils, and some herbs and spices. Although these products do exist in nature, these compounds are processed in some way to make them available for use in commercial foods. The most common naturally derived antioxidants include mixed tocopherols (vitamin E compounds), ascorbic acid (vitamin C), rosemary extract, and citric acid.

Alpha-tocopherol has the strongest biological function on tissues but is a poor antioxidant in foods. Delta and gamma tocopherols both have low biological activity but are more effective than alpha-tocopherol as antioxidants. Tocopherols used in foods are obtained primarily from distillation of soybean oil residue. Tocopherols are rapidly decomposed as they protect the fat from oxidation; for this reason, foods preserved with mixed tocopherols have a shorter shelf life compared with foods preserved with a mixture of antioxidants.

Ascorbic acid (vitamin C) is a water-soluble antioxidant and is not easily soluble with the fatty portion of foods. It does work synergistically with other antioxidants, such as vitamin E and butylated hydroxytoluene. Ascorbyl palminate is similar in structure to ascorbic acid; although it is not normally found in nature, when hydrolyzed, it yields ascorbic acid and the free fatty acid (FFA) palmitic acid, both of which are natural compounds.

Rosemary extract is obtained from the dried leaves of the evergreen shrub *Rosemarinus officinalis*. It is effective as a naturally derived preservative in high-fat diets and has been shown to enhance antioxidant efficiency when combined with mixed tocopherols, ascorbic acid, and citric acid. A lot of processing of the plant oil is needed before adding it to foods due to the taste associated with the oil altering the taste of the food.

Citric acid is found in citrus fruits, such as oranges and lemons, and is often included in combination with other naturally derived antioxidants.

These compounds are costly and therefore are frequently used in conjunction with synthetic antioxidants as preservatives in pet foods. It is difficult to attain the necessary level of naturally derived antioxidants without the cost becoming prohibitive.

Synthetic antioxidants are more effective than naturally derived antioxidants and withstand the heat, pressure, and moisture better during food processing; this is called "carry-through." Increased effectiveness helps better preserve the fat-soluble vitamins A, D, and E for activity in the body rather than in the food.

Synthetic antioxidants include butylated hydroxyanisole (BHA), butylated hydroxytoluene (BHT), tertiary butylhydroquine (TBHQ), and ethoxyquin. BHA and BHT are approved for use in both human and animal foods and have a synergistic antioxidant effect when used together. BHA and BHT also have good carry-through; they have high efficiency in the protection of animal fats but are slightly less effective when used with vegetable oils. Ethoxyquin was approved for use in animal feeds more than 40 years ago and has been used since in human and pet food manufacturing. Ethoxyquin has good carry-through and is efficient in protecting the fats in foods. Ethoxyquin is more efficient as an antioxidant than BHA or BHT and allows lower levels to be used. It is especially effective in the protection of oils that contain high levels of polyunsaturated fatty acids (PUFAs). However, many pet food manufacturers have discontinued the use of ethoxyquin, BHA, and BHT because of client demand for more "natural" preservatives.

If the use of synthetic antioxidants causes concern in clients, they should be educated that most canned foods do not contain antioxidants and that many commercially prepared dry foods use naturally derived antioxidants. No studies have supported the contention by owners that synthetic antioxidants in general and ethoxyquin in particular are responsible for the variety of health problems reported to the FDA. The proper use of antioxidants

prevents the occurrence of rancidity and the production of toxic peroxide compounds in foods. In most cases, synthetic antioxidants are the best choice because of their efficacy, good carry-through, and low cost. In contrast, poor carry-through, instability, and high levels needed for effective protection make naturally derived antioxidants not ideal for use as the sole source in pet foods.

Natural

Natural pet foods claim to avoid any chemically synthesized ingredients. The term "natural" most often is associated with preservatives used in dry products (moist foods usually do not need added preservatives as the sealed cans prevent spoilage). Some consumers wish to avoid chemical preservatives but find natural preservatives, such as vitamin E, to be acceptable. At the present time, many pet foods that claim to be "all natural" contain added vitamins, minerals, and trace nutrients that are chemically synthesized. As described earlier, many nutrients must be added to pet foods to meet minimum requirements, because animal and plant food sources alone may not supply the correct amounts. Also, raw ingredients may have been preserved with "artificial chemicals" before arriving at the pet food processing plant. One example is fish, which always must be preserved between the time it is caught and when it is made into pet food. The claim of being "natural" should therefore be regarded with some skepticism and, in fact, most pet food companies have substituted "natural" preservatives for "artificial" chemicals to meet perceived consumer demand.

Organic

Organic pet foods generally refer to those that use food ingredients that are not exposed to insecticides, pesticides, or, in the case of animals, medications such as antibiotics or growth promoters. At present, no complete and balanced pet food can be considered 100% organic because of the need to add inorganic vitamins, minerals, and trace nutrients. Although organic products appeal to consumers who try to avoid artificial chemicals, no evidence currently suggests that organic foods are by definition healthier or more nutritious.

Holistic

"Holistic" is a more recent product claim seen on certain pet food labels. There is no official definition or general agreement on what the term *holistic* means. In medical practice, holistic often implies consideration of the health of the whole person or animal instead of just a single aspect or symptom. Some health care professionals claim to practice "holistic medicine," and pet foods marketed as "holistic" may appeal to those professionals and the pet owners they serve.

Raw

Raw pet foods and ingredients are marketed to those consumers who believe that food in its natural, uncooked state is healthier than when cooked or to those who think that nutrients are destroyed during processing, leading to unhealthy products. Some people attempt to eat only raw foods themselves for the same reasons. Proponents of raw feeding claim that dogs and cats in the wild eat uncooked food sources, and therefore pets should do the same. The main problem with offering raw foods to pets is that most of the meats and even some of the plant food sources sold in stores are contaminated by pathogenic bacteria. Raw or undercooked meat is a frequent cause of food poisoning, and outbreaks of foodborne illness in humans are common. Dogs and cats are likewise susceptible to illness from bacterial contamination of raw food. Animals can also acquire harmful bacteria from raw food and can spread disease to humans, even if the animals themselves remain apparently healthy. Another issue with raw foods is that overall diets are often incomplete and unbalanced unless they come from reputable companies that ensure the nutritional value of their products. Feeding of bones is recommended by many raw food feeders but, depending on size and type, bones can cause GI upset, obstruction, slab fractures of teeth, and even perforation and death. Frozen and refrigerated raw foods for pets are available, but owners should be advised to take as much care in preparing and handling these products as they would raw beef or raw chicken in their kitchen.

TECHNICIAN NOTE

The main problem with offering raw foods to pets is that most of the meats and even some of the plant food sources sold in stores are contaminated by pathogenic bacteria. Raw or undercooked meat is a frequent cause of food poisoning, and outbreaks of foodborne illness in humans are common.

Home-Prepared Pet Food

Many pet owners feed "human" foods in addition to or instead of commercial dog and cat diets. In a telephone survey of pet owners in the United States and Australia, owners reported they fed table scraps, leftovers, or homemade foods to 30% of dogs and 13% of cats in the study (635 dogs and 469 cats were included). However, greater than 93% of dogs and cats received at least half their diet as commercial pet food. Pet owners feed human foods for a variety of reasons.

Including or Avoiding Specific Ingredients. Some owners believe that their pets need a certain food or type of food. Various meat and dairy products, eggs, grains, vegetables, fruits, or supplements are added to commercial foods or are substituted for part of the diet. If there is an inexpensive convenient source of food, such as venison after deer season, owners may want to feed that instead of commercial pet food. Another motivation is that some owners perceive "organic" or "natural" foods to be better, so they seek out special types of foods to feed their pets. In contrast to wanting to include certain foods, owners may wish to avoid other foods or additives because of the perception that they are harmful or are not nutritionally beneficial.

Homemade Recipe Formulation. Home recipes can be formulated appropriately if potential problems are identified and managed. The first step in preparing a home diet is to evaluate the animal and determine the reason a home diet is requested or necessary. Complete medical and diet histories should be reviewed so that previous commercial or home foods can be evaluated and medical problems can be identified. The diet for a healthy 2-year-old large-breed dog will be very different from the diet for a sick 15-year-old toy-breed dog. Age, breed, activity level, food preferences, and owner commitment to the process should be assessed before the process of formulating a home diet is begun. The basic reasons why home diets are considered are that commercial diets are not palatable or acceptable, health or medical issues preclude regular diets, and/or owners prefer home diets.

Because of the complexity of accurately formulating home diets, trained veterinary nutritionists should be consulted whenever possible. Veterinarians who have advanced training in nutrition and experience with home diets often offer consulting services to other veterinarians and owners so that appropriate recipes can be formulated. Although the Internet is full of people claiming to be able to prepare home diets, it is best to check their credentials before requesting a consultation. Some are not veterinarians, others have no training or education in nutrition, and still others claim to have dubious degrees and certifications. The only current certification for veterinarians in the United States is diplomate status conferred by the American College of Veterinary Internal Medicine (ACVIM). Nutrition is one of the six subspecialties of the ACVIM. The ACVIM is the international certifying organization with advanced knowledge and training for veterinary specialists in cardiology, large animal internal medicine, neurology, nutrition, oncology, and small animal internal medicine, with over 3000 members worldwide.

Life Stage Nutrition for Cats and Dogs

Gestation and Lactation

Proper feeding and management will increase the chances of a healthy pregnant bitch or queen and an uneventful whelping. Poor nutrition can negatively affect reproductive performance in bitches and queens. Females undergo large extremes in the need for nutrients when considering the entire reproductive cycle. Pregnancy and lactation need specific nutrients and levels of nutrients. Malnutrition, caused by too much or too few nutrients, can affect pregnancy and lactation. Obesity at the end of pregnancy may result in a difficult delivery and may prolong labor, resulting in low oxygen or low blood sugar in puppies or kittens.

Body condition before breeding and good nutrition throughout gestation and lactation play a large role in a successful nursing outcome between the bitch/queen and the litter. Throughout the nursing period, nutrient requirements are linked to milk production. Production of milk is dependent on the number in the litter. The nursing stage has the highest nutrient requirement than any other adult life stage and, in some instances, may be equal to or higher than nutrient requirements for growth.

Technicians need to remind pet owners about the importance of water—in all stages of pregnancy and puppyhood/kittenhood. Water is the first nutrient needed for lactation. Water is needed in large quantities to produce milk. Water requirements in milliliters are roughly equal to energy requirements in kilocalories. It is important to put this in perspective—a 35-kg bitch nursing a large litter may require 5 to 6 liters of water per day during the nursing stage. Thus it is important that clean, fresh water be always available throughout pregnancy and nursing.

During pregnancy, energy requirements may be as high as 30% above adult maintenance for bitches with smaller litters. Energy needs for bitches with larger litters may increase by 50% to 60%. Energy needs are highest during weeks 6 to 8 of the pregnancy. However, food intake is limited by abdominal fullness as the puppies are growing in the uterus. It is also important to remember that giant breeds may find it difficult to eat enough food and maintain their BW even earlier than the last week of gestation. Enough energy should be provided to the bitch during the early weeks of pregnancy. Pregnancy is not an ideal time to lose body condition; thus the food should be high in energy density. After whelping, the bitch's energy requirement progressively increases, with the highest point being between 3 and 5 weeks. This point requires two to four times the energy for nonnursing adults. The energy requirement returns to maintenance levels about 8 weeks after whelping.

In cats, poor food intake over the course of the queen's pregnancy may impair weight gain, nursing, and kitten health. The recommended energy allowance for gestation is 25% to 50% above adult levels or approximately 90 to 110 kcal/kg BW per day, although total caloric intake may increase as much as 70% above maintenance. The increased need for energy can be met by providing 1.6 × RER at breeding with a gradual increase to 2 × RER when the kittens are born.

Just as with humans and dogs, energy requirements at times may exceed the recommended energy allowance in individual cats, especially those with large litters. Free-choice feeding allows queens to adjust food intake as needed to meet the energy requirement for pregnancy.

As the pregnant bitch nears the birthing time, her protein requirement increases by 40% to 70%. To improve the overall health of the newborn puppies and minimize neonatal mortality, the protein quality should also be higher. The minimum recommended crude protein allowance for foods for gestation and lactation in bitches ranges from 20% to 22%. For optimal reproductive health, foods for gestation and lactation should contain between 25% and 35% DM crude protein.

For queens, protein quality and quantity are important factors to consider. Cats need proteins that provide essential amino acids for healthy fetal growth and development. The minimum recommended protein level is 21.3% DMB, although 30% DM dietary protein is recommended, because it results in optimal weight gain in queens during gestation and kittens during lactation. Because of the fluctuating nutrient availability in typical pet food ingredients, protein levels at or above 35% DM are recommended for gestating queens. Remember cats are obligate carnivores and thus require animal-based proteins as the major source of dietary protein. These are often more digestible and have more desirable amino acid profiles. Protein deficiency during pregnancy may result in low birth weights, neonatal death, and impaired immune function in kittens.

Fat provides EFAs and boosts absorption of fat-soluble vitamins. Increasing fat levels in foods improves digestibility and provides energy. Feeding a food containing approximately 19% fat (DMB) usually meets this recommendation. It is important to remember that the fat level may need to be changed, depending on litter size, body condition of the bitch, food intake of the bitch, and so on. The minimum recommended allowance for fat in foods intended for late gestation and peak lactation is 8% to 8.5% DM. To ensure the best health during pregnancy, especially later in the pregnancy and for lactating bitches with fewer than four puppies, at least 20% crude fat (DMB) is recommended. This amount is also recommended for giant-breed bitches throughout pregnancy and nursing. The omega-3 fatty acid docosahexaenoic acid (DHA) should also be part of the nutritional profile of nursing bitches. Foods for pregnancy and nursing should contain the minimum recommended allowance of DHA plus eicosapentaenoic acid (EPA) of at least 0.05% (DM). Therefore DHA needs to be at least 40% of the total DHA plus EPA, or 0.02% DM.

> **TECHNICIAN NOTE**
>
> The omega-3 fatty acid docosahexaenoic acid (DHA) should also be part of the nutritional profile of nursing bitches.

To optimize reproductive performance in queens, foods during pregnancy and nursing should contain at least 18% DM fat (range

of 18%–35%, DMB). Nutrients in the food would then need to be balanced to the higher energy content of energy-dense foods (>4.5 kcal/g DM).

When discussing EFAs, the need for DHA during growth in foods for kittens may be even more important than in foods for puppies, because the ability to convert shorter-chain fatty acids to DHA is significantly lower in cats. DHA should be included in foods fed to lactating queens and can be found in such ingredients as fish and poultry meal. For queens in late pregnancy and those that are nursing, the minimum recommended allowance of DHA plus EPA is at least 0.01% DMB. Thus DHA needs to be at least 40% of the total DHA plus EPA, or ≥0.004% DM.

Feeding a carbohydrate-free food to pregnant bitches is not recommended as it potentially may result in weight loss, decreased food intake, reduced puppy birth weight and stillbirth, and increased risk of hypoglycemia and ketosis during late pregnancy. It is recommended that foods for lactation provide at least 10% to 20% of the energy intake in the form of digestible carbohydrate to support normal lactose production and at least 23% DM digestible carbohydrate.

In queens, digestible carbohydrates protect against weight loss in queens that are lactating. Digestible carbohydrates spare protein necessary to sustain blood glucose concentrations in queens and provide a substrate for lactose during milk production. Providing some digestible carbohydrate improves lactation performance even with an abundant supply of dietary protein. At least 10% DMB digestible carbohydrate should be included in foods for lactating queens.

Foods for gestation and lactation in dogs should contain 1% to 1.7% calcium and 0.7% to 1.3% (DM) phosphorus. The calcium-phosphorus ratio should be 1.1:1 to 2:1. Calcium supplementation is not necessary and should not be recommended during pregnancy or nursing when an appropriately balanced commercial food is fed.

> **TECHNICIAN NOTE**
>
> Calcium supplementation is not necessary and should not be recommended during pregnancy or nursing when feeding an appropriately balanced commercial food. The minimal recommended dry matter (DM) allowances for dietary calcium and phosphorus for queens in late gestation and peak lactation are 1.08 and 0.76%, respectively. Recommended levels for foods for feline gestation and lactation should be within the ranges of 1.1 to 1.6 for calcium and 0.8 to 1.4 for phosphorus DM. These levels can be found in commercial cat foods. The calcium-to-phosphorus ratio should be between 1:1 and 1.5:1.

It must be remembered that the pet needs nutrients in foods that are highly available because of the high nutritional demands during late gestation and lactation. Late in the bitch's/queen's pregnancy, the ability to ingest adequate amounts of food may surpass food intake capacity, especially if the food is not highly digestible. It is important to recommend foods with above average digestibility during the reproductive process.

The amount fed to the bitch throughout the nursing phase should be offered three times per day or free choice. Free-choice feeding is especially important for lactating bitches with more than four puppies. Some bitches are nervous throughout lactation, and free-choice feeding will allow them to eat on their schedule.

The goal of a feeding plan for puppies and kittens is to create a healthy adult. This means nutrition should be designed to achieve healthy growth, optimize trainability and immune function, and minimize obesity and developmental orthopedic disease. Nutrition plays a role in the health and development of growing dogs and cats and directly affects the immune system, body composition, growth rate, and skeletal development.

TECHNICIAN NOTE

The goal of a feeding plan for puppies and kittens is to create a healthy adult.

Feeding Puppies

The requirements for all nutrients are increased during growth. Most nutrients supplied in excess of that needed for growth cause little to no harm. However, excess energy and calcium are of special concern; these concerns include energy for puppies of small and medium breeds (for obesity prevention) and energy and calcium for puppies of large and giant breeds (for skeletal health).

Energy requirements for growing puppies consist of energy needed for maintenance and growth. During the first weeks after weaning, BW is relatively small and the growth rate high; puppies use about 50% of their total energy intake for maintenance and 50% for growth. Gradually, the growth curves reach a plateau as puppies become young adults. The proportion of energy needed for maintenance increases progressively, whereas the part for growth decreases. Energy needed for growth decreases to about 8% to 10% of the total energy requirement when puppies reach 80% or more of adult BW. A puppy's DER should be about three times its RER until it reaches about 50% of its adult BW. Thereafter, energy intake should be about 2.5 times the RER and can be reduced progressively to 2 times the RER. When approximately 80% of adult size is reached, 1.8 to 2 times the RER is usually sufficient.

$$RER \ (kcal \ / \ day) = 70 \times BW \ (kg)^{0.75}$$

or

$$RER \ (kcal \ / \ day) = (BW \ (kg) \times BW \ (kg) \times BW \ (kg))$$

These factors are general recommendations or starting points to estimate energy needs. Body condition scoring should be used to adjust these energy estimates for individual puppies.

Prevention of obesity is essential and should start at weaning. Too much food intake during growth may contribute to skeletal disorders in large-breed and giant-breed puppies. If too much weight is carried into adulthood, the risk for several important diseases is increased. These include hypertension, heart disease, diabetes mellitus, osteoarthritis, and exercise intolerance. Feeding a food with a very low energy density and low digestibility may not supply enough energy and nutrients to support optimal growth. This can lead to intake of large quantities of the food, which can overload the GI tract and result in vomiting and diarrhea. Consequently, energy and food intake and body condition should be monitored starting at an early age.

TECHNICIAN NOTE

Prevention of obesity is essential and should start at weaning.

Protein requirements of growing dogs differ quantitatively and qualitatively from those of adults. Quantitatively, during puppyhood, protein requirements are highest at weaning and decrease progressively. For example, the level of crude protein in bitch's milk is 33% DM. Bitch's milk is a highly digestible food, with an energy density of 6.4 kcal/g DM. This level is equivalent to 21%

highly digestible protein in a commercial food with 4 kcal/g DM. For puppies 14 weeks and older, the minimum recommended allowance for crude protein is 17.5% DM. The recommended protein range in foods intended for growth in all puppies (small, medium, and large breeds) is 22% to 32% DM. Most dry commercial foods marketed for puppy growth provide protein levels within this range.

Protein levels above the upper end of this range have not been shown to be detrimental but are well above the level in bitch's milk. Protein requirements of growing dogs differ from those of adults. An important difference is that arginine is an essential amino acid for puppies, whereas it is only conditionally essential for adult dogs. Foods formulated for adult dogs should not be fed to puppies. Although protein levels may be adequate, energy levels and other nutrients may not be balanced for growth.

Dietary fat serves three primary functions: (1) a source of EFAs, (2) a carrier for fat-soluble vitamins, and (3) a concentrated source of energy. Growing dogs have an estimated daily requirement for EFAs (linoleic acid) of about 250 mg/kg BW, which can be provided by a food containing between 5% and 10% DM fat. The fat source must be carefully chosen when low-fat foods (<10% DM fat) are fed to ensure that enough linoleic acid are provided. Studies indicate that DHA is essential for normal neural, retinal, and auditory development in puppies. Inclusion of fish oil as a source of DHA in puppy foods improves trainability. Thus adding a source of DHA should be considered essential for growth. The minimum recommended allowance for DHA plus EPA is 0.05% DM; EPA should not exceed 60% of the total. The DHA needs to be at least 40% of the total DHA plus EPA, or 0.02% DM. Fat contributes greatly to the energy density of a food; however, excessive energy intake can cause overweight/obesity and developmental orthopedic disease, as discussed above. The minimum recommended allowance of dietary fat for growth (8.5% DM) is much less than that needed for nursing but more than is needed for adult maintenance (5.5% DM). To provide a DM energy density between 3.5 and 4.5 kcal/g, between 10% and 25% DM fat is required. This range of dietary fat is recommended from the postweaning period to adulthood.

Although growing dogs need more calcium and phosphorus compared with adult dogs, the minimum requirements are relatively low. Puppies have been successfully raised when fed foods containing 0.37% to 0.6% DM calcium and 0.33% DM phosphorus.

Foods for large-breed and giant-breed puppies, as represented in Fig. 9.7, should contain 0.7% to 1.2% DM calcium (0.6%–1.1% phosphorus). Foods with a calcium content of 1.1% DM provide more calcium to puppies just after weaning than if bitch's milk is fed exclusively.

Because small-sized to medium-sized breeds are less sensitive to slightly overfeeding or underfeeding calcium, the level of calcium in foods for these puppies can range from 0.7% to 1.7% DM, (0.6%–1.3% phosphorus) without risk. The phosphorus intake is less critical than the calcium intake, provided the minimum requirements of 0.35% DM are met and the calcium-to-phosphorus ratio is between 1:1 and 1.8:1. For large-breed and giant-breed dogs, the calcium-to-phosphorus ratio should be between 1:1 and 1.5:1.

The ability of 11-week-old puppies to digest foods is less than at 60 weeks of age. If puppies are fed foods low in energy density and digestibility, they will need to eat larger quantities of food to achieve growth. This will increase the risk of flatulence, vomiting, diarrhea, and the development of a "pot-bellied" appearance.

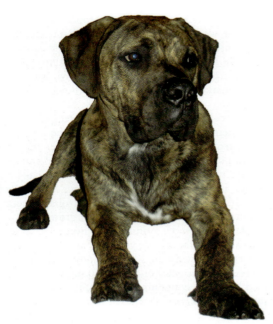

• **Fig. 9.7** Giant-breed puppy. (Copyright Kara M. Burns.)

Foods recommended for puppies should be more digestible compared with typical adult foods. An indirect indicator of digestibility is energy density. Foods with a higher energy density are likely to be more digestible.

The level of digestible (soluble) carbohydrates for growing puppies is recommended to be approximately 20% (DMB). This level is believed to optimize the health of the puppy.

Feeding Kittens

Kittens have high energy requirements to meet the needs of a rapid growth rate, thermoregulation, and maintenance. It is not unusual for kittens to grow at rates from 14 to 30 g/day during the rapid growth phase. As with other species, excessive energy intake may lead to obesity. It should be remembered that an overweight kitten has an increased risk of becoming an overweight adult cat.

> **TECHNICIAN NOTE**
>
> It is not unusual for kittens to grow at rates from 14 to 30 g/day during the rapid growth phase.

After neutering, it is recommended that food intake be limited and/or a food with a lower energy density be fed to prevent excessive weight gain. The energy density of the food fed to rapidly growing kittens should be between 4.0 and 5.0 kcal ME/g (16.7–20.9 kilojoules [kJ] ME/g). A higher energy density allows smaller volumes of food intake to satisfy caloric needs. It is also recommended that foods with energy densities toward the lower end of this range should be fed to neutered kittens, especially those with a body condition score (BCS) of 4/5 or greater. The prevalence of obesity increases dramatically after 1 year of age.

Protein requirements of kittens reflect their essential amino acid requirements and minimal nitrogen needs. Protein also provides sulfur-containing amino acids, which are required in greater amounts in kittens than in other species. Protein requirements are high at weaning, then decrease gradually to adult levels as the

kitten's growth slows. In kittens, the recommended range of crude protein for foods for healthy kitten growth is 35% to 50% DMB.

As in the case of puppies, dietary fat serves three primary functions in growing kittens: fat (1) supplies EFAs, (2) acts as a carrier for fat-soluble vitamins, and (3) provides a concentrated source of energy in food. It should be remembered that too much fat and too many calories may predispose young kittens to obesity. Kittens and adult cats require linoleic and AA, and they also require omega-3 (n-3) fatty acids (DHA, 20:6n-3). DHA has been shown to be necessary for normal neural, retinal, and auditory development in kittens. The percentage of fat in kitten foods should be in the range of 18% to 35% fat. This will aid in enhancing palatability, meeting EFA needs and maintaining the energy density of the food. DHA levels should be at least 40% of the total (DHA plus EPA), or 0.004% DMB.

Feeding Adult Cats and Dogs

Water accounts for approximately 56% of an adult dog's BW (73% of lean body mass). Water deprivation will result in death more quickly than withholding any other nutrient and should be considered the most important nutrient for cats and dogs. Total water intake is dependent on such factors as environment, physiologic state, activity, disease processes, and food composition. Dogs usually self-regulate water intake according to physiologic need. Healthy adult dogs and cats need approximately the equivalent of their energy requirement in kcal ME/day, expressed in milliliters per day (mL/day). Dogs and cats should be offered free access to clean, fresh water. The technician should remember to discuss the importance of water with pet owners.

Fats are an excellent source of energy, but the real requirement for fat is to supply EFAs. In addition, fat serves as a carrier for the absorption of fat-soluble vitamins. Fat is also a palatability enhancer. The minimum recommended allowance for dietary fat in foods for normal, healthy adult dogs is 8.5%, with at least 1% of the food as linoleic acid (DM). Depending on the type/source of fat, increasing the amount of fat in foods increases palatability and EFA levels; however, energy content also increases. The recommended range of fat for foods intended for young adult dogs is 10% to 20% (DM). Lower levels of dietary fat are recommended for obesity-prone adult dogs (7%–10% DM).

The minimum recommendation of fat in adult cat foods is 9% DMB. However, fat levels above 9% DMB are recommended for most cats. It has been shown that cats prefer foods with fat levels near 25% DM fat versus foods containing 10% or 50% fat DM. Technicians need to remember the correlation between high-fat foods and an increased incidence of obesity in cats. The majority of domestic cats today do well when fed foods containing 10%–30% fat DMB. Cats prone to obesity, however, should be fed foods with lower levels of dietary fat (9%–17% DM).

> **TECHNICIAN NOTE**
>
> Dietary fat and fiber levels in pet foods indicate the food's energy density.

Dietary fat and fiber levels in pet foods indicate the food's energy density. Fat provides more than twice as much energy compared with carbohydrate or protein. High-fat foods have increased energy density; however, low-fat foods have decreased energy density. Fiber is not a good source of energy for dogs and cats; thus as the fiber content of foods increases, energy density decreases. Dietary fiber does help promote satiety. In pet foods, fiber is listed as crude fiber, which is an imprecise measure, because most soluble fiber is omitted. A better measure would be total dietary fiber. Up to 5% fiber DMB seems appropriate for adult dogs and cats. Obesity-prone dogs may benefit from higher levels—around 10% crude fiber DM, with fat between 7% and 10%. As with dogs, increased levels of dietary fiber in cat foods reduce energy density and can induce satiety. The recommendation for obesity-prone cats is 5% to 15% crude fiber DMB. Also, adding fiber to the cats' diet has shown a benefit in cats that are susceptible to hairballs.

The level of protein in adult dog foods varies widely—anywhere from 15% to 60% protein DMB. More protein is not necessarily better for dogs. Dogs need to meet their amino acid requirements. After these are met, adding more protein to the diet provides no known physiologic benefit. However, owners believe that dogs are carnivores and need more protein. This is not true, as dogs are omnivores. Today's dogs' digestive and metabolic physiology are that of an omnivore. Excess dietary protein above the amino acid requirement is not stored as protein but rather, is deaminated by the liver. The kidneys excrete the excess which, in turn, causes an increased workload on the kidneys. The minimum crude protein content of food depends on digestibility and quality. The recommendation of crude protein DM for foods for adult dogs is between 15% and 30%.

> **TECHNICIAN NOTE**
>
> Excess dietary protein above the amino acid requirement is not stored as protein in cats and dogs but rather, is deaminated by the liver. The kidneys excrete the excess which, in turn, leads to increased workload on the kidneys.

Meeting the minimum protein needs of cats is critical, because they have minimal capacity to adapt to low levels of dietary protein. Protein in excess of the requirement is rapidly catabolized and used to provide energy and maintain blood glucose levels. Any excess energy will be stored as fat; therefore there appears to be little benefit to feeding large excesses of protein to cats. Cats should not be fed "vegetarian" diets. Cats are obligate carnivores and need to ingest animal protein for proper nutrients and overall nutrition and health. The recommended amount of protein for both normal weight and inactive/obesity-prone adult cats is 30%–45% DMB.

Feeding Mature and Elderly Cats and Dogs

Nutritional management of mature adult cats and dogs focuses on:

- Maintenance of optimal nutrition
- Risk factor management
- Disease management (i.e., slowing the progression of certain chronic diseases)
- Improvement in the quality and length of life

Older dogs and cats are more susceptible to dehydration, especially if they are prescribed diuretics or have chronic renal disease. In cats, aging impairs thirst sensitivity even further than previously known for cats. The importance of access to fresh, clean water must be emphasized with pet owners, and water intake should be routinely monitored.

As dogs age, they become slower and less active and can lose muscle mass and strength, including atrophy of the temporal muscles. Fig. 9.8 shows this temporal muscle atrophy in a senior mixed-breed dog.

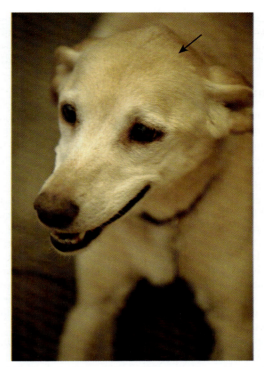

• **Fig. 9.8** Senior mixed-breed dog with temporal muscle atrophy, indicated by the *black arrow*. (Copyright Kara M. Burns.)

Thus it may be appropriate to feed a more energy-dense food to very old dogs. Because of the potential for mature dogs to have different energy needs, energy densities in foods recommended for this age group may vary from 3.0 to 4.0 kcal/g DMB. In mature cats, the energy density of foods should range from 3.5 to 4.5 kcal/g DMB.

Fat levels for the majority of mature dogs should fall between 7% and 15% DMB. For cats, this level should range between 10% and 25% fat DMB. EFA requirements should also be met, as previously discussed with adult cats and dogs.

Constipation is a common finding in mature dogs and cats because of reduced water intake, limited activity, and reduced motility in the colon. Fiber helps combat these issues and normalize the GI tract. Also, fiber added to foods for obesity-prone mature dogs and cats dilutes calories. The recommended levels of crude fiber in foods to be fed to mature dogs are at least 2% (DM), and for cats ≤%DMB or less.

> **TECHNICIAN NOTE**
>
> Constipation is more common in mature dogs and cats as a result of reduced water intake, limited activity, and reduced motility in the colon. Fiber helps combat these findings and normalize the GI tract.

Healthy mature dogs and cats should receive enough protein to ensure that protein energy malnutrition does not occur. Older pets may begin to lose muscle mass; therefore increasing protein in the diet may be warranted. However, older pets are also at increased risk for renal disease, in which case higher levels of protein are not recommended. Improving protein quality rather than increasing the amount eaten can provide sufficient protein for the older pet. Dietary protein should not be restricted in healthy mature adult cats. Adequate protein and energy intake are needed to sustain lean body mass, protein synthesis, and immune function. For healthy mature dogs, the protein percentage recommended is 15% to 23% protein DMB. For healthy mature cats, moderate levels of dietary protein—30% to 45% DMB—are recommended.

Feeding Working and Performance Dogs

Nutrition can play a major role in the success and long-term health of performance dogs. In general, all working dogs have energy requirements higher than those of an adult dog during times of normal activity. The type of work being done and the intensity of the work may necessitate modifications in the nutrient composition of the food and the feeding schedule.

Exercise requires the transfer of chemical energy into physical work. ATP is the sole source of energy for muscle contraction.

The two primary fuels used by the body for working muscles are muscle glycogen and free fatty acids. Dogs rely more heavily on free fatty acids for energy generation when exercising, regardless of the level of exercise. Therefore feeding a higher-fat diet to endurance-trained and intermediate-trained athletes prepares the muscles to efficiently mobilize and use free fatty acids for energy. It also exerts a glycogen- sparing effect that can help prolong glycogen use during work.

In canine athletes, no dietary requirements for carbohydrates truly exist except during pregnancy. Carbohydrates fed to canine athletes should be highly digestible to decrease fecal bulk in the colon.

Amino acids provide approximately 5% to 15% of the energy used during exercise. The majority of this energy comes from the branched-chain amino acids (leucine, isoleucine, and valine). It should be remembered that these are essential amino acids and cannot be synthesized from other amino acids; thus they must be included in the diet. Muscle and organ meat–based proteins have the highest level of essential amino acids and are also the most digestible and most bioavailable.

Amino acids are not stored as proteins in the body but are deaminated (broken down) to ketoacids. These ketoacids are either oxidized for energy or converted to fatty acids and/or glucose and stored as adipose tissue (fat) or glycogen.

> **TECHNICIAN NOTE**
>
> Remember, water is the most important nutrient in the body.

It should be remembered that water is the most important nutrient in the body. This is especially true of performance athletes, because water acts as a transport medium for nutrients, wastes, and heat; absorbs physical shock; and lubricates various internal and external surfaces. Heat is the primary by-product of muscle contraction, and the respiratory tract, through panting, is responsible for dissipation of this heat. Because evaporative heat loss is the primary way the bodies of dogs dissipate heat, ensuring adequate hydration is crucial for the maintenance of normal body temperature. Depending on the type of work done and environmental conditions, water losses during exercise can increase 10 to 20 times above normal.

A diet needs to be highly digestible to limit the total volume of food consumed at each meal. An ideal diet would provide increased levels of high-quality protein to meet anabolic requirements and enough nonprotein-energy nutrients (fats and carbohydrates) to meet energy requirements. The food needs to be calorically dense and palatable, highly digestible, and practical so

that the dog can physically consume enough to meet its caloric requirements.

Timing of meals is important to allow the most availability of nutrients to the athlete. Ideally, the timing of feeding the canine athlete is one meal at least 4 hours before exercise, one meal within 2 hours after exercise, and, if necessary, small amounts during exercise. The largest meal should be given after exercise. It is also very important to allow access to plenty of fresh, clean water to prevent dehydration.

The recommended caloric distribution for canine athletes is as follows:
- Calories from protein: 30% to 35% ME
- Calories from fat: 50% to 65% ME
- Calories from carbohydrate: 10% to 15% ME

Feeding Overweight Cats and Dogs

Pet obesity is widespread throughout the United States and Canada. It is likely that approximately 40% of adult pets and 50% of pets over age 7 years are overweight or obese. The definition of obesity states an increase in fat tissue mass sufficient to contribute to disease. Dogs and cats weighing 10% to 19% greater than the optimal weight for their breed are considered overweight; those weighing 20% or greater above the optimal weight are considered obese. Obesity has been associated with several disease conditions and reduced lifespan. A combination of excessive caloric intake, decreased physical activity, and genetic susceptibility are associated with most cases of obesity, and the primary treatment for obesity is reduced caloric intake and increased physical activity. Obesity is one of the leading preventable causes of illness/death. With the dramatic rise in pet obesity over the past several decades, weight management and obesity prevention should be among the top health issues discussed with every pet-owning customer.

> **TECHNICIAN NOTE**
>
> Dogs and cats weighing 10% to 19% greater than the optimal weight for their breed are considered overweight; those weighing 20% or greater above the optimal weight are considered obese.

Obesity is caused by an imbalance of energy intake and energy expenditure. It is very simple: too many calories in, not enough calories out! There are several risk factors that affect energy balance. Today, indoor pets (in North America) are often neutered. Although there are many positive health benefits associated with neutering, it is important that metabolic impacts and energy intake are addressed as well. Other recognized risk factors for obesity include breed, age, decreased physical activity, and type of food and feeding method.

It is important to talk to owners about what their pets eat daily. Revisit Fig. 9.1. In this way, veterinary technicians can find out specifically what type of food (all food) is fed. They can also learn about the feeding method (how much and how often), who is responsible for feeding the pet, and any other sources of energy intake (no matter how small or seemingly unimportant).

> **TECHNICIAN NOTE**
>
> To acquire the nutritional information you need, an excellent question to ask pet owners is this: "If you are going on vacation and I am watching your pet(s), tell me everything I need to do to feed your pet just as you do."

The strategy for weight loss in overweight dogs and cats, as in humans, is to decrease the daily calories eaten and increase the amount of exercise. Most typical maintenance-type pet foods are balanced according to their energy density and the expected ingestion required to support a given BW. Remember, if energy restriction is attempted by having the pet owner feed less of the currently provided food, the intake of all nutrients is restricted, not just energy. A deficiency in energy and other nutrients may occur if the amount of a maintenance food being fed is reduced to produce weight loss.

However, it would be more beneficial to use energy-restricted food. A properly formulated restricted-calorie food will be complete with all nutrients except energy. Therefore protein, EFAs, vitamins, and minerals will be present in amounts sufficient to support normal physiologic processes and retention of lean body tissue, even when calorie intake is insufficient to maintain BW. The goal of a weight-management food should be to *restrict energy* but not other nutrients. Pet foods sufficiently restricted in energy content are more suitable for weight management. It should be remembered that pet foods marketed as restricted in calories can vary widely in caloric content, including the proportion of nutrients contributing calories, fiber, and digestibility.

The recommended upper limit for dietary fat for dogs is 9% DMB; for cats, it is 10% DMB. For dogs that are on weight reduction plans, it is 9% DMB; for cats, it is 10% DMB. When maintaining the ideal weight and preventing weight regain, 9% DMB should be used. The upper limit of dietary fat in dogs is 14% DMB; for cats it is no greater than 18% fat DMB. The range for fiber content of dog foods intended for weight loss should fall between 12% and 25% DMB and for cats between 15% and 20% DMB. To maintain weight loss, the fiber range for dogs should be between 10% and 20% DMB and for cats, between 6% and 15% DMB. An important client communication point is that increased fiber in the diet may lead to increased frequency of defecation and increased likelihood of loose stools.

Protein in the diet affects weight loss in a few ways. It can cause both muscle and adipose reduction. Increased dietary protein and amino acids are therefore necessary for pets on a weight loss program to prevent loss of lean body mass. Dog foods for weight loss should contain at least 25% crude protein DMB (higher is better) to help combat loss of lean body mass. Dog foods intended for prevention of weight regain should contain at least 18% crude protein DMB (higher is better). Cat foods for weight loss should contain at least 35% crude protein DMB (again, higher is better) for the same reason. These values are also suggested for preventing regaining of lost weight in cats. It should be kept in mind that the *amount* of protein and the *quality* of protein are *both* important in protecting against the loss of lean body mass during weight loss programs.

The maximum amount of carbohydrates in foods for weight loss in dogs is 40% DMB; in cats, it is 35% DMB. To maintain weight loss and to prevent regaining of weight, the maximum amount of dietary carbohydrates should not exceed 55% DMB. In cats, carbohydrates should not exceed 40% DMB.

L-carnitine is a vitamin-like amino acid that can be found in all cells of animals. L-carnitine is involved in fat metabolism and the production of energy. It is responsible for helping fat being converted to lean tissue. The recommended level of L-carnitine (DM) in foods intended for weight loss in dogs and cats is at least 300 parts per million (ppm) and at least 500 ppm, respectively. The same amount is recommended for weight maintenance in dogs and cats as well.

Therapeutic Nutrition for Cats and Dogs

Veterinary technicians are directly involved in assisting pet owners with creating and implementing a nutritional plan for healthy dogs and cats and for those pets that do not fall into the "healthy" life stage categories (growth, maintenance, and reproduction). Pets are often identified as having medical conditions or health issues in which nutrition can play a critical role. It is important to realize that nutrition can be the cause of an illness. But it can also be an immediate cure for a nutritionally based disorder and a means of supportive care for the sick and the injured.

Assisted Feeding

Providing excellent nutrition is necessary when caring for sick veterinary patients with a wide array of aberrant conditions. Excellent nutrition supports immune system function, tissue healing, and proper GI function, to name only a few. Historically, in both human medicine and veterinary medicine, sick patients often were not fed or were allowed to remain anorectic (with poor to no appetite) in the belief that "resting" the GI system (and other systems) would be beneficial. However, research and clinical experience have shown that withholding food often leads to worsening of diseases and raises the rates of morbidity and mortality. Intentional starvation of patients during illness or hospitalization should no longer be practiced by conscientious health care providers.

> **TECHNICIAN NOTE**
>
> Feed sick and injured animal patients as soon as possible to avoid worsening of the disease symptoms and rate of mortality.

A nutritional assessment should be performed on all sick, injured, and hospitalized dogs and cats. A medical and dietary history can be obtained from owners and used to improve the patient's condition. This information gives important insight, historical information about the illness, and current and previous dietary and feeding plans. A complete physical examination of the patient is necessary to determine the extent of the medical problem, and the initial BW and BCS should be recorded. For hospitalized patients, daily examination and body weigh-in data help guide nutritional therapy. Vomiting, diarrhea, oral disease, and other such problems can complicate the feeding of sick animals, but there are modalities that can be utilized to get nutrients into patients as soon as possible. Medical therapy is always indicated first to correct fluid and electrolyte imbalances, decreased perfusion (shock), infection, pain, and other significant problems. Assisted feeding is generally delayed until the patient has been stabilized. Indications for assisted feeding include 72 hours (at most) of hospitalization without eating, 10% or greater weight loss (or 5% in young animals), and presentation of the animal in a debilitated condition. It should be remembered that these are only guidelines, and each patient should be assessed individually.

> **TECHNICIAN NOTE**
>
> Assisted feeding is generally delayed until the patient has been stabilized. Indications for assisted feeding include no longer than 72 hours (at most) of hospitalization without eating, 10% or greater weight loss (5% in young animals), and presentation of the patient on arrival in a debilitated condition.

Malnutrition in veterinary patients increases morbidity and mortality in a number of ways. In the GI tract, malnutrition increases transit times and decreases absorption as the villi atrophy. At the same time, the risk of bacterial translocation increases. In the kidneys, excretion of urinary calcium and phosphorus increases, and the ability to excrete acid decreases. Gluconeogenesis increases, and glomerular filtration rate decreases in the kidneys. Malnutrition has been documented to decrease humoral immunity and barrier function (skin and mucosal surfaces), inflammatory response, leukocyte motility, and bactericidal activity. Patients are at risk for pulmonary complications because of decreased response to hypoxia, decreased lung elasticity, secretion production, altered permeability, and decreased tidal volume. Cardiovascular complications include increased incidence of arrhythmias and decreased weight of the heart muscle. Protein malnutrition may also alter the normal or expected metabolism of certain drugs, which may increase or decrease their therapeutic effect, even when given at recommended dosages.

The GI tract needs to be fed. The gut receives an overwhelming percentage of its nutrition from chyme passing through it. In the small intestine, enterocytes use lumenal glutamine preferentially as their source of metabolic fuel. The colonocytes prefer butyrate, a short-chain fatty acid formed by fermentation of lumenal carbohydrates. In the absence of these fuel sources, growth and replication of the gut epithelium slow down, resulting in atrophy, necrosis, and increased risk of bacterial translocation across the now abnormal gut barrier. A key to prevention of this potentially serious problem is providing nutritional support to the gut. The rule of nutritional support is "If the gut works, use it."

Force feeding sick, hospitalized animals creates food aversions. It is an inefficient feeding method that results in more nutrients on the patient and the health care team member, rather than in the patient. Typically, force feeding will not provide a significant percentage of needed calories and will lead to a false sense of accomplishment and continued inadequate intake.

> **TECHNICIAN NOTE**
>
> Force feeding sick, hospitalized animals creates food aversions.

The use of indwelling feeding tubes is the method of choice in enteral assisted feeding. After an indwelling tube has been placed, feeding is easier and less stressful. Nasoesophageal (NE), esophagostomy, **gastrostomy**, and jejunostomy feeding tubes are the most commonly used. In animals undergoing laparotomy, placing gastrotomy or jejunostomy feeding tubes should be considered. The choice of one tube over another is based on the anticipated duration of nutritional support (e.g., days vs. months); the need to circumvent certain segments of the GI tract (e.g., oropharynx, esophagitis, pancreatitis); clinician experience; and the patient's ability to withstand anesthesia (very critical animals may only tolerate placement of NE feeding tubes).

Feeding Tube Options

- NE tubes are generally used for 3 to 7 days. Polyurethane tubes and silicon tubes may be placed in the caudal esophagus or stomach. An 8-French (Fr) tube will pass through the nasal cavity of most dogs. A 5-Fr tube is more comfortable in cats. Anesthesia or tranquilization is not necessary (use topical ophthalmic anesthetics to numb the nasal cavity). These tubes can be used in patients considered anesthetic risks.

- Pharyngostomy and **esophagostomy tubes** range in size from 8- to 16-Fr and may be placed in patients with disease or trauma to the nasal or oral cavity. These tubes can be used for the long term in hospital or home feedings. Gastrostomy (mushroom-tipped, 16- to 22-Fr) can be placed either intraoperatively or percutaneously. Refer to Figs. 9.9 and 9.10.

- Any tube that has been placed in the esophagus or stomach generally allows for bolus-type meal feeding, except in patients that vomit after each feeding. These patients will benefit from a slow, continuous drip administered via a pump or gravity.

- Jejunostomy tubes (J-tubes; 5- to 8-Fr) are placed within the small intestine either surgically or endoscopically and are appropriate for cases in which the stomach and proximal duodenum must be bypassed. Ideally, food is administered at a slow, continuous drip delivered via a pump.

Feeding Horses and Other Livestock

Equine

The feeding of horses is an intricate science that requires feeding the precise and balanced amount of nutrients. Horses have long been domesticated and are considered companion animals.

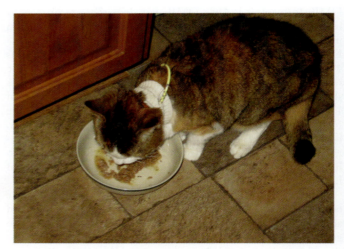

• **Fig. 9.9** Feline with a percutaneous esophagostomy (PEG) tube. (Copyright Ann E. Wortinger.)

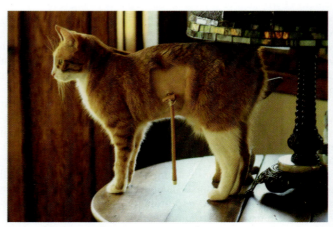

• **Fig. 9.10** Feline with percutaneous esophagostomy (PEG) tube. (Copyright Ann E. Wortinger.)

Companion horses consume a variety of feeds ranging, in physical form, from forage with a high content of moisture to cereals with a high amount of starch and from hay in the form of physically long fibrous stems to salt licks and water. Horses are nonruminant herbivores that naturally spend 60% to 75% of their day grazing. Horses ingest approximately 2% of their BW (DMB) per day while grazing.

TECHNICIAN NOTE

Horses are nonruminant herbivores that naturally spend 60% to 75% of their day grazing.

With domestication of the horse came alterations in feed, feeding times, and feeding methods—more in line with domesticated canines and felines. The horse is "meal fed," and unfamiliar materials, such as starchy cereals, protein concentrates, and dried forages, have been introduced. Horses are confined most of the time in stalls or smaller pastures, are fed one to two times per day and, as a result, spend less time of the day, approximately 40%, eating.

The diets formulated for horses contain, on average, 5% fat and 7% to 12% protein, with carbohydrates being the major source of energy ($\approx$80%). This results from the evolution of the eating patterns in horses to eating grass and other forages. Thus grass and hays serve a strong foundation for the feeding of horses. Protein, however, is required mainly in the building and replacement of tissues, and although some may consider protein to be an expensive source of energy, dietary protein and fat can contribute to meeting the physiologic energy demands of the horse. Protein converts the carbon chain of amino acids to intermediary acids and some of the carbon chains to glucose. Fat can aid in meeting energy demands after its hydrolysis to glycerol and fatty acids. Subsequently, the glycerol can be converted to glucose, and the fatty acid chain can be broken down by a stepwise process called *beta oxidation* in the mitochondria, which yields ATP and acetate or acetyl coenzyme A and requiring tissue oxygen.

Carbohydrate digestion and fermentation yield mostly glucose and acetic, propionic, and butyric volatile fatty acids. The portal venous system collects these nutrients, and a proportion of them are removed from blood as they pass through the liver. Both propionate and glucose contribute to glycogen (liver starch) reserves, and acetate and butyrate bolster the fat pool and constitute primary energy sources for many tissues.

Nutritional Physiology

The nutritional physiology of the horse differs from that of the cat or the dog. Multiple compartments make up the digestive tract of the horse, and each compartment has its own function in terms of using the ingested feed. The oral cavity is responsible for physically processing foods into smaller particles ($\approx$1.6 mm), allowing for passage through the esophagus and increasing the surface area for the small intestine enzymatic action. Also, the oral cavity breaks down structural carbohydrates for bacterial fermentation in the large intestine. The horse averages 60,000 chews per day, and it is only during chewing that the salivation process is activated. However, due to the increased chewing in the equine species, a horse will average 5 to 10 L/day of saliva which, in turn, acts as a lubricant for passage into the esophagus.

The stomach is responsible for approximately 8% of the total capacity of the equine GI tract, but retention time can range from 2 to 18 hours. The fundus and the pylorus are the two main regions of the stomach. The pyloric region secretes 10 to 30 L/day

of gastric juice. The small intestine of the horse measures 50 to 70 feet long and has a volume of 40 to 50 L. The transit time of the small intestine is, on average, 2 to 8 hours. At the anterior end of the small intestine, pancreatic juice aids in the digestion of lipids, protein, and nonstructural carbohydrates. Also, the small intestine is lined with microvilli that increase the surface area of the gut. As mentioned earlier, digestion in the small intestine is dependent on oral processing and the types of feed (forage is less digested than processed feed). The large intestine has capacity for large volume (100 L) and has a very slow transit time ($\approx$50 hours). The large intestine is responsible for the fermentation of structural carbohydrates to volatile fatty acids, which is responsible for 50% of ME. The large intestine absorbs roughly 80 L/day of water. B vitamins are produced by the bacteria that are absorbed in the large intestine. It is also important to note that nonprotein nitrogen is not used well in the large intestine.

Key Nutritional Factors for Adult Horses

The main nutrients that veterinary nutritionists consider for the horse are water, energy, protein, minerals, and vitamins. Water is the most important nutrient in any mammalian species. There should always be fresh, abundant water available. Horses will drink on average 25 L/day. In conditions of extreme heat or stress on the horse, the amount it will drink increases to 100 L/day. Also, it is necessary for technicians to remind owners that the more grain ingested by the horse, the more water will be needed by the horse.

TECHNICIAN NOTE

Water is the most important nutrient in any mammalian species. Horses will drink on average 25 L/day of water.

Energy is measured in terms of DE and fed in kilocalories. The amount of DE horses need depends on various factors: physiologic state, activity level, environment, and the size of the individual horse. Most of the energy used by the horse is from carbohydrates that are ingested through the horse's natural feed. (Refer to Table 9.1 for the amount [in kcal/kg] in various carbohydrate feeds.)

Fats provide the horse with high-density energy. In equines, fat should not exceed 20% of the total diet or 30% of concentrate. Exceeding these percentages will likely result in decreased palatability and loose stools.

Protein amounts are typically expressed as "crude protein" (CP) and are expressed as % dry matter (% DM). Again, the amount of protein needed by an individual horse is dependent upon several factors: physiologic state, type of diet, age, quality of diet. The closer the proportions of each of the various indispensable amino acids in the dietary protein conform to the proportions in the

TABLE 9.1 Equine Carbohydrates

Feed	Kcal/kg
Oats	3000
Alfalfa (early bloom)	2100
Bermuda grass hay	1800
Corn cobs	1250

mixture required by the tissues, the higher is the quality of the protein.

Calcium and phosphorus are considered together because of their interdependent roles as the main elements of the crystal apatite, which provides the building blocks for the skeletal system. The requirements of calcium and phosphorus are dependent on the physiologic state of the horse. The average adult horse weighing approximately 500 kg will need about 20 g of calcium and 14 g of phosphorus per day. It is important to balance the ratio of calcium to phosphorus, with a mature horse needing a ratio of 1.1:1 to 6:1. The recommended ratio for a growing horse is 1.1:1 to 3:1.

Sodium is the principal determinant of the osmolarity of extracellular fluid and, as a result, the volume of that fluid. Chloride concentration in extracellular fluid is directly related to that of sodium. Rarely do companion animals have an excess or deficiency of sodium or chloride; however, both these conditions should be closely watched for. Daily sodium requirements are recommended to be approximately 0.18% to 0.36% DM. If the requirements for sodium are met, seldom will a deficiency of chloride occur. Good sources of sodium and chloride can be found in grains with premixes and salt blocks.

Potassium is the main intracellular cation. Deficiency of potassium is rare in equines, and excess is rarely a problem. However, excess potassium can lead to *hyperkalemic periodic paralysis*, a syndrome of episodic weakness in horses accompanied by elevated serum potassium concentration. This syndrome appears to occur only in descendants of the American Quarter Horse. Forages contain approximately 1% to 4% potassium, with cereals being relatively poor sources of potassium.

Selenium is a trace element needed for antioxidant defense. Selenium forms an integral part of the glutathione (GSH)-Px molecule. Selenium catalyzes peroxide detoxification in body tissues, during which reduced GSH is oxidized. It is closely involved in the activity of alpha-tocopherol (vitamin E), which protects PUFAs from peridoxication. The requirement is 1 to 2 mg/day for a 500-kg horse, or 0.1 to 2 ppm. Selenium deficiencies cause pale, weak muscles in foals and yellowing of the depot fat, known as *white muscle disease*. It is imperative that pregnant mares receive adequate amounts of selenium in the diet. Selenium is highly toxic to animals, with the minimum toxic dose through continuous intake being 2 to 5 mg/kg feed. Skin, coat, and hoof abnormalities result from excess selenium.

Grazing horses derive their vitamin A from the carotenoid pigments present in herbage. The principal one is beta-carotene, with 1 mg of beta-carotene equating to approximately 400 international units (IU) of vitamin A. Horses that graze for 4 to 6 weeks build up a 3- to 6-month supply of vitamin A in the liver (Table 9.2).

Requirements for vitamin A during certain life stages are as follows: mature horses require 30 IU/kg BW; the gestation/lactation stage requires 60 IU/kg BW; and the growth stage requires approximately 50 IU/kg BW.

Vitamin E functions as a cellular antioxidant in conjunction with vitamin A and is required for normal immune function. Fresh green forage and the germ of cereal grains are rich sources of vitamin E. Adult horses require 80 to 100 IU/kg DM. Although deficiencies are rare, two neurologic disorders of horses have been recognized to involve the alpha-tocopherol status: equine degenerative myeloencephalopathy and equine motor neuron disease. These diseases typically are seen in horses that do not have access to pastures and consume poor-quality hay, and in horses with low concentrations of circulating levels of alpha-tocopherol.

Types of Feed

There are three types of feed to consider for horses: **roughages**, concentrates, and **complete feeds**. Roughages include grasses and forage legumes cut for hay. Most common species of grass are suitable for horses, but the preferred ones are the more popular and productive grasses, such as rye grasses, fescues, timothy, and cocksfoot. Other species found in permanent pastures are satisfactory as well, and these include meadow grasses, brome, bent grass, and foxtails. Legumes used are red, white, alsike, and crimson clovers and trefoils; lucerne; and sainfoin. Roughages are relatively low in energy and have greater than 18% crude fiber. Roughages are considered the foundation of an equine feeding program. Quality hay can provide energy to meet the maintenance requirements of the horse. Legumes and nonlegume grasses that are well managed and fertilized (proteinaceous roughages) provide greater than 10% CP as opposed to carbonaceous grasses (those that are not well maintained or fertilized), which provide less than 10% CP. Veterinary technicians can educate clients on the quality of roughage using the following guidelines:

- Free of mold
- Soft and pliable to touch
- Leafy with fine stems (⅔ E, ¾ protein)
- Pleasant, fragrant aroma
- Bright green, not brown or yellow

Another key point to communicate to owners is the fact that excess handling of roughages can result in loss of one-quarter of the leaves, loss of one-quarter to one-third energy and protein, and loss of 90% of beta-carotene.

TECHNICIAN NOTE

It is important to communicate to owners the fact that excess handling of roughages can result in loss of one-third of the leaves, loss of one-quarter to one-third of energy and protein, and loss of 90% of beta-carotene.

Concentrates are typically cereal grains that may or may not have supplemented protein, minerals, and vitamins. Concentrates are high in energy (typically, >50% compared with forage) and are less than 18% crude fiber. Often, concentrates are used as supplements if forage is insufficient in nutrients—especially energy and protein. Concentrates are needed more often in certain life stages, such as gestation (especially later in the gestation period), lactation, and growth, and in work horses. A rule of thumb would be to not exceed a concentrate-to-roughage ratio of 50:50 (wt:wt). As always, anything new should be introduced and transitioned slowly. It is important for health care team members and owners alike to be cognizant of the fact that excess concentrate may lead to laminitis, rhabdomyolysis, developmental orthopedic disease, and obesity.

TABLE 9.2	Carotene Levels in Herbage
Carotene Levels mg/kg DM	**Amounts**
Pasture grass/alfalfa	300–600
Good hay	20–40
Poor hay	4–5

DM, Dry matter.

Complete feeds are typically a mixture of roughage and concentrate—usually a mixture of 80% roughage and 20% concentrate. Complete feeds are manufactured by grinding the food and formulating it into pellets, thus making it easier (all in one) for the owner; at the same time, it potentially increases the cost. Because the complete feed is pelleted or wafered, careful consideration must be given to the potential risks associated with inadequate particle size; these risks include colic, choking, wood chewing, and coprophagy, to name a few.

When discussing nutritional management with clients, the technician should remember to emphasize that fresh water should always be available. ME can be met entirely with quality hay, but it may be supplemented with concentrate if necessary. However, it should be ensured that the horse is not supplemented more than 50% by weight with concentrate. Good-quality green roughage should supply adequate amounts of vitamins A and E. It should be remembered that nutrition is one area of equine veterinary medicine that affects every horse and should be discussed every time on every visit.

Pediatric Equine Nutrition

The goal of a feeding plan for foals and young horses is to create a healthy animal and thus a healthy adult horse. The specific objectives of a feeding plan for a young horse are to achieve healthy growth, optimize trainability and immune function, and minimize obesity and developmental orthopedic disease. Growth is a complex process involving interactions among genetics, nutrition, and environmental influences. Nutrition plays a role in the health and development of growing horses and directly affects the immune system, body composition, growth rate, and skeletal development.

Foals should be assessed for risk factors before weaning for implementation of recommendations for appropriate nutrition. A thorough history and physical evaluation are necessary. Additionally, the BCS provides valuable information about nutritional risks. Growth rates of young horses are affected by the energy density and amount of food fed. It is important that horses be fed to grow at an optimal rate for physiologic development and body condition rather than at a maximal rate.

Nutritional requirements and dietary composition of foals change markedly from the time they are transitioned from neonate to weanling. The foal is transitioning from a continuous supply of nutrients from the dam in utero to sporadic absorption of ingested nutrients after birth. Concurrently, the neonate's metabolism no longer is dependent on maternal glucose concentration to maintain normal glucose levels, and the pancreas initiates the regulation of glucose homeostasis. This alteration in energy metabolism is dramatic and does not always occur smoothly, leading to limited energy reserves (glycogen and fat) in the neonatal foal. Even in the "normal" neonatal foal, hypoglycemia occurs frequently, and veterinary health care teams must be aware of this fact. In the sick foal, severe hypoglycemia will result if the foal is deprived of energy for even a short period.

The neonatal foal has a high metabolic rate, and thus frequent ingestion of high volumes of milk to meet its energy requirements for maintenance and growth are needed. During the first week to months of the foal's life, caloric needs are as follows:
- First week: approximately 150 kcal/kg per day
- Three weeks: approximately 120 kcal/kg per day
- One to 2 months: approximately 80 to 100 kcal/kg per day

Healthy foals less than 7 days of age will nurse approximately seven times per hour for approximately 1 to 2 minutes a time. After 7 days, there is a decrease in the number of times a foal will nurse, but conversely, there is an increase in the duration of nursing. On average, the mare's milk contains about 64% sugar (as lactose), 22% protein, and 13% fat. Thus the main source of energy for the foal is glucose.

After the first 24 hours, foals will start to eat small amounts of hay, grass, and grain, along with the mare's feces. It is understood that the feces provide the initial microbial flora the foal needs to aid in the digestion of the hay, grass, and grain. Until several weeks of age, the roughage and grain are not well digested by the foal. It is at this time that transitioning from weaning (a milk-based diet) to a forage-based diet is occurring gradually. The milk amount produced by the mare peaks after approximately 2 months of lactation, and then the amount of milk produced begins to decline. Shortly thereafter, the foal will be weaned from the mare and rely on solid feed for an increasing proportion of its nutritional requirements. Complete maturation of hindgut function will occur around age 3 or 4 months.

Energy Requirement of Growing Horses

The energy requirement of growing horses is determined by calculating the total energy required for maintenance in addition to the energy required for growth or gain. DER is dependent on several factors: the environment, the foal's age, the desired **average daily gain** (ADG), and the individual characteristics of the specific foal. The individual characteristics that health care team members must consider when calculating DER include metabolic and health characteristics. Researchers and scientists have yet to determine the optimal growth rate for horses; therefore it is difficult to determine the exact energy requirement. If horses grow too quickly and too much weight is added, skeletal integrity and longevity may be adversely affected. However, inadequate energy intake will result in poor and slower growth rates, and young horses will look unhealthy.

> **TECHNICIAN NOTE**
>
> The daily energy requirement (DER) of foals is dependent on several factors: the environment, the foal's age, the desired average daily gain (ADG), and the individual characteristics of the specific foal.

Most nutritionists and equine specialists follow the formula recommended by the National Research Council (NRC). This formula calculates the DER of growing horses in the following manner:

$$DE\left(Mcal/day\right) = \left(56.5x^{-0.145}\right) \times BW + \left(1.99 + 1.21x - 0.021x^2\right) \times ADG$$

(x is age in months; ADG is average daily gain; BW is body weight in kilograms)

Most owners feed their horses aiming to achieve an ADG of 1.1 to 1.4 kg/day, with some owners aiming slightly higher. Both veterinary health care team members and owners must be cognizant of what feed is being given, how much, other feedstuffs that are being added to the diet, and the energy concentration for total diets consumed. The team must perform a nutritional assessment prior to initiating a feeding plan and on every subsequent patient visit (whether farm visit or hospital visit). The average energy concentration for the total amount of feed (on an as-fed basis) given to a growing horse can range from 2.5 Mcal/kg, with diets consisting of 70% concentrate and 30% hay, to 0.72 Mcal/kg for certain pasture-fed growing horses. Young horses have been found to gain enough energy from pasture feeding to sustain adequate growth. Many factors must be taken into consideration—whether the horse is pasture fed or concentrate and roughage fed. These factors would include the type and quality of forage (if pasture fed), training level, environmental conditions, body condition, and health of the growing horse. Again, the feed or pasture must also be evaluated for protein level, protein quality, vitamin and mineral level, etc. All of these factors will influence the desired growth rate in young horses. Restrictions in protein have a direct correlation to restrictions in the growth rate of a young horse.

CP requirements for the growing horse can be calculated by using the following equation:

$$CP\,requirement = (BW \times 1.44\,g\,CP/kg\,BW) + ([ADG \times 0.20]/E) \div 0.79$$

The E in the equation represents the efficiency of the use of dietary protein. Estimates from the NRC for the efficiency of use of dietary protein in the young horse are as follows:
- ≈50% for 4- to 6-month-old horses
- ≈45% for 7- to 8-month-old horses
- ≈40% for 9- to 10-month-old horses
- ≈35% for 11-month-old horses
- ≈30% for 12-month-old horses and older horses

It is important also to remember that the quality of protein, as defined by amino acid composition, plays a significant role in the nutrition of the growing horse, and that poor-quality protein sources can have deleterious effects on growing horses. Also, the amount of dietary energy consumed will be inadequate if the feed is too low in either DE or protein, even though plenty of feed may be available. Thus the growth rate in the young horse will decrease with inadequate intake of dietary energy or protein. A slower growth rate has the potential to mask other nutritional deficiencies and, if growth is slowed significantly, it may reduce the body size of the horse at maturation. With a fast growth rate, deficiencies in minerals may result. If a deficiency of calcium, phosphorus, zinc, or copper occurs, developmental orthopedic disease may result. Conversely, if dietary protein and energy intake are too high in the young horse, a rapid growth rate may occur, increasing the risk of developmental orthopedic disease and obesity.

During the feeding of the young horse, from nursing to maturity, fresh, clean water should always be available. Veterinary health care team members often need to remember to mention the importance of this key nutrient.

Owners should weigh growing horses as often as possible (biweekly is recommended), using a weight tape if scales are not available, and record BW and food intake. A BCS should also be obtained at least every 2 weeks (Fig. 9.11). This level of attention to body condition scoring is important to the development of a healthy growing horse. Also, regularly assessing body condition provides immediate feedback about optimal nutrition. This will prepare the owner to continue to make these observations throughout the life of the horse. Horses receiving such attention would be less likely to experience skeletal diseases and overweight or obesity and the myriad of related problems as adults. Veterinary health care team members should reassess growing horses during farm calls and work in conjunction with the owners to detect the potential for or the occurrence of under- or overnutrition. Reassessment should include BW and body condition assessment, food assessment, and calculations of correct feed amounts.

Critical Care Nutrition in Equines

As in other species, nutrition in critically ill horses can be administered enterally or parenterally. It is imperative that nutrition be assessed and administered throughout the entire hospitalization of the critically ill equine patient. Enteral nutrition (EN) is considered less expensive and more physiologic, or more natural, for the patient. EN is also believed to provide enhanced immunity to the horse and is somewhat easier to administer. The technician should remember the adage "If the gut works, use it." This adage was formulated because of studies in a variety of species demonstrating that EN helps support organ function, improves organ blood flow, improves immune function, and helps the patient gain weight. Current guidelines suggest the use of EN whenever it is tolerated by the horse instead of or in combination with parenteral nutrition (PN). Veterinary technicians play a large role in the management of nutrition in critically ill horses and should understand that early EN with parenteral supplementation (if necessary) is the standard for critically ill horses.

Nutritional support should be considered in patients that have or are at risk for increased metabolic rate. This would include equines that are growing, have experienced a history of malnutrition or hypophagia, have an underlying metabolic abnormality that has the potential to worsen if food is withheld, have experienced trauma or sepsis, or have an increased energy demand. The healthy adult horse can withstand food deprivation (simple starvation) for 24 to 72 hours with little systemic effects. However, in stressed and injured animals, food deprivation has a deleterious effect.

> **TECHNICIAN NOTE**
>
> Nutritional support should be considered in equine patients that have or are at risk for increased metabolic rate.

Stressed or injured horses have an increased resting metabolic rate and use their own protein reserves as the principal energy source. This is known as *catabolism*. Increased metabolic rate and catabolism in the equine patient leads to accelerated body wasting. Total body protein synthesis is reduced, because the body is using amino acids for energy. Subsequently, the horse has increased metabolic demands, uses protein for energy, develops insulin resistance and glucose intolerance, exhibits poor wound healing and decreased immune function, and becomes extremely weak. Despite protein supplementation, the critically ill horse will continue to experience protein catabolism. Therefore simply providing protein is not the answer; rather, nutritional supplementation will help minimize protein loss; provide essential and conditionally essential amino acids, vitamins, and minerals; and subsequently decrease morbidity.

Enteral Nutrition in Horses

EN can be composed of normal feed, slurry diets made primarily from the patients' normal feed, and liquid diets containing micro- and macrominerals. Typically, the normal feed is not tolerated by the horse because appetite has decreased significantly, and nutrition must be given through a nasogastric (NG) tube. When using an NG tube, making a slurry from a complete pelleted feed is advantageous, because it is relatively inexpensive and is well balanced for an adult horse. Also, these formulations contain fiber, which aids in GI activity, colonic blood flow, and colonic mucosal cell growth and absorption. However, a slurry made from the feed may not easily pass through the NG tube. If a slurry is to be made, 1 kg of pelleted complete feed should be soaked in 6 L of water and administered through a large-bore NG tube using a marine supply bilge pump; if a pump is not available, the pellets should be pulverized before water is added. Great care and caution should

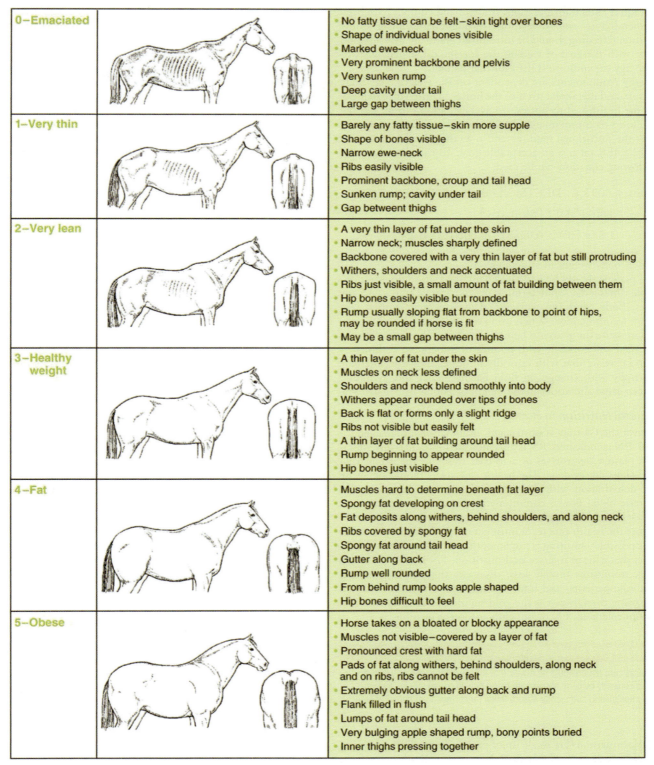

0–Emaciated		• No fatty tissue can be felt—skin tight over bones • Shape of individual bones visible • Marked ewe-neck • Very prominent backbone and pelvis • Very sunken rump • Deep cavity under tail • Large gap between thighs
1–Very thin		• Barely any fatty tissue—skin more supple • Shape of bones visible • Narrow ewe-neck • Ribs easily visible • Prominent backbone, croup and tail head • Sunken rump; cavity under tail • Gap betweent thighs
2–Very lean		• A very thin layer of fat under the skin • Narrow neck; muscles sharply defined • Backbone covered with a very thin layer of fat but still protruding • Withers, shoulders and neck accentuated • Ribs just visible, a small amount of fat building between them • Hip bones easily visible but rounded • Rump usually sloping flat from backbone to point of hips, may be rounded if horse is fit • May be a small gap between thighs
3–Healthy weight		• A thin layer of fat under the skin • Muscles on neck less defined • Shoulders and neck blend smoothly into body • Withers appear rounded over tips of bones • Back is flat or forms only a slight ridge • Ribs not visible but easily felt • A thin layer of fat building around tail head • Rump beginning to appear rounded • Hip bones just visible
4–Fat		• Muscles hard to determine beneath fat layer • Spongy fat developing on crest • Fat deposits along withers, behind shoulders, and along neck • Ribs covered by spongy fat • Spongy fat around tail head • Gutter along back • Rump well rounded • From behind rump looks apple shaped • Hip bones difficult to feel
5–Obese		• Horse takes on a bloated or blocky appearance • Muscles not visible—covered by a layer of fat • Pronounced crest with hard fat • Pads of fat along withers, behind shoulders, along neck and on ribs, ribs cannot be felt • Extremely obvious gutter along back and rump • Flank filled in flush • Lumps of fat around tail head • Very bulging apple shaped rump, bony points buried • Inner thighs pressing together

• **Fig. 9.11** Body condition scoring of the horse. (From Holtgrew-Bohling K. *Large Animal Clinical Procedures for Veterinary Technicians.* 2nd ed. St. Louis, MO: Mosby; 2011.)

be taken when administering the slurry, and the technician should be cognizant of the horses' reaction during the procedure. The slurry should be administered very slowly. Each feeding should not exceed 6 to 8 liters, because the stomach volume of an adult horse (weighing ≈450 kg) ranges from 9 to 12 L. If prolonged feeding is required (i.e., dysphagia; head, neck, or oral trauma; prolonged anorexia with a functional GI tract), an indwelling esophagostomy tube is considered a better option for enteral feeding. Longer-term intubation with use of a smaller-bore tube will not be conducive to administration of the aforementioned slurry diets. Liquid enteral formulations (human and equine) have been recommended in enteral feedings through an esophagostomy tube. Enteral feeding should be introduced gradually over a period of days, with the goal of feeding the specific calculated DER or daily energy expenditure (DEE) for that patient.

Energy requirements are dependent on the weight, age, body condition, and metabolic stress of the horse. Maintenance requirements for healthy adult horses, on average, are 33 to 40 kcal/kg per 24 hours or approximately 18,000 kcal/day. When attempting to meet the nutritional requirement in a critically ill horse, using the DEE/DER ratio is an acceptable goal. To calculate the ratio, the following equation can be used:

$$\text{Horses} \leq 600\,\text{kg} : \text{DEE (Mcal / day)} = 1.4 + (\text{BW} \times 0.03)$$

$$\text{Horses} \geq 600\,\text{kg} : \text{DEE}\left(\text{Mcal / day}\right)$$
$$= 1.82 + \left(\text{BW} \times 0.0383\right) - \left[0.000015 \times \text{BW}\right]$$

(BW = body weight in kilograms)

The patient should be evaluated daily (and, in some instances, multiple times a day) to determine the nutritional status and any changes. Body condition scoring and measurement with weight tapes are recommended. When using the weight tape, technicians should measure the girth just behind the elbow. The circumference determined will correlate with pounds or kilograms. Technicians need to be aware that with critically ill horses, BW can fluctuate dramatically with changes in fluid balance. Diet and hydration status can cause alterations in the weight of a horse by 5% to 10%.

Parenteral Nutrition in Horses

Whenever the GI tract is obstructed, dysfunctional, damaged, or painful, PN is indicated. PN is also indicated if there is any alteration in plasma electrolytes or acid-base status to the extent that clinical signs are evident. The health care team should be aware that if dehydration with or without shock is evident clinically, mesenteric blood flow is commonly inadequate for the intestines to sufficiently absorb fluids for correction of dehydration or shock. Therefore the health care team must get nutrition into the horse as soon as possible—waiting is not an option. Studies suggest that in patients that cannot tolerate oral nutrition, PN improves wound healing, minimizes muscle loss, decreases the weight loss seen in catabolic patients, and improves immune function. As stated above, using the GI tract is the gold standard, but in times when EN is not tolerated, PN must begin as soon as possible.

> **TECHNICIAN NOTE**
>
> The health care team should be aware that if dehydration with or without shock is clinically evident, mesenteric blood flow is commonly inadequate for the intestines to sufficiently absorb fluids for correction of dehydration or shock.

PN formulations are made up of protein in the form of amino acids, carbohydrates in the form of dextrose, and lipids in the form of long-chain fatty acids. Electrolytes, minerals, and vitamins also can be added to the formulation. The carbohydrates and lipids in PN meet the energy needs of the horse, break down the autologous protein for energy, and work synergistically with the protein for wound healing and increased immune function.

PN is administered for short periods of time, multiple times a day. *Total parenteral nutrition* is a misnomer in veterinary medicine versus human medicine. Human medicine has a greater ability to prepare nutritional supplementation per individual patient and includes a wider range of microminerals compared with what is available in veterinary medicine. To begin, the goal is to provide 30% to 40% of the solution's calories with lipids and 60% to 70% with protein. Lipid supplementation may be increased to approximately 60% in those equines that need prolonged PN feeding.

When administering PN, technicians should be aware of the risk of thrombophlebitis and administer the solution via a central vein or the jugular vein of a horse. Administration of PN solutions should be through a dedicated catheter placed in an aseptic manner. Whether the solution can be administered via a peripheral catheter or a central line is directly related to the osmolarity of the solution. Catheters composed of silicone, polyurethane, or tetrafluoroethylene are also recommended to avoid thrombophlebitis. PN solutions are typically administered as a constant rate infusion over a 24-hour period. Once the solution is warmed to room temperature, it is recommended that the entire solution be used up in this time frame to prevent contamination and lipid particle destabilization. It is imperative that the health care team reevaluate the nutritional plan every day while administering PN. If the patient is not improving with use of this modality over several days and remains anorectic, the decision to institute EN should be considered.

It is important for nursing care to include calculating the patient's caloric requirements. This is important, because feeding more food than necessary has the potential for causing metabolic complications. A general rule to remember is that most patients tolerate the food or solution that meets their RER. Equine patients that are hospitalized have metabolic rates very near their DER. The DER of hospitalized patients can be estimated by using the equations given above. Feeding patients at DER is a safe and rational approach as opposed to doubling basal requirements, since this has been shown to result in overfeeding and potential complications including hyperglycemia, hyperammonemia, and hyperlipidemia. At a minimum, veterinary technicians should perform daily nutritional assessments to guide any needed adjustments to the nutritional plan for the hospitalized patient. Often, a critically ill equine patient may require more frequent assessments.

Potential complications with PN administration can be classified into three main categories: mechanical, metabolic, and septic. Mechanical complications usually involve catheter-related problems. Examples include occlusion, premature removal, line disconnection/breakage, and/or thrombophlebitis. These problems can be avoided by the technician's strict adherence to aseptic technique and careful monitoring of patients. Metabolic complications are more likely to occur with PN solutions formulated to deliver total caloric requirements. The most common metabolic complication in equines is hyperglycemia and decreases in plasma electrolyte concentrations—especially potassium. Other complications include hypertriglyceridemia, hyperammonemia, or electrolyte changes consistent with refeeding syndrome (e.g., hypokalemia, hypophosphatemia, hypomagnesemia). Reformulation of the PN solution is required if any of these problems occur. The most serious and potentially life-threatening complication is sepsis. Technicians need to use strict antiseptic techniques when placing a catheter. Nursing management of catheters carrying hyperosmolar solutions containing amino acids requires special attention, because the solution type is highly susceptible to colonization of bacteria. Antiseptic techniques and focused nursing care should be the same for all types of fluid administration but is especially important in patients receiving PN. If signs of sepsis develop without an identifiable source, contamination of the solution and/or intravenous catheter should be suspected. Culture and sensitivity tests for both should be considered. It is because of this potential complication that many veterinarians recommend having the PN solution compounded at an outside facility.

In summary, EN and PN are viable nutritional choices for critically ill equine patients. When applicable, combined EN and PN is recommended to prevent intestinal hypertrophy and to facilitate healing by promoting intestinal growth. Proper nursing care and aseptic technique are also crucial to a positive patient outcome in both EN and PN. Nutritional requirements of hospitalized patients should be carefully monitored by the veterinary technician. With complete understanding of some of the potential complications, the effectiveness of EN and PN can be enhanced.

> ### TECHNICIAN NOTE
> Enteral nutrition and parenteral nutrition (EN and PN) are viable nutritional choices for critically ill equine patients. When applicable, combined EN and PN is recommended to prevent intestinal hypertrophy and to facilitate healing by promoting intestinal growth.

Nutritional Histories of Large Animal Patients

Every herd and every animal should have a nutritional history performed by the veterinary health care team. The nutritional history provides the background for the veterinary health care team and is necessary to ascertain the information on the quantity and quality of the diets that the animals have been receiving. The nutritional history provides very useful information and assists the team in determining whether the nutrient requirements for that species are being met.

Pasture-fed Livestock

Livestock maintained on pastures differ significantly from stall-fed livestock in that the diet of the former is not easy to control and subsequently may be much more difficult to evaluate. In animals that graze, the risks for parasitic infestation and infectious diseases are much greater.

Questions to ask regarding pasture fed livestock are related to the following:
- Composition of the pasture
- Nutritive value
  - Recent changes brought about by rain or drought
  - Whether rotational grazing is practiced
  - Fertilizer program
  - Potential for minerals and trace elements to be provided by top-dressing or mineral mixtures
- Mineral supplementation (i.e., phosphates, which may contain excess fluorine)
- Homemade mixtures (which may have excessive quantities of certain ingredients)
- Authentic examination of the pasture area versus owner descriptions

Hand-fed and Stall-fed Large Animals

Hand-fed or stall-fed animals have access to a relatively controlled feed supply. However, the potential for human error exists with stall feeding, because of the potential for mistakes in dietary compositions. Therefore when taking a nutritional history of stall-fed animals, it is important to ask for the following information:
- Types and amounts of feeds
- Sources of the dietary ingredients

- Grains from certain areas may be much heavier and may contain a greater proportion of starch to husk versus grains from other areas.
- When feed is measured as opposed to being weighed, the risk of overfeeding or underfeeding is significantly increased.

Several diseases are associated with inadequacies in hand-fed diets, and these include:
- Osteodystrophia fibrosa—in equines on feeds composed of excess grain
- Azoturia—in equines fed carbohydrate-heavy diets during periods of rest
- Lactic acid indigestion—in cattle introduced to high-level grain diets too rapidly

Other considerations for the veterinary health care team to keep in mind with hand-fed livestock include the following:
- Use of nonmilk sources of carbohydrates and proteins (as in milk replacers) may result in indigestion and nutritional diarrhea. Physiologically, the digestive enzyme capacity of newborn farm animals is most efficient in the digestion of whole milk versus milk replacers.
- Exotic diseases (e.g., anthrax, foot-and-mouth disease, hog cholera) have the potential to be introduced via feed materials.
- Although not common, food preparation may result in significant variations in feed.
  - Foods that are pelleted or cooked have the potential for a reduction in the vitamin content.
  - Poisoning by chlorinated naphthalene compounds may be the result of the use of lubricating oil in the production line.
  - Pressure extraction of linseed has the potential to leave residue of hydrocyanic acid in the residual oil cake.
- Feeding practices may, in themselves, cause disease, for instance, large numbers of pigs being fed in inadequate trough spaces or calves being fed in communal troughs. Contamination with lubricating oil can result in overeating or inanition. High-level feeding and consequent rapid growth may create deficiencies due to increased requirements for other nutrients.

In all animals, changes in diets should be carefully noted. Health care team members should document the following in the nutritional history:
- Movement of animals from one field to another
- Change from pasture to cereal grazing
- Change from unimproved to improved pasture
- Periods of bad weather or transportation
- Change to new/unfamiliar feeds
- Changes occurring rapidly versus gradually, especially in pregnant and lactating ruminants, increasing the risk of metabolic diseases (i.e., hypocalcemia, hypoglycemia, hypomagnesemia)
- Availability of drinking water

Assessment of Nutritional Status

In addition to a nutritional history taken from the owner, large animal patients should undergo a physical examination to assist in determining nutritional needs. It is important for health care team members to evaluate potential systemic, mechanical, or neurologic diseases that may be associated with or contributing to poor nutrition. Examples would include foreign bodies, abscesses, botulism, and so on.

All patients should have BW and BCS measured and recorded. BW measurements should be taken when the large animal patient presents to the hospital or to the health care team. If the animal is hospitalized, BW should be taken frequently throughout the patient's hospitalization. The health care team will often have to obtain the weight with no access to a scale. In these instances, the health care team member should use a weight tape or length and girth measurements to estimate the patient's weight.

Another valuable tool to evaluate nutritional status is BCS, which allows for subjective assessment of endogenous protein and lipid stores in a large animal patient. BCS tools for various species are described in the following: Figs. 9.11 and 9.12A and B, Table 9.3, Figs. 9.13 and 9.14.

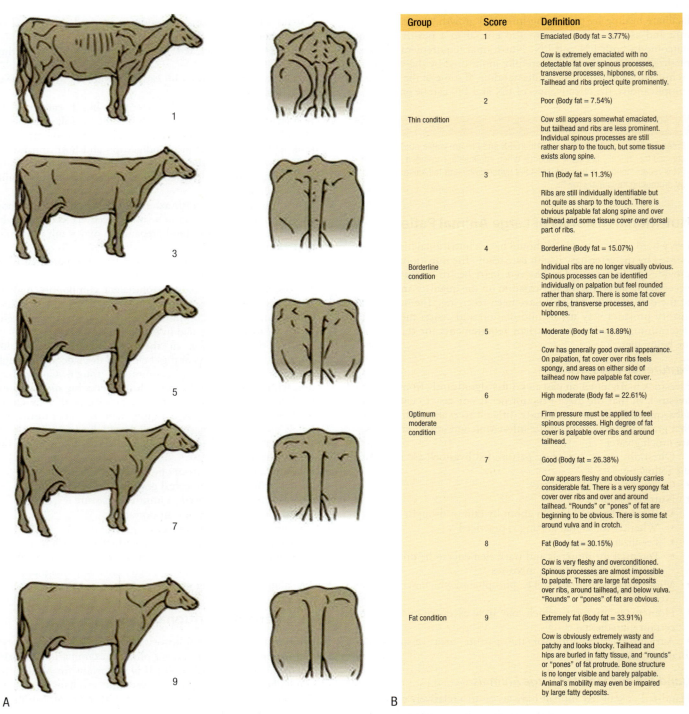

Group	Score	Definition
	1	Emaciated (Body fat = 3.77%)
		Cow is extremely emaciated with no detectable fat over spinous processes, transverse processes, hipbones, or ribs. Tailhead and ribs project quite prominently.
Thin condition	2	Poor (Body fat = 7.54%)
		Cow still appears somewhat emaciated, but tailhead and ribs are less prominent. Individual spinous processes are still rather sharp to the touch, but some tissue exists along spine.
	3	Thin (Body fat = 11.3%)
		Ribs are still individually identifiable but not quite as sharp to the touch. There is obvious palpable fat along spine and over tailhead and some tissue cover over dorsal part of ribs.
Borderline condition	4	Borderline (Body fat = 15.07%)
		Individual ribs are no longer visually obvious. Spinous processes can be identified individually on palpation but feel rounded rather than sharp. There is some fat cover over ribs, transverse processes, and hipbones.
	5	Moderate (Body fat = 18.89%)
		Cow has generally good overall appearance. On palpation, fat cover over ribs feels spongy, and areas on either side of tailhead now have palpable fat cover.
Optimum moderate condition	6	High moderate (Body fat = 22.61%)
		Firm pressure must be applied to feel spinous processes. High degree of fat cover is palpable over ribs and around tailhead.
	7	Good (Body fat = 26.38%)
		Cow appears fleshy and obviously carries considerable fat. There is a very spongy fat cover over ribs and over and around tailhead. "Rounds" or "pones" of fat are beginning to be obvious. There is some fat around vulva and in crotch.
	8	Fat (Body fat = 30.15%)
		Cow is very fleshy and overconditioned. Spinous processes are almost impossible to palpate. There are large fat deposits over ribs, around tailhead, and below vulva. "Rounds" or "pones" of fat are obvious.
Fat condition	9	Extremely fat (Body fat = 33.91%)
		Cow is obviously extremely wasty and patchy and looks blocky. Tailhead and hips are buried in fatty tissue, and "rounds" or "pones" of fat protrude. Bone structure is no longer visible and barely palpable. Animal's mobility may even be impaired by large fatty deposits.

• **Fig. 9.12** (A) Body conditioning scoring (BCS) in the bovine and (B) BCS description. (A, From Holtgrew-Bohling K. *Large Animal Clinical Procedures for Veterinary Technicians.* 2nd ed. St. Louis, MO: Mosby; 2011. B, From Spitzer JC. Influences of nutrition on reproduction in beef cattle. In Morrow DA, ed. *Current Therapy in Theriogenology.* Philadelphia, PA: Saunders; 1986; and modified from National Research Council (NRC). *Nutrient Requirements of Beef Cattle,* 7th ed. Washington, DC: National Academy of Sciences, NRC; 1996.)

TABLE 9.3	Body Condition Scoring in Goats

Score Appearance

0 No subcutaneous tissue seen

1 Dorsal aspect of vertebral column forms a continuous ridge with hollow flank, ribs easily seen. Sternal fat easily moved laterally. Chondrosternal joints easily palpable. No muscle or fat between ribs or bones. Transverse process of lumbar vertebrae easily visualized and articular processes easily palpable.

2 Sternal fat movable but 1 to 2 cm thick. Tissue visible between skin and chondrosternal joints. Some tissue around transverse process of lumbar spine, but it is more difficult to palpate than in Score 1. Need slight pressure to palpate articular processes.

3 Dorsal aspect of vertebral column is less prominent. Sternal fat is thick and barely movable. Chondrosternal joints are difficult to palpate. Lumbar vertebrae have thick tissue covering. Articular process of transverse process not palpable.

4 Sternal fat, costochondral fat, and rib fat are continuous. Transverse process is difficult to palpate. Spinous process is not palpable.

5 Sternal fat and rib fat bulges between pressed fingers. Spinous and transverse processes are not palpable.

From Santucci PM, Branca M, Napoleone R, et al. Body condition scoring of goats in extensive conditions. In Morand-Fehr P, ed. *Goat Nutrition*. Wageningen, Netherlands: Pudoc; 1991.

It is very common for alterations in the animals' weight to occur, or BCSs may not be noticeable because of the day-to-day interactions with the patient. As mentioned, the BCS charts are available, but the specific needs of certain species should be noted. Palpation of the animal (ribs, dorsal vertebral processes) is necessary in sheep with heavy fleece, camelids with long fiber, and horses with a thick winter haircoat. Animals with a low BCS (1–3 of 9; 1–1.5 of 5) have minimal protein and lipid stores and are at greater risk for protein-calorie malnutrition after a period of anorexia. Large animal patients with a high BCS (7–9 of 9; 3.5–5 of 5) that are anorectic may have an increased risk for complications (hyperlipemia, hepatic lipidosis) from abnormal lipid metabolism. It is imperative that dietary therapy be initiated in a large animal patient that has lost 3% to 5% of its primary BW or whose BCS diminishes by one grade or greater.

Another part of nutritional assessment to be performed by the large animal health care team would be laboratory testing, specifically biochemical analysis. Although few biochemical tests assess protein malnutrition in large animals, physiologic response indicative of anorexia manifests as endogenous protein catabolism. Therefore performing a BCS is critical. Anemia and hypoproteinemia (hypoalbuminemia) may be seen in cases of malnutrition, but typically, these are associated with other disease processes (e.g., parasitism or protein-losing enteropathy). Abnormally low serum urea nitrogen (SUN) concentrations in horses and ruminants may also be linked to severe protein malnutrition. Liver disease may decrease the formation of urea nitrogen and therefore should be ruled out by the health care team when assessing the animal's condition. Protein malnutrition can result in an increase in the urinary excretion of 3-methylhistidine, a myofibril amino acid that is not metabolized. In the future, measurement of this metabolite may be a useful tool to monitor protein catabolism in large animal patients.

Cattle

The fact that cattle are ruminants and are herbivores has already been established. Herbivores have the ability to convert such products as cellulose in plants into meat products for human consumption. Approximately 42.5 gallons can be held in the rumen of a cow (see Table 9.4).

It is also in the rumen that microbial digestion occurs through the action of bacteria and protozoans. During fermentation, poor-quality forage and NPN (i.e., urea) produce volatile fatty acids, amino acids, vitamins B and K (used by the body), and methane and CO_2, which are released from the body. Cattle are also able to manufacture their own vitamin C. The pH of the rumen is recommended to be maintained between 6.2 and 7.2. However, it is important for health care team members to remember that if livestock are fed a high-grain diet, it may result in a more acidic rumen. Dietary fiber is key when talking about nutritional factors for cattle, because it is the fiber in the diet that is necessary to keep the microorganisms alive.

The honeycomb reticulum is responsible for regurgitation of food during rumination and can hold up to 2.5 gallons. The omasum can contain up to 4 gallons and is responsible for getting the fluid out of the ingested food. The peptic digestion of proteins in cattle begins in the abomasum (the true, glandular stomach). The abomasum may hold up to 5 gallons. The small intestine is approximately 150 feet long and can hold about 16 gallons, with the cecum measuring approximately 3 feet long and responsible for about 2.5 gallons. Finally, the GI tract in cattle also includes the large intestine, measuring 33 feet long and holding 7.5 gallons.

Key Nutritional Factors in Cattle

It cannot be stated often enough that water is of utmost importance for all animals. The health care team must remind livestock owners to provide water ad libitum. Mature cattle in good physical condition require 10 to 14 gallons of water per day. Dairy cows require 3 to 5 gallons of water to produce 1 gallon of milk. Therefore a cow at peak lactation may need an estimated 45 gallons of water per day.

Cows in good health and condition can be fed good-quality hay or pasture. Pregnant cows can remain on this hay feed regimen until approximately 2 weeks prior to calving. Cows in their last trimester characteristically gain the amount of weight which they innately predict to be lost during calving. Obese cows are at risk for complications and health issues as much as underweight cattle. Obesity can cause reproductive problems and predispose the cow to ketosis. As with other species, obesity may put cows at risk for a multitude of disease conditions.

Again, as with other species, lactation requires the highest energy needs in cattle. Feed that is fully balanced and has proper dry matter intake (DMI) is essential for optimal milk production. It should be remembered that feed concentrates supply the highest energy level; however, it is important to balance concentrates with roughages. This balance will help circumvent such problems as obesity, digestive disorders, and decreased milk production.

Cattle are typically fed by a method known as *challenge feeding,* which is based on the level of milk production of which they are capable. It has been found that the size of the cow does not appear

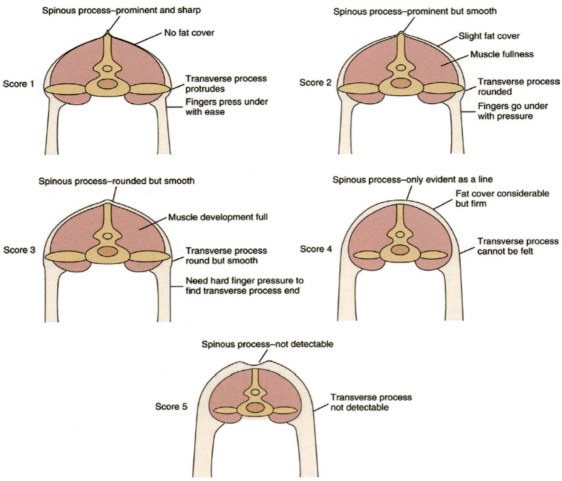

Spinous process–prominent and sharp

No fat cover

Score 1

Transverse process protrudes

Fingers press under with ease

Spinous process–prominent but smooth

Slight fat cover

Muscle fullness

Score 2

Transverse process rounded

Fingers go under with pressure

Spinous process–rounded but smooth

Muscle development full

Score 3

Transverse process round but smooth

Need hard finger pressure to find transverse process end

Spinous process–only evident as a line

Fat cover considerable but firm

Score 4

Transverse process cannot be felt

Spinous process–not detectable

Score 5

Transverse process not detectable

• **Fig. 9.13** Body conditioning scoring in sheep. (From Santucci PM, Branca M, Napoleone R, et al. Body condition scoring of goats in extensive conditions. In: Morand-Fehr P, ed. *Goat Nutrition.* Wageningen, The Netherlands: Pudoc; 1991.)

to have much effect on the efficiency of milk production; therefore most cattle are often challenge fed.

TECHNICIAN NOTE

As with other species, lactation requires the highest energy needs in cattle.

It is recommended that beef calves be creep fed. *Creep feeding* involves feeding small amounts of grain in a location that the dam does not have access to. The creep feeding method has been associated with less weaning stress and allows the calves to start to digest the feed that they will be eating after weaning. Upon weaning, a 50-lb weight advantage has been shown through use of the creep feeding method.

Meat, bone meal, and other animal by-products from mammals are not recommended to be fed to cattle and other ruminants. This rule was established by the FDA in 1997 to minimize the risk of spread of transmissible bovine spongiform encephalopathy. Exclusions to this rule are tallow, blood by-products, gelatin, and milk products. These are acceptable for use in ration or ruminant formulation.

Iodized salt aids in preventing deficiency of iodine; subsequently, cattle are recommended to have free access to sodium and chloride. Iodine deficiencies are most often seen in pregnant animals and have been correlated with increases in stillbirths. In ruminants, calcium deficiency occurs when they are fed high-grain diets. When this deficiency is uncovered, limestone can typically correct it. When discussing phosphorus, the amount available to the animal is directly related to the amount in the soil. Phosphorus deficiencies in young animals manifest as poor appetite, slow growth, and an overall unhealthy appearance. Lactating animals may have fragile bones and a poor appetite. Only small amounts of cobalt are stored in the body, so owners and health care team members must be vigilant, because cobalt deficiency could occur rapidly. Typical signs of cobalt deficiency to look for are listlessness, ocular discharge, anemia, ketosis, abortions, decreased milk production, and decreased appetite. It is recommended that cobalt be fed with trace mineralized salt. Conversely, feeding too much cobalt can lead to cobalt toxicity. Signs of cobalt toxicity to watch for are decreased growth rates, incoordination, elevated hemoglobin, and elevated packed cell volume levels. Diets that are deficient in copper may result in neurologic signs, diarrhea, lameness, and anemia. Copper toxicity signs include liver and kidney disease, increased occurrence of respiratory disease in calves, hemorrhagic diarrhea, and gastroenteritis. Selenium levels vary in the soil. Selenium should also be fed in a trace mineralized salt. Growing cattle

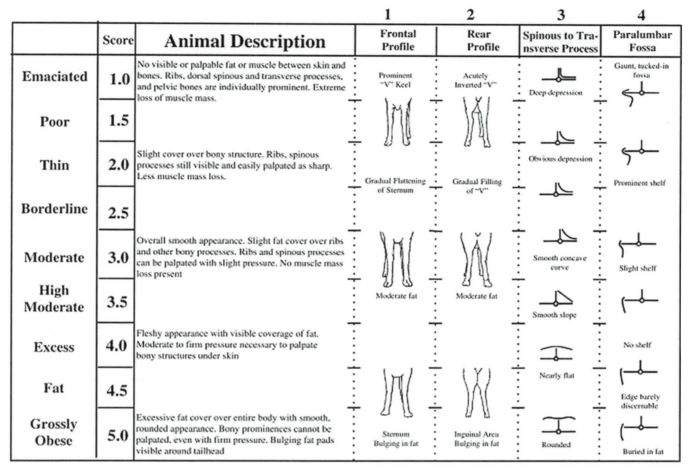

	Score	Animal Description	1 Frontal Profile	2 Rear Profile	3 Spinous to Transverse Process	4 Paralumbar Fossa
Emaciated	1.0	No visible or palpable fat or muscle between skin and bones. Ribs, dorsal spinous and transverse processes, and pelvic bones are individually prominent. Extreme loss of muscle mass.	Prominent "V" Keel	Acutely Inverted "V"	Deep depression	Gaunt, tucked-in fossa
Poor	1.5					
Thin	2.0	Slight cover over bony structure. Ribs, spinous processes still visible and easily palpated as sharp. Less muscle mass loss.	Gradual Flattening of Sternum	Gradual Filling of "V"	Obvious depression	Prominent shelf
Borderline	2.5					
Moderate	3.0	Overall smooth appearance. Slight fat cover over ribs and other bony processes. Ribs and spinous processes can be palpated with slight pressure. No muscle mass loss present	Moderate fat	Moderate fat	Smooth concave curve	Slight shelf
High Moderate	3.5				Smooth slope	
Excess	4.0	Fleshy appearance with visible coverage of fat. Moderate to firm pressure necessary to palpate bony structures under skin			Nearly flat	No shelf
Fat	4.5					Edge barely discernable
Grossly Obese	5.0	Excessive fat cover over entire body with smooth, rounded appearance. Bony prominences cannot be palpated, even with firm pressure. Bulging fat pads visible around tailhead	Sternum Bulging in fat	Inguinal Area Bulging in fat	Rounded	Buried in fat

• **Fig. 9.14** Body condition scoring of camelids. (Used with permission from Van Saun RJ. Feeding the alpaca. In: Hoffman E, ed. *The Complete Alpaca Book.* 2nd ed. Santa Cruz, CA: Bonny Doon Press; 2003:179-232; and from Anderson DE, Whitehead CE. *Veterinary Clinics of North America: Food Animal Practice: Alpaca and Llama Health Management.* Philadelphia, PA: WB Saunders; 2009.)

TABLE 9.4	Cattle Gastrointestinal Anatomy and Fluid Volume	
Anatomic Structure	**Volume (Gallons) Held**	
Rumen	42.5	
Honeycomb reticulum	2.5	
Omasum	4	
Abomasum	5	
Small intestine	16	
Cecum	2.5	
Large intestine	7.5	

rates, reduced immune response, bone irregularities, decreased appetite, decreased wound healing, and hoof problems. Young male animals need higher levels of zinc to ensure normal testicular development. An essential component of hemoglobin is iron. Iron deficiency rarely occurs in adults, but may be seen in a calf fed an all-milk diet. Treatment includes iron dextran injections in calves.

Camelids

Key Nutritional Factors

Camelids are not classified as ruminants but are considered *functional ruminants.* In functional ruminants, roughage is converted to usable nutrients, just as in ruminants. Camelids are extremely efficient in their ability to convert forages to energy and do best when allowed to graze on pasture freely. Feed consumption is based on a percentage of BW and is higher in smaller animals and lower in larger animals. Concentrates are rarely needed; if provided, they should be given carefully, because obesity is common in overfed camelids.

Protein requirements for camelids are very similar to those in sheep and goats. When CP is calculated on a DMB, camelids require 10% CP for maintenance and 16% for pregnancy, lactation, and growth.

fed low-protein diets may require more selenium and vitamin E in the diet to avoid deficiencies. Selenium deficiency predisposes cattle to reproductive problems and immunosuppression. Deficiency of selenium in pregnant cows may result in the birth of calves that have white muscle disease. Zinc should be added to trace mineralized salt to avoid growth retardation, reduced conception

Water should be provided ab libitum to camelids. Camelids require water in the amount of 9% to 13% of their BW (in kg). When providing water to camelids in cold weather, it is important to know that they will not break through ice to get to a water source. Trail llamas most often drink water in the evening and refuse to drink during the day. When water is withheld or is unavailable to lactating camelids, milk production is often decreased or stopped altogether. In extreme cases of water deprivation, camelids may become hyperthermic. Camelids have oval erythrocytes that can swell up to 240% of their normal size without lysing, whereas round erythrocytes in other animals can only swell up to 150% without lysing.

The camelid diet should contain no greater than 0.3% calcium on a DMB. The calcium-to-phosphorus ratio should be no less than 1.2:1. Camelids are sensitive to copper. Copper toxicity can be a problem and is thought to be a factor in the failure to thrive syndrome seen in crias. Zinc deficiency in llamas and alpacas may present as dermatitis. All other mineral requirements are like those in other ruminants.

Sheep and Goats

As mentioned earlier, nutrition is believed to have the most profound effect on the general health of both the individual animal and the flock or the herd. This also holds true for sheep and goats. The veterinary health care team must remember that the goal in proper nutrition goal is healthy animals and herds. In sheep and goats, proper nutrition is reflected in productivity, reproduction, and performance.

Sheep and goats can convert forages (and other feedstuffs) considered into usable animal products (e.g., meat, milk, fiber) or to reach peak performance (e.g., pet, show, breeding). Sheep and goats have increased mobility of the tongue and the lips, which allows for discrimination in the diet (Table 9.5).

Goats do less well on flat, monoculture pastures compared with sheep or cattle. However, goats do thrive when grazing in areas featuring browse or numerous plant species. Meat goats (e.g., Kiko, Spanish, Boer, Tennessee Wooden Leg) typically do very well on a diet of 15% to 20% grasses and 80% to 85% browse.

Goats are very particular creatures, especially where their diet is concerned. Goats may refuse to eat feeds that have been soiled. Goats are also commonly used for brush management throughout the world. It is important for veterinary health care team members to monitor goats used in brush control for alterations in BW, BCS, and haircoat and be on the lookout for signs of toxicosis. Browse foraging may lead to greater mineral ingestion versus grass foraging.

Key Nutritional Factors

Water is the most important nutrient for all animals, and sheep and goats are no exception. They should always have easy access to fresh, clean water, especially because sheep and goats are very particular about their water quality. Paving the surface 8 to 10 feet around the water tanks will help prevent unsanitary conditions, thus reducing the risk of sheep or goats contracting foot rot. Adults generally drink 1 to 1.5 gallons daily, with fat lambs and kids drinking approximately 0.5 gallons per day. High-protein diets, increased mineral consumption, and summer months all have the tendency to increase water consumption.

Energy

The energy requirements for sheep and goats are dependent on the production level and stage, activity level, and the intended use of the animals. Energy requirements can most often be met through the feeding of medium- to high-quality forage. The exception to this would be found in those animals where rapid growth rates are desired or in animals where maximum milk production is desired.

Diets that are deficient in energy have the potential for sheep and goats to experience the following:
1. Reduced growth rates
2. Lower BCS
3. Decreased fiber production
4. Reduced fiber diameter
5. Diminished immune function
6. Increased vulnerability to parasitic diseases and other pathologic conditions

The greater part of the energy that is used by sheep and goats comes from the breakdown of structural carbohydrates from roughage. Thus roughage should constitute the bulk of their diet. Energy can be expressed in terms of the NE system (calories) or in terms of **total digestible nutrients** as a percentage of the feed (%TDN). The %TDN of various feedstuffs is shown in Table 9.6.

Good to excellent forage should be offered, but in instances where this is not available, energy supplementation may be required, especially in certain life stages or activity level (e.g., lactating ewe). The health care team and livestock owner typically have several energy supplementing choices. Cereal grains, with corn being very common, are a consistent choice. Corn is a dense energy source, with most of the energy coming from starch. Energy from the corn will assist in keeping the energy level of the goat or sheep higher, even if a decrease in foraging occurs.

Cereal grains, such as oats, grain sorghum, barley, and so on, may also be used as an energy supplement for ruminants consuming forage-based diets; however, corn remains the highest source of energy density.

Soybean hulls and wheat middlings have also been recommended; however, they are not often used. The outermost layer of the soybean is the soybean hull, which is high in digestible fiber. The advantage of soybean hulls versus corn is that fiber digestion is not suppressed, and an increase in hay digestibility may result.

TABLE 9.5	Grazing Preferences of Sheep and Goats Based on Differences in the Anatomy of Their Oral Cavities	
Sheep	**Goats**
Roughage grazer	Active forager
Grass	Highly digestible grass parts
High-quality plant parts	Flowers, fruits, leaves

TABLE 9.6	Total Daily Nutrition (TDN) of Various Feeds	
Feed	**% TDN**
Grass hay (perennial)	50%–54%
Cereal grains	80%–90%
Green vegetation forage	62%–70%
Lesser quality hay (↑stems)	<50%

Similar responses are found in wheat middlings, which are a by-product of wheat milling. Beet pulp, citrus pulp, and brewer's grains may also be effective in sheep and goat feeds and have been found to be more cost effective compared with corn. The veterinary health care team should analyze the composition of by-product feeds and use them accordingly in diet formulation.

Fat

Fat can also be used as an energy source. However, the health care team must remember the risks associated with an animal being overweight in any life stage or lifestyle. Consequently, the total fat content should not exceed 8% of the sheep or goat diet, or 4% to 5% as supplemental fat. Cotton production is widespread in the southern portion of the United States, and it has been established that whole cottonseed (which contains approximately 24% fat) is used as an energy supplement for both sheep and goats. Not greater than 20% of the daily intake should be whole cottonseed in sheep and goat feeds being supplemented. This percentage will need to be lower if there are other sources of fat in the diet.

Protein

In sheep and goats, a minimum of 7% dietary CP is necessary for normal rumen bacterial growth and proper rumen function. Protein levels less than 7% will suppress forage intake and digestibility. Deficiency in protein manifests as the following: decreased fiber production, retarded growth, poor immune function, anemia, lethargy, edema, and even death. CP content varies in sheep and goat feed (see Table 9.7).

As plants age, their protein content declines. CP requirements also vary, depending on the sheep's or goat's life stage or production. For maintenance, ewes and does of most weight classes require a diet containing 7%–% protein. Lactating ewes and does require 13%–15% CP in the diet. Health care team members should consider the potential for protein deficiency if grass hay is being fed. Signs of protein deficiency to watch for in lactating animals are poor weight gain or slow growth in their lambs or kids, particularly those with multiple offspring.

Protein supplementation in sheep and goats include the following:
- Oilseed meals as in cottonseed meal or soybean meal
- Commercially blended supplements with natural protein and NPN
  - Range cubes
  - Pellets
  - Molasses-based products
- By-products
  - Whole cottonseed
  - Corn gluten feed
  - Dried distiller's grains

In sheep and goats, protein should be fed to meet requirements. Too much protein may lead to excessive cost and higher rates of disease (e.g., heat stress, pizzle rot). NPN is an economical

way to increase the protein concentration. As discussed earlier, NPN is nitrogen in the nonprotein form. The commonly used type is urea. Whenever NPN is used, the diet should have appropriate amounts of highly fermentable energy components. Feeding grain with NPN can result in a decrease in rumen pH. This altered environment may depress the ability of the ruminal urease enzyme to ferment urea. This depression then results in a sluggish release of or breakdown to ammonia and CO_2. Slowing this metabolic pathway allows more efficient protein synthesis by the rumen microbes. Conversely, poor-quality roughage diets result in a higher rumen pH and enhanced urease activity. If NPN is added to the diet, feeds containing a urease enzyme (e.g., raw soybeans, wild mustard) should be severely limited or avoided.

When urea is fed as a protein source:
1. Urea should not be more than one-third of the protein in the diet or greater than 3% of the grain portion of the diet.
2. A highly fermentable source of carbohydrates (e.g., corn, milo) should be fed with NPN.
3. Urea should not be introduced into the diet suddenly; at least 8 to 10 days should be allowed for its introduction.
4. Feed should be properly mixed whenever urea is used.
5. When crude protein of the diet is greater than 14% of the dietary TDNs, NPN is of little value.
6. NPN is best used in sheep or goats with BCSs greater than 2.5 and should be avoided in animals with BCSs less than 2.
7. If NPN is used in feeding animals, it should be ensured that it is fed daily; less is used for protein synthesis if the supplement is fed less frequently.

Fiber

Fiber is another key nutritional factor for sheep and goats and is an important dietary consideration for ruminants. Normal rumination cannot occur without adequate amounts of fiber. Sheep will resort to "wool pulling" as they search for a roughage source if they are fed a concentrate-based diet low or limited in fiber. The dietary fiber content of feeds for sheep and goats should be greater than 50%. This level will help promote a healthy rumen.

Fiber is also required in the diet to maintain acceptable levels of milk fat. The particle size of the fiber is important. It is generally accepted that a minimum particle size of 1 to 2.5 cm is appropriate to stimulate normal rumination, although the effect of smaller particles is not well documented in sheep and goats. Pelleted roughage does not meet the requirement for fiber size. Animals that are fed pelleted forage or lush pasture should be offered hay.

Minerals

Key nutritional factors in clinical nutrition for sheep and goats should also include minerals—macrominerals and microminerals. Macrominerals are expressed as a percentage of the diet. Microminerals are expressed as parts per million or milligrams per kilogram.

Macrominerals important to the overall health of sheep and goats are calcium, phosphorus, sodium, chlorine, magnesium, potassium, and sulfur. The eight microminerals that are important to the overall health of sheep and goats are copper, molybdenum, cobalt, iron, iodine, zinc, manganese, and selenium. Although not very common, trace mineral deficiency may occur, and the health care team needs to be aware of the potential for mineral deficiency.

Calcium and Phosphorus

Calcium and phosphorus are interrelated and work synergistically. Most calcium and phosphorus in the body can be found

TABLE 9.7	Protein % in Various Feed
Feed	**% Protein**
Grass hay (perennial)	<6% to >12%
Legumes (vegetative state)	≥28%

in skeletal tissues. Lack of calcium and phosphorus deficiency in young lambs and kids results in slow growth and development of and predisposition to metabolic bone diseases (e.g., rickets, osteochondrosis). A severe reduction in milk production is also a result of calcium and phosphorus deficiencies in lactating ewes and does; therefore supplemental calcium and phosphorus may be needed to meet high demands for milk production. Serum phosphorus concentrations are recommended to be between 4 and 7 mg/dL for sheep and between 4 and 9.5 mg/dL for goats. The most common mineral deficiency found in range- or winter-pastured animals is phosphorus deficiency. Most forage, especially legumes, are high in calcium and low in phosphorus. Beet pulp and legumes (e.g., clover and alfalfa) are good to excellent sources of calcium. Phosphorus serum concentrations of less than 4 mg/dL are indicative of phosphorus deficiency. Phosphorus deficiency manifests in slow growth, lethargy, an "unkempt" appearance, and depraved appetite, or pica.

High-grain or high-concentrate diets fed to sheep and goats often require supplemental calcium and but not additional phosphorus. This is because grains are relatively low in calcium but contain moderate to high concentrations of phosphorus. It has been found that serum concentrations consistently below 9 mg/dL are indicative of chronic calcium deficiency. Another disease condition that may lead to a decrease in calcium and phosphorus is chronic parasitism. Calcium supplementation can be achieved by adding oyster shells and limestone to the feed. Defluorinated rock phosphate is an excellent source of phosphorus. Dicalcium phosphate or steamed bone meal are good sources of calcium and phosphorus. In sheep and goats, the calcium-to-phosphorus ratio should be 1:1 and 2:1.

Sodium and Chloride

Sodium and chloride are essential components for many functions in the body. Salt (sodium chloride) is the carrier for most ad libitum mineral supplements. Salt should be offered ad libitum for overall health. Otherwise, it is necessary to add salt into feed at a level of 0.5%. Salt blocks are commonly used to promote salt intake because adults consume roughly 10 grams of salt a day. Sodium is primarily an extracellular ion and is important for normal water metabolism, intracellular and extracellular functions, and acid-base balance. Conversely, chloride is an intracellular ion, functions in normal osmotic balance, and is a component of gastric secretions. Signs for the health care team to look for in sheep or goats that are deficient in salt include wood chewing, soil licking, or consuming other unlikely plants or debris. The salt [NaCl] content of feeds may be increased to 5% to aid in increasing water intake and reducing urolithiasis.

TECHNICIAN NOTE

Salt (sodium chloride [NaCl]) is the carrier for most ad libitum mineral supplements. Salt should be offered ad libitum for overall health.

Magnesium

Magnesium is an important mineral that aids in the normal functioning of the nervous system. Magnesium is also necessary for many of the enzymatic reactions in the body. If an animal is deficient in magnesium, skeletal magnesium would be used up by the animal; however, the skeletal magnesium reserve is much smaller compared with the calcium reserve. Many fast-growing, heavily fertilized cereal grains or grass pastures are deficient in magnesium. High levels of plant potassium or rumen ammonia may suppress magnesium absorption. Livestock owners who are looking for a good source of magnesium will find it in legume pastures and legume-grass mixed pastures. Deficiency of magnesium may lead to a clinical manifestation known as *grass tetany* in sheep and goats. Magnesium toxicity is very rare.

Potassium

Potassium is required for normal acid-base balance and is an integral component of many enzymatic pathways; it functions as an intracellular ion. Depending on the stage and level of production, the requirement for potassium is between 0.5% and 0.8% of the diet. Most grains have less than 0.4% potassium, although fresh green forages generally contain greater than 1%. Deficiencies or toxicities of potassium in sheep and goats are rare. However, the health care team should watch for deficiency in stressed animals strictly fed grain diets. Therefore it is prudent to recommend supplemental potassium for stressed animals (i.e., weaning) fed mostly grain.

Sulfur

Sulfur makes up many bodily proteins. Higher concentrations are seen in wool and mohair, in keeping with the large amounts of sulfur-containing amino acids (cystine, cysteine, and methionine) in keratin. Deficiency of sulfur in Angora goats, specifically, can lead to reduced mohair production. It is recommended that a 10:1 nitrogen-to-sulfur ratio be maintained in sheep and goat diets. In both sheep and goats, sulfur deficiency may result in the following:

- Anorexia
- Reduced weight gain
- Decreased milk production
- Decreased wool growth
- Excessive tearing
- Excessive salivation
- Death
- Depressed digestion
- Decreased microbial protein synthesis
- Decreased use of NPN
- Lowered rumen microbial population

If signs of marginal trace mineral deficiencies are noticed in sheep or goats, owners and health care team members should measure the sulfur concentrations in the forage. Too much dietary sulfur can lead to a variety of trace mineral deficiencies (e.g., copper, zinc) without causing any overt toxicity problems.

Copper

Copper deficiency can occur because of low dietary intake or because of high concentrations of molybdenum, sulfur, and/or iron or other substances in feedstuffs. In the rumen, copper, molybdenum, and sulfur form thiomolybdates, which reduce the availability of copper. This results in clinical signs of deficiency. High concentrations of dietary cadmium, iron, selenium, zinc, and vitamin C and alkaline soils all interfere with copper absorption. Zinc supplementation in the diet (to a concentration >100 ppm) will reduce the availability and liver stores of copper. Plants with roughage grown on fertilized and limed pastures is more likely to be deficient. Adding lime decreases the amount of copper uptake by plants, and many fertilizers contain molybdenum. Good-quality lush grass forages have less available copper compared with that typical for most hays, and legumes have more available copper compared with most grasses. Copper reserves in the liver last up to 6 months in sheep.

Signs of copper deficiency seen in sheep and goats include the following:

- Microcytic anemia
- Decreased milk production
- Faded hair color
- Poor-quality fleece
- Heart failure
- Infertility
- Decreased immune function
- Slow growth
- Enlarged joints
- Lameness
- Gastric ulcers
- Diarrhea

To aid in prevention of copper deficiency, copper supplementation may be instituted using oral supplements, copper needles, trace mineral mixtures, or, in some instances, injectable copper. Additionally, an appropriate dietary copper-to-molybdenum ratio must be maintained. Dietary copper for sheep and goats should range between 4 and 15 ppm. Copper toxicity happens more often in sheep than in goats. Goats are considered closer to cattle than to sheep regarding copper toxicity. With sheep, the difference between copper deficiency and copper toxicity is quite small. Copper toxicity may result from mixing errors during the formulation of mineral premixes or from feeding mineral mixes formulated for species other than sheep. Toxicity may be intensified by the ingestion of toxic plants (e.g., lupines, alkaloid-containing species) and stress.

Copper toxicity signs to be cognizant of include the following:

- Increased respiration
- Depression
- Weakness
- Hemoglobinuria
- Icterus
- Sudden death

Cobalt

Cobalt is used by rumen bacteria to assist in the formation of vitamin B_{12}. Organic or poorly drained soils may be low in cobalt. Cobalt deficiency in sheep or goats manifests as classic B_{12} deficiency, resulting in signs and symptoms ranging from decreased appetite to emaciation ("wasting disease"), anemia, pale skin, and excessive ophthalmic discharge. Cobalt deficiency is associated with white liver disease, although phosphorus and copper deficiencies and chronic parasitism also play roles in pathogenesis. Again, an evaluation of the diet must be performed. Typically, a diet with a cobalt concentration of 0.1 ppm is adequate in most instances. Cobalt level in the diet below 0.06 ppm is insufficient. The discovery of cobalt deficiency should lead the health care team to feed a cobalt-supplemented trace mineral mixture ad libitum. In North America, cobalt toxicity typically is not of great concern in sheep and goats.

Iron

Iron deficiency in sheep and goats is rare, especially when the herd grazes. The dietary iron requirement generally is 30 to 40 ppm.

Iodine

Deficiencies in iodine are seen in certain geographic locations—particularly the northern parts of North America. The winter months seem to be the time when iodine availability in the body is at its peak.

Rubidium, arsenic, fluorine, calcium, and potassium are known to interfere with iodine absorption, so health care team members must take these minerals into consideration when discussing nutrition. Signs of iodine deficiency to watch for include goiter, poor growth, depressed milk yield, pregnancy toxemia, and reproductive abnormalities (e.g., abortion, stillbirth, retained placentas, irregular estrus, infertility). Lambs or kids with enlarged thyroid glands are often born to iodine-deficient dams. Recommendations for treatment include three to six drops of iodine (Lugol solution) every day for 7 days.

Zinc

Zinc deficiency has been seen in sheep and goats. Vitamin C, lactose, and citrate in the diet help increase zinc availability, whereas the following suppress zinc availability: oxalates; phytates; and large dietary concentrations of calcium, cadmium, iron, molybdenum, and orthophosphate. Zinc concentrations are found to be higher in legumes than in grasses. However, legumes invariably contain large concentrations of calcium, which we determined can depress zinc availability. Zinc does not appear to be readily available in cereal grain feeds. Signs of zinc deficiency include the following:

- Dermatitis and parakeratosis
- Decreased milk production
- Diminished appetite
- Inability to use the nutrients
- Delayed growth
- Susceptibility to foot rot
- Reduced hair growth on legs and head
- Joint swelling
- Decreased reproduction
- Reduced testicular development
- Weakened vitamin A metabolism
- Increased vitamin E requirements

About 20 to 50 ppm of zinc in the diet should be sufficient, except in those animals consuming a high percentage of legumes in their diets. For these animals, a chelated form of zinc is indicated. Providing trace mineral-salt mixes with 0.5% to 2% zinc usually prevents deficiency. Zinc toxicity is very rare.

Selenium

The absorption of selenium from the small intestine is enhanced by adequate dietary levels of vitamins E, A, and histidine. Conversely, the absorption of selenium can be inhibited when the diet has large quantities of arsenic, calcium, vitamin C, copper, nitrates, sulfates, and unsaturated fats. Legumes are a better source of selenium compared with grasses, and grasses are a better source than cereal grains.

The health care team must be cognizant of signs of selenium deficiency, including the following:

- Nutritional muscular dystrophy (skeletal and cardiac muscles of fast-growing young lambs or kids)
- Retained placentas
- Slow growth
- Weakness
- Premature birth of lambs or kids
- Depressed immune function
- Mastitis
- Metritis

Selenium deficiency is seen most often in lambs between birth and age 8 weeks.

In the diet, 0.1 to 0.3 ppm of selenium is recommended. Those regions that are low in selenium should use mineral-salt mixes with approximately 24 and 90 ppm of selenium. Selenium toxicity is rare, but signs to look for include wool break, anorexia, depression, incoordination, and death.

Vitamins

Animals with healthy rumen function only need the fat-soluble vitamins A, D, E, and K in their diets.

Several body functions require vitamin A, such as growth, reproduction, appropriate skeletal development, vision, and epithelial tissue integrity. The liver can store vitamin A for 4 to 6 months. Signs to watch for in vitamin A deficiency include weight loss, depressed immune function, night blindness, decreased fertility, and hair loss. Sheep and goats need 105 IU/kg of BW/day to meet their vitamin A requirement. This can be attained through the ingestion of green vegetative forage. Vitamin A requirement increases in late gestation and lactation to 150 IU/kg per day, and 175 IU/kg per day, respectively.

Vitamin D requirement can be met in pasture animals through exposure to sunlight. Feeding operations that are mostly performed indoors and in overcast or cloudy conditions/regions should supplement vitamin D. Obviously, during the winter months, with more overcast conditions and shorter sunlight exposure, blood vitamin D levels may be low. In addition to calcium and phosphorus, as discussed earlier, vitamin D is important for normal bone growth and structure. The condition rickets is commonly seen in vitamin D deficiencies. The requirement for vitamin D in sheep is 5 to 6 IU/kg of BW/day. Early weaned lambs have a slightly higher requirement of 6 to 7 IU/kg per day.

Cell membrane integrity is the major role of vitamin E. Vitamin E is similar in mode of action to selenium. As with selenium, deficiencies in vitamin E in sheep and goats can cause white muscle disease, decreased immune function, and depressed fertility. Daily intake of vitamin E is imperative, because vitamin E is not stored well in the body. Alfalfa meal, cottonseed meal, and brewer's grains have abundant vitamin E. However, it should be noted that corn, feeds containing high levels of sulfur, and onions will decrease the availability of vitamin E. For small ruminants, 5.3 IU/kg of BW/day of vitamin E is recommended.

Vitamin K plays a significant role in proper blood clotting and normal vision. Vitamin K should not need to be supplemented, because it is produced in sufficient quantities in the rumen and lower gut of healthy livestock.

Nutrition is vital to the health and well-being of all animals. Nutrition is also the one area of veterinary medicine that affects every animal. Proper nutrition and feeding management form the foundation on which healing and the maintenance of health rests. The veterinary health care team, especially the veterinary technician, should be well versed in the differences in key nutritional factors for the various large animal species. Appropriate nutrition and the proper feeding of livestock will help increase the quality of life for the animal, extend the life of the animal, and help increase productivity individually and in the overall herd.

Nutrition for Birds and Small Mammals

Avians

As we have discussed thus far, there are three important components that affect the health of an animal—genetics, environment, and nutrition. Health is directly correlated to the quality of life and life span of the avian species. Nutrition is the one factor on which the veterinary health care team can have a great impact.

Proper nutrition and feeding management form the foundation upon which healing and the maintenance of health rests.

Each species of bird has specific nutritional requirements, typically determined by individual physiology. As in other species, nutrition must be viewed in life stages, as nutritional requirements in birds vary from neonate to adult to senior—with other life stage variations in between (Fig. 9.15).

A balanced diet should be provided for optimal health. To achieve a complete and balanced diet, it is recommended that a commercially formulated food be fed to companion birds. These formulated foods come in a variety of forms, with the most popular being (1) pellets, (2) extruded diets with a pellet appearance, and (3) whole grains and/or seeds with added pelleted material.

One other option would be a seed-based food with a vitamin-mineral mix coated on the outside of the seed. However, seeds are often not hulled. Thus when the bird dehulls the seed, essential vitamins and minerals are removed and, as a result, a nutritional imbalance is created, and the bird's health is jeopardized.

Process of Pellet Manufacturing

Two processes are used when pelleted diets are manufactured—bound and extruded. In manufacturing grains, such as corn, soybean, and oat, groats are ground. After the grinding process, vitamins, minerals, and other components are added to make a balanced food (according to the manufacturer's formula). The grinding process produces a consistent pellet that makes it difficult for birds to pick out only their favorite parts of the diet. With bound pellets, in general, the food material is not cooked, and the food has a longer fiber chain length. Bound pelleted diets may not be as palatable as extruded diets.

Extruded pellets are composed of finely ground grains, which are mixed with vitamins, minerals, and so on until a balanced formulation is reached. This pellet mixture is then forced through an extruder under pressure and at high temperatures. The mixture will take on the shape of the "die" in the extrusion process, like the way a cookie cutter works. This allows for extruded pellets to be made into different shapes and colors.

Extruded pelleted diets come in a variety of sizes and should be selected based on the species and sizes of birds. Owners must be instructed to monitor their birds to prevent them picking out

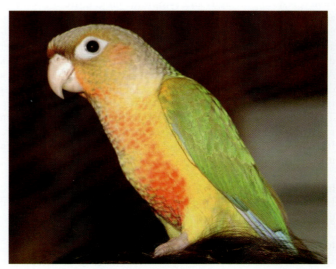

• **Fig. 9.15** Side view of Green-Cheek Conure shows an array of colors that includes green-colored wings, red patches on the belly with yellowish surrounding, and a pointed white beak. (Copyright Kara M. Burns.)

certain colored pellets and ignoring others. Owners should not choose colors or shapes because their birds "like these," because this can be expensive and wasteful. Companion birds are healthier when they are psychologically stimulated, and this can occur by presenting multicolored pellets in an assortment of shapes.

Historically, diets for birds have included seed-based diets. Although pelleted diets have allowed bird owners to provide a better-balanced diet without vitamin and mineral supplementation, not every bird will eat such foods. Also, as discussed earlier, each species has different nutritional requirements. For example, certain canary and finch species require seeds in their base diet. However, for the psittacine species, seeds are not included in the recommended diet, and a balanced pelleted food is advised as the appropriate base diet. Overall, many seed diets are high in fat and lower in other essential nutrients and therefore should be considered a treat. As with any species, treats should be offered in small quantities, or the bird will be at risk for malnutrition—most likely, obesity.

Transition from a seed diet to a pellet is believed to be difficult. However, this is not the case, even in older birds. Health care team members must educate owners regarding what to look for when transitioning a bird from seeds to pellets. Owners should ensure that their pet is ingesting the food and not simply crushing the pellet looking to find a kernel inside. Two signs that indicate that the bird is eating the pellets are the production of fecal material and a color change of the fecal material associated with the pellet color being ingested.

To aid owners in transitioning their birds from seeds to pellets, formed seed products have been manufactured (i.e., Nutri-Berries; Lafeber Co., Cornell, IL). These products are composed of whole grains and seeds, which are mixed with additional components and are stuck together. Refer to Fig. 9.16, which shows a Meyers parrot using a Nutri-Berry to transition to pellets. This product is similar to pellets but is not ground. The bird must pick off the seeds to eat them.

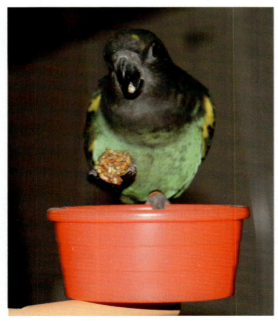
• **Fig. 9.16** Meyers Parrot using a Nutri-Berry to transition to pellets. (Copyright Kara M. Burns.)

Owners can also learn to transition their birds from seeds to pellets through the slow introduction of increased pellets in the seed mixture over a period. The transition is recommended to be done over 7 to 14 days, with the final diet consisting of 100% pellets.

Water

Water is the most critical nutrient, and all birds should always have access to fresh, clean water. Water should be changed daily (or more often if soiled), and the health care team is responsible for emphasizing this important part of husbandry with owners. Birds typically accept municipal tap water, but if using well water, it is recommended that it be boiled before allowing the bird to drink freely. This recommendation is made, because well water can be contaminated easily by bacterial colonies in the pipes leading to the faucet.

Protein and Amino Acids

Protein requirements differ among species. The minimum recommended protein allowance for maintenance in granivorous companion birds is 12%.

As with all foods, the quality of the protein is dependent on bioavailability and essential amino acid content. Bird food formulations must avoid excess and deficiency of proteins and amino acids. For most companion birds, the following amino acids are considered essential: arginine, isoleucine, lysine, methionine, phenylalanine, valine, tryptophan, and threonine. Budgies also require glycine.

Too much protein in the diet of birds has been associated with renal disease, behavioral changes (biting, feather picking, nervousness, rejection of food), and regurgitation. Poor weight gain, poor feathering, stress lines on feathers, plumage color changes, and poor reproductive performance are clinical signs associated with protein and amino acid deficiencies.

> **TECHNICIAN NOTE**
> Too much protein in the diet of birds has been associated with renal disease, behavioral changes (biting, feather picking, nervousness, rejection of food), and regurgitation.

Fats and Essential Fatty Acids

Fats are a more concentrated source of energy in a diet. EFAs (linoleic and arachidonic) are required in birds for the following: the formation of membranes and cell organelles, hormone precursors, and the basis for psittacofulvins (i.e., feather pigments found in psittacine species). The typical recommended fat allowance for granivorous companion bird diets is approximately 4%. Health care team members should note that in birds, lipogenesis takes place primarily in the liver. Pet birds fed high-energy diets may develop illness associated with hepatic lipidosis. This is heightened if the bird has limited exercise.

As with other companion animals and humans, too much fat in the diet may result in obesity, congestive heart failure, diarrhea, and oily feather texture. Increased fat levels may also interfere with the absorption of other nutrients, such as calcium. Low amounts of fat in the diet may lead to weight loss, reduced disease resistance, and overall poor growth, especially when coupled with restriction of other energy-producing nutrients.

Carbohydrates

Carbohydrates are another energy source and, in the bird's liver, carbohydrates can be converted to fat and vice versa. Glucagon is the major component of carbohydrate metabolism in birds. The result of inadequate carbohydrates in the diet is the use of glucogenic amino acids to manufacture carbohydrates. The process involves amino acids being shifted away from growth and production and instead being used in glucose synthesis.

Carbohydrates are the only source of energy usable by the nervous system; therefore neurologic abnormalities may indicate a deficiency in the diet that is otherwise adequate in **kilojoule** content.

Calcium

Calcium is an important dietary element for companion and caged birds. Calcium is essential for bone and eggshell formation. Calcium is also necessary for blood coagulation and nerve and muscle function. It is recommended that all birds have calcium supplementation in their cages, regardless of the type of diet they are eating. This is especially true for birds fed a seed diet. Calcium supplementation can be provided in the form of cuttlebones, mineral blocks, crushed oyster shells, or baked crushed eggshells. Birds will eat the calcium if provided and when needed to meet physiologic demands. Cuttlebones should be placed in the cage, with the soft side of the bone facing the bird. Cuttlebones are strictly a calcium source and are not beak-sharpening devices. It should also be noted that high levels of phosphorus in the diet can negate the adequate amounts of calcium in the diet. High phosphate levels will interfere with calcium absorption from the intestinal tract. The calcium-to-phosphorus ratio should range from 1:1 to 2:1.

Vitamins and Minerals

Vitamin requirements for companion birds are similar to those of companion mammals, the major exception being that the active form of vitamin D required by birds is vitamin D_3 (cholecalciferol) as opposed to vitamin D_2 (ergocholeciferol). Vitamin C is most important in specific fruit-eating species. However, vitamin C has been suggested to assist debilitated birds, because the ability to create vitamin C is reduced and these patients' requirements are greater.

If the bird is prescribed antibiotics, the health care team should monitor the patient closely, because vitamin deficiencies may result from the antibiotics interfering with normal intestinal microflora. Intestinal infections (e.g., giardiasis) may block vitamin absorption from the intestine (e.g., vitamin E, vitamin A). Hypervitaminosis has become an increasing problem, because clients may oversupplement formulated food or multivitamin preparations, thereby causing renal failure resulting from hypervitaminosis D. Hypervitaminosis A can also result in diseases, especially in nectarivorous birds.

Fruits and Vegetables

Fruits and vegetables are typically presented as supplementation to the pet birds' commercial diet. Fruits are made up of mainly sugars and water and thus should not be offered in excess. Fruit is a necessary part of the diet for some psittacine species, such as eclectus and lories, but these are exceptions. Fruits should not be fed more than a couple of times in a 7-day period.

Companion birds receive greater nutritional benefit from vegetables versus fruits. As much as possible, fresh or cooked dark green, red, and orange vegetables should be offered daily. One vegetable that should *not* be offered is comfrey. Consumption of comfrey, a green leaf herb especially popular in canary aviaries, may result in liver damage. Proper husbandry is of the utmost importance. The health care team should educate owners to place fruit and vegetables in a separate container and leave the container in the cage no longer than 30 minutes. Time restriction will help decrease the likelihood of growth of microorganisms.

Optimal feeding practices of companion birds are constantly being evaluated. Health care team members must understand the key nutritional factors in avian nutrition. This will allow for proper recommendation and education regarding nutrition to bird owners. Pet bird owners influence their bird's diet and therefore have a major impact on their bird's health and longevity. Educating the owner on proper nutrition is one of the most important roles of the veterinary health care team.

Feeding Small Mammals

Small mammals are extremely popular pets, and many of them are brought to veterinary hospitals for advice about proper care, including nutritional management and treatment of medical disorders. Each species of small mammal presents its own unique nutritional challenges. Nutritional management of all small mammals, just as with the species we have discussed above, should be dependent on life stage, level of physical activity, and state of health. Pet owners of small mammals will need to be educated about proper feeding to meet the needs of maintenance, growth, reproduction, or stress. Disorders in these mammals may result from an improper diet or poor husbandry.

As with all species, nutritional management starts with assessment of the pet, the animal's food, and the method of feeding. From this assessment, the health care team can begin to formulate a feeding plan. The nutritional assessment is like that performed in other species. It begins with a detailed history of the animal, a nutritional history, husbandry practices, and the animal's environment. A systematic physical examination should be performed and the BCS and weight of the pet recorded. The five-point BCS system appears to be most useful in assessing the condition of small mammals. BCS should be obtained at every visit and documented in the medical record. With small mammals, husbandry, diet, and/or disease may lead to loss of body fat, which is suggestive of starvation. Excessive loss of muscle is indicative of advanced starvation, forced inactivity, or altered metabolic states.

Ferrets

Ferrets are popular pets because of their low maintenance needs, their relatively small size, and their fun, inquisitive nature. Ferrets are strict carnivores and have a very short, simple GI tract, which lacks the cecum and the ileocolic valve. As a result, ferrets' GI transit time is rapid—approximately 3 to 6 hours. Highly digestible foods containing large amounts of protein and fat should be offered. Also, the nutritional composition should include minimal digestible (soluble) carbohydrate and fiber.

Ferrets are obligate carnivores, and as with other carnivorous species, young ferrets imprint on food by smell and develop strong food preferences by the time they are a few months old. Consequently, ferrets should be exposed to a variety of food tastes, textures, smells. Providing experience with a variety of protein sources when they are juveniles will assist in diet flexibility in adulthood. This can be extremely helpful when ferrets experience medical conditions that may require restricted or altered diets at an older age.

Foods with higher animal fat for energy, higher amounts of good-quality meat (not plant) protein, and minimal carbohydrate and fiber are recommended for ferrets. Whole-prey diets are appropriate, but owners typically do not want to feed a whole-prey diet. Dry kibble is commonly the diet fed to ferrets. Dry foods are recommended for ferrets, because these products are more energy efficient, cost less, and are easier to store and feed than moist foods or whole-prey diets. Health care team members should familiarize themselves with the ingredients listed on the package and be prepared to educate owners. The CP for a ferret should be 30% to 35% DMB and composed primarily of high-quality meat sources. The fat content should be 15% to 20% DMB. Growing kits need 35% protein DMB and 20% fat DMB, and lactating females require 20% DMB fat and twice the calories required by a ferret that is not pregnant.

Ferrets find commercial grocery store cat foods very palatable, because of the animal fat coating on the kibble. However, these foods may not be nutritionally adequate for the various life stages. Minimally stressed ferrets may live on these foods for years, but nutritional deficiencies may occur, especially in breeding animals. Pelleted ferret food is the preferred diet, although premium dry kitten food is generally acceptable for meeting the ferret's nutritional requirements for growth and reproduction. Feeding moist/ canned food as the major part of the diet should be avoided as ferrets are unlikely able to consume enough protein and fat on a DMB.

The specific amino acid requirements for ferrets are not known, but the assumption is that the requirements are like those of cats. It should be noted that strict carnivores need proteins of high biological value. Therefore nutritional protein for ferrets should come from animal-based ingredients.

As discussed, ferrets do well when eating commercial foods containing 15% to 20% fat DMB. Ferrets are assumed to require linoleic and AAs in their diets. Linoleic acid is abundant in vegetable oils. AAs are found in animal-based ingredients. Fatty acid requirements should be met by providing meat-based commercial cat or mink foods.

It is believed that ferrets do not have dietary requirement for carbohydrates, including fiber, as is seen in other obligate carnivores. Glucose is provided through gluconeogenesis in the liver, with the use of amino acids. Dietary fiber is a factor in weight control and reduction. It is also considered to play a role in certain specific GI disorders. The short digestive tract of ferrets dictates hydrolysis of most dietary fuels, with little or no hindgut fermentation of fiber. The intestinal tract of ferrets is relatively deficient in brush border enzymes, causing inability to absorb calories from carbohydrates. Generally, foods with additional fiber should not be fed to healthy or lactating ferrets or young kits.

The technician should remember to educate the ferret owner to offer their pets a variety of food items throughout life. This may include a minimum of weekly whole-prey foods, daily high-quality ferret kibble, and small amounts of high-quality canned cat food or other meat-based treats fed two to three times a week. This variety would be mentally enriching for the ferret. Ferrets are intelligent animals and will need environmental enrichment to keep them stimulated. This feeding strategy would also increase the variety of the ferret's diet preferences.

Ferrets should not be fasted for longer than 3 hours because of their short GI tract and the short GI transit time. It is common to see ferrets over 2 years of age develop insulinoma. Fasting a ferret with insulinoma for longer than 3 hours could result in a serious hypoglycemic condition.

As with all species, owners should provide clean, fresh water and ensure it is always available. The best method for providing water to ferrets is with a sipper bottle or a heavy crock-type bowl. Ferrets are fun-loving animals and especially love to play in the water, so the health care team must educate owners to provide bowls that are not easily tipped over.

Rabbits

Rabbits are popular pets because they are small, relatively easy to care for, fastidious, and quiet-mannered, and can be litterbox trained (Fig. 9.17). Two pairs of upper incisor teeth differentiate rabbits from rodents. The smaller, second upper incisors (peg teeth) are found behind the first. These peg teeth lack a cutting edge. Rabbit teeth are hypsodont. Malocclusion and overgrowth commonly occur with the incisor teeth, because these can grow 10 to 12 cm a year during the rabbit's life. Rabbit teeth are developed for a high-fiber, herbivorous diet. Rabbits are herbivorous hindgut fermenters and have a GI system like that of horses. Rabbits' GI tracts consist of a noncompartmentalized stomach and a large cecum. The simple stomach has thin walls and indistinctly separated glandular and nonglandular areas. It is important to explain to owners that rabbits are unable to vomit because of the presence of a well-developed cardiac sphincter.

Nutritional management of a rabbit should be aimed at providing sufficient fiber to support normal GI motility and to ensure that sufficient amounts and types of digestible nutrients are available to the cecal microflora for fermentation. Rabbits also need enrichment, and thus the diet should stimulate normal foraging behavior throughout the day.

Rabbits derive amino acids directly from the foods they ingest and from cecotrophs. Essential amino acids in the rabbit include arginine, glycine, histidine, isoleucine, leucine, lysine, methionine, phenylalanine, threonine, tryptophan, and valine. Grasses tend to contain limited amounts of methionine and isoleucine; however, they are abundant in arginine, glutamine, and lysine. Synthetic amino acids are regularly added to commercial mixes for rabbits, because these cereals are often low in methionine and lysine. Conversely, legumes are high in lysine and may be used to balance low lysine levels in cereal-based diets. Rabbits could digest forage-based protein because of the increase in protein digestibility that occurs due to cecotrophy. An appropriate protein level for pet rabbits is 12% to 16%

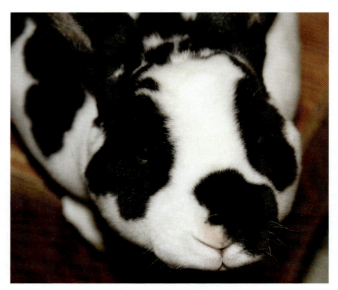

• **Fig. 9.17** Pet rabbit. A black and white rabbit lies down on its feet. (Copyright Kara M. Burns.)

DMB. For lactating does, the level may increase to 18% to 19% protein DMB.

Although simple sugars and starches can be used for energy, excessive levels of these should not be fed. Lagomorphs have a rapid gut transit time, resulting in starches and simple sugars being incompletely digested in the small intestine. These are then directed into the cecum, where they may be used for fermentation by the cecal microorganisms. Carbohydrate overload in the cecum predisposes to enterotoxemia, especially in young animals. Low-energy grains, such as oats, are recommended for the rabbit's diet, as opposed to corn or wheat. Care should be taken to not process the grains too finely.

An essential nutrient for the maintenance of GI health in rabbits is fiber. Additionally, fiber helps promote normal dental attrition and encourages normal foraging behavior, thus decreasing the potential for behavioral issues. The digestion of fiber in rabbits overall is poor; however, indigestible fiber is essential for stimulating gut motility and to help control gut transit time. Manufacturing processes play a role in the digestibility of commercial rabbit foods. For example, the finer the grinding, the longer the gut transit and cecal retention times, leading to greater potential for cecal dysbiosis.

The dietary management of rabbits requires a balance between providing enough indigestible fiber to maintain normal motility, cell regeneration, secretion, absorption, and excretion and providing enough digestible fiber for sufficient bacterial fermentation in the gut. The total dietary fiber levels recommended for pet rabbits is 20% to 25% DMB. Health care team members should educate owners to provide an ad libitum source of indigestible fiber (e.g., grass and/or hay). Also, owners should ensure that the amounts of other dietary components are limited. This will ensure that the rabbit eats the primary fiber source. Commercial foods used as a portion of the diet should preferably have a crude fiber content greater than 18% DMB, with indigestible fiber greater than 12.5% DMB.

Fat provides another source of energy and increases palatability. Fat also decreases dustiness and crumbling of commercially manufactured pellets. As with other species, rabbits are prone to obesity. Rabbits are also at risk for hepatic lipidosis. Consequently, high-fat diets must be avoided. The recommended level of fat for rabbits is 2.5% to 4% DMB.

> **TECHNICIAN NOTE**
>
> The dietary management of rabbits requires a balance between providing enough indigestible fiber to maintain normal motility, cell regeneration, secretion, absorption, and excretion and providing enough digestible fiber for sufficient bacterial fermentation in the gut.

In the nutritional management of rabbits, vitamins A, D, and E are important and should be part of the dietary composition. Gut bacteria synthesize B-vitamins in sufficient quantities, so adding B-vitamins to commercial foods may be unnecessary. Vitamin K synthesis in the gut is not as efficient. Therefore vitamin K is often added to the commercial formulation by rabbit food manufacturers. Vitamins A and E are readily destroyed by oxidation, so it is imperative that food preparation and storage methods prevent losses caused by excess light or heat. The recommendation is to store rabbit feed at 15°C (60°F) and feed within 90 days of milling. If the food is composed of greater than 30% alfalfa meal, there should be sufficient vitamin A in the form of the precursor beta-carotene. However, if the alfalfa has been stored for longer than a year after harvest, vitamin A deficiency can occur. Vitamin recommendations for pet rabbits include:

- 7000 to 18,000 IU vitamin A/kg food
- 40 to 70 mg vitamin E/kg food
- 2 mg vitamin K/kg food

Calcium regulation and the role of vitamin D in it differ in rabbits from those in other species. The presence of vitamin D is not required for the intestinal absorption of calcium. Vitamin D is important for the metabolism of phosphorus. Vitamin D deficiency can lead to hypophosphatemia and osteomalacia. Husbandry education should include proper cage placement, because sunlight is necessary for endogenous synthesis of vitamin D in rabbits. Commercially prepared rabbit pellets are supplemented with vitamin D. For pet rabbits, a level of 800 to 1200 IU/kg is recommended.

Guinea Pigs

Guinea pigs make wonderful pets—for people of all ages. Guinea pigs are herbivores with simple stomachs (Fig. 9.18).

The teeth of guinea pigs are open rooted and erupt continuously. Unlike other rodents, which typically have yellow incisors, a distinguishing factor of guinea pigs is white incisors. The guinea pig digestive tract is long and has a gastric emptying time of roughly 2 hours. The total GI transit time ranges from 8 to 20 hours. The normal flora found in the GI tract includes mainly *Lactobacillus* and occasionally *Streptococcus* spp., yeast, and soil bacteria. The majority of the digestive process happens in the cecum. The cecum of a guinea pig is a thin-walled sac divided into several lateral pouches by smooth muscle bands (taenia coli). The cecum is normally found on the central and left side of the abdomen and may contain as much as 65% of the GI contents. Guinea pigs exhibit coprophagous behavior, a fact which is important to convey to owners.

Guinea pigs dislike change. They develop dietary preferences early in life and do not adjust readily to changes in type, appearance, or presentation of their food or water. Guinea pig owners are encouraged to expose their pets to small amounts of different

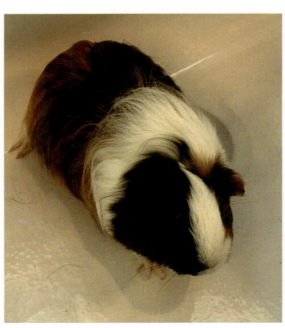

• **Fig. 9.18** Guinea pig. (Kara M. Burns.)

foods and vegetables while their pet is young. This will help the pet to accept variety in its feedstuffs. The reluctance to change can be a dangerous characteristic of guinea pigs; therefore it is important to educate owners to be cognizant of this fact and to gradually transition guinea pigs when introducing something new in the diet. In this way, client education may prevent a self-imposed fast by a pet guinea pig that is fed new food.

A CP level of 18% to 20% DMB is sufficient for growth and lactation in the guinea pig. The recommended minimum level of crude fiber is 10% DMB.

Guinea pigs require a dietary source of vitamin C (ascorbic acid), because they lack the enzyme involved in synthesizing glucose to ascorbic acid. This enzyme is L-gulonolactone oxidase. Nonbreeding adult guinea pigs require 10 mg/kg daily of ascorbic acid, with higher levels needed for growing and pregnant animals; 30 mg/kg daily is recommended during pregnancy.

The recommended diet for pet guinea pigs consists of guinea pig pellets and grass hay, supplemented with fresh vegetables. Good-quality grass hay should always be available. A variety of leafy greens can be offered in handfuls, because guinea pigs like greens. The technician should remember to advise owners to wash and prepare fresh foods. Also, it is important to advise owners that fresh foods should not be left in the cage and should be removed after a few hours if not eaten. Fruits, rolled oats, and dry cereals should be offered only in very small quantities, if at all, as treats. Any additions or changes to the diet should be made gradually.

Guinea pig foods that are commercially prepared typically contain 18% to 20% CP DMB and 10% to 16% fiber DMB. Pellets are fortified with ascorbic acid, but almost half the initial vitamin C content may be oxidized and lost 90 days after the diet has been mixed and stored at 22°C. Many commercially prepared guinea pig diets are now available with stabilized vitamin C, and these diets should be stored in a cool, dry area (<70°F [22°C]). Foods can be refrigerated or frozen but should be protected from condensation and increased storage temperature and humidity in vegetables and fruits or in the drinking water. Foods with higher levels of ascorbic acid include the following:

- Red and green peppers
- Broccoli
- Tomatoes
- Kiwi fruit
- Oranges

Many types of leafy greens (kale, parsley, beet greens, chicory, spinach) are high in vitamin C, but many contain high levels of calcium or oxalates; these should be offered in only small amounts. Vitamin C can be added to the water at 1 g/L. In an open container, water with added vitamin C loses greater than 50% of its vitamin C content in 24 hours. Water must be changed daily to ensure adequate activity of the vitamin.

Miscellaneous Small Mammals

Hamsters, gerbils, mice, and rats are very popular pets. These pets belong to the rodent family and are known for naturally hoarding food items. This behavior makes it difficult to determine how much food is truly being ingested. The role of the veterinary health care team is to educate owners on the natural hoarding tendencies of rodents. Although owners need to be aware when the food dish of these small mammals is empty, consistently filling the bowl may result in obese small mammals.

Most rodents are omnivorous. They typically eat grasses, seeds, grains, and occasionally invertebrates in the wild. Pet small mammals' dietary needs are best met by providing a formulated diet supplemented with small amounts of fresh foods and seeds for variety and interest. Seed mixtures are popular choices for small mammals; however, seed mixtures regularly lead to selective feeding—they pick out what they like and leave important nutrients. A nutritional imbalance can result from small mammals eating high-calorie seeds (sunflower) while ignoring the formulated pellets. Many rodents have short lifespans, so determining a nutritional deficiency is rare. The most common form of malnutrition in rats is obesity. Studies show an increase in length of life and a decrease in certain disease conditions in rats fed a calorie-restricted diet. Gerbils exhibit sensitivity to high-fat, high-cholesterol diets, resulting in changes in the gerbils' levels of blood cholesterol.

Protein requirements for rodents range from 14% to 17% DMB in hamsters, from 14% to 16% DMB in rats and mice, and up to 22% DMB in gerbils. Nutritional management of hamsters, rats, mice, and gerbils should ensure that these ranges are followed. Nutritional management of reproducing small mammals should contain higher levels of protein.

As discussed earlier, water is of the utmost importance, and small mammal owners should be educated about the importance of providing fresh, clean water always. Typically, water bottles are used, because they help prevent bedding from getting wet and are often preferred by small mammals. However, over time, water bottles may become clogged or start to leak. It is best for the health care team to educate owners to change the water and to check water bottles every day.

Feeding Reptiles

Health care team members should always consult comprehensive feeding guidelines specific to each species of reptile, because there is tremendous variability in their dietary requirements. Husbandry plays a huge role in the health and prevention of nutrition-related disorders. Dietary deficiencies are not commonly seen in snakes that eat whole animals; however, a variety of dietary deficiencies are commonly seen in lizards, turtles, and crocodilians that scavenge. One of the most common disorders seen in reptiles is metabolic bone disease, which is caused by inappropriately low calcium or low vitamin D_3 intake or excessive intake of phosphorus. This disease may be prevented by feeding a species-appropriate diet and by regularly exposing the animal to ultraviolet (UV) light (natural or artificial). It is essential that reptiles, especially lizards, have full-spectrum lighting available during the normal daylight hours. Animals with metabolic bone disease must be treated very gently, because their bones are prone to pathologic fractures. In addition, vitamin A deficiency is commonly seen in turtles and tortoises and usually manifests as an overgrown beak, palpebral edema, and conjunctivitis.

Many captive lizards are omnivores and will eat mealworms, crickets, grasshoppers, waxworms, and an array of plants. However, most insects are nutritionally deficient, particularly in calcium. Therefore it is important to feed lizards nutritional supplements and to include calcium-rich plants and supplements in the diet. In the wild, however, lizards are primarily carnivorous, eating invertebrate or vertebrate prey. In general, captive lizards require vitamin and mineral supplementation, with an emphasis on variety in food. Juvenile lizards should be fed one to two times a day, with adults requiring feeding two to three times per week. Most lizards are diurnal and require day feedings and time to bask in natural or UV light.

Herbivorous lizards, such as the green iguana, require a varied diet to ensure adequate nutritional balance. Recommended diets for herbivores include leafy greens (e.g., romaine lettuce, collard greens), mustard greens, and clover. Vegetables, including green beans, okra, carrots, and squash, are also adequate dietary substances. It is important to note that certain vegetables, such as spinach, cabbage, peas, and potatoes, contain substances that bind calcium and other trace minerals, inhibiting their absorption.

Commercial iguana food is available to provide a base diet for these animals. Commercial diets do not require additional supplementation if the captive lizard is fed a diet based primarily on such purchased food. Homemade diets of vegetables and fruit should always be supplemented with appropriate vitamins and minerals. Technicians can advise lizard owners to purchase a good-quality reptile vitamin product containing vitamin D_3 to be administered one to two times a week if a good diet is provided. Common iguanas also require protein for normal growth and development. Juvenile iguanas in captivity generally need more protein and calcium compared with adults. Common protein sources include dark green leafy vegetables, such as collards, turnip greens, kale, bok choy, and broccoli with leaves. Iguanas should never be fed a meat-based diet or any commercial food other than iguana food. Commercial dog or cat food should never be fed to iguanas, because this will cause renal disease and death.

Snakes are carnivores, and they feed on whole prey. Eating the entire prey provides added nutrients, such as calcium. Snakes will excrete via feces those parts of the prey they do not use. As mentioned, supplementation is typically not necessary when feeding whole prey, such as rats, mice, and so on.

Water should be provided in a bowl for bathing and drinking. Note that some lizards (e.g., chameleons) will drink water only if it is in the form of droplets on plant leaves, similar to dew. Therefore it is important to spray or mist the animal's enclosure several times a day. In addition, most lizards should be sprayed with water or allowed to bathe to prevent skin problems associated with low humidity.

Recommended Readings

AAHA Nutrition Guidelines https://www.aaha.org/aaha-guidelines/2021-aaha-nutrition-and-weight-management-guidelines/home/.

Fascetti AJ, Delaney SJ, Larsen JA, Villaverde C. *Applied Veterinary Clinical Nutrition*. Ames, IA: Wiley Blackwell; 2012.

Hand MS, Thatcher CD, Remillard RL, et al. *Small Animal Clinical Nutrition*. 5th ed. Mark Morris Institute; 2010.

Towell TL. *Practical Weight Management in Dogs and Cats*. Ames, IA: Wiley Blackwell; 2011.

World Small Animal Veterinary Association Global Nutrition Committee. *Nutrition Toolkit*. WSAVA website. http://www.wsava.org/nutrition-toolkit; Accessed 08.19.

Wortinger A, Burns KM. *Nutrition and Disease Management for Veterinary Technicians and Nurses*. Ames, IA: Wiley Blackwell; 2015.

10
Animal Reproduction

JUSTIN T. HAYNA

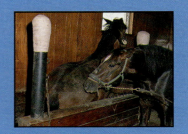

CHAPTER OUTLINE

LEARNING OBJECTIVES

When you have completed this chapter, you will be able to:

1. Pronounce, define, and spell each of the key terms in this chapter.
2. Locate the anatomic parts of the reproductive system, including endocrine organs in the cranium.
3. Describe hormonal changes that occur during the estrous cycle and pregnancy.
4. Compare and contrast the processes of oogenesis and spermatogenesis.
5. Explain the process of fertilization and embryo development, including the anatomic locations of these events.
6. Compare and contrast canine, feline, and equine estrous cycles, gestation, and parturition, and describe the collection process and interpretation of canine vaginal cells and state the importance of vaginal cytologic examination in breeding dogs.
7. Compare and contrast the bovine, ovine, caprine, and camelid estrous cycles, gestation, and parturition.
8. Identify and put in order the important aspects of a breeding soundness examination in a male and a female animal.

KEY TERMS

Allantois
Amnion
Anestrus
Artificial insemination
Barrow
Buck
Calf
Calving
Camelids
Capacitation
Caslick's surgery
Chorioallantois membrane
Colostrum
Corpus hemorrhagicum
Corpus luteum
Cria
Cryptorchidism
Cumulus
Diapedesis
Diestrus
Diffuse

Doe
Embryo
Estrogen
Estrus
Fetal membranes
Follicle
Follicle-stimulating hormone
Gonadotropin-releasing hormone
Luteinizing hormone
Oocyte
Oxytocin
Parturition
Pineal gland
Placenta
Progesterone
Prolactin
Relaxin
Seasonally polyestrous
Superfecundation
Superfetation

Introduction

Theriogenology is the branch of veterinary medicine concerned with the management of animal reproduction and is a cornerstone of all herd health programs. Although unique differences exist in the reproductive systems of domestic animal species, there are many similarities. A working knowledge of normal reproductive anatomy and physiology, including hormone interactions, spermatogenesis, fertilization, pregnancy, and birth, is essential. When the normal process is understood, the abnormal process is more easily recognized. Furthermore, knowledge of normal and abnormal processes in one species can help recognize normal and abnormal processes in other species.

This chapter provides an overview of female and male reproductive systems, followed by a review of the most important aspects of reproduction in the canine, feline, equine, bovine, ovine, caprine, and camelid species. Reproduction is an extremely intricate and complex process, with ongoing research constantly adding to and changing what we think we know. For more in-depth and current information, consult other sources of information, including veterinary endocrinology texts, specialty journals, and referenced articles.

Overview of Female Reproduction

Reproduction in female mammals is an elegantly coordinated cyclic interaction of reproductive hormones produced by the hypothalamus, the anterior and posterior pituitary glands, the ovaries, and the tubular genitalia (oviducts, uterus, and vagina). These hormones control ovulation, mating, pregnancy, birth, and the nurturing of offspring. Refer to Fig. 10.1 and Table 10.1.

Hormones from other glands, including the pineal, thyroid, and adrenal glands, also affect reproduction. The **pineal gland** is particularly important. Both the pineal gland and the hypothalamus are part of the limbic system, which is the part of the

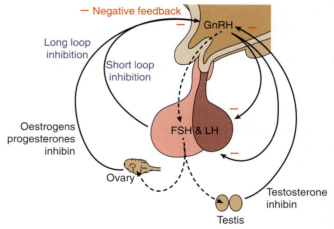

• **Fig. 10.1** Diagram of hormonal control of ovarian and testicular activity. *FSH*, Follicle-stimulating hormone; *GnRH*, gonadotropin-releasing hormone; *LH*, luteinizing hormone.

brain that regulates autonomic and endocrine functions (Fig. 10.2). The pineal gland produces melatonin, which is secreted in response to the dark and inhibited by light. Melatonin is important in the regulation of seasonal and diurnal rhythms, including the seasonal breeding cycles of long- and short-day breeders, such as cats and horses and sheep and goats, respectively.

TECHNICIAN NOTE

Estrous, the adjective, refers to the type of cycle. *Estrus*, the noun, refers to the part of the estrous cycle when the female is in "heat" and sexually receptive. Puberty occurs when the first ovulation occurs, whether or not the female has had signs of heat. Sexual receptiveness is brought about by the ratio of estrogen to progesterone.

TABLE 10.1 Summary of Female Reproductive Glands, Secretions, and Functions

Organ	Location	Hormone Produced	Target Organ	Function
Hypothalamus	Part of brain (see Fig. 10.2)	Gonadotropin-releasing hormone (GnRH)	Anterior pituitary gland	Stimulate release of gonadotropins (FSH, LH)
Anterior pituitary gland	Ventral to hypothalamus (see Fig. 10.2)	Follicle-stimulating hormone (FSH)	Ovaries	Stimulates growth of ovarian follicles and estrogen secretion
		Luteinizing hormone (LH)	Ovaries	Stimulates ovulation, conversion of follicles to the corpus luteum (CL), and secretion of progesterone
		Prolactin	Mammary glands	Stimulates milk production
Posterior pituitary gland	Ventral to hypothalamus (see Fig. 10.2)	Oxytocin	Uterus	Increases frequency of uterine contractions
			Mammary glands	Stimulates milk letdown from mammary glands into the nipples
Ovarian follicle CL	On ovary	Estrogen Progesterone	Uterus, vagina	Prepare for implantation of fertilized ova and development of the embryo
Ovarian CL	On ovary	Progesterone	Hypothalamus	Inhibits GnRH, resulting in less secretion of FSH and LH
Ovary	Abdomen	Inhibin	Hypothalamus Anterior pituitary	Inhibits GnRH from hypothalamus and FSH and LH from anterior pituitary
Uterus	Abdomen	Prostaglandin F2alpha	Ovarian CL	Lysis of CL (luteolysis)

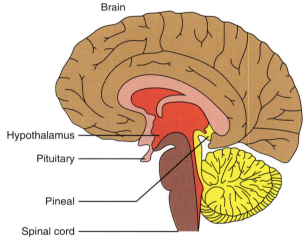

Brain

Hypothalamus

Pituitary

Pineal

Spinal cord

• **Fig. 10.2** Sketch of the brain, locating the hypothalamus, pituitary glands, and pineal glands.

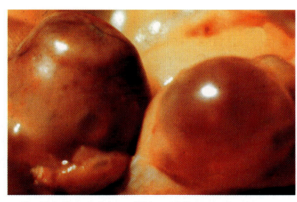

• **Fig. 10.3** Corpus luteum (CL) and follicle on a bovine ovary.

Gonadotropin-releasing hormone (GnRH), secreted by the hypothalamus, stimulates the secretion of **follicle-stimulating hormone** (FSH) from the anterior pituitary. FSH, in turn, stimulates the development of the ovarian **follicle** and **estrogen** secretion (see Table 10.1).

Folliculogenesis is the process of growth and development of immature germ cells into fully fertilizable germ cells. FSH is related to the stimulation and development of this process. Immature germ cells undergo a two-step process called *meiosis*, forming mature sperm and **oocytes** (ova). Like somatic cells, primary oocytes are diploid, with two sets (2n) of homologous chromosomes. The first meiotic division of a primary oocyte occurs in the fetus and produces secondary oocytes with the diploid number (2n) of chromosomes plus a small polar body. The second meiotic

division generally occurs around the time of ovulation. This is a reduction division without duplication of the chromosomes. It results in an oocyte with a haploid number of chromosomes (n = 1) and a polar body. The polar bodies have no function except as part of the reduction process. There are species-specific variations in the timing of the division.

Ovulation of a mature follicle (Fig. 10.3) is caused by an increase in **luteinizing hormone** (LH) from the anterior pituitary. LH also triggers the conversion of the follicle into a progesterone-secreting **corpus luteum** (CL). Increasing progesterone levels inhibit hypothalamic secretion of GnRH (negative feedback) and, consequently, pituitary FSH and LH secretion decrease. In some species, lower LH levels result in lower progesterone levels unless fertilization has occurred, but this is not true for all species.

After ovulation, the empty follicular sac fills with clotted blood, forming the **corpus hemorrhagicum** (CH), which

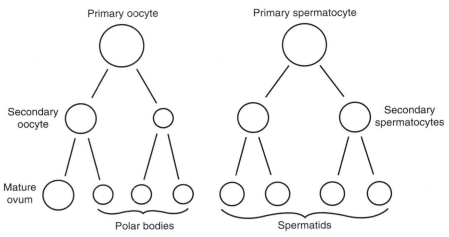

• **Fig. 10.4** Diagram of oogenesis and spermatogenesis (meiosis).

TABLE 10.2   Placentation and Passage of Immunoglobulin G (IgG) for Domestic Species

Species	Placenta Type	Maternal Layers	Contact Points	Transplacental IgG
Horses, swine	Epitheliochorial	All 3	Diffuse	No
Ruminants	Epitheliochorial	All 3	Cotyledonary	No
Dogs, cats	Endotheliochorial	1 endothelium	Zonary	Limited
Humans, rodents	Hemochorial	0	Discoid	Yes

provides a nutritional matrix for the rapid development of the surrounding cells. The CH becomes a progesterone-producing CL (see primary spermatocyte, Fig. 10.4). This process can be quite fast for horses or take a few days for cattle. **Progesterone** helps prepare and maintain the uterus for implantation and pregnancy. The CL is maintained for a predetermined time after ovulation in most species, whether fertilization occurs or not. If fertilization does not occur and there is no embryonic signaling to the dam, prostaglandin F2alpha (PGF2alpha) produced by the uterus causes luteolysis, regression of the CL, and a rapid drop in progesterone.

When an oocyte is released from an ovarian follicle, it is covered with the cumulus cells that surround it within the follicle. These cells supply nutrition to the oocyte as it matures. After ovulation, the layer of cells serves as a roughened surface, which helps the oocyte move through the oviduct toward the uterus. Fertilization, which involves penetration of the ovum (mature oocyte) by a single sperm, occurs in the last part of the oviduct.

The fertilized ovum (zygote) then passes through the isthmus into the uterus, where it implants itself. Once the zygote reaches the uterus, it releases an early conception factor (ECF) chemical signal. ECFs are species dependent and only partially understood for some species. They generally have mechanisms to prevent uterine release of PGF2alpha, as well as immunosuppressive and growth factor properties that protect the zygote from being targeted as foreign.

As the zygote develops into an **embryo**, the outermost cells become the **placenta**. The remaining cells form the inner cell mass. These cells differentiate into three layers. The *endoderm*, or inner layer, becomes the intestines, liver, and lungs. The *mesoderm*, or middle layer, becomes the cardiovascular, musculoskeletal, and

reproductive systems. The *ectoderm*, or outer layer, becomes hair, skin, and the nervous system.

The uterine-placental attachment varies in the number of layers separating maternal and fetal blood and the distribution of contact points. The placenta is an organ of fetal origination that interfaces with the maternal uterus for nutrient exchange. Three maternal and three fetal layers are associated with this uterine-placental interface. These are the vascular endothelium, connective tissue (mesoderm), and epithelium, and all three layers are present in the fetal component. The outermost of these is the chorionic epithelium, which is in direct contact with the maternal component. Depending on the species, some of the maternal layers are lost (Table 10.2). The number of placental layers affects immunoglobulin G (IgG) antibody transfer from the mother to the fetus, and whether the newborn has antibody protection at birth or solely depends on the colostrum consumed after birth for maternal antibodies. The number of maternal layers present and that which is in closest approximation to the fetal placental layers is the basis of one of the classification schemes of placenta. This might be epitheliochorial or endotheliochorial, depending on the number of layers and on the species.

The placenta is also classified according to the shape and distribution of contact points (Fig. 10.5). The placenta is *diffuse* if the contact is evenly distributed over most of the placenta, and it is *cotyledonary* if the contact is between fetal cotyledons and maternal caruncles that together form placentomes. The number of maternal caruncles is fixed at birth, and they do not regenerate if damaged. The placental attachment is *zonary* if the contact area takes the form of a band or ring around the fetus, and it is *discoid* if the contact is limited to a single disk-shaped area.

Overview of Male Reproduction

The primary anatomic structures involved in the reproductive processes of males include the hypothalamus, pituitary, testicles (testes), accessory sex glands (prostate, bulbourethral gland, ampulla, and vesicular glands), and the tubular genitalia (vas deferens and urethra). The pineal gland regulates seasonal cycles and circadian rhythms (see Fig. 10.1 and Table 10.3).

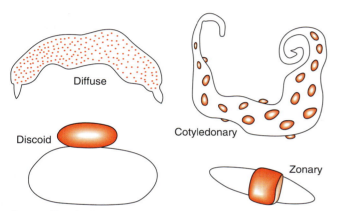

• **Fig. 10.5** Sketch of placenta types based on distribution of contact areas between fetal and maternal components.

During early embryonic and fetal development, the testicles are in the abdomen. As the fetus develops, the testicles, covered by a capsule of connective tissue (tunica albuginea), are drawn into and migrate through the inguinal rings into a pouch of skin outside the body wall (scrotum). The external location maintains the testicles 1°C to 2°C cooler than the body core. A lower temperature is required for sperm production but not to produce testosterone. **Cryptorchidism** refers to males with one or neither testicle descended. Fertility is compromised and dependent on whether one or both testicles are retained. Cryptorchids have normal testosterone levels and secondary sex characteristics and are at an increased risk of testicular cancer in the retained testicle(s).

The testes are organized into lobules, each containing many seminiferous tubules that empty into central collecting ducts. The tubules are lined by primordial germ cells (immature sperm cells) and Sertoli cells. The Sertoli cells surround the developing sperm cells, isolating them from the immune system, which might consider them foreign and destroy the developing sperm. This is the basis of the blood-testis barrier. Interstitial (Leydig) cells, located in the spaces between tubules, produce testosterone, which is necessary for sperm production.

During early development and differentiation of sperm cells, meiosis occurs. This two-step process results in immature germ cells with half the number of chromosomes (haploid) compared with normal somatic cells, which have the full complement of chromosomes (diploid). Once these haploid spermatids are formed, additional morphologic changes occur, including developing a flagellum (tail) and an acrosome, eliminating excess cytoplasm and chromatin condensation. These changes ultimately make the sperm capable of independent streamlined movement, penetration of the ovum membrane and surrounding structures, and delivery of the genetic material for completion of fertilization.

TABLE 10.3 Summary of Male Reproductive Glands, Secretions, and Functions

Organ	Location	Hormone Produced	Target Organ	Function
Hypothalamus	Part of brain over brainstem	Gonadotropin-releasing hormone (GnRH)	Anterior pituitary	Stimulate release of gonadotropins (FSH, LH)
Anterior pituitary	Ventral hypothalamus	Follicle-stimulating hormone (FSH)	Testicles	Formation of sperm
		Luteinizing hormone (LH)	Testicles	Secretion of testosterone
Testicles	Outside of abdominal wall in scrotum Temperature 1°C–2°C degrees less than body temperature	Sperm Testosterone		Fertilization of ovum Sperm formation Develop/maintain reproductive tract Sex drive and male behavior Secondary male characteristics, muscles
Seminal vesicles		Produce viscous fluid containing: Fructose—energy for sperm PGF2alpha—motility and viability of sperm Proteins—slight coagulation after ejaculation		60% of semen volume
Prostate	Near urinary bladder	Thin, milk-colored, alkaline fluid	Enhance sperm motility	Slightly less than 40% semen volume
Bulbourethral (Cowper) glands		Alkaline mucuslike fluid		Neutralize residual urine acidity Lubricate tip of penis

Spermatogenesis is completed when spermatozoa (singular is spermatozoon) move into the lumen of the seminiferous tubule. Although spermatogenesis is completed within the testicle, sperm maturation is not achieved until the spermatozoa pass through the epididymis. In the canine, this takes 12 to 14 days. From the start of spermatogenesis to ejaculation, formation of a mature sperm cell in dogs and many other species takes about 62 days.

Sperm and testosterone production is controlled by hormones produced by the hypothalamus, anterior pituitary, and gonads (see Table 10.3). LH from the pituitary stimulates testosterone production. As testosterone increases, it inhibits secretion of GnRH from the hypothalamus and consequently LH from the pituitary. This is a classic example of negative feedback. The decrease in GnRH and LH decreases testosterone production. As less testosterone is produced, the production of GnRH and LH increases and again stimulates testosterone production. GnRH also triggers pituitary FSH release from the hypothalamus. FSH acts on Sertoli cells to increase the division of primordial sperm cells and to release more sperm cells that are embedded in Sertoli cells.

As in the female, the interplay of hormones controls the reproductive processes in males. It results in relatively constant sperm production and testosterone levels. There are other hormones that are involved in reproduction. These include inhibin, activin, follistatin, **relaxin**, etc. They stimulate or inhibit hormone release at different levels of the hypothalamic-pituitary-ovarian axis. This is an active area of investigation, and new hormones are being hypothesized and identified frequently.

After sperm is released from Sertoli cells, they move through the tubules and into the head of the epididymis. Within the epididymis, the sperm acquires motility and the preliminary ability to fertilize ova. Movement through the epididymis to the tail of the epididymis is relatively constant and not affected by the number or frequency of ejaculates. The sperm cells are stored in the tail of the epididymis, where they may be ejaculated or voided through urine.

Ejaculation through the penis is the final process in sperm production and delivery. In most domestic species, the penis comprises cavernous blood tissue surrounded by a firm covering, or tunic. An erection occurs when the male is sexually stimulated, when parasympathetic innervation causes increased blood flow into the cavernous portions of the penis. As blood flow to the penis is increased, muscles around the proximal penis contract to prevent blood outflow. Because the cavernous portions of the penis are contained within the tunic, pressure increases, resulting in penile erection.

During erection, sperm cells in the tail of the epididymis are moved from the ductus deferens into the ampulla through a process called *emission*. Once sperm are present in the ampulla, stimulation of the penis during mating causes ejaculation, the forceful expulsion of semen through the penis. The force comes from sympathetic nerves, causing smooth muscle contractions in the urethra. During ejaculation, sperm are mixed with fluid from the accessory sex glands (ampulla, prostate, vesicular glands, and/or bulbourethral glands). Fluids from these glands add various components to the ejaculate, increase the volume, and stabilize the sperm cell membrane. When sperm are mixed with accessory sex

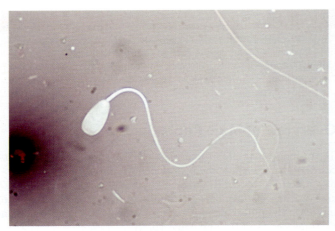

• **Fig. 10.6** Photomicrograph of normal sperm.

gland fluid, the result is called *semen*. Once sperm enter the female reproductive tract, the sperm cell membrane undergoes a physical and biochemical change, called *capacitation*, which makes sperm capable of fertilization (Fig. 10.6). Uterine contractions move sperm rapidly to the oviduct, where fertilization occurs.

Canine Reproduction

Estrous Cycle

The canine estrous cycle consists of four stages: proestrus, **estrus** (ovulation occurs), diestrus, and **anestrus**. Refer to Table 10.4 for information on reproductive terminology and estrous cycles for all species discussed in this chapter.

The period between the canine estrous cycles averages 6 to 7 months but varies from less than 4 months to greater than 1 year. Serum levels of progesterone (P4) and LH are commonly used to pinpoint the time of ovulation and calculate optimal breeding times in dogs that are exhibiting signs of estrus. Microscopic evaluation of cells from the vagina and observation of changes in behavior of the bitch are also helpful methods of identifying optimal breeding times. However, the latter approaches are more time consuming and less precise than monitoring P4 and LH levels in the blood. Refer to Box 10.1 for information about vaginal cytology.

At puberty and during the last month of anestrus thereafter, GnRH is secreted by the hypothalamus and stimulates the secretion of FSH from the pituitary. FSH, in turn, stimulates the growth of ovarian follicles and estrogen secretion. Under the influence of increasing estrogen, the endometrium (uterine lining) becomes highly vascularized and engorged with blood. Some blood leaks through capillary walls (diapedesis) and into the uterine cavity. It drains into the vagina and out through the vulva as a serosanguinous bloody discharge. Increased estrogen levels cause hyperemia and swelling of the vulva.

Proestrus. The presence of a bloody discharge from the swollen vulva marks the start of proestrus. Males are attracted to the bitch, but she will not allow them to mount. Breeders have traditionally used the appearance of blood to estimate when to start teasing the stud. The length of this stage is variable but averages around 9 days.

Estrus. This stage of the estrous cycle is classically described as the time when the female begins accepting the male. It is a time

TABLE 10.4

Summary of the Canine Estrous Cycle

Stage	Bitch's Behavior	Clinical Signs	Duration	Physiology	Cytology: Predominant Cell Types
Proestrus	Attracts male Will not stand for breeding	Serosanguinous discharge Hyperemic, swollen vulva	9 days (range 3–17 days)	Estrogen levels increase Uterus engorged with blood, seen in vaginal discharge Vaginal epithelium proliferates	*Early:* Nondegenerated neutrophils, mixture of parabasal, intermediate, and superficial epithelial cells Some bacteria *Late:* Number of neutrophils decrease, and superficial cells increase
Estrus	Seeks males Stand for coitus	Clear discharge Less vulvar swelling	9 days (range 3–18 days)	Luteinizing hormone (LH) surge Ovulation Estrogen decreases Corpus luteum (CL) produces progesterone	Less than 90% cornified epithelial cells Bacteria attach to superficial cells
Diestrus	Stops accepting male	Little discharge Very little vulvar edema	60 days (range 60–90 days)	CL produces progesterone Cervix constricts Vaginal secretions tacky	Decreased superficial and increased intermediate cells Neutrophils contain phagocytized red blood cells (RBCs) and bacteria Can resemble proestrus
Anestrus	No specific sexual behavior	Scant discharge No vulvar edema	4 months (range 2–8 months)	Reproductive system at rest Secretions scant Cervix closed Vaginal mucosa pale	Parabasal and intermediate cells No superficial cells

of shifting hormone profiles that affect behavior and physiology. Hormonally, there is a rapid increase in LH, called an "LH surge," that occurs at the start of estrus (Fig. 10.7). Ovulation occurs approximately 2 days after the surge and is followed by conversion of the follicle into a progesterone-producing structure called the corpus luteum, or CL. Younger bitches tend to ovulate slightly earlier and older bitches slightly later. Canine ova are not mature at the time of ovulation and require an additional 2 days to fully mature in the oviducts. Once mature, they can remain fertilizable for 3 or more days.

Diestrus (Metestrus). The start of diestrus is dependent upon what is being used to determine hormone activity. When using vaginal cytology, diestrus is identified by a sharp change from superficial cells to parabasal cells. Superficial cells are cornified, with a folded appearance, and resemble cornflakes in appearance. Parabasal cells have large amounts of cytoplasm and small, dark nuclei. These have been described as looking like "fried eggs." Hormonally, this is when progesterone rises above 2 ng/mL. Diestrus ends when a pregnant bitch whelps or a nonpregnant bitch's progesterone drops to below 1 ng/mL. Prostaglandin (PGF2alpha) does not appear to be important as a natural controller of CL regression in the bitch, but it can be used therapeutically to lyse (cause to regress) a CL. **Parturition** occurs within 24 hours after the CL is no longer functional and progesterone is less than 1 ng/mL.

Anestrus. This is the period of least reproductive activity. The uterus is regenerating from the changes that occurred during pregnancy or during the estrous cycle. Uterine involution after whelping or in the nonpregnant bitch is not complete until about 120 days after ovulation. There is no ovarian activity until close to the end of anestrus, when the next estrous cycle begins.

TECHNICIAN NOTE

The canine estrous cycle averages 6 to 7 months but varies from less than 4 months to greater than 1 year. Serum levels of progesterone (P4) and luteinizing hormone (LH) are used to pinpoint the time of ovulation and calculate optimal breeding times. Changes in behavior and in vaginal secretions, although less precise, are also helpful indicators of times to breed.

Breeding

Breeding can be performed using natural service or **artificial insemination** (AI). With either method, inseminations occur during estrus. The bitch in estrus will flag, with the tail raised and held to one side. At the beginning of the "courtship," she may play with the male and establish a behaviorally friendly relationship. She will stand for the male to mount and breed. If natural breeding or service occurs, it is normal for the male and female to be "locked" together (tied) for half an hour or more. The tie is caused by the engorgement of the bulbus gland, which is located at the base of the penis. such engorgement occurs immediately after penetration and by the contraction of circular muscles in the vagina preventing withdrawal.

AI can be done through vaginal, transcervical, or surgical approaches by using fresh or frozen semen. Timing needs to be precise when cryopreserved (frozen) semen is used. Although frozen semen can be stored indefinitely in liquid nitrogen, it has a

• BOX 10.1   Vaginal Cytology

Until the widespread availability of cageside serum hormone assays, behavior and vaginal cytology were the primary methods used for staging the estrous cycle for breeding dogs. It is still useful in areas without ready access to specialty practices with imaging and laboratory support. It takes some practice to become proficient at the use of this method.

Materials Needed

- Nonsterile examination gloves
- Cotton swabs on 6-inch sticks
- Sterile saline
- Glass microscope slides
- Methanol or a spray fixative
- Diff-Quik or Giemsa-Wright stain
- Lugol solution or no stain

Obtaining the Sample

Moisten the swab, gently part the lips of the vulva, and push the swab in while rotating it. Gently pull the swab out and roll it on a clean slide. The specimen can be dried and fixed, air dried and stained without fixing, or examined wet.

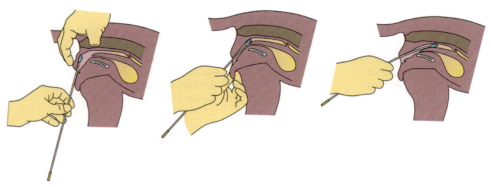

A diagram demonstrating cell collection for vaginal cytologic preparation and examination. (From Eilts BE. Determining estrous status. *NAVS Clin Brief* 2007;5:40.)

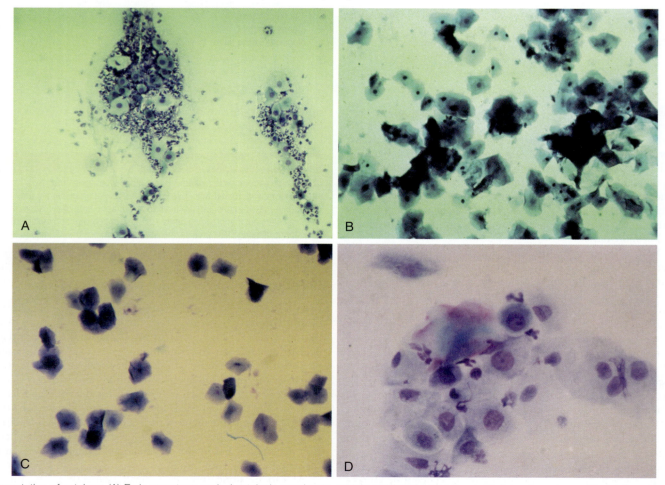

Interpretation of cytology. (A) Early proestrus: vaginal cytologic specimens contain parabasal and a few epithelial cells and a multitude of neutrophils and red blood cells, mucus, and debris. (B) Late proestrus: superficial, nucleated epithelial cells predominate, and the amount of mucus is decreased. (C) Estrus: nucleated and anucleated superficial cells are visible. Stark absence of all other cell types is evident. (D) Diestrus: many parabasal and superficial epithelial cells are visible, with no neutrophils, red blood cells, mucus, or debris.

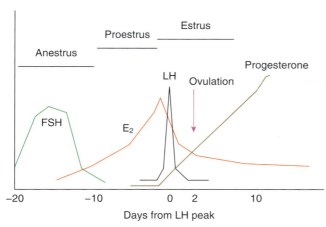

• **Fig. 10.7** Hormonal changes during the estrous cycle of the bitch. Luteinizing hormone *(LH)* surge is followed by ovulation in 2 days. *FSH,* Follicle-stimulating hormone.

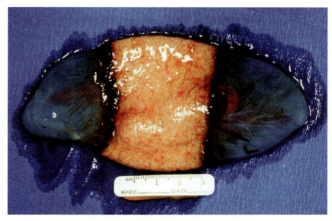

• **Fig. 10.8** Zonary placentation of the bitch.

very short lifespan once it is thawed. Ideally, fertilization should occur within 12 hours after thawing. Fresh semen delivered by natural service or by AI stays fertile for 3 to 5 days. Insemination should be precisely timed and only done once. Natural service is best done after progesterone reaches a serum concentration of 2 ng/mL or on day 2 to day 4 after the LH surge. This is the basis of what can be called the 2:2:2 rule. When progesterone reaches 2 ng/mL, then ovulation is likely to occur in 2 days, and insemination should occur 2 days after that.

Progesterone measures about 5 ng/mL at the time of ovulation and greater than 10 ng/mL during the fertile period. Until the concentrations exceed 10 ng/mL, the progesterone level is highly useful for predicting when to inseminate. At higher levels, the predictive value is lost. Vaginal cytology and the bitch's behavior become more accurate for making breeding decisions. The reappearance of white blood cells and noncornified epithelial cells indicates estrus is over. If service is natural, male and female reluctance to breed is an excellent indication that estrus has ended.

PUT INTO PRACTICE

When working with clients who want to breed their pets, time spent with your client explaining the importance of caring for their pets during pregnancy and during parturition is a vital role for the veterinary nurse/technician. In addition, the importance of caring for mothers and babies after they have given birth is another important role for you.

Pregnancy Diagnosis

Pregnancy examination by palpation is possible in most bitches at 21 to 30 days of gestation. Ultrasonography is used to diagnose pregnancy and confirm that embryos are alive. The optimal timing for initial ultrasound examination is commonly 28 days post ovulation. Normal heart rates are higher than 220 beats per minute (average 230 bpm). An assay test (WITNESS, Relaxin Rapid Test, Zoetis, NJ) that measures relaxin, a hormone produced by the placenta, can confirm pregnancy from 3 to 4 weeks to term.

Radiography can be used to detect signs of pregnancy as early as 21 days. At this early stage, no fetal structures are usually seen,

but a distended, fluid-filled uterus can be noted. Fetal skeletal calcification of the spine and skull starts about 43 to 46 days after the LH surge. Further calcification of scapula, femur, and tibia starts about 46 to 51 days after the LH surge. Each of these methods can be helpful in determining fetal count, the size of fetuses in relationship to the dam's pelvis, and presentation of the first fetus to be delivered. Fetal counts are likely best determined with later-gestation radiography. It should always be noted that counts using either method are full of issues that can over- or underestimate the actual number of offspring at parturition. Radiography may also be helpful during cases of dystocia.

Hormonal analysis is also possible but less reliable for pregnancy diagnosis. The bitch does not produce a pregnancy-specific hormone, like some other species. Progesterone is elevated throughout diestrus, which is similar in most species. Relaxin will increase in the bitch starting at 20 days after LH peak. **Prolactin** has been shown to increase starting at day 30 of gestation. FSH and urine estrogen concentrations have also been examined. One must also recognize that these hormones are not necessarily produced by the fetus and thus false-positives and/or pregnancy losses can occur. Radiography and ultrasonography are currently the best methods for pregnancy diagnosis.

Gestation

Gestation in the bitch lasts approximately 60 days from fertilization. The 63 days of gestation are related to LH surges and progesterone levels. The placenta type is endotheliochorial, with a zonary attachment area (see Table 10.2, and Figs. 10.5 and 10.8). This means that there are only four layers of tissue barriers between the maternal and fetal blood supplies. There is some potential discrepancy, but most authors describe the reduction of tissue layers to occur on the maternal side. This feature of canine placentation means that more maternal antibodies are transmitted to the fetuses in utero. There are many factors associated with the care of the pregnant bitch that are beyond the scope of this chapter, and the reader is referred to other texts for this information.

Parturition (Whelp)

Parturition or delivery of the neonate from an internal maternal environment to an external one is a stepwise process. Commonly, this is referred to as whelping in the dog. The process of parturition is divided into three stages.

Stage I

In this stage, uterine contractions without an abdominal component begin. Stage I lasts 6 to 12 hours but can last longer, up to 36 hours. The bitch is usually restless and shows nesting behavior. She appears nervous, pants, and trembles. Body temperature drops 1°C to 3°C to 37.2°C (99°F) about 24 hours before stage II in about 85% of bitches. This temperature drop is related to the abrupt decrease in progesterone and is a signal that whelping is imminent. The temperature should be taken at the same time each day, preferably in the morning before any activity.

Stage II

Puppies are delivered (whelped) (Fig. 10.9) at this stage. It usually takes 20 to 60 minutes per puppy. In general, no more than 2 hours should elapse between puppies. Whelping usually lasts 3 to 6 hours but may take up to 24 hours. There are normal appearances and discharges with delivery of each neonate. Outer placental membranes generally rupture once the neonate enters the vagina. There can be clear or blackish-green discharge that is normal during parturition, as it comes from the sites of placental attachment. However, if fluids appear prior to the first puppy or there is no puppy present shortly thereafter, it can be a strong indicator of dystocia or difficulty with the birthing process.

Stage III

This is the portion of delivery that relates to expulsion of the placenta/**fetal membranes**. In the bitch and most litter-bearing species, this occurs concomitantly with stage 2 as each neonate is delivered and for a period just after the last neonate is produced. This process lasts about 5 to 15 minutes after delivery of each neonate.

Dystocia

Guidelines for recognizing dystocia (difficult birth) include strong continual contractions for 30 minutes without progress; weak, infrequent contractions for 2 hours without progress; a prolonged interval between pups; and a "stuck" puppy because of malpositioning or large size. Approximately 60% of puppies come out in the anterior presentation, with the forelegs and the head first. The other 40% come out in the posterior presentation, with the hind limbs first. Presentation with the hindquarters first and the hind limbs folded back against the body is called *breech presentation*. Professional assistance or cesarean section is required if the pup gets stuck. Uterine inertia, due either to inherent breed factors or from prolonged parturition, is also an important cause of dystocia. Prompt veterinary consultation and examination is warranted if birthing is not progressing normally.

Ultrasonography can be used to assess fetal viability at any point, but radiography is the only reliable method for accurately determining the number of pups in utero, their relative sizes, and their positions.

Feline Reproduction

See the Comparative General and Reproduction Summary tables (Tables 10.5 and 10.6).

Estrous Cycle

The estrous cycle of the cat is distinctly different than other species, although it shares the same phases as dogs: prophase, estrus, diestrus, and anestrus. Queens have two distinct factors that affect their cycles. They are photoperiod dependent and are induced ovulators. Queens are long-day breeders, meaning light stimulates the pineal gland, and there is a reduction in melatonin. This allows for increased hypothalamic activity, thus stimulating the gonadotropins, which drive the estrous cycle.

> **TECHNICIAN NOTE**
>
> Queens are long-photoperiod breeders, and ovulation is induced by copulation.

Proestrus is a very short part of the cycle and is not always noted by owners. It is a time of increasing estrogen and behavior by the queen. Most of these behaviors are head and neck rubbing on objects. The queen will not accept the male at this time. It lasts from day 0 to 2 days.

Estrus is longer and more easily recognized than proestrus. The queen often has increased vocalization, and she may roll, demonstrate lordosis, and tread in place. This behavior intensifies with handling. Anorexia and urine spraying may occur, and no vulvar discharge is evident. Owners who have not had the experience of observing estrus behavior in cats may think it is abnormal and seek veterinary assistance for their seemingly distressed pet. Estrus can last from 2 to 19 days, with an average of about 8 to 9 days. The outcome of estrus depends upon coital contact and ovulation. The possible outcomes of estrus when breeding occurs are pregnancy (CL formed), nonpregnancy (CL formed), and no ovulation (no CL). Although mating occurs, ovulation is not always induced. If no ovulation occurs after breeding or if there is no breeding, the CL is not formed and progesterone is not produced. The queen will return to estrus in about 3 to 14 days. If ovulation occurs, but there is no pregnancy, the CL is maintained for about 5 to 6 weeks.

Diestrus refers to the phase after estrus where ovulation does occur and progesterone levels are increased. It can occur with or without pregnancy, and its time is different in either physiologic state. The act of copulation stimulates LH surges in the pituitary to cause ovulation. Greater LH peaks are caused with greater duration and frequency of mating. LH is released within minutes of copulation and lasts up to 24 hours. However, less than 50% of queens ovulate after a single mating. If ovulation does occur without

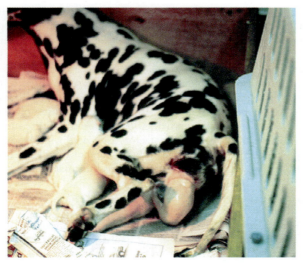

• **Fig. 10.9** A puppy delivered during a normal canine parturition.

TABLE 10.5 Reproductive Terminology for Species, Age, Sex, and Birthing

Species	Immature	Age at Puberty	Female Mature	Female Neutered	Male Mature	Male Neutered	Birthing
Canine: dog	Puppy, pup	7–12 months	Bitch, dam	Ovariectomized, spayed	Dog, stud	Castrated, neutered	Whelping
Feline: cat	Kitten	4–12 months Female 5–6 lb	Queen	Ovariectomized, spayed	Tom	Castrated, neutered	Queening
Equine: horse	Foal 0–6 months Weanling 6–12 months Yearling 1–2 years	Filly 1–2 years Colt 3 years	Mare, filly 0–2 years	Ovariectomized, spayed Uterus rarely removed	Stallion, stud Colt less than 3 years	Gelding	Foaling
Bovine: cow	Calf	10–12 months, 50%–60% adult weight	Cow, heifer less than 2 years old		Bull	Steer, ox	Calving
Porcine: pig, swine	Piglet	6–7 months	Sow Preparous—gilt	Spayed, yelt	Boar	Barrow	Farrowing
Ovine: sheep	Lamb	5–12 months 60%–70% adult weight	Ewe		Ram	Wether	Lambing
Caprine: goat	Kid	3–7 months Greater than 40% adult weight	Doe		Buck	Wether	Kidding
Camelid: llama, alpaca	Cria	10–12 months 65% adult weight	Female, hembra dam		Male, macho, stallion		Unpacking

TABLE 10.6 Reproductive Cycle Characteristics for Common Domestic Species

Species	Cycle Type	Cycle Length	Estrus Length	Ovulation	Best Time to Breed	First Postpartum Estrus	Gestation
Canine	Monoestrous all year	6 months (range 4–12 months)	9 days (range 3–21 days)	2 days after luteinizing hormone (LH) peak	2 days after ovulation	4–5 months	63 days from day of ovulation
Feline	Seasonally polyestrous spring to fall	14–19 days (range 4–30 days)	10 days	Induced 24–48 hours post breeding	Daily from day 2 of estrus	4–6 weeks	63 days (range 58–70 days)
Equine	Seasonally polyestrous spring to fall	21 days (range 19–23 days)	5–7 days	1–2 days before end of estrus	Last days of estrus before ovulation	9 days (range 4–14 days)	330 345 days (11 months)
Bovine	Polyestrous all year	21 days (range 18–24 days)	18 hours (range 6–24 hours)	10–12 hours after estrus	Midestrus to 6 hours after end	20–60 days	279–283 days (9 months)
Porcine	Polyestrous all year	21 days (range 19–23 days)	40–60 hours	40 hours after start of estrus	Daily during estrus	4–10 days after weaning	112–115 days
Ovine	Seasonally polyestrous fall to winter	17 days (range 14–20 days)	36 hours	24–30 hours after start of estrus	18–20 hours after start of estrus	Next fall	145–152 days
Caprine	Seasonally polyestrous fall to winter	21 days	24–48 hours	24–30 hours after start of estrus	Daily during estrus	Next fall	145–152 days
Camelid: llama, alpaca	Polyestrous	NA	2–8 days Up to 36 days	Induced	When large follicle is present	15–20 days	340–350 days

conception, then the diestral phase will last about 40 days. If pregnancy occurs, diestrus/gestation will last about 60 to 63 days. Progesterone is the hormone of dominance, and levels above 2 ng/mL are suggestive of functional luteal tissue. Progesterone from corpora lutea (plural of corpus luteum) increases 2 to 3 days after breeding and peaks between 21 and 30 days. By day 45, the placenta produces progesterone, which decreases near parturition. If the queen did not achieve ovulation during estrus, estrus will end without entrance to diestrus. This period has been termed postestrus. Since there is no CL formation, metestrus is a poor term. This phase lasts about 8 to 10 days and represents a time where the previous group of follicles regress and another will start to back up. The queen will then enter proestrus, and the process will begin anew.

> **TECHNICIAN NOTE**
>
> Fertilization of oocytes occurs in the oviduct—*not* in the uterus for all species covered in this chapter. Implementation likewise occurs in uterine structures.

Gestation

Fertilization in the queen occurs in the oviducts, and the fertilized eggs then migrate to the uterine horns, where they implant. The type of placentation is zonary endotheliochorial, as in other carnivores (see Table 10.2). The fetal heartbeat is detectable with the use of ultrasonography at approximately day 16. The range of gestation may vary because of multiple breeding and because ovulation may not occur when suspected. When parturition occurs before day 60 of gestation, the fetuses are considered premature and generally do not survive.

Observable signs of pregnancy include increased size of the teats by weeks 2 to 3 and increased mammary enlargement throughout term. Weight gain is obvious by mid-gestation and depends on the age of the queen, previous litters, and the size of the litters. Pregnancy can be diagnosed by abdominal palpation of the uterus about 18 days after fertilization. By days 32 to 35, the amniotic vesicles coalesce and are no longer individually discernible.

Ultrasonography provides clear results, starting at day 15, and can be used through to term. Radiographic diagnosis is possible from day 40 until term and is most useful for fetal counts around 60 days.

In the pregnant queen, concentrations of free estrogen increase before parturition, sensitizing the uterus to the effects of oxytocin. Prolactin is increased during the last half of gestation, and a significant increase is seen 3 days before parturition. It remains increased during lactation. Relaxin is produced by the fetoplacental unit and is responsible for relaxing the pelvic connective tissue before parturition. Concentrations are detectable by day 25 of pregnancy and plateau at approximately day 35. PGF2alpha is secreted by many tissues and both sustains homeostatic function and is a mediator of inflammatory reactions. The placenta and endometrium are major sources within the reproductive tract. Concentrations of PGF2alpha start to rise at day 30 of gestation and plateau at day 45. PGF2alpha concentrations increase greatly before delivery and improve uterine contractility at term. PGF2alpha has been used to induce abortion in queens.

Parturition

Queens usually build nests. Parturition can last from a couple of hours to over a day with survival of the fetuses. Queens can return to estrus and get pregnant while nursing a litter of kittens.

Stage I begins with uterine contractions without abdominal contractions. Decreased general activity is seen, with behavioral changes, including the queen becoming more or less social. Fetal movements are increased, lactational secretion is evident, and relaxation around the perineal area occurs. Stage I ends when the chorioallantois membrane ruptures. Stage II is when fetuses are delivered. Stage III is when the placenta has passed. Uterine size returns to normal rapidly, but re-epithelialization of the endometrium takes a few weeks. After parturition, the queen enters anestrus, depending on the time of year.

Dystocia

This is uncommon in the queen, and most cases occur in purebreds. The queen is the only animal commonly seen in a veterinary practice that can assist itself during dystocia. If the fetus is exposed through the vulva, she grasps the membranes or the fetus with her teeth and pulls. At the same time, she pushes with uterine and abdominal contractions. Fetal causes of dystocia are large fetus size, lateral deviation of the head, and breech presentation. Dystocia can often be managed successfully but takes longer. Delayed delivery can result in fetal death. Maternal causes of dystocia include uterine torsion, primary and secondary uterine inertia, and small pelvic size, often resulting from poor nutrition or an extremely young age. Radiographs taken within a few days of delivery can determine the number of fetuses and their presentations. If the most posterior fetus is positioned properly, oxytocin (2 international units [IU] intramuscularly, per cat) can be administered and repeated in 20 to 30 minutes. A cesarean section should be considered if parturition does not progress within a reasonably short time or if the queen and/or the fetus is distressed.

Equine Reproduction

See the Comparative General and Reproduction Summary tables (Tables 10.5 and 10.6).

Estrous Cycle

Horses are long-day breeders—estrus occurs with lengthening photoperiod. The peak of estrus activity occurs near June 21 (the longest day of the year), and the least activity occurs near December 21 (the shortest day of the year). This is mediated by decreased melatonin secretion from the pineal gland in response to decreased darkness (increased light).

Puberty occurs at age 1 to 2 years. Severe stress, including that caused by poor nutrition and heavy workloads, can stop normal estrous cycling in females. Fillies younger than 3 years have an increased abortion rate of up to 50%.

Estrus

Behavioral signs of estrus include frequent urination; a raised tail; winking of the vulva, exposing the clitoris; decreased kicking; forward ear position; and leaning toward the stallion. Stallion receptivity and allowing the stallion to mount would be a cardinal sign of estrus. The ear position of horses is a good indicator of disposition and attitude.

A stallion exhibits the *flehmen response* when he approaches a mare in heat. He curls his upper lip, exposing his vomeronasal organ to the female's pheromones (Fig. 10.10). Various methods are used to tease mares to check for heat. Teasing is the term used to expose a mare to a stallion to assess her behavior and subsequent stage of the estrous cycle. The mare can be held outside the

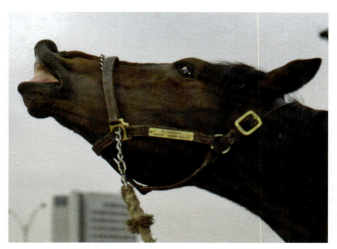

• **Fig. 10.10** Flehmen response of a stallion.

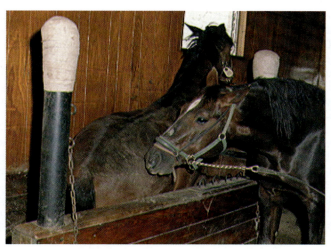

• **Fig. 10.12** Stallion *(right)* teasing a mare *(left)* in stocks.

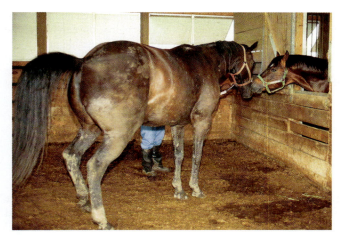

• **Fig. 10.11** Stallion *(right)* teasing a mare *(left)* through a Dutch doorway.

stallion's stall, or the stallion can be held outside the mare's stall. The stallion can be allowed inside the teasing stall, or he can be walked through the mare's field (Figs. 10.11 and 10.12). Inability to control the stallion may rule out some of these methods. Another option to decrease the risk of injury to horses and people is to use a pony stallion. A teasing system that includes vocalization, sight, smell, and physical contact of the stallion and mare will give the best results.

Estrus is about 5 to 7 days in the mare and is dominated by estrogen and is a time of follicular growth. Compared with other species, a mare's follicles grow to a much greater extent, ranging from 35 to 50 mm, with up to 60 mm not uncommon or necessarily pathologic. The mare will ovulate during estrus about 48 hours before the end of behavioral estrus. Ovulation is different in the mare due to its inverted ovarian structure. All ovulations occur via a point called the ovulatory fossa, as opposed to "surface ruptures," possibly seen in species like cattle.

Diestrus

Signs of diestrus when the mare is out of heat may include clamping or swishing of the tail; increased kicking, striking, and biting; keeping the ears back, and moving away from the stallion. These behaviors might even be seen in maiden mares in heat, in recently foaled mares, and if an overly aggressive teaser is used. Diestrus

is dominated by the presence of progesterone and lasts about 14 to 17 days. It ends if there is no establishment of pregnancy with luteolysis. Luteolysis is caused by PGF2alpha, which is secreted by the uterus.

> **TECHNICIAN NOTE**
>
> The flehmen response occurs when a stallion curls the upper lip, exposing the vomeronasal organ inside the nose so that it is easier for the him to smell the pheromones from the mare.

The mare does not really have the phases of proestrus or metestrus like some other species. The mare's estrous cycle is different, mainly in that it has a much longer estrus phase than other species. Some other aspects that affect breeding management strategies are described below.

Ovulation can occur with no obvious signs of heat, particularly in mares that have recently foaled, maiden mares, and mares being teased with an aggressive teaser. It is also common for mares to show signs of heat without being in physiological estrus. This occurs primarily in late winter, early spring, or late fall. Estrus behavior is a submissive behavior and can also be expressed from mare to mare as part of their social strata.

Twin ovulations occur about 18% of the time in equines. It is a genetic trait, and the rate is higher in some families of horses. Usually one of the twin fetuses dies, so the live birth of twins is rare.

Variability in the length of the estrous cycle and estrus makes predicting the exact time of ovulation difficult. Fertility is highest within 12 hours of ovulation and then decreases rapidly. It is best if sperm are present within the oviduct before ovulation occurs or if the mare is inseminated within 12 hours after ovulation. Sperm usually remain fertile for at least 48 hours, but this is stallion specific. The ovum is mature at ovulation, and fertilization can occur immediately if sperm are present. Ovulation can be induced when a nearly mature follicle is present by using human chorionic gonadotropin (hCG) or deslorelin, a GnRH analog developed for use in equine reproduction.

Once ovulation occurs, the follicle converts to CH and then to CL very rapidly. CL produces progesterone and is fully functional by day 2 of ovulation (8 to 9 days from the start of estrus).

Under normal conditions, the CL would be maintained and continue to produce progesterone until about 14 days after ovulation. The ovaries continue to have follicular activity and occasionally, ovulation occurs 8 to 10 days after the initial ovulation. The cervix should be closed after estrus. If it is not closed, progesterone levels may be low or the cervix may be injured. At 14 days after ovulation, progesterone concentrations begin to decrease. By day 17, the progesterone concentration reaches baseline (<1.0 ng/mL) and the mare returns to heat. If pregnancy is established, the CL continues to produce progesterone for about 60 days.

The breeding season in North America runs from approximately February 1 to July 15. The reason for the early start is that the Thoroughbred registry and other registries have set January 1 as the universal birthdate of all foals. Foals born on or before December 31 are considered yearlings the next day on January 1. The goal is to have foals born in January or February, thus making them the oldest in their age group, but not on or before December 31, which would make them the youngest, only a few days old on their first birthday. The desire to have the mare foal in January or February creates many equine reproductive management problems, because the mares are made to conceive earlier in the year before their peak estrus activity. For example, for a February foaling with an 11-month gestation period, the mare would need to conceive in March.

Mares can be induced into estrus earlier in the year with the use of artificial lighting. The light does not need to be bright or kept on for a long time. The light can be from any type of bulb (incandescent, fluorescent, LED, or mercury vapor). It is the quality of light that is important, not the quantity. Several lighting programs can be used. For example, the flash system turns lights on for a 2-hour window of time between 1:00 AM and 4:00 AM. It requires 60 days for this system to initiate follicular activity and another 30 days for the estrous cycle to become stabilized.

The use of progestogens may shorten the period from follicular development to ovulation. Mares will need to be treated for 10 to 14 days, and this treatment will need to be performed after there has been significant follicular growth. It will not cause a deeply anestrus mare to cycle. Progestogens work only if sufficient follicular activity is present. Administration of hCG will induce ovulation of follicles if sufficient follicular activity is present to permit CL formation. Other hormonal methods of enhancing follicular development have not been very successful. Melatonin has been fed experimentally to mares and has induced earlier cycling activity. However, this program must be initiated 5 months before the breeding season begins, which is not practical. Other hormones have been used to initiate follicular development but have not been successful in maintaining the CL after ovulation. PGF2alpha is effective in bringing a mare into heat only if CL is present on the ovary and is at least 5 days old.

Examination of the Reproductive Tract

Palpation of the mare's reproductive tract via the rectum and examination with ultrasonography are used to determine the stage of the estrous cycle, monitor follicular growth, determine pregnancy, and detect abnormalities. The internal anatomy of the mare is slightly different that other species. Of note, the position of the broad ligament prevents uterine manipulations that are available in the cow. The reproductive tract is freely palpable, including the uterine horns, body, cervix, and both ovaries. The reproductive tract changes dramatically in response to the major hormones of the estrous cycle, estrogen, and progesterone. During estrus there is decreased or very little uterine tone, relaxation of the cervix, and increased follicle size. During diestrus, when progesterone is dominant, uterine tone increases and the cervix tightens up and is quite prominent.

Vulvar conformation is important, and the external vulva is also especially important as it is a primary barrier to infection from external sources. A more vertical orientation decreases the amount of fecal contamination. The dorsal opening of the vulva should be at or below the pubic bone. Abnormal angles of the vulva may allow air and fecal material to enter the vagina, resulting in infection. The surgical repair for this condition is called *Caslick's surgery* or vulvoplasty.

Visual examination of the vagina is done to gain additional information on the estrous status and to help detect the presence of infection or abnormalities. To avoid contamination of the reproductive tract, the area should be prepared and cleaned as described in the section "Female Breeding Soundness Examination" at the end of this chapter. A sterile vaginal speculum, lubricated with sterile lube, is inserted into the vestibule. The speculum is pushed gently upward and forward until the transverse vestibular fold is encountered. Once in contact with the fold, care should be taken to confirm how intact the tissue is. Additional pressure anteriorly and parallel to the ground will get the speculum or gloved hand through this tissue. Once the speculum is in the vagina, the cervix and the vaginal wall are easily visualized with the aid of a flashlight.

> **TECHNICIAN NOTE**
> Think safety first! When working around horses, their hindquarters can be particularly dangerous. Tranquilization should be used, when necessary, to protect both the workers and the animals.

Breeding

Breeding can be done by natural cover or AI. Natural cover may be as simple as putting the mare and the stallion together in a field with handlers in attendance. When handlers are involved, the tail is usually wrapped and the perineal area washed. The male's penis also is also washed. Care is taken to ensure that all products used are nonspermicidal. When AI is used, the tail is wrapped and tied to one side. The area is prepped as described in the section "Breeding Soundness Examination" at the end of this chapter, or by following the inseminator's standard protocol. A syringe is used to fill the AI pipette. The pipette containing the semen is inserted into the vagina and through the cervix by using sterile technique. Then, the semen is deposited directly into the uterus. If "deep" intrauterine insemination is performed, special tubing is passed up the uterine horn to the opening of the oviduct (papilla) and the semen is deposited. This technique is used with frozen semen when sperm numbers are low and/or the semen quality is poor.

Gestation

Pregnancy is dependent on progesterone. Progesterone production is from multiple sources in the mare, including the initial CL from ovulation, the secondary CL, and from other sources. The initial CL lasts about 60 days and the secondary CL from approximately day 37 to day 120 of gestation. Secondary CL are derived from follicles stimulated by *equine chorionic gonadotropin* (eCG). eCG is produced by endometrial cups formed from embryonic cells that migrate from the embryo and invade the uterine lining. eCG was originally named *pregnant mare serum gonadotropin* (PMSG), because that was where it was first identified. It has superovulatory effects in most species but not in the equine. eCG is identical to pituitary LH and is even encoded by the same gene, which explains the luteinizing effect on the secondary ovarian follicles. When progesterone from the primary and secondary CL decreases, placental progestins are sufficient to maintain pregnancy.

Pregnancy diagnosis via ultrasonography is more accurate and can diagnose pregnancy earlier than transrectal palpation. Most portable units provide accurate results from day 12 after ovulation. It is useful to repeat the procedure after a few days in case of a negative result. Ovulations may occur later than anticipated, and it allows a second check for twins. Twins have a poor survival rate during and after gestation. Usually, one of the embryos is removed by pinching, which destroys one embryo and allows the other to develop normally.

Parturition

Parturition normally occurs between 325 and 365 days. The fetus needs to be mature to survive, and techniques to gauge fetal maturity in the horse are lacking. This is a primary reason that induction of parturition is rarely performed in this species. Immature foals often have insufficient surfactant in their lungs, which makes breathing difficult and may result in the death of the foal. If induction is necessary, problems associated with the delivery and foal are high, so referral to a hospital setting is recommended.

There are commercially developed tests available to determine colostrum electrolytes, which may correlate with preparedness for parturition. These test kits are akin to hard water tests for home use and are not always accurate. *Waxing*, or drying of a mammary secretion at the teat orifice, may occur several weeks or days before parturition. It is not a reliable sign of foal maturity or impending parturition.

Udder secretions, or "milk" pH, has been looked at as an indicator of parturition in the horse. A small number of secretions are tested and the pH of these secretions drops from an elevated level approximately 48 hours prior to parturition. In very general terms, udder secretions will have a pH of about 8 and then fall towards 6 prior to delivery. It has been noted that these readings may be less accurate in sick or debilitated patients and maiden mares.

Parturition is rapid and strenuous (Fig. 10.13). For purposes of review, parturition is divided into three stages.

Stage I

This is a preparatory stage that involves fetal movements for proper alignment of the body. This can be seen as maternal restlessness,

pawing, up/down behaviors, and sweating. Timing of this stage is variable and ends with rupture of the chorioallantois.

Stage II

This is the time of fetal expulsion and is characterized by very forceful uterine contractions. This process is very quick, with purposeful progression of delivery of the fetus occurring within 15-minute increments. After the chorioallantois ruptures, if the forefeet and head are not in the vagina, there may be a problem. During checking for proper fetal presentation of a muzzle and two forefeet, it is paramount to detect dystocia as early as possible.

Stage III

This stage of parturition is about expelling the placenta. This commonly occurs within 30 minutes to 3 hours after delivery of the foal. If the placenta is not passed within 3 hours, it is considered retained and veterinary advice should be sought.

After delivery, the mare may be quite defensive of its foal, so care should be taken. The foal should commonly rise within 1 hour of delivery and nurse within 2 hours. The antibody levels of the colostrum should be checked, especially if the mare has been leaking a significant amount before parturition, to determine whether supplementation is needed. Foals do not get IgG transplacentally. They must get it within a few hours of birth from colostrum. Foals commonly have their umbilicus dipped shortly after birth and are checked for a cleft palate and good suckle reflex. Foal IgG levels can be checked from 12 to 24 hours after birth. A simple 1-2-3 rule can be applied when the foal is born. Foals should stand about 1 hour after birth, they should nurse by about 2 hours, and the placenta should pass about 3 hours after birth.

The first postpartum estrus is called *foal heat* and occurs within 18 days of foaling. This heat is generally fertile, and breeding on them helps maintain a foaling interval of 12 months. Waiting until a subsequent heat results in an open season every few years and the economic losses of no foal crop and maintaining the mare. There are hormonal ways to address breeding outside of foal heat that do not lead to a loss of season.

A female is born with all the ova she will ever have. Each time she cycles and as she ages, ova are used up and eventually exhausted. The number of ova in the mare is estimated to be 70,000 to 120,000. When they are all gone, the mare stops cycling but may exhibit signs of heat related to estrogen and progesterone originating from the adrenals.

TECHNICIAN NOTE

Foal heat occurs within 18 days of parturition and is a fertile heat in many mares.

Bovine Reproduction

See the Comparative General and Reproduction Summary tables (Tables 10.5 and 10.6).

General

In the United States and other developed countries, cattle are raised for beef and milk production for the human population. There are specific breeds of cattle that have been developed over hundreds of years that are extremely efficient in their production capability.

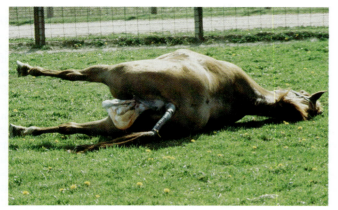

• **Fig. 10.13** Parturition in the mare with fetal head, limbs, and amnionic membrane exposed.

When raising food-producing animals, efficient reproduction is an essential part of an economically viable operation that caters to the consumer at a reasonable cost. Efficient reproduction requires an environment that maximizes comfort and minimizes stress. Optimal nutrition, health management, and excellent record keeping are also essential.

Reproduction

The onset of puberty depends on the breed and level of nutrition. Well-nourished animals reach puberty at a younger age. In general, puberty occurs at around 10 to 12 months and at 50% to 60% of adult body weight. Gestation occurs at roughly 9 months. The desired age at first calving is about 2 years. This means that a heifer needs to be pregnant by 15 months of age or 3 to 5 months after puberty. With dairy cows, a 12-month interval between calving is generally considered ideal.

Estrous Cycle

Hormonal control of the estrous cycle in cows is like that of other species. The estrous cycle lasts about 21 days. It is commonly divided into follicular (proestrus and estrus) and luteal (metestrus and diestrus) stages. Estrus or behavioral heat is short, lasting only 7 to 8 hours. Unobserved estrus is a major cause of reduced reproductive efficiency, which affects the farmer's profitability and the costs of beef and milk for everyone.

Observation of the herd for heat should be performed three times a day by an astute record-keeping observer to minimize the number of unobserved heats. It should be done when the cows are not eating, being milked, or being moved. Cows in heat are generally restless, anxious, walking around, and bellowing. They may go off feed, and milk production may decrease in dairy cows. Pedometers, linked to computers via telemetry, have been used to detect estrus based on increased movement. It is normal for cows to mount other cows. However, only cows that are in heat will stand to be mounted by other cows or a bull. A clear, stringy, vaginal discharge may be present. A blood-tinged vulvar discharge, which is referred to as metestrus, may be noted within 3 days after heat. The terms metestrus and discharge are not necessarily related, as metestrus is related to the time it takes for a CL to form and become functional.

> **TECHNICIAN NOTE**
> Because of cows' very short estrus, barn personnel should check for heat three times a day.

The LH surge occurs at the start of estrus, and ovulation occurs 24 hours later, which is 8 to 12 hours after the cow goes out of standing heat. Oocytes are viable for only about 12 hours after ovulation.

During estrus, increasing levels of estrogen increase uterine tone, making it feel turgid and tightly coiled when palpated. It has been compared with the feel of a double-walled rubber hose. After ovulation, the follicle becomes the *ovulation depression* (OVD) and then the corpus hemorrhagicum (CH) as it fills with blood. On rectal palpation, the CH is sometimes confused with an immature follicle. As the CL forms, the site of ovulation is readily palpable as the crown of the CL. Diestrus is the longest portion of the estrous cycle. The CL will remain functional until day 17. If the cow is not pregnant, the uterus releases PGF2alpha, the CL regresses, and the progesterone level falls.

Breeding

Natural mating by bulls happens very fast. The bull mounts, gives a single thrust forward, and ejaculates. AI should be done before ovulation and 12 hours after standing heat is seen. Poor conception rates, especially with cryopreserved semen, occur particularly if cows are bred too early.

Missed heats that result in cows not being bred are a major problem. Heat detector patches are dye packets that are placed on the dorsal sacral vertebral area of cows. If another cow or a teaser bull mounts the cow, the dye will be visible, even though no one sees the exact time of mounting. Bulls with lateral deviation of the penis and which have been vasectomized to decrease the spread of venereal disease can be used as teaser animals. The bulls have chin ball markers that release easy-to-see chalk or dye after a cow is mounted.

Teaser bulls are used more in beef operations than in dairy operations. Bulls can be hard to handle and pose a danger to workers. This is more of a problem in dairy operations, where there are more workers moving the cows around and involved in milking. Because dairy cows are used to being around people and handled often, performing procedures, such as blood and milk sampling, ultrasonography, and palpation, is easier than in beef animals. This allows the use of other methods of heat detection besides behavior.

With advances in estrous control, AI of beef and dairy cattle has become even more practical. Currently, controlled internal drug release (CIDR) preparations containing progesterone are used. There are different synchronization protocols that are similar, but each generally adds injections before and after the CIDR insertion. The CIDR device is inserted into the cow's vagina, and progesterone is absorbed through the vaginal wall until the CIDR insert is removed in 5 to 7 days and the cow receives an injection of PGF2alpha. AI is performed 60 to 66 hours later, and a second GnRH injection is given. The pregnancy rate is reported to exceed 55%, which significantly increases the number of animals pregnant than using other estrus-detection methods.

> **TECHNICIAN NOTE**
> The number of caruncles is determined by the time of birth. The cow has an average of 75 to 120 caruncles; once damaged or destroyed, they are not replaced.

Gestation

Pregnancy is diagnosed primarily by palpation, but the use of ultrasonography is increasing. Rectal examination is performed after 28 days. Ultrasonography can be performed a few days sooner, with a higher degree of accuracy.

Udder enlargement begins weeks to months before parturition and depends on whether the pregnancy is the first or not. Udder edema may be present and should be treated if severe. Before parturition, the pelvic ligaments relax and the tail head and hips tilt, increasing the size of the pelvic opening. The vulva becomes edematous and elongated. Colostrum, the antibody-rich first secretion of the udder, should be fed to all calves, or they should be allowed to nurse.

Parturition

Stage I

The cervix relaxes to a width of 6 to 10 centimeters about a week before delivery. Uterine contractions begin when the cervix allows a hand to pass through it. The contractions force fetal fluid in the allantoic sac (**allantois**) into the cervix, dilating the lumen. This starts with the *Ferguson reflex*, which is a neuroendocrine cyclic reflex. Dilation of the cervical lumen stimulates oxytocin release, which further dilates the cervix until the fetus passes. Cervical dilation in the bovine with annular cervical rings is slower than in species with longitudinal cervical folds. Abdominal discomfort is present, with restlessness and weight shifting. Cows try to isolate themselves from the rest of the herd. The average length of stage I of labor is 6 hours, which may last up to 24 hours.

Stage II

The fetus is delivered during this stage and it begins with rupture of the chorioallantois membrane (Fig. 10.14). Strong abdominal and uterine contractions occur. Dilation of the cervix by the fetus causes the release of oxytocin, followed by the release of PGF2alpha to aid in uterine contractility. The cow will be up and down. If dilation does not continue between two manual examinations spaced 30 minutes apart, delivery has slowed significantly or stopped, and a cesarean section may be required. The **amnion** may appear at the vulvar opening during this stage. It will rupture instead of being passed around the fetus because of attachments with the chorioallantois membrane. Cows may be sternal or in lateral recumbency at the time of delivery. A standing delivery can occur, but it is rare. The average length of stage II is 2 to 4 hours, but for some cows, it can take up to 6 hours up to 12 hours for heifers.

Stage III

The placenta is passed, and the uterus begins its return to normal. Major myometrial contractions continue for approximately 3 days after parturition. Continued reduction in uterine size resulting from contraction persists for weeks. Nursing stimulates continued periodic release of oxytocin, which aids in uterine contraction. The effectiveness of oxytocin is of greatest clinical significance during the first 24 hours after parturition. After the first 24 hours, the uterus has reduced sensitization to estrogen, and oxytocin does not have the same clinical effectiveness as when estrogen is present. PGF2alpha is more effective than oxytocin after 24 hours.

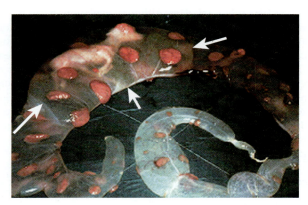

• **Fig. 10.14** A bovine fetus is visible within the amnion *(arrows)*, which is within the chorioallantois.

Small Ruminant (Sheep And Goat) Reproduction

See the Comparative General and Reproduction Summary tables (Tables 10.5 and 10.6).

Estrous Cycle

Sheep and goats are **seasonally polyestrous**, with cyclic activity occurring from late summer to early winter as the photoperiod shortens. The decreasing photoperiod increases the release of melatonin from the pineal gland in the brain. In these species, melatonin stimulates the release of GnRH. This in turn increases secretion of pituitary FSH and LH, starting the estrous cycle. The estrous cycle consists of four stages: proestrus, estrus, metestrus, and diestrus. The estrous cycle of the ewe is approximately 18 days, while the doe is 21 days. Estrus is the stage when the female is receptive to the male and lasts 12 to 24 hours. Ovulation commonly occurs at the end of estrus or within 24 hours. Diestrus is the longest phase and is dominated by progesterone production from a functional CL. Females stop cycling (anestrus) during spring as the photoperiod lengthens.

Depending on the breeding program, lambs and doelings may be bred during the fall of their first year or held over for breeding as yearlings. There are pros and cons for both systems, and the choice depends on the use of the animals and the preference of the owner. With proper nutrition and parasite control, early breeding does not have major adverse effects. Lambs and doelings bred in the fall of their first year generally have earlier and higher lifetime production levels compared with those first bred as yearlings. The cost of maintaining weanlings for the first year with no return on investment is a big incentive for early breeding programs.

> **TECHNICIAN NOTE**
>
> Breeding sheep and goats in the fall of their first year as weanlings can be an economically sound practice, provided that good nutrition and parasite control have been ensured.

Body condition scores (BCSs) should be noted before breeding, and those with scores lower than 2.5 on a scale of 1 to 5, with 5 being "overconditioned," should be flushed. Flushing and feeding a higher level of nutrition before breeding increases the number of oocytes and results in multiple births. Flushing females with BCSs greater than 2.5 does not increase production. Females with BCSs greater than 3.5 are overweight, which may decrease their reproductive success primarily by increasing the rate of dystocia caused by large fetuses and the occurrence of metabolic diseases, such as pregnancy toxemia and milk fever.

Signs of estrus in sheep and goats include a raised tail with frequent flicking from side to side. The vulva and surrounding area become slightly swollen and hyperemic (red). The females will seek out males and urinate more often in their presence.

Both species respond to male pheromones, which can shorten anestrus by a week or more. Bucks have scent glands, found around the base of the horn, that produce a very pungent odor. The urine is also a source of pheromones. Bucks urinate on their hind limbs, increasing their appeal for females.

Breeding

Breeding occurs toward the end of estrus. If bred naturally, semen deposited at the beginning of heat will still be capable of fertilizing the oocyte after ovulation. Mating behavior of rams and bucks is short and fast. It includes pawing at the side, a flehmen response, mounting, one or two thrusts forward, and ejaculation. A marking harness on the male helps detect which females have been bred. The harness positions a crayon between the forelimbs. When the male mounts, he leaves a mark on the female's back, showing that she is in heat and has been bred (Fig. 10.15). Vasectomized males wearing harnesses are often used as part of an AI breeding program to indicate which females are in heat and ready to be inseminated.

Use of intravaginal CIDR inserts that release progesterone allows estrus synchronization. Treated females will come into estrus within 2 to 3 days of removing the CIDR inserts.

Pregnancy Detection

Pregnancy can be determined by changing the marking chalk color on the ram and noting which ewes do not return to estrus. Ultrasonography can be used to determine pregnancy and provides the added advantage of determining the number of fetuses. This is helpful when determining the nutritional needs of each female and of the flock or herd. Ultrasonography is performed rectally at 25 days and transabdominal examination at 35 days or later in gestation.

Gestation

Pregnancy establishment and maintenance is based upon progesterone secretion and the embryonic signals to the dam. This signal is through the secretion of a product called interferon-tau. The interferon causes changes in the uterus of the dam, so that it does not produce PGF2alpha and kill the CL.

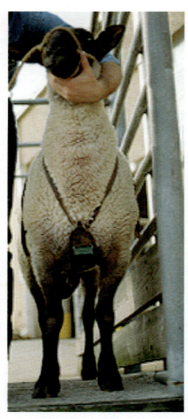

• **Fig. 10.15** A ram fitted with a marking harness to detect estrus.

The ewe and doe have similar lengths of gestation. The doe is about 150 days and the ewe 152. Although progesterone is needed for maintenance of pregnancy, the doe and ewe achieve this differently. The doe uses the original CL for progesterone production for the entire gestation. The ewe uses the original CL but then shifts to a placental-fetal interaction for progesterone production in later gestation.

Abortion rates in sheep and goats are generally low. Noninfectious causes include plant toxins, dietary deficiencies, and certain drugs. Major infectious causes include leptospirosis, toxoplasmosis, and *Chlamydophila* (formerly *Chlamydia*) *abortus* infection and *Campylobacter* spp.

Camelid Reproduction

See the Comparative General and Reproduction Summary tables (Tables 10.5 and 10.6).

Breeding

Waves of developing ovarian follicles start to occur at age 10 to 12 months, when the female reaches puberty. Puberty can be associated with seasonality, but in North America, this does not seem to occur. This is likely due to the nutritional quality of farm-raised operations in this country. One follicle becomes dominant every 12 to 14 days and will grow from 4 to 5 mm to a mature size of 7 to 12 mm in the last 3 to 6 days of development. The dominant follicle remains for 2 to 8 days or until mating. Like the cat, the biggest difference in estrous cycles is that ovulation is induced by copulation in camelids. If mating does not occur, the follicle regresses and another follicle becomes dominant. CL is not formed, and progesterone is not produced unless copulation occurs.

The male can produce sperm at age 10 to 12 months; however, preputial adhesions prevent erection and copulation until age 18 to 30 months. Llamas generally reach sexual maturity by age 30 months. It tends to occur slightly later in alpacas.

Females in heat will adopt a position of sternal recumbency ("kushing") and allow breeding shortly after a male is introduced. While mounting, the male will typically begin making an "orgling" sound. This may be a neural stimulus for LH release and ovulation. The male llama has also been shown to have a "conception factor" present in the semen. This factor, the act of copulation, and the auditory cues all contribute to successful ovulation in the female camelid.

Gestation

Gestation lasts about 350 days. Although ovulations occur equally from both ovaries, pregnancies occur primarily in the left horn. Pregnancy is dependent on a functional CL. The range of embryonic loss is 10% to 50%, which is higher than in most domestic species. Most of the losses occur within the first 60 days. After the first 2 months, the rate of abortion drops to about 5%. Although twin ovulations may occur, delivery of twins is rare. Infectious causes of abortion as in sheep and goats include leptospirosis, toxoplasmosis, and *C. abortus* infection.

Parturition

Stage I takes about 1 to 2 hours. Stage II, with expulsion of the fetus, takes 20 to 30 minutes. Stage III, including expulsion of the placenta, takes 1 to 4 hours. If the placenta is not passed within 6 hours, it is assumed to be retained, and treatment with oxytocin

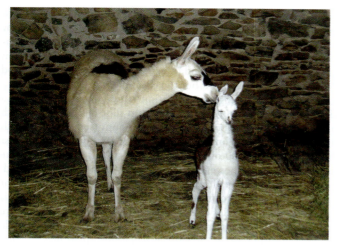

• **Fig. 10.16** Mother llama and her 1-day-old cria.

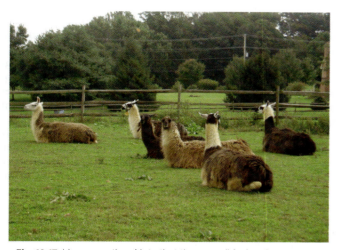

• **Fig. 10.17** Llamas resting. Note that they are all facing the same way.

is indicated. The placenta should not be removed manually. Cria (young animals), like other grazing species, are up and running with the herd within 1 hour of birth (Figs. 10.16 and 10.17).

Early postpartum rebreeding should be done shortly after the female becomes receptive at about 20 days after parturition. If the female is not rebred then, she may stop cycling because of high milk production or production of a hormone that prevents follicular maturation.

> **TECHNICIAN NOTE**
>
> Camelids, including alpacas and llamas, are induced ovulators. They do not cycle regularly; rather, copulation induces ovulation.

Breeding Soundness Examination of the Male

General

The purpose of a breeding soundness examination (BSE) in males is to determine potential fertility without breeding. The

examination includes physical reproductive characteristics, semen quality, attitude, disposition, libido, and any system abnormalities that could influence reproductive performance. An example of a system abnormality is lack of hind limb soundness.

The examination begins with identification of the animal. This should be done with permanent markers such as microchips, tattoos, brands, or color markings, if unique. Identification is followed by obtaining a complete history, with emphasis on reproductive performance. The history includes age, previous injuries or illnesses, temperament, reason for the BSE, previous fertility, method of breeding, number of females serviced, number of matings per week, and the results of any previous BSEs. Complete physical examination, including detailed examination of external genitalia, is done. The scrotum and both testes are examined for symmetry, normal epididymis, and vas deferens, and absence of palpable abnormalities. The testicular or scrotal size should be recorded, because there is a link between size and sperm production. Scrotal circumference is used in ruminants and testicular size in other species.

The internal genitalia are examined in large animals. The bull and stallion have seminal vesicles, a prostate, and a bulbourethral gland. The seminal vesicles are important in the bull and the stallion, because these parts are responsible for most clinical problems in these species. The dog only has a prostate, which is palpated rectally. The internal inguinal rings in stallions and bulls are examined during rectal examination. If possible, the male's libido should be assessed.

> **TECHNICIAN NOTE**
>
> The purpose of a breeding soundness examination (BSE) in males is to determine potential fertility without breeding. Males of all species should have a BSE before they are used for breeding.

When semen is being collected by using an artificial vagina, a condom, or electroejaculation, the male should be observed for a time, noting any difficulty in protrusion of the penis, obtaining an erection, and ejaculating. Electroejaculation can be used in boars and stallions but is usually not used, because these animals require general anesthesia to undergo this procedure. Electroejaculation is commonly done in bulls, rams, and bucks. The process is performed by placing a probe in the rectum of the animal and applying the minimum electrical current in pulses needed (Fig. 10.18) to produce an erection and ejaculation. The penis is cleaned before semen collection from the stallion; however, no cleaning is performed in other domestic species. The penis and the prepuce should be checked to ensure that they appear normal. A warm water jacket should be used on the artificial vagina when collecting semen from bulls, rams, boars, and stallions (Fig. 10.19). When an artificial vagina is used to collect semen from a dog, no water jacket is required, because stimulation and ejaculation are not dependent on the use of the artificial vagina.

> **TECHNICIAN NOTE**
>
> In an examination of semen, rapid, forward progressive movement indicates excellent motility. A finding of 70% or more of progressively motile sperm is desirable.

Semen Analysis

Semen is examined first for motility. A small drop of semen is placed on a warm slide and coverslip using a warm pipet and

- Embryo transfer
- Superovulation to increase ovum from desired females
- Embryo cryopreservation
- Embryo sexing
- Intracytoplasmic sperm injection (ICSI)
- Follicular aspiration/ovum pick-up

Recommended Readings

Carleton C, ed. *Blackwell's Five Minute Veterinary Consults: Clinical Companion—Equine Theriogenology*. New York: Williams & Wilkins; 2008.

Ettinger SJ, Feldman EC, eds. *Textbook of Veterinary Internal Medicine*. St. Louis, MO: Saunders; 2009.

Root Kustritz MV. *The Practical Veterinarian: Small Animal Theriogenology*. St. Louis, MO: Butterworth-Heinemann; 2003.

Root Kustritz MV. *Clinical Canine and Feline Reproduction: Evidence-Based Answers*. Ames, IA: Wiley-Blackwell; 2010.

Vet Partners. http://www.veterinarypartner.com/.

Veterinary Information Network (VIN). https://www.vin.com/vin/.

Youngquist RS, Threlfall WR, eds. *Current Therapy in Large Animal Theriogenology*. St. Louis, MO: Saunders; 2007.

11

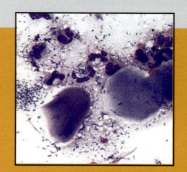

Hematology and Cytology

ORETA M. SAMPLES

CHAPTER OUTLINE

LEARNING OBJECTIVES

When you have completed this chapter, you will be able to:

1. Pronounce, define, and spell all key terms in this chapter.
2. Describe proper collection techniques, handling of blood samples, and components of a complete blood count (CBC).
3. Describe the advantages, disadvantages, and capabilities of automated hematology analyzers.
4. Do the following regarding blood counts:
    • Compare and contrast procedures used to determine red blood cell (RBC) mass (packed cell volume [PCV], hematocrit [HCT], hemoglobin, and RBC count) and discuss the causes and significance of abnormal values.
    • Describe methods used to calculate RBC indices and RBC distribution width (RDW) and discuss the causes and significance of abnormal values.
    • Describe methods used to determine plasma protein concentration and discuss the causes and significance of abnormal values.
    • Describe methods used to determine the white blood cell (WBC) count and the platelet count.
5. Do the following regarding blood smears:
    • Describe the technique used to prepare a stained blood smear, list factors that influence smear quality, and discuss the evaluation process.
    • Describe normal and abnormal morphology of RBCs, WBCs, and platelets in each species as they appear on a blood smear.

• Discuss the causes and significance of RBC, WBC, and platelet abnormalities commonly observed on a blood smear.
• Describe the procedure used to perform a differential WBC count and calculate absolute values.
6. Do the following regarding coagulation testing:
    • Explain normal primary and secondary hemostasis, including intrinsic, extrinsic, and common pathways.
    • Discuss bleeding time, activated clotting time (ACT), activated partial thromboplastin time (APTT), and prothrombin time (PT), and the uses and significance of each.
    • Discuss tests used to evaluate fibrinolysis, including fibrin(ogen) degradation products (FDPs), D-dimer tests, and fibrinogen tests.
7. Do the following regarding cytology:
    • Explain uses for and limitations of cytology.
    • Describe procedures used to evaluate the cytology of solid tissue masses, enlarged organs, thoracic and abdominal effusions, and synovial fluid.
    • Discuss procedures used to submit cytology samples to a reference laboratory.
    • Describe collection and preparation of otic cytology samples and identify common findings on normal and abnormal otic cytology preparations.

KEY TERMS

Activated clotting (coagulation) time (ACT)
Activated partial thromboplastin time (APTT)
Agglutination
Anisocytosis
Band neutrophil
Basophil
Blood smears
Coagulation cascade
Complete blood count (CBC)
Cytology
D-dimers
Eosinophils
Fibrin(ogen) degradation products (FDP)
Fibrinolysis
Hematocrit (HCT)
Hemocytometer
Hemoglobin
Hemostasis
Heterophil
Left shift
Lymphocyte
Mast cells
Mean corpuscular hemoglobin concentration (MCHC)

Mean corpuscular hemoglobin (MCH)
Mean corpuscular volume (MCV)
Monocyte
Neoplastic lymphocytes
Neutrophils
Packed cell volume (PCV)
Pelger-Huet anomaly
Plasmin
Platelets (thrombocytes)
Prothrombin time (PT)
Reactive lymphocytes
Red cell distribution width (RDW)
RBC indices
Red blood cells (also called *erythrocytes*)
Refractometer
Reticulocyte
Rouleaux formations
Segmented neutrophil
Specific gravity
Spherocytes
Toxic changes
White blood cells (also called *leukocytes*)

Introduction

Laboratory testing is an integral component of patient evaluation to assess health at a time of crisis, establish a diagnosis, and monitor response to treatment. Inaccurate results may lead to an incorrect diagnosis, unnecessary testing, and ineffective, often costly treatment; it is therefore critical for laboratory results to be accurate. Whether samples are submitted to a reference laboratory or analyzed within the practice, veterinary technicians should be knowledgeable about proper collection, handling, and processing of samples, along with other sample requirements, and the routine maintenance, calibration, and quality control procedures necessary for each instrument being used. A basic understanding of the principles of each instrument is helpful in knowing how to determine when an instrument is not functioning properly, and in troubleshooting, and recognizing when sample quality or pathologic abnormalities might interfere with the determination of accurate results.

If samples are sent to a reference laboratory, the veterinary technician should contact the reference laboratory for information about proper specimen collection, storage, and submission requirements prior to the collection process. Veterinary reference laboratories are recommended over human reference laboratories, because veterinary reference laboratories have instruments specifically designed and calibrated for processing blood from a variety of animal species and are staffed by technicians and pathologists with the appropriate expertise. Accurate interpretation of laboratory results requires species-specific reference levels, ideally determined by the laboratory performing the test, because results may vary depending on the instrument and the reagents used.

The **complete blood count** (CBC) is one of the most commonly performed laboratory tests, because it provides information about **red blood cells** (RBCs or *erythrocytes*), **white blood cells** (WBCs or *leukocytes*), **platelets (thrombocytes)**, and plasma protein concentration, all components that can be helpful in determining health or disease and in monitoring therapeutic response. **Cytology**, the study

of cells, is frequently used to evaluate superficial masses, abnormal tissues, and fluid accumulation due to relative inexpensive timely turn around. This chapter will focus on techniques used for the CBC and cytology as points of interest that a veterinary technician should be familiar with rather than on strict interpretation of blood smear evaluation, although common abnormalities are included.

Hematology

Complete Blood Count

Blood samples necessary for a CBC are collected in a tube containing an anticoagulant. The preferred anticoagulant for mammals and most nonmammalian species is ethylenediaminetetraacetic acid (EDTA), which prevents clotting by binding calcium. EDTA preserves cell morphology unless samples are stored for extended periods, at which time cells may begin to break down. There are other anticoagulants that may be used; for some nonmammalian species, heparin is the preferred anticoagulant, because EDTA causes RBC lysis (cell rupture). However, heparin typically causes artifacts in cell morphology and may lead to false interpretations of blood smear results. For those species, it is recommended that a blood smear be made from a drop of whole, nonanticoagulated blood at the time of sampling and stained for examination. All samples should be clearly labeled with an identification number or the name of the animal and the date and time of collection. Other anticoagulants are utilized for specific tests and are directed by universally recognized cap colors (Table 1).

Commercially available lavender-top blood collection tubes contain EDTA, and green-top tubes contain heparin; both are available in various sizes. The 2-mL blood collection tubes are used most, often because this volume is sufficient for a CBC and smear preparation. It is important to fill the collection tubes with the correct volume of blood, because overfilling or underfilling can cause erroneous results caused by incorrect ratio of blood to

TABLE 11.1	Color Designation of Anticoagulants	
Cap Color	**Preservative**	**Usage**
Black	Sodium citrate	Sedimentation rate
Blue (light)	Sodium citrate	Coagulation
Blue (royal)	No additive	Lead
Gold	Gel separator	Chemistries
Gray	Potassium oxalate and sodium fluoride	Blood alcohol and/or glucose
Green	Heparin	Chemistries
Lavender	EDTA	Hematology and A1c
Red	Clot activator	Chemistries
Red/gray	Clot activator	Chemistries
Tan	EDTA	Lead

anticoagulant. Samples should be inspected grossly for small clots before a sample is processed for a CBC and, if clots are present, a new sample should be collected. It is important to gently invert the tube several times after collection to make sure the blood sample thoroughly mixes with the anticoagulant without damage to the blood cells. The tube should be inverted 10–15 times before the blood is processed through an automated hematology analyzer. A microhematocrit tube is also filled for further testing, such as a manual comparative reading of hemoglobin or clotting time, and **blood smears** are made for staining and visualization.

TECHNICIAN NOTE

Blood in ethylenediaminetetraacetic acid (EDTA) tubes should be mixed after collection and before the packed cell volume is determined, the blood smear is made, or the sample is processed through an automated hematology analyzer.

The CBC typically includes a PCV (**packed cell volume**, or **hematocrit** [HCT]), RBC count, **hemoglobin** concentration, **mean corpuscular volume** (MCV), **mean corpuscular hemoglobin concentration** (MCHC), RBC distribution width (RDW), platelet count, WBC count, and WBC differential. Newer instruments with direct laser measurement may include RBC hemoglobin content (CH), hemoglobin content of **reticulocytes** (CHr), corpuscular hemoglobin concentration mean (CHCM), hemoglobin concentration distribution width (HDW), mean cell volume of reticulocytes (MCVr), platelet volume distribution width (PDW), and plateletcrit (PCT). The CBC also may include determination of plasma protein concentration and examination of a blood smear to evaluate cell morphology and perform a manual differential WBC count. It is important to use species-specific reference intervals for interpretation of results, whether they are generated manually or by automated instruments.

Automated Hematology Analyzers

Hematology analyzers designed for processing blood samples from animals are most commonly used in practice settings to count RBCs, WBCs, and platelets; determine hemoglobin

concentration; and calculate **RBC indices**. These instruments also determine cell size and evaluate other cell parameters, such as the granularity of the cytoplasm and the shape of the nucleus for WBCs. Compared with manual methods, thousands of cells are counted, instead of hundreds, making results more accurate and reproducible in a short time. Larger instruments can be loaded with multiple samples, allowing the technician time to perform other tests while the samples are being processed. However, despite the convenience of automatic hematologic measurements, technicians should endeavor to continue to master the manual test procedures that measure hemoglobin and other factors and allow for performance of manual blood cell counts to perform secondary examination of blood components or for confirmatory testing. Manual examination of blood smears also is invaluable in cases of many blood-borne parasites.

PUT INTO PRACTICE

You should strive to become proficient in manual hematological examination before learning the mechanical methods. In times of emergency or in the field, the manual methods will yield quick results that can be confirmed later by automation.

These instruments use light scatter from a focused laser beam, impedance technology, and various staining methods to count and evaluate cells. Cells are directed through a small aperture, and each cell is individually evaluated. With light scatter methods, cells scatter light from a laser beam in different directions and at different angles, depending on the physical properties of the cell. This allows the instrument to count RBCs and determine their size, count WBCs, generate a WBC differential, and count platelets and determine their size. With impedance methods, cells interfere with an electrical current, and the sizes of the cells are proportional to the deflection of the current. Special stains also can be used to further distinguish different populations of cells.

Instrument settings for the size of each cell type are important and may vary depending on the patient species, which is why instruments designed for human samples often do not generate accurate results for veterinary samples. Newer automated hematology analyzers are manufactured with computer software that adjusts for analysis of blood from a variety of animal species. Many of these analyzers are easy to use and provide reliable results, especially for healthy animals with normal CBCs. However, manual evaluation of a blood smear is strongly recommended if the animal is anemic, thrombocytopenic, or leukopenic or exhibiting moderate to marked leukocytosis. Each instrument should be validated by the laboratory for each species being evaluated, and an adequate quality control program that includes regular analysis of commercially available control material should be established by the user. Reference laboratories and those in academic settings often establish criteria for evaluating blood smears as part of the CBC. In some laboratories, all blood smears are evaluated as part of the quality assurance program and because important morphologic changes and some blood-borne parasites are detected only by microscopic examination.

Red Blood Cell Mass Evaluation

PCV (or HCT), RBC count, and hemoglobin concentration are used to evaluate RBC mass, which is an indication of the oxygen-carrying capacity of blood. In veterinary medicine, PCV is the most used parameter to assess RBC mass, because it can be measured manually. Determination of PCV is quick, inexpensive to perform, and often done to assess hydration and to monitor fluid therapy, even if a CBC is not performed.

PCV is the percentage (%) of RBCs in a specific volume of blood. PCV is determined manually by filling a plain microhematocrit tube two-thirds to three-quarters full of EDTA-preserved blood, sealing one end with a sealant clay, and centrifuging the sample in a microhematocrit centrifuge for a specified length of time and speed, according to the manufacturer's recommendations. Longer centrifugation periods may be required for blood samples from cattle, sheep, and goats, because their RBCs are smaller than those from dogs and cats. During centrifugation, RBCs are tightly packed toward the sealed end of the microhematocrit tube. After centrifugation, three components of blood are visible in the microhematocrit tube: (1) a column of packed RBCs at the bottom, (2) a buffy coat layer of WBCs and platelets just above the packed RBCs, and (3) plasma at the top (Fig. 11.1). PCV is determined by using a special wheel or card chart with a grid to measure PCV (Fig. 11.2).

Automated hematology analyzers calculate HCT by multiplying MCV by the RBC count. Although values are determined by different methods, the terms *PCV* and *HCT* often are used interchangeably. They should be numerically similar, and both are accurate indicators of RBC mass. However, errors in determination of HCT and PCV can occur; if the blood collection tube has been inadequately filled, excess anticoagulant will cause RBCs to shrink, falsely decreasing the PCV. When the sample is processed by the automated hematology analyzer, the diluent allows the RBCs to expand to their normal volume; therefore HCT is a more accurate indication of RBC mass. If agglutination of RBCs is noted, as occurs in immune-mediated hemolytic anemia, the RBC count from the automated instrument will be falsely low because of clumping of RBCs. This falsely decreases the HCT that

was calculated using the RBC count. In this case, the manually spun PCV is a more accurate indication of RBC mass.

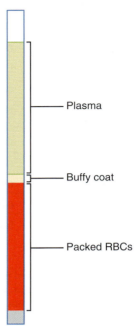

• **Fig. 11.1** Microhematocrit tube after centrifugation. The plasma is in the upper portion, and packed red blood cells (RBCs) are in the lower portion and are separated by the buffy coat, containing white blood cells (WBCs) and platelets. (Illustrated by Tim Vojt, Biomedical Media, The Ohio State University College of Veterinary Medicine [OSU-CVM]. Copyright The Ohio State University.)

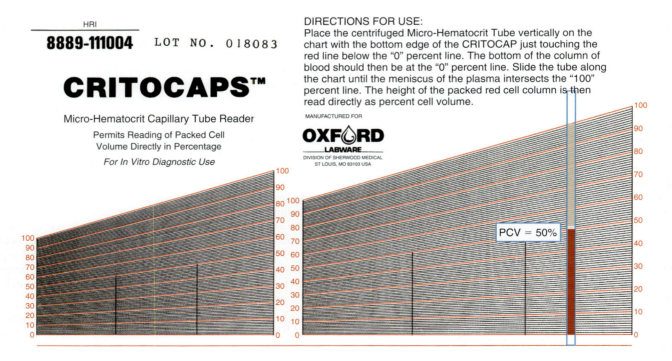

• **Fig. 11.2** A card with a grid can be used to determine packed cell volume (PCV) from a centrifuged microhematocrit tube by following the instructions indicated on the card. The PCV in this patient is 50%. (Illustration by Tim Vojt, Biomedical Media, OSU-CVM. Copyright The Ohio State University.)

• BOX 11.1 Calculation of RBC Indices

$$MCV(fL) = \frac{HCT\% \times 10}{RBC\ count \times 10^{12}/\mu L}$$

Example: HCT = 42%, RBC count = $6 \times 10^{12}/\mu L$

$$MCV = \frac{42 \times 10}{6} = 70fL$$

$$MCHC\left(\frac{g}{dL}\right) = \frac{Hemoglobin\ g/dL}{HCT\%} \times 100$$

Example: Hemoglobin = $\frac{15g}{dL}$, HCT = 45%

$$MCHC = \frac{15}{45} \times 100 = 33g/dL$$

Red Blood Cell Count

RBCs can be counted accurately by automated instruments using laser or impedance technology. The RBC count is reported as the number of RBCs $\times 10^{12}/L$ (or $\times 10^6/\mu L$). Manual RBC counts are not very accurate compared with automation; however, they should not be discounted, because manual observation may demonstrate abnormal cellular findings that may not otherwise be detected. such as infection by erythrocytic parasites (e.g., *Anaplasma* spp.). Because changes in RBC count usually are proportional to changes in PCV and HCT, most clinicians use PCV and HCT to evaluate RBC mass. However, the RBC count is useful in calculating RBC indices (see later), which aids in classifying anemia and in measuring hemoglobin concentration.

Hemoglobin Concentration

Hemoglobin is the protein in RBCs that carries oxygen from the lungs to tissues. Hemoglobin concentration, reported as grams per deciliter (g/dL), is determined by automated analyzers that employ several different methods. Manual hemoglobin measurement is somewhat subjective and cannot be performed accurately. Changes in hemoglobin concentration usually are proportional to changes in PCV (or HCT). In most species, except camelids (camels, llamas, alpacas, vicunas), PCV (or HCT) divided by 3 is a good estimate of hemoglobin concentration.

Red Blood Cell Indices

MCV is used as an indicator of the average size of RBCs and is reported in femtoliters (fL; $1\ fL = 10^{-15}\ L$). The analyzer measures the volume of each RBC counted and determines the mean volume for the RBC population. MCV also can be calculated from a manually determined PCV and RBC count (Box 11.1), but manual RBC counts are not very accurate. There are marked species differences in MCV. RBCs with normal MCV are called *normocytic*, those with an increased MCV are called *macrocytic,* and those with a decreased MCV are called *microcytic*. MCV often increases in regenerative anemias associated with hemorrhage or hemolysis but usually is normal in nonregenerative anemias associated with inflammation, chronic renal failure, and primary bone marrow disease. MCV may be decreased in iron-deficient anemia resulting from chronic external blood loss.

MCHC is the average amount of hemoglobin in a specific volume of blood and is calculated from the hemoglobin concentration

and HCT as determined by the automated instrument. In most species, MCHC is 32 to 36 g/dL, but in camelids, MCHC ranges from 41 to 45 g/dL. MCHC is increased if there is intravascular hemolysis or in vitro hemolysis associated with sample collection or handling. Lipemia and large numbers of Heinz bodies can interfere with measurement of hemoglobin concentration, resulting in falsely increased MCHC. RBC agglutination may cause a falsely decreased HCT and thus an increased MCHC. If MCHC is increased, it is helpful to examine the plasma to determine whether hemolysis or lipemia is present and to evaluate a blood smear to see whether Heinz bodies or agglutinated RBCs are evident. In the absence of hemolysis, lipemia, or Heinz bodies, an increased MCHC may indicate instrument error, at which time quality control measures should be implemented and a repeat analysis done with a fresh sample. RBCs with normal MCHC are described as *normochromic,* and those with decreased MCHC are referred to as *hypochromic*. RBCs often are normochromic in health and in nonregenerative anemia. Hypochromic RBCs occur in marked regenerative anemia and in some animals with severe iron deficiency.

Mean corpuscular hemoglobin (MCH), the average amount of hemoglobin in each RBC, is reported in picograms. MCH is calculated from the hemoglobin concentration and the RBC count as determined by the automated instrument. Although not used, a low MCH indicates iron deficiency, while a high MCH demonstrates poorly oxygenated blood.

Red Cell Distribution Width

RDW is a mathematical index that describes variation in RBC size or **anisocytosis**. It is the coefficient of variation of RBC size determined by the automated analyzer and calculated by dividing the standard deviation of RBC volume (size) by the MCV. In most species, the distribution of RBC size is that of a Gaussian distribution or bell-shaped curve with a consistent RDW for each particular species. An increased RDW may indicate regenerative anemia or early iron deficiency anemia. This can be visualized as widening of the bell-shaped curve generated by the analyzer or by evaluation of a blood smear for anisocytosis. A decreased RDW is not clinically relevant but should be reported.

Plasma Protein Concentration

Plasma protein concentration can be determined by refractometry of the plasma portion of the spun microhematocrit tube and reported in grams per deciliter (g/dL). Plasma in the microhematocrit tube should be evaluated for clarity and color before plasma protein concentration is determined. Plasma from healthy dogs and cats is clear and colorless, whereas plasma from horses and cows often is clear and light yellow because of dietary differences. Changes in color and clarity may be important indicators of disease and should be reported as part of the CBC.

> **TECHNICIAN NOTE**
>
> Changes in color and clarity of the plasma may be important indicators of disease and should be recorded and reported to clinicians.

The centrifuged microhematocrit tube is carefully broken slightly above the buffy coat, the tube is inverted, and the unbroken end is used to fill the window of a **refractometer** by capillary action with the cover on the window closed. Tapping the end

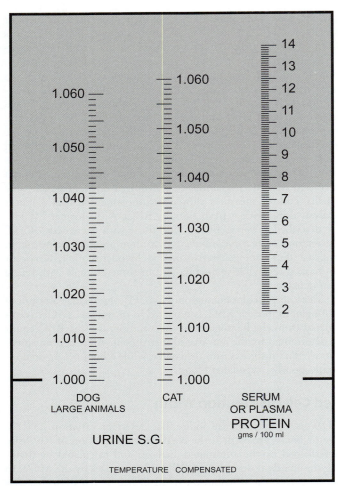

• **Fig. 11.3** Protein concentration is determined by visualizing where the distinction between the darker portion at the top and the lighter portion at the bottom intersects the scale. In this patient, the total protein concentration is 7.5 g/dL. (Illustration by Tim Vojt, Biomedical Media, OSU-CVM. Copyright The Ohio State University.)

of the microhematocrit tube directly on the face of the window may scratch the surface and should be avoided. Plasma protein concentration is determined through the eyepiece by visualizing the intersection, which is the horizontal distinction between the darker stained region at the top and the lighter stained region at the bottom for plasma protein concentration (Fig. 11.3).

Plasma protein concentration determined by refractometry is accurate if the plasma is clear and of normal color for the species. If the plasma is lipemic or excess anticoagulant is present, plasma protein concentration may be falsely increased and should be repeated with a newly drawn sample. Plasma protein concentration also can be falsely increased from marked hyperglycemia or azotemia (increase in blood urea nitrogen [BUN]). Marked hemolysis and bilirubin can falsely increase plasma protein but often, the increase is minimal. Plasma protein concentration usually is slightly higher than serum protein concentration because of the presence of fibrinogen. Plasma fibrinogen concentration sometimes is used as an indicator of inflammation in horses and cattle and can be determined semiquantitatively by using a heat precipitation method (Procedure 11.1) or quantitatively by using coagulation analyzers.

PROCEDURE 11.1

Determination of Fibrinogen by Heat Precipitation

- Fill two microhematocrit tubes 2⁄3 to 3⁄4 full with EDTA-anticoagulated blood.
- Centrifuge both tubes in a microhematocrit centrifuge, according to the manufacturer's recommendations for determination of packed cell volume (PCV).
- Carefully break one microhematocrit tube slightly above the buffy coat and use the unbroken end to fill the prism of a hemocytometer.
- Read the total protein (TP) in grams per deciliter (g/dL) by using the scale for plasma protein concentration.
- Heat the second microhematocrit tube in a 56°C (132.8°F) water bath for 3 minutes to precipitate fibrinogen.
- Recentrifuge the heated microhematocrit; the precipitated fibrinogen will settle just above the buffy coat.
- Carefully break the microhematocrit tube above the buffy coat and determine the TP in g/dL.
- Calculate the fibrinogen concentration:

(TP of unheated microhematocrit tube – TP of heated microhematocrit tube) × 100 = Fibrinogen concentration in mg/dL

White Blood Cell Count

WBCs can be counted manually or by automated instruments or from the examination of buffy coat layer or blood smear. For manual WBC counts, a **hemocytometer** and commercially available reagent such as Leuko-TIC 1:20 "blue" (bioanalytic GmbH, Umrich/Freiburg, Germany) system may be used. A hemocytometer such as the Neubauer hemocytometer is a specialized counting chamber with a surface that contains a pair of etched counting grids and a special weighted, reusable cover glass. The detailed manufacturer's instructions must be followed carefully for accurate results. Briefly, 20 µL of blood is diluted with a fluid, causing RBCs to be lysed; a small volume of diluted blood is added to the hemocytometer by capillary action underneath the coverslip. WBCs are counted in the four large corner squares of the grid; the number of WBCs is multiplied by 50 to determine WBCs/µL (Fig. 11.4). Diminishing the light by lowering the substage condenser may enhance contrast to make it easier to visualize the WBCs. Both grids of the hemocytometer should be filled with the same sample and counted. WBC counts from each grid should be within 10% of each other if the procedure has been performed accurately. If not, the sample should be reloaded and recounted.

TECHNICIAN NOTE

Follow the manufacturer's detailed instructions carefully when using commercially available reagents and a hemocytometer to achieve the most accurate WBC counts by manual methods.

WBC counts determined by automated hematology analyzers often are more accurate and precise than manual WBC counts, because the instrument counts thousands of cells. The WBC count can be estimated by quantitative buffy coat (QBC; Becton Dickinson, Franklin Lakes, NJ) analysis, in which the buffy coat layer is measured in a specialized microhematocrit tube with a float that expands the buffy coat region for optical scanning. The WBC count also can be estimated by evaluation of a stained blood

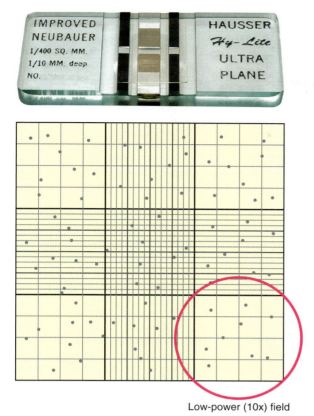

• **Fig. 11.4** An improved Neubauer hemocytometer is shown on the top and the counting chamber is shown at the bottom. The pink circle indicates a corner square, which can be visualized through the ×10 objective. In this patient, 36 cells are seen in the four corner squares and the WBC count is 36 × 50 = 1800/µL. (Illustration by Tim Vojt, Biomedical Media, OSU-CVM. Copyright The Ohio State University.)

Low-power (10x) field

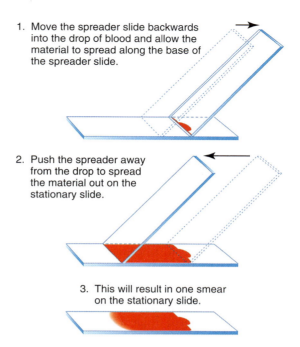

1. Move the spreader slide backwards into the drop of blood and allow the material to spread along the base of the spreader slide.

2. Push the spreader away from the drop to spread the material out on the stationary slide.

3. This will result in one smear on the stationary slide.

• **Fig. 11.5** To create a blood smear, a drop of blood is placed on one end of a glass slide that is held stationary on a flat surface, and a second spreader slide is used to push the drop forward in a smooth, even motion, resulting in a blood smear that is evenly distributed across the stationary slide. (Illustration by Tim Vojt, Biomedical Media, OSU-CVM. Copyright The Ohio State University.)

smear (see below). Species-specific reference levels should be used to interpret the WBC count.

Birds and reptiles have nucleated RBCs (nRBCs); this interferes with WBC counts as determined by some instruments and the manual method described previously for mammalian species. Some newer hematology analyzers can determine WBC counts of birds and reptiles, or WBCs can be determined indirectly using a different reagent system such as Thrombo-TIC or Ery-TIC (bioanalytic GmbH, Umkrich/Freiburg, Germany). Other protocols using methyl violet, phloxine B dye, or Natt and Herrick solution have been described. Because of the amount of blood that can be reasonably collected from small reptiles and/or birds, a stained smear may be needed to perform a manual cell count.

Platelet Count

The platelet count determined by automated hematology analyzers is accurate for most species unless macroplatelets or platelet clumps are present, as occurs most commonly in cats. The number of platelets can be estimated from the blood smear or counted manually by using commercially available reagent systems such as Thrombo-TIC (bioanalytic GmbH, Umkrich/Freiburg, Germany) and a hemocytometer. There are marked species differences in platelet counts.

Preparation of Blood Smears

Microscopic evaluation of a blood smear is an important component of a CBC, because some hematologic abnormalities are recognized only on the blood smear. Examination of the blood smear is an important quality control measure for confirmation of quantitative information obtained from automated hematology analyzers or manual cell counts and for qualitative evaluations for extracellular parasites and so on. The numbers of RBCs, WBCs, and platelets can be estimated from a blood smear, and the morphology of all cell types can be evaluated. Infectious agents and circulating neoplastic cells sometimes can be detected. If samples are being sent to a reference laboratory for analysis, it is recommended that an unstained blood smear be included, especially if a delay in transit is anticipated, to help determine whether any changes are pathologic or caused by sample processing. The sample should be packaged separately from any formaldehyde or formalin-preserved samples. Smears from blood samples should be made immediately after blood is collected for optimal preservation of cell morphology.

Preparation of high-quality blood smears is a technical skill that requires practice. Blood smears should be made with new, clean microscope slides. Most commonly, a small drop of blood is placed close to one end of a microscope slide that is held stationary on a flat surface (Fig. 11.5). A second "spreader" slide is held at a 30- to 45-degree angle in front of the drop of blood and is moved backward to contact the front edge of the drop of blood. A short hesitation allows the blood to flow by capillary action along the edge of the spreader slide before the spreader slide is pushed forward in a smooth, even motion with minimal downward pressure until the end of the stationary slide is reached. This should result in a blood smear that is evenly and thinly distributed across half to three-quarters of the stationary slide. If the drop of blood is too small, the spreader slide is pushed too slowly, or the angle of the spreader slide is too obtuse, the smear will be too thin or too short. If the drop of blood is too large, the spreader slide is pushed too quickly, or the angle of the spreader slide is too acute, the smear may be too thick or too long.

Blood smears should be dried quickly before staining to prevent RBC artifacts. Slides should be labeled at one end with the date and the animal's name or identification number. Ideally, slides should be stained within a few hours. A lapse longer than 48 hours may result in inadequate staining. Unstained smears being sent to a reference laboratory should be stored at room temperature, not in a refrigerator or freezer, because water condensation will damage the cells. All smears should be stored away from formalin fumes and shipped separately from surgical biopsy samples that have been placed in formalin, because formalin vapors inhibit optimal staining. The reference laboratory should be contacted for instructions about how to properly package and ship blood smears to avoid breakage or damage.

Romanowsky-type stains, such as Wright or Wright-Giemsa stain, provide optimal staining but can be labor intensive, require distilled water, and may need frequent filtering. Several commercially available staining procedures that mimic Wright or Wright-Giemsa staining have been described. Diff-Quik (Baxter Scientific Products, McGraw Park, IL) is commonly used in veterinary practices; similar stains are available. These stains are relatively inexpensive and convenient to use. Although they may overstain nuclei, blur chromatin detail, and fail to stain cytoplasmic granules in some cells, they are adequate for determining a leukocyte differential and for evaluating most morphologic abnormalities, if used properly.

Blood Smear Evaluation

Despite the mechanization of veterinary laboratories, a properly maintained, high-quality microscope is a good investment for evaluating smears and cytology samples. The microscope should be binocular, with adjustable oculars, an adjustable substage condenser, and planachromatic ×10, ×40 (high dry), and ×100 (oil immersion) objectives. If additional objectives are an option, some prefer to have ×4, ×20, and ×50 (oil immersion) objectives. The technician should be familiar with optimizing the light by adjusting the condenser, iris diaphragm, and diffuser, depending on the sample being evaluated. For evaluation of blood and cytology smears, the substage condenser should be in a relatively high position, and the iris diaphragm should be open. Use of the ×40 objective requires mounting a coverslip onto the slide for optimal visualization, but the oil immersion objective is recommended for blood smear evaluation. For oil immersion objectives, a drop of immersion oil is placed on the slide to achieve optimal optics. Oil immersion objectives and the slides should be gently wiped clean after use. All other objectives should be kept free of immersion oil.

Accurate evaluation of blood smears requires a systematic procedure for examination and expertise in identifying normal cells, morphologic abnormalities, and artifacts. A blood smear consists of three regions: body, counting area, and feathered edge (Fig. 11.6). The *body* is the area where the drop of blood was first placed. In the body, the blood smear is thick and cells are piled on top of each other, so it is difficult to identify cells or evaluate cell morphology. The *counting area*, between the body and the feathered edge, appears progressively thinner as it approaches the feathered edge. The counting area contains a monolayer of cells. In

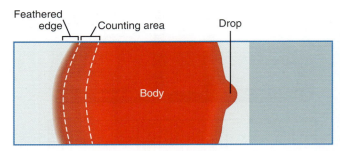

• **Fig. 11.6** The blood smear is made up of regions: the body, counting area, and feathered edge are shown. (Illustration by Tim Vojt, Biomedical Media, OSU-CVM. Copyright The Ohio State University.)

this region, RBCs, WBCs, and platelets can be identified and their morphology adequately evaluated. The *feathered edge* is the end of the blood smear, farthest away from the drop. At the feathered edge, many of the cells may be broken, distribution of cells may be uneven, and RBCs often lose their central zone of pallor. Cell morphology should therefore not be evaluated at the feathered edge.

The blood smear should be evaluated initially with the ×10 objective. In the body of the smear, RBCs can be evaluated for **rouleaux formation** or agglutination appearing as RBCs in chains resembling a stack of coins (Fig. 11.7). In horses and cats, rouleaux formation is common, whereas in dogs, rouleaux formation may be an indication of inflammation or may be an artifact of smear preparation. **Agglutination** refers to irregular, variably sized clumps of RBCs that form because of excess antibodies bound to the surface of RBCs. This occurs in immune-mediated hemolytic anemia (IMHA), which is most common in dogs (Case Presentation 11.1). It may be difficult to distinguish rouleaux formation from agglutination on the blood smear. A saline dispersion test often is performed by adding 10 drops of saline to one drop of EDTA-anticoagulated blood and gently mixing the sample. A drop of the diluted blood is added to a clean glass slide, and the sample is observed by using ×10 or ×40 magnification. A coverslip can be added but is not necessary. Saline disperses rouleaux but not agglutination.

The counting area of the blood smear can be located using the ×10 objective by recognizing the region in which a monolayer of evenly dispersed cells can be seen between the body and the feathered edge. The counting area of the smear should be evaluated with the ×100 oil immersion objective by using a systematic approach to estimate platelet number, evaluate cell morphology, and perform a differential WBC count. Always evaluate platelets, RBCs, and WBCs in the same order. The order is not critical, but using the same order for each blood smear is an important part of a systematic approach to avoid missing something important.

The ×10 objective also should be used to scan the feathered edge for platelet clumps, microfilaria, and large, abnormal cells (Fig. 11.8A and B). It is important to recognize platelet clumps, because these may falsely decrease platelet counts, whether determined manually, by an automated analyzer, or by microscopy at higher magnification. Although more sensitive methods may be used to detect microfilaria, their presence on a blood smear should be noted as few or many. Recognition of abnormal cells at the feathered edge is helpful because they may be present in low numbers and missed if only the counting area is examined. The WBC count can be estimated from several fields in the counting area using the ×10 objective. An average of about 10 to 30 WBCs should be present per ×10 field for a normal WBC count in most

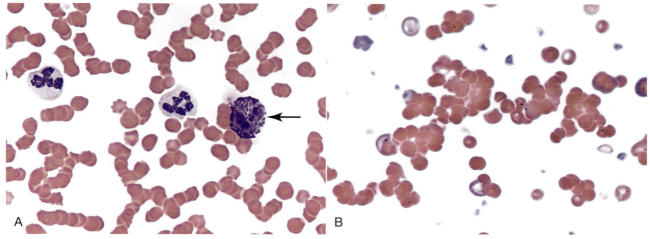

• **Fig. 11.7** Rouleaux and agglutination. (A) Rouleaux formation is normal in horses and is shown at low magnification. The red blood cells (RBCs) appear like a stack of coins. Two neutrophils are present on the left and a basophil on the right *(arrow)*. (B) RBC agglutination occurs most commonly in dogs with immune-mediated hemolytic anemia. The RBCs are in irregular clumps of various sizes.

CASE PRESENTATION 11.1

Immune-Mediated Hemolytic Anemia and Thrombocytopenia

Signalment: 6-year-old spayed female Collie
History: acute onset of severe lethargy
Physical examination: pale, icteric mucous membranes; tachypnea; enlarged spleen
This case illustrates the importance of evaluating a blood smear.

CBC	Patient		Reference Interval
Plasma protein, g/dL	7.6	H	5.7–7.2
Plasma appeared clear and moderately yellow.			
HCT, %	17	L	36–54
Hemoglobin, g/dL	5.0	L	11.9–18.4
RBCs, ×10^{12}/L	2.2	L	4.9–8.2
MCV, fL	80	H	64–75
MCHC, g/dL	29.1	L	32.9–35.2
RDW	19.1	H	13.4–17.0
Reticulocytes, ×10^9/L	477.5	H	<60

RBC morphology: There is marked agglutination that did not disperse with saline. Moderate anisocytosis, marked polychromasia, and numerous spherocytes are observed. Numbers of Howell-Jolly bodies and nucleated RBCs (nRBCs) are increased.

Platelets, ×10^9/L	94	L	106–424
WBCs, ×10^9/L	34.6	H	4.1–15.2
nRBCs, ×10^9/L	10.9	H	0.0
Band neutrophils, ×10^9/L	8.2	H	0.0–0.1
Segmented neutrophils, ×10^9/L	28.2	H	3.0–10.4
Lymphocytes, ×10^9/L	1.8		1.0–4.6
Monocytes, ×10^9/L	7.3	H	0.0–1.2
Eosinophils, ×10^9/L	0.0		0.0–1.2

WBC morphology: Moderate numbers of Döhle bodies and moderate cytoplasmic basophilia and vacuolation are interpreted as toxic change.

Interpretation
RBCs

A marked macrocytic hypochromic anemia is present that is markedly regenerative, based on the increased reticulocyte count. Reticulocytes are less-mature RBCs and are characterized by macrocytic hypochromic indices. The increased numbers of Howell-Jolly bodies and nRBCs likely are part of the regenerative response. Marked agglutination (not rouloux formations) and the presence of numerous spherocytes are hallmarks of IMHA, especially when there is no history of blood transfusion.

Platelets

Platelets appear mildly decreased on the blood smear, and no platelet clumps are noted. Some dogs with IMHA also may have immune thrombocytopenic purpura (ITP). However, other causes of thrombocytopenia cannot be excluded. Disseminated intravascular coagulation (DIC) is a serious complication that occurs in some dogs with IMHA, resulting in thrombocytopenia secondary to consumption of platelets.

WBCs

Moderate to marked neutrophilia with a left shift and monocytosis is typical for dogs with IMHA. These animals do not really have inflammatory disease but likely have increased concentrations of cytokines that stimulate increased production of WBCs and RBCs (aka "toxic changes"). The toxic changes in the neutrophils are the result of rapidly increased proliferation of neutrophils in bone marrow. Some dogs with IMHA also have lymphopenia, which is caused by superimposed stress leukography and treatment with corticosteroids, but this dog has normal numbers of lymphocytes.

Summary

Evaluation of the blood smear is important in establishing a diagnosis of IMHA. Key features that are present in many (but not all) dogs with IMHA include the following:
• RBC agglutination (does not disperse with saline)
• Spherocytes (remember to look only in the counting area)
• Anisocytosis, polychromasia, Howell-Jolly bodies, and nRBCs
• Leukocytosis caused by neutrophilia with a left shift and monocytosis
• Thrombocytopenia and macroplatelets in dogs with concurrent ITP

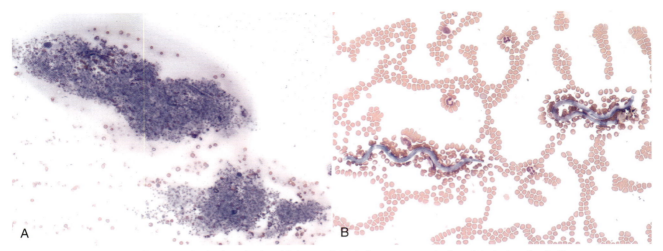

• **Fig. 11.8** Scanning the feathered edge. (A) Large platelet clumps are most often detected on the feathered edge during ×10 scan of the blood smear and, if present, may falsely decrease the platelet count or estimate. (B) Two microfilaria are present in this field.

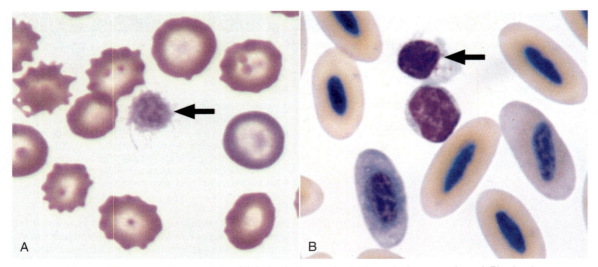

• **Fig. 11.9** Platelets and thrombocytes. (A) A platelet from a dog is shown in the center *(arrow).* Platelets in mammals do not have nuclei, and the cytoplasm appears granular. (B) A thrombocyte from a bird is shown in the upper center *(arrow),* just above the small lymphocyte. In birds and reptiles, thrombocytes often are round to oval and have round to oval nuclei. The cytoplasm may appear vacuolated and may contain several small granules, as shown in this thrombocyte.

species. The number of WBCs/×10 field multiplied by 100 can be used to estimate the number of WBCs/μL.

> **TECHNICIAN NOTE**
>
> Blood smears should be examined with ×10 and ×100 oil immersion objectives in a systematic manner for adequate evaluation.

Platelets

In mammals, platelets are nonnucleated fragments of cytoplasm released from megakaryocytes in bone marrow. In most mammals, platelets are smaller than RBCs. The cytoplasm stains light blue and contains small, light purple granules (Fig. 11.9A). Platelets may not stain as well in horses, and platelets from llamas and alpacas are very small compared with those from other species. In birds and reptiles, platelets have nuclei and are called *thrombocytes* (Fig. 11.9B). Platelets that approach the size of RBCs are called

macroplatelets and, in some species, may indicate increased platelet production. Macroplatelets may be normal in cats and in Cavalier King Charles Spaniels. For this reason, an estimate of the platelet count from the blood smear of Cavalier King Charles Spaniels may be more accurate than an automated platelet count, and they have normal coagulation protein activity. Other morphologic abnormalities are unusual and should be noted.

In general, automated platelet counts are more accurate than manual platelet counts. The platelet count can be estimated on the blood smear by determining the number of platelets in several oil immersion fields. On average, 6 to 15 platelets per oil immersion field indicates a normal platelet count. The average number of platelets can be multiplied by 15,000 or 20,000 to estimate the number of platelets per microliter. If the platelet count is decreased or if platelets appear decreased on the blood smear, make sure the feathered edge is examined for the presence of platelet clumps. A decreased platelet count is called *thrombocytopenia;* if

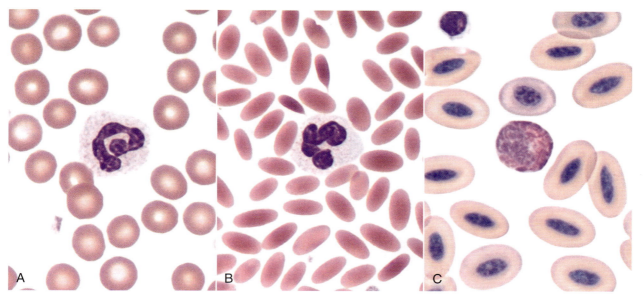

• **Fig. 11.10** Red blood cells (RBCs) in various species. (A) RBCs in dogs have a prominent central zone of pallor. (B) (RBCs in camelids are oval. Several teardrop-shaped RBCs (dacrocytes) are seen in this field. (C) RBCs in birds and reptiles are oval and have oval nuclei.

marked, this condition may be associated with abnormal bleeding. Increased platelet counts, called thrombocytosis, are less common and typically do not cause clinical signs unless the thrombocytosis is pronounced.

Red Blood Cells

RBC morphology varies among species (Fig. 11.10). In most mammals, RBCs circulate as biconcave disks and appear round and flat, with varying degrees of central pallor on a blood smear. The central zone of pallor is most prominent in RBCs from dogs and is least apparent in RBCs from cats, horses, and goats. RBCs from camelids are oval, whereas those of birds and reptiles are oval and have nuclei. There are obvious species differences in RBC size. Of commonly evaluated domestic animals, RBCs from dogs have the largest diameter (7 μm), and RBCs from goats have the smallest diameter (3.2 μm). RBCs from cattle display anisocytosis (variation in RBC size), whereas RBCs from dogs typically have very little anisocytosis. Increased anisocytosis occurs in regenerative anemia as a result of increased numbers of larger, less-mature RBCs and in iron deficiency anemia because of increased numbers of microcytic RBCs. Several breed differences in RBC size have been recognized in dogs. Some Poodles have macrocytic RBCs, some Japanese breeds have microcytic RBCs, and macrocytic RBCs have been reported in some cats infected by feline leukemia virus.

Numerous morphologic changes can occur in RBCs, some of which have clinical relevance (Fig. 11.11A–F). Sometimes these changes are subjectively reported as slight or 1+, moderate or 2+, or marked or 3+ or 4+. *Poikilocytosis* refers to variation in RBC shape but, if possible, a more specific term should be used. *Leptocytes,* RBCs with increased surface area, often appear as target cells (*codocytes*). Target cells have a round area of hemoglobin in the central zone of pallor and usually have minimal clinical relevance (see Fig. 11.11C). *Stomatocytes* appear to have a clear, mouthlike area near the center of the RBC. These often are an artifact of smear preparation, although stomatocytosis has been reported as an inherited defect in several breeds of dogs, including

the Alaskan Malamute, Drentse Patrijshound, Miniature/Standard Schnauzer, and Pomeranian.

Crenated RBCs, also called *echinocytes*, have evenly distributed, short, blunt to pointed projections from the surface (see Fig. 11.11A). Echinocytes most often are an artifact of slow drying of the smear but have been associated with renal disease, lymphoma, rattlesnake envenomation, and chemotherapy in dogs and have been noted postexercise in horses. Acanthocytes have longer, blunt, or club-shaped projections that are unevenly distributed on the RBC surface (see Fig. 11.11B). Acanthocytes can occur in dogs with hemangiosarcoma and in cats with hepatic lipidosis. If physical or chemical injury to RBCs occurs (e.g., iron deficiency), small vacuoles may form in the RBC membrane. If the vacuole ruptures, these projections resemble horns. If two projections are present, the RBC is called a *keratocyte* (see Fig. 11.11C); if only one projection is visible, the RBC is called an *apple stem cell*. Fragments of RBCs, called *schistocytes,* can occur with diseases that cause intravascular trauma to the RBCs, such as disseminated intravascular coagulation, hemangiosarcoma, or heartworm disease (see Fig. 11.11D).

Spherocytes are RBCs that lack a central zone of pallor and often appear slightly smaller and denser than normal RBCs (Fig. 11.12A). Spherocytes result from antibody binding to the RBC surface and removal of a portion of the membrane by macrophages in the spleen. This occurs in IMHA, which is most often recognized in dogs. It is difficult to recognize spherocytes in horses and cats, but IMHA is much less common in these species. Recognizing spherocytes on a blood smear is an important part of the diagnosis of IMHA, and care should be taken to evaluate only the counting area of the blood smear. Almost all RBCs resemble spherocytes near the feathered edge, and it is much more difficult to recognize spherocytes in thicker portions of the smear. Small numbers of spherocytes may be present if oxidative damage or microvascular injury occurs and after a blood transfusion.

Oxidative damage results in several morphologic abnormalities in RBCs. *Eccentrocytes* are RBCs in which the hemoglobin has shifted to one side of the cell, creating a clear area outlined by a

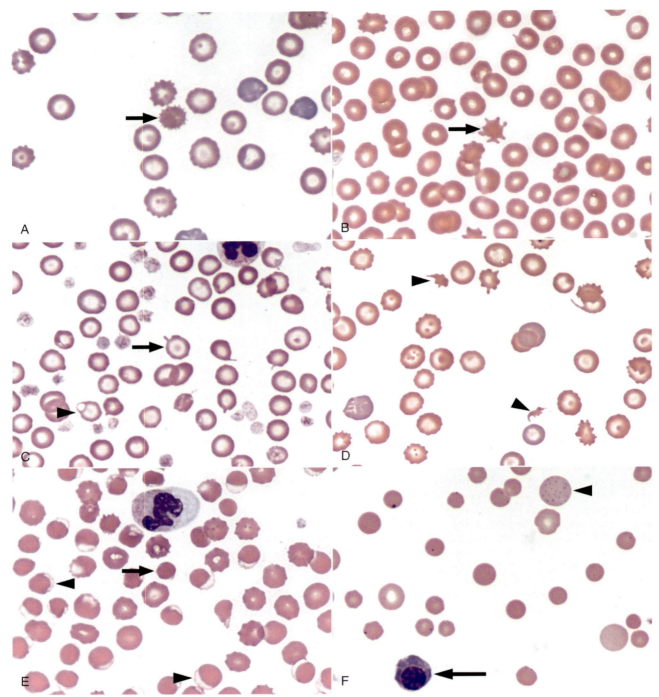

• **Fig. 11.11** Red blood cell (RBC) abnormalities. (A) Crenated RBCs have numerous sharp, evenly distributed projections on the surface and often are an artifact of drying. The cell in the center *(arrow)* has sharp projections, but several echinocytes in this field have projections that are not quite as sharp. (B) Acanthocytes have several blunt projections that are not evenly distributed on the surface. An acanthocyte can be seen in the center *(arrow)* of this blood smear from a dog with hemangiosarcoma. (C) Keratocytes have two portions of membrane that project from the surface of the RBC, resembling horns *(arrowhead)*. Several apple stem RBCs have only one projection *(arrow)*. This smear is from a dog with iron deficiency anemia, so the RBCs appear hypochromic, and the platelets are increased. (D) Several RBC fragments *(arrowheads)* in a blood smear from a dog with hemangiosarcoma. (E) Numerous eccentrocytes *(arrowheads)* can be seen in this blood smear from a dog. The hemoglobin is pushed to one side of the cell, leaving a clear portion of the cytoplasm with a thin rim of membrane. A pyknocyte is noted in the center *(arrow)*; this is an eccentrocyte that has lost the portion of cell with minimal hemoglobin, so it appears as a small, dense RBC. (F) An RBC with basophilic stippling *(arrowhead)* appears as *small blue dots* throughout the cytoplasm. This blood smear is from a cow with regenerative anemia. Several cells with Howell-Jolly bodies are also present, and a nucleated RBC is evident at the bottom of the field *(arrow)*.

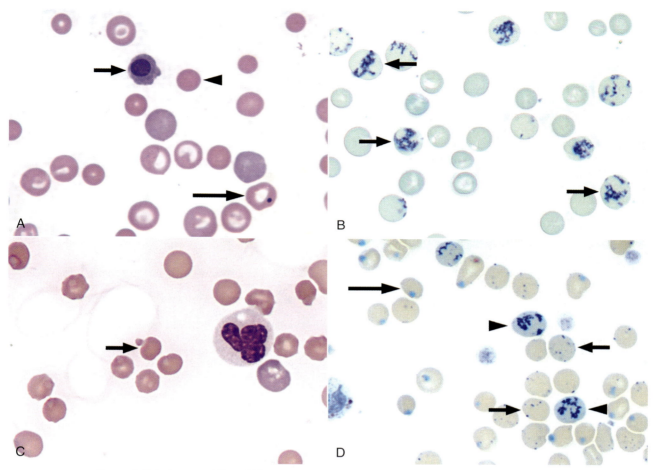

• **Fig. 11.12** Polychromatophilic red blood cells (RBCs) and reticulocytes. (A) Spherocytes *(arrowhead)* appear slightly smaller and denser than normal RBCs. Several larger polychromatophilic cells are characterized by more basophilic cytoplasm in this blood smear from a dog with regenerative anemia resulting from immune-mediated hemolytic anemia (IMHA). These same cells would be reticulocytes if they were stained with new methylene blue (NMB). A nucleated RBC *(short arrow)* and an RBC with a Howell-Jolly body *(long arrow)* are seen. (B) This blood from a dog with IMHA has been stained with NMB. Numerous aggregate reticulocytes are shown *(arrows)*. (C) This blood smear is from a cat. An RBC with a protruding Heinz body is seen in the center *(arrow)*. Heinz bodies are evident in many of the other RBCs. They appear as lighter-staining structures if they do not protrude from the RBC, in which case they are more difficult to see. (D) This blood, from a cat with Heinz body hemolytic anemia, has been stained with NMB. Only aggregated reticulocytes *(arrowheads)* would be counted as reticulocytes to determine whether the anemia is regenerative; punctate reticulocytes *(short arrows)* would not be counted. Heinz bodies are the larger, blue-staining structures that often protrude from the RBC *(long arrow)*. A and C have been stained with Wright stain (NMB).

thin rim of membrane (see Fig. 11.11E). Pyknocytes form if the thin region is disrupted, leaving a slightly irregular, dense portion of RBC (see Fig. 11.11E). Eccentrocytes occur because of oxidative damage to the RBC membrane. Heinz bodies occur with oxidative damage to hemoglobin, which binds to the inner surface of the membrane, creating a pale structure that may protrude from the surface (Fig. 11.12C). When stained with new methylene blue (NMB), Heinz bodies appear blue and are easier to visualize (Fig. 11.12D). Heinz bodies are often found in RBCs from sick cats but are interpreted as significant if they are numerous or large or if multiple Heinz bodies per RBC are present. Heinz bodies in other species are abnormal and may be associated with exposure to many different oxidative compounds, including ingestion of onions, garlic, and zinc-containing objects in dogs and wilted red maple leaves in horses.

Occasional nRBCs or metarubricytes can be seen in peripheral blood from healthy animals. Increased numbers of nRBCs can occur in markedly regenerative anemia (see Figs. 11.11F and 11.12A), but increased nRBCs in animals with nonregenerative anemia may indicate primary bone marrow disease. Increased nRBCs along with basophilic stippling in animals that are not anemic may indicate lead toxicity. Some splenectomized animals will have increased nRBCs and Howell-Jolly bodies. nRBCs may be erroneously counted as WBCs by manual methods and by some automated hematology analyzers, resulting in falsely increased WBC counts. If nRBCs are included in the WBC count, this should technically be reported as a total nucleated cell count. The simplest way to enumerate nRBCs is to include them in the differential and report them as nRBCs per microliter. However, the WBC count can be corrected for the presence of nRBCs. When a differential leukocyte count is performed, nRBCs are tallied separately and are expressed as nRBCs per 100 WBCs. The corrected WBC count = (total nucleated cell count × 100) ÷ (# nRBCs + 100). However, this correction is not necessary unless large numbers of nRBCs are present or unless WBCs are counted by using automated hematology analyzers that cannot distinguish nRBCs from WBCs.

Howell-Jolly bodies are nuclear remnants that appear as small, round basophilic structures in RBCs and sometimes are increased in animals with regenerative anemia (Fig. 11.12A). Basophilic stippling appears as numerous small basophilic dots from aggregated ribosomes. Basophilic stippling may occur in lead toxicity and in regenerative anemia in cattle and horses or in intense regenerative responses in dogs and cats (see Fig. 11.11F).

Polychromasia is the term used to describe RBCs with cytoplasm that is more basophilic than that of normal RBCs (see Fig. 11.12A). These cells usually are larger and have more ribonucleic acid (RNA) and less hemoglobin compared with mature RBCs. Polychromatophilic RBCs usually account for less than 1% of the RBCs in healthy animals. Increased numbers of polychromatophilic RBCs occur in regenerative anemia, indicating an appropriate bone marrow response. The regenerative response by the bone marrow can be more quantitatively evaluated by performing a reticulocyte count (Procedure 11.2). Dogs have only aggregate reticulocytes (Fig. 11.12B), but cats have aggregate and punctate reticulocytes (see Fig. 11.12D). Aggregate reticulocytes have clumps of reticulum and are a more accurate indication of the bone marrow response than punctate reticulocytes, which have small, single dots of reticulum and are not indicative of active regeneration. Only aggregate reticulocytes are counted. Calculating the absolute reticulocyte count, reported as reticulocytes per microliter, is recommended; this value is reported by most large reference laboratories. The percentage of reticulocytes or the corrected reticulocyte percentage (CRP) (see Procedure 11.2) can be used to assess regeneration if the RBC count is not available.

Several RBC parasites can be identified from blood smear evaluation. Many of these parasites cause anemia but other than the hemotropic *Mycoplasma* species in cats, most are uncommon in the United States. Species-specific hemotropic *Mycoplasma* organisms have been described in dogs, cats, pigs, cows, llamas, and alpacas. Hemotropic *Mycoplasma* organisms appear as small basophilic cocci or rings on the RBC surface or free in the background if the organisms have detached from the cell (Fig. 11.13). These structures often resemble stain precipitate, so care should be taken to evaluate a blood smear with minimal stain precipitate. *Anaplasma marginale* infects bovine RBCs and appears as a dark, round structure, 1–2 micrometers in diameter, within RBCs, sometimes near the edge. *Babesia* organisms, most commonly seen in dogs, may be single or paired teardrop-shaped structures several microns in diameter, or they may be much smaller, irregularly shaped structures, depending on the species. Deoxyribonucleic acid (DNA)–based and serologic tests are available for many of the hemotropic parasites to confirm infection. Additional reference texts can be consulted for identification of other hemotropic parasites.

TECHNICIAN NOTE

Recognition of ribonucleic acid (RBC) morphologic abnormalities can be helpful in establishing a list of differential diagnoses.

White Blood Cells

Most WBCs have distinctive morphologic features that allow them to be identified by using routine staining procedures (Fig. 11.14A–J).

PROCEDURE 11.2

Reticulocyte Count

1. Add several drops of new methylene blue (NMB) stain to several drops of EDTA-anticoagulated blood in a small test tube.
2. Incubate for 10 minutes at room temperature.
3. Make a conventional blood smear from the NMB-stained blood and allow the smear to dry in ambient air.
4. Count a total of 1000 red blood cells (RBCs) as reticulocytes, which contain clumps of dark-staining aggregated organelles (see Fig. 11.12) or as normal RBCs.
5. Calculate the *percentage of reticulocytes* by dividing the number of reticulocytes counted in Step 4 by 1000. A *corrected reticulocyte percentage* (CRP) can be determined when the RBC count is not available to calculate an absolute reticulocyte count (Step 6).

$$CRP = \frac{\% \text{ reticulocytes } \times \text{ Patient's PCV}}{45(\text{dog}) \text{ or } 37(\text{cat})}$$

6. Calculate the *absolute number of reticulocytes* by multiplying the percentage of reticulocytes determined in Step 5 by the RBC count as determined by the automated hematology analyzer. Absolute reticulocytes are reported as the number of reticulocytes × 10^9/L or as the number of reticulocytes per microliter.
   Example: reticulocyte count = 200
   RBC count = 2.2 × 10^{12}/L
   Percentage reticulocytes: 200/1000 = 20%
   Absolute reticulocytes: (0.20) × (2.2 × 10^{12}/L) = 440,000/µL

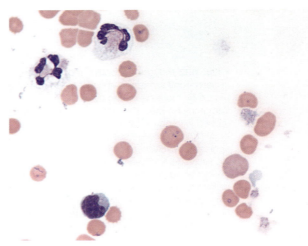

• **Fig. 11.13** *Mycoplasma haemocanis.* Although uncommon in dogs, the red blood cell (RBC) in the center shows a small, rod-shaped form on the upper edge, small cocci on the lower edge and in the center, and several ring forms in the cytoplasm. Several other RBCs have similar parasites. In dogs, *M. haemocanis* sometimes forms chains of organisms (see RBC in the *lower left*).

Determination of the numbers of each type of WBC can be helpful in establishing a list of differential diagnoses. A differential WBC count is performed by identifying and enumerating a minimum of 100 leukocytes in the counting area of the blood smear. At least 200 cells should be counted if the WBC count is increased. WBCs are classified as **segmented neutrophils**, **band neutrophils**, **eosinophils**, **basophils**, **lymphocytes**, **monocytes**, or abnormal cells to determine the percentage of each cell type. Neutrophils, eosinophils, and basophils collectively are called *granulocytes*, because they have cytoplasmic granules visible upon routine staining. Lymphocytes and

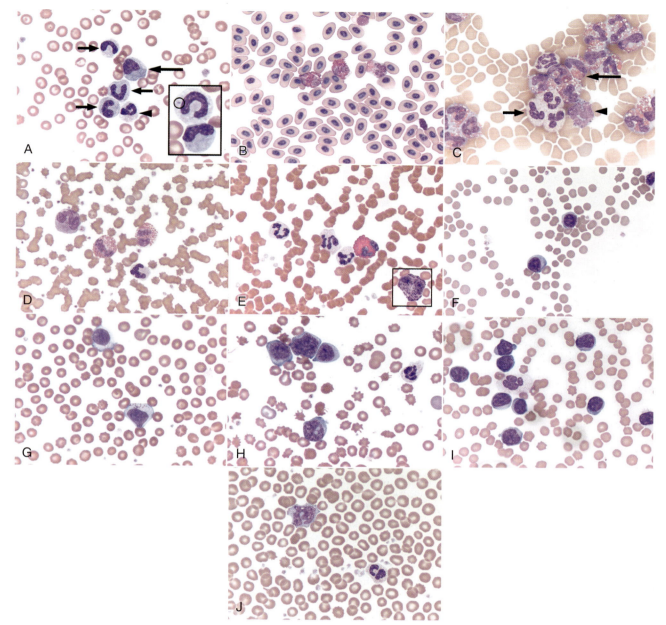

• **Fig. 11.14** White blood cells (WBCs) from various species. (A) This blood smear, with a degenerative left shift, is from a dog. A segmented neutrophil *(arrowhead)*, three bands *(short arrows)*, and a metamyelocyte *(long arrow)* can be seen. The bands have C- or U-shaped nuclei, with relatively condensed chromatin and basophilic cytoplasm. The metamyelocyte has an indented nucleus with less condensed chromatin, and the cytoplasm is basophilic. *Inset,* The band neutrophil has basophilic cytoplasm that appears vacuolated. The *pale blue* structures are Döhle bodies *(open circle)*. Toxic changes are associated with marked inflammation. (B) Two heterophils on the left have granules that are larger, more irregular or seed shaped, and darker red than the granules in the eosinophil on the *right*, which are round and stain brighter red. The smaller cell with dark nucleus in the *lower right* is a thrombocyte in this blood smear from a bird. (C) There are several neutrophils *(short arrow)*, numerous eosinophils *(long arrow)*, and one basophil *(arrowhead)* at the feathered edge of this blood smear from a dog. Note the small, dark-blue granules in the cytoplasm of the basophil compared with the larger, reddish granules in the cytoplasm of the eosinophils and the pale neutral-staining granules in the cytoplasm of the neutrophils. (D) A basophil with lavender granules *(left)*, two eosinophils with reddish granules *(center)*, and a segmented neutrophil with inconspicuous granules *(lower center)* are seen in this blood smear from a cat. (E) Three segmented neutrophils and an eosinophil can be seen in this blood smear from a horse. In horses, eosinophils have numerous large granules, so they are easy to identify. *Inset,* Basophils in horses and cows have numerous dark-staining granules that may obscure the nucleus. (F) A normal lymphocyte is shown in the upper portion and a reactive lymphocyte in the lower portion of this blood smear from a cat. The reactive lymphocyte has abundant basophilic cytoplasm with a perinuclear clear area. (G) Two large granular lymphocytes (LGLs) in a blood smear from a dog with chronic lymphoid leukemia (CLL). LGLs have several azurophilic granules in the cytoplasm. (H) Several neoplastic lymphocytes from a dog with acute lymphoid leukemia (ALL). Neoplastic lymphocytes are larger than normal lymphocytes and have abundant basophilic cytoplasm. Nuclei have less condensed chromatin and may have one to several nucleoli. A neutrophil is shown on the right for comparison. Normal lymphocytes are smaller than neutrophils. (I) In this blood smear from a horse with chronic lymphocytic leukemia, most of the cells are neoplastic lymphocytes. The lymphocytes are smaller than the neutrophils and have minimal cytoplasm and nuclei, with condensed chromatin and inconspicuous nucleoli. (J) There is a monocyte *(upper left)* and a neutrophil *(lower right)* in this blood smear from a dog. Monocytes appear similar in most mammalian species and are characterized by abundant basophilic cytoplasm that often contains clear vacuoles. Nuclei are indented or irregular in shape and have moderately condensed chromatin that appears unevenly dispersed.

monocytes do not have granules and are referred to as *agranulocytes*. Percentages of each cell type are relative numbers and have minimal diagnostic utility. The WBC differential should be interpreted based on absolute numbers of each cell type, determined by multiplying the percentage of each cell type (expressed as a decimal) by the total WBC and reported as the number of each cell per microliter of blood (or per liter of blood—the international unit for cell enumeration). For example, if 60% neutrophils (0.6 expressed as a decimal) are present and the total WBC count is 10,000/µL (10×10^9/L), the absolute number of neutrophils is 6000/µL (6.0×10^9/L). The morphology of the leukocytes is evaluated, and any abnormalities are noted.

Neutrophils

Neutrophils are the predominant circulating WBCs in dogs, cats, and horses but in cattle, sheep, and goats, lymphocytes are the predominant circulating WBCs. In pigs, about equal numbers of neutrophils and lymphocytes are present. An increased number of neutrophils is called *neutrophilia* and often occurs with inflammation. Mature neutrophils, called *segmented neutrophils,* or "segs," are about 12 µm in diameter and are characterized by a segmented nucleus that often has three to five lobes. The condensed chromatin stains darkly and, in most domestic animals, the cytoplasm is relatively clear, with poorly visible, neutral-staining granules (see Fig. 11.14A). The granules are slightly eosinophilic, appearing more prominent in neutrophils from cattle. In some species, neutrophils are called **heterophils** because of the intense staining of the granules. Heterophils are the most abundant granulocytes in rabbits and in some nonmammalian species. The granules are larger, typically rod or seed shaped and may appear oval or round in some species. The granules appear dark orange or reddish-brown with routine stains and may obscure the nucleus (see Fig. 11.14B).

Although it is rare to see giant neutrophils, less-mature neutrophils sometimes are released from bone marrow during inflammation. Band neutrophils, often called "bands" or "stabs," have a C-shaped or S-shaped nucleus with parallel sides or minimal nuclear constriction. Bands may be slightly larger than segmented neutrophils, and the cytoplasm may appear slightly more basophilic (see Fig. 11.14A). In more intense inflammatory reactions, metamyelocytes and occasionally myelocytes can be released from bone marrow. Metamyelocytes have an indented nucleus and are slightly larger and have more cytoplasmic basophilia than bands. Myelocytes have a round nucleus and are slightly larger and more basophilic than metamyelocytes. The chromatin is progressively less condensed in less-mature cells, so it stains lighter (see Fig. 11.14A). An increased number of circulating band neutrophils (and metamyelocytes and myelocytes) is called a *left shift* and indicates that bone marrow is releasing immature cells to meet demand. If the number of band neutrophils (and metamyelocytes and myelocytes, if they are present) exceeds the number of segmented neutrophils, this is called a *degenerative left shift* and often indicates a poor prognosis.

Several morphologic abnormalities, known as "**toxic changes**," indicate intense stimulation of neutrophil production and shortened maturation time but do not necessarily imply an association with a toxin. Nuclear features of toxic change may be more subtle and include vacuolation, hyposegmentation, ring formation, and fragmentation. Toxic changes can be subjectively reported as mild, moderate, or marked, depending on the percentages of cells affected and the severity of the change. Döhle bodies are whorls of rough endoplasmic reticulum that appear as grayish-blue, round to irregularly shaped aggregates in the cytoplasm (see

Fig. 11.14A). Small Döhle bodies may be normal in some healthy cats. Cytoplasmic basophilia is the result of retention of rough endoplasmic reticulum with vacuolation because of degranulation of lysosomes or disruption of cell membrane integrity. Toxic granules are coarse, pink or reddish granules in the cytoplasm; they are primary granules with increased staining permeability.

Several other abnormalities in neutrophil morphology sometimes are noted. Hypersegmented nuclei are seen with increased endogenous or exogenous corticosteroids. Pelger-Huet anomaly is a congenital or acquired defect in nuclear segmentation of neutrophils and eosinophils, most often seen in dogs. Most of the granulocytes resemble bands, metamyelocytes, and myelocytes, which can be misinterpreted as a left shift. However, the chromatin is condensed, and the cytoplasm is relatively clear, like mature segmented neutrophils. This is an incidental finding in dogs, and most are otherwise healthy. Healthy, prominent neutrophil granules are seen as a breed variation in Birman cats and also are reported in some rare inherited storage diseases such as Chediak-Hihashi disease. Infectious agents, such as bacteria, fungal elements, viral inclusions, and rickettsia inclusions, occasionally can be observed. Neutrophils with intracellular infectious agents may be easier to detect at the feathered edge than in the counting area.

Eosinophils

Eosinophils circulate in low numbers in health. As important mediators of hypersensitivity reactions, they contain substances that can damage and kill some parasites. Increased numbers or *eosinophilia* can occur with allergic reactions and in some parasite infections. *Eosinopenia* (decreased eosinophils) occurs in response to corticosteroids. Marked species variation in eosinophil morphology has been noted. In most species, nuclei are segmented and have condensed chromatin. The prominent feature is the presence of numerous pink to reddish granules in the cytoplasm. In dogs, the granules are round and intermediate in size and number (Fig. 11.14C). In Greyhounds, the granules often do not stain but appear instead as clear structures in the cytoplasm. In cats, the granules are numerous, small, and rod shaped (Fig. 11.14D). Eosinophils in cows have numerous, small, round, brightly staining granules, whereas in horses, the granules are numerous, brightly staining, and much larger than in other species (Fig. 11.14E). Eosinophils from most nonmammalian species have numerous round, brightly eosinophilic granules, although in some species, the granules may be oval or elongate. In a few nonmammalian species, the granules stain light blue.

Basophils

Basophils circulate in very low numbers; often, none are encountered during routine evaluation of blood smears from healthy animals. Increased numbers of basophils (called *basophilia*) may be present in hypersensitivity reactions or parasite infections, similar to eosinophils. The morphology of basophils is species dependent. In dogs, basophils appear slightly larger than neutrophils and have a twisted or irregularly shaped nucleus with less condensed chromatin (see Fig. 11.14C). The cytoplasm is more basophilic than in neutrophils and there may be several dark-blue granules or no visible granules, in which case the cells are more difficult to identify. In cats, basophils have numerous lavender granules (see Fig. 11.14D). Basophils from horses and cows typically have numerous dark bluish-purple granules and may resemble mast cells, but the nucleus is segmented (see Fig. 11.14E). Basophils from most nonmammalian species have round nuclei with numerous dark purple granules that may obscure the nucleus, like mammalian mast cells. In some species of turtles, basophils may be the most abundant circulating leukocytes.

Lymphocytes

Lymphocytes are the predominant circulating cell in cattle, sheep, and goats, but they are less numerous than neutrophils in other species. Most circulating lymphocytes are smaller (9 μm in diameter) than a neutrophil. A round nucleus with condensed chromatin almost fills the cytoplasm, resulting in a high nucleus-to-cytoplasm ratio. In many lymphocytes, only a narrow crescent of pale blue cytoplasm is visible (see Fig. 11.14F). In cows, up to 50% of lymphocytes may be intermediate to large, even in the absence of disease. Lymphocytes from most nonmammalian species resemble lymphocytes from mammals. In most species, a small percentage of circulating lymphocytes have a few azurophilic granules in the cytoplasm. These cells are called *large granular lymphocytes* (LGLs). Increased numbers of LGLs occur with some types of chronic inflammation and in some forms of chronic lymphocytic leukemia (CLL; see Fig. 11.14G). Lymphocytes can have abnormal granules from inherited storage diseases, but these are rare.

Intermediate- to large-sized lymphocytes, known as "reactive lymphocytes," sometimes circulate secondary to antigenic stimulation and have more abundant, more intensely basophilic cytoplasm that may contain a perinuclear clear area (see Fig. 11.14F). It may be difficult to distinguish reactive lymphocytes from neoplastic lymphocytes that circulate in acute lymphoid leukemia (ALL) and in some animals with lymphoma. Nuclei in reactive and many neoplastic lymphocytes have less condensed chromatin, but reactive lymphocytes usually do not have visible nucleoli. The number of reactive lymphocytes usually is low, whereas the number of neoplastic lymphocytes may be very high.

Lymphocytosis can occur with antigenic stimulation and is often seen in young animals. Transient lymphocytosis resulting from epinephrine release is common in cats and horses that become excited during blood collection. Lymphoid neoplasia is associated with persistent lymphocytosis. Many animals with ALL have marked lymphocytosis, whereas animals with lymphoma and circulating neoplastic lymphocytes have mild to moderate lymphocytosis. The neoplastic lymphocytes in ALL and lymphoma usually are large and have abundant basophilic cytoplasm, fine chromatin, and prominent nucleoli (see Fig. 11.14H). In CLL, mild, moderate, or marked lymphocytosis may occur, but the lymphocytes typically are small and appear well differentiated (see Fig. 11.14I). In dogs with CLL, the most common neoplastic cells are LGLs (see Fig. 11.14G).

Monocytes

Monocytes usually circulate in relatively low numbers and appear similar in most species, including birds and reptiles (see Fig. 11.14J). Monocytes are larger than neutrophils and have abundant gray-blue cytoplasm. The cytoplasm sometimes contains several clear vacuoles and/or fine magenta granules. Nuclei are round, oval, indented, or variable in shape and have less condensed chromatin than neutrophils. Monocytes in tissues become macrophages but in blood, it is unusual to see phagocytized material in the cytoplasm. It may be difficult to differentiate monocytes from bands or metamyelocytes with toxic changes. Monocytosis can occur with inflammation or hemolysis. Reactive monocytes are characterized by more deeply staining cytoplasm with a perinuclear clearing and may occur with some types of chemotherapy and in some inflammatory responses.

TECHNICIAN NOTE

Evaluation of a blood smear can be very helpful because of marked species differences in the morphology of some leukocyte types; clinically relevant changes in the white blood cell (WBC) differential may not be detected by some automated instruments.

Other Cells

Mast cells sometimes can be detected on blood smears from animals with inflammatory disease or mast cell tumors. Mast cells are large, round cells with round nuclei and abundant basophilic cytoplasm that contains numerous purple granules. Because of their larger size, mast cells may be most readily detected on the feathered edge. Similarly, neoplastic hematopoietic cells often are large compared with normal circulating leukocytes and can be detected at the feathered edge. These cells should be noted and, if questions about cell identification arise, smears can be sent to a reference laboratory for further evaluation. Broken cells, sometimes called *smudge cells,* can occur if too much pressure is used to make the blood smear or if too much time has elapsed between collecting blood and making the smear. Poorly preserved cells with pyknotic nuclei may be present if the sample has been exposed to heat or if a delay between blood collection and smear preparation occurs. Broken or poorly preserved cells should not be counted in the differential; if high numbers are present, a differential will not be accurate, and a fresh sample should be collected.

Coagulation Testing

Hemostasis (or clotting of blood) requires interaction between blood vessels, platelets, and coagulation factors. When a blood vessel is damaged, endothelial cells lining the vessel are disrupted, and subendothelial proteins such as collagen are exposed. Platelets then adhere to the subendothelial collagen, forming a platelet plug to slow bleeding. Formation of the initial platelet plug is termed *primary hemostasis*. At the same time, tissue factors that activate the coagulation cascade or secondary hemostasis are released. Coagulation factors are plasma proteins that undergo stepwise activation, ultimately resulting in conversion of prothrombin to thrombin. Thrombin then converts fibrinogen to fibrin. A meshwork of fibrin forms in and around the platelet plug, stabilizing the plug and preventing it from being washed away by the flow of blood. If the fibrin clot does not form, a patient may initially stop bleeding as the platelet plug forms but may begin to bleed again as the primary platelet plug is dislodged. As the blood vessel heals, fibrinolytic pathways, such as plasmin, are activated and the clot is dissolved. Abnormalities in the hemostatic system can result in bleeding or thrombosis.

A variety of tests can be used to evaluate hemostasis. A coagulation panel typically includes a platelet count and tests used to evaluate coagulation factors. The platelet count is performed on blood collected in EDTA. Using laboratory testing, the coagulation cascade can be divided into two pathways that result in formation of thrombin: *intrinsic* and *extrinsic* pathways. Factors shared by the two pathways are part of the "common" pathway. Depending on clinical indications, tests for fibrinolysis and platelet function also may be performed. A few tests can be done within the clinic setting, but others are more specialized, requiring shipping samples to a reference laboratory. For accurate testing for hemostasis, it is critical to strictly follow the procedures indicated on the test kit or by the reference laboratory.

Two tests that can be performed in-house are bleeding time and activated clotting (coagulation) time (ACT). Bleeding time measures the time it takes for the primary platelet plug to form. If the platelet number is normal, this test may be used to screen for abnormal platelet function. A one-eighth- to one-quarter-inch slit is made using a #11 scalpel blade or a commercially available lancet in a nonhaired area of skin, such as the gingiva or the inside of an inverted lip. Filter paper is used to remove blood drops every 30 seconds, making sure not to touch the wound. The time until bleeding stops is recorded. Normal animals should stop bleeding in 1–5 minutes. ACT evaluates intrinsic and common pathways of the coagulation cascade and requires a special tube that contains diatomaceous earth to activate clotting factors. The ACT tube must be prewarmed to 37°C (98.6°F) before filling with exactly 2 mL of whole blood. The tube is inverted five times and is incubated at 37°C (98.6°F) for 1 minute. The tube is then checked by inverting every 5–10 seconds to determine the time it takes for a clot to form. Abnormalities in the coagulation cascade prolong the time until clot formation. This test should not be done on animals that are severely thrombocytopenic (<10,000 platelets/μL). ACT can also be performed using a point-of-care instrument (iSTAT; Abaxis, Union City, CA).

Two common tests of the coagulation cascade are **activated partial thromboplastin time** (APTT) and **prothrombin time** (PT). APTT evaluates the intrinsic and common pathways, whereas PT evaluates the extrinsic and common pathways. Instruments that perform these tests measure the time it takes for fibrin to form by using optical endpoint or electrical impedance methods. These tests will be prolonged when a deficiency of clotting factors results from consumption (clot formation), decreased production, or genetic abnormalities. Because APTT and PT methods must be specifically adapted for use in animals, it is best to have them performed in a veterinary reference laboratory, not a human laboratory. In-house analyzers designed for the veterinary market are available. APTT and PT tests require citrated plasma and careful adherence to collection and processing requirements. Venipuncture must be clean, because trauma to the vessel will release tissue factor that can activate coagulation. Likewise, blood samples should not be taken from a heparinized catheter, because heparin will interfere with testing. Whole blood must be added to a blue-top (citrate) tube in exactly a 9:1 ratio of blood to 3.8% trisodium citrate and well mixed. The vacuum present in the blue-top vacutainer tube should result in correct filling of the tube. Underfilling or overfilling of the tube will produce erroneous results. After centrifugation, the plasma is removed and is stored in plastic (not glass) tubes. Plasma should be refrigerated if samples are to be run within hours for APTT or within 24 hours for PT. If samples are to be shipped to a reference laboratory, they should be frozen and transported on enough ice to keep them frozen until arrival to the laboratory. It is important to communicate with the reference laboratory before obtaining samples from the patient to ensure compliance with all sampling and shipping requirements. Other tests of the hemostatic system may have additional requirements, which should be determined ahead of time.

TECHNICIAN NOTE

Blood must be added to a blue-top tube in exactly a 9:1 ratio of blood to trisodium citrate. Underfilling or overfilling of the tube will produce erroneous results.

Fibrinolysis can be evaluated by measuring **fibrin(ogen) degradation products** (FDPs) or **D-dimers**. FDPs form when fibrin or fibrinogen undergoes proteolysis by plasmin. D-dimers are specific products of fibrin proteolysis and are more reflective of active degradation of clots. The Thrombo-Wellco test (Remel, Lexexa, KS) is used to measure FDPs and may be performed in-house. Blood from a clean venipuncture is added to a tube provided by the test kit that contains a clot accelerator. Serum from the tube is collected and mixed with latex particles that are coated with antibodies against FDPs. The presence of FDPs is indicated by macroscopic agglutination of the latex beads. D-Dimer tests are run in reference laboratories and usually require citrated plasma.

Fibrinogen is the most abundant coagulation factor. Decreases in fibrinogen occur when clot formation (consumption) is excessive, or when production is decreased because of liver failure or genetic factors. Fibrinogen production increases with inflammation. Fibrinogen can be measured using tests of fibrin clot formation (e.g., thrombin time), immunologic methods, or heat precipitation. Although easy to perform in-house (see Procedure 11.1), the heat precipitation test is not very accurate at low concentrations of fibrinogen; more sensitive methods are recommended if hypofibrinogenemia is suspected.

Cytology

Cytology refers to microscopic examination of cells that have exfoliated from tissues or have accumulated in fluid. Cytology may be helpful in establishing a provisional or definitive diagnosis for inflammatory or neoplastic lesions involving many types of tissues. Sample collection is relatively noninvasive, and the equipment needed for sample collection and processing is inexpensive and readily available in most veterinary practices. Most samples can be collected on an outpatient basis, and results often are available the same day if samples are interpreted in the veterinary practice or within 24 hours if samples are sent to a reference laboratory. Samples can be collected from a wide variety of sites and from different tissues. However, important limitations include inability to evaluate surgical margins, vascular invasion, organization of cells within the mass, and association of cells with normal tissues—all of which require histopathology. The definitive diagnosis of many neoplasms and the grading of some tumors also require histopathology. High-quality preparations are essential for adequate interpretation of cytology samples, so attention to detail in sample collection and processing should be a high priority. Hemodilution may limit cytologic interpretation, and some tissues do not exfoliate readily when sampled by fine-needle aspiration (FNA). Complications are rare but include hemorrhage, infection, injury to adjacent structures, and dissemination of neoplastic cells.

TECHNICIAN NOTE

Cytology may be helpful in determining whether inflammation or neoplasia is present and, in some cases, can be used to establish a definitive diagnosis.

Solid Tissue Masses and Enlarged Organs

Samples are most often obtained by FNA by using a 21- to 25-gauge needle with a 12- to 20-mL syringe. Preparation of superficial sites is similar to that for venipuncture; however, sterile surgical preparation should always be performed when internal masses and organs are sampled. The mass is identified by palpation, radiography, or ultrasonography and is manually isolated. Ultrasonography is useful for guiding the needle for aspiration of internal organs to increase the likelihood of a diagnostic sample and to decrease the risk of complications. It is important to minimize the presence of the ultrasound gel before sample collection to avoid contamination of the sample, because this can interfere with staining and preclude adequate evaluation of the stained smear.

Once the lesion has been identified and isolated, the needle is introduced into the lesion and suction is applied several times. Depending on the tissue and the size of the lesion, the needle is redirected several times and suction is reapplied to ensure adequate sampling. Suction is released before the needle and the syringe are withdrawn to minimize contamination with blood or cells from surrounding tissue. Frequently, only a small volume of aspirated material is present in the needle or hub of the syringe and is usually adequate to obtain several smears.

For small skin masses and aspiration of some internal masses, sometimes only the needle is used to poke the lesion repeatedly several times without using a syringe to apply negative pressure. The sample is collected only by the cutting action of the needle. The needle can then be attached to a syringe before the smears are made. If only a small amount of material has been collected by this technique or by the more conventional aspiration technique, the needle is detached, air is aspirated into the syringe, the needle is replaced, and a small amount of material is carefully expelled onto several clean glass slides. While working quickly, a spreader slide and a pull or push technique is used to disperse the cells (Fig. 11.15). Failure to disperse the cells on the slide results in smears that are too thick for interpretation (Fig. 11.16, *top slide*). This is one of the most common errors in preparation of cytology samples. Too much pressure during slide preparation results in broken cells, a relatively common error. Application of minimal pressure during slide preparation usually results in slides that are of acceptable quality (Fig. 11.16, *bottom slide*).

Impression smears can be made from ulcerated masses or from a small portion of a biopsy sample before formalin fixation for histopathology. Before sampling, blood and superficial debris should be gently blotted from ulcerated lesions by using absorbent paper. For biopsy samples, tissue fluid should be blotted from a freshly cut surface, taking care not to damage the tissue or disrupt surgical margins. Clean glass slides are touched to the surface of the ulcerated lesion or biopsy sample using minimal pressure. Several touch impressions often can be made on a single slide. For some dense, firm masses that may not exfoliate cells easily, a sterile scalpel blade can be gently scraped across the surface of the lesion and the material spread on a slide, but this often results in broken cells. Using the scalpel to make a crosshatch pattern on the surface of the tissue before making impression smears is an alternate method that may result in better cell exfoliation with less cell breakage.

Smears made from FNA or impression smears should be labeled with the patient's name or identification number and date and allowed to dry in ambient air before staining. It is not necessary to fix the slides with heat or acetone for routine staining. Slides should not be exposed to formalin fumes or packaged with samples that have been fixed with formalin. This is important, because formalin fumes prevent adequate staining. Slides should not be stored in a refrigerator, because water condensation will lyse cells and prohibit adequate staining. Slides can be sent unstained to a reference laboratory or stained for in-house interpretation.

Thoracic and Abdominal Effusions

Fluid can be collected from thoracic and abdominal effusions. Sterile technique should be used to avoid infection or sample contamination. Fluid should be placed in collection tubes containing EDTA to prevent clotting in case the sample is contaminated with blood. If the sample clots, cell counts will be inaccurate. EDTA tubes are not sterile, so a separate portion of the fluid should be set aside and kept sterile if culture will be performed. Fluid samples can be processed and interpreted in the veterinary practice or sent to a reference laboratory.

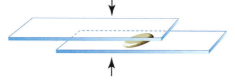

1. Place a drop of cytologic specimen close to the center of one of the slides. Invert one slide, touch the slides together, and allow the material to start to spread.

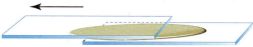

2. The top slide is used to disperse the sample.

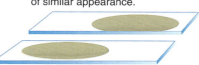

3. This will result in two pull smears of similar appearance.

• **Fig. 11.15** Technique for making cytology smears. A small drop of aspirated material is placed near the center of one slide. A second slide is used to gently disperse the material. (Illustration by Tim Vojt, Biomedical Media, OSU-CVM. Copyright The Ohio State University.)

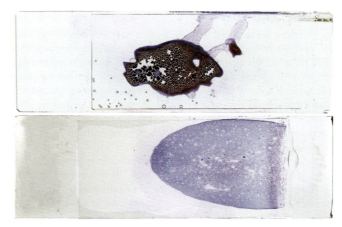

• **Fig. 11.16** A too-thick, poorly dispersed smear *(top)* and adequately dispersed cells *(bottom)* from fine-needle aspirates.

The clarity and color of the fluid should be described, because they may be important indications of disease processes. Normal thoracic and abdominal fluid is clear and colorless in small animals but may have a yellow tint in large animals. Cloudy samples may indicate increased cells or protein concentration or the presence of lipid. Samples that are cloudy from lipid may remain cloudy after centrifugation, whereas the supernatant will be clear in samples that are cloudy from increased cells. Hemorrhagic samples or samples contaminated by blood appear pink to red, depending on the amount of blood. If hemorrhage is suspected, a PCV evaluation can be performed to determine the severity of hemorrhage. Samples that are white or tan often contain lipid or high numbers of inflammatory or neoplastic cells. Fluid may appear brown if there has been previous hemorrhage or if leakage of bowel contents has occurred. A greenish discoloration may be seen with a ruptured bile duct. Yellow fluid may be noted if hemolysis and icterus are present, if there has been previous hemorrhage, or if the bladder has ruptured.

Total protein concentration and specific gravity are determined by refractometry, like plasma protein concentration. This information will be used to determine whether the fluid is a transudate, a modified transudate, or an exudate; this may be helpful in establishing a differential diagnosis. Cells should be enumerated manually using a hemocytometer or an automated instrument, or the number can be estimated from a direct smear. Automated instruments provide accurate cell counts if the count is high but may not be accurate for the low cell counts that often are present in transudates, cerebrospinal fluid, or synovial fluid. If the cell count is greater than $10,000/\mu L$ or if the fluid is turbid or bloody, direct smears should be made using the pull or push technique, as described earlier. If the fluid is relatively clear, the cell count will be low; cytologic interpretation is more readily accomplished if the cells are concentrated. Cells can be concentrated by using a cytocentrifuge or by using techniques similar to those used in preparing urine sediment. Slides are air dried and are sent to a reference laboratory or stained for in-house interpretation. If a fluid sample is to be sent to a reference laboratory, air-dried direct and sediment smears should be made and submitted with the fluid. Cell degeneration and bacterial overgrowth can occur during transport and inhibit adequate evaluation of cell morphology. Slides made at the time the sample was collected are useful for the clinical pathologist in assessing cell morphology and determining whether any bacteria that are present are clinically significant.

Synovial (Joint) Fluid

Synovial fluid is evaluated in animals that have swollen joints, joint pain, or fever of undetermined origin. Samples often are collected in EDTA to prevent clotting. However, EDTA may interfere with evaluation of viscosity and the mucin clot test; therefore a portion is placed in a red-top tube, which does not contain anticoagulant. Normal joint fluid is clear and colorless, very light yellow or straw colored. Normal joint fluid is very viscous, because it contains a protein called *mucin*. A mucin clot test is performed to evaluate mucin quality by adding equal volumes of joint fluid to 2.5% glacial acetic acid. If a normal amount of mucin is present, a tight white clot forms, often reported as "good." If the mucin has been degraded by bacterial or cellular enzymes or diluted by an effusive process, the clot will be soft or less distinct (fair or poor) or absent.

Viscosity also can be evaluated by subjectively determining how long of a strand forms when a wooden applicator stick is placed in the fluid and withdrawn slowly. A strand of 2–3 cm is normal; shorter strands are reported as "decreased." The number of large mononuclear cells are very low in normal synovial fluid; counts can be performed using a hemocytometer or by estimating from a direct smear. Neutrophils are increased in animals with joints infected by bacteria and in cases of immune-mediated polyarthritis. WBC reagent kits (e.g., Leuko-TIC 1:20 'Blue'; bioanalytic GmbH, Umkrich/Freiburg, Germany) that use acetic acid as a diluent cannot be used because the mucin will precipitate, rendering counts inaccurate; oxalate diluents should be used. Automated instruments can be used to determine cell counts, but the results may be inaccurate if the count is very low. When an automated instrument is used for cell counts, synovial fluid samples can be pretreated with hyaluronidase to prevent the sample from clogging the aperture and thus ensure accurate cell counts. Most of the cells in normal synovial fluid are large mononuclear cells.

Stains, Immunophenotyping by Flow Cytometry, and DNA-Based Testing

Wright stain, Wright-Giemsa stain, or commercially available quick stains, such as Diff-Quik, are most used for cytology smears.

Most commercially available quick stains are a modification of the Wright or Wright-Giemsa stain and are inexpensive and easy to use. These stains provide good color contrast, the cytoplasmic details are good, the nuclear details are acceptable, and most infectious agents are stained permanently, which is an advantage for practitioners who interpret cytology results in-house and want a second opinion from a clinical pathologist. Mast cell granules and granules in some lymphocytes stain purple with Wright and Wright-Giemsa stains, whereas some commercially available quick stains do not consistently stain these granules (Fig. 11.17). This is important, because cutaneous mast cell tumors are found commonly in dogs, and LGLs (neoplastic cell type) are found in some cats with gastrointestinal lymphoma or dogs with CLL. These tumors may be misdiagnosed by cytology if only commercial quick stains are used. Special stains sometimes are used to determine cell lineage or to identify causative agents. These stains usually are available at commercial reference laboratories or academic institutions. Immunophenotyping by flow cytometry and DNA-based testing may be useful in the diagnosis of some neoplastic diseases and can be performed on cytology samples by some laboratories. The laboratory should be contacted for information on requirements for sample submission.

Submission of Samples to a Reference Laboratory

The reference laboratory should be contacted to obtain information about sample submission prior to collection if possible. Many reference laboratories provide special containers for submitting glass slides and fluid samples to minimize slide breakage and sample degradation. In general, all cytology specimens should be labeled and submitted to the reference laboratory with the following information: identification name or number, species, age, sex, a brief history, relevant physical examination findings, previous therapy, a summary of results of previous pertinent diagnostic tests, differential diagnoses, and the site from which the sample was collected. If a mass is present, it is useful to describe the size of the mass and whether it is superficial or deep, firm or soft, freely movable or firmly attached to surrounding tissue. Although commonly omitted, this information is very helpful to the clinical pathologist in making an interpretation and providing the most complete information for optimal patient care.

Otic Cytology

Cytology frequently is performed on samples collected from the external ear canal by using clean cotton-tipped swabs, which then are rolled onto clean glass slides to prepare a thin layer of exudate material. Samples collected from the horizontal portion of the ear canal should be collected by using an otoscope. For evaluation of inflammation, infectious agents, and neoplasia, slides are air dried and stained routinely. Pathogenic bacteria and yeast stain adequately with Wright stain. Samples prepared to check for the presence of mites usually are examined unstained before the slide is allowed to dry. A drop of immersion oil can be added before a coverslip is applied to prevent the slide from drying. Some practices keep two sets of stains—one for otic cytology and fecal samples (regarded as "dirty" stain), and one for blood smears and other cytology samples (regarded as "clean" stain)—to avoid contamination of stains.

Smears prepared from normal external ear canals are minimally cellular and often, only a small amount of poorly staining cerumen is present. Low numbers of keratinized anucleate squamous epithelial cells (Fig. 11.18A) and small numbers of cocci or yeasts (*Malassezia pachydermatis*) may be observed. *Malassezia* organisms measure 2 to 6 μm by 4 to 7 μm and have a characteristic peanut

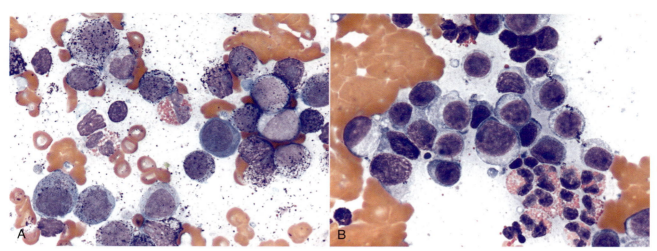

• **Fig. 11.17** Anaplastic mast cell tumor stained with Wright stain (A) and Diff-Quik (B). Note that purple mast cell granules and eosinophilic granules from the eosinophils *(center)* are apparent on the slide stained with Wright stain. The mast cell granules are unstained and only the eosinophil granules are apparent on the slide stained with Diff-Quik. Although the eosinophils are an indication that this could be an anaplastic mast cell tumor, the diagnosis would be much more difficult with the slide stained with Diff-Quik.

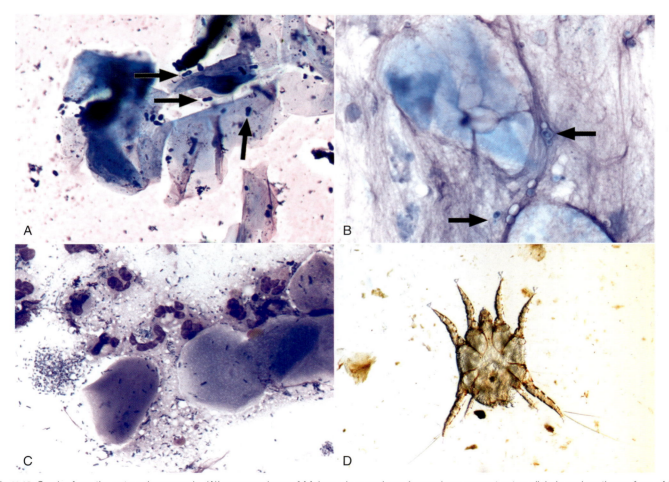

• **Fig. 11.18** Swabs from the external ear canals. (A)Large numbers of *Malassezia* organisms *(arrows)* are present extracellularly and on the surface of the anucleate squamous epithelial cells. No inflammatory cells are present, which is not unusual in some dogs with *Malassezia* overgrowth (Wright stain). (B) There are several budding yeasts from a dog with otitis caused by *Candida* spp. (C) Swab from the external ear canal of a dog with neutrophilic inflammation caused by bacterial infection. Large numbers of bacteria that include rods and cocci are present extracellularly and within the degenerate neutrophil in the center. Several anucleate squamous epithelial cells are present (Wright stain). (D) *Otodectes* mite from the external ear canal of a cat (unstained).

or footprint shape because of the broad-based budding that occurs during replication (see Fig. 11.18A). *Candida* spp., another yeast, replicates by narrow-based budding (Fig. 11.18B). Large numbers of bacteria (>15–25/high-power field) or yeasts (>10/high-power field), mixed populations of rods and cocci, inflammatory cells, and intracellular bacteria (Fig. 11.18C) support a diagnosis of infection, especially in conjunction with clinical signs, patient history, and culture results. *Otodectes cynotis* infection, the most common parasitic infestation of the external ear canal, occurs more commonly in cats than in dogs. Both mites and eggs can be present (Fig. 11.18D). Numerous benign and malignant neoplasms involving the external ear canal have been described. FNA may be helpful in a presumptive diagnosis of neoplasia, but biopsy may be required for a definitive diagnosis.

Recommended Readings

Hematology

Thrall MA. *Veterinary Hematology and Clinical Chemistry.* Baltimore, MD: Wiley-Blackwell; 2012.

Weiss DJ, Wardrop KJ. *Schalm's Veterinary Hematology.* 6th ed. Ames, IA: Wiley-Blackwell; 2010.

Cytology

Cowell RL, Tyler RD. *Diagnostic Cytology and Hematology of the Horse.* 2nd ed. St. Louis, MO: Mosby; 2002.

Raskin RE, Meyer DJ. *Canine and Feline Cytology: A Color Atlas and Interpretation Guide.* 3rd ed. St. Louis, MO: Elsevier; 2015.

Valenciano AC, Cowell RL. *Cowell and Tyler's Diagnostic Cytology and Hematology of the Dog and Cat.* 4th ed. St. Louis, MO: Mosby; 2014.

12

Clinical Chemistry, Serology, and Urinalysis

LORI L. STOSE

CHAPTER OUTLINE

LEARNING OBJECTIVES

When you have completed this chapter, you will be able to:

1. Pronounce, spell, and define all key terms in this chapter.
2. Do the following regarding clinical chemistry:
   - Explain the purpose of the clinical chemistry profile and list the preanalytical and analytical factors that can affect clinical chemistry testing.
   - Compare and contrast the use of chemistry analyzers in veterinary medicine and human medicine.
   - Define a calibrator and a control and describe how they are used in quality control.

3. Describe the general principles of serologic testing and discuss the most common methods of serologic testing.
4. Do the following regarding urinalysis:
   - Describe proper collection techniques and handling of urine samples.
   - List and describe methods for the physical and biochemical evaluation of urine.
   - Describe the preparation of urine for microscopic evaluation, list the cellular elements that can be found in the urine sediment, and identify the three most common urine crystals.

KEY TERMS

Aciduric
Alanine aminotransferase
Alkaline phosphatase
Alkaluric
Aspartate aminotransferase
Azotemia
Calibrator
Control
Creatine kinase
Creatinine
Crystalluria
Cylindruria
Cystocentesis
ELISA
Glucose

Electrolytes
Hemolysis
Icterus
Immunoglobulins
Isothenuric
Levey-Jennings chart
Lipemia
pH
Pyuria
Quality control
Refractometer
Sorbitol dehydrogenase
Spectrophotometry
Urine specific gravity (USG)

Introduction

Evaluation of most patients will include a minimum database consisting of a complete blood count (CBC; see Chapter 11), chemistry profile, and urinalysis. In addition, serology may be used as an adjunct to routine diagnostic testing, especially if the patient is suspected of having endocrine or infectious disease. Chemistry panels, urinalyses, and serologic tests may be either analyzed in the clinic or sent to a reference laboratory. Regardless of where the samples are analyzed, accurate and reliable results depend on careful attention to preanalytical and analytical factors. It is critical that a veterinary technician is knowledgeable about proper sample collection, sample processing and storage, and quality control (QC) to ensure accurate and reliable results.

This chapter overviews common methods and instrumentation employed in biochemical, serologic, and urinalysis testing. Emphasis is on understanding preanalytical and analytical factors that can affect the reproducibility and accuracy of test results. Because the veterinary technician is usually responsible for maintaining and troubleshooting instrumentation, an overview of the principles of operation of common instruments is given.

Clinical Chemistry

The clinical chemistry profile is essential to the basic database used to evaluate most patients. It can be used to screen for disease in a healthy-appearing individual (e.g., geriatric profiles), assess risk before surgery, distinguish between differential diagnoses, or assess the severity of disease. With the use of serial sampling, it may be possible to monitor the progression of disease or response to therapy, including potential adverse drug reactions. The routine chemistry panel is typically run on serum and often measures 10 to 20 constituents (Case Presentation 12.1). Some calculated values, such as anion gap or osmolality, may be provided. In addition, indices for common interferences, such as hemolysis, lipemia, or icterus, may be included. The clinical chemistry profile is most valuable when interpreted in conjunction with the complete clinical picture, such as the history, physical examination findings, CBC, and urinalysis. It is generally most helpful in making interpretations if all samples, including those for the CBC, chemistry profile, and urinalysis, are obtained from a patient within the same time frame. In the perfect scenario, all samples needed for analysis are obtained at the same veterinary visit and prior to all potential treatments.

The chemistry panel is not a direct measure of individual organ or cellular function. However, organ or cellular functional integrity can be inferred by changes in constituents in the blood that reflect leakage from damaged cells, failure to clear waste products, or failure to regulate electrolytes or other various metabolites. Constituents of a routine chemistry panel can be grouped to look for patterns that suggest specific organ or cellular dysfunction; for example, increases in blood urea nitrogen (BUN) and serum creatinine (CREA) indicate azotemia (increased nitrogenous wastes in the blood). However, BUN and CREA must be interpreted in conjunction with patient hydration status and a concurrent urine specific gravity (USG) to distinguish prerenal azotemia (dehydration) from renal azotemia (impaired kidney function). If a dehydrated patient has normally functioning kidneys, increases in BUN and CREA should be accompanied by high USG, indicating that the kidneys can concentrate urine to conserve as much water as possible. In patients with renal azotemia, the kidneys fail to adequately concentrate urine and USG is lower than expected to compensate for dehydration.

CASE PRESENTATION 12.1

Preoperative Panel on a Young Dog

Signalment: 10-month-old mixed-breed male dog
History: A preoperative chemistry panel was run before orthopedic surgery

	Units	Sample 1		Sample 2		Reference Interval
BUN	mg/dL	13		13		5–20
Creatinine	mg/dL	0.8		0.9		0.6–1.6
Phosphorus	mg/dL	5.2		6.4		3.2–8.1
Calcium	mg/dL	0	L	11.5		9.3–11.6
Sodium	mEq/L	139	L	152		143–153
Potassium	mEq/L	47.3	H	4.7		4.2–5.4
Chloride	mEq/L	98	L	111		109–120
Anion gap	mEq/L	68	H	21		15–25
Osmolality (calculated)	mOsm/kg	277	L	303		285–304
Bicarbonate	mmol/L	20.4		25		16–25
ALT	IU/L	21		25		10–55
AST	IU/L	23		28		12–40
AlkP	IU/L	0	L	35		15–120
CK	IU/L	97		131		50–400
Cholesterol	mg/dL	144		166		80–315
Total bilirubin	mg/dL	0.3		0.4		0.1–0.4
Total protein	g/dL	4.9	L	5.4		5.1–7.1
Albumin	g/dL	3.3		3.6		2.9–4.2
Globulin	g/dL	1.6	L	1.8	L	2.2–2.9
A:G ratio		2.1		2.0		0.8–2.2
Glucose	mg/dL	91		112		77–126

A:G, Albumin-to-globulin; *AlkP*, alkaline phosphatase; *ALT*, alanine aminotransferase; *AST*, aspartate aminotransferase; *BUN*, blood urea nitrogen; *CK*, creatine kinase; *H*, high; *L*, low.

Interpretation:

This is a typical menu of constituents for a baseline biochemical panel. When the first sample produced unrealistic results, some of which were not compatible with life, it was noted that plasma from a purple-top (ethylenediaminetetraacetic acid [EDTA]) tube had been used. Sample 2 was drawn in a red-top tube, and serum was obtained. Most parameters were now within the reference interval. The low globulins may have been the result of the young age of the dog. This case illustrates the importance of using the correct tubes and samples for analysis and the critical role of the veterinary technologist in ensuring high-quality laboratory results.

Serum enzymes can be used to detect hepatocellular injury, cholestasis, or muscle damage. In dogs and cats, increases in alanine aminotransferase (ALT) and aspartate aminotransferase (AST) indicate hepatocellular damage, whereas levels of AST and sorbitol dehydrogenase (SDH) are used for that purpose in horses and cattle. AST also may increase with muscle damage, so it is often interpreted with creatine kinase (CK), an enzyme released from muscle but not from the liver. Other enzymes increase with cholestasis, including alkaline phosphatase (AlkP) and gamma-glutamyltransferase (GGT). Increases in bilirubin usually accompany increases in AlkP and GGT if cholestatic disease is present. However, AlkP is not specific for cholestasis and may be induced by corticosteroids or other drugs, especially in dogs. Likewise, bilirubin is not specific for cholestasis and may increase with hemolysis. If bilirubin is increased, the hematocrit and a blood smear should be evaluated to look for anemia and causes of hemolysis.

Increased serum glucose may indicate diabetes mellitus, excitement, or stress. Excitement-induced hyperglycemia should be transient, and glucose should return to normal once the animal settles. However, in excitable animals, this distinction may be more difficult. Additional tests, such as serum fructosamine or urinalysis, may help distinguish the causes of hyperglycemia.

TECHNICIAN NOTE

Serum fructosamine is especially useful in cats as it reflects the average blood glucose over the past 7 to 14 days. A urinalysis may help distinguish the cause of hyperglycemia as glycosuria (glucose in urine) is not generally a finding of stress hyperglycemia.

Electrolytes include sodium, potassium, chloride, bicarbonate, calcium, and phosphorus. Electrolyte concentration in blood reflects extracellular fluid concentrations but may not be a good indicator of intracellular or total body content. Electrolyte disturbances may result from altered function of the gastrointestinal (GI) tract, kidney, skin, and endocrine systems and may fluctuate with and play a role in regulating water balance and acid-base status.

Total or serum proteins are composed of albumin and globulins, with albumin being the serum protein normally found in the highest concentration. Total protein and albumin are measured, while globulins are determined by subtracting albumin from the total protein concentration. Species differences have been noted in the binding of albumin to the test reagent used in some analyzers, so it is important for laboratories to establish reference intervals for individual species. Rabbits often have higher albumin measurements than total protein because of enhanced dye binding. Albumin acts as a transporter for various serum constituents; for example, calcium binds to albumin, and hypoalbuminemia (decreased albumin) will be accompanied by a decrease in total calcium (hypocalcemia). Globulins comprise the remainder of the total protein and contain immunoglobulins and other factors that can increase with inflammation (acute-phase proteins). Albumin and globulins (hyperproteinemia) increase with dehydration, whereas globulins increase with inflammatory diseases and some lymphoid neoplasms. Hypoalbuminemia may develop from loss through the kidney or GI tract, or from decreased production because of liver failure. Both albumin and globulin can decrease with hemorrhage.

See Case Presentation 12.1 for an illustration of some of the constituents found in a basic biochemical panel. Specialty panels of few or more analytes are often available from reference laboratories or may be designed for use with in-clinic analyzers to be more cost effective. Additional specialized tests are becoming increasingly available at reference laboratories, diagnostic laboratories, and universities to further aid in diagnosis.

The veterinary technician is a key player in ensuring high-quality and accurate results of laboratory tests. Accuracy and reliability of biochemistry tests depend on preanalytical and analytical factors. Preanalytical factors can affect the quality of the sample before the biochemical tests are actually run. Analytical factors are those factors that are directly involved in performing the biochemical assay.

Preanalytical Factors

Preanalytical factors that can affect the quality of test results include precollection and collection procedures, sample labeling, sample handling and processing, and shipping procedures. Patient variables, such as age, breed, or diet, may also affect sample quality. Lipemia caused by the presence of circulating triglycerides and

hemolysis resulting from rupture of red blood cells (RBCs) are commonly encountered interferences. Ideally, if the patient's life stage and disease state allow, dogs and cats should be fasted 12 hours before obtaining samples to avoid lipemia that may occur after a meal. Fasting is not required for ruminants, because continual digestion in the rumen eliminates significant postprandial changes. Difficult venipuncture, excessive pressure on the syringe, rough transfer of blood to the collection tube, or vigorous mixing may result in hemolysis. Minimal equipment needed to obtain a sample for a biochemical profile includes needles, syringes, appropriately sized blood collection tubes, sample storage tubes with caps, and a centrifuge. All equipment should be clean and in working order. The use of the correct sampling tube is essential (see Case Presentation 12.1); all blood collection tubes should be filled with the correct blood volume to prevent iatrogenic dilution errors.

Biochemical profiles are typically performed by using serum or heparinized plasma. Serum is often preferred and is obtained by collecting blood in a red-top tube, which does not have an anticoagulant. If multiple samples are collected through the same needle, it is best to fill the red-top tube first, followed by the sodium citrate tube (blue-top tube, if used), and finally the ethylenediaminetetraacetic acid (EDTA) tube (purple-top tube). This helps avoid serum contamination with anticoagulants, which may interfere with analysis. The red-top tube is set in the upright (vertical) position in a test tube rack, and blood is allowed to clot for 15 to 30 minutes at room temperature. The tube is then centrifuged for 10 minutes at a relative centrifugal force of 1000 to 2000 g to separate the serum from cellular components and fibrin. Consult the centrifuge manufacturer's guide to determine the settings needed for the correct speed. When the upper serum layer is removed from the tube, it is important to avoid pulling up cells from the clot into the serum. Some red-top tubes contain a serum separator gel to aid in clean removal of serum. Refrigeration of the sample during the clotting procedure is not recommended, because it will delay clot formation, which will result in an incompletely clotted sample or formation of a fibrin clot above the cells in the serum portion of the sample. Fibrin can clog analyzer tubing or falsely alter the analyte results, so the serum should be separated as soon as a firm clot has formed. Leaving serum on the clot for longer than 1 hour will decrease the glucose concentration due to glucose utilization by cells in the sample. Alterations in serum electrolytes and enzymes may result from cell leakage or lysis, and hemolysis may occur. Stored serum samples should be refrigerated (unless otherwise specified by laboratory protocols) and capped to prevent evaporation, which would falsely increase the concentrations of serum constituents.

In some cases, it may be preferable to use heparinized plasma collected in a lithium heparin (green-top) tube. Heparinized samples are often used when sample size is limited, such as those from birds or other small pets. Heparinized plasma or whole blood may be the preferred sample type for some benchtop analyzers or point-of-care instruments. As with all other blood collection tubes, it is important that the green-top tubes be filled to the correct volume. An advantage of heparinized samples is that both hematology and chemistry data can be obtained from a single green-top tube. One note of caution is that cell morphology and the staining quality of blood smears made from heparinized samples could be better (see Chapter 11). Similar considerations apply for rapid and clean removal of plasma, as described previously for serum. Additional specific sample requirements may apply for some assays performed by reference laboratories, so it is important to contact the reference laboratory before sample collection and submission.

Visual inspection of the serum or plasma may indicate the presence of some common interfering substances (Fig. 12.1). Normal serum from dogs and cats should be clear and colorless, whereas serum from horses and ruminants is light yellow in color. Hemolysis is characterized by red discoloration of the sample, whereas bilirubin imparts a yellow-to-orange color. Lipemia (Fig. 12.2) is characterized by increased turbidity of the sample, ranging from haziness to a milky appearance, and is often accompanied by in vitro hemolysis, giving the sample a pink, milky appearance. Some drugs can interfere with an assay, so it is important to know about all the medications that the animal has received. Information on the effects of interfering substances on individual biochemical tests should be provided by the reference laboratory or by the test kit instructions supplied by the manufacturer for in-clinic assays.

Every sample should be clearly identified through all steps of the process to avoid sample mix-up. Information on labels might include the names of the owner and the patient, medical record number, age, breed, and sex. When a sample is sent to a reference laboratory, the unique identifying information for the patient and the clinic's name and phone number should appear on the tube and submission sheet. Reference laboratories often have standardized submission forms, which should be completed with all requested information. Reference laboratories should provide specific instructions for proper shipping of samples.

Because of stringent preanalytical requirements for sample handling, blood gas analysis must be performed in-house and cannot be shipped to a reference laboratory. Whole blood to be treated with heparin may be drawn from a vein or artery in both small and large animal species (see Chapters 18 and 19). The sample should be drawn anaerobically, and air bubbles within the syringe should be immediately expelled. Exposure to air will result in a gradual decrease in the partial pressure of carbon dioxide (PCO_2), whereas the pH increases. Venous blood partial pressure of oxygen (PO_2) will increase, whereas the partial pressure of oxygen in arterial blood (PaO_2) of an animal on oxygen therapy will decrease. Blood cells continue metabolizing glucose in the syringe, so analysis should be done as soon as possible to avoid a rise in PCO_2 and lactate and a decrease in PO_2 and glucose. Clinically significant changes occur after 1 hour, and these effects may be exaggerated if the patient has a leukocytosis.

Analytical Factors

Analytical factors involve actual performance of biochemical assays and include the analyzer and other equipment, test methods and components, QC, and operating and maintenance procedures. Proper maintenance of equipment, attention to assay methods, and QC are essential both in a large reference laboratory and in a veterinary practice setting using benchtops or point-of-care analyzers.

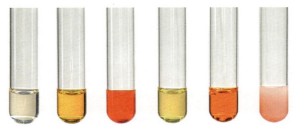

• **Fig. 12.1** Examples of normal serum and of serum with substances that may interfere with some analyses on a chemistry panel. *From left to right:* normal serum in a cat, normal serum in a horse, hemolysis in a dog, hyperbilirubinemia in a dog, hyperbilirubinemia in a horse, and lipemia with mild hemolysis in a dog.

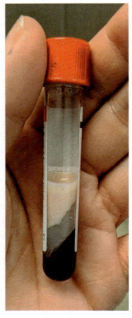

• **Fig. 12.2** Example of severe lipemia in a cat with severe pancreatitis.

Chemistry Analyzers

Chemistry analyzers vary regarding the analytical method, speed of sample processing, cost per sample, and maintenance requirements. In commercial laboratories, many analyzers that were designed for use with human samples have been adapted for use with veterinary samples. Although some tests designed for humans may be used without alteration, others require significant modification because of the differences between humans and animals (i.e., cell size, etc.). Veterinary reference laboratories go through extensive test validation to ensure accurate measurement of analytes and establishment of species-specific reference intervals. If a laboratory that analyzes primarily human samples will be used as a reference laboratory, it is important to check with the laboratory first to determine whether an appropriate method of validation has been used to ensure accurate results with veterinary samples. Analyzers marketed for veterinary practices often come with manufacturer-established reference intervals. However, it is important to keep in mind that what is considered "normal" may be influenced by many factors, such as age, breed, or even location (e.g., high altitude).

Most analyzers found in reference laboratories use liquid reagent–based chemistry and spectrophotometric methods.

Addition of the patient sample to the liquid reagent results in a chemical reaction and subsequent development of a colored product. Light of a specific wavelength is passed through the sample, and a photodetector measures the change in color. Color development is proportional to enzyme activity or the analyte's concentration. Because measurement depends on light transmittance, liquid reagent methods are susceptible to interferences that may add color or increase sample turbidity. Common interferences include bilirubin, hemolysis, and lipemia. Some systems use blanking methods to minimize the effects of interfering substances. Reports often give a numeric estimation of the level of interference in the sample, such as the icteric index, the hemolytic index, or the lipemic index. Manufacturers of tests or the reference laboratory should be able to provide interference guides that relate the index level at which interference becomes significant and the direction of the effect the interference has on an analyte (e.g., whether the analyte is falsely increased or decreased).

Dry reagent systems use reflectance photometry and are more commonly found in small analyzers designed for use in veterinary practices (e.g., Heska Element DC5X, Loveland, CO; IDEXX Catalyst One Chemistry Analyzer, Westbrook, ME). This type of analyzer has a lower throughput, but reagent management is simpler. The patient sample is added to a test strip or pad that is impregnated with reagents, resulting in a chemical reaction. Color development is measured by the amount of light reflected off the surface of the reagent pad and is correlated with the amount of analyte in the sample. These methods are less sensitive to lipemia, hemolysis, or icterus interference. Reconstituted chemistry systems combine dry reagents with **spectrophotometry** (e.g., Zoetis VetScan VS2, Kalamazoo, MI), and reagents are lyophilized in prepackaged assay tubes or rotors. Addition of the patient sample reconstitutes the reagents, and developed color is measured by a photometer.

Total electrolytes, ionized electrolytes, and blood gases are measured by using electrochemical methods (potentiometry or amperometry). These methods are used in many blood gas and point-of-care analyzers (e.g., iSTAT Alinity v, Zoetis; VetStat, IDEXX). A sample is placed in contact with a semipermeable membrane that prevents the ion being measured from equilibrating across both sides of the membrane. This generates an electrical difference or current proportional to ion concentration that can be measured by using electrodes.

TECHNICIAN NOTE

Proper calibration; routine maintenance; and running of daily, weekly, and monthly controls are essential components of good quality control (QC) and of production of accurate and reliable results. As technology continues to improve, interferences in sample analysis are becoming less common, but interference may require dilution of the sample for the analyzer to properly read test values.

Quality Control

Good quality control (QC) is essential if a laboratory is to produce accurate and reliable results. A QC system is designed to detect problems before test results are reported. The veterinary technician needs to have a working knowledge of QC procedures to ensure that all components of a testing system are functioning correctly and to recognize when something is amiss and take corrective action. Errors may occur if deterioration of reagents is caused by expiration or improper storage and handling. Components

of an analyzer may fail, presenting as a sudden change, as when tubing becomes clogged or breaks. Failure of other components may be more gradual, resulting in a drift of control values over time. Detailed maintenance records are important in tracking issues with an instrument and for making decisions as to when an instrument needs to be repaired or replaced. It is important to have a standard operating procedure (SOP) for each instrument. An SOP is a detailed, step-by-step description for performing a test, performing QC, or operating an instrument. Use of an SOP ensures that the test is performed in a uniform fashion every time, whether the same technician or multiple technicians perform the assay. All reagents, controls, and calibrators should be dated when opened or reconstituted and properly stored. Reagents and controls should be discarded appropriately on the expiration date.

Most manufacturers provide recommendations for instrument calibration. Instruments should be calibrated every 6 months, after a major service, or as part of troubleshooting, as recommended by the manufacturer, when QC values are out of range. Calibration is the process whereby the instrument is adjusted using a standardized material, called a *calibrator*. A **calibrator** contains a known, standard amount of a reference material, and the instrument is adjusted such that the instrument reading matches the known amount of reference material in the calibrator. Calibrators are commercially available, usually through the manufacturers of the instruments. For some instruments, a representative from the manufacturer may calibrate the instrument as part of a routine maintenance call. For other instruments, the veterinary technician will have this responsibility. Instruments that need to be properly calibrated will yield accurate results. All calibrations should be recorded in an instrument log.

PUT INTO PRACTICE

To ensure that equipment remains functional, make sure to run QC tests on all machines monthly. Also, get to know your sales reps; they are a great resources when troubleshooting issues.

Controls are different from calibrators. Routinely running controls is an integral part of good QC, because **controls** are used to monitor the performance of a test to ensure that the instrument and/or test procedure is working correctly and consistently. A control contains a known quantity of the analyte being tested. Calibrators are also used to set up and adjust the instrument and/or procedure to perform correctly and to desired specifications. Controls are used on a regular and frequent basis to independently monitor the performance of the instrument or the analytical procedure in its entirety, including the calibration procedure, and to assess consistency over time. With good QC practices, calibrator material that is used to set up an instrument or procedure should not be used as the control material. If the calibrator material is used as a control, errors in the calibration procedure or shifts resulting from degradation of the calibrator might be missed.

Controls are commercially available and may be provided with test kits or purchased separately. For chemistry instruments, running at least two control levels (normal and abnormal) is recommended. In some cases, low, normal, and high controls may be run if both high and low values of the analyte are clinically important. For small in-house laboratories, a minimum of one abnormal control should be run. Controls should be run at least daily and before patient samples are run. In large reference laboratories, controls are often run more frequently, as at the beginning of each new shift. Even in small laboratories, where an instrument may not be used every day, a control should be run daily. Running controls just before analyzing a patient sample is the absolute minimal requirement. Control values should be recorded in a log and compared with targeted values provided with the individual lot of control material. It is helpful to plot the results on a graph (e.g., Levey-Jennings chart) to quickly determine whether an individual control value is out of the acceptable range or if an unacceptable trend is developing over a 20- to 30-day period (Fig. 12.3). Some analyzers come with software to record, graph, and analyze control data. Usually the acceptable variation in controls is within ±2 standard deviations of the mean. This means that less than 5% of the time, a control may be slightly out of the acceptable range. If this is an isolated incident, no further action is required. In some cases, controls can be repeated immediately, or the technician may choose to wait until the next regularly scheduled time to run the controls. If one or several controls fall significantly outside the acceptable range, immediate action should be taken to troubleshoot and correct the problem. A pattern of controls consistently falling on one side of the mean, especially if values are near the assay limits, suggests a need for calibration of the instrument. A pattern of control values that are progressing toward the upper or lower acceptable limits suggests deterioration of control materials, reagents, or instrument components. (See the Recommended Readings section at the end of the chapter for additional information on QC.)

Some point-of-care instruments (e.g., iSTAT Alinity v, Zoetis) that use single-use, self-contained cartridges and electrochemical methods for measurement do not require in-house calibration, because each cartridge is calibrated during manufacture. Electronic checks are done to ensure QC. When a patient sample is run, the instrument reads electronic signals from the cartridge to determine whether the sample is correctly loaded and the cartridge is functioning properly. These instruments require proper attention to preanalytical factors, such as correct shipping and storage of cartridges, handling of cartridges, blood collection, and loading of cartridges.

Serology

Serology is commonly used for endocrinologic testing, detection of infectious agents, or drug testing. In endocrinologic and drug tests, the antigens are a hormone and a drug, respectively. For infectious agents, the test may detect antigens from the pathogen. A serologic test uses antibodies to detect an antigen. Examples include tests for feline leukemia virus antigen and parvovirus antigen. More commonly, the serologic test detects antibodies produced by the patient as part of the immune response against an infectious agent. A single positive serologic test for antibodies will indicate that an animal has been exposed to the infectious agent and may, in some cases, be adequate for diagnosis. For example, equine infectious anemia (EIA) virus results in lifelong infection with ongoing antibody production, so a single test is adequate for diagnosis. The exception to this is an uninfected foal that acquired antibodies to EIA by ingestion of colostrum from an infected mare. Maternal antibodies result in a positive EIA test result until the antibodies are cleared by the foal around 6 months of age, at which time the foal will become negative if not infected.

For other diseases, paired samples (convalescent titers) are taken 1 to 3 weeks apart to diagnose an active infection because of the time it takes for an animal to mount a humoral immune response. The first sample is taken when the patient initially shows clinical signs. Antibody titers should rise over the next 2

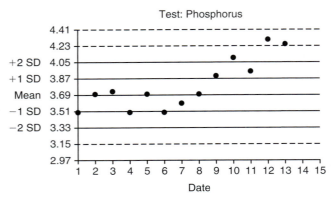

• **Fig. 12.3** Levey-Jennings chart illustrating daily control measurements for phosphorus. Information provided with the control lot included the mean, ±1 standard deviation (SD), and ±2 SD. An upward trend is noted for the control data, which eventually results in data points >2 SD from the mean. Both the upward trend and the presence of multiple data points above the 2 SD limit indicate the need for immediate troubleshooting of this assay.

to 3 weeks, after which the second sample is taken. Typically, a fourfold increase in antibody titer is expected if the patient has an active infection. This contrasts with an animal with antibodies from previous exposure to the pathogen, in which case antibody titers should not rise. Antibodies resulting from vaccination may interfere with some serologic tests. Laboratories conducting the tests or the manufacturer's instructions should provide information concerning the extent of this problem.

Types of Serologic Tests

Serology can be performed using a variety of techniques including enzyme-linked immunosorbent assay (ELISA), radioimmunoassay (RIA), immunoradiometric assay (IRMA), western blot analysis, agar gel immunodiffusion (AGID), virus neutralization, hemagglutination inhibition, and complement fixation, all of which have been used to detect antigens from or antibodies against infectious agents. Many of these tests use serum or plasma, but other types of samples, such as saliva or fecal swabs, can be used, depending on the organism. Hormones are more likely to be measured in serum or plasma by using RIA, IRMA, or ELISA. Studies have shown that the gel in serum separator tubes may interfere with the measurement of some antibodies, drugs, and hormones, so it is best to check with the reference laboratory to determine the ideal collection method. With all of these methods, the basic principle is to link the binding of antigen and antibody to a detection system (Fig. 12.4). Common detection systems result in the production of a colored substrate, emission of light (chemiluminescence), or capture of a radiolabeled substance. Because of the requirements for validating and carrying out these types of assays, most are performed in diagnostic laboratories, which can provide information on the type of sample, proper handling, shipping requirements, and interpretation of results.

An example of an ELISA assay is shown in Fig. 12.4. An antibody against the antigen of interest is bound to a solid matrix. The patient sample is mixed with reagent containing an enzyme-labeled antibody against the antigen. The mixture containing the enzyme-labeled antibody-antigen complex is added to a chamber containing the matrix-bound antibody, which captures the enzyme-linked antibody-antigen complex. Unbound antigen and enzyme-labeled antibody are washed away. A colorless chemical

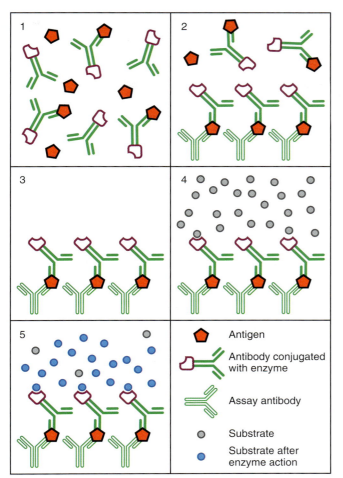

• **Fig. 12.4** Example of an enzyme-linked immunosorbent assay (ELISA). (1) An antibody that is conjugated with an enzyme is incubated with the patient sample, allowing binding of the antigen of interest and the labeled antibody. (2) The sample containing the antigen-/enzyme-labeled antibody complexes is incubated with the fixed second antibody. This fixed antibody binds to the antigen. (3) The sample is washed, removing any unbound labeled antibody and antigen. (4) A chemical substrate for the enzyme is added. (5) The chemical reaction between the substrate and the enzyme results in a color change that is proportionate to the amount of antigen. (Illustration by Tim Vojt, Biomedical Media, The Ohio State University College of Veterinary Medicine. Copyright The Ohio State University.)

Legend:
- Antigen
- Antibody conjugated with enzyme
- Assay antibody
- Substrate
- Substrate after enzyme action

substrate is added and is acted on by the enzyme to generate a colored substance that is read spectrophotometrically, allowing quantitative measurement of the antigen. Other "qualitative" platforms have the user visually evaluate the test for the presence of a colored spot or line on the test unit; positive and negative controls are included with the assay. When these types of tests are performed, it is critical to follow all QC guidelines and instructions. Variations in temperature, incubation times, and washing can interfere with the accuracy of the test.

ELISA methods can quantify the amount of antigen by automated testing. An example is the Immulite Immunoassay System (Siemens, Deerfield, IL), which uses chemiluminescence as the detection system to measure hormone levels. This is a very sensitive method that can detect hormone concentrations at picogram and femtogram levels. In this system, the solid matrix is a bead that captures antigen (hormone)/enzyme–labeled antibody complexes. After washing, a chemiluminescent substrate is added, and it emits light when acted on by the enzyme. Light photons are read by a photomultiplier to determine the concentration of the hormone.

SNAP tests based on ELISA technology have become increasingly available for in-clinic use, are often used to screen for infectious agents, and can be designed to detect antigen or antibody. Tests can be packaged to screen for more than one organism at a time. An example is the SNAP4Dx Plus test (IDEXX), which screens for heartworm antigen, along with antibodies against *Borrelia burgdorferi* (Lyme disease), *Ehrlichia canis/Ehrlichia ewingii*, and *Anaplasma phagocytophyllum/Anaplasma platys*. This type of test yields a qualitative positive or negative result. With tests that detect antibodies to an infectious agent, a positive test indicates that the animal has been exposed to the pathogen and has developed an immune response. Further testing may be needed to confirm an active infection. A positive result for an antigen from an organism usually indicates infection by that organism. An advantage of these in-house tests includes results within approximately 8 to 10 minutes versus a typical turnaround time of 1 to 3 days if the sample were sent to an outside reference laboratory.

Urinalysis

Urinalysis is an essential part of the baseline data obtained from most patients. To maximize its usefulness in interpreting all patient laboratory data, a urine specimen should be collected within a short time relative to blood collection for the chemistry panel and CBC. In addition to labeling the specimen with identifying information as described earlier, the method of collection should be noted, because this can affect interpretation regarding the presence of bacteria, blood, or epithelial cells. Collection methods include free catch, cystocentesis, catheterization, or collection from the floor or cage. Collection from the floor or cage is the least desirable because of the likelihood of environmental contamination of the sample. Samples should be collected in a clean and preferably sterile syringe, glass, or plastic container. To avoid contamination, sampling for bacterial culture should be done before the rest of the urinalysis is performed.

Ideally, urine should be examined within 30 minutes of collection. Because of the potential effects of storage on urine composition, the times of collection and analysis should be included with the sample. If analysis is delayed, the sample should be protected from exposure to ultraviolet (UV) light, which may result in deterioration of some constituents, such as bilirubin. Containers should be tightly capped to prevent evaporation or loss of volatile constituents, such as ketones. The urine sample can be stored in the refrigerator, but the stability of urinary constituents is variable. Recommendations for maximum storage time at refrigeration temperature range from 6 to 24 hours. Initial pH, concentration, and the presence of bacteria can significantly affect urine stability. Crystals can form or dissolve, depending on length of storage and pH. Refrigerated samples should be allowed to come to room temperature before analysis.

Equipment and Collection

Free catch is a simple method of collecting urine, but it requires that the animal void spontaneously or in response to gentle manual compression. The point of the stream at which the sample is caught should be noted on the specimen. Care should be taken if manual compression is used. If the bladder is fragile, as may occur with urethral obstruction, manual compression may cause additional damage or even rupture of the bladder. A disadvantage of this method is contamination from the urethra, from areas around the urethral opening, and from the lower genital tract. Contamination may be lessened by catching urine midstream. Samples collected via this method should not be used for bacterial culture.

Catheterization of the bladder can be used to collect a urine sample, avoiding contamination from the urethra and genital tract. The size of the catheter must be matched to the size of the urethra to avoid damage during catheterization. Equipment should be sterile, and care must be taken to perform this procedure in a sterile manner to avoid introducing bacteria into the bladder. Catheterized samples often contain squamous epithelial cells from the urethra and may contain blood if the procedure traumatizes the urethra or bladder. "Traumatic catheterization" is a technique for sampling bladder masses, such as transitional cell carcinomas.

Cystocentesis is performed by inserting a needle attached to a syringe through the ventral body wall directly into the bladder. Sterile preparation of the body wall should be done before the procedure is begun. Urine is aspirated directly from the bladder, thus avoiding the effects of urethral contamination, and is the preferred method for obtaining urine samples for bacterial culture. A disadvantage of this method is that often some iatrogenic hemorrhage contributes RBCs and leukocytes to the specimen.

Analysis of the urine specimen requires glass or plastic pipettes, clean conical centrifuge tubes, a centrifuge, a **refractometer**, urine chemical test strips (dipsticks), microscope slides, coverslips, and a microscope. Urine sediment stains may be used to assist with microscopic evaluation.

Color and Turbidity

Visual examination of the urine includes color and turbidity. This should be done by using a mixed sample before centrifugation. Normal urine is yellow to amber in color. Red to reddish brown coloration indicates the presence of RBCs (hematuria), hemoglobin from lysed RBCs (hemoglobinuria), or myoglobin from muscle damage (myoglobinuria). Hematuria and hemoglobinuria may be distinguished grossly by letting the sample sit or by centrifuging the sample. RBCs settle to the bottom of the tube, whereas hemoglobin and myeloglobin remain in solution. Additional testing is needed to distinguish myoglobin from hemoglobin, because these cannot be distinguished by visual inspection or chemical test strips (Procedure 12.1). Bilirubin imparts a dark yellow, yellow-brown, or yellow-green color to urine. Unusual discoloration may result from drug treatment.

In most species, normal urine should be clear. Exceptions are equine urine, which is normally cloudy because of the presence of calcium carbonate crystals, and normal rabbit urine, which is densely turbid as the result of mucus and calcium carbonate crystals. If clear urine is allowed to sit or is refrigerated, it may become cloudy because of precipitation of salts and crystals. Increased turbidity of urine may be caused by the presence of epithelial or inflammatory cells, blood, mucus, casts, crystals, or microorganisms. Microscopic inspection will help determine the cause.

Urine Specific Gravity

USG is related to the number and molecular weight of particles in urine and is used as an indicator of the concentrating ability of the kidney. A refractometer is a quick and simple way to measure USG. Refractometry measures the bending of light as it passes through a solution and is related to the density (number of particles) of a fluid. Urine should be obtained before initiation of

---

PROCEDURE 12.1

Ammonium Sulfate Test to Differentiate Myoglobinuria from Hemoglobinuria

- Centrifuge the urine sample. Observe the color, or test with a dipstick.
  - Red/brown color of the supernatant or a positive dipstick result for blood/heme indicates the presence of hemoglobin or myoglobin.
  - Red blood cells (RBCs) should be in the sediment.
- Slowly add 2.8 g ammonium sulfate to 5 mL of urine and mix well.
- Pour urine through a filter paper.
- Observe the filtrate for color, or test the filtrate with the blood/heme pad on a dipstick.
  - If the filtrate remains red/brown or the dipstick remains positive, this indicates the presence of myoglobin.
  - Hemoglobin should precipitate and be trapped by the filter paper.

---

treatment with fluids, diuretics, corticosteroids, or other drugs that will affect USG. To determine USG, a drop of urine is placed on the window of the refractometer, and the USG is read from the appropriate scale. It is best to use a refractometer designed for veterinary patients, because there is a special scale for cats. USG can be performed on a turbid sample with or without centrifugation, but sometimes it is easier to use a centrifuged sample, because particulate material can obscure the scale on the instrument. Maintenance of the refractometer is straightforward. The window should be cleaned with water and wiped with a soft cloth. Care should be taken to avoid scratching the window, because this would interfere with the ability to read the scales. Accuracy of the refractometer should be periodically checked by using distilled water, which should show a USG of 1.000.

Reference intervals are not used for USG, because an appropriate USG would vary with the hydration status of the animal. A healthy kidney should be able to concentrate urine in the face of dehydration or dilute urine to prevent overhydration. USG less than 1.008 indicates that the kidneys are functioning and can actively dilute urine. The USG should reach or exceed minimal levels in dehydrated animals if the kidneys are functioning normally. The minimal USG in dehydration is 1.030 for dogs, 1.035 for cats, and 1.025 for horses and cattle. USG that is lower than the minimal USG for a dehydrated adult animal indicates impaired kidney function. Urine with USG in the range of 1.008 to 1.012 is **isothenuric** and indicates that urine is being neither concentrated nor diluted compared with plasma. This may be normal in a well-hydrated animal but is evidence of kidney dysfunction if the patient is dehydrated or overhydrated. Quantities of other substances in the urine must be interpreted in conjunction with USG; for example, 4+ protein in urine with a USG of 1.010 represents more severe proteinuria than 4+ protein in concentrated urine with a USG of 1.045.

Chemical Evaluation

A variety of tests using chemistry reagent strips are routinely performed. Urine should be at room temperature when tested and does not need to be centrifuged unless it is turbid. Urine is placed on reagent pads, or the test strip is dipped in the urine sample. Chemical reactions result in color changes of the pads. Directions accompanying the reagent strips indicate the appropriate incubation time, with readings typically occurring between 30 seconds and 2 minutes. The color change of the strips is visually compared with a key usually found on the container of the strips, or the strip may be read by an automated reader. Reagent pads for leukocytes and USG that are designed for use with human samples do not work in the case of animal samples and therefore should not be used. Reagent strips are sensitive to storage conditions, such as temperature, humidity, and light, so the containers should be recapped and stored immediately after a strip is removed.

In-clinic urine chemistry analyzers automate the process of reading urinalysis strips. These machines are fast, easy to use, and are often integrated into a clinic's in-house laboratory workspace. Urine is added to the test strip and placed in the analyzer tray. Results are read by the machine, reducing subjectivity and decreasing misinterpretation of color changes on the test pads. Examples of such machines include the VetScan UA Urine Analyzer, Zoetis, and the Vetlab UA Analyzer, IDEXX.

TECHNICIAN NOTE

Urine that has been stored in the refrigerator should be brought to room temperature before undergoing chemical analysis. Urine should not be refrigerated for longer than 24 hours.

pH

pH is a measure of the concentration of hydrogen ion (H^+). As H^+ concentration increases, pH decreases. A pH of 7 is neutral, whereas a pH less than 7 is **aciduric** (or acidic) (increased H^+), and pH above 7 is **alkaluric** (or alkaline) (decreased H^+), according to diet and acid-base status of the patient. Normal urine pH of carnivores, such as dogs and cats, is 5.0 to 7.5, whereas that of herbivores, including horses, cattle, sheep, and camelids, is 7.5 to 8.5. Omnivores, such as pigs, may have acidic or alkaline urine. Because the kidney is responsible for maintaining normal blood pH by regulating H^+ and bicarbonate ion (HCO_3^-) excretion, urine pH often reflects acidosis or alkalosis in the patient.

Urine pH should be measured shortly after sample collection. As urine stands, its pH will increase because of loss of CO_2. The presence of urease-positive bacteria in urine caused by urinary tract infection or contamination can cause urinary pH to increase as the result of ammonia production. Various drugs may alter urinary pH, so it is important to know what medication the patient is currently receiving.

Protein

Reagent strips measure proteinuria from negative to 4+ (1000 mg/dL). Normal urine can have a trace to 1+ reading, especially if urine is concentrated. Alkaline urine (pH >8) can result in a false-positive protein level, whereas acidic or very dilute urine can result in a false decrease in the amount of protein detected. Reagent strips are most sensitive to albumin and poorly detect globulins, Bence Jones proteins (may be present in certain types of cancer), hemoglobin, myoglobin, or mucoproteins. Special tests are needed for accurate measurement of globulins and Bence-Jones proteins. Inflammation or hemorrhage in the urinary tract will cause proteinuria. If proteinuria is accompanied by inactive urine sediment, this may help localize the source of the protein-uria to the kidney. Glomerular diseases often result in selective loss of albumin, and sensitive tests are available to measure small amounts of albumin in urine.

Sometimes it is clinically helpful to quantify urine protein excretion by performing a urine protein-to-creatinine ratio. In this case, protein and creatinine in the urine are measured by using a chemistry analyzer. Urine should be obtained by cystocentesis or midstream catch and centrifuged before analysis. The ratio is calculated by dividing protein (mg/dL) by creatinine (mg/dL). In dogs, a urine protein/creatinine ratio is normally less than 0.5, whereas a ratio greater than 1.0 is abnormal, indicating significant proteinuria.

Glucose

Normal urine should not contain glucose. When blood passes through the glomerulus, an ultrafiltrate of the plasma is formed that contains many of the same constituents found in plasma, including glucose. Normally, the tubules reabsorb all glucose from the ultrafiltrate. Glycosuria occurs if glucose in the glomerular ultrafiltrate exceeds the ability of the renal tubules to reabsorb the glucose. This occurs if blood glucose levels exceed renal thresholds of 180 mg/dL for dogs, 300 mg/dL for cats, or 100 mg/dL for horses and cattle. Glycosuria can be transient, as when an animal has a drug-induced hyperglycemia or a metabolic condition such as diabetes mellitus. In general, the chemical reaction is specific for glucose, but the reagent pads are prone to degradation, limiting the shelf life of the reagent strips. If refrigerated, urine should be brought to room temperature to avoid falsely low results. Oxidizing cleaning products, such as peroxide and hypochlorite, may produce false-positive reactions, whereas formaldehyde or vitamin C may cause false-negative reactions.

Ketones

Ketonuria occurs with metabolic diseases involving increased lipid or impaired carbohydrate metabolism, such as diabetic ketoacidosis in dogs and cats, ketosis in cattle, or starvation. Ketones (acetoacetate, acetone, and beta-hydroxybutyrate) may be detectable in urine before reaching readily detectable levels in blood. Reagent test strips are most sensitive to acetoacetate and acetone, whereas beta-hydroxybutyrate is not detected. Thus ketonuria may not be detected at some stages of diabetic ketoacidosis. Because ketones are volatile and may be lost upon exposure to air, urine samples should be tested immediately, or the sample container should be tightly capped until testing. Bacteria from infection or contamination can decrease acetoacetate.

Bilirubin

Bilirubin results from the metabolism of hemoglobin and is normally excreted in bile. Serum bilirubin may increase with hemolytic disease or cholestasis. Intact male dogs may have small amounts of bilirubin in concentrated urine samples normally, whereas neutered male dogs and female (altered or unaltered) do not. The renal threshold for bilirubin is low in dogs, so bilirubinuria may be detected before icterus can be discerned. Bilirubin is not detected in normal urine in cats, so bilirubinuria in this species indicates disease. Urine should be tested within 30 minutes of collection. At room temperature and upon exposure to air, bilirubin will be metabolized to biliverdin, which is not detected by dipstick. Bilirubin is also light sensitive, so urine should be stored away from light (i.e., in amber containers or in the refrigerator) if analysis will be performed later.

Blood or Heme

The dipstick test for blood (sometimes labeled "heme") is based on the ability of hemoglobin or myoglobin to act as a peroxidase to generate a colored chemical substrate. The test is designed to detect the presence of blood that is not discernible to the naked eye, so the sensitivity of dipsticks is very high, becoming positive with as few as 5 RBCs/mL. This test cannot distinguish among intact RBCs (hematuria), free hemoglobin (hemolysis or hemoglobinuria), and myoglobin, so the results must be interpreted in conjunction with microscopic examination of urine sediment for intact RBCs. Urine should be mixed before testing is done with the reagent pad. The presence of RBCs in urine sediment (see later) accompanied by a negative blood dipstick test can occur if urine is centrifuged or is allowed to settle before testing. Some urinary acidifiers, such as ascorbic acid, may cause a false-negative result. Oxidizing disinfectants may produce a false-positive result. Hemolysis may occur with alkaline urine or with dilute urine (USG <1.008).

Microscopic Examination

To aid in interpretation, urine samples should be prepared using a standardized method. Samples should be gently mixed, and 5 or 10 mL should be added to a conical centrifuge tube. The sample should be centrifuged at 1500 to 2000 revolutions per minute (rpm; relative centrifugal force of 400–500 g) for 5 minutes. The supernatant should be removed by pipetting or decanting, leaving 0.5 mL of supernatant with the pellet in the tube. The pellet is gently resuspended and stain added, if desired. The sample may be examined with and without staining. When using stain, a consistent number of drops of stain should always be added to avoid the effects of variable dilution on interpretation. A drop of the urine sediment is placed on a microscope slide, which is then covered with a coverslip. Improved contrast of the wet mount can be achieved by lowering the condenser and partially closing the iris diaphragm. Results are recorded as the number of elements per low-power field (LPF or ×100 magnification) or high-power field (HPF or ×400 magnification). LPF is used to identify and enumerate casts and to look for crystals, cells, sperm, mucus, and lipid droplets. HPF is used to enumerate RBCs, leukocytes, and epithelial cells, and to identify microorganisms and crystals.

With the help of technology and artificial intelligence, interpretation of urine sediment can now be automated using machines such as the SediVueDx Urine Sediment Analyzer by IDEXX, the Element AIM by Heska (Loveland, CO), or the VetScan SA Sediment Analyzer by Zoetis. With the SediVue Analyzer and Element AIM, urine is dispensed into a cartridge, placed into the analyzer, and the machine reads the sediment, comparing captured images to a database with the help of artificial intelligence. The VetScan Analyzer uses a probe to obtain the urine sample directly from the collection tube. These machines differentiate cells, bacteria, casts, and crystals found in the sample. Results include pictures captured during the testing process and a report of the results. All images should be reviewed by a trained technician. In some instances, results should be verified by performing a manual "dry" preparation of urine sediment and examining it microscopically.

Cellular Elements

The numbers and types of cellular elements depend, in part, on the collection method. Squamous epithelial cells are larger polygonal cells with small nuclei that originate from the urethra, vagina, or prepuce (Fig. 12.5A). Squamous cells are found in free-catch or catheterized urine samples, are absent in cystocentesis, and have no clinical significance. Transitional epithelial cells are medium sized and may be found singly or in clusters (see Fig. 12.5B and C). They can occur in larger numbers or in sheets in samples obtained by catheterization, appearing as round to oval; elongated

or caudate in shape, and lining the renal pelvis, ureters, bladder, and proximal urethra. Atypical-appearing transitional epithelial cells or large rafts of cells may be seen with transitional cell carcinoma (see Fig. 12.5D). Dry preparation of a sediment smear stained with Wright stain or a quick stain may aid in differentiation between cancer and hyperplasia, especially if inflammation is present (see Fig. 12.5E). Renal tubular epithelial cells are small round cells that may be seen with tubular degeneration.

Occasional leukocytes and RBCs are found normally in urine, each with 0 to 8 per HPF expected in a voided sample, 0 to 5 per HPF in a catheterized sample, or 0 to 3 per HPF in a cystocentesis sample (see Fig. 12.5A, B, and F). Higher numbers of RBCs can be seen with traumatic catheterization or with cystocentesis if traumatic hemorrhage has occurred. The presence of leukocytes or RBCs does not localize the regional source of the cells within the urinary tract, and it may not be possible to distinguish between genital and urinary tract origins with voided and catheterized samples. Increased numbers of leukocytes indicate **pyuria**, inflammation in the urinary tract. Pyuria is frequently associated with infection (see Fig. 12.5F), and a careful examination for microorganisms and a culture should be performed. The presence of leukocyte casts (see later) indicates inflammation in the kidney. RBCs may lyse in very dilute urine or may shrink (crenate) in highly concentrated urine.

Casts

Casts consist of protein with entrapped cells and debris that form in the distal renal tubules, where flow is slowest and acidity and solute concentration are highest, favoring precipitation of protein. The presence of casts localizes the problem to the kidneys, but the number of casts does not reflect the severity of disease. A few hyaline casts (0–2/LPF) (Fig. 12.6A) and granular casts (0–1/LPF) (see Fig. 12.6B) are considered normal, whereas cellular, waxy, and fatty casts are always abnormal. Increased numbers of casts are called **cylindruria**. Hyaline casts are protein casts that appear homogeneous and colorless, are difficult to see (see Fig. 12.6A), and may be found in healthy animals and with increased protein leakage or tubular protein secretion. Hyaline casts may dissolve in dilute or alkaline urine. Cellular casts contain cells that have been trapped within the protein matrix. Leukocyte casts indicate inflammation, whereas RBC casts occur with hemorrhage. Tubular epithelial cells can slough and become entrapped in cases of tubular necrosis or pyelonephritis (see Fig. 12.6C). Granular casts can be coarsely or finely granular and result from degeneration of cellular casts (see Fig. 12.6B). Waxy casts are the result of continued degeneration of granular casts and indicate a chronic renal lesion. Waxy casts are smooth with blunt ends and folds or cracks (see Fig. 12.6D). Fatty casts contain lipid droplets that accumulated in cells before becoming part of the cast.

Crystals

Crystals in the urine are defined as **crystalluria**. They form or dissolve in urine, depending on pH, concentration, and temperature. Crystalluria is often of no clinical significance; however, crystalluria may be associated with risk for urolithiasis (stone formation), may indicate abnormal metabolism of a substance, or may be a response to diet composition. Crystals, such as struvite (see Fig. 12.7A), calcium phosphate (see Fig. 12.7B), and calcium oxalate (see Fig. 12.7C), are commonly found in the urine of healthy dogs and cats. Horses normally have calcium carbonate crystals (see Fig. 12.7D), especially if they are on forage with high calcium content, such as alfalfa. Dihydrate and monohydrate

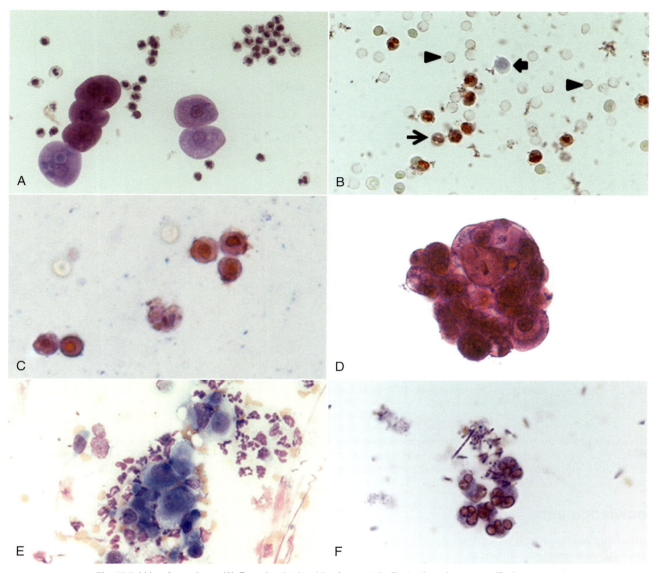

• **Fig. 12.5** Urine from dogs. (A) Sample obtained by free catch, illustrating six noncornified squamous epithelial cells originating from the urethra and many neutrophils. Note the large size of the squamous epithelial cells compared with the neutrophils. (B) Size comparison of a normal transitional epithelial cell *(thick arrow)*, neutrophils *(thin arrow)*, and red blood cells (RBCs) *(arrowhead)*. (C) Normal transitional epithelial cells. (D) A cluster of atypical-appearing transitional epithelial cells, suggestive of transitional cell carcinoma. (E) Wright-stained smear of urine sediment from a dog with transitional cell carcinoma. Note the variation in nuclear and cellular size, the stippled chromatin pattern, multiple nucleoli, and basophilic cytoplasm. These characteristics of neoplastic epithelial cells are often easier to see with Wright stain than with Sedi-Stain or unstained preparations. Neutrophils, RBCs, and bacteria also are present. (F) Neutrophils and rod-shaped bacteria. (A–D and F, Sedi-Stain.)

forms of calcium oxalate (see Fig. 12.7C) may be normal or may be associated with urolithiasis or increased urinary calcium loss. The hippuric acid–like form of calcium oxalate monohydrate has been associated with ethylene glycol (antifreeze) toxicity (see Fig. 12.7E). Bilirubin crystals may form in patients with bilirubinuria (see Fig. 12.7F). Ammonium biurate and other urate crystals may be seen in Dalmatians as the result of an inherited error of metabolism and in some dogs with portosystemic shunts (see Fig. 12.7G). Cystine crystals occur in dogs with inherited defects in amino acid transport (see Fig. 12.7H). Drugs and their metabolites that are excreted by the kidney may form crystals (e.g., sulfonamides).

Microorganisms

The significance of microorganisms in a urine sample must be interpreted in conjunction with the collection method and whether there is an associated inflammatory response (see Fig. 12.5F). Cystocentesis samples should be sterile, but samples obtained through voiding or catheterization may be contaminated by organisms in the lower urinary and genital tracts. These organisms will readily grow at room temperature, causing deterioration of the cellular and chemical constituents. It is important to make sure that equipment used for urinalysis, including stains, is free of contamination, because this will confound microscopic

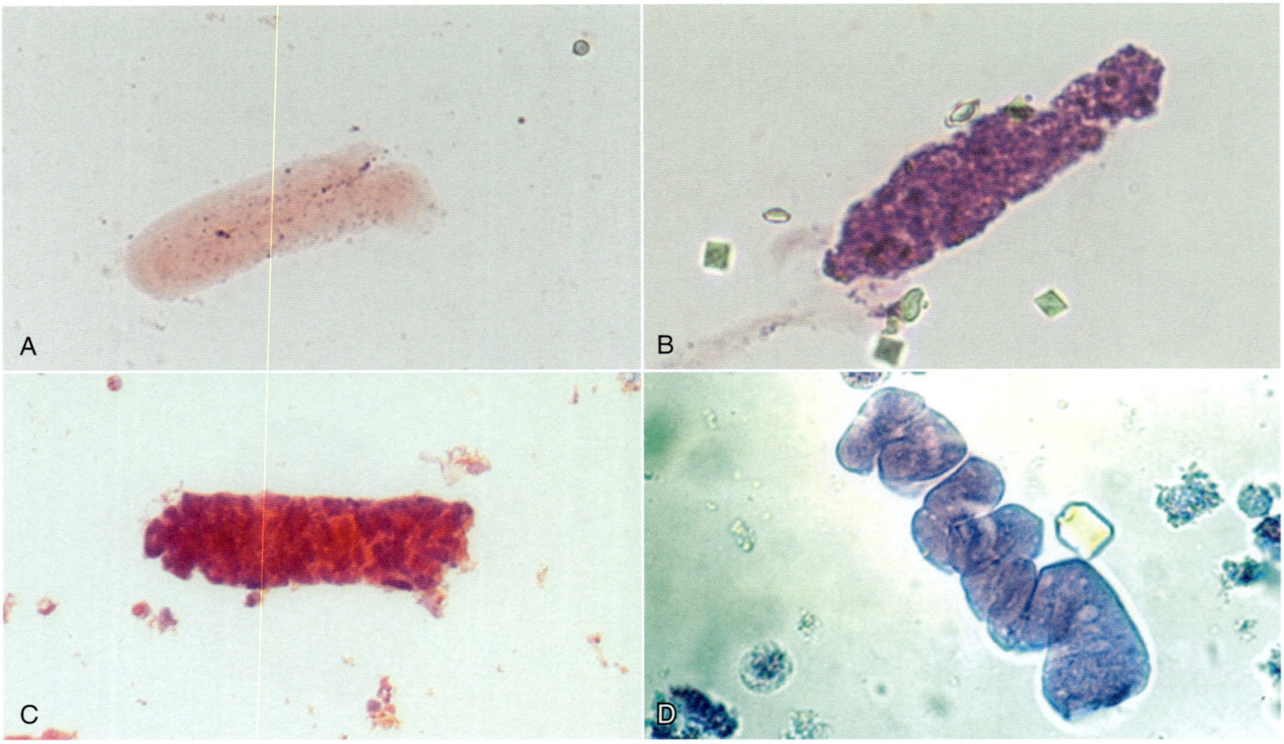

• **Fig. 12.6** Urine from dogs (Sedi-Stain). (A) Hyaline cast. (B) Granular cast and calcium oxalate crystals. (C) Cellular cast. (D) Waxy cast with the typical smooth appearance and well-defined edges and folds.

interpretation and culture results. Bacteria are the more common urinary tract pathogens, but fungal infections may also occur. Absence of microorganisms in urine sediment does not exclude infection as a cause of urinary tract inflammation.

Acknowledgments

The author and publisher wish to acknowledge the contributions of Oreta Samples to previous editions of this chapter.

Recommended Readings

Chemistry
Rifai N, Horvath AR, Wittwer CT. *Tietz Fundamentals of Clinical Chemistry and Molecular Diagnostics.* St. Louis, MO: Elsevier Saunders; 2020.
Kaneko JJ, Harvey JW, Bruss ML. *Clinical Biochemistry of Domestic Animals.* Burlington, MA: Elsevier; 2008.

Thrall MA, Weiser G, Allison RW, Campbel TW. *Veterinary Hematology and Clinical Chemistry, and Cytology.* 3rd ed. Baltimore, MD: Wiley-Blackwell; 2022.

Quality Control
The American Society of Veterinary Clinical Pathology: *Quality Assurance and Laboratory Standards Guidelines.* Available at: http://www.asvcp.org.
Westgard QC: Tools, technologies, and training for healthcare laboratories. Available at: http://www.westgard.com.

Serology
Zimmerman KL, Crisman MV. Diagnostic equine serology. *Vet Clin North Am Equine Pract.* 2008;24:311–334.

Urinalysis
Chew DJ, DiBartola SP. *Interpretation of Canine and Feline Urinalysis: Nestle-Purina Clinical Handbook Series.* Wilmington, DC: The Gloyd Group Inc; 1998.
Chew DJ, DiBartola SP, Schenck P. *Canine and Feline Nephrology and Urology.* 2nd ed. St. Louis, MO: Elsevier Saunders; 2011.

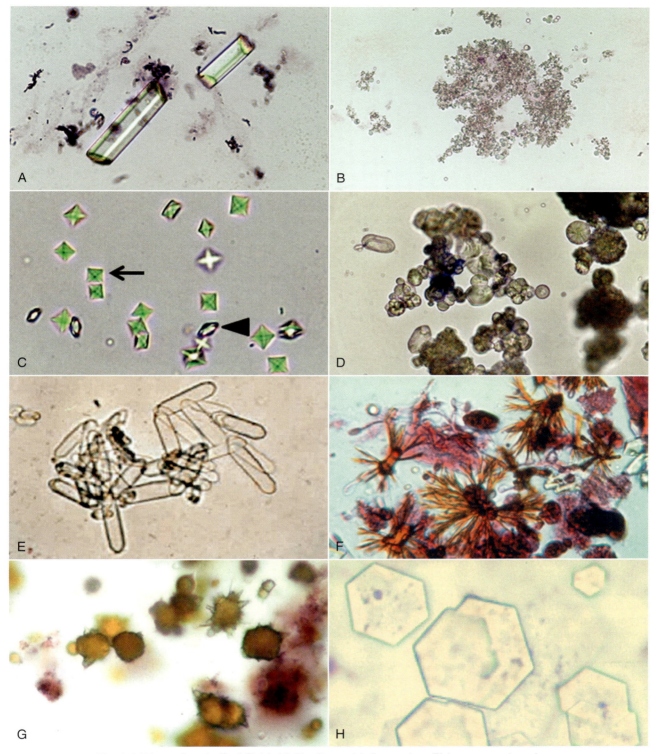

• **Fig. 12.7** Urine sediments (Sedi-Stain). (A) Struvite crystals from a dog. (B) Low-power view of amorphous calcium phosphate crystals from a dog. (C) Calcium oxalate dihydrate *(arrow)* from a dog. Several calcium oxalate monohydrate "hemp seed" morphology crystals are present *(arrowhead)*. (D) Calcium carbonate crystals from a horse. These crystals are a normal finding and exhibit a variety of shapes. (E), Calcium oxalate monohydrate crystals with hippuric acid–like morphology. (F) Bilirubin crystals from a dog. (G) Ammonium biurate crystals from a dog. (H) Cystine crystals from a dog.

Parasitology

ORETA M. SAMPLES

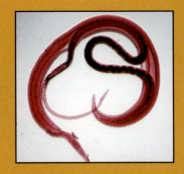

CHAPTER OUTLINE

LEARNING OBJECTIVES

When you have completed this chapter, you will be able to:

1. Pronounce, define, and spell all key terms in this chapter.
2. Identify the common name, affected species, key clinical signs, methods of diagnosis, life cycle, zoonotic potential, treatment, prevention, and control of ectoparasites (arthropods, flies) and endoparasites (protozoans, cestodes, nematodes, trematodes) of veterinary importance.
3. Describe the origin and clinical signs of *visceral larval migrans*, *ocular larval migrans*, *neurologic larval migrans*, and *cutaneous larval migrans*, including risk factors for and methods of preventing these zoonotic diseases.
4. Identify the common name, affected species, key clinical signs, methods of diagnosis, life cycle, zoonotic potential, treatment, prevention, and control of the pentastomes (snake parasites) of veterinary importance.
5. Do the following regarding collection and examination of fecal samples for the diagnosis of endoparasites:
   - Describe the principles of collection, storage, and examination of fecal samples and necessary safety precautions.
   - Describe indications for and procedures used to examine feces by direct fecal smear, fecal flotation, and sedimentation.
6. Do the following additional tasks regarding the diagnosis of endoparasites:
   - List the special procedures used to detect the coccidian parasites *Giardia*, *Cryptosporidium* spp., and *Cystoisospora* spp., including safe handling.
   - Describe how necropsy findings are utilized to diagnose parasitism.
   - Explain how samples are prepared and shipped to an outside laboratory for parasite diagnosis.
   - Explain how the Baermann technique is set up and used to detect nematode larvae in feces and tissues.
   - Compare and contrast the blood examination and concentration techniques used to diagnose *Dirofilaria immitis* from other similar nematode species.

KEY TERMS

Aberrant/erratic parasite
Acanthocephalans
Acariasis
Ascariasis
Arthropod
Bradyzoite
Brood capsule
Cestode
Cutaneous larva migrans
Cysticercoid
Definitive host
Digenetic fluke
Ectoparasites
Egg packet
Endoparasite
Giardia
Germinal membrane
Hermaphroditic
Heterogonic life cycle
Homogonic life cycle
Hexacanth embryo
Hypobiosis
Intermediate host
Many-host tick
Merozoite
Metacestode
Microfilaria (microfilariae, pl.)
Miracidium
Multilocular hydatid cyst

Myiasis
Nematodes
Neurologic larval migrans
Ocular larval migrans
One-host tick
Oocyst
Operculated egg
Otoacariasis
Paratenic host/transport host
Parthenogenesis
Plerocercoid
Procercoid
Proglottid
Protozoan
Pseudoparasite
Pseudotapeworm
Pyrethrin
Schistosome
Seed ticks
Sparganosis
Sparganum
Tachyzoite
Three-host tick
Trematode
Trombicula species
Trophozoite
Two-host tick
Unilocular hydatid cyst
Visceral larval migrans

Introduction

Parasites, simply defined, are organisms that live on or within other "host" organisms and derive such benefits as nutrition, habitation, or mobility from place to place. Some may require multiple hosts during their lifetime, depending on current life stage. Parasitism severely affects animals younger than 1 year of age but may affect animals of any age, with damage being exacerbated by such factors as parasite load, location within the host, toxin production, and interference with normal physiologic processes such as breeding and milk production. Clinical signs may include anemia, hypoproteinemia, diarrhea, vomiting, weight loss, intestinal obstruction, and death.

Parasites are subdivided into two large groups: **endoparasites** (internal parasites), which include **nematodes**, **cestodes**, **trematodes**, **protozoa**, and **acanthocephalans**; and **ectoparasites** (external parasites), which include fleas, lice, ticks, mites, chiggers, biting flies, and **myiasis**-inducing flies. Endoparasites spend most of their life within the body of their host, while ectoparasites live on the surface of a host body or in some cases, briefly mature within superficial layers of the body (i.e., bots). Ectoparasites may even serve as vectors for endoparasitic life cycles. While some parasites are host specific, others can infect a broad range of species. Modes of transmission vary considerably and are often affected by environmental conditions. Transmission ranges from direct transmission (one host to another) to multiple hosts through an extremely complex life cycle.

This chapter focuses on the major parasites and accompanying conditions that may be encountered within the treatment of common small and large animal species in North America. Parasites of zoonotic potential will be covered, including information that the veterinary technician should convey to clients in a public health effort to educate regarding parasites that may affect the pet and associated humans.

Parasitic Diseases of Large and Small Animal Species and Public Health

Considering the various professional responsibilities noted in the Veterinarian's Oath, it is easy to focus on the health and welfare of animals. However "the promotion of public health" is highlighted in the oath. The role of veterinarians and veterinary technicians to promote public health is often overlooked and yet is vital to client protection against zoonotic diseases.

The veterinary technician acts crucially in client education and must understand the life cycle, diagnostics, treatments, and prevention for different parasites, especially those causing zoonotic disease. It is important to understand the life cycles of these parasites in order to explain the risks, methods of prevention, and reasons for specific treatment intervals to clients. Understanding the life cycle of *Ancylostoma caninum*, the "canine hookworm," reminds us that at least two consecutive treatments with pyrantel pamoate, 2 weeks apart, are essential for eradication of all life stages. Puppies or dogs must be treated to kill the adult worms, eggs, and larvae.

PUT INTO PRACTICE

Consider taking Continuing Education (CE) credits or attending sessions on parasitology at conferences to learn about parasites in ones home geographic location. One never knows when an unlikely flea, tick, or worm will hitch a ride in or on traveling pets.

This requires effective communication with clients using words that clients can understand, such as "egg" instead of "ova." Because today's clients will often perform extensive Internet searches in advance of an appointment, understanding the details of these parasites will better prepare the veterinary technician for dialogue with clients to ensure that information they have researched is accurate and relevant. Case Presentation 13.1 illustrates the importance of effective client communication.

Ectoparasites of Veterinary Importance

Ascarides (Mites and Ticks)

Sarcoptes scabiei

- Parasite's common name: "scabies mite"
- Pronunciation: "Sar-*cop*-tes" "*skay*-bee-eye"

Species Affected

Almost all species of mammals are infested by a distinct variety of this tunneling mite; for example, humans are infested by *S. scabiei* variety *hominis*, and dogs are infested by *S. scabiei* variety *canis*. Although *S. scabiei* variety *felis* is rare, cats are infested by a similar tunneling mite—*Notoedres cati*. Infestation by mites (or ticks) is called *acariasis*, hence infestation by *S. scabiei* is referred to as *sarcoptic acariasis*. The

CASE PRESENTATION 13.1

Hookworm and Roundworm Infection in a Litter of Puppies

History

A litter of 5-week-old American Staffordshire Terrier puppies (three males and one female) was presented for evaluation of an acute illness. Two puppies had been lethargic and anorexic for a day before presentation. On the morning of the office visit, one male was recumbent and not responsive. There was no history of deworming, and the dam was not on a heartworm preventive or intestinal anthelmintic. The other two puppies were bright and alert, still playful, and had a good appetite.

The clients were a young couple with two young children. They reported that the puppies were fine until the previous day, but when they found one puppy unresponsive that morning, they called to make an appointment right away. They were very concerned, with only $100 for treatment.

Physical Examination of Puppy #1

This puppy was laterally recumbent, unresponsive, and appeared underweight. His temperature did not register on the thermometer. Pulse was 85 beats per minute (normal bpm = 100–180 bpm), and respiratory rate was 12 breaths per minute (normal = 18–34 breaths per minute). White, tacky mucous membranes, severe abdominal distension, and a body weight of 3 pounds was noted. His limbs were cold, hair coat was dull, and he was estimated to be 10% dehydrated.

Physical Examination of Puppy #2

This puppy was depressed but responsive with a temperature of 101.2°F (normal = 100.5°F–102.5° F), pulse: 180 bpm (normal= 100–180 bpm), and respiratory rate of 48 breaths per minute (normal = 18–34 breaths per minute). The mucous membranes were white, PCV was 20% (normal = 26%–36%) and capillary refill time (CRT) could not be determined. The puppy's abdomen was severely distended, hair coat was dull, and the weight was 3 pounds, with an estimated 8% dehydration.

Diagnostics

Fecal centrifugation was positive for roundworms and hookworms. Puppy #2 had a bowel movement, with feces consisting mostly of roundworms and very little fecal material.

Diagnosis

- Parasitism—hookworms (*Ancylostoma caninum*) and roundworms (*Toxocara canis*)
- Anemia and dehydration

Outcome

Based on the poor prognosis for puppy #1 and the limited financial resources available, it was recommended that puppy #1 be euthanized and resources directed to saving the remaining pups. A necropsy was performed on puppy #1 to reveal a perforated duodenum, ascites, anemia, intestines filled with roundworms and hookworms, and roundworms penetrating through the perforation and extending into the abdominal cavity.

Treatment

Puppy #2 was given subcutaneous fluids and pyrantel pamoate. Puppy #3 and puppy #4 were also given pyrantel pamoate. All three puppies were sent home with a second dose of pyrantel to be given in 2 weeks.

Discharge

The owners of the puppies were very concerned and confused as the puppies lived indoors, and they were unsure where the puppies had contracted the worm infestation. The clients thought that the puppies perhaps had one or two worms and did not understand how puppy #1 had gotten sick so fast. They wondered what steps they should take as owners.

Analysis of the Case and Client Communication

1. Be mindful of the gravity of the situation by first demonstrating empathy; these owners just had to euthanize a puppy. Remember that they did the best they could with the information they had and acted as soon as they knew something was wrong.
2. Be thoughtful as you share information about the life cycle of these parasites, explaining that these puppies likely became infected in utero and while nursing, causing puppy #1 and puppy #2 to become very sick. Use language that the clients will understand, avoid medical jargon, and provide small chunks of information gradually. Pause periodically to check that the clients understand and to answer any questions they may have.
3. The dam needs to be examined and treated immediately and, to prevent both heartworms and intestinal worms in subsequent pregnancies, she should be put on a combination monthly heartworm intestinal worm preventive. The puppies should be dewormed every other week starting at 2 weeks of age.
4. The clients should be told that their children are susceptible to infection by these parasites through fecal-oral contamination. Remind them of the importance of good hygiene and daily removal/disposal of all fecal material to decontaminate the environment.
5. Reassure the clients that you are available if they have other questions and emphasize their role in the puppies' survival.

This case illustrates the value of effective communication and client education concerning parasitic zoonoses and the important public health role those veterinary technicians play.

mite is spread by direct contact, so one infested dog in the household environment can transmit the parasite to all uninfested dogs in the home. Clinically, *S. scabiei* produces extreme pruritus (itching) and alopecia (loss of hair) in all infested animals.

Laboratory Tests for Detection of Mites
The detection of each type of mite generally involves collection of the mites via swabs (*Otodectes* sp.), skin scrapings (dermatophytes), or use of a flea comb (*Cheyletiella parasitivoax*). Mites collected by swab or skin scraping are placed within a drop of mineral oil on a microscope slide to view, beginning at the lowest ocular power by microscopy. The detritus and mites collected by grooming with a flea comb may be placed on a black piece of paper for visualization of *Cheyletiella*, where they appear as "walking dandruff." Superficial skin scrapings obtained with a scalpel blade of crusts from affected areas often are most diagnostic for certain mite species. *S. scabiei* mites are round to oval, and they possess jointed legs. At the end of some of the legs is a long, unjointed pedicel (straight stalk) with a tiny sucker on its end (Fig. 13.1). The eggs of *S. scabiei* are oval and may contain a developing larval mite. *Demodex* sp. are cylindrical in shape.

Abbreviated Life Cycle
Four developmental stages are noted in the life cycle of *S. scabiei*—egg, larva, nymph, and adult. Initially, adult male and female mites live on the skin surface, but postcopulation, the female mite burrows into the skin, tunneling within the epidermis while laying her eggs within the tunnel shaft. Once the eggs hatch, released larvae penetrate the wall of the tunnel and themselves make new tunnels that are perpendicular to the initial main shaft, producing the extreme pruritus associated with *S. scabiei*.

Zoonotic Potential for Clients
Common transmission to humans occurs from direct contact with infested dogs, a contaminated environment, and fomites. Mites can be readily transmitted between dogs (and to cats) from direct contact with or from sharing beds, a habit that should be discouraged.

Treatment
Animals should be bathed in an antiseborrheic shampoo, removing debris and crusting scabs, followed by a parasiticidal macrocyclic lactone dip or a spot-on imidacloprid-moxidectin formulation that is used monthly such as selamectin, moxidectin, milbemycin oxime, or ivermectin (off-label). Amitraz is also recognized as an effective scabicide in research studies, although its use is extralabel at a dosage of 0.025% solution used as a dip at 1- to 2-week intervals for a total of 6 weeks. Animals should be monitored for any abnormal reactions when extra-label usage is employed using Amitraz and reported to the veterinarian immediately. Extra-label usage of such preparations should not be employed without veterinary consultation to avoid negative impact. Confirmatory testing should be conducted after the treatment period to confirm efficacy of treatment. Amitraz in any form is not recommended for use in cats.

Prevention and Control Techniques
Because of their zoonotic potential, lesions on affected animals should not be held or touched directly, and the hospital environment should be decontaminated with **pyrethrins**. Therapeutic trials using dependable acaricides are essential to confirm or rule out scabies in pruritic dogs with negative skin scrapings. Remove all animal bedding and cloth toys from the home to prevent continued exposure. Veterinary staff should take precautions during the handling of suspected cases, using disposable personal protective equipment (PPE), including gloves and lab coats/aprons.

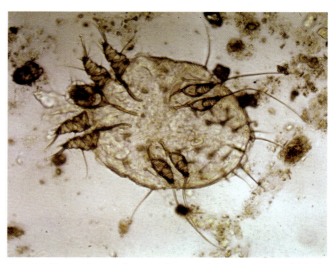
• **Fig. 13.1** Deep skin scraping revealing an adult *Sarcoptes scabiei* mite.

> ### TECHNICIAN NOTE
> The phylum Arthropoda includes all **arthropods** such as centipedes, millipedes, crustaceans, insects, mites, and ticks. Shared characteristics of these include jointed appendages and feet.

Otodectes cynotis
- Parasite's common name: "ear mite"
- Pronunciation: "Oh-toe-*deck*-teez" "sigh-an-*oh*-tiss"
- Species affected: dogs, cats, and ferrets

Dogs, cats, and ferrets are species commonly affected by ear mites. Clinical signs include head shaking, head tilt, scratching at ears, and dark, odorous cerumen in the outer ears.

Abbreviated Life Cycle
The life cycle of this parasite is about 3 weeks from the egg stage to adulthood. The female mite lays approximately five eggs per day in the ear, where they mature into larvae within 4 days before hatching into nymphs. The nymphs undergo two developmental stages before they emerge as adults approximately 1 week after hatching. Adult mites live for approximately 2 months.

Laboratory Identification of *Otodectes cynotis*
During ear collection, cerumen is collected for examination. Similarly to sarcoptiform mites, ear mites are round to oval, and they possess jointed legs. At the end of some of the jointed legs is a short, unjointed pedicel (stalk) with a tiny sucker on its end. This morphologic feature is diagnostic of *O. cynotis* (Fig. 13.2).

Zoonotic Potential
There have been few cases of *O. cynotis* in humans reported in the past 40 years, and these may well be coincidental in nature.

Treatment
Treatment begins with cleaning ear canals to remove debris and cerumen so that topical treatments may be effectively applied. Treatment for ear mites may occur via topical application (either in both ear canals or on skin as a transdermal application) or by injection. Alternative treatments (i.e., home remedies) such as mineral oil should be discouraged. Table 13.1 demonstrates treatment options for ear mites in cats and dogs.

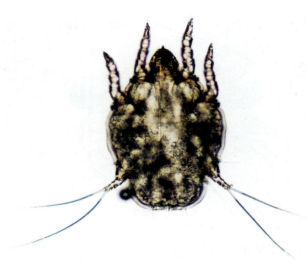

• **Fig. 13.2** Adult *Otodectes cynotis* retrieved from the external ear canal of a dog.

TABLE 13.1	Treatment of Ear Mites	
Species	**Treatment**	**Mode of Treatment**
Cat	Ivermectin	Apply to ear (otic)
Cat and dog	Milbemycin oxime	Apply to ear (otic)
Cat and dog	Imidacloprid + moxidectin	Apply to skin (transdermal)
Cat	Moxidectin + fluralaner	Apply to skin (transdermal)
Cat	Selamectin + sarolaner	Apply to skin (transdermal)
Cat and dog	Selamectin	Apply to skin (transdermal)
Cat	Fluralaner	Apply to skin (transdermal)
Dog	Fluralaner	Apply to skin or give orally
Dog	Sarolaner	Oral

Prevention and Control Techniques

All animals within a household where affected pets live should be treated for *O. cynotis*, even if the test results are negative and the animals' ear canals are mite free.

Demodex sp.

- Parasite's common name: "skin mite," "mange mite," "dog mite"
- Pronunciation: "*dee*-moe-decks"

Species Affected

All mammalian species may be affected; infestation is common in dogs and cats.

Abbreviated Life Cycle

Mites dwell in hair follicles and sebaceous glands and, although they are not a sarcoptiform mite, they produce localized or generalized alopecia. This type of **ascariasis** is nonpruritic unless

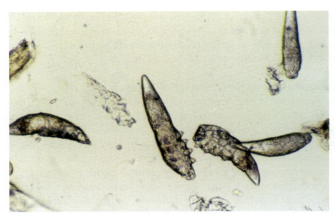

• **Fig. 13.3** Deep skin scraping reveals adult *Demodex canis*, the follicle mite of dogs that are carrot-shaped in appearance.

complicated by secondary bacterial infection. Canine demodicosis can be contracted only through intimate body contact between an infested dam and her puppies during the nursing process.

Laboratory Identification of *Demodex* sp.

Demodectic ascariasis is also associated with immunodeficiency in infected adult dogs older than 18 months of age and is diagnosed using deep skin scrapings or plucked hair. The unique morphological shape is a long and slender carrot-shaped body that resembles an eight-legged alligator (Fig. 13.3). It is possible to identify mites from pustules squeezed to release exudate. The appearance of the mite results from its predilection site—the long, thin, confining hair follicle. Use of PPE is advised when managing suspected cases.

Zoonotic Potential

Demodex in humans is rare and considered an obligate parasitic infection, although *D. folliculorum* and *D. brevis* are species found in humans and treated with topical and systemic medications. Clients suspected of being infected should be referred to a dermatologist.

Treatment

A parasiticide shampoo is used before dipping. Amitraz (Mitaban) remains the only FDA-approved dipping solution for treatment in dogs (*never* used in cats) and should be administered 1 to 2 weeks apart until skin scrapings demonstrate absence of the parasite. Extralabel use of ivermectin (*never* used in Collies) and milbemycin have been reported effective in cases of resistance. Care should be taken with the use of these products due to their adverse effects.

Prevention and Control Techniques

All dogs have a small number of *D. canis* residing in their hair follicles. Prevention and control techniques aimed at this parasite are not realistic outside of treatment when overgrowth of the mites occurs.

Cheyletiella parasitivorax

- Parasite's common name: "walking dandruff mite"
- Pronunciation: "Shay-leh-tea-*el*-lah" "pear-ah-sit-ah-*vor*-ax"

Species Affected

Dogs, cats, and rabbits are primarily affected by this parasite, and clinical signs include intense pruritus. Bitches and queens are often asymptomatic carriers of these parasites. If any dandruff is observed in rabbits, *C. parasitivorax* should be considered. *Cheyletiella yasguri* is seen in dogs with lesions that appear as dry, scaly dermatitis with dandruff, with or without pruritus, located on the dorsum above the tail and the neck. Cats may develop miliary dermatitis (allergic dermatitis with lesions resembling millet seeds) due to *Cheyletiella blakei*. These mites produce a skin condition in which excess keratin debris (dandruff) is seen. If parting the hair coat of infested animals with a fine-toothed comb, the observer will be able to detect these mites as they "walk" along the skin surface, appearing as "walking dandruff."

Abbreviated Life Cycle

Cheyletiella has a 21-day life cycle involving five stages: egg, prelarva, first and second nymphs, and adult. The female attaches eggs to the host's hair, where they hatch into six-legged prelarvae that mature into nymphs, then adults (both of which possess eight legs). If the mite leaves the host, it will die, as it requires a host to survive. The mite is extremely contagious and has been found on fleas, flies, lice, and, of course, mammalian species, which further explains ease of transmission.

Laboratory Detection of *Cheyletiella*

Mites can be detected on the skin surface or within the hair coat of animals by performing flea combing. Mites are approximately 0.5 mm in length and have a unique appearance—a bell pepper shape with a pair of accessory hooks on its capitulum (head). At the end of each leg is a tiny, comblike structure (Fig. 13.4). It is possible to see mites or eggs upon fecal flotation in animals that are fastidious groomers. Veterinary personnel should use PPE, especially gloves and disposable lab wear, when overseeing suspected cases. All clinical areas visited by patients require sanitizing/disinfecting after the visit due to the ability of this mite to survive on fomites for up to 10 days. These patients should be quarantined or kept in a singular waiting area to avoid contamination of the waiting room environment or other clients/patients.

Zoonotic Potential for Clients

Owners should be especially concerned if their dog, cat, or rabbit is diagnosed with *Cheylatiella* species, because this mite is highly contagious. If the infested animal remains in the home or is frequently handled by its owners, the mite is readily transferred to humans, even during brief periods of exposure. Clinically, infestation in rabbits may be mild; however, infestation in humans can be severely pruritic. When diagnosed in pets, the zoonotic potential should be strongly emphasized to the client, as the mite can live up to 10 days off-host within the environment and is spread through direct contact and fomites (consider replacing all bedding and toys).

Treatment

Infested pets should be bathed with seborrheic shampoo to remove crusts and debris before being treated with pyrethrin to aid in absorption. Systemic treatment with ivermectin, selamectin, or moxidectin for 6 weeks is also recommended.

Prevention and Control Techniques

Although *Cheyletiella* species are susceptible to most insecticides, environmental control of this parasite is impractical unless the service of a professional exterminator is used.

Infested animals should be isolated and treated to prevent the spread of disease. Owners should wear protective clothing and gloves when managing infested animals. All animals in direct contact with infected animals should be treated. The use of disposable bedding is encouraged until the animal is cleared of the infection.

Trombicula species (Chiggers)

- Parasite's common name: "chiggers," "jiggers," "red bugs"
- Pronunciation: "Trom-*bic*-you-lah"

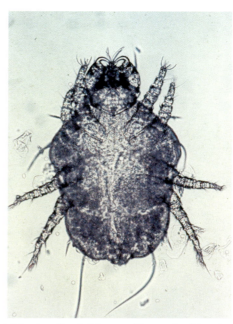

• **Fig. 13.4** Adult mite, *Cheyletiella parasitivorax*, "walking dandruff." Mites are approximately 0.5 mm in length, with a unique appearance—a bell pepper shape, with a pair of accessory hooks on its capitulum (head). At the end of each of the eight legs is a tiny, comblike structure (replacing claws) and two long stalks in the tail region.

Species Affected

Warm-blooded animals, both avian and mammalian, and reptiles, including snakes, may harbor chiggers. The six-legged larval chigger (Fig. 13.5) is the only stage of this mite that is considered parasitic. Larval chiggers typically attach to the skin of the infested host, on which they feed before dropping off. Contrary to widespread belief, these mites *do not* burrow into the skin. Clinical signs become enhanced when these larval mites attach themselves to the host's skin, into which they inject their saliva. This saliva liquefies the host's tissues, allowing the chiggers to suck up this liquid "food," causing skin irritation.

Abbreviated Life Cycle

There are four developmental stages in the life cycle of *Trombicula species*—egg, six-legged larva, eight-legged nymph, and eight-legged adult. This mite is unusual in that *only* the six-legged larva is parasitic. All other stages (nymph and adult) are free living in nature and nonparasitic.

Laboratory Identification of *Trombicula* species

Because these mites normally rigidly attach to the host, they can be observed on/collected from the skin of an infested host. The morphologic details (six-legged larva) of this common mite can be observed by compound microscopy as round to oval, slightly hairy, and possessing six jointed legs.

Zoonotic Potential for Clients

Once attached to a canine host, chiggers rarely transfers to a human host; however, it is possible for them to be "riding aboard" pet hosts and mechanically transfer/attach themselves to human hosts to feed.

Treatment

Dogs or cats infested by chiggers must be bathed immediately in pyrethrin-based shampoos. All pet bedding and cloth toys should be discarded as potentially contaminated fomites.

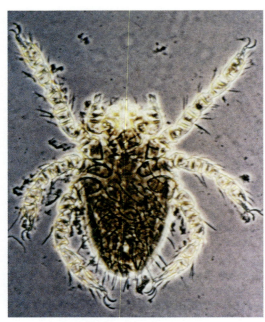

• **Fig. 13.5** The six-legged larval mite of the *Trombicula* species has oval shape. Two legs are folded toward its tail region. The legs in the head region are straight. The larval chigger is the only parasitic stage in the life cycle of this ectoparasite.

Prevention and Control Techniques

Restrict pets from accessing areas frequented by chiggers (wooded areas and undergrowth). Humans should prevent exposure of bare skin to chiggers when in such areas by using insect spray.

> **TECHNICIAN NOTE**
>
> Because of the potential for transmission, technicians should practice stringent sanitation measures, including use of disposable bedding, cage liners, and disposable PPE associated with patients suspected of having a *Sarcoptes, Cheyletiella,* or *Trombicula* infestation.

Ticks (Various Species)

- Common species: *Dermacentor, Rhipicephalus, Ambylomma, Ixodes*
- Parasite's common name: "dog tick," "spotted tick"
- Pronunciation: *Dermacentor* ("Derma-ah-*cen*-tor"); *Rhipicephalus sanguineus* ("Rip-ah-*cef*-ah-lus" "san-*gwen*-e-us"); *Amblyomma* ("Am-blee-*oh*-mah"); *Ixodes* ("Ick-*zoo*-dees")

Species Affected

Almost all species of warm-blooded animal (mammals and birds) and *poikilothermic* (having a body temperature that changes with the outside temperature) animals (e.g., snakes, other reptiles) can serve as host for some type of ticks. Humans are susceptible, particularly after spending time in an outdoor environment where ticks are prevalent. Infestation by ticks (or mites) is referred to as *acariasis*. Ticks produce an infestation, inhabiting areas of the skin (both haired and nonhaired areas) and especially the external ear canal (**otoacariasis**). Ticks are voracious blood feeders, capable of producing significant anemia in all species of domestic and wild animals and "tick paralysis," which is an ascending flaccid motor paralysis that may affect mammals, including humans. Tick paralysis may result from a salivary toxin produced in the tick's mouthparts or from an ovarian toxin secreted by a gravid

adult female tick. Ticks also serve as intermediate hosts for several protozoan parasites and as vectors for many bacteria, viruses, chlamydial agents, spirochetes, and other assorted pathogens, many of which are zoonotic.

Abbreviated Life Cycle

There are four developmental stages in the life cycle of the tick—egg, larva, nymph, and adult stages. After copulation and incubation, the adult female tick will drop off the host and lay her eggs in the external environment, where they hatch, producing the six-legged larvae (i.e., **seed ticks**). The larva crawls up a blade of grass to attach to its first host, usually a small mammal, to feed on before dropping off the host and molting into an eight-legged nymph. The nymph crawls up a blade of grass and attaches to its second host, usually a larger mammal. After feeding, the nymph drops off to molt to the final developmental stage—the eight-legged adult stage, again ascending a blade of grass to encounter a host to begin the life cycle again. The number of hosts vary among the many genera that occur throughout the world, including **one-host ticks**, **two-host ticks**, **three-host ticks**, and **many-host ticks**.

> **TECHNICIAN NOTE**
>
> The one-host tick feeds on a single animal or a single species of animal. One-host ticks often attach to the host immediately after hatching from the egg while in the six-legged larval stage and molt to the eight-legged nymph stage, followed by the eight-legged adult stage (e.g., *Boophilus annulatus*, the Texas cattle fever tick). The two- and three-host ticks involve two or three different hosts that the tick feeds on during different life stages (example of a two-host tick: *Rhipcephalus*; examples of a three-host tick: *I. scapularis*).

Laboratory Identification of Tick Species

Most veterinary practices are not interested in the speciation of ticks commonly found on patients. Some diagnostic laboratories are capable of rendering generic or specific identification of ticks by using a dichotomous key, if requested.

Unengorged male and female ticks should be submitted because it is difficult to identify engorged female ticks. Box 13.1 lists common zoonotic diseases and associated ticks.

Zoonotic Potential for Clients

Ticks can transmit a variety of zoonotic diseases from animals to humans (Table 13.2). Clients should be educated on the pathogenicity of many of these zoonotic conditions and the need for rigorous tick-control programs and correct tick removal, as well as encouraged to seek medical attention should they experience symptoms after discovering attached ticks.

Treatment

Pyrethrin, permethrins, fipronil, and amitraz are commercially available tick treatments and preventive agents for dogs. Fipronil and selamectin, two main tick preventives, are also safe for use in cats. Most topical monthly preventive treatments target both fleas and ticks and their eggs, and are marketed for use in dogs or cats; however, canine products should *never* be applied on cats.

Prevention and Control Techniques

Dogs are very susceptible to tick bites and tickborne diseases. Vaccines are not available for many of the tickborne diseases of dogs; the use of commercial products will reduce the risk of zoonotic disease spread. Prophylactic 30-day use of flea and tick preventives is an excellent way to prevent exposure, although pets should be examined daily for the presence of ticks (in the ears, axillary regions, and anal area), especially after they have been outdoors. When ticks are found on an animal, the entire tick should be removed and destroyed. Tick habitats in yards can be eradicated through proper landscaping and lawn maintenance. Owners should sanitize bedding regularly and inspect living areas for ticks, dead or alive.

• BOX 13.1	Tickborne Diseases and Associated Microbes	
Disease	**Microbe**	**Tick Association**
Anaplasmosis	Anaplasma phagocytophilum	*Ixodes scapularis, Ixodes pacificus*
Babesiosis	*Babesia microti, Borrelia burgdorferi, Borrelia mayonii*	*Ixodes scapularis*
Lyme disease	*Borrelia burgdorferi, Borrelia mayonii*	*I. scapularis*
Colorado tick fever	Coltivirus	*Dermacentor andersoni*
Ehrlichiosis eauclairensis	*Ehrlichia chaffeensis, Ehrlichia ewingii, Ehrlichia muris*	*Ambylomma americanum*
Powassan disease	Flavivirus	*Ixodes scapularis, Ixodes cookei*
Rickettsiasis	*Rickettsia rickettsii*	*Ambylomma maculatum, Dermacentor occidentalis* (California only)
Rocky Mountain spotted fever	*Rickettsia rickettsii*	*Dermacentor variabilis, D. andersoni, Rhipicephalus sanguineus*
Southern tick–associated disease (STAD)	*Borrelia lonestari* (unconfirmed)	*A. americanum*
Southern tick–associated rash illness (STARI)		
Tularemia	*Francisella tularensis*	*D. variabilis, D. andersoni, A. americanum*

When removing a tick, it is important to ensure that residual tick mouthparts are not left in the pet's skin, as secondary infections may result. It is also important to use disposable gloves and if available, tick "tweezers" to avoid squeezing the tick during the removal process, as pathogens may be regurgitated from the tick into animal or the owner's bare skin.

Fleas

Ctenocephalides sp.

- Common species: *Ctenocephalides canis, Ctenocephalides felis, Pulex* species
- Parasite's common name: "flea"
- Pronunciation: "ten-ō-sə-ˈfal-ə-ˌdēz"

There are over 2500 species of fleas; all are wingless yet are prolific jumpers. They are blood suckers, taking their first blood meal to trigger maturation of the ovaries (females) and dissolution of the testicular plug (males). They are associated with the spread of tapeworms and more dangerous zoonotic diseases such as plague.

Species Affected. Mammalian species and humans.

Abbreviated Life Cycle

Fleas have a four-part life cycle. Eggs are shed by the female into the environment to hatch into larvae within 3 to 4 days and feed on organic debris. The larva forms the pupa, which takes 3 to 4 weeks to mature; then the adult flea hatches from the pupa and seeks a mammal to feed on.

TABLE 13.2 Characteristics of Common Tickborne Diseases

Disease/Cause	Clinical Signs	Diagnosis	Treatment	Zoonotic Potential	Technician Tips
Rocky Mountain spotted fever/*Rickettsia rickettsii*	Fever, depression, anorexia, lymphadenopathy, coughing or dyspnea, abdominal pain, and edema of face or extremities	Presumptive through serologic testing with IFA test (showing fourfold rise between acute and convalescent titers), along with clinical signs	• Doxycycline is treatment of choice • Chloramphenicol in pregnant bitches or puppies younger than 6 months	• Direct transmission from dogs to people does not occur • Dogs are short-term reservoirs and sentinels for the disease	• Disease occurrence highest from April to September • Ticks removed from pets must not be crushed by unprotected fingers to prevent exposure
Q fever/*Coxiella burnetii*	• Goats, sheep, and cattle are primary domestic reservoirs, and unapparent infection is typical, because clinical signs rarely develop in infected livestock • Can cause abortion and abortion storms in sheep and goats when infection passes through previously uninfected flock or herd	• Serologic testing is diagnostic tool of choice with complement fixation and ELISA • Microscopic demonstration of *Rickettsia* in impression smears from placenta also diagnostic	• Tetracycline antibiotic treatment is effective • Separation of pregnant animals and burning or burying of infective reproductive tissues/fluids can reduce spread	• *C. burnetii* is transmitted via inhalation, direct, or indirect contact with infected animals, or direct or indirect contact with their dried excretions • Humans are not typically infected by tick bites	• In the United States, Q fever outbreaks have resulted mainly from occupational exposure involving veterinarians, slaughterhouse workers, sheep and dairy workers, livestock farmers, and laboratory workers

TABLE 13.2	Characteristics of Common Tickborne Diseases—cont'd				
Disease/Cause	**Clinical Signs**	**Diagnosis**	**Treatment**	**Zoonotic Potential**	**Technician Tips**
Tularemia/*Francisella tularensis*	• Varies with species infected • Rabbits, hares, rodents—naturally infected, most often found dead • Sheep—high fever, lethargy, anorexia, rigid gait, diarrhea, polyuria, weight loss, tachycardia, tachypnea, dyspnea • Clinical disease occurs occasionally in cats and rarely in dogs	• Definitive diagnosis through bacterial culture from clinical specimens, such as blood, exudates, or biopsy • Can also be confirmed by demonstration of organism with PCR or IFA tests	• Streptomycin and tetracycline are antibiotics of choice for treating wild and domestic animals • Early treatment should prevent death	• Most cases of tularemia in United States are associated with bites of infected ticks, mosquitoes, and biting flies or with handling of infected rodents, rabbits, or hares • Another source is contaminated wild rabbit meat	• Tularemia is extremely infectious and is readily transmitted from infected animals to humans • Strict protective measures should be used in handling animals, their bedding, and all laboratory samples
Ehrlichiosis (canine monocytic ehrlichiosis)/*Ehrlichia canis* (rarely caused by *Ehrlichia chaffeensis*)	• Fever, depression, anorexia, lymphadenopathy • Thrombocytopenia, bleeding episodes	• Blood smear and serology using IFA is best • ELISA can also be used • Clinical signs and response to therapy can be presumptive diagnosis before definitive diagnostic answers are received	• Doxycycline is preferred method of therapy • Early treatment is critical	• Most *Ehrlichia* spp. may be infectious to humans, but dog-to-dog or dog-to-human transmission does not occur • Dogs can, however, bring vectors into the human environment	• Low platelet numbers might increase bleeding time after blood sample collection • Most cases occur during highest tick activity—April to September • Infected dogs pose little to no hazard to humans as long as ticks are well controlled
Tick paralysis/salivary neurotoxin produced by certain female ticks	• Hindlimb weakness rapidly progressing to generalized weakness, then complete flaccid paralysis • Dogs become recumbent in 24–72 hours, and death can occur as a result of paralysis of respiratory muscles	• Diagnosis rests entirely on finding of ticks on an animal with compatible clinical signs, removal of ticks, and rapid clinical improvement within 24–48 hours	• Tick removal can be curative • Use insecticide if ticks are not found • Whole-body shave, if necessary • Supportive care until clinical signs resolve	• Some ticks may cause tick paralysis in humans; animal-to-animal or zoonotic transmission does not occur	• Delay in finding and removing ticks can affect prognosis significantly • Remember to remove the entire tick head, because toxin resides in salivary glands • Tick paralysis can also affect cats, lambs, calves, goats, and foals
Cytauxzoonosis/*Cytauxzoon felis*	• Anorexia, lethargy, dyspnea, icterus and fever, pallor, and death • Anemia and leukopenia	• ID of organism on blood smear or from tissue aspirates in acute cases • PCR can be used to confirm presence of organism in cats that are subclinical	• Atovaquone and azithromycin used in combination are the most current therapy	• No evidence of human infection has been found	• Clinical suspicion and early diagnosis through identification of organism on blood smear or from tissue aspirates have resulted in successful response to treatment • Outdoor cats in areas where bobcats roam are at risk for this deadly disease

ELISA, Enzyme-linked immunosorbent assay; *ID,* identification; *IFA,* immunofluorescence assay; *PCR,* polymerase chain reaction.

Courtesy of Hendrix C, Sirois M. *Laboratory Procedures for Veterinary Technicians.* 5th ed. St. Louis, MO: Mosby; 2007.

Laboratory Tests

Visual identification on pets or pet environments.

Zoonotic Potential for Clients

The cat flea has the potential to spread *Bartonella henselae* to humans via its fecal matter. In humans, this is the source of a disease called *cat scratch fever*. Symptoms of this disease include lymphadenopathy, which is self-limiting and clears with 2 to 4 weeks in healthy individuals. However, in those with compromised immune systems, vasoproliferative tumors can develop, further compromising health.

Plague, caused by *Yersinia pestis*, is a zoonotic disease of historical importance and identified as a "flea-borne" disease found worldwide, except for Australia and Antarctica. Most cases in the United States are located in New Mexico, Arizona, Colorado, California, Oregon, and Nevada. There are three types of plague caused by *Y. pestis*: bubonic, septicemic, and pneumonic. Pneumonic plague is the only form that can spread from human to human, while all three forms are zoonotic.

> **TECHNICIAN NOTE**
>
> To differentiate "flea dirt" from environmental dirt, place a small amount of the debris on white paper and sprinkle with water. If it resembles blood, this dirt is actually flea feces.

Treatment

Pets may be dosed with a monthly preventive to kill eggs, larvae, adult fleas; other ectoparasites (i.e., mites and ticks); and specific endoparasites (heartworm, roundworms, etc.). In cases of extreme infestation, appropriate flea shampoos and/or dips may be used according to the manufacturer's instructions; the instructions should be carefully reviewed to ascertain when monthly preventives should be started after treatment with shampooing. Due to a strong risk of toxic overdose, shampoos, dips, and preventives should not be started simultaneously.

Prevention and Control

Through *integrated pest management* (IPM), the pet and all the environments that it encounters are treated to eradicate fleas. Additionally, the home environment should be cleaned thoroughly, including vacuuming of all rugs and carpets, with the vacuum bag discarded outdoors after each vacuuming to remove the pests from the house completely. Bedding should be washed regularly and the animals inspected for fleas or flea dirt. If fleas are noted in yards or grassy areas, clients should be directed to their local hardware store to determine the best application for their situation.

Lice

Pediculus sp.

There are nearly 5000 species of lice, an obligate parasite of most bird and mammalian life forms. The species is divided into two types, chewing and sucking lice, based on their feeding habits. They are also regarded as a one-host parasite that cannot survive off-host.
- Common species:
  - Large animals: *Bovicola* spp.; *Linognathus vituli, Solenopotes capillatus, Haematopinus* spp.
  - Small animals: *Trichodectes canis, Trichodectes felis, Linognathus setosus*
- Parasite's common name: lice
- Pronunciation (small animals): trik′ō-dek′tēz, li-nog′nă-thŭs

Abbreviated Life Cycle

Female lice lay up to eight eggs per day; the terms *nit* and *egg* are synonymous. Eggs hatch in 1 week, then the nymph emerges to attach to a hair shaft to undergo three molts over 7 days. Adults are about the size of a sesame seed. Lice feed several times daily and will die without a blood meal. They will not survive on a dead host and may utilize "phoresis" to gain transport on scavenging flies to reach a new host.

Laboratory Tests

Lice can be visually identified with the use of a flea comb and, for differentiation, a dissecting scope and a parasitology text.

Zoonotic Potential for Clients

There are two species of lice affecting humans: the head and body louse (subspecies of *Pediculus humanus*) and the pubic louse (*Pthirus pubis*). Clients who are concerned about possible infestation should visit a dermatologist or a general physician for diagnosis and treatment, as veterinary personnel should never attempt to diagnose and treat human body lice.

Treatment

In extreme cases of lice infestation, the animal's hair coat should be shaved to reduce the parasite burden; however, if that is not possible, a flea comb should be used to remove all live and dead lice from the hair coat before beginning pharmaceutical treatment. Fipronil, imidacloprid, and selamectin are recognized as effective agents, although most parasiticides will kill lice.

Prevention and Control

In addition to treatment of the affected animals, bedding and environments must be treated to rid the premises of lice. Bedding, toys, and stalls can be washed in hot, soapy water frequently to control the infestation. The use of disposable bedding, if possible, is advised until the infestation has been eliminated.

Flies and Mosquitoes

Although flies and mosquitoes may not be regarded as "veterinary parasites," they play a role in negative veterinary health outcomes by spreading other endoparasites or bacterial infections during feeding on animals.

Fly Strike

A condition in which flies lay eggs on animals, oftentimes in or around a wound. Once eggs hatch into maggots, they feed on fresh or necrotic flesh. This may occur in a variety of mammalian species causing infection and, in cases of domestic livestock and poultry, negative financial consequences.

Cattle Bot Fly

The fly *Hypoderma bovis* (also known as a "heel fly") causes cattle to run, stampede, and otherwise jump wildly to escape the insect. Larvae, known as bots, burrow into the skin to mature; once matured the bot-turned-fly will exit the skin. This causes damage, economically devaluing the hide or pelt. Bots are also found in the nasal cavity of sheep and goats; the legs, shoulders, or flanks of horses; and heel areas of cattle (before migrating up the leg to the back). They may occasionally be seen in dogs and cats around the face or other loose skin.

Mosquitoes

The vector for the spread of heartworm disease in dogs; there are more than 20 species of mosquitoes that carry infective larvae.

Because mosquitoes can survive in both favorable and unfavorable weather seasons, canines should be treated year-round with monthly preventives.

Treatment and Prevention

To treat medical issues, the "attractant" that is encouraging flying insects must be addressed. If this is open wounds, diarrhea, food bowls, etc., the medical issues should be addressed, as well as providing the recovering patient with a fly-proof environment, if possible. If flies are attracted to unsanitary environmental conditions, stringent cleaning, manure removal/composting, and use of chemical deterrents will aid in decreasing the population.

To decrease mosquitoes, remove all standing water sources from the environment and treat drains with larvicidal packets regularly. Ensure that dogs are on 12-month (year-round) preventive heartworm protection programs and tested at least once yearly.

Endoparasites of Veterinary Importance

Cestodes and Metacestodes of Veterinary Importance

Cestodes are adult tapeworms, whereas metacestodes are the larval forms. These flatworms parasitize a wide variety of domesticated and wild animals. Adult cestodes are often associated with parasites of the intestinal tract; however, their larvae may be found in a wide variety of extraintestinal sites. Diagnosis often occurs through sightings of gravid tapeworm **proglottids** filled with **egg packets** on the animal's hindquarters near and around the anus.

Tapeworms are parasites with a long and flat body, which is made up of three basic parts: the scolex, neck, and strobilus, which is composed of proglottids. A **metacestode** is the larva of a tapeworm, usually found outside of the intestinal tract within the intermediate host (extraintestinal site). There are several metacestode stages, including the cysticercoid, cysticercus, coenurus, hydatid cyst, and the **sparganum**. (See Box 13.2 for cestodes of veterinary and zoonotic importance.)

Dipylidium caninum (Cucumber Seed Tapeworm, Double-Pored Tapeworm)

- Parasite's common name: "double-pored tapeworm," "cucumber seed tapeworm"
- Pronunciation: "*dip*-ah-*lid*-ee-yum" "kay-*nine*-num"

Species Affected

Tapeworms are found in many animals, including the small intestines of dogs, cats, and ferrets (Fig. 13.6). Humans, especially small children, may also become infected with the adult tapeworm. Dogs and cats are most often asymptomatic, but the owner may report that they frequently drag their anus along the ground because of pruritus. The most common clinical sign is the presence of gravid tapeworm proglottids (tapeworm segments) on top of or adjacent to the host's voided feces (Fig. 13.7) or clinging to the area around the anus of infected host. Dried tapeworm segments resembling dry, uncooked white rice (Fig. 13.8) may be found clinging to hair, on the bedding of the pet, and even on the owner's bed sheets if the pet usually sleeps with the owner. The *Taenia* species of tapeworms have gravid proglottids, similar to those of *D. caninum*; however, each proglottid has only one set of male and female reproductive organs connecting to a single lateral genital pore (Fig. 13.9A and B).

BOX 13.2	Species Affected by Various Cestodes	
Host(s)	**Cestode Species**	**Life Cycle**
Canines	*Echinococcus granulosus*	Adults
Sheep, cattle	*E. granulosus*	Larvae
Cats, foxes	*Echinococcus multilocularis*	Adults
Rodents	*E. multilocularis*	Larvae
Humans	*E. granulosus* and *E. multilocularis*	Larvae and adults

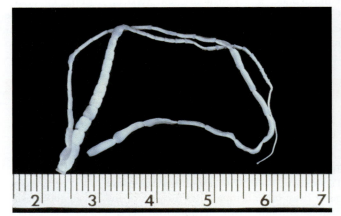

• **Fig. 13.6** Mature tapeworm of dogs and cats. Note the multiple mature segments.

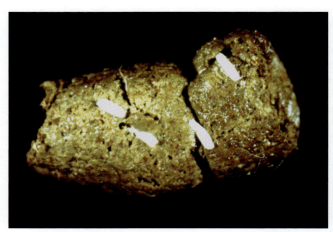

• **Fig. 13.7** Segments of *Dipylidium caninum* in fresh dog feces.

Life Cycle

Cestodes have a total of three stages within their life cycle: ova, larvae, and adult. Adults lay eggs within the intestines of the host, where they are excreted in fecal matter. Once in the environment, they are ingested by an organism in which the egg hatches into larvae. The larvae then encyst within the host's muscle or organs. Once this intermediate host is itself eaten as prey, the parasite is released from the cyst to form an adult tapeworm capable of reproduction (Fig. 13.10).

Among tapeworm proglottids, both cross fertilization and self-fertilization can occur. A mature proglottid has functioning male and female reproductive organs, but older gravid proglottids contain a uterus filled with thousands of egg packets (Fig. 13.11), with each packet containing 20 to 30 individual hexacanth (six-toothed) embryos (Fig. 13.12). As a result of the expanding uterus, both sets of reproductive organs atrophy until the only organ remaining in the segment is the uterus. Individual gravid proglottids are released into the external environment via host feces, eventually rupturing to release egg packets which, in turn, break open, releasing the individual hexacanth embryos. The hexacanth embryo is eaten by the larval cat flea *C. felis* (Fig. 13.13), the intermediate host for this tapeworm, after which the ingested hexacanth embryo develops into a cysticercoid, which is the infective larval stage of the tapeworm (Fig. 13.14).

Each **cysticercoid** found within the body of the flea contains one immature tapeworm scolex that matures into one adult tapeworm. During the grooming process, the dog or the cat ingests adult fleas containing cysticercoids, which are then released into the host's body where adult tapeworm will form. The scolex within each cysticercoid attaches to the lining of the small intestine, and an entirely new tapeworm begins to grow, producing the aforementioned three types of proglottids.

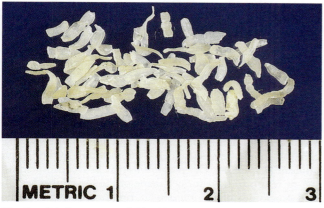

• **Fig. 13.8** Dried segments of *Dipylidium caninum* from the bedding of a dog. (Courtesy Hendrix CM, Robinson E. *Diagnostic Parasitology for Veterinary Technicians.* 4th ed. St. Louis, MO: Mosby; 2012.)

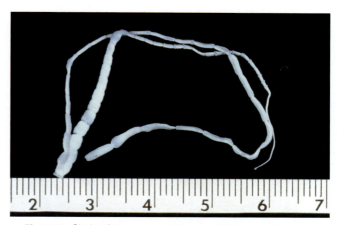

• **Fig. 13.10** Chain of tapeworm segments, which are easily broken.

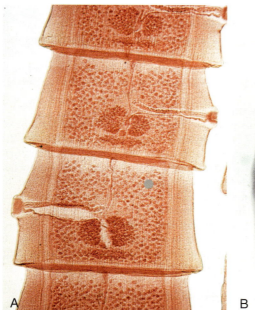
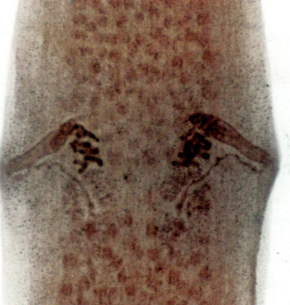

• **Fig. 13.9** (A) *Taenia pisiformis,* a canine taeniid, possesses a single set of both male and female reproductive organs, located laterally, next to the single lateral genital pores. (B) *Dipylidium caninum,* the double-pored tapeworm, possesses two sets of both male and female reproductive organs, located laterally, next to the two lateral genital pores.

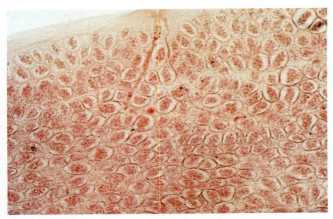

• **Fig. 13.11** Microscopic view of a gravid proglottid of *Dipylidium caninum* containing thousands of egg packets (rough oval structures with a dark patch inside).

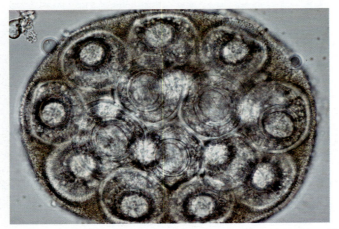

• **Fig. 13.12** A single egg packet of *Dipylidium caninum* containing 20 to 30 individual hexacanth embryos.

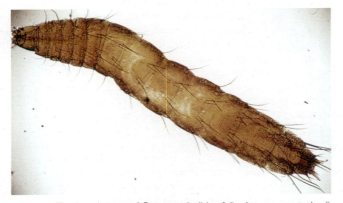

• **Fig. 13.13** The larval stage of *Ctenocephalides felis* shows a curved cylindrical structure with body segments and sparse bristles. The maggotlike larval stage ingests the egg packets and serves as the intermediate host for *Dipylidium caninum* (when it becomes an adult flea).

Laboratory Test(s) Used to Diagnose the Infection

D. caninum may be confused with *Taenia pisiformis* ("*Tee*-nee-ah" "*pie*-sah-form-iss") in the dog, and with *Taenia taeniaformis* ("*Tee*-nee-ah" "*tee*-nee-ah-form-iss") in the cat. *T. pisiformis* is commonly found in hunting dogs, because the intermediate host is usually a rabbit or a hare. *T. taeniaformis* is found in cats that

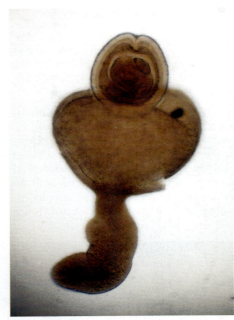

• **Fig. 13.14** Infective stage of the tapeworm life cycle known as cysticercoid.

frequently consume rodents (intermediate hosts). The veterinary technician should be able to identify both motile and dried proglottids of *D. caninum*. Dry proglottids may be reconstituted with water to return to their former shape of the "cucumber seed." If gravid proglottids of *D. caninum* are ruptured during defecation by the dog or the cat, it may be possible to observe the egg packets on fecal flotation; however, this is a rare occurrence, so this test cannot to be relied on. Egg packets are usually observed using a compound microscope when a gravid proglottid is teased open, releasing egg packets.

Zoonotic Potential for Clients

If there are small children in the home, clients should be warned of the zoonotic potential of this parasite. If a child ingests a flea containing an infective cysticercoid, it is possible for the child to harbor adult *D. caninum* and to require the care of a pediatrician.

Treatment

Praziquantel is the treatment of choice for tapeworms at a dose of 7.5 mg/kg body weight orally once daily for 2 days, although epsiprantel, at 5 mg/kg body weight, may alternatively be used. Flea preventive and control techniques are necessary to prevent reinfection, but it should be stressed to clients that the correct products should be used on the specific animal species. All pets in the home environment must be treated for both tapeworms and fleas and all bedding washed thoroughly. The use of disposable bedding would be wise until both flea and tick infections have cleared. Clients are discouraged from sharing their own bedding areas with pets.

Prevention and Control Techniques

Species-specific anthelmintics should be administered routinely to all pets in the home environment. Flea populations in the home must be controlled and eradicated. After vacuuming, the bag should be disposed of in outdoor trash after each session to remove flea eggs, larvae, and adults from the home environment.

Echinococcus granulosus/Echinococcus multilocularis

- Parasite's common name: *Echinococcus granulosus*—the uni-locular hydatid cyst tapeworm of dogs; *Echinococcus multi-locularis*—the multilocular hydatid cyst tapeworm of cats and foxes, seen recently in canines.
- Pronunciation: "Ee-*kine*-oh-*cock*-us" "gran-you-*low*-sus"; "Ee-kine-oh-*cock*-us" "mull-tee-*lock*-you-*lair*-riss"

> **TECHNICIAN NOTE**
>
> Upon diagnosis of *Echinococcus* species, a reportable disease, it is important to advise clients of the zoonotic potential of this parasite. Care should be exercised in handling suspected samples to prevent personnel infections.

Species Affected

The **unilocular hydatid cyst** for *E. granulosus* is encased in a thick, fibrous cyst wall containing a single large, fluid-filled cyst lined by a thin germinal membrane that forms brood capsules containing protoscolices. The **multilocular hydatid cyst** for *E. multilocularis* has, in contrast, a very thin cyst wall which contains highly invasive, multicompartmentalized fluid-filled cysts lined by a thin germinal membrane that forms brood capsules containing proto-scolices. Each protoscolex matures into one tapeworm. Adult *E. multilocularis* are normally found in the posterior portion of small intestines. Clinical signs in the intermediate host range from being asymptomatic to exhibiting severe symptoms indicative of infection of the organ or organ systems in which the hydatid cysts develop.

> **TECHNICIAN NOTE**
>
> *Echinococcus granulosus* = unilocular hydatid cyst = enveloped cyst
> *Echinoccocus multiloculus* = multilocular hydatid cyst = nonenveloped cyst

Abbreviated Life Cycle

The ova pass in the feces of the final host to the outside environ-ment, where a suitable intermediate host must ingest the ovum. Each ovum ingested by a suitable intermediate host produces one hydatid cyst. Cyst encapsulation occurs within the new host. With *E. multilocularis*, no similar cyst wall is produced; therefore gen-erational formation of cysts occurs (mothers produce daughters which produce grand-daughters, etc.). This type of external bud-ding can go on indefinitely and, with no cyst wall to contain it, the cyst will become invasive, destroying normal host tissues and causing eventual host death, after which the hydatid cyst must be ingested by the definitive host. Each protoscolex within the hydatid cyst that is ingested by the definitive host produces one adult tapeworm within the small intestines. Unlike most other tapeworms, these tiny tapeworms have only a scolex plus three segments: immature, mature, and gravid proglottids.

Laboratory Test(s) Used to Diagnose the Infection

Identification of adult *Echinococcus* or their proglottids in the definitive host is difficult because of their small size. Routine fecal examinations do not allow for distinction of *Echinococcus* spe-cies from other tapeworm eggs, although flotation in a modified Sheather sugar solution followed by centrifugation will yield ova. An *Echinococcus* immunoglobulin G ELISA test is available com-mercially for detection via serum antigen–antibody detection.

Zoonotic Potential for Clients

E. granulosus is most prevalent in areas where sheep are raised, although the most common source of human infection is contact with an infected dog or their feces. On sheep farms, lack of regular preventive anthelmintic therapy for dogs living on the premises causes infection when they consume infected sheep viscera or feces containing unilocular hydatid cysts. In the United States, most cases of human echinococcosis are seen in immigrants from geo-graphic areas where cystic echinococcosis is endemic. *E. multilocu-laris* is found in areas in the United States from eastern Montana to central Ohio to Alaska, and is present in Canada where foxes and wild rodents are plentiful and often fed on by outdoor cats. Most human cases have been found in Alaskan Native Americans, with the zoonotic transmission of *E. multilocularis* occurring via canines that have patent intestinal infections.

Treatment

The cysts, if located, can be surgically removed or drained by use of a needle, after which salt solution can be injected into the cyst. Albendazole should be given before and after surgical procedures for up to 6 months after drainage. Praziquantel (5 mg/kg body weight) can also be used. In ruminants, surgical excision of hyda-tid cysts is followed by long-term albendazole treatment, during which time the animal should be kept confined.

Prevention and Control Techniques

Dogs should be discouraged from eating sheep viscera or carcasses and rodents. All dogs should be tested and treated to eliminate adult tapeworms, especially dogs that are in frequent contact with sheep. Vaccination for *E. granulosus* should be considered in sheep. Proper hygiene when handling dogs, cats, and foxes and their feces should be emphasized. Careful handling of fox carcasses (i.e., GI tract) is encouraged when preparing taxidermy specimens.

Spirometra mansonoides

- Parasite's common name: "zipper tapeworm," "sparganosis" tapeworm
- Pronunciation: "spy-row-*meet*-tra" "man-sun-*oid*-ees"

Species Affected

These adult tapeworms are found in the small intestines of both dogs and cats, and adult tapeworms produce very little pathology, including nonspecific GI signs. If the metacestode form of this adult tapeworm infects the dog or the cat, a single sparganum is usually produced subcutaneously, resulting in very little pathol-ogy; however, if the sparganum begins to multiply asexually, fatal, rapid proliferative **sparganosis** may ensue. The parasite at this point is refractory to treatment.

Abbreviated Life Cycle

Adult **pseudotapeworms** (i.e., *Spirometra*) are found within the small intestine of the canine or feline definitive host. *Spargano-sis* refers to infection of humans by the **plerocercoid** stage. This tapeworm is called the "zipper tapeworm," because the proglottids may divide in the middle of the tapeworm and then reunite—much like a zipper coming unzipped. Proglottids seldom break from this tapeworm's strobila; instead, operculated eggs exit the centrally located uterus through the associated uterine pore. Upon contact with water, these operculated eggs "hatch," releasing the coracidium, a motile, ciliated hexacanth embryo stage. The cora-cidium is covered with tiny moving hairs and spins about in the water and must be ingested by the first intermediate host, a micro-scopic aquatic crustacean, to develop into the next metacestode stage, the **procercoid**. The crustacean, in turn, is ingested by the second intermediate host, an amphibian (frog), a reptile (snake), or a small mammal (mouse), where the second intermediate host, the procercoid, develops into the next metacestode stage—the plerocercoid (sparganum). The pleurocercoid entwines within the subcutaneous tissues or the musculature. The definitive host becomes infected by ingesting the second intermediate host containing the plerocercoid/sparganum, which then emerges from the tissue site, attaching itself to the mucosa of the stomach to mature into an adult. If a dog or a cat ingests the aquatic crustacean containing the procercoid or the second intermediate host containing the parasite, the plerocercoid/sparganum may migrate to the animal's subcutaneous tissues or muscles. In these sites, the plerocercoid/sparganum may undergo uncontrolled multiplicative asexual reproduction (i.e., one becomes two, two become four, four become eight, etc.) to the point that these plerocercoids/spargana multiply throughout the dog's body, causing a fatal condition known as *proliferative sparganosis* in which the spargana literally overtake the host's body, at which point treatment is futile.

Laboratory Test(s) Used to Diagnose the Infection
Fecal flotation may reveal an operculated egg, the characteristic egg type produced by a pseudotapeworm; however, this test cannot be relied on. It is possible to identify the egg by using molecular technology; this egg is very similar in form to that of a digenetic trematode.

Zoonotic Potential for Clients
This parasite has also been reported in humans and is a severe zoonotic condition. There are three ways in which humans can become infected: (1) drinking water containing the procercoid-infected copepod (first intermediate host), thus becoming the second intermediate host containing the plerocercoid stage in their subcutaneous tissues; (2) ingesting the second intermediate host (e.g., a raw frog), which contains the plerocercoid stage, which would migrate to and infest the human's subcutaneous tissues; and (3) if a poultice made from an infected second intermediate host (e.g., a frog), containing the plerocercoid or sparganum stage, were applied to an open wound. The sparganum could migrate from the frog's tissues to human tissues and produce a subcutaneous sparganum.

Treatment
There are no products currently approved for treatment of *Spirometra* spp. in dogs and cats. However, praziquantel has been used extralabel at a dose of 25 mg/kg orally. Treatment over 2 consecutive days is indicated as well as preventing further ingestion of infected prey animals. It is also possible to treat cats with praziquantel at a dosage of 30 mg/kg by the subcutaneous (SQ), intramuscular (IM), or per os (PO) route. Mebendazole has also been reported to be successful at a dosage of 11 mg/kg PO. If spargana are found before death in the subcutaneous tissues of a cat or a dog, they may be surgically removed from the tissues for examination. Proliferative sparganosis in canines has no known treatment and normally has a fatal outcome.

Prevention and Control Techniques
Dogs and cats should be prevented from drinking water from infected lakes, streams, or ponds and from predation and carrion consumption.

Nematodes—Roundworms of Zoonotic Importance
Nematodes are commonly referred to as *roundworms* because of a unique feature—they are round when observed on cross section.

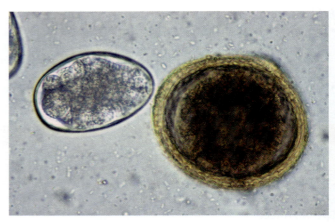

• **Fig. 13.15** Unembryonated egg of *Toxascaris cati*.

Nematodes come in all shapes (from cylindrical to round) and sizes (from the tiny *Strongyloides stercoralis* to the giant kidney worm, *Dioctophyme renale*). Roundworms can parasitize an assortment of domesticated and wild animals and are found in a variety of body organs and systems, including the GI tract, the circulatory system, the respiratory tract, the urogenital system, and the eye. Diagnosis often involves finding characteristic eggs on fecal flotation, microfilariae on examination of peripheral blood smears, with the use of ELISA testing, by observation of unique larvae in tracheal or bronchial washes, or through a variety of other diagnostic techniques.

TECHNICIAN NOTE

Some common species of canine nematodes are *Toxocara canis*, *Ancylostoma caninum*, *Trichuris vulpis*, and *Dirofilaria immitis*. Some common species of feline nematodes are *Toxocara cati*, *Ancylostoma tubaeforme*, and *Dirofilaria immitis*.

Toxocara canis, Toxocara cati, and Toxascaris leonina (Ascarids and Roundworms)
- Parasite's common name: "canine ascarid/roundworm," "feline ascarid/roundworm," "canine and feline ascarid/roundworm"
- Pronunciation: "*Tocks*-oh-care-ah" "*kay*-niss"; "Tocks-oh-care-ah" "*cat*-eye"; "*Tocks*-ass-care-riss" "lee-oh-*nine*-ah"

Species Affected
Adult *T. canis* and *T. cati* are found in the small intestine of dogs and cats, respectively (Fig. 13.15). Adult *T. leonina* are found in the small intestine of dogs and cats. The life cycle of these roundworms is varied and very complex, with these worms often relying on a variety of mammals as **paratenic** or **transport hosts** (a host in which a parasite does not undergo further development), where it remains encysted or in "suspended animation" (i.e., hypobiosis), serving as a source of the definitive host when the definitive host ingests the paratenic host. For example, the atypical hosts, rats and mice, may eat the infective eggs of *T. canis*; then the infective second-stage larva will hatch to migrate to an extraintestinal tissue site to encyst or rest. If the mouse is ingested by a dog, the larva will excyst in the intestine of the dog, continuing its development to the adult stage in the canine definitive host. When humans act as paratenic hosts (most often to *T. canis*), the conditions that result from this infection are known as *visceral larval migrans* (VLM) and **ocular larval migrans** (OLM).

Symptoms of *T. canis* in young puppies include diarrhea, vomiting, an enlarged abdomen, constipation, flatulence, and poor growth rate. Clinical signs, except for diarrhea, are not as common in adult dogs. *T. cati* infections in young kittens are often asymptomatic, but heavy infections can cause diarrhea, abdominal distention, rough hair coat, and dehydration. *T. leonina* causes similar signs in kittens and puppies, whereas adult cats tend to be asymptomatic.

Abbreviated Life Cycle

Among these three parasite species, the life cycles differ greatly; to further expediency, only the life cycle of *T. canis* will be discussed here. Adult male and female ascarids are found in the small intestine of the canine host. After copulation, the female produces unembryonated eggs that pass into the external environment in the dog's feces, which under warm and humid environmental conditions allow the ascarid egg to begin to embryonate (division of central mass). Eventually, a first-stage larva may be found within the ascarid egg, where the larva will molt and develop into the second-stage larva (Fig. 13.16). It is during this infective stage that the canine host must ingest the egg for the life cycle to continue. Tracheal migration occurs in dogs younger than 3 months of age, and the larva hatch in the small intestine, enter the bloodstream, and migrate through the liver and into the lungs. The developing larva is then coughed up, swallowed, and returns to the small intestine, where it eventually matures to the adult stage. In canines older than 3 months of age, somatic migration occurs and involves larval hatching in the small intestine, where the larvae enter the bloodstream to be carried to somatic sites (e.g., muscles, kidney, mammary gland) throughout the dog's body. The now-encysted, second-stage larvae undergo no further development and remain in suspended animation.

In female dogs older than 3 months of age that ingest the egg containing the second-stage migrating larva, the somatic migration route is followed, where the larva becomes encysted within extraintestinal tissues. During the height of canine pregnancy, the larva will migrate from the mother to a developing fetus, residing in the liver. Soon after birth, the larva will migrate from the liver to the lungs of the neonate, where it will be coughed up and swallowed to return to the small intestine, where it will mature to the adult stage. This series of development uses somatic migration in the dam and tracheal migration in the puppy. Alternatively, the migrating larva may encyst within the mammary gland where during lactation, the encysted larva may become activated and passed to the puppy in the milk to develop directly to the adult stage within the puppy's small intestine.

If the egg containing the second-stage larva is ingested by a mouse (a paratenic host), the migrating larva follows the somatic migration route and becomes encysted within the mouse's extraintestinal tissues. If a dog ingests the paratenic host (mouse), the encysted larva will exit the mouse to grow into an adult in the dog's small intestine.

Laboratory Test(s) Used to Diagnose the Infection

Ascarid infections in dogs and cats may be diagnosed using fecal centrifugation/flotation techniques employing a variety of solutions

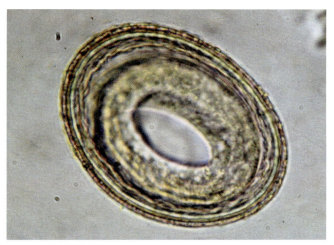

• **Fig. 13.16** Infective stage of *Toxocara canis*; an egg containing a second-stage larva.

for the identification of unique egg types (see Figs. 13.15 and 13.16). Adult worms may also be visualized in vomit or fecal material.

Zoonotic Potential for Clients

These parasites can produce two serious zoonotic conditions: VLM and OLM. Young children living near infected kittens or puppies or adult pets not on preventive regimens are at risk, especially if they ingest ascarid eggs containing infective second-stage larvae (fecal-oral route). After ingestion, the larva undergoes extensive migration through the liver or the lungs (in the case of VLM) or the eyes (in the case of OLM) within the child, who serves as a paratenic host. Parents should be warned to use caution regarding uncovered sandboxes, playgrounds, or beaches contaminated by dog/cat feces or other sites where the infective eggs might be picked up and ingested by the child.

Treatment

Commonly used anthelmintics include fenbendazole, milbemycin, moxidectin, piperazine, and pyrantel, as well as most monthly heartworm preventive agents, such as moxidectin and milbemycin oxime. Selamectin is also approved for use in cats and kittens for this purpose. Deworming of puppies and kittens should begin at age 2 weeks and repeated at 2-week intervals to eliminate shedding of *Toxocara* eggs. Deworming dams (or administering monthly heartworm/anthelmintic preventives) before breeding is another important preventive measure. The Companion Animal Parasite Council (CAPC) recommends year-round treatment of all dogs and cats with broad-spectrum heartworm anthelmintics that also have activity against other endoparasites with zoonotic potential.

Prevention and Control Techniques

Daily removal of feces and cleaning of kennels is essential for preventing *Toxocara* infection. Sandboxes should be covered when not in use and inspected to ensure that cats are not using them as areas for defecation. Furthermore, VLM and OLM in humans can be prevented by having pets strategically dewormed, removing feces from the environment, enforcing leash laws, practicing proper hygiene, discouraging pica and geophagia in children, and teaching them the importance of hand washing, especially before eating.

Baylisascaris procyonis—Neurologic Larva Migrans

- Parasite's common name: "raccoon roundworm"
- Pronunciation: "Bay-liss-*ass*-care-riss" "prosigh-*own*-niss"

Species Affected

Baylisascaris procyonis (raccoon roundworm) is a common parasite of the North American raccoon that is like *Toxocara* species affecting dogs and cats, although typically, the adult *B. procyonis* produces little pathology and is asymptomatic in the raccoon, which harbors the parasite in the small intestines. It produces significant clinical pathology in other animals (i.e., hunting hounds) or in humans (i.e., hunters, taxidermists, trappers) who might ingest an egg containing second-stage larvae. These infective larvae can migrate to the intestinal wall of the paratenic host before migrating through the brain and other neural tissues such as the spinal cord (**neurologic larval migrans** [NLM]). Such migration will produce severe neurologic symptoms and even death. Children in rural settings are considered a high-risk population if indulging in geophagia or pica while outdoors.

Abbreviated Life Cycle

Adult male and female *B. procyonis* reside in the small intestine of the raccoon, the definitive host. Under warm and humid environmental conditions, embryonation occurs within the egg, where larva will molt and develop into the infective second-stage larva. A raccoon must ingest this egg for the life cycle to continue, ending with adult ascarids found in the raccoon's small intestine. Ultimately, the eggs will be excreted into the environment in established raccoon "latrine" areas, such as gutters, crawlspaces, firewood stands, and other protected areas. If a mammalian or avian paratenic host ingests the egg containing the second-stage larva, the larva migrates through neural tissues (e.g., brain and spinal cord). Although the paratenic host is a dead-end host, it usually succumbs to this highly pathogenic zoonotic parasite, which normally produces a fatal outcome due to tissue damage to the central nervous system (CNS).

Laboratory Test(s) Used to Diagnose the Infection

B. procyonis may be diagnosed in the definitive host by using routine fecal flotation in various solutions. In humans, it is diagnosed through biopsy normally taken at autopsy (postmortem). Care should be taken by clinicians while handling feces to avoid accidental ingestion or contamination with parasitic eggs.

Zoonotic Potential for Clients

Should a child ingest the *B. procyonis* egg containing the infective second-stage larva, neurologic larval migration may result, involving migration of the larva to the brain and spinal cord of the child, an almost-certain fatal condition. If suspected ingestion has occurred, immediate medical care is imperative.

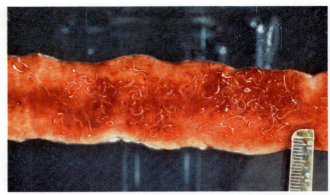

• **Fig. 13.17** Adult *Ancylostoma caninum* in the small intestine of a dog.

Treatment

Keeping raccoons as pets or as captives is not recommended; therefore treatment is not encouraged. If dogs or cats become infected with the adult *B. procyonis*, the same treatment as for *Toxocara* species is indicated (i.e., pyrantel pamoate, fenbendazole, piperazine). Hunting hounds engaged in the sport of "coon hunting" should be tested regularly and maintained on anthelmintic regimens to prevent infection and possible zoonotic transmission to humans. Monthly preventive measures with anthelmintics are successful in the eradication of this parasite in canines.

Prevention and Control Techniques

In areas where raccoons are prevalent, maintaining an outdoor environment around the home that is inhospitable to raccoons by removing food sources and securing areas that commonly attract raccoons, such as garbage cans and possible latrine sites, such as crawlspaces, basements, and attics, are excellent preventive measures. Hunters, trappers, and taxidermists should practice rigorous sanitation measures and good hand hygiene when handling raccoon carcasses to prevent contamination and when field dressing or preparing carcasses. This should include wearing gloves when handling a carcass and avoiding eating, chewing tobacco, or dipping snuff when carrying out field dressing or skinning an animal to avoid accidental ingestion of eggs. Hunters should discourage hounds from chewing or eating racoon carcasses during hunting activities. Use of carcasses as training aids for hunting hounds should be discouraged.

Ancylostoma caninum, Ancylostoma braziliense, Ancylostoma tubaeforme, and *Uncinaria stenocephala* (Hookworms)

- Parasite's common name: "hookworm"
- Pronunciation: "An-sea-los-*toe*-mah" "kay-*nine*-num"; "An-sea-los-*toe*-mah" "brazil-ee-*inn*-sea"; "An-sea-los-*toe*-mah" "two-buh-*four*-me"; "Unsin-*air*-ee-ah" "sten-oh-*cef*-ah-lah"

Species Affected

Hookworms are found in the small intestine of dogs, cats, other carnivores, and occasionally rats and cattle (Fig. 13.17). As a group, hookworms may produce a zoonotic condition in humans known as *cutaneous larva migrans* (CLM). Canine hookworms are voracious blood feeders, with their unique teeth and large buccal cavity (Fig. 13.18). Pale mucous membranes and hydremia (watery blood) are conditions signaling anemia, particularly in young puppies. Diarrhea may also be observed—blood-tinged or black and tarry. Symptoms of chronic infections in puppies include being underweight, a distended abdomen, poor hair coat, and inappetence. Although *A. braziliense* causes only mild diarrhea and GI upset, this is a significant hookworm due to its zoonotic nature and associated CLM in humans. In *A. tubaeforme* infection, cats are often asymptomatic unless heavily infected and then may demonstrate regenerative anemia and weight loss. *U. stenocephala* causes signs like those of *A. caninum* but with dermatitis associated with larval migration in the skin.

Life Cycle

Among these four parasites, the life cycles differ greatly. To expedite an overall understanding, only the life cycle of *A. caninum* will be discussed here. Adult male and female hookworms, which are voracious bloodsuckers, are found in the canine small intestine, firmly attached to the mucosa. After copulation, the female produces unembryonated eggs that pass into the external environment in the dog's feces. In warm and humid environmental conditions and moist soil, the hookworm egg will begin to embryonate (division of internal morula), producing a first-stage larva within the egg. This egg will hatch in the external environment to molt, developing into the actively feeding second-stage larva, which will molt to the third stage without shedding the cuticle of the second-stage larva. The unsheathed third-stage larva is infective when it penetrates the skin of the canine definitive host. For a dog younger than 3 months of age, the larva will then migrate into the bloodstream and pass through the body and into the lungs, where tracheal migration begins via the developing larva being coughed up and swallowed to eventually reach the small intestine to mature into adult hookworms. In a dog older than 3 months of age, the larva will migrate via somatic migration into the bloodstream and will travel to assorted somatic sites (e.g., muscles, kidney, mammary gland) throughout the dog's body to become an encysted second-stage larva. At this point, the encysted larva undergoes no further development and is in a state of **hypobiosis.** If the infective larva penetrates the skin of a female dog older than 3 months of age, the migrating larva follows the somatic migration route and becomes encysted within the extraintestinal tissues.

During the height of pregnancy, larvae may migrate from the dam to the developing fetuses, where they will reside in the liver. Soon after delivery of the fetuses, the larvae will migrate from the liver to the lungs, where they will be coughed up and swallowed to return to the small intestine to mature to the adult stage. This series of development involves somatic migration in the dam and tracheal migration in the puppy, which is a rare sequence of events in the canine hookworm life cycle. More commonly, the migrating larva may become encysted within the mammary gland (somatic migration). During lactation, the encysted larva may become activated and pass to the puppy via milk. As with the infectious route of *Toxocara* species, the larvae develop directly to the adult stage within the puppy's small intestine (somatic migration: pregnant female; no migration: puppy).

Laboratory Test(s) Used to Diagnose the Infection

Fecal flotation using a variety of solutions, with sodium nitrate solution being the most common method, will demonstrate ova (Fig. 13.19).

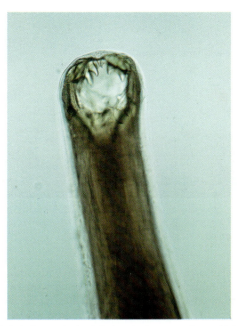

• **Fig. 13.18** Anterior end of adult *Ancylostoma caninum*. Note the three pairs of ventral teeth and the large buccal cavity.

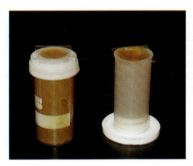

• **Fig. 13.19** Ovassay Plus Zoetis) *(left)* and Ovatector *(right)* are two examples of commercial fecal flotation kits.

Zoonotic Potential for Clients

Canine hookworms (especially *A. braziliense*) are zoonotic parasites. If a hookworm larva penetrates the skin of a human, the migrating larva causes CLM (Fig. 13.20). Skin penetration can occur upon contact, so walking barefoot in areas of possible larval contamination predisposes humans to infection. This condition is characterized by raised, erythematous, pruritic, tortuous tracts in the skin and may be prevented by wearing shoes in suspect areas. The public health significance must be considered, especially in households with an infected puppy or kitten and young children, something of which clients should be warned. This is one of the main reasons dogs are often prohibited from public beaches and swimming areas.

Treatment

Treatment may be carried out by using fenbendazole, moxidectin, pyrantel, or milbemycin for *A. caninum*. Monthly preventives treat heartworm and other parasites and are effective in controlling canine hookworm.

Prevention and Control Techniques

Bitches should be free of hookworms before breeding and should be kept out of potentially contaminated areas during pregnancy;

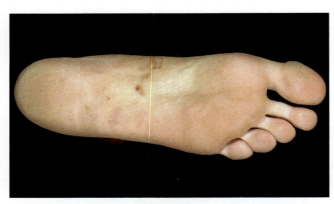

• **Fig. 13.20** Cutaneous larva migrans caused by *Ancylostoma braziliense* in the sole of a human foot. This zoonotic skin condition is also known as *creeping eruption*, *sandworms*, or *plumber's itch*.

sandy or clay areas should be sanitized with sodium borate. Whelping should always take place in sanitary quarters with frequent bedding changes. Litters should be treated with an age-appropriate anthelmintic at ages 2, 4, 6, and 8 weeks.

> **TECHNICIAN NOTE**
>
> Hookworms should be considered in any puppy or kitten that presents with signs of anemia or gastrointestinal (GI) problems. *Ancylostoma caninum* infection can quickly be fatal in young puppies due to anemia. Obtaining an adequate fecal sample for proper identification of ova is key to a definitive diagnosis. Routine deworming should be scheduled for all puppies and kittens not on monthly preventive agents. Clients with children must be warned of the zoonotic potential.

The HOT Complex

This complex includes three stomach worms found in domestic ruminant species. The three nematode parasites are *Haemonchus contortus*, *Ostertagia ostertagi*, and *Trichostrongyles*. The three parasites share similar life cycles and contribute to such physiological manifestations as bottle jaw (edema seen under the lower jaw) and hypoproteinemia. Symptomatically, while *Haemonchus* presents with constipation, *Ostertagia* and *Trichostrongyles* manifest symptoms of watery diarrhea.

Species Affected

The HOT complex affects cattle, sheep, goats, and swine. Other animal species may be infected by various species of each genus individually.

Laboratory Tests

Members of the HOT complex may be detected by fecal flotation, fecal culture, and use of the McMasters technique for enumeration of eggs per gram (EPG).

Abbreviated Life Cycle

These parasites share a similar life cycle in which the adults live in the abomasum and intestines, feeding off blood, and females pass eggs through the feces of the host into the environment, where they hatch into larval form. The larvae crawl up stalks of grass seeking hydration, where they are ingested by grazing ruminants and continue their maturation in the host. Because the three species often represent a mixed infection in animals, they are difficult to individually identify, a task that is often left to fecal culturing techniques in commercial laboratories.

Prevention and Control

In order not to discourage anthelmintic resistance, animals should be tested and only dewormed if there is a presence of parasites, rather than conducting a blanket deworming program. The following anthelmintics are effective in ruminants: albendazole, fenbendazole, ivermectin, levamisole, and moxidectin.

Zoonotic Potential

Of the three parasites that make up the HOT complex, only *Ostertagia* and *Trichostrongyles* pose a zoonotic threat to humans. Strict attention to hygiene when handling animals and their fecal material is key to avoiding contamination or infection by these organisms. Because the eggs must be ingested, smoking, drinking, or eating in proximity of animals being handled, sampled, or treated should be avoided.

Trichuris vulpis (Whipworms)—Trichuriasis

- Parasite's common name: "whipworm"
- Pronunciation: "Try-*cure*-iss" "*vulp*-iss"

Trichuris vulpis resembles a whip; hence its name, whipworm. For identification of whipworms, a fresh fecal sample is best. The veterinary technician must be able to recognize the whipworm's unique whiplike shape (fat posterior handle with long, filamentous anterior end) and its unique trichinellid egg type. The symptomology of severe whipworm infestations can be mistaken for hypoadrenocorticism (i.e., Addison disease). For this reason, a definitive diagnosis is required prior to treatment.

Species Affected

T. vulpis is found in members of the canine family such as dogs and foxes. *Trichuris campanula*, the feline trichurid, is found in cats, usually outside of North America. There are also trichurids that parasitize ruminants and pigs; the only domestic animal species that does not serve as a definitive host for trichurids is the horse. Trichurids are associated with the cecum and portions of the large intestine. This parasite is a bloodsucker, with a tiny mouth at its anterior end and a tiny stylet just inside the opening. The whipworm "threads" its anterior end through the mucosa, much like a needle and thread passing through cloth. The fat posterior "handle" of the whipworm is found within the intestinal lumen. Adults use the lashlike anterior end to tunnel into the large intestinal mucosa while "threading" the anterior end into the tiny blood vessels and using a styletlike mouthpart to cannulate the vessel, ingesting whole blood. Dogs can tolerate large burdens of whipworms and show little clinical effect, although anemia may be evidenced by blood in feces. It is only when worms number in the hundreds or thousands that they may produce diarrhea, weight loss, or unthriftiness.

Abbreviated Life Cycle

The bioperculate, symmetric, yellow, football-shaped eggs of *T. vulpis* (Fig. 13.21A and B) are passed to the environment in feces. Under warm and humid environmental conditions, the whipworm egg will begin to embryonate until eventually, a first-stage larva may be found within the egg, where it will molt again to develop into the infective second-stage larva. It is important to note that at this infective stage, eggs are extremely resistant to adverse environmental conditions and can remain viable in the environment for years. Once the canine host ingests the eggs, the

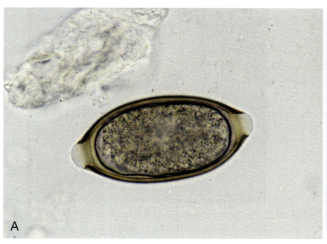
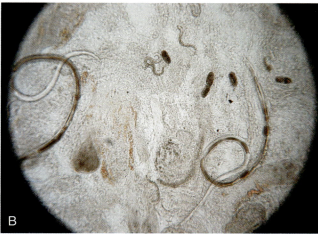

• **Fig. 13.21** (A) A bioperculate, symmetric, yellow, football-shaped egg of *Trichuris vulpis*. (B) Whip-shaped adult of *Trichuris vulpis*, with its thin anterior end and its fat posterior end.

larvae penetrate the anterior small intestine and then move to the cecum and the large intestine, where they develop to the adult stage. It takes approximately 12 weeks for the infective larva to develop to the sexually mature, egg-producing adult.

Laboratory Test(s) Used to Diagnose the Infection
These include fecal centrifugation/flotation using Sheather sugar solution of fresh feces, egg identification, and a commercial ELISA test that detects antigen–antibody reactions. Fecal flotation as a diagnostic tool can be problematic, because the eggs are often shed in low amounts and they do not float well.

Zoonotic Potential for Clients
If a child ingests the infective whipworm eggs, the eggs could develop to the adult stage within the cecum and the large intestine; however, this is an extremely rare occurrence. Clients should be advised to seek medical attention for children suspected of being infected.

Treatment
Fenbendazole is given initially for 3 days, is repeated in 3 weeks, and is again used for a final treatment in 3 months to ensure that all life stages of the parasite have been eradicated. Some monthly heartworm-preventive agents, including milbemycin and moxidectin, also help to treat *T. vulpis* infections.

Prevention and Control Techniques
To adequately control whipworm infection, rigorous hygiene is paramount. Dog kennels and exercise runs should be constructed with concrete flooring and should be cleaned and disinfected regularly and allowed to dry completely in sunlight. Because eggs can survive in soil for months to years, access to contaminated areas should be avoided.

TECHNICIAN NOTE

Feline trichurids (*Trichuris campanula*) are extremely rare in North America, but sometimes trichurid eggs may be observed on flotation of feline feces. These eggs are probably pseudoparasites; that is, species of trichurids that parasitize a cat's prey—birds, rats, and mice.

Strongyloides stercoralis and Strongyloides cati; Aelurostrongylus abstrusus
- Parasite's common name: "intestinal threadworms" (*S. stercoralis* and *S. cati*); "feline lungworm" (*A. abstrusus*)
- Pronunciation: "Stron-gee-*lloyd*-ees" "stir-co*ral*-iss"; "Stron-gee-*lloyd*-ees" "*cat*-eye"; "A-lure-oh-*stron*-gee-lus" "ab-*stru*-sus"

Species Affected
Threadworms infect many domestic species of animals including dogs, cats, horses and cattle. *S. stercoralis* is the only species that is zoonotic. Bloody, mucoid diarrhea leading to dehydration may be seen in very young puppies and kittens. Infection can result in emaciation and stunted growth in small animals; however, *S. cati* is nonpathogenic in adult cats. *A. abstrusus*, the feline lungworm, typically produces a mild, chronic cough in infected cats. These two parasites are closely associated, because they both produce first-stage larvae in the feces of infected cats.

Abbreviated Life Cycle
Intestinal threadworms are unusual parasites; only the female worm is parasitic and found buried in the mucosa of the small intestines. The parthenogenetic female produces three types of eggs, which are morphologically identical: N, 2N, and 3N eggs. The "adverse environmental" homogonic cycle allows survival of 3N eggs, whereas the "optimal environmental" heterogonic cycle allows not only the 3N eggs but also the 2N and N eggs to survive.

A tiny worm, the parasitic females are triploid (3N) with regard to chromosome count; the organism has three times the "normal" number of chromosomes. Females can produce similar triploid eggs without having been fertilized by a male worm—this is essentially a "virgin birth" process, called *parthenogenesis*. The parasite's egg-to-larval development is dependent on environmental temperatures, with extreme temperatures causing the eggs to embryonate until a first-stage larva is formed within the threadworm egg. Upon hatching, this larva will molt, develop into the second-stage larva, and molt again before developing into third-stage larva. This larva has the same chromosome count as that of the parasitic female; it cannot survive in a "free-living" environment and *must* reenter its host oral mucosa by penetration, after which it enters the systemic circulation, eventually returning to the gut as an adult parthenogenetic female. This type of life cycle is called the *homogonic life cycle* (prefix "*homo-*" meaning "same"; suffix "*-gonic*" meaning "egg"; hence "same egg type").

Alternatively, in moderate temperatures, a **heterogonic life cycle** (prefix "*hetero-*" meaning "different"; suffix "*-gonic*" meaning "egg"; hence "different egg type") takes place that involves the eggs embryonating in the environment before developing into a third-stage larva. Larvae hatching from the N eggs are free-living male larvae, while larvae that hatch from the 2N eggs will be free-living female larvae. These larvae mature to free-living adult threadworms that copulate with the free-living female and produce 3N eggs. Because the 3N larva has the same chromosome count as that of the parasitic female, it cannot be free-living and *must* reenter its host by penetration of the oral mucosa, entering the systemic circulation before returning to the gut as an adult parthenogenetic female.

> **TECHNICIAN NOTE**
>
> The main difference between the homogonic and heterogonic cycles lies in the environmental temperatures during the time when the cycle occurs. A fair and moderate temperature is conducive to the heterogenic cycle, whereas more extreme temperatures promote the homogonic cycle.

Laboratory Test(s) Used to Diagnose the Infection

First-stage larvae may be detected both in fresh fecal samples as well as mucosal scrapings using the Baermann technique. Mucosal scrapings made postmortem may reveal adult female parasites, eggs, and first-stage larvae (Fig. 13.22). When these larvae are detected on feline fecal flotation, a practitioner's first instinct is to diagnose feline strongyloidiasis, an uncommon occurrence in cats, as opposed to a more correct diagnosis of lungworm infection with *A. abstrusus*. Confirmatory testing using the *Strongyloides* IgG antibody test is required to make an accurate diagnosis.

Zoonotic Potential for Clients

Strongyloidiasis is encountered more frequently during the hot, humid months of summer. The disease is endemic in the Appalachian United States, especially in eastern Tennessee, Kentucky, and West Virginia. Humans become infected by the fecal–oral route; infection can be prevented by ensuring proper sanitation and hand washing. There are also species-specific varieties of *S. stercoralis* that parasitize humans and canines, therefore thorough hand washing is recommended.

Treatment

Recommended treatment includes ivermectin at a dosage of 0.2 mg/kg SQ or PO with a second dose 4 weeks later of 0.08 mg/kg; fenbendazole at a dosage of 50 mg/kg PO for 5 days, repeated 4 weeks later; or thiabendazole at a dosage of 100 to 150 mg/kg/day PO for 3 days, repeated weekly until no larvae are detected through testing. Cattle may be treated using pour-on doramectin.

Prevention and Control Techniques

Thorough washing of impervious surfaces with steam or concentrated salt or lime solutions, followed by rinsing with hot water, effectively destroys *Strongyloides* species. The infected animal's bedding should be disposable until the infection has cleared. Humans should avoid skin-to-soil contact by not walking barefoot in areas of suspected contamination and practice strict sanitation measures.

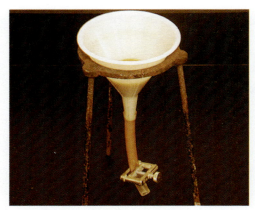

• **Fig. 13.22** The Baermann apparatus is most useful in recovering larvae of lungworms and consists of a funnel supported by a stand.

> **TECHNICIAN NOTE**
>
> First-stage larvae of *Aelurostrongylus abstrusus* are often confused with the larvae of *Strongyloides cati*; however, first-stage larvae of lungworms possess a prominent dorsal appendage on the tail, distinguishing them from the larvae of *Strongyloides* species, which has no appendages.

Dirofilaria immitis

- Parasite's common name: "canine heartworm"
- Pronunciation: "dye-row-phil-*air*-e-ah" "*em*-meh-tus"

Species Affected

Adult heartworms are usually found within the pulmonary arteries and right ventricle of dogs, cats, and ferrets; however, they may be aberrant or erratic parasites, capable of traveling to a variety of ectopic sites. **Microfilariae** (Fig. 13.23A and B) are usually found in the peripheral blood of the canine host. Dogs may be asymptomatic early on; as the disease advances, weight loss, decreased exercise tolerance, and cough are seen. In advanced cases, dyspnea, fever, ascites, cyanosis, and periodic collapse may occur. Cats can also be infected and may be asymptomatic. A poor host, in cats, heartworms typically die within 3 to 4 months postinfection. They still may cause disease and damage to the animal such as sporadic vomiting and mild signs of respiratory illness (chronic cough, wheezing, and inappetence); this is referred to as *heartworm-associated respiratory disease* and may result in acute respiratory distress syndrome or sudden death. Cats may also present with ectopic infection, with adult worms presenting in the CNS, eyes, or subcutaneous tissues. Clinical signs are often demonstrated when immature adult heartworms have reached the pulmonary vasculature, where they die, or when mature adult worms die. This may occur 2 to 4 years postinfection. Ferrets are less likely to be infected if kept inside; however, owners should consider preventive treatment (selamectin or ivermectin) for animals allowed outside.

> **TECHNICIAN NOTE**
>
> An *aberrant/erratic parasite* is limited to a single parasite that has wandered into an organ or location where it is not normally found. For example, *Dirofilaria immitis*, the canine heartworm, may wander "off track" during its migration to the heart and become established in the anterior chamber of the dog's eye.

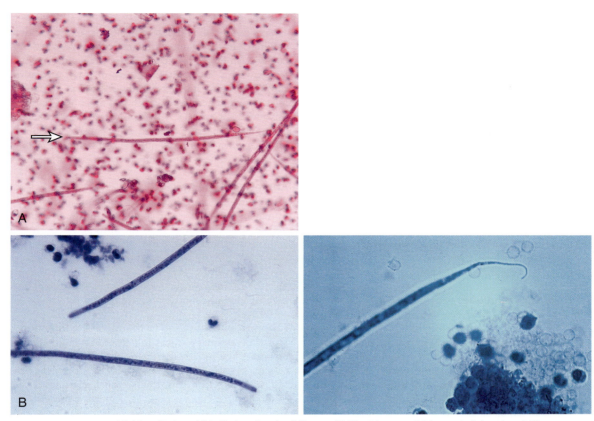

• **Fig. 13.23** (A) Microfilariae of *Dirofilaria* using the Difil test. (B) The blunt cranial (or cephalic) end and (C) the needlelike caudal end of a *Dipetalonema reconditum* microfilaria.

Abbreviated Life Cycle

A female mosquito (intermittent hosts) must take a blood meal, ingesting microfilariae, after which larval development takes place. Microfilariae (310 μm long, tapered anterior end, straight tail) are initially found in the mosquito's midgut but migrate to the mosquito's kidneys. Here they develop into first-stage larvae before molting to become second-stage larvae and finally to a third-stage larval molt. These larvae exit from the kidneys, migrating to the mosquito's proboscis (mouthparts). When the infected adult female mosquito takes a blood meal from an uninfected dog, third-stage larvae will emerge onto the host's skin surface from the mosquito's proboscis, penetrating the puncture wound to migrate through the subcutaneous tissues and molt into fourth-stage larvae. Eventually, migration to the pulmonary arteries occurs, with higher worm burdens spilling over into the right ventricle, where they molt to fifth-stage larvae—the adult stage. It takes approximately 6 months for maturation from the third stage to the adult stage. After copulation, the female produces microfilariae, and the life cycle begins again. *Acanthocheilonema reconditum* (a-canth-oh-*kyle*-low-nee-ma reh-con-*dye*-tum), previously called *Dipetalonema* (dye-peh-tal-low-*nee*-ma) *reconditum*, parasitizes dogs; its microfilariae (290 μm long, blunted anterior end, buttonhook tail) are sometimes confused with the microfilariae of *D. immitis*; the difference lies in the blunted anterior end and buttonhook tail of *D. reconditum*. This nematode is found subcutaneously and uses the flea, *C. felis*, as its intermediate host.

TECHNICIAN NOTE

The intermediate host for *D. immitis* is the female mosquito (the intermediate host for *D. reconditum* is the flea).

Laboratory Test(s) Used to Diagnose the Infection

Commercially available canine and feline ELISA serologic tests and immunochromatographic tests (100% specificity and 85% sensitivity) are used to detect both adult and microfilarial antigens. In microfilaremic dogs, the direct blood smear analysis has approximately 5% to 10% accuracy; the modified Knott test is still relied on to demonstrate the presence of microfilariae, as well as examination of the buffy coat of a packed cell volume (PCV)-filled tube (Fig. 13.24). However, all these tests are less accurate compared with ELISA. Thoracic radiography and ultrasonography may also confirm the presence of microfilariae, especially when examining the right ventricle or the pulmonary artery.

In cats, the antigen test is the most accurate test for detecting mature female worms that are producing microfilariae, but it does not detect males or immature worms, which is problematic. The antibody tests that are available currently detect the presence of infections—past and present—by male or female worms but do not necessarily tell if the cat is currently infected; hence antigen testing and antibody testing should be done simultaneously to confirm parasitic infection. If these tests are inconclusive, radiography and echocardiography may be helpful in arriving at a diagnosis.

Zoonotic Potential for Clients

Humans rarely serve as incidental hosts for *D. immitis* as they are dead-end hosts. Human dirofilariasis usually manifests as pulmonary "coin lesions" within the lungs, or aberrant worms may be found in the brain, eyes, or testicles. The parasite is incapable of reproducing, therefore the infection cannot be spread further.

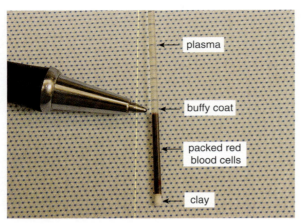

• **Fig. 13.24** Buffy coat in a hematocrit tube lies between the plasma above and packed red blood cells below and is an area of visualization of heartworm larvae.

Prevention and Control Techniques

To assist in the prevention of new heartworm infestation, macrocyclic lactones are given 2 months before the treatment begins. Then, prior to treatment beginning, a course of doxycycline (10 mg/kg twice daily [BID] for 4 weeks) will stop bacterial infection with *Wolbachia*, a gram-negative, obligate bacteria. If doxycycline is not available, the drug minocycline may be substituted. Once the course of treatment against *Wolbachia* is completed, melarsomine may be administered as deep-muscle IM injections per the manufacturer's label. Animals should be kept quiet and on strict confinement with minimal activity throughout the treatment and recovery period.

Macrolide agents, which include ivermectin (not to be used in Collies), milbemycin oxime, moxidectin, and selamectin, are the drugs of choice as monthly preventive agents for all dogs and cats to be given every 30 days, year-round. Instructions must be strongly emphasized when educating clients to give their pets heartworm-preventive treatment "every 30 days as opposed to monthly, which may be confusing." Dogs should be tested yearly to ensure that preventive medications are effective in protecting the animal. Clients should be advised to note on a calendar the date that the medication is given as most preventive packages come with decorative calendar reminder stickers to help keep up with the date of administration. Pausing preventives in winter months is not encouraged, as mosquitoes can still be present and feeding.

> **TECHNICIAN NOTE**
>
> During the heartworm infection process, the female mosquito deposits the larvae within a pool of hemolymph on the skin surface, and the larvae make their way into the puncture wound; they are not "injected" by mosquito.

Enterobius vermicularis—Enterobiasis

- Parasite's common name: "human pinworm"
- Pronunciation: "En-tear-*oh*-bee-us" "ver-mick-you-*lair*-us"

> **TECHNICIAN NOTE**
>
> Dogs and cats are *never* infected by pinworms but remain incriminated as sources of infection by some pediatricians. Because pinworms do not parasitize carnivores, if found in dogs and cats, they are regarded as "pseudoparasites."

Species Affected

E. vermicularis, the human pinworm, is seen in children. Parents of children infected by pinworms are frequently advised by physicians to take the family pet to the veterinary clinic and have that pet treated for pinworms. However, the pinworm is not a parasite of the "true carnivore", rather it infects omnivores such as humans, primates and mice as well as herbivores which includes horses and cattle; therefore this advice is erroneous. This parasite is found in the cecum and colon of humans, especially children. This parasite is of public health significance; the technician should be knowledgeable about it to provide client education and dispel any myths surrounding the family pet.

Abbreviated Life Cycle

Adult pinworms are found in the cecum and ascending colon of humans, particularly children. During the evening hours, adult female pinworms migrate to the anus and deposit their eggs with a pruritic gluelike secretion on the child's perianal or perineal region. Within a day or two, the eggs become infective. Because the glue is pruritic, the child will often scratch the area. Within 2 months after ingestion of eggs, mature worms will be found in the cecum, appendix, and ascending colon.

Laboratory Test(s) Used to Diagnose the Infection

It is the veterinary team's job to educate and inform the public regarding the intricacies of this common childhood parasite and to refer parents to a physician who may perform the Scotch tape test, as recommended by the National Institutes of Health (NIH), to identify the characteristic asymmetric ovum of *E. vermicularis*.

Zoonotic Potential for Clients

E. vermicularis may be found in primates, so owners should be advised of this malady and the potential for zoonotic transmission, especially to children.

Treatment

Infected primates should be treated with pyrantel pamoate (250 mg/5 mL). The veterinary staff should refer owners to their physicians if contamination is suspected.

Prevention and Control Techniques

Technicians working with primate colonies should take precautions and employ PPE to prevent infection during sample collection and testing and cleaning of cages.

> **TECHNICIAN NOTE**
>
> *Enterobius vermicularis* infection is the most common worm infection in the United States and may be incorrectly blamed on the household pet; however, humans are the primary means of transmission. Clients with concerns about pinworms should be properly educated/redirected to their physician for assistance.

Trematodes (Flukes) of Veterinary Importance

Fasciola hepatica

- Common Species: *Fasciola hepatica*, *Fasciola gigantica*
- Parasite's common name: "flukes"
- Pronunciation: fah-*see*-oh-la ha-pat-*ee*-ka
- Species affected: sheep, cattle, horses, pigs, goats, llamas, deer

Trematodes (digenetic flukes) are flatworms that parasitize a variety of domesticated and wild animals and are often associated with diseases of the intestinal tract. Some digenetic flukes parasitize the respiratory passages (e.g., *Paragonimus kellicotti*) or the blood vasculature (e.g., **schistosomes**). Diagnosis occurs through discovery of operculated ova in the feces of infected animals.

Abbreviated Life Cycle

Eggs are laid in the biliary duct and shed via feces into watery environments where they embryonate, releasing miracidia. The miracidia invade a snail as the intermediate host, which plays host to the sporocysts, rediae, and cercariae. The snail releases cercariae to encyst as metacercaria on water plants, which are then eaten by mammals, to excyst in the duodenum, migrating through the intestinal wall, peritoneal cavity, and liver parenchyma before beginning a new cycle in the biliary duct.

Laboratory Tests

Fecal sedimentation tests utilizing a high-density sucrose solution and necropsy examination of the liver and the bile ducts are useful to identify ova. Currently, ELISA testing is not approved in the United States, although the gamma glutamyl transferase level will be elevated if damage to the bile duct has occurred. Further confirmatory testing using radiographs and ultrasound are recommended as well as possible liver biopsy.

Zoonotic Potential

Dogs and cats that are infected by trematodes do not pose a threat to humans, although humans can be affected by *F. hepatica* and suffer from "fascioliasis." The parasite affects approximately 50 million people worldwide and is caused by ingestion of contaminated leafy vegetables or undercooked, contaminated fish or frog legs.

Treatment

There are no specific products labeled for eradication of trematodes in dogs and cats, although praziquantel, epsiprantel and fenbendazole have been used in extralabel fashion against these parasites. In the United States, only clorsulon and albendazole may be used in cattle, goats, and sheep, although each species requires different dosages.

Prevention and Control

Ideally, in addition to treating animals to remove fluke infestations, reducing the populations of snails in water sources will "theoretically" control this problem. However, most molluscicides are toxic to livestock, which are frequently infested with trematodes.

> **TECHNICIAN NOTE**
>
> Most of the parasitic flukes of domesticated animals are **digenetic flukes**. The prefix "di-" means "two." The suffix "gen-" means "beginning," hence "two beginnings." The digenetic flukes of most domesticated animals have two intermediate hosts in addition to the **definitive host**.

> **TECHNICIAN NOTE**
>
> **Hermaphroditic** flukes are those with both male and female reproductive organs present to produce **operculated eggs** (eggs with a tiny doorlike structure at one end). When an egg encounters water, the operculum opens, releasing a free-swimming ciliated larva, known as a **miracidium**, into the environment.

Pentastomids of Veterinary Importance

Pentastomes

- Parasite's common name: "pentastomes," "tongue worms"
- Pronunciation: "*pen*-tah-stomes"

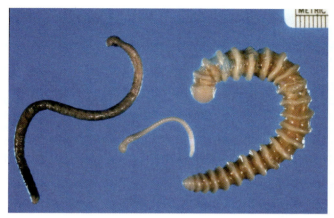

• **Fig. 13.25** Assorted pentastomes from the respiratory passages of snakes.

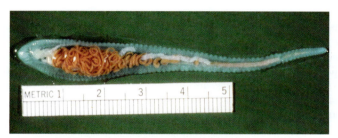

• **Fig. 13.26** *Linguatula serrata*, the canine pentastome, from the nasal passages of a dog.

Species Affected

Reptiles and mammals are affected (Fig. 13.25).

Abbreviated Life Cycle

Only one adult pentastome parasitizes mammals: *Linguatula serrata* (pronunciation "lin-gwat-you-lah" "ser-ah-tah"). The canine pentastome is found in the nasal passages of the dog, causing sneezing and nosebleeds. Nymph-stage pentastomes may be found in a variety of internal organs (liver, spleen, lymph nodes), while adult pentastomes are associated with a portion of the respiratory tract (e.g., nasal passages, lungs, air sacs). Larval pentastomes are associated with mesenchymal tissues (e.g., liver, spleen, lymph nodes) (Fig. 13.26). Female pentastomes produce eggs that are passed to the environment through fecal matter. Each egg contains a mitelike larva, with four or six jointed legs with hooklike claws on the end, and may be ingested by a rat or a rabbit. Within the intermediate host, the mitelike larva migrates to various mesenchyme tissues (e.g., liver, spleen, lymph nodes, and omentum), where it develops into the nymph, resembling a "C"-shaped, grublike creature. Dogs are infected by adult pentastomes by ingesting the nymph-infected intermediate host. Nymphs bore through the wall of the intestine and the diaphragm; when they reach the lungs, they migrate up the bronchial tree to the nasal passages, where the parasites reside as adults.

Laboratory Test(s) Used to Diagnose the Infection

Diagnosis may be made by fecal flotation or respiratory secretions and through organ examination for cysts at necropsy using a dissecting microscope. Pentastome eggs are unique in that they are round and contain mitelike larvae, complete with jointed legs that end in claws. The nymphs within parenchymal tissues have a characteristic "C" shape in situ that can be identified in a histopathologic tissue section. Infected snakes and reptiles are usually asymptomatic; adult pentastomes are usually incidental findings at necropsy.

Zoonotic Potential for Clients

Clients who own snakes and reptiles should be advised that they are capable of serving as the intermediate host for pentastomes, which might infect their cold-blooded pets. Should the client ingest the mitelike larva, the nymph may develop within the person's liver, spleen, omentum, or other tissue. Clients should be educated as to proper hygienic practices regarding cages and animal handling practices.

Treatment

There is no "recognized" treatment for pentastomes. Praziquantel at an extralabel dosage of 8 mg/kg or ivermectin at 5 to 10 times the normal dosage has been shown to reduce ova numbers but does not eradicate the worms.

Prevention and Control Techniques

Owners of snakes and reptiles should wash their hands after contact with the feces or saliva of the snakes or reptiles because of the potential for zoonotic infection. In addition, handling feces-contaminated water, dishes, and other equipment within the herpetarium may result in accidental transmission. Feed captive snakes and reptiles only prey that is pentastome-free.

> **TECHNICIAN NOTE**
>
> Precautions should be taken by all veterinary personnel when handling reptiles and snakes presented for care. PPE should be worn when cleaning the habitats and cages of reptiles and snakes to avoid accidental parasitic contamination.

Diagnosis and Identification of Ectoparasites

Most ectoparasites, including fleas, mites, ticks, and lice, can be identified upon sight; however, identification of the genus, species, and larval or nymph stages may require the benchside use of a dissecting scope, microscope, dichotomous key, and a parasitology manual. One should also be knowledgeable about disease-causing microbes that may be carried by various ectoparasites, especially those that may be zoonotic.

Ectoparasites are easily identified by their appearance to the naked eye, although some small species of mites or lice will require microscopic examination. Fig. 13.27 illustrates a comparative view of common parasites. Endoparasites are often identified by the shape of the eggs or larvae found in feces or other biological samples.

Collection and Preservation of Ectoparasites

Ectoparasites pose special problems in collection, because they may still be alive when being collected and prone to jumping/crawling to their escape. They are also fragile due to their jointed appendages and body parts, so care is required in removing them from animals to avoid leaving mouthparts attached to the host. One method of trapping live insects involves placing them on a piece of tape to prevent escape and allow for humane visualization. For longer preservation (i.e., for shipping), securing the parasite in a vial or tube with alcohol or glycerin is a humane method of kill/collection.

Diagnostic Identification of Endoparasites

Endoparasites can infect the oral cavity, esophagus, stomach, small and large intestines (i.e., gastrointestinal nematodes), and other internal organs of domesticated animals. They can also infest or briefly inhabit environments where animals/humans live during certain life stages and may contribute to animal infection, especially domestic livestock.

Collection of Fecal Samples

Fecal samples collected for routine examination should be as fresh as possible. Specimens that cannot be examined within a few minutes of defecation should be refrigerated or preserved with 10% formalin to stop parasitic development. The need for fresh feces stems from the fact that eggs, oocysts, and other life cycle stages may be altered by development, making diagnosis extremely difficult. Nonfresh fecal samples may also harbor pseudoparasites (due to contamination), which may cause confusion.

The deposition of feces by large animals in open environments can present challenges regarding preservation of freshness due to

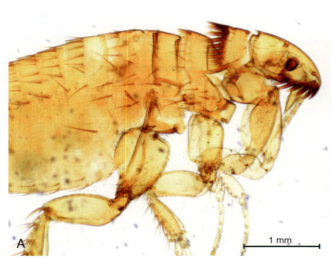
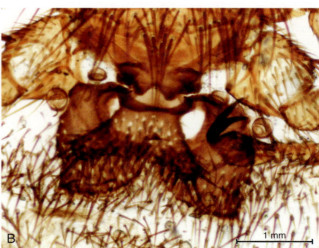

• **Fig. 13.27** Comparison of (A) flea and (B) lice mouthparts.

possible insect or pollen contamination. Samples should be collected as soon as possible after elimination to avoid contamination. The ideal fecal collection in equine and ruminant species is via digital rectal collection directly from the animal. Alternatively, collection from the ground is acceptable if this is done immediately after visualized defecation. Place fecal samples in a sealed bag for transport or invert the glove of the hand used to collect and tie closed.

Small Animal Fecal Samples

Clients should be encouraged to bring fecal samples, if possible. An owner may collect a fecal sample immediately after the animal has defecated, storing the sample in any type of container (zippered plastic bag or clean plastic bowl with a tight lid); alternatively, the clinic may provide a container as only a small amount of feces (1 teaspoon) is required for examination. All specimens are properly identified with the owner's name, animal's name, species, and date and time of collection. Veterinary personnel should collect and preserve all feces or urine that is excreted during clinic visit in the event it is needed. Never discard any sample before checking to see if it is needed for testing. Common exam procedures utilizing a thermometer or gloved digits may yield sufficient fecal mass for a direct or fecal flotation exam. Because of the small fecal amount collected with a fecal wand, analysis should be carried out immediately.

Large Animal Fecal Samples

For best results, fecal samples collected from pastures or stalls should be fresh and free of grass, plant detritus, or insect contamination. Picking up the sample in a gloved hand or by rectal collection, inverting the glove, and tying it off will ensure that the sample is "stored" for transport to the laboratory (label with identifiers). Refrigeration is necessary to prevent further maturation of parasites until analysis can be completed.

Examination of Fecal Samples

Several precautions should be taken during fecal examination:
- Handle the sample with care, because it may contain zoonotic parasites, bacteria, or viruses. Appropriate clothing, such as a clean laboratory coat or jacket and latex or nitrile gloves, should be worn during the laboratory examination. Upon examination and degloving, hands should be washed with soap and warm water to avoid the spread of infection.
- Exam tables and the laboratory area should be sanitized after fecal collection and examinations are completed. Eating, drinking, and applying makeup or contact lenses should never happen in the laboratory or the examination room.

If testing multiple fecal specimens, it is helpful to use a numbering system to keep the samples in order; to minimize errors, a number is assigned to the patient, and that number is written on the corresponding centrifuge tube/slides with a marking pen.

Gross Examination of Feces

Several characteristics of feces should be recorded for review by veterinarian:
- *Consistency:* Fresh feces should be somewhat formed, depending on the species of animal. Diarrhea (loose stool) or constipation (hard, dry stool) could be the result of a parasitic infection and should be noted.
- *Color:* Fecal color may be affected by food or drugs an animal has ingested. Also, malabsorption or a parasitic infection may alter the color of feces.

PROCEDURE 13.1

Microscope Calibration

1. Start at low power (×10).
2. Focus on the 2 mm line.
3. 2 mm = 2000 μm.
4. Rotate the eyepiece so that the marks are horizontal and parallel to the stage micrometer scale (0 is aligned).
5. These steps are repeated at every magnification (×10, ×40, ×100). The information is recorded on a label that is attached to the calibrated microscope. For example:

Objective	Distance Between Hash Marks (μm)
×10	12.5
×40	2.5
×100	1.0

- *Blood:* Blood may impart a dark reddish-brown color to feces. Blood may also appear as bright red streaks in feces or impart a dark, tarry appearance (digested blood). This indicates a severe parasitic infection or serious intestinal disease and is an important clinical finding to be brought to the attention of the veterinarian.
- *Mucus:* Mucus in feces can be a result of digestive disorders such as colitis or a parasitic infection and should be reported.
- *Gross parasites:* The segments of two common tapeworms infecting a large animal appear as follows: adult roundworms resemble strings of spaghetti, whereas tapeworm segments resemble pieces of cooked rice..

Occasionally, a client may submit dried tapeworm segments to be identified. This may be done by soaking the segments in saline for 1 to 4 hours to rehydrate them. Once rehydrated, they may be identified based on their unique size, shape, morphologic features, and egg presence. Segments of some tapeworm species do not contain eggs, and some segments may have expelled the eggs before the examination. In either case, a tapeworm segment may be identified by finding small mineral deposits (calcareous bodies) within the segment by crushing the segment between two glass slides and examining it under a microscope, or the segments may be sent to a commercial lab.

The Microscope and the Fecal Examination

Accurate measurements are obtained easily with the use of a calibrated eyepiece on the microscope. Individual calibration of each objective must be performed on the microscope to be used (Procedure 13.1). The stage micrometer is a microscope slide etched with a 2-mm line marked in 0.01-mm (10-μm) divisions (Fig. 13.28) and is useful for size determination.

Microscopic Examination of Feces

Microscopic examination of feces is the most reliable method to detect parasitic infection. A compound microscope with ×4, ×10, and ×40 objectives is required for proper examination of a fecal specimen and should have a mechanical stage and a micrometer for best results.

Fecal specimens should be examined routinely using the ×10 objective, beginning at one corner of the slide and ending at the opposite corner, moving over the slide in a systematic pattern (Fig. 13.29). The microscope should be focused continually with the fine-tuning knob during the examination, with the initial plane of focus being

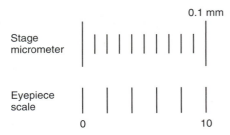

• **Fig. 13.28** Stage micrometer *(upper scale)* and eyepiece scale *(lower scale)* used to calibrate the microscope.

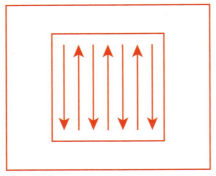

• **Fig. 13.29** Schematics indicating the direction to completely scan and examine a microscope slide.

air bubbles, as most helminth eggs are found in this plane. The more powerful objectives can be used to examine material more closely.

> ### TECHNICIAN NOTE
>
> A stage micrometer is represented as 1 micron (μ) = 0.001 mm.
>   The eyepiece scale is a glass disk etched with equally spaced hash marks; it fits into and remains in one of the microscope eyepieces and is used to determine the distance in microns between the hash marks for each objective lens of the microscope being calibrated.

To measure an object, such as a parasite egg, one end of the egg is placed on the zero mark of the ocular scale, and the number of divisions on the other end of the egg is counted and multiplied by the calibration factor for the objective being used. Example: a *Trichostrongyles* egg is 24 divisions long and 13.5 divisions wide when measured with the ×40 objective.

The calibration factor for the ×40 objective is 2.5. Therefore the egg is:

$24 \times 2.5 = 60$ μm long and $13.5 \times 2.5 = 33.75$ μm wide.

Round parasite eggs are measured through the middle of the egg at the greatest diameter. To measure microfilariae, the head (anterior end) is aligned with the zero mark of the ocular scale, and the number of divisions to the end of the tail (posterior end) is counted using the higher objective (×40 instead of ×10).

Direct Smear Fecal Examination

A sample of feces is taken from a fecal loop or thermometer, placed on a slide, and stained with Romanowski stain (wet mount), or a simple dry mount is used to rapidly estimate an animal's parasite burden and detect motile protozoa.

The advantages of direct smears include short preparation time and minimal equipment required, while the disadvantage is the small amount of feces examined, often insufficient to detect a low

parasite burden, and the amount of extraneous fecal debris seen on the slide, often confused with parasitic material.

Concentrated Methods for Fecal Examination

The concentration technique makes it possible to examine large amounts of feces quickly. Two types of procedures are commonly used in veterinary hospitals: flotation and sedimentation.

Fecal flotation methods rely on the specific gravity (ratio: weight of an object compared with the weight of an equal amount of water) of parasitic material and fecal debris. The specific gravity of most parasite eggs is between 1.100 and 1.200 g/mL, whereas the specific gravity of water is 1.000 g/mL. To allow for flotation of parasite eggs, oocysts, and other life cycle stages, the flotation solution must have a specific gravity higher than that of the parasitic material and water. Several salt and sugar solutions work well for flotation with a specific gravity of 1.200 to 1.250; this allows heavy fecal debris to sink and parasitic material to rise to the top of the solution for easy collection.

Sodium nitrate solution is the most common fecal flotation solution used in veterinary hospitals. This solution is efficient for floating parasite eggs, oocysts, and larvae but forms crystals and distorts eggs if allowed to sit longer than 20 minutes. It is supplied in commercial diagnostic test kits or individual aliquots. If purchased in gallon containers, the cost is reasonable. Another common flotation solution is saturated sugar solution, which is also inexpensive and does not crystallize or distort eggs with a long shelf life; a sticky substance to work with, it may be removed with warm, soapy water to avoid attracting insects.

Zinc sulfate solution is more commonly used in diagnostic laboratories to float protozoal organisms with the least amount of distortion. It generally is used in combination with one of the previously mentioned solutions to identify a variety of parasites.

The least desirable solution used is saturated sodium chloride solution as it corrodes laboratory equipment, forms crystals, and severely distorts parasite eggs. Saturated sodium chloride solution is also a poor flotation medium as the maximum specific gravity obtainable is 1.200, allowing heavier eggs to remain submerged.

> ### TECHNICIAN NOTE
>
> To make solutions in-house:
>
> **Magnesium Sulfate Solution (1.25 SG)**
> 8 quarts of warm water
> 10 pounds of Epsom salts
> Mix until the salt is dissolved; it will need to be shaken to remix occasionally if left sitting for an extended period (weekends).
>
> **Sugar Solution (1.27 SG)**
> 1 pound of granulated sugar
> 1.5 cups of warm water
> 6 mL of formaldehyde
> Dissolve the sugar and water over low heat, then once cooled, add formaldehyde and mix. May occasionally need to be remixed if left sitting for an extended period; keep in a lidded container to avoid attraction of ants and other insects.
>
> **Zinc Sulfate Solution**
> 336 g of zinc sulfate ($ZnSo_47H_2O$)
> 1000 mL of distilled water
> Dissolve the zinc sulfate in water and store in a lidded container. May need to be remixed if left to sit for an extended period.

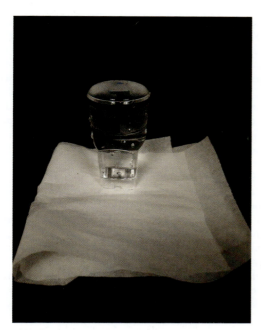

• **Fig. 13.30** Vial filled with flotation solution, showing a positive meniscus.

TABLE 13.3	Trophozoites and Movement	
Trophozoite	**Appearance**	**Movement Pattern**
Giardia spp.	Tear-shaped, 5–8 flagella	Jerky
Trichomonads	Long, slender, single flagella	Gliding
Amoeba	Amorphous	Flowing

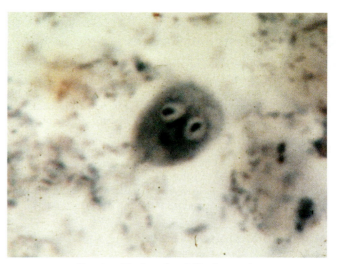

• **Fig. 13.31** Trophozoite of *Giardia* species.

Standard Fecal Flotation

The standard fecal flotation is one of the most common flotation techniques used in veterinary hospitals. Using a test tube or vial, feces and flotation solution are mixed with enough solution to form a positive meniscus (Fig. 13.30); a coverslip or microscope slide is placed on top of the test tube, and the unit is allowed to sit undisturbed for 5 to 10 minutes. Any parasite eggs dislodged float to the top, adhering to the underside of the coverslip/microscope slide. The coverslip/slide is then removed and microscopically examined for parasitic material, beginning at ×10 magnification before moving to ×40.

Commercial flotation kits use the same principle as the standard flotation technique and are constantly updated to improve validity. These kits contain a vial with a filter and prepared flotation solution. Examples of commercial flotation kits include Ovassay Plus (Zoetis), Fecal Ova Float Kit (Jorgenson Lab), Fecatector (Med-Vet), and Ovatector (BGS Medical Products, Venice, FL), to name a few. These kits come ready to use but are more expensive compared with the simple flotation technique. Some practices reduce expense by washing and reusing the vials and filters; this practice should be discouraged because of the risk of possible cross contamination.

Centrifugal Flotation

Centrifugal flotation of parasite eggs, oocysts, and other parasitic material is the most efficient detection method available, requiring less time to perform either individually or in batches. The only drawback is the requirement of a centrifuge with a horizontal (nonfixed) rotor that can hold 15-mL centrifuge tubes.

Fecal Sedimentation

Fecal sedimentation concentrates parasite eggs, oocysts, and other parasitic material that does not float by allowing settlement to the bottom of a tube of liquid, usually water. The fluid is decanted and remaining drops of sediment are retrieved and examined. A disadvantage of this technique is difficulty separating fecal debris and parasite material, which are often mixed, making microscopic examination somewhat difficult.

Detection of Protozoans in Feces

Some protozoans do not form cysts; rather, they pass out of the host in trophozoite form, a one-cell, motile organism that lacks the rigid walls of cysts. Flotation without distortion or death of the trophozoite is impossible. Protozoal cysts and trophozoites may be identified by wet mounts and stained preparations of fresh stool sample. However, while cysts may be seen via concentrated methods with or without staining, trophozoites are not demonstrated. The direct smear technique, using saline and a stain, is the preferred procedure to examine a fecal sample from protozoal organisms. In a direct smear, trophozoites may be recognized by their movement (Table 13.3 and Fig. 13.31).

If a protozoan parasite cannot be identified on direct smears, fecal smears containing protozoan trophozoites can be dried, stained with Diff-Quik, Wright, or Giemsa stain, and sent to a diagnostic laboratory for identification. Stains such as Lugol iodine and new methylene blue are helpful in the recognition of structural characteristics of trophozoites and cysts. They do not preserve the slide but do facilitate easier laboratory examination of the specimen.

Special Staining for Coccidian Parasites

Several coccidian parasites require special staining techniques for identification. *Cryptosporidium* sp. require acid-fast staining of a fecal smear, which involves fixation of the sample with absolute methanol, staining with carbol fuchsin, an alcohol rinse, and staining with malachite green before a final rinse with distilled water. The second procedure, Diff-Quik staining, is used to identify *Cystoisospora* species, a coccidian found in the gastrointestinal (GI) tract (especially the jejunum) of many animals. This parasite can cause the death of many piglets before any oocysts are found through flotation of feces. Postmortem intestinal mucosal scraping is necessary for staining and examination to detect the diagnostic stages. To identify schizonts or merozoites, the mucosa of the jejunum must be scraped with material placed on microscope slides, dried, and stained with Diff-Quik before examination via oil immersion.

For diagnostic accuracy, several samples should be examined. If not possible, samples of feces or intestines may be sent to a diagnostic laboratory.

Commercial Tests and Services

Commercial antigen tests, such as enzyme-linked immunosorbent assay (ELISA) kits for detection of *Giardia* and *Cryptosporidium*, are available. However, it has been noted that *Giardia* antigens persist in feces for some time after successful treatment has occurred. Most commercial laboratories are equipped for performing indirect immunofluorescence assay (IFA), which detects both *Giardia* and *Cryptosporidium* species. Polymerase chain reaction (PCR) testing is available via commercial laboratories for the examination of genetic material of parasites and viruses and the detection of drug-resistant markers in certain parasites such as *Ancylostoma* spp. (hookworms) and other species.

Sample Collection at Necropsy

Necropsy (postmortem examination) is an important method of diagnosing many diseases including parasitism and is often used to preserve the surviving herds and litters. Examination of the types of lesions produced by immature parasites, the presence of adult parasites found in the body cavity and tissues, and histopathologic examination of infected tissues are solid diagnostic tools. The veterinary technician's role in a necropsy involves sample collection, preservation, proper labeling, documentation, and shipping. Necropsy techniques are further covered in Chapter 16. Aseptic technique and use of PPE should be practiced whenever handling necropsy samples involving suspected parasites.

Digestive Tract Necropsy

Two methods may be used to recover parasites from the digestive tract at necropsy are the decanting method and sieving method. With either method, the veterinary technician separates the different parts of the digestive tract for rinsing, saving the contents of each part to recover parasite eggs, larvae, or adults.

The decanting method involves placing all ingesta from one organ (i.e., the abomasum) into a bucket and scrubbing lightly to remove worms before discarding the organ. Mix the ingesta with 3 quarts of warm water, allowing the sample to rest for 5 minutes before decanting to remove the supernatant, retrieving the sediment. Place a small amount of sediment in a Petri dish and examine, using a stereomicroscope or a dissecting microscope. Active worms should be easily seen and may be gently removed for closer examination or preservation. Likewise, the sieving method requires processing through decanting to collect sediment, which is then rinsed over a sieve to detain larvae for collection/identification.

Parasites obtained through decanting or sieving may be preserved in 70% alcohol or 10% neutral buffered formalin for later identification or shipping. Occasionally, bladder worms or cysticercus may be found attached to the viscera of domestic animals. A bladder worm is a fluid-filled, balloonlike structure which is, in fact, a larval tapeworm. These samples should be handled with care, because the fluid is often allergenic and zoonotic. If an in-hospital diagnosis is not possible, the samples may be preserved as previously described and sent to a diagnostic laboratory for identification.

Shipping Parasitology Specimens

Any parasitology specimen shipped to a diagnostic laboratory should be preserved with 70% alcohol or 10% neutral buffered formalin, unless otherwise directed by laboratory personnel. All specimen containers should be labeled correctly, noting the site from which the specimen was obtained; the owner's name; the animal's species, name, or identification number; and the referring veterinarian (including telephone number and address). There should be three layers of protection between the specimen and the courier. Place paperwork in a sealed plastic bag.

Miscellaneous Procedures for Detection of Endoparasites

Baermann Technique

The Baermann technique is used to recover nematode larvae from feces, tissues, or soil. The technique uses warm water to stimulate larvae to move and be freed from the sample to sink to the bottom of the funnel for collection and identification.

The apparatus (Figs. 13.22 and 13.32) consists of a ring stand and a ring holder, a funnel with a piece of rubber tubing on the end, a clamp, and cheesecloth folded to fit the bottom of the funnel. The sample is placed on the cheesecloth and warm water added to cover the sample. All air bubbles are allowed to flow from the tube of the funnel and are discarded by releasing the clamp. The apparatus, once loaded, should be allowed to sit undisturbed for 12 to 24 hours.

After 24 hours, the first drop of fluid from the bottom of the funnel is removed and placed on a microscope slide. If any larvae are found swimming on the slide, the slide is heated with a match, rendering the larvae immobile for possible staining. A fresh sample yields success; if not fresh, various parasitic and nonparasitic larvae and adults may be seen, yielding erroneous results. Larvae should be identified using a parasitology text.

Examination of Blood Samples

Blood samples are commonly examined for such bloodborne parasites as *Trypanosoma*, hemoplasmas, anaplasmosis, babesia, ehrlichiosis, and *D. immitis* (canine heartworm), which is regarded as one of the most important parasites of the vascular system in domestic animals in the United States.

Direct Blood Smear Examination

Direct examination of the blood, a simple procedure, may be used to detect movement of microfilariae and other parasites present among erythrocytes (RBCs). As with direct examination of feces, direct examination of blood requires only one drop. However, unless parasites are present in large numbers, they may be missed; therefore the direct smear is not always a reliable technique for diagnosing heartworm-associated microfilariae, and a confirmatory antigen–antibody test is needed. There are several ELISA

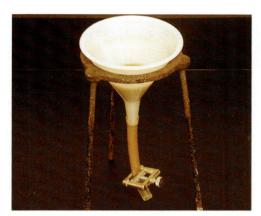

• **Fig. 13.32** Baermann apparatus used to recover larvae of roundworms (especially lungworms) from feces, soil, or animal tissues. This apparatus is most useful in recovering larvae of lungworms.

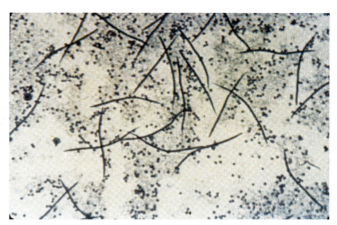

• **Fig. 13.33** Microfilariae of *Dirofilaria immitis*, identified with the modified Knott test.

kits available through veterinary supply companies at a range of prices. These use antigen-specific antibodies to identify the antigens associated with parasites such as *D. immitis* and require a short amount of time.

Differentiation between *Dirofilaria* species and *Dipetalonema* species is extremely important, because treatment for heartworms is expensive, physiologically stressful, and involves the use of organic arsenic compounds. In a direct blood smear, microfilariae of *Dirofilaria* species coil and uncoil, whereas those of *Dipetalonema* species may glide smoothly across the slide, with the number of microfilariae of *Dirofilaria* species in a sample being greater than *Dipetalonema* species (although this is not always the case). Direct examination of blood is useful only to determine the presence of microfilariae, not species identification. To identify microfilaria "types," the modified Knott test stains microfilariae while lysing RBCs to make the microfilariae more visible (Fig. 13.33 [*Dipetalonema reconditum*]). Table 13.4 lists the characteristics that may be assessed to identify microfilariae.

Thin Blood Smear

The thin blood smear is prepared and stained similar to a blood smear for a differential white blood cell (WBC) count. Occasionally, when performing a differential WBC count, microfilariae may be found along the feathered edge. Differentiation of microfilariae is not possible in a thin blood smear and requires further testing. Trypanosomes, protozoans, and rickettsia also may be found among or within cells. As with the direct smear procedure, a small blood sample is used and mild parasitic infections may be missed, requiring confirmatory testing.

Thick Blood Smear

A thick blood smear examines a slightly greater volume of blood compared with a thin blood smear. Microfilariae may be seen but cannot be differentiated easily by this method.

Concentration Techniques
Buffy Coat Method

The buffy coat method is used on a small volume of blood as a quick technique to be performed along with PCV and total protein (TP) evaluation. Centrifugation of blood (separation into three layers occurs: plasma, WBC layer [buffy coat], RBC layer) in a microhematocrit tube is done to determine the PCV (Fig. 13.34). Motile microfilariae can be found on the surface of the buffy coat layer; however, differentiation is not possible.

TABLE 13.4	Differentiations of Microfilariae Using the Modified Knott Technique	
Characteristic	*Dirofilaria immitis*	*Dipetalonema reconditum*
Body length	310 μm	290 μm
Midbody width	6 μm	6 μm
Head	Tapered	Blunt
Tail	Straight	Hooked[a]

[a]Artifact of formalin fixation.

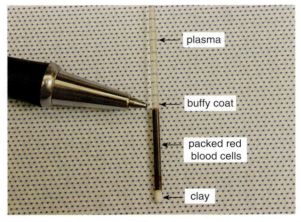

• **Fig. 13.34** Three tests may be performed with a single centrifuged microhematocrit tube: packed cell volume (PCV), total protein (TP), and microfilariae confirmation.

Modified Knott Technique

The modified Knott technique is explained above under the subheading "Direct Blood Examination."

Filter Techniques

Filter techniques remain one of the most utilized in veterinary practices for the detection of microfilariae in blood by using commercial kits with filters, lysing solution, and stain. It should be noted that a negative result does not necessarily rule out heartworm infection, and differentiation is possible but difficult. The kits require 1 mL of whole blood, which is mixed with nine parts of lysing solution in a syringe and passed through a filter. The filter is removed and placed on a slide on which a drop of stain is added before a coverslip is applied to microscopically examine the filter for microfilariae.

Protozoans of Veterinary Importance

A protozoan is a unicellular (one-cell) organism. Some protozoans are parasitic to humans and wild and domestic animals. Protozoans can be classified into several types based on their means of locomotion: ciliates (use tiny beating "hairs"), flagellates (use one or more whiplike flagella), amoebae (use pseudopodia), and apicomplexans (by gliding).

Giardia Species

- Parasite's common name: "tennis racket with eyes"
- Pronunciation: "Gee-*ard*-dee-uh"

Species Affected

Giardia is the most common intestinal parasite affecting humans, virtually all domestic species, and many wild species of animals. Several species of *Giardia* are recognized (Table 13.5). Infected animals may be asymptomatic, and clinical disease in cats is uncommon. Affected animals may experience weight loss secondary to diarrhea, with diarrhea being characteristic and common in puppies and kittens, animals that are stressed, immunosuppressed, or housed in groups.

Abbreviated Life Cycle

The life cycle begins with a noninfective cyst being voided in the feces of an infected animal. The cyst is highly resistant to environmental factors (i.e., heat, cold, dehydration) and possesses four prominent nuclei. When a host ingests the cyst, the motile tear-shaped **trophozoite** emerges from the cyst and begins to feed within the gut (see Fig. 13.31).

> ### TECHNICIAN NOTE
> Trophozoites (literally "a tiny, moving organism") are defined as fast-growing organisms in developmental stages occurring as cysts in the life cycle of *Toxoplasma gondii* and other similar apicomplexan parasites.

Motile trophozoites cover the tops of intestinal epithelial cells, limiting absorption. They multiply through longitudinal binary fission to form a trophozoite, then a cyst before passing through the digestive system into the external environment via defecation; while trophozoites may be found in feces, only the cysts can survive outside of the host.

Laboratory Test(s) Used to Diagnose the Infection

Both cysts and trophozoites (Figs. 13.35 and 13.36) may be identified on direct fecal smear or direct saline preparation; however, a negative result does not rule out infection. Zinc sulfate or sugar flotation medium in combination with centrifugation should be subsequently used, with serial fecal samples necessary over a period of 3 to 5 days for prompt diagnosis. Fecal IFA, fecal antigen ELISA, and fecal PCR assay are also useful, and a combination of these tests may be needed to confirm infection.

TABLE 13.5	*Giardia* Species and Hosts Affected
Giardia spp.	Host(s)
Giardia canis	Canines
Giardia lamblia	Humans, mammals
Giardia muris	Mice, mammals
Giardia ardeae	Avian
Giardia psittaci	Avian
Giardia agilis	Amphibians
Giardia microti	Voles

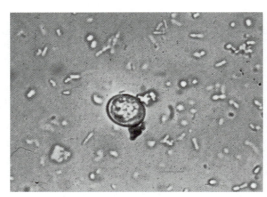

• **Fig. 13.35** Cyst of *Giardia* species.

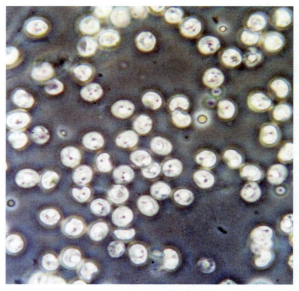

• **Fig. 13.36** A fecal floatation showcases the oocysts (eggs) of *Toxoplasma* species.

Zoonotic Potential for Clients

The veterinary technician should always consider this parasite as zoonotic, especially if present in a dog or a cat with diarrhea. *Giardia* has not been shown to be highly host specific and therefore may be spread from dogs and cats to humans. Because this organism is spread through fecal–oral contact, young children and immunocompromised humans as a population are most at risk. Clients should be advised of hygienic measures needed in the home to minimize infection.

Treatment
Currently, in the United States, no drugs are approved by the FDA for the treatment of *Giardia*. The CAPC recommends metronidazole (10–25 mg every 12 hours for 3–5 days) or a combination therapy of fenbendazole (50 mg/kg every 24 hours) and metronidazole (25 mg/kg every 12 hours for 5 days).

Prevention and Control Techniques
Prompt removal and disposal of feces from cages, runs, and yards help prevent environmental exposure. Cysts can be inactivated by most quaternary ammonium compounds—a 1:32 dilution of household bleach, steam, or boiling water. Grassy areas should be considered contaminated for at least 1 month after contamination by infected dogs and avoided. Cysts contaminating the hairs of dogs and cats may be a source of reinfection, so regular shampooing/rinsing of the animal's coat is important to limit disease spread. Use of disposable bedding is needed until fomite-associated infection has been cleared. Animals should not share owners' sleeping areas.

> **TECHNICIAN NOTE**
> Although *Giardia* species are not highly host specific and can be spread from domestic animals to humans, a more common source of infection is contaminated water bodies. In addition, infants and children in childcare facilities may be at increased risk for infection. While pets are often the primary suspect in human giardiasis, other sources of infection must be considered, especially in young children.

Toxoplasma gondii
- Parasite's common name: "toxo"
- Pronunciation: "Tox-oh-*plaz*-ma" "*gon*-dee-eye"

Species Affected
The *only* host harboring this parasite in its sexual stages is the feline host as an asymptomatic definitive host. All other warm-blooded mammals may serve as intermediate hosts for this protozoan parasite. Kittens infected transplacentally or during nursing are often the most severely affected patients, showing signs of lethargy, depression, ascites, fever, and sudden death. Older cats with clinical illness may present with symptoms including fever and anorexia to more specific symptoms involving any body system that is affected by the spread of **tachyzoites** or **bradyzoites** throughout the body.

> **TECHNICIAN NOTE**
> A *bradyzoite* is defined as a slow-growing organism in the developmental stage.
> A *tachyzoite* is defined as a fast-growing organism in the developmental stage.

Abbreviated Life Cycle
The life cycle of *T. gondii* has two phases: a sexual phase and an asexual phase. The sexual phase occurs only in domestic and wild cats as definitive hosts and is found within intestinal cells. Macrogametes are fertilized by microgametes, forming tiny oocysts that have undergone sporulation. The asexual phase takes place in any warm-blooded animal (intermediate hosts), including mammals

and birds, where the parasite invades cells, forming intracellular cysts that contain slow-dividing cysts. The cysts are called *bradyzoites* and are found in muscles and brain tissue. Because the host's immune system does not recognize these cysts as being "foreign," the bradyzoites multiply to the point that the infected cells containing them burst open and release tachyzoites (rapidly dividing forms). These tachyzoites form more cysts containing bradyzoites or tachyzoites. Cysts are ingested by a cat when it feeds on an infected mouse and digested before they infect the cells of the small intestine, where they undergo sexual reproduction to form oocysts that are shed in the feces of the cat (see Fig. 13.36). Infection occurs when oocysts are ingested by animals and humans (e.g., by eating unwashed vegetables contaminated by cat feces or improperly cooked meat contaminated with tissue cysts); after this, the parasites enter the macrophages in the lining of the intestine and are distributed via the bloodstream throughout the body.

Laboratory Test(s) Used to Diagnose the Infection
Diagnosis of *T. gondii* is usually presumptive based on clinical signs consistent with *T. gondii* infection and positive serologic testing (ELISA), clinical response to medications, and exclusion of other causes for the clinical signs (i.e., rule-outs). Although uncommon, confirmation is possible by organism identification in tissues and body fluids upon necropsy or through biopsy.

Zoonotic Potential for Clients
Minimizing the feline shedding of oocysts in feces into the environment is important. This parasite is of greatest concern to pregnant women due to the possibility of transplacental transmission of infection to the developing fetus, a serious zoonotic consequence.

Treatment
Clindamycin is the treatment of choice for dogs and cats, at a dosage of 10 to 40 mg/kg and 25 to 50 mg/kg, respectively, for 14 to 21 days. Certain drugs, such as diaminodiphenylsulfone, atovaquone, and spiramycin, have been used to treat toxoplasmosis in difficult cases. Clients should be referred to their physician if they suspect they have been infected.

Prevention and Control Techniques
Litter boxes must be cleaned daily, because oocysts need a minimum of 1 to 3 days to sporulate and become infective, a time frame that is dependent on temperature and gets longer as the temperature gets colder. Litter boxes should be disinfected with boiling water at least once weekly. Outdoor sandboxes should be kept covered to prevent their use as litter boxes and inspected before children use them to prevent zoonotic infection. Immunocompromised individuals need not necessarily be separated from their cats, but care must be taken to ensure pet health to avoid disease spread. Pregnant women must avoid contact with soil, cat litter, raw meat, and cats excreting oocysts. All persons should wash hands and surfaces thoroughly after handling raw meat or cleaning litter boxes.

> **TECHNICIAN NOTE**
> Although humans can be infected by oocysts that are shed in cat feces, they are more often infected by eating raw/undercooked meat (i.e., lamb, venison, pork) or shellfish (i.e., clams, mussels, or oysters) that contains the cysts. Pregnant women are most at risk of fetal injury if contaminated with this parasite. The parasite is considered a dangerous zoonotic parasite.

Cryptosporidium parvum

- Parasite's common name: "crypto," "cryptosporidiosis"
- Pronunciation: "Crypt-oh-spore-*rid*-ee-yum" "*par*-vum"

Species Affected

Cryptosporidium species infects all species of domestic animals—especially calves, dogs, and cats—but also rodents and humans. Cryptosporidiosis usually occurs in dogs that are younger than 6 months of age. This tiniest of protozoan parasites is found on the tips of the villi of the small intestine.

Cryptosporidiosis can be asymptomatic or symptomatic, with GI symptoms such as acute, watery diarrhea with mucus of a few weeks' duration. Many asymptomatic dogs recover spontaneously from cryptosporidiosis. Other dogs may develop only mild diarrhea; in dogs with weakened immune systems, cryptosporidiosis can cause chronic diarrhea and subsequent dehydration, something that is life-threatening and requires treatment and support.

Abbreviated Life Cycle

Oocysts of *C. parvum* may be found in untreated surface water, contaminated water supplies, cattle manure, and on objects that have been contaminated by human feces. If ingested by a suitable host, oocysts pass through the stomach, entering the small intestine. Within the intestine, oocysts will excyst ("hatch"), releasing four motile, arc-shaped sporozoites that adhere to the external cell wall of the intestinal cells, where they begin to multiply, producing the next parasitic stage—the merozoite stage (which is neither male nor female). Six to eight merozoites are produced from one sporozoite through asexual multiplication and may break out of the host's cells and invade new cells, repeating the process. At some point, some of these merozoites develop into both male and female gametocytes, which can unite to form gametes and develop between the cell wall layers, becoming oocysts. These oocysts break out to be excreted in fecal matter, at which time the host is likely to become symptomatic, exhibiting profuse diarrhea, carrying the oocysts out of the body. Some of the oocysts mature very quickly and release their sporozoites before being deposited into the external environment, where they invade the intestinal cells, multiplying and beginning the process anew. In a healthy animal, the immune system will respond and recovery occurs, but in immunocompromised individuals, infection with *Cryptosporidium* will persist and turn into a vicious and deadly cycle as infective oocysts are passed into the external environment. Because oocysts are quite resilient, unaffected by cold, chlorine, and other chemicals added to water for disinfection, they can survive for long periods in moist conditions. They will perish if they dry out but if ingested, the infectious process will begin anew.

Laboratory Test(s) Used to Diagnose the Infection

Cryptosporidium is diagnosed using fecal smears stained with modified acid staining or iodine (wet mount), fecal flotation, sedimentation, ELISA, fluorescent-labeled antibodies, and PCR. Brightfield microscopy is not effective for viewing the oocysts; however, phase-contrast and immune-fluorescent microscopy are. The following commercial microfluorescent products used include: Merifluor or Cryptosporidium/Giardia (Meridian Diagnostics), Detect IF Cryptosporidium (Shield Diagnostics), and Crypto/F Kit (Tech Lab). All kits are approved for testing of both human and veterinary patients. Commercial serologic tests are available to identify antibodies against *C. parvum* in the dog's blood; a positive test result indicates exposure but not necessarily current infection.

Zoonotic Potential for Clients

C. parvum causes chronic diarrhea and severe dehydration in humans with HIV/AIDS and can easily develop into a life-threatening secondary infection in people with compromised immune systems. Clients suspecting infection should consult their physician for diagnosis and treatment.

Treatment

No reliable treatment is available for enteritis caused by *C. parvum* in dogs; in most cases, dogs recover from cryptosporidiosis spontaneously. Symptomatic treatment includes broad-spectrum antibiotics and a high-fiber diet to help relieve the symptoms of diarrhea associated with the infection and supportive therapy (e.g., fluid replacement) to address dehydration.

Prevention and Control Techniques

Contaminated areas in the dog's environment must be disinfected with a solution of 1:10 bleach and water and allowed to completely dry due to oocyst resistance to chlorine and the ability to thrive in moist environments. The pet's bedding should be discarded in favor of disposable bedding to be changed regularly. The infected dog must be isolated from other pets, children, and especially individuals with compromised immune systems until cleared of infection.

TECHNICIAN NOTE

Because of medical privacy issues, members of the veterinary team should never make inquiries regarding the client's medical information (e.g., HIV/AIDS). However, in case of a diagnosis of cryptosporidiosis in dogs, the severity of the zoonotic potential must be communicated to every pet owner or client so that they are well educated on their options.

14

Clinical Microbiology

ORETA M. SAMPLES, LEIAH BROOKS, AND KAREN CAPPS-MCMULLAN

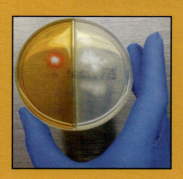

CHAPTER OUTLINE

LEARNING OBJECTIVES

When you have completed this chapter, you will be able to:

1. Pronounce, define, and spell all key terms in the chapter.
2. Identify circumstances under which dangerous microorganisms (i.e., select dimorphic fungi) should not be cultured in a private practice setting.
3. Do the following regarding the collection of samples:
   - Describe methods used to collect and preserve representative samples.
   - Describe the special collection and handling procedures used to culture samples from tissues, urine, the respiratory tract, blood, joints, milk, and feces. Identify appropriate transport media and packing conditions that must be met for safe transport to an outside laboratory through shipping.
4. Do the following regarding sample processing:
   - Identify staining procedures used to for direct microscopic examination of prepared slides such as Gram stain, acid-fast stain, modified acid-fast stain, and spore staining.
5. Do the following regarding bacterial culture and identification:
   - Describe the principles of bacterial culture, including safe disposal of microbiological laboratory waste and basic equipment used for microbiological cultures.

- Describe the differences between nutrient, enrichment, selective, and differential media; describe how to inoculate for biochemical testing, and primary isolation of bacterial pathogens.
- Explain how examination of growth on a culture plate is used to identify pathogens and guide clinical decisions.
- Describe the roles that catalase, oxidase, coagulase biochemical tests, and hemolysis patterns play in preliminary grouping of gram-positive and gram-negative bacteria.
- List common bacterial flora and pathogens, identifying the classification of each and associated diseases.
6. Do the following regarding antimicrobial susceptibility testing:
   - Explain the reasons for susceptibility testing for performing and interpreting antimicrobial susceptibility tests.
   - Describe the procedures for and principles of interpretation of the broth dilution test and the disk diffusion test.
7. Do the following regarding fungal culture (mycology):
   - Describe the methods used to collect dermatophytes, inoculate dermatophyte test medium and Sabouraud dextrose agar, and interpret culture results.

8. Do the following regarding the molecular detection of pathogens:
   List the methods commonly used to detect pathogens in patient samples via enzyme-linked immunosorbent assay (ELISA), virus isolation (VI), fluorescent antibody (FA), electron microscopy (EM), immunohistochemical staining, polymerase chain reaction (PCR) and deoxyribonucleic acid (DNA) sequencing.
9. Do the following regarding nosocomial infections:
   - Demonstrate an understanding of agents and their method of causing nosocomial infections.

KEY TERMS

Abscess
Acid-fast staining
Actinobacillus spp.
Aeromonas spp.
Anaerobe
Antimicrobial susceptibility testing
Bacillus anthracis
Bordetella bronchiseptica
Brucella spp.
Catalase
Coagulase
Corynebacterium pseudotuberculosis
Cytochrome oxidase
Dermatophyte
Differential media
Disk diffusion
DNA sequencing
Enterococcus spp.
Erysipelothrix rhusiopathiae
Escherichia coli
Enrichment media

Fastidious
Gram stain
Hemolysis
Indigenous flora
Listeria monocytogenes
Minimum inhibitory concentration
Nosocomial infection
Opportunistic infection
Oxidase
Pasteurella multocida
Proteus spp.
Polymerase chain reaction (PCR)
Rhodococcus equi
Salmonella spp.
Selective medium
Staphylococcus pseudintermedius
Streptococcus spp.
Transport media
Trueperella
Yeasts
Zone of inhibition

Introduction

The veterinarian relies on clinical microbiology to provide information rapidly and accurately about the presence of infectious agents (bacteria, fungi, and viruses) in patient samples, providing guidance and support for making decisions regarding treatment of infections. The veterinary technician will have a direct impact on the success of identification of infectious agents through correct collection, labeling, and handling of appropriate samples, and by the culture, testing, or timely submission of those samples to a diagnostic laboratory.

Increasingly, veterinary practices rely on diagnostic laboratories to examine patient samples for bacteria and fungi for several reasons. First, it may not be safe to culture certain samples in a veterinary practice. By sending samples to diagnostic laboratories, the veterinarian reduces the risk to veterinary personnel, patients, and clients. Second, some expertise is required to recognize bacterial and fungal pathogens and to differentiate them from indigenous flora. Additionally, it is necessary to do regular quality control testing on media and antibiotics to avoid erroneous conclusions that could have a negative impact on patients. If tests or cultures are performed infrequently, it may be more cost effective to submit the samples to a diagnostic laboratory than to maintain media and reagents not utilized. Finally, regulatory issues, such as those outlined by the Centers for Disease Control and Prevention (CDC), make it advantageous to submit samples to diagnostic laboratories whose personnel understand these regulations. After isolating an organism, sending it to a laboratory for confirmatory testing may also be necessary. Some private practices routinely perform point-of-care (POC) microbiological testing, including mastitis testing in dairy practices, cultures of the reproductive tract in equine practices, and dermatophyte testing of companion animals, as these are inexpensive and some yield immediate results.

This chapter describes current methods used in veterinary microbiology, with a focus on practical clinical application. Testing, such as mass spectrophotometry or DNA sequencing, is not done within the clinical setting; commercial reference laboratories have the capabilities to perform these tests. Currently, in-house laboratories are restricted to culturing techniques and some POC tests that are less expensive but still identify bacterial and fungal pathogens.

Microbiological Safety

When preparing to culture a patient, it is important to consider whether it is safe to handle the sample in-house, as some bacterial and fungal agents can be dangerous because of their highly infectious nature. Use of personal protective equipment (PPE) (masks, gloves, and face shields) is necessary, as is a biological safety hood for protection of personnel against infectious agents. Such agents may be classified by governments as "select" agents or "agents of interest" because of their potential use as biological weapons (i.e., Anthrax). Many of these organisms are endemic to certain parts of the United States and may be encountered in veterinary patients. Because of the risk to personnel handling these cultures, testing is best left to specialized laboratories with the appropriate safety equipment; no attempt should be made to culture these agents in private practice. Identification of such agents must also be reported to appropriate regulatory agencies and include *Bacillus anthracis*, *Brucella abortus*, *Francisella tularensis*, and *Yersinia pestis*. Examples of select fungal agents include the dimorphic fungi *Histoplasma capsulatum* and *Blastomyces dermatididis*.

TABLE 14.1   Indigenous (Normal) Flora

Aerobes	Obligate Anaerobes
Skin, Ear	
Staphylococcus, Micrococcus, Streptococcus	
Mouth, Nasopharynx, Oropharynx	
Micrococcus, Staphylococcus, Streptococcus (alpha- and beta-hemolytic), *Bacillus*, coliforms, *Proteus, Pasteurella, Actinobacillus, Haemophilus, Mycoplasma*	*Bacteroides, Prevotella, Porphyromonas, Fusobacterium, Actinomyces,* spirochetes
Trachea, Bronchi, Lungs	
Only transient contaminants	
Stomach, Small Intestine	
Streptococcus	*Lactobacillus*
Large Intestine	
Streptococcus, Escherichia coli, Klebsiella, Enterobacter, Proteus, Enterococcus	*Clostridium, Fusobacterium, Bacteroides, Porphyromonas, Prevotella,* spirochetes, *Lactobacillus*
External Genitalia (Vulva, Prepuce)	
Micrococcus, Staphylococcus, Corynebacterium	
Conjunctiva, Uterus, Mammary Glands	
Occasionally may contain small numbers of insignificant bacteria	

Sample Collection and Preservation

The results of microbiological culture depend on the quality of samples collected. It is important to remember that the skin, mucous membranes, conjunctiva, respiratory tract, urogenital tract, and particularly, the gastrointestinal (GI) tract are inhabited by a variety of normal bacterial species, often called *indigenous flora* (Table 14.1). One of the challenges of bacterial culture is differentiating pathogens from indigenous flora, which can cause **opportunistic infections**. Although these organisms are usually harmless, they can cause disease under certain circumstances, such as in immune-compromised patients (Table 14.2).

The first step in collecting samples for culture is to determine the best specimen to collect, given clinical signs in the patient and the pathogens that are suspected to be present. The samples most commonly collected are urine, blood, feces, washes of infected sites (transtracheal washes or bronchoalveolar lavage fluids), hair, tissues (biopsy, necropsy specimens), and swabs of exudates. When collecting samples, contamination from normal flora should be avoided by aseptically preparing the sample collection sites (Fig. 14.1).

It is best to collect samples early in the disease process before initiation of antimicrobial therapy, which interferes with pathogenic isolation. In a patient receiving antimicrobial therapy, it is best to collect the sample just before the next drug dose is given, when antimicrobial drug concentration will be lowest.

If stained slides are to be prepared along with cultures, sufficient material must be collected for both. Anticoagulants, such as ethylenediaminetetraacetic acid (EDTA), heparin, and sodium citrate, prevent bacterial growth and therefore should not be used for preservation. It is critical to correctly label samples with the patient's name and collection date and time; multiple samples from the one patient should be labeled with the site of collection, the date, and the time.

Blood and joint fluids are often submitted to the laboratory in blood culture bottles that contain broth. The broth aids in recovery of bacteria that are difficult to grow or are slow growing, and it also dilutes antimicrobial proteins from the animal that will inhibit bacterial growth. It takes only one viable bacterial cell to turn a broth culture positive, so contamination of these cultures with indigenous flora of the skin, such as *Staphylococcus epidermidis*, or environmental organisms, such as *Bacillus* spp., is to be avoided.

> **TECHNICIAN NOTE**
>
> A broth culture can be contaminated at several different points: when collecting the sample with indigenous flora from the patient's skin, during culture inoculation, or in the clinical laboratory.

Special Collection and Handling Procedures

Tissue samples can be collected aseptically during surgery, biopsy, or necropsy. The conditions surrounding collection dictate the amount of tissue collected and how the specimen is submitted. Samples collected at surgery and considered aerobic should be placed in a sterile labeled container with a few drops of sterile non-bacteriostatic saline for submission. Samples collected at necropsy should contain representative lesions and should be sufficiently large to allow decontamination of the external surface of the tissue by using alcohol or flame before culture. Anaerobic cultures should be placed in a transport container approved for anaerobic culture (i.e., anaerobic swab collection system). Tissue samples should be refrigerated or placed on ice for shipment to prevent degradation.

Use of swabs is a convenient method for sample collection; such swabs are commercially available. It is important to match swab type (aerobic or anaerobic) to the sample being collected. Determination of presence of indigenous flora at the collection site is necessary; such flora can interfere with results. Some sites, including skin, may be inhabited by several different organisms (incidental and nonpathogenic organisms); therefore, biopsy may be preferable to swabs. It should be confirmed that the sample was aseptically collected and submitted. Most commercial anaerobic swab systems have an oxygen indicator that enables the user to confirm aerobic maintenance of sample. Swabs are often used to collect samples from abscesses (infectious pockets containing purulent material such as bacteria, neutrophils, and macrophages). When collecting samples from abscesses, it is tempting to collect purulent material (i.e., dead bacteria or cells), but it is generally better to collect the sample from the leading edge or capsule of the abscess to sample actively growing bacteria.

> **TECHNICIAN NOTE**
>
> When using swabs to prepare stained slides and bacterial cultures, set up cultures before preparing slides by using separate swabs for each purpose, as glass slides are not sterile.

TABLE 14.2   Bacteria Associated With Infections

Canine	Feline	Equine	Porcine	Ruminants
Conjunctivitis/Corneal Ulcer				
Staphylococcus Streptococcus Pseudomonas	Staphylococcus Pasteurella Chlamydophila	Often fungal Streptococcus Staphylococcus	Streptococcus Staphylococcus	Moraxella bovis/bovoculi Branhamella Streptococcus Staphylococcus Mycoplasma E. coli
Central Nervous System				
Rare	Rare	Streptococcus Actinobacillus Escherichia coli	Streptococcus E. coli	Histophilus somni Listeria monocytogenes E. coli Pasteurella
Gastroenteritis				

Salmonella
Clostridium perfringens
Campylobacter
Clostridium difficile
	Salmonella	Salmonella
		Clostridium perfringens
		Clostridium difficile
		E. coli
		Actinobacillus
		Rhodococcus equi
			Salmonella
			E. coli
			Clostridium perfringens
			Clostridium difficile
			Brachyspira hyodysenteriae
				Salmonella
				E. coli
				Clostridium perfringens
				Mycobacterium
				  avium, subspecies
				  paratuberculosis

Genital Tract				
Brucella canis E. coli Streptococcus Staphylococcus Mycoplasma	Streptococcus Pasteurella E. coli	Streptococcus E. coli Klebsiella Pseudomonas	Brucella suis Streptococcus Leptospira	Brucella Listeria monocytogenes Trueperella pyogenes Campylobacter Mycoplasma
Mastitis				
Staphylococcus	Staphylococcus	Streptococcus	Streptococcus Staphylococcus E. coli Actinobacillus Trueperella pyogenes	Streptococcus Staphylococcus Trueperella pyogenes Mycoplasma Mycobacterium E. coli Klebsiella Nocardia
Musculoskeletal				
Staphylococcus E. coli Pseudomonas Brucella canis Anaerobes	Rare	Streptococcus Actinobacillus E. coli Rhodococcus equi Clostridium Staphylococcus	Streptococcus Mycoplasma E. coli Erysipelothrix Trueperella pyogenes	Clostridium Trueperella pyogenes E. coli Streptococcus Erysipelothrix Histophilus somni Mycoplasma
Otitis				
Staphylococcus Pseudomonas Streptococcus Malassezia Corynebacterium Actinomyces canis	Rare	Rare	Streptococcus	Streptococcus Pasteurella Trueperella pyogenes Mycoplasma
Upper Respiratory Tract				
Bordetella bronchiseptica	Pasteurella multocida	Streptococcus equi	Bordetella bronchiseptica Pasteurella multocida	Histophilus somni Trueperella pyogenes

TABLE 14.2 Bacteria Associated With Infections—cont'd				
Canine	**Feline**	**Equine**	**Porcine**	**Ruminants**
Pneumonia				
Bordetella bronchiseptica	Rare	*Streptococcus*	*Bordetella bronchiseptica*	*Histophilus somni*
Pasteurella	*Pasteurella multocida*	*Actinobacillus*	*Pasteurella multocida*	*Trueperella pyogenes*
Klebsiella	*Chlamydia*	*Rhodococcus equi*	*Mycoplasma*	*Mannheimia baemolytica*
E. coli	*Bordetella*	*Pasteurella*	*Haemophilus parasius*	*Pasteurella multocida*
Mycoplasma		*Staphylococcus*	*Actinobacillus*	*Fusobacterium*
Streptococcus		*Klebsiella*	*pleuropneumoniae*	*Mycoplasma*
Staphylococcus		*Pseudomonas*	*Streptococcus*	
Anaerobes		*Bordetella bronchiseptica*		
Pleuritis				
Anaerobes	Anaerobes	*Streptococcus*	*Actinobacillus*	*Mannheimia*
Actinomyces	*Pasteurella*	Anaerobes		*Pasteurella*
	Nocardia			*Trueperella pyogenese*
Skin Wounds, Abscesses				
Staphylococcus	*Pasteurella multocida*	*Streptococcus*	*Streptococcus*	*Trueperella*
Streptococcus	*Streptococcus*	*Corynebacterium*	*Staphylococcus*	*(Arcanobacterium)*
Pseudomonas	*Staphylococcus*	*pseudotuberculosis*	*Trueperella pyogenes*	*pyogenes*
Nocardia	Anaerobes	*Pseudomonas*		*Dermatophilus*
Actinomyces		*Dermatophilus*		*Actinomyces*
Anaerobes		*Staphylococcus*		*Actinobacillus*
				Staphylococcus
				Corynebacterium
				pseudotuberculosis
Urinary Tract				
E. coli	*Staphylococcus*	*Streptococcus*	*Actinobaculum suis*	*Corynebacterium renale*
Proeus	*E. coli*	*E. coli*	*Streptococcus*	*Trueperella pyogenes*
Staphylococcus	*Enterococcus*			
Enterococcus				
Streptococcus				
Klebsiella				
Pseudomonas				
Mycoplasma				

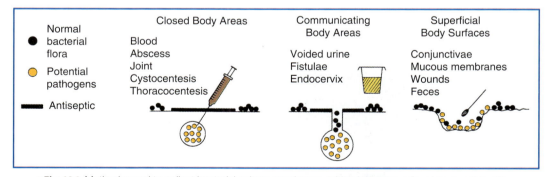

• **Fig. 14.1** Methods used to collect bacterial culture specimens, taking indigenous flora into consideration.

Cystocentesis is the preferred collection method for urinary culture due to the presence of indigenous flora of the external genitalia. In some animal species, it is not anatomically possible to perform cystocentesis; one might catch urine as it is voided (free catch) or collect it by using an indwelling urinary catheter. Ideally, free-catch urine samples should be collected "midstream" after the patient has already begun to urinate. This sample typically includes bacteria, so immediate evaluation of the number of bacteria in the sample to determine whether an infection is present is critical. Regarding cultures, it is important to inform the laboratory staff which collection method was used, as organisms present in low amounts of a free-catch sample reflect indigenous flora from the external genitalia.

An ideal sample for urine culture equals at least 0.5 mL of urine collected by cystocentesis and submitted in a urine transport system. Sterile tubes designed for submission of serum (red-top tubes) are also used for this purpose and may be refrigerated (never frozen) until inoculation. Because bacteria can die during transport, it is preferable to use systems designed for bacterial maintenance without promoting their growth or allowing their death. All cultures and tests should be completed as soon as possible.

Samples of bronchoalveolar lavage and transtracheal wash are collected aseptically by introducing a small amount of sterile saline or other sterile wash fluid into the bronchus or trachea and then removing it through aspiration. Such samples are directly examined by microscopy and cultured. The ideal sample consists of at least 0.5 mL of fluid in a sterile container (e.g., a red-top tube), which is shipped under refrigeration. For direct microscopic examination, a smear is made and stained with Wright or Diff-Quik stain.

Localized infections that have spread to multiple organs are called *disseminated infections* or *systemic infections* in which bacteria are transported from a site of local infection throughout the body by blood or lymph. Infection of blood is called *bacteremia* and requires performance of a blood culture for diagnosis of systemic disease. Because bacteremia is transient, bacteria may or may not be present in blood at the time that a sample is collected. To increase the chances of detecting bacterial presence, a total of three blood samples should be collected from the patient at different times (at least 30 minutes apart) from a different vein over a 24-hour period. Before inoculation, the skin over the vein should be aseptically prepared, akin to a surgical prep, removing possible contaminants to prevent false-positive results. Samples are collected from separate veins to avoid contamination by bacteria of the skin. This contamination is not harmful to the patient but can cause false-positive culture results and impede an accurate diagnosis. If aerobic and anaerobic cultures are desired, separate samples should be collected. Samples should not be collected from veins used for intravenous (IV) fluids, because blood will be diluted. If possible, IV fluid therapy should be stopped for 15 to 20 minutes before collection.

Joint fluid typically is submitted in a blood culture medium for the recovery of organisms. Samples may also be submitted in sterile vials (red-top tubes) or on swabs in which sodium polyanethol sulfonate is used as an anticoagulant. Anticoagulants, such as heparin or EDTA, which interfere with bacterial culturing, should not be used.

In patients with suspected mastitis but no clumps noted in milk, testing via the California mastitis test (CMT) helps confirm the presence of subclinical mastitis. For the CMT, the udder is cleaned and about 2 mL of milk is expressed from each teat into the CMT paddle (Fig. 14.2). Each of the four wells of the CMT paddle has two raised rings. The outer ring is the level to which milk is added. After milk has been collected, the CMT reagent is added to the level of the inner ring. Milk is then swirled horizontally in the paddle for 10 seconds, then assessed for the presence of clumps, indicating the severity of subclinical mastitis, and may be noted as 1+, 2+, 3+, or 4+. The CMT reagent package instructions should be closely followed. A description of test interpretation is provided in Table 14.3.

Milk culture is useful in identifying the causative agent in cases of clinical or subclinical mastitis. Clinical mastitis demonstrates obvious clumps of fibrin and other material in milk without staining. For milk culture, collection is done before milking the animal; gloves should be worn when cleaning and drying the udder. Beginning with the teats on the far side of the udder, the teat opening is scrubbed thoroughly (10–15 seconds) with cotton balls or gauze moistened with 70% isopropyl alcohol. It is important not to touch the teat end once cleaned, and collection should start at the closest teats. The first two streams of milk from each teat are discarded, and 1–2 mL of milk is collected in a sterile vial, without touching the vial with the teat. The sample is labeled with the animal identifier and the quarter collected (i.e., left front [LF], left rear or right front [LR/RF], right rear [RR]). It is acceptable to combine milk from all teats, but this must be noted as a "bulk sample," on both the sample and the submission form. It is also important to collect milk before administering any antibiotic treatment and maintain it on ice or refrigerate for transportation to the laboratory within 24 hours. Any samples to be held for longer periods before culturing should be frozen; milk fats will preserve the bacteria. Teat dipping should be done after testing.

About 1–10 grams of fresh feces is collected in a clean, tightly lidded container and shipped to the laboratory, refrigerated or on ice. Selective media that exclude the growth of most organisms are used for fecal cultures. Organisms most expected in feces in cases of diarrhea are *Salmonella, Campylobacter, Clostridium perfringens, Clostridium difficile,* and *Mycobacterium avium* subsp. *paratuberculosis.*

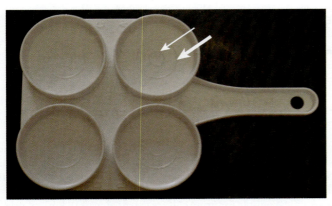

• **Fig. 14.2** Performance of the California mastitis test (CMT) using the CMT test paddle and reagent for detection of subclinical mastitis. The outer ring *(large arrow)* is the level to which the paddle is filled with milk, whereas the inner ring *(small arrow)* is the level to which the paddle is filled with CMT reagent.

TABLE 14.3   Interpretation of the California Mastitis Test

Score	Interpretation	Description
0	Negative	Mixture remains liquid with no clotting.
T	Trace	Slight thickening or precipitation forms but disappears within 10 seconds.
1	Weakly positive	A distinct precipitate but no gel formation.
2	Distinctly positive	The mixture thickens immediately, with some gel formation.
3	Strongly positive	A gel is formed that causes the surface of the mixture to become convex. Viscosity is increased, and the gel tends to adhere to the bottom of the cup.

There are several types of commercial transport media ideal for transport to the veterinary laboratory or for shipping out to a reference laboratory. As a rule, these media contain buffers and salt but do not contain nutrients, because this would encourage growth and possible replication, which may skew diagnoses related to disease severity. Table 14.4 lists common media and their intended purposes.

Preservation and Shipping Procedures

Sample preservation and transportation are critical components for good results from culture. It is important to use transport systems and media appropriate for the sample (Fig. 14.3). When shipping, one must consider what will happen to a sample during transportation and ship in accordance with federal shipping regulations. Other than milk samples, which may be frozen after collection, samples should not be frozen as freezing and thawing can kill bacteria. Three layers of protection are needed between the sample and the courier as a public health safety measure.

TABLE 14.4	Purposes for Specific Media
Media and Purpose	**Reactions and Interpretation**
Blood agar plate (trypticase soy agar with 5% sheep blood)	Primary isolation medium used for colony isolation.
Brucella blood agar plate	Primary isolation medium used for colony isolation.
MacConkey agar plate	Used to select gram-negative organisms used for colony isolation; allows differentiation of lactose fermentation (see Fig. 14.5).
Hektoen enteric agar	Used for direct isolation of *Salmonella* spp. from feces and colony isolation.
Selenite or tetrathionate broth	Used to enrich samples to detect *Salmonella* spp.
Salt mannitol agar	Used to differentiate species of *Staphylococcus* based on mannitol fermentation.
Triple sugar iron (TSI) agar slant	Used to determine the ability of an organism to use glucose, sucrose, and lactose and to produce hydrogen sulfide (see Figs. 14.7 and 14.9).
Lysine iron agar slant	Differentiates *Salmonella*.
Christensen urea agar slant	Determining whether an organism produces urease.
Motility media	Determining motility via flagella (see Fig. 14.8).
Indole test media	Determining the ability of an organism to split indole from tryptophan.
Citrate test media Differentiate *Enterobacteriaceae*	Determines presence of *Enterobacteriaceae*.

Safety and Disposal

It is imperative to conduct all microbiological collections, preservation, and testing with care and regard for the safety of not only the animal but the veterinary personnel involved. This includes the use of PPE (gloves and masks) when handling microbiological samples, which is important when handling dimorphic fungi. These samples are sent to commercial reference laboratories because of the zoonotic potential of these specimens. The clinical laboratory should have approved methods of disposal, including broken glass disposal boxes for slides/coverslips, sterilization bags for sterilizing testing materials that have been exposed to pathogenic microbes or body fluids, and sharps containers for the disposal of scalpel blades or other sharps, with attention to regular disposal. It is useful to have a separate autoclave for sterilization of microbiological waste prior to disposal, because these items should not be sterilized in the same autoclave used for surgical instruments. Most large laboratories steam sterilize (autoclave) laboratory waste materials. In a small practice setting, this may not be possible as practices have only one autoclave for sterilizing surgical and other equipment. Commercial contractors will dispose of biological waste for a fee; a quick Internet search will help identify disposal companies in the area, such as SHARPS Assure, Maine Labpac, BioMed Regulated Waste Disposal, and Safe Klean.

The M31-A3 document of the Clinical and Laboratory Standards Institute (CLSI) establishes breakpoints for each organism and each drug. A *breakpoint* is the number—either **minimum inhibitory concentration** (MIC) or diameter of the zone of inhibition—at which an organism should be called *susceptible* or *resistant* to a drug.

Regular testing of controls to ensure that laboratory equipment is functioning accurately is essential so that when a problem arises during testing, it is possible to identify the source of the problem. Simple measures, such as keeping a thermometer in an incubator to record daily temperatures, can help prevent erroneous test results that affect patient care.

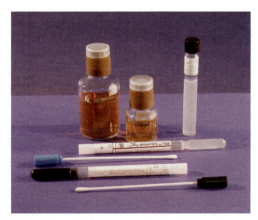

• **Fig. 14.3** Culturette swab transport systems with transport media (black medium is Amies transport medium with charcoal), Port-a-Cul Anaerobic Transport Tube (BD Diagnostic Systems, Franklin Lakes, NJ), and blood culture bottles. Swabs are used to collect culture inoculum to place into transport medium for preservation for transportation. Blood culture bottles are inoculated with blood to prevent coagulation and contamination during transport.

Quality assurance testing is essential in susceptibility testing to ensure that all tests and reagents perform appropriately. Drugs and media that exceed the expiration date should not be used, because testing an improperly stored drug that is inactive may lead to the erroneous conclusion that an isolate is resistant. It is also important to understand the interpretive criteria that are used to evaluate the results of a test and determine whether bacteria are susceptible or resistant to specific drugs.

> **TECHNICIAN NOTE**
>
> Local, state, and federal regulations on biological waste disposal should be considered before a laboratory is set up. Waste can be disposed of through a commercial contractor or by the laboratory using approved methods.

Direct Examination of Microbial Specimens

There are different ways to prepare a microbiological sample for immediate examination, including wet mounts, dry mounts, or stained specimens. A wet mount is prepared by placing a drop of water on a concave slide and mixing the sample with water (to preserve). The slide is then covered with a coverslip to view under the microscope. For dry mounts, the swab is rolled on a slide to adhere the sample to the slide before heat-fixing or applying a coverslip for viewing. Stained slides involve "fixing" of slide before staining.

Microscopic Examination

Direct examination of specimens from patients can be helpful when contemplating therapy. It is particularly helpful to examine exudates, material from draining tracts, and thoracic fluid from patients with pneumonia. However, it can be difficult to prepare adequate slides from samples that contain a high concentration of protein or large numbers of neutrophils or other leukocytes. Several slides should be prepared and examined, because slide-to-slide variation may be noted. For the quantity of bacteria to sufficiently allow visualization on a prepared slide, approximately 10^5 bacteria per milliliter of fluid are needed. Examining slides from samples with low bacterial numbers can be frustrating; it is also important to remember that infection may be present in the absence of bacteria.

> **TECHNICIAN NOTE**
>
> Stains may contain alcohol and other flammable liquids and should be contained in special flammable liquid cabinets away from flames. Maintain proper storage of all stains and ensure safety data sheet (SDS) labeling of all secondary containers (i.e., dropper bottles, dipping trays, etc.) and accessible SDS information as a public health measure.

Before examining prepared slides, one should confirm that the microscope is properly aligned for Köhler illumination, ensuring that stains appear as the correct color. Köhler illumination uses a collector lens, field diaphragm, condenser diaphragms, and a condenser lens to provide indirect illumination of samples, resulting in an even field of light to prevent artifacts from interfering with the image. Preparing control slides simultaneously with specimen slides is valuable to evaluate the performance of any stain. Control slides are helpful and may be commercially purchased or made in-house.

Stain Types

Simple stains are basic dyes, such as methylene blue, Gram safranin or Gram crystal violet, and nigrosin (i.e., negative stain) stains.

They are used to determine cell size, shape, and arrangement (i.e., clusters, chains, etc.). Differential stains are complex mixed stains, such as Gram, acid-fast (i.e., Ziehl-Neelsen or Kinyoun), and spore stains used for specific diagnostic purposes.

> **PUT INTO PRACTICE**
>
> Treat your stains as if they are pharmaceuticals, ensuring that they are used within date and replaced when compromised.

Staining Procedures

Gram stain, a commonly used stain, is named after its developer Hans Christian Gram (1853–1938). This technique uses dyes to distinguish between bacterial cell walls. Gram-positive organisms have cell walls composed of peptidoglycan; gram-negative organisms have cell walls that consist of a double-lipid bilayer comprising inner and outer cell membranes with a space in between, called the *periplasmic space* (Fig. 14.4 and Procedure 14.1).

The presence of neutrophils, other cells, or protein can alter the pH or the physical and chemical properties that are important for accurate Gram staining, thus making it difficult to know how the fluid will stain; it is advisable to run a control slide with the sample to be tested to evaluate a successful staining procedure. It can be difficult to get an adequate slide utilizing thick, viscous fluids, because such samples can retain stains. Additionally, these fluids tend to dry as a uniform sheet, fail to decolorize adequately, and will wash off the slide during washing. There is no simple solution for this except for dilution of viscous fluids with sterile saline and creating several slides with varying thickness of fluid for evaluation.

> **TECHNICIAN NOTE**
>
> It is important that the sample on the slide is thin enough for microscopic visual examination. Viscous fluids may be diluted with sterile normal saline to appropriate thickness before staining.

To examine the Gram-stained slide through a microscope, the slide is scanned first at low magnification before switching to the oil immersion lens. Do not get oil on lenses not designed for oil; all lenses should be cleaned with solvent (90% alcohol, acetone, or xylene) after examining specimens to avoid contamination of other samples.

Consider the control slide when interpreting the sample slide and how well it has stained; this helps interpret the sample slide, determining whether there is a need to stain another. Consider the sample source and the likely organisms that may be encountered when choosing a Wright-based stain (e.g., Diff-Quik stain) for comparison with the Gram-stained slide.

> **TECHNICIAN NOTE**
>
> Create two stained slides, one to determine Gram status and one to differentiate cells, organisms, parasites, etc.

Acid-Fast Staining Procedures

Acid-fast staining is required to determine the identity of organisms, such as *Mycobacterium* species and *Nocardia* species, whose cell walls contain mycotic acid (Procedure 14.2). Different procedures are used for acid-fast staining, most commonly the

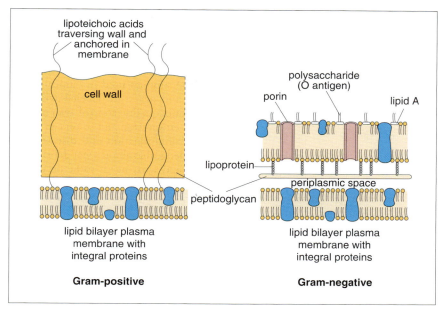

• **Fig. 14.4** Structure of the cell walls of gram-positive and gram-negative bacteria. Note the difference in the composition of the cell walls of gram-positive bacteria (which are largely made up of peptidoglycan) and the cell walls of gram-negative bacteria (which have a double-lipid bilayer composed of inner and outer cell membranes with a space in between called the *periplasmic space*). The gram-positive organisms retain crystal violet stain and appear purple, whereas gram-negative organisms do not retain crystal violet but counterstain with safranin and appear pink. (From Goering R, Dockrell H, Zuckerman M. *Mim's Medical Microbiology.* 4th ed. St. Louis, MO: Mosby; 2008.)

PROCEDURE 14.1

Gram Staining and Interpretation*

1. On a glass slide, prepare a thin, air-dried sample of the material to be examined.
2. If a sample will also be cultured, be sure to collect separate material for Gram staining and for the culture. The glass slide is not sterile, so the sample used for Gram staining cannot subsequently be used to inoculate culture media.
3. Flood the dry specimen with absolute methanol for 1 minute or with heat by passing it through the flame of a Bunsen burner for 5 to 10 seconds. Heating to 60°C (140°F) for 3 minutes should be sufficient to kill the bacteria and fix them to the slide.
4. Flood the slide with crystal violet solution and let stand for 1 minute, then rinse with tap water.
5. Flood the slide with Gram iodine solution and let stand for 1 minute, then rinse with tap water.
6. Decolorize the sample with Gram decolorizer (25% acetone, 75% isopropanol) for 1 to 5 seconds and immediately rinse the slide with tap water.
7. Flood the slide with safranin counterstain for 30 seconds to 1 minute and rinse with tap water.

*Perfecting this stain requires trial and error with known positives and negatives. Even experienced users have difficulty with some organisms. When results are inconclusive, it is best to run a control slide side-by-side with the sample.

PROCEDURE 14.2

Acid-Fast Stain Procedure (for detection of acid-fast organisms, such as *Mycobacterium* spp.)

1. Suspend a small amount of the sample in saline on a slide. When using feces, tissue, or exudates, make a direct preparation of this material, if possible.
2. Air dry and heat fix the slide.
3. Flood the slide with carbol fuchsin for 5 minutes and rinse with tap water.
4. Decolorize the sample with acid alcohol for 3 minutes and rinse with tap water.
5. Counterstain the sample with malachite green for 1 minute and rinse with tap water.
6. Blot the slide dry with bibulous paper or use a slide dryer.

Ziehl-Neelsen procedure or a variant of the acid-fast stain called the *partial* or *modified acid-fast stain, modified Ziehl-Neelsen stain,* or *Kinyoun acid-fast stain.* Organisms that are stained by acid-fast methods tend to have waxlike, almost impermeable cell walls, and the smear must be heat fixed before staining. As a result of mycolic acid, fatty acids, wax, and complex lipids in cell walls, carbol fuchsin as a primary stain is added by heat to aid in penetration, and methylene blue is used as a counterstain for cells undergoing decolorization.

After preparing an acid-fast stain, the control slide is examined first to confirm that the positive and negative controls are appropriately stained before examining the slides prepared from patient samples. Acid-fast organisms stain bright pink to red. Nonacid-fast organisms and the background should stain green.

With acid-fast staining of fluids, cytologic samples and feces, it can be difficult to see *Mycobacterium* species because the organism is minute; therefore it is important to be absolutely certain before calling a slide positive, because consequences for the patient are significant regarding treatment. Negative findings have low predictive value and additional testing is needed if test results are questionable regarding *Mycobacterium*.

The Kinyoun modified Ziehl-Neelsen acid-fast stain is used for identification of partially acid-fast organisms, such as *Nocardia* spp. (Procedure 14.3). The slides stained by this method are examined as described for acid-fast staining. Partially acid-fast organisms stain bright pink to red. Nonacid-fast organisms and the background should stain blue-green.

Acid-fast–stained samples from pure cultures are normally easy to interpret due to the bright pink to red coloring if positive. Background material in patient specimens may cause difficulty in interpretation. Difficulty can also arise with "partially" acid-fast organisms, because nonacid-fast organisms may stain purple instead of blue-green. With questionable results, a new sample should be stained and counterstained with malachite green for a longer time (up to 3 minutes), allowing for proper color development and ease of interpretation.

Bacterial Culture and Identification

Equipment and Supplies

The primary item of equipment needed for routine bacterial culture is a good-quality light microscope with low power and oil immersion lenses and an incubator that will maintain culture materials at a constant temperature (usually 35°C [95°F] to 37.5°C [99.5°F]). Some organisms are **fastidious** in their growth requirements, needing specialized atmospheric conditions or nutrients to grow. Typically, clinical microbiology laboratories use incubators supplied with carbon dioxide (CO_2) gas (providing a 5% CO_2 atmosphere) to enhance fastidious bacterial growth (non-CO_2 incubators are not effective). This equipment can be expensive and is beyond the routine needs of most veterinary practices.

The supplies used in clinical microbiology are often disposable, and agars are labeled with expiration dates. One must maintain quality control over the laboratory, because expired agars, culturettes, and so on can cause erroneous results. To prevent contamination and disease spread, technicians should be knowledgeable about what debris can be disposed of in the clinic trash and what needs to be decontaminated or sterilized before disposal.

Culture Media

The medium used for a particular culture is dependent on the sample being tested and the needs of the pathogens expected to be identified, given the anatomic site and the patient species. Obtaining details of the patient's signalment and a brief history is necessary for selection of the appropriate medium for the culture. Isolation of pathogens from samples collected from anatomic sites that have significant indigenous flora, such as the GI tract, relies on selective media that will inhibit the growth of most organisms and **enrichment media** that will inhibit the growth of some organisms while promoting the growth of likely pathogens.

Culture media can be liquid broth, solid agar plates, tubes (liquid), or tube slants (solids). For initial isolation of organisms, solid agar plates are typically used, because they allow isolation of individual bacteria. Broth cultures started directly from patient samples usually contain a mixed bacterial population, which must be subcultured onto agar plates one or more times before identification or susceptibility testing is performed. Tests performed on mixed cultures (two or more types of bacteria mixed) will give erroneous results interfering with clinical diagnosis; it is important to work from pure cultures derived from individual bacterial colonies.

Most laboratories use a combination of a nutrient-rich medium, such as trypticase soy agar plates with 5% blood added (blood agar plate), which will allow the growth of most bacteria, and a **selective medium**, such as MacConkey agar plates, which will allow the growth of gram-negative enteric organisms such as *Escherichia coli* while inhibiting gram-positive organisms. Many media options are commercially available for culture as ready-to-use prepared media or dehydrated media to be reconstituted and prepared as needed (see Table 14.4). For the small laboratory, it is generally more efficient and cost effective to purchase prepared media that include quality control measures.

Isolates requiring definitive identification can be subcultured on agar slants to prevent breakage and shipped out to reference laboratories. Swabs also work well for shipping isolates. A key challenge for the practitioner is deciding when cultures should be submitted to an outside laboratory.

Enrichment, Selective, and Differential Media

Enrichment media enhance the recovery of organisms that are difficult to grow or occur in low numbers in the presence of indigenous flora. Selective media prevent the growth of some types of organisms while facilitating isolation of organisms from mixed cultures. MacConkey agar is an example of a selective medium with bile salts to inhibit the growth of some bacteria, containing an indicator that allows for identification/differentiation between organisms regarded as lactose positive and lactose negative (Fig. 14.5). Some media serve as both enrichment and selective media such as selenite broth and tetrathionate broth, both of which are used to enhance the growth of *Salmonella*, which (unlike many enteric bacteria) can grow in both media. These media inhibit the growth of organisms that cannot grow in the presence of sulfur compounds. **Differential media** (i.e., blood-based agar [BBA]) contain ingredients/chemicals that distinguish whether or not microbial specimens possess a specific biochemical process, allowing the user to differentiate among various organisms. BBA allows determination of whether the microbe can break down erythrocytes. Table 14.4 lists examples of different media.

Inoculation of Media

Most microbiological culture work is performed by using Petri dishes containing solid agar that includes a specific medium. Before use, quality control of all media should be done by using known organisms to confirm that the media work properly, are free of contamination, and that contamination is prevented when media and patient samples are handled. Biochemical reactions are tested by using differential media in tubes containing agar or broth. With a permanent marker, the culture plate (not the lid) should be labeled with the date, the patient identifier, and the sample. In diagnostic laboratories, each sample is given a unique identifying number (accession number), allowing the culture to be followed from start to finish and to track results.

Examples of inoculation of plate and tube media are shown in Figs. 14.6–14.9. When plate media are inoculated, the sample should be aseptically placed in the first quadrant of the plate. Then the plate should be struck for isolation by passing the loop two or three times over the primary quadrant containing the sample without piercing the media. This is repeated in the second, third, and fourth quadrants until all four quadrants are inoculated (see Fig. 14.6). If using a metal loop, sterilize between quadrants or use sterile plastic loops.

Tube media may or may not have a slant. The slant is formed by tilting the tube while the medium is in molten form and leaving it in this position until it solidifies. A slant inoculation is formed by carefully streaking the surface of the slanted agar without breaking. Motility media are inoculated by using an inoculating needle to stab the butt of the tube and carefully withdrawing the needle along the stab line (see Figs. 14.7 and 14.8).

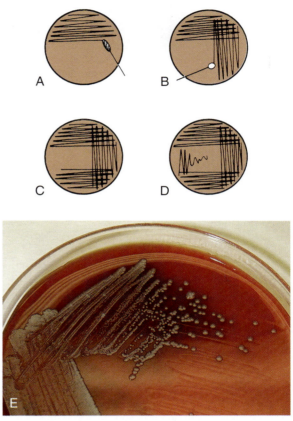

• **Fig. 14.6** Inoculation procedure for agar plate media and streaking method for isolation of bacterial colonies. (A) Inoculate with swab, covering one-fourth to one-third of the plate. (B) Streak lightly, overlapping the previous area. (C) Flame loop, allowing to cool, and streak next area. (D) Repeat as in C. (E) Well-isolated colonies.

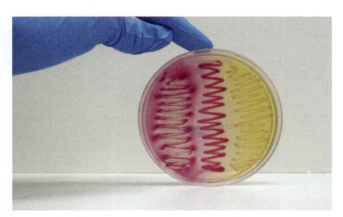

• **Fig. 14.5** MacConkey agar plate inoculated with lactose-positive *Escherichia coli* with bile salt precipitation on the far left *(pink with hazy precipitate)*, lactose-positive *E. coli* in the middle *(pink)*, and lactose-negative *Proteus mirabilis* on the far right.

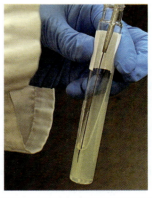

• **Fig. 14.7** The inoculation procedure for agar tube media may be done by stab maneuver. The needle is stabbed into the agar, then withdrawn and agar loosely capped before incubation.

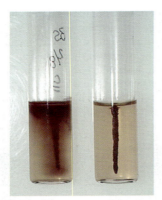

• **Fig. 14.8** Inoculation procedure and results for motility media. (A) To inoculate motility test medium, the inoculation needle is stabbed into the medium and is withdrawn along the same tract. (B) Motile bacterial growth in the left tube and nonmotile growth in the right tube.

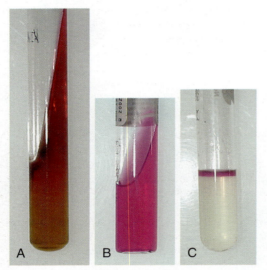

• **Fig. 14.9** (A) Alkaline slant and acid butt reaction (K/A) in triple sugar iron (TSI). (B) Positive urease reaction after slant inoculation. (C) Positive indole test.

Incubation Conditions

Plates must be incubated in an inverted position (lid down) to prevent moisture from collecting on the lid, dripping onto the agar surface to contaminate culture, or mixing the bacteria on the plate surface. After inoculation, plates and biochemical tests should be incubated overnight at 35°C (95°F) to 37.5°C (99.5°F) or, for fastidious organisms, in the presence of 5% CO_2. For some susceptibility tests, the length of the incubation time is critical (see the section "Antimicrobial Susceptibility Testing"). Screwcaps for tube media should be left loose during incubation for air exchange.

It is important to inspect plates at least once daily, noting any findings. If no bacteria grow from a specimen in which organisms were observed on direct microscopy, the plates should be held and examined for 3 days before reporting "no growth." Cultures from patients receiving antimicrobial therapeutics may be held for an additional period of 2 days to allow bacteria weakened by the drugs to grow. It is usually unnecessary to hold cultures beyond this time, and culture of slow-growing organisms should not be attempted in a small laboratory, because specialized media are required for both isolation and identification. Contamination is problematic for cultures held for long periods due to slow growth.

Routine Culture Systems

There are several commercially available culture systems designed for ease of aseptic collection and culture of samples for diagnostic purposes. Some are complete kits that allow for quick diagnosis, while others allow for collection before sending to commercial laboratories (Hardy Diagnostics, Thermo-Fisher Scientific, and Rapid-Bac). Universities housing veterinary schools often have diagnostic reference laboratories that offer testing services.

Primary Isolation Media

Selection of media for initial inoculation of samples depends on the site of collection. A sample should be plated initially on blood agar and/or MacConkey agar plate. For anaerobic cultures, an additional blood agar plate can be inoculated and incubated in an anaerobe jar using a commercially available system, such as the one by Anaerobe Systems, Inc. Suspect anaerobes can be subcultured to plates to be aerobically and anaerobically incubated before evaluation. Comparisons are made of the plate results; while identification and susceptibility testing of anaerobes are possible, it is generally not cost effective for a small laboratory to perform these tests.

In some practices, enriching the growth of fastidious organisms is done by using a trypticase soy or a brain-heart infusion broth tube; both media support the growth of fastidious organisms. Unfortunately, broth enrichment cultures can be easily contaminated, and care must be exercised in determining the significance of organisms that grow only on the enriched culture. Examples of primary isolation media may be found in Table 14.4.

Preliminary Evaluation of Cultures

Evaluating a culture accurately after 24–48 hours of incubation is important for accurate and timely documentation of the culture results. The first step in this process occurs before plating, when the technician evaluates the appropriateness and quality of the sample, deciding which media to inoculate and whether indigenous flora are likely to be present. Culture of samples collected from sites that are normally sterile are the simplest to evaluate because, in most cases, only one or two organisms or colony types are present on the culture plates. Evaluation of cultures collected from sites where indigenous flora are present such as skin, the GI tract, the external genitalia, and the respiratory tract may be difficult to read due to mixed cultures (see Table 14.1). It is not necessary to identify every organism present in cultures from sites where indigenous flora are likely and can be distracting and misleading to the reviewer; only the most prevalent should be identified.

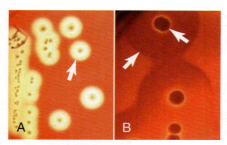

• **Fig. 14.10** Patterns of hemolysis observed in blood agar plates. (A) Complete hemolysis (also named beta-hemolysis if the organism is *Streptococcus*). (B) Double-zone hemolysis as produced by *Staphylococcus intermedius*.

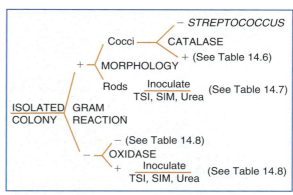

• **Fig. 14.12** Flow chart for bacterial identification procedure.

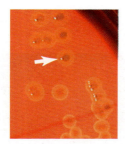

• **Fig. 14.11** Alpha-hemolysis produced by some strains of *Streptococcus*.

After overnight incubation of the plates, they should be visually inspected, taking care not to contaminate the sample. The technician should determine the number of different organisms present, which of those organisms are predominant, the number of colonies of each organism present, the appearance of the colonies, and how the organisms affect surrounding media. Changes to the media can include **hemolysis** (clearing of media around the colony), a possible indication of virulence (Figs. 14.10 and 14.11).

Bacteria are microscopically identified by their cell wall structure, shape, and growth characteristics. It is important to note the amount of time an organism took to grow and the number of quadrants on which it is present. The level of growth on the blood agar plate can indicate the degree of infection. A common tool for relative quantification of the number of organisms present in a culture is noting the number of quadrants in which the organism grew. The scale typically used is 1+ to 4+, where 4+ indicates that the organism grew on the entire plate, compared with 1+, which indicates that the organism grew only in the primary or first quadrant of the plate.

The following is a comparison of how one might interpret multiple or singular colonies on a plate. *Pseudomonas aeruginosa* is a virulent pathogen that tends to be resistant to several classes of antimicrobial agents, but it can also be present in feces as indigenous flora. Hence a single colony of *P. aeruginosa* in a urine sample collected by cystocentesis is important to note and should be potentially tested for susceptibility to antimicrobial drugs, whereas a single colony found in fecal sample is not important.

New technicians will find it necessary to perform biochemical tests to adequately identify organisms. With experience, it becomes easier for the technician to recognize pathogens on the basis of their growth characteristics and to evaluate cultures. However, even experienced technicians find it helpful to routinely perform some biochemical tests for bacterial identification and should identify a "go-to" reference manual to keep at the bench.

Recording, Interpreting, and Reporting Results

It is important to record all observations regarding a culture (e.g., biochemical and susceptibility tests) as these results become part of the patient's medical record and legal documents to be maintained. In general, a worksheet that follows a consistent format for reporting cultures is helpful, making it easier for anyone in the laboratory or the practice to evaluate a culture that is in progress and decrease reliance on one technician. This worksheet should list collection sites and briefly summarize initial findings and daily observations until the culture is complete. Each entry should be initialed/dated by the person performing the observations to avoid miscommunication.

Identification Procedures

After preliminary evaluation, the next step is to isolate and identify significant organisms. If isolated colonies are present on initial culture plates, it is possible to work directly from these plates. It is helpful to subculture organisms to a new blood agar plate for further workup of isolates. The subsequent steps are documented in flow charts based on colony morphology and Gram stain reaction results (Fig. 14.12).

Biochemical Tests for Identification

Catalase Test

The **catalase** test is based on the ability of bacteria to convert 3% hydrogen peroxide to water and oxygen gas and tests for the presence of the enzyme catalase and differentiates between staphylococcus (Cat+) and streptococcus (Cat−). To perform this test, a sample of an isolated colony is placed on a glass slide by using an inoculating loop or sterile wooden stick; then a small drop of hydrogen peroxide is placed on the bacteria and the colony observed. Formation of bubbles indicates a positive test (*Staphylococcus*) (Fig. 14.13); absence of bubbles indicates a negative test (*Streptococcus*).

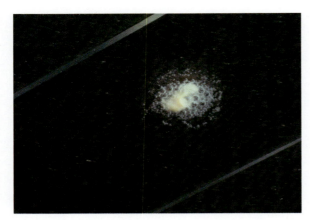

• **Fig. 14.13** Positive catalase test. Catalase produces bubbles in the presence of hydrogen peroxide for a positive result.

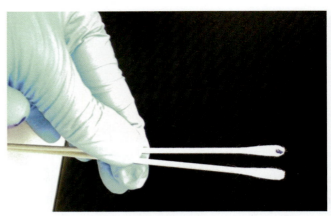

• **Fig. 14.14** Oxidase test. Oxidase reagent turns blue in the presence of bacteria with cytochrome oxidase for a positive result.

> **TECHNICIAN NOTE**
>
> Hydrogen peroxide degrades over time, so it is best to put a small amount in a properly labeled (i.e., name and expiration date) brown glass dropper bottle and to store it in the refrigerator. Hydrogen peroxide should be tested periodically with a known *Staphylococcus* isolate to confirm that it is active.

Oxidase Test

This test is used to identify bacteria containing the respiratory enzyme **cytochrome oxidase** and is commercially available in several different types. It is commonly used to differentiate gram-negative bacteria. A colony is picked from a blood agar plate and tested with the **oxidase** reagent using a wood or plastic loop, as iron from inoculating loops or needles can give a false-positive result. A positive test is indicated by the formation of blue coloration; a negative test result is colorless and occurs in less than 30 seconds. Some organisms, such as *Pasteurella*, may take up to a minute for positive results (Fig. 14.14).

Presumptive Identification

Once the Gram stain reaction and morphology have been determined and subsequent preliminary tests, such as oxidase and catalase tests, have been performed, an organism can be grouped and subjected to appropriate differential tests (see Fig. 14.12).

Gram-positive cocci are categorized by catalase-negative (*Streptococcus* and *Enterococcus*) or catalase-positive (*Staphylococcus* and *Micrococcus*) organisms. Streptococci are differentiated by the pattern of hemolysis that they produce (see Figs. 14.10 and 14.11). Although alpha-hemolytic *Streptococcus* isolates are generally considered to be normal flora except when seen in sterile anatomic site, beta-hemolytic streptococci are generally considered pathogenic. Beta-hemolytic streptococci, such as *Streptococcus agalactiae*, are further differentiated by the ability to produce a synergistic hemolysis with *Staphylococcus aureus* in the CAMP test (Fig. 14.15). Enterococci were previously categorized as fecal alpha-hemolytic streptococci. They typically grow in the presence of bile and salt and are only considered pathogenic when found on a normally sterile site, such as the urinary bladder, manifesting as a urinary tract infection. Unlike alpha-hemolytic streptococci, they are positive for bile esculin and can grow in the presence of 6.5% sodium chloride.

Catalase-positive, gram-positive cocci include *Staphylococcus* and *Micrococcus* isolates. *Micrococcus* is usually nonpathogenic, oxidase positive, and a weakened to non-glucose fermentor on

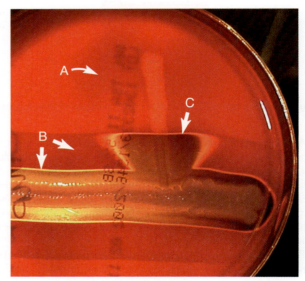

• **Fig. 14.15** Cyclic adenosine monophosphate (cAMP) test for *Streptococcus agalactiae*. The isolate (A) to be tested is inoculated perpendicular to a stock strain of double-zone hemolytic *Staphylococcus* (B), producing a synergistic triangle of hemolysis (C) as a positive cAMP test result.

triple sugar iron (TSI) slants. *Staphylococcus* isolates are differentiated on the basis of their production of **coagulase**. Coagulase converts fibrinogen in rabbit plasma to fibrin and has historically been a measure of virulence. Coagulase-negative staphylococci are typically indigenous flora and often are considered nonpathogenic unless they are accidentally transferred to normally sterile sites during medical procedures (hip replacement and intravenous catheter placement) to become a nosocomial infection.

> **TECHNICIAN NOTE**
>
> *Staphylococcus schleiferi* subsp. *schleiferi* is associated with pyoderma and otitis and can present as antibiotic resistant.

Small gram-positive rods (i.e., bacilli) are differentiated by catalase activity, colony morphology, and results when exposed to TSI slants, urea agar, and motility testing. Gram-positive branching rods should be tested for catalase production and stained with acid-fast stain to differentiate between *Mycobacterium* spp. or *Nocardia* species.

Gram-negative organisms are subgrouped according to their ability to produce oxidase. Oxidase-negative, gram-negative bacteria are typically members of the family Enterobacteriaceae, also identified by using biochemical tests and most commercial identification systems. Oxidase-positive, gram-negative organisms of veterinary importance can be differentiated by using colony morphology, TSI slants, urea agar, and motility testing. Weakly oxidase-positive organisms (*Pasteurella* spp.) can be difficult to identify.

Definitive Identification

Small laboratories are not set up for definitive identification as this requires extensive testing and can be labor intensive; confirmatory testing needs referral to commercial laboratories for sequencing.

Commercial Identification Kits

The development of commercially available identification kits has simplified the identification of isolates by small, in-house laboratories. Most kits consist of a series of biochemical tests within a single unit to be inoculated. Once inoculated with an isolated organism (i.e.,"isolate"), incubation is carried out for a time period under specific conditions. Results are recorded and compared with a database of biochemical test results from known bacteria to determine the isolate identity.

These kits can be an accurate, cost-effective alternative to pre-pared media or "send-outs," owing to their long shelf life, their requirement of minimal storage space, and for providing results that are easy to interpret. The manufacturer's directions and expiration dates should be strictly adhered to, because failure to do so can lead to inaccurate identification and treatment. It is important to remember that such commercial kits are designed for humans and may not have an adequate database for veterinary isolates. Oxidase-positive, gram-negative bacteria; oxidase-negative, gram-negative enteric bacteria; and catalase-positive, gram-positive rods can be identified via commercial kits.

Special Culture Procedures

Fecal Culture

Feces are cultured to identify diarrhea-causing pathogens, with the most common being *Salmonella*, *Campylobacter jejuni*, *C. perfringens*, and *C. difficile*. In the case of *C. perfringens* and *C. difficile*, disease is caused by *toxins* produced by bacteria, not the presence of *organisms*. Enzyme-linked immunosorbent assay (ELISA) is typically used to detect the presence of such toxins. Additional causes of diarrhea include *Yersinia enterocolitica*, *M. avium* subsp. *paratuberculosis*, and *Lawsonia intracellularis*. Isolation of pathogens from fecal material requires enrichment and/or selective media for identification. *Salmonella* is identified through overnight incubation in selenite or tetrathionate broth, after which the broth enrichment cultures are subcultured onto Hektoen enteric agar or MacConkey agar and incubated overnight at 35°C (95°F). Subsequently, they are examined for the presence of suspect colonies, which are confirmed using biochemical tests including TSI agar slants, lysine iron agar slants, urease agar, and indole test media. Other media, such as xylose tergitol agar, can also be employed to recover *Salmonella*. *C. jejuni* can be difficult to culture, requiring an oxygen-reduced environment for growth and possibly a specialized *Campylobacter* medium incorporating an antimicrobial agent to reduce the growth of other organisms. *Campylobacter*

cultures are typically incubated at higher temperatures, such as 42°C (107.6°F), for 48–72 hours. Suspect *Campylobacter* colonies are gray, flat, and nonhemolytic, with an irregular edge, displaying gram-negative small, curved bacteria.

Blood Cultures

Blood culture media are inoculated immediately upon collection with care taken to avoid contamination, as a single organism can yield a positive culture result. Aerobic samples are typically vented by using a blood culture venting needle and should be incubated at 37°C (98.6°F) before being subcultured onto agar plates at least twice over a 10-day period. Blood cultures are typically held up to 14 days before a negative result is reported. Automated incubator systems alert the user when a bottle turns positive; owing to costs, these are not common in veterinary practices.

Quantified Urine Cultures

When urine is cultured, the number of organisms predicates the likelihood and severity of infection. The number of organisms present in a 1-mL urine sample can easily be quantified by using commercially available, disposable calibrated inoculating loops (available as 1-μL or 10-μL loops).

> ### TECHNICIAN NOTE
>
> Microscopic analysis of urine sediment should not be used as a substitute for culture in suspected urinary tract infections, because bacilli may be detected, but the cocci in the sample may be missed.

Samples are inoculated onto separate blood agar plates in a pattern that makes it easy to count the colonies (Fig. 14.16). Each plate should be labeled with the patient information and the dilution. The 1μL loop holds the equivalent of a 1:1000 dilution of urine (1000 μL of urine = 1 mL). In contrast, the 10-μL loop holds the equivalent of a 1:100 dilution of urine (1 mL of urine = 100 10-μL). To determine the number of bacteria present in each milliliter of urine, the number of colonies on the plate is multiplied by the dilution factor of the plate. For example, if 54 colonies of *E. coli* are present on the 1:1000 plate, this represents 54,000 *E. coli* per milliliter of urine (54 × 1000). By convention, this number would be reported as 54,000 colony-forming units (CFUs) of *E. coli* per milliliter of urine (54,000 CFU/mL). The term *CFU* is used to describe the number of bacterial colonies, because it is not possible to know whether more than a single bacterium formed the colony growing on the plate. If more colonies are present than can be counted or greater than 100 colonies are seen on the 1:1000 dilution plate, the culture is reported as "greater than 100,000 CFU/mL." The 1:1000 dilution plate should have approximately $\frac{1}{10}$ as many bacteria as the 1:100 dilution plate. If it does not, the technician should evaluate their technique.

MacConkey agar plate should also be inoculated and incubated for 24 hours at 37°C (98.6°F), because enteric gram-negative organisms preferring this agar commonly cause urinary tract infection and can be rapidly isolated and identified.

Milk

Milk culture, similarly to urine culture, must be quantified for bacteria. Plates are inoculated by using calibrated inoculation loops and are labeled accordingly (i.e., animal number and udder location = 101 = RF and RR; LF and LR). The most significant organisms to cause contagious mastitis are *S. aureus*, *S. agalactiae*,

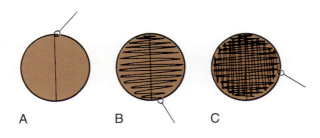

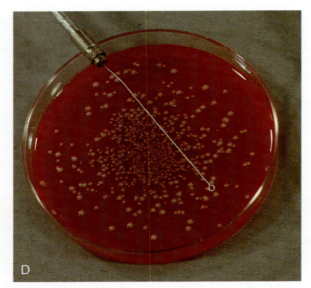

• **Fig. 14.16** Procedure for inoculating media for semiquantitative bacterial colony counts when culturing urine or milk. (A) Primary inoculation with calibrated loop. (B) Streak at right angles to primary inoculation. (C) Streak at right angles to previous streak. (D) Photo illustrates a plate with more than 100 colonies resulting from inoculation with a 1-μL loop.

and *Mycoplasma* species. Mastitis caused by environmental organisms, such as coliforms and alpha-hemolytic streptococci, also occur and should be quantified; this may be done to confirm positive CMT results.

Common Bacterial Species

Gram-Positive Cocci

Staphylococcus spp. are catalase-positive, gram-positive cocci normally inhabiting the skin and mucous membranes. *S. aureus* is a normal skin inhabitant of humans, cats, and large animals. *Staphylococcus pseudintermedius* (formerly *S. intermedius*) is a normal inhabitant of the skin of dogs. It should be noted that *S. intermedius* is still an appropriate name, and this organism is found in species other than dogs (birds, horses, etc.). For practical purposes, *S. pseudintermedius* and *S. intermedius* are identified by using common biochemical tests, with little clinical benefit in attempting definitive identification because they are not normally disease-causing pathogens.

Streptococcus spp. are catalase-negative, gram-positive cocci normally inhabiting the mouth and the skin, where they may cause infection or generalized infections, including septicemia. In rare cases, it is responsible for necrotizing fasciitis (i.e., flesh-eating disease).

Enterococcus spp. (previously called *group D streptococci*) are catalase-negative, gram-positive cocci that can grow in the presence of bile salts. Members of this genus are normal inhabitants

of the GI tract and are associated with opportunistic infections, particularly urinary tract infections.

Gram-Positive Rods

Bacillus spp. are ubiquitous gram-positive rods commonly found as culture contaminants, although some are associated with diseases such as mastitis. The most important member of this genus is *Bacillus anthracis*, the causative agent of anthrax; the organism should not be cultured due to ease of aerosolization and potential lethality to humans. It is also a select agent designated by the US government as an agent of biowarfare and is a reportable disease in humans and animals. Suspect samples should be sent to the appropriate diagnostic facility.

Corynebacterium spp. are pleomorphic in shape, cause a variety of diseases, and consist of many organisms, some of which are indigenous flora. *Corynebacterium pseudotuberculosis* is an important veterinary pathogen that causes caseous lymphadenitis in sheep and goats and abscesses and ulcerative lymphangitis in horses. Colonies of this organism are typically small with a dry, waxy appearance and take 48 hours for colony formation (1 mm in diameter).

Trueperella (*Arcanobacterium*) *pyogenes* was previously classified as a *Corynebacterium* and subsequently as *Actinomyces* before it was assigned to the genus *Arcanobacterium*. In 2011, this organism was reclassified as *Trueperella*, an opportunistic pathogen and common inhabitant of the skin and mucous membranes of cattle and other ruminants. It is catalase negative and produces a small hemolytic colony (<1 mm in diameter) after 48 hours of culture.

Erysipelothrix rhusiopathiae causes disease in swine, turkeys, and marine mammals. This small, catalase-negative rod forms pinpoint colonies with partial hemolysis on blood agar plates and produces hydrogen sulfide along the stab line when inoculated into TSI agar. It is difficult to differentiate from alpha-hemolytic streptococci and should be sent for confirmation to a reference laboratory.

Listeria monocytogenes is a cause of foodborne illness and a causative agent of listeriosis in ruminants. A small catalase-positive rod, it is motile at room temperature and can cause septicemia in neonatal animals, abortion, and encephalitis. Isolation of this organism can be difficult because of its zoonotic potential; utilize a reference laboratory for safety reasons.

Rhodococcus equi is a soil-borne, aerobic, nonmotile, cyclic adenosine monophosphate (cAMP)–positive, gram-positive rod that causes pneumonia in foals and, rarely, disseminated disease in adult horses.

Gram-Negative Bacteria

Gram-negative bacteria are divided based on production of cytochrome oxidase and ability to grow on MacConkey agar. Initially, the oxidase test is performed when these organisms are identified. Members of the family *Enterobacteriaceae*, which includes *E. coli*, are oxidase negative. Coliforms (*E. coli*, *Klebsiella*, *Enterobacter*) are normal inhabitants of the GI tract and frequently are opportunistic pathogens causing urinary tract and wound infections, enteritis, and septicemia in neonatal animals. These organisms may be present in infections of the respiratory tract and reproductive tract and vary in their susceptibility to antimicrobial drugs. If they are isolated, susceptibility testing should be conducted.

Salmonella causes diarrhea and septicemia in a variety of animal species and is commonly isolated from reptiles and amphibian feces. A zoonotic organism and an agent of nosocomial infections, it is important to practice good hand hygiene and to disinfect equipment, cages, and stalls in suspected cases. Clients owning reptile and amphibian species as pets should be educated to prevent zoonotic infection.

> ### TECHNICIAN NOTE
>
> *Proteus* spp. can readily swarm a plate, overwhelming other, slow-growing organisms unless selective media is used. Urinary tract infections and opportunistic infections of wounds, skin, and ears are associated with this bacterium.

Other enteric organisms (*Serratia, Citrobacter, Edwardsiella, Hafnia*) are less commonly isolated but can present as opportunists and as indigenous flora with a potential for antimicrobial resistance.

Aeromonas is frequently found as an infection in aquatic animals (fish and amphibians) and occasionally septicemia in mammals. These oxidase-positive, gram-negative rods are commonly found in soil and water.

Actinobacillus spp. are oxidase-positive, small, gram-negative rods that typically grow on MacConkey agar and may be present as normal respiratory flora in adult horses. Similar to *Pasteurella*, it often isolates from foals with septicemia or joint infection and is part of the indigenous flora of the mouth and upper respiratory tract. Visualized as oxidase-positive, short, fat rods (i.e., *coccobacilli*), the organism ferments glucose, although not well, on TSI agar slants and often do not grow on MacConkey agar. *Pasteurella multocida*, one of the most isolated members of this genus, is associated with cat bites, feline abscesses, and infection in most other mammals. Many animals carry *P. multocida*, yet strains are not typically passed between species; as a zoonotic disease, *P. multocida* can cause rapidly progressing cellulitis in humans bitten by cats. For this reason, it is imperative that medical attention be sought without delay if bitten by a cat to determine its rabies vaccination status and to follow the legal requirements for reporting animal bites to appropriate regulatory officials.

> ### TECHNICIAN NOTE
>
> Clients disclosing suffering from cat bites should be advised to seek medical attention. Humans should never be treated by veterinary staff.

Haemophilus spp. are oxidase-positive, small coccobacilli, commonly inhabiting the oronasal mucosa and are important respiratory pathogens. These organisms may be difficult to cultivate as they require enriched media such as lysed blood cells and additional CO_2 for growth. They can grow as satellite colonies around colonies of *Staphylococcus* spp. and may be seen in initial culture sample cultures from the respiratory tract. They may fail to grow when subcultured without enriched conditions, and are best left to reference laboratories for identification.

Pseudomonas spp. are oxidase-positive rods commonly found in soil and water that are generally opportunistic yet significant pathogens due to resistance to several antimicrobial agents. When cultured, they are often hemolytic, secreting a green pigment (*pyocyanin*) into the media surrounding the colonies, appearing metallic on blood agar plates and lactose negative on MacConkey agar.

Bordetella spp. are small, oxidase-positive coccobacilli that cause infection of the respiratory and reproductive tract. They test urease positive within 4 hours and can be associated with reproductive failure and abortion. *B. bronchiseptica* is a causative agent of canine tracheobronchitis (e.g., "kennel cough"), a disease prevented through vaccination.

Brucella spp. are small, oxidase-positive coccobacilli that test urease positive within 10 minutes and are associated with abortion and reproductive failure (i.e., brucellosis). They typically grow over several days, requiring increased atmospheric CO_2. Some are select agents, and culturing is best left to reference laboratories with appropriate safety equipment to prevent spread.

Acid-Fast Bacteria

Mycobacterium spp. have cell walls that include mycolic acid, which does not retain Gram stain but stain positively with carbol fuchsin. These are typically slow-growing organisms, sometimes taking weeks to grow sufficiently before colonies are seen. Their culture is best left to reference laboratories for safety reasons (especially *M. tuberculosis*); however, staining specimens, such as fluids, impression smears, and feces, can aid in making a presumptive diagnosis of mycobacterial infection while awaiting confirmation. It is important to evaluate staining technique by simultaneously staining a control slide and the sample being tested.

Colonies of *Nocardia* spp. have the appearance of white chalk. Gram staining reveals the presence of long, branching, gram-positive rods that are partially acid fast when stained with the Kinyoun acid-fast staining procedure, with rods having a "beaded" appearance. They may be described as "rough" or "dry," and take up to 5 days to grow under standard culture conditions.

> ### TECHNICIAN NOTE
>
> Diseases suspected of being zoonotic should not be cultured in-house; instead, specimens should be sent to a reference laboratory for confirmatory testing.

Anaerobes

Many important anaerobic pathogens have been identified; however, the culture of obligate anaerobes should be left to reference laboratories with specialized equipment and media. Anaerobic pathogens can be gram-negative or -positive rods or cocci and are part of the indigenous flora of the GI tract, but they may be found in abscesses or mixed infections. Some of the common gram-negative anaerobic rods are members of the genera *Bacteroides, Dichelobacter, Fusobacterium, Porphyromonas,* and *Prevotella*. Among the anaerobic gram-positive cocci, *Peptostreptococcus* is the most common genus. The most important anaerobic gram-positive rods are of the *Clostridium* spp.; those of veterinary significance can be detected in tissues using serologic techniques, but identification is best left to reference laboratories. The two organisms of greatest importance for a small laboratory are *C. perfringens* and *C. difficile*, both indigenous flora of the GI tract, which may be cultured using anaerobic techniques to diagnose specific toxins.

Spirochetes and Curved Bacteria

Several significant veterinary pathogens are spirochetes (i.e., curved bacteria). These organisms are difficult to culture and are potentially zoonotic; using a reference laboratory for their identification is advised. Diagnosis includes serologic or molecular testing rather than culture. The most important spirochetes are *Leptospira* spp., *Borrelia burgdorferi, Brachyspira hyodysenteriae,* and *Campylobacter* spp. *Leptospira* spp. are shed in the urine of affected animals and cause febrile illness, renal disease, abortion, and infertility. *B. burgdorferi* is the causative agent of Lyme disease and arthritis and associated lameness in dogs. *B. hyodysenteriae* causes diarrhea and dysentery in pigs and typically is diagnosed by identification of large spirochetes in gram-stained, direct smears made from necropsy-provided, colonic mucosa. *Campylobacter* spp. may also cause gastroenteritis and abortion in bovines.

> ### TECHNICIAN NOTE
>
> Spirochetes represent several significant and zoonotic veterinary pathogens; therefore samples are sent to reference laboratories.

Mycoplasma

Mycoplasma spp. lack cell walls and therefore are not visible on Gram staining; they are difficult to culture and require specialized transport media. They are associated with mucous membranes and can cause urinary tract infections in dogs and cats; joint and respiratory infections in cattle, pigs, and sheep; and mastitis in cattle. Currently, this bacterial species can be detected by ELISA and polymerase chain reaction (PCR) testing; samples should be sent to a reference laboratory for analysis.

Obligate Intracellular Organisms

Obligate intracellular bacteria will not grow on standard culture media and, similar to viruses, they require cultured animal cells to grow. Infections with these organisms are often diagnosed using serologic or molecular testing. Important genera include *Anaplasma*, *Chlamydia*, *Chlamydophila*, *Coxiella*, *Ehrlichia*, *Rickettsia*, and *Neorickettsia*; many are causative agents of tickborne diseases.

Methods of Antimicrobial Susceptibility Testing

Antimicrobial agents include both antibiotics and synthetic agents that inhibit microbial growth. Antimicrobial susceptibility testing is performed to assist in selection of appropriate antimicrobial drugs to treat bacterial infections (see Case Presentation 14.1). Several tests are available to determine bacterial antimicrobial susceptibility or resistance. They are highly standardized to be performed in accordance with the guidelines of the US Food and Drug Administration (FDA) and the CLSI (formerly National Committee for Clinical Laboratory Standards [NCCLS]). It is important to use the appropriate concentrations of bacteria during testing, because using too many bacteria can lead to the erroneous conclusion of drug resistance when this is not the case. Microbiology laboratories use the McFarland concentration standards to estimate bacterial numbers, with the 0.5 McFarland standards used in susceptibility testing, equivalent to approximately 1.5×10^8 bacteria per milliliter of diluent.

Broth Dilution or Microbroth Dilution

This method of susceptibility testing uses dilution of antimicrobial agents in liquid culture (broth) to determine the lowest amount of antimicrobial to inhibit growth of the bacterium being tested in a pure sample or culture. Commercial systems are available for this type of testing, and manufacturer's instructions should be followed carefully. For microbroth dilution methods, cultures are adjusted to a final concentration of 1×10^5 bacteria per milliliter. For each day tests, a series of twofold dilutions of antimicrobial agent encompassing a clinically relevant range of concentrations is prepared. After inoculation, the dilutions are incubated overnight at 37°C (98.6°F), and the MIC is then determined (Fig. 14.17A and B).

CASE PRESENTATION 14.1

Urinary Tract Infection

History

Bailey, a 6-year-old female mixed-breed dog, was presented for inappropriate urination. The owner reported that during the previous week, Bailey had several "accidents" in the house and seemed to need to go outside more frequently. After she was housetrained as a puppy, Bailey had never urinated indoors until recently. The owner also reported that when cleaning up the urine from the "accidents," the urine smelled bad. Physical examination revealed no abnormalities, although Bailey tensed when abdominal palpation was attempted; it was not possible to do a thorough abdominal examination. Acute cystitis with a possible bacterial infection was suspected, and urine was collected via cystocentesis for urinalysis, culture, and sensitivity testing.

Laboratory Results

The dog's urine was cloudy, and urinalysis indicated the presence of leukocytes, erythrocytes, and glucose. Because beta-lactam antibiotics concentrate in urine and are effective against most common organisms associated with urinary tract infection (UTI), the attending veterinarian prescribed amoxicillin with clavulanate for 10 days while awaiting culture results. Three days later, culture results showed *Enterobacter cloacae* in the urine sample at greater than 100,000 CFUs/mL. The minimum inhibitory concentrations (MICs) of the antibiotics tested were as follows: amoxicillin with clavulanate, >32 µg/mL; ampicillin, >16 µg/mL; ceftiofur, 1 µg/mL; cephalexin, >16 µg/mL; enrofloxacin, <0.5 µg/mL; tetracycline, <2 µg/mL; and trimethoprim with sulfonamide, <0.5 µg/mL. Based on of the evaluation of the MIC of each drug, the organism was considered resistant to beta-lactam antibiotics (amoxicillin with clavulanate, ampicillin, ceftiofur, and cephalexin but was considered susceptible to enrofloxacin, tetracycline, and trimethoprim with sulfonamide.

Outcome

The veterinarian decided, based on results, to prescribe enrofloxacin, and directed the owner to discontinue amoxicillin with clavulanate and start the new antibiotic instead. This change causes Bailey's UTI to resolve quickly. Additional testing demonstrated diabetes mellitus, which may have predisposed Bailey to the UTI and, with careful management of her diabetes, there were no recurrences.

Conclusion

This case illustrates the value of bacterial culture and sensitivity testing in selecting the appropriate antimicrobial treatment for patients with bacterial infections. Without the data provided by these tests, Bailey's infection probably would not have been eliminated. By using the data to guide treatment, the attending veterinarian was able to eliminate Bailey's UTI, relieving her discomfort and decreasing the likelihood of complications from this infection.

Disk Diffusion (Kirby-Bauer Method)

The disk diffusion method uses bacterial growth in the presence of antibiotic-saturated paper disks on agar plates to determine susceptibility of organism to an antimicrobial agent. Mueller-Hinton agar plates are inoculated with a solution of the bacterium diluted to be equivalent to the McFarland 0.5 standard, and a paper disk (impregnated with the antimicrobial agent at a specific concentration) is placed on the surface of the inoculated plate before incubating for 18–24 hours at 37°C (98.6°F). Some organisms require a full 24 hours of incubation. If the bacterium is inhibited by the antimicrobial agent, a clear zone (i.e., zone of inhibition) will be present around the paper disk, where the bacterium cannot survive (see Fig. 14.17C and D; Procedure 14.4). The diameter of

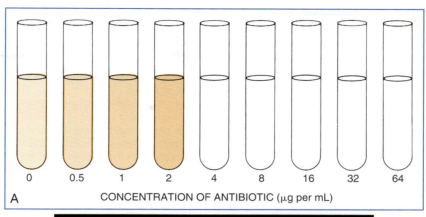

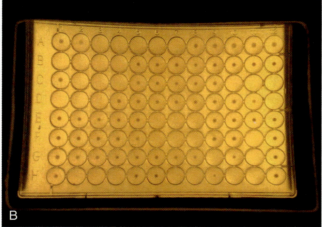

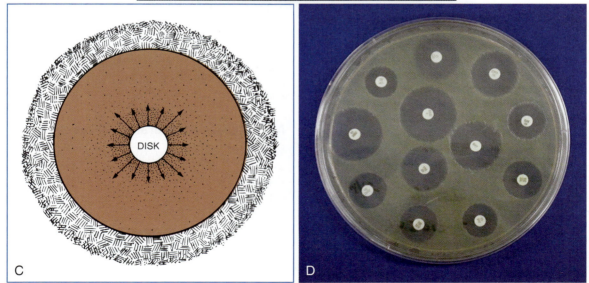

• **Fig. 14.17** Antimicrobial susceptibility testing. (A) Broth dilution susceptibility test. The organism grew in broth containing antibiotic in the amounts of 0.5, 1, and 2 µg/mL, but growth was inhibited in the tube containing 4 µg/mL. Therefore the minimum inhibitory concentration (MIC) is 4 µg/mL. (B) Picture of broth dilution test results using a 96-well plate format; wells A1 through A7 contain a twofold dilution series consisting of 0.25, 0.5, 1, 2, 4, 8, and 16 µg/mL of ampicillin. Growth was noted in wells 1 and 2 but not in well 3, so the MIC is 1 µg/mL. (C) As antibiotic diffuses from the disk, the concentration of antibiotic is highest near the disk and is logarithmically diluted as it diffuses radially into a larger area. At some point, the antibiotic is diluted to less than the MIC for the test organism; this allows the organism to grow (D).

PROCEDURE 14.4

Basic Protocol for Performing Disk Diffusion Testing

1. Using a sterile swab, pick three to five isolated colonies that are less than 48 hours old and are cultured on a tryptic soy agar plate supplemented with 5% sheep's blood (blood agar plate).
2. Mix the bacterial colonies in tryptic soy broth until a concentration equivalent to a 0.5 McFarland concentration standard is achieved.
3. Within 15 minutes of adjusting the bacterial suspension to the appropriate concentration, dip a sterile swab into the solution and rotate the swab against the tube wall to remove excess liquid from the swab.
4. Inoculate the dry surface of a Mueller-Hinton agar plate, streaking the swab over the entire surface. Repeat the streaking process two more times, rotating the plate 60 degrees each time.
5. Disks should be placed on the agar surface using a commercially available dispenser or sterile forceps. Gently press up to 12 disks (no more than 9 for *Streptococcus*) to ensure their adherence to the agar surface.
6. Invert the plate and place in an incubator for 18–24 hours at 37°C (98.6°F). Some organisms, including staphylococci, require a full 24 hours of incubation.
7. Remove the plate from the incubator; measure the zones of inhibition by using a ruler or a caliper (see Fig. 14.18D).
8. Compare the diameter with the guidelines (breakpoints) established in CLSI M31-A3.

the zone is measured by using a caliper or ruler. This value is then compared with the breakpoints for that drug to determine whether the organism is susceptible or resistant or somewhere in-between (intermediate).

TECHNICIAN NOTE

Several methods are available for determining susceptibility or resistance of bacteria to antimicrobial drugs. Broth dilution (microbroth dilution) is used to determine the MIC of various antimicrobials. Disk diffusion (Kirby-Bauer method) is used to determine susceptibility based on zones of inhibition.

Fungal Culture (Mycology)

Safety

It is best to perform fungal cultures in a biological safety hood to protect workers who are handling samples and cultures. The only fungal cultures commonly performed in a veterinary practice are **dermatophyte** cultures, yet it is common for the veterinarian to ship inoculated media to a diagnostic laboratory for fungal identification, especially highly infectious dimorphic fungi such as *Coccidioides immitis*, *Histoplasma capsulatum*, and *Blastomyces dermatididis*, all occurring as **yeasts** in veterinary patients. The more infectious mycelial or hyphal form of the fungus grows at room temperature and samples from patients suspected of harboring such infections should never be cultured but rather, submitted to a diagnostic laboratory, with the risk clearly stated on the submission form as an alert.

Standard Dermatophyte Culture

Specimen Collection and Media Inoculation

Dermatophytes are fungi that invade hair, nails, and the superficial layers of the skin and often are detected with a Wood lamp as 75%

of dermatophytes will fluoresce under long-wavelength ultraviolet light. To culture dermatophytes, hair should be gently plucked or collected by brushing the lesion or the patient's haircoat with a new toothbrush. Nails can be collected by using sterilized nail clippers. Gently push plucked hairs or nails into the surface of the agar to inoculate dermatophyte test medium (DTM), Sabouraud dextrose agar (SDA), or DTM slant before incubating (Fig. 14.18).

TECHNICIAN NOTE

Never attempt to culture suspected dimorphic fungi in-house; submit it to a reference laboratory in a clearly marked container to reduce accidental exposure. Ensure that there are three layers of protection between the sample and the courier.

These media are commercially available in a variety of forms, including a system containing both media and DTM slants (see Fig. 14.18A). This plate should be labeled with patient information and the date of sample collection, placed in a loosely sealed plastic bag, and incubated at room temperature for up to 3 weeks. DTM agar contains phenol red, which turns the media red upon dermatophyte growth. Dermatophytes are not the only organisms that will initiate the media color change; microscopic examination is required to identify the organism involved. The red coloration may be observed as early as 3–5 days after inoculation. SDA is also inoculated to encourage sporulation by dermatophytes that are inhibited from sporulating on the DTM agar. Most dermatophyte colonies will be white to yellowish tan (see Fig. 14.18B), and darkly pigmented colonies are considered contaminants.

Microscopic Examination of Dermatophyte Cultures

A thin line of lactophenol aniline blue or lactophenol cotton blue stain is placed on a clean glass slide. A piece of clear adhesive tape is torn off, pressed onto the surface of the colony, and then peeled away to be placed gently over the line of stain and observed under high (×40), dry magnification. The organism is identified by comparing the conidia with reference manual pictures (See Recommended Reading). Discard slides in an antifungal disinfectant.

Microscopic Appearance of Yeasts

Yeast can be easily observed in patient samples such as during cytologic examination of an exudate. Dimorphic fungi are infectious, and samples should be sent to a reference laboratory that has appropriate safety equipment and protocols. The most important yeasts of veterinary concern are described below.

Malassezia pachydermatis

M. pachydermatis is frequently found in patients with otitis externa and can also be seen in dermatitis, particularly in immunosuppressed patients with underlying diseases such as diabetes mellitus or hypothyroidism. This organism is readily observed in Diff-Quik–stained slides prepared from swabs of the external ear and does not require culture; its shape may be described as resembling a "footprint" or a "snowman" (Fig. 14.19A).

TECHNICIAN NOTE

Even if only one ear or eye shows a positive sign of infection, both the right and left should be treated to stop the spread of infection.

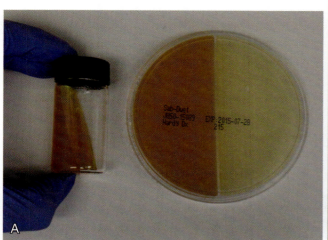
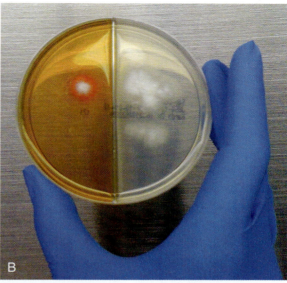

• **Fig. 14.18** (A) Examples of commercially available dermatophyte test medium. (B) *Microsporum canis* growing on dermatophyte test medium *(orange)* and Sabouraud dextrose medium *(clear)*.

Candida albicans

C. albicans is an opportunistic fungal organism associated with human vaginitis but may be present in a variety of veterinary clinical specimens, including samples from avian respiratory and GI tracts, canine and feline skin, and the equine reproductive tract. Cytologic examination of this organism reveals a single-celled, ovoid organism that is approximately 4–6 μm in size and may be budding (Fig. 14.19B). The yeast will stain positive on Gram staining, although definitive identification requires culture, utilizing SDA and incubating it at room temperature or at 37°C (98.6°F) for 2–5 days.

Coccidioides immitis

C. immitis is a dimorphic fungus typically found in the San Joaquin Valley in California. A related fungus, *Coccidioides posadasii*, is found throughout the desert regions of the southwestern United States. Both organisms cause respiratory lesions, draining tracts, and osteomyelitis in dogs, horses, and other animals. In the mammalian host, the reproductive form or arthroconidium enlarges and forms a spherule (20–100 μm in diameter), which can be visualized in cytologic specimens (Fig. 14.19C). Samples of dimorphic fungi should be sent directly to a reference laboratory for confirmatory testing due to safety concerns.

Cryptococcus neoformans

C. neoformans is identified by the abundant capsular material surrounding a yeast cell, approximately 2–20 μm in diameter. India ink is used to stain impression smears of lesions taken from animals suspected of having this infection, such as cats with rhinitis (Fig. 14.19D). Identification is confirmed by culture on SDA and is best left to a reference laboratory.

Blastomyces dermatididis

B. dermatididis is a dimorphic fungus presumptively diagnosed by cytologic examination of prepared patient specimens. The presence of broadly budding yeast measuring approximately 5–20 μm is indicative of infection (Fig. 14.19F). In dogs, this infection is multisystemic, with clinical signs of dyspnea, cutaneous lesions

such as draining tracts, anorexia, and lameness with osteomyelitis. Confirmatory testing should be done by a reference laboratory.

Sporothrix schenckii

S. schenckii is a zoonotic, dimorphic fungus that grows on decaying plant material, causing cutaneous and disseminated lesions (common) in cats and humans. Sporotrichosis in cats is diagnosed through cytologic evaluation of impression smears made from lesion exudates or abscess aspirates and should be confirmed by a reference laboratory.

Virology

Within the reference laboratory, several methods may be used to detect viruses in patient samples, including ELISA, virus isolation, electron microscopy, immunohistochemical staining of histopathologic samples, and molecular tests. In diagnostic laboratories, antigen-antibody–based tests to detect viral antigen loads and molecular methods to detect viral nucleic acid are mostly used in veterinary patients. In most clinical, in-house laboratories, virus detection is limited to antigen-antibody–based tests, such as ELISA, and specialized equipment is not required.

Antigen-Antibody–Based Tests

ELISA can be used for detection of antibodies or antigens. For viral detection, an antibody specific for a viral protein or viral antigen (e.g., *primary antibody* or a *capture antibody*) is bound to a solid carrier, such as the plastic well in a 96-well plate or a cellulose or nylon membrane. Because a solid carrier is used, these tests are sometimes called *solid-phase immunoassays*. The patient sample (e.g., blood, serum, feces) is incubated on the membrane or in the well, allowing the primary antibody to bind with the viral antigen present in the patient sample. The membrane or well is washed, and then an enzyme-labeled secondary antibody that is also specific for the viral antigen is added to the well or the membrane and incubated per instructions for binding. The well or the membrane is again washed, and enzyme substrate is added for a visible color change. The amount of enzyme activity is reflected by

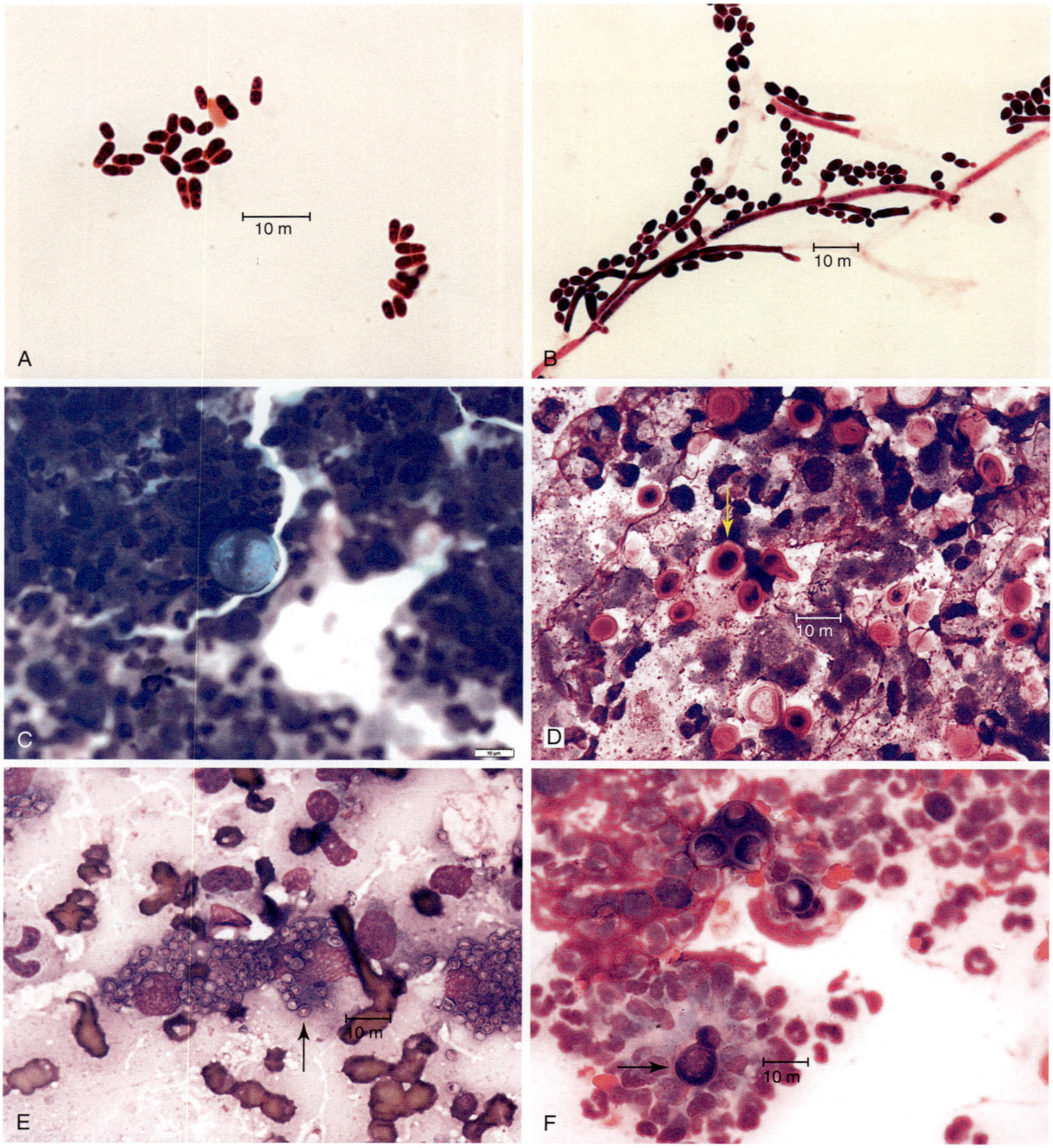

• **Fig. 14.19** Cytologic pictures of yeasts in patient specimens stained with Wright-based stain. (A) *Malassezia pachydermatis.* Note the characteristic "footprint" or "snowman" shape. (B) *Candida albicans.* Note the single-celled, ovoid organism measuring approximately 4 to 6 μm that may be budding. (C) *Coccidioides* spp. Note the spherule (20–100 μm in diameter). (D) *Cryptococcus neoformans* (2–20 μm in size). (E) *Histoplasma capsulatum.* (F) *Blastomyces dermatididis.* (Photos courtesy Dr. Gwendolyn Levine.)

the intensity of the color change and is directly related to the virus amount present in the patient sample. ELISA is commonly used to detect feline leukemia virus antigen in blood, canine parvovirus in feces, and influenza virus in respiratory tract secretions.

Virus isolation from tissue or body fluid samples may be performed directly on patient samples or by culturing virus using cultured human or animal cells. Culturing of animal cells requires specialized equipment, such as tissue culture

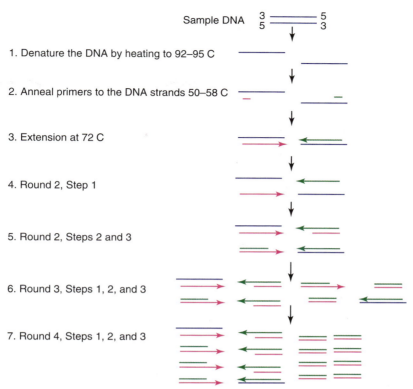

Sample DNA

1. Denature the DNA by heating to 92–95 C

2. Anneal primers to the DNA strands 50–58 C

3. Extension at 72 C

4. Round 2, Step 1

5. Round 2, Steps 2 and 3

6. Round 3, Steps 1, 2, and 3

7. Round 4, Steps 1, 2, and 3

• **Fig. 14.20** Depiction of polymerase chain reaction (PCR) process and products. PCR consists of making multiple copies of a deoxyribonucleic acid (DNA) template by using a three-step process. This process is commonly called *DNA amplification*, because it can be used to detect a small amount of DNA by making more copies. These DNA copies are called *PCR products.* In this graphic depiction of the three-step process, the original sample (template) DNA is shown in *blue*, and primers and PCR products are shown in *pink* and *green*.

hoods that protect cells from contamination by bacteria, and incubators, which can supply CO_2 in the proper concentration (usually 5% of the atmosphere). This is not something normally done in a veterinary hospital but rather, sent to a laboratory.

Molecular Detection of Pathogens

Molecular detection of pathogens is normally carried out in reference laboratories due to the high cost and types of specialized equipment needed. For this reason, this topic will be covered minimally within the scope of this chapter. Pathogens may be detected through testing of vectors in which they are harbored. For instance, it is possible to extract the DNA of tickborne diseases through molecular testing of the crushed parasite to achieve a diagnosis. It is also possible to perform confirmatory testing through PCR testing in which the microbe's messenger ribonucleic acid (mRNA) may be detected through testing of the parasite that harbors it.

DNA Sequencing

DNA sequencing can be used to identify pathogens and rapidly identify bacteria, fungi, and viruses. Although still an expensive test that is not yet routinely performed in veterinary laboratories, it provides a way to definitively identify most organisms. It is now possible to identify the families of bacteria (i.e., microbiomes) present in complex samples by DNA sequencing.

Polymerase Chain Reaction

Polymerase chain reaction (PCR) has revolutionized pathogen detection and phylogenetic analysis in the reference laboratory. With the advent of PCR testing, it is no longer necessary to grow a bacterium or a virus to obtain sequence information as a way to identify obligate intracellular bacteria or viruses (e.g., *Ehrlichia canis* or *Rickettsia rickettsii*) that cannot be cultured using standard methods. PCR testing can also be used to rapidly detect slow-growing organisms such as *M. avium* subsp. *paratuberculosis* and to perform diagnostic tests without the need to maintain viral or bacterial stocks (Fig. 14.20)

Nosocomial Infections

Nosocomial infections are infections that hospitalized patients acquire from the hospital environment, another patient, or a health care provider. These are not to be confused with infections incubating within the patient at the time of admission that become apparent while the patient is hospitalized; such infections are called *community-acquired infections*. These are not to be confused with zoonotic transmission of organisms transmitted from animal patients to human personnel. These infections can have serious consequences; strict precautions must be taken to protect hospital personnel and clients through education, sanitation, and use of PPE.

Hospitalized patients typically are stressed by their illness, unfamiliar surroundings, underlying disease conditions, and therapies (chemotherapy), which can suppress the immune system by increasing susceptibility to infection. Antimicrobial therapy can predispose the patient to infection by altering or reducing the normal flora that prevent pathogen colonization. It is frequently common practice to require certain vaccinations before boarding otherwise healthy animals to prevent the spread of diseases such as "kennel cough" caused by *B. bronchiseptica*.

Both virulent pathogens and opportunistic organisms can be spread by nosocomial transmission. Opportunistic infections are often associated with nosocomial transmission because of increased patient susceptibility for reasons previously noted. Nosocomial agents can also be transmitted on *fomites* (i.e., physical items) such as food bowls, cage mats, clippers, toys, and thermometers. It is important to clean and disinfect/sterilize these items to prevent possible transmission between patients and not allow sharing of such items. Additionally, hospitalized patients are often housed close to one another, increasing the opportunity for potential spread of organisms directly from patient to patient, especially airborne respiratory pathogens.

Finally, pathogens can be transmitted between patients by hospital personnel during treatment. Although animal-to-human transmission is most common, human-to-animal transmission can also occur. Transmission of a zoonotic agent is frequently through direct contact, so hand washing and the use of PPE are important methods of preventing pathogen transmission. Hand sanitizers are useful, but they should not replace washing with soap and water. It is also important to wear PPE and to change laboratory coats or coveralls after treating patients with infections that are easily spread.

TECHNICIAN NOTE

Good hygiene is critical to inpatient care and can be as simple as consistent hand washing, which can significantly reduce the risk of transmission of pathogens between patients and between patients and caregivers.

Agents of Nosocomial Infections

Bacteria are commonly associated with nosocomial infections, although viruses, fungi, and some parasites can also be transmitted from patient to patient. Bacterial agents that infect the respiratory tract, GI tract, and skin are common causes of nosocomial infections, such as *S. equi* subsp. *equi (S. equi)*, *Salmonella* spp., *C. perfringens*, and *C. difficile*, partly because of the types of disease that they cause. *S. equi* is a respiratory pathogen of horses, but the other three agents can cause diarrhea in susceptible patients. Drug-resistant organisms, the most common being methicillin-resistant *Staphylococcus aureus* (MRSA), are frequently transmitted to patients, often through contact with health care providers. Vancomycin-resistant enterococci and multidrug-resistant gram-negative organisms such as *E. coli*, *Salmonella*, *Klebsiella*, *Enterobacter*, and *Pseudomonas* may colonize a patient, causing disease after the animal returns home and necessitating further care.

Viruses are the second most likely cause of nosocomial infections and include canine distemper virus, canine parvovirus, feline panleukopenia virus, equine influenza virus, and equine herpesvirus. Respiratory viruses are frequently implicated, because they are readily transmitted among healthy animals through aerosols.

Recognition and Control of Nosocomial Infections

The most common indicators of nosocomial infection in a hospital include a sudden increase in the number of patients with similar clinical signs specific to the suspected agent and increased isolation of a single agent in samples from multiple patients. Early recognition of possible nosocomial infection is the key to reducing patient morbidity and preventing further pathogenic spread. Once the technical staff knows that transmission is occurring, the next step is to identify the likely sources of the infection (e.g., fomites, inadequate hand washing, faulty sterilization of equipment, patient-to-patient spread) and implement the proper interventions. Most commonly, several interventions are implemented simultaneously; however, routine disinfection of animal housing areas, equipment, and treatment areas must be done, with a monitoring system in place ensuring that pathogens do not thrive.

TECHNICIAN NOTE

An increase in the numbers of patients with clinical signs specific to the suspected agent and increased isolation of a single agent from multiple patients may be indicators of nosocomial transmission, and all practices and potential sources should be investigated.

Recommended Readings

Clinical and Laboratory Standards Institute (CLSI), CLSI document M31-A3. In: *Performance Standards for Antimicrobial Disk and Dilution Susceptibility Tests for Bacteria Isolated from Animals, Approved Standard*. Wayne, PA: Clinical Laboratory Standards Institute; 2013.

Giguère S, Prescott JF, Baggot JD, et al. *Antimicrobial Therapy in Veterinary Medicine*. 5th ed. Ames, IA: Blackwell Publishing; 2013.

Greene CE. *Greene's Infectious Diseases of the Dog and Cat*. 5th ed. Philadelphia, PA: WB Saunders.

Markey B, Leonard F, Archambault M, et al. *Clinical Veterinary Microbiology*. London, UK: Mosby.

McVey DS, Kennedy M, Chengappa MM. *Veterinary Microbiology*. 3rd ed. Ames, IA: Blackwell Publishing.

Zimbro MJ, Power DA, Miller SM, et al., eds. *Difco and BBL Manual*. 2nd ed. Franklin Lakes, NJ: BD Diagnostic Systems; 2009. Available from: https://www.trios.cz/wp-content/uploads/sites/149/2016/08/DIFCO-A-BBL-MANUAL-2.pdf.

15

Diagnostic Imaging

RACHEL McGINTY

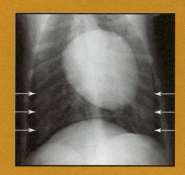

CHAPTER OUTLINE

LEARNING OBJECTIVES

When you have completed this chapter, you will be able to:

1. Pronounce, define, and spell all key terms in this chapter.
2. Do the following regarding the production of x-rays:
   - Describe the properties of x-radiation.
   - Describe the parts of the x-ray tube and machine and discuss the role each part plays in the generation of x-radiation.
   - Explain the production of useful x-ray beam and scatter radiation and discuss the negative consequences of scatter radiation.
3. Do the following regarding x-ray equipment:
   - Describe the features of and uses for portable, mobile, and stationary x-ray equipment.
4. Do the following regarding image production and exposure factors:
   - Explain how *milliamperage, exposure time, kilovoltage,* and *focal–film distance* is set to produce a high-quality diagnostic radiograph.
   - Discuss the purpose of a grid, filtration, and collimation.
5. Explain the purpose of a technique chart.
6. Do the following regarding image formation with film screen systems:
   - Explain the principles of image formation using the film screen system and the purpose of cassettes and screens.

7. Do the following regarding film processing:
   - Discuss the purpose of the darkroom in film processing and safe film handling practices.
8. Do the following regarding digital radiography:
   - Describe the features, advantages, and disadvantages of and the uses for computed radiography and digital radiography equipment.
   - Discuss the difference between computed radiography and digital radiography.
9. Describe common digital radiography artifacts, including how to identify and prevent each one.
   - Explain the roles of digital imaging and communications in medicine (DICOM), picture archiving and communication system (PACS), radiology information system (RIS), and teleradiography in the production and management of digital radiographs.
10. Do the following regarding radiographic image quality:
    - Explain how radiographic density, contrast, and detail are controlled by changing milliamperage and kilovoltage to optimize image quality.
    - Describe types of geometric distortion, such as magnification and elongation.

- List the common technical errors and artifacts that affect image quality.
11. List and describe methods for labeling and storing radiographic images.
12. Do the following regarding radiation safety:
    - Describe the hazards of radiation and explain the role of beam filtration in minimizing its damaging effects.
    - Discuss the methods used to monitor radiation exposure and the units for measuring radiation.
    - Understand ALARA and the three main concepts of radiation safety, including time, distance, and shielding.
    - Explain the principles and practices used to minimize exposure to radiation, including the use of personal protective equipment (PPE).
13. Explain the principles of patient positioning for radiographic studies, including the importance of appropriate restraint.
14. Do the following regarding radiographic contrast agents:
    - List the commonly used positive and negative radiographic contrast agents and explain how they are used in the production of a diagnostic contrast study.
    - Describe the contrast procedure used to image the upper gastrointestinal (GI) tract.
15. Do the following regarding ultrasonography:
    - Describe the indications for and characteristics of ultrasonography in diagnostic imaging.
    - Describe the basic principles of production of an ultrasound image, including the appearance of various tissues and organs on a finished image.
    - Describe how a patient is prepared for ultrasound imaging and the procedure used to conduct an ultrasound examination.
    - Discuss the equipment used to produce B-mode, M-mode, and Doppler ultrasound images.
    - Describe the appearance of an ultrasound image and the appearances and causes of common artifacts.
16. Discuss the indications and use of endoscopy, along with basics of endoscope use and care.
17. Describe indications for and characteristics of fluoroscopy, computed tomography, magnetic resonance imaging, diagnostic nuclear medicine, and positron emission tomography.

KEY TERMS

Anechoic
Anode
B-mode
Cassette
Cathode
Computed radiography (CR)
Computed tomography (CT)
Cradle
Diagnostic ultrasonography (DUS)
Digital fluoroscopy (DF)
Digital imaging and communication in medicine (DICOM)
Digital radiography (DR)
Doppler ultrasonography
Dosimetry
Elongation
Endoscopy
Exposure time
Fluoroscopy
Foreshortening
Gray (Gy)
Grid
Heel effect
Hertz (Hz)
Hyperechoic

Hypoechoic
Intensifying screen
Ionizing radiation
Isoechoic
Kilovolt peak (kVp)
Magnetic resonance imaging (MRI)
Magnification
Maximum permissible dose (MPD)
Milliamperage (mA)
M-mode
Nuclear medicine (NM)
Picture archival computing system (PACS)
Positron emission tomography (PET)
Radiographic detail
Radiographic contrast
Radiographic density
Radiology information system (RIS)
Rotating anode
Scatter radiation
Sievert
Source image distance (SID)
Stationary anode
Teleradiology
X-rays

Introduction

Radiology and ultrasonography are the primary diagnostic imaging techniques available to the veterinarian, but to arrive at a correct diagnosis, high-quality images must be available. The responsibility to provide useful diagnostic images falls to the veterinary technician or nurse. It is essential for the veterinary technician or nurse to produce images of diagnostic quality, understand the factors that go into producing such images, and the physics behind the production of x-rays and ultrasound.

Many different types of imaging equipment are available to veterinarians and technicians, and various exposure factors can be adjusted to produce an image with the appropriate qualities. Patient preparation and positioning also contribute greatly to image quality. In some cases, exposing a regular radiograph of a patient may not give sufficient diagnostic information. In this case, contrast materials may be used to show anatomic areas of interest more readily, or other methods of imaging may be used, such as ultrasonography, endoscopy, fluoroscopy, computed tomography (CT), magnetic resonance imaging (MRI), diagnostic nuclear scintigraphy, and positron emission tomography (PET).

Radiology

Definition of X-rays

X-rays are a form of electromagnetic radiation that have characteristics similar to those of visible light, radio, and television signals but with much shorter wavelengths. This gives the x-ray beam more energy compared with visible light and makes it capable of penetrating tissues and affecting x-ray detectors and fluorescent screens. The interaction of the x-ray with the detector and screen make it possible for a radiographic image to be produced.

X-ray Production

X-rays used in diagnostic radiography are produced when fast-moving electrons collide with a target. There are five essential components that are needed to create an x-ray beam provided by the x-ray tube: (1) a source of electrons, (2) a method of accelerating those electrons, (3) an obstacle-free path to allow electrons to move at top speed, (4) a target for the electrons to interact with, and (5) a vacuum environment.

The x-ray tube is composed of a negatively charged cathode and a positively charged anode and is enclosed in a vacuum environment maintained by a glass envelope. The glass envelope is then surrounded by a metal casing or housing (Fig. 15.1).

The process of x-ray production begins on the cathode side of the tube, where a coiled wire filament sits on the inside of a hollowed-out wall, called the *focusing cup*. When the filament is heated up to a critical temperature, electrons are boiled off and create an electron cloud within the focusing cup. The amount of heat that is applied to the filament determines the number of electrons that are produced.

The electrons formed in the focusing cup are attracted to the positive anode. Energy is applied to the electrons to accelerate them across the tube at high speed. The energy packed in the rapidly moving electrons comes to an abrupt stop by hitting the target, creating heat (99%) and x-rays (1%). The x-rays are then directed downward through the tube housing window as a controlled beam.

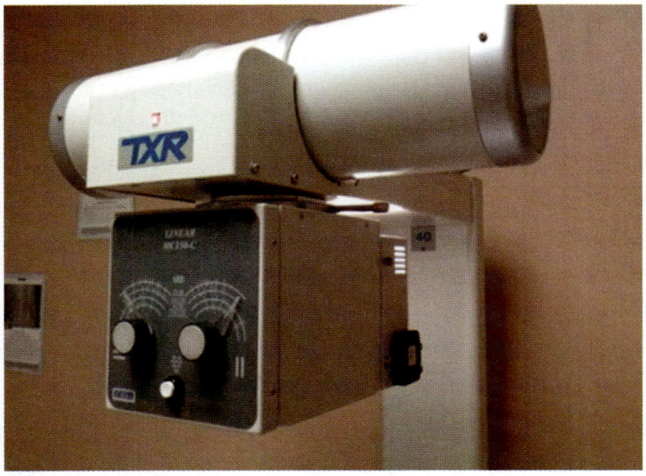

X-ray Tube Components

Tube Housing

Everything inside of the tube is enclosed within metal housing to prevent the escape of stray x-rays. X-rays that are produced in the tube should leave through a window in the bottom of the tube as a controlled x-ray beam.

Glass Envelope

The job of the Pyrex glass envelope is to house the cathode and the anode and to also maintain a vacuum environment. Electrons need to travel at top speed across the tube to have high-energy impacts with the anode to produce x-rays. A vacuum environment prevents the electrons from colliding with air molecules, which will slow them down.

Cathode

The **cathode** is the negatively charged side of the tube that contains one or two filaments enclosed in the focusing cup (Fig. 15.2). The filament, much like one inside a light bulb, is made of up tungsten alloy, a metal which has a high atomic number and a high melting point. The high atomic number allows for more electrons to be produced when the filament is heated up, and the high melting point allows for the filament to be heated to a high temperature without evaporating. A larger filament contains more tungsten than a small filament and can therefore produce more electrons. The more electrons produced on the cathode, the higher the number of potential x-rays that can be produced from the x-ray tube.

The filament is heated by a low-voltage, or **milliamperage (mA)** circuit. This circuit contains a step-down transformer, which reduces the voltage to the filament so it does not overheat while also allowing enough voltage to the filament to allow for electrons to be boiled off and create an electron cloud. The more mA applied to the filament, the more electrons that can be produced.

For the electrons produced by the filament to hit the anode target with great force, they must be accelerated across the tube. The

• **Fig. 15.1** X-ray tube assembly. The cathode and anode encased in the glass envelope are surrounded by a metal housing. The tube is suspended above the table by the tube stand and a collimator attached under the tube to control the dimensions.

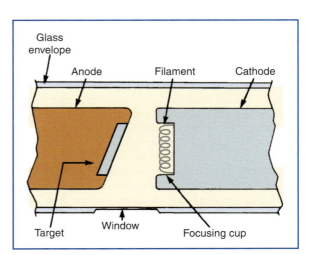

• **Fig. 15.2** Stationary anode x-ray tube. Diagram shows the relationship of the anode to the cathode. (From Eastman Kodak Company. *The Fundamentals of Radiography*. 12th ed. Rochester, NY: Eastman Kodak, Radiographic Markets Division; 1980.)

acceleration is controlled by **kilovolt peak (kVp)** applied between the cathode and the anode.

kVp is produced by a high-voltage circuit that contains two types of transformers. The step-up transformer increases the incoming voltage to thousands of volts (kVp) to move the electrons with great speed. The autotransformer controls the amount of kVp that is applied to the electrons. Because kVp controls the speed and energy of the impact, it then controls the energy level or the penetrability of the x-rays that are produced.

> **TECHNICIAN NOTE**
>
> The energy of the x-ray beam is determined by the energy of the impact the electrons have at the target, which is controlled by the amount of kilovoltage. Increasing kilovoltage will allow x-rays to pass through thicker tissues. Milliamperage heats the filament and produces electrons, which have the potential to become x-rays. The more electrons produced, the more potential x-rays are produced.

Anode

The **anode** is the positive side of the tube that attracts the negative electrons. It contains a tungsten alloy target where the electrons collide and x-ray production occurs. A tungsten alloy is used as the target material, because it has a high atomic number, which allows the target to absorb the electrons and heat up without overheating.

The area of the target where electrons collide is called the *focal spot*. The size of the focal spot is important because of its effect on the detail of the film. A small focal spot produces an image with good clarity and sharpness.

The target of the anode is oriented at a 20-degree angle, which allows the x-rays produced to be redirected out of the tube toward the patient. The effective focal spot is the area of the focal spot that is visible from the tube housing window (Fig. 15.3). In other words, it is the tightly packed, focused primary x-ray beam that exits the tube window.

The anode in the x-ray tube serves two purposes: (1) it supports the target area where all electrons hit, and (2) it helps dissipate some of the heat that is produced by the electron interaction with the target. The anode heat reduction allows for the focal spot size to be small without causing heat damage to the target and providing more detail of the image. There are two types of anodes: stationary and rotating.

Stationary anodes are found in older equipment; dental equipment; small portable units, such as those used in large-animal extremity radiology; and fluoroscopy. Stationary anodes are constructed such that the tungsten target is embedded in a block of copper. Copper is used to absorb and diffuse the tremendous amount of heat generated by the interaction of the electron beam with the target area. However, the amount of heat that is dissipated pales compared with the amount of heat produced during x-ray production, so the technician must pay close attention to the indicators on the machine to ensure that enough heat has been dissipated between exposures. These types of anodes are primarily used when radiographing thinner tissues, because these anodes are not capable of producing a powerful enough beam to penetrate thicker body areas. The inability to dissipate enough heat requires the machine to have a lower mA capacity to avoid producing too many electrons. These anodes also do not allow for shorter **exposure times** that are needed to expose thoracic radiographs without respiratory motion artifacts.

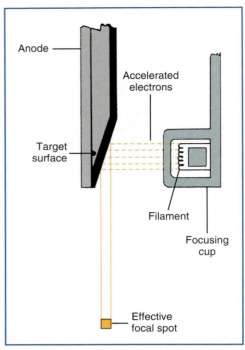

• **Fig. 15.3** Effective focal spot. The surface area is decreased when the target area is constructed at a 20-degree angle to the electron beam.

Rotating anodes (Fig. 15.4) can use much higher currents, shorter exposure times, and smaller focal spots. This will impart a higher quality to the radiograph, because the electrons deposit their energy over a larger target area when the anode is rotating, allowing more heat to be dissipated without losing image detail. This is especially helpful when more electrons are required for an adequate exposure, such as when radiographing thicker tissues.

The rotating anode is a tungsten alloy bonded to molybdenum or graphite to help diffuse the tremendous amount of heat that is generated by a high-powered x-ray machine. The apparatus used to rotate the anode and dissipate the heat must be of highest quality and perfectly balanced to prevent the tube from wobbling, which can lead to a loss of image quality and tube destruction (Fig. 15.5). Anodes may rotate at speeds varying from 3600 revolutions per minute (rpm) to 10,000 rpm. Rotating anode x-ray machines have a two-step exposure switch. The first step of the switch starts the anode rotating, and the second step of the switch activates the high-voltage circuit, accelerating the electrons across the tube and allowing for x-ray production.

Heel Effect

When an x-ray beam leaves the tube, it has an uneven x-ray photon distribution. This phenomenon is related to the angle of the target area and to absorption by the anode target material. As a result, the x-ray beam is more intense at the side of the cathode than at the center of the beam or on the anode side. This phenomenon is called the **heel effect** (Fig. 15.6).

This feature can be used to great advantage in veterinary radiology when radiographing parts of uneven thickness—a common problem when radiographing deep-chested dogs. By placing the thickest part of the patient toward the cathode side of the x-ray tube, a more uniform density (amount of exposure) can be obtained on the radiograph.

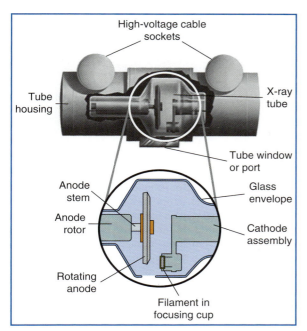

• **Fig. 15.4** Modern rotating anode radiographic tube. Exploded schematic view demonstrates the relationship of the filament to the rotating target. (From Eastman Kodak Company. *The Fundamentals of Radiography.* 12th ed. Rochester, NY: Eastman Kodak, Radiographic Markets Division; 1980.)

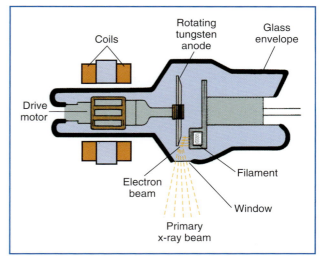

• **Fig. 15.5** Rotating anode tube. Heat is better dissipated by placing the target material at the circumference of a high-speed rotating disk.

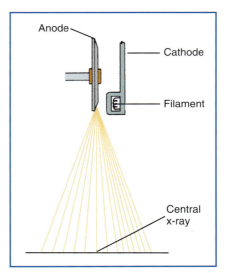

• **Fig. 15.6** Heel effect, produced by uneven intensity of the primary beam. Intensity decreases rapidly toward the anode.

> **TECHNICIAN NOTE**
>
> Always place the thickest part of the area being radiographed toward the cathode side of the x-ray tube.

Tube Rating Chart

The tube rating chart provides information from the manufacturer on the maximum safe exposure time that can be used with specific mA and kVp settings. If longer than designated exposure times are used, tube damage may occur. The chart is of utmost importance when radiographing large-sized patients that require more radiation exposure and when using older x-ray–generating equipment.

Scatter Radiation

Scatter radiation is lower energy x-ray photons that have undergone a change in direction after interacting with structures in the patient's body or anything else in the path of the primary beam (Fig. 15.7). Scatter radiation is of concern, because it decreases image quality and increases radiation exposure for personnel involved in restraining the patient as the radiograph is exposed. Scatter radiation will contribute to overall image darkness or radiographic density but does not contribute to the useful image. The result is reduced subject contrast or an overall "grayish" appearance of the image called *image fogging.* Scatter radiation is the primary source of radiation exposure for technicians who manually restrain patients. It increases with an increase in the following three factors: kilovoltage, thickness of the part being radiographed, and size of the x-ray field (Fig. 15.8).

Careful collimation with beam-limiting devices and close attention to technical factors to avoid the need for retakes are the best ways to decrease exposure from scatter radiation. Beam-limiting devices, correct kVp settings, compression radiography, and grids help to control scatter radiation. Other methods of decreasing technician scatter radiation exposure will be discussed later in the chapter.

> **TECHNICIAN NOTE**
>
> Scatter radiation coming from the area of the patient exposed during radiography is the main source of radiation exposure for the veterinary technician.

X-ray Equipment

Because technicians may be working with a large-animal practitioner or a small-animal practitioner in a large corporate practice or in a veterinary teaching hospital, it is necessary to be familiar with the various types of x-ray units found in such practices.

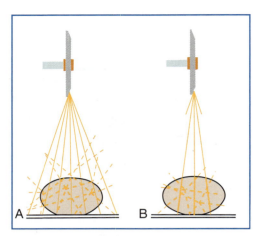

• **Fig. 15.7** Scatter radiation. (A) Scatter radiation is produced when the primary beam is redirected after interacting with structures in the patient's body. (B) Reduction in the amount of radiation produced when the primary beam is restricted by a diaphragm or a collimator.

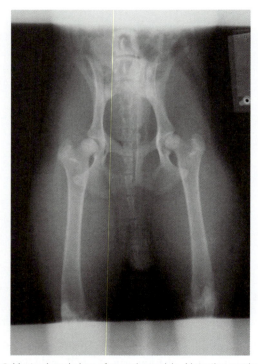

• **Fig. 15.8** Ventrodorsal view of a canine pelvis. Note the graying around the collimated field, with anatomic areas of the patient that have been exposed by scatter radiation. This is called *extra-focal radiation*.

Regardless of type and model, most x-ray machines share many features. For small-animal radiology, an x-ray machine must have a table on which the animal can be positioned (Fig. 15.9A and B). For larger animals, portable x-ray units are often used with image receptor holders (Fig. 15.10). The control panel of x-ray machines may have varying selection features. Many x-ray machines have a common selector control for mA and time of exposure— milliamperage × time in seconds (mAs). This automatically sets the highest mA and the fastest time to provide the requested mAs, controlling the number of x-ray photons produced by the x-ray tube.

Three types of x-ray machines are generally used in veterinary practice: portable units, mobile units, and stationary units.

Portable Units

As the name implies, *portable units* can be carried from one location to another, such as between farms. These units are generally used on blocks or on custom-made stands and weigh 15 to 45 lb or greater (Fig. 15.11). From a safety perspective, they should never be held in the hand. This recommendation especially applies to lighter models with a thinner lead metal in the tube housing, which permits more radiation leakage, potentially exposing the technician. Holding an x-ray machine in the hand not only places the operator close to the x-ray tube, thus increasing the technician's radiation exposure, but also decreases image quality because of tube motion during exposure.

Most portable units are used in equine extremity radiography. Portable units are smaller versions of a traditional x-ray tube. They have lower mA, kVp, and exposure time capacity but are still powerful enough to produce diagnostic images of the equine limb and foot. Portable units also have a collimator with an adjustable light source to illuminate and limit the field size to the same size as the image receptor. Some portable units are battery operated, which is ideal for on-site radiography.

Mobile Units

Mobile units are medium-powered, wheel-mounted units that can be moved around the hospital (not to be confused with portable units). In many small-animal practices, these units are used as fixed units and remain in one room. They are also popular in mixed practices, because the same unit can be used for both large and small animals.

These units are powered when plugged into a 220-volt (V) or 110-V outlet. The 220-V units require more extensive electrical wiring if they are to be moved within the practice setting and require long, heavy power cords, which can pose safety hazards to staff and patients. The 110-V units are lighter, with a smaller power cord, and thus easier to move around the practice setting. These units are of great advantage when radiographing equine extremities. However, because they are less powerful, these units may need more power for radiographing thicker anatomic structures.

Stationary Units

Stationary units are more powerful and are found in most small- and large-animal hospitals. Stationary units commonly seen in small-animal veterinary practices are of the 50 to 300 mA type with an exposure time of 1/30 seconds to 1/120 seconds. All these units can hold an image receptor under the table, with or without the use of a grid, which will be discussed later in the chapter.

Customized large-animal x-ray units and radiography rooms are found mainly in veterinary teaching hospitals. These units are among the most powerful diagnostic x-ray units installed, with a maximum mA of 2000 and maximum kVp of 150. The x-ray tube may be suspended from the ceiling or attached to a floor stand support, with the potential to move or rotate around the patient.

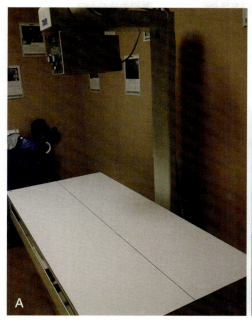

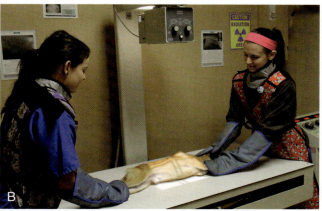

• **Fig. 15.9** (A) A 300-mA x-ray machine commonly used in small-animal practice. (B) Canine patient correctly positioned on an x-ray table for a lateral thoracic radiograph.

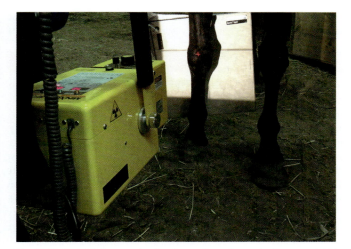

• **Fig. 15.10** Portable large-animal radiography unit, used with a special film cassette holder for equine extremities.

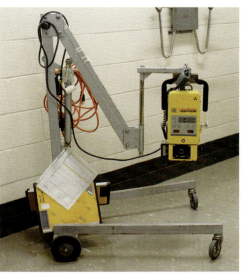

• **Fig. 15.11** Portable x-ray unit commonly used in large-animal extremity radiography. This unit has a lighted collimator and a mobile operating stand.

These tubes also have a heavy-duty collimator to change the field size of the radiation exposure, thus reducing scatter radiation to the patient, the image receptor, and the technician.

Producing an Image Using Exposure Factors

The veterinary technician is responsible for selecting an x-ray technique to produce a diagnostic radiograph. Factors that must be selected include the length of exposure, mA, and kVp. As previously mentioned, most x-ray machines have a common dial for exposure time and mA, called the *mAs setting*. The selection of each factor is based on an accurate technique chart.

Digital imaging has made the selection of adequate exposure factors more straightforward. The digital system provides preset exposure parameters when the patient species, anatomic area of interest, and view of study are entered into the computer software program. The technician may need to adjust the preset exposures to produce a better-quality image of patients with varying tissue thickness or specific medical conditions.

Milliamperage (mA)

The mA setting controls the quantity of electrons boiled off the filament in the x-ray tube, which affects the number of x-rays produced on the anode. Most diagnostic units used in small-animal radiology are operated at settings from 50 to 300 mA. The smallest portable x-ray unit commonly used in large-animal practices may use settings as low as 10 or 20 mA, whereas larger units used in veterinary teaching hospitals may have mA settings of up to 2000.

Adjustments of the mA setting on an x-ray machine allow control of the quantity of x-rays produced. The mA setting is based on how many x-rays are needed to reach the image receptor. This means mA is directly related to the density—the degree of darkness—on the radiograph. When mA is increased, radiographic density—or image darkness—is increased; conversely, when mA is decreased, a reduction in radiographic density—or a lighter image—results.

Exposure Time

Exposure time is when electrons are released from the focusing cup and accelerated across the tube for x-ray production to occur. The longer the exposure time, the greater the number of electrons that flow from the cathode to the anode and the greater the number of x-ray photons that are produced. By using the highest mA setting, the number of electrons in the focusing cup is maximized so that the time of their release from the cathode to the anode can be reduced to create the desired number of x-ray photons.

> **TECHNICIAN NOTE**
>
> Because both exposure time and mA affect the number of photons created and because the shortest exposure time possible is desired to decrease patient motion blur, the highest mA setting and the lowest time setting should be used to achieve the desired mAs.

To understand this concept, consider the following example: an exposure made at 100 mA and at 1/10 seconds should produce an image of equivalent density as an exposure made at 200 mA and 1/20 seconds. In both cases, the mAs factor (milliamperage × time) is the same (10 mAs). Shorter exposure times reduce the problem of motion artifacts that reduce image detail. For this reason, a thoracic radiograph of a dog or a cat should be taken at 1/20 to 1/60 seconds to prevent blurring because of respiratory motion.

When using the highest mA, however, one must be cautious not to overheat the filament and cause it to evaporate. To prevent this, the operator should prevent heating the filament prematurely before the exposure or excessively heating the filament with multiple retakes.

Kilovoltage (kVp)

Kilovoltage is the quality factor that regulates the energy, or the penetrating power, of the x-ray beam. This setting regulates the voltage differential applied between the anode and the cathode in the x-ray tube. The higher the voltage, the faster the acceleration of the electrons and the greater the energy of the x-ray beam, increasing the amount of patient tissue that can be penetrated. Increasing the kVp will also increase radiographic density (i.e., image darkness) because of increased x-ray photons passing through the patient. The kVp setting most often used in diagnostic radiology ranges from 40 to 150 kVp.

The kVp setting affects the contrast scale on a radiograph more than controlling the density. Contrast is necessary to differentiate the anatomic structures seen in an image. The *scale of contrast* refers to the number of shades of gray that can be seen. If no contrast existed, everything would have the same radiographic opacity. Using low kVp settings produces a higher contrast image (blacker and whiter with few grays), because such a beam is more discriminating than a beam with a high kVp. More contrast will be created, because thicker or denser tissues absorb radiation, and thinner or less dense tissues are penetrated. The use of a high kVp setting results in a darker image, which shows little difference in opacity among bone, soft tissue, and fat (low contrast). This is caused by more x-rays passing through thicker structures, making all the structures, whether thick or thin, darker on the image, creating more shades of gray. The kVp setting must be high enough to penetrate the patient's tissues but not so high as to decrease contrast.

> **TECHNICIAN NOTE**
>
> The technician can change the density of the image by changing the total number of x-ray photons (milliampere per second [mAs]) or the energy of the x-ray (kilovolt peak [kVp]). The film's contrast can be increased or decreased by changing the x-rays' penetrating power or energy (kVp).

The kVp, or penetrating power, needed for adequate contrast depends on the tissue's thickness being radiographed. To calculate the correct kVp, the tissue thickness is measured in the direction the beam will pass through it in centimeters (Fig. 15.12A and B).

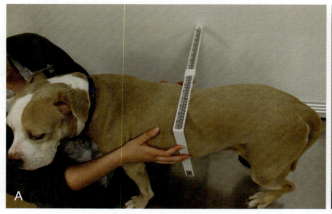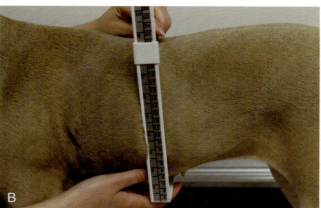

• **Fig. 15.12** A caliper is used to measure the thickness of the anatomic area in the direction that the beam passes through the patient. If multiple views are required, multiple measurements are needed. (A) Measurement of a patient's abdomen for a lateral view. (B) Abdomen measurement from dorsal to ventral.

To estimate the amount of kVp needed, a mathematical equation known as *Sante's rule* is used:

$$2 \times \text{thickness of tissue in cm} + \text{distance} = \text{kVp}$$

This equation assumes that the technician has measured the patient correctly and that the image receptor is placed on top of the table. With the thickness of the patient and the distance the x-rays have to travel accounted for, an x-ray of suitable energy will be produced.

Source Image Distance (SID)

The term source image distance (SID) refers to the distance between the target in the x-ray tube and the surface of the x-ray detector. This factor is normally kept constant from one exposure to another at 70 to 85 cm (28–34 inches) for large-animal radiology and 90 to 105 cm (36–42 inches) for small-animal radiology.

It is important to keep the SID constant from one exposure to the next, because it significantly influences exposure factors. An increase in distance decreases the number of x-rays that reach the image receptor. If you double the SID, the number of x-rays that reach the receptor will be reduced by a factor of four. This is often referred to as the *inverse square law*, which states that the intensity (quantity) of the x-ray beam at a given point is inversely proportional to the square of the distance from the x-ray source. Therefore the results of changing the SID are similar to changing the mAs.

TECHNICIAN NOTE

If you double the image receptor distance from the x-ray source, you will decrease the x-ray beam intensity to one-fourth of the original strength. Small changes in source image distance (SID) can result in big changes in radiographic density.

It sometimes is necessary to change the SID to obtain proper patient positioning. The following simple calculation will help you choose the new mAs setting when the distance is changed:

$$\frac{mAs_{new}}{mAs_{old}} = \frac{SID^2_{new}}{SID^2_{old}}$$

For example, if an x-ray taken at 10 mAs at 100 cm must be taken at 50 cm, by using the formula given the new mAs setting can be calculated as follows:

$$mAs_{new} = mAs_{old} \times \left(\frac{SID_{new}}{SID_{old}} \right)^2$$

This new mAs setting should produce an image of radiographic density like that produced by the original setting of 10 mAs.

One must also consider the kVp when changing the distance that the x-ray must travel. As the distance increases, the energy of the beam must be increased as well. Recall Sante's rule: (2 × thickness in centimeters) + distance = kVp.

Another reason to keep the SID constant is its effect on image detail. Reducing the SID will decrease the image detail. Using an SID that is too small will result in "unsharpness" of the image, making it more challenging to reach a diagnosis. Increasing the SID will enhance the details. However, the technician will then need to increase the radiation coming out of the tube to generate an image of the correct density. It must be kept in mind that this will also result in increased exposure for the patient and technician.

Summary of Exposure Factors

Choosing the exposure factors that work for the patient being radiographed is much like preparing for a bowling game. In bowling, the objective is to knock down the pins. To do that, one must choose a bowling ball of the correct weight, decide how much power to put behind the ball's roll, and stand at a certain distance from the pins. If the ball is not heavy enough or not rolled with enough force, the pins will not be knocked down. The correct combination must be used. If more force is placed behind the ball or the ball is heavier, it is more likely that the pins will be knocked over. The ball is released from a certain distance from the pins. If the distance were decreased, the bowler would not need as much force behind the ball to knock over the pins.

If this principle is applied to radiography, the weight of the ball represents the number of x-rays coming from the tube, the force behind the ball represents kVp, the distance from the bowler to the pins represents the SID, the pins represent the patient, and the ball represents the x-ray beam. The goal, however, is only to have some of the pins knocked down, not all of them; hence some x-rays need to be absorbed. You must use the correct combination of mAs, kVp, and distance, according to patient size. If there were more pins or larger pins, more weight or more force would be needed, just as for larger patients.

Grids, Filtration, and Collimation

When x-rays enter a patient, some pass straight through to the image receptor, but a great many are scattered or redirected along a different path before exiting the patient. The purpose of a grid is to control scatter radiation before it reaches the x-ray receptor and causes unwanted exposure to the image. A **grid** is constructed of a sheet of lead strips interfaced with radiolucent spacers made of plastic or aluminum. These strips are encased in a protective aluminum cover for durability. Grids come in various sizes and are placed directly between the animal and the receptor or, more commonly, mounted under the x-ray table above the image receptor (Fig. 15.13).

The purpose of a grid is to allow only the primary x-ray beams to pass through, thereby preventing scatter radiation from reaching the film. Fig. 15.14A shows how a grid absorbs scatter and prevents it from reaching the film. The grid is constructed in such a way as to absorb all radiation that does not pass between the lead strips. The grid is most useful when producing images of body parts that cause considerable scatter; this includes thick body areas

• **Fig. 15.13** Cassette tray positioned under the table top of a stationary unit.

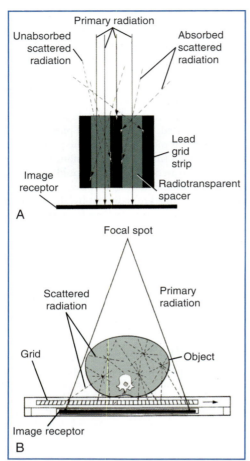

• **Fig. 15.14** Cross section of a grid. (A) Diagram of a small section of a grid showing how a large proportion of the scatter radiation is absorbed and image-forming primary radiation passes through to the image detector. (B) Diagram of focused Potter-Bucky diaphragm being moved toward the right. (Modified from Eastman Kodak Company. *The Fundamentals of Radiography.* 12th ed. Rochester, NY: Eastman Kodak, Radiographic Markets Division; 1980.)

(e.g., thorax, abdomen, skull) and joints and bones greater than 10 cm in thickness.

The amount of scatter radiation the grid can absorb depends on the grid ratio and its lines per centimeter. The term *grid ratio* refers to the relationship between the height of the lead strips and the space between them. For example, if the height of the lead strips is 12-times greater than the space between them, the grid ratio will be 12:1, and if it is 10 times greater, the ratio will be 10:1. The greater the ratio, the more scatter radiation the grid will be able to absorb. Fig. 15.14A shows a grid ratio of 5:1.

Another method of identifying a grid is by the number of lines (strips) per cm. Because the grid is made of lead, which can absorb radiation, the thickness and the number of lead strips will determine whether the grid will absorb too much radiation, causing the lead lines to appear on the image. Thicker lead strips will absorb more scatter radiation, but they will also be more likely to appear on the image. Thinner lead strips will not be as likely to show up on the image but will also not absorb as much scatter. To compensate for the decreased amount of scatter absorbed with thinner lead strips, grids can contain more strips placed closer together,

thus increasing the lines per centimeter. In veterinary medicine, a grid with a ratio of 8:1 at 103 lines per 2.5 cm is recommended.

The disadvantage of using a grid is that some absorption of the primary beam will also occur. To compensate for reduced radiation reaching the receptor, the exposure time used must be increased to produce the correct amount of density on the image. Since grids are mounted under the tabletop, the kVp will also need to be modified to allow the beam to have enough energy to move through the table and an acceptable amount of radiation to be able to move through the grid lines.

Grids can also be described by how their lead lines are oriented. Grids may be parallel or focused. A parallel grid is constructed with strips that are parallel to each other. A *focused grid* is one in which the lead strips and spacers are gradually angulated from the center to the periphery of the grid. The distance from the point of convergence, or the focal point, is called its *focal distance*. The advantage of a focused grid is that it allows unobstructed amounts of radiation to pass through it at the center and at the edge of the grid as long as the radiation is parallel to the axis of the lead strips. Such grids can be used only at an SID specified by the manufacturer. If distances above or below the SID are used, grid cutoff will occur; that is, part of the primary beam will be absorbed by the grid. With grid cutoff, the resulting radiograph will contain large, incompletely exposed areas.

Grids can be stationary or moving (Potter-Bucky diaphragm) (Fig. 15.14B). The moving of a grid horizontally across the x-ray beam during exposure ensures that the grid lines are not visible on the image. However, these grids are not generally used in veterinary medicine due to the loud sound that they create, which startles the patient and creates motion artifacts.

Filtration provides greater image contrast by decreasing lower energy, less-penetrating x-rays from the x-ray beam. Inherent filtration includes materials that filter "soft x-rays" that are manufactured within the tube, such as the glass envelope. Added filtration are things that can be added to the primary beam to increase image quality. These filters can be added to the collimator to filter lower energy x-rays from the beam prior to reaching the patient and image receptor. Filters are also important when it comes to reducing scatter radiation exposure to the technician, as discussed in the radiation safety section of the text. Other materials, such as large saline bags, bags of rice, or beanbags, that absorb the low-energy x-rays, may also be placed next to the patient on the table. Leaded rubber or lead gloves may also be used. However, cautious placement is required to ensure that there is no overlap with the anatomic area of interest.

As mentioned previously, collimation will also decrease scatter radiation and enhance image quality. The collimator is the beam-limiting device attached to the tube window, the area where the x-ray beam exits the tube. The lead shutters inside of the collimator control the dimensions of the primary beam, limiting the exposure to just the area of interest and decreasing exposure.

TECHNICIAN NOTE

Always use a grid between the patient and the image receptor when the body part being radiographed is greater than 10 cm thick.

Technique Chart

A technique chart provides suggested exposure factors to use based on the anatomic part being radiographed, the thickness of the tissue, and the position of the patient. It provides the technician with predetermined exposure settings for various radiographs to be taken

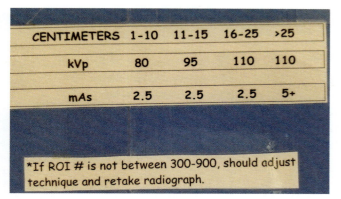

CENTIMETERS	1-10	11-15	16-25	>25
kVp	80	95	110	110
mAs	2.5	2.5	2.5	5+

*If ROI # is not between 300-900, should adjust technique and retake radiograph.

• **Fig. 15.15** The best diagnostic radiographs in digital imaging are acquired with a technique that is representative of the patient parameters. This digital x-ray technique chart is simple compared with the technique chart of a film-screen system due to the dynamic range of the image receptor and the ability to process the image postexposure. (Courtesy of Jessica Vorndran, BSAn.Sc, RVT, MedVet Medical and Cancer Centers for Pets.)

to receive an image of good diagnostic quality. When using a technique chart, no calculations for determining kVp and mAs need to be performed. The technician must only measure the anatomic thickness of the patient and refer to the chart for the exposure values.

Technique charts are usually produced by the manufacturer of the x-ray machine and provided when the machine is purchased. Each x-ray machine must have its own specified technique chart because of variations in output from one machine to the next. Likewise, a technique chart for a digital system is simplified in comparison to a technique chart for a film screen system due to variation in exposure required, the dynamic range of the digital receptor, and postimage processing (Fig. 15.15). Therefore a technique chart formulated for another x-ray machine should never be used without making appropriate changes. If you select exposure factors from a good technique chart, consistent radiographic examinations of diagnostic quality will be obtained.

Many types of technique chart may be available, each one using the maximum potential for that particular x-ray machine. The most popular type of technique chart used by veterinarians is a variable kilovoltage chart. Table 15.1 is an example of a variable kVp technique chart. However, combined use of technique charts with variable kilovoltage and mAs is recommended, because they take into consideration the need to adopt the appropriate chart for different anatomic structures.

There are times when a technique chart may not provide adequate exposures of correct density or contrast. In this case, the technician may have to change the exposure setting suggested on the chart or may even have to re-create a chart that provides suitable exposure factors for all exposures. For a more extensive discussion on how to prepare different technique charts with examples of each, refer to the works by Han and Hurd (2005), Brown and Brown (2022), and Morgan (1993) (see the "Recommended Readings" section).

Capturing the Image

Once x-rays can be produced, there are two ways that an image can be captured: (1) by using a cassette with film, and (2) by using a computer to receive a digital image. With advances in imaging technology, digital image capturing is preferred; the image, x-ray tube, table, and auxiliary instruments used are the same for both.

Image Formation With Film Screen Systems

When an x-ray beam penetrates a body system and reaches the film, a latent image is produced that will be revealed when the film is processed chemically. Several factors are involved in the formation of a high-quality latent image.

X-ray Cassettes. **Cassettes** (film holders) used for veterinary radiography (Fig. 15.16) must be of good quality to ensure uniform contact between the x-ray film and the screen and to prevent light leakage that could fog the film. Most cassettes have a solid front made of plastic or light metal. The cassette back may be made of steel and can sustain moderate patient weight without being damaged.

Cassettes should be handled with care. If dropped, they may warp, or if the cover is forced closed, the hinges may be damaged, resulting in a cassette that does not close properly. If film contact is not perfect along the surface of the screen, distortion of the x-ray image will occur.

Intensifying Screens. **Intensifying screens** are the smooth, shiny, white inner surfaces of the film cassette. They are made of layers of tiny crystals bonded together on a plastic support and covered with a protective coating. These crystals fluoresce, or emit light, after exposure to x-rays. Screens are mounted into the cassette, and the x-ray film is sandwiched between. The use of fluorescent intensifying screens dramatically decreases the amount of radiation needed to produce a film of diagnostic radiographic density, because the film is more sensitive to light exposure than to radiation exposure. Thus intensifying screens allow for much lower mAs settings. This has three advantages: (1) it prolongs the life of the tube; (2) it decreases the amount of exposure to patients and technicians; and (3) it reduces the risk of patient motion.

Intensifying screens are usually mounted in pairs in an x-ray cassette. They are made of the four components (Fig. 15.17): (1) the *backing*, which is made of cardboard or plastic, most commonly Mylar; (2) the *reflecting layers*, which reflect light from the active layer toward the x-ray film; (3) the *active layer*, which contains light-emitting rare-earth phosphor crystals that produce light when struck by x-ray radiation, causing exposure of the film; and (4) a *plastic coating*, which reduces static electricity and provides a protective covering that can be cleaned. The screens must be cleaned on a regular basis or whenever artifacts are noted on a radiograph. Artifacts occur when material falls between the screen and the film and blocks light from getting to the film. The surface of the screen must be thoroughly dry before an x-ray film is inserted; otherwise the film will stick to the screen and will permanently ruin it. Any stain on the screen's surface will also interfere with transmission of light from the screen to the film, causing an artifact. If a patient is likely to urinate or defecate while being placed on the table, the cassette should be wrapped in a

TABLE 15.1	Variable kV Technique Chart for an X-ray Machine of 300 mA, 125 kV, 1/120 Second Timer With FFD of 40 Inches					
Thickness, cm	kV	mA	Seconds	mAs	Grid	
4	48	300	1/120	2.5	No	
5	50	300	1/120	2.5	No	
6	52	300	1/120	2.5	No	
7	54	300	1/120	2.5	No	
8	56	300	1/120	2.5	No	
9	58	300	1/120	2.5	No	
10	63	300	1/60	5	Yes	
11	65	300	1/60	5	Yes	
12	67	300	1/60	5	Yes	
13	69	300	1/60	5	Yes	
14	71	300	1/60	5	Yes	
15	73	300	1/60	5	Yes	
16	75	300	1/60	5	Yes	
17	77	300	1/60	5	Yes	
18	79	300	1/60	5	Yes	
19	81	300	1/60	5	Yes	
20	84	300	1/60	5	Yes	
21	87	300	1/60	5	Yes	
22	90	300	1/60	5	Yes	
23	93	300	1/60	5	Yes	
24	96	300	1/60	5	Yes	
25	99	300	1/60	5	Yes	
26	102	300	1/60	5	Yes	
27	105	300	1/60	5	Yes	
28	99	300	1/30	10	Yes	
29	102	300	1/30	10	Yes	
30	105	300	1/30	10	Yes	

Radiographs were taken with Kodak Lanex Regular screens and Kodak TML x-ray film. *FFD,* Focal–film distance; *kV,* kilovolts; *mA,* milliampere; *mAs,* milliamperes per second.

plastic bag to prevent urine or feces from getting on the screen. *Screen speed* refers to converting absorbed x-ray energy into visible light. *Screen speed* is a relative term that refers to the amount of radiation required by that screen to produce a film of diagnostic radiographic density. Table 15.2 gives different screen speed characteristics and uses.

> **TECHNICIAN NOTE**
>
> The use of a screen is advantageous for veterinary radiography, because fewer x-rays are required to produce a diagnostic radiograph. Lower exposures mean lower radiation doses to the patient and technician, fewer retakes because of patient motion, and longer x-ray tube life.

X-ray Film. X-ray film is prepared from a suspension of light-sensitive silver halide crystals, which are x-ray–sensitive granules that are embedded in a gelatin emulsion coating a polyester base. There are different film speeds depending on the size of the crystal, just like screens. The gelatin layer must be durable yet flexible

enough for the film to go through an automatic processor without being damaged. The gelatin matrix is protected by a thin covering called the "*supercoat.*"

X-ray films can be classified into two categories: screen film and nonscreen film. Screen film is sensitive primarily to light emitted from intensifying screens and is primarily used in practices still using film-based imaging. It is less sensitive to ionizing radiation, reducing exposure to the patient and scatter radiation to the technician. Nonscreen films are designed for direct exposure to x-ray and are relatively insensitive to light from screens. Nonscreen films provide superb detail and are especially good for intraoral examination of the nasal cavity, dental studies, and examination of bony extremities.

> **TECHNICIAN NOTE**
>
> Be sure that the x-ray film used is sensitive to the spectrum of light that the screen is emitting. Rare-earth screens should be used with film sensitive to green light.

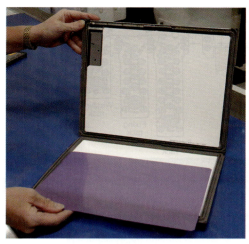

• **Fig. 15.16** An open rigid cassette containing film sandwiched between two intensifying screens. The screen film is manufactured for the special purpose of being used with image-intensifying screens. When used with the proper screen, such film will drastically reduce x-ray exposure time.

TABLE 15.2	Screen Speed Characteristics and UseFast	
Screen		**Slow Screen**
Thicker phosphor layer and larger phosphor crystals to increase x-ray absorption		Thinner phosphor layer and smaller phosphor crystals leading to decreased x-ray absorption
Produces more light for film exposure		Produces less light for film exposure
Requires less mAs for adequate exposure Shorter exposure time = less radiation		Requires more mAs for adequate exposure Longer exposure time = more radiation
Produces an image with less resolution (detail)		Produces an image with more resolution (detail)
Used for anatomic areas with more physical density and thickness		Used for anatomic areas with less physical density and thickness

mAs, Milliamperes per second.

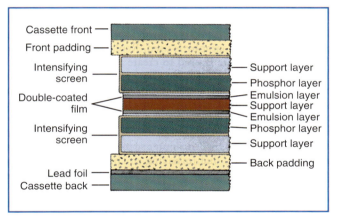

• **Fig. 15.17** Cross section of a cassette-intensifying screen system.

The Darkroom

Film radiography begins and ends in the darkroom, where films are loaded into cassettes for exposure and returned for processing into a finished radiograph. It is essential that the darkroom be lightproof, clean to prevent artifacts, and have adequate ventilation and temperature control. A safelight is an important feature of the darkroom to allow visibility for the technician but must have the correct characteristics to not expose the film. The darkroom should be organized into wet and dry areas to reduce any chemical exposure to the film and cassettes.

Unexposed x-ray film and preprocessed exposed film is very sensitive. Unexposed x-ray film should be stored upright in a safe, dry, cool environment, such as a film bin. Because film is very sensitive to damage, it is important that it be handled only by the corners or the edges to reduce the risk of damage to the area where the image is located. Care must be taken to prevent static electricity, bending, creasing, or scratching when the x-ray film is transferred from the bin to the cassette and from the cassette to the automatic processor.

Automatic processors are manufactured in different shapes and sizes (Fig. 15.18). It is necessary to maintain fresh developer, fixer, and wash solution and to ensure that the solutions are flowing properly within the processor. Automatic processors allow for fast, standardized film processing but do require regular maintenance and proper ventilation.

> **TECHNICIAN NOTE**
>
> Old radiographs (those stored for 3 years or longer) used to fix solution must be recycled, because the silver crystals inside of them are environmental pollutants.

Digital Radiography

Digital imaging techniques are commonly used for **digital fluoroscopy** (DF), **computed tomography (CT)**, **diagnostic ultrasonography** (DUS), **nuclear medicine** (NM), **magnetic resonance imaging** (MRI), **digital radiography** (DR), and **computed radiography** (CR). The components for generating the x-rays may vary depending on the image receptor used, but the x-ray production process is the same. There are three types of image receptors commonly used in digital imaging: CR, indirect digital imaging, and direct digital imaging receptors (DDRs).

A digital x-ray unit uses the same x-ray tube, collimator, and table used in film screen imaging (Fig. 15.19). In DDR, an x-ray tube coupled to a specialized detector panel that changes x-rays into electrical signals is used. The analog image is digitalized and displayed on a computer screen. The same is true for indirect imaging, except that x-rays are first converted to light and then to electrical signals to form the image on the computer screen. Creating an image as an electronic signal allows for postproduction digital enhancement, including magnification, rotation, annotation and measurement of images, contrast, brightness, and zoom. The main advantage of the ability to alter the image is a decrease in the number of retakes, which saves time and reduces exposure to the patient and the technician.

• BOX 15.1 Digital Artifacts

Lucent Halo Around Metal Implants
- Uberschwinger artifact or rebound effect (an artifact of digital processing that may be mistaken for bone lysis). This can be caused by computer image processing.

Linear Striations Seen in the Background of the Image
- Planking artifact (caused by plate saturation or overexposure)

Disappearance of Thin Tissues or Soft Tissues Surrounding Bone
- Overexposure

Grainy Appearance (quantum mottle or noise)
- Underexposure

Nonuniform Appearance of the Image (seen mostly with computed radiography [CR] systems)
- Improper use of the heel effect
- Contrast media on table or detector

Ghost Images
- Taking an image quickly after a previous image that required a very high exposure. Occurs with digital radiography (DR) systems when previous exposure is still on the detector panel.
- Double exposures (CR only since the CR plate acts similarly to a cassette).
- Failure to erase a CR plate in the reader so exposure is still left on the plate.

Fogging
- CR plate exposed to radiation from any source: through wall if storage room adjacent to x-ray room or cassette left in x-ray room while exposure is made.

White Spots
- Scratches on CR imaging plate.
- Hair, dirt, or other particles trapped in the CR cassette.

Digital artifacts can occur for many different reasons. Box 15.1 lists digital artifacts that can occur. The technician's responsibility is to identify the cause of the artifact and contact the correct persons to remedy it.

DICOM, RIS, PACS, and Teleradiology

DICOM. Medical image distribution and archiving has changed significantly since the beginning of the digital imaging movement, primarily the usage of **digital imaging and communication in medicine (DICOM)**. DICOM is a universal digital image format that has allowed digital images to be shared among software from various vendors. This makes sending electronic images to other locations (teleradiology), hospitals, or specialists much more efficient.

Each DICOM image file contains image information and patient identification, modality used (CT, DUS, MRI, etc.), date and time of the examination, and display formats. Imaging modalities that operate on the DICOM standard include CT, DR or CR, MRI, DUS, and secondary capture (SC; e.g., from a film scanner). DICOM functionality enables image storage, query (searching), retrieval, display, and manipulation.

Within DICOM, each image is given a tag. The tags are read by computer software, which organizes them automatically into groups according to date, modality, study, and series. DICOM

functions also allow generation of a worklist, which can help communicate with the hospital information system (HIS) or the radiology information system (RIS) so that the images become part of that patient's digital hospital record.

RIS. The **radiology information system (RIS)** is a computer software program that allows all patient data to be made available, coupled with digital imaging data. The advantage of the RIS is that when patient identification information or results of a test are entered by any individual in the hospital, this information is "coordinated" with all other hospital forms and records, such as radiology forms.

PACS. The **picture archival computing system (PACS)** is used to store data permanently and to move images around to different computer workstations within a single hospital or between hospitals. The benefits of PACS include the following: (1) it eliminates the need to generate and store film hard copies; (2) communication with other veterinarians is improved; (3) tracking down lost films is no longer an issue; and (4) multiple users can view the images at the same time. As with any computer system, there are disadvantages. When computer systems go down, become blocked, or lose connectivity, productivity may decrease and data can be lost. It is a good idea to make backup copies of all digital files.

TECHNICIAN NOTE

A technician using the digital radiology (DR) system should have sufficient working knowledge of the computer system to be able to troubleshoot and maintain a picture archival computing system (PACS).

Three components of the PACS that may be used by the technologist are the server, the workstation, and the monitor. The server receives the images and catalogs them into a database, allowing for a search of the image when it is needed for viewing. The workstation consists of a computer with imaging software that allows images to be exported, received, and manipulated (contrast, brightness, magnification, etc.), and measurements (length, width, circumference, angle, etc.) to be made. Images can then be viewed on high-quality monitors, printed, and/or digitally shared with other veterinarians.

Teleradiology. **Teleradiology** allows transmission of digital data across the Internet from private practices to referral centers. Specialists can receive images almost instantly, interpret them, and quickly send back a written report. There is no longer the need to package and label films to be sent by mail carriers, which also delays response time. Digital data, including MRI, CT, DUS, DR, and CR images, can be sent directly.

Radiographic Image Quality

It is of utmost importance to produce radiographs of excellent quality to achieve an accurate radiographic diagnosis. An image of good diagnostic quality should provide optimal density, correct scale of contrast, and excellent detail (Fig. 15.21).

Radiographic Density

Radiographic density refers to the degree of darkness on the image. If an image has increased radiographic density, it means that it is darker. When the image receptor is exposed to x-ray radiation, these exposed areas will become darker after processing. Likewise, if a portion of the image receptor is not exposed, it will be lighter and have less radiographic density.

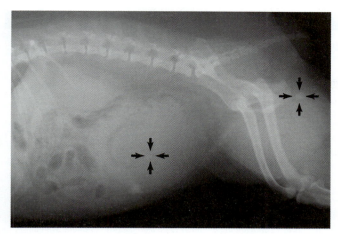

• **Fig. 15.21** Lateral radiograph showing good radiographic detail and contrast. Round, opaque mineral structures (uroliths) are seen within the urinary bladder *(arrows near the middle)*. The urinary bladder is large as the result of obstruction by another stone within the urethra *(arrows on the right)*.

The primary factor affecting density is the mAs setting. As has been discussed, mAs is the factor that regulates the quantity of x-rays produced. If more x-rays reach the image receptor, the image will be darker. Therefore it can be stated that high mAs settings will increase radiographic density and that low mAs settings will reduce radiographic density.

Another factor affecting density is kilovoltage. Inside the x-ray tube during activation, kVp is responsible for accelerating electrons from cathode to anode. The faster the electrons move, the more energy they will have. More powerful x-rays can penetrate the patient, hitting the image receptor and making the image darker and increasing the radiographic density. Although kVp does influence density, it controls contrast more.

The distance from the focal spot (where the electrons hit and produce x-rays) to the surface of the image receptor is another important factor in film density. A change in distance can cause significant overexposure (if the distance is reduced) or underexposure (if the distance is increased). This effect can be dramatic, because the intensity of the radiation is reduced or increased as the square of the distance is changed. This effect is discussed further in the section "Source Image Distance" on inverse square law and emphasizes the need for consistency and accurate measurement of distance.

The anatomic part's thickness and density will also affect radiographic density. Thicker or denser portions of the patient's body, such as bone, will absorb x-rays, blocking exposure to the image receptor and resulting in low radiographic density (a white coloration). Thinner tissues or areas containing gas (lungs) will allow x-rays to penetrate easily, resulting in more exposure to the image receptor and increasing radiographic density (making it darker) (Case Presentation 15.1).

Radiographic Contrast

Radiographic contrast refers to the difference in radiographic density, or the shades of white and black, between two areas on the radiograph. Contrast on the image is mostly influenced by the kVp setting. A higher kVp setting allows more x-rays to penetrate tissues, making absorption of the x-ray beams more uniform among various tissues. This causes more shades of gray to appear on the image, giving it lower contrast. A radiograph with lower

contrast is said to have long latitude. *Latitude* refers to the range of different densities on the radiograph. In this case, a radiograph with more shades of gray is said to have long latitude.

High radiographic contrast, or an image with short-scale latitude, would have whiter and blacker areas versus shades of gray (Fig. 15.22). High contrast is achieved by using a lower kVp setting. The low kVp setting allows for thicker areas of the body to absorb the x-rays, making them appear white on the image, and thinner areas to be penetrated by x-rays, making them darker.

The type of radiographic contrast desired depends on the subject contrast of the anatomic area being viewed. Subject contrast refers to the difference in density between two adjacent anatomic structures. Thoracic or abdominal views require more shades of gray, because the thicker tissues in those parts of the body require a higher kVp. More shades of gray—lower subject contrast—occurs because these tissues have roughly the same physical density and absorb the same amount of x-rays. Thinner tissues of the body, such as the extremities, require a lower kVp setting. The bone of the extremity can absorb much of the beam and the thinner tissues next to the bone are penetrated, resulting in higher subject contrast. Subject contrast affects the overall radiographic contrast of the image. Higher subject contrast increases radiographic contrast.

Radiographic Detail

Radiographic detail refers to the degree of sharpness that defines the edge of an anatomic structure. It represents the best possible reproduction of an organ. Detail is influenced by every possible factor, but geometry and motion factors are more influential than others.

SID is one important factor in the loss of detail. If the focal spot is too close to the part being radiographed, the image will appear larger than normal in size and will have a lack of distinction at the margins of the structure. Therefore it is important to maintain an SID as long as possible without significantly reducing x-ray beam intensity.

Movement in veterinary radiology is a constant problem. Motion of the patient, x-ray tube, or image receptor will cause blurring of images. Movement can be caused by respiration, intestinal movement, and patient movement. Sedation may be necessary to prevent lack of detail caused by patient movement and the mAs setting adjusted to prevent blurring caused by respiratory and bowel movement. It is difficult to produce diagnostic images of the thorax with a unit that does not have a minimum exposure time of at least $\frac{1}{30}$ seconds and ideally, $\frac{1}{120}$ seconds. Movement is a constant problem in large-animal radiology when small portable units are used. Using shorter exposure times will reduce potential motion artifacts and increase the radiographic detail.

In digital radiography, many factors that affect detail are mitigated due to image-enhancing software and reduced technical errors. In film screen imaging, poor radiographic processing contributes most to poor detail. However, poor film screen contact and over- or underexposure will also reduce detail.

> ### TECHNICIAN NOTE
> A radiograph of good diagnostic quality should have optimal density, the correct scale of contrast, and excellent detail.

Geometric Distortion

Geometric distortion occurs with improper positioning of the patient, image receptor, or x-ray tube. **Magnification** is most common and occurs when the anatomic area is not close enough

CASE PRESENTATION 15.1

Radiographic Study of a Patient with Gastric Dilatation-Volvulus

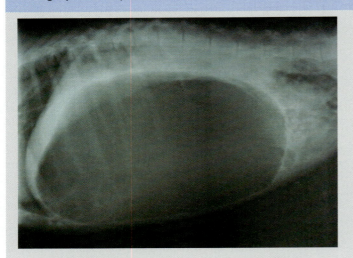

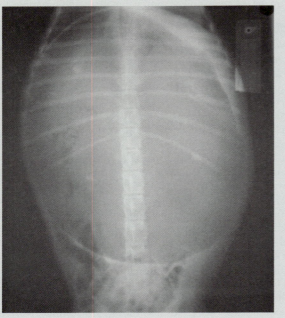

Clem, a 6-year-old spayed female hound mix was presented after being found in lateral recumbency and in respiratory distress in her kennel. Physical examination findings included increased capillary refill time (CRT); pale mucous membranes; tachycardia; shallow, rapid breathing; and a significantly distended abdomen. The veterinarian ordered abdominal radiographs to definitively diagnose gastric dilatation-volvulus (GDV). The veterinary technician exposed ventrodorsal (VD) and lateral abdominal views for evaluation of the abdominal structures. After evaluating the radiographs, the veterinarian concluded that the patient did have GDV. What do you think the veterinarian observed in the radiographs that confirmed this diagnosis?

Answer
The radiographs showed the stomach to be significantly distended with air. Air is radiolucent, meaning that it allows more x-rays to pass through it and interact with the image receptor, causing it to appear darker. A right lateral view can be used to determine the position of the pylorus to differentiate between gastric distension ("bloat") and GDV.

Follow-up
Clem was stabilized, and emergency surgery was performed to decompress the stomach and rotate it back to its normal position. A gastropexy was then performed to attach the stomach to the abdominal wall to prevent the recurrence of torsion.

to the image receptor. The further the anatomic area is from the image receptor, the larger and more diffuse the final image becomes. Magnification can also occur if SID is reduced. In some cases, magnification may be beneficial to the radiographer, especially when radiographing smaller structures or exotic or pocket pet patients.

Another type of geometric distortion that may occur is **elongation**, where the image appears longer than normal size. This occurs when the x-ray beam and the structure are not centered to each other. The same effect happens with our shadow and the sun. If it is 12 o'clock noon, the sun hits you from directly above, and your shadow is an exact replication underneath you. As the sun sets and hits your body from a different angle, your shadow extends out alongside you and is longer than your actual length. To avoid elongation, it is important to center the patient directly under the beam.

Foreshortening occurs if one portion of the patient is lifted from the image receptor while another part is in contact with the image receptor, causing the image to appear shorter than the actual size of the object. This commonly occurs when radiographing a patient's femur or humerus. Because of the different thicknesses of the soft tissues surrounding these bones, the distal end of the limb can be held parallel to the image receptor to reduce foreshortening. Elongation and foreshortening can be useful in cases such as dental imaging. However, both potentially cause loss of detail and poor diagnostic quality.

Motion is generally not of benefit to the overall quality of the image. Voluntary or involuntary motion from the patient will reduce the sharpness of the image. Therefore adequate restraint of the patient and proper timing to reduce involuntary motion is of utmost importance. However, blur from patient motion may

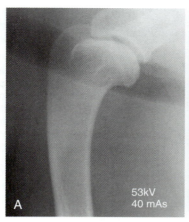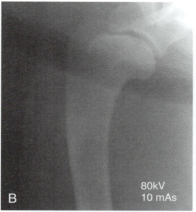

A   53kV
     40 mAs

B   80kV
     10 mAs

• **Fig. 15.22** Mediolateral radiograph of the shoulder showing high (A) and low (B) contrast. In (A) the kVp is set at 53, whereas in (B) it is set at 80. In (B), little difference in opacity between bone and soft tissue leads to a low-contrast image.

• BOX 15.2   Technical Error Artifacts

Increased Radiographic Density
Severely high mAs or kV settings
Too-short FFD
Equipment malfunction

Decreased Radiographic Density
Severely low mAs or kV settings
Too-long FFD
Equipment malfunction

Distorted or Blurred Radiograph
Motion: patient, image receptor, or machine
Excessive object-film distance, causing magnification and distortion
Poor centering of primary x-ray beam

Miscellaneous Artifacts
Collimation of edges, causing underexposed margins
Target damage, resulting in inconsistent image density: requires tube replacement
Double exposure
Faulty equipment

---

prove useful when imaging anatomy that is obscured by overlying structures. Blur is particularly useful in CT.

Technical Errors and Artifacts

As previously discussed, there are few artifacts that can occur with digital imaging. Artifacts may still be produced by the imaging plate, grid, mechanical system, and the software. Human errors often are responsible for artifacts, such as over- or underexposure, which can be resolved with proper digital processing of the image. Software problems resulting in reduced image quality should be addressed quickly to ensure all images exposed are of diagnostic quality. Technical errors may still contribute to poor quality radiographs when digital software cannot compensate for the problem (Box 15.2).

Most artifacts occur during film-based imaging, particularly during film processing. It is important that standard procedures be implemented when handling and storing film, and especially during processing, to keep artifacts from reducing image quality.

Legal Records and Film Identification

Radiographs are part of the legal medical record and must be correctly identified and carefully labeled (position, anatomical feature, etc.). Identification should include the patient and owner identification, date of examination, and the practice name and location.

> **TECHNICIAN NOTE**
>
> Radiographs are part of the legal medical record and must be correctly identified and carefully labeled. Proper storage is also important for radiographs to be easily retrieved for comparison views or follow-up studies.

Several methods of film labeling are available. In one method, leaded numbers and letters are placed onto a lead blocker, which is then placed on top of the cassette next to the patient during the time of exposure. The lead numbers and letters absorb the radiation, causing them to appear white on a finished radiograph. A second method involves the use of a special lead-impregnated tape. The desired information is written or typed on it, and the tape is then placed on the cassette or on a lead blocker next to the patient during exposure. One of the better film identification methods is photo imprinting, which is a simple and inexpensive system. The required information is typed on a card that is placed in the imprinter. This system requires placement of a small lead blocker in the upper left-hand corner of the film cassette, which prevents exposure to that part of the film. The card is placed in the light flasher in the darkroom. The unexposed left-hand corner of the exposed radiograph is placed underneath the card and the light flashed through the card. The information recorded on the card is exposed into the x-ray film and will be visible when the radiograph is developed.

In DR, the patient information is part of the DICOM tag. The owner's name, animal's name, clinic name, examination date, species, breed, weight, gender, region examined, and other pertinent information is added to the study using vendor software. This information is ultimately linked to the digital information that forms the radiograph and is visible on each radiograph taken for that patient to make it part of the permanent record for legal purposes.

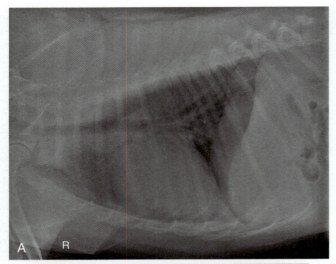

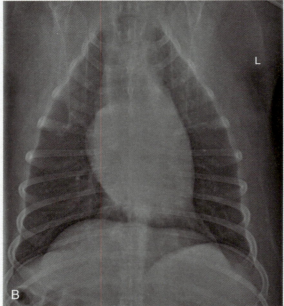

• **Fig. 15.23** (A) Right lateral thorax view labeled with an "R," indicating the patient is in right lateral recumbency. The label is placed cranially and ventrally to the patient. (B) Ventrodorsal thorax view with an "L" placed on the left side of the patient, indicating the left side and placed cranially in the field of view. (Courtesy of Jessica Vorndran, BSAn.Sc, RVT, MedVet Medical and Cancer Centers for Pets)

In addition to the legal identification on the image, it is necessary to identify the body part radiographed at the time of exposure. Leaded right and left markers should be placed appropriately at the time of exposure to identify the extremity being examined or the side on which the animal is positioned for examination (i.e., right or left lateral recumbency) (Fig. 15.23A and B). Box 15.3 discusses proper label positioning for common radiographic views. Timing markers are used in contrast studies, such as upper GI studies, to indicate when the image was obtained in relation to when the contrast medium was administered.

Filing of the Radiograph

Like all medical records, film radiographs must be kept for 3 years by a method that facilitates retrieval for further diagnostic review

or follow-up comparison. The radiographs from each examination should be placed in a 14 × 17-inch, patient-specific x-ray envelope. The envelopes should be filed in an upright position according to the filing system used for other hospital records (i.e., by last name or case number).

As previously discussed in digital imaging (radiography, DUS, CT, MRI), the DICOM tag allows for the image to be stored in the patient's electronic medical record. The image can then be retrieved and viewed using the hospital's PACS or transferred digitally to other radiologists or physicians for consultation. When archiving digital images on a computer, it is important to ensure that sufficient back-up methods are established to mitigate loss of patient records should computer systems fail.

Radiation Safety

Many diagnostics in medicine and surgery are aided by the use of diagnostic imaging. Therefore the technicians should be aware of the hazards of using x-rays or any other type of ionizing radiation. Ionizing radiation causes the loss of an electron from an atom, changing the atom's electrical charge. It must be kept in mind that all tissues are made of atoms and thus can be damaged by ionization. It is the entire veterinary medical staff's responsibility to ensure that proper radiation safety measures are observed in the hospital. The practice should provide instruction on the proper use of all X-ray–generating equipment and safety devices and ensure that the design of the x-ray room meets state regulations.

All animal tissues are sensitive to radiation, and absorption of radiation doses above a certain amount will change or alter the tissue. The following tissues (not in order of sensitivity) are most readily affected by ionizing radiation: skin, lymphatics, hematopoietic and leukopoietic tissues, breast, thyroid, bone, and the germinal epithelium or gonads. These tissues are sensitive to all forms of ionizing radiation, especially those that are composed of rapidly dividing cells, such as gonadal tissue. All animal species are affected, including humans, which means that it is important to consider the safety of the patient and of the clinic personnel exposed to radiation.

There are two major concerns regarding the technician's exposure to x-rays. The first is called *stochastic effects*, which result from accumulation of radiation doses over a period of time. The damage may not be evident right away but may take years of exposure for effects to manifest. Some examples of this damage are malignancies, anemias, sterility, and cataracts. It is also possible for technicians to experience *deterministic effects*, or effects seen shortly after exposure, such as sunburns; however, these are uncommon.

The second concern is *genetic effects*, which occur when radiation damages the DNA of the recipient's reproductive cells. This damage is generally not seen in the lifetime of the recipient but in future generations, including grandchildren. These effects occur not only in humans but also in the animals being radiographed. Therefore the safety of both the patient and the technician is of utmost importance. Although cases of death from radiation exposure resulting from medical imaging have not been documented, the risk of damage caused by radiation must be considered.

Radiation Exposure

Technician exposure occurs in three ways. The first is exposure to the *primary beam* as it comes out of the tube. Technicians should be trained to avoid exposure to this higher energy x-ray beam, even if lead shielding is worn. Lead does not absorb the higher energy, allowing the primary beam to pass through and cause exposure. Thus lead does not protect the technician from primary radiation. Using a collimator that has a light source to illuminate the area of study can be helpful in ensuring that human restrainers are outside of the primary field.

The second method of exposure is from *scatter radiation*, which is the main culprit behind exposure of technicians to radiation. Scatter is produced when an object, usually the patient, interacts with the path of the primary beam. Because scatter is produced in all directions, it can travel to the technician, causing exposure. Lead shielding is worn to absorb scatter radiation before it enters the technician's body. Collimating to the smallest field size possible will also be effective in reducing the amount of scatter radiation produced.

The third method of exposure is to *leakage radiation*. This very rarely occurs with newer machines, which provide adequate filtration of lower level x-rays coming from the tube.

Radiation Filtration

The x-ray beam is a spectrum of x-ray photons of various energy levels. The useful portion of the x-ray beam (the portion that passes through the patient to interact with film and screens) is the upper two-thirds of the energy levels. The lower third of the x-ray beam energy is too weak to pass through the patient. This radiation is called *soft radiation*. It is of no use for image formation and only causes increased radiation exposure for the patient and potentially the technician. Insertion of a 2.5-mm aluminum filter into the path of the primary beam at the window of the x-ray tube is essential to filter out the soft x-rays. By absorbing this soft radiation, the filter reduces the amount of radiation absorbed by the patient. Increased aluminum filtration also generally improves contrast and detail by improving the quality of the x-ray beam, as previously discussed.

Radiation Measurement

To understand radiation safety and radiation dose units of measurement, it is necessary to define a few terms commonly used in the measurement of radiation exposure: *absorbed dose* and *dose equivalent*.

Absorbed Dose. The previously used unit of absorbed dose of ionizing radiation is the rad. It is the energy imparted by ionizing radiation to a unit mass of irradiated material. The number of rads

deposited in tissue varies with the energy of the x-ray beam and with the composition of the absorber. A newer unit has recently replaced rad to measure this radiation, called *Gray (Gy)*. To convert from Gy to rad, use the following conversion factor: 1 Gy = 100 rad. This unit, however, is more likely to be used when encountering higher doses of radiation.

Dose Equivalent. *Rem* is an abbreviation (for "roentgen equivalent man") used to refer to the equivalent dose, which is more commonly used to measure radiation exposure of persons, such as veterinary technicians, who encounter minimal amounts through the course of their work. It is the product of the dose in rads and the relative biological effectiveness of the radiation used. This unit of measurement makes allowance for the fact that the effect of radiation on different tissues varies with the type of radiation or the relative biological effectiveness. A rem is equal to the absorbed radiation dose in rads multiplied by a quality factor:

$$Rem = Rads \times Qualityfactor$$

The unit *rem* has more recently been replaced by the unit *Sievert* (Sv). To convert from rem to Sievert, use the following conversion: 1 Sv = 100 rem

Maximum Permissible Dose. The **maximum permissible dose (MPD)** is the maximum dose of radiation a person is allowed to receive during occupational exposure over a specified time. If an individual receives more than the MPD, they are more likely to have physical effects from radiation exposure. The MPD for occupational personnel is 0.05 Sv per year. The MPD for nonoccupational personnel should be no greater than 0.005 Sv per year. Embryo or fetus exposures are reduced to 0.5mSv/month to allow for minimal exposure to the rapidly dividing fetal cells.

The technician should remember that in the United States, MPD is determined by the International Commission of Radiological Protection (ICRP) and the National Council of Radiation Protection and Measurements (NCRP) as the dose not harmful to the person receiving it during their lifetime. MPD is the maximum occupational exposure allowed by law; technicians should try to keep radiation exposure as low as possible by carefully following radiation safety practices. Many other governing bodies, including the Occupational Safety and Health Administration (OSHA) and state health departments, aid in the regulation of proper safety measures.

Personal Monitoring Dosimetry. **Dosimetry** is the measurement of personal radiation exposure. To protect staff members from overexposure, the radiation that each person receives can be measured on a personal dosimeter.

There are two types of personal dosimeters commonly used in veterinary medicine. The first is a *thermoluminescent dosimeter* (TLD). The TLD can store collected measurements over an extended period and can be reused after being read. The TLD contains a chamber of specialized compounds such as lithium and calcium fluoride. When exposed to ionizing radiation, the electrons of the fluoride move to a higher energy state and remain in the higher state until the badge is processed. During processing, the badge is heated, which allows the electrons to return to the ground state, causing the emission of visible

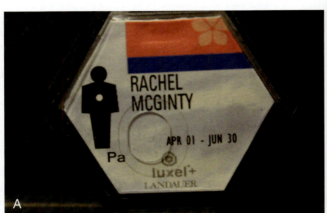

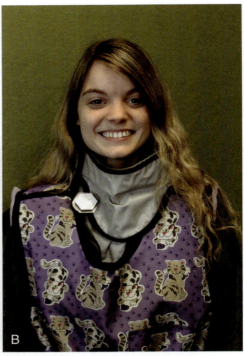

• **Fig. 15.24** (A) The optically stimulated luminescence (OSL) badge is a method of dosimetry used to monitor radiation exposure. Each technician working in radiology should have one. (B) The film badge should be worn outside the lead apron at the level of the upper neck. This technician wears a thyroid shield in addition to gloves and an apron when radiographic exposures are taken.

light or fluorescence. The amount of fluorescence relative to the temperature is used to determine the dose of radiation the badge received.

The second type of dosimeter is the optically stimulated luminescence (OSL) dosimeter (Fig. 15.24). OSL dosimeters operate much like a TLD but use aluminum oxide inside of the chamber rather than lithium fluoride, creating a different type of fluorescence during processing. During processing, a laser rather than heat is used to stimulate the exposed aluminum oxide. When the laser is directed at the aluminum oxide, it becomes luminescent in proportion to the amount of exposure received.

These dosimeters are mailed back to the manufacturing company and are analyzed/reported on a monthly, quarterly, or biannual basis. To ensure that there has been no lapse in monitoring, the badge service will send a replacement badge when it is time to return the one that is worn. Technicians operating imaging equipment using radiation should insist that the practice provide them with a radiation-monitoring device.

TECHNICIAN NOTE

A dosimeter should be worn outside the collar of the apron or on the thyroid collar (see Fig. 15.24B) every time the technician is potentially exposed to ionizing radiation.

Protection Officer. Every veterinary hospital should have a designated employee who is responsible for ensuring radiation safety. The employee's tasks should include maintaining dosimeters, ensuring that the x-ray machine is properly calibrated, and maintaining a good exposure control system that includes an updated technique chart. Low-exposure techniques that provide quality diagnostic radiographs should be the goal. Safe, reliable radiography equipment that is clean and, in the case of digital equipment, calibrated correctly, with software that is regularly updated and has a server that can handle the quantity of data necessary to efficiently operate the veterinary practice, is imperative. A reliable shielding program *requiring* all staff to follow the ALARA ("As Low As Reasonably Achievable") principle whenever an image is being exposed is equally important. The employee in charge of this essential part of the veterinary practice must ensure that compliance with all government regulations is strictly maintained.

PUT INTO PRACTICE

Becoming your practice's protection officer offers you a way to become an invaluable asset for your practice and ensures the safety of your coworkers and patients.

Protection Practices

- Always collimate to the smallest field size possible for the anatomic area of interest (Fig. 15.25) to reduce scatter radiation and limit the exposure area.
- A 2.5-mm aluminum filter should be used to reduce exposure to low-energy x-rays coming from the tube.
- Retakes must be prevented by setting correct exposure factors and properly positioning the patient the first time.
- The technician should never permit any part of the body, whether shielded or not, to encounter the primary beam.
- The technician should always wear a well-maintained apron, thyroid shield, and gloves (Fig. 15.26) when restraining an animal. Gonadal shields and lead glasses should also be available to all relevant personnel.

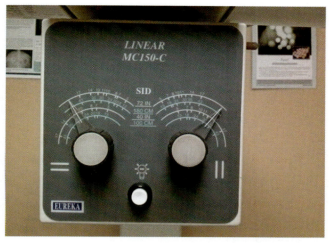

• **Fig. 15.25** A collimator is used to limit the size of the x-ray beam to the part to be examined. By coning down on the area of interest, the amount of scatter radiation can be drastically reduced, improving image quality and decreasing technician exposure.

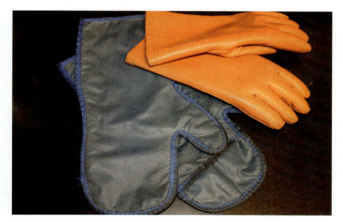

• **Fig. 15.26** Lead gloves should have a minimum of 0.5 mm of lead equivalent; 1 mm of lead equivalent is ideal. They should always be worn when restraint is needed for examination.

- The technician should use accessory equipment designed to reduce radiation exposure whenever possible, such as image receptor holders for large-animal extremity radiography and restraint and positioning devices for small-animal radiography (Fig. 15.27).
- Anesthesia or tranquilization of the patient should be provided every time an animal cannot be controlled easily and adequately for a given examination.
- Only required personnel should be in the x-ray room at the time of exposure. Personnel assisting with radiographic exposures should also be rotated to reduce personal exposure.
- Individuals younger than 18 years of age should not be permitted in the x-ray room during exposures as they have cells that are constantly going through mitosis and are much more sensitive to ionizing radiation.
- Pregnant women should make efforts to reduce radiation exposure to the embryo or fetus. The use of a monthly fetal dosimeter, worn under the lead apron at waist level, will help to monitor fetal exposure.

- While restraining animals manually, personnel should always look away and stand up straight at the end of the table to increase the distance from the primary beam.
- *Dose creep* is a term used in DR to describe the incremental increases in technique made to reduce the amount of noise adversely affecting the quality of the image. This increases exposure to personnel and the patient. Good-quality fast screens should be used to lower the mAs settings as much as possible.
- The x-ray tube should never be held in the hand while it is being activated, nor should it be aimed directly at personnel or adjacent occupied rooms.
- The x-ray machine should be calibrated on a regular basis to ensure proper amounts of exposure from the tube.
- Radiation safety codes for the state of residence must be followed.

Radiation safety is a habit that requires awareness of the danger of radiation. It is easy to become careless about radiation, because it is invisible, tasteless, and odorless, and produces no external stimulation at diagnostic levels. Technicians should always remember that radiation is dangerous to one's health and can destroy all living tissue if the absorbed doses are high enough.

The big three methods of radiation protection to keep in mind are (1) time, (2) distance, and (3) shielding. *Time* means avoiding retakes; the rule to keep in mind is "Do it right the first time." The time of exposure should be minimized; the mAs setting should be as low as possible but still produce diagnostic radiographs. Decreasing exposure time decreases the number of x-rays leaving the tube and minimizes overall exposure. *Distance* means staying as far away as possible from the patient and the x-ray beam. This decreases the intensity of the beam, reducing exposure. Standing up straight at the end of the table, looking away from the beam, or not being in the room at all will help keep a safe distance. *Shielding* refers to having a lead barrier between the source of the radiation and oneself. In some types of imaging, this may be a lead wall or window; however, in veterinary medicine, this is only possible when manual restraint of the patient is not needed, such as when the patient is anesthetized for CT. When restraining a patient in a situation where no wall is possible, it is important to always wear an apron, gloves, and a thyroid collar with a 0.5-mm lead equivalent to ensure effective protection from scatter radiation. Use of lead eyewear is becoming common practice in veterinary medicine to decrease damage to the lens of the eye. Most practices provide PPE to technicians, or technicians may purchase these items themselves.

It is important to take care of the apron and gloves. Aprons and thyroid collars should be hung carefully after use and never folded (Fig. 15.28), because this can cause the lead to bend and then crack, allowing radiation to get through to the technician. Gloves should also be hung vertically so that there is air flow through the interior of the gloves. If hanging the glove is not possible, cut-end soup cans may be inserted into the glove to allow for air flow when the gloves are laid down in the horizontal position.

TECHNICIAN NOTE

When working in radiology, always remember the three main components of radiation safety:

1. Time. Reduce retakes by doing it right the first time and use the minimal exposure time whenever possible.
2. Distance. Stay as far away as possible from the patient who produces scatter and the x-ray beam. Increasing distance = reduced exposure.
3. Shielding. Keep lead barrier between the radiation source and oneself, such as a lead wall, aprons, thyroid collars, and gloves.

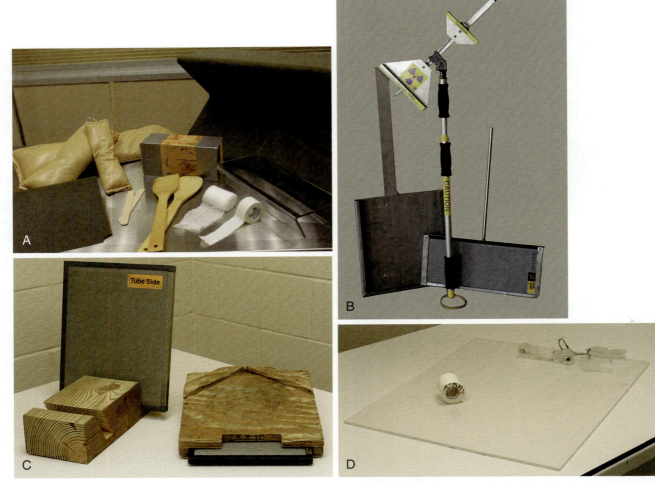

• **Fig. 15.27** Several commercially available positioning devices can be used to help position animals and reduce the time needed to perform the examination. (A) Various foam wedges and sandbags used to position small animals, along with tape, tongue depressors, wood blocks, wooden spoons, and gauze. (B) Cassette holders for large-animal examinations. (C) Wood blocks for examination of large-animal feet. (D) Lucite tray with neck restraint holder for avian radiology. Porous tape is used to position the wings of anesthetized birds.

PPE should be inspected periodically for any signs of wear and tear (inconsistencies in the lead) and should be checked before every use. All lead protective devices should be radiographed annually to check for any cracks more thoroughly.

Positioning

Proper positioning of the patient is essential to obtain diagnostic radiographs and avoid misdiagnoses. With improper positioning, retake of the radiograph is necessary, increasing radiation exposure to the patient and the restrainers. Veterinary technicians work to ensure that patients are positioned properly for diagnostic views.

> **TECHNICIAN NOTE**
>
> Proper positioning is essential to obtain diagnostic radiographs.

Principles of Positioning

Because radiographs are two-dimensional images of three-dimensional structures, the technician should remember that two views at right angles are necessary to obtain a diagnostic image. Exceptions to this rule include examinations in traumatized or debilitated animals when only lateral views can be taken without causing undue stress.

Another principle that should be kept in mind is the importance of centering the primary beam on the area of interest. This is especially important in orthopedic cases. For example, fracture healing may look different when the x-ray beam is centered over the fracture line as opposed to a short distance away from it. Placing the area of interest under the primary beam also helps the technician ensure that all anatomic structures required for diagnosis are included and that tight collimation can be completed to include only the necessary anatomy.

It is important to use an image field that is sufficiently large to completely capture the area to be examined. When radiographing large dogs, it may be necessary to take two exposures of the abdomen, one of the cranial abdomen and the other of the caudal abdomen, to include all anatomic areas needed for diagnosis. When radiographing long bones, the joints both proximal and distal to the bone should be included. When radiographing joints,

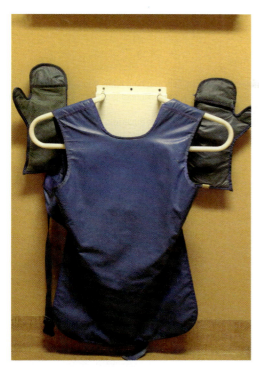

• **Fig. 15.28** Aprons and gloves on a holder. It is important to keep the apron on a stand and the gloves well aerated when not in use. The apron should have a minimum of 0.5 mm of lead equivalent.

one-third of the long bones proximal and distal to the joint should be included. In some cases, the limb opposite to the limb of interest is radiographed for comparison views.

The area of interest should also be positioned as close to the image receptor as possible to minimize distortion. The thickest portion of the anatomic area should be placed under the cathode side of the tube to take advantage of the heel effect. These principles are basic but essential. It is not the intent of this chapter to discuss positioning at length. Tables 15.3 and 15.4 provide basic guidelines for positioning patients for common views in veterinary practice. Refer to excellent discussions on this topic by Brown and Brown (2022), Butler et al. (2008), Han et al. (2005), Morgan (1993), and Sirois et al. (2010) (see the "Recommended Readings" section). Proper positioning is achieved through practice. A positioning reference textbook, such as those listed above, should be available in the radiology room of every veterinary practice.

Large-animal radiography is mostly performed in the field, often on equine limbs, by using portable x-ray units. The horse should be kept in the natural standing position with minimal restraint, when possible, or in stocks. Sedation may be required to keep the patient calm during the procedure. The limb should be dry and clean of artifactual debris. When radiographing the foot, the shoe is removed, the sole cleaned, and the frog packed with Play-Doh. Table 15.3 lists the common radiographic projections used when radiographing the equine limb. Ancillary and oblique views are extremely important in equine radiography to ensure visibility of all anatomic structures in need of evaluation. Refer to earlier text for more details.

Patient Preparation and Restraint

Before the patient is radiographed, the technician should remove anything that contains metal, such as a collar, leash, or harness, from the patient. If possible, bandages and splints should be removed from the patient, along with any debris that may be on the patient's haircoat, which leaves artifacts that may be seen over anatomic areas of interest on the radiograph. When performing abdominal views, it may be necessary to make sure that the patient is free of ingesta before placing the animal onto the table. This may be done by walking the patient outside or potentially administering an enema before radiographic exposure.

Many types of restraint may be used, including manual, mechanical, and chemical restraints. For radiation safety, manual restraint should be avoided as a routine procedure to reduce exposure to personnel. In some states, manual restraint of the patient during radiography is prohibited. However, when it is essential to be in the room with the animal, lead protective gear should be worn by the technician, and the x-ray beam should be limited to the area of interest through proper collimation.

Mechanical restraint is available in various forms. One of the most useful and inexpensive devices for use with dogs is a simple muzzle, which often has a calming effect. Sandbags, gauze, tape, wooden spoons, foam wedges, compression bands, V-troughs, and U-troughs can also be used to obtain excellent positioning. Once the animal has been positioned properly, it is most important to perform the exposures rapidly to reduce patient motion artifacts.

Chemical restraint can be achieved with tranquilizers, analgesics, or anesthetics and should be used every time total immobility or relaxation is required for proper positioning. In many circumstances, tranquilization is adequate to control most animals and is excellent for control of frightened or aggressive animals. Positioning aids used with chemical restraint allow reduction of exposure to the technician, because manual restraint may no longer be required (Fig. 15.29). It must be kept in mind that in some instances, the patient may not be medically stable enough to undergo chemical sedation for radiographic procedures, and the welfare and comfort of the patient should be given more importance than achieving perfect positioning. Often, diagnostic-quality images can still be achieved.

> **TECHNICIAN NOTE**
>
> Chemical restraint has contributed greatly to the progress made in radiology by allowing positioning that otherwise would be impossible to achieve. Chemical restraint used with positioning devices also allows for a "hands-off" approach to positioning, reducing technician exposure.

Radiographic Contrast Agents

In many radiographic examinations, natural or inherent contrast of the anatomy is insufficient for a diagnosis to be made; this is especially true in gastrointestinal (GI), urogenital, and spinal cord diseases. Furthermore, contrast agents may also be utilized in other diagnostic imaging modalities such as fluoroscopy, CT, and MRI. In veterinary medicine, two groups of contrast media are used: positive and negative.

Positive contrast media are those that appear white or radiopaque on the image (Fig. 15.30). Negative contrast media appear black or radiolucent (Fig. 15.31). Adding a contrast medium to a structure increases the density difference between that structure and the surrounding structures, giving the image higher contrast and increasing the likelihood of correct image interpretation.

TABLE 15.3 Positioning Tips for Common Radiographic Views

Area of Interest	Routine Views Exposed	Positioning Tips
Abdomen	*Most common views:* • VD • Right lateral *Ancillary views:* • DV views: for compromised patients and contrast studies • Left lateral views: for vomiting patients and contrast studies	• Forelimbs extended cranially and hind limbs caudally • Include areas just cranial to the xiphoid process and just caudal to the greater trochanters • VD: spine and sternum should be superimposed • Lateral: spine and sternum positioned parallel to the x-ray table • Expose during the expiratory pause
Thorax	• Right and/or left lateral views • Ventrodorsal or dorsoventral views Thorax notes: • VD view preferred for imaging the lungs and mediastinal area and evaluation of pleural effusion • DV view preferred for imaging the heart and dorsal lung fields, diagnosing pneumothorax, and imaging patients in respiratory distress • Three views of the thorax may be required for proper diagnosis; views included are left lateral, right lateral, and a DV or VD view	• Forelimbs extended cranially and hind limbs caudally • Include the thoracic inlet and just caudal to the 13th rib. Include spine and sternum on lateral views. • VD/DV: spine and sternum should be superimposed • Lateral: spine and sternum positioned parallel to the x-ray table • Expose views during full inspiration

Forelimb
• Scapula, shoulder and humerus
• Elbow and radius/ulna
• Carpus/metacarpals and digits
	• Lateral (mediolateral): affected side down
	• Caudocranial
	Ancillary views:
	• CrCd views of the humerus may be exposed as an alternative to CdCr
	• Lateral (mediolateral): affected side down
	• Craniocaudal
	Ancillary views:
	• Hyperflexed lateral views of the elbow are used in evaluation of elbow dysplasia, osteochondrosis, and nonunited anconeal processes
	• Lateral (mediolateral): affected side down
	• Dorsopalmar
	Ancillary views:
	• Hyperextended and hyperflexed lateral views of the foot are used to evaluate joint laxity and lesions that may not be visible on regular lateral views. The use of a wooden spoon or tape will allow for holding the extension or flexion. Be careful to not extend/flex beyond the patient's normal range of motion.
		• Lateral: head extended slightly dorsally, affected limb extended cranioventrally, and contralateral limb extended caudoventrally
		• CdCr: position in dorsal recumbency, extend both forelimbs as cranially as possible to keep the forearm at full extension and as parallel as possible to the table, position head lateral from affected limb
		Include:
		• Scapula: caudal border of the scapula and the shoulder joint
		• Shoulder: distal third of the scapula to proximal third of the humerus
		• Humerus: shoulder and elbow joints
		• CdCr views of the humerus will show some distortion due to the humerus not being parallel to the image receptor
		• Lateral: head positioned slightly dorsally, affected limb extended cranially, contralateral limb extended caudodorsally
		• Craniocaudal: position in sternal recumbency, head pulled dorsally or abducted from view, forelimbs extended cranially, unaffected limb abducted from view. It is important for the limb to be at full extension with the olecranon between the humeral condyles.
		• Include:
		  • Elbow: distal third of the humerus to the proximal third of the radius/ulna
		  • Radius/Ulna: elbow to the carpus
		• Lateral: Head positioned slightly dorsally, affected limb extended cranially, contralateral limb extended caudodorsally
		• Dorsopalmar: Position in sternal recumbency, head positioned dorsally or lateral to the affected limb, limb of interest extended cranially, elbow abducted slightly so carpus rests directly on the table, contralateral limb abducted from the view
		• Include:
		  • Carpus: distal radius/ulna to the proximal third of the metacarpals
		  • Metacarpals/digits: Proximal carpus to the distal phalanges

• Pelvis	• Lateral: affected side down • VD extended views: • Commonly used to evaluate for hip dysplasia and OFA certification *Ancillary views:* • VD: frog-leg positioning can be used in cases of fractures or trauma where the patient is too painful for limb extension	• Lateral: place the affected side down in a true lateral position (positioning wedges may be necessary) head in a natural position, forelimbs pulled cranially, slightly scissor the hind limbs so the limb closest to the table is slightly cranial to the contralateral limb, slightly flex the stifles • VD: position in dorsal recumbency, with the head and forelimbs extended cranially and the hind limbs extended caudally until resistance is felt Holding the tarsus, rotate the femurs and stifles medially. The tail should be aligned with the rest of the spine. • Proper positioning of the VD is imperative. Ensure that the pelvis is without rotation and symmetric on either side, the femurs are parallel to one another, the patellae lie in the trochlear grooves • Include: tip of the iliac wings to the distal patellae

TABLE 15.3   Positioning Tips for Common Radiographic Views—cont'd

Area of Interest	Routine Views Exposed	Positioning Tips

Pelvic limb
• Femur
• Stifle and tibia/fibula
• Tarsus, metatarsal, and digits
	• Lateral (mediolateral): affected limb down
	• Craniocaudal
	Ancillary views:
	• Caudocranial
	• Lateral (mediolateral): affected side down
	• Caudocranial
	Ancillary views:
	• Craniocaudal: can be used as an alternative; however, distortion of stifle occurs
	• Lateral (mediolateral): affected limb down
	• Plantar–dorsal
	Ancillary views:
	• Flexed/extended lateral of the tarsus
	• Dorsoplantar: distortion is possible on the distal third of the tibia/fibula
		• Lateral: place affected side down, hind limbs scissor positioned with affected limb extended slightly cranioventral and slightly flexed, contralateral limb flexed and abducted out of the view
		• Craniocaudal: Position in dorsal recumbency; extend both femurs caudally until resistance is felt; holding the tarsus, rotate the femurs medially so patellae lie in trochlear grooves. Center the beam over the femur of interest.
		• Include the coxofemoral joint to the stifle
		• Lateral: place affected side down, position affected limb extended slightly cranioventral and slightly flexed, contralateral limb flexed and abducted out of the view
		• Caudocranial: sternal recumbency, extend the affected limb caudally, rotate the limb medially so the patella is centered in the trochlear groove, with the contralateral limb flexed and abducted out of the view
		• Include:
		  • Stifle: distal third of the femur to the proximal third of the tibia/fibula
		  • Tibia/fibula: stifle to the tarsus
		• Lateral: place affected side down, position affected limb extended slightly cranioventrally and slightly flexed, contralateral limb flexed and abducted out of the view
		• Plantar–dorsal: sternal recumbency, extend affected limb caudally, rotating the limb medially to align the foot with the femur, stifle and tibia/fibula
		• Include:
		  • Tarsus: distal third of the tibia/fibula and proximal third of the metatarsals
		  • Metatarsals and digits: tarsus and distal phalanges

Vertebral column	• Lateral
	• Ventrodorsal
	  • VD views are preferred to prevent distortion
	Note: Dorsoventral views are not recommended due to the possibility of distortion.
	Ancillary views:
	• Hyperextended and hyperflexed views may be beneficial when radiographing the cervical and lumbosacral spine
		• Lateral: lateral recumbency, forelimbs extended cranially, hind limbs extended caudally, head extended cranially, and tail caudally
		• It is important to keep the vertebral column as parallel to the table as possible by placing foam under the muzzle and cervical lumbar vertebra and between the hind limbs
		• VD: dorsal recumbency, forelimbs extended cranially at even extension, position the head so the nose is parallel to the table, hind limbs kept in a natural position
		• It is important to ensure the patient is in a true VD position with the spine and sternum superimposed
		• Include:
		  • Cervical: base of the skull to T1
		  • Thoracic/lumbar/sacral: one vertebra cranial and caudal to the area of interest
		  • Caudal spine (tail): full tail or 4–5 vertebra cranial and caudal to area of interest

Skull	• Lateral: affected side down • Dorsoventral: preferred view for better symmetry • *Ancillary views:* used to evaluate various regions of the skull and are chosen based on the study required	• Lateral: lateral recumbency with affected side down, head in a natural position, and forelimbs extended caudally. Ensure proper symmetry of the skull by having the mandible perpendicular to the table. • Dorsoventral: sternal recumbency, head and neck extended with the ears lateral to the head, forelimbs extended cranially alongside the head and out of the view. Ensure proper symmetry of the skull. • Include: the tip of the nose to the base of the skull

CrCd, Craniocaudal; *CdCr*, caudocranial; *DV*, dorsoventral; *OFA*, Orthopedic Foundation for Animals; *VD*, ventrodorsal.

Positive Contrast Materials

Many types of positive contrast agents can be used in diagnostic imaging. The agent of choice depends on the area of interest. Positive contrast agents include barium sulfate and organic iodide agents, including both ionic and nonionic iodides.

Barium sulfate has a high atomic number and absorbs a large amount of radiation, resulting in greatly increased radiographic opacity (whiteness). It is used almost exclusively for upper and lower GI tract examinations. Barium sulfate is inert, nonabsorbed, and soothing to the GI tract. It does not alter the physiologic function of the GI tract, which makes it useful for

TABLE 15.4	Common Equine Limb Views
Area of Interest	**Common Views**
Carpus/tarsus and distal limb	• Dorsopalmar/plantar and lateromedial views *Ancillary views:* • Specific anatomic areas require flexed, extended, and oblique views
Radius and elbow	• Craniocaudal and lateromedial views *Ancillary views:* • Caudocranial and oblique views
Shoulder	• Lateromedial *Ancillary views:* • Oblique views
Stifle	• Lateromedial • Caudocranial *Ancillary views:* • Craniocaudal and oblique views

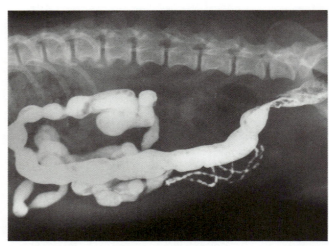

• **Fig. 15.30** Barium, a positive contrast material, is used to perform an upper gastrointestinal (GI) study of a canine patient. Barium is radiopaque and absorbs x-rays, causing the area of interest to show up white on the radiograph and increasing the contrast of the GI tract.

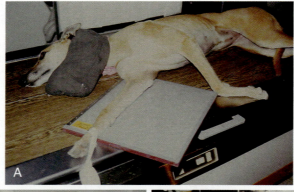

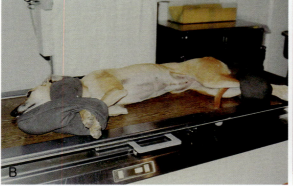
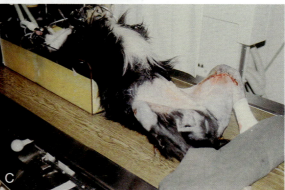

• **Fig. 15.29** (A) Sandbags and porous tape can help position tranquilized patients for some extremity radiographs. (B) Sandbags can take the place of manual restraint for lateral thoracic and abdominal radiographs. (C) The use of Lucite or Plexiglass positioning trays and sandbags can often take the place of manual restraint in postoperative radiography.

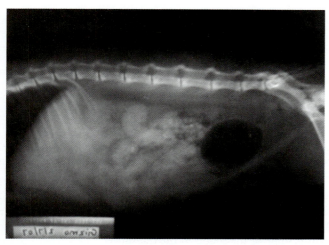

• **Fig. 15.31** Air, a negative contrast material, is used to perform a pneumocystogram on a feline patient. The air is radiolucent, allowing for more x-rays to penetrate through the urinary bladder, causing it to appear darker. This increases the contrast of the bladder to allow for enhanced visualization of smaller stones or clumps of crystals.

viewing serial images that show GI function. It coats the GI mucosa better compared with organic iodides, improving visualization of the luminal surface. Barium sulfate is available in powder, paste, or liquid form, and can be administered orally or rectally to the patient. Contraindications for use include severe constipation and upper or lower bowel perforations. Because barium is insoluble, the body cannot break it down if the barium travels outside of the GI tract. If this occurs, the barium should be surgically flushed out of the peritoneal cavity. As with all oral contrast media, care should be taken when treating patients with a high risk of aspiration.

Soluble radiopaque ionic contrast media include iothalamate and diatrizoate. These products can be used orally for GI examinations; intravascularly for venous or arterial studies and excretory urography; in the peritoneal cavity, bladder, and urethra; intra-articularly; in draining wounds for fistulography; and in salivary ducts for sialography. Ionic organic iodides should not be used in the respiratory tract, nor should they be used intrathecally for myelography. Ionic iodides are essentially hyperosmolar salt solutions, so when used intravascularly, they can cause an increase in intravascular fluid volume followed by osmotic diuresis. The hyperosmolarity can cause diarrhea when ionic iodides are administered orally. Because of these properties, these agents are contraindicated in dehydrated patients and in patients with known iodine sensitivity.

The newest class of positive contrast agents includes the nonionic organic iodides, represented by iohexol, iopamidol, and iotolan. These agents can be used in a similar manner to ionic organic iodides but offer the advantage of not dissociating into positively and negatively charged ions in solution. This allows the agents to be used intrathecally for myelography and everywhere ionic iodides can be used. These contrast agents are also hyperosmolar but much less so than the ionic organic iodides. They appear to have a lower incidence of adverse effects and contrast reactions but with the disadvantage of increased costs. Organic iodides (both ionic and nonionic) may cause serious reactions or adverse effects when given intravenously, intra-arterially, or intrathecally. These reactions are much less likely when the agents are used orally. Contrast reactions include nausea and vomiting, hypotension, cardiac

arrest, and anaphylaxis. These reactions occur infrequently, but it is advisable to have a catheter in place and to have rapid access to fluids, oxygen, endotracheal tubes, and cardiopulmonary resuscitation drugs during organic iodide contrast procedures.

> **TECHNICIAN NOTE**
> Whenever using organic iodides for contrast studies, constant monitoring of the patient for adverse reactions is required throughout the procedure.

Negative Contrast Materials and Double Contrast

Radiolucent gases absorb very small amounts of radiation, resulting in images of increased radiographic density. Examples of these gases include air, nitrous oxide, oxygen, and carbon dioxide. Gases are generally used to distend hollow structures in the body but do not produce as much mucosal detail as positive contrasts can. Caution must be used when inflating structures with gas, because overinflation may cause the structure to rupture, with release of gas into compartments of the body. If room air is used and rupture occurs, an embolism may result. Oxygen or carbon dioxide are safer options.

Some studies may require the use of double contrast. This method uses both positive and negative contrast media for better views of structures. The negative medium is introduced first to inflate the structure, followed by the positive medium to delineate better mucosal detail. Double contrast is used in gastrography and cystography.

Radiographic contrast studies are no longer commonplace in private practice due to advanced methods of imaging, such as DUS and endoscopy; all allow for quicker visual and functional assessment of anatomic areas. However, one radiographic contrast study that is still commonly performed in practice is the upper GI study. This study is outlined in Procedure 15.1. For a thorough discussion of contrast media and procedures, see "Recommended Readings".

Ultrasonography

Ultrasound imaging has become an essential diagnostic tool in veterinary practice. The equipment is portable; the use of ionizing radiation is not required; and the procedure is noninvasive, well tolerated by patients, and accepted by clients. Veterinary technicians should familiarize themselves with the basics of DUS but must remember that ultrasonography is user dependent—image quality and interpretation are only as good as the skills of the person performing the examination. For this reason, supplemental training is usually required. This text covers the basics of ultrasonography. Refer to "Recommended Readings" for further discussion on veterinary ultrasonography.

Ultrasonography Basics

Sound is a mechanical pressure wave made up of a series of compressions and rarefactions transmitted through a medium that encompasses ultrasonography. Sound waves are characterized by wavelength or distance between compressions, frequency in cycles per second, and velocity or speed of transmission (Fig. 15.32). These characteristics are integrated by the following formula:

$$\text{Velocity} = \text{Wavelength} \times \text{Frequency}$$

For simplicity, assume that the speed of sound in the body is 1540 m per second. As the frequency of sound increases, the

PROCEDURE 15.1

Upper Gastrointestinal Positive Contrast Study

An upper gastrointestinal (GI) study allows for increased contrast of the stomach, small intestine and, if desired, the large intestine.

Indications

Unresponsive vomiting, diarrhea, melena, hematemesis, anorexia, suspected foreign body or obstruction, wall distortions and lesions, abdominal organ displacement, persistent weight loss or abdominal pain, and observation of GI function.

Precautions

- In cases of suspected rupture of the GI tract, water-soluble iodide should be used in place of barium.
- Iodides should be used only in well-hydrated patients.
- The use of tranquilizers or other sedatives may increase transit time. Acepromazine may be used in dogs and ketamine may be used in cats if sedation is required for restraint.
- In compromised patients or those with specific GI abnormalities, such as gastric dilatation-volvulus (GDV) or ileus, other methods of imaging, such as endoscopy or ultrasonography, should be considered.

Patient Preparation

- Exposure of survey images, including ventrodorsal (VD) and lateral abdominal views.
- The patient should be free of ingesta.
  - Fasting for 12–24 hours is recommended in patients that are not anorexic or vomiting.
  - Enemas may be considered at least 2–4 hours prior to the study.
- Barium may be administered orally into the buccal pouch, mixed with food for patient consumption, or given through an orogastric tube.
- Contrast:
- Barium sulfate 60% weight/volume (w/v):
  - Dogs:
    - <20 kg: 8–12 mL/kg
    - >20 kg: 5–7 mL/kg
  - Cats:
    - 12–20 mL/kg
- Water-soluble organic iodide (Brown and Brown [2018], see Recommended Readings):
  - Dogs: 2–3 mL/kg
  - Cats: 1–3 mL/kg

Procedure

- Immediately after administration of contrast, expose VD, dorsoventral (DV), left lateral, and right lateral views.
  - Four views are recommended for complete evaluation of the stomach. Fewer views may be sufficient if study is focused more on the intestines.
- Subsequent views (VD and right lateral) should be exposed at 15 minutes, 30 minutes, and 60 minutes after barium administration.
- VD and right lateral views are repeated hourly after barium administration until the barium reaches the colon.

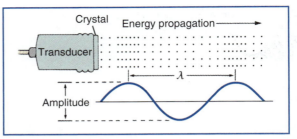

• **Fig. 15.32** Sound wave with wavelength = λ. *Closely spaced dots*, compressions; *widely spaced dots*, rarefactions. The amplitude is proportional to the loudness.

is produced from the transducer and transmitted into the patient. The sound wave strikes an echogenic surface in the patient and returns some of the sound to the transducer. The strength of the returning sound wave determines the brightness of the image, and the time it takes for the sound to travel into the patient and back to the transducer determines where the echo will be seen on the screen.

Ultrasound production and reception are based on the piezoelectric effect. A piezoelectric crystal will change shape or thickness when subjected to a voltage pulse. Rapid pulses of electrical energy are converted into mechanical energy or sound waves by the vibrating crystal. Returning sound waves cause the crystal to vibrate, and that mechanical energy is converted into electrical energy by the transducer, which is then transformed into the grayscale image on the screen. The transducer acts as both the sound transmitter and the receiver. The operating frequency of the transducer is partially determined by the thickness of the piezoelectric crystal. The thinner the crystal, the higher the transducer frequency. The transducer transmits sound 0.01% of the time. It receives returning sound waves 99.9% of the time.

TECHNICIAN NOTE

Ultrasound production and reception are based on the piezoelectric effect. As the piezoelectric crystal changes in thickness, the frequency of the sound waves changes, increasing or decreasing image resolution and imaging depth.

Ultrasound-tissue Interaction

To better understand the ultrasound image, it is important to understand the interaction of ultrasound within tissues. As the sound wave proceeds through the body, it is progressively attenuated or weakened. This attenuation limits the depth of penetration of the sound wave and thus limits the depth of structures that can be effectively imaged. The ultrasound beam is attenuated or weakened by absorption, reflection, scattering, refraction, and diffraction. Reflection is a redirection of the sound beam back to the transducer and is the basis for the diagnostic image. Absorption is sound energy converted to heat within the tissues. Scattering is the intertissue microreflection of sound, which is responsible for much of the echo texture of various organs. Refraction and diffraction are the result of bending of the sound beam as it crosses areas of differing tissue densities. Refraction attenuation is important in the generation of several ultrasound artifacts.

Sound reflection or echo production forms the basis of the ultrasound image. An echo is produced whenever the ultrasound beam crosses an acoustic interface. An acoustic interface is the

wavelength decreases. Shorter sound waves produce increased image resolution but decreased patient penetration. The frequencies used in veterinary DUS generally range from 2.5 to 12 megahertz (MHz). A **hertz (Hz)** is 1 cycle per second. Therefore typical ultrasound frequencies range from 2.5 million to 12 million cycles per second.

Real-time grayscale ultrasonography is based on the pulse-echo principle. A short pulse of sound, usually two or three cycles long, boundary between two tissues of differing acoustic impedances, or Z.

$$\text{Acoustic impedance (Z)} = \text{Density(P)} \times$$
$$\text{Speed of sound}$$
$$(C) \text{ or } Z = P \times C$$

If we assume that the speed of sound in soft tissue is constant at 1540 m per second, then the main factor that influences acoustic impedance is the density or composition of tissue. Thus the more different two adjacent tissues are, the greater the echo reflection between them. This is why homogeneous populations of cells (those of lymphomas, lymph nodes, or regenerative liver nodules) produce few echoes and are generally hypoechoic (darker). If the acoustic interface difference is small, only a small percentage of sound will be reflected. If the difference is large, a large portion of sound will be reflected.

Interface	% Reflection
Fat/muscle	0.94
Fat/bone	49.00
Tissue/air	100.00

By looking at this list, one can see that the acoustic impedance (Z) between fat and muscle is low, whereas the acoustic impedance between fat and bone and between soft tissue and air is high. This property is the reason why ultrasound cannot be used to image through bone or gas. Too much of the sound beam is reflected from bone and gas interfaces because of the large change in density.

Patient Preparation

Patient preparation is important, because all of the sound is reflected when the ultrasound beam intersects air. Hair traps air, so if an ultrasound beam is passed through hair, most of the beam is reflected before it ever enters the animal. Clipping the hair, removing dirt and scales, and applying alcohol to the area of interest will increase the image quality. A generous volume of ultrasound gel is beneficial for displacing air and coupling the transducer to the skin. Small animals are placed in dorsal or lateral recumbency for abdominal examination and in lateral or sternal recumbency for cardiac examination. A special cardiac table with large and small holes in it is helpful for echocardiography. The animal is placed in lateral recumbency, with the chest area positioned over the hole of appropriate size; this allows better access for the ultrasound transducer. Most small animals tolerate abdominal and cardiac examinations well and rarely require tranquilization. Patient movement can negatively affect diagnostic ability, so patients that tense up, pant, or resist restraint should be sedated. Large-animal examinations are done in the standing, tranquilized animal.

TECHNICIAN NOTE

Hair traps air and, if not clipped, most of the ultrasound beam is reflected before it even enters the animal. This is why good patient preparation is critical.

Ultrasound Display Modes

The returning echo can be displayed in several ways. **B-mode**, or brightness mode, forms the basis for two-dimensional imaging. Returning echoes are displayed as dots on the image screen. The brightness of the dot is a function of the strength of the returning echo. The placement of the dot is a function of the time it took for the echo to return to the transducer. The cross-sectional image is formed through data storage. The sound beam is automatically swept across the patient while the transducer is held steady and is moved slowly over the area of interest. Rapid collection of images is called *real time*. This permits direct observation of moving structures, such as a beating heart or the movement of a fetus in a pregnant female. With B-mode real-time equipment, images are displayed in gray scale, a technique in which various echo strengths are displayed in numerous shades of gray from black to white.

M-mode, or "motion mode," is produced by passing a narrow sound beam across a body part. Each echo interface is presented as a dot. The motion of the body part is displayed by sweeping the image across the screen or image recorder. M-mode can be thought of as a thin sector of B-mode displayed as a function of time. M-mode is used primarily in echocardiography. This aids in determining the thickness and diameter of ventricular walls and valve motion. The ideal ultrasound equipment for veterinary practice would include a real-time B-mode scanner with M-mode capabilities (Fig. 15.33).

Doppler ultrasonography is used to demonstrate the flow of blood or other fluids and to measure their velocity. There are four types of Doppler techniques: (1) color Doppler illustrates the flow and the direction of blood. In most cases, the color blue is used to track blood flow away from the transducer and red is used to track blood flow toward the transducer. (2) Power color Doppler is used to track the flow of blood; however, it does not specifically identify its direction. (3) Pulse wave Doppler transducers alternate between sending and receiving signals and do well at illustrating blood flow for smaller vessels. (4) Continuous-wave Doppler can consistently send and receive signals and is useful in conditions where higher-velocity blood flow is more common.

Other modes of imaging include harmonic mode, which is used when performing ultrasound examination of larger-sized patients or those that are obese. Three- and four-dimensional modes are also available, but these are not as commonly used in veterinary medicine.

The selection of an appropriate transducer is critical when ultrasound equipment is purchased. Transducers vary in type, size, style, shape, and frequency. Linear array transducers are made with several piezoelectric crystals stacked side by side. The crystals are fired in rapid sequence to produce a rectangular cross-sectional image. Linear array transducers are used primarily for transrectal reproductive examinations in cattle and horses. Small-footprint convex array transducers are used most for small-animal imaging.

Sector scanners produce a triangular field. The crystal is swept across the area by mechanical or electronic means, and the transducer generally has a small contact area. More expensive transducers may incorporate annular array and dynamic focusing technology. These transducers form the ultrasound beam by adding together many small beams from an array of small crystals. Dynamic focusing allows the operator to place any portion within the beam into maximum resolution without having to change transducers.

Determining the frequency of transducer to use is easy. It must be remembered that the higher the frequency of the transducer, the shorter the sound wavelength and the better the resolution. However, as the frequency increases, the depth of sound beam penetration decreases. For abdominal ultrasonography in small dogs ($\leq$15 kg) and cats, a 7.5-MHz transducer is ideal. For medium- to large-sized dogs and nonreproductive large-animal imaging, a 5-MHz transducer works well. A 3- and 5-MHz linear array transducer is

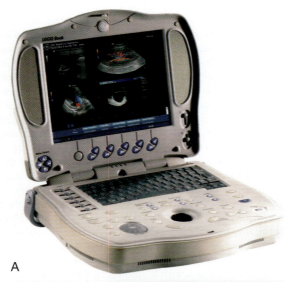

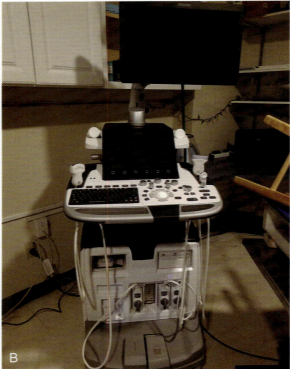

• **Fig. 15.33** (A) Portable notebook-style, real-time B-mode (brightness), M-mode (motion), and dedicated color Doppler veterinary ultrasound unit that can be used on both large and small animals. (B) Larger mobile veterinary ultrasound unit most commonly used in small-animal practices. ([A] Courtesy Sound Technologies, Inc., Carlsbad, CA. [B] Courtesy of Jessica Vorndran, BSAn.Sc, RVT, MedVet Medical and Cancer Centers for Pets.)

used extensively for transrectal reproductive ultrasonography in large animals.

> **TECHNICIAN NOTE**
>
> High-frequency transducers have increased resolution and attenuation but cannot penetrate deeper tissues. Low-frequency transducers have decreased resolution and attenuation but can penetrate deeper tissues.

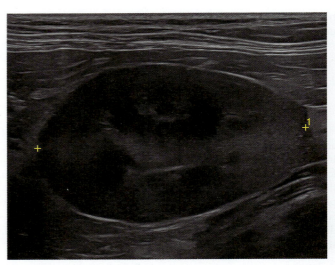

• **Fig. 15.34** Diagnostic ultrasound of a left kidney demonstrating varying echogenicity of the kidney structures, allowing for distinction of structures. (Courtesy of Jessica Vorndran, BSAn.Sc, RVT, MedVet Medical and Cancer Centers for Pets.)

Ultrasound equipment controls vary from machine to machine, but a time-gain compensation (TGC) control is deemed universal. The echoes coming from acoustic interfaces close to the transducer are stronger than those returning from farther away from the transducer. Time-gain amplification compensates for progressive attenuation of the ultrasound beam with increasing depth. TGC is operator dependent and is set for the best-looking and uniform image. TGC controls most often consist of a series of slide pods on the front of the machine. The top pod is the near field of the image, and the lowest pod is the far field, or bottom, of the image.

The Ultrasound Image

The ultrasound image is a thin, cross-sectional slice through the body in a new or different orientation. It aids in standard image orientation, in which the head or the front of the animal is placed on the left in the sagittal or longitudinal view and the animal's right on the left of the screen on the transverse or axial view.

Ultrasound terminology is easy to remember. *Echogenicity*, a relative term, refers to the strength or amplitude of the returning echoes (Fig. 15.34). A structure that is echogenic (bright) produces echoes. A structure that is **anechoic** (dark) produces few or no echoes. A structure is **hyperechoic** (brighter) if it produces more echoes than adjacent structures. A structure is **hypoechoic** (darker) if it produces fewer echoes than surrounding structures. A structure is **isoechoic** (same) if it has a level of echogenicity like that of adjacent structures. Any structure can be made bright by adjusting machine control settings. Organs are compared at the same depth and control settings to prevent misinterpretation of relative echogenicities.

Ultrasound Artifacts

Many technicians fail to take the time to fully understand what ultrasound artifacts are. They ignore artifacts because, by definition, an artifact does not contribute useful image information. This, however, is not true of ultrasound artifacts; they provide accurate clues to the makeup of the ultrasound image.

Reverberation Artifact

A reverberation artifact occurs when the ultrasound beam hits gas or air. Because of the large drop in acoustic impedance, the entire ultrasound beam is reflected to the transducer. A portion of the reflected beam bounces off the transducer surface and re-enters the patient's body, where it hits the soft tissue–air interface again. The sound bounces from patient to transducer repeatedly and appears on the screen as a set of bright parallel lines that are the same distance from each other and represent the distance between the transducer-gas interface. Reverberation artifacts can also be referred to as *comet tails* (Fig. 15.35). This artifact commonly occurs in areas of gas pockets, such as in the GI tract, or off of metal objects, such as foreign bodies or biopsy needles.

Shadowing

A shadowing artifact occurs because of inadequate sound beam penetration through a highly reflective or sound-absorptive substance. Acoustic shadowing is an area of darkness or hypoechogenicity that occurs within deep to dense material, such as bone, calcium, or calculi. Small objects cast an acoustic shadow only if they are within the focal zone of the ultrasound beam.

Acoustic Enhancement

Acoustic enhancement occurs when the ultrasound beam passes through a structure with low attenuation, such as the fluid-filled gallbladder. As sound travels through the surrounding liver tissue, it is attenuated, or slowed. The sound traveling through the gallbladder is attenuated less, so the echo returning to the transducer is more intense when the sound hits the opposite side of the gallbladder, causing an increase in echogenicity (Fig. 15.36). This artifact is seen deep to fluid-filled structures.

Refraction or Edge Artifact

Refraction is a hypoechoic band or stripe at the margin of a curved structure caused by refraction or redirecting of the sound beam. The sound beam is deflected from its true path and never returns, with an effect similar to shadowing. An edge artifact is helpful in identifying smooth round structures, such as the urinary bladder and cysts. It appears as a hypoechoic shadow on the forefield of the curved surface of a fluid-filled structure with a solid side.

Mirror Image Artifact

The ultrasound machine places the returning echo on the viewing screen as a function of the time it takes the echo to return. If the sound wave reverberates within a highly echogenic structure before returning to the transducer, the image will be duplicated on the screen distal to the original image and is commonly seen as a duplication of the gallbladder in mirror image on the other side of the diaphragm.

Slice-Thickness Artifact

If the width of the ultrasound beam cuts through the edge of a cystic structure and solid tissue, the solid tissue may look as if it is layered within the cyst. This artifact is responsible for the erroneous appearance of debris within the urinary bladder and gallbladder, although no debris may be present. The erroneous appearance is the result of volume averaging of tissue by the ultrasound machine.

The Ultrasound Examination

When ultrasonography is used for a quick answer to a question, such as whether a female patient is pregnant or has a pyometra, the examination will be shorter. When it is used for diagnosis of abdominal disease, a complete examination should be performed every time and can last 20 to 30 minutes. It is important to remember that *echogenicity* is a relative term, so organs should be compared at similar control settings and similar depths to determine normal tissue from abnormal tissue and to avoid misinterpretation.

> **TECHNICIAN NOTE**
>
> It is important to have a thorough understanding of the normal appearance of various abdominal organs on ultrasound before trying to identify abnormalities associated with disease.

Clinical Use

Ultrasonography is used almost as frequently as radiography. Traditional cardiac and solid abdominal organ examinations are most commonly performed, but ultrasonography can be used to find answers for hundreds of clinical questions in a wide variety of species. Box 15.4 lists common applications of ultrasonography in both large and small animals.

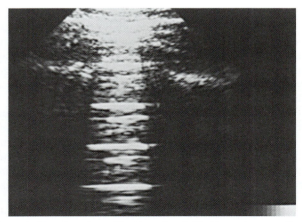

• **Fig. 15.35** Reverberation artifact from the air-filled lung of a normal horse. Parallel, evenly spaced echogenic bands represent reverberation between the transducer and the pleural surface.

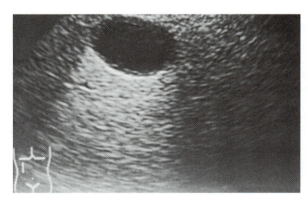

• **Fig. 15.36** The bright echogenic band beneath the gallbladder represents acoustic enhancement. The ultrasound beam is not attenuated as much as it traverses the fluid-filled gallbladder as it is in the surrounding liver.

- Tendon injury evaluation and response to surgery or therapy
- Diagnosis of tendon sheath infections, adhesions, and foreign bodies
- Evaluation of joint effusions, intra-articular injury, osteomyelitis, and neoplasms
- Evaluation of congenital and acquired cardiac disease and response to therapy
- Diagnosis of pleural effusion, pleuritis, and pleuropneumonia
- Evaluation of lung and mediastinal masses
- Evaluation of soft tissue, neck, thyroid, parathyroid, tongue, and mediastinal disease
- Evaluation of hepatic, renal, splenic, adrenal, urinary bladder, gallbladder, and biliary disease
- Diagnosis of abdominal and peripheral vascular malformations
- Peritoneal and pleural fluid assessment and sampling
- Evaluation of abdominal masses of unknown origin
- Diagnosis of intestinal foreign bodies, intussusceptions, infiltrative disease, and neoplasia
- Testicular and prostate evaluation and location of retained testicles
- Pregnancy diagnosis, fetal evaluation, twin removal, and complete fertility evaluations
- Evaluation of soft tissue neoplasia, granulomas, abscesses, and foreign bodies
- Diagnosis of umbilical infections and persistent and patent urachus
- Ocular and orbital evaluation
- Vascular thrombosis and catheter foreign body evaluation
- Guidance for fine-needle aspiration, drain placement, biopsy, and culture

Endoscopy

Endoscopy Use

Endoscopy has become common in private practice as a vital aid in patient diagnosis, treatment, and surgical procedures. It is commonly used to view the internal mucosae and intraluminal contents of hollow organs, such as the esophagus, stomach, colon, intestine, joint cavities, and the abdominal cavity of patients. Endoscopy provides a less invasive method of viewing internal structures without making a surgical incision.

An endoscope is composed of a rigid or flexible tube that contains a high-density fiberoptic camera. Ancillary equipment, such as flexible forceps for tissue biopsy and cytology, microbiology brushes, aspiration needles, and foreign body removal forceps, can be introduced through the tube to perform a variety of procedures.

Endoscope Care and Storage

Because endoscopy equipment is costly and delicate, proper care, use, and storage, according to the manufacturer's instructions, are important. Equipment should be inspected prior to use. Caution must be taken to not drop, kink, or overtwist the tubing, and to keep sharp objects from contact with the endoscope.

It is critical to clean the equipment after every use to avoid spreading infectious agents between patients. The scope should be cleaned with a nonabrasive enzymatic detergent, followed by a high-level disinfectant. The water and air channels of the scope should be flushed by suctioning through the enzyme solution, followed by water to remove biological and organic contaminants. The electrical components of the scope should be covered by the caps provided by the manufacturer.

The outside of the scope can then be cleaned by using gauze dampened with the enzyme cleaner and then wiped down with water-dampened gauze. A leak test should always be performed before and after cleaning, and all ancillary equipment should be cleaned as well.

After the scope is cleaned, it is important to properly store it to reduce the risk of damage. The scope should be hung vertically in a safe area. Storing the scope in its original box is not recommended, because this increases the potential for bacterial growth and poses health risks to patients.

A log of endoscopic procedures should be kept ensuring that the equipment functions properly for every procedure. The log should also document proper cleaning and leak checking of the scope and proper cleaning of ancillary equipment. For further discussion on endoscopy see Cox (2016) in the Recommended Readings.

Alternative Imaging Modalities

Alternative imaging modalities are advanced methods of diagnostic imaging that are not practiced in the private sector but rather, are used more commonly in specialty referral centers or teaching hospitals. Compared with radiography, these modalities provide more in-depth details of the architecture of organs and, in some cases, functional assessment of structures. Contrast agents may also be used to allow for better contrast and visualization of anatomy.

Fluoroscopy

Fluoroscopic units are better suited to the study of moving structures and dynamic processes compared with x-ray images. Although images exposed close together in time provide some information about these structures and processes, an image that is continuous in time is required for maximum information. The presentation of a continuous image is called *fluoroscopy*; it involves directing the x-ray beam through the patient and onto an image intensifier. The image intensifier amplifies the x-rays coming through the patient, thus reducing the amount of radiation needed for continuous exposure. The resulting images can be recorded for analysis and stored as part of the permanent medical record.

Fluoroscopy can be used in GI studies, tracheal studies, surgical situations such as fracture reductions and the placement of catheters or stents, and myelography, and is essential for heart and vascular studies. Fluoroscopy is commonly used to view the changing diameter of the trachea during inspiration and expiration that occurs in patients with tracheal collapse and to view esophageal motility in animals that experience regurgitation. Contrast agents may also be added for a better view of anatomic structures and their movements during the study (Fig. 15.37).

Fluoroscopic equipment is available only in larger veterinary specialty hospitals and referral centers. Equipment consists of an x-ray tube, much like the tube used in radiography, and an image intensifier, along with a monitor. The x-ray tube and image intensifier are mounted on a "C"-shaped arm that can be moved in all directions around the patient (Fig. 15.38). The patient is placed on a free-standing table that is clear of obstruction above and below it. The C-arm must be able to move either the intensifier screen or the tube under the table, when needed, for the study. This also means that a table made of a radiolucent material must be used.

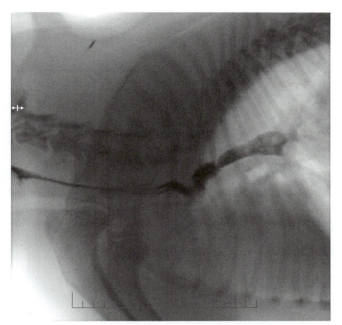

• **Fig. 15.37** Fluoroscopy provides real-time images of structures to show anatomy and function. In this illustration, barium is used to highlight esophageal anatomy and function. (Courtesy of Jessica Vorndran, BSAn. Sc, RVT, MedVet Medical and Cancer Centers for Pets.)

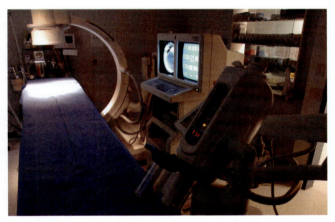

• **Fig. 15.38** Fluoroscopy equipment. The C-arm can be moved around the patient to observe multiple angles of anatomic structures. (Courtesy MedVet Medical and Cancer Centers for Pets.)

As the patient is positioned on the table, kVp, mAs, and time may be set. Time, however, is controlled by the veterinary professional performing the study. When the foot pedal is depressed, the tube is activated, and x-rays are emitted. Care should be taken to limit exposure times to avoid overheating the fluoroscopy tube, which contains a stationary anode. A timer alerts the radiographer about how much time has elapsed so that the study can be ended. The image can then be reviewed or recorded for diagnostic interpretation.

There are some minor safety concerns that should be kept in mind when using fluoroscopy. Radiation burns may occur in patients if they are positioned too close to the unit. Radiographers must also follow safety procedures to prevent personal exposure to the continuous x-ray beam. Lead aprons, gloves, and dosimeters should be worn during the procedure.

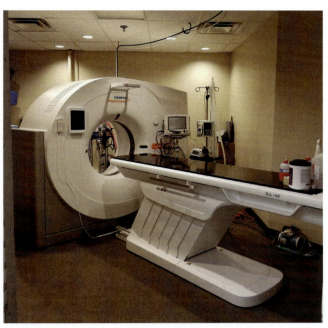

• **Fig. 15.39** The large, circular gantry houses the x-ray tube and detectors. The table moves the patient through the gantry in precise, measured, incremental steps. Technicians control the CT from outside of the shielded CT room to minimize exposure. (Courtesy MedVet Medical and Cancer Centers for Pets.)

Computed Tomography

Most veterinary schools and some specialty practices have access to CT (Fig. 15.39). A CT scan is obtained by passing a thin x-ray beam transaxially through the patient and measuring the x-ray attenuation (drop-off) at multiple sites in a thin slice of the patient's anatomy. The computer then reconstructs the transmitted x-ray data into a cross-sectional image on a monitor. Images can also be reconstructed by the computer in different ways to aid in the diagnosis of the patient, including two- and three-dimensional views.

Advantages of CT over standard radiography include greatly improved radiographic contrast and spatial resolution, both of which eliminate the problem of superimposition of structures, because it is shown in cross sections. The cross-sectional image is not a whole-body view but a sagittal view of one portion of the body. Imagine taking a whole loaf of bread, slicing it into sections, and then removing one piece and laying it flat on the counter (Fig. 15.40A and B). The most common uses of CT in veterinary medicine include head and spinal examinations for neurologic disease and radiation treatment planning. It can also be useful in the visualization of musculoskeletal, thoracic, abdominal disorders, and vascular abnormalities.

When CT is performed, the patient is placed in the ventrodorsal, dorsoventral, or lateral position on the long, narrow, movable CT table called the *cradle*. The cradle then moves the patient through the circular gantry that houses the x-ray tube and detectors. In older units, the table moves in a measured stepwise fashion. During each table step, the CT scanner obtains a single cross-sectional slice of data. Modern scanners have what is called a *helical scan mode* such that the x-ray tube turns 360 degrees around the patient while the table moves slowly through the gantry. This results in spiral or helical acquisition of the images, which

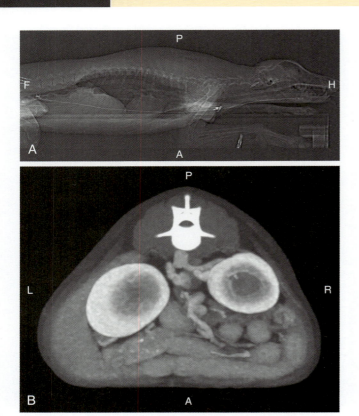

• **Fig. 15.40** (A) A scout computed tomography scan is completed in the patient, illustrating the anatomy of the entire abdomen prior to contrast being administered. (B) A cross-sectional image of the abdomen after contrast material has been administered. (Courtesy of Jessica Vorndran, BSAn.Sc, RVT, MedVet Medical and Cancer Centers for Pets.)

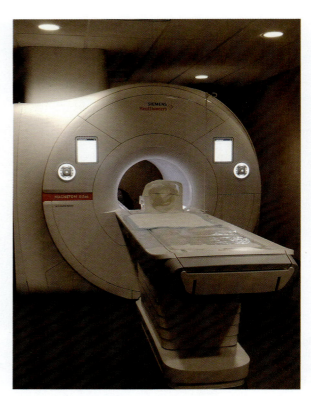

• **Fig. 15.41** A high-field superconductor magnet that allows for increased image resolution, which is needed when imaging the brain. (Courtesy of Jessica Vorndran, BSAn.Sc, RVT, MedVet Medical and Cancer Centers for Pets.)

then are reconstructed instantaneously by the computer to appear as conventional transverse images. Helical scanners are faster and, because of their speed, are excellent for moving regions like the thorax. The entire thorax of even a large dog can be scanned during a single short breath-hold performed under anesthesia.

During CT, the patient must be heavily sedated or placed under general anesthesia to prevent any movement and must be positioned perfectly straight. Because patients are sedated or under general anesthesia, the imaging technician must remain close by to monitor the patient but can stand behind a leaded window to reduce exposure. Most studies are performed twice on the same animal. The first study is performed without contrast, and the second is performed after intravenous administration of iodinated contrast. Contrast will highlight vascular structures, and some neoplasms will have a characteristic contrast enhancement pattern, aiding in the visualization of problem areas in the patient.

> ### TECHNICIAN NOTE
>
> When computed tomography (CT) studies are performed, the same contrast agents are used as for radiographic contrast procedures but at much lower concentrations, because CT is much more sensitive than radiography for detecting the presence of contrast agents.

Magnetic Resonance Imaging

MRI (Fig. 15.41), much like CT, is not performed in a regular private practice but only in teaching hospitals and specialty practices.

MRI is likened to CT in that the image is a thin slice of cross-sectional anatomy, but it differs from CT in that it uses no ionizing radiation to create the image. Instead, MRI represents the intensity of a radio wave signal from tissue in which hydrogen nuclei have been disturbed by a characteristic radiofrequency pulse. MRI is superior to CT in image resolution, anatomic definition, and sensitivity to tissue composition differences. Because of this, MRI is vastly superior to CT for imaging of the brain and spinal cord and is currently used primarily for head and spine evaluation (Fig. 15.42). It can also be used for soft tissue structures, such as ligaments and articular cartilage. One disadvantage of MRI is the much longer scan time required compared with CT.

> ### TECHNICIAN NOTE
>
> Magnetic resonance imaging (MRI) differs from computed tomography (CT) in that it uses no ionizing radiation to create the image. MRI is vastly superior to CT for imaging of the brain and spinal cord and is currently the state-of-the-art modality for head and spine evaluation.

A disadvantage of MRI is the strong magnetic field in the vicinity of the machine. One cannot use anything made of metal in or around the magnet. The magnetic field will rapidly and forcefully pull these objects into the magnet, potentially injuring anyone or anything in its path. Such objects include gas anesthetic machines, oxygen tanks, intravenous poles, clipboards, ink pens, leashes, and collars. Nonmagnetic products are available for use during MRI, but generally, they are cost prohibitive for most veterinary hospitals. Plugging the animal's ears with cotton is essential for maintaining sedation and protecting hearing because of the loudness of the

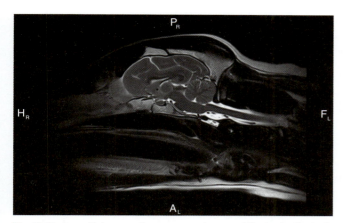

• **Fig. 15.42** A sagittal magnetic resonance image of the brain, illustrating enhanced detail of the brain tissue. (Courtesy of Jessica Vorndran, BSAn. Sc, RVT, MedVet Medical and Cancer Centers for Pets.)

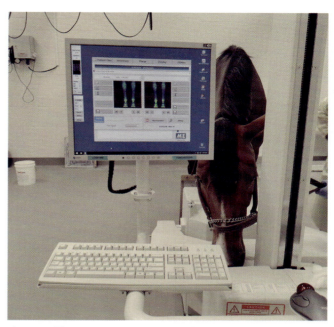

• **Fig. 15.43** The computer generates the bone scan image as the emitted gamma rays from the patient are detected by the scintillation camera. (Courtesy of Paige Allen.)

magnet during scanning. Personnel remaining in the room to monitor anesthesia must also use ear protection. The interaction of the magnet and radiofrequencies also produces heat. Because animals cannot dissipate the heat produced like humans can, it is important to apply cooling packs to larger dogs with less surface area. Patients must be absolutely still for MRI, because any motion will severely degrade the image. This can become complicated, because it is often difficult to carefully monitor animals during the examination owing to the narrow tubular shape of some magnets and the inability to use mechanized monitoring devices. MRI examinations can be performed with or without paramagnetic intravenous contrast.

In addition to the need for anesthesia and the monitoring difficulties created by the high magnetic field, the personal safety of the technician is a concern, so precautions must be taken. It is important to remember that even though no images are being produced and the MRI technician is not at the controls, the magnet is always still on at full power. Credit cards and watches may be permanently damaged if carried too close to the high magnetic field. Any devices that deliver a radiofrequency signal, such as televisions, radios, or cell phones, cannot be close to an MRI unit. In addition, technicians with cardiac pacemakers, aneurysm or intracranial hemoclips, neural stimulators, metallic fragments within the orbits, or hearing aids should not be involved with patient care during MRI. Likewise, patients with metallic implants may not be good candidates for MRI, because these items may move out of their desired positions when the magnet is activated.

> **TECHNICIAN NOTE**
>
> The high magnetic field in a magnetic resonance imaging (MRI) unit is always active. It is never safe to bring anything made of metal, including medical equipment and personal belongings, close to the machine.

Nuclear Medicine (NM)

Many veterinary schools and some progressive specialized veterinary practices have NM capabilities. NM involves the use of unsealed radioactive isotopes for diagnostic or therapeutic purposes. Radioactive isotopes are in an abnormally excited state created by an unstable nucleus. In effort to regain stability, these atoms emit particles (alpha, beta, or gamma) and energy to transform themselves into different atoms, a process called radioactive decay. The time it takes for half of the atom to decay is called the

half-life. Diagnostic NM involves administering radioactive isotopes to the patient and measuring the radiation emitted (alpha, beta, or gamma radiation) as the isotope goes through the process of radioactive decay. NM does not generate visual images equivalent to those of diagnostic radiography, but it can detect functional or physiologic, pharmacologic, and kinetic patient data from the image. There are two main types of diagnostic NM utilized in veterinary medicine: nuclear scintigraphy and PET. Pregnant individuals should not work with patients that are undergoing these procedures.

Nuclear Scintigraphy

Nuclear scintigraphy involves the injection of a radionuclide that goes through gamma decay (emits gamma particles) and detection of the electromagnetic radiation emitted from the animal with a gamma scintillation camera (Fig. 15.43).

> **TECHNICIAN NOTE**
>
> Therapeutic nuclear medicine (NM) involves the administration of radioactive iodine (^{131}I) for the treatment of hyperthyroidism and thyroid tumors.

Common clinical uses of nuclear scintigraphy in veterinary medicine include bone scanning for detection of tumor metastasis and radiographically undetectable bone injury or infection, lung scanning for detection of pulmonary embolism and as a pulmonary function test, renal scanning for assessment of kidney perfusion and function, and thyroid scanning for characterization of hyperthyroidism and detection of metastasis.

The most used radionuclide is technetium 99m (^{99m}Tc). Technetium is administered in an ionic form as $^{99m}TcO_4$ (pertechnetate) or is bound to a specific organ-localizing pharmaceutical agent before administration. Technetium is the radiopharmaceutical of choice because it has a 6-hour physical half-life and emits a 140-kiloelectron–volt (keV) gamma ray, appropriate for most

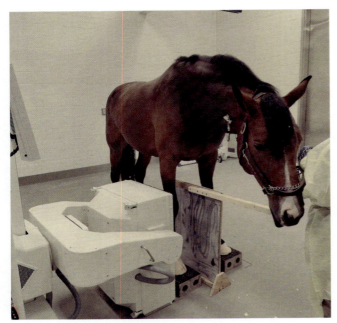

• **Fig. 15.44** A sedated horse dosed with Tc-99 positioned in front of the scintillation (gamma) camera for a bone scan. The lead backstop is positioned between the extremities to allow for imaging of the limb of interest. (Courtesy of Paige Allen.)

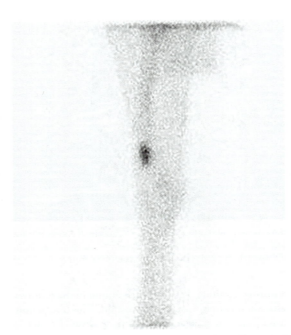

• **Fig. 15.45** Equine limb bone scan image illustrating a "hot spot" (black area), an area of increased gamma ray emission. This occurs when there is increased blood flow to an area of bone inflammation or injury. Increased blood flow allows for more Tc-99 accumulation, resulting in more gamma ray emission and detection in the area of abnormality. (Courtesy of Paige Allen.)

imaging studies. The primary route of radionuclide administration to veterinary patients is intravenous.

Shortly after administration of technetium, the patient is scanned with the gamma scintillation camera (Fig. 15.44). The emissions of gamma photons are detected and recorded. The camera can then be moved to different angles around the area of interest to collect the most information possible. Any areas that have higher radiation emission show up darker on the screen and are called "hot spots," indicating increased blood flow to the area (Fig. 15.45). "Cold spots," or areas that show up lighter on the screen, are areas with low gamma emissions, indicating decreased blood flow or necrosis.

Radiation safety practices are important in NM, and pregnant individuals should not participate in testing or care of patients undergoing this procedure. Latex examination gloves, laboratory coats, disposable boots, and dosimeters should be worn during radionuclide administration, and careful injection techniques should be used to ensure that the entire dose is delivered intravenously. Technetium is excreted primarily in urine, with a lesser amount excreted in feces. Animals should be housed in a separate restricted area of the hospital, and their stool and urine should be carefully collected and held for decay until levels are below exempt quantities. Appropriate PPE, as listed earlier, should be worn, and contact with patients limited to only that necessary for their care. Animals should be held in restricted areas and scanned using a Geiger counter to ensure they pose no radiation threat to their owners or to the general population prior to leaving, as determined by state health regulations.

TECHNICIAN NOTE

The technician must wear appropriate PPE when administering a radionuclide intravenously, including gloves, lab coat, and, potentially, eye protection. Dosimeters should be worn during administration and during patient care. Geiger counters should be kept on hand to detect any radionuclide that may potentially contaminate dosing personnel or facilities.

Positron Emission Tomography

Positron emission tomography (PET) is another type of NM that demonstrates the function of a structure rather than the anatomic structure. Just like with nuclear scintigraphy, PET utilizes the injection of a radioisotope that emits gamma rays during radioactive decay. PET imaging aids in the diagnosis of brain and heart abnormalities and detection of various types of cancer. It is a useful tool in planning radiation, chemotherapeutic, and surgical procedures.

Fluorodeoxyglucose (FDG) is the most common isotope used in PET imaging. The fluorine in the FDG molecule acts as the position-emitting radioactive tracer, known as fluorine-18 or ^{18}F. FDG is administered intravenously to the patient 30 to 45 minutes before imaging and acts as a "tag" as it attaches to other compounds in the body. For example, the glucose in the FDG is metabolized by the brain and cancerous tissue. As the ^{18}F gets metabolized by those tissues, it begins to go through radioactive decay. The positrons collide with the electrons in the body and create gamma photons. A gamma camera detects the gamma photons, creating areas of "hot spots" like in nuclear scintigraphy. Other isotopes may also be used in PET imaging, such as ammonia when performing cardiac imaging. Isotopes used in PET imaging are generated in a cyclotron and generally have short half-lives. This means that the isotopes must be produced, delivered, and administered in a timely manner to ensure that radioactive decay does not occur before delivery to the patient.

In most cases, PET imaging is combined with CT or MRI. The CT or MR image is performed first, and the PET image is superimposed to illustrate both the function and anatomy of a structure. Since the patient must remain still during the CT or MRI and scanning may take up to an hour, general anesthesia is recommended. Radiation safety practices like those mentioned with nuclear scintigraphy should be followed to reduce exposure to the veterinary staff.

Acknowledgment

The author and publisher wish to acknowledge Beth Paugh Partington and Lorrie Gaschen for their contributions to previous editions of this textbook, and Jessica Vorndran, BSAn.Sc, RVT, along with MedVet Medical and Cancer Centers for Pets for their illustration contributions to the text.

Recommended Readings

Barr F, Gaschen L. *BSAVA Manual of Canine and Feline Ultrasonography*. Gloucester, UK: British Small Animal Veterinary Association; 2012.

Berry, Clifford R. *The Handbook of Veterinary Nuclear Medicine*. North Carolina State University, College of Veterinary Medicine; 1996.

Brown LC, Brown M. *Lavin's Radiography for Veterinary Technicians*. 7th ed. St. Louis, MO: Elsevier; 2022.

Butler JA, et al. *Clinical Radiology of the Horse*. 4th ed. Oxford, UK: Wiley-Blackwell; 2017.

Cox S. *Endoscopy for the Veterinary Technician*. Ames, IA: John Wiley and Sons; 2016.

Curry TS, Dowdey JE, Murry RC. *Christensen's Introduction to the Physics of Diagnostic Radiology*. 4th ed. Philadelphia, PA: Lea & Febiger; 1990.

Drost WT, Reese DJ, Hornof WJ. Digital radiography artifacts. *Vet Radiol Ultrasound*. 2008;49(Suppl 1):S48.

Hall EJ, Giaccia AJ. *Radiobiology for the Radiologist*. 8th ed. Philadelphia, PA: Wolters Kluwer; 2019.

Han CM, Hurd CD. *Practical Diagnostic Imaging for the Veterinary Technician*. 3rd ed. St. Louis, MO: Elsevier; 2005.

Kealy JK, McAllister H, Graham J. *Diagnostic Radiology and Ultrasonography of the Dog and Cat*. 5th ed. St. Louis, MO: Saunders; 2011.

Kodak Company Eastman. *The Fundamentals of Radiography*. 12th ed. Rochester, NY: Eastman Kodak; 1980.

Morgan JR. *Techniques of Veterinary Radiography*. 5th ed. Ames, IA: Iowa State University Press; 1993.

Nyland TG, Mattoon JS. *Small Animal Diagnostic Ultrasound*. 4th ed. St. Louis, MO: Elsevier; 2020.

Penninck D, d'André M. *Atlas of Small Animal Ultrasonography*. 2nd ed. Ames, IA: John Wiley & Sons; 2015.

Rantanen NW, McKinnon AD. *Equine Diagnostic Ultrasonography*. Baltimore, MD: Williams & Wilkins; 1998.

Schwatrz T, Saunders J. *Veterinary Computed Tomography*. West Sussex, UK: John Wiley & Sons, Ltd; 2011.

Sirois M, Anthor E. *Handbook of Radiographic Positioning for Veterinary Technicians*. Clifton Park, NY: Delmar Cengage Learning; 2010.

Thrall DE. *Textbook of Veterinary Diagnostic Radiology*. 8th ed. St. Louis, MO: Elsevier; 2018.

16

Basic Necropsy Procedures

MOGES WOLDEMESKEL AND MICHELE D. COARSEY

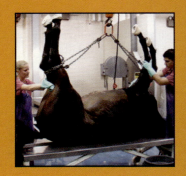

CHAPTER OUTLINE

LEARNING OBJECTIVES

When you have completed this chapter, you will be able to:

1. Pronounce, define, and spell all key terms in the chapter.
2. List and discuss the indications for a necropsy.
3. List and discuss the role of a veterinary technician in the necropsy process.
4. Explain how to write a necropsy report, including how to describe lesions.
5. Discuss sample collection for laboratory testing, including the uses for the following collections: fixed tissue, fresh tissue, swabs, and whole blood, serum, fluids, and feces, and performance of rabies procedure.
6. Discuss the public health importance of correctly shipping diagnostic specimens.
7. Describe the facilities, instruments, and supplies needed to perform a necropsy, including protective clothing and other personal protective equipment (PPE).
8. Do the following regarding the necropsy procedure for a small mammal:

- Describe how to open the carcass.
- Explain the principles of preliminary and external examination of the carcass.
- Describe the initial steps of a necropsy dissection, including reflection of the skin and limbs and examination of superficial organs and body cavities.
- Describe the steps for dissection and examination of the skull and brain, neck and thoracic viscera, abdominal cavity, female and male urogenital tracts, abdominal aorta, rectum, and anal glands, vertebral column, and spinal cord.
- Outline all of the steps for an entire necropsy procedure.
9. Do the following regarding necropsy variations:
- Describe variations in necropsy procedure specific to ruminants, horses, pigs, fetuses, birds, and laboratory animals.
- Explain the differences between a complete necropsy and a cosmetic necropsy.

KEY TERMS

Abomasum	Irritant
Appendicular skeleton	Laminae
Atlas	Lesions
Atrioventricular (AV) valve	Mediastinum
Autolysis	Meninges
Axis	Myocardium
Diaphragm	Necropsy
Duodenum	Omentum
Foramen magnum	Pathogenesis
Forestomach	Pathology
Gross pathology	Pituitary gland
Histopathology	Prosector
Hydronephrosis	Pulmonary artery
Hyoid bone	Sciatic nerve
Idiopathic	Sternum
In situ	

Introduction

Necropsy is the examination of an animal after it has died to determine cause of death and abnormal and disease-related changes that occurred during its life. The term *necropsy* originated from the Greek *nekros* (dead) and *-opsis* (sight) and means "viewing the dead." Necropsy is also known as *autopsy* (from Greek) in human medicine, which means "seeing with one's own eyes."

Before beginning the discussion about necropsy, it is important to understand the meaning of the terms used frequently in this chapter. Pathology, for example, is the study of disease and disease processes to determine the causes and development of abnormal conditions and death. *Gross pathology* refers to pathologic changes in tissue that are visible to the unaided eye, whereas *histopathology* refers to pathologic changes in tissue that can be seen only with the use of a microscope. Lesions are abnormalities in a tissue (pathologic changes), and pathogenesis is the sequence of events that leads to or underlies a disease.

Necropsy

A necropsy is often done on an animal for the following reasons:
- To determine the cause of death, which can be caused by infections (bacteria, viruses), parasites, toxins, trauma, neoplasia, nutritional deficiencies, metabolic diseases, and congenital or hereditary diseases, or it can be simply idiopathic in nature.
- To determine the disease process or processes that led to the animal's death.
- To determine the association of the clinical diagnosis with the lesions.
- To evaluate the positive and negative effects of therapeutic measures.

In situations in which more than one animal is at risk, as in multiple-animal households, farms, and laboratory animal facilities, a necropsy is helpful in determining whether other animals are at risk for infection, inherited conditions, or injury caused by toxins or environmental hazards. In addition, the necropsy gives the technicians the opportunity to increase their knowledge about the anatomies of various animal species each time one is performed. (See Case Presentation 16.1.)

Successful performance of a necropsy requires knowledge of anatomy and gross pathology and a systematic procedure for examination of the animal's body.

CASE PRESENTATION 16.1

Boots, a 3-year-old neutered, male domestic shorthair cat, was presented for necropsy after dying suddenly and unexpectedly. The owners asked their veterinarian to examine the body, because this was their second cat that died unexpectedly within the previous month. The owners had several cats that lived mostly outdoors, and they were worried that a neighbor (who was hostile to the cats because of predation of birds at his bird feeder) might have "done something bad" to them. Other than the owners' perception that Boots was sluggish for 2 days before death, no significant clinical findings were reported.

Methodical dissection of the cadaver revealed no evidence of trauma, such as bruising or fractured bones. Tissues were fresh; abdominal viscera were grossly normal, and no stomach contents were found. When the chest cavity was opened, 5 mL of cloudy gray-green fluid was noted in the right pleural space. A culture swab was inserted into the fluid to obtain a sample before proceeding further. The lungs and the heart were then extracted. The pleural surfaces on the right side retained a thin sheet of velvety yellow fibrin. The right lung lobes were compressed and firmer than the normal-appearing left lung lobes. The lung samples were placed in a bottle containing 10% buffered formalin, and culture swab and tissue samples were forwarded to a reference laboratory. The carcass was bagged and frozen.

One week later, the histopathology report was received, and it stated that the lung samples showed evidence of severe acute pleuropneumonia and bacteria. *Pasteurella multocida* was recovered from the aerobic culture.

This case demonstrates how a necropsy can be used to determine the cause of death. In this case, the necropsy, coupled with two simple tests (histopathology and culture), showed that a natural disease process (severe bacterial pleuropneumonia) caused this patient's death. Although it was not clear how the patient got this infection, *P. pleuropneumonia* is a documented disease entity that could not have been the result of any actions on the neighbor's part. A visit to the veterinarian at the onset of the signs might have saved Boots' life.

Generally, technicians trained in necropsy techniques and supervised by a veterinarian can and should perform necropsies. Necropsies should be

CASE PRESENTATION 16.1—cont'd

performed frequently enough that the techniques are familiar to the technician and to the supervising veterinarian.

Before beginning to describe the necropsy procedure, several important things must be considered. First, the practice should confirm that the owner's written permission has been obtained before the necropsy is performed. Second, it must be ensured that the animal scheduled for necropsy is correctly identified. The signalment (species, breed, sex, age) and identifying tags or tattoos should be carefully matched with the information on the owner's permission form and the medical record. This step is critical to prevent necropsy being performed on the wrong animal. If the animal has a radiofrequency identification device (RFID, also called a *microchip*), the device can be collected for verification. In addition, the owner's preference for disposition of the body (e.g., cremation, private cremation, burial) should be determined before the necropsy, if possible. Cosmetic necropsy, in which the internal organs are removed for examination without disrupting the external body, may be conducted if the owner requests it.

The signalment, history, and clinical findings should be reviewed before the necropsy is begun. The record should include the owner's name, address, and telephone numbers; names of other veterinarians involved with the case; the animal's signalment, name, or identification; and the hospital record number. The history should include vaccination history, the clinical signs, treatment used, length of illness, and the number of other animals at risk. The clinical findings should include results of the physical examination and clinical tests (e.g., complete blood count [CBC], clinical chemistry panels, radiography), surgical procedures, and the date and time of death or euthanasia. It is important that the time of death and the time of necropsy be recorded.

It is important to perform the necropsy as soon as possible after the animal's death to avoid decomposition (autolysis). If the necropsy must be delayed, the body should be refrigerated as soon as possible. The body *must not be frozen,* because freezing and subsequent thawing cause postmortem artifacts and, in the case of suspected aerobes, will render organs

diagnostically useless. This is especially important regarding suspected cases of rabies, which legally cannot be diagnosed from frozen tissue.

Small animals should be placed in thin plastic bags with identification tags secured on both the body and the outside of the bag. Decomposition occurs most rapidly in large, obese animals at high temperatures. It is particularly troublesome in large animals that rely on gut fermentation for their nutrients, because the rumen continues to generate heat long after the animal's death.

Before opening the carcass for necropsy, the clinical history, including the clinical findings and herd health if applicable, should be reviewed, because this gives a clue as to which organ or tissue is mainly affected. For example, the brain and the spinal cord should be carefully examined in cases of animals that died after showing neurologic signs. The animal should be weighed, and the weight should be recorded in grams or kilograms.

After reviewing the history, the next step is external examination of the carcass (Figs. 16.1A and B, and 16.2). This includes examination of skin for wounds, lacerations, and external parasites and an evaluation of the mucous membranes of the eye, nostrils, mouth and the vulva in females, before opening the carcass. During the necropsy, all abnormalities and lesions must be recorded and described. All organs that are abnormal in size or shape must be measured and/or weighed. Appropriate samples are collected for histopathology, cytology, bacteriology, virology, parasitology, and toxicology as needed. The samples should include both formalin-fixed and fresh tissues from major organs and grossly observed lesions, along with swabs, fluids, smears, and feces to determine the definitive diagnosis and the cause of death; all must be clearly labeled accordingly. Descriptions of gross findings must be recorded and included in the report and submitted together with the animal's signalment. All samples collected at necropsy must be packaged in the correct manner to reach the laboratory in the best condition possible for testing. Samples that are submitted to the laboratory for further testing should be packaged with a copy of the report and digital photos of lesions, if available. The report should be added to the animal's record, together with the other reports.

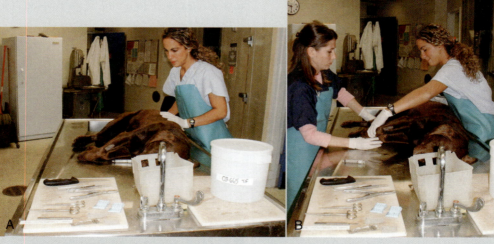

• **Fig. 16.1** (A) and (B) Prosector ready to begin a small animal necropsy.

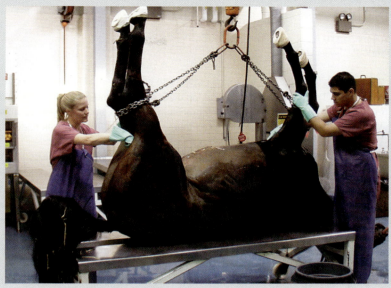

• **Fig. 16.2** Prosector ready to begin a large animal necropsy.

Necropsy Reports

As the necropsy is being performed, all abnormalities must be described and recorded. Once completed, a report, including tentative conclusions (diagnoses), must be written (Fig. 16.3).

All lesions are described and recorded by using the following criteria (examples are given in parentheses):

- Location (caudal, cranial, dorsal, ventral, left, right)
- Number (one, two, hundreds)
- Color (red, green, yellow-tan)
- Size (e.g., 3 × 5 × 4 cm, or weights for liver and heart)
- Shape (round, flat, spherical, stellate)
- Distribution (focal, focally extensive, multifocal, diffuse)
- Consistency (soft, firm, hard, rubbery)
- Odor (sweet, sour, ammonia)

Findings are usually recorded in the order in which they were encountered during the necropsy. The descriptions should be as specific as possible without drawing conclusions, because this may erroneously influence the diagnosis. For example, "There are multiple dark red 1- to 4-mm diameter soft nodules in all lung lobes," rather than using the term *hemangiosarcoma*. Based on the descriptions, the veterinarian formulates a morphologic diagnosis, which includes severity, duration, distribution, lesion, and anatomic site. An example of such a diagnosis might be "severe acute multifocal interstitial pneumonia."

Sample Collection for Laboratory Testing

Before samples are collected for examination to be completed by the microbiology, parasitology, and toxicology departments, the laboratory should be contacted for specific advice on which samples to collect, and how they should be collected, packaged (preserved) and submitted. This minimizes potential errors and provides the laboratory with the best possible specimens, especially in samples that must be shipped out to the laboratory. Description of fresh and fixed tissue samples collection to be submitted to the laboratory is given below.

Fixed Tissues

Fixed tissues are tissues preserved in fixative solutions to prevent further decomposition (autolysis) after sample collection or death of the animal. Histopathology routinely requires that fixed tissues must be handled carefully before fixation and properly labeled (identified). Tissue sections should not be squeezed, stretched, or rinsed with water, and epithelial surfaces should not be rinsed or rubbed with fingers or instruments before obtaining samples for histopathology. Tissues become rigid with fixation so if there is a need to retain the flatness of the tissue (e.g., a nerve or a section of skin), the tissue should be placed on a piece of cardboard to which it remains adhered after immersion in formalin. Sections from paired organs may be trimmed differently to distinguish them from one another. For example, the left kidney may be sectioned

Owner: Brown
Clinic #: 01-34567
Animal name: Ralph
Clinician: Smith
Date/time of death: 01/17/17 (9 AM)
Date/time of necropsy: 01/17/17 (11 AM)

This is a 3.0-kg, 7½-year-old, spayed, female seal-point Siamese cross cat in adequate postmortem and emaciated nutritional condition. There is a clipped area on the distal aspect of the right front leg with an electrocardiogram (ECG) lead taped in place. The left antebrachium is clipped, and a catheter is in the left cephalic vein. The ventral cervical area and the ventral and lateral abdomen are clipped. There is little body fat, and the muscle mass is reduced.

There is approximately 100 ml of yellow stringy fluid in the abdomen. There are multifocal, 2- to 10-mm, yellow-tan clots of fibrin throughout the abdomen and loosely adherent to abdominal organs. There are white-tan, multifocal to confluent, 1- to 5-cm diameter plaques on the surface of the liver, spleen, small intestine, omentum, mesentery, diaphragm, and body wall. The small intestine and colon are dilated (1 to 2 cm in diameter), and the wall of the small intestine is multifocally thickened. In the most severely affected area, at the jejunoileal junction, the serosa is corrugated and the wall is 3 to 5 mm thick. The abdominal and sternal lymph nodes are enlarged (0.5 to 2.0 cm in diameter) and white on the capsular surface. On section, they have a normal lymph node architecture with a thick white cortex.

The lungs are heavy, wet, and red-purple, and they sink in formalin. There is approximately 5 ml of serosanguineous fluid in the pericardium.

Gross Findings

Lungs: moderate to severe acute pneumonia, presumptive
Abdomen: severe fibrinous peritonitis
Small intestine and colon: severe chronic enteritis and colitis, presumptive
Pericardium: moderate serosanguineous effusion
Abdominal and sternal lymph nodes: severe reactive hyperplasia, presumptive

Gross Diagnosis

- Euthanasia
- Feline infectious peritonitis (FIP)
- Severe enteritis and colitis, presumptive
- Severe pneumonia, presumptive

Comment

I am not sure if the changes in the small intestine and colon are due to FIP or some other process. The lung lesion is also not typical for FIP. Impression smears of the peritoneal surface lesions reveal a mixed population of inflammatory cells, including neutrophils, lymphocytes, plasma cells, and macrophages, consistent with the diagnosis of FIP.

Samples of lung and small intestine are submitted for bacterial culture. Samples of lymph nodes, small intestine, colon, lungs, liver, and spleen are submitted for histologic-examination.

• **Fig. 16.3** Sample necropsy report.

longitudinally, and the right kidney may be cut transversely. In addition, sections can be labeled with clip-on laundry tags for identification. If there is any possibility that a section of tissue may lose its identity (i.e., be difficult to distinguish) when mixed with other specimens, the sections should be tagged with clip-on laundry tags or stored separately. If tissue samples are small, they may be placed in separate labeled containers, such as tissue cassettes. The pituitary gland of a small animal, for example, is well differentiated from other tissues when placed in a small tissue cassette.

Buffered formalin (10%) is the most widely used fixative for the preservation of tissues for histopathology. Slices of tissue (generally no thicker than 1 cm) should be placed in large volumes of formalin (10 times as much formalin solution as tissue by volume). The fixative solution is available from commercial companies and is also easily prepared. It is made by mixing nine parts water with one part commercially available formaldehyde solution (37%–40%). The addition of 6.5 g of dibasic anhydrous sodium phosphate and 4 g of monobasic sodium phosphate per 1000 mL of solution creates neutral buffered 10% formalin. This is an excellent general purpose fixative and is somewhat more desirable than plain (acidic) 10% formalin. The addition of buffers to formalin (and all fixatives) is important, because this will eliminate the formation of undesirable hematin pigment in tissue sections. Formalin should be handled with care, because it is a contact **irritant** and a carcinogen; therefore protective plastic gloves (preferably nitrile composition) and eye protection should always be worn when fixatives or fixed tissues are handled. Containers with fixatives must be kept tightly closed except when placing tissues in them, and fixatives must be handled and used in a well-ventilated space.

For the preservation of whole brains, intact spinal cords, and bones, 50% formalin, which is made by mixing one part 10% buffered formalin with one part commercial formaldehyde (37%–40%), is superior to the 10% solutions. The 50% solution penetrates and fixes the large tissue mass more rapidly and thoroughly compared with 10% formalin. Formalin fixation of tissues is usually completed within 24 hours (large brains may take 48 hours). Tissues fixed in 10% formalin are traditionally stored in 10% formalin, but storage in 70% alcohol is superior.

Bouin solution is less widely used than 10% formalin but is often preferred because it produces less tissue shrinkage and better preservation of cellular detail. Fetal tissues, intestinal epithelium, eyes, testes, endocrine glands, and the inclusion bodies associated with viruses are particularly well preserved with commercial Bouin solution.

In all cases, it is desirable to save sections of critical tissues for histopathologic examination. These include lung, myocardium, liver, spleen, pancreas, stomach, small intestine, kidneys, lymph nodes, whole brain, endocrine organs, urinary bladder, colon, and muscle. Ten percent buffered formalin (10%; i.e., 10:1 formalin-to-tissue ratio) is the most widely used fixative for the preservation of tissues. All containers (not lids) of fixed tissue samples should be clearly labeled. Appropriate caution should be used in handling, shipping, and disposing of all fixatives.

Fresh Tissues

Fresh tissues are tissues collected for suspected microbiological (bacteria, virus, fungus) contamination and other biological organisms and toxicologic examinations without the addition of preservatives. Tissues and other specimens (fresh, never frozen) for bacteriology, mycology, and mycoplasma culture are collected aseptically, placed in culturettes or sterile containers without preservatives, and submitted to the laboratory without delay. Sterilized instruments are used to collect samples for microbiological testing. If the surface of the tissue is contaminated, sear it with a flamed spatula, cut with a sterile blade, and insert a culturette or needle attached to swab or aspirate the tissue for testing. Fresh tissues submitted for laboratory testing need to arrive at the diagnostic laboratory in optimal condition. Collected tissue samples must be placed in clearly labeled, leak-proof containers and kept refrigerated until the time for shipping to a diagnostic laboratory. Depending on the desired testing, some tissues could be stored in a freezer. Specimens collected for microbiology always must include the primary site of disease. Other samples may include

heart, blood, lung, liver, spleen, stomach contents of aborted fetuses, placenta, exudates, synovia, brain, and small intestine as needed. When an intestinal sample is submitted, a 10-cm segment of intestine is tied off at each end to prevent leakage of internal contents and contamination. The instruments used to do this are heavily contaminated by the microbes exposed at the cut ends. For this reason, the sample must be collected last and placed in a separate container to prevent contamination of other tissue samples. Tissue sections of 2 × 3 × 1 cm and fluid specimens of 3 to 5 mL are desirable. If possible, disposable instruments should be used. Samples must be shipped to the laboratory with ice packs to protect against excessive heat and shipped overnight or, if possible, delivered directly to the laboratory.

Tissues for virus isolation are collected aseptically and in a sterile container and frozen. Fresh, refrigerated tissue immersed in virus transport medium (available from the virology laboratory) is the preferred method of tissue submission. Lung, liver, spleen, kidney, and brain are prime specimens; sections need to measure 5 × 5 × 10 mm. Contact the virology laboratory for the appropriate technique and preferred shipment packaging.

For toxicology, blood, liver, stomach contents, kidney, fat, brain, and urine may be saved. Blocks of tissue 10 × 5 × 4 cm (approximately 200 g), 10 to 20 mL of blood, and 50 to 100 mL of fluid are desirable. Unlike many samples, these samples may be frozen.

PROCEDURE 16.1

Rabies-Related Necropsy Procedure

Technicians and clinicians must be familiar with the policies and guidelines of their specific states regarding rabies-related necropsy. In all cases where rabies is suspected, animal carcasses must be handled only by clinicians and technicians who are preimmunized against rabies, have a serum titer greater than 1:5, and are wearing proper PPE. In the case of small animals, the prosector must double-glove and wear protective masks and goggles. In the case of animals larger than large dogs, personnel must wear rubber boots, a scrub suit, an apron, double gloves (the outer glove is heavy vinyl with gauntlets), and a face shield for splash protection. Pathology personnel who decapitate and extract brains must use the additional protection of a Tyvek coverall or a surgical gown and apron. Use of a high-efficiency particulate air (HEPA)–filtered helmet and face shield are suggested when working on equine carcasses because of concerns about aerosolization of West Nile virus.

In suspected cases of rabies, the head must be carefully removed by disarticulation at the atlanto-occipital junction using a disposable scalpel or knife, double-bagged, placed in a refrigerated container (with ice packs, *not* dry ice), and sent overnight to the appropriate laboratory for fluorescent antibody testing. Brain samples should NEVER be frozen, as this will negate the value of the sample due to changes in tissues. The remaining carcass must be double-bagged in a red biohazard bag, labeled as a rabies suspect, and disposed of as biologically hazardous material.

Some states require removal of the brain before submission to the laboratory for animals larger than a large dog (horses, cattle, etc.). To remove the brain of a large animal for rabies testing, a special head vise is used, or the head is held on the table (eyes may be removed to facilitate head holding). As much of the hide and flesh is removed over the calvaria as possible. The rostral transverse cut through the skull is made behind an imaginary line connecting the lateral canthi of the eyes. Lateral saw cuts start at the dorsolateral notch of the occiput and just miss the dorsal projection of the coronoid process. A small hatchet, inserted into the saw cuts, can be used to lever the calvaria. Next, the cranial nerves and the meningeal attachments can be severed and the brain removed. Hemisection, parasagittal section, or selective subsection of the brain should

PROCEDURE 16.1—cont'd

Rabies-Related Necropsy Procedure

be performed for the rabies specimens submitted to the laboratory, as directed by the state testing laboratory.

In cases where a human has been bitten or exposed to saliva through open wounds and rabies is not on the differential list or the animal did not have neurologic signs, either the whole head or two transverse slices of the brain (one involving the medulla and cerebellum bilaterally and the other involving the hippocampus bilaterally) should be submitted for rabies testing. The necropsy can be performed in the usual manner.

In all cases, tables and instruments must be carefully disinfected and cleaned. Disposable scalpels are placed in a sharps container, and other instruments must be cleaned and disinfected.

All submitted tissue specimens must be accompanied by a completed state rabies questionnaire.

If rabies is suspected, the animal's head should be sent to the appropriate laboratory for testing, according to the guidelines and laws of the state (Procedure 16.1). In cases in which rabies is suspected, decapitation or other necropsy procedures should not be attempted unless the technician has been specifically trained to perform the procedure because of zoonotic potential. A necropsy should be performed on the rest of the carcass only if the rabies test result for the brain is negative. Head or brain specimens should never be frozen.

For cytologic examination, smears are made either by scraping the cut surface of the specimen with a new, sterile scalpel blade before spreading the scraped material onto a slide or by lightly pressing small pieces of tissue against the surface of a clean slide. Several impressions are made across the slide. Slides are generally submitted fixed and unstained to the laboratory, or they can be stained and examined at the time of the necropsy.

TECHNICIAN NOTE

Fresh tissues for laboratory examinations must be collected aseptically. If rabies is suspected, the animal's head must be sent to the appropriate laboratory for testing, according to the guidelines and laws of the state.

Swabs

Swabs may be taken of an infected area for bacterial culture, viral growth, and molecular testing, such as polymerase chain reaction (PCR). Swabs should be collected aseptically to be kept and shipped in a similar way to fresh tissues. Swabs must not be allowed to dry out; it is useful to use a culturette with gel in the bottom or place the swab in a plain red-top tube with a few drops of sterile saline. Ship swabs to the laboratory the same way as shipping fresh tissues.

Whole Blood, Serum, Fluids, and Feces

Before collection occurs, contact the diagnostic laboratory for specific advice on which samples to collect and how they should be collected, packaged, and submitted. Blood samples taken before the death of the animal may be an invaluable diagnostic tool. Certain diseases may be confirmed with blood tests that require serum or whole blood. In addition, fluids may be collected from body cavities (thoracic, abdominal, pericardium) for various tests. Collect all fluids aseptically, placing them in red-top serum tubes for storage and transport to the laboratory. On the tubes, one should clearly mark from which cavity the fluid was recovered. Similarly, feces may be collected for laboratory tests. An adequate sample of fecal material, about 15 g or one tablespoon, placed in a leak-proof, labeled container is an easy sample to collect.

Shipping Diagnostic Specimens

The rules for shipping diagnostic samples, technically referred to as *clinical specimens*, have changed in recent years. Senders can be fined if containers break or specimens leak during normal transit conditions. Correct labeling is important, and a special packaging symbol (UN 3373) is required. Although most courier companies abide by International Air Transportation Association (IATA) rules, which impose the highest packaging and labeling standards, it is best to contact the courier to request specific packaging requirements.

In general, all clinical specimens must be shipped in rigid, leak-proof primary containers. Excess formalin can be removed if the specimen has been fixed. The primary container is enclosed in a secondary container, usually a sturdy, sealable plastic bag. Primary and secondary containers must be labeled. The plastic bag should contain absorbent material in case there is any leakage. This package then goes inside a rigid shipping box. The contents of the shipping box should be cushioned; styrofoam shipping boxes with outer cardboard shells are ideal. Formalin-fixed material need not be refrigerated, but bacterial cultures and fresh or frozen tissues need to be placed in freezer packs, *not* in ice. Submission forms must not be placed in the primary containers and should be in a dedicated plastic bag for extra protection.

Facilities and Instruments

Necropsies should be performed in a well-lit, well-ventilated space, ideally outside the usual surgical and treatment areas. The area should be easy to clean and disinfect, have adequate drainage for fluids and water, and be large enough to comfortably move around in (Fig. 16.4). When necropsies are performed in the field (outdoors), contamination, inappropriate disposal of tissues, and inadvertent spread of disease become public health concerns.

The person performing the necropsy (i.e., **prosector**) should wear protective clothing, such as a plastic apron, a laboratory coat, or scrubs, which can be removed and either discarded or cleaned after the necropsy (Fig. 16.5). Latex or other protective plastic gloves should always be worn, and a mesh glove should be worn on the nondominant hand when dissecting the carcasses of large animals. In addition, a surgical mask and goggles should be worn

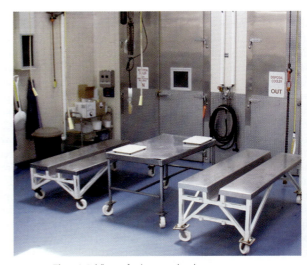

• **Fig. 16.4** View of a large animal necropsy room.

when dealing with the bodies of animals that have died as a result of infectious diseases that can be spread through aerosolization. Protective footwear (boots or booties) should be worn at all times during necropsy.

Necropsies do not require specialized equipment or instruments; most equipment can be obtained from surgical suppliers and hardware stores (Figs. 16.6 A–C, and 16.7). Box 16.1 lists the instruments used in a typical necropsy.

> ### TECHNICIAN NOTE
>
> All equipment and instruments must be thoroughly cleaned and disinfected after each necropsy. Instruments should be dedicated for necropsy use only to prevent the spread of pathogens. Labeling such instruments helps avoid confusion.

Necropsy Procedure for a Small Mammal

The procedure described below is appropriate for dogs, cats, ferrets, rodents, and rabbits. A brief outline of this procedure is provided in Procedure 16.2.

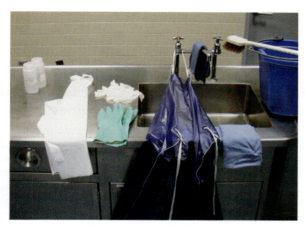

• **Fig. 16.5** Personal protective clothing (PPE) and equipment commonly used in a large animal necropsy.

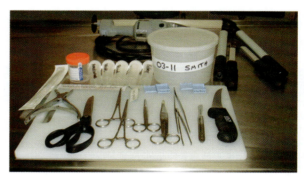

• **Fig. 16.7** Instruments and equipment commonly used in a small animal necropsy.

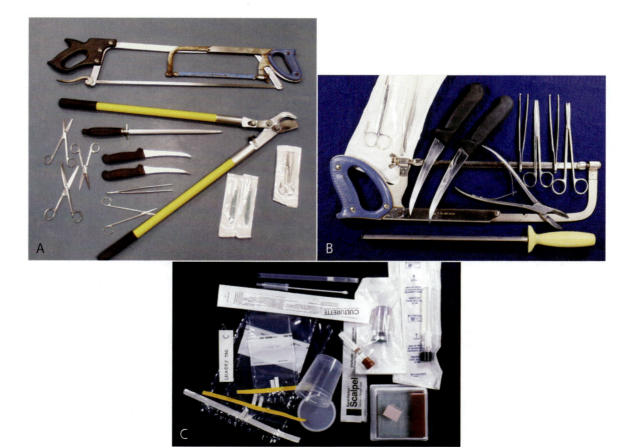

• **Fig. 16.6** (A) and (B) Instruments commonly used in a large animal necropsy. (C) Equipment commonly used in a large animal necropsy.

Preliminary Observation

Before the necropsy is begun, the prosector should confirm identity and client permission for performance of necropsy and then review the signalment (species, breed, color, sex, age, weight, and animal identification), the clinical history, and available laboratory data.

External Examination

The exterior of the animal is examined for any abnormality or lesion and external parasites, such as ticks and lice. The body conformation, hair coat, skin, nose, mouth (lips, cheeks, gums, teeth, and tongue), eyes (eyelids, conjunctiva, cornea, sclera, anterior chamber, iris, and lens), ears, mammary gland, penis, prepuce, scrotum, vulva, anus, and feet should be examined and the findings noted.

Because the retina decomposes rapidly after death, dissection begins with the eyes. The upper and lower eyelids are examined and excised. The *membrana nictitans* is grasped with tissue forceps, the globe is lifted, and soft tissue attachments to the bony orbit are incised with scissors or a scalpel in a 360-degree arc. As the globe is freed from the orbit, care must be taken to avoid application of excessive tension to the optic nerve. The optic nerve is carefully severed at the optic canal. The excised globe is examined before the extraocular muscles, fascia, fat, conjunctiva, and *membrana nictitans* are dissected from the globe. The interior of the eye can be examined by immersing the globe in clear, cool water. The sclera is examined, and the unopened globe is immersed in Bouin solution or 10% buffered formalin.

Reflections of Skin and Limbs and Examination of Superficial Organs and Body Cavities

The animal is placed in left lateral recumbency and a midline incision is made, beginning at the right axilla and extending cranially to the mandibular symphysis (Fig. 16.8). The incision is continued in the opposite direction caudally as a median or paramedian incision, passing between the mammary glands and around the penis, prepuce, and scrotum to the perineum (Fig. 16.9). The upper forelimbs are reflected by dissection between the scapula and the ribs. Fat, fascia, and superficial muscles are reflected, together with the skin. The skin of the ventral aspect of the neck, throat, and abdomen is reflected. The hindlimbs are reflected by extending the incision into the coxofemoral (hip) joints. The carcass is now moved into dorsal recumbency (Fig. 16.10).

Skin incisions are extended down the cranial medial aspects of both hindlimbs, with the skin reflected. As they are exposed during dissection, superficial organs are examined and samples from these organs are collected: lymph nodes (mandibular, superficial cervical, prescapular, axillary, inguinal, and popliteal), mammary glands, testes, and skin.

In all necropsy examinations, the coxofemoral joints are opened and examined during the initial incision. The

---

• BOX **16.1**   **Instruments Used in a Typical Necropsy Procedure**

- Necropsy knives (sturdy and capable of being sharpened) and honing steel
- Scalpel handle and blades
- Scissors (large and small operating, Mayo, or Metzenbaum scissors work well)
- Forceps (large- and small-toothed)
- Serrated, all-purpose, plastic-handled utility scissors
- Bone-cutting forceps
- Hacksaw, meat saw, or Stryker saw (for brain removal)
- Lopping (pruning) shears for cutting ribs and bones
- String or hemostats for closing off bowel ends
- Labeled plastic buckets or screw-top plastic containers containing formalin
- Tissue cassettes (for small tissues) and clip-on laundry tags for identifying tissues
- Labeled, sealable, plastic bags and plastic vials or bottles for refrigerated and frozen samples
- Culturettes for aerobic and anaerobic cultures

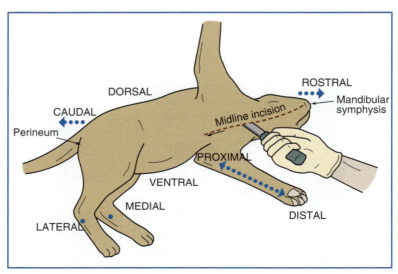

• **Fig. 16.8** The necropsy begins with the animal placed on its left side. A midline incision is made from the mandibular symphysis.

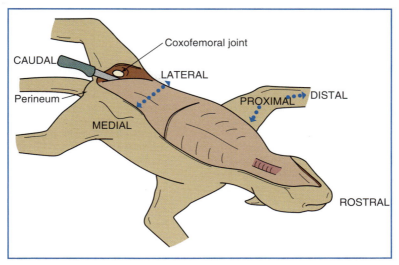

• **Fig. 16.9** The forelimbs are reflected by making incisions between the ribs and the scapulae. The hindlimbs are reflected by incising the coxofemoral (hip) joints.

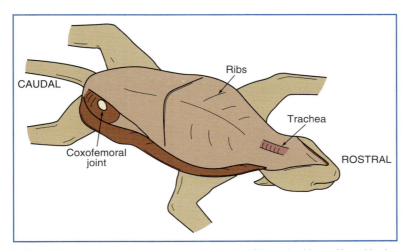

• **Fig. 16.10** After all four limbs have been reflected, the body of the animal is positioned in dorsal recumbency (i.e., on its back).

scapulohumeral and stifle joints are also examined during all routine necropsies. The atlanto-occipital joint will be examined when the head is removed.

Samples of the **sciatic nerve**, synovium with patella, and skeletal muscle are collected. Bone marrow samples for impression smears or histopathologic examination should be collected by cracking the upper midshaft femur with pruning shears.

At this point, eyes, lymph nodes, testes or mammary glands, skin, synovium, sciatic nerve, skeletal muscle, and bone marrow have already been collected.

Next, the three major body cavities (peritoneal, pleural, and pericardial) are opened, and organs are examined in situ, with any abnormalities noted. The abdomen is opened via a midline incision.

All routine tissues and organs and all lesions are collected, described, and measured and weighed, if appropriate. All necessary samples for microbiology, cytology, and toxicology, and formalin-fixed tissues for histopathology are collected for every necropsy.

> ### TECHNICIAN NOTE
>
> The history and preliminary findings are reviewed with the clinician. The thyroid, parathyroid, adrenal glands, and thymus should be identified and removed. The adrenal glands should then be sectioned to note the corticomedullary ratio. The mandibular salivary glands, parotid salivary glands, parotid lymph nodes, jugular veins, and parapharyngeal and retropharyngeal lymph nodes are examined.

Dissection (Opening Carcass)

The method of dissection described here is a standard technique that can be applied to all mammalian species and is based on the following two precepts:

1. In stepwise fashion, each part of the carcass is examined **in situ** (naturally, as lies undisturbed and in place in the body); sections can then be isolated from the carcass and examined as a whole and, finally, before being dissected for examination.

PROCEDURE 16.2

Necropsy Procedure Outline

1. Before you begin dissection, make sure you have the owner's permission, the correct animal's body, disposition instructions, body weight, labeled formalin container, instruments, cassette for bone marrow, tag for the brain, cardboard for nerve and skin, and an understanding of the clinical history.
2. Weigh the animal and perform the external examination; remove the eyes and then place the body in left lateral recumbency; make a midline skin incision extending into axillary and inguinal areas to reflect limbs; extend the incision rostrally to the mandibular symphysis and caudally to the perineum.
3. Dissect and examine, section, and collect (DESC) skin, lymph nodes, salivary glands, and testes or mammary glands. Open coxofemoral, stifle, and scapulohumeral joints. DESC the synovium, skeletal muscle, sciatic nerve, and bone marrow.
4. Cut the sternum to the symphysis pubis and incisions laterally from the sternum along both caudal costal margins. The abdominal wall is then reflected laterally exposing the abdominal cavity (Fig. 16.11).
5. The diaphragm is now punctured to check for negative pleural pressure (Fig. 16.12) before being cut away from the ventral and lateral rib cage. The ventral rib cage is removed by cutting the ribs bilaterally on both sides, midway between the costochondral junction and the vertebral column (Fig. 16.13) by using utility scissors or pruning shears. The pleural surface of the rib cage is examined first. In young animals, the costochondral growth plate may be examined and saved for histopathology. Next, the pericardial sac is opened to examine the exterior of the heart.
6. Open the abdomen (midline), puncture the diaphragm, open the chest (bilateral, cutting ribs) and the pericardium, collect microbiological samples aseptically, and examine organs and vessels in situ. DESC the thyroid, parathyroid, and adrenal glands.
7. Remove the tongue from the oral cavity and reflect the tongue, tonsils, larynx, and esophagus caudally. Cut the spinal cord and the vertebral column at the atlanto-occipital joint, remove skin and muscle from the calvaria, cut the calvaria with a Stryker saw in the hood, and remove the caudal-dorsal calvaria and the dorsal meninges. Transect the cranial nerves and remove the brain and the pituitary gland. Open the tympanic bullae. Section the head longitudinally and examine the nasal and oral cavities.
8. Remove the tongue, tonsils, esophagus, trachea, lungs, heart, and thoracic aorta together. Serially section the tongue and open the esophagus and the trachea. Open the right atrium, followed by the right ventricle, and then follow the pulmonary arteries, isolate the heart, and open the left atrium, left ventricle, and thoracic aorta. Weigh the heart. Collect the whole heart in cats and small dogs and three sections of the heart in larger animals. Serially section the lungs, saving one section from each lobe.
9. Remove the distal duodenum, jejunum, ileum, colon, and mesenteric lymph nodes together by stripping from the mesentery (open later unless critical). Remove the liver, duodenum, pancreas, stomach, and spleen. Serially section the spleen, open the stomach and duodenum, express the gallbladder, weigh the liver, and serially section the liver (collect one section of each lobe). Open the gallbladder, stomach (collect fundus and pylorus), duodenum, and pancreas (one section of right lobe with duodenum and one section of left lobe). Collect samples from all tissues.
10. Remove the floor of the pelvis and DESC the right kidney and ureter, left kidney and ureter, urinary bladder, urethra, prostate, testicles, ovaries and uterus, cervix and vagina, rectum, anal glands, and abdominal aorta, and then DESC the small intestine, colon, and mesenteric lymph nodes.
11. Remove the spinal cord, if necessary.

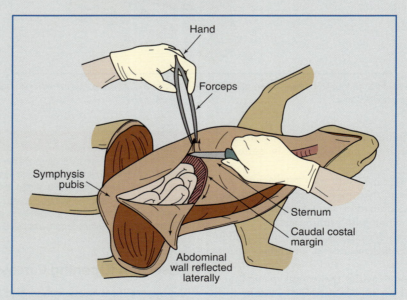

• **Fig. 16.11** The abdominal wall is incised with a midline incision. The right and left halves of the abdominal wall are reflected laterally by making incisions from the sternum along both right and left caudal costal margins.

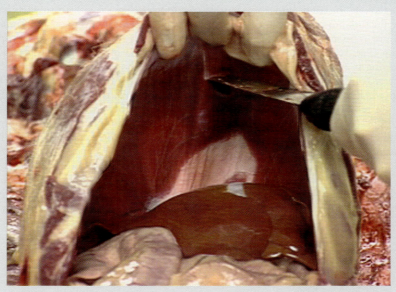

• **Fig. 16.12** The diaphragm is punctured to test for negative pressure in the pleural cavity.

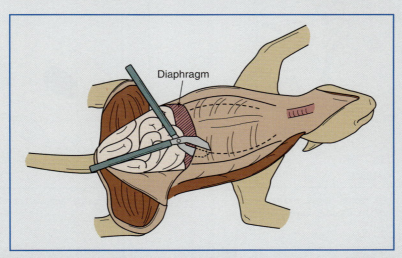

Diaphragm

• **Fig. 16.13** The ventral portion of the rib cage is removed by cutting the ribs bilaterally (on both sides) with heavy pruning shears.

2. Once a part has been taken from the body, it is dissected to completion (except for tissues from the gastrointestinal [GI] tract, brain, spinal cord, and eyes). Sections for histologic or laboratory examination are collected before further dissection is undertaken.

This method is direct contrast to those that call for "evisceration now and dissection later" methods, which disrupt the entire carcass all at once and might lead to forgotten or lost tissues. Immediate and complete dissection of one part at a time reduces the possibility of lost or forgotten parts while leaving the remainder of the carcass intact. In this way, if the findings in one organ suggest that another part or parts of the carcass should be explored

in situ, this is still possible and has not been precluded by previous dissection.

Examination of Skull and Brain

The oral cavity is examined by stretching the tongue out of the oral cavity and then reflecting the tonsils, larynx, trachea, and esophagus caudally (Fig. 16.14). An incision is made through the intermandibular muscles along the medial surface of the ramus of each mandible from the angle to the symphysis. The frenulum of the tongue is incised, and the tongue is pulled ventrally between the rami to use as a handle; right and left paramedian incisions are extended from the larynx to the thoracic inlet, exposing the length of the trachea and esophagus. It is necessary to cut or disarticulate the **hyoid bones** dorsal to the pharynx to free the tongue, larynx, pharynx, trachea, and esophagus as a unit.

The spinal cord is transected via incision into the ventral atlanto-occipital joint while the atlanto-occipital membranes, ligaments, and joint capsule are transected, disarticulating the head from the vertebral column (Fig. 16.15A and B). The skin is removed from the head by leaving it attached to the skin of the body and peeling the head forward out of the skin. The superficial muscles of the head are removed. External ears are opened and examined. Temporal muscles are removed, exposing the calvaria (skull cap) (Fig. 16.16).

The calvaria and caudal wall of the cranial cavity are removed from the skull as a unit, exposing the dorsum of the brain. This requires three cuts made with a Stryker saw, a hacksaw, or a meat saw. First, the transverse cut through the frontal bones is made immediately caudal to the orbits. Care is taken to make the cut just deep enough to transect bone but not deep enough to engage the brain beneath. The second and third cuts are made through the side walls and the caudal wall of the cranial cavity; at 45-degree angles to the longitudinal **axis** of the skull, cuts extend from the lateral ends of the transverse cut to the medial faces of the occipital condyles (Fig. 16.17). In small animals, the bone may be broken away piecemeal, progressing cranially from the **foramen magnum**, with scissors, bone-cutting forceps, or postmortem shears. The calvaria and the caudal wall as a unit are pried loose from surrounding bones and removed to examine the **meninges** and the surface of the brain in situ (Fig. 16.18).

To remove the brain, the dorsal meninges are removed, and the cranial nerves are transected, to progress rostrally from the foramen magnum. The brain is examined, tagged, and immersed in 50% formalin to be thoroughly fixed in formalin before slicing or sectioning.

The **pituitary gland** is removed from its fossa with the brain and examined. The middle ears (tympanic bullae) are opened ventrally by using rongeurs. For examination of the nasal septum, turbinates, and frontal or maxillary sinuses, the skull is sectioned longitudinally with a saw. The oral cavity is also examined.

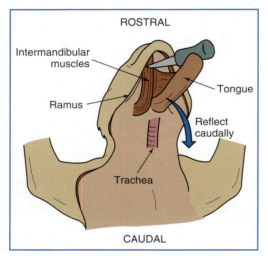

• **Fig. 16.14** Examination of the tongue, tonsils, larynx, and esophagus are reflected caudally after the intermandibular muscles have been incised.

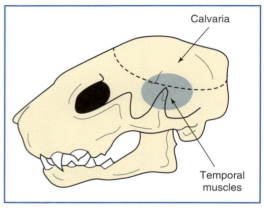

• **Fig. 16.16** The temporal muscles are removed to reveal the skull cap or calvaria.

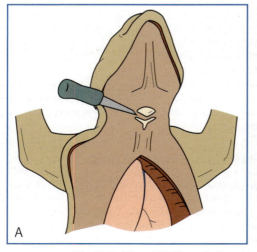
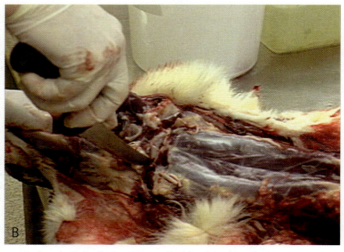

• **Fig. 16.15** (A) and (B) The spinal cord is transected ventrally by first making an incision into the atlanto-occipital joint. The head is disarticulated from the vertebral column.

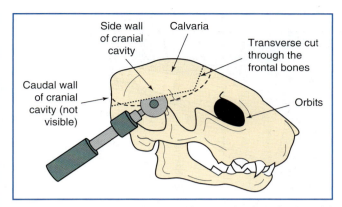

• **Fig. 16.17** The cranial cavity is opened by removing the calvaria and the caudal wall as a unit.

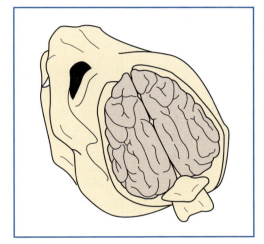

• **Fig. 16.18** The meninges and the surface of the brain are examined in situ.

Dissection and Examination of Neck and Thoracic Viscera

To remove and examine the cervical and thoracic viscera, the trachea and the esophagus, as a unit, are used as a handle, and the thoracic organs are removed from the body by cutting between the dorsal **mediastinum** and the vertebral column from the thoracic inlet back to the diaphragm. The dorsal incision is directed above the aorta. At the diaphragm, the aorta, the postcava, and the esophagus are transected, and the throat, neck, and thoracic viscera and tissues are removed as a unit. This unit is dissected and examined from tongue to aorta. The tongue is examined and is sliced transversely. The pharynx is opened middorsally with scissors to examine the pharynx and tonsils. The esophagus is opened longitudinally via a middorsal incision, and the larynx is opened middorsally with utility scissors or a knife with incision extended through the trachea to the lungs. The lungs are examined and palpated (for "fine fixation," the lung may be "inflated" with 10% formalin).

The right side of the heart and the pulmonary arteries are examined before the lungs are cut. The heart is held in such a way that the right side is on the prosector's left and the left side is on the right. The right auricle is incised with the incision extended away from the prosector to the far end of the right atrium (Fig. 16.19A).

The incision is then directed downward through the right **atrioventricular (AV) valve** and along the interventricular septum to the apex of the right ventricle. The incision is continued up along the interventricular septum through the pulmonic valve into the **pulmonary artery** (Fig. 16.19B). The right free wall of the heart is reflected to examine the valves and endocardial surfaces. The pulmonary arteries are opened into each lung lobe (Fig. 16.19C). The air passages and the transected lung tissues are examined. Sections of lung are squeezed gently to assess fluid content, and the bronchial lymph nodes are examined and sliced longitudinally.

The heart and major vessels are then separated from the lungs and held in such a way that the right side is on the prosector's left and the left side is on the right. The left auricle is incised, and the incision is extended away from the prosector to the far end of the left atrium (Fig. 16.20A). The incision progresses downward through the left AV valve and along the center of the left ventricular free wall to the apex of the left ventricle (Fig. 16.20B). The aortic valve and aorta are examined by cutting up through the septal leaflet of the left AV valve and into the aorta (Fig. 16.20C). The valves, endocardium, and endothelial surfaces are then examined. The heart may be weighed after all major vessels have been removed at the base of the heart. Next, the **myocardium** is sliced longitudinally for examination, and samples are collected. Small-sized hearts should be fixed whole after they have been opened.

Dissection and Examination of Abdominal Cavity

Examination of the abdominal cavity begins with examination of the portal vein as it enters the liver and removal of the intestinal tract. The intestine is removed by stripping the mesentery from the small intestine and colon. The **duodenum** is clamped or tied and transected distal to the tail of the pancreas, whereas the colon is transected at the pelvic inlet, and the intestinal tract is clamped and removed for later examination.

The stomach, liver, spleen, pancreas, and duodenum are removed by cutting the attachments between these organs and the ventral body wall. The spleen is examined and sectioned. The stomach is opened along the greater curvature, and the duodenum is opened. The gallbladder is squeezed to determine the patency of the bile duct. The stomach, duodenum, and pancreas are dissected from the liver, examined, and sectioned. A section of the right side of the pancreas is collected with the duodenum, and a section of the left side is collected separately. The liver is then examined and sectioned. Multiple slices (approximately 1 cm apart) are made in the liver, and samples, including lesions observed, are collected from each lobe.

The intestinal tract is examined, usually at the end to avoid contamination, by laying it out on the table and examining the serosal surface. The tract is then opened from the duodenum through the colon by using scissors. The mucosa is examined, and sections are taken from the jejunum, ileum, and colon, including lesions. The mucosa should be handled carefully to prevent creation of artifacts. Once sections have been taken, the mucosa can be gently rinsed with water to reveal mucosal details. This water may be saved/decanted to look for parasites later.

Dissection and Examination of Female and Male Urogenital Tracts

The floor of the pelvis should be removed to facilitate examination and removal of the urogenital tract. This is accomplished

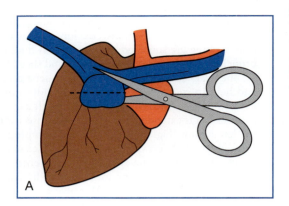
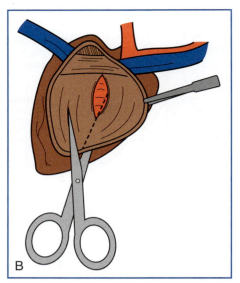
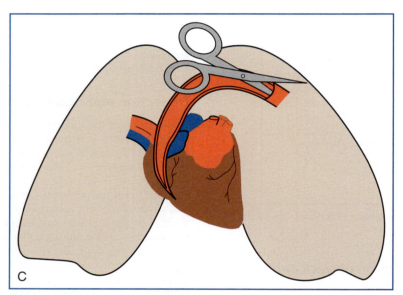

• **Fig. 16.19** (A) Dissection of the heart begins with an incision into the right auricle. (B) The heart is incised through the right atrium and ventricle after incising the interventricular septum. The incision is then continued into the pulmonary artery. (C) The pulmonary artery is incised, and the incision is continued into each lung lobe.

by making paramedian cuts through the obturator foramina on the floor of the pelvis. The mesovarium, mesosalpinx, and mesometrium are examined. Ovaries, oviducts, and uterus are freed from mesentery, reflected toward the pelvis, and removed with the cervix, vagina, and vulva as a unit. Large ovaries are sliced longitudinally, oviducts are examined and palpated, and the uterus, cervix, vagina, and vulva are opened with scissors or a knife. The serosa, contents of the uterus, endometrium, cut surfaces, cervical folds, and luminal surfaces of the vagina and vulva are examined.

The kidneys are dissected free from the abdominal wall but remain attached to the ureter. It is sliced longitudinally, and the capsule is peeled from one-half of the kidney (Fig. 16.21). The surface, cortex, medulla, and pelvis are examined, and the ureters are examined and palpated. If the ureters or the renal pelvis is dilated, the ureters are opened from the kidney to the bladder with scissors. The ureter is cut near the bladder, and the kidney is removed. Kidney sections are taken from the middle of both halves—one with the capsule intact and one without the capsule. Samples are also collected from any renal lesions before the urinary bladder is incised and opened (Fig. 16.22). The bladder serosa, mucosa, and cut surfaces are examined, avoiding rubbing the mucosal surfaces. The urethra is opened and examined, and the prostate is examined and sectioned.

TECHNICIAN NOTE

Care should be taken to avoid rubbing the mucosal surfaces of tissues during examination.

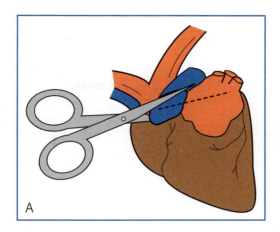

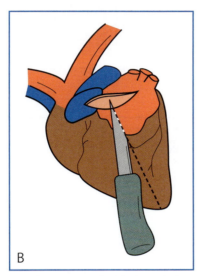

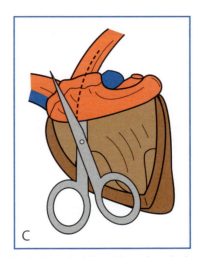

• **Fig. 16.20** (A) The second half of the heart is dissected by incising the left auricle and continuing the incision into the left atrium. (B) From the left atrium, the incision is continued through the left atrioventricular (AV) valve into the left ventricle to the apex. (C) The incision is then continued into the aorta.

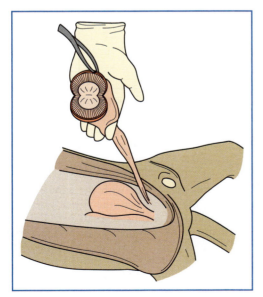

• **Fig. 16.21** The kidney is dissected with a longitudinal incision. The renal capsule is then peeled away to reveal the renal surfaces.

Dissection and Examination of Abdominal Aorta, Rectum, and Anal Glands

The abdominal aorta is opened longitudinally, examined, and a section is taken for histologic examination. The rectum is opened, and the anal sacs are examined.

Dissection and Examination of Vertebral Column and Spinal Cord

The manner and extent to which the vertebral column is dissected depends on the history and size of the animal. For more extensive examination of the vertebral column and spinal cord, the remaining rib cage, the four limbs, and most of the dorsal spinal musculature are removed from the vertebral column and the pelvis. Dorsal laminectomy is performed to demonstrate ventral or lateral impingements on the spinal cord of small animals. The spinal cord is covered dorsally by the vertebral arches; each arch consists of a right and a left lamina, which unite to form the dorsal spinous process. Beginning at the **atlas**, the right and left **laminae** of each vertebra are cut with bone shears or the Stryker saw (larger specimen). Once several dorsal arches have been freed, the connected arches are held as a handle and are used to reflect succeeding

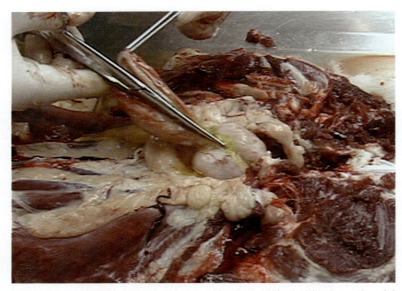

• **Fig. 16.22** The urinary bladder is incised and opened in situ, and the incision is continued through the prostate and urethra.

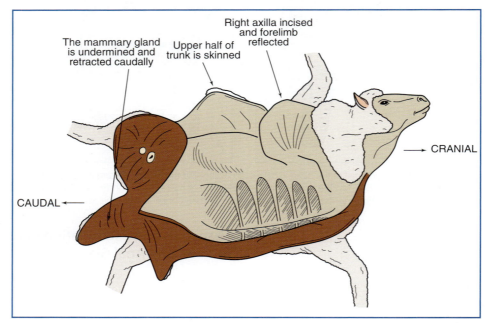

• **Fig. 16.23** The ruminant is positioned in left lateral recumbency, a position that allows the rumen to be on the "down side" and facilitates access to the abdominal organs.

arches dorsally and caudally. When the entire roof of the vertebral canal has been removed, the meninges, spinal cord, and vertebrae are examined in situ. The spinal cord and meninges are removed by cutting spinal nerve roots, and the floor of the vertebral canal and the intervertebral disks are examined.

Necropsy Variations

The sections that follow describe variations on the basic small mammal necropsy procedures that are useful in dealing with ruminants, horses, pigs, fetuses, farm animals, birds, and laboratory animals.

Ruminants

Necropsy of a ruminant is done with the animal in left lateral recumbency, with the rumen on the lower side to facilitate removal of the abdominal organs (Fig. 16.23). The right inguinal area is incised, and the coxofemoral joint is penetrated. The muscles near the pelvis are severed, and the right hindlimb is reflected away from the body. Each mammary gland is detached from its body wall attachment and retracted caudally. The mammary glands should remain attached to the body by the perineal skin so that gland position can be identified when they are serially sectioned. The right axilla is incised so that the entire forelimb can

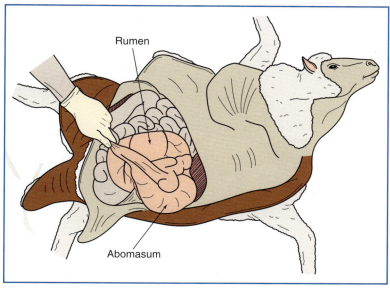

• **Fig. 16.24** Access to the abdominal cavity is achieved by making an incision along the midline, followed by cuts along the last ribs.

be reflected away from the body before the upper half of the trunk is skinned.

Abdominal entry is initiated by cutting the body wall behind the last rib and along the midline and upper flank to permit exposure of the cavity (Fig. 16.24). After an in situ inspection, the **omentum** is stripped from the **forestomach**; double-string ligatures are placed on the duodenum (near the pylorus) and the rectum, and a single ligature is placed around the esophagus near the reticulum to prevent leakage. If the rumen is severely distended with gas, making a tiny nick in the wall or piercing with a sterile needle will release the gas without excessive contamination. The intestines are opened, examined, and sampled while still attached to the mesentery (Fig. 16.25). The entire intestinal tract is removed by severing the mesenteric root and cutting the dorsal attachments to the rumen so that the forestomach and the **abomasum** are rolled onto the floor. Ruminoreticular contents should be examined/sampled for foreign objects or undesirable plant material.

Thoracic contents are readily removed via an abdominal cavity approach. The large size of the chest cavity, coupled with the difficulty of cutting ribs of mature animals, encourages use of this procedure. The **diaphragm** is incised along its costal attachment, and the caudal and ventral mediastinal attachments are severed. The tongue, larynx, trachea, and esophagus are then freed of their attachments. Disconnecting the hyoid-laryngeal apparatus can be difficult, requiring bold knife cuts medial to the mandible to expose the lateral surfaces of hyoid bones. Next, the knife is inserted medial to the hyoid bones and pulled forward parallel to the larynx, forcing the knife through one of the hyoid bone joints. The thoracic inlet connective tissues are severed by rimming the knife medial to the first ribs. The tongue is threaded into the chest and the entire unit—tongue, larynx, trachea, esophagus, lungs, and heart—is pulled into the abdominal cavity.

In ruminants, various circumstances (e.g., legal mandates or the presence of neurologic disease) may require sample collection for prion disease testing (Box 16.2). In such cases, the brainstem, pharyngeal lymph nodes, and sometimes the tonsils are collected. The remainder of the ruminant necropsy is like that described for the small mammal.

Horse

Left lateral recumbency is the preferred body position for necropsy of a horse. Reflect the right forelimb and the right hindlimb, as described for the ruminant. The trunk is skinned and the abdomen entered. The intestines are removed in the following multistep process:

1. Retract and drape the free portion of the large colon over the horse's body to facilitate access to the abdominal viscera.
2. Sever the ileum at the ileocecal junction and remove the small intestine by cutting along the mesenteric insertion.
3. Cut the duodenum where it wraps around the mesenteric root; a string ligature here will reduce contamination by digesta.
4. Next, remove the small intestine mesentery.
5. Cut the small colon near the pelvic inlet and detach along the mesocolon.
6. With careful blunt dissection, peel the soft connective tissue and pancreas adhering to the large colon near the mesenteric root. With one hand, hold the mesenteric root, advancing the knife to cut as close to the aorta as possible.
7. Obtain samples from the large colon and cecum and empty them of their contents. Rinse and examine the mucosal surfaces; liquid may be retained for examination for parasites later.

The remainder of the necropsy is like the procedure done on ruminants and small mammals. Special attention should be given to the guttural pouches and jugular veins.

All of the joints of the **appendicular skeleton** should be opened. Joints are best approached from the medial and cranial aspects after the skin has been reflected. The coffin joint is the most difficult joint to access, but access is easier if the foot can be split (with a saw), which also facilitates examination of the hoof wall lamina.

Spinal cord removal is extremely tedious without access to a meat cutter's band saw. Alternatively, the cervical cord can be extracted by disarticulating the cervical vertebrae one by one. As much muscle as possible is removed before disarticulating at the facets and annulus fibrosus. Sever the nerve roots by advancing a pair of thin, long-handled scissors along the wall of the spinal

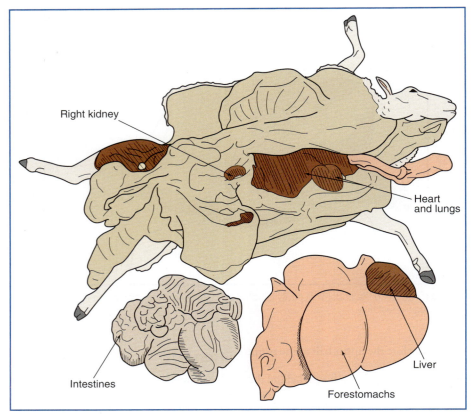

• **Fig. 16.25** After the omentum is examined in situ, it is stripped from the forestomach. The duodenum, rectum, and esophagus are ligated, and the entire intestinal tract is removed by severing the mesenteric root.

canal. The cord is grasped by its dura mater, and every effort is made to avoid crushing the soft central nervous system tissue.

Pig

For necropsy of a pig, small mammal procedures apply. Because enteric disease is a frequent reason for necropsy, attention should be focused on collecting the freshest possible gut tissues. It is customary to examine both nasal turbinates of market-weight pigs. This is accomplished by making a cut of the snout with a transverse saw at the level of the second and third premolars. Mature swine have sinus bone covering much of the calvaria. Brain removal is best accomplished by hemisectioning the head.

Fetus

Fetuses are often severely autolyzed, sometimes mummified as a result of in utero retention after death. Nevertheless, sample collection is justified. Placental membranes should be carefully examined, with all abnormal-appearing sites sampled. Equine fetal membranes are examined for completeness, whereas fetuses from cattle and horses are measured and weighed (if possible) to estimate gestational age. Crown-to-rump length (the distance from the poll to the tail base along the dorsum) is determined with a flexible tape measure.

The fetus is placed in right lateral recumbency, because fetal abdominal organs are more easily sampled from the left side. The left limbs are removed, and the body wall is skinned. The

abdominal wall is incised without touching the underlying viscera or allowing the body wall to drop onto the viscera behind the rib, with the incision extended along the ribs, sublumbar flank, and midline. The left hemidiaphragm and costosternal cartilage are cut with the tip of the knife and, as in the abdominal approach, the rib cage is retracted (ribs may break along vertebral column) without touching the underlying tissues.

Organs are sampled in situ by using sterile tools and aseptic technique. The organs of greatest interest for viral cultures are the lungs, liver, kidneys, and lymphoid tissue (e.g., spleen, thymus), whereas the organs of greatest interest for bacterial culture are the stomach (for fluid), lungs, and liver. The body can now be routinely examined for anatomic correctness and samples collected for histopathologic examination. The umbilical stump and brain should always be examined and collected.

Birds

Birds suspected of having infectious or zoonotic diseases, such as psittacosis, should be submitted (whole carcass) to a diagnostic laboratory for necropsy. If avian necropsies are done, the prosector should wear a mask, in addition to protective clothing, and gloves. The carcass should be dampened by immersing it in warm, soapy water or disinfectant to decrease the spread of infectious agents and to reduce the quantity of irritating, aerosolized dander and feathers. After external examination, the bird carcass is placed in dorsal recumbency, and the feathers are parted along the ventral midline. In the case of small birds, one wing may be

Prion Disease Surveillance

Prions are unconventional infectious agents that are proteins (i.e., neither bacterial nor viral) with an insidious mode of transmission. Abnormal prions are the cause of fatal neurodegenerative diseases collectively known as *transmissible spongiform encephalopathies* (TSEs). Species-specific diseases include chronic wasting disease (CWD) of deer, scrapie of sheep and goats, and bovine spongiform encephalopathy (BSE, "mad cow disease"), which affects cattle and humans. State departments of agriculture and state wildlife agencies rely on technicians to collect tissues from the brains of targeted species. Because testing is regulated by state and federal entities, technicians must be certified by demonstrating that they can properly document and collect the required specimens.

Pharyngeal lymph nodes and brainstem are required samples. Procedural details are beyond the scope of this text, because sample collection is not as straightforward a task as it might initially seem. For example, the brainstem is typically harvested with a "brain spoon," which is a modified tablespoon with sharpened edges that is inserted through the foramen magnum, advanced, and twisted and retracted, pulling out an intact brainstem. A skilled technician can collect brainstems with the spoon more quickly than by any other technique. Lymph nodes are concealed in the loose connective tissue and fat around the pharynx. Species variability in lymph node location has been noted, and salivary glands are occasionally collected in error because of their similar size, shape, and color. Tonsils are included in some sampling protocols and are not always of a distinctive anatomic structure; therefore anatomic landmarks are needed for consistent site selection. Skill is required to collect samples efficiently and intact, without undue crushing or slashing. Samples are fixed in formalin, although some surveillance programs also include fresh tissues. An Internet search will generate numerous sources of information about TSE, and some of these sites provide detailed instructions and photos for sample collection.

Basic PPE (examination gloves and apron) is usually sufficient. However, animals known to have neurologic disease or that appear to have been unhealthy should be handled as though they are rabies suspects, with attention to prevention of zoonotic diseases.

pinned to a corkboard or cardboard for easier dissection. A skin incision extending from the beak to the vent is made, and the skin is reflected. The legs are reflected laterally by cutting into and exposing the coxofemoral joint. The abdomen is opened, as in the small mammal necropsy, and the **sternum** and lateral ribs are removed by cutting through the sternum, ribs, coracoid bones, and clavicles with scissors, utility scissors, poultry shears, or pruning shears, depending on the size of the bird. The air sacs and the thoracoabdominal contents are examined and sampled for examination by a microbiologist, if necessary.

For small birds (e.g., hummingbirds, finches), the entire carcass can be fixed after the body cavities have been opened. For larger birds, the joints, nerves, muscles, eyes, brain, and spinal cord can be examined as in the small mammal necropsy technique. The thyroid and parathyroid glands, located at the thoracic inlet adjacent to the carotid arteries, are removed, as is the heart. The entire GI tract, liver, pancreas, and spleen are removed, beginning with the esophagus, for examination and specimen collection. The tongue, trachea, and lungs are then removed, examined, and samples are collected. The gonads (only the left ovary is present in birds) and adrenal glands are removed and fixed whole in small birds, and then the kidneys are removed, examined, and sampled.

The spinal cord in small birds is difficult to remove without damage. The entire vertebral column with the spinal cord inside should be collected and fixed once the limbs, the head, and the

muscles surrounding the vertebral column have been removed. The vertebral column and the spinal cord can be submitted to be decalcified and trimmed by the pathology laboratory.

TECHNICIAN NOTE

Birds suspected of having infectious or zoonotic diseases, such as psittacosis, should be submitted to a diagnostic laboratory for necropsy.

Laboratory Animals

The necropsy technique for small mammals can be used for most laboratory animals, including rodents; however, for evaluation of the health status of laboratory animal colonies, more extensive testing is required. Complete health monitoring includes serology, bacteriology, parasitology, genetic monitoring, gross pathology, and histopathology. It is beyond the scope of this chapter to include techniques for blood collection for serology, bacteriologic sampling techniques, techniques for ectoparasite and endoparasite examinations, and genetic monitoring. Many laboratories provide complete diagnostic services and health monitoring for laboratory animals and should be contacted before specimens (live animals or dead, from necropsies) are submitted to them.

The technique for small mammals is used, except for the variations for small rodents, as follows. An entire hindlimb can be removed at the coxofemoral joint, the skin can be removed, and the limb can be fixed whole for bone, bone marrow, synovium, nerve, and skeletal muscle samples. For small rodents (e.g., mice, hamsters, gerbils), the lungs should be gently inflated with formalin until they fill the thorax by using a 5- to 10-mL syringe with a small- to medium-bore needle filled with formalin and threaded caudally for a few millimeters from the middle of the trachea; the trachea is then clamped with a hemostat rostral to the needle insertion site. This is done before the lungs and the heart are removed from the thorax. The heart is often too small to open easily; before fixation, it can be cut longitudinally through the middle of the right and left ventricles.

The intestinal tract can be opened in a few places and then infused with formalin by using a 5-mL syringe and a small-bore needle, or the entire tract can be opened up and pinned to cardboard before fixation. The kidney and adrenal gland on each side can be removed as a unit and left together for fixation once the kidney has been incised longitudinally to evaluate the renal pelvis for **hydronephrosis**. The uterus and the ovaries in female animals or the testes and the seminal vesicles in male animals can be removed, along with the urinary bladder, and fixed whole without sectioning.

The spinal cord in small animals is difficult to remove without damage. The entire vertebral column with the spinal cord inside should be collected and fixed after the limbs, head, and muscles surrounding the vertebral column have been removed. The vertebral column and the spinal cord can be submitted whole to be decalcified and trimmed at the pathology laboratory.

TECHNICIAN NOTE

The necropsy technique for small mammals can be used for most laboratory animals. However, for evaluation of the health status of laboratory animal colonies, more extensive testing is required.

Cosmetic Necropsies

Cosmetic necropsies can be performed when disease processes are limited to the abdomen and the chest. A midline incision is made in the ventral abdomen from the xiphoid to the pubis. The abdominal organs are examined in situ, and the diaphragm is cut away from the ventral rib cage. The colon and the urethra are tied off at the pelvic inlet and are transected caudal to the tie. By reaching up through the diaphragm, the prosector can grasp and transect the trachea and esophagus at the thoracic inlet. Thoracic and abdominal contents are removed as a unit and are dissected and described as in a noncosmetic necropsy. Body cavities are examined before being filled with paper towels, and the ventral abdominal incision is sutured.

TECHNICIAN NOTE

Cosmetic necropsies can be performed when disease processes are limited to the abdomen and the chest.

Recommended Readings

King JM, Dodd DC, Roth L, et al. *The Necropsy Book*. 5th ed. Gurnee, IL: Charles Louis Davis DVM Foundation; 2003.

Latimer KS, Rakich PM. Necropsy examination. In: Richie BW, Harrison GJ, Harrison LR, eds. *Avian Medicine: Principles and Application*. Lake Worth, FL: Wingers Publishing; 1994.

17

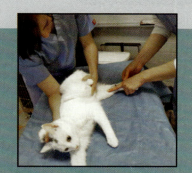

Diagnostic Sampling and Therapeutic Techniques

LORI L. STOSE

CHAPTER OUTLINE

LEARNING OBJECTIVES

When you have completed this chapter, you will be able to:

1. Pronounce, define, and spell each of the key terms in this chapter.
2. Compare and contrast patient preparation, positioning, and procedures for blood collection in small animals using venipuncture and arterial blood sampling techniques.
3. List and describe general guidelines for the collection of samples for laboratory testing and exhibit proficiency in the administration of medication to small animals:
   - Describe the indications and methods for administration of medication to cats and dogs using each of the following approaches: oral, orogastric, transdermal, ophthalmic, aural, intrarectal, intranasal, intradermal, subcutaneous, intramuscular, intravenous (IV), intratracheal, intraosseous, and intraperitoneal.
   - Compare and contrast placement of IV catheters in the peripheral and jugular veins in cats and dogs. Describe the specific steps to carry out placement of through-the-needle (TTN), over-the-needle (OTN), and multilumen catheters.
4. List and describe procedures for collection of urine samples in cats and dogs, including the advantages and limitations of each method.
5. Describe the indications, materials needed, and procedures for performing thoracocentesis and abdominocentesis on small animals.
6. Describe diagnostic peritoneal lavage (DPL) and list its indications and contraindications.
7. Compare and contrast percutaneous and endotracheal lavage techniques.
8. Describe the indications, materials needed, and procedures for different methods of performing transtracheal wash on small animals. Explain sample handling and interpretation.
9. Define arthrocentesis and list indications for performing it in the cat or the dog, list the materials needed, and explain the procedure.
10. Explain the procedure of collecting bone marrow aspirate samples, including indications, contraindications, and potential complications; compare and contrast the procedure if the sample is obtained from the ilium, humerus, or femur; and explain how the procedure of fine-needle aspiration differs from other procedures.
11. Describe the methods of orally administering medication to large animal species.
12. Compare and contrast the procedures for administering large volumes of medication via nasogastric tubes in horses and orogastric tubes in ruminants and swine.
13. Do the following regarding IV administration of medication in the large animal:
   - Describe the procedures in the horse for IV administration of medications using the jugular vein and IV catheterization utilizing the cephalic vein and the lateral thoracic vein.
   - List the indications for the use of specific veins for IV administration of medication in ruminants and swine.
   - Compare and contrast the materials needed and procedures for placing IV catheters in camelids and food animal species.
14. List the possible sites of intramuscular administration for each large animal species and describe limitations and contraindications.
15. Compare and contrast the methods used for administration of medication to horses and food animal species using each of the following approaches: subcutaneous, intradermal, intraperitoneal, intranasal, intramammary (cows only), ophthalmic, epidural, transdermal, intrasynovial, rectal, and intramuscular, including limitations and contraindications in food animals.
16. Compare and contrast venous and arterial blood collection techniques in equine, camelid, and food animal species.
17. List and describe procedures for collecting urine and fecal samples in equine, camelid, and food animal species, and list the advantages and limitations of each method.
18. Describe procedures for collection and evaluation of milk samples from dairy animals.
19. Describe procedures for collection of rumen fluid in large animals.
20. Describe the indications, materials needed, and procedures for performing a thoracocentesis, transtracheal wash, bronchoalveolar lavage (BAL), abdominocentesis, and cerebrospinal fluid collection in equine, camelids, and food animal species.

KEY TERMS

Abdominocentesis
Analgesia
Anorexia
Arthrocentesis
Ascites
Bone marrow aspirate
Bronchoalveolar lavage
Cerebrospinal fluid tap
Chronic productive cough
Coupage
Cystocentesis
Diagnostic peritoneal lavage
Epidural
Extravasation

Fine-needle aspiration
Foley catheter
Hematuria
Intraosseous
Jugular vein
Lameness
Leukocytosis
Mastitis
Neutropenia
Osmolality
Pancytopenia
Percutaneously
Phlebitis
Pleural effusion

Pneumothorax
Polymerase chain reaction
Rumen
Sarcoidosis
Seizure
Skin mass

Thoracocentesis
Thrombocytopenia
Thrombophlebitis
Thrombosis
Vasodilatation

Introduction

The veterinary technician plays a vital role in the preparation, collection, and submission of diagnostic samples and in the diagnosis and therapeutic interventions that may be required. Veterinary technicians commonly begin their careers by first developing their skills in basic techniques, such as administering medications, and then progress to more advanced sampling techniques. Therefore the contents of this chapter will describe the proper sample collection and administration of medication to both small and large animals.

Given the advances in veterinary nursing, it is incumbent on the veterinary technician to have the knowledge, skills, and ability to collect diagnostic samples and perform therapeutic techniques. When assisting with procedures, veterinary technicians should be aware of the reasons for performing the procedure, the equipment needed, the correct technique to be used, potential complications of the procedure, and postprocedural nursing care. Knowing potential complications or risks during a procedure will place the veterinary technician in a position to be proactive rather than reactive to the problem(s) that may arise. The technician should be able to assess the patient, identify the problem(s), and act on a "game plan" to address the problem(s) immediately.

Technicians should have expertise in a range of diverse procedures, including blood, urine, and feces sample collection, intravenous (IV) and arterial catheter placement, and fluid and medication administration.

Basic Guidelines

All supplies needed for medicating patients, collecting diagnostic samples, and performing therapeutic procedures should be gathered beforehand. Samples should be collected and stored in appropriate containers with the patient's name, hospital identification number, sample type, method of collection if indicated, and date printed on each label.

Pretreatment blood and urine samples should be obtained before administering fluids and/or medications. Administration of fluids, certain medications, and recent high-fat or high-protein meal ingestion may alter blood or urine laboratory values.

Whenever a needle is inserted through the skin as a part of a treatment (e.g., subcutaneous [SC] injection) or a sampling procedure (e.g., bone marrow aspiration), the skin should be properly prepared and free of apparent inflammation and infection as microbes and other contaminants present on the skin surface may be introduced into the underlying tissue when the needle is inserted. Needles and IV catheters from which the protective coverings have been removed should remain sterile and handled only at the hub (e.g., the shaft should not be touched or set down on a nonsterile surface).

Knowing potential risks or complications will place the veterinary technician in a position to be proactive rather than reactive to problems. The technician should be able to assess the patient, identify problems, and act with a game plan in mind to address problems. For example, a technician who is knowledgeable in IV catheter complications is performing IV catheter care and notices that the catheter insertion site is erythematous, swollen, painful, and warm to the touch. The veterinary technician assesses the problem as **thrombophlebitis**, determines that a new catheter is needed, and removes the old one before identifying a new site.

TECHNICIAN NOTE

Pretreatment blood and urine samples should be obtained before administration of fluids or medications.

Sampling Techniques in the Small Animal

Blood Sample Collection

Veterinary technicians perform venipuncture on a routine basis to collect blood samples for laboratory tests or to inject a drug. The collected samples must be acquired with minimal trauma to the vessel and minimal stress and discomfort to the patient, because stress in the patient can alter several laboratory test results (e.g., leukogram, cortisol, and glucose concentrations) (Procedure 17.1). As such, to minimize these types of errors, proper animal restraint during venipuncture is of great importance, along with distension and immobilization of the vessel. (Refer to Chapter 6 on "Restraint and Handling of Animals" for performing proper restraint technique.)

PROCEDURE 17.1

Venous Blood Collection

- Attach a 20- to 25-gauge needle to a 1- to 6-mL syringe.
- Occlude the vein with a tourniquet or digital pressure.
- Wipe the skin and hair on top of the vein with an alcohol-soaked cotton ball to help identify the vein.
- Insert the needle with the bevel facing up through the skin and into the vein at a 25-degree angle.
- Slowly retract the syringe plunger and collect a blood sample.
- Release the pressure on the vein and release the syringe plunger when a sufficient volume of blood has been collected.
- Remove the needle from the vein.
- Apply digital pressure to the venipuncture site as soon as the needle is removed until hemostasis occurs.

Before the veterinary technician performs any venipuncture, sufficient knowledge and understanding of such procedures should be gained to acquire the best diagnostic sample(s) for the requesting veterinarian. Background knowledge, along with a thorough understanding of the procedure, will aid in acquisition of the best diagnostic sample(s) possible. These objectives are most easily accomplished when two people work together.

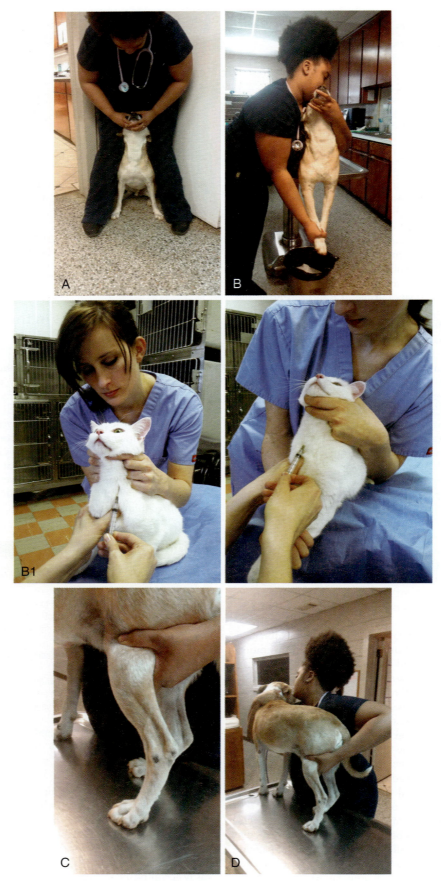

• **Fig. 17.1** (A) Floor restraint of a dog for jugular venipuncture. (B) Table edge restraint of a dog for jugular venipuncture. (B1) Two styles of restraining a cat for jugular venipuncture; note the position of the restrainer's hands. (C) Standing restraint for lateral saphenous venipuncture. (D) Manual restraint on table of dog for lateral saphenous venipuncture.

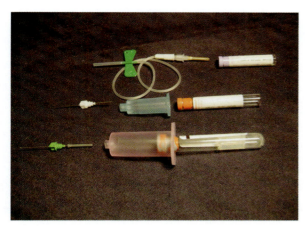

• **Fig. 17.2** Tools of the trade utilized for venipuncture include a Vacutainer set-up and butterfly syringe set-up. The Vacutainer blood collection system is used to collect blood samples directly into the collection tubes. The system consists of a needle, a holder, and collection tubes. (From Hendrix CM, Sirois M, ed. Laboratory Procedures for the Veterinary Technician. 5th ed. St. Louis, MO: Mosby; 2007.)

TABLE 17.1	**Small Animal Collection Sites**
Canine	**Feline**
Cephalic	Cephalic
Jugular	Jugular
Lateral saphenous	Femoral
	Medial saphenous

General Facts and Knowledge Regarding Venipuncture

I. The successful venipuncture technique requires proper restraint of the animal and visualization and immobilization of the vessel. Venipuncture should only be attempted if the vessel is clearly delineated; blind venipuncture often fails and leads to unnecessary patient discomfort. If the technician cannot locate the vessel upon visual inspection or digital palpation, the way the vessel is distended or immobilized must be changed (Fig. 17.1A–D).

II. Venipuncture procedures are performed with a needle and syringe, butterfly catheter with a syringe or Vacutainer, or a Vacutainer collection system, which consists of a double-pointed needle, a plastic holder, and blood collection tube(s) with or without anticoagulant (Fig. 17.2).

III. The collection site, method of collection, and needle gauge selected depend on the vessel size, amount of blood (sample) required, and the intended use of the sample, as well as the veterinary technicians' preference. The amount of negative pressure applied to aspirate blood into the syringe must not be excessive, because this may lead to the vein collapsing or hemolysis of the red blood cells (RBCs) as they pass through the needle, with the potential of erroneous laboratory results.

IV. Small-gauge needles (25-gauge to 28-gauge) are usually utilized when blood is collected from smaller, fragile vessels and/or multiple/frequent venipunctures (i.e., during blood glucose curves).

V. Medium-gauge needles (22-gauge) are usually utilized during venipunctures performed on cats and small dogs, and larger gauge needles (20-gauge and 18-gauge) are often utilized in large-breed dogs and most farm animals. For any venipuncture technique, the needle should always be inserted into the vein with the bevel facing upward.

VI. Blood collected must be placed into a specific colored-top tube for holding before diagnostic testing. However, these tubes must be filled in a certain order, known as the "order of draw," which allows for minimal contamination or "carryover" between tubes. Carryover may yield both test error and reduction in the effect of microclot formation within the utilized tubes.

VII. The collected blood is placed into the appropriate tube(s) by removing the needle from the collection apparatus and the stopper from the tube. The blood is *gently* expelled from the blood collection device into the tube by allowing the blood to flow down the side of the collection tube to the fill line, located on the side of the collection tube. If the tube contains an additive such as an anticoagulant, proper filling is necessary to achieve the correct blood-to-anticoagulant ratio. The tube is then gently rocked back and forth a number of times to ensure adequate mixing of the tube's contents. Vigorous mixing of the blood and the tube's contents, shaking, and forcefully ejecting the collected blood though the needle of the collection device may cause hemolysis of the collected blood sample and potentially affect the results.

VIII. Blood is never poured from one tube into another tube.

IX. All collection tubes should be labeled with the patient's first and last name, collection date, and the owner's first and last name.

X. Sterile gloves should be worn when blood is collected for bacterial culture. The venipuncture site should be shaved and aseptically prepared prior to collection of samples to avoid contamination of the blood collected for culturing.

XI. When collecting blood for coagulation profiles (i.e., activated clotting time [ACT], prothrombin time [PT], and activated partial thromboplastin time [APTT]), the needle of the collection device is ideally inserted within the skin so that it penetrates the vessel at the first attempt. This will minimize the amount of tissue fluid entering the collected samples (thromboplastin), which could cause a clotting cascade. Multiple attempts to redirect the needle under the skin, also known as *fishing* for the vessel, is not warranted during coagulation studies and should be avoided due to tissue trauma and venous stasis, which may affect the results of blood tests.

XII. If the initial venipuncture attempt is unsuccessful, reinsert the needle proximal to the previous entry site. For jugular venipuncture, the initial attempt is made in the caudal region of the jugular vein. Subsequent venipuncture attempts can be made in a more cranial region. If the vessel is damaged in the distal portion of the vein, a more proximal region is still patent and usable for blood collection.

Refer to Procedure 17.1 for step-by-step instructions.

See Table 17.1 for appropriate collection sites for canines and felines.

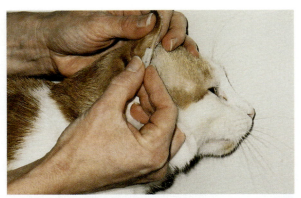

• **Fig. 17.3** Restraint and preparation for venipuncture of a marginal ear vein.

Various Venipuncture Sites and Methods of Collection in Small Animals

Quite a few locations on the body of a small animal may be used for venipuncture to obtain a blood sample for diagnostic purposes. However, some sites are more advantageous than others. For example, if large blood samples are needed, the jugular vein may be the venipuncture site of choice, because it is a rather large vessel compared with others; blood collection is faster, preventing clotting within the sample, and often yields larger quantities of blood. Conversely, if small blood samples are needed, the medial or lateral saphenous veins may be the venipuncture sites of choice, because they are smaller vessels than others and yield smaller quantities of blood. Therefore knowing the locations of all small animal venipuncture sites is very useful to veterinary technicians to be able to provide the best diagnostic samples possible for the requesting veterinarian.

Beginning with the head and ending with the tail, the venipuncture sites of small animals that will be discussed within this section are the marginal ear vein, cephalic vein, jugular vein, lateral saphenous vein, and medial saphenous vein (femoral). For arterial blood collection, the dorsal pedal artery, dorsal metatarsal artery, and femoral artery are commonly used. Techniques and procedures on how to properly obtain diagnostic samples from each of these locations are discussed below.

Marginal Ear Vein and Venipuncture Technique

The marginal ear vein in small animals is anatomically located coursing around the periphery of the lateral aspect of the pinna. This venipuncture collection site is often utilized when the smallest amounts of blood are required to obtain diagnostic results. Such tests include but are not limited to blood glucose readings in patients with diabetes mellitus and/or parasitic organism evaluation, such as *Babesia* spp. or *Mycoplasma* spp.

To collect blood from the marginal ear vein, the patient's ear is warmed with a heated cloth, a light source, a technician's hand, or a sock filled with rice that has been warmed in the microwave oven for a few seconds, all of which aid in **vasodilatation** of the vein. Once the heated material is removed (approximately 30 seconds after application), the site of venipuncture is wiped with a cotton ball soaked in 70% isopropyl alcohol. A 25-gauge × ¾-inch needle or lancet (technician's choice) is utilized to nick the skin of the pinna and the vein. Once blood appears at the skin's surface, the pinna is massaged until a sufficient sample of blood is obtained, after which direct pressure should be applied to staunch the bleeding for approximately 15 seconds (Fig. 17.3).

If the collected sample is to be used for a blood glucose reading, the glucometer test strip, which has already been loaded into the glucometer, can be placed directly next to the animal to receive the blood drop from the pinna of the ear as the blood moves via capillary action directly onto the test strip. Blood glucose results are obtained within seconds. (*Note:* It must be ensured that the glucometer is set for capillary, not venous, blood samples; that the glucometer strips are compatible with the glucometer type; and that the appropriate glucometer code is set on the glucometer.)

If the collected sample is to be used for examination of erythron parasites, the blood should be collected into a heparinized capillary tube. The blood-filled tube is used in preparing peripheral blood smears that will be evaluated microscopically for erythron parasites. In either instance, it is important to ensure that the patient does not move its head or flick its ear, or the blood sample may be lost.

Cephalic Vein and Venipuncture Technique

The cephalic vein in small animals is anatomically located along the cranial aspect of the foreleg and extends medially just above the carpus, and the accessary cephalic vein branches off laterally. Although blood may be acquired from either of these vessels, it should be noted that the medial aspect of the cephalic vein is the best choice for IV catheter placement, which will be discussed later.

This venipuncture collection site is often used when small quantities of blood from both cats and dogs are needed for diagnostic testing. Such tests include but are not limited to occult heartworm antigen test, feline leukemia virus (FeLV) antigen and feline immunodeficiency virus (FIV) antibody combination test, packed cell volume (PCV), etc.

To collect blood from the cephalic vein, the patient is positioned in sternal or lateral recumbency, preferably at the end of an examination table, which is recommended for beginners. The veterinary assistant restrains and positions the patient on the table by reaching over the patient's back and gently grasping the desired foreleg with their hand at the patient's elbow. The forearm and elbow of the assistant is positioned along the patient's body and is used in a "huglike" action to bring the patient close to the assistant's body to ensure minimal movement. The other hand of the veterinary assistant is gently placed under and around the patient's neck to pull the animal's head away from the venipuncture site and within proximity to the assistant. Once the patient is properly restrained, the vessel is occluded with a tourniquet by placing and tightening it just above the elbow, or the veterinary assistant may occlude the vessel using the thumb or forefinger and wrapping it around the patient's foreleg at the level of the elbow to occlude the cephalic vein. The patient's skin is then rotated outward, rolling the vein to the top of the foreleg (Fig. 17.4). This action should result in visualization of the cephalic vein.

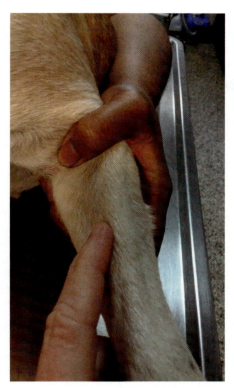

• **Fig. 17.4** The cephalic vein must be held off and identified in a fixed position for positive venipuncture to occur.

Once the vein has been properly occluded and visualized by the veterinary technologist, they should break the seal of the syringe plunger by pulling the plunger until the manufacturer's seal is broken. Then the technician grasps the desired forelimb of the patient with their nondominant hand at the level of the carpus or metacarpus and wipes the venipuncture site with a cotton ball soaked in 70% isopropyl alcohol. This action will aid in the removal of superficial contaminants and microbes and avoid introducing them into the underlying tissue during venipuncture, assist with vasodilation, and allow improved visualization of the vessel. Flexing the carpus may also aid in visualization of the vessel.

Once the veterinary technician has digitally palpated the vessel, the thumb of their nondominant hand should rest parallel to the vessel to aid in immobilization while the needle of the syringe is gently inserted, bevel side up, directly along the other side of the vessel. (This action aids in trapping the vessel between the nondominant thumb and the needle attached to the collection device.)

The initial puncture into the skin is the most painful part of the procedure and may cause the animal to react and move. During the insertion process, the needle of the syringe should be inserted parallel to the vessel and gently redirected into the vein, if it is not a clean stick into the vessel on initial puncture. If blood does not flow into the syringe upon gentle aspiration, then the needle should be slightly redirected and aspiration repeated. Once the needle has entered the vessel, a "flash" of blood should be noted within the hub of the needle. At this point, further insertion should discontinue and gentle pulling of the syringe plunger should allow for filling of the syringe with a predetermined amount of blood.

Once the desired quantity of blood has been collected, the needle should be removed from the skin slowly while gently aspirating. The veterinary assistant should apply direct digital pressure on the venipuncture site for a minimum of 15 to 30

seconds while the veterinary technician places the collected sample into the proper blood collection tube(s) for analysis. The venipuncture site should be evaluated for bleeding and/or hematoma formation for several minutes. If bleeding continues, a pressure bandage should be applied and the delay in clotting should be reported to the attending veterinarian in case clotting factors need to be evaluated.

If an IV injection is the purpose of the venipuncture, the procedure is the same as described above, except instead of collecting a blood sample, a medication is injected into the vein. The proper dose of the medication is loaded into an appropriate syringe. The vein is held off by the assistant as described above. The veterinary technician wipes the venipuncture site with 70% isopropyl alcohol, inserts the needle into the cephalic vein, aspirates to make sure that the needle is inserted into the vein by visualizing a flash of blood into the syringe, and then injects the medication at an appropriate rate for the type of medication being delivered. After the injection is complete, the veterinary technician will remove the needle from the leg, and the assistant will apply digital pressure for 15 to 30 seconds, or a pressure bandage may be applied to the leg.

Jugular Vein and Venipuncture Technique

The jugular vein of small animals is anatomically located along the lateral aspect of the neck, where it lies superficially within the jugular groove, leading up toward the head. This venipuncture site is used when large samples of blood are required for diagnostic testing. Such tests include but are not limited to complete blood cell counts, chemistry profiles, endocrine testing, and serology.

There are several different restraint techniques that may be used to collect blood from the jugular vein in small animals. Often, the size and tolerance of the animal will dictate the method of restraint required. For example, large, heavy dogs are often restrained on the floor by backing them into a corner, whereas smaller dogs or cats are placed onto an examination table and restrained for blood collection (refer to Fig. 17.1A and B).

Large dogs may be positioned in sternal or lateral recumbency or may be more comfortable seated on the floor. If seated on the floor, the patient can be backed into a corner to prevent them from backing up during blood collection (see Fig. 17.1A). For those restrained on the exam table, the assistant will grasp the forelimbs with one hand at the level of the carpal joint while stretching the legs over the edge of the table (see Fig. 17.1B) and the head towards the ceiling by grasping underneath either side of the patient's jaws. During this action, care should be taken not to compress the trachea, impair breathing, or overextend the neck, because this will lead to vein collapse.

Once the patient is properly restrained, the veterinary technician should break the seal of the syringe and occlude the vessel by applying digital pressure in the jugular groove at the thoracic inlet. With optimal positioning, the vessel is easily visualized and palpated with minimal mobility. However, at this point during the visualization process, the head of the patient may need to be turned in one direction or the other or lowered slightly for easy visualization of the vein. The veterinary technician (blood collector) will dictate in which direction the head should be moved, if needed. In sternal positioning, venipuncture is usually performed in the cephalad direction (toward the head); in lateral positioning, venipuncture is generally done in a caudal direction.

Once the vein has been properly occluded and visualized and the skin wiped with 70% isopropyl alcohol by the veterinary technologist, the needle of the collection device should be inserted directly into the skin, bevel side up, in the same manner as described above for cephalic venipuncture. Once the appropriate amount of blood has been collected, the needle should be removed from the skin slowly while gently aspirating. Direct pressure should be applied to the venipuncture site by the veterinary assistant for 15 to 30 seconds while the veterinary technologist places the collected blood within the appropriate blood collection tubes.

To collect blood from the jugular vein in cats and small dogs, the patient is often restrained, preferably at the end of an examination table, in sternal or lateral recumbency; sternal recumbency is recommended for beginners (refer to Fig. 17.1B1) by gently reaching over its back with the dominant hand and arm. The outer forearm and elbow of the assistant are positioned along the patient's body that is the furthest from the restrainer and are used to mimic a hug like action to bring the patient close to the assistant's body to ensure minimal movement. This hand is gently placed along under the jaw to pull the head up toward the ceiling. At the same time, the other hand of the veterinary assistant pulls and holds both forelegs of the patient over the end of the examination table. Again, care should be taken not to compress the trachea, impair breathing, or overextend the neck, because this will lead to vein collapse or struggling of the patient.

Once the cat or the small dog has been restrained properly, and the manufacturer's seal of the syringe plunger has been broken, the veterinary technologist once again should apply direct digital pressure on the jugular vein by pressing into the thoracic inlet to aid in vein distention and visualization. Once the vein is visualized, venipuncture may commence, as described above, followed by proper hemostasis. Collected blood should be placed into the appropriate and properly labeled collection tubes.

Lateral Saphenous Vein and Venipuncture Technique

The lateral saphenous vein of small animals is anatomically located on the lateral aspect of the hind limbs and runs from the craniomedial side of the talus to the popliteal notch. This venipuncture collection site is often used when blood is needed in small to medium amounts from aggressive, shy, and/or anxious patients, because this venipuncture site places the veterinary technician farthest away from the animal's head, thus minimizing potential injury from bites

This method is more commonly used for canine blood collection, whereas the medial saphenous is more commonly used for felines.

To collect blood from the lateral saphenous vein, both canine and feline patients alike are positioned in lateral recumbency. For lateral saphenous blood collection in dogs, the restrainer lays their forearm gently but firmly across the patient's neck just caudal to the pinna while applying downward pressure. The hand of the arm is used for holding both forelegs at the carpus (especially the lower limb) to ensure that the patient does not try to stand during the collection process. The other hand of the restrainer is placed on the hind limb furthest from the table, where circumferential pressure is applied at the level of the stifle to occlude and distend the vein. For larger dogs, the lateral saphenous vein can also be accessed in a patient standing on all four limbs.

Once the lateral saphenous vein is clearly delineated, the veterinary technician should grasp the leg with their nondominant hand at the level of the metatarsus. The vein is then aseptically wiped with 70% isopropyl alcohol. Just prior to needle insertion, the thumb of the veterinary technician's nondominant hand may be placed parallel and just to the side of the distended vessel. This will aid in immobilizing the vessel during the venipuncture process. Venipuncture should then be performed as described above (Fig. 17.5A and B).

To collect blood from the lateral saphenous vein in cats, the restraint technique is slightly modified to decrease the likelihood of injury to all personnel. Again, the cat is placed in lateral recumbency, with the restrainer "scruffing" the patient's neck gently backward with their nondominant hand while the forearm is placed parallel to and snugly along the backbone of the patient. The dominant hand of the restrainer grasps the upper hind limb with the thumb just cranial to the patella, while the index finger resides at the level of the stifle on the caudal aspect of the hind limb. Upward digital circumferential pressure is placed behind and caudal to the patella to aid in distention of the medial saphenous vein. (*Note:* Clipping the hair in the stifle area, just cranial to the tarsal bone, may aid in visualization of the vein.) (Fig. 17.6).

Once the vein has been properly positioned and delineated, the veterinary technician should grasp the upper hind limb of the

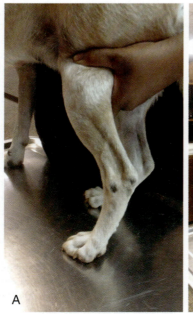
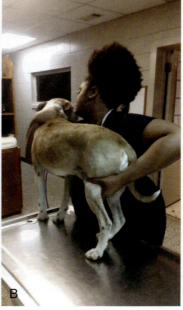

A B

• **Fig. 17.5** Restraint and holding off of the lateral saphenous vein.

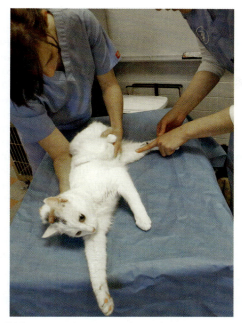

• **Fig. 17.6** Tabletop restraint of a cat for venipuncture of the right lateral saphenous vein.

patient, with their nondominant hand at the level of the metatarsals. The vein is then aseptically wiped with 70% isopropyl alcohol. Just prior to needle insertion, the thumb of the veterinary technician's nondominant hand may be placed parallel and just to side of the distended vein. This will aid in immobilizing the vessel during the venipuncture process. Venipuncture should then be performed as described above.

Medial Saphenous Vein and Venipuncture Technique

The medial saphenous vein, often called the *femoral vein*, is anatomically located along the medial aspect of the hind limbs in cats and dogs. This is often the vessel of choice when small volumes of blood are needed, especially in feline patients. Such diagnostic tests include but are not limited to those for FeLV and FIV.

To collect blood from the medial saphenous vein in canine patients (although rarely performed), the patient is positioned in lateral recumbency and the restrainer lays their forearm gently but firmly across the patient's neck just caudal to the pinna while applying gentle, firm downward pressure. The hand of the same arm is utilized for holding both forelimbs at the carpus (especially the lower limb) to ensure that the patient does not try to stand during the collection process. The other hand of the restrainer is used for applying pressure to the lower leg at the stifle while abducting and flexing the upper leg proximally toward the patient's body. Pressure is applied proximal to the stifle area of the leg closest to the table to occlude the vessel. Once the vessel has been visualized and immobilized, venipuncture may commence as described above.

To collect blood from the medial saphenous vein in feline patients (often the preferred site), the patient is positioned in lateral recumbency. The dominant hand of the restrainer is utilized for "scruffing" the neck and for pulling the head gently backward while the forearm is placed parallel to and snugly along the backbone of the patient. The nondominant hand of the restrainer is used for grasping the upper hind limb of the patient so that it can be abducted and flexed to expose the medial surface of the bottom leg. Pressure is applied with the side of the abducting hand along the inguinal area of the bottom leg in a "karate chop" fashion. This will aid in occluding and distending the vessel running along the medial surface of the leg.

Once the vein has been delineated, the veterinary technician should grasp the lower hind limb of the patient with the nondominant hand at the level of the metatarsals. The vein is then aseptically wiped with 70% isopropyl alcohol. Venipuncture should then be performed as described above (see Fig. 17.4).

> **TECHNICIAN NOTE**
>
> Cephalic veins should be the last site of choice for collection of diagnostic samples, because these vessels need to be maintained for intravenous (IV) catheter placement, if warranted.
>
> Jugular venipuncture should not be used in patients that have sustained head trauma, possible heatstroke, clotting abnormalities, and/or snake bites.

Arterial Blood Collection Sites and Techniques in Small Animals

Arterial blood samples are samples collected from the arteries, not veins, and are commonly used for *arterial blood gas (ABG) samples*. These samples are used for evaluation of a patient's pulmonary function, gas exchange within the lungs, measurement of the partial pressure of oxygen (PaO_2) and carbon dioxide ($PaCO_2$) levels in the blood, and the pH levels of blood. Such data aids the veterinarian in identifying kidney disease, heart failure, and uncontrolled diabetes mellitus (called diabetic ketoacidosis). The measurement of ABGs gives the best insight into the patient's ability to ventilate and oxygenate.

> **TECHNICIAN NOTE**
>
> One of the best ways to assess pulmonary function is through measurement of arterial blood gases (ABGs).

As the term implies, *arterial blood samples* may be collected from any of the arteries that run throughout the body. However, the four most common arterial blood collection sites in dogs and cats are the dorsal pedal artery, the dorsal metatarsal artery, the femoral artery, and/or the lingual artery. However, it should be noted that both the femoral artery and the lingual artery are most often used on unconscious or anesthetized patients (http://veterinarymedicine.dvm360.com/arterial-blood-gas-analysis-and-interpretation-anesthetized-patients). Techniques and procedures on how to correctly obtain diagnostic samples from each of these locations are discussed below.

For collection of an arterial sample, the internal lining of a 1- or 3-mL syringe (with a 25-gauge needle) is coated with lithium or sodium heparin (1000 units/mL); the excess is expelled from the syringe. The collection site should be swabbed with 70% isopropyl alcohol prior to puncture. In addition, a Vacutainer tube cork and a thermometer will be needed if the sample analysis will be delayed or sent to an outside laboratory. When the sample is collected, care should be taken to avoid introducing air or applying excessive negative pressure, both of which can affect the measurement of partial pressure of oxygen as dissolved in plasma or PaO_2. Once the sample collection is complete, the needle is withdrawn and digital pressure applied over the puncture site for at least 1 minute; in addition, one should monitor for bleeding or hematoma formation for another 4 minutes. Air is expelled from the syringe, and the syringe is capped with the cork and placed in an ice water bath for transport to the laboratory. Blood gas samples may stay in an ice water bath for several hours if testing cannot be done immediately before metabolism alters pH or blood gas values.

Dorsal Pedal/Dorsal Metatarsal Artery Collection Techniques

The dorsal pedal artery of small animals is anatomically located along the dorsomedial aspect of the metatarsals just distal to the hock, where it branches off into three dorsal metatarsal arteries that run parallel to that of the phalanges. Even though these two types of arteries are smaller in diameter compared with that of the femoral artery, the interstitial connective tissue around the dorsal arteries are much tighter than those that surround the femoral arteries, thus facilitating the vessel's positioning and minimizing postpuncture hematoma formation. Both the dorsal pedal artery and the dorsal metatarsal artery are known to be the most used sites for acquisition of an ABG sample.

To obtain an ABG sample from the dorsal pedal artery and/or the dorsal metatarsal artery, all the necessary supplies and equipment need to be collected near the patient, which is then positioned in lateral recumbency (or in a standing patient if they are resistant to being in lateral recumbency) while the pulse of the desired artery (either the dorsal pedal artery or the dorsal metatarsal artery) is palpated with one or two fingers of the veterinary technician's nondominant hand. Once the pulse has been successfully palpated, the patient's hair is gently clipped and that area is aseptically prepped (Fig. 17.7). It may be helpful to tape the paw to the table or sandbag to help isolate the position. If a visual pulse is not observed within the prepped area, the veterinary technician should then repalpate the clipped area with the nondominant hand to locate the pulse again.

Once the pulse has been located, the needle of an ABG self-filling syringe coated with lithium heparin or a 3-mL syringe that has been coated with lithium heparin and a 22-gauge or 25-gauge needle attached should be gently inserted with the bevel side up directly into the skin. After the patient has settled from the initial stick (the puncture into the skin is the most painful part of the procedure), the fingers palpating the pulse are used as a guide, and the needle is inserted parallel to the artery at a 45-degree angle. If the arterial puncture is unsuccessful, the needle can be either advanced further or withdrawn into the SC position and the arterial puncture reattempted.

Upon entering the artery, a flash of blood should be observed within the hub of the needle. If an ABG self-filling syringe has been used, the syringe will automatically fill to a predetermined volume set prior to venipuncture. If using a lithium heparin-coated syringe and needle, the veterinary technician will have to gently pull back on the syringe plunger to acquire the desired amount of blood, which is usually 1 to 1.5 mL. Once the desired amount of blood has been collected, the needle is removed while the veterinary assistant applies direct pressure to the venipuncture site for 1 to 5 minutes to minimize hematoma formation.

Once the desired sample amount has been obtained, all air is removed from the collection syringe and a rubber stopper is placed on the end of the needle to decrease the likelihood of atmospheric oxygen and carbon dioxide entering the sample as this could lead to inaccurate results. The sample is then immediately taken to a diagnostic laboratory and processed without delay. It is ideal for the sample to be run in-house using a commercial analyzer to decrease the risk of exogenous changes to the sample. Inexpensive point-of-care instruments have been developed for in-house use, and these analyzers are cost effective and easy to use.

Femoral Artery

The femur of small animals, also known as the *thigh bone*, is anatomically in the proximal portion of the hind limb of small animals and is located between the hip and the knee joint. Along the medial aspect of the hind limb, parallel to the femur, is the femoral artery, which runs the length of the femoral bone down into the distal portions of the hind limbs. During an ABG sample draw, this vessel should not be confused with the medial saphenous vein. (*Hint:* the femoral artery is located more medially than the femoral vein, and a pulse can be felt over the artery.)

To properly collect an ABG sample from the femoral artery in both cats and dogs, the patient should be positioned in lateral recumbency and restrained in the same manner as when blood is being collected from the medial saphenous vein. However, during patient restraint, the bottom part of the hind limb should be extended caudally, whereas the top hind limb should be positioned such that it is completely out of the way for femoral arterial puncture (see Figs. 17.5 and 17.6). After the puncture site has been prepared properly, the first and middle fingers of one hand are used to locate the artery, and the leading edge of the same hand can be used to slide the skin and underlying SC tissues toward the inguinal region. The femoral artery must be immobilized properly to prevent it from rolling away from the needle. The syringe is held at a 45-degree angle over the site where the pulse is strongest. As previously described, the needle is advanced through the skin and the sample collected (see Fig. 17.7).

Arterial Catheter Placement

Arterial catheters are inserted for continuous measurement of direct arterial blood pressure and for collection of multiple arterial blood samples. The most common artery selected for catheterization is the dorsal metatarsal artery, which offers many advantages over the femoral artery. The cylindrical nature of the tarsus allows the catheter to be taped rather than sutured. Risk of hematoma formation and hemorrhage is reduced because of the tight SC tissues, and it is easier to maintain the catheter position, because the catheter does not move and bend within the SC tissues.

A 20- or 22-gauge over-the-needle (OTN) catheter may be placed in the dorsal metatarsal artery. The catheter is flushed with heparinized saline. The patient is placed in lateral recumbency

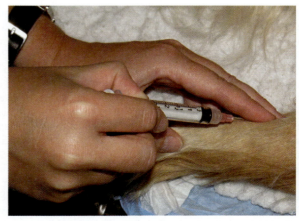

• **Fig. 17.7** Palpating the dorsal metatarsal artery for arterial blood sampling; note the position of the hand in relation to the syringe.

with the hock extended; it may be helpful to tape the paw to a table or a sandbag. The insertion site is clipped and aseptically prepared. The artery to be catheterized is palpated with one or two fingers of one hand. The end of the needle is inserted through the dermis with the beveled edge of the needle (without entry into the artery). The catheter is positioned SC above the artery with the bevel side up. The needle tip and the artery are palpated simultaneously with the finger(s) of the opposite hand. The catheter is inserted into the artery steeply at first, just so that the tip of the needle penetrates the upper wall of the artery, and then flat against the skin surface and parallel to the longitudinal axis of the artery, so that the bevel of the needle and the end of the catheter lie in the lumen of the artery. A "flash back" of blood should be seen in the hub of the needle; the catheter is gently advanced into the artery to its full length. The needle is replaced with a T-connector and stopcock. The catheter is taped in place and flushed with heparinized saline. Refer to the section "Peripheral Vein Catheterization" for further details.

The catheter may be attached to a continuous flush system or flushed with heparinized saline every 2 hours. The toes should be checked for warmth every 2 to 4 hours. If the toes are cool, the catheter may need to be removed. Catheter care is performed every 48 hours.

Urine Sample Collection

A urine sample may be obtained by using several methods, and the veterinary technician should be familiar with the various techniques. Urine is most often collected for gross and microscopic analyses and for culture, if indicated. Common collection techniques include obtaining urine from the patient as the animal naturally voids, from manual expression of the bladder, by cystocentesis, and from catheterization of the bladder. Most references advocate a volume of 7 to 10 mL for a quantitative urinalysis; however, smaller samples are sufficient for culture or spot assays for ketones or glucose. Every effort should be made to collect as much urine as possible.

Urine collected is stored in clean, dry containers, and samples for culture are collected and submitted in sterile containers. Samples that are not analyzed within 30 minutes of collection are refrigerated in secured sealed containers. Urine samples are returned to room temperature before analysis.

Voided Collection

A naturally voided sample is easy to collect and is most easily obtained from canine patients by walking the dog outdoors and catching a midstream sample. These samples are adequate for routine urinalysis. A free-catch sample is not acceptable for culture as it may contain bacteria, cells, and debris from the skin, hair, and genitourinary tract. The initial void of urine contains the greatest concentration of contaminants and should be excluded from collection. Most dogs stop urinating if a person gets too close, but innovative collection devices can be easily made to catch urine from a voiding dog. Examples are devices made with a long handle or a straightened clothes hanger with a loop at one end for holding a disposable cup or container. Commercial collection devices are available through veterinary distributors.

TECHNICIAN NOTE

Urine is most easily obtained from a dog by walking it outdoors and catching a midstream sample.

Hospitalized patients or small dogs can be elevated on a raised grate in a clean cage. Urine is collected from the cage floor with a syringe after the animal urinates.

With cats, fresh voided urine samples are obtained from litter boxes that are clean and empty. Lining the litter box with a plastic bag or with clear plastic food wrap facilitates collection of the sample. For cats that prefer litter in boxes, shredded wax paper and specialty nonabsorbent litter made of plastic beads, such as NOSORB (Catco, Inc., Cape Coral, FL), are options. After the cat urinates in the litter pan, urine is collected immediately by syringe or poured into a clean container.

Manual Bladder Expression

Urine collected by manual expression of the bladder can be used for routine urinalysis but should not be used for culture, because urine obtained by this method will contain contaminants from the lower urinary tract, skin, and hair. Bladder expression can be difficult to accomplish in some patients, because transabdominal compression causes the pressure inside the bladder to increase, but the urethral sphincter may not relax simultaneously. Manual expression of the urinary bladder is warranted in patients with neurologic impairment when the animal cannot initiate voluntary urination or does not have the ability to completely empty the bladder.

To perform manual expression of the urinary bladder, the technician should place a hand on either side of the caudal abdomen of a patient that is standing or in lateral recumbency. Isolate the bladder between the palmar surfaces of the fingers and apply firm and steady nonaggressive pressure until urine is produced. In small-breed dogs and in cats, it is possible to do this using only one hand.

If urine cannot be produced by manual expression with moderate compression, an alternative method of emptying the bladder or obtaining a sample must be employed. The technician should not apply too much pressure. Extreme caution is exercised in patients with an overly distended bladder in the presence of urethral obstruction, such as that seen in male cats with an obstruction. Urethral or vesicular rupture may occur in these patients.

Cystocentesis

Cystocentesis is the percutaneous aspiration of urine from the bladder and is indicated to obtain a sterile urine sample for analysis and/or culture and sensitivity testing. Aspiration of a sample renders it free of bacteria, cells, and debris from the lower urinary tract as well as minimizing iatrogenic urinary tract infection caused by catheterization, especially in patients with preexisting disease of the urethra and/or urinary bladder. Cystocentesis sampling can also aid in localization of hematuria, pyuria, and bacteriuria. Cystocentesis is used as a last resort to empty an overly distended bladder (i.e., male feline with a blockage) when a urethral obstruction prevents urinary catheterization. The common contraindication for cystocentesis is attempting to perform the procedure when urine in the bladder is inadequate or when the patient resists restraint and abdominal palpation. Waiting until sufficient urine is present in the bladder or seeking ultrasound guidance is recommended, along with proper physical and chemical restraint, if necessary. Although statistically rare, laceration of the bladder and laceration of the bowel resulting in peritonitis are additional complications. Patients having recent abdominal surgery or trauma, suspected bleeding disorders, pyometra, or suspected caudal abdominal or bladder tumors should not undergo cystocentesis procedures.

Supplies needed to perform a cystocentesis in canine and feline patients include a 22-gauge, 1- to 1.5-inch needle attached to a 12-mL or larger syringe. The patient can be standing, in lateral recumbency, or in dorsal recumbency. The site allows ventral or ventrolateral insertion into the bladder wall, depending on the patient's positioning. When cystocentesis is performed, most (but not all) of the urine should be removed from the bladder. Excessive pressure from a full bladder might lead to extravasation of urine from the puncture site when the needle is withdrawn. However, removal of the entire volume of urine increases risk of contact between the needle and the bladder wall, which may result in damage to the bladder. Thus it is ideal to insert the needle a short distance cranial to the trigone region of the bladder. Having the needle a short distance cranial to the junction of the bladder with the urethra, rather than at the apex of the bladder, allows removal of urine and decompression of the bladder without the need for reinsertion of the needle into the bladder lumen. If the needle is placed into or adjacent to the apex of the bladder, it may not remain in the bladder lumen, because of the decrease in bladder size after aspiration of urine. The technician should position the needle at about a 45-degree angle through the bladder wall, creating an oblique needle tract. When the needle is directed in this fashion, the elasticity of the vesicle musculature and the interlacing arrangement of individual muscle fibers will provide a better seal of the small pathway created by the needle when it is removed. Use of ultrasonography as an imaging tool to identify the location and the size of the bladder is becoming common practice, because it offers visualization of the needle as it enters the bladder wall. Procedures for ventrolateral (Fig. 17.8) and ventral cystocentesis (Fig. 17.9) are outlined in Procedure 17.2. It should be noted that in male dogs, the prepuce and the penis are diverted laterally, and the needle is inserted on the ventral midline or slightly paramedian. If blood enters the needle, another cystocentesis attempt is made with a different needle and syringe in a different location. The needle should never be redirected once it is in the abdominal cavity, because accidental laceration of viscera may occur. Last, the technician needs to remember to always release negative aspiration pressure on the plunger of the syringe before withdrawing the needle-and-syringe apparatus. Urine samples collected via this route may have elevated RBC counts due to needle puncture into the bladder.

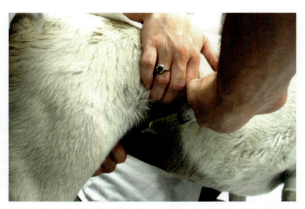
• **Fig. 17.8** Positioning for ventrolateral cystocentesis.

Catheterization

Indications for urinary catheterization include collecting a urine sample, emptying the bladder, relieving a urethral obstruction, allowing access to the urinary tract for radiographic studies, and treating patients with conditions for which an indwelling urinary catheter is indicated. Complications of urinary catheterization include urinary tract infection, particularly with indwelling catheters or in patients with immunosuppression. Even though aseptic techniques are used for catheter placement, these approaches may induce urethral inflammation, bacterial urinary tract infection, urethral and bladder irritation, and trauma. Trauma from catheterization may cause increases in RBC count, protein, and transitional epithelial cells in the sample, although urine samples

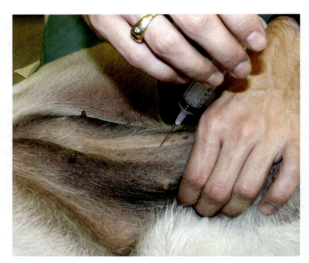
• **Fig. 17.9** Note the placement of hands to restrain and complete ventral centesis of a dog.

PROCEDURE 17.2

Intravenous Injection

- Occlude the vessel with digital pressure or a tourniquet.
- Grasp the extremity and pull the skin tautly in a distal direction.
- Wipe an alcohol-soaked cotton ball over the hair and skin, covering a distal section of a peripheral vein.
- Insert a 22- to 25-gauge needle attached to a syringe, with the bevel facing up through the skin and into the vein.
- Aspirate a small volume of blood into the syringe to ensure that the needle is within the vein.
- Release the pressure from the vein.
- Inject the contents of the syringe into the vein slowly and steadily.
- Remove the needle and apply digital pressure to the needle insertion site for 30 to 60 seconds until hemostasis occurs.
- If a hematoma occurs when the needle is inserted, remove the needle and apply digital pressure over the hematoma until the bleeding subsides. Make another injection attempt proximal to the initial site or in a different vein.

may contain contaminants from the genital region and the urethra. Urine obtained by catheterization is acceptable for bacterial culture if a sample cannot be obtained by cystocentesis.

Indwelling urinary catheters are placed in patients at risk for recurrence of urethral obstruction, such as male cats that have recently had urethral calculi removed or patients with neurologic impairment or traumatic conditions that interfere with normal urination. Catheterization is also an important part of quantifying the urinary output. It is essential to practice aseptic technique when placing urinary catheters.

The prepuce or the vulva is gently rinsed twice with a warm antimicrobial solution and water before drying. Sterile gloves are worn to detach the catheter or connect it to extension tubing or a collection system. A closed system is created by connecting the catheter to IV extension tubing that is connected to a sterile collection bag. The collection bag serves as a urine reservoir. Its contents must be measured and emptied periodically. Commercial urinary collection bags are available on the market, or an empty sterile fluid bag can be used.

Indwelling urinary catheters should be inspected for occlusion and the patient monitored for adequate urine output. A normotensive, normovolemic patient with intact renal function should produce 1 to 2 mL of urine per kilogram of body weight per hour. If urine in the reservoir bag is not adequate, the patient's urinary bladder should be palpated for distention and the urinary catheter inspected for obstructions or kinks. The bladder can be gently compressed to determine whether urine will flow through the catheter. A small volume of sterile 0.9% saline solution can be gently flushed through the catheter to relieve obstruction.

Indwelling urinary catheters should be removed as soon as possible to reduce inflammation of the urinary tract and catheter-induced infections. If catheterization is required on a long-term basis, a new catheter should be placed every 4 to 5 days.

Urinary catheters are available in French (Fr) sizes. See Table 17.2 for general guidelines for catheter selection. Note the length of available urinary catheters on the market. Many catheters that are manufactured for human medicine do not possess the length needed for large-breed canine male anatomy.

Long catheters should be premeasured externally on the patient and excessive lengths not advanced in smaller patients, because the catheter can tie itself in a knot within the urinary bladder, making withdrawal impossible without surgical intervention. Therefore measurement is made to the caudal portion of the bladder with placement being verified via radiographs.

Male Dog

Placement of a urinary catheter in a male dog is not difficult unless a urethral obstruction is present. Polypropylene urinary catheters are rigid and easy to pass into the urinary bladder for a sample collection or for emptying of the bladder. For indwelling catheters, a softer, flexible feeding tube or a silicone self-retaining Foley catheter is more desirable and comfortable for the patient.

The dog is placed in lateral recumbency with the upper leg abducted. Any long hairs around the preputial orifice are carefully clipped. The prepuce is flushed with a dilute antiseptic solution and rinsed with warm sterile saline solution or water. An assistant retracts the prepuce so that the tip of the penis is exposed and maintains this position. The tip of the penis is gently washed with an antiseptic solution and rinsed with warm saline solution or water. Sterile gloves are donned by the person who will pass the urinary catheter. The catheter is taken aseptically out of the packaging, and the distal tip of the catheter is lubricated with a sterile water-soluble lubricant or sterile lidocaine ointment. If sterile gloves are not worn, the catheter should be kept wrapped so that it can be handled aseptically as it is advanced through the urethra. Sterile scissors can be used to cut a movable butterfly tab at the end of the packaging. The tab is then used to feed the catheter into the bladder; this allows the operator to avoid touching the sterile catheter.

Insertion and advancement of the catheter into the urethra should be done smoothly; the catheter should never be forced. If the catheter cannot be passed, a smaller catheter should be used. It is common to feel some resistance at the level of the os penis—the portion of the urethra that curves around the ischial arch—and at the level of the prostate gland in older intact males; steady, gentle pressure should overcome this slight resistance. The catheter can be guided around the curvature at the ischial arch by applying digital pressure on the perineum externally or by pressing the catheter with an index finger placed in the rectum.

Urine should flow into the catheter as it enters the neck of the bladder. The catheter is then advanced 1 cm further or to the predetermined measurement. A sterile syringe is attached to the catheter and urine is slowly aspirated from the bladder (Fig. 17.10). The first few milliliters of urine suctioned from the catheter should be discarded, because it may contain contaminants and should not be submitted for urinalysis or culture. Collected urine should be stored in a sterile capped tube and labeled.

The catheter may be withdrawn from the bladder when the desired procedure is completed. The catheter must be secured if it is to remain in the bladder. If the catheter is a self-retaining Foley catheter, the appropriate volume of sterile saline or water is injected into its distal balloon cuff via the one-way valve at the proximal end of the catheter. The catheter must be secured in the following fashion (optional for a Foley catheter): two stay suture loops are made through the skin on two sides of the distal prepuce with 3-0 or 4-0 nylon suture material. An adhesive tape butterfly tab is folded around the catheter and over on itself at the location where the catheter exits the penis. A suture is passed through one side of the tape and then through the nylon loop in the prepuce. This is repeated on the other side of the tape and

TABLE 17.2	Sizing Chart for Urethral Catheter Selection: General Guidelines for Selection of Urethral Catheters			
Animal	**Sex**	**Weight**	**Urethral Catheter Size**
Canine	Male	<9 kg	3.5 Fr
	Male	9–23 kg	5 or 8 Fr
	Male	>23 kg	10 or 12 Fr
	Female	<9 kg	5 Fr
	Female	9–23 kg	8 or 10 Fr
	Female	>23 kg	10 or 12 Fr
Feline	Male	All weights	3.5 Fr
	Female	All weights	3.5 Fr

Fr, French.

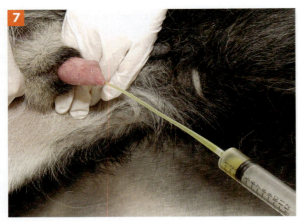

• **Fig. 17.10** Retraction of the penis for insertion of a catheter that is connected to a syringe for ease of extracting urine.

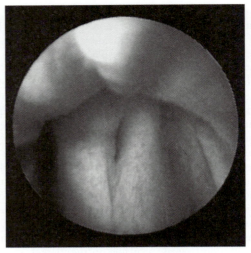

• **Fig. 17.11** Visualization of the urethral opening.

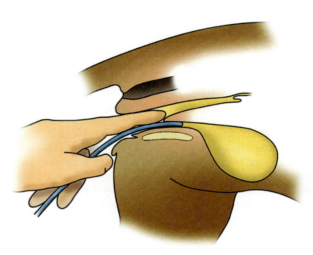

• **Fig. 17.12** Example of a method to perform digital palpation and guidance of a urinary catheter in a female dog that is restrained in a standing position.

with the other nylon loop in the prepuce. This secures the catheter to the prepuce so that it remains in place. Stay suture loops remain in place in the prepuce, allowing catheter adjustments or changes without the need to pass another needle through the prepuce.

Female Dog

Urinary catheterization is more challenging in the female dog than in the male. Catheterization can be accomplished with the patient in the standing position, in lateral recumbency, or in sternal recumbency with the hind limbs dangling from the end of the table. With a conscious dog, it is preferred that the dog stand with its hindquarters positioned at the end of an examination table. The assistant should support the patient under the abdomen to prevent lowering of the hindquarters during catheterization. Excessive long hairs are clipped from the vulvar area. The vulvar and perineal areas are gently washed with a dilute warm antiseptic solution and rinsed with sterile saline solution or water. The ventral vaginal floor is instilled with 1.0 mL of sterile 2% lidocaine jelly. The two techniques required to pass the catheter include: (1) visualization with a sterile speculum and a light source (light vaginal speculum, Killian nasal speculum, otoscope, laryngoscope blade), and (2) a blind technique in which a digit is used to palpate and guide the catheter. The speculum of choice is gently inserted into the vagina. Caution should be exercised to avoid the clitoral fossa. After donning sterile gloves, the speculum is inserted vertically and then straightened to horizontal when the pelvic canal is entered (2–4 cm inside the vagina). With the aid of a light, locate the urethral papilla and the urethral opening and insert a lubricated catheter (Fig. 17.11). The catheter is advanced until urine is obtained or at the premeasured length. If a speculum is not available, the blind technique can be performed. With sterile gloves on, a lubricated finger is placed into the vagina and slid 2 to 5 cm along the ventral floor until the papilla and the external urethral orifice are located. The catheter is introduced into the vagina and guided into the urethral orifice by the finger in the vestibule. Proper placement is acknowledged by palpating the catheter within the urethral orifice, not in the cranial vestibule (Fig. 17.12). The catheter is advanced until urine is obtained or until the premeasured length is reached. A sterile syringe is attached to the catheter and gentle negative pressure applied to obtain the desired sample. If the catheter is to remain in place, it is ideal to select a self-retaining Foley catheter. Once the catheter is placed in the bladder, the balloon cuff is inflated with the appropriate

volume of sterile saline or water to prevent the catheter from slipping out of the bladder. Then the catheter is taped to the tail to prevent the dog from stepping on it. Place a closed collection system on the free end of the Foley catheter.

TECHNICIAN NOTE

The most common reason for catheterizing a male cat is to relieve a urethral obstruction.

Male Cat

Routine catheterization of male cats for urine collection is rare. The most common reason for catheterizing a male cat is to relieve a urethral obstruction, and catheterization of male cats often warrants cautious use of sedation or general anesthesia. Cats that have had an obstruction for a long period are often obtunded and hyperkalemic and therefore should be carefully evaluated and monitored before anesthetic agents are administered. The cat is placed in lateral or dorsal recumbency with its hind limbs drawn cranially, and the prepuce is retracted to expose the glans of the penis (Fig. 17.13). The perineum is prepared aseptically,

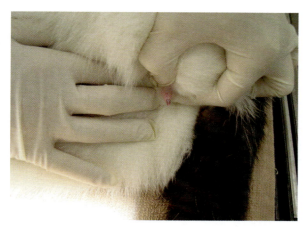

• **Fig. 17.13** Retraction of the prepuce to expose the penis for feline urinary catheterization.

as described for male canine catheterization, and the penis is extended dorsally so that the urethra is parallel to the vertebral column. An evaluation of the tip of the penis of a cat with an obstruction should be done at this time. With gloves on, the tip of the penis is first palpated to check for the presence of a distal urethral plug or calculus. If an obstruction is present in the tip of the penis, the penis is gently massaged between the thumb and the forefinger to attempt to dislodge the plug. If this is unsuccessful, proceed with catheterization. With sterile gloves, a 3.5-Fr polypropylene or silicone Tomcat catheter is lubricated and passed into the urethra. If resistance is met, the catheter is slightly withdrawn and readvanced with slight rotation. If the catheter cannot be easily advanced, a small volume of sterile saline is injected through the catheter. Extreme care should be exercised when attempting retropulsion of a urethral calculus. Excessive force or volume of fluid should be avoided, because it could result in significant urethral trauma or rupture of the urinary bladder. Once the catheter has been placed and urine flow is good, the catheter is secured in place in the same fashion as described for the male dog. The cat should be fitted with an Elizabethan collar to prevent removal of the catheter and the urine collection system.

Female Cat

Routine catheterization of female cats for urine collection is rarely if ever performed due to difficulty and sedation requirements. The cat is placed in sternal recumbency, and the perineal region is prepared aseptically. The technician uses sterile gloves, and the lips of the vulva are pulled caudally before a sterile 3.5-Fr catheter is inserted into the vagina. Keeping midline, the catheter is advanced. The urethral papilla is located about 0.7 to 1.0 cm within the vagina. The catheter should pass into the urethra with little resistance. When urine flows out of the catheter, a syringe is attached. The first 1 to 2 mL of urine that flows is discarded (as contaminated) before obtaining a second sample for analysis. The catheter is removed or secured in place, and a closed urine collection system is attached, as previously described.

Fecal Sample Collection

Fecal samples are commonly collected from the ground, floor, cage bottom, or litter box after defecation. Alternative methods include a lubricated fecal loop or a gloved finger inserted into the rectum to remove feces. Gross and microscopic examinations of

feces for mucus, blood, intestinal parasites, and ova are commonly performed in veterinary practices. Fresh fecal samples are placed in a sealed container or bag. If samples are to be checked for parasites but are not examined for several hours, they should be refrigerated to slow further parasitic development. Refer to Chapters 13 and 17 for additional information on sample collection for parasitic examination.

Administration of Medication in the Small Animal

Multiple routes are available for administration of fluids and medication. Selection depends on many factors including but not limited to the patient's condition and temperament, types of medication or fluid, urgency involved in administering fluid or medication, cost, ease of administration, and whether a systemic or local effect is desired.

Oral Administration

The administration of medication by direct placement into the oral cavity is frequently and easily performed. Technicians should be adept at administering oral medications to animals and capable of demonstrating techniques for education of pet owners.

> **TECHNICIAN NOTE**
> Technicians should be adept at administering oral medications to animals and able to demonstrate techniques for pet owners.

Oral medications are usually administered in liquid, capsule, or tablet form. Liquids are easy to administer through a dropper or syringe. Pulverized tablets and the contents of capsules can be mixed with a small volume of food, water, or flavored liquid. When liquids must be administered with a syringe or dropper, the patient's lower lip is pulled out at the commissure. The tip of the syringe or dropper is placed between the cheek and the gums, and small volumes of liquid are dispensed. The muzzle should be held at a neutral angle and not elevated. Hyperextension of the neck or movement by the patient during administration may result in fluid aspiration into the trachea. If the patient struggles or coughs or if fluid spills out of the mouth, the patient should be allowed to rest before further administration attempts are made. Flavored liquid compounds are also a viable method, especially for cats that may react with hypersalivation because of the unpleasant tastes or bitterness of some medications.

A tablet or capsule is most easily administered to a dog if it is hidden in meat, cheese, or a "meatball" of canned pet food. There are also commercially available flavored treats in which tablet and capsule medications can be hidden. Cats rarely consume pills hidden in food, but it is worth trying a small amount of butter or cream cheese to hide a pill. Cats may meticulously eat the food that surrounds the pill and leave the medication. If a patient has a diminished appetite, it may not consume the entire amount of medication-laced food and will receive an insufficient dose of medication.

An animal that will not consume baited food is medicated by tilting the head back, gently prying open the jaws, and placing the pill as far back in the mouth as possible (Fig. 17.14). The tablet will be expelled if it is not placed far enough back in the pharynx. The technician holds the muzzle closed, rubs under the animal's

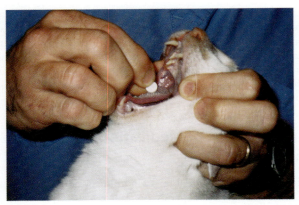

• **Fig. 17.14** Restraint of a cat for the purpose of administering a pill, also known as "pilling."

chin, taps the tip of the nose, or blows air into the nostrils to stimulate the animal to swallow. When the animal licks its nose, it can be assumed that the tablet has been swallowed. However, some dry pills or capsules, such as doxycycline, can take minutes to hours to travel the length of the esophagus before reaching the stomach. This prolonged contact between medication and the delicate lining of the esophagus can cause irritation and esophageal strictures. Therefore to avoid complications, it is beneficial to follow administration of dry pills with liquid via a syringe. Flavored liquids, such as chicken broth or tuna juice, may be appreciated by the patient.

A specially designed device is available for administering tablets to fractious cats and dogs. The tablet is secured in the flexible tip of a specially designed plastic syringe that is inserted into the back of the mouth. The plunger is quickly depressed and the pill dispensed into the back of the pharynx. Technicians can demonstrate use of the "pill popper" to owners for administration of medication at home (Fig. 17.15).

Orogastric Intubation

Sometimes it is necessary to administer medication, food, or fluids through a tube passed through the mouth and directly into the stomach. This technique is used to administer activated charcoal solutions or to lavage the stomach of animals that have ingested toxins. Orphan or weak neonates that cannot nurse can be fed milk replacer via a tube passed through the mouth and into the distal esophagus or stomach. An orogastric tube (OGT) is also passed to decompress a patient with gastric dilatation (bloated stomach). Dogs usually permit OGT placement, showing only moderate resistance. Cats, apart from neonates, usually require sedation.

The length of 10- to 22- Fr plastic or rubber tube required to extend from the tip of the nose to the 13th rib is measured and marked on the tube with tape or ink (Fig. 17.16). If the tube is to be placed in the distal esophagus to feed an animal, the distance between the tip of the nose and the eighth rib is marked. Water-soluble gel is used to lubricate the tip of the tube. The animal is restrained in sternal recumbency or in the standing or sitting position. A roll of tape, a plastic or wooden speculum with a hole in the middle, or a plastic syringe case with smooth ends is placed behind the canine teeth to hold the mouth open. The muzzle is kept in a normal position and is held so that the mouth speculum does not become dislodged.

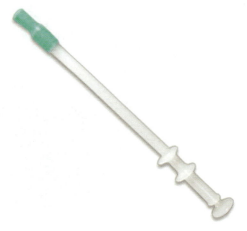

• **Fig. 17.15** Example of a plastic pilling syringe that may be used for dogs and cats.

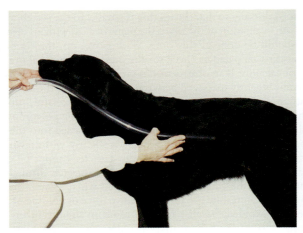

• **Fig. 17.16** It is important to measure the length of tubing that is necessary before intubating an animal.

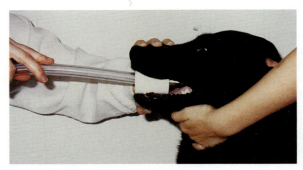

• **Fig. 17.17** A speculum is required to prevent animals from chewing or biting tubing. A roll of tape or piece of polyvinyl chloride (PVC) pipe that has been filed to smooth away rough edges to protect the animal's mouth may be used.

The tube is slowly passed through the speculum (Fig. 17.17). Swallowing will be noted as the tube passes over the base of the tongue and into the esophagus. If the animal coughs, the tube may have entered the trachea and should be removed. Once the tube is in the esophagus, it is advanced the premeasured length until it enters the stomach.

Correct placement of the tube in the gastrointestinal (GI) tract should always be verified before the introduction of any medications or fluids. Refer to the discussion on nasoesophageal tubes and nasogastric tubes (NGTs) and the placement of enteral feeding tubes found in Chapter 9, "Animal Nutrition," for instructions on how to check tube placement.

Fluid is added to the tube with a 60-mL syringe, a metal drench pump, or a funnel. After the fluid has been administered, the tube is bent to occlude it and then is withdrawn in a downward direction. This technique prevents a backflow of fluid from entering the trachea.

Transdermal Administration

Certain medications applied topically to the skin have systemic and local effects. Many drugs commonly administered via the oral route, such as prednisone or methimazole, can be formulated into an ointment for transdermal application. Other medications, such as nitroglycerin, are manufactured as a cream to be applied directly to the skin.

Medications dispensed in this form may be absorbed by the individual applying them; disposable gloves should be worn to prevent absorption. A small quantity of ointment is applied to a sparsely haired region, such as the pinna of the ear, the groin, or a shaved area on the ventral thorax. If gloves are unavailable, the ointment can be applied to a small piece of wax paper and wiped onto the patient's skin. The treated area is covered with a light bandage to avoid accidental contact. A note is placed on the front of the patient's cage specifying the medication used, the site to which the medication has been applied, and the duration of time that must pass before the application site can be safely touched.

Many topical medications are dispensed in a liquid or aerosol form to control fleas, ticks, mites, heartworms, and intestinal parasites. Depending on the product, the medication may be sprayed on the haircoat, on the entire body, or applied to the skin between the shoulder blades. Manufacturers' directions regarding application, including use of gloves, should be followed closely, and the site of administration should not be touched for a specified period after application.

Transdermal application of analgesics may also be used. One analgesic manufactured in a form specifically for transdermal application is fentanyl citrate. A fentanyl-impregnated self-adhesive patch is placed directly onto a shaved, dry region of the skin. The technician should not touch the adhesive side of the patch containing the fentanyl, because the medication can be absorbed topically. Gentle pressure is applied with the palm of the hand over the patch application site for 1 minute to allow patch adherence to the patient's skin. Each patch can be applied only once, because it may not adhere to the skin and deliver the complete dose of fentanyl if it is removed and reapplied. The patch can be covered with tape on which the date and time of placement can be recorded.

It is important to place the fentanyl patch in a location from which the animal cannot remove it, such as on the intrascapular region. It should not be applied to an area of the skin that will be in contact with a heating pad, a heat lamp, or another external heat source, because the rate of drug delivery is increased when the skin beneath the patch warms and the cutaneous vessels vasodilate.

Topical application of creams (e.g., EMLA [eutectic mixture of local anesthetics] cream, lidocaine, prilocaine) desensitizes the skin so that a venipuncture is more comfortable for the patient. This topical anesthetic must be in contact with the skin for at

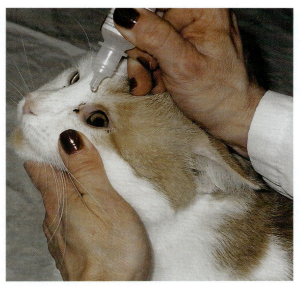

• **Fig. 17.18** Restraint of the head is important when administering eye drops to small animals.

least several minutes (ideally, 30–60 minutes) for it to reach its maximal effectiveness.

Topical Ophthalmic Administration

Administration of topical ophthalmic medications are commonly used to treat ocular diseases. In some instances, vaccines may also be administered by intraocular delivery in compliance with manufacturer labeling. To successfully place a medication onto the surface of the eye, the technician must ensure good restraint of the patient. Control of the forelimbs of the patient is essential, along with minimization of movement of the animal, to prevent the medication from being inadvertently placed on the eyelids or the face. If necessary, an additional person may be needed to assist with restraint; if administering medication to a small dog or cat, the patient may be wrapped in a towel to prevent movement and use of the forelimbs. Eye medication for a patient should be used exclusively on that patient and not used on any others to prevent transmitting ocular infection. The tip of the medication dispenser should not come into direct contact with any surface of the eye, including the cornea, to prevent contamination and trauma to the eye. If an ophthalmic medication in solution form appears cloudy, contains particulate matter, or has a color change, it should not be used and discarded.

Ophthalmic medications should be administered slightly warm or at room temperature. The technician can place refrigerated medications in the palm of the hand for 1 to 2 minutes before administration to ensure patient comfort. The eyelids are held open with the thumb and index finger of one hand, with the hand holding the medication resting on the patient's head as one drop of the medication is deposited onto the sclera (Fig. 17.18). For ointments, the lids are held open with the thumb and index finger of one hand, and a 3- to 5-mm strip of ointment is squeezed onto the upper sclera or the lower palpebral border. The ointment dissipates across the cornea when the animal blinks.

If the patient requires multiple topical ophthalmic medications in the same eye, these should be applied 3 to 5 minutes apart to allow sufficient absorption. When both a solution and an ointment need to be administered, the solution should be placed in the eye 3 to 5 minutes before the ointment as the ointment, if applied first, may coat the cornea and interfere with absorption of the solution.

Aural Administration

The key to successfully medicating an ear is to have the medication in contact with the epithelium of the ear canal to enhance its absorption and effectiveness. It is important to check the instructions supplied with the medication as some require removal of debris prior to application, whereas others do not recommend cleaning prior to use. Heavy debris can be removed using a dry cotton swab if needed. Some aural cleansers change the pH and should not be used at the same time as certain aural medications.

When medication is placed into the ear canal, the pinna is grasped and pulled upward and slightly out laterally, like the motion of introducing an otoscope cone for an otoscopic examination. This helps straighten the ear canal. The tip of the medication dispenser is placed into the vertical ear canal and the dispenser is squeezed. The base of the ear is massaged to distribute the medication.

Intrarectal Administration

The mucosa of the large intestine is capable of absorbing medications delivered intrarectally. Medications delivered by this route may have both local and systemic effects. Absorption is most effective when the intestine is free of fecal material. Antiemetic tablets or suppositories can be administered intrarectally to vomiting patients that cannot be medicated orally. A gloved, lubricated finger is used to insert the tablet into the rectum a distance of at least 5 cm. The medication is then gradually absorbed.

Antiseizure drugs, such as diazepam, can be given intrarectally if IV or intranasal (IN) administration is difficult to perform. A lubricated short rubber feeding tube or a urinary catheter is inserted 8 to 10 cm into the rectum. Diazepam is placed into a syringe and is injected through the catheter. Several milliliters of warm water are then flushed into the catheter to disperse the drug. Diazepam can also be injected directly into the rectum with a needleless syringe.

Enemas are also administered per rectum. A syringe containing the enema is lubricated and inserted into the rectum. After the enema has been injected, the animal should be placed in an area where it can defecate, such as outdoors or near a litter box. Warm-water enemas are administered through lubricated plastic tubing inserted through the rectum and into the large intestine. Water is funneled or injected into the end of the tube held in a raised position. The tube is moved back and forth and is slowly advanced up the intestinal tract as fecal material is expelled.

When a medication, such as lactulose, is added to the enema solution, it must be retained within the large intestine for a specified length of time. The solution is injected into a urinary catheter or feeding tube placed into the descending colon. The rectum is held closed with a gloved hand to prevent the expulsion. After the allotted time has passed, the catheter is removed, and the intestine is evacuated.

Intranasal Administration

Certain vaccines, including feline viral rhinotracheitis-calici-panleukopenia and canine infectious tracheobronchitis, are formulated for IN administration. The patient's muzzle is held in one hand and elevated slightly. The tip of the vaccine dispenser is placed into the nostril and the dispenser is compressed. Alternatively, the patient's head can be tilted back and the pipette containing the vaccine can be squeezed to dispense the liquid onto the plane of the nose. The vaccine runs into each nostril as the animal inhales. This method frequently results in less sneezing after administration than when the dispenser tip is placed directly into the nostril.

Diazepam can be administered intranasally for the immediate treatment of status epilepticus if intravascular access cannot be obtained. Diazepam is absorbed more rapidly into the systemic circulation by the IN route than by the intrarectal route.

Intradermal Administration

Intradermal (ID) injections are performed to desensitize the skin with a local anesthetic or to perform allergy skin testing. Most animals will not tolerate skin testing unless they are sedated. The hair on the lateral aspect of the trunk is shaved with a #40 clipper blade. The skin is carefully wiped with a water-moistened gauze sponge. Vigorous scrubbing or use of an antimicrobial cleaning solution is contraindicated, because possible skin irritation interferes with reading of the test. For an ID injection, a fold of skin is lifted and a 25- to 27-gauge needle attached to a 1-mL syringe is inserted, bevel side up, into the dermis. A 0.1-mL volume of allergen is injected. The injection site will look like a translucent lump if the injection is performed correctly. The skin is then examined at intervals for tissue reaction based on the allergy testing protocol.

Subcutaneous Administration

SC injection is easily and frequently performed and is the most common route for administering vaccines, isotonic fluids, and some types of injectable medications. Except for delayed absorption in obese animals, the SC route for injection, in general, offers relatively rapid absorption rates for most injectables. However, the SC route is not recommended in severely dehydrated or critically ill patients when immediate absorption is required. During an emergency situation, the IV or **intraosseous** (IO) route provides much faster absorption, with the IV route preferred when large volumes of fluid must be administered.

Moderate volumes of isotonic fluids can be injected under the skin to rehydrate animals if IV or IO access is unavailable or impractical. Approximately 50 to 100 mL or more of body-temperature fluids can be injected per site, depending on the patient's size. Owners of patients that may require long-term fluid supplementation at home (e.g., those with chronic renal disease) can be instructed on how to administer SC fluids.

The preferred site for most SC injections is the dorsolateral region from the neck to the hips. The dorsal region of the neck and back should be avoided because of the difficulty involved in treating any abscesses or masses that may occur after an injection. When vaccines are administered, especially to feline patients, the intrascapular region should be avoided because of the incidence of vaccine-induced tumors. Feline vaccination should be administered distally on an extremity. The following sites are recommended for feline vaccination: right forelimb, rhinotracheitis-calici-panleukopenia; right hind limb, rabies; and left hind limb, feline leukemia. The intrascapular area should also be avoided for insulin injections because of the relatively poor absorption of insulin from that site and the fibrosis that may occur upon repeated injections. Insulin should be injected into alternating sites along the dorsolateral or ventrolateral aspect of the trunk.

When an SC injection is administered, a fold of skin is tented, and the needle is inserted at the base of and parallel to the long axis of the fold. If the needle is inserted perpendicular to the long axis, the needle may penetrate both sides of the skin, and the syringe contents may be accidentally deposited onto the patient's hair. The syringe plunger is retracted slightly and the needle hub checked for blood before injection. If no blood appears, injection should be performed steadily; if blood appears in the hub, a vessel has been penetrated, and the needle should be removed and reinserted in another location. After the injection, the skin is briefly massaged to facilitate drug distribution. If multiple vaccinations or medications are administered, injection sites should be a minimum of several centimeters apart.

Intramuscular Administration

The intramuscular (IM) route is appropriate for the injection of small volumes of medication most often administered in the lumbosacral musculature lateral to the dorsal spinous processes or in the semimembranosus or semitendinosus muscles of the hind limb. Deep lumbar injections in the third to fifth lumbar region are used to administer heartworm (adulticide) treatment. Placement of the needle in the lumbosacral muscles is not recommended in very thin animals. When injections are made into the semimembranosus or semitendinosus muscles, the needle should enter the lateral aspect of the muscle and be directed caudally to prevent contact with the sciatic nerve, which causes pain and lameness. In well-muscled animals, the cranial thigh and even the gastrocnemius are used. Occasionally, the triceps muscles on the caudal aspect of the forelegs are used as injection sites. The neck is never used as a site for IM injections.

When an IM injection is performed, the muscle is isolated between the fingers and thumb, and a 22- to 25-gauge needle attached to a syringe is embedded into the muscle. As with SC injections, the plunger is retracted and the needle hub is checked for blood before medication is administered to ensure that a vessel is not inadvertently penetrated. If blood is observed, the needle is removed and inserted into another site. Once placement within the muscle has been verified, the drug is slowly injected. The site is massaged for a few seconds after the injection to help distribute the substance.

Intravenous Administration

Many medications are administered directly into a vein. IV injection is used for drugs or fluids that must rapidly reach high blood concentration levels or that would be irritating to tissue or insufficiently absorbed if given by another route (Procedure 17.3). Certain anesthetics, chemotherapeutic agents, anticonvulsant drugs, and drugs used in cardiopulmonary resuscitation, among others, are given IV. If an extremely rapid onset of action is required, the IV or IO route is chosen.

The most frequently used sites for IV injection in the dog are the cephalic and lateral saphenous veins. IV injections in the cat are typically administered in the cephalic, medial saphenous, or femoral veins. The jugular vein is used to administer injections in both large and small animals if an IV jugular catheter is in place. Refer to Procedure 17.3 for step-by-step instructions for IV injections.

PROCEDURE 17.3

Procedure for Cystocentesis

Ventrolateral Cystocentesis

- Place the patient in lateral recumbency or in the standing position.
- Palpate the abdomen to determine the size and location of the bladder.
- Hold the syringe with the needle in one hand and stabilize the bladder from below with the free hand. The bladder should be pressed dorsally and caudally to immobilize it against the pelvis.
- Wipe the area of insertion with alcohol.
- Insert the needle into the abdominal cavity and bladder, angling caudomedially at a 45-degree angle to the bladder wall and toward the trigonal region, as previously described.
- Aspirate urine in the syringe. After the desired sample volume is obtained, stop aspiration or release negative pressure on the plunger of the syringe before withdrawing the needle from the bladder and abdominal cavity.

Ventral Cystocentesis

- Place the patient in dorsal recumbency. This may take two assistants to accomplish this, especially in large-breed or deep-chested dogs.
- Palpate the abdomen to determine the size and location of the bladder.
- Wipe the area of insertion with alcohol. Stabilize the bladder against the pelvis with one hand.
- Insert the needle into the abdomen, staying on midline, into the bladder. The needle should be positioned at a 45-degree angle and directed caudally.
- Aspirate the desired sample. Release negative pressure on the syringe plunger before withdrawing the needle.

Intravenous Catheter Placement

Temporary venous access is often required for administration of medications, fluids, and electrolyte replacement therapy, or for transfusion of blood products. Medications and fluids with an osmolality of 600 milliosmoles (mOsm) or less may be safely administered via a peripheral vein. Site selection depends on available vessels and the condition of the vessels, as well as the patient and the urgency of the situation. The veterinary technician should be familiar with various types of catheters, placement techniques, and catheter maintenance.

A variety of catheters are commercially available. The length and gauge (diameter) of the catheter to be used are dependent on the species and size of the patient, the veins available, and their condition. Four general categories of IV access devices are available: winged needle (butterfly catheter), over-the-needle (OTN), through-the-needle (TTN), and multilumen catheters (Fig. 17.19).

The winged needle is for short-term use in animals not moving around or that are easily restrained. Applications might include blood collection or administration of nonirritating medications, because it is easy for the indwelling sharp needle to puncture the vessel wall, resulting in SC infiltration of fluids or medications. Plastic wings on the shaft facilitate placement and taping into place. Plastic tubing of various lengths extends from the needle to the syringe connector port, allowing for some movement of the patient while preventing the needle from being dislodged from the vein.

The OTN catheter is the most common type of catheter used today and is used primarily for peripheral vein catheterization. This type of catheter is fitted outside or over a steel needle, with

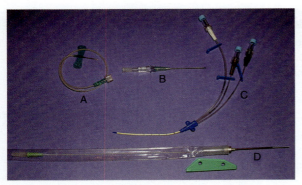

• **Fig. 17.19** Examples of four types of intravenous catheters. (A) Butterfly catheter; (B) over-the-needle (OTN) catheter; (C) multilumen (triple-lumen) catheter; and (D) through-the-needle (TTN) catheter.

the needle point extending approximately 1 mm beyond the catheter tip for entry into the vein.

Catheters passed through the needle are called *TTN catheters*. TTN catheters are usually longer than OTN catheters (8–12 inches) and are used primarily in the jugular vein. A plastic sleeve to prevent contamination protects the catheter. Once the catheter is placed and the needle has been withdrawn from the insertion site, a needle guard is closed to protect the needle from sticking the animal and shearing the catheter; these can be bulky in small animals.

Multilumen catheters have two to three separate lumina in one catheter. Multilumen catheters allow simultaneous infusions at a single catheter site. Although one catheter is placed, the multilumen catheter provides the same functions as two or three separately introduced single-lumen catheters. Catheter placement is usually completed **percutaneously** via a guidewire; they are more expensive than commonly used IV catheters and typically used in specialty practices.

Although slight variation may be noted, the set-up for venous (peripheral and jugular) or arterial catheterization is essentially the same, no matter what type of catheter is being placed. The veterinary technician will gather a catheter (butterfly, OTN, TTN, or multilumen); a syringe filled with heparinized saline flush; an injection cap or T-port connector; tape and/or nonabsorbable suture; bandage material; clippers; and antiseptic scrub and solutions. It is essential to gather all supplies before the procedure to ensure smooth catheterization. Case Presentation 17.1 provides an example of a case requiring placement of a multilumen jugular catheter.

Peripheral Vein Catheterization

Common peripheral insertion sites include the cephalic, medial (cat), and lateral (dog) saphenous veins. There is a tendency to insert a lateral saphenous catheter into the vessel as it traverses the hock; as an alternative, it might be preferable to insert the catheter into the lateral saphenous vein on the caudal surface of the leg because it is easier to secure in this location.

The area of the insertion site is generously shaved and aseptic preparation is performed using antiseptic scrub and solution. Aseptic technique is important to prevent indwelling catheter-related infection. Taking care to avoid veins, a facilitative incision or cut-down reduces skin tension and friction against the catheter. The cut-down is a 0.5- to 1-mm incision made directly over the vessel with a #11 blade or 20-gauge needle to cut through the dermis.

A facilitative incision is indicated in severely dehydrated patients and in patients with tough skin. Care should be taken to avoid the vessel when making the relief incision. Local anesthetic blocks are rarely needed. The vein is occluded proximal to the insertion site by a tourniquet or digital pressure by an assistant. The distal portion of the patient's leg is grasped in the palm of the hand of the veterinary technician placing the catheter, and the patient's leg is extended to tense and immobilize the vein. Although use of the thumb to stabilize the vein is not recommended because this compresses and collapses the vein, the thumb and the vein may be aligned side by side to stabilize the vein. Flexion of the carpus will stretch the vessel improving vessel immobilization, especially in achondroplastic breeds (i.e., Dachshund, Basset Hound).

With the bevel side up, the catheter is inserted through the skin or cut-down at approximately a 15-degree angle. The catheter is advanced into the vessel; when blood appears in the flash chamber (hub), the needle and the catheter are advanced together as a unit for an additional 1 to 4 mm. This ensures that the end of the catheter is entirely inside the lumen of the vessel. Then, with the needle held steady and longitudinal tension maintained on the leg, the catheter is advanced from the needle (which is removed) and into the vessel lumen. The catheter is capped with an injection cap or a T-port connector before flushing with heparinized saline. A ½-inch (1.3-cm) strip of adhesive tape is wrapped around the circumference of the hub of the catheter and leg to secure the catheter. A 2 × 2–inch gauze pad is placed over the insertion site. A 1-inch (2.54-cm) second piece of tape is placed sticky side down underneath the catheter before wrapping around the leg. Roll gauze is wrapped around the catheter and leg proximal and distal to the insertion site. Finally, tape is applied to the top and bottom of the gauze, where it interfaces with the skin.

Jugular Vein Catheterization

Placement of the jugular catheter provides several advantages over use of a peripheral catheter. It (1) allows safe administration of fluids that have **osmolality** greater than 600 mOsm/L and constant-rate infusions of drugs known to cause **phlebitis**, such as diazepam, pentobarbital, and mannitol; (2) enables measurement of central venous pressure; (3) facilitates frequent aspiration of blood samples; and (4) is necessary for the administration of total parenteral nutrition.

The key to successful jugular vein catheter insertion is patient positioning and vessel immobilization. If the patient is not positioned properly, it can be difficult to visualize and immobilize the vein. Jugular catheters are placed antegrade, with the tip of the catheter always directed toward the heart. Placement of the jugular catheter is best done with the patient in lateral recumbency so that the patient's head is extended and its forelimbs pulled caudally by an assistant. Sedation of uncooperative patients is recommended. Placement of a bag of fluids, a sandbag, a roll of gauze,

CASE PRESENTATION 17.1

Patient With Diabetic Ketoacidosis and Aspiration Pneumonia

History

Reb, a 26-kg, 10-year-old castrated male Labrador Retriever, is brought to the clinic with a 2-week history of vomiting. The owner reports that the dog vomited two to three times a day in the first week but was not exhibiting any lethargy at the time. However, the vomiting continued, and Reb became lethargic 2 to 3 days before presentation. He progressively became worse and developed partial anorexia 4 days before and complete anorexia 2 days before admission. The owner reported increased water consumption and increased frequency of urination before the onset of vomiting. The dog is not given any medications and is up to date on its immunizations.

Significant Physical Examination Findings

The veterinarian performed an initial physical examination and found the following:

Patient was depressed but responsive; temperature = 103.8°F; respiratory rate = 60 breaths per minute; body condition score is 3/9 with diffuse and symmetric muscle atrophy, decreased skin elasticity, and tacky mucous membranes; estimated level of dehydration = 8%; quiet lung sounds except in the left cranioventral region; abdominal palpation revealed large, firm intestines and a painful mid-abdomen; the patient's breath had an acetone smell; and a pulse oximeter reading of 92%.

Veterinarian's Orders

Based on the history and physical examination findings, the veterinarian ordered the following:

1. Complete blood count (CBC) to evaluate evidence of an infectious or inflammatory process.
2. Serum chemistry panel (including electrolytes) to rule out metabolic and electrolyte derangements.
3. Urinalysis and culture to rule out glycosuria, ketonuria, and infection.
4. Arterial blood gas sample to assess oxygenation, ventilation, and acid-base status.
5. Chest radiography to rule out pulmonary parenchymal disease.
6. Abdominal ultrasonography to further define the source of abdominal pain.
7. Placement of a multilumen jugular catheter and initiation of fluid therapy.

Nursing Care Plan

It is the technician's responsibility to carry out the veterinarian's orders and to independently develop a nursing plan of care. This plan should include the following interventions:

1. Perform regular physical assessments of the hospitalized patient.
2. Place a multilumen jugular catheter using aseptic technique. The technician should ensure that they take steps to minimize the risk for bacterial contamination when placing and caring for any indwelling catheter.
3. Per the veterinarian's instruction, develop a fluid plan utilizing lactated Ringer solution (LRS; see Box 25.1), assuming 8% dehydration; correct the dehydration over 8 hours and replace abnormal losses as they occur.

Calculation of Reb's Fluid Therapy Plan

1. Replacement volume (26 kg × 0.08) = 2.1 L
2. Maintenance volume = 1.5 L
3. Total volume = 3.6 L or 3600 mL
4. 2100 mL × 8 hours = 263 mL/hour LRS
5. 1500 mL/24 hours = 63 mL/hour LRS
    *   Administer 326 mL/hour (263 mL + 63 mL) over 8 hours, then decrease to 63 mL/hour for remaining 16 hours.
    *   Make up abnormal losses (vomiting, diarrhea, and polyuria) by adding previous hour's abnormal losses to next hour's fluid input.
    *   Reevaluate patient at frequent intervals to determine desired end point.

6. Obtain laboratory samples prior to starting fluid therapy or delivery of any medications. Steps are taken to avoid unnecessarily stressing the patient and gathering samples using proper sample collection techniques to avoid preanalytical error.
7. Obtain an arterial blood gas sample, making sure to minimize the risk of preanalytical error, such as an anticoagulant-dilutional problem, introduction of air into the sample, or improper storage of the sample.
8. Take diagnostic thoracic radiographs and assist with abdominal ultrasonography while minimizing stress to the patient.

Diagnostic Test Results

1. Serum chemistry profile: demonstrated an elevated serum glucose of 741 mg/dL. In addition, patient was hypokalemic (2.1 mEq/L), exhibiting hypophosphatemia (2.9 mg/dL), and had metabolic acidosis (pH 7.32, bicarbonate [HCO_3] 14.1 mEq/L).
2. Arterial blood gas analyses revealed that the patient was hypoxemic; Reb's partial pressure of oxygen in arterial blood (PaO_2) was 74.7 mm Hg while breathing room air.
3. Complete blood count showed leukocytosis (37,500 μL) with left shift (750 μL metamyelocytes and 9750 band) and marked toxicity and hemoconcentration (hematocrit [HCT] 50%, total protein [TP] 9.6 g/dL).
4. Urinalysis showed glycosuria and ketonuria.
5. Thoracic radiography and abdominal ultrasonography results were consistent with aspiration pneumonia and pancreatitis, respectively.

Veterinarian's Problem List

1. Diabetic ketoacidosis
2. Pancreatitis
3. Aspiration pneumonia
4. Hypoxemia

Veterinarian's Second Set of Orders

*   Initiate regular insulin therapy—5.2 units intramuscular (IM) initially, then 2.6 units IM every 2 hours (q2h). Measure arterial blood gas (ABG) q2h, supplement fluids with dextrose to 2.5% when blood gas approaches 250 mg/dL and notify clinician.
*   Supplement LRS with 40 mEq/L of K^+ (split with potassium chloride [KCl] and with dipotassium phosphate [K_2PO_4]); based on serum potassium measurements, adjust potassium concentration per protocol; split with KCl and with K_2PO_4.
*   Place nasal prongs for oxygen supplementation with oxygen flow rate of 50 to 200 mL/kg/minute; adjust to maintain peripheral capillary oxygen saturation (SpO_2) or PaO_2 greater than 95% or 85 mm Hg, respectively.
*   Check serum electrolytes every 4 hours; notify clinician if potassium is <2.0 or >5.5 mEq/L.
*   Check ABG every 24 hours.
*   Check venous blood gas at 1600 and 2400.
*   Obtain temperature, pulse, and respiration rates every 4 hours (q4h) × 6 and then every 6 hours (q6h) if vitals are within normal limits.
*   Measure SpO_2 q4h.
*   Nebulize and coupage patient q4h.
*   Post patient NPO (nothing by mouth) status.
*   Administer ampicillin 22 mg/kg intravenous (IV) every 8 hours (q8h).
*   Administer enrofloxacin 10 mg/kg every 24 hours (q24h).
*   Administer famotidine 3 mg IV q24h.
*   Administer 0.05 mg/kg oxymorphone IM q4h for pain.

Nursing Concerns and Plans

*   Neutral protamine Hagedorn (NPH) insulin to be administered twice daily by owner.

Continued

CASE PRESENTATION 17.1—cont'd

- Administer proper dose of insulin by using the correct insulin syringe. Have the dose verified by a colleague before administration.
- Verify compatibility of various drugs and take steps to ensure that they are not mixed in the IV line during administration.
- Ensure that those drugs that require dilution are diluted correctly and that all drugs are administered at the proper rate.
- Verify that potassium orders do not exceed the maximum safe administration rate of 0.5 mEq/kg/hour; inform the clinician if it does.
- Monitor patient for resolution of dehydration and restoration of intravascular blood volume.
- Monitor patient for resolution of hyperglycemia and ketonuria.
- Monitor and document input and output of fluid. Does input (IV fluids) exceed output (urine production) or vice versa?
- Provide IV catheter care as per protocol.
- Assess patient regularly and monitor specifically for development of the following complications. Consider possible interventions for these complications:
  1. Pain

  2. Fluid overload (skin elasticity—"jellylike," acute increase in body weight, increase in respiratory rate and/or effort, auscultation of crackles, urine output should not exceed 2 mL/kg/hour [assuming no renal disease])
  3. Hypoglycemia
  4. Evidence of infection
  5. Hypokalemia or hyperkalemia
  6. Catheter-related problems (phlebitis, thrombosis, perivascular fluid infiltration)

Outcome

Reb's glucose reached 220 mg/dL within 12 hours, and the ketonuria subsequently resolved. Dextrose (50%) was added to the patient's fluids to make a 2.5% solution. Reb was started on long-acting insulin. Metabolic acidosis resolved by day 2. Aspiration pneumonia resolved based on thoracic radiographs taken on day 4 and normal ABG readings. Oxygen therapy was therefore discontinued on day 4. The patient was discharged on day 6 and was prescribed the appropriate diet to assist in maintaining normal glucose levels.

---

or a rolled towel under the neck may be helpful to flex the neck, making the vessel more accessible and stable. The assistant should hold off the vein by pressing into the thoracic inlet; this should cause the vein to engorge and "stand up." The other end of the vein is immobilized by extending the head.

TECHNICIAN NOTE

Placement of a bag of fluids, a sandbag, a roll of gauze, or a rolled towel under the neck helps to make the vessel more accessible and stable for jugular catheter placement.

The area of the insertion site is generously shaved. Aseptic preparation is performed with antiseptic scrub and solution. To place a TTN catheter, the catheter needle should be introduced SC. The needle tip is positioned over the vein and aligned as close as possible to the longitudinal axis of the vein. It may be necessary to angle the needle somewhat to pick up the superficial vein wall before inserting needle tip into vein. Once it is estimated that the entire needle tip is within the lumen of the vein, the needle is stabilized and the catheter is threaded through the lumen of the needle into the vein (Fig. 17.20). Once the catheter is fully advanced into the vein, pressure is applied over the venous puncture site to stop the bleeding, and the needle is backed out before securing the needle guard around the needle. The plastic protective bag and stylet are removed; aspiration is performed to confirm proper placement of the catheter and to clear the catheter of air. It is then flushed with heparinized saline. The catheter should be capped with an injection cap or a T-port connector and again is flushed with heparinized saline. The catheter is sutured or stapled to the skin close to the insertion site before covering with a sterile 2 × 2–inch gauze pad, and the catheter site is bandaged.

The Seldinger guidewire technique facilitates placement of a multilumen catheter. The Seldinger technique uses a smaller catheter or *trocar* and a guidewire to safely gain venous access. Before the procedure is begun, the required distance for catheter insertion is premeasured with the aim of having the tip of the catheter lie within the thoracic cavity, just cranial to the right atrium. This distance is commonly estimated by measuring the distance from the intended insertion site to the caudal edge of the

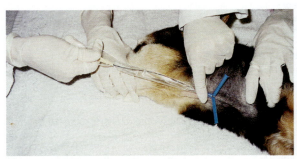

• **Fig. 17.20** The catheter is threaded into the jugular vein through a protective sleeve.

triceps muscle. The insertion site is widely clipped and aseptically prepared. Infiltration of the intended insertion site with a local anesthetic is recommended in alert animals under aseptic sterile conditions. The use of sterile gloves, a surgical cap or bonnet, a mask, and a sterile gown may also be appropriate. The distal port of the multilumen catheter is identified as the port that terminates at the very tip of the catheter and is the one through which the guidewire will be passed. All ports of the multilumen catheter are flushed with heparinized saline, and all ports apart from the distal port are capped. The insertion site is draped to avoid contamination of the guidewire, which is long and flimsy.

TECHNICIAN NOTE

The required distance for jugular vein catheter insertion is estimated by measuring the distance from the intended insertion site to the caudal edge of the triceps muscle.

A small relief incision is made through the dermis with a scalpel blade at the site of the intended insertion. The introducing needle or short OTN catheter enters the skin through the relief incision and is inserted into the underlying vessel. The guidewire is threaded through the insertion needle or catheter into the vein (Fig. 17.21). The distal end of the wire has a flexible J-tip to prevent puncturing through the vessel wall. In some instances, when it is difficult to pass the J-tip along the vessel, it may be

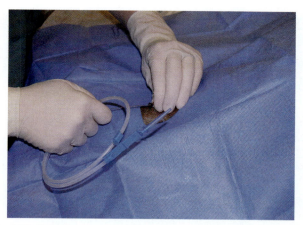

• **Fig. 17.21** Note the use of a guidewire to place the catheter; the guidewire is removed and discarded once catheter is in place.

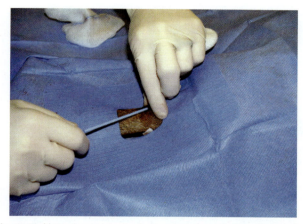

• **Fig. 17.22** Note the guidewire is inserted through fenestrated drape, ensuring continued surgical sterility.

advantageous to use the straight end of the guidewire instead. To prevent embolism of the guidewire, the technician should always maintain a firm grasp on the wire. Once the guidewire has been inserted approximately two-thirds to three-quarters of its length into the vessel, the introducing needle or catheter is removed, and a vessel dilator is threaded over the wire (the skin entry site may need to be enlarged with a #11 blade to accommodate the dilator). The dilator is grasped near the distal tip and, with a forward twisting motion, is advanced into the vessel (Fig. 17.22). Pressure is applied over the insertion site with aseptic gauze pads as the dilator is removed, preventing blood loss and leaving the guidewire in place. In the case of a sheath introducer, the dilator is incorporated into the sheath and is removed once the sheath is in place. The multilumen catheter is threaded over the guidewire until the proximal end of the guidewire protrudes from the hub of the catheter. If an excessive length of the guidewire was advanced into the vessel, it will be necessary to back the guidewire out of the vessel to achieve proper placement. Finally, while the proximal end of the guidewire is held, the catheter is advanced into the vessel the desired distance, as determined by premeasurement (Fig. 17.23A–D). The wire is removed and aspiration is performed in all ports to remove any air and to ensure that blood is easily drawn through the catheter. If necessary, the catheter may be repositioned to allow effective aspiration of blood; aseptic technique must be maintained throughout this time. All ports are then flushed with

heparinized saline. The catheter is sutured in place, and the insertion site is covered by aseptic gauze and bandaged appropriately.

Intravenous Catheter Maintenance

IV catheter care should be performed every 48 hours or on an as-needed basis. The catheter dressing should be removed and the site inspected for signs of phlebitis, infection, or **thrombosis** (Table 17.3). When signs of phlebitis or thrombosis are apparent, the catheter should be removed and a new one placed at a different site. While the catheter is flushed with heparinized saline, the insertion site should be observed for leaking of fluid at the insertion site and pain upon injection. If either is observed, the catheter should be removed and replaced with a new one. If any portion of the catheter is exposed, it should not be reinserted, and this should be documented in the medical record. If the catheter site looks good, the site should be cleaned with an iodophor or chlorhexidine solution. When the catheter site is dry, cover the insertion site with a sterile 2 × 2–inch pad before rebandaging. Traditionally, it has been recommended that a catheter not be left in place for longer than 72 hours, as recommended in human medicine.

IV catheters should be observed several times a day. If the catheter bandage is found to be wet, the reason should be identified and the bandage should be changed. Swelling distal to the catheter is usually indicative of a tight bandage, whereas swelling proximal to the catheter may be caused by infiltration of surrounding tissue by extravasation of fluids. If the patient is disturbing its bandage, the reason should be investigated; there may be a problem with the catheter or the bandage. Catheters that are not used continuously for fluid administration should be flushed with 4 units/mL of heparinized saline (1000 units/250 mL normal saline) every 4 hours. Bags of heparinized saline should be discarded every 12 to 24 hours to minimize the risk of contamination. If a catheter is not going to be used for a prolonged period, a heparin lock ("heplock") should be considered, which involves filling the dead space of the catheter with 100 units/mL heparin every 12 hours. The concentrated heparin solution is never flushed into the patient; rather, heparin is aspirated before medication is administered or before the hep-lock is renewed. The catheter should be clearly labeled to prevent inadvertent flushing of concentrated heparin into the patient.

Intravenous Chemotherapy Administration

The veterinary technician should be familiar with chemotherapy administration protocols and safety precautions, because the use of chemotherapeutic agents to treat neoplasia is becoming more common in companion animal practices. Refer to Chapter 20, "Veterinary Oncology," and Chapter 28, "Pharmacology and Pharmacy," for information on safe handling of chemotherapeutic drugs. Because many chemotherapeutic agents are carcinogens, it is advisable to minimize human exposure to these drugs during administration. Latex gloves, safety glasses, masks, and nonpermeable and long-sleeved, elastic-cuffed gowns should be worn by technicians at the time of administration. For maximum protection, chemotherapeutic material should be drawn up in an oncology hood, and a needleless administration system should be used to avoid inadvertent human exposure (Figs. 17.24 and 17.25A–D). Materials used for chemotherapy administration should be gathered in advance of administration and thereafter discarded in leakproof hazardous waste containers. If a regular needle system is to be used, drug aerosolization can be minimized by placing an alcohol-soaked gauze sponge over the injection cap during administration.

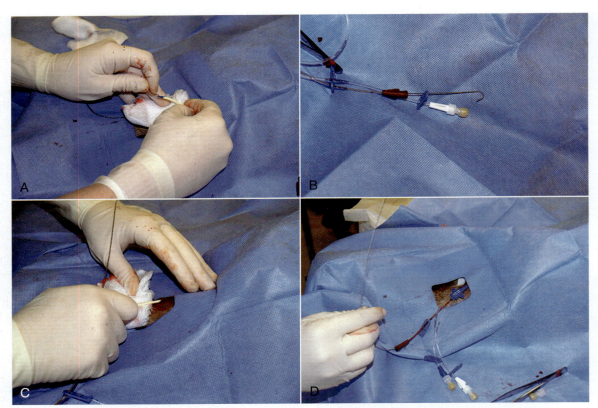

• **Fig. 17.23** The proximal end of the guidewire is threaded up the catheter (A) until it comes out at the distal catheter hub (B). The wire is then grasped, and the catheter is threaded into the vessel (C). The wire is then removed from the catheter (D).

TABLE 17.3	**Catheter-Induced Pathology**	
Phlebitis	**Infection**	**Thrombosis**
Erythema	Erythema	Veins stand on their own
Swelling	Swelling	Cord like feeling in veins
Tenderness	Tenderness	
Increased skin temperature	Increased skin temperature	
	Purulent discharge	

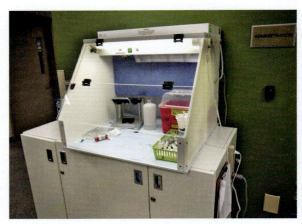

• **Fig. 17.24** Example of a needleless hematologic system.

IV catheters are used to administer cytotoxic solutions, especially those that cause tissue irritation when injected extravascularly. Examples of such drugs, which are termed *vesicants*, include doxorubicin, vincristine, vinblastine, and actinomycin D.

IV chemotherapy catheters must be placed with extreme care. The catheter should be placed in a peripheral vein and the vessel must be punctured only once during placement. If a "clean stick" is not achieved on the first placement attempt, a different vein should be used. This prevents tissue irritation caused by drug leakage from the previous puncture site. The catheter should be flushed with nonheparinized 0.9% sterile saline solution when using specific chemotherapy drugs that precipitate when mixed with heparin (e.g., doxorubicin).

Catheters used for drug administration should be frequently evaluated for patency. The area proximal to the catheter site should be freely visible so that extravasations may be observed. Signs that the chemotherapeutic agent has leaked out of the vein

include loss of catheter patency, redness or swelling at or proximal to the injection site, and vocalization or signs of discomfort exhibited by the patient.

If extravasations occur, as much of the drug as possible should be removed from the site by aspirating 5 mL of blood back through the catheter. The tissue surrounding the site should be infused with saline solution, corticosteroids, or 2% lidocaine, and warm or cold compresses should be applied, depending on the chemotherapy drug being administered.

When chemotherapy administration is complete, the catheter is flushed with several milliliters of sterile nonheparinized 0.9%

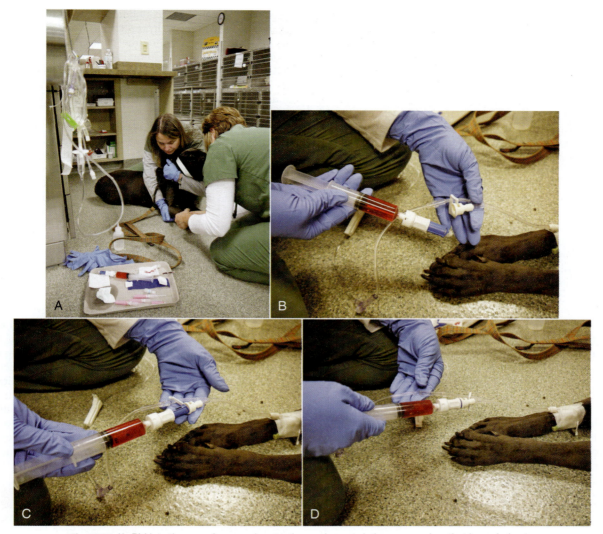

• **Fig. 17.25** (A–D) Note the use of personal protective equipment during a procedure that is carried out on the floor for the comfort of the patient and the protection of the technical staff.

saline solution. An alcohol-soaked gauze sponge covers the catheter as it is removed from the vein. The skin puncture site is covered with an antibiotic-treated gauze pad and is securely bandaged.

When less than 2 mL of a chemotherapeutic drug, such as vincristine, is injected IV, a 23- or 25-gauge butterfly catheter is often used. After the drug has been administered, the catheter is flushed with several milliliters of saline solution. The tubing is crimped to prevent fluid from leaking back out of the catheter, and the needle is removed from the vein. The needle is covered with an alcohol-soaked gauze pad as it is removed from the skin and the venipuncture site is bandaged.

> **TECHNICIAN NOTE**
>
> Care should be taken to appropriately dispose of needles and catheters used in chemotherapeutic dosing.

Intratracheal Administration

In an emergency, such as during cardiopulmonary resuscitation, drugs can be injected directly into the trachea of an unconscious animal. The absorption by this route is extremely rapid.

When an intratracheal (IT) injection is performed, a polypropylene urinary catheter or rubber feeding tube is inserted into the trachea, either directly or through an endotracheal tube. The drug contained in a syringe is forcefully injected through the urinary catheter or feeding tube. Approximately 10 mL of air or 3 to 10 mL of sterile saline solution is injected through the catheter or tube immediately afterward to disperse the drug. The acronym ALE (e.g., atropine, lidocaine, or epinephrine) is useful to remember which drugs can be administered via the endotracheal tube at a dosage that is usually twice the IV dosage. Drugs that are caustic cannot be given via this route.

Intraosseous Administration

Needles are placed directly into the bone marrow cavity to deliver fluids, drugs, and blood products when IV catheterization is not possible or cannot be performed rapidly. The IO route is often overlooked and may be useful in emergency situations. Medications and fluids quickly enter the central circulation via intramedullary vessels in the marrow cavity. IO placement of a needle or catheter allows rapid fluid delivery to neonates, small and exotic animals, and patients with circulatory collapse. IO needles are removed as soon as IV access is established.

Placement of an IO needle or catheter is contraindicated in patients with sepsis. Catheters are not placed in bones that are fractured or infected. The skin overlying the insertion site should be rendered free of infection through surgical scrub preparation so that skin surface pathogens are not introduced into underlying tissue or bone during IO needle placement. If the bone cortex is punctured multiple times during insertion attempts, a different bone should be used; fluid that is administered may leak from the bone into SC tissue.

Sites for IO administration includes the tibia, femur, humerus, and occasionally, the iliac wing or the ischium. The IO catheter or needle should have a stylet to help prevent the needle from bending or becoming occluded with a core of bone as it is inserted. Needles used include 15- to 18-gauge bone marrow needles specially designed for IO access. If IO access is needed in a neonate, an 18- to 22-gauge hypodermic needle can be used. If the hypodermic needle plugs with a core of bone, it can sometimes be flushed out with saline solution. A 22-gauge, 3.75-cm needle can be nested inside an 18-gauge, 2.5-cm needle to serve as a stylet during placement.

When an IO catheter or needle must be placed into the femur, the hip region is shaved and aseptically prepared. The patient is placed in lateral recumbency and the technician stands at the dorsum of the patient. The trochanteric fossa of the femur of the leg on the top is identified on the medial aspect of the greater trochanter of the proximal femur.

Approximately 0.5 to 1.0 mL of 2% lidocaine is injected into the skin, the SC tissue, and the periosteum over the trochanteric fossa to provide local anesthesia. A stab incision is made through the skin to grasp the femur so that the hip is held in a flexed position. The IO needle is introduced medial to the greater trochanter and parallel to the femoral shaft, with the needle inserted through the skin incision and into the femur by using firm, steady pressure as the wrist is rotated back and forth. Insertion of the needle through a skin incision helps decrease the likelihood that skin contaminants will be carried into the bone. During needle insertion, care is taken to prevent piercing the sciatic nerve, which is posteromedial to the greater trochanter of the femur. When the needle enters the marrow cavity, the needle will feel firmly embedded. Placement is confirmed by aspiration of bone marrow into a syringe attached to the needle hub.

Once placed, the needle is secured by wrapping a butterfly tab of tape around it as it exits the skin. The tape is sutured to the skin. A povidone-iodine ointment–treated gauze pad is applied to the skin entry site before applying a bulky gauze bandage around the needle for further stabilization. Patency of the IO needle is maintained by flushing every 6 hours with 1 to 2 mL of heparinized 0.9% saline solution. Although the needle may remain in place for up to 3 days, it is difficult to maintain in an ambulatory patient.

Intraperitoneal (IP) Administration

The intraperitoneal (IP) route involves placement of substances directly into the abdominal cavity and is used occasionally to administer noncaustic fluids, blood products, or medications. It may be used in neonates when intravascular or IO access is difficult to obtain. Specific chemotherapy drugs, such as asparaginase, can be given IP. Body-temperature fluids may be infused into the abdominal cavity to lavage the abdomen in animals with peritonitis or pancreatitis. Warm or cool fluid IP lavage may be used to help treat patients with severe hypothermia or hyperthermia.

Substances injected into the peritoneal cavity are absorbed more rapidly than those administered SC but more slowly than those given by the intravascular or IO route. When a drug or fluids must be administered into the peritoneal cavity, the ventral abdomen between the umbilicus and the bladder is shaved and aseptically prepared.

An 18- to 22-gauge needle or catheter is inserted into the abdominal cavity on the ventral midline a few centimeters caudal to the umbilicus, after which a syringe is attached and aspiration performed. If the needle is in the proper location in the peritoneal cavity, no blood or fluid will be aspirated into the syringe. If blood or fluid enters the syringe tip, the needle may have punctured a vessel or an abdominal organ. The needle is removed and a new needle is inserted into a different site. If the syringe remains empty when negative pressure is applied, the medication or fluids can be injected.

Thoracocentesis

Thoracocentesis is a procedure that may be used to diagnose or treat pleural filling defects (**pneumothorax** or **pleural effusion**). Air and fluid, which may compress the lungs within the pleural cavity, can be removed via thoracocentesis, allowing the lungs to re-expand. Pleural filling defects should be considered when the patient has tachypnea; short, shallow breaths; respiratory distress; open-mouth breathing; and/or cyanosis. Chest auscultation may reveal diminished or absent breath sounds and muffled heart sounds. If a pneumothorax or pleural effusion is suspected, oxygen should be administered and a thoracocentesis should be performed to stabilize the patient before the patient becomes stressed by radiography.

> **TECHNICIAN NOTE**
>
> Pleural filling defects should be considered when the patient has tachypnea; short, shallow breaths; respiratory distress; open-mouth breathing; diminished breath sounds; and/or cyanosis.

Materials Needed

- Sterile gloves
- OTN catheter: 2 to 5 inches (5.08–12.7 cm)
- IV extension tubing
- Three-way stopcock
- Syringe
- Scalpel blade #15
- Lidocaine 2%
- Clippers
- Antiseptic scrub and solution
- Vacutainer blood tubes: lavender-top EDTA and red-top clot tubes
- Culture transport media

Procedure

Thoracocentesis is performed at the seventh to eighth intercostal space. An area several inches in diameter is clipped and aseptically prepared. It is best to prepare an area on the thorax dorsally for collection of air and ventrally for fluid. Lidocaine (1–2 mL) is injected into and around the intended insertion site.

After donning sterile gloves, the equipment is assembled. It is helpful to add two or three small fenestrations to the catheter with the scalpel blade. The stopcock is attached to the syringe and the extension tubing is attached to the stopcock (Fig. 17.26). An additional extension tube can be added to the free port of the stopcock and the end of the tube placed in a bowl or a graduated cylinder to collect the pleural fluid.

The patient may stand or be placed in sternal or lateral recumbency. Intercostal vessels and nerves run along the caudal aspect of each rib; therefore the catheter will be inserted just *cranial* to the rib and in the caudal aspect of the intercostal space. With the catheter perpendicular to the chest wall, the catheter is advanced gradually through the chest wall until a flash of fluid is seen in the hub or a pop is felt. Once in the thoracic cavity, the catheter is advanced over the needle a few millimeters so that the needle no longer extends beyond the catheter; the needle and the catheter together are then directed ventrally, staying close to the thoracic wall to avoid lung tissue. When in position, the catheter alone is advanced and the needle removed before attaching extension tubing. In cats, a butterfly catheter can be used instead of extension tubing and catheter and in this instance, the needle is inserted in a direction that is parallel to the long axis of the rib, with the bevel facing the thoracic cavity. Ultrasonography may be useful in determining the end point for the procedure. If the thoracocentesis is nonproductive, it may be necessary to withdraw a few millimeters and redirect the catheter or needle. Using gentle pressure, aspiration should be performed until achieving slight negative pressure on the plunger or until the patient's condition improves.

Complications include pneumothorax, lung laceration, and laceration of an intercostal vessel or internal thoracic artery, leading to hypovolemia secondary to hemothorax. Postthoracocentesis nursing care includes close observation, respiratory rate

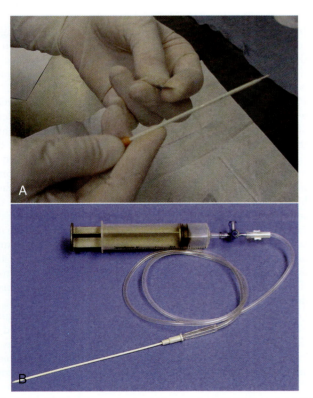

• **Fig. 17.26** (A) The stopcock should be used when there is a need for administration of a variety of drugs during a procedure that may necessitate changing syringes. (B) Note the set-up that is required for use with a syringe and catheter.

measurement, auscultation of lung sounds, and measurement of oxygen saturation with a pulse oximeter. Laboratory samples may be submitted for cell count, total protein (TP), cytologic examination, biochemical analysis (e.g., triglycerides, glucose, lactate), and culture and sensitivity.

Abdominocentesis

Abdominocentesis is a procedure that involves aspiration of fluid from the abdominal cavity for diagnostic and therapeutic purposes. It can aid in the diagnosis of hemoabdomen or uroabdomen, peritonitis, or ascites (from cardiac or hepatic causes) but is not indicated in patients suffering from a penetrating abdominal injury or suspected of having a pyometra.

This procedure has a high incidence of false-negative results. Large volumes (5–7 mL/kg) of peritoneal fluid are necessary to obtain adequate results. Use of a syringe can increase the likelihood of false-negative results due to occlusion of the needle with omentum or viscera. If the abdominocentesis result is negative, a diagnostic peritoneal lavage (DPG) may be indicated.

The veterinary technician sets up for the procedure by gathering sterile gloves, two to four 20- or 22-gauge needles, a syringe, clippers, antiseptic scrub and solution, and laboratory tubes (EDTA and clot tubes and culture transport media). The abdominocentesis is performed at the right midabdominal region to avoid the liver, spleen, and urinary bladder, and local anesthesia is not usually necessary. An area several inches in diameter is clipped and aseptically prepped. The patient may be standing or may be placed in sternal or lateral recumbency. Using aseptic technique, the needle is gently introduced into the peritoneal cavity. Fluid is gently aspirated or allowed to flow from the hub into the collection tubes. Rotation of the needle or placement of a second needle into the abdomen 2 cm from the first can stimulate fluid flow. If no fluid is retrieved, the procedure should be repeated in one or two other locations. As an alternative, abdominocentesis can be performed with an 18- to 20-gauge OTN catheter.

Postprocedure nursing care includes monitoring of vital signs and observation for pain, abdominal distention, and continued bleeding or bruising of the insertion site. Laboratory samples may be submitted for cell count, PCV, TP, cytologic examination, biochemical analysis (e.g., creatinine, potassium, bilirubin, lactate), and culture and sensitivity.

Diagnostic Peritoneal Lavage

Diagnostic peritoneal lavage (DPL) consists of infusion of fluid into the abdomen followed by retrieval of the fluid for laboratory analysis. This procedure has greater diagnostic accuracy than abdominocentesis and may be considered when the abdominocentesis result is negative. DPL has the same contraindications as abdominocentesis and is not indicated when historical, physical, or radiographic evidence suggests the need for an exploratory laparotomy. Caution should be exercised in patients with respiratory distress, because instilled fluid will place pressure on the diaphragm, potentially impairing ventilation.

Materials Needed
- Peritoneal lavage catheter or a long OTN catheter
- IV administration set
- Isotonic crystalloid solution
- Basic surgical set
- Sterile gloves

- Vacutainer blood tubes: lavender-top EDTA and red-top clot tubes
- Culture transport media
- Lidocaine 2%
- Surgical prep materials

Procedure

The bladder is emptied and the patient is placed in lateral recumbency. The skin of the ventral abdomen is clipped and aseptically prepared caudal to the umbilicus. The skin and the abdominal wall are infiltrated with lidocaine. If a peritoneal lavage catheter is used, the veterinarian may make a small midline incision just caudal to the umbilicus through the skin, SC tissue, and superficial abdominal fascia. As an alternative, the veterinarian may make the incision just to the right of the umbilicus to minimize risk of trauma to the spleen and descending colon. If an OTN catheter is used, the veterinarian will make a stab incision to insert the catheter through the incision to be directed caudally and dorsally. Gentle aspiration is performed; if a diagnostic sample is obtained, there is no need to perform the lavage. If a diagnostic sample is not obtained, approximately 20 mL/kg of warmed crystalloid solution is infused into the abdomen. The patient is gently rocked from side to side. The fluid is allowed to flow freely from the catheter or gently aspirated and placed into collection tubes for analysis. If the fluid is clear, the catheter is removed; otherwise, it is sutured in place temporally for serial evaluations. Post-DPL nursing care is the same as for abdominocentesis.

Transtracheal Wash

It has been proved that culture swabs of the pharynx and the tonsil region are unreliable in evaluating lower respiratory tract disease because of contamination of the samples with oral flora (*Bordetella* may be an exception). Appropriate sampling is obtained more consistently by using techniques that completely bypass the mouth and oropharynx. Transtracheal lavage and aspiration provide a means of obtaining samples from the tracheobronchial tree that is uncontaminated by the oral cavity for culture and cytologic examination. The technique is simple and clinically useful and can be accomplished within a relatively short time.

The veterinarian makes the decision to perform a transtracheal lavage based on clinical, radiographic, and hematologic findings. Patients often have a chronic productive cough, and the examiner can elicit a cough easily by external palpation of the laryngeal area. There are many pulmonary conditions in which this procedure is indicated, because it can identify a wide spectrum of diagnostic clues, such as inflammation and inflammatory cells (eosinophils, neutrophils, etc.); parasitic eggs and larvae; infectious agents (bacteria, fungi); and abnormal tracheobronchial cells, such as neoplastic cells. Culture and sensitivity studies are frequently performed on the fluid extracted from transtracheal lavages. Patients that are not ideal candidates for transtracheal lavage procedures include those with severe respiratory distress and those that are compromised when manipulated. Patients with coagulopathy conditions may require plasma transfusions before the procedure or may be best suited for a tracheal lavage procedure through a sterile endotracheal tube (see Endotracheal Lavage section).

Risks and complications relative to the procedure include post-procedural hemorrhage, SC emphysema, acute dyspnea, pneumomediastinum, pneumothorax, and iatrogenic infection.

Note that it is best to have the patient awake with a cough reflex present; heavy sedation or a general anesthetic is not advised for the procedure. An oxygen source, including a face mask, should be on hand at all times; therefore preoxygenation of the patient via a face mask is advised, even in eupneic animals.

Percutaneous Technique
Method 1: Two-Catheter System
Materials Needed
- OTN catheter: firm, 16-gauge × 2-inch indwelling OTN catheter
- Polypropylene urinary catheter: 3.5-Fr catheter*
- 20-mL or 35-mL syringe filled with sterile nonbacteriostatic saline (approximately 0.5–1.0 mL/kg of body weight)
- Three-way stopcock (optional)
- Scalpel blade #11 (optional)
- Sterile gloves
- Lidocaine 2% drawn up in a syringe
- Bandage material: sterile 2 × 2–inch gauze with antiseptic gel, gauze roll, and tape

Procedure
1. *Positioning:* The animal is restrained in the sitting position or sternal recumbency, with the animal's head extended and nares pointed toward the ceiling. Large-breed dogs are managed better on the floor and in a corner of a room.
2. *Site:* Cricothyroid ligament or intertracheal membrane (through trachea between cartilage rings). For the latter approach, generally, a lower site near the thoracic inlet is used in large-breed dogs to ensure that the catheter tip will reach the tracheal bifurcation (dependent on catheter length).
3. *Preparation:* Standard clipping of hair and aseptic prep over the area. Infiltration with 2% lidocaine is done up to the level of the ligament. Alternatively, a 14-gauge OTN catheter and a 5-Fr urinary catheter may be used.
4. *Incision:* Stab incision (2–3 mm) is optional. No suturing is required. Alternatively, tenting of the skin and introduction of the catheter through the skin before positioning and advancing through the cricothyroid ligament or intertracheal membrane is advised.
5. *Placement of catheters:* A rigid 16-gauge indwelling catheter with stylet in place is inserted through SC tissues to the level of the ligament. The trachea is steadied with one hand and the catheter held with the other hand; with firm action, the catheter is passed through the ligament and into the lumen of the trachea. The catheter should be placed at 45 degrees once inside the tracheal lumen, pointing down toward the tracheal bifurcation. The catheter is advanced over the stylet and the stylet removed while always keeping a hand on the hub of the catheter. Placement is verified by attaching a syringe to the catheter in place in the trachea and aspirating small amounts of air. The urinary catheter may now be passed through the indwelling catheter to a predetermined level (measured from the larynx to the caudal border of the scapula to approximate distance to tracheal bifurcation) (Fig. 17.27).
6. *Obtaining sample:* A sterile 20-mL or 35-mL syringe containing no more than 10 mL of nonbacteriostatic saline is attached to the urinary catheter. Saline is rapidly infused, and fluid is aspirated while slightly moving the urinary catheter gently back and forth within the trachea. It may be helpful to coupage the animal's chest at this time, because the greatest amount of material will be aspirated if suction is applied while the animal

---

*Alternatively, a 14-gauge OTN catheter and a 5-Fr urinary catheter may be used.

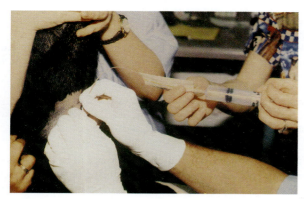

• **Fig. 17.27** Passing of urinary catheter into the trachea for a transtracheal wash.

coughs. This procedure is repeated until the fluid in the syringe is cloudy or contains visible clumps of mucus. The presence of the optional stopcock allows air to be evacuated from the syringe without disrupting the assembly. The aspiration procedure is repeated with a new syringe for two samples, one for a culture and one for cytology. Once the procedure is complete, cap the syringe containing the laboratory samples with a new needle. *Note:* one should not expect to retrieve all the saline infused through the catheter. A yield of 20% to 25% is common.

7. *Patient monitoring:* The patient is closely monitored during sample collection. Oxygen can be delivered directly through the catheter or by face mask, if necessary.

8. *Removal of catheters:* The urinary catheter is removed first, followed by the indwelling catheter. This will prevent contamination of soft tissues with the catheter tip.

9. *Bandage placement:* A light pressure wrap with a sterile 2 × 2–inch gauze square with antiseptic dressing applied to the entry site is sufficient to prevent excessive bleeding or SC emphysema.

Method 2: TTN Catheter
Materials Needed
- TTN catheter, 19-gauge × 12 inches
- 20-mL syringe filled with 10 mL of nonbacteriostatic saline
- Three-way stopcock
- Scalpel blade #11 (optional)
- Sterile gloves
- Lidocaine 2% drawn up in a syringe
- Bandage material: sterile 2 × 2–inch gauze with antiseptic gel, gauze roll, and tape

Procedure
1. Positioning, site preparation, and incision (steps 1–4) are performed as in method 1.
2. The trachea is stabilized with one hand while the catheter is held with the other hand. The needle of the catheter is placed through the SC tissues until it contacts the ligament. The angle of the needle is perpendicular to the trachea, with the bevel side pointing down. With a firm action, the needle is introduced through the ligament; then the angle of the needle is changed to 45 degrees, pointing downward toward the tracheal bifurcation to prevent the catheter from feeding back through the larynx and causing chewing or gagging. The catheter is advanced through the needle, with the catheter sliding down the enclosed plastic housing. After the catheter is advanced to its full length,

the needle is withdrawn from the trachea and skin, leaving the catheter in place. If the needle is left in the trachea and the animal begins to move, the catheter may be severed off by the needle tip, leaving the catheter as a foreign body in the trachea. The needle guard provided with the catheter should be placed over the needle at this point to prevent injury to the animal or cutting of the catheter with the exposed sharp tip.

3. The sample is obtained and the patient monitored, as described in method 1 (steps 6 and 7).

4. The catheter is withdrawn and removed from the trachea and the skin, making sure to avoid cutting the catheter with the needle.

5. Bandage placement is the same as described in method 1 (step 9).

Endotracheal Lavage
Materials Needed
- Sterile endotracheal tube suitable for the patient's size
- Polypropylene urinary catheter: 5-Fr or larger
- 20-mL syringe filled with sterile nonbacteriostatic saline
- Three-way stopcock
- Sterile gloves
- Lidocaine 2% (for feline patients to facilitate intubation and reduce laryngeal spasms)
- Laryngoscope
- Gauze roll to secure endotracheal tube
- Anesthetic agents necessary to achieve intubation with endotracheal tube

Procedure
1. *Anesthetic plan:* This should be established for each individual patient. It is necessary to induce anesthesia in the animal just to the depth necessary to cleanly place a sterile endotracheal tube. Care should be taken not to contaminate the tip of the endotracheal tube within the oral cavity. Laryngeal spasms may be reduced, especially in the feline patient, with the use of a few drops of 2% lidocaine placed on the arytenoids before intubation. Anesthetic agents commonly used include ketamine hydrochloride and diazepam, and propofol. The animal should be monitored closely, because apnea is a common occurrence with propofol used as an induction agent. Once the endotracheal tube has been placed and secured with gauze, the animal can be allowed to recover from the induction dose to a lighter plane of anesthesia, allowing a cough response to be elicited when the procedure is performed. It is necessary to hold the head of the patient to prevent chewing of the endotracheal tube. Ideally, the patient should be placed in ventral recumbency.

2. *Placement of catheter:* With sterile gloves, the polypropylene urinary catheter is advanced to a predetermined distance to the tracheal bifurcation (measure from larynx to the caudal border of the scapula to approximate the distance to tracheal bifurcation).

3. *Obtaining the sample:* This is the same as in step 6 of method 1.

4. *Removal of the polypropylene catheter.*

5. *Monitoring and recovery of the patient:* Supplemental oxygenation is provided through the endotracheal tube as needed while monitoring the patient's respiratory effort and signs for distress. Thickened mucous secretions may occlude the airway and should be removed by suction of the endotracheal tube with an aspiration catheter. The endotracheal tube is removed when the patient regains the swallowing reflex and no longer tolerates the tube in place. Monitoring of the patient should continue until it becomes ambulatory.

Sample Handling

Tracheal lavage samples are commonly submitted for both culture and cytologic examination. Aerobic and anaerobic cultures are often requested by the clinician. If a reference laboratory is used, the technician should check with the laboratory for its protocols on sample handling as the laboratory itself may provide the transport media. If samples are submitted in a syringe, the needle should be sealed with a rubber stopper and the sample refrigerated and cultured within 12 hours. If smears for cytologic examination are made before shipment, they should be made from both supernatant and sediment after centrifugation. The technician must be sure to make monolayer smears and to air dry them before packing in a protective container for shipment. If an on-site cytology examination is preferred, suitable stains include Romanovsky and Giemsa-type stains.

Cytologic Sample Interpretation

Material obtained from deep transtracheal lavage procedures includes cellular elements normally lining the tracheobronchial tree; cells infiltrated from inflammatory, hemorrhagic, congestive, neoplastic, or other pathologic processes; and background material derived from mucus, proteinaceous exudate, or cellular fragments. Causative agents, including bacteria, fungi, or parasites, may also be observed.

Arthrocentesis

Arthrocentesis is the aspiration of fluid from a joint. Disorders involving joints are etiologically diverse, ranging from congenital, developmental, and acquired disorders to various infectious and immunologic diseases. Depending on the specific disorder, joint disease may be a primary or a secondary symptom. To establish and differentiate the diagnosis of joint disease in the dog or cat, synovial fluid analysis is essential.

Indications for joint fluid analysis include persistent or cyclic fever (especially fever of unknown origin [FUO]), and/or generalized stiffness or limb lameness associated with systemic signs of illness, fever, leukocytosis, neutrophilia, hyperfibrinogenemia, malaise, and anorexia. Palpation may indicate localized pain and/or joint swelling, along with a change in stability or range of motion involving one or more affected joints.

Contraindications for joint fluid collection include moderate-to-severe pyoderma or lick granuloma over the affected joint, because there is a potential for inoculation of the joint from the infected skin. Risks and complications include joint trauma with or without hemorrhage, especially when degenerative changes involving the joint are present, making access difficult; patients can be uncooperative and unable to be properly immobilized. Iatrogenic contamination or inoculation of the joint is a complication prevented by good aseptic technique.

Joint Fluid Collection of Distal Joints in the Dog and Cat

Equipment needed for arthrocentesis includes the following: ¾-inch or 1-inch, 25-gauge needles and 3-mL syringes; 1-inch or 1½-inch, 22-gauge needles and 3-mL syringes; clean microscope slides and coverslips; sterile gloves; clippers; and aseptic surgical preparation supplies.

Patient restraint is essential. Joint fluid can sometimes be obtained from the distal joints without sedation or any type of anesthetic if the patient is not in pain, but proper restraint is essential. Sedation or light tranquilization and the use of analgesics are necessary for uncooperative patients and/or for those experiencing pain.

Patient preparation includes placing the animal in lateral recumbency. The sites are prepared by clipping the animal's hair and proceeding with aseptic surgical preparation.

With sterile gloves donned, the joint space to be entered is palpated with the index finger before introducing the needle attached to the syringe. The syringe is held in such a manner as to easily aspirate with slight negative pressure without having to reposition hands on the syringe. A steady hand is essential to minimize joint trauma and to produce a noncontaminated (bloody) sample (Fig. 17.28). The suction should always be released before the needle is withdrawn to prevent contamination (blood) from the skin, SC tissues, and synovium. An adequate sample often includes just enough fluid to fill the needle hub.

Common sites for arthrocentesis in the dog and cat include the distal joints, including carpus, tarsus, and stifle (Fig. 17.29A1–C2).

Carpus

The joint is held in flexion. The needle can be inserted into any palpable intercarpal space, although the medial radiocarpal joint is most used to avoid the cephalic vein, which courses over the carpal joint. The needle is inserted perpendicular to the skin to avoid the articulating surfaces.

Tarsus

The hock is held in partial flexion at 90 degrees with the metatarsals and the tibia. The joint may be approached medially or laterally. During a lateral approach, care must be taken to avoid the caudal branch of the saphenous vein as the needle is inserted just caudal to the lateral malleolus and dorsal to the tibial tarsal bone before being directed under the lateral malleolus, where it forms a lip over the fibular tarsal bone. The syringe and the needle are kept parallel (flat), with the metatarsal bones advancing the needle in the direction of the animal's toes. A ¾-inch, 25-gauge needle is often inserted and advanced to its full length before fluid is obtained from a medium- or large-sized dog.

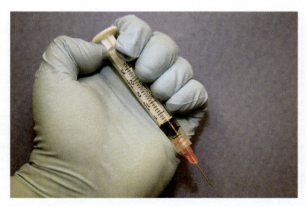

• **Fig. 17.28** Note the use of gloves and the method of holding a syringe in preparation for arthrocentesis. Hold the syringe in such a manner that you can easily aspirate back on the plunger without having to reposition your hands. The shown "dart" technique is preferred by many clinicians and technicians.

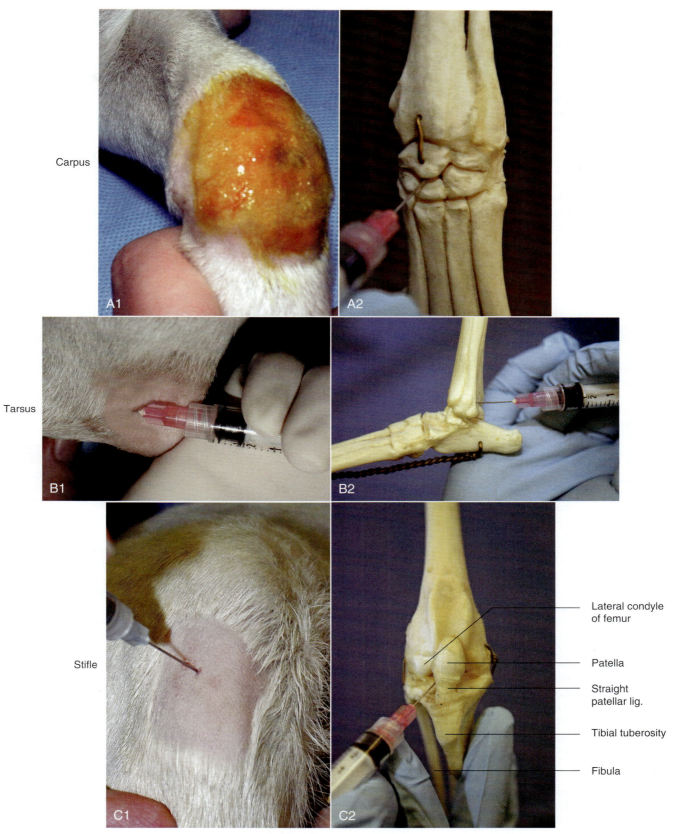

Carpus

A1   A2

Tarsus

B1   B2

Stifle

Lateral condyle
of femur

Patella

Straight
patellar lig.

Tibial tuberosity

Fibula

C1   C2

• **Fig. 17.29** Sites of arthrocentesis.

Stifle

The stifle joint is partially flexed during the procedure with the patella, the straight patellar ligament, the tibial tuberosity, and the lateral condyle of the femur providing landmarks for tapping the stifle. These landmarks form a triangle that aids in entering the joint space. A 1-inch to 1.5-inch needle is inserted just lateral to the straight patellar ligament and directed medially (at an approximately 35–45-degree angle) and slightly upward into the origin of the cruciate ligaments between the femoral condyles.

Joint Fluid Analysis

A single drop of synovial fluid is sufficient for gross and histologic examination. The synovial joint analysis is complete with an additional drop of synovial fluid for a bacterial culture (including aerobic, anaerobic, and *Mycoplasma*). Samples of synovial fluid may be submitted to a reference laboratory in a small EDTA tube. When synovial fluid is minimal, excess EDTA should be decanted from the EDTA collection tube to minimize a diluting effect.

Gross Appearance

A normal synovial fluid sample consists of a small volume of about 0.05 mL to 0.3 mL colorless, clear, and viscous (thick, sticky) fluid. An increased volume of synovial fluid can be observed in both noninflammatory and inflammatory joint diseases. A bloody tap because of trauma during the collection procedure can usually be distinguished from hemarthrosis because blood is incompletely mixed with the synovial fluid. Blood can be aspirated from inflamed and/or septic joints. Yellow-tinged fluid is a result of previous hemorrhage with release of hemoglobin pigments into the joint fluid (as seen in inflammatory, degenerative, and traumatic joint disease). If RBCs or white blood cells (WBCs) or both are present in excess, an increase in turbidity or lack of clarity is observed. Viscosity can be subjectively evaluated by observing the fluid exiting the needle and moving onto a microscope slide. A normal joint sample will form a long string between the needle and the slide; occasionally, poor viscosity is observed in degenerative or traumatized joints. In addition, the drop on the slide should remain formed, rather than dispersing over the slide. A thin, runny consistency is a frequent, consistent finding in inflammatory disorders.

Culture

Aerobic, anaerobic, and *Mycoplasma* cultures are most often negative in polyarthritis. A negative culture therefore supports a noninfectious inflammatory polyarthritis disorder.

Histologic Appearance

Normal values are noted in Box 17.1. Absolute cell counts can be done with a hemocytometer. Joint fluid samples are often small, and cell counts are often estimated in a clinical setting. This can be accomplished by recording the number of nucleated cells per microscopic field and comparing the counts with a peripheral blood smear of known concentration of nucleated blood cells.

Examples of Joint Fluid Analysis

1. Blood smear = 6 WBCs/high-power field (hpf) from a blood sample containing 18,000 WBCs/μL
2. Synovial fluid smear = 0 to 1 WBC/hpf
3. Estimated count = 0 to 3000/mm³
4. The estimated count and zero to an occasional observed WBC suggest a normal joint

---

• **BOX 17.1**   **Normal Values for Synovial Fluid**

Cell count
    Red blood cells—rare
    Nucleated cells/mm³—250–3000
Differential for nucleated cells
    Mononuclear—94%–100%
    Neutrophils—0%–6%

---

5. Blood smear = 6 WBCs/hpf from a blood sample containing 20,000 WBCs/μL
6. Synovial fluid smear = 12 WBCs/hpf
7. Estimated count = 40,000/mm³
8. The estimated count and frequent appearance of WBCs on the smear suggest a markedly elevated nucleated cell count.

Differential. Normal synovial fluid contains a mixture of small and large mononuclear cells, and the absolute number of mononuclear cells varies. Therefore the subclassification and absolute count of mononuclear cells provide limited diagnostic information, although elevations tend to occur with traumatized or degenerative joints, chronically inflamed joints, and joints with osteochondrosis.

Polymorphonuclear Neutrophils (PMNs). Polymorphonuclear neutrophils (PMNs) are generally absent; if present, they should account for less than 10% of the nucleated cell count. An increase in the relative (normal cell count) or absolute number of PMNs indicates inflammation of the synovial joint lining. Generally, more severely inflamed joints will contain a greater concentration of WBCs with a greater percentage of PMNs.

TECHNICIAN NOTE

Common sites for bone marrow aspiration include the iliac wing, femur, and humerus.

Bone Marrow Aspiration

Bone marrow aspiration is performed to evaluate the cells in the bone marrow. Bone marrow aspirations for cytologic examination or a core biopsy are safe, easily performed techniques that may yield valuable information about the cause or pathogenesis of many disease processes.

Indications for bone marrow aspiration include patients with nonresponsive anemia, thrombocytopenia, neutropenia without suspicion of infection (i.e., sepsis), pancytopenia, suspected hematopoietic malignancies (i.e., myelogenous leukemia), polycythemia, and inappropriate RBC response, such as the presence of nucleated RBCs in peripheral blood without the presence of reticulocytes or without anemia. Patients that are suspected to have neoplasia, such as lymphoma or multiple myeloma, often undergo bone marrow aspiration procedures. Clinical staging of lymphoma and the presence of mast cell tumors are additional indications.

Contraindications include clotting factor abnormalities as well as severe thrombocytopenia, which is a relative contraindication and may require the administration of plasma or platelet-rich plasma before the procedure is begun.

Complications include infection at the site if aseptic technique is not maintained, especially in patients with leukopenia; damage to soft tissue structures; and hematoma formation if a coagulopathy or thrombocytopenia is present.

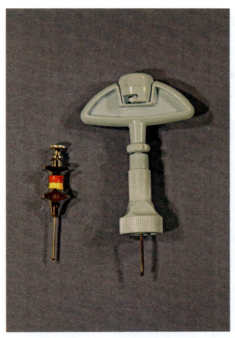

• **Fig. 17.30** Bone marrow aspiration needles: 18-gauge stainless steel Rosenthal needle; 16-gauge Illinois-style needle with depth stop.

TECHNICIAN NOTE

Stainless steel Rosenthal bone marrow aspirate needles are manufactured with a matched stylet. The stylet and the needle have matching identification numbers that identify them as a unit.

Supplies needed to perform bone marrow aspiration include a bone marrow aspiration needle. This needle may be purchased from a variety of manufacturers, but types commonly used in a small animal practice include 18-gauge, 1-inch Rosenthal needles with a matched stylet and 16-gauge, {15/16}-inch Illinois needles with a matched stylet and depth stop (Fig. 17.30). Other equipment required consists of a #11 scalpel blade; a 12-mL or 20-mL syringe; sterile gloves; a sterile drape; local anesthetic, such as 2% lidocaine in a syringe with a needle; clean glass slides; and an EDTA collection tube. A complete blood count (CBC) with reticulocyte count is done within 24 hours before or after the aspiration so that peripheral and marrow cell populations can be compared. The bone marrow aspiration procedure is a very painful procedure requiring heavy sedation with good analgesic agents in combination with a local infiltrate anesthetic or general anesthetic. Bone marrow aspirations are most performed in the ilium, humerus, and femur in small animal patients (Fig. 17.31A–C). The patient's size, age, and conformation determine which site is used. It is important to remember that the bone marrow of aged patients is less active in long bones than in flat bones; therefore in geriatric patients, a higher success rate for a cellular diagnostic sample is attained with a flat bone, such as the ilium. Bone marrow aspiration procedures are performed by using strict aseptic technique. The hair over the site is clipped, and the skin is surgically prepared. A sterile drape is placed, and sterile gloves are worn by the person performing the aspiration.

Iliac Aspiration

The patient is placed in sternal or lateral recumbency with its legs drawn forward for better palpation of the wings of the ilium. The hair is clipped from the procedure site and the skin is prepared for aseptic surgery. Local infiltration of 2% lidocaine is done by injecting into the skin, the SC tissue, and periosteum of the bone. A stab relief incision is made into the skin over the iliac crest with a #11 scalpel blade. The stylet of the bone marrow needle is inspected to confirm that the stylet is perfectly occluding the distal tip to avoid plugging the needle with cortical bone. If a Rosenthal needle is used, the operator must hold the needle in such a fashion that the stylet does not back out by placing counterpressure on the stylet with an index finger or the palm of the hand. One hand is placed on the ilium to stabilize it while the bone marrow needle and stylet are advanced through the skin incision and into the bone. The needle is advanced into the bone by rotary motion with the wrist twisted in a clockwise-to-counterclockwise motion while the elbow remains immobilized. The goal is to keep a single axis and to avoid wobbling of the needle. Considerable force is typically required as the needle is advanced into the bone 1 to 1.5 cm or until the needle is well seated.

Once the needle is well seated and stabilized in the bone, the stylet is removed from the needle and is placed on the sterile field. A 12-mL or 20-mL syringe is firmly attached to the bone marrow needle, and negative pressure is applied to the syringe plunger. Aspiration should be very quick, and negative pressure should be immediately discontinued once 0.1 mL to 1.0 mL of sample has been obtained. Actual aspiration of the marrow fluid is the most painful part of the procedure for the patient, and the conscious sedated patient may show signs of discomfort. Performing the procedure on unanesthetized patients is not recommended. Restrainers of conscious patients should be prepared for the patient to react with a yelp, a cry, or movement. Once the bone marrow enters the syringe and negative pressure is released, the syringe is removed from the bone marrow needle and the sterile stylet is reinserted into the needle. Six to eight fresh smears are made immediately by placing a drop of the sample on tilted microscope slides or by putting some of the sample into a Petri dish and tilting the dish so that blood separates from the marrow particle. Bone marrow is usually more viscous than blood, is a deeper red, and contains bony spicules and fat globules (Fig. 17.32). Bone marrow particles can be picked up with the tip of a hypodermic needle or a microhematocrit tube and transferred to a microscope slide. A pull slide is made with each sample by placing a clean glass slide on top of the slide containing the sample and pulling the slides apart to create two slides for cytologic analysis. The excess bone marrow sample should be immediately placed in an EDTA collection tube. It is helpful to do this exercise simultaneously with someone making the slides and another person placing the excess sample into the anticoagulant EDTA collection tube. If this collaboration cannot be done, it is recommended to have the collection syringe precoated with an anticoagulant, such as 2.5% to 3.0% EDTA solution.

While the patient still has the bone marrow aspiration needle in place, one of the pull slides is quickly examined by adding one drop of new methylene blue stain and a coverslip and examined to determine whether bone marrow elements are present (Fig. 17.33). If the sample is not adequate, another sample can immediately be obtained, therefore preventing the need for another invasive procedure, and the veterinarian will not be delayed in getting a result and a diagnosis.

Once the sample has been determined to be adequate, the bone marrow needle is removed in the same fashion it was placed by using a clockwise-to-counterclockwise motion to pull out the

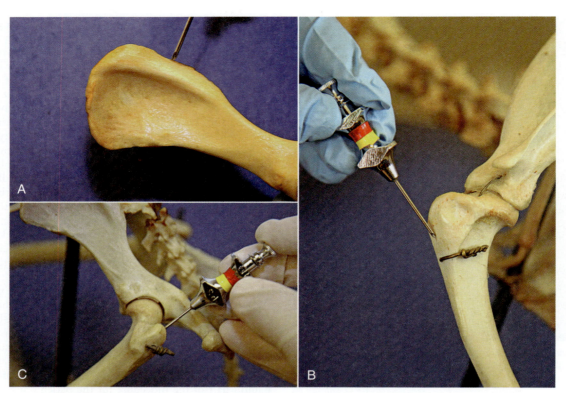

• **Fig. 17.31** Common sites for bone marrow aspiration in dog and cat patients. (A) Wing of the ilium. (B) Greater tubercle of the proximal humerus. (C) Trochanteric fossa of the femur.

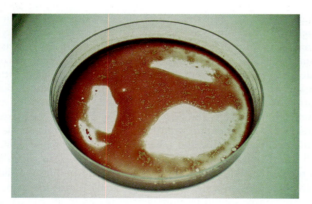

• **Fig. 17.32** Bone marrow aspirate sample displayed in a Petri dish. Note the bone spicules.

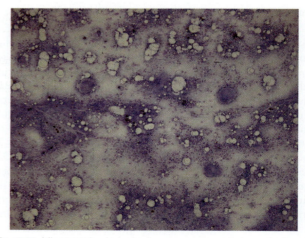

• **Fig. 17.33** Microscopic view of a bone marrow aspirate under low 10× power stained with new methylene blue. Note the nucleated precursor cells and large megakaryocytes.

bone marrow needle. Once removed, pressure is held on the site until hemostasis occurs.

The dried unstained smears, along with the excess sample in the EDTA collection tube, are packaged in a protective container for shipment to a reference laboratory.

Humeral Aspiration

The humerus is an excellent bone site for marrow aspiration, with the insertion site being the craniolateral aspect of the greater tubercle of the proximal humerus. The advantage of this site is that it consists of less tissue, fat, and muscle overlying the bone. When a patient is heavily muscled or overweight, the dorsal iliac crest is difficult to palpate; this site is always palpable and superficial

in animals with this conformation. The humerus is also advantageous to use in animals with narrow iliac wings, such as small, toy-breed dogs and cats.

The patient is placed in lateral recumbency, and the presenting proximal humerus is clipped, surgically prepped, and infiltrated with a local anesthetic as described for iliac aspiration. The bone marrow needle is placed perpendicular to the humeral shaft as the elbow is flexed, and the shoulder is rotated or abducted externally. The assistant holding the limb in position should concentrate on using pressure points, such as the elbow and the blade of the scapula, as the operator advances the needle with constant pressure and force. Squeezing the soft tissues while maintaining the position of a limb should be avoided, because this causes severe bruising of the patient with thrombocytopenia. Techniques for site preparation, needle placement, bone marrow aspiration, and slide preparation are identical to those described for iliac bone marrow aspiration.

Femoral Aspiration

The femur can be used in small-breed dogs and in cats for bone marrow aspiration. Site preparation, needle placement, marrow aspiration, and slide preparation procedures are identical to those described for bone marrow aspiration from the ilium.

The patient is placed in lateral recumbency, and the presenting hip region is surgically prepared over the palpable greater trochanter of the femur. Once aseptically prepped, 2% lidocaine is injected into the skin, SC tissue, and periosteum over the trochanteric fossa. A stab incision is made through the skin. The operator grasps the femur, and the hip is held in a flexed position. The bone marrow aspiration needle is introduced medial to the greater trochanter and parallel to the femoral shaft. Once the needle is well seated within the shaft of the femur, the sample is taken and is processed as described previously.

Fine-Needle Aspiration

Fine-needle aspiration (FNA) is a quick procedure performed routinely in veterinary practices to acquire a sample of fluid or tissue cells from an accessible mass in the dermis, viscera, or lymph node. These cytologic samples aid in differentiation between inflammation and hyperplasia of structures, such as lymph nodes or mammary glands, as well as diagnosing inflammation, neoplasia, and hyperplasia of the skin, SC, or other superficial masses. Complications of FNA procedures, although minor, include minor hemorrhage, tissue damage, and infection.

Supplies needed to perform a FNA include 25- to 20-gauge needles of lengths determined by the depth of the mass to be sampled. Other supplies include 3- to 6-mL syringes, clean glass microscope slides, and surgical scrub or alcohol for skin preparation.

The animal is restrained so that the mass to be aspirated is accessible. The skin over the underlying mass may be surgically prepped (for visceral aspirates) or wiped with alcohol to remove superficial contaminants. The mass is secured with the free hand and a 22- or 20-gauge needle is introduced into the mass with the other. With large masses, the needle is directed into peripheral parts of the lesion to avoid the necrotic center. The needle is redirected within the tissue once or twice and is removed. A syringe containing at least 1 mL of air is attached to the needle. The syringe plunger should be depressed quickly, because expulsion should be rapid and forceful to remove all material from the needle lumen onto a clean microscope slide. If the aspirated material is liquid, a push slide can be made; if the material is more viscous, a pull smear is made.

An alternative technique for performing FNA involves the use of a 3- to 12-mL syringe attached to the needle. After the needle has been inserted into the mass, suction is applied to the syringe plunger to aspirate cells into the needle. During this process, the needle may be redirected once or twice; however, negative pressure is released before the needle is withdrawn from the mass. The needle is then detached from the syringe, and the operator aspirates 1 to 2 mL of air into the syringe and reattaches the air-filled syringe onto the needle. The syringe plunger is then forcefully depressed

as described before to expel the contents of the needle onto a clean microscope. Slides can be made by a push technique or a pull technique.

Administration of Medication in the Large Animal

Oral Administration

Medications to be administered orally (per os [PO]) are available in a variety of forms, including tablets, capsules, powders, pastes, and liquids.

The simplest way to administer oral medications to all large animal species is by placing them in food or water. For a variety of reasons, this route may not always be feasible if the patient is NPO (nothing by mouth), the patient detects a bitter substance in their food or water, refuses to be baited, has a decreased appetite associated with illness, or when multiple animals are housed and fed communally. The oral route has slower absorption than IV or IM administration, but it is the only route that can be used for certain medications; however, it may be unreliable for ascertaining the amount ingested. Oral absorption of medications is often unpredictable in ruminants due to the complexity of their GI anatomy. Oral medications are administered by a variety of methods, including syringes, drenching, balling guns, and nasogastric and orogastric intubation.

Syringes

Many commercially available products come in a paste form in premeasured dosing syringes, which make accurate dosing and administration easy. Other oral medications are provided in tablet form and need to be crushed and mixed with water or simply dissolved in water over time or hidden in commercial treats. The easiest way to do this is by placing the tablets in a 60-mL catheter tip syringe, adding water, and letting the tablets dissolve. The technician should always be aware of the medications that are in use and should use safe handling practices. For some medications (e.g., chloramphenicol), use of a mask, safety glasses, and gloves while preparing and administering the medication is advised. It is good practice to assume that oral medications will be unpalatable to the patient and therefore there is a need to add molasses, Karo syrup, maple syrup, or thin applesauce to the mixture to aid in administration. Proper restraint of the head should be used with the syringe method, with the free arm cradling the head and reaching around so that the hand is up over the muzzle. The technician then inserts the syringe into the mouth at the commissure of the lips near the diastema (space between the incisors and premolars), between the cheeks and teeth, and advances it as far back into the mouth as possible (Fig. 17.34). With firm pressure, the medication is given slowly to avoid aspiration or drooling before the syringe can be withdrawn. Lifting the head slightly and gently blowing on the nose may encourage the animal to swallow rather than spit out the medication.

The technician should be conscious of the probability of the patient's spitting out the material and getting it on the skin or mucous membranes of personnel. Hands and skin that have been in contact with the medication should always be washed immediately.

Oral medications should be administered carefully to neonatal foals to prevent squirting the medication out the other side of the mouth or into the trachea. If the patient is laterally recumbent,

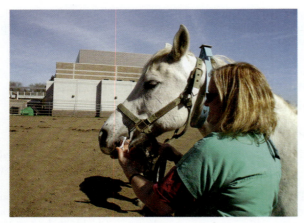

• **Fig. 17.34** Administering oral medication to an equine using a syringe.

it should be moved into a sternal position to ensure that medication administered into the mouth gets past the epiglottis and into the esophagus; keeping the patient in a sternal position for at least 1 minute reduces the possibility of aspiration. The technician should restrain neonates that are ambulatory and standing by holding the animal close to their own body, with one arm around the patient's chest and the other arm reaching over the neck, and placing the syringe into the side of the mouth opposite the technician (Fig. 17.35). The technician should use caution, making sure not to place their own face close to the foal's head to avoid getting hit in the face or head if the foal tosses its head. No pressure should be placed on the poll of the foal, because the foal may push back against the pressure and rear up. This is very risky for foals, because they can fall backward and suffer severe injury or death from hitting their head on the ground.

Drench (Dose Syringe)

Liquid medication or small volumes of fluid can be administered by using a dose syringe. For calves, sheep, and goats, a catheter tip syringe can be used, whereas a large-dose syringe is appropriate for adult cattle (Fig. 17.36). Drenching in sheep and goats should be limited to small volumes of fluid (no greater than 30 mL). The animal is held with the nose slightly elevated and pulled toward the handler; the tip of the dose syringe is inserted into the diastema, and the fluid is slowly dribbled onto the tongue.

> **TECHNICIAN NOTE**
>
> Mineral oil should never be given via drench, because it can be fatal if aspirated.

Balling Guns (Pilling)

For cattle, sheep, and goats, balling guns are commonly used to accomplish oral tablet administration. Several sizes are available, and the appropriate size should be selected in accordance with the size of the patient. Use of a large balling gun on a small calf, goat, or sheep can result in splitting of the soft palate and rupture of the pharynx. The balling gun should have a smooth end, preferably made of rubber, to limit the trauma that can be caused to the back of the mouth, including the soft palate, pharynx, and esophagus. The gun should be inspected before each use to make sure that no sharp edges have formed. All food should be removed from the patient's mouth before dosing. For cattle, placing the patient in

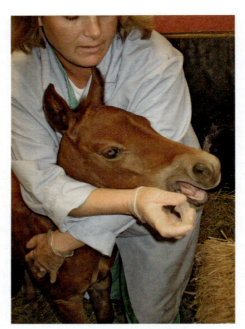

• **Fig. 17.35** Administering oral medication to a foal; note the method of gentle restraint.

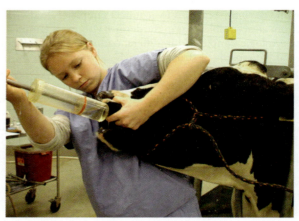

• **Fig. 17.36** Using a dosing syringe to administer liquid medication to a cow.

a head gate will help restrain the animal for the procedure. The technician should stand next to the animal's head while facing the same direction as the animal. The arm nearest the animal reaches over and grasps the mouth at the diastema (interdental space) and opens the animal's mouth by pressing on the hard palate. Alternatively, placing a finger in one nostril and the thumb in the other, then pulling the nose dorsally will encourage cattle to open the mouth. The balling gun is inserted into the mouth and gently worked back to the pharynx. Once the thumb rings of the gun are at the commissure of the lips, the plunger is depressed (Fig. 17.37). The animal's head should be kept down to prevent loss of medication. Cattle will lick their nostrils once they swallow the pill.

When working with sheep and goats, back them up to a wall and straddle the shoulders. Insert a hand into the diastema (interdental space) at the commissure of the lips, open the mouth, and insert the balling gun to the back of the throat before depressing

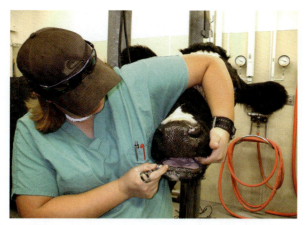

• **Fig. 17.37** Using a balling gun to administer medication in pill form to a cow.

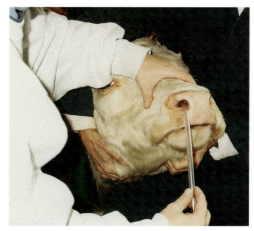

• **Fig. 17.38** Nasogastric intubation of a cow with a foal stomach tube.

the plunger. If the balling gun is not inserted far enough, the medication may be chewed by the animal and spit out. If the balling gun is inserted too far, serious damage to the pharynx and larynx may occur. To decrease the chance of aspiration of the medication, the head of the animal should not be overly elevated, and the neck should not be overextended.

> ### TECHNICIAN NOTE
> Read labels carefully because certain medications can cause severe complications for staff members if they are mishandled. For example, chloramphenicol tablets should not be crushed, because inhaling the powder has been shown to increase the risk of fatal aplastic anemia in humans.

Nasogastric and Orogastric Intubation

When large volumes of an oral medication need to be given (mineral oil, fluids, bismuth) or when oral fluid therapy or enteral feeding is required for extended periods, an OGT (for cattle, sheep, goats, pigs, and camelids) or a NGT (for horses, cattle, adult sheep and goats, and neonatal camelids) is indicated. Nasogastric intubation is a procedure that is commonly used in equine patients. Cattle, sheep, goats, and camelids have small nasal passages and, although nasogastric intubation (with small-diameter tubes) can be done (Fig. 17.38), the usual method for these species is placement of an OGT.

Nasogastric Intubation

Tubes of many different sizes can be used; the choice depends on the size of the patient and the thickness of the solution that needs to be given (or retrieved, if that is the intent of the procedure). An estimation should be made of the length of the tube required from the entrance of the nostril to the point of the stomach or **rumen** (nostril to the last rib). For horses, it is helpful to mark the tube at a point where the tube should reach the pharynx (Fig. 17.39A and B). This is helpful, because the tube can be rotated upward when it reaches the pharynx to deflect it into the esophagus, rather than down the trachea. If the tube is cold, soaking it in warm water will make it more pliable for insertion. The tube should be lubricated with water-soluble lubricant or warm water to aid in easy passage. The patient is restrained as outlined earlier and, with a hand over the muzzle and thumb placed into the nostril, the tube is passed in a ventral manner through the ventral nasal meatus and nasopharynx. Resistance is felt when the tube passes into the esophagus.

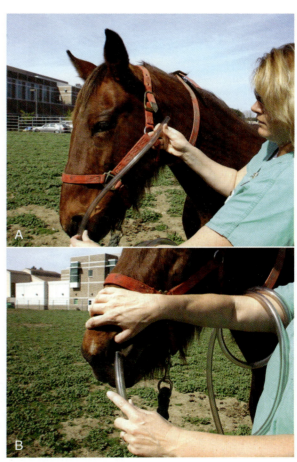

• **Fig. 17.39** Nasogastric tube (NGT) secured to the halter of a horse for repeated NGT procedures.

Once the tube has passed into the esophagus and traveled down to the rumen or stomach, the premeasured mark made on the tube should be checked and presence in the rumen or stomach confirmed. Most patients will cough if the tube is placed into the trachea, but at times, a cough will not be elicited (small-diameter tubes; flexible, soft tubes used in neonates; comatose patients that are lacking cough reflex, etc.); therefore it is essential that proper placement is confirmed before medication is administered. When the tube is passing through the esophagus,

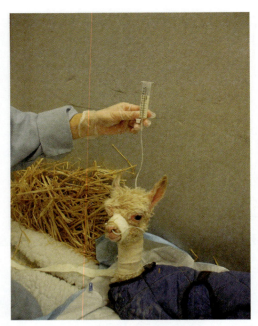

• **Fig. 17.40** Passing an orogastric tube (OGT) in an alpaca.

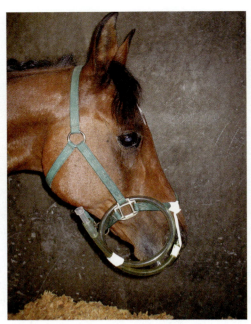

• **Fig. 17.41** Placement and securing of a nasogastric tube in an equine. Note the stabilization of the tube to the side of the horse's face using the halter.

it is often possible to visualize tube advancement and feel the tube (one should feel two firm tubular structures, one being the trachea and the other the esophagus with the NGT present). This view can be enhanced by moving the tube in and out a bit and looking at the neck for the movement. For all patients, blowing into the tube should elicit gurgles from the tube or rumen or the smell of stomach fluid, and if an assistant places a stethoscope over the area of the rumen or stomach, they should be able to hear bubbling as air passes over the fluid. Aspirating on the tube should reveal negative pressure (this should not be the only check as the opening of the tube may be up against tissue). Placing one's mouth on the distal end of the tube and sucking back may result in getting an unpleasant mouthful of gastric fluid, which has the potential to cause illness in humans if enteric bacteria are present and therefore is discouraged.

Once the position of the tube has been verified, the patient is checked for gastric reflux. If no abnormal amount of gastric fluid is noted, medication, fluids, and so forth can be administered by using a stomach pump, a dose syringe, or gravity flow (Fig. 17.40). For neonates, a 60-mL syringe is placed on the end of the tube, and aspiration is performed to check for reflux. For some patients requiring repeated administration of medications or food, the NGT should be left in place. This can be accomplished in adult equines by coiling and then taping the tube to the halter of the patient (Fig. 17.41). A syringe case, tube cap, or another adaptor should be placed on the end of the tube to prevent entry of foreign material. In neonatal patients, tubes can be secured into place by using elastic tape around the muzzle of the patient and then coiling the tube off to the side of the mouth (while making sure it does not interfere with the action of the mouth). A 1-inch piece of butterflied tape can be secured to the tube at the base of the nostril, then sutured to the elastic tape around the muzzle. This method of securing the tube is preferred over suturing the tube directly to the nostril because direct suturing is irritating to the patient, causing it to rub at the tube possibly pull it out (Fig. 17.42).

After administration of fluids via NGT, the pump is removed from the end of the tube and the tube is held up above the patient's head to deliver any remaining medication from the tube into the stomach/rumen. A small amount of water or air can gently be pumped into the tube to clear the tube; forceful pumping should be avoided. When ready to remove the tube from the patient, the end of the tube is covered with the technician's thumb and kinked and, in gentle, long motions, the tube is pulled out. Complications from removal of the tube can include nosebleed or aspiration of any residual fluid or medication. The patient should be closely monitored after medication is delivered in this fashion for colic symptoms, bloat, or respiratory problems.

NGTs are routinely passed in horses to relieve gastric distention. The tube is passed as described earlier, and once placement in the stomach has been established, a predetermined amount of water is pumped into the tube, causing a siphon, and gastric fluid and contents are collected back from the tube into a bucket. The tube is manipulated as needed and the procedure repeated while fluid is collected. If significant gastric fluid is retrieved, the tube can be secured in place by coiling it and taping it to the halter. This is less stressful for the patient than repeated passing of the tube and more efficient for the staff. If a syringe casing is placed in the end of the tube, gastric reflux can be very accurately quantified. If a large amount of gas is present, the veterinarian may decide it is prudent to leave the tube in place with no cap to provide continuous decompression and relief to the patient.

NGTs may also be inserted to provide gastric lavage. This may be helpful in relieving feed impactions. Water is pumped into the

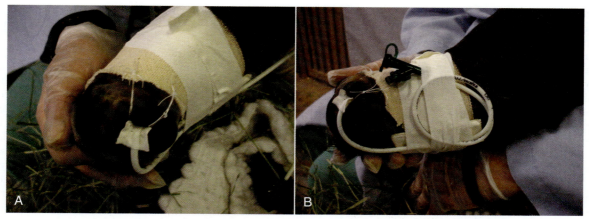

• **Fig. 17.42** (A) Placing suture loops in tape that is adhered to the muzzle of a foal allows the tube to be secured without causing irritation to the nares, as occurs when sutures are placed directly through the skin. (B) Nasogastric tube (NGT) well secured to the foal, easily accessible, and very likely to stay in place, even with movement of the foal.

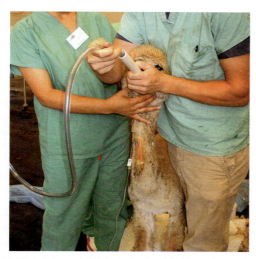

• **Fig. 17.43** Technician administering enteral feeding via gravity flow into the nasogastric tube (NGT) of an alpaca cria.

tube and gastric contents collected, as described earlier. If the water that is inserted is being retrieved, more water can be inserted, and so on, to attempt to dilute the impacted material.

Orogastric Intubation

As a result of small nasal passages, OGT is the routine choice for food animals and camelids by using the restraint techniques described earlier (Fig. 17.43). OGT is used to deliver medications and oral fluids, for transfaunation of rumen contents, enteral feeding, and for relief of some bloats. OGT can be passed into large ruminants and into sheep restrained while set up on their rumps, and piglets can be lifted by the back of the head and neck. A ⅝- to 1-inch-diameter tube can be passed in adult cattle, whereas a 9.54-mm–diameter tube is appropriate for adult sheep and goats. Small-diameter 10- to 18-Fr tubes are useful for neonatal kids, lambs, and crias. The technician should hold the tube next to the animal and place a mark at the point estimated to reach the rumen (from mouth to last rib). A speculum should be used in the animal's mouth to prevent the patient from biting down on the tube, although neonatal kids, lambs, and crias do not require use of a speculum. A wide assortment of items can be used as speculums,

ranging from a roll of tape for small patients to polyvinyl chloride (PVC) pipe or a piece of garden hose to a metal Frick speculum for cattle. The speculum needs to be inserted over the tongue root in the middle of the mouth. In cattle, "popping" or "give" will be felt when the speculum passes into the pharynx. At this point, the tube is passed through the speculum and down the esophagus into the rumen. Slight resistance should be felt when the tube enters the esophagus. It is essential to make sure the tube is in the rumen, not the trachea, before any medication is administered. This can be done by blowing on the end of the tube and listening for gas crackles, feeling negative pressure, and noting the smell of rumen fluid. In ruminants, placing a tube into the rumen may stimulate regurgitation through and around the tube; therefore sucking on the tube is discouraged.

Once placement has been confirmed, medication can be pumped into the patient or by gravity flow, as used for smaller patients and neonates. Medications should not be forcibly pumped or administered as this may rupture the rumen or cause damage to the esophagus. When finished, the end of the tube is covered with a finger and kinked before it is gently pulled out.

> ### TECHNICIAN NOTE
>
> Occluding the end of the tube and kinking it prevents any residual fluid from entering the trachea when the tube is removed from the patient.

Intravenous Administration

IV injections are commonly performed on large animal patients. Drugs administered via the IV route are very rapidly absorbed. Some medications are quite caustic, and injecting them into the vein dilutes the drug, making it less damaging than it would be if it were administered by the IM or SC route.

Equine

With most horses, minimal restraint (halter and lead rope) can be used to successfully administer medication by this route. If the patient is uncooperative, aggressive, or sensitive to needles, placing the animal in the stocks or using a second person and a twitch may ease the procedure, reducing the likelihood of injury to personnel and complications associated with misdirected puncture.

Jugular Vein

The jugular vein is the most common site for IV administration in equine patients. The right or left jugular vein is chosen, using the most cranial half of the neck. This is preferred because of the muscle layer that lies in the upper half of the neck and protects the underlying carotid artery from the risk of puncture. The right jugular vein is preferred because in most horses, the esophagus lies within the left jugular furrow and could potentially be tapped with an aggressive venipuncture. The site is then wiped down with alcohol before digital pressure is applied to the jugular furrow below the intended puncture site to distend the vein. For adult horses, a 1.5-inch needle is used (18-, 19-, or 20-gauge is adequate). With the free hand, only the needle is inserted into the vein in an upward direction (toward the head). Once blood drips from the hub of the needle, the needle is advanced until just the hub is visible. It is critical to identify that the needle is in a vein, not in an artery, because medication accidentally injected into the artery goes directly to the brain and may result in a serious, violent reaction that may prove fatal. If certain substances are injected perivascularly (e.g., phenylbutazone), they can cause severe necrosis to the surrounding tissue. When a large-bore needle is inserted, arterial blood will forcibly pulse out of the hub of the needle with each heartbeat and tends to be bright red, whereas venous blood will steadily drip from the hub of the needle and tends to be darker red.

> ### TECHNICIAN NOTE
> Arterial blood will forcibly pulse out of the hub of the needle and tends to be bright red, whereas venous blood will steadily drip from the hub of the needle and tends to be darker red.

The syringe with medication can now be attached to the needle, making sure not to move the needle outside of the vein. Before any substance is injected, confirmation of placement needs to be reestablished through gentle aspiration to confirm that blood enters the syringe and that it is not bright red in color (indicating arterial puncture). Remove digital pressure from the jugular furrow and administer the medication in a slow and continuous fashion. Once all medication is administered, remove the needle and syringe, applying digital pressure over the site for a couple of minutes to reduce potential hematoma formation.

IV injection of a medication may result in an anaphylactic reaction (mild to severe) that may include sweating, urticaria (hives), anxiety, agitation, difficulty breathing, and even collapse. If the technician notes any of these responses, the remainder of the drug in the syringe should not be given, the technician should move safely away from the animal, and the veterinarian should be notified of the situation. An injection of epinephrine may be necessary, and the technician should have prior arrangements with the veterinarian regarding the amount to administer if an anaphylactic emergency occurs when the veterinarian is not immediately available.

> ### TECHNICIAN NOTE
> Administration of a drug by any route can result in an anaphylactic reaction, and treatment with epinephrine may be indicated.

Other sites for IV injection include the cephalic vein and the lateral thoracic vein; however, these sites are usually reserved for catheter placement instead of routine injection of medications, because they are more awkward to access on the patient.

Equine Intravenous Catheterization

For repeated IV drug injections or when large volumes of IV fluids are required, an indwelling catheter should be placed in the jugular vein. If the jugular vein is not accessible due to thrombosis or trauma or if the horse pesters the jugular catheter, it may be necessary to catheterize the cephalic vein (Fig. 17.44) or the lateral thoracic vein. Many different types of catheters are available; selection should be made based on the length of time the catheter will be in place and the number of ports that may be necessary. For adult equine patients when OTN catheters are used, 14-gauge × 5.25 inches is sufficient, but for neonates, small ponies, or miniature horses, 16-gauge × 3.25 inches may be preferred. Miniature horse neonates may require a smaller catheter, and an 18- to 20-gauge × 3-inch catheter may be used, with the realization that the size of the catheter will dictate the fluid administration rates that can be achieved (Box 17.2).

> ### TECHNICIAN NOTE
> Polyurethane and silastic catheters are less thrombogenic compared with catheters made of Teflon and can be maintained in veins for longer periods.

The site chosen is shaved and surgically scrubbed to remove all debris. A final wipe with Betadine solution is then made over the area and left to dry. A "bleb" of lidocaine (ID administration using a 25-gauge needle and approximately 2 mL of lidocaine) should be administered over the intended catheter site, including above the site, to desensitize an area for suturing the catheter in place. A sterile field is created by opening a package of sterile gloves and aseptically laying the desired catheter on the gloves. All necessary items should be placed on the sterile field or kept readily accessible nearby.

With sterile gloves on, the technician grasps the catheter with the dominant hand and uses the other gloved hand to apply digital pressure to the jugular furrow. The catheter is inserted through the skin (into the bleb) at approximately a 45-degree angle and should be inserted toward the heart, with the direction of blood flow. Once the lumen of the vein has been accessed (identified by the flash of blood at the hub of the catheter), the catheter is aligned more perpendicular to the vein and is advanced 1 cm more. If the catheter is still in the vein (as indicated by flash back blood coming from the catheter), digital pressure is released to grasp the top of the stylet portion of the catheter before sliding the catheter all the way into the vessel, and the stylet is removed at the same time. The placement is rechecked to make sure that it is still inside the vein by applying digital pressure below the tip of the catheter and watching for blood to drip from the hub before attaching an intermittent infusion plug (PRN adaptor) or T-port and suturing the catheter into place (see Fig. 17.44A–E).

> ### TECHNICIAN NOTE
> Once the stylet has been withdrawn from the catheter, it should not be reintroduced, because the sharp tip may cut through the catheter, causing a small piece to be dislodged into the vein or make a very jagged edge on the catheter. Discard in a sharps container.

If the carotid artery is catheterized, bright red blood will forcibly pulse out of the catheter. If this should occur, the catheter

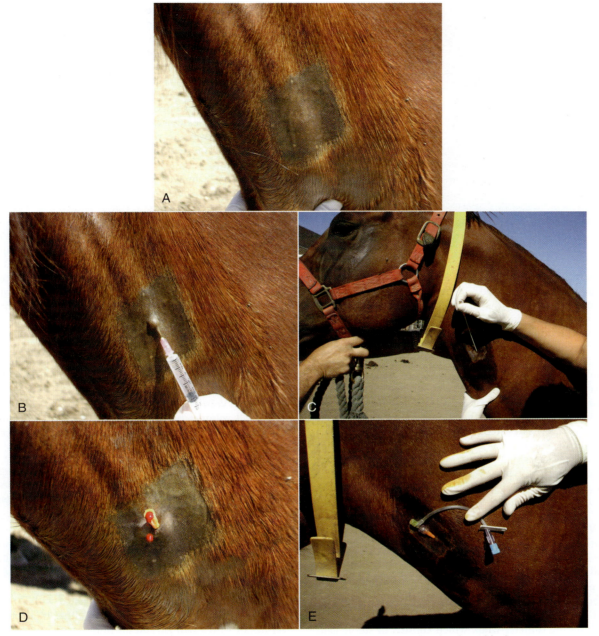

• **Fig. 17.44** (A–E) Catheter placement of the cephalic vein in the equine. Note the site shaved for intravenous catheterization of the equine cephalic vein.

• BOX 17.2	**Materials Needed for Catheter Placement**

Catheter of choice
Heparinized saline (flush) with syringe and needle
T-port
PRN adaptor (intermittent infusion plug)
Razor
Surgical soap
Suture material
Sterile gloves
Betadine-soaked gauze
Alcohol-soaked gauze
Wrap materials (antibiotic ointment, Elastikon, gauze)

---

should be immediately removed and digital pressure applied over the site for a minimum of 5 minutes to prevent the formation of a hematoma. Neck wraps or stents can be placed over catheters to stabilize them and to prevent the patient from rubbing them out. A common practice is to apply a small amount of antibacterial ointment before placing a wrap over the catheter. If the catheter remains in place for a long period, the ointment used can be alternated (e.g., Nolvasan, Betadine, triple antibiotic) to reduce the chance of a drug-resistant *Staphylococcus* infection at the catheter site. Foals and adult horses that spend a considerable amount of time in recumbency should have wraps placed over the catheter to protect the site from bedding, urine, and manure. When IV catheters are placed in recumbent neonatal foals, it is helpful to place a rolled-up towel under the neck to enhance the view of

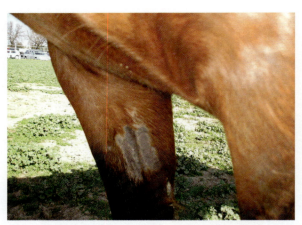

• **Fig. 17.45** Preparation of a horse's leg for insertion of a catheter. Note the width of the shaven area to allow for aseptic catheterization.

the jugular vein and stretch the skin. Making a small nick in the skin (cut-down) at the insertion site with a needle or a blade will facilitate insertion of the catheter. It is extremely helpful to have an assistant stretch the skin while digital pressure is applied, thus maintaining distention while the catheter is advanced.

When administering fluids or medications into an IV catheter, the technician should always clean the injection port with isopropyl alcohol before and after administration to prevent bacterial contamination.

The use of a guidewire-type catheter requires the same steps for preparing and placing the catheter, but use of guidewire-type catheters entail a few extra steps (refer to the Seldinger guidewire technique for small animals, as described above, or read directions on individual packages). The most important point to remember when placing these types of catheters is to *never* let go of the guidewire until the catheter has been successfully placed and the guidewire fully removed.

Cephalic Vein

For IV catheterization of the cephalic vein (Fig. 17.45), aseptic technique is observed before inserting catheter proximal to the carpus and upward. A 14- to 16-gauge × 3.25- to 5.25-inch catheter is an appropriate choice for an adult equine. Placement of a T-port is beneficial; in some cases, a piece of IV extension tubing is connected to the catheter so that IV infusions can be made without disturbing the catheter wrap, which consists of sterile gauze and elastic wrap covering the catheter.

Lateral Thoracic Vein

The site is shaved and standard preparation is performed. The IV catheter is inserted in a cranial direction (toward the head). This large-diameter vein is deeper than other veins and can accommodate a large-bore catheter, if necessary. A wrap is placed over the catheter and around the body of the horse.

Bovine Intravenous Administration

Jugular Vein

The jugular vein is the most commonly used vein for administration of IV medication or fluids to a bovine patient. Proper restraint of the animal is critical for the safety of the animal and the staff. For adult bovines, the head should be haltered and ideally, the animal should be placed in a head gate or stanchion. The head is lifted slightly and pulled away from the side to be used and tied with a

quick-release knot. This will give the technician a good visual of the area and will prevent the animal from swinging its head into the technician. Calves may be restrained while standing, with the handler holding the calf up against their body or in recumbency. Once the animal has been sufficiently restrained, the injection site is cleaned with 70% isopropyl alcohol until all organic material and debris are removed. The fingers or a fist may be placed into the jugular groove to occlude the vessel while performing a venipuncture with the other hand. Ballottement of the vessel (stroking with a finger over the vein in a downward direction) will help make the vein more prominent and will assist with visualization. For the jugular vein, a 16- to 18-gauge × 1½-inch needle should be used. The technician introduces the needle into the skin at a 45-degree angle using strong, committed motion because of the toughness of the skin. Success is noted when blood drips from the needle hub. Placement in the vein, not in an artery, is confirmed as described for horses, before the needle is inserted all the way to the hub (arterial blood pulses, while venous blood drips). At this time, the syringe containing the medication to be administered can be attached to the needle, with aspiration performed to reconfirm that the needle is still in the vein. If no blood is obtained, the needle should be redirected without being completely removed from the skin. Once in the vein, pressure applied to the jugular groove for occlusion can be removed and the medication can be administered. After the entire amount has been administered, the needle and syringe are removed, and digital pressure is applied over the access site to prevent hematoma formation.

Coccygeal Vein

For small volumes (up to approximately 5 mL) of nonirritating (xylazine, acepromazine, oxytocin) medication, the coccygeal vein can be used.

> **TECHNICIAN NOTE**
>
> Administering irritating drugs into the coccygeal vein can cause thrombosis of the vein and sloughing of the tail and should be avoided.

All cattle (dairy and beef) should be placed in a chute for the safety of personnel. An 18- to 20-gauge × 1.5-inch needle is appropriate for tail vein injections. The midline of the ventral surface of the tail is palpated to determine the location of the second or the third coccygeal vertebra. The site is cleaned with 70% isopropyl alcohol before insertion of the needle, either independent of the syringe or with a syringe, and the plunger is withdrawn slightly to check for placement in the vein. Once in the vein, the medication is injected (Fig. 17.46).

Subcutaneous Abdominal Vein

The SC abdominal (milk or mammary) vein is rarely used to administer IV injections; use of this vein is strongly discouraged, as noted in the section on blood sample collection. It is hazardous to the animal and dangerous for the technician.

Auricular Vein

This ear vein is not typically used for IV injections but could be used for very small volumes. The head should be secured to limit movement.

Bovine Intravenous Catheterization

When large volumes of fluids are to be administered or repeated IV injections are performed, a catheter should be placed in the

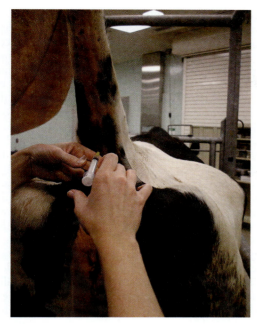

• **Fig. 17.46** Intravenous injection into the coccygeal vein of a cow.

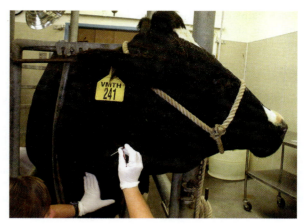

• **Fig. 17.47** Inserting a needle into the jugular of a cow. Note the restraint of the head to prevent injury to the technician.

jugular vein to avoid trauma to the vessels from repeat venipuncture. To place an IV catheter, the restraint techniques outlined previously should be used. The site is clipped and surgically prepared and an antiseptic, such as Betadine solution, is wiped onto the site and left to dry. Because of the thickness of cattle skin, a cut-down using a #15 scalpel blade or puncture through the skin with a needle the same size as the catheter will allow easier insertion of the catheter. If a blade is used to cut the skin before catheter insertion, a local anesthetic bleb should be placed into the proposed site. A 12- to 16-gauge × 5¼-inch catheter is used on adult cattle while a smaller size, such as 15- or 18-gauge × 3¼ inch, can be used for calves (Fig. 17.47 and Box 17.2).

The cephalic vein can be used for catheter placement if the jugular veins are inaccessible. In addition, the caudal auricular vein (ear vein) may be used for small-gauge catheters, but these are difficult to maintain because the animal often has a propensity to rub the catheter or shake the head and displace it.

Camelid

Although the jugular vein is the most common site of catheterization and IV injection in llamas and alpacas, it is not as easily accessed as it is in other large animal species. Injections can be given high on the neck or low on the neck, but not in the middle portion of the neck. Each of these sites (high or low) has potential for complication. Refer to "Camelids" in the section "Sampling Techniques in the Large Animal" for details about locating the high and low landmarks around the jugular vein.

Camelid Intravenous Catheterization

To complicate matters further, camelids have very thick skin (up to 1 cm in adult males), and the large transverse processes of the cervical vertebrae offer protection of the underlying jugular vein. To place a catheter in the jugular vein, use the upper or lower third of the neck and not the middle third. A 14-gauge × 5¼ inch catheter is acceptable for adults, and a 16- to 20-gauge × 3¼-inch catheter can be used for crias. The process outlined earlier for the bovine should be used to place a catheter in the camelid. In adult

animals, it is beneficial to make a cut in the thick skin where the catheter will be inserted. The cephalic vein can also be used, but placement and maintenance may be difficult because of the camelid's propensity for lying down in sternal recumbency ("kushing").

TECHNICIAN NOTE

The thick skin and large transverse processes of the cervical spine help protect camelids from exsanguination (being drained of blood) caused by bites from fighting males.

Ovine and Caprine

As with the other large animal species already discussed, the most common route for IV administration in the goat or sheep is the jugular vein. Proper restraint is essential for administering medications. It is possible for one person to perform the procedure, but the procedure will go more smoothly with assistance. For both sheep and goats, after backing the animal up against a wall, the technician straddles the patient over the shoulders facing the head and gently grasps under the mandible, lifting the head up and away from the vein to be punctured. The technician should not underestimate the strength of these animals. If caught off guard, the technician may end up "riding" the neck of the animal. For sheep, the wool should be parted, not cut or shaved, for visualization of the skin. Sheep can be set up on their rump and veins accessed as described for blood collection. The area is wiped down with isopropyl alcohol and digital pressure is applied in the jugular furrow to distend the vein before inserting a needle into the vessel (20-gauge × 1 inch for adults; 22-gauge × 1 inches for kids and lambs). Once the vein has been punctured and it has been established that it is venous blood, attach the syringe with medication and aspirate back for confirmation before slowly injecting the substance. After all medication has been delivered, the needle is removed and digital pressure applied for 2 to 3 minutes to prevent hematoma formation.

Ovine and Caprine Intravenous Catheterization

The jugular vein is the most suitable site for placing a catheter, but the cephalic vein can be used if jugular access is not an option. The procedure for placing a catheter in the goat or sheep is the same as described previously for other large animal species. For adults, 14- to 18-gauge × 3.5- to 5.25-inch catheters are appropriate, and for lambs and kids, 18- to 22-gauge × 1.5- to

3.25-inch catheters are used. It is helpful to nick the skin at the insertion site with a needle for easy insertion of the catheter through the skin.

Porcine

IV administration to pigs is accomplished by using the auricular veins, located on the dorsal aspect of the pinna. Three veins are present, and the one used most for injection is the lateral vein. The pig should be restrained by using a snare or a chute; however, an assistant can hold smaller animals against their body. Pigs have very sharp teeth and strong jaws; proper restraint is essential to prevent the possibly of a serious bite. The ear should be cleaned with an alcohol-soaked gauze and the base of the ear occluded with digital pressure. A small-gauge needle is inserted into the vessel at a very shallow angle. The needle should be attached to the syringe before insertion because of the very fragile nature of these vessels. Very gentle aspiration is performed to confirm venous placement and to release any occlusion, and then the medication is injected with steady pressure. The needle and syringe should be removed and digital pressure applied. The cephalic vein can also be used in adult pigs, but in small piglets, the jugular vein should be used due to the small diameter and difficulty accessing the cephalic and ear veins at that age.

Porcine Intravenous Catheterization

To catheterize the ear vein, a 19- or 21-gauge butterfly catheter or an 18-gauge OTN catheter can be used. The dorsal aspect of the pinna is aseptically prepared and the base of the ear is occluded with digital pressure or by using a rubber band tourniquet. The catheter is then inserted toward the base of the ear into the vein, as described previously for injecting into the vein, and the tourniquet or pressure is released. The catheter is then capped with a PRN injection port and secured to the ear using glue. To provide support, a roll of gauze is placed against the inside of the pinna, and the margins of the ear are bent around the gauze and secured with strips of adhesive tape (Fig. 17.48A–D).

Complications of IV catheterization include phlebitis, thrombophlebitis, and local cellulitis. Septicemia may result if a venipuncture is made through dirt or fecal material. This can occur in veins that have been injected or catheterized, and thrombophlebitis can result in life-threatening conditions in the animal, especially in those that are highly compromised, despite excellent cleanliness and technique. If veins are rendered unusable, it may become impossible to administer needed fluids and medications. The technician should be attentive to any changes in the appearance of the vein including swelling, heat, mucopurulent discharge, a thick-corded feel to the vein, or the appearance of fluid from the

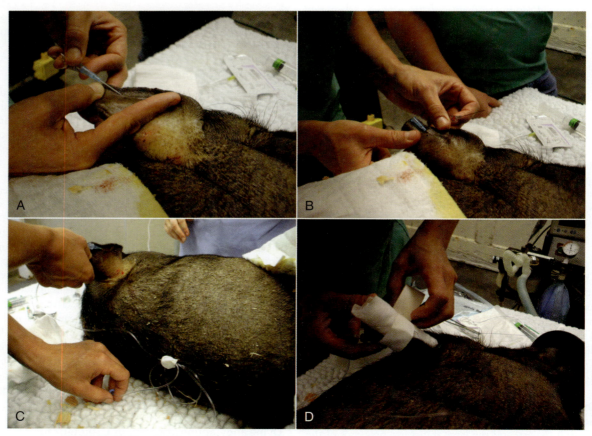

• **Fig. 17.48** (A) All materials needed to administer chemotherapy to a patient are gathered before administration is attempted. Veins are examined. (B) A needleless connection system is used to administer chemotherapeutic agents safely. (C) A locking system allows the syringe to be attached to the injection hub. The connecting system allows for administration of medication without the risk of inadvertent self-injection by the technician. (D) Forward pressure advances the white "female" portion of the connector system over the blue "male" portion. Injection of the chemotherapeutic agent is then safely administered. ([A] Courtesy Dr. Joanna Bassert.)

catheter site, and should promptly inform the veterinarian when these signs are noticed.

Intramuscular Administration

Drugs that are administered directly into the muscle are absorbed relatively quickly and provide more rapid drug absorption compared with the SC route and slower absorption compared with the IV route. The standard procedure for IM injection involves restraint of the animal as needed based on its size and temperament and cleaning the injection site with 70% isopropyl alcohol or another appropriate disinfectant to remove all dirt and debris. Selection of needle size is determined by the viscosity of the drug, the size of the muscle, and the volume to be administered. The needle is inserted without the syringe attached into the muscle all the way to the hub, taking care to touch only the hub. If the needle is inserted with the syringe attached, the added weight of the syringe may cause the needle to come out of the muscle if the animal moves. The syringe containing the drug to be delivered should then be attached and gentle aspiration performed to confirm that the needle is in a muscle and has not inadvertently hit a vessel. If a vessel has been punctured, the needle should be removed, the procedure started with a new needle, and the process repeated.

> ### TECHNICIAN NOTE
>
> Always use a new needle for each attempt at intramuscular (IM) injection. *Never* reuse a needle.

After confirming that the needle is in the muscle, the substance is injected with steady, nonaggressive pressure. Forcing the solution into the muscle may cause the syringe to detach from the needle, spraying medication everywhere, and the technician would be unable to determine the exact amount of drug delivered to the patient. Some substances that are injected can prove harmful to personnel if they encounter mucous membranes (eyes, mouth, etc.). Once the medication has been delivered, the technician should remove the syringe and needle. Pressure should be applied if any blood comes from the injection site and the area massaged gently.

If repeated IM injections are required, various sites should be used to minimize muscle damage and pain.

Equine

Several locations can be used for IM administration of therapeutics to equine patients. These sites include the lateral cervical (neck), semimembranosus and semitendinosus, and pectoral and gluteal muscles on both the left and right sides of the animal. When choosing the location for IM injections, the technician should consider the volume to be delivered, the viscosity of the solution, potential injury to personnel, and the potential for complications with the muscle chosen. Minimal restraint with a halter and lead rope must be used whenever an injection is given. Placing a horse in stocks will greatly reduce the likelihood that the animal will move once the needle is introduced and will prevent injury to personnel who work outside of stocks. Animals that are reactive while in stocks may suffer injuries; careful observation is important. Individual horses respond differently to injections. Some respond only slightly or not at all, and others may respond violently. One method used to desensitize the injection site just before a needle insertion consists of rubbing the site very firmly and rapidly back and forth using an alcohol-soaked cotton swab

or piece of gauze and then immediately inserting the needle. Some technicians prefer to tap the horse firmly with the edge of the fist just before inserting a needle into the muscle, because they believe this desensitizes the area before insertion, while others believe that tapping in this manner alerts the horse that something is about to happen. Technicians should use whatever method proves to be a good approach for them and the animals under their care.

Lateral Cervical (Neck) Muscles

IM injections into the neck protect the safety of personnel and small volumes (<10 mL in an adult horse) can be delivered into the lateral aspect of the neck. The technician should choose a spot in the triangular space that is bordered dorsally by the nuchal ligament, ventrally by the cervical vertebrae, and caudad about one hand's width in front of the cranial border of the scapula (Fig. 17.49). An 18- to 22-gauge needle is appropriate for most horses. The skin next to the injection site is grasped and pulled up before the needle is inserted; with a quick thrust of the needle, the injection is administered, and the skin is released back into place. This method results in a needle hole in the skin a few inches away from the needle hole in the muscle. When the skin is released, it acts as a barrier, preventing leakage of the drug. The neck muscles are not recommended for IM injections in foals, because soreness caused by the injections may make the foals reluctant to nurse.

Semimembranosus/Semitendinosus Muscles

Semimembranosus and semitendinosus muscles are located on the caudal aspect of the hind limb between the point of the buttock and the hock, and are often used with minimal complications. Particular attention needs to be paid to the sciatic nerve that runs down the lateral aspect of the leg, because inadvertent injection into the nerve can cause paralysis. The technician should stand facing the tail end of the animal, with their body next to the hip of the horse (never behind the horse). Positioning the body closely pressed into the horse's hip will lessen the impact if the animal chooses to kick. If the technician is tall enough, they can reach across the horse and insert the needle into the opposite leg (Fig. 17.50A and B). This reduces the chance of being kicked, because a horse that kicks in response to insertion of the needle will usually kick with the leg that has received the injection.

An 18- or 19-gauge × 1.5-inch needle should be inserted with swift action into this muscle group. Once the animal has stopped

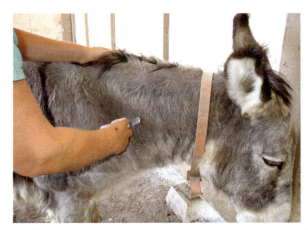

• **Fig. 17.49** Intramuscular injection in the neck of a donkey. A needle is placed in an imaginary triangular area of the lateral neck to avoid the cervical vertebrae, the scapulae, and the ligamentum nuchae.

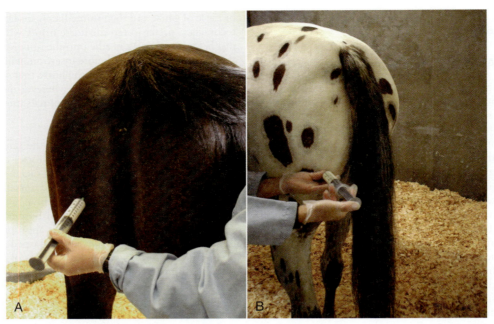

• **Fig. 17.50** (A) A technician positioned on the opposite side of the injection for an intramuscular injection into the semitendinosus muscle group of a horse. (B) A technician positioned on the same side as the injection.

moving, the syringe is attached and the procedure continued as described previously. If injecting large volumes of medication, it is preferable to detach the syringe from the needle after 15 mL has been administered; the needle is then withdrawn slightly and redirected within the muscle. There is no need to remove the needle completely, but care should be taken to avoid side-to-side movement, because moving the needle can cause trauma to the tissue. Once the needle has been redirected, the syringe is reattached, aspiration performed, and the substance injected, as described earlier. This process is continued until all solution has been administered.

Excessive distention caused by injection of large volumes of medication can result in tissue necrosis. When repeatedly injecting into these muscle groups, it is advisable to alternate between right and left sides to minimize muscle soreness and decrease the likelihood of puncturing a vessel. The large size of the muscles in this area makes them a good choice for IM injections in foals, because injections may be given with the foal standing and restrained or in recumbency. Repeated IM injections in the hind limbs may cause soreness that appears as lameness, which usually lasts for only a few days after the last injection. Repeated injections may lead to increased vascularization in the area, making it more difficult to insert the needle without encountering blood.

Pectoral Muscles

The pectoral muscles are located between the forelimbs. Just as with the rear end, there is a need for observation of safety to avoid being kicked. A needle insertion at this site usually elicits less reaction compared with an injection into the hind limbs, but the technician should assess the temperament of the animal and be prepared for the horse to move forward, jump to the side, strike, or rear. The technician should stand next to the shoulder of the horse, facing the head. Reaching around with the hand farthest from the horse, insert the needle all the way to the hub. An 18- to 20-gauge × 1- to 1.5-inch needle is appropriate (Fig. 17.51). The

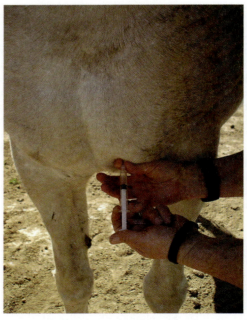

• **Fig. 17.51** Intramuscular injection into the pectoral muscles of a horse.

pectoral muscles are relatively small, and repeated IM injections at this site may cause pain and swelling as well as edema that may be temporarily unsightly and of concern to owners, depending on the planned use of the horse.

Gluteal Muscles

The gluteus, or rump, of the horse is the largest muscle mass on the hindquarters. It is located high on the rear limb, lateral to the spine and caudal to the point of the hip (Fig. 17.52). It can accommodate large volumes and repeated injections but is not

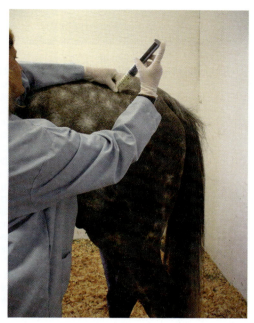

• **Fig. 17.52** Intramuscular injection into equine gluteals.

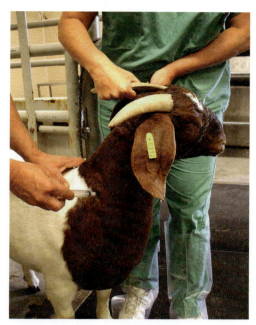

• **Fig. 17.53** Site for intramuscular injection in the neck of a goat.

often chosen as the site for IM injections because of difficulty detecting inflammation, abscess formation, and difficulty in adequate drainage of this area. If the gluteus is used, the technician should stand close to the hip of the horse and insert the needle with a quick thrust, as for other IM sites.

Bovine

Because the meat of most cattle is eventually consumed by humans, IM injections are highly discouraged to avoid causing damage to muscles. In accordance with beef industry quality assurance guidelines, the needle must be clean and sharp, the injection procedure should be smooth so as not to cause too much muscle damage, and no greater than 10 mL of substance should be administered in one spot at any one time. If it is necessary to give an IM injection, the muscles of the neck should be used, with the animal restrained in a head gate or a squeeze chute, with a halter applied. The borders are the same as those described for equine patients (cervical spine, nuchal ligament, and scapula). The needle should be inserted with a quick thrust into the muscle.

The semitendinosus, semimembranosus, shoulder, and gluteal muscles should not be used for IM injections in cattle, because any damage to these muscles would result in these areas being condemned, resulting in expensive loss of high-value cuts of meat.

Ovine and Caprine

Sheep and goats have small muscle masses. As with cattle, the semitendinosus, semimembranosus, and shoulder muscles should not be used as injection sites in meat animals. The neck is commonly used for IM administration, although significant soreness and head drooping may result (Fig. 17.53). This can be particularly problematic in kids and lambs, because they may become too sore to nurse. The gluteal and triceps can be used for very small volumes. Once the muscle to be used has been identified, the standard procedure described for large animals is followed. For adult sheep and goats, an 18- to 20-gauge × 1-inch needle should be used. A 20- to 22-gauge × 1-inch needle is appropriate for lambs and kids.

Porcine

IM injections in pigs can prove to be complicated because of the thickness of the skin, the tendency to store a thick layer of SC body fat, the difficulty involved in restraining them, and the potential for damage to muscle (meat). Generally, the cervical neck muscles just caudal and ventral to the ear are used. In adults, a maximum volume of 5 to 10 mL per site is recommended. Piglets can receive 1 to 2 mL per site. For adults, a long needle (at least 1.5 inches) should be used to avoid the fat, because injecting into the fat will delay drug absorption. The needle gauge can range between 20-gauge for piglets and 16- gauge for larger stock. The gluteal, semimembranosus, and semitendinosus muscles can be used but not in animals intended to be used for meat. Drug residues in various muscles will reduce the market value of the animal. In accordance with quality assurance guidelines, as mentioned earlier for cattle, the technician grasps the skin in this area and will pull cranially. With a firm motion, the needle is inserted at a perpendicular angle to the skin. Once the needle is in the syringe is attached, aspiration is performed and the substance injected.

Camelid

IM injection sites for llamas and alpacas are generally the same as for other large animal species; however, the neck should not be used because of the risk of causing soreness. These animals do not have a large muscle mass in any one place, so SC is the preferred route for administration of large volumes or potentially irritating substances. The semimembranosus and semitendinosus muscles are good choices for IM injection in these animals (Fig. 17.54). For adults, an 18- to 20-gauge × 1-inch needle is appropriate. Twenty-gauge to 22-gauge × 1-inch needles are recommended for crias.

Subcutaneous Administration

In all species, SC injections can be given anywhere that the skin can be lifted and tented (Box 17.3). Medications that are administered by the SC route are absorbed less rapidly compared with

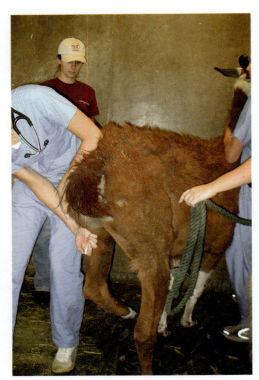

• **Fig. 17.54** A llama receiving an intramuscular injection into the semitendinosus. Note the restraint techniques.

• **BOX 17.3** **Subcutaneous Injection Sites and Restraining**

Animal	Supporting Figure	Site of Injection	Restraint Method
Equine	17.55	Base of neck	Depends on temperament of animal; at a minimum, use of a halter is advised
Bovine		Neck Behind elbow	Use of cattle chute with head control (standing)
Llamas	17.56	Behind elbow	Manual restraint with halter in standing position
Caprine	17.57	Behind elbow Axillary region Flank fold	Manual restraint, standing position
Ovine	17.58	Axillary region Inguinal area Flank fold	Set sheep on rump for access to unwooled areas
Porcine		Axillary region Inguinal region Caudal to base of ear	Piglets: Hold by hind limbs to expose flank and abdominal wall Adults: Use hog snares or chutes

the IV or IM routes but more rapidly compared with those given orally or ID. Therapeutic agents that are administered SC includes vaccines, local anesthetics, small volumes of other medications, and fluid therapy, which may be administered via the SC route for some large animal patients. SC injections may be preferred for show animals, because a noticeable adverse reaction is less likely at the injection site with SC injections versus IM injections. To reduce damage to the meat and economic loss that can occur because of IM injections, the meat industry recommends that drugs be administered by the SC route. Strict regulatory requirements have been put forth for administration of pharmaceuticals to cattle; the medications must be administered per label, and most of those used in cattle are labeled for SC administration.

SC injections are administered by inserting a needle between the skin and muscle of the animal. The site selected should have loose skin that is easily grasped. It is wiped with 70% isopropyl alcohol and the skin is grasped and pulled away from the muscle of the animal before the needle is inserted into the base of the tented skin. The needle size used will depend on the viscosity of the substance to be administered, the size of the animal, and the thickness of its skin. A 20- to 25-gauge needle of 1 inch or less should be used for SC injections in horses. An 18- to 22-gauge × 1.5-inch needle is a common choice for calves, sheep, goats, and pigs. Adult cattle may require a 16- to 18-gauge needle. Before injecting the solution from the syringe, aspirate back to make sure that a vessel has not been punctured. Once needle placement in the SC space has been confirmed, gently inject the medication. The solution should be ejected easily from the syringe, and a bleb or bump is often visible under the skin. A slow flow of solution may indicate that the needle is placed ID. If resistance is felt, the needle should be repositioned before the injection is continued. After the needle and syringe have been removed, the injection area

should be gently rubbed to lessen the bump that has been created and to increase circulation in the area, promoting absorption of the medication. If an SC injection is given into edematous tissue, a bump is not likely to be observed (Figs. 17.55–17.58).

> **TECHNICIAN NOTE**
>
> When injecting the *Brucella* vaccine, the technician should refrain from tenting the skin to ensure that no drug is accidentally injected into the person administering the vaccine.

When administering injections to piglets, the skin is grasped and pulled dorsally, making sure that the injection is shallow, with the needle being inserted at an approximately 10-degree angle. Larger pigs should be restrained with the use of a hog snare or a chute to access the loose skin just caudal to the ear.

Intradermal Administration

ID administration is the injection of a substance between the dermis and the epidermis (skin layers). This route results in very slow absorption. ID injections are performed primarily for the purposes of skin testing, allergen identification, and provision of local anesthesia.

ID administration is used in horses for allergy testing and to treat nodular skin lesions and sarcoidosis (a common tumor affecting the skin of horses). The selected site should be clipped, cleaned, and allowed to dry. Depending on the purpose of the injection, use of an antiseptic agent may be contraindicated, because it may interfere with test results, so the technician preparing for the procedure should be clear about the intent of the veterinarian. The skin is grasped between the thumb and the forefinger

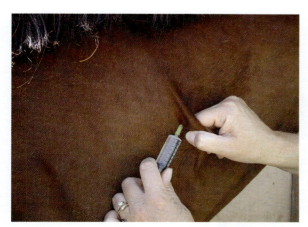

• **Fig. 17.55** Subcutaneous injection into loose skin on the lateral neck of a horse.

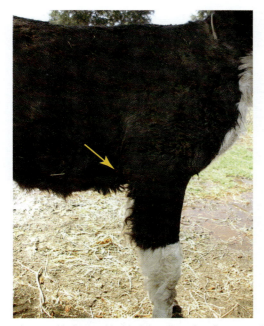

• **Fig. 17.56** Loose skin located behind the elbow in a llama can be a site for subcutaneous injection.

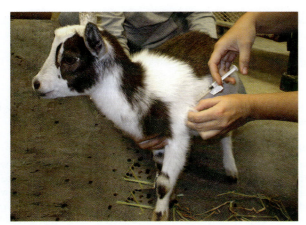

• **Fig. 17.57** A goat kid receiving a subcutaneous injection behind the elbow.

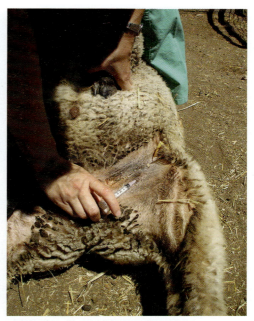

• **Fig. 17.58** A technician administering a subcutaneous injection to a sheep.

and is pulled up from the body. A small needle (25–27-gauge × ⅝ inch) is placed parallel to the site, with the bevel directed up and inserted at a slight angle. The syringe plunger is withdrawn slightly to aspirate and to make sure that no vessels have been penetrated before the solution is slowly injected. Resistance should be felt if the needle is correctly placed in the dermis. A noticeable bleb should appear as the solution is injected. If no bleb is visible, the needle has been placed too deep. The site should not be massaged after ID injections, because the solution is intended to remain localized.

For goats, sheep, and swine, a 25- to 22-gauge × ¾- to 1-inch needle is used. Cattle have very thick skin, so a 20- to 22-gauge × 1.5-inch needle is more appropriate.

Intraperitoneal Administration

Equine

In the equine patient, IP administration of fluids and medication is usually accomplished through an abdominal lavage system. The drain system is inserted surgically by the veterinarian during abdominal surgery or with the animal in the standing position when peritonitis is suspected and general anesthesia is not necessary. The technician will not be involved in the surgical procedure but will be responsible for care and maintenance afterward. To lavage the abdomen, latex tubing is attached to the desired fluids and is connected to the drain system by using a five-in-one connector. The desired amount of fluid (routinely 10 L for an adult equine patient, adjusted for smaller patients) is administered, along with any medication (heparin, antibiotics, etc.), the latex tubing is clamped off, and the patient is walked. This is done to attempt to distribute the fluid and medication throughout the abdominal cavity while washing internal organs and breaking up any adhesions. The latex tubing is then unclamped and fluid is allowed to drain out of the abdomen back into the original fluid bag (Fig. 17.59A–C). Ideally, the amount returned is equal to the amount originally administered. This process can be repeated several times per

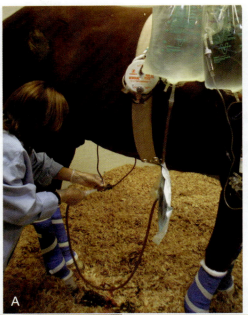
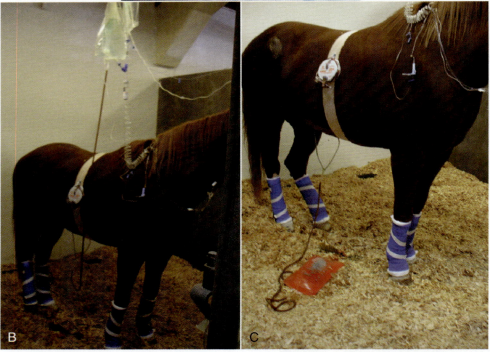

• **Fig. 17.59** (A) A technician attaches latex tubing from an intravenous fluid bag to abdominal drain tubing from an animal for equine abdominal lavage. (B) The fluid bag is raised to allow fluid to flow through the tubing and into the abdominal cavity. (C) The empty fluid bag is lowered to the ground to retrieve peritoneal fluid from the abdominal cavity.

day. When the drain system is handled, gloves should be worn and the technician should pay careful attention to keeping the system clean while not introducing any contaminants during administration.

Bovine

IP injections may be indicated if IV administration is not possible and for treatment of peritonitis. If an IP injection is administered in cattle, the site selected is usually in the paralumbar fossa. Care must be taken when on the left side to prevent puncturing the rumen and when on the right side to prevent puncturing the intestine or dilated or displaced internal organs.

Caprine and Ovine

IP injections are usually reserved for neonatal kids and lambs with umbilical infection or hypoglycemia. After lifting the neonate by its forelimbs, a 20-gauge needle attached to the syringe filled with medication is inserted just to the left of the umbilicus up to a depth of 1 cm. The medication is aspirated to verify that a vessel or an internal organ has not been hit. Once placement is confirmed, medication is injected into the peritoneal cavity and then the needle and syringe removed.

Porcine

In neonatal pigs, fluids are generally administered by the IP route because of the impracticality of placing IV catheters and administering fluids by that route. Fluids should be given at body temperature and be nonirritating and isotonic. The site used needs to be prepared by using aseptic technique to ensure that contaminants are not introduced. The piglet is held up by the hind limbs, and an 18-gauge × ¾- to 1-inch needle is inserted paramedially between the midline and the flank. The needle is stabilized to prevent damage to internal organs. To perform this procedure in a mature pig in the standing position, preparation guidelines should be followed and a 16- to 18-gauge × 3-inch needle inserted through the paralumbar fossa.

Complications from IP administration include peritonitis, abscess, and injury to internal organs.

Intranasal Administration

Certain vaccines and local anesthetics are administered IN. IN anesthetics may be used before other procedures involving the nasal cavity are performed. The head of the patient needs to be secured. Small piglets can be held, whereas a hog snare should be used to restrain larger pigs. A halter and lead rope (and a head gate for adult cattle) may provide sufficient restraint for most large animals. The technician uses their free hand to steady the head.

An easy method is to bring the free arm under the mandible and reach around while placing the hand on top of the muzzle area. Any nasal discharge should be wiped away from the nares by using damp gauze sponges. While the head is slightly lifted, a needleless syringe containing the medication is introduced into the nostril and the substance is injected, preferably during the animal's inspiration. The patient may sneeze afterward, causing the medication to spray. The technician should take precautions to prevent having their own mucous membranes being exposed to the spray from the sneeze.

Oxygen can be administered intranasally to help with certain conditions, such as pneumonia or hypoxic ischemic encephalopathy. Oxygen may be administered to periparturient females that are considered to have a high-risk pregnancy to increase the oxygen content of circulating blood in both the dam and the fetus.

While using a commercially available product (AirLife O_2 Catheter; Cardinal Health, Dublin, OH) or a small rubber feeding tube, the distance from the medial canthus of the eye to the entrance of the nostril is determined. This is how far the catheter will be inserted into the nostril. The catheter is gently inserted ventrally into the nasal passage to the point that was premeasured. To maintain the catheter in the nostril for the long term, it is beneficial to first wrap adhesive tape (Elastikon by Johnson & Johnson, New Brunswick, NJ, works very well) loosely around the muzzle. Then the catheter, with a piece of butterflied 1-inch adhesive tape attached, can be secured using suture material to connect the butterflied piece of tape to the Elastikon. The end can be hooked up to an oxygen source, providing the desired oxygen flow in liters per minute.

Intramammary Administration

Intramammary infusion of antibiotics is used routinely to treat or control mastitis in cows and is also performed on goats and sheep. Because of the high risk of introducing contaminants (organic debris, yeast, or other opportunistic organisms) during this process, the procedure must be performed aseptically. Minimal restraint is usually required, but a TailJack restraint may be necessary for some cows.

The udder is completely milked out and manually stripped as residual milk will dilute the medication. The teats are cleaned with a teat dip and then thoroughly dried, using a separate cloth for each teat. Each individual teat is wiped with an alcohol-soaked sponge and air dried. The teats on the far side from the technician are cleaned before those on the near side to prevent transmission of contaminants from dirty teats to clean teats.

Teats on the near side are infused first. The teat is grasped at the base and a sterile teat cannula or disposable mammary infusion cannula on an antibiotic syringe is partially inserted into the teat (up to 4 mm); the antibiotic is injected slowly into the canal. For goats and sheep with a very small teat orifice, a sterile Tomcat catheter can be used. The technician then proceeds to the next teat with the new cannula and syringe, and then moves to the teats on the far side and repeats. It is recommended that the end of the teat be occluded, and the teat and udder be gently massaged to distribute the medication. After the teats have been infused, teat dip is reapplied and left to dry. In very cold (0°C) conditions, chapping and frostbite can occur, so the animal should not be moved outside until the udders are dry.

> **TECHNICIAN NOTE**
>
> Partial insertion of the cannula into the teat canal delivers fewer contaminants to the udder than would occur with full insertion.

Topical Ophthalmic Administration

To treat ocular diseases or conditions (ulcers, abrasions, lacerations, keratitis), topical ophthalmic ointment and solutions are routinely administered to the eyes. Hands should be cleaned thoroughly or gloved. When medication is provided in ointment form, a small amount is applied directly into the eye. Proper restraint of the head must be employed to deliver the intended amount successfully into large animal patients (both adults and neonates). The lower eyelid of the eye that needs medicating is pulled down slightly and the ointment is applied without touching the surface of the eye. The lid is then released and the blinking action distributes the medication. Another method of ointment application involves wearing sterile gloves and placing a small ribbon of ointment on a gloved finger. The ointment on the finger is then applied directly to the eye. This eliminates the risk of scratching the eye with the end of the ointment tube in fractious animals.

Ophthalmic solution can be applied by gently pulling the lower eyelid out slightly and placing drops into the lower conjunctival sac. Drops may come directly from a plastic bottle with a dispenser or may be administered using a small sterile syringe—with no needle attached.

When both ointment and solution need to be applied, the technician should apply the solution, wait 5 minutes, then apply the ointment. This is because ointment may prevent absorption of solution.

Most patients tend to be averse to repeated applications into the eye, and many eye conditions are quite painful, so it may be necessary to place a long-term lavage system to properly treat the disease or condition.

Two types of lavage systems are available to supply medication to the eye. The subpalpebral lavage system is inserted through incisions made into the upper or lower eyelids (Fig. 17.60). The narrow rubber tubing is inserted through the incision(s) of the eyelid to open directly in the conjunctival sac and away from the cornea. Because the tubing is very narrow, liquid solutions are delivered through the system instead of ointments. Once the tubing is placed, the system is secured to the skin above the eye and is extended over the poll (IV extension tubing is attached to make the appropriate length to extend up and over the head). A PRN adaptor (intermittent infusion plug) is attached to the end of the system and should be changed every 24 hours or more often if it becomes friable from repeated injections. The medication to be delivered should be warm enough to avoid causing discomfort to the patient and the lines should be cleared after the administration using a very slow bolus of air (1–2 mL). The injections should be given very slowly. If resistance is felt when solution is injected into the lavage system, the veterinarian should be notified so that the tube can be cleared of any debris. If air is used, the patient may be startled when air hits the eye, so the technician should be prepared for any reactions.

The second type of lavage system is placed through the nasolacrimal duct (tear duct). The tubing is inserted into the nasal punctum, and a small stab incision is created through the nostril to pass the tubing through and attach it to the skin. This will prevent the tubing from moving inside the nostril and will prevent the patient from rubbing it out. The method of medication delivery described previously is used. This approach requires a greater volume of medication than is given by the subpalpebral lavage method.

The veterinarian may choose to provide protection to the eye in the form of protective eye cups or hoods, especially in large animals (Eye-Saver, JorVet, Jorgensen Labs, Loveland, CO; Guardian Mask, Guardian Mask Company, Burnet, TX) (Fig. 17.61). These provide protection from sunlight and serve as a mechanical barrier, preventing the animal from rubbing the eye and keeping it free of debris.

Epidural Administration

Epidural administration deposits drugs into the epidural space and is a procedure used to provide anesthesia or for pain control. Epidural injection of analgesics or local anesthetics provides complete analgesia and muscle relaxation caudal to the block. For all species, proper restraint is required for the success and safety of this procedure. Two locations may be used for epidural administration. The cranial epidural is located at the lumbosacral junction (between L6 and S1), and the caudal epidural (sacrococcygeal or first and second coccygeal intervertebral space) is located between S5 and Cd1 or C1 and Cd2. The veterinarian will choose the location for the epidural, depending on the effect that they wish to achieve. Lidocaine, mepivacaine, xylazine, and morphine are commonly administered as epidurals.

Equine

The horse should be restrained in stocks and a twitch applied. Some horses will require the administration of a sedative. The

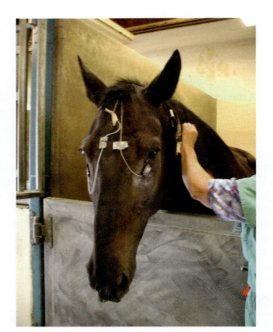

• **Fig. 17.60** Subpalpebral lavage system in an equine patient.

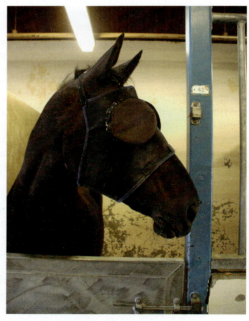

• **Fig. 17.61** Guardian Mask (Guardian Mask Company, Burnet, TX) placed on the head of the horse to provide protection to its eyes.

technician should prepare the supplies necessary, including sterile gloves, local anesthetic, a sterile 12-mL syringe, and a 19-gauge × 1.5-inch sterile needle (3.5 inches for very large horses) or an 18-gauge epidural catheter with stylet. Before the procedures, a 3-inch–square (approximately) area over the first and second coccygeal vertebrae should be clipped, shaved, and aseptically prepared. This area is usually close to where the coarse tail hairs originate. A SC bleb of local anesthetic is placed. This site can be identified by lifting the tail up and down with one hand while feeling for the vertebral space with the other hand (Fig. 17.62). The technician should attempt to have the horse stand still and

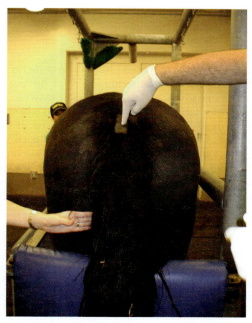

• **Fig. 17.62** Locating the site for equine epidural injection.

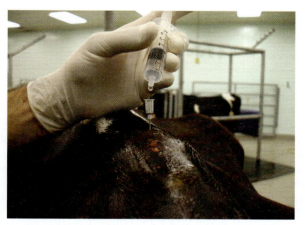

• **Fig. 17.63** A technician performing an epidural injection in a bovine patient.

squarely (even distribution of weight on both hind limbs) on its legs to ensure an even distribution of the drug into both sides of the epidural space.

> **TECHNICIAN NOTE**
>
> To hand the sterile syringe to the veterinarian, open the plastic syringe casing and gently slide the syringe into the sterile gloved hand of the veterinarian without touching the outer casing to the glove. To provide the veterinarian with a sterile needle, remove the cap covering the hub and, while holding the needle cover tightly, point the hub toward the veterinarian, so that they may use sterile gloved fingers to pull the needle from the cover.

Directing the needle slightly cranially and ventrally into the epidural space at an approximately 45-degree angle to the rump, an 18- to 19-gauge × 1.5-inch needle is inserted about 1 inch in adult horses. When the needle enters the epidural space a slight pop is felt, and resistance to the passage of the needle is lessened. The drug is injected and the needle may be left in place to facilitate an additional injection. An epidural catheter may be placed and secured to the skin to facilitate repeated drug administration. When the needle or catheter is removed, antibiotic ointment is applied to the site. The technician should be aware that hind limb instability may occur following epidural anesthesia.

Bovine

Both dairy and beef cattle must be securely restrained. To locate the site, the tail is moved up and down by using one hand while using the other hand to feel the top of the vertebrae to find the first movable joint (Cd1 and Cd2). Clip, shave, and aseptically prep a 3 × 3-inch area. An 18-gauge × 1.5- to 3-inch needle is inserted perpendicular to the spine and into the vertebral space between S1 and S2 (Fig. 17.63). A pop is felt when the space is entered. The epidural space is a relative vacuum compared with atmospheric conditions, and the medication will be sucked into the space; 3 mL of 2% lidocaine are commonly used for bovine epidurals.

Camelid

The tail is moved up and down to locate the intervertebral space between S5 and Cd1. In most llamas and alpacas, this will be the first movable joint, because the five sacral vertebrae are usually fused. The site is clipped and surgically prepared. Owners may object to clipping of the fiber, so efforts should be made to shave only a small site and secure surrounding fibers away from the site with adhesive tape. A 20-gauge × 1.5-inch needle is inserted. The veterinarian will confirm successful insertion, as described for other large animals.

Ovine and Caprine

According to the procedure guidelines for cattle, an 18- to 21-gauge × 1- to 1.5-inch needle is inserted at a 45-degree angle. Sheep and goats are very sensitive to local anesthetics and should be monitored closely after the procedure.

Porcine

The site used for epidural injection in pigs is different from the site described earlier for other large animal species. The lumbosacral junction (between L6 and S1) is accessible for porcine epidurals. This is considered a cranial epidural as opposed to a caudal epidural. To locate the site, an imaginary line is drawn vertically up from the patella to the back, and a dorsal midline site is clipped and surgically prepared. An 18- to 20-gauge spinal needle may be used; the length is determined by the size of the animal. The procedure is the same as previously mentioned.

Transdermal (Cutaneous, Topical) Administration

Application of medication through the skin is done primarily in the form of an impregnated patch that is placed directly on the skin and is left there for the medication to be absorbed. Fentanyl, scopolamine, nitroglycerin, and estrogen are common medications that can be delivered in this fashion. When any type of impregnated patch is applied to the skin, gloves should be worn so that the technician does not absorb any of the medication themselves. The location for patch placement should be shaved and the area cleaned with an alcohol-soaked gauze and dried before the patch is applied.

When it is time to remove or replace the patch, gloves need to be worn in case any residual medication is left on the patch, and the area should be wiped with a gauze sponge to remove any excess product. The patch should then be disposed of according to local guidelines (fentanyl has strict legal disposal requirements).

Many other ointments, solutions, and creams may be applied topically without the need to bandage the area. With these treatments, gentle application of the desired medication via gauze sponges, swabs, or directly from the gloved hand to the affected area will be effective. Before application, the area should be cleared of any debris. In some instances, such as severe burns or wounds, the outer perimeter will be debrided first. The technician should always wear gloves when using topical or transdermal products to limit the potential for contaminants to be added to the medication and to prevent accidental self-administration of the medication.

Intrasynovial Administration

Patients may require administration of medication, such as antibiotics or anesthetic agents, directly into a joint. Intrasynovial administration affords high drug levels localized in the joint compared with levels that would result from systemic drug administration. Veterinarians commonly perform intrasynovial injections on equine patients, and the procedure may be performed on other large animal species as well. Although the technician usually does not perform the injection, they may be asked to prepare the joint that will be infused and to assist with the procedure.

The site that is to be injected needs to be surgically scrubbed and cleaned to minimize the chance of introducing a contaminant into the joint. The technician lays out sterile gloves of appropriate size, several needles of the requested gauge and length (18- or 19-gauge × 1.5 inches is common for adult horses), and the syringe with the solution to be injected. These items must be handled in an aseptic fashion.

Proper restraint of the patient is necessary to ensure the safety of personnel and of the patient. In horses, the use of a twitch in addition to a halter and lead rope lessens the likelihood of movement during the procedure. In addition, chemical sedation should be used to prevent movement and subsequent trauma while the needle is introduced into the joint.

Once the injection is complete, the needle and the syringe are withdrawn and pressure can be applied to the site to prevent leakage of the solution from the joint. The patient should be monitored for pain, heat, or swelling over the joint.

Joint flushing (joint irrigation, joint lavage) is commonly performed with the animal under general anesthesia, but it is also performed on young animals that have received injectable anesthetics or very heavy sedation (because of the risk involved, heavy sedation is not commonly used). Two needles are placed at different sites on the affected joint capsule, and sterile flush forced through one needle exits through the other. Joint lavage may be followed by intrasynovial injection of antibiotics after the exit needle is removed.

Rectal Administration

Rectal administration of therapeutics in large animals is used as a method of delivering medication to a patient that cannot tolerate oral medication because of ileus or regurgitation, or to deliver an enema to a patient with constipation.

Rectal Medications

It may be necessary to remove feces from the rectum before medications are administered. The technician must discuss this with the veterinarian in advance, because it may or may not be necessary, and risk of injury to the animal is increased when a hand is inserted into the rectum. Rectal tears can be fatal. If instructed to do so, the technician must have fingernails clipped short and should remove rings and watches. If fecal evacuation is necessary, a well-lubricated rectal sleeve is placed and the technician gently inserts the hand a short distance into the rectum and will gently remove obvious feces present before the tube is inserted. To deliver medication per rectum, a tube of appropriate size should be selected based on the size of the patient. A Harris enema tube (24-Fr) or a fenestrated tube (multiple holes along the distal end) is appropriate for adult animals, foals, and calves, whereas smaller diameter soft rubber tubes can be used for lambs, kids, and crias. The fenestrated tube may provide better distribution of the medication, but the fenestrations on some tubes may be rough and may cause irritation to the rectal mucosa. The technician should always check the tube for any rough edges and should discard any tube that is not smooth. The distal end of the tube is lubricated with a water-soluble solution (e.g., K-Y Jelly) and the tube is inserted 1-12 inches into the rectum. This distance is determined by the size of the patient. Appropriate restraint, tailored to the individual species and age of the animal, is used. For standing animals, the technician should take precautions to stand to the side of the animal to avoid getting kicked.

Medications are dissolved in a small amount of water or, at the veterinarian's request, in another solution (e.g., dimethyl sulfoxide [DMSO]) and are injected gently via a catheter tip syringe into the tube; this is followed by a small amount of water (or air) to ensure that all medication is evacuated from the tube. The tube is then gently removed.

The veterinarian may administer 2% lidocaine per rectum to facilitate performance of a rectal examination by reducing patient straining. A 60-mL syringe containing lidocaine is attached to rubber tubing or to IV extension tubing that is inserted into the rectum, and the drug is injected. Sedation may be given via the epidural route for patients that are straining to prevent potential problems, such as rectal tears, during the examination.

Enema Administration

Enemas are administered to animals with constipation to facilitate defecation, and they can be safely administered to animals of any age or species. The tube used and the volume and composition of fluid administered will vary with the size and condition of the animal. Fluids should be nonirritating and warmed to room temperature but should not be warmed above body temperature.

Neonates

A common practice of many horse owners is to routinely administer a prepackaged human enema to newborn foals to facilitate passage of meconium (feces that has accumulated in the foal while in utero). Warm-water enemas and enemas containing other agents, such as gentle soap, mineral oil, or other lubricants, are administered using a tube and gravity flow. Retention enemas are routinely used in hospitalized neonatal patients. Excessive enema volume and repeated enemas can be harmful to the patient. The technician must be aware of variation in patient size. For example, the standard 120 to 180 mL of fluid delivered for an equine neonate would be far too much for a cria.

The tip of the tube is well lubricated with a water-soluble lubricant and the tube is gently advanced into the rectum. Once the tube is inserted the desired distance into the rectum, a 60-mL catheter tip syringe, a funnel, or an enema bucket can be attached to the end and the desired amount of solution delivered. Gravity flow is preferred to pumping of fluid, because this method lessens the risk of tearing the rectum. If a syringe is used, gentle pressure is applied until all enema solution has been delivered. After all solution has been administered, the end of the tube is capped off with the thumb and the entire length of tubing gently removed.

Retention Enemas

Retention enemas involve insertion into the rectum of a well-lubricated Foley catheter with a balloon. The tube is inserted a few inches (usually 2–4 inches) into the rectum, and the balloon is inflated using a syringe containing air or water. The enema solution (often Mucomyst [acetylcysteine]) is infused, after which the catheter is clamped off by using a hemostat and is left in place for at least 15 minutes. The hemostat is then removed, the balloon deflated, and the catheter removed (Fig. 17.64A–D).

Enema Administration to Adult Animals

To facilitate enema administration in adult animals, the animal is properly restrained; the technician stands to the side of the patient, inserts a well-lubricated tube (an NGT can be used for enema administration to adult large animals), and delivers the enema solution. The technician administering the enema may benefit from preparing in advance of the procedure by cutting one hole in the center of the bottom of a large plastic trash bag (for their head) and cutting a hole on either side of the bottom of the bag (for their arms) to wear as a disposable coverall in the event of rapid projectile expulsion of fluid and feces.

Sampling Techniques in the Large Animal

Venous Blood Sample Collection

Blood sampling is a simple method that is used routinely to gather a large quantity of diagnostic data. The choice of blood collection tube (or syringe with anticoagulant added) will determine which laboratory parameters can be evaluated. Some tests require serum (centrifugation after clotting of a whole blood sample), some require plasma (centrifugation of unclotted blood yielding serum and fibrinogen) obtained by using an anticoagulant, and some require whole blood for analysis. Blood sample tubes containing an anticoagulant should be filled to ensure the correct blood-to-anticoagulant ratio. Insufficient blood mixed with the anticoagulant may lead to erroneous laboratory results. Once collected, the sample should be gently inverted (not shaken) several times to ensure adequate mixing of the blood with the anticoagulant.

For all sites and species, the hair and/or skin should be cleaned with isopropyl alcohol to remove any obvious debris. In addition to providing cleansing, alcohol facilitates visualization of the vein and acts as a local vasodilator. If blood cultures are desired, full sterile preparation (as described earlier) is required.

> **TECHNICIAN NOTE**
>
> Cleaning the hair and/or the skin with isopropyl alcohol facilitates visualization of the vein.

The choice of vein depends on the appearance of the vessels, the position of the animal, and the disposition of the animal. If repeated samples will be required, the technician should start first with a more distal venipuncture site, with subsequent samples taken progressively more proximal on the vein. The bevel-up position of the needle facilitates venipuncture and is less traumatic to the skin and the vein upon puncture. If the need to collect multiple samples is anticipated, placement of an IV catheter should be considered.

A syringe and needle or a Vacutainer needle and collection tube may be used. When a needle and syringe are used, the needle may be inserted first and then the syringe attached, or in some cases, the needle may be attached to the syringe before insertion. The Vacutainer system (consisting of a plastic hub and needle) can be used by inserting the long end of the double-ended needle into the vein and then slipping a blood collection tube over the needle. Alternatively, the tube may be placed on the double-ended needle before injection by inserting the tube into the holder and pressing the rubber stopper against the metal end of the needle until the top of the rubber stopper is aligned with the circumferential score on the tube holder. It should not be pushed farther until the needle is inserted into the lumen of the vein. Once in the lumen, the tube is pushed fully onto the needle. If the tube is pushed fully onto the needle before the other needle end is in the vein, the vacuum is broken and blood will not flow into the tube. Multidraw, rubber-capped Vacutainer needles are more sanitary to use than uncapped needles with regard to blood leakage.

Equine

The horse should be restrained as necessary depending on its behavior. A halter and lead rope may be the only restraint required, but additional restraint is necessary in some horses.

Jugular Vein

To occlude and distend the vein, pressure is placed on the jugular furrow in the lower third of the neck. With an alcohol-soaked sponge or cotton ball, ballottement of the vessel is performed (stroked several times in a downward direction). A 19- to 25-gauge × ⅝- to 1.5-inch needle is inserted into the lumen of the vessel, and blood is aspirated using a syringe or a Vacutainer tube (Figs. 17.65 and 17.66).

Some animals violently resist needle insertion. For these patients, if the needle is inserted first and the animal jumps, twitches, or otherwise moves, the needle is more apt to remain in place without the weight of the syringe. Once the animal settles, the syringe is attached and the blood sample aspirated.

Transverse Facial Vein

The transverse facial vein runs transversely beneath the facial crest and above the transverse facial artery and can be located midway between the medial canthus of the eye and the rostral end of the facial crest (Fig. 17.67A–C).

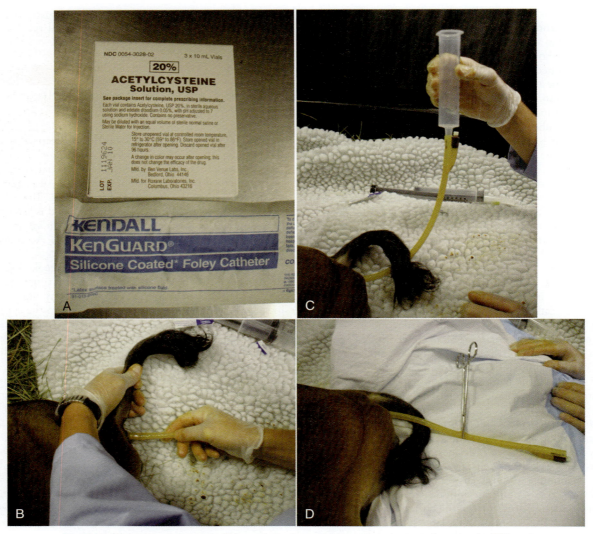

• **Fig. 17.64** (A) Acetylcysteine and a Foley catheter for a retention enema in an equine neonate. (B) Inserting a well-lubricated Foley catheter into the rectum. (C) Administering an enema solution via gravity flow. (D) The Foley catheter is clamped off to allow for retention of the enema.

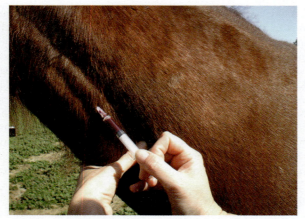

• **Fig. 17.65** Needle and syringe placement for drawing blood from the equine jugular vein.

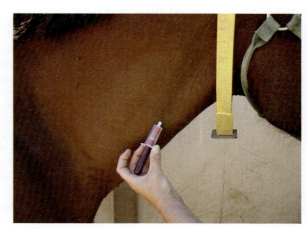

• **Fig. 17.66** Use of a Vacutainer set-up for drawing blood from an equine jugular vein.

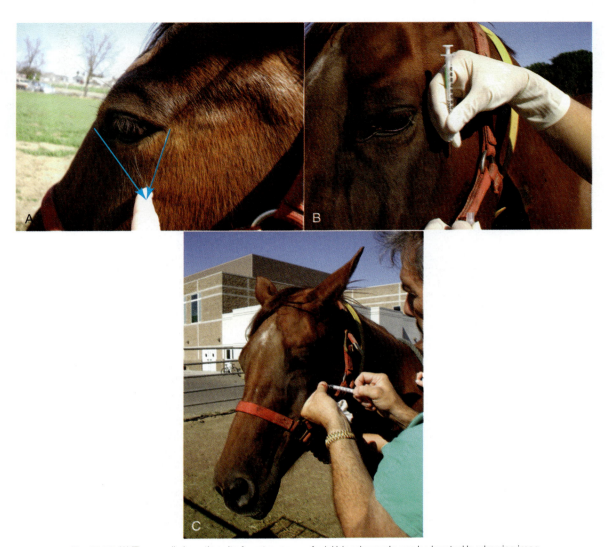

• **Fig. 17.67** (A) The needle insertion site for a transverse facial blood sample can be located by drawing imaginary lines from the medial canthus and the lateral canthus, intersecting them at the facial crest, and inserting the needle just below the facial crest. (B) Holding the syringe to protect the eye in case the horse moves while the technician is preparing to insert the needle. (C) Blood collection from the transverse facial vein.

TECHNICIAN NOTE

To locate the site, the technician may place the thumb at the medial canthus and the index finger at the lateral canthus and draw an imaginary V shape diagonally down to the facial crest.

This vein is commonly used in nonfractious horses to collect small volumes of blood. There is no need to occlude the vein. A 22- to 25-gauge × ⅝- to 1-inch needle is inserted perpendicular to the skin beneath the facial crest and is advanced until bone is felt. The syringe is then attached, and the needle is withdrawn slowly during aspiration. When blood enters the syringe, placement is maintained until collection is complete. A very minimal risk for hematoma formation or bleeding from this site has been noted. Horses rarely object to needle insertion at this site. Caution must be used when handling needles around the face of the horse, because carelessness can lead to puncture of the eye. The hand that holds the needle should always be cupped, protecting the eye from the needle.

Cephalic Vein

The cephalic vein is located on the medial aspect of the forelimb and can be safely accessed in many horses. The site is cleaned with a rubbing alcohol wipe, which also enhances visibility of the vein. The vein is occluded above the needle insertion site (as with all veins, blood flows back toward the heart). A 20- to 22-gauge × 1- to 1.5-inch needle is inserted (Fig. 17.68). Horses may quickly lift up the foot when the needle is inserted, so it is beneficial to insert the needle first and then attach the syringe once the horse has placed the foot back on the ground to reduce the likelihood of the needle coming out of the vein. Because this is a low site on the animal's body, the risk for hematoma formation is increased; therefore after removal of the needle, the technician must make a concerted effort to apply pressure to the site. If the technician is completing other work on the patient, a cotton ball may be placed on the site and adhesive tape wrapped around the limb, but this can be left on only very briefly, because circulation can be compromised. The technician must remove the tape before leaving the patient.

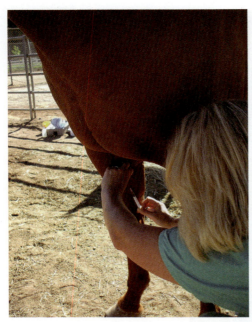

• **Fig. 17.68** Injection into a skin fold on equine patient. Note the position of the technician, ensuring safety against kicks.

Saphenous Vein

The saphenous vein is located on the medial aspect of the hind limb. It is unsafe for the technician to use this site in nonanesthetized adult horses. It can be used successfully in recumbent neonates. Care needs to be taken to apply sufficient digital pressure after removal of the needle.

Bovine

Jugular Vein

The animal is restrained, with its head elevated slightly and tied securely. If necessary, nose tongs may be applied for additional restraint. The jugular vein is distended by placing pressure low in the jugular furrow. The bovine jugular vein is very large, and the palm of the hand should be used to occlude the vessel. Firmly wiping the jugular groove several times in a downward direction with an alcohol-soaked sponge facilitates visualization of the vein. The needle (16–18-gauge × 1.5 inch) should be thrust into the vein with the needle tip directed cranially at an approximately 45-degree angle (Fig. 17.69). Distention of the vein is maintained while collecting the blood; then digital pressure is applied at the site when the needle is removed for 5 minutes to staunch the bleeding.

Coccygeal Vein (Tail Vein)

The tail vein is commonly used when blood samples are collected from many cattle during one visit and when the jugular vein of an individual patient is thrombosed or inaccessible. The animal should be restrained in a chute or stanchion, and a TailJack restraint applied, both as restraint and to position the tail for venipuncture. With one hand, the tail is lifted up and toward the spine of the animal until it is vertical. The ventral surface of the tail is cleaned with 70% isopropyl alcohol to remove dirt and fecal material. An 18- to 21-gauge × 1.5-inch needle is attached to a syringe. The diameter of the coccygeal vein is considerably smaller than that of the jugular vein, so larger needles are inappropriate. The soft space between two vertebrae is located by palpating

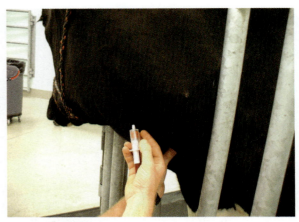

• **Fig. 17.69** Blood collection from a bovine jugular vein.

between two bony prominences. These are *hemal processes*, which are bony canals on the ventral aspect of the vertebral bodies that protect the artery and vein. The needle is inserted perpendicular to the midline until bone is felt, and then the needle is slowly backed out slightly from the bone while applying suction to the syringe. Blood should flow freely into the syringe (Fig. 17.70).

After sample collection is complete, the needle is withdrawn, the tail lowered, and pressure applied to the site for approximately 15 seconds to discourage hematoma formation. The coccygeal artery lies near the coccygeal vein and may be inadvertently punctured. If this is done, digital pressure should be applied to the site for at least 1 minute to prevent hematoma formation.

Subcutaneous Abdominal Venipuncture (Milk Vein)

The right and left milk veins are located along the ventrolateral body wall of the thorax and abdomen and may appear deceivingly enticing for venipuncture. These provide major venous drainage of the udder. Use of these veins for venipuncture can result in life-threatening conditions for the cow. Milk veins are very large and are prone to prolonged and pronounced bleeding and large hematoma formation; they are at great risk for infection because they are easily contaminated by feces, dirt, and other material when the animal is recumbent. Thrombosis of the milk vein may lead to insufficient circulation to the udder, and collateral circulation is inadequate to overcome the problem and thus economic loss. *It is recommended that these veins never be used for venipuncture.*

On very rare occasions and as a last resort, a veterinarian may direct the technician to collect a blood sample from the milk vein. If no other vein is available for sampling and the veterinarian has deemed it necessary to collect a sample from the milk vein, the animal must be restrained adequately in a chute or stanchion with a TailJack or a leg restraint applied.

An accessible site should be selected and the technician should stand next to the shoulder of the cow, facing the tail or close to the flank, facing the head. The technician should then bend just enough to insert the needle while keeping their head up to avoid contact when the cow kicks to the side (there is a strong likelihood that the animal will kick when the needle is inserted). The technician then cleans with isopropyl alcohol, stabilizes the vein with one hand, holds the skin taut, and inserts the needle (18–22-gauge × 1.5-inch needle) in either direction (the blood flows cranially) with the syringe attached. Alternatively, a Vacutainer collection needle may be inserted and a Vacutainer collection tube attached. After the needle has been removed, prolonged

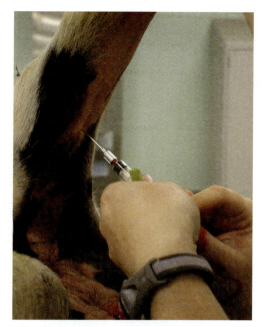

• **Fig. 17.70** Blood collection; note the position of the hands to steady the needle and syringe.

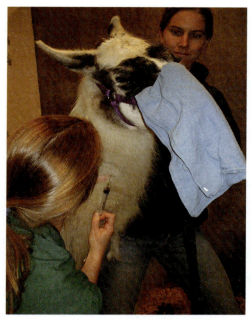

• **Fig. 17.71** Blood collection from an alpaca jugular vein using a needle and syringe; note the restraint applied by a secondary person. A towel can be draped loosely through the halter on the bridge of the nose to protect personnel from being spit upon if the animal is resistant.

digital pressure must be applied over the puncture site (for several minutes); however, this vein should only be used as a last resort.

Camelid (Llama, Alpaca, Lamoid, South American Camelid)

Jugular Vein

Jugular venipuncture in llamas and alpacas can be challenging. In adult animals, visualization of the jugular vein is not possible. No jugular groove is visible, the skin over the jugular vein is thick (in males it can be 1 cm thick), and fibers are long. The transverse process of a cervical vertebra has a ventral projection that curves around the jugular furrow, and llamas and alpacas have valves in the jugular vein that function to keep blood flowing toward the heart, rather than allowing backflow when the head is lowered.

A jugular venipuncture can be performed at a high or a low site. The high site can be located by creating an imaginary line along the ventral border of the mandible and dropping an imaginary line vertically down from just in front of the ear. The intersection of these two lines provides a guide for locating the vein. In some animals, a fluid wave may be visualized by occlusion and ballottement of the vein (stroking the vein toward the occluding hand). The skin is thickest at this point, but the jugular vein is separated here from the carotid artery by a muscle, making the likelihood of arterial penetration at this site less than at the lower neck site (Fig. 17.71).

The low position is located by palpating the ventral projection of the transverse process of the sixth cervical vertebrae (this is close to the thorax and prominent) and occluding the vein just above the transverse process (Fig. 17.72). As with the high neck site, ballottement of a fluid wave can help identify the vein. Although the skin is thinner at this location and movement of the head is less of a problem than with the high neck site, fibers are thicker. The carotid artery and the jugular vein are located close to this area; therefore arterial penetration is more likely.

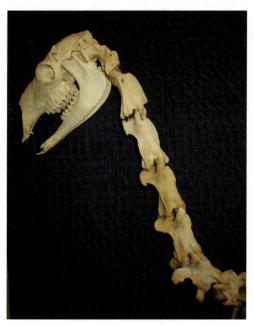

• **Fig. 17.72** Skeleton displaying the skull and cervical vertebrae of a llama. The sixth cervical vertebra is used as a landmark for lower neck venipuncture.

Saphenous Vein

The saphenous vein is superficial and is found on the medial aspect of the stifle. This vein can be used in recumbent animals and lies in proximity and cranial to the artery.

Auricular (Ear) Vein

The ear vein can yield small amounts of blood, sufficient for many laboratory tests, with the use of a butterfly needle. Digital pressure is usually sufficient to raise the vein; however, an elastic band can be wrapped temporarily around the base of the ear as a tourniquet.

Middle Coccygeal Vein

The middle coccygeal vein is located as in cattle but is more superficial in camelids—just under the skin.

Cephalic Vein

The cephalic vein lies similar in placement to that of dogs and can be accessed in adults when the animal is in sternal recumbency (i.e., in the "kushed" position).

Neonatal Camelids (Crias)

Veins commonly used in neonates include the jugular, cephalic, and saphenous veins, and occasionally the ear vein. The jugular vein is much easier to use in the neonate than in the adult, because the skin is thin and the jugular vein can be easily distended and visualized.

Ovine and Caprine

Jugular, cephalic, and femoral veins are commonly used in sheep and goats. The ear vein also provides an accessible site for blood sampling.

Most sheep will be restrained in a "set-up" position on the rump, with the back side leaning up against the handler as this reduces the effort needed to accomplish tasks (as opposed to standing position [Figs. 17.73–17.75]). Jugular, cephalic, femoral, and ear samples can be taken from this position. The jugular, cephalic, and ear veins can be easily accessed in goats while they are standing. The handler can restrain the animal by backing it into a corner and then straddling the goat with the handler's legs tight on either side of the neck, or they can push the goat up against a wall. When straddling the animal, the handler should not underestimate the strength of the animal and must be prepared so that an inadvertent "ride" is avoided. The femoral vein is accessible when the goat is in lateral recumbency.

Porcine

Blood collection from swine is more difficult than from other large animals. Restraining these animals is challenging; they have thick jowls, short legs, and tough skin, and have excessive SC fat. Sampling can be done with the animal restrained or under anesthesia. The technician should be aware that in addition to commercial hogs, many pigs that are receiving veterinary care are beloved pets, and the handling and restraint required for venipuncture and other procedures should be explained well to the owner.

Veins commonly used for venous blood collection in pigs include the cranial vena cava, jugular, auricular, cephalic, and peripheral leg veins, and occasionally the orbital sinus or tail vein.

Cranial Vena Cava

The cranial vena cava may be used for collection of blood from commercial pigs when a large volume of blood is desired; for example, for collection of blood to be used in transfusions or for health certificates. It is not used on pot-bellied or other pet pigs because of risk of death resulting from the procedure. The cranial vena cava rests in the thoracic inlet between the first pair of ribs. The right side of the animal should be used to prevent damage to the phrenic nerve, which is anatomically more protected on the right side of the animal than on the left. Hitting the phrenic nerve may alter the function of the diaphragm and can result in life-threatening cardiac or respiratory problems. For piglets, a

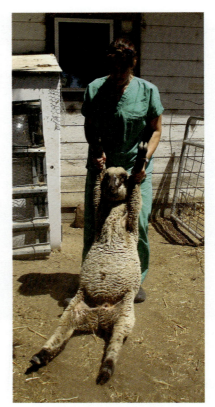

• **Fig. 17.73** The correct positioning of a sheep when "setting" it up for medical procedures. Note the position of the technician for support of the animal and safety and protection of the handler's back.

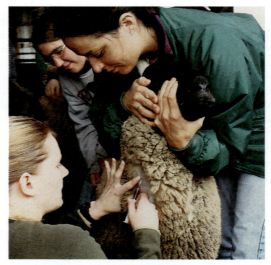

• **Fig. 17.74** Blood collection from the jugular vein in a sheep.

20-gauge × 1.5-inch needle is used. An 18- to 20-gauge × 1- to 1.5-inch needle is appropriate for small pigs (up to approximately 25 kg). For pigs weighing greater than 25 kg, an 18- to 20-gauge × 1.5- to 3.5-inch needle is used. Large adults require a 16- to 18-gauge × 4- to 4.5-inch needle.

When blood is collected from a small pig, the animal is placed on its back (dorsal recumbency) on a 45-degree incline, with the head lower than the hips. The head is extended and the forelimbs pulled caudally. The jugular furrow is visualized, and the needle

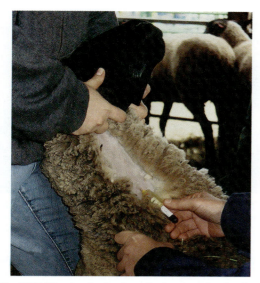

• **Fig. 17.75** Blood collection from the jugular vein of a sheep.

with a syringe attached is inserted into the furrow lateral to the manubrium of the sternum. The needle is pointed toward the caudal aspect of the top of the opposite shoulder blade. As the needle is inserted, the syringe plunger should be pulled slightly to maintain negative pressure. When blood enters the syringe, the needle is held in place while the desired amount of blood is aspirated.

Blood can also be collected with the animal well restrained in the standing position and with the head slightly elevated. Larger hogs are restrained with the use of a hog snare. The person with the syringe crouches in front of the right side of the pig, facing the body of the pig, or can crouch to the side of the right shoulder, facing the neck. The needle is inserted into the right jugular furrow lateral to the manubrium (Fig. 17.76), directed toward the shoulder. The cranial vena cava in large pigs is deep (4 inches may be required to reach the lumen) and care should be taken to avoid injury by tusks.

Jugular Vein

The jugular vein can be used for blood sample collection in commercial pigs of any age. It is not recommended for collection from pot-bellied or other pet pigs because of the risk of death caused by the procedure. The vein is in the jugular furrow and is not as deep as the vena cava, so fewer potential complications are associated with its use. The jugular vein has a smaller diameter than the vena cava and is more difficult to access, especially in large or heavy pigs. The needle size selected depends on the size of the animal. A jugular venipuncture in piglets can be done with a 20-gauge × 1.5-inch needle. Large pigs may require 16-gauge × 3- to 3.5-inch needles. To prevent puncture of the phrenic nerve, the right side of the animal should be used when possible. The needle should be inserted cranial to the manubrium where the jugular furrow appears deepest. The animal is restrained as for a vena cava venipuncture. An imaginary horizontal line that passes through the shoulders and the manubrium sterni is visualized. A second line is visualized that extends from the manubrium sterni to the scapula at an angle of 45 degrees to the first line. The needle is inserted perpendicular to the skin at the intersection of the second line with the deepest part of the right jugular fossa before being directed caudodorsally but should not be angled toward either scapula. Because the vein is superficial, the syringe plunger should be retracted slightly as

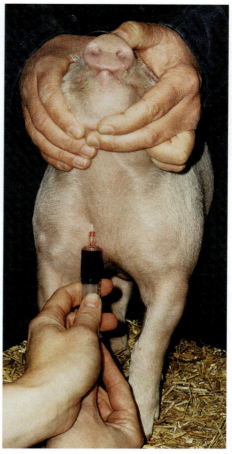

• **Fig. 17.76** Restraint of a pig for blood draw. Note that the venipuncture is performed as a blind stick while the head is pulled back to present access. Venipuncture is performed by using the right anterior vena cava in a small pig; note the needle directed into the jugular fossa, just lateral to the manubrium sterni.

soon as the needle penetrates the skin. The needle is advanced until blood is aspirated into the syringe. Once a sufficient volume of blood has been collected, the needle is removed.

The technician should be aware that fewer complications and lower risk for incidental injury to the animal are associated with venipuncture of the more distal veins, discussed next.

Auricular Vein

The auricular vein is located near the lateral border of the pinna of the ear. It is easily visualized on the dorsal side of the ear and can be seen even more clearly by placing digital pressure at the base of the lateral surface of the ear. The ear is held and digital pressure (or a rubber band tourniquet) applied at the base of the ear to distend the vein. A needle with a syringe attached can be inserted into the vein while gently pulling back on the plunger. To prevent collapse of the vein with aspiration, some technicians prefer to insert the needle and allow the blood to drip from the needle hub directly into the uncapped collection tube while gently mixing; the use of a butterfly needle may also be preferred. For most pigs, a 20-gauge × 1-inch needle is appropriate. For large adult pigs, an 18- to 19-gauge × 1-inch needle may be used. Vacutainer collection needles and tubes may apply too much suction and, as in the case of excess pressure on the syringe plunger, they tend to cause the vein to collapse and therefore are discouraged. When

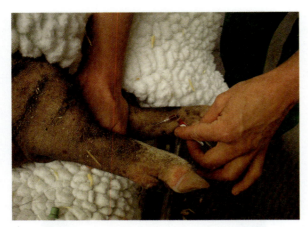

• **Fig. 17.77** Blood collection in a pig for a peripheral capillary sample.

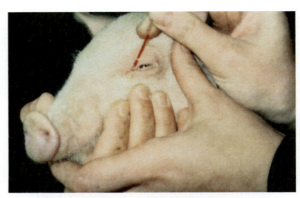

• **Fig. 17.78** Small quantities of blood can be collected from the orbital sinus of a pig.

an adequate blood sample has been collected, pressure is released from the base of the ear, the needle removed, and pressure applied to the insertion site. For repeated sampling, placement of an IV catheter should be considered.

Peripheral Leg Veins

The cephalic vein on the forelimb, the saphenous vein on the hind limb, and branches of veins located on the lower limbs are accessible in small pigs and can be used for venous sampling. These veins can be visualized and are readily accessible in anesthetized pigs. To prevent collapse of the vein the needle is inserted and blood is allowed to drip from the hub of the needle into the open collection tube (Fig. 17.77). Collection of blood from the standing and restrained pig can be done by placing hand pressure or a tourniquet above the collection site to distend the vein. A 20-gauge × 1- to 1.5-inch needle is inserted at an approximately 45-degree angle to the skin in the direction of the body. If anticoagulants are used, care must be taken to prevent clotting.

Coccygeal Vein

Although this site is not commonly used in commercial pigs, it is frequently used for blood sample collection from pot-bellied pigs as well as adult pigs with intact (not docked) tails. A 20-gauge × 1-inch needle is inserted at the ventral midline of the tail perpendicular to the skin.

Orbital Sinus (Medial Canthus of the Eye)

The orbital sinus is adjacent to the medial canthus of the eye and can be used for collection of small volumes of blood. A 20- to 22-gauge × 1-inch needle can be used for piglets. Sampling on larger pigs may require a 16- to 18-gauge × 1.5-inch needle. The needle is inserted into the medial canthus deep into the third eyelid (nictitating membrane) and is advanced at a 45-degree angle toward the opposite jaw until bone is felt. The needle is then rotated between the fingers until blood enters the hub. The syringe is attached and blood collected with gentle aspiration. When collection is complete, the needle is removed and digital pressure applied over the medial canthus with the head elevated. A microcapillary tube with the end broken to form a rough point can be used in lieu of a needle (Fig. 17.78).

Arterial Blood Sample Collection (ABG)

Arterial blood gas (ABG) samples are commonly obtained for blood gas analysis, which provides information on oxygen and

carbon dioxide content, pH, base deficit, and bicarbonate. This information is used to evaluate the respiratory status of the patient. If the data include base deficit and bicarbonate, the analysis is also used to assess metabolic (acid-base) status. Arterial blood reflects the ventilation status of an animal more accurately than venous blood, because arteries carry freshly oxygenated blood from the heart to the body, whereas veins carry blood back to the heart for circulation to the lungs, where oxygen is replenished and carbon dioxide is released. Because ABG samples are frequently obtained intraoperatively when the animals are under general anesthesia, arterial catheters are commonly placed to facilitate sequential blood sampling. Values obtained from the sample analysis allow close monitoring of anesthesia.

Arterial samples are routinely collected in alert foals and crias and are less frequently taken from adult equines and camelids. Arterial sampling in cattle, sheep, goats, and pigs is rarely done on nonanesthetized animals.

The smallest gauge needle possible should be used to minimize trauma to the vessel. For most sample sites, a 25-gauge needle and a 1- or 3-mL syringe are used. A very small amount of heparin (enough to fill the needle and appear in the hub) is aspirated into the needle, and the plunger is pulled back on the syringe to coat the syringe. The needle is removed and a new 25-gauge needle placed on the syringe; the heparin is then expelled from the syringe through the new needle. This eliminates the needle that was dulled by puncturing the rubber stopper on the heparin vial and allows use of a sharp needle for arterial sample collection. The heparin residue that remains in the syringe is sufficient to prevent coagulation but is not enough to alter laboratory results. Some veterinarians prefer to use commercially prepared blood gas syringes containing powdered heparin (Fig. 17.79).

Some veterinarians prefer to have the sites for arterial puncture shaved before cleaning with alcohol (this is often the case with arterial samples on neonatal patients). The area is palpated to find a pulse and determine the location of the artery. The selected artery site is given a surgical prep or is at least cleaned well with 70% isopropyl alcohol before insertion of the needle. It is not necessary to occlude arteries as is done with venous blood sampling. Depending on the patient's behavior and the site selected, the needle may be inserted first and the syringe attached when blood comes from the hub, or the needle may be inserted with the syringe attached. When the needle enters the artery, bright red blood pulses from the needle hub into the syringe. With most arterial samples, blood will rapidly fill the syringe. Very little force is placed on the plunger of the syringe, because the blood in the artery is under pressure and

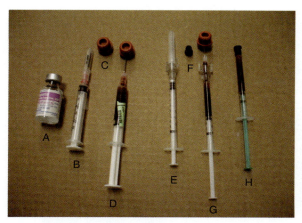

• **Fig. 17.79** Syringes for blood gas sample collection. (A) Sodium heparin (1000 units/mL). (B) A 3-mL syringe with the barrel coated with heparin. (C) Rubber stopper. (D) Blood sample in syringe. (E) Commercial preheparinized syringe (Micro ABG, Marquest, Englewood, CO). (F) Stopper. (G) Micro ABG syringe with a needle inserted into the rubber stopper. (H) Micro ABG syringe with cap.

will flow rapidly. A minimum of 1 mL of blood should be collected into the syringe that has been lined with liquid heparin to ensure results with diagnostic value. Smaller volumes can be taken using commercial blood gas syringes, because these syringes are designed to eliminate errors in dilution. When the needle is withdrawn, firm digital pressure should be applied immediately to the puncture site and should be maintained for several minutes. Arteries are far more susceptible to hematoma formation compared with veins. The technician must make sure to apply sufficient pressure long enough to stop bleeding and prevent formation of a hematoma. If care is taken with this step, the artery will be preserved and can be used for repeated sampling. If insufficient pressure and time are taken to hold off the collection site, the artery will become damaged and may become unusable for future sampling; the related area may suffer from impaired circulation, thus compromising the condition of the patient.

> **TECHNICIAN NOTE**
>
> Following the collection of arterial blood samples, firm digital pressure should be applied immediately to the puncture site and maintained for several minutes.

Any bubbles present in the syringe are expelled and the tip of the needle is inserted into a rubber stopper to occlude the needle tip and prevent air from entering the syringe. Samples for blood gas analysis must remain anaerobic (not contaminated by atmospheric air), because exposure to air will modify oxygen and carbon dioxide values. The syringe should be rolled between the palms to ensure distribution of anticoagulant throughout the sample. If the sample is not analyzed promptly, it should be placed in an ice water bath. Placing the sample in a freezer or on ice (with no water added) can damage the sample and affect the results of the analysis.

> **TECHNICIAN NOTE**
>
> Samples for blood gas analysis must remain anaerobic (not contaminated by atmospheric air), because exposure to air will alter the laboratory values obtained.

Equine

Arteries commonly used for blood sampling in horses include facial (most often used in anesthetized animals), transverse facial, carotid, and metatarsal (in recumbent foals and anesthetized animals). In addition to these sites, arterial sampling on foals can include brachial and palmar (digital) arteries.

The facial artery is accessible in the area under the mandible to the facial crest. This site is commonly used for arterial catheterization in anesthetized animals (Fig. 17.80A–D).

The transverse facial artery lies caudal to the lateral canthus of the eye (Fig. 17.81). Some technicians prefer to inject 0.25 mL of 2% lidocaine into the skin over the artery prior to sample collection, but often, there is little or no objection from horses when this site is used without a lidocaine block.

The carotid artery is accessible in the lower third of the neck in the dorsal aspect of the jugular groove and is deeper than the jugular vein. The artery feels like a cord, and a pulse is normally not palpable. An 18- to 19-gauge × 1.5-inch needle is directed into the artery at a 90-degree angle.

The dorsal metatarsal artery is located on the lateral aspect of the third metatarsal bone (cannon bone on hind limb) and is the preferred site of sampling in recumbent foals (Fig. 17.82). A pulse is usually easily palpable. If a pulse is not obvious, the technician may put firm digital pressure proximal to the selected site, slowly release pressure, and feel for the pulse; this often enhances the pulse quality distally. The pulse may not be felt in very sick neonates with poor blood pressure. In these patients, it is helpful to place a warm water bottle or compress over the artery to enhance pulsation of the artery. The technician sits with the foal's hind hoof secured between the knees. The artery is palpated with one hand, and the needle inserted with the other hand. The foal's leg can be secured by holding it between the technician's legs. Some patients require additional handler assistance; the technician should make use of available help to complete procedures more quickly and with less stress to the patient and less risk for injury to personnel. The behavior and condition of some foals allow the procedure to be done by the technician with no additional restraint; however, this decision depends on the patient and the experience and skill of the technician. Many foals will accept this procedure if the needle is slowly and smoothly inserted into the skin, although some foals will violently resist needle insertion and will jerk and kick the leg. In these foals, the needle is quickly inserted and the syringe is attached after the foal's leg is again secured in place.

The palmar (digital) artery is palpable on the abaxial surface of the fetlock. This site is more difficult to access, because the artery moves around quite a bit, and the location precludes restraining the foal's leg between the technician's legs.

The brachial artery may be palpated where it crosses the medial aspect of the proximal forelimb and may yield a sample when attempts at other sites have been unsuccessful.

Camelid

The auricular (ear) artery is often used in llamas and alpacas for arterial sampling (Fig. 17.83).

Bovine, Ovine, and Caprine

Arteries used for sampling in these animals include the transverse facial, carotid, auricular, and dorsal metatarsal. As noted previously, collection of arterial samples from these animals is usually restricted to anesthetized individuals or neonatal patients.

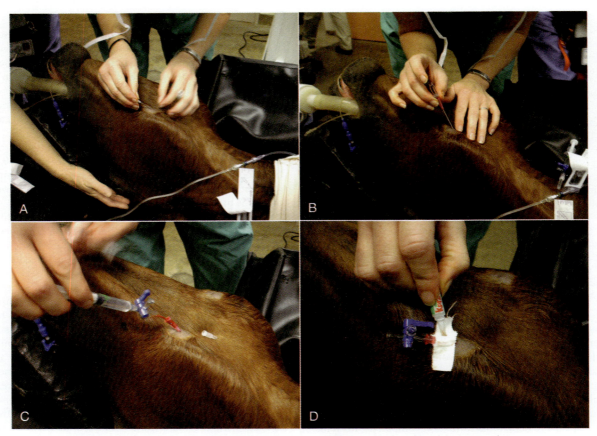

• **Fig. 17.80** (A–D) Placement of a catheter in an equine patient; note the location of the stopcock.

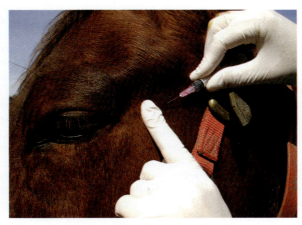

• **Fig. 17.81** Collection of blood from the orbital sinus of a horse.

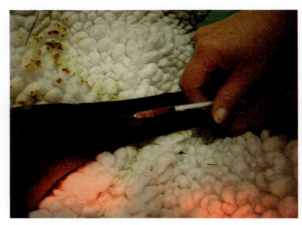

• **Fig. 17.82** Use of a tuberculin syringe for arterial blood collection.

Arterial Catheterization

A short OTN catheter can be placed in the artery of an anesthetized patient. Arteries commonly catheterized in the horse include the transverse facial and dorsal metatarsal arteries. Arteries commonly catheterized in food animals include the transverse facial, dorsal metatarsal, and auricular arteries. The procedure for placing arterial catheters is the same as for IV catheters; only the location and use differs.

Urine Sample Collection

Urine is collected from patients to screen for systemic (e.g., rhabdomyolysis, azoturia) or urinary tract disease. Urine is routinely analyzed in race and performance horses for drug detection purposes. Cleansing of the external genital area is not necessary when urine is collected for drug testing. Urine can be collected for urinalysis from all large animal species in a free-catch midstream sample. Catheterization is recommended for samples that will be cultured but, as described later, bladder catheterization is not always possible. Cystocentesis may be performed by some veterinarians on small ruminants but is not practical in horses because of the inability to stabilize the bladder and the risk for intestinal perforation with the needle.

For all urine samples, the sample should be collected in a dry, clean container (sterile if a culture is desired and catheterization is performed). A midstream sample should be collected, because the

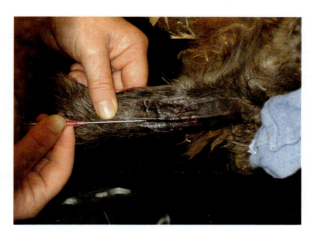

• **Fig. 17.83** Insertion of an arterial catheter. Note the position of the hands steadying the vessel as the catheter is advanced.

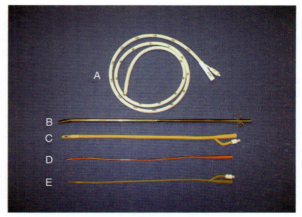

• **Fig. 17.84** Urinary catheters. (A) Stallion catheter. (B) Mare Chambers catheter. (C) 28-French (Fr) Foley catheter. (D) 12-Fr red rubber feeding tube. (E) 12-Fr Foley catheter.

initial stream often contains bacteria, mucus, and cellular debris compared with the rest of the urine and does not as accurately reflect the actual content of the urine. Bacterial contamination in free-catch samples is significant. Urine samples degrade rapidly, so samples should be analyzed promptly (within 20 minutes) or refrigerated for no longer than 2 days.

> **TECHNICIAN NOTE**
> Urine samples degrade rapidly, so they should be analyzed promptly or refrigerated for no longer than 2 days.

Complications of urinary catheterization include infection of the urinary tract if sterile technique is not followed, mucosal irritation, slow and painful urination, and bacterial contamination of the sample.

Equine
Free-Catch Method
Urination may be encouraged by placing the horse in a freshly bedded stall. Sometimes making the horse stand on a grassy area will encourage urination. Other suggestions include running water on cement and tickling the prepuce with a piece of straw. Some race and performance horses have been conditioned to urinate by whistling to them. Recumbent neonates will frequently urinate when they are assisted to stand. The technician should be prepared by having a plastic urine collection container within reach when helping a foal to rise or supporting it in the standing position.

> **TECHNICIAN NOTE**
> A midstream sample should be collected for analysis to avoid sample contamination.

Urinary Catheterization
Materials Needed
• Urinary catheter: tube with the smallest outer diameter possible used to minimize trauma to the urethra (Fig. 17.84)
• Adult males: urinary (Foley) catheter 24- to 28-Fr with 6- to 9-mm outer diameter and approximately 140 cm long
• Colts: red rubber catheter 12-Fr
• Adult females: Chambers catheter or Foley catheter 30-Fr
• Fillies: Foley catheter 12-Fr

• A 60-mL catheter tip syringe
• Sterile gloves
• Gentle antimicrobial soap and 70% rubbing alcohol or other disinfectant cleanser (povidone-iodine solution and scrub)
• Soft cotton
• Sterile lubricant
• Sterile collection containers (for urinalysis, cytologic examination, and culture)
• Sedation

Male Horses. Sedation is usually required when stallions and geldings are catheterized for restraint and extension of the penis from the prepuce. The technician should be positioned cranially to avoid being kicked. The prepuce is retracted, the penis grasped gently but firmly caudal to the glans penis (hold steady as the horse may attempt to retract the penis), and the penis washed with dilute antibacterial soap. Care must be taken to cleanse the urethral process and the urethral diverticulum (a blind pouch located dorsal to the urethral opening), making sure to remove any smegma ("beans") present in the diverticulum, followed by rinsing with water. This must be done to prevent introduction of bacteria that are present at the urethra and prepuce into the bladder and to prevent bacterial contamination of the urine sample. With sterile gloves on, the technician applies sterile, water-soluble lubricant to the tip of a flexible urinary catheter. The penis is held with one hand and the other hand is used to gently advance the catheter through the urethra and into the bladder. A curvature is present around the ischial arch (just ventral to the anus), and slight force may be necessary to advance the catheter past this point. The horse will characteristically raise its tail and flag when the catheter passes over the ischial arch just before it reaches the bladder.

If urine does not flow from the catheter, a syringe can be attached to gently aspirate the sample. Excessive negative pressure must not be used, because it may cause minor hemorrhage and can alter the sample composition. A small volume of air can be injected into the catheter, or the catheter can be repositioned, if necessary, to encourage flow.

Female Horses. Wrap the tail and tie it out of the way to prevent hair from entering the vagina or touching the glove or catheter, thereby introducing contaminants.

The vulva and the perineum should be thoroughly cleaned. With sterile gloves on and using sterile, water-soluble lubricant, the technician locates the urethral orifice on the ventral aspect of the vaginal vault. The orifice is approximately 10 to 12 cm from the ventral commissure of the vulvar lips. A small Chambers catheter, stallion catheter, or Foley catheter can be used to catheterize female horses. Lubricate the catheter and use a finger to slide the catheter down into the urethral orifice; the catheter is advanced 5 to 10 cm (2–4 inches) until it enters the bladder (Fig. 17.85A–D). The flow of urine can be facilitated as described earlier.

Camelid

Free-Catch Method

Llamas and alpacas urinate and defecate on communal dung piles, so the animal should be led to a dung pile, if possible. Attaching a collection cup to the end of a broom or dowel facilitates collection without requiring personnel to be close enough to distract the animal. Both males and females urinate in a caudal direction while in a squatting position. Complete urination usually takes 30 to 60 seconds.

Urinary Catheterization of Llamas and Alpacas

In addition to the sigmoid shape of the penis, which makes passage of urinary catheters extremely difficult, male llamas and alpacas have a membranous flap at the ischial arch that prevents passage of urinary catheters into the bladder, so this procedure cannot be done in male camelids.

Materials Needed for Urinary Catheterization of Female Llamas and Alpacas

- Sterile gloves
- Sterile, water-soluble lubricant

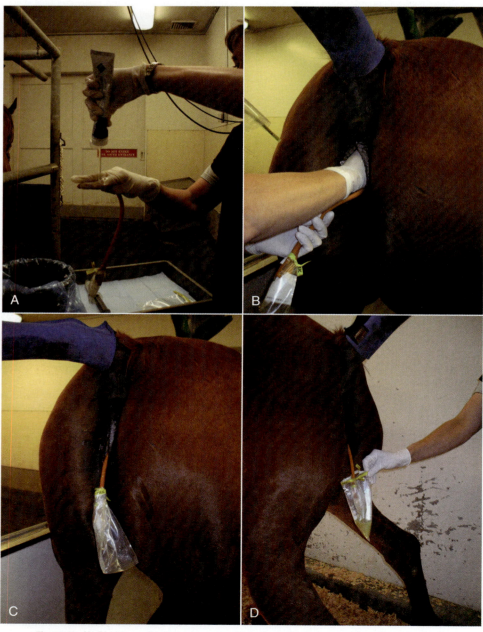

• **Fig. 17.85** (A–D) Urine collection on a mare. Note the collection vessel for collection of urine.

- A 60-mL catheter tip syringe
- Red rubber tube or polypropylene catheter, 5-Fr
- Gentle antimicrobial soap or other cleanser
- Soft cotton
- Sample collection containers (sterile if culture desired)
- Sedation, if necessary

The llama or the alpaca is restrained, the lips of the vulva are cleaned, and the area is dried. With sterile gloves on, the technician places a small amount of lubricant on the glove. A finger is inserted into the vulva and the external urethral orifice located. This is felt as a groove on the floor of the vulva. When located, the technician withdraws the finger slightly and slides the catheter along the dorsal aspect of the index finger into the orifice. Sliding the catheter along the finger in this manner avoids insertion into a blind ventral urethral diverticulum, which is located just caudal to the orifice of the urethra. The catheter is slowly advanced. For most adult llamas or alpacas, the catheter is inserted about 25 cm from the vulvar lips to enter the bladder. A free-flowing sample is collected into a sterile container or a syringe is attached and the fluid gently aspirated.

Bovine
Free-Catch Method
The animal is placed in a chute or stanchion and allowed to relax. Urination in cows may be encouraged by lightly massaging the vulvar tip and the skin beneath the vulva or tickling with a blade of grass or straw. The technician may try repeated parting of the lips of the vulva to elicit urination. Steers and bulls may urinate if the prepuce is massaged and splashed with warm water. Urine is best collected into a plastic container or, depending on the required analysis, a urine dipstick (litmus paper test strip) can be held directly in the stream of urine. This technique is often used to monitor urine pH and ketones.

Urinary catheterization in male cattle is nearly impossible because of the anatomy and therefore is not performed by the technician.

Cows can be catheterized with a small-diameter (0.5-cm) catheter with techniques like those used for mares. The perineal region is gently scrubbed with an antiseptic solution and rinsed well with warm water. A sterile gloved and lubricated hand is inserted into the vagina and is slid forward along the floor of the vagina (approximately 10 cm in an adult), where a finger is inserted into the suburethral diverticulum; the catheter tip is then guided over the diverticulum and into the external urethral orifice. Urine will flow through the catheter when it has reached the bladder.

> **TECHNICIAN NOTE**
> Always use a plastic collection vessel to avoid breakage and possible injury to animals or the technician.

Ovine and Caprine
Free-Catch Method
Both ewes and does tend to urinate immediately after rising from a period of recumbency. Therefore the technician should be prepared to collect a urine sample when the animal stands. This is the easiest approach and causes the least stress to the animal.

Urination may be induced in ewes by occluding the nostrils for up to 45 seconds while the animal is standing. This causes stress to the animal and may be unpleasant for the owner to view. This should be taken into consideration and the technique should be clearly explained to the owner. The animal will indicate discomfort by struggling, and as the nostrils are released and the animal is allowed to breathe again, it will urinate. The use of this method in does seldom results in urination. Providing clean bedding or a newly cleaned pen may elicit urination and may be an easy way to encourage urination. Male ruminants may respond to manual stimulation of the prepuce; the technician should be prepared with a plastic collection container and should make every effort to collect a sample when the animal urinates.

Urinary Catheterization
Males. As with male cattle, the anatomy of male sheep (rams) and male goats (bucks) makes catheterization of the bladder extremely difficult, and the procedure is not commonly attempted. Catheterization of the urethra (not completely into the bladder) is commonly performed on blocked goats (obstruction of the flow by urinary stones). The urethra opens 1 to 2 cm beyond the tip of the glans penis through the urethral process and it is difficult to enter this narrow structure with a catheter. The S-shaped curvature of the penis (sigmoid flexure) provides another obstacle to passage of a catheter. In addition, a urethral diverticulum (a blind sac) near the ischial arch prevents the catheter from entering the bladder. In male goats, the catheter can be directly inserted into the bladder from the body wall through an ultrasound-guided procedure. This is done to allow the urethra to heal or to release pressure caused by accumulation of urine.

Females. The animal should be properly restrained and the tail held or tied out of the way during the procedure to prevent contamination. The vulva is cleansed as described for other large animal species. With sterile gloves on, the technician applies sterile, water-soluble lubricant to the fingers, and the fingers are inserted into the vagina. The urethral opening is found midline on the ventral surface within 5 to 10 cm of the vulva (depending on the size of the animal). The vulvae of ewes and does are quite small. A small animal vaginal speculum may be helpful in allowing visualization of the urethral opening. A 5- to 12-Fr urinary catheter is inserted. Female ruminants have a small suburethral diverticulum (blind sac) that extends from the ventral aspect of the urethra. If the catheter is inadvertently fed into the diverticulum, resistance will be felt, and the catheter should be pulled out slightly and redirected more dorsally. When the catheter is in the bladder, urine is likely to flow spontaneously; however, gentle aspiration with a sterile syringe may be necessary.

Porcine
The technician should be ready with a collection cup, because free-catch urine is necessary for a urinalysis in swine. It is common for adult swine to urinate two or three times a day.

Males should be confined and observed; when the animal is calm, the prepuce may be stroked with a warm, wet towel or a soft brush. Stimulating the vulva by stroking with fingers, a soft brush, or dry straw can be attempted in females. Male pigs cannot be catheterized because of the difficulty accessing the penis and the small diameter of the urethra.

Females can be catheterized with the aid of a vaginal speculum and a canine catheter, but this procedure is not routinely performed.

Fecal Sample Collection

Fecal samples are collected for gross visual inspection; to check for the presence of mucus, sand, or blood (frank or occult); for microscopic examination to check for intestinal parasites; and for microbiological culture or **polymerase chain reaction** (PCR) assay. Occasionally, feces may be evaluated for osmolality and electrolyte concentration (to determine the presence of an osmotic diarrhea). The technician should be familiar with the normal character (content, consistency, color, and odor) and volume of feces for each species.

Feces contain a variety of bacteria that are normal and nonpathogenic. Fecal samples are cultured for specific microorganisms (e.g., *Salmonella*) by inoculating the feces onto an enrichment medium that is designed to inhibit growth of many normal bacteria while encouraging growth of the specific bacterium to be identified. Some PCR assays that are now available are more sensitive, providing results more quickly compared with microbial culture for specific pathogens. Fresh feces should be collected and placed in a clean container. Fresh feces will yield more accurate diagnostic information for parasite identification and an accurate culture result. Feces may be collected with a gloved hand from the ground or directly from the rectum. If the animal is not producing feces, a rectal swab may be collected for culture.

> ### TECHNICIAN NOTE
> Fresh feces will yield more accurate diagnostic information for identification and culture of parasites.

If feces are to be collected directly from the equine rectum, the person performing the collection must have short fingernails and should remove rings and watches. The horse is restrained (preferably in stocks), and the technician should wear an obstetric sleeve with generous amounts of lubrication gel applied to the sleeve. The technician will stand slightly to the side of the horse, touch fingertips together forming a cone, and insert the coned hand slowly and gently just far enough into the rectum to collect a handful of feces. The glove or sleeve can be turned inside out and tied in a knot to store the sample. The utmost care must be taken by the technician because rectal tears that may be life-threatening can occur via this method of collection.

If sand colic is suspected in a horse, fecal sedimentation may be used as a diagnostic test. Feces can be mixed with water in the glove or in the sleeve. The sleeve can be hung up to allow solid material to settle, and sandy material may be seen or felt through the fingers of the glove.

> ### PUT INTO PRACTICE
> To keep fecal samples preserved and viable when collecting from large animals, consider taking a small cooler with you to the field or barn, complete with a cold pack to prohibit continued maturation of organisms.

Milk Sample Collection

Milk samples are routinely collected from dairy animals to test for the presence of *mastitis*, which is inflammation of the mammary gland that is commonly caused by bacterial infection. Inflammation may be present without a bacterial component if the teat or udder has received a traumatic injury (kicked, stepped on, cut). *Clinical mastitis* refers to the presence of obvious clinical signs, including a hard, hot udder; abnormal appearance or smell of the milk; and pain. Subclinical, sometimes asymptomatic, mastitis must be confirmed through diagnostic testing of the milk. Colostrum samples are frequently collected from mares and cows and tested to determine the quality of colostrum present.

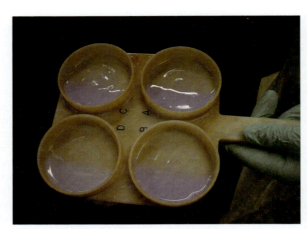

• **Fig. 17.86** California Mastitis Test (CMT) paddles containing milk samples.

Sterile Milk Sample

Hands should be thoroughly washed and dried before cleaning the teat end of the udder with an alcohol-soaked cotton swab, starting on the udders furthest away from the technician. The process is repeated until the cotton is clean after rubbing the end of the teat and is allowed to dry. Using clean, dry hands, the technician removes the top of a culture tube. Each quarter of the cow's udder (each half in small ruminants) is collected individually. If milk from more than one teat is collected, the teats closest to the milker should be sampled first to prevent contamination of the far-side teats by the arm of the milker. The tube is held in such a manner that no dirt or debris will fall into the tube and nothing is allowed to touch the opening of the tube. The first few squirts of milk are discarded, and then a stream of milk is squirted directly into the collection tube and the top replaced. The sample can be refrigerated for up to 24 hours before laboratory processing.

Nonsterile Milk Sample

Samples for California Mastitis Test

The California Mastitis Test (CMT) is commonly used to identify the presence of mastitis in cows, does, and ewes. This test involves the use of a white plastic test paddle with four cups labeled A to D and a reagent fluid (Fig. 17.86).

The teats are cleaned and dried. It is not necessary to clean the entire udder. If washed completely, the risk of introducing contaminants from the udder into the teat orifice is increased. A small amount of milk is stripped and the first stream discarded before collecting the sample to avoid a false-positive result. The paddle may be held with the handle in a caudal direction to strip a small amount from one teat into one well of the paddle. The same is done for the remaining teats, and the technician notes which teat was milked into each well (Fig. 17.87). An equal volume of CMT reagent solution (one part milk to one part reagent solution) is added to each well, the paddle is gently moved to swirl the milk, and the resultant solution is graded based on gel formation. The number indicates the severity of infection.

0 = No gel.

Trace = Precipitate disappears with continued movement of the sample.

1 = First visible precipitate does not disappear.

2 = First visible gel—mixture moves toward the center of the cup, leaving the bottom of the outer edge of the cup exposed.

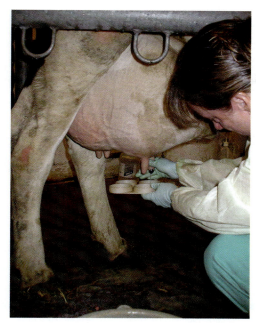

• **Fig. 17.87** Note the position of the California Mastitis Test (CMT) paddles for testing of milk from each quadrant of the udder.

3 = Egg yolk–type clot sticks to the bottom of the plate and may have the appearance of cottage cheese.

Colostrum Sample

Colostrometers provide a measure of the quality of colostrum by comparing the density of the colostrum to immunoglobulin G (IgG) concentration. Colostrum may be submitted for laboratory analysis, including IgG content and an antierythrocyte alloantibody determination. Sterile samples are not required.

The mare's udder should be washed well with soft cotton saturated with gentle soap and warm water and rinsed well before milking after foaling. The technician should be familiar with the use of a colostrometer and should collect the appropriate volume (usually 5–10 mL) of colostrum. Samples can be milked directly into a collection tube or poured from another container into the necessary tubes.

Rumen Fluid Collection

Rumen fluid is collected and analyzed for diagnosis of diseases of the forestomachs (reticulum, rumen, and omasum) in large and small ruminants. Characteristics of interest include color, pH, odor, microbial organisms and numbers, and electrolyte levels. Rumen fluid may also be collected for therapeutic purposes. When collected from a healthy animal, it may be used for transfaunation (inoculation of the sick animal's rumen with normal rumen flora needed to aid digestion).

Oral Gastric Tube (Orogastric Tube, Ororumen Stomach Tube) Method

Tubes are inserted orally (through the mouth) into the rumen in cattle. The nasal passages of cattle have a smaller diameter than those of horses; this significantly limits the diameter of tube that can be placed nasally.

Materials Needed

- Stomach tube: for adult cattle, medium- to large-diameter stomach tubes with an internal diameter no less than 1.5 cm, because a smaller size is more likely to become obstructed with ingesta; for calves, sheep, and goats, small- and medium-sized foal stomach tubes
- Water-based lubricant
- Frick speculum (cattle)
- PVC pipe "speculum," a block of wood with a hole cut in the center, roll of tape (sheep, goats)
- Dose syringe
- Sample collection container

> **TECHNICIAN NOTE**
>
> A Frick speculum is commonly used on cattle to pass OGTs. For small ruminants, a short piece of PVC pipe may be used as a mouth speculum.

Bovine

The animal is restrained to sufficiently limit movement of the head, which should not be overly elevated during this procedure. Ruminants may regurgitate fluid around the tube, and an overly elevated head increases the likelihood of fluid aspiration.

The length of tube needed to reach the rumen is estimated by measuring the tube outside the animal from the mouth to the rumen. The restrainer wraps one arm around the muzzle and places nose tongs (or places one finger into one of the animal's nostrils and a thumb into the other nostril) and pulls the nose upward to open the mouth. Standing to the side of the animal, the technician inserts the speculum (to prevent biting of the tube) over the root of the tongue in the center of the mouth. A popping or a "give" feeling is felt as the speculum passes over the root of the tongue and into the pharynx.

The tip of the tube is lubricated with a water-soluble lubricant or water before inserting through the speculum. Resistance is usually felt when the tube reaches the back of the pharynx. As the animal swallows, advance the tube down the esophagus. If the tube is not easily advanced, it may be necessary to slightly withdraw and rotate the tube and try again. Blowing into the tube dilates the esophagus and may ease passage of the tube. Proper placement of the tube in the esophagus is confirmed by palpating (the trachea and tube may be felt as two distinct tubular structures) or visualizing the tube in the esophagus and feeling mild resistance as it is passed. Coughing may indicate that the tube is in the trachea, and feeling air pass out of the tube when the animal exhales may indicate erroneous placement into the trachea.

Placement of the tube within the rumen can be confirmed by blowing into the tube and listening for gurgling from the end of the tube, or by blowing into the tube with an assistant auscultating the abdomen with a stethoscope over the rumen (left paralumbar fossa) while listening for gurgles. Air should be heard bubbling in the rumen. Additional confirmation of placement may be done by smelling the exposed end of the tube, which should yield a distinctive odor of fermented gas. Aspiration of rumen fluid (rumen juice) clearly confirms placement of the tube and should be saved for assessment of microbial health (Fig. 17.88).

A dose syringe is used to collect the rumen fluid sample. The initial fluid is discarded because it often contains an excessive amount of saliva, which may cause erroneously elevated pH measurement of the fluid. When the process is complete, the tube is kinked and withdrawn with a smooth downward motion. This

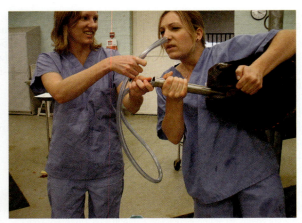

• **Fig. 17.88** Checking for odor emanating from the stomach tube will assist in confirming correct placement of the tube.

prevents rumen contents from leaking out of the tube and entering the trachea as the tube is withdrawn. The pH of the sample should be measured immediately after the sample is obtained. Rumen fluid begins to degrade immediately upon removal; therefore testing should be performed immediately.

Small Ruminant

The animals should be restrained as necessary. Sheep may be backed into a corner and straddled or "set up" on the rump; goats may be pushed against a wall or backed into a corner and straddled. A speculum is placed between the lower incisors and the dental pad. A short piece of PVC pipe or a block of wood with a hole in the center or even a roll of tape may be used as a speculum (Fig. 17.89). Whatever is used must be long enough to reach the back of the mouth so that the tube is not deflected to the side, where it can be bitten or chewed by the animal.

A tube of suitable size and length (outside diameter of approximately ⅜ to ½ inch) is selected and the necessary length estimated as described for cattle; tube passage is then performed as described previously.

Rumenocentesis

This method is seldom used because of the ease and safety of the stomach tube method described earlier; however, if used, it should only be attempted by a veterinarian.

The ventral abdomen caudal to the xiphoid process and left of the ventral midline is clipped and surgically prepared. The veterinarian inserts a needle with a syringe attached (14-gauge needle for cattle, 16–18-gauge needle for small ruminants) through the skin and into the rumen. Rumen fluid is aspirated into the syringe and then used for requested diagnostic testing.

Thoracocentesis (Thoracentesis, Pleurocentesis, Chest Tap, Pleural Tap)

Thoracocentesis is the aspiration of fluid from the thoracic cavity. It is performed in large animals to obtain pleural fluid samples for diagnostic purposes and therapeutically to drain fluid, air, or exudate from the pleural cavity. Pleural fluid is produced by the cells of the pleura, which line the pleural cavity and the surface of the lungs. Fluid volume and character change with the presence of disease in the pleural cavity or lungs. In the normal animal, little or no fluid is obtained from the thorax; however, large volumes

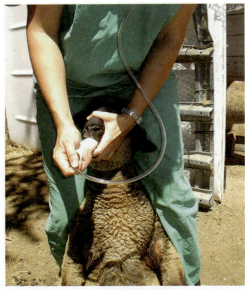

• **Fig. 17.89** Polyvinyl chloride (PVC) pipe used as a mouth speculum in sheep for orogastric tube (OGT) insertion. The speculum prevents the animal from biting the tube.

of fluid may be obtained in diseased animals. Gross analysis of the fluid includes color, opacity, and the presence of fibrin material, mucopurulent debris, and odor. Laboratory analysis includes cytologic and microbiological examinations as well as pH, lactate, and glucose levels. Occasionally, PCR analysis is done to identify certain pathogens.

This procedure is generally performed by the veterinarian and the technician is called upon to set up, prepare, and assist with the procedure. If facilities allow, the technician may perform the laboratory analysis of the sample. When an indwelling chest tube is placed, the technician will be expected to maintain the drain and monitor the patient (Fig. 17.90).

Equine and Bovine
Materials Needed
- Sterile gloves
- Ample collection tubes
  - EDTA (for cytologic examination)
  - Serum (for microbiological examination)
  - Heparin (for pH, lactate, and glucose determination) or fluoride (for pH and glucose assessment), depending on specific laboratory analyzer requirements
- Instrument of veterinarian's choice
  - Needle (minimum 3 inches) with large gauge *or*
  - 14- to 16-gauge IV catheter *or*
  - Sharp trocar and cannula *or*
  - Teat cannula *or*
  - Bitch catheter
- 2% lidocaine, 3 to 5 mL
- A 6-mL syringe with 20- to 22-gauge × 1-inch to 1.5-inch needle
- Scalpel blade #15
- Sterile 35- to 60-mL Luer tip syringe
- Three-way stopcock
- IV extension tubing
- Suture material, needle drivers, and scissors
- Ultrasound machine, if available and requested by veterinarian

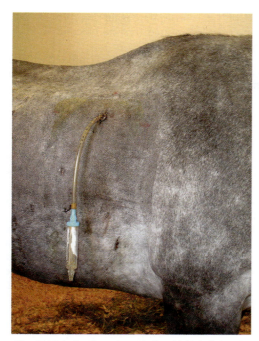

• **Fig. 17.90** Indwelling chest drain with Heimlich valve.

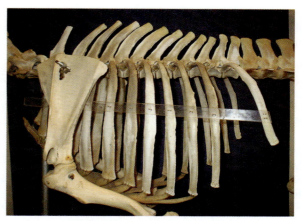

• **Fig. 17.91** Side view of alpaca ribs.

The horse is restrained and sedation administered as needed. The veterinarian will select the appropriate site on the right or left lateral thorax and may use ultrasonography to identify the most appropriate site. The patient may require thoracocentesis on both left and right sides, with each side of the thorax yielding different laboratory results because of diseases of the plural cavity causing blockage of normal communication between right and left sides. It is possible that abnormal fluid may be present on one side, with the other side remaining essentially normal.

> ## TECHNICIAN NOTE
>
> A patient may require thoracocentesis on both the left and right sides, because each may yield different laboratory results.

A large area from the point of the olecranon back to the tenth intercostal space and from the point of the shoulder to well below the olecranon is shaved and aseptically prepared. The needle will be inserted into the ventral portion of the sixth and seventh intercostal (between the ribs) space, 10 to 12 cm dorsal to the olecranon, above the lateral thoracic vein, and below the anticipated level of fluid. The site can also be determined with the use of ultrasonography, if indicated. Inject 5 mL of 2% lidocaine into the skin SC to make a bleb on the cranial aspect of the rib and deep enough into the intercostal muscles to include the parietal pleura. A stab incision is made into the anesthetized bleb with a scalpel blade. The entrance of air during the procedure should be avoided. A teat cannula (12–14-gauge × 3 inch) can be used to remove small volumes of air or fluid. A wider-bore sterile metal bitch catheter or a human thoracic drainage cannula may be needed if a large volume of fluid is present or if the fluid is thick. The needle, catheter, or cannula, along with extension tubing and a three-way stopcock, is inserted cranial to the rib border and is advanced through the parietal pleura. This approach is done to prevent damage to the intercostal vessels and nerves that run along the caudal border of the ribs. The heart,

pericardial sac, and lateral thoracic vein must be avoided. Once in the pleural cavity, a syringe is attached to the stopcock and fluid is aspirated. When the fluid has been collected, the veterinarian may stitch a purse-string suture around the stab incision and tighten the suture as the cannula is removed.

Camelid

The preferred site for thoracocentesis is at the sixth or seventh intercostal space, 10 to 15 cm dorsal to the sternum (Fig. 17.91). The area is clipped and surgically prepped. Any long fibers that may contaminate the shaved site should be taped back out of the way. Local anesthetic is injected as described for equines. A 14- to 16-gauge × 2-inch needle or teat cannula with a syringe attached is inserted near the cranial border of the rib. The pleural space is entered approximately 2 to 3 cm under the skin. Once the sample is aspirated into the syringe, the needle is withdrawn and antibiotic ointment applied to the procedure site.

Thoracocentesis in other large animals is like the procedure described for camelids and equines; the cannula size is dependent on the animal's size.

Complications of thoracocentesis include pneumothorax, dyspnea, and iatrogenic infection. Careful monitoring postprocedure is necessary to identify any complications early so proper interventions can be performed.

Transtracheal Wash (Tracheal Wash, Trach Wash)

Transtracheal aspiration is the collection of fluid from the lower respiratory tract (bronchi, bronchioles, and alveoli) for cytologic and microbiological analyses; it is performed to assist the diagnosis of lower airway and lung disease. The fluid is a mixture of secretions and cellular material that has collected in the distal portion of the trachea.

Equine Transtracheal Aspiration

The two methods used for this procedure are the percutaneous and endoscopic methods. Both procedures are also carried out in bovine and other large animal species in the same manner.

Percutaneous Method

The horse should be restrained appropriately. The animal may require mild sedation (heavy sedation should be avoided because it may suppress the cough reflex). A site on the midline of the neck, directly over the trachea about one-third of the way down the neck, is selected. An area approximately 4 × 4 inches is clipped or shaved, sterile preparation done, and the necessary materials set up.

Materials Needed

- Sterile gloves
- Surgical blades: #20 to #30 for adults; #15 to #20 for foals a few months old
- Syringes of sodium chloride (NaCl): one or two 60-mL syringes containing 30 mL of 0.9% NaCl (bacteriostatic saline should not be used); the syringe should be placed back into the case
- Commercially available equine tracheal wash kit (Jorgensen Laboratories, Loveland, CO)
- Needles: one or two 25-gauge needles for capping the collection syringe after the sample is obtained

Procedure

1. Inject approximately 1 to 2 mL of 2% lidocaine ID and SC over the selected site on the trachea and apply a final aseptic preparation.
2. Open the tracheal wash kit and, while wearing sterile gloves, remove the long catheter. Tie the long catheter in a loose half-hitch knot. This will allow the catheter to stay completely on the sterile field (created by the open sterile glove package) and will make it easier to control the distal tip to prevent contamination by accidental touching of something before or during insertion.
3. After the sterile preparation procedure, make a stab incision with the scalpel blade through the skin between the tracheal rings. Grasp the cannula from the kit with one hand. Stabilize the trachea with the other hand, palm side up; use fingers and thumb placed on each side of the trachea and hold firmly.
4. Insert the distal tip of the needle with bevel side down through the incision and advance it into the tracheal lumen. If resistance is felt, redirect the tip of the needle between the tracheal ring spaces and then advance the needle into the trachea. A burst of air will exit the needle when it penetrates the lumen of the trachea.
5. Remove the stylet. This prevents possible laceration and loss of catheter tubing. Place on a sterile field in case it is needed again.
6. Insert the catheter until it reaches the thoracic inlet.
7. Attach the 60-mL syringe and retract the plunger. Air is aspirated if the catheter is in the tracheal lumen. If no air is aspirated, reposition the catheter as it may be bent or occluded against the tracheal wall.
8. Once air has been aspirated, infuse 30 mL of NaCl and immediately try to aspirate a 5-mL or larger fluid sample (only a small portion of the fluid that is instilled will be retrieved). A 5-mL sample should be sufficient for microbiological and cytologic examinations.
9. Continue aspirating while slowly withdrawing the catheter. Stop withdrawing when fluid for aspiration is evident and collect as much as possible with a catheter at that location.
10. Withdraw again as needed to continue collection of the fluid (do not reinsert the catheter). If fluid is not obtained, infuse 10 mL of NaCl and aspirate again (Fig. 17.92A–D). The total volume of saline infused (first and second attempts) should not exceed 50 mL.

Some horses will cough while saline is infused, which may have the positive effect of increasing the yield of mucopurulent material. Unfortunately, coughing may also cause the catheter to kink cranially, which may prevent collection of any sample. With a sample syringe, the catheter is removed while keeping the cannula in place. This helps avoid an SC infection by preventing the contaminated catheter from coming into direct contact with tissue at the insertion site as it is removed. The cannula is removed, pressure applied to the site, any bleeding controlled, and a 4 × 4-inch piece of gauze with antiseptic ointment placed over the incision for 24 hours. A sterile needle is used to cap the syringe containing the sample for transport to the laboratory.

Cellulitis or SC abscessation at the tracheal puncture site is the most common complication. If swelling occurs, warm compresses are applied. Other complications include SC emphysema around the trachea, pulmonary foreign body because of the presence of a catheter piece in the airway, acute dyspnea, tracheal laceration, minor SC hemorrhage, and iatrogenic infection.

Endoscopic Method

Use of an endoscope is considered noninvasive and allows visual examination of the upper airways, trachea, carina, and primary and secondary bronchi; however, presence of the endoscope leads to questionable accuracy of the microbial samples recovered with this technique. An endoscope is inserted through the nasal cavity to the tracheal lumen. Special tubing (polyethylene tubing or endoscopic microbiological aspiration catheter) is placed through the biopsy channel of the endoscope, and fluid is injected and aspirated for collection of the sample. Use of these specialized sample collection items decreases the risk of contamination from the pharynx or the endoscope, which would otherwise occur with the endoscopic approach. It is usually necessary to infuse saline, as described for the percutaneous approach, to aspirate a fluid sample from the trachea.

Bronchoalveolar Lavage

Bronchoalveolar lavage (BAL) is a procedure used to collect fluid samples from the lower airway. BAL provides fluid samples that are better for cytologic assessment compared with samples obtained by transtracheal aspiration, but the fluid samples are representative of only a limited area of the lung and are subject to contamination caused by passing the tube through the nares. BAL is performed by inserting a sterile tube into the nares and trachea. To prepare for the procedure, the technician should have sterile BAL tubing, a syringe containing 50 mL of 2% lidocaine, and three syringes, each containing 60 mL of sterile saline (not bacteriostatic saline). The veterinarian may choose to use varying amounts of saline, so the technician should check before the procedure to be sure that the desired amount of saline is available in the syringes.

The horse should be sufficiently restrained and may require sedation. While the tube is passed into the trachea, 2% lidocaine is injected into the tube whenever the horse coughs. This acts as a local anesthetic to the bronchi and helps decrease the cough reflex. It is not uncommon to use the entire 50 mL of lidocaine before the procedure is complete. Sterile saline (previously drawn up into three separate 60-mL syringes) is injected and aspirated (as is done through the transtracheal aspiration procedure).

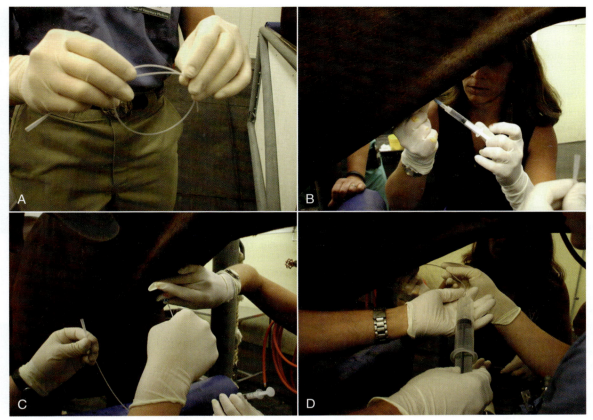

• **Fig. 17.92** Transtracheal aspiration of an equine patient. (A) Coiling the catheter to keep it sterile and easily controlled. (B) Aspirating air to confirm placement in the tracheal lumen. (C) Inserting a catheter into the trachea. (D) Aspirating a sample.

> **TECHNICIAN NOTE**
>
> While the bronchoalveolar lavage (BAL) tubing is passed into the trachea, 2% lidocaine may be injected into the tube whenever the horse coughs to decrease the cough reflex.

This procedure can also be done with the use of an endoscope, with sterile tubing passed through the biopsy channel of the scope so that saline can be injected and fluid samples aspirated. This method is preferred for sample collection when bronchial and/or alveolar disease is suspected. Use of the endoscope allows sampling from specific areas of the lung, but a limited sample is obtained rather than the pooled secretions that are obtained when a transtracheal aspiration is done.

If the veterinarian intends to perform both percutaneous transtracheal aspiration and BAL, the transtracheal aspiration should be performed first. This will allow fluid samples to be obtained before any contamination is introduced via passage of the BAL tubing (or endoscope). Often, the cough reflex is intentionally suppressed for the BAL, whereas a cough may be desirable during the transtracheal aspiration procedure.

Abdominocentesis (Abdominal Tap, Peritoneal Tap, Paracentesis, Belly Tap)

Peritoneal fluid obtained by abdominocentesis can provide valuable diagnostic information as this fluid is produced by the cells of the peritoneum. These cells line the abdominal cavity and the outer surfaces of abdominal organs, and the composition of this fluid is determined by the condition of the abdominal organs. Analysis focuses on gross appearance, laboratory results, and the volume of fluid present. Accumulation of fluid in the abdominal cavity is abnormal (i.e., ascites).

> **TECHNICIAN NOTE**
>
> The composition of peritoneal fluid is determined by the condition of the abdominal organs.

Abdominocentesis is commonly performed on horses, camelids, cattle, sheep, and goats. The veterinary technician may be asked to prepare for and assist with the procedure or to perform the procedure themselves. Several variations on the procedure may be performed, and the technician will be directed by the veterinarian as to which approach is preferred. With any of these techniques, it must be ensured that the sample is not contaminated, that no contaminants are introduced into the patient, that as little trauma as possible is inflicted upon the patient, and that personnel are not injured while the sample is obtained.

Indications for abdominocentesis include colic, suspected peritonitis, weight loss, abdominal distention, chronic diarrhea, signs of internal hemorrhage, abnormal ultrasonographic findings, and FUO.

For all species:
- Gather all required supplies (include alternates in case use of first-choice instruments is unsuccessful).

- Appropriately restrain the patient.
- Clip or shave the area.
- Perform sterile prep.
- Wear sterile gloves and maintain sterility throughout the procedure.

Equine Abdominocentesis

Many horses require minimal restraint for the procedure and, if possible, should be restrained in standing stocks. A handler should remain at the horse's head and a twitch should be applied or sedation administered, depending on the nature of the horse and the degree of discomfort the horse is exhibiting.

When preparing the site and performing the procedure, the person should squat next to the horse, adjacent to the forelimbs and facing the rear of the horse. This position reduces the likelihood of the person being kicked with the horse's hind limb. The person should take care to keep their head up and safely away from the belly and legs of the horse and should be prepared to move back quickly, if necessary, to remain safe. If the technician is assisting with the procedure and will be collecting the fluid into tubes, they should be positioned similarly on the opposite side of the animal (if space permits) or should wait until the instrument has been inserted, then should squat or bend over next to the veterinarian (being prepared to move quickly, if necessary), using an outstretched hand to place the collection tube under the needle or cannula.

The site for the tap is determined, and the lowest portion of the abdomen and the ventral midline are located. This is usually 2 to 4 inches caudal to the xiphoid. Abdominocentesis can be performed at the ventral midline, but use of a paramedian site 1 to 2 inches to the right of midline reduces the likelihood of tapping the spleen (in horses) or the rumen (in ruminants). Abdominocentesis should not be performed through skin abrasions or surgical lesions and, whenever possible, tapping through edema should be avoided. The clinician may use ultrasonography to assist in determining the most desirable site for abdominocentesis and to prevent penetration of organs.

TECHNICIAN NOTE

Safety must always be observed during abdominocentesis—expect the unexpected and be prepared to move away from the animal quickly.

Teat Cannula or Female Canine Urinary Catheter (Bitch Catheter) Method

Use of a blunt-tipped bovine teat cannula or stainless steel female canine urinary catheter reduces the risk of bowel penetration; therefore this method may be chosen over the needle method for animals with abdominal distention or bowel distention (as identified by rectal examination performed by a veterinarian). This method requires the use of local anesthesia.

An area approximately 2 inches square is shaved and a sterile preparation performed. The technician then aspirates 2 mL of 2% lidocaine into a 3-mL syringe. Local anesthesia is achieved by infusing the skin and SC tissue with approximately 1 mL of lidocaine using a 25-gauge needle. The needle is inserted into the center of the shaved area (avoid any obvious cutaneous vasculature), aspiration is performed to check for blood, and then the lidocaine is infused. The 25-gauge needle is removed and a 19-gauge × 1.5-inch needle placed directly into the center of the SC bleb. The needle should be inserted completely to the hub, and

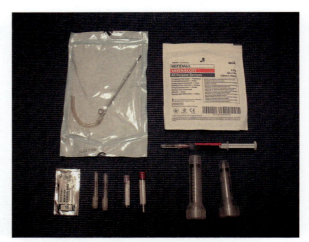

- **Fig. 17.93** Supplies for abdominocentesis. Bitch catheter, 4 × 4-inch sterile gauze sponges, #15 scalpel blade, 19-gauge × 1.5-inch needles, 2-mL EDTA tube, 3-mL plain tube, 3-mL syringe with 25-gauge × 1-inch needle containing 2% lidocaine, 12-mL syringe, and 6-mL syringe.

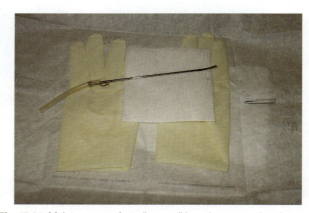

- **Fig. 17.94** Maintenance of sterile conditions in preparation for procedures should be maintained. The established sterile field is shown with sterile supplies for abdominocentesis.

the remaining 1 mL of lidocaine is injected while slowly removing the needle from the patient. This is done to block the parietal peritoneum.

The sterile preparation is completed with a final swab of Betadine solution (or an alternative antiseptic).

Materials Needed. (See Fig. 17.93.)
- A 4-inch teat cannula or bitch catheter
- #15 scalpel blade
- A 2-mL EDTA tube
- A 3-mL serum tube
- Heparin tube or syringe (depending on laboratory capabilities)
- Sterile 4 × 4-inch gauze sponges
- 12- and 6-mL syringes

Procedure
- Create a sterile field by opening a pair of sterile gloves and placing the teat cannula (or bitch catheter or needle), scalpel blade, and sterile gauze (4 × 4 inches) onto the field (Fig. 17.94).
- Put on sterile gloves.
- Puncture the center of one gauze 4 × 4-inch sponge with the scalpel blade and put the teat cannula through the gauze. This

will help prevent contamination of the sample with blood or dust.

- Using the scalpel blade, make a stab incision through the skin. Hold the blade with about ⅜ inches exposed. Using the back of the gloved hand, gently touch the horse's belly, then insert the scalpel blade straight into the bleb and pull it straight out. Avoid cutting the musculature.
- Slowly but firmly, insert the teat cannula through the incision perpendicular to the musculature. The muscle will feel gritty and a slight pop will be felt when the peritoneum is punctured. A decrease in resistance is felt when the abdomen has been entered. If firm resistance is felt at this point, it may indicate contact with an organ, and care must be taken if further manipulation on the cannula is required.
- Once the cannula is in, expect to wait while the horse takes a few breaths before fluid begins to flow from the cannula. If fluid does not immediately flow, the cannula can be gently flicked with a finger to encourage flow, and the cannula can be moved around slightly, rotated, or redirected. If necessary, a syringe may be attached to the cannula and aspiration may be attempted (Fig. 17.95A–C).

- The first few drops of fluid may contain contaminants, so these drops should be discarded. Collect the sample by gravity flow into collection tubes, with the EDTA tube being collected first, because most of the desired laboratory tests will require this sample. The tube should be filled as much as possible to ensure the correct ratio of EDTA to abdominal fluid. If less than 1 mL of abdominal fluid is collected, results of the laboratory analysis may be inaccurate; in this case, a common practice involves removing the rubber stopper from the EDTA tube and shaking the tube to remove a bit of the EDTA before the fluid sample is collected for cytologic analysis, protein measurement, and PCV (if fluid appears bloody).

When refractometry is performed, excessive EDTA in relation to sample size will result in false elevation of the protein reading. A serum sample should be collected in a plain clot tube for bacterial culture, with as little as one drop of fluid being sufficient for this purpose. Some facilities have the capability to perform pH, gas, lactate, and glucose analyses on abdominal fluids. The technician should be familiar with laboratory capabilities and required anticoagulants. Many analyzers that perform these additional tests require heparin as the anticoagulant of choice. Some facilities will require

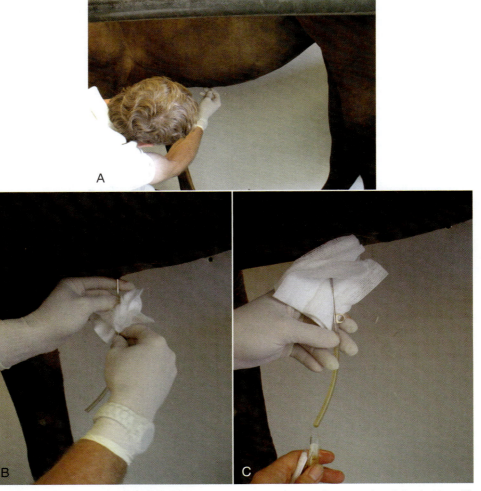

- **Fig. 17.95** (A) Incision on a prepped and blocked ventral midline area for an equine abdominal tap. (B) Insertion of a bitch catheter through an incision. (C) Collection of abdominal fluid through a bitch catheter into collection tubes. Note the technician's position of safety when performing the procedure on the abdominal region of the equine patient.

a sodium fluoride tube for glucose and lactate measurements. If unsure, it is best to contract the laboratory for confirmation.

When removing the cannula, the technician should be aware that some of the omentum may be attached to the cannula and can follow it out when the cannula is pulled from the site. To prevent it from being exteriorized, care should be taken to use fingers to guard close to the insertion site when the cannula is removed. As a result of incidental perforation of skin vessels, slight bleeding is common after removal of the cannula. Bleeding may be stopped by applying manual pressure to the site, although the veterinarian may suture or staple the site if needed. The centesis site should be cleaned gently and antibiotic ointment applied daily for a couple of days.

18- to 22-Gauge × 1.5-Inch Needle Method

Local anesthetic is usually not required for this method, but this varies depending on the individual horse. The needle is held midway between thumb and forefinger and is inserted through the skin, avoiding superficial veins. The fingers are moved slightly to grasp the hub of the needle for gradual advancement as the needle is advanced at slight intervals, pausing to notice whether a scratching sensation is felt. The scratching sensation indicates that bowel is rubbing over the tip of the needle. The fingers should be removed from the needle periodically to watch for rotary or flicking movement of the needle, which indicates bowel contact. Periodic back-and-forth movement of the needle in time with respiration is normal. If no bowel is encountered, the needle is advanced slowly to the hub until fluid is obtained. If abdominal fluid is not seen in the needle hub, the needle can be repositioned and rotated, and a syringe may be used to attempt aspiration of a sample. If fluid is not obtained, 1 to 2 mL of air (in a sterile syringe) may be injected to dislodge any material that might be occluding the needle. Another option to encourage the flow of fluid is to insert a second or third needle a few centimeters from the first (while leaving the first needle in place) to release negative pressure in the abdomen.

18-Gauge × 3.5-Inch Spinal Needle Method

This long needle may be required in very large horses, draft horses, and obese individuals. Some clinicians report that this long needle is also useful in Arabian horses to facilitate penetration beyond the abdominal wall and the subperitoneal fat layer. Local anesthesia is not usually necessary for this method, but this varies depending on the individual horse.

With the stylet in place, the needle is inserted to a depth of approximately one-quarter of an inch. The stylet is removed before further advancement and the procedure is continued as is done with a standard needle.

Equine Abdominocentesis (Foal)

This procedure is safer for the patient and for personnel if sufficient human assistance is provided for physical restraint and positioning of the foal, although sedation is usually indicated.

For neonates younger than 1 month or for actively colicky foals, abdominocentesis can be done with the sedated foal restrained in lateral recumbency. A 20-gauge × 1- to 1.5-inch needle is inserted caudal to the xiphoid on the midline or the right paramedian (off center but near the midline). Foal intestine is thin and fragile, and care must be taken to avoid contacting the bowel. A blunt-ended, small-diameter teat cannula or a canine bitch catheter can be used, because it poses less risk for intestinal laceration compared with a needle, but local anesthesia and a stab incision are needed to facilitate cannula insertion. Lack of subperitoneal fat in foals increases the risk for laceration of the bowel with a scalpel blade when a stab incision is made. The blade should be held up near the tip of the blade to maintain control and ensure that it is not inserted too deeply. For foals older than 1 month, an 18- to 20-gauge × 1.5-inch needle, a teat cannula, or a bitch catheter would be appropriate, with the procedure being performed as for younger foals.

Camelid Abdominocentesis (Adult)

Two sites are commonly used for abdominocentesis in camelids: a ventral midline site and a right paracostal (near the ribs) site. The paracostal site is easier to tap because camelids frequently choose to drop to sternal recumbency ("kushed" position) when being resistant, thus making the ventral midline site unavailable. The midline site is also complicated by a thick subperitoneal fat layer on either side of the linea alba, and visualization may be obscured by a long-fiber coat hanging from the sides of the animal.

Appropriate restraint is achieved by using a camelid chute or by having a handler push the left side of the animal up against a wall or fence. Chemical sedation may be required for some animals.

The paracostal abdominal tap site is located on the right side of the animal, about 4 inches behind the caudal most curve of the ribs (approximated by placing the palm of the hand behind the last rib) about one-third of the way up between the ventral abdomen and the spine (Fig. 17.96). A 3- to 4-inch–square area is clipped or shaved and long fibers in the surrounding area taped back, away from the site. A sterile preparation of the site is performed. Using a 22- to 25-gauge needle, 1 to 3 mL of 2%

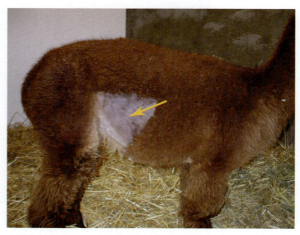

• **Fig. 17.96** Note the region that has been clipped *(arrow)* in preparation for surgical scrub in a nonrestrained animal in lateral recumbency.

lidocaine is injected into the skin and SC tissue before performing a final sterile site preparation. With a #11 or #15 scalpel blade, a stab incision is made into the anesthetized area; then with a quick, controlled thrust, a 4-inch blunt-ended teat cannula is inserted perpendicular to the abdomen, which is then advanced slowly into the abdomen. If fluid does not flow, the tip of the cannula can be gently repositioned, a syringe may be attached, and negative pressure may be applied, or a few milliliters of air can be injected into the abdominal cavity.

For the ventral midline approach, the lowest site, which is just caudal to the umbilicus, is selected. To avoid the retroperitoneal fat pads on either side of the linea alba (which will obstruct the cannula and prevent a sample collection), the site chosen should be directly on the linea alba. A 3- to 4-inch area is clipped, a sterile preparation performed, and a small amount of local anesthetic (as described earlier) injected before final sterile preparation. Using a scalpel blade, create a small stab incision to insert a teat cannula as described for an equine abdominal tap.

Camelid Abdominocentesis (Neonatal)

The cria can be mildly sedated as needed and should be restrained in lateral recumbency. A teat cannula or a 20-gauge × 1-inch needle may be used at the same site as for the standing adult camelid.

Bovine Abdominocentesis (Adult)

The animal is placed in a head gate, stocks, or a chute that will allow access to the right side of the animal. A TailJack restraint may be sufficient, but chemical sedation may be necessary, depending on the behavior of the animal and the site used.

An 18-gauge × 1.5-inch needle is sufficient for abdominocentesis in most adult cattle, although some very large individuals may require a 3-inch needle. A teat cannula can be used instead of a needle. If "hardware disease" (traumatic reticulitis from ingestion of heavy foreign objects) is suspected, the site selected should be just caudal to the xiphoid and to the right of the midline, as described for horses. The person performing the tap should stand by the animal's forelimbs facing backward and should be aware of the risk of being kicked. If general effusion or widespread disease is suspected, alternate sites can include the flank fold on the right side of the animal or the ventral abdomen at the lowest point, approximately 2 to 4 inches to the right of the umbilicus. Tapping the abdomen through the flank fold can be done successfully without local anesthesia.

Bovine Abdominocentesis (Neonatal)

Abdominal taps on calves can be done with the animal standing or in left lateral recumbency. Appropriate restraint is necessary; sedation should be considered to keep the animal still. A ventral midline site about 4 cm (approximately 1.5 inches) cranial to the umbilicus or a paramedian site approximately 4 cm to the right of the umbilicus can be used, with abdominocentesis performed by a needle or a teat cannula.

Ovine and Caprine Abdominocentesis

Abdominocentesis in sheep and goats may be performed to investigate abdominal distention, poor forestomach motility, and suspected uroabdomen (caused by urinary tract obstruction or ruptured bladder). A ruptured bladder is common in male goats (bucks) secondary to obstructive urolithiasis and leads to the accumulation of urine in the abdominal cavity.

The animal is manually restrained and sedated, if necessary. The procedure can be done with the animal standing. A site at the lowest point of the abdomen 2 to 4 cm to the right of the ventral midline (to prevent tapping the rumen) is selected. Care is taken to avoid the mammary veins (milk veins or SC abdominal veins) of females and the penis and prepuce in males. An 18- to 20-gauge × 1.5-inch needle or teat cannula can be used. Local anesthesia is necessary when a stab incision is needed if the use of a teat cannula is required, and may be desirable even if a needle is used. If peritonitis is suspected, the veterinarian may choose to tap multiple sites to increase the chances of confirming a diagnosis. Additional sites include those caudal to the xiphoid, medial to the right and left milk veins, and slightly cranial to the mammary gland on the right and left of the midline.

The most common complications associated with abdominocentesis are failure to obtain a sample and slight skin hemorrhage. Protrusion of omentum through the site of puncture in the abdominal wall can also occur. More serious complications of abdominocentesis in large animals include penetration of the bowel, penetration of the spleen, damage to the xiphoid process if the centesis site is too cranial, and introduction of bacteria leading to peritonitis or cellulitis. SC abscessation and cellulitis are uncommon when an unremarkable abdominocentesis procedure is performed, but risk for these complications increases markedly when the intestine has been punctured, when abdominocentesis is done through edematous tissue, or when animals have septic peritonitis.

Cerebrospinal Fluid Collection (Spinal Tap, CSF Tap)

CSF may be collected from patients when central nervous system disease is suspected. CSF analysis includes gross visualization of color, clarity, and the presence of particulate matter, as well as TP, cytologic examination, and chemistry evaluation. The technician will be expected to prepare the site, restrain the patient, assist the veterinarian as they perform the procedure, and secure appropriate samples for testing.

Equine

Atlanto-occipital Site (AO Tap)

This site is located at the dorsal midline just caudal to the poll. Collecting spinal fluid from this site requires general anesthesia and placement of the animal in lateral recumbency. The area is surgically clipped and a complete sterile prep is performed. Once preparations have been completed, the nose is directed down toward the front feet to flex the head and neck. The head should be at a right angle to the neck. The veterinarian inserts an 18-gauge × 3-inch spinal needle into the atlanto-occipital (AO) space (about 5–7 cm deep). Once inside the space, the trocar (stylet) is removed and placed onto the sterile field. A sterile syringe is attached to the needle for gentle aspiration of the sample. Alternatively, fluid may be collected directly into a tube by free flow. If the fluid is blood tinged, a few milliliters of fluid is aspirated and then a new syringe is attached. The technician should be ready with additional syringes for multiple sampling. The trocar (still sterile) is replaced in the needle, and the needle is withdrawn. After removal of the needle, any blood present can be cleaned from the site, and an antiseptic-soaked gauze sponge can be placed at the site.

The AO tap in neonates is done with a 20-gauge × 1.5-inch needle directed at the mandible. Fluid should drip from the needle hub for collection of approximately 3 to 6 mL of fluid.

Lumbosacral Site (LS Tap)

Sedation is required for this procedure, and use of a twitch for restraint is indicated because the animal must remain very still. The horse should be placed in stocks. Identify the tap site by making an imaginary line across from the caudal edge of each tuber coxae and another line at the dorsal midline. A slight depression can be palpated by using firm pressure at the intersection of these imaginary lines, just caudal to the sixth lumbar spinal process (L6). A large area is surgically clipped and a sterile preparation is performed. A local anesthetic is injected into the skin and SC tissue. The patient should be standing as squarely as possible, because an asymmetric stance makes collection more difficult (Fig. 17.97A–F). The veterinarian inserts a 6-inch (15-cm) × 18-gauge spinal needle perpendicular to the midline (about 11–15 cm, or 4.5–6 inches). For some draft and warm-blooded horses, longer needles (up to 8 inches) may be needed. When the needle reaches the subarachnoid space, the patient may respond with movement. The trocar is removed from the needle and is placed onto the sterile field. The technician places a sterile syringe in the veterinarian's sterile gloved hands for collection; the initial sample may be contaminated by blood, so a second or third filled syringe of fluid may be collected if enough is aspirated. The veterinarian may instruct assistants to occlude both jugular veins to increase intracranial pressure upon completion. The sterile trocar is replaced into the needle, and the needle is removed.

The lumbosacral CSF tap in neonates can be done with the foal standing, in sternal recumbency, or in lateral recumbency, using a 3-inch × 20-gauge spinal needle.

Complications that may result from CSF taps include trauma to the spinal cord during needle placement, herniation of the cerebellum (which can occur with high intracranial pressure or as the result of aggressive aspiration), and iatrogenic meningitis. These complications can lead to the death of the patient. The chances of these complications occurring are minimized by having the patient sufficiently restrained and following strict sterile technique throughout the procedure.

Camelid

CSF collection from llamas and alpacas follows the same procedure guidelines as described for horses.

The AO site is located midline as it intersects the wings of the atlas. In adults, a 20-gauge × 2.5-inch spinal needle is used, and the subarachnoid space is usually reached at a depth of 4 cm.

The lumbosacral site is midline about 2 cm caudal to the dorsal spinal process of the seventh lumbar vertebra. Landmarks used to locate the site include the tuber sacrale of the pelvis and the dorsal spinal process of the last lumbar vertebra. The site is cranial to the tuber sacrale. An 18- or 19-gauge × 3.5-inch spinal needle is appropriate for most adult llamas and alpacas.

Acknowledgments

The author and publisher wish to acknowledge the contributions of Oreta M. Samples and Dana M. Smith to previous editions of this chapter.

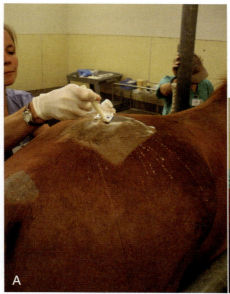
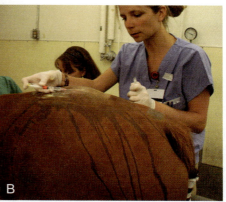

• **Fig. 17.97** (A) Shaving the area for a lumbosacral (LS) spinal tap. (B) Injecting 2% lidocaine for local anesthetic block.

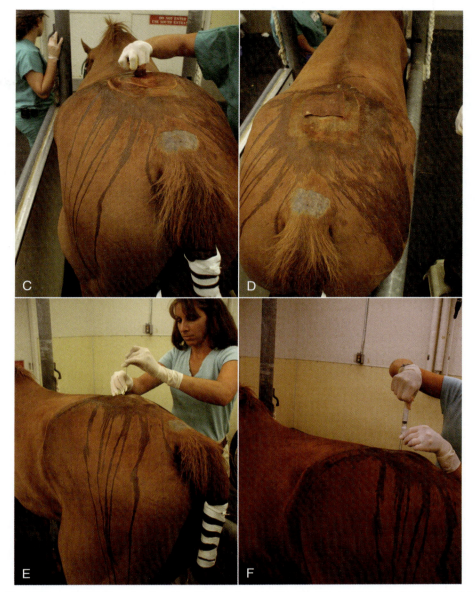

• **Fig. 17.97, cont'd** (C) Prepping the site with Betadine solution. (D) Site covered with Betadine-soaked gauze. (E) Inserting a spinal needle. (F) Aspirating a spinal fluid sample.

References

Hanie EA. *Large Animal Clinical Procedures for Veterinary Technicians*. St. Louis, MO: Mosby; 2006.

Recommended Readings

Bowden C, Masters J, eds. *Textbook of Veterinary Medical Nursing*. London, UK: Butterworth Heinemann; 2003.

Busch SJ, ed. *Small Animal Surgical Nursing*. St. Louis, MO: Mosby; 2006.

Colville T, Bassert JM, eds. *Clinical Anatomy and Physiology for Veterinary Technicians*. 3rd ed. St. Louis, MO: Mosby; 2016.

Ettinger SJ, Feldmen E, eds. *Textbook of Veterinary Internal Medicine*. 8th ed. Philadelphia, PA: Saunders; 2017.

Fowler ME. *Medicine and Surgery of South American Camelids*. Ames, IA: Iowa State University Press; 1998.

Frandson RD, Wilke WL, Fails AD. *Anatomy and Physiology of Farm Animals*. Baltimore, MD: Lippincott Williams & Wilkins; 2003.

Hanie EA. *Large Animal Clinical Procedures for Veterinary Technicians*. St. Louis, MO: Mosby; 2006.

Hendrix CM, Sirois M, eds. *Laboratory Procedures for the Veterinary Technician*. 6th ed. St. Louis, MO: Mosby; 2015.

House JK, Smith BP, Van Metre DC, et al. Ancillary tests for assessment of the ruminant digestive system. *Vet Clin North Am Large Anim Pract*. 1992;8:203.

Kopcha M, Schultze AE. Peritoneal fluid. II. Abdominocentesis in cattle and interpretation of nonneoplastic samples. *Compend Contin Educ Pract Vet*. 1991;13:703.

Lawhorn B. A new approach for obtaining blood samples from pigs. *J Am Vet Med Assoc.* 1988;192:781.

Macintire DK, Drobatz KJ, Haskins SC, et al. *Manual of Small Animal Emergency and Critical Care Medicine.* Baltimore, MD: Lippincott Williams & Wilkins; 2005.

McKenzie EC. *Abdominocentesis in Large Animals: Methods and Interpretation of Results, Proceedings of the 25th Forum of the American College of Veterinary Internal Medicine.* Seattle: ACVIM; 2007:27.

Orsini JA, Divers TJ. *Manual of Equine Emergencies.* 3rd ed. St. Louis, MO: Saunders; 2008.

Radostits OM, Gay CC, Blood DC, et al., eds. *Veterinary Medicine, A Textbook of the Diseases of Cattle, Sheep, Pigs, Goats and Horses.* 10th ed. Oxford, UK: Saunders; 2007.

Rockett J, Bosted S. *Veterinary Clinical Procedures in Large Animal Practice.* Clifton Park, NY: Thomson Delmar Learning; 2007.

Rose RF, Hodgson DR. *Manual of Equine Practice.* 2nd ed. Philadelphia, PA: Saunders; 2000.

Sirois M. *Principles and Practice of Veterinary Technology.* 4th ed. St. Louis, MO: Mosby; 2016.

Smith BP. In: *Large Animal Internal Medicine.* St. Louis, MO: Mosby; 2015.

Smith MC, Sherman DM, eds. *Goat Medicine.* Philadelphia, PA: Lea & Febiger; 1994.

Taylor FGR, Hillyer MH, eds. *Diagnostic Techniques in Equine Medicine.* Philadelphia, PA: Saunders; 1997.

Terry C, Rashmir-Raven A, Linford RL. Placing an intravenous catheter in horses. *Vet Tech.* 2000;4:207–212.

Williams CSF. Routine sheep and goat procedures. *Vet Clin North Am Large Anim Pract.* 1990;6:737–758.

18

Small Animal Medical Nursing

LIZA WYSONG RUDOLPH AND AMY NEWFIELD

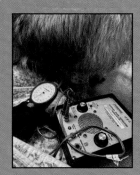

CHAPTER OUTLINE

LEARNING OBJECTIVES

When you have completed this chapter, you will be able to:

1. Pronounce, define, and spell all key terms in this chapter.
2. Explain the relationship between the "Five Freedoms of Animal Welfare" and the veterinary technician's responsibilities.
3. List in order the four steps that constitute the veterinary technician practice model and describe what is involved in carrying out each step of the nursing process.
   - List the four steps of SBAR (Situation, Background, Assessment, Recommendation) and explain the importance of a clear and concise communication method and how it supports patient care.
4. Explain the relationship between etiology, pathogenesis, and clinical signs; list and describe the most common forms seen in cats and dogs regarding:
   - Respiratory diseases. Explain the clinical relevance of upper versus lower disease and the role of inflammation in clinical signs.
   - Cardiovascular diseases. Explain the significance of determining if a patient has situational, idiopathic, or secondary hypertension.
   - Gastrointestinal and hepatobiliary diseases. Define vomiting versus regurgitation and list the clinical signs associated with small versus large bowel diarrhea.
   - Urinary diseases. Explain the differences between acute kidney injury (AKI) and chronic kidney disease (CKD), and the importance of International Renal Interest Society (IRIS) staging/grading in patient care.
   - Endocrine disease. Explain the importance of client education and support for successful long-term disease management.
   - Immune-mediated disease. Explain the importance of client education and support for successful long-term disease management.
5. Do the following regarding infectious diseases in dogs and cats:
   - Discuss the etiology and pathogenesis of infectious diseases.
   - List and describe special protocols needed to provide nursing care for dogs and cats with infectious diseases.
   - Explain how to educate clients about stopping the spread of infectious diseases.

KEY TERMS

Acquired kidney disease (CKD)
Acute kidney injury (ACI)
Amyloidosis
Anorexia
Azotemia
Barrier nursing
Cachexia

Cardiomyopathy
Chronic tubulointerstitial nephritis (CTIN)
Colitis
Constipation
Cough
Diarrhea
Dyspnea

Escherichia coli
Etiology
Feline lower urinary tract disease
Glomerulonephritis
Hematemesis
Hematochezia
Hematuria
Hemoptysis
Hemorrhagic
Hepatic encephalopathy
Hepatitis
Hyperphosphatemia
Hyperthermia
Hypoalbuminemia
Hypokalemia
Hypoxemia
Hypoxia
Immune-mediated hemolytic anemia (IMHA)
Melena
Mucoid
Mucopurulent
Nasal and sinus congestion
Nausea

Orthopnea
Pathogenesis
Pleural effusion
Polyarthropathies
Polycystic kidney disease (PKD)
Polydipsia
Polyuria
Portosystemic shunts
Primary immune-mediated hemolytic anemia
Pyelonephritis
Regurgitation
Rounds
Secondary immune-mediated hemolytic anemia (IMHA)
Serous
Stertor
Stridor
Systemic hypertension
Technician assessment
Tenesmus
Urolith
Vomiting
Zoonoses

Introduction

Providing nursing care to injured and sick animals is a core function of the credentialed veterinary technician. A strong foundation in veterinary nursing principles is essential for the veterinary technician to be an effective animal care provider. The basic tenets of animal welfare are upheld by veterinary technicians when providing nursing care. These were succinctly classified by the Farm Animal Welfare Council (now known as the *Animal Welfare Committee*) of the United Kingdom as the "Five Freedoms of Animal Welfare." These include the following:

1. *Freedom from Hunger and Thirst:* by ensuring ready access to fresh water and a diet to maintain full health and vigor.
2. *Freedom from Discomfort:* by providing an appropriate environment, including shelter and a comfortable resting area.
3. *Freedom from Pain, Injury, or Disease:* by prevention or rapid diagnosis and treatment.
4. *Freedom to Express Normal Behavior:* by providing sufficient space, proper facilities, and company of the animal's own kind.
5. *Freedom from Fear and Distress:* by ensuring conditions and treatment that avoid mental suffering.

During the care of veterinary patients, the goal is to meet all these basic patient needs. These guiding principles serve as important benchmarks for veterinary technicians to reach. In each medical or nursing intervention, whether administering a deep intramuscular injection or walking outside, veterinary technicians should constantly reflect on the freedoms of the patients impacted.

To ensure that excellent care is provided consistently, veterinary technicians should aim to practice a disciplined, planned approach for every patient. This discipline is encapsulated by the veterinary technician practice model, which is relevant to all veterinary patients, particularly those hospitalized.

A Veterinary Technician Practice Model: The Nursing Process

The veterinary technician practice model is a cyclical, structured discipline that ensures that consistently excellent care is provided to every patient and that information about the patient's changing status is communicated to other members of the veterinary health care team and the client. This model is based on a structured, systematic approach to nursing care called the *nursing process*, which was initially introduced to human nursing in 1958 and is considered a significant step forward for the ability of registered technicians to assess the individual needs of patients, rather than making assumptions based on a diagnosis. Veterinary technicians work closely with attending veterinarians to ensure that any patient status changes are addressed promptly, as needed (Fig. 18.1).

TECHNICIAN NOTE

The veterinary technician practice model provides a structured nursing process to ensure that consistently excellent care is provided to every patient.

PUT INTO PRACTICE

Implementing the veterinary technician practice model for every patient provides consistent care among all shifts at your hospital. While it may seem complicated, it is what we do every day in our jobs, and if you start naming the steps (assessment, planning, implementation, evaluation) with each patient, you will find it may greatly improve patient care.

The following four steps comprise the veterinary technician practice model.

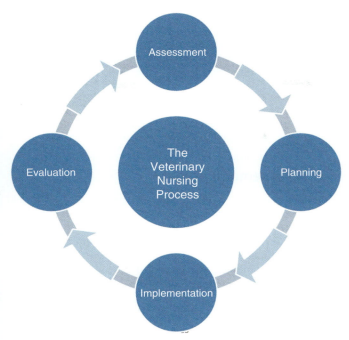

• **Fig. 18.1** The veterinary nursing process comprises four steps: patient assessment, planning, implementation, and evaluation of results. Each step of the nursing process is addressed separately, but depending on the patient case dynamic, these steps may occur concurrently, overlap, or even occur out of sequence.

Step 1: Assessment

The veterinary technician gathers subjective and objective patient data to recognize actual and potential health problems, then records and communicates that information to the veterinary health care team. Subjective data collection might be described as the "art of nursing," because this is any information that is based on opinion, emotion, or interpretation (e.g., level of consciousness, general demeanor, or pain). Objective data are often collected by applying a clinical skill (e.g., blood pressure measurements, heart rate, body temperature). As objective data are measurable and factual, collecting them may be considered the "science of nursing." When gathering information, it is essential to prioritize establishing what is normal—particularly for that individual patient.

> **TECHNICIAN NOTE**
>
> It is recommended that assessment tools, such as body condition scores (BCS), muscle condition scores (MCS), and validated pain, should be utilized whenever possible to lend a degree of objectivity to subjective data, facilitate communication, and promote continuity of care.

Information gathered during the assessment phase becomes part of the patient record, and this collection is accomplished in the following ways:

1. Gathering the initial medical history from the owner or reviewing this information in the patient's chart if the initial history has been gathered by the veterinarian or another veterinary technician.
2. Reviewing the medical record for past historical information.
3. Performing a physical examination.
4. Reviewing laboratory results and diagnostic, surgical, and medical reports.

5. Consulting with the attending veterinarian regarding any questions about the case not mentioned in the medical record.

In addition to collecting information and recording the above findings, having a verbal exchange of information or **rounds** when patient care transfers to another technician will facilitate communication between the veterinary health care team and promote continuity of care. Many different communication tools can facilitate the conveying of information. One such method adopted by the US Navy for health care is the SBAR (Situation, Background, Assessment, Recommendation) method. This communication tool is typically used to convey clear and concise information but can be modified to suit the need for relaying varying levels of detail. The Situation part is a short summary of the problem. The Background part provides the context for the situation. The Assessment describes the relevant subjective and objective data from the patient database. The Recommendation part describes proposed action(s) to address the Situation (Box 18.1).

Step 2: Planning

Based on the patient information gathered in the assessment phase of the nursing process, the veterinary technician analyzes the database and makes a clinical judgment regarding the physiological and psychological needs of the patient. This judgment is called *technician evaluation* and is based on the technician's independent critical thinking in identifying actual (current) problems, potential problems, and any additional factors, such as the level of client knowledge and/or coping abilities that may or may not impair at-home care of the pet (Tables 18.1, 18.2, and 18.3).

For example, for a patient with tachypnea, cyanosis, dyspnea, and a low pulse oximetry measurement (the data), a technician may determine that it is hypoxic through the evaluation performed. This assessment is separate from the veterinarian's medical diagnosis, which focuses on the cause of the problem, such as congestive heart failure (CHF). The technician observes the patient's physiologic response to CHF and assigns evaluations independently based on the data gathered. Additionally, technician evaluations may include information on the owner's level of knowledge regarding the care of the pet and the owner's ability to cope with the responsibility. Technician evaluations intuitively consider the five freedoms, compared with a systems approach veterinarians use to diagnose a patient's medical condition.

<table>
<tr><td colspan="3">**TABLE 18.1**   **Physical Parameters of the Cat and the Dog**</td></tr>
</table>

Parameter	Adult Cat	Adult Dog
Rectal temperature, °F (T)	100–102.2	100–102.2
Heart rate (HR), beats/minute	140–220	60–160 (smaller breeds may have higher rate)
Respiratory rate (RR), breaths/minute	20–42	16–32
Mucous membrane quality	Moist	Moist
Capillary refill time (CRT), seconds	<2	<2
Skin turgor/snap, seconds	Immediate/<2	Immediate/<2
Systolic blood pressure (SBP), mm Hg	120–160	130–160
Intraocular pressure (IOP), mm Hg	15–25	15–25
Oxygen saturation (SaO_2)	>95%	>95%
Urine volume, mL/kg body weight/day	10–20	20–100

TABLE 18.2   **Mucous Membrane Color Assessment**

Color	Physiology
Pink/pale pink	Normal
Pale/white	Inadequate blood volume or low hemoglobin concentration
Blue/purple (cyanotic)	Inadequate oxygenation of tissues
Yellow (icteric)	Hyperbilirubinemia
Brick red (injected)	Endotoxemia, shock

TABLE 18.3   **Lung Auscultation Sounds and Their Associations**

Sound	Association
Wheeze (musical, high or low pitched)	Bronchial disease
Crackles (popping)	Pleural disease, pulmonary disease
Absent lung sounds/muffled heart sounds	Space-occupying problem: effusions, diaphragmatic hernia

Once a list of technician evaluations has been generated for the patient, each evaluation is prioritized in terms of importance to the patient's life, and interventions can be planned. For example, let us imagine that a patient with cyanosis and dyspnea has a body condition score (BCS) of 5/5. A technician might document "**hypoxia**" and "overweight" as two separate technician evaluations. However, it is more important for the patient to breathe than to have an ideal body weight. Hence the technician evaluation "hypoxia" takes precedence over the technician evaluation "overweight" when the nursing plan is devised and implemented. Refer to Table 3.2 in Chapter 3 for technician evaluations listed in order of importance.

TECHNICIAN NOTE

Technician evaluations are clinical judgments that the veterinary technician makes regarding the physiologic and psychological needs of the patient.

Step 3: Implementation

Once the technician has evaluated the patient and identified and prioritized any concerns or observations, each should have a desired outcome. In our patient with hypoxia, for example, the desired outcome is adequate oxygenation and comfortable breathing, which would be evidenced by the resolution of the dyspnea and tachypnea, the return of mucous membranes to their normal pink color, and a normal pulse oximetry measurement. One or more interventions or actions accompany each technician evaluation to help achieve the desired patient outcome. Technician interventions number in the hundreds; Box 18.2 gives some examples of common technician interventions employed in small animal medical nursing. A technician intervention can be something seemingly simple, such as a nail trim, but when taken in the context of a feline patient who has forelimb paralysis and cannot use the scratching post to maintain healthy nails, a nail trim is an integral part of patient care, because it prevents the nails from growing into the pads, causing an infection.

The nursing care plan refers to the entire list of interventions specific to each technician evaluation for a particular patient. Table 18.4 and Table 18.5 provide examples of technician interventions for selected technician evaluations.

Step 4: Evaluation

The care plan is continuously revised based on the patient's response (positive or negative) to the interventions, and the technician will continuously evaluate the patient and update the patient's status. The evaluation step is crucial, because it focuses on a patient-centered approach and evaluates each patient's response to therapy instead of a "one size fits all" approach. Developing a nursing plan allows the veterinary health care team to set specific parameters and goals. If these goals are unmet, the veterinary health care team will review the current interventions, assess the patient, determine whether the goals were appropriate, and make any necessary adjustments. In some cases, additional data, such as laboratory and imaging study findings, are required to fully assess the patient's response to nursing interventions and the treatment the attending veterinarian prescribes. In this way, the first phase of the veterinary technician practice model is repeated, underscoring its cyclical pattern. Case Presentation 18.1 provides an example of a nursing care plan.

TECHNICIAN NOTE

Veterinary technicians are often the first caregivers to observe subtle clinical changes in hospitalized veterinary patients. The veterinary technician's role as an equal partner in providing quality patient care cannot be overstated.

• BOX 18.2 Examples of Veterinary Technician Interventions (Relevant to Internal Medicine)

Basic Patient Care

Ensuring that the patient can breathe
Providing access to proper amounts of food and water
Providing access to a clean litter box or ensuring frequent walks outside
Providing adequate, comfortable, clean housing
Providing patient hygiene—grooming, bathing, clipping
Providing exercise for mobile patient
Providing patient safety
Providing relief from pain and discomfort

Medication Administration and Catheter Placement

Medication/fluid administration: oral, subcutaneous, intravenous, intraosseous, and/or intramuscular
Medication administration: topical—eye, ear, nose, and/or skin
Catheter placement: intravenous, intraosseous, and/or urinary

Tube Management

Tracheostomy tubes
Chest tubes
Feeding tubes

Patient Monitoring

Basic patient monitoring: temperature, pulse, respiration, capillary refill time, mucous membranes, skin turgor, body weight, mentation, appetite, urination, defecation
Advanced monitoring of critical patients may include thoracic auscultation, pulse oximetry, capnography, arterial blood gases, measurement of fluid losses/output, central venous pressure, electrocardiography, blood pressure
Monitoring laboratory values as they pertain to the disease process and medical therapies
Monitoring for pain
Monitoring for desired/adverse effects of medical therapy
Monitoring for desired/adverse effects of fluid therapy
Monitoring for desired/adverse effects of electrolyte replacement

Client Education (Addressing Client Knowledge Deficit)

Pet selection
Kitten and puppy care and training
Reproduction and neonatal care
Nutritional recommendations
Grooming care
Problem behavior management
Preventive care: vaccinations, parasite control, dental care
Drug therapies: indications, dosing, side effects
Drug therapies: handling and storage
Drug therapies: the importance of compliance
Drug therapies: the importance of follow-up diagnostics
Medication administration techniques
Subcutaneous fluid administration
Feeding tube management and meal administration
Wound management/bandage care
Disease pathophysiology
Infectious disease control
Chronic pain management

Client Support

Hospice care
Grief counseling

The Medical Record

All patient data, technician evaluations, interventions, and nursing care plans are recorded in the medical record using the SOAP (subjective, objective, assessment, and plan) format or by entering the data into the medical record (refer to Chapter 3 for detailed information). Specific flow sheets for hospitalized patients may be used for ease of recording technician interventions, such as administration of medication and fluid therapy and monitoring of vital signs.

Small Animal Diseases

The development of a disease begins with etiology, or cause, such as an infectious agent or injury (Box 18.3). This, in turn, leads to the development of adverse physical changes or lesions that subsequently manifest in patients as clinical signs. The development of disease can therefore be summarized as follows:

$$\text{Etiology} \rightarrow \text{Pathogenesis} \rightarrow \text{Lesions} \rightarrow \text{Clinical Signs}$$

Part of the **pathogenesis** of heartworm disease, for example, involves the physical presence of the heartworm, which irritates the lining of the pulmonary vessels, causing inflammation. Continued inflammation of the pulmonary vasculature leads to coughing—a well-known clinical sign of heartworm disease. Remember that the technician evaluation involves observing the patient's physiologic response to disease. This is why it is essential for the technician to have a basic grasp of the pathogenesis of common small animal medical diseases. The information presented in this chapter on pathogenesis is, by necessity, very brief and focuses on the diseases most commonly seen in cats and dogs. The recommended reading list at the end of the chapter supplies more comprehensive information.

It is worth noting that not all patients with disease show outward signs of illness. Patients with heart disease, for example, are often devoid of outward signs of disease. Their body makes physiologic adjustments that enable their heart to continue functioning despite their altered cardiac health. The patient may appear outwardly healthy. CHF results when homeostatic mechanisms fail. Only then does the patient show overt signs of illness. The same applies to a patient with well-controlled diabetes mellitus (DM) that is not overtly ill. Thus much of a veterinary technician's work is that of a detective searching for clues that link the clinical signs with the illness. In small animal veterinary medicine, some diseases are more prevalent in dogs than in cats and are more common in certain breeds and at certain life stages than others.

Respiratory Disease

Most respiratory tract diseases ultimately result in inflammation, irritation, and obstruction or restriction of the airway (see Table 18.6). Each of these processes causes an array of clinical signs. The veterinary technician must be familiar with all the clinical signs, because they help direct the nursing process. A technician familiar with the signs of respiratory disease, for example, will be more focused when taking a history, completing a physical examination, performing technician evaluations, and carrying out diagnostic and therapeutic interventions.

Clinical Signs of Respiratory Disease

Animals are aerobic, meaning all cells need oxygen to function best. When an animal patient experiences respiratory distress, there is a lack of oxygen delivered to cells. Signs of respiratory

TABLE 18.4	Selection of Technician Evaluations and Interventions			
Veterinary Technician Evaluation and Definition	Potential Physiologic Consequences	Clinical Findings	Desired Patient Outcome	Veterinary Technician Interventions
Anorexia Complete or partial loss of appetite	Poor immune function Decreased wound healing Dehydration Electrolyte imbalance Hypoalbuminemia Hepatic lipidosis Cachexia Hypoglycemia Hypothermia Seizures Death	Loss of appetite for >2 days Prolonged diminished appetite	Sustained return of appetite and intake of an appropriate number of daily calories	Administer doctor-prescribed appetite stimulants, antiemetics, antacids Encourage patient to eat on their own: • Coax/socialization • Novel, odoriferous foods • Stress-free eating area • Patient hygiene • Assisted feeding: syringe, orogastric tube Avoid food aversion Feeding tube management and meal administration Monitor calorie intake Basic patient monitoring*
Dehydration Loss of total body water	Decreased renal perfusion Electrolyte imbalance Hypothermia	Tacky/dry mucous membranes Delayed skin turgor Enophthalmos Decreased urine output Increased PCV and TP Hyperalbuminemia Increased urine concentration	Restoration of normal hydration: • Moist mucous membranes • Normal skin turgor • Normal urine output	Administer fluid therapy per doctor's orders Basic patient monitoring Monitor fluid intake and output Monitor for signs of fluid overload: • Presence of lung crackles • Presence of new heart murmur • Presence of edema • Increasing body weight • Increased serous nasal discharge • Increased central venous pressure Treat/prevent electrolyte imbalance
Hypovolemia Loss of intravascular fluid	Decreased perfusion of vital organs: kidneys, heart, and brain Hypothermia Shock End organ failure Death	Dry mucous membranes Pale to white mucous membranes Prolonged CRT Tachycardia Weak pulses Altered mentation Hemorrhage Increased or decreased PCV Hypoalbuminemia Hypotension	Restoration of normovolemia: • Pink/moist mucous membranes • Normal CRT • Normotensive • Normal cardiac function	Administer fluid therapy per doctor's orders Basic patient monitoring Monitor fluid intake and output Monitor for signs of fluid overload: • Presence of lung crackles • Presence of new heart murmur • Presence of edema • Increasing body weight • Increased serous nasal discharge • Increased central venous pressure Administer blood transfusion per doctor's orders Monitor for signs of transfusion reaction: • Anxiety • Nausea, vomiting, diarrhea • Fever • Pruritus • Skin erythema • Urticaria
Hyperthermia Elevated body temperature	Increased metabolism Dehydration Electrolyte imbalance Shock Coagulopathies CNS abnormalities Death	Temperature >103°F Panting (dog) Warm skin Tachypnea Tachycardia Altered mentation	Restoration and maintenance of normal body temperature/ Thermoregulation	Cool patient: Provide cool environment Apply ice packs to the groin Cool-water bath Administer fluid therapy per doctor's orders Basic patient monitoring* Treat/prevent dehydration Administer doctor-prescribed antipyretics

TABLE 18.4 Selection of Technician Evaluations and Interventions—cont'd

Veterinary Technician Evaluation and Definition	Potential Physiologic Consequences	Clinical Findings	Desired Patient Outcome	Veterinary Technician Interventions
Hypothermia Decreased body temperature	Decreased metabolism Decreased tissue perfusion Ischemia Shock Death	Temperature <99°F Shivering Altered mentation Prolonged CRT Bradycardia Decreased respirations Cyanosis	Restoration and maintenance of normal body temperature/ Thermoregulation	Provide heat support: • Warm-water circulating blanket • Bair Hugger blanket (3M Medical, St. Paul, Minnesota) • Incubator • Warmed IV fluids Severely hypothermic patients must be warmed slowly Basic patient monitoring Oxygen therapy
Pain Unpleasant sensation	Increased stress response leading to: • Increased metabolism • Tachycardia • Hypertension • Nausea • Vomiting • Anorexia • Immunosuppression	Refer to pain scales Changes in behavior, posture, and reaction to palpation Clinical signs of *acute* pain also include: • Tachycardia • Tachypnea • Hypertension	Resolution or reduction of pain to an acceptable level as evidenced by decreasing pain score	Administer doctor-prescribed analgesics Monitor for breakthrough pain Basic patient monitoring Monitor for signs of adverse reaction to analgesics: • Vomiting and diarrhea • Melena • Decreased respiratory rate • Constipation • Agitation (cats) Physical therapy Provide comfortable environment Educate owner on changes to patient lifestyle and environment (chronic pain)
Electrolyte imbalance Abnormal plasma electrolyte levels	Dehydration Nausea, vomiting Polyuria/polydipsia Muscle weakness Seizures/tremors Cardiac abnormalities Altered mentation Coma Death	Depending on specific electrolyte, may see: • Bradycardia • Tachycardia • Arrhythmias • Muscle weakness • Muscle tremors • Seizures	Normal electrolyte concentrations	For deficiencies: • Administer doctor-prescribed supplementation For elevations: • Administer doctor-prescribed medications • Fluid diuresis Basic patient monitoring Monitor ECG Provide padded bedding for patients with muscle tremors, seizures
Urethral obstruction Unable to void a normal stream of urine because of occlusion of the urethra	Buildup of toxins in the bloodstream Dehydration Electrolyte imbalance Bladder rupture and urine peritonitis Coma Death	Stranguria Full, turgid bladder on palpation with inability to express urine Vomiting Altered mentation	Normal elimination of urine	Urinary catheterization per doctor's orders Administer doctor-prescribed medications Monitor urine output, urine stream Manual bladder expression (neurologic patients) Basic patient monitoring Treat/prevent dehydration Treat/prevent electrolyte imbalance Educate client on technique for manual bladder expression (neurologic patients)
Cardiac insufficiency Inadequate cardiac output necessary for tissue perfusion	Ischemia Necrosis Fluid accumulation Hypoxia Hypovolemia End organ failure Death	Tachypnea Tachycardia Abnormal heart sounds Prolonged CRT Pale or cyanotic mucous membranes Weak or asynchronous pulses Exercise intolerance Syncope Signs of ATE† (cats) Signs of CHF† ECG abnormalities Hypotension or hypertension	Adequate cardiac output: • Normal CRT • Pink mucous membranes • Normal heart rate • Normal respirations • Normotensive	Oxygen therapy Basic patient monitoring Monitor for signs of CHF/ATE Monitor ECG, oxygen saturation Monitor blood pressure Monitor fluid intake and output Administer doctor-ordered medications Monitor for adverse effects of medications Low-sodium diet

Continued

TABLE 18.4 **Selection of Technician Evaluations and Interventions—cont'd**

Veterinary Technician Evaluation and Definition	Potential Physiologic Consequences	Clinical Findings	Desired Patient Outcome	Veterinary Technician Interventions
Hypoxia Inadequate oxygenation	Tissue ischemia Death	Cyanotic mucous membranes Dyspnea Tachypnea Altered mentation Decreased oxygen saturation (SaO_2) Altered arterial blood gas (ABG) values ($\downarrow PaO_2$)	Adequate oxygenation: • Pink mucous membranes • Normal respirations • Normal oxygen saturation • Normal ABG values	Oxygen supplementation Basic patient monitoring Monitor oxygen saturation with pulse oximetry and arterial blood gas analysis
Overweight Excessive intake of nutrients	Obesity is a predisposing factor to a wide variety of small animal diseases	Body condition score (BCS) of 4+ out of 5	BCS of 3/5, ideal body weight	Determine ideal body weight and daily calorie requirement Develop a nutritional weight loss and exercise plan for patient Educate owner on health consequences of obesity and importance of plan implementation Monitor patient's progress to ensure appropriate degree of weight loss
Underweight Inadequate intake or absorption of nutrients to meet metabolic demands	Malnutrition leads to: • Multisystemic organ dysfunction • Dehydration • Electrolyte imbalance • Vitamin deficiency	BCS of 1–2 out of 5	BCS of 3/5, ideal body weight	Determine ideal body weight and daily caloric requirement Develop nutritional plan for weight gain Treat electrolyte imbalance Treat vitamin deficiency Treat anorexia, if present Avoid refeeding syndrome Client education regarding feeding plan Monitor patient's progress to ensure appropriate degree of weight gain
Vomiting Forceful expulsion of contents from the stomach and/or intestines	Anorexia Dehydration Electrolyte imbalance Malnutrition Weight loss	Nausea Vomiting Abdominal pain	Resolution of vomiting	Isolate patient if contagion is suspected Administer doctor-prescribed medications Limited fasting Provide nutritional support/dietary therapy (e.g., small, frequent meals of bland food) Basic patient monitoring Decrease smell of strong odors (trigger nausea/vomiting) Prevent/treat dehydration Treat electrolyte imbalance Treat anorexia
Diarrhea Frequent passage of loose, unformed stool	Dehydration Electrolyte imbalance Malnutrition Weight loss	Diarrhea Abdominal pain	Passage of normally formed stool	Isolate patient if contagion is suspected Administer doctor-prescribed medications Prevent/treat dehydration Basic patient monitoring Ensure patient hygiene: • Clip away matted fur • Clean perineal area with warm water and a mild soap • Thoroughly dry patient after bathing Provide nutritional support/dietary therapy
Constipation Infrequent and often difficult passage of hard stool	GI toxin buildup Anorexia Vomiting Electrolyte imbalance Rectal prolapse	Abdominal distension Abdominal pain Altered mentation Palpation of large amounts of hard stool in colon	Easy passage of normally formed stool at least once a day	Ensure adequate hydration Administer enema Basic patient monitoring Treat anorexia Feed high-fiber or low-residue food

*Basic patient monitoring as listed in Tables 18.1–18.3.

†See text.

ATE, Arterial thromboembolism (saddle thrombus); *CHF,* congestive heart failure; *CNS,* central nervous system; *CRT,* capillary refill time; *ECG,* electrocardiography; *PCV,* packed cell volume; *TP,* total protein.

TABLE 18.5   A Selection of "At-Risk" Veterinary Technician Evaluations

Veterinary Technician Evaluation	Characteristics of an At-Risk Patient	Veterinary Technician Intervention
Risk of aspiration	Loss of gag and swallow reflexes • Patient is sedated or anesthetized • Altered mentation • Damage to cranial nerves • Megaesophagus	Feed gruel-consistency foods Elevate food and water bowls Maintain elevation of head and forelimbs for 10 minutes after eating Feeding tube meals Do not feed patients recovering from anesthesia until they can swallow
Risk of infection	Compromised immune system function • Naïve • Immature • Suppressed • Deficient Break in physiologic barriers to infection • Skin lacerations, burns • Change in acidity of GI tract • Change in normal GI tract flora • Decreased urine concentration	Monitor for signs of infection, including: • Fever • Swelling, discharge, erythema • Pain • Change in lung sounds (pneumonia) • Decreased blood glucose (sepsis) • Increased white blood cell count Administer doctor-prescribed prophylactic antibiotic therapy Prevent both contagious and nosocomial infections • Reverse isolation • Proper aseptic technique when handling patient
Risk of infectious disease transmission	History of exposure Clinical signs of a potential contagious disease • Fever • Cough • Vomiting/diarrhea • Sneezing, nasal discharge, conjunctivitis Any patient with confirmed contagious infectious disease	Treat as outpatient when possible Institute standard hospital isolation protocols Educate owner regarding at-home isolation procedures and disease transmission to other household animals
Risk of self-trauma	Patients with pruritic or inflammatory disease Patients with localized pain (e.g., feline declaw) Patients with: • IV catheter • Urinary catheter • Feeding tubes • Chest tubes Patients with skin sutures or staples	Administer doctor-prescribed medications to alleviate pruritus, inflammation, and pain and to treat underlying disease process (e.g., topical corticosteroids) Administer doctor-prescribed medications to treat underlying disease process (e.g., topical flea control) Sedate patient Deter patient from area: • Bandage site (catheters, tubes) • Sweater/t-shirt (pruritus) • E-collar • BiteNot collar
Risk of pain	Patients needing an invasive medical procedure known to be painful (chest tubes, bone marrow aspiration) Patients with severe inflammatory disease (acute pancreatitis) Patients undergoing surgical procedures	Pre-emptive analgesia as prescribed by veterinarian Monitor for breakthrough pain

distress can be minimal or catastrophic. Patients may present with changes in breathing, cyanotic mucous membranes, poor pulses, disorientation, lethargy, anorexia, and an inability to walk. Depending on the cause of the respiratory distress, the patient may have a fever and nasal discharge.

Nasal discharge results from inflammation or irritation of the nasal mucosa and can be serous (clear liquid), mucoid (opaque and sticky), mucopurulent (green-yellow and mucoid), or hemorrhagic (bloody). The technician must note the type and whether the discharge is unilateral or bilateral. When a medical history is obtained, it is important to ascertain the duration and progression of the nasal discharge. Nasal and sinus congestion is caused by inflammation of the epithelial tissue that lines the nasal and sinus passages. Vasodilation of capillaries, fluid leakage from these vessels into surrounding parenchyma, and increased mucus production by epithelial cells lead to narrowing of the nasal and sinus passages, causing partial or, in severe cases, complete obstruction. Clinically, the patient presents with a "stuffy nose." Nasal discharge and edema can compromise airflow, leading to open-mouth breathing in some patients. Additionally, the diminished sense of smell may

CASE PRESENTATION 18.1

Veterinary Nursing Care Plan

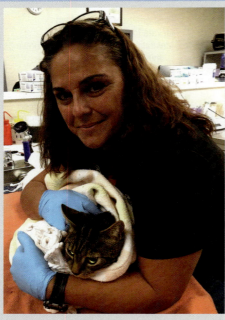

Jonesy, a 3-year-old neutered male Domestic Shorthair (DSH) tabby cat, presents with lethargy and anorexia.

Signalment: Jonesy, a 3-year-old neutered male Domestic Shorthair (DSH) tabby cat

Chief complaint: Owner reports that Jonesy is lethargic and has not been eating well since yesterday.

Pertinent history: Owner has three cats and one litter box, so it is difficult to know whether Jonesy is urinating and defecating normally. Owner meal-feeds an appropriate amount of high-quality commercial dry and wet food. Usually, Jonesy runs over to eat during mealtimes, but the past day, the owner has noticed he has yet to come and eat and is hiding in unusual locations.

Physical Examination:

Body weight: 13 pounds (5.9 kilograms); body condition score: 3/5; muscle condition score: normal; temperature: 101.5°F; heart rate: 160 beats per minute, sinus rhythm; synchronous and strong pulses; respiration: 22 breaths per minute, lungs clear; mucous membranes: pink and moist; capillary refill time: <2 seconds; skin turgor: normal; skin and haircoat:

normal; ears, eyes, and nose: normal; gastrointestinal system: large amounts of firm stool in colon, no reaction to palpation; urogenital system: normal; musculoskeletal system: normal.

Medical diagnosis (by veterinarian): Uncomplicated constipation

Technician evaluations: Constipation; client knowledge deficit

Nursing Care Plan

1. Constipation

Intervention	Rationale
Fluid therapy: 100 mL balanced isotonic crystalloid subcutaneously per veterinarian orders	Address potential dehydration: fluid loss may occur due to enema administration and/or vomiting following enema administration
Enema: preparation and administration	Soften stool: facilitates bowel evacuation
Housing: large cage with two litter boxes	Promote defecation: allows for patient movement and ample space to defecate; stimulates evacuation
Basic patient monitoring: avoid rectal temperature	Vomiting and bradycardia: can be vagally induced via enema administration
	Abdominal palpation: ensure complete evacuation of stool
Patient hygiene: bathing of perineal region, hind limbs, and tail	Maintain cleanliness: reduce skin irritation and staining

2. Client knowledge deficit

Intervention	Rationale
Litter box management: - Four litter boxes is ideal for three cats, with at least one box on each floor of the home - Daily cleaning	Patient's constipation is likely related to inadequate access to clean litter boxes for normal daily elimination
Hydration: - Fresh water access at all times; consider multiple access points or water fountain - Increase wet food offered or add water to existing food options	Patient's constipation may be compounded by insufficient access to fresh water

---

cause **anorexia**, particularly in cats. The following clinical signs may be noted in patients suffering from respiratory distress:

Sneezing: Frequent, rapid bouts of sneezing are abnormal. Sneezing is most often seen in dogs inhaling foreign material; in cats, it is most often associated with an upper respiratory tract viral infection. Until proven otherwise, sneezing patients, particularly cats, should be treated as if they are contagious, and isolation procedures should be instituted.

Facial swelling: A patient with nasal discharge, congestion, and/ or sneezing should be closely examined for facial swelling that can accompany the causative disease, such as a tooth root abscess, migration of nasal foreign bodies, neoplasia, or fungal infection.

Stertor/stridor: Obstruction of the pharynx or larynx can cause *stertor*, a loud snoring or snorting sound, or **stridor**, a high-pitched inspiratory wheeze. The presence of either sound justifies a thorough examination of the upper airways, and steps must be taken to ensure an open airway.

Cough: A *cough* is a forceful expulsion of air from the lungs through the mouth. It may be a reflexive or conscious action resulting from irritation or inflammation to the pharynx, larynx, trachea, bronchi, or pleura. A cough may be productive, meaning that mucus, fluid, or blood is brought up from the airway (usually swallowed), or nonproductive, sometimes called a "dry cough." **Hemoptysis**, the coughing up of blood, can be seen in heartworm disease and other cardiac diseases, such as CHF. The owner often confuses a productive cough, particularly in

• BOX 18.3 Understanding Etiology and Pathogenesis

Etiology is the study of the causation or origination of disease. For example, the etiologic agent or cause of heartworm disease is the bloodborne parasite *Dirofilaria immitis.* Many causes of disease are known, including infectious agents, toxins, physical trauma, nutritional deficits, genetic defects, aging, and psychological stress. If the cause of a disease is unknown, it is termed *idiopathic.*

Pathogenesis is the mechanism of disease development; it can be acute or chronic. Regardless of whether the pathogenesis of a disease is acute or chronic, complex or simple, it ultimately leads to injury to cells and body tissues, which may be visible as gross and microscopic lesions. Examples of common pathologic mechanisms that lead to disease include inflammation, cell injury (e.g., infectious, toxic, and physical), cell growth abnormalities (e.g., neoplasia, hypertrophy, and hyperplasia), metabolic disturbances, and immune system dysfunction. The veterinary technician may see the body's response to these pathologic events as clinical signs.

TABLE 18.6 Examples of Common Respiratory Diseases

Obstructive	Inflammatory/ Infectious	Pleural Space Disease
Laryngeal paralysis	Heartworm disease	Pneumothorax
Tracheal collapse	Pneumonia	Pleural effusion
	Asthma	

cats with asthma, with retching or vomiting, so careful questioning is indicated when a medical history is gathered. Palpation of the trachea may elicit a cough in patients with tracheal irritation. Thorough auscultation of the thoracic cavity is necessary to detect abnormal lung sounds or heart abnormalities (coughing can be seen in dogs with CHF).

Pleural effusion: **Pleural effusion** is excessive fluid accumulation within the thoracic cavity. Causes include fluid overload, infection, lymphatic obstruction, coagulopathies, and trauma. In some patients experiencing respiratory distress, pleural effusion may occur. For various reasons, pleural effusion may occur, but no matter the cause, fluid shifting or buildup occurs within the lungs, resulting in fluid within the pleural space. Pleural effusion restricts normal breathing. Fluid in the thoracic cavity causes compression of the lung tissue and inadequate lung expansion. It can be a life-threatening condition, because it results in the patient being unable to ventilate appropriately. Clinically, patients often present in respiratory distress, with increased inspiratory effort. On examination, lung sounds are decreased, and heart sounds are muffled. Cats may have noticeably decreased chest compliance, with significant amounts of fluid.

Pleural effusion can be confirmed via thoracocentesis, radiography, or ultrasonography. For a patient in respiratory distress, thoracocentesis may be performed immediately after auscultation or ultrasonographic assessment and before radiography to restore normal intrapleural pressure and cause re-expansion of the lungs. If pleural effusion is highly suspected, it is often safer to perform a thoracocentesis first rather than stress the patient to obtain a radiograph.

Dyspnea: **Dyspnea**, or respiratory distress, is difficulty breathing, characterized by increased respiratory rate or effort, often with an abdominal component to the breath. Patients often also exhibit **orthopnea**, the inability to breathe except in the upright position; dogs tend to stand with their necks extended and their elbows abducted, whereas cats prefer sternal recumbency. Normally, cats do not pant; therefore open-mouth breathing with noticeable chest movement equates to dyspnea and is an urgent situation. Any interruption of normal airflow (e.g., upper or lower respiratory tract obstruction), inadequate lung inflation (e.g., pleural effusion, pneumothorax), or alveolar gas exchange (e.g., pneumonia) can cause dyspnea.

Respiratory pattern: The respiratory pattern can yield some clue to the location of the problem. Patients with upper airway disease tend to exhibit increased inspiratory effort and take slow, deep breaths; patients with lower airway disease typically exhibit increased expiratory effort and have shallow, rapid breaths. Patients with dyspnea are in a critical condition, and demonstration of a patent airway and provision of oxygen is required immediately (refer to Chapter 25, "Emergency and Critical Care Nursing"). If pleural effusions or pneumothorax are present, thoracocentesis is performed as quickly as possible to help stabilize the patient. Stressing a dyspneic patient can result in death. Therefore thorough examination and diagnostic tests begin once the patient's condition has been stabilized. Even then, patient interactions may need to be performed in stages, using low-stress handling techniques and allowing the patient to have frequent breaks. Additionally, patients need to be closely monitored by the veterinary technician during these procedures for signs of hypoxia and commonly need oxygen support throughout the diagnostic procedures.

Hypoxia: Hypoxia is defined as deficient oxygenation of tissues. Hypoxia can result from reduced blood flow (e.g., CHF), decreased oxygen-carrying capacity (e.g., anemia), hypoventilation (e.g., pleural effusion), or ventilation-perfusion mismatch (e.g., pneumonia). Pulse oximetry yields an estimate of the saturation of hemoglobin, which provides some information about tissue oxygenation and oxygen delivery. In a normal patient, this value should be greater than 95% when the patient is breathing room air (21% fraction of inspired oxygen [FiO_2]). Hypoxia manifests clinically as tachypnea, tachycardia, cyanosis or pallor, and dyspnea. Nursing care for the hypoxic patient is presented in Table 18.4.

Hypoxemia: **Hypoxemia** refers to a decrease in the partial pressure of oxygen in arterial blood (PaO_2) as measured by arterial blood gas analysis.

Diagnostic procedures for respiratory diseases include rhinoscopy, bronchoscopy, radiography, ultrasonography, computed tomography (CT), and magnetic resonance imaging (MRI); cytologic examination and cultures of secretions, exudates, and effusions; biopsy; arterial blood gas analysis; serum fungal titers; and parasitological tests. Table 18.7 summarizes the general therapeutic approach to a patient with respiratory disease. Table 18.8 lists common respiratory diseases and their specific treatments.

TECHNICIAN NOTE

Unduly stressing a patient with dyspnea can cause respiratory arrest. Ensure a patent airway and provide oxygen immediately. Do not perform diagnostic tests until the patient has been stabilized. Even then, patient interactions may need to be performed in stages, using low-stress handling techniques and allowing the patient to have frequent breaks.

TABLE 18.7	Therapeutic Approach to Patients With Respiratory Disease
Treatment	**Rationale**
Ensuring open airway: • Intubation • Positioning patient to alleviate pressure on airway • Administering bronchodilators • Removal of foreign body	Prevents respiratory arrest
Ensuring adequate patient oxygenation: • Providing supplemental oxygen	Treats/prevents hypoxia
Decreasing stress in dyspneic patients: • Minimal handling • Staged interventions • Quiet environment • Sedation	• Stress causes an increased demand for oxygen, which a dyspneic patient may not be able to meet • Leads to respiratory decompensation and possible respiratory arrest
Thoracocentesis	Immediate removal of pleural effusion will allow for proper lung inflation
Airway humidification • Vaporizer • Nebulization • Steam therapy (outpatient) • Saline nasal drops • Systemic hydration	• Mucous membranes lining respiratory tract must be moist to function properly • Dry mucous membranes promote inflammation, increase mucus, decrease mucociliary clearance, and decrease local immune function and barrier protection
Antitussives	Control nonproductive cough
Expectorants	Thin mucous secretions and encourage productive cough
Prophylactic antibiotics	Prevent bacterial infection secondary to compromised respiratory tract function
Anti-inflammatories	Reduce inflammation of the airways
Antibiotics	Treat primary infection
Antiparasitics	Treat primary infection
Antifungals	Treat primary infection

Heartworm-associated Respiratory Disease (HARD)

Diagnosis of canine heartworm disease is based on a positive serum test result for heartworm antigen. Feline heartworm disease often goes undiagnosed, and antigen testing alone is unreliable, because unisex infection is common in cats. A positive heartworm antibody titer, the presence of basophilia and eosinophilia on a complete blood count (CBC), and enlarged pulmonary vessels on radiography support the diagnosis; the presence of a worm on echocardiography confirms it.

Treatment of canine heartworm disease consists of adulticide therapy, with microfilaricide therapy started 3 to 4 weeks later. In some cases, surgical removal of worms from the right atrium is necessary as a lifesaving procedure; adulticide therapy is started a few weeks postoperatively once the patient's condition has stabilized.

Adult heartworms die slowly over 2 to 30 days. Patients are at risk for pulmonary thromboembolism (PTE) during this time. Clinical signs of PTE include dyspnea, tachypnea, coughing, hemoptysis, and possibly fever. To minimize the risk of PTE, it is essential to restrict exercise for 3 to 4 weeks after administration of adulticide therapy. Patients with a high worm burden and severe cardiopulmonary disease are at high risk for PTE and must be stabilized before the adulticide is administered. Treatment for feline heartworm disease is unrewarding, because a safe and effective adulticide protocol has yet to be found. Treatment focuses on supporting the patient through the natural course of the infection and eventual self-cure, which occurs in about 80% of patients. The death of just one heartworm can trigger anaphylactic shock or cause PTE, both of which can result in sudden death. Feline patients in crisis can be treated with steroids, oxygen, and bronchodilators as prescribed by the veterinarian.

In dogs and cats, the key to treating heartworm disease is preventing infection; this is achieved by using any of several approved macrolide preventive agents.

Cardiovascular Disease

Heart Disease and Congestive Heart Failure

Heart disease is a pathologic abnormality that affects the myocardium, the valves, rhythm conduction, the pericardium (the sheath covering the heart), or the overall structure of the heart (shunts). In cats, myocardial disease accounts for most cases of heart disease; in dogs, valvular disease accounts for most cases of cardiac disease. The body has incredible compensatory mechanisms to maintain cardiac output when faced with an abnormally functioning heart; therefore many patients are asymptomatic at home or owners may miss subtle clinical signs, such as mild exercise intolerance, lethargy, or tachypnea. Early detection of heart disease relies on thorough annual physical examinations and, for predisposed breeds, screening echocardiography. On physical examination, a patient with heart disease may exhibit tachycardia; a weak, bounding, or asynchronous pulse; a heart murmur; and/or arrhythmia. The animal may also exhibit signs of hypoxemia, as described above.

Diagnosis of heart disease relies on diagnostic imaging of the heart via radiography, echocardiography, and electrocardiography (ECG). In recent years, serum cardiac biomarkers, such as B-type natriuretic peptide, have become available to aid in diagnosis. With the notable exception of some congenital disorders that may be corrected with surgery (e.g., patent ductus arteriosus), no efficacious treatments are currently available to slow the progression of heart disease to heart failure, so it is recommended that asymptomatic patients be closely monitored. This includes periodic echocardiography and, perhaps more importantly, education of owners to monitor the resting respiratory rate at home for tachypnea—one of the earliest signs of heart failure. As time progresses, the compensatory mechanisms sustaining cardiac output eventually fail, causing *heart failure* and inadequate tissue perfusion.

A patient with heart failure has clinical signs referable to the perfusion deficit: tachypnea, exercise intolerance (dogs), syncope, weakness, prolonged capillary refill time (CRT), cough, and pale mucous membranes. Sudden death can also occur. Clinical signs in cats with heart failure are more often nonspecific and include anorexia, depression, and weight loss. However, cats can undoubtedly present in CHF crisis with tachypnea, dyspnea, and other signs pointing to impaired gas exchange. Patients diagnosed with heart failure are treated with medications to reduce afterload, improve contractility, treat volume overload (diuretics), and sometimes prevent blood clots. These medications include angiotensin-converting enzyme (ACE) inhibitors, beta-blockers, positive inotropes, diuretics, calcium channel blockers, antihypertensives, and antiarrhythmic drugs. Low-sodium diets, stress reduction, and exercise restrictions are recommended.

Heart disease can be valvular, myocardial, arrhythmogenic, and pericardial in nature. As an example, large- and giant-breed dogs (namely Newfoundlands, Irish Wolfhounds, Great Danes) may suffer from atrial fibrillation (rapid and chaotic atrial depolarization), which may (or may not) lead to structural heart disease. Additionally, dogs and cats may suffer from pericardial diseases such as neoplasia. This may lead to pericardial effusion (fluid accumulation in the pericardial sac) and life-threatening pericardial tamponade, where the pressure within the pericardial sac affects cardiac output.

TABLE 18.8 **Small Animal Respiratory Diseases**

Disease	Pathogenesis	Clinical Signs	Diagnostics	Treatments
Rhinitis/sinusitis	Inflammation of the mucosa of the nasal passages and sinuses caused by viral, bacterial, or fungal infection; foreign bodies, allergies, neoplasia, or tooth root abscess	Nasal discharge Nasal/sinus congestion Sneezing Facial swelling Open-mouth breathing	History and clinical signs Determination of infectious agent Radiograph Computed tomography (CT)/magnetic resonance imaging (MRI) scans	Airway humidification Treat underlying cause: • Foreign body removal • Antifungal therapy • Tooth extraction • Allergy relief • Antibiotics • Anti-inflammatories
Brachycephalic airway syndrome	Upper airway obstruction seen in brachycephalic breeds caused by a constellation of anatomic deformities, including stenotic nares, elongated soft palate, hypoplastic trachea, and laryngeal collapse	Voice change Stertor Stridor Exercise intolerance Hypoxia	Signalment Physical examination Direct visualization of upper airway Radiography	Emergency treatment of dyspnea Weight management Avoid overheating Exercise restrictions Surgical correction of anatomic deformities
Laryngeal paralysis	Damage to the recurrent laryngeal nerves resulting in paralysis of the arytenoid cartilage	Change in voice Stridor Exercise intolerance Gagging or coughing with eating or vocalization Dyspnea	Direct visualization of larynx	Maintaining open airway (intubation) Emergency treatment of dyspnea Surgery—laryngoplasty
Feline bronchitis (feline asthma)	Irritation and inflammation of the bronchi causing bronchial constriction, hypertrophy of bronchial smooth muscle, and increased production of mucus. Varied causes: allergic, fungal, bacterial, parasitic, idiopathic.	Cough Wheezing Dyspnea	Radiography Cytologic examination and culture of fluid from tracheal wash or bronchoalveolar lavage Fecal analysis for lung parasites Heartworm test	Emergency treatment of dyspnea Maintenance: • Bronchodilators • Corticosteroids • Improve indoor air quality to decrease inhaled allergens • Infections/parasites
Pneumonia	Inflammation of the lung caused by bacterial, viral, fungal infection, or by aspiration of a foreign body or stomach contents	Cough Hypoxia Crackles heard on lung auscultation Fever Anorexia Weight loss	Radiographs Bronchoscopy Cytologic examination and culture of tracheal wash Viral and fungal serology	Oxygen therapy Airway hydration Changing patient positioning frequently Coupage Bronchodilators Antibiotics Antifungals
Diaphragmatic hernia	A congenital or acquired rent in the diaphragm, allowing abdominal organs to enter the thoracic cavity	Dyspnea Tachypnea Lethargy Anorexia Decreased lung sounds Muffled heart sounds	Radiographs	Emergency treatment of dyspnea Surgical hernia repair
Pyothorax	Pus in the pleural cavity caused by bacterial infection secondary to foreign bodies (grass awns in dogs), penetrating wound to the chest wall (bite wounds in cats), or progression of lung infection	Hypoxia Cough Fever Lethargy Anorexia Decreased lung sounds Muffled heart sounds Pleural effusion	Pleural fluid analysis, cytologic examination	Oxygen therapy Drainage of effusion • Thoracocentesis • Chest tubes Antibiotics Analgesia for patients with chest tubes

Continued

TABLE 18.8   Small Animal Respiratory Diseases—cont'd

Disease	Pathogenesis	Clinical Signs	Diagnostics	Treatments
Chylothorax	Accumulation of chyle in the pleural cavity, resulting from decreased lymphatic drainage (obstructed thoracic duct) or increased lymphatic flow	Cough Hypoxia Decreased lung sounds Muffled heart sounds Pleural effusion	Pleural fluid analysis, cytologic examination	Oxygen therapy Thoracocentesis Treatment of underlying disease Feeding low-fat diet Benzopyrone medication Thoracic duct ligation
Pneumothorax	Air in the pleural cavity caused by trauma to the thoracic cavity (blunt force, penetrating wounds) or secondary to underlying pulmonary disease; can be idiopathic	Hypoxia Decreased lung sounds Muffled heart sounds	Radiography	Oxygen therapy Drainage of air • Thoracocentesis • Chest tubes with continuous suction Treatment of underlying disease Analgesia for trauma cases, patients with chest tubes

---

TECHNICIAN NOTE

One of the first signs that heart disease has progressed to heart failure is tachypnea. Therefore teaching the owner to monitor the patient's resting respiratory rate at home is an essential strategy for early detection.

CHF results when decreased cardiac output causes poor venous return to the heart. This leads to fluid overload (congestion) in tissues and impaired pulmonary gas exchange. The patient becomes hypoxic, and a worsening situation ensues. If the left side of the heart is afflicted, this condition is classified as *left-sided CHF*. In this condition, fluid builds up in the pulmonary vasculature (pulmonary edema) into the pleural space (pleural effusion) in dogs and cats. Clinical signs are consistent with respiratory compromise and hypoxia; dyspnea, tachypnea, cyanosis, and abnormal respiratory sounds, including crackles, wheezes, and decreased lung sounds, are all heard on thoracic auscultation. Coughing is commonly seen in dogs but not in cats. If the right side of the heart is afflicted, the condition is classified as *right-sided CHF*, with venous congestion occurring in the abdominal and thoracic cavities. Clinical signs include edema, jugular distention, abdominal distention caused by ascites, hepatomegaly, and pleural and pericardial effusions. Nursing care for patients with CHF is presented in Table 18.4 under the associated technician assessments "hypoxia" and "cardiac insufficiency."

TECHNICIAN NOTE

Coughing is a common sign of congestive heart failure (CHF) in dogs but not cats.

Cardiomyopathy. *Cardiomyopathy* is a disease of the heart muscle and can be primary or secondary. Primary cardiomyopathies are not caused by any other cardiovascular or systemic disease. They are classified as hypertrophic, dilated, arrhythmogenic right ventricular (Boxer cardiomyopathy), restrictive, or unclassified. Hypertrophic cardiomyopathy and, to a much lesser degree, restrictive and dilated cardiomyopathies are seen in cats; the most noted form in dogs is dilated cardiomyopathy. Secondary cardiomyopathies result from an underlying disease process, for example, ventricular hypertrophy secondary to feline hyperthyroidism or dilated cardiomyopathy secondary to canine parvovirus infection.

Hypertrophic cardiomyopathy (HCM), the most common form of feline cardiomyopathy, is characterized by increased thickness of the left ventricle wall and a small ventricular lumen. The presence of these abnormalities on echocardiography confirms the diagnosis. Treatment commences once the patient is in heart failure and may include diuretics, ACE inhibitors, beta-blockers, and/or calcium channel blockers. Cats with HCM (or any cardiomyopathy) are at risk for feline arterial thromboembolism (FATE), in which blood clots form in the heart and lodge in the arterial vasculature, most commonly the abdominal aortic trifurcation, disrupting the blood supply to the hind limbs. Clinical signs of femoral arterial thromboembolism include hind limb paresis or paralysis and severe pain, cyanotic toe pads, absent or poor femoral pulses, and coolness of the affected limb. However, clots can lodge in any vascular system, including the cerebral, renal, and hepatic systems. Cats with undiagnosed HCM may first present with signs of arterial thromboembolism. The prevention of thromboembolism formation is an important goal when feline cardiomyopathy is treated but, unfortunately, it is difficult to achieve because no single drug has proven effective. However, many new antithrombolytic medications are being researched to prevent this life-threatening complication. Feline patients are often prescribed aspirin or clopidogrel (Plavix) to reduce further thromboembolic complications.

Dilated cardiomyopathy (DCM), the most common canine cardiomyopathy, is characterized by extreme atrial and ventricular dilatation, with decreased contractility. Primarily, the left side of the heart is damaged; however, right-sided DCM can be seen. Diagnosis is confirmed by using radiography, ECG, and echocardiography. Treatment commences once the patient is in heart failure and may include the use of diuretics, ACE inhibitors, and positive inotropes.

Degenerative Atrioventricular Valve Disease. *Degenerative atrioventricular valve disease* affects the cardiac valve leaflets or cusps and is characterized by the thickening of the tissue. It primarily affects dogs, with approximately 60% of cases involving only the mitral valve and 30% involving both mitral and tricuspid valves; only the tricuspid valve is affected in 10% of patients. Degenerative changes lead to insufficient functioning of the valves; therefore these diseases are referred to as *mitral valve* or *tricuspid valve insufficiency*. Mitral valve insufficiency has been documented in cats, but it is uncommon. On physical examination, localizable heart murmurs are evident. Diagnosis is made based on valvular changes shown by echocardiography. Treatment commences once the patient is in heart failure and may include the use of diuretics, ACE inhibitors, positive inotropes, and antihypertensives. Arrhythmias are common sequelae in the advanced stages of this disease; if present, an antiarrhythmic medication is added to the treatment regimen.

Heartworm Disease

Heartworm disease is a mosquito-borne infectious disease that affects both cats and dogs. (See Chapter 13 regarding the life cycle of *Dirofilaria immitis* and diagnostic testing.) Clinical signs of heartworm disease in cats and dogs differ (Box 18.4). These differences in clinical signs reflect the worm burden and the longevity of the adult worm. In dogs, large numbers (≥30) of adult worms can be present in the pulmonary arteries, the right atrium and ventricle, and the caudal vena cava, and they can live for up to 7 years. The presence of up to several hundred heartworms has been reported in large dogs with heavy heartworm burdens. In cats, heartworm infection generally consists of one to three worms that can survive up to 3 years. They live primarily in the pulmonary arteries but can migrate to the right atrium. The heartworms may not reach adulthood, but even immature worms cause significant damage in cats.

Systemic Hypertension

Systemic hypertension is defined as an increase in systemic blood pressure. In small animals, hypertension is classified by its inherent risk of causing organ damage, with a repeatable measurement in a calm patient of 150 mm Hg or greater.[1] Systemic hypertension may be classified as situational, idiopathic, or secondary. Situational hypertension is a temporary rise in blood pressure in response to the stressors associated with being in a veterinary environment, including obtaining blood pressure measurements. Identifying systemic hypertension can be challenging for the veterinary practitioner; therefore we must be mindful of evaluating the whole patient. The presence of a disease process in a patient associated with systemic hypertension can increase the likelihood that the patient truly requires antihypertensive medications.

Hypertension secondary to another disease process is still the most diagnosed form, representing most cases. CKD, hyperthyroidism, hyperadrenocorticism (HAC), and DM are most often associated with secondary systemic hypertension. Hypertension can cause or exacerbate cardiac disease, so the veterinary technician must know how to obtain a blood pressure reading in a patient with a risk factor for hypertension or as part of routine screening. Most hypertensive patients are asymptomatic; therefore early detection is important, and routine blood pressure screening is recommended for patients with predisposing disease. Because

of the high incidence of CKD and hyperthyroidism in cats, the American Association of Feline Practitioners (AAFP) recommends routine screening of patients 10 years of age and older. It is not unusual for the diagnosis of systemic hypertension to be made first, leading to the diagnosis of the primary disease.

If systemic hypertension cannot be correlated to a disease process, a diagnosis of idiopathic hypertension (formerly known as primary or essential) may be reached. Idiopathic hypertension is more frequently recognized in small animals now than in the past; however, it is possible that some of these patients may have an undetectable subclinical disease (e.g., kidney disease) that limits the ability to identify secondary hypertension.

Additionally, patients presenting with cardiac disease should have their blood pressure monitored. Routine funduscopic examinations should be performed in at-risk patients, because enlarged retinal vessels and retinal hemorrhage are early warning signs of impending retinal detachment resulting from hypertension. Unfortunately, one of the most common presenting signs in a patient with undiagnosed severe hypertension is acute blindness caused by retinal detachment. Once hypertension has been diagnosed, treatment with antihypertensive medication (calcium channel blockers, ACE inhibitors) is begun immediately. The goal is to gradually lower blood pressure to normal without a dramatic drop. Frequent blood pressure monitoring begins early to help titrate the medication dose and ensure normotension. The successful treatment plan also includes diagnosing, treating, and monitoring underlying disease in patients with secondary systemic hypertension. Proper blood pressure monitoring is essential in making and validating the readings and subsequent diagnosis. Refer to Chapter 25, "Emergency and Critical Care Nursing."

TECHNICIAN NOTE

Systemic hypertension is often secondary to another disease, such as chronic kidney disease (CKD), hyperthyroidism, or hyperadrenocorticism (HAC).

Digestive and Hepatobiliary Diseases

Gastrointestinal Tract

Most stomach and small intestine diseases ultimately result in local inflammation or infection, with or without the obstruction of the gastrointestinal (GI) tract, with each of these pathologic processes causing a finite array of clinical signs. Canine patients are more susceptible to GI disorders as they are more prone to ingesting nonfood items. When a canine patient is "sick," it often involves the GI tract. The veterinary technician needs to be familiar with the most common clinical signs, because this knowledge can help focus medical history questions, identify the anatomic location of the problem, develop technician evaluations, and direct diagnostic and therapeutic approaches.

Regurgitation is the passive expulsion of material (usually food or fluid) from the esophagus due to various obstructive diseases or functional abnormalities. Apparent signs of nausea and abdominal contractions are not typically seen. Patients can exhibit difficulty eating (dysphagia), hypersalivation, and gagging. Regurgitated material typically consists of undigested or partially digested food and can occur immediately or hours after eating. Patients are at risk for esophagitis and aspiration of stomach contents, subsequently resulting in aspiration pneumonia. The underlying cause must be determined as nursing care, diagnostics, and treatment will vary greatly depending on the cause. Postoperative patients without control of their airway are at particular risk for regurgitation and subsequent aspiration pneumonia.

TABLE 18.9	Small Bowel Versus Large Bowel Diarrhea	
	Small Bowel Diarrhea	**Large Bowel Diarrhea**
Volume of feces	Increased	Normal or decreased
Mucus in feces	Uncommon	Common
Blood in feces	Melena may be seen	Hematochezia may be seen
Frequency of bowel movements	Normal	Increased
Tenesmus	Rare	Common
Weight loss	Common	Rare

Nursing care may include elevating food and water bowls, keeping the patient's head and forelimbs elevated for 10 to 30 minutes after a meal, changing the form of food (gruel, meatballs), and monitoring for signs of aspiration, in addition to administering medical therapies to treat the underlying cause and motility issue.

Vomiting is the forceful ejection of contents from the stomach and the upper small intestine (duodenum); it is an active process requiring abdominal contraction to expel contents forcefully. Retching involves abdominal contraction without expulsion of contents. It may be a precursor to vomiting but typically does not result in any vomiting. Signals of nausea often precede vomiting, including anxiety, hypersalivation, vocalization, and lip smacking. Vomitus can comprise any combination of undigested or digested food, hair, mucus, bile, and gastric secretions. Patients may vomit intestinal parasites (e.g., roundworms) or pieces of foreign material that they ingested (yarn, ribbon, tennis balls, plastic bags, etc.) or even blood. This is called **hematemesis** if the patient is vomiting fresh or digested blood. When the medical history is obtained, the owner must be asked about the amount and content of the vomitus, and the duration, severity, and frequency of vomiting. The owner must also be asked to confirm the occurrence of vomiting at home. Owners may present the pet for vomiting when the patient was only regurgitating (especially noted in dogs). With cats, owners must be carefully questioned to help distinguish "trying to bring up a hairball" (retching) from coughing. It must be remembered that vomiting can have non-GI causes, and a full system review is always indicated. Vomiting causes patients to be prone to dehydration and electrolyte imbalance, whereas retching does not; monitoring for and treating these secondary problems is essential in ensuring complete patient care. Nursing care for the vomiting patient is summarized in Table 18.4.

> **TECHNICIAN NOTE**
>
> It is important to distinguish between vomiting and regurgitating, which often appear the same to the owner. Remember that one is active (vomiting), in which the pet is forcefully expelling contents, and one is passive (regurgitating), in which contents are ejected out of the mouth without active abdominal contraction.

Diarrhea is characterized by frequent passage of loose, unformed, often watery feces. When a medical history of a patient with diarrhea is obtained, it is crucial to question the owner about the duration, severity, frequency, amount, and quality. This information can assist in localizing diarrhea involving the small or large bowel (Table 18.9). Knowing the duration of the problem—acute versus chronic—helps the clinician to determine the proper diagnostic testing. Patients with diarrhea are prone to dehydration, so monitoring for and treating dehydration is vital in ensuring complete patient care. Nursing care for the patient with diarrhea is summarized in Table 18.4.

Constipation is characterized by the infrequent and often difficult passage of hard stool. In establishing the history of constipation, questioning the owner about when the last normal bowel movement was observed is essential. Constipation can be a primary GI problem caused by bowel obstruction or diminished bowel motility; however, it can also occur secondary to orthopedic pain (i.e., inability to posture for defecation), environmental stressors (e.g., poor litter box maintenance), and dehydration. Completing a full system review when obtaining a medical history is essential to evaluate all potential causes. Nursing care for the constipated patient is summarized in Table 18.4.

Hematochezia is the presence of blood in the stool and will appear red, indicating fresh blood. It can be seen with diarrhea or as blood streaks outside normally formed stool and usually indicates a problem with the colon or the rectum.

Melena is defined as the presence of digested blood in feces. The stool is characteristically a tarry black color. Melena may be seen in patients with upper GI bleeding resulting from endoparasites, ulcerations, neoplasms, coagulopathies, etc.

Tenesmus is defined as painful straining at urination or defecation. A thorough medical history and physical examination must be completed to determine which body system is involved. Tenesmus of GI origin is usually the result of colonic disease, often accompanying diarrhea or constipation.

The diagnostic approach to a patient with stomach or intestinal disease primarily involves fecal analyses (e.g., flotation, cytologic examination, virus detection, cultures), plain and contrast radiography, ultrasonography, endoscopy, surgical exploration, and biopsy of the GI tract. A minimum database (CBC, serum chemistry, urinalysis [UA]) helps document secondary problems, such as electrolyte imbalance and inflammation, but independently is unlikely to lead to a definitive diagnosis.

Treatment of a patient with GI disease is multimodal; it involves medical management of clinical signs and treatment of the primary cause and can include medical and/or surgical approaches. Tables 18.10 and 18.11 summarize medical therapies for GI clinical signs and common diseases and disorders of the GI tract in cats and dogs. Selected diseases of the GI tract include gastritis, gastroenteritis, acute hemorrhagic diarrhea syndrome (i.e., hemorrhagic gastroenteritis), inflammatory bowel disease (IBD), colitis, and emergent conditions, such as gastric dilatation-volvulus (GDV) and foreign bodies causing intestinal obstruction.

Exocrine Pancreas

Pancreatitis— Acute and Chronic. Pancreatitis occurs when the digestive enzyme trypsin is prematurely activated within the pancreatic tissue instead of within the duodenum as is expected. Trypsin in the pancreas causes autodigestion of pancreatic tissue, resulting in local inflammation, necrosis, and peritonitis. Pancreatitis may be acute or chronic; acute disease is seen more commonly in dogs, and chronic disease is more common in cats. Most cases of acute pancreatitis are idiopathic; however, risk factors for the development of acute pancreatitis include dietary indiscretion (dogs), blunt force trauma, pancreatic hypoperfusion, and the use of pancreotoxic drugs. In most cases, the

TABLE 18.10	Medical Management of Gastrointestinal Clinical signs
Treatment	**Rationale**
Limited fasting	A 12–24-hour fast will lessen clinical signs by allowing the gastrointestinal (GI) tract to rest; indicated for vomiting and/or diarrhea.
Fluid therapy	Treat or prevent secondary dehydration. Ensure patient hydration in patients with chronic constipation. Treat electrolyte imbalances.
Dietary therapy	• Bland diets: easier to digest, gentler on the GI tract. Generally fed as small, frequent meals. Ideal for patients with nonspecific vomiting or diarrhea. • Hypoallergenic diets: novel proteins and carbohydrates for patients with food allergies or intolerance. Reduce inflammation. • Fiber-rich diets: helpful in patients with diarrhea or constipation. Fiber helps normalize colonic health. • Low-residue diets: helpful for patients with chronic constipation. • Feeding tube placement: to feed around the problem (e.g., esophagitis, pancreatitis) and/or to treat severe anorexia.
Probiotic therapy	Helps normalize proper concentration and composition of GI bacterial flora.
Antiemetics	Control vomiting.
Antacids	Decrease gastric acidity. Indicated for patients with or at risk for ulcerative diseases. Can also help decrease nausea.
Mucosal protectants	Protect the mucosal lining of the GI tract. Used in patients with or at risk for ulcerative disease.
Promotility drugs	Used to promote stomach emptying and intestinal peristalsis, which is helpful in reducing vomiting in select patients. Used to increase colonic motility for feline patients with idiopathic megacolon.
Antidiarrheal drugs	Decrease GI transit time, which is helpful in the treatment of diarrhea.
Enemas, laxatives, stool softeners	For the treatment of constipation.
Antibiotics	For patients with specific antibiotic-responsive diseases or for patients at risk for sepsis or aspiration pneumonia.
Anthelmintics	For patients with diagnosed or suspected endoparasites.
Anti-inflammatories	Reduce GI inflammation.

cause of chronic pancreatitis is unknown. However, because cats have only one pancreatic duct, which joins the common bile duct before emptying into the duodenum, an association with concurrent bile duct or liver inflammation (cholangiohepatitis) and/or IBD has been noted in this species. Clinical signs of acute pancreatitis include anorexia, vomiting, abdominal pain, diarrhea, and fever. Clinical signs associated with chronic pancreatitis include anorexia, lethargy, weight loss, hypothermia, and vomiting. Patients with severe acute disease may go on to develop hypotension, disseminated intravascular coagulation (DIC), acute renal injury (AKI), and multiorgan failure. A presumptive diagnosis is commonly made and relies on a constellation of laboratory work (e.g., CBC, serum chemistry, UA, and pancreatic lipase immunoreactivity [PLI] concentrations) and diagnostic imaging findings. Treatment of acute pancreatitis includes administering intravenous fluid therapy, analgesics, antiemetics, mucosal protectants, and feeding an ultra-low–fat diet to dogs. Fat restriction is not recommended for cats because of the high requirement of arachidonic acid in their diet; however, novel protein sources or hypoallergenic diets are often helpful in managing the feline patient with chronic pancreatitis. Evidence shows that early nutritional intervention is associated with improved outcomes and shorter hospital stays. Therefore feeding tube placement is often recommended to provide appropriate nutritional support for small animal patients.

Patients with chronic pancreatitis have a history of recurrent, intermittent, milder episodes of clinical signs, making diagnosis more difficult. Chronic pancreatitis can lead to exocrine pancreatic insufficiency (EPI) or DM. Symptomatic treatment of GI clinical signs, identification and treatment of concurrent disease, and treatment of EPI or DM, if present, are the mainstays of the therapeutic plan.

Exocrine Pancreatic Insufficiency. EPI is caused by insufficient production and secretion of pancreatic digestive enzymes. In dogs, this is most commonly the result of pancreatic acinar atrophy. In cats, EPI is commonly caused by chronic pancreatitis. Loss of digestive enzymes leads to maldigestion and malabsorption of ingested nutrients, causing clinical signs of polyphagia, weight loss, and chronic diarrhea with pale, fatty, and voluminous feces, referred to as *steatorrhea*. A greasy haircoat may result from poor absorption of fatty acids from the diet. EPI also leads to cobalamin (vitamin B_{12}) deficiency, particularly in cats, which contributes to weight loss and diarrhea. Documentation of a low serum trypsinlike immunoreactivity (TLI) concentration confirms the diagnosis of EPI. Treatment consists of oral replacement of pancreatic digestive enzymes given at mealtimes and parenteral supplementation of cobalamin.

Hepatobiliary System
Liver and gallbladder disease leads to various physical and laboratory abnormalities, depending on the location, chronicity, and severity of the disease process. Patients with severe hepatobiliary disease may develop hepatic encephalopathy (HE). HE results when the brain is exposed to GI toxins, such as ammonia, due to decreased liver function or portosystemic shunts, which compromise the normal functioning of liver detoxification or enterohepatic circulation. Clinical signs of HE includes altered mentation, head pressing, hypersalivation, circling, ataxia, seizures, blindness, behavior changes, lethargy, and coma.

Treatment of HE focuses on addressing any seizure activity resulting from increased intracranial pressure and decreasing the amount of ammonia in the systemic circulation; this can be achieved by decreasing ammonia production in the intestines. Therapies include oral lactulose, which decreases ammonia absorption; small, frequent meals of a diet that contains a moderately restricted amount of highly digestible proteins; antibiotic therapy to reduce ammonia-producing bacteria; and administration of probiotics to encourage the growth of beneficial intestinal bacteria. Management of acute HE also includes fluid therapy, treatment of electrolyte imbalance, administration of lactulose enemas, and treatment of seizures.

TABLE 18.11	Small Animal Gastrointestinal Diseases			
Disease	Pathogenesis	Clinical Signs	Diagnostics	Treatments
Esophagitis	Inflammation of the esophagus caused by administration of certain medications, gastroesophageal reflux, chronic vomiting, ingestion of caustic agents May lead to ulcers and stricture	Regurgitation Excessive drooling Anorexia Vomiting	History and clinical signs Plain and contrast radiographs are helpful Endoscopy ± biopsy is definitive	Antacids Promotility drugs Mucosal protectants Antibiotics Gastrostomy feeding tube Analgesics
Acute gastritis	Inflammation of the stomach mucosa often caused by ingestion of spoiled food, toxic plants, foreign objects, or irritating drugs	Acute vomiting Hematemesis Abdominal discomfort Anorexia	History and clinical signs Radiography Minimum database	Appropriate symptomatic therapies Removal of foreign body Treatment of toxicity
Gastrointestinal (GI) obstruction	Obstruction of the stomach or intestines Potential causes include intussusception, foreign body, neoplastic mass	Acute, severe, intractable vomiting Abdominal pain Diarrhea Sepsis Shock	History and clinical signs Plain and contrast radiography Ultrasonography Minimum database	Appropriate symptomatic therapies Treatment of shock Surgical correction of cause
GI ulcers	Defect in the mucosal layer caused by administration of nonsteroidal anti-inflammatory drugs, neoplasia, and liver disease	Anorexia Vomiting Hematemesis Melena	History and clinical signs Endoscopy, direct visualization, and biopsy	Appropriate symptomatic therapies Eliminate underlying cause
Acute enteritis	Inflammation of the intestinal mucosa often caused by infectious agents (viral, bacterial, parasitic), dietary changes, or indiscretions	Small bowel diarrhea ± vomiting Abdominal pain Fever Anorexia	Fecal analyses Serum viral testing	Appropriate symptomatic therapies
Canine antibiotic-responsive enteropathy (ARE)	Abnormal host immune response to an elevated number of bacteria in the small intestines	Diarrhea Weight loss	History, clinical signs, and response to treatment Routine fecal analysis to rule out parasites	Empirical broad-spectrum antibiotic therapy
Inflammatory bowel disease	Idiopathic intestinal inflammation; antigenic hypersensitivity is currently believed to the main cause	Chronic, recurrent pattern of weight loss, vomiting, diarrhea, and/or anorexia Thickened bowel loops on palpation	Exclude all other causes of clinical signs Full-thickness biopsy of the intestines	Appropriate symptomatic therapies Nutritional management Cobalamin supplementation in cats Immunosuppressant therapy for severe cases
Colitis	Inflammation of the colon caused by parasites, diet, bacteria	Large bowel diarrhea	Fecal analyses Endoscopy and biopsy for severe and/or prolonged cases	Appropriate symptomatic therapies
Feline idiopathic megacolon	Dysfunction of the colonic smooth muscle that results in a dilated and hypomotile colon Cause unknown	Chronic constipation Tenesmus Vomiting Abdominal pain Weight loss	Radiography demonstrates megacolon	Appropriate symptomatic therapies Subtotal or total colectomy

Diagnosing hepatobiliary disease involves laboratory analyses, diagnostic imaging (radiography and ultrasonography), and histopathologic examination. Serum assays may reveal increases in liver enzymes, hyperbilirubinemia, hyperammonemia, bile acids, hypoglycemia, and hypoalbuminemia. Abnormal UA findings include bilirubinuria and the presence of bilirubin crystals and ammonium biurate crystals. Treatment is specific to the diagnosed disease and often includes nutritional support, antioxidant therapy, antibiotics, and/or anti-inflammatories.

Feline Hepatic Lipidosis. *Feline hepatic lipidosis* (FHL) is characterized by the accumulation of lipids or fats within the cytoplasm of greater than 80% of hepatocytes. As hepatocytes swell, cholestasis and hepatic damage result. Hepatic lipidosis is caused by a lipid metabolism derangement associated with prolonged anorexia. Obese cats are predisposed to FHL; however, any cat experiencing prolonged anorexia is at risk for developing the disease. FHL is idiopathic and secondary to environmental stressors or concurrent diseases that promote prolonged anorexia (e.g., other hepatobiliary diseases, pancreatitis, or IBD). In addition to anorexia, clinical signs of FHL include recent, dramatic weight loss; lethargy; vomiting; icterus, dehydration; and palpable hepatomegaly; some patients develop HE. A definitive diagnosis of FHL requires a liver biopsy. A presumptive diagnosis is made based on history, physical examination, diagnostic imaging, and serum chemistry results. Additional diagnostics may be necessary to diagnose a concurrent disease process. FHL is a potentially lethal disease; however, early and aggressive treatment, particularly nutritional support, greatly improves patient survival.

TECHNICIAN NOTE

Hepatic lipidosis is a predominantly feline condition caused by a lipid metabolism derangement associated with prolonged anorexia. Obese cats that are anorexic have a high risk of developing the syndrome.

Canine Chronic Hepatitis. *Hepatitis* is defined as inflammation of the liver parenchyma. Chronic hepatitis (CH) indicates a history of liver disease for a prolonged period—usually longer than 4–6 months. Causes of CH include viral infection, leptospirosis, copper storage disease, and hepatotoxic drugs. However, most cases are idiopathic and have a suspected autoimmune component. The progression of the disease is characterized by hepatocyte swelling and necrosis, loss of hepatic mass and subsequent loss of liver function, hepatic fibrosis, portal hypertension (high blood pressure in the portal veins), and cirrhosis (liver fibrosis). Clinical signs are generally nonspecific, including vomiting, diarrhea, anorexia, weight loss, **polyuria/polydipsia**, and occasionally **icterus**.

Portal hypertension may occur with some diseases or injuries. Blood pressure in the portal vein and surrounding smaller vessels becomes elevated, increasing pressure on the liver. Patients with portal hypertension often exhibit ascites, evidence of GI ulcerations, and/or HE.

Clinical signs of CH are usually not apparent until 75% of the liver mass is lost, making early detection of liver dysfunction imperative. At annual examinations, routine screening of liver enzymes, particularly for predisposed breeds, is the best approach. A definitive diagnosis of CH is made based on liver biopsy; however, clinical signs, persistently elevated serum liver enzymes, abnormal liver function assays, and diagnostic imaging of microhepatica support a presumptive diagnosis.

Portosystemic Shunt. A *portosystemic shunt* (PSS) is an extra vessel that develops in or outside the liver. This unnatural vessel shunts (diverts) blood from the liver, which results in blood bypassing the liver either partially or wholly, causing abnormal liver function. Many puppies with liver shunts will be smaller than the rest of the litter and fail to thrive as they age. While it can occur in any breed of dog or cat, toy and small breed dogs are overrepresented. Extrahepatic shunts are congenital and typically involve one or two vessels that connect the portal vein to the vena cava. Intrahepatic shunts can be congenital or acquired secondary to portal hypertension and are multiple small shunts within the hepatic parenchyma.

Clinical signs include HE, polyuria/polydipsia, and signs of bladder irritation secondary to urate stone formation. Lethargy, anorexia, and seizures may occur as the patient experiences hypoglycemia and high ammonia levels owing to the undeveloped liver. Patients can also present with neurologic signs after eating a meal or hypoglycemic episodes. Young patients with congenital PSS are often unthrifty and have a poor BCS and dull haircoats.

Diagnosing a PSS is based on elevated serum postprandial bile acids, hyperammonemia, and direct visualization of the shunting vessel(s) via diagnostic imaging or during surgery. Congenital PSS is generally diagnosed in cats and dogs younger than 2 years of age. Acquired PSS is typically seen in older dogs as sequelae of CH. For extrahepatic PSS, surgical ligation of the shunt is the treatment of choice. Medical management of HE is required immediately before and for 2 months after surgery. Surgical ligation of intrahepatic shunts is not achievable, so treatment relies on the medical management of HE.

Feline Cholangitis/Cholangiohepatitis. *Cholangitis* refers to inflammation of the bile ducts. In some cases, inflammation spreads to the liver, termed *cholangiohepatitis*. Cholangitis/cholangiohepatitis can be acute or chronic. Acute cholangitis is caused by an ascending bacterial infection from the small intestines and is characterized by neutrophilic inflammation. Clinical signs include fever, vomiting, lethargy, icterus, and abdominal pain. Chronic cholangitis is characterized by lymphocytic-plasmacytic inflammation; the cause is unknown. Immune-mediated disease, progression of acute cholangitis, and liver fluke infection have been implicated in the development of chronic cholangitis. Clinical signs include anorexia, weight loss, lethargy, and icterus. Diagnosis and differentiation between the two forms rely on history, clinical signs, blood work, diagnostic imaging, bile culture, and liver biopsy. Treatment is primarily the same for both forms of the disease: fluid therapy, antioxidants, antibiotics, ursodiol (prescription bile acid), nutritional support, and vitamin supplementation. Glucocorticoid therapy may be added for the treatment of chronic cholangitis.

Urinary Disease

The International Renal Interest Society (IRIS) has proposed a five-tier system for staging acute kidney injury (AKI) and a four-tier system for staging CKD based on serum creatinine concentration. In addition to creatinine, CKD staging also includes evaluating serum symmetric dimethylarginine (SDMA) levels. This system also provides for substages of CKD based on the presence and severity of proteinuria and systemic hypertension. Table 18.12 summarizes the CKD staging system and provides a correlation with urine specific gravity (USG), percentage of remaining kidney function, and clinical signs. AKI may be subgraded based on the presence of oliguria or anuria and if renal replacement therapy is required. Staging and grading of AKI and CKD helps direct patient treatment, monitor plans, and determine prognosis. Further information can be found on the IRIS website.

Clinical signs of kidney disease relate to impairment of fluid homeostasis, uremia (the buildup of toxins in the bloodstream), and electrolyte abnormalities that result from diminishing kidney function. Diagnosis of renal disease is based on serial documentation of **azotemia**. *Azotemia* refers to serum elevations of the protein metabolites creatinine and blood urea nitrogen (BUN). USG measures the concentration of urine and reflects patient hydration status and kidney function. Less than adequate USG in a well-hydrated patient indicates the impaired urine-concentrating ability of the kidney.

Acute Kidney Injury

AKI results from a dramatic, quick decrease in glomerular filtration (GF) rate and is often reversible if diagnosis and subsequent treatment are made early.

Three groups characterize AKI causes: prerenal (before the kidneys), intrinsic (inside the kidneys), and postrenal (after the kidneys). Prerenal azotemia is not caused by primary kidney disease but rather by decreased cardiac output, resulting in inadequate blood supply to the kidneys. Intrinsic damage to the kidneys occurs from damage to the renal parenchyma, specifically to the

TABLE 18.12   IRIS CKD Staging in Dogs and Cats

A. IRIS CKD STAGE			
Stage		Dogs	Cats
Stage I	Creatinine	<1.4 mg/dL (<125 mcmol/L)	<1.6 mg/dL (<140 mcmol/L)
	SDMA	<18 ng/dL	<18 ng/dL
Stage II	Creatinine	1.4-2.8 mg/dL (125-250 mcmol/L)	1.6-2.8 mg/dL (140-250 mcmol/L)
	SDMA	18-35 ng/dL	18-25 ng/dL
Stage III	Creatinine	2.9-5.0 mg/dL (251-440 mcmol/L)	2.9-5.0 mg/dL (251-440 mcmol/L)
	SDMA	36-54 ng/dL	26-38 ng/dL
Stage IV	Creatinine	>5.0 mg/dL (>440 mcmol/L)	>5.0 mg/dL (>440 mcmol/L)
	SDMA	>54 ng/dL	>38 ng/dL

A. SUBSTAGING BY PROTEINURIA		
URINE PROTEIN-TO-CREATININE RATIO		
Substage	Dogs	Cats
Proteinuric (P)	>0.5	>0.4
Borderline proteinuric (BP)	0.2-0.5	0.2-0.4
Nonproteinuric (NP)	<0.2	<0.2

I. SUBSTAGING BY BLOOD PRESSURE		
Blood Pressure Substage	Systolic Blood Pressure (mm Hg)	Risk of Target Organ Damage
Normotensive	<140	Minimal
Prehypertensive	140 to 159	Low
Hypertensive	160 to 179	Moderate
Severe hypertensive	≥180	High

CKD, Chronic kidney disease; *IRIS*, International Renal Interest Society; *SDMA*, symmetric dimethylarginine.
Used with permission from http://www.iris-kidney.com/pdf/2_IRIS_Staging_of_CKD_2023.pdf. © Copyright 2023 International Renal Interest Society.

vasculature, glomeruli, tubular epithelium, and interstitium of the kidney. In cats, the most common causes occur from toxins, infectious diseases, and ischemic causes (such as heatstroke, pancreatitis, and DIC). The kidney is particularly vulnerable to toxins because of its high blood filtration rate. Postrenal causes occur from obstruction or rupture of the urinary tract system.

Lily Intoxication
Lilies are a common toxicity in cats and, while the principal toxic factor is still unknown, it is known that all parts of the plant are toxic, including pollen. After initial ingestion of the plant, cats may exhibit GI signs such as nausea and vomiting. Signs develop within 12 hours, but the plant may still affect the body for 2 to 5 days after ingestion. Although the exact amount needed to produce a toxic effect is unknown, it is known that even a single bite can cause clinical signs, which is why any cat exposed to a lily plant should be treated as if it were going to suffer nephrotoxic effects.

Pyelonephritis
One of the most common diseases that causes AKI in cats is pyelonephritis. Pyelonephritis (inflammation of the kidneys) most commonly occurs secondary to a lower urinary tract infection

(UTI). Clinical signs may include fever, vomiting, anorexia, and abdominal pain upon palpating the kidneys. Most commonly, *Escherichia coli* (*E. coli*) is the isolated organism. Antibiotics that are specific to the organism isolated should be administered as a treatment along with treating the AKI clinical signs.

Urethral Obstruction
Another common AKI insult is urethral obstruction. It is most seen in young to middle-aged male cats. Cats with feline interstitial (idiopathic) cystitis (FIC) are more likely to become obstructed. AKI may occur in cats that have been obstructed for an extended period. When a cat becomes obstructed, the pressure within the urethra and urinary bladder will continue to increase, affecting the ureters and nephrons. Eventually, the pressure alters the GF until the rate is zero. Early detection and treatment are imperative to correct azotemia.

Obstruction may also occur because of bilateral or unilateral obstruction of a kidney from nephroliths or ureteroliths (most commonly calcium oxalate). Cats with unilateral ureteral obstruction may be asymptomatic, and clinical signs may occur only when the kidney becomes enlarged due to hydronephrosis. Bilateral ureteral obstruction will result in more clinical signs, including azotemia, vomiting, hematuria, and anorexia.

diagnostics may be required in some patients to reach a diagnosis, including measurement of the free T_4 concentration, T_3 suppression tests, and thyroid scintigraphy. Three-view chest radiographs are recommended to rule out the possibility of metastatic thyroid carcinoma. Secondary thyrotoxic hypertrophic cardiomyopathy and systemic hypertension are commonly seen, as well as concurrent CKD. These disease processes must be monitored for, diagnosed, and managed as part of overall patient care.

Treatment of hyperthyroidism falls into two categories: curative and palliative. Palliative treatment consists of antithyroid medication, typically methimazole, given once or twice daily to block thyroid hormone synthesis, thus decreasing the levels of circulating thyroid hormones. The dose is titrated to effectiveness based on frequent monitoring of T_4 levels and resolution of clinical signs. Curative treatment involves surgical removal of the thyroid gland or radioactive iodine (^{131}I) treatment. Thyroidectomy may involve the removal of one or both thyroid lobes. ^{131}I therapy, the treatment of choice for patients with healthy renal function, is provided at specialized, licensed treatment centers and typically consists of a single subcutaneous injection of ^{131}I, which is preferentially absorbed into abnormal thyroid tissue and destroys it.

Hypothyroidism

Hypothyroidism is a disease that primarily affects dogs and rarely cats, although a rare congenital form can be seen in kittens. Patients with this disease have an underactive thyroid, resulting in subnormal circulating levels of thyroid hormones, which causes a subsequent decrease in metabolic rate. In dogs, the most common causes of hypothyroidism include immune-mediated destruction and idiopathic atrophy of the gland. Clinical signs are varied, with the most common signs being weight gain, exercise intolerance, altered mentation, and lethargy caused by the decreased metabolic rate. Hypothermia, bradycardia, truncal alopecia, and seborrhea may be noted on physical examination. The diagnostic confirmation includes documenting low serum T_4 and free T_4 levels and elevated thyroid-stimulating hormone levels, evaluating CBC and a full serum chemistry panel. Treatment of hypothyroidism consists of oral T_4 replacement therapy, titrated to effectiveness based on frequent monitoring of T_4 levels and resolution of clinical signs.

Diabetes Mellitus

DM may result from insufficient production of insulin by pancreatic beta cells (type 1 or insulin-dependent) or from dysfunctional beta cells and insulin resistance characterized by the body's inability to respond appropriately to endogenous insulin (type 2 or noninsulin-dependent). Dogs tend to develop type 1 DM, but cats are prone to type 2 DM. Clinical signs include polyphagia, weight loss (often in a previously obese patient), polyuria, and polydipsia. Feline patients with an advanced form of the disease often present with a plantigrade stance; dogs may present with cataracts. Diagnosis consists of documenting persistent elevated blood glucose (hyperglycemia) with concurrent glucose in urine (glycosuria). Cats are particularly prone to stress-induced hyperglycemia, so elevated fructosamine levels are often used to help confirm DM in this species.

PUT INTO PRACTICE

The success of managing diabetes mellitus with your patients can depend on communication between your clinic and the client. Understanding the disease process and good communications skills on your part can be very helpful to your clients and their pets.

Treatment of patients with DM involves subcutaneous insulin injections, normally twice daily; dietary changes; and maintenance of a healthy BCS. As with many other hormone therapies, the insulin dose must be titrated for effectiveness through monitoring glucose levels (via serial blood glucose curves—inpatient or in the home), periodic fructosamine testing, and urine glucose monitoring. Based on these results and clinical response, the veterinarian will adjust the insulin dose. In some newly diagnosed cats, achieving tight glycemic control with insulin may lead to spontaneous remission within 3 to 4 months and subsequent discontinuation of insulin therapy, though not always. Dogs, however, need lifelong treatment. Recommendations for dietary change vary, but cats are generally given a high-protein/low-carbohydrate diet, and dogs are given a higher-fiber diet. The technician plays a vital role in client education and supporting patients with DM. Owners must be educated on monitoring for and treating hypoglycemia, properly handling and administering insulin, and performing in-home glucose curves.

Uncontrolled or undiagnosed DM will progress to *diabetic ketoacidosis* (DKA). As the patient's body remains unable to use glucose, an alternative pathway for carbohydrate metabolism is used. By-products of this pathway are ketones, which are toxic metabolites. Their presence in the urine (ketonuria) is a hallmark finding in DKA, as is a symptomatic fruity odor to the breath imparted by ketones. Patients with DKA are critically ill and can present with anorexia, depression, polyuria, polydipsia, weight loss, and vomiting. On physical examination, they are often dehydrated and hypothermic, have altered mental status, and possibly cardiac arrhythmias. Clinicopathologic abnormalities include hyperglycemia, glycosuria, ketonuria, metabolic acidosis, and decreased serum potassium, phosphorus, and sodium. Treatment of a patient with DKA is very complex and focuses on insulin therapy, fluid replacement therapy, and correction of electrolyte abnormalities and acidosis.

Hyperadrenocorticism

HAC, or Cushing syndrome, is a disease that primarily affects dogs and is characterized by elevated circulating levels of cortisol (hypercortisolemia) produced by the adrenal cortex. The cause can be a functional anterior pituitary tumor, which secretes large quantities of adrenocorticotropic hormone (ACTH), or a functional adrenal tumor, which secretes large quantities of cortisol. In some patients, both types of tumors are present. Pituitary-dependent HAC is the most common form of the disease. Cushing syndrome in the feline is rare and, when diagnosed, is almost always seen with concurrent DM. Clinical signs result from hypercortisolemia and include increased appetite, weight gain, lethargy, muscle weakness, polyuria, polydipsia, skin and haircoat abnormalities, and a pot-bellied appearance. The patient often is prone to secondary skin and urinary infections. Diagnosis of HAC is multifactorial, considering findings on physical examination, the minimum database, and the results of specialized endocrine function tests and diagnostic imaging of the brain and adrenal glands. Specialized tests that assess adrenal gland function include the ACTH stimulation test, the low-dose dexamethasone suppression test, the high-dose dexamethasone suppression test, and endogenous ACTH levels. (Refer to Chapter 12, "Clinical Chemistry, Serology, and Urinalysis.")

Treatment of patients with pituitary-dependent HAC consists of pharmacologic intervention to decrease the amount of cortisol produced by the adrenal glands. This can be achieved by using a drug that promotes the complete or partial destruction of adrenal cortex tissue (mitotane) or one that inhibits the synthetic pathway of cortisol production (trilostane). The treatment of choice for adrenal-dependent HAC is the surgical removal of the adrenal tumor(s). The patient is placed on glucocorticoid (in some cases, mineralocorticoid) replacement therapy immediately after surgery. If both adrenal glands are removed, this therapy continues lifelong. If only one gland is removed, replacement therapy can usually be discontinued within 3 months as the remaining adrenal gland regains normal functioning. Adrenalectomy is the treatment of choice in feline patients with either form of the disease.

Hypoadrenocorticism

Hypoadrenocorticism, or Addison disease, primarily affects dogs and is caused by adrenal gland atrophy or destruction, resulting in inadequate secretion of glucocorticoids and mineralocorticoids, primarily cortisol and aldosterone. Common historical information on these patients includes episodic events of anorexia, vomiting, diarrhea, polyuria, polydipsia, weakness, and collapse—especially during periods of stress. Weight loss, bradycardia, weak femoral pulses, altered mentation, and prolonged CRT can be seen on physical examination of a patient experiencing a hypoadrenocortical (addisonian) crisis. Common clinical pathologic abnormalities in these patients include anemia, azotemia, hypoglycemia, and elevated serum potassium (hyperkalemia), with a concurrent decrease in sodium (hyponatremia). Definitive diagnosis is made based on an ACTH stimulation test that reveals low cortisol levels before and after administration of ACTH. Treatment of the acute patient is a medical emergency and focuses on treating dehydration and electrolyte imbalance, managing GI clinical signs, and administering glucocorticoids. Long-term disease management is achieved through mineralocorticoid supplementation, with some dogs also requiring glucocorticoid replacement therapy.

Immune-mediated Disease

Immune-mediated diseases are those in which the immune system of an animal fails to adequately recognize its own tissues and cells as "self." Consequently, the animal's immune system labels cells and tissues with antigens, triggering an immune response against parts of the animal's body. Autoimmunity may be primary (idiopathic) or secondary (resulting from an underlying disease process). Secondary immune-mediated disease can result from infection, cancer, vaccine administration, or exposure to certain drugs or toxins.

TECHNICIAN NOTE

Immune-mediated diseases are those in which the immune system has lost tolerance of self and perpetuates damage to the body's organs.

Immune-mediated Hemolytic Anemia

Hemolytic anemia is characterized by RBC destruction. One cause of hemolytic anemia, and the most common cause in dogs, is the destruction of RBCs by the immune system. *Immune-mediated hemolytic anemia (IMHA)* may be primary or secondary, although alternative terminology (nonassociative and associative, respectively) has been proposed by the 2019 American College of Veterinary Internal Medicine (ACVIM) consensus statement on the diagnosis of IMHA in dogs and cats.[2] Primary IMHA is idiopathic and occurs in most cases in dogs, whereas IMHA secondary to blood parasite infection is more common in the cat. In primary IMHA, the immune system targets RBCs as foreign (an antigen) and develops autoantibodies against RBC membrane components which, in turn, are targeted for destruction. Secondary IMHA, such as a *Babesia* spp. or *Mycoplasma* spp. infection, is responsible as an underlying cause for the massive immune response and can often be treated. Clinical signs of IMHA include lethargy, exercise intolerance, pale or yellow mucous membranes, tachycardia, heart murmur, splenomegaly, hepatomegaly, fever, and abdominal pain. Diagnosis is based on CBC findings consistent with hemolytic anemia and evidence of autoimmunity: autoagglutination and a positive Coombs test result. A Coombs test is less frequently run in practice (see Chapter 11). Once the diagnosis of IMHA is made, the search for an underlying disease is undertaken, although if no underlying disease can be documented, primary IMHA is diagnosed. Treatment for IMHA includes immunosuppressive therapy, judicious use of blood transfusions, fluid therapy, and treatment of any underlying disease. Patients with acute, severe anemia will be hypoxic and may benefit from oxygen supplementation, at least until a transfusion can be performed to increase oxygen-carrying capacity. Although glucocorticoids are almost always used in these patients, combination therapy (e.g., azathioprine, cyclosporin, mycophenolate, or leflunomide) is often required to achieve remission. Thromboembolism is a common and often fatal complication of IMHA; therefore anticoagulant treatment is also instituted. Treatment of IMHA can be both intensive and costly, requiring significant owner commitment. Most patients will require at least 3 to 6 months of immunosuppressive therapy; some may require a much longer duration of treatment. Client education and communication with the veterinary health care team is imperative for successfully managing these cases.

PUT INTO PRACTICE

Good communication skills are imperative when a technician engages in client communication. Practice active listening skills and support your clients when they ask questions. Let the clients lead you to what they need.

Immune-mediated Polyarthritis

Patients with polyarthropathies often display lethargy, lameness, stiffness, spinal pain, or reluctance to walk due to inflammation of multiple joints. A diagnosis of immune-mediated polyarthritis (IMPA) is one of exclusion. It can only be reached after the possibility of septic arthritis and infectious agents, such as vector-borne agents, have been excluded. Patients often have a fever of unknown origin and may show signs of systemic illness (e.g., anorexia, weight loss, etc.). On physical examination, determining if one or multiple joints are involved is often difficult, and arthrocentesis from multiple joints is recommended. Fluid analysis and cytology will be consistent with sterile inflammation, and the carpal and tarsal joints may be more affected. Immunosuppressive treatment with glucocorticoids is typical, but secondary agents such as cyclosporin, mycophenolate, or leflunomide may be required to achieve remission. The minimum recommended duration of therapy is 4 months, but some patients may require more long-term management. A strict medication schedule should be discussed with the pet owners in detail, as a rapid tapering of immunosuppressive drugs can increase the chance of patient relapse.

Acquired (Immune-mediated) Myasthenia Gravis

Myasthenia gravis (MG) is a disorder of neuromuscular transmission that causes muscle weakness. Acquired MG is caused by an immune system dysfunction that produces autoantibodies against acetylcholine receptors in the postsynaptic membrane. This is differentiated from congenital MG, an inherited deficiency of these receptors. Acquired MG is more common in dogs than in cats. The main clinical sign is a generalized weakness that is worsened by exercise and resolves with rest, although megaesophagus is a common finding. If the patient has megaesophagus due to the disease, hypersalivation and regurgitation are evident. The presence of autoantibodies against acetylcholine receptors in the serum confirms the diagnosis. The presence of megaesophagus is determined by using radiography with treatment including the administration of immunosuppressive drugs and anticholinesterase inhibitors, prolonging the action of acetylcholine at the synapses by blocking the enzyme (acetylcholinesterase) that degrades the acetylcholine, thereby improving muscle strength. Patients with megaesophagus and regurgitation are at risk for aspiration (refer to Table 18.5); appropriate nursing care for regurgitation is instituted.

Infectious Disease

Infectious diseases are caused by pathogenic micro-organisms that invade and colonize the tissues and fluids of an individual animal (host). Infectious diseases are prevalent in cats and dogs and involve many pathogens, such as viruses, bacteria, fungi, and rickettsia (see Chapter 13, "Endoparasites" section). The required components and steps of infection are as follows (Fig. 18.2):

1. *The pathogen:* Must be able to avoid host defense systems, reproduce in the host, and cause disease.
2. *Reservoir:* Can be an animal, insect, or fomite (inanimate objects, such as water bowls, cages, clipper blades, instruments, towels, scrubs, etc.) in which the pathogen can survive.
3. *Portal of exit (from the animate reservoir):* Where/how the pathogen leaves the reservoir, often related to clinical signs of the disease process (e.g., sneezing).
4. *Mode of transmission:* How the pathogen travels to the next host:
   a. Direct transmission is immediate and requires direct contact of skin or mucous membranes with an infected animal or its secretions or excretions (e.g., nose-to-nose contact can transmit feline herpesvirus), ingestion of virus (e.g., ingestion of parvovirus-laden feces), or inhalation of virus (e.g., inhalation of aerosolized canine parainfluenza virus).
   b. Indirect transmission is delayed and requires contact with a contaminated fomite (e.g., transmission of ringworm through contaminated clipper blades) or is transmitted via a biological vector, usually an insect (e.g., heartworm disease transmitted via mosquito bite). The hands of veterinary personnel can also be considered a vector.
   c. Transplacental or transmammary transmission.
5. *Portal of entry (route of infection):* Where/how the pathogen gains entry into the new host.
6. *Host susceptibility:* Exposure to a pathogen does not guarantee infection and disease. The host must be susceptible to the pathogen due to a naïve, immature, suppressed, or deficient immune system and is unable to kill the pathogen. However, other considerations, such as species specificity (dogs cannot contract feline herpesvirus), opportunity for exposure (a city-dwelling dog that never leaves an apartment and is not taken to areas where other dogs congregate is less likely to be exposed to canine influenza virus), and geographic location of the host (specific tick vectors are found only in particular areas), could be listed here.

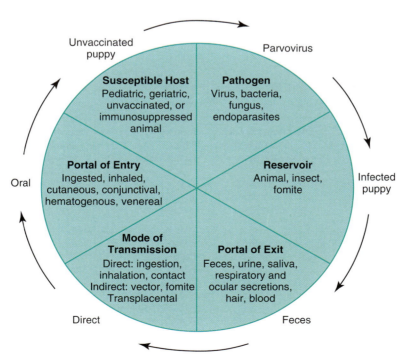

• **Fig. 18.2** Required steps for infection of transmissible diseases.

It is helpful to classify transmissible infectious diseases. Infectious pathogens transmitted directly between animals or indirectly through fomites contaminated with animal secretions are considered contagious (e.g., canine infectious respiratory disease). Infectious diseases that require a biological vector are termed *vector-borne* (e.g., Lyme disease). Zoonoses are infectious diseases transmitted directly from animals to humans (e.g., rabies virus). Infectious agents that can infect a human or an animal via a common vector (fleas, ticks) are called *shared-vector zoonoses*. *Reverse zoonoses* are infectious diseases transmitted from humans to animals (e.g., dermatophytosis).

Control of transmissible infectious diseases involves interrupting the process of infection:

1. Kill the pathogen while it is in the host or animate reservoir: Antibiotic, antiviral, or antiparasitic medication.
2. Kill the pathogen while living on a fomite: Sanitation, disinfection, sterilization.
3. Kill the pathogen while living in/on a vector: Preventive antiparasitic medication, environmental pesticide, soap and water. (Wash your hands between patients!)
4. Strengthen host defense systems:
   a. Administer vaccination (see Chapter 8).
   b. Maintain proper health and nutrition.
5. Decrease host exposure:
   a. Limit exposure of immunodeficient and immunosuppressed individuals, for example, by a change in lifestyle (e.g., cats with feline immunodeficiency virus should be housed indoors).
   b. Follow proper isolation protocols for contagious animals to prevent the spread of disease.

Nursing Care

Patients with infectious diseases often require extensive nursing care and support while the patient's body fights the infection. This is especially true of infections in which there is no direct way to destroy the pathogen (e.g., antibiotics), as occurs with viral infections. Supportive care requires attending to the patient's basic needs and treating clinical signs, such as nasal discharge, vomiting, or dehydration. Many infectious diseases compromise the function of the immune system, putting patients at risk for secondary infection. Monitoring these patients for signs of secondary infections while administering prescribed prophylactic antibiotic therapy is essential (Table 18.5).

Client Education

Veterinary technicians have a critical role in educating and supporting the owner of a pet with a transmissible infectious disease. Many infectious diseases can be prevented with vaccines. Most infectious diseases can be treated on an outpatient basis, with the bulk of care falling to the owner when a pet becomes ill. The veterinary technician must provide oral and written instructions on patient care, demonstrate medication administration techniques, educate the owner on isolation procedures to control the spread of the disease to other animals in the household, zoonotic potential (e.g., ringworm), and provide information about household disinfection protocols. The veterinary technician must provide support throughout this process, which can be overwhelming and frustrating for pet owners. Frequent phone calls and in-office visits will ensure owner support and compliance, thereby completing patient care.

Small Animal Infectious Diseases

Barrier nursing refers to a set of infection control practices designed to limit the transmission of infectious agents. It may involve the use of physical barriers, such as gloves, gowns, and masks, to prevent direct contact and exposure to potentially harmful micro-organisms. Barrier nursing is particularly essential when dealing with highly contagious diseases or patients with compromised immune systems and is of vital importance to prevent the spread of disease. It is beyond the scope of this chapter to provide detailed information on all infectious diseases seen in small animals; instead, focus is placed on clinically relevant contagious diseases and important zoonotic diseases seen in the clinical setting (see Tables 18.14–18.19).

TABLE 18.14	Contagious Diseases of the Respiratory Tract				
Disease and Pathogen	**Mode of Transmission**	**Pathogenesis**	**Clinical Signs**	**Diagnostics**	**Treatments**
Feline upper respiratory tract disease Feline herpesvirus-1 (FHV-1)*	Direct: contact with mucosal secretions Indirect: contaminated fomites	Viral replication in the mucosal lining of the upper respiratory tract, conjunctiva, and tonsils Secondary infections ensue Infection usually leads to asymptomatic carrier state with chronic flare-ups	Rhinitis Conjunctivitis Anorexia Fever Corneal ulcers	History and clinical signs Virus isolation and detection can be performed but is generally reserved for chronic cases	Relieve nasal congestion Airway humidification Treat anorexia Treat corneal ulcers Treat conjunctivitis Treat dehydration Antibiotics for secondary infection Decrease stress
Feline upper respiratory tract disease Feline calicivirus (FCV)*	Direct: contact with mucosal secretions Indirect: contaminated fomites	Viral replication in the epithelial lining of the upper respiratory tract, conjunctiva, and tongue Secondary infections ensue Infection usually leads to asymptomatic carrier state with chronic flare-ups	Rhinitis Conjunctivitis Fever Gagging, hypersalivation due to lingual and oral ulcers Anorexia Joint pain	History and clinical signs Virus isolation and detection can be performed but is generally reserved for severe cases	Airway humidification Treat conjunctivitis Treat anorexia Relieve oral ulcer pain: Systemic analgesics Topical diluted lidocaine Antibiotics for secondary infection Decrease stress

TABLE 18.14 Contagious Diseases of the Respiratory Tract—cont'd

Disease and Pathogen	Mode of Transmission	Pathogenesis	Clinical Signs	Diagnostics	Treatments
Canine infectious respiratory disease (kennel cough, infectious tracheobronchitis) Multifactorial: canine adenovirus type 2 (CAV-2); canine herpesvirus 1 (CHV-1); canine parainfluenza virus (CPIV); *Bordetella bronchiseptica*	Direct: contact with mucosal secretions or environmental fomites Direct: inhalation of airborne virus *Note:* Cats are also susceptible to *B. bronchiseptica*	Viral replication in the respiratory epithelium	Acute, harsh cough Gagging/retching Nasal/ocular discharge Tracheal sensitivity Hyporexia	History and clinical signs	Avoid exercise and excitement Decrease pressure on trachea: harness versus collar Maintain hydration ± Antibiotics ± Antitussives

*FHC-1 and FCV are common coinfections present in up to 80% of patients with clinical signs.

TABLE 18.15 Contagious Diseases of the Digestive and Hepatobiliary Systems

Disease and Pathogen	Mode of Transmission	Pathogenesis	Clinical Signs	Diagnostics	Treatments
Feline panleukopenia Feline parvovirus (FPV)	Direct: ingestion of feces (fecal-oral) Indirect: contaminated fomites Transplacental	Replication of the virus within the intestinal crypts, bone marrow, and lymphoid tissue Secondary sepsis common	Anorexia Lethargy Fever Vomiting Dehydration Abdominal pain ± Diarrhea Septic shock Cerebellar hypoplasia	History Clinical signs CBC: leukopenia Fecal parvovirus antigen ELISA test	Control vomiting Treat dehydration and electrolyte imbalance Treat anorexia Treat hyperthermia Antibiotics to treat/prevent secondary bacterial infections Monitor for sepsis
Canine parvoviral enteritis Canine parvovirus (CPV-2)	Direct: ingestion of feces Indirect: contaminated fomites	Replication of the virus within the intestinal crypts, bone marrow, and lymphoid tissue Secondary sepsis and protein-losing enteropathy common	Anorexia Lethargy Fever Vomiting Diarrhea, often bloody Dehydration Abdominal pain Septic shock	History Clinical signs CBC: leukopenia Fecal parvovirus antigen ELISA test	Control vomiting Treat dehydration and electrolyte imbalance Treat anorexia Administer plasma to treat hypoalbuminemia Antibiotics to treat/prevent secondary bacterial infection Monitor for sepsis
Canine infectious hepatitis Canine adenovirus type 1 (CAV-1)	Direct: ingestion of saliva, feces, urine	Infection begins in the tonsils and spreads to the liver, spleen, kidneys, lungs, and vascular endothelial cells	Fever Injected mucous membranes Petechiation Enlarged tonsils Anorexia Dehydration Prolonged bleeding Signs of hepatitis	History and clinical signs Virus isolation	Treat dehydration Administer blood products Prophylactic antibiotic therapy

CBC, Complete blood count; *ELISA,* enzyme-linked immunosorbent assay.

TABLE 18.16   Polysystemic Contagious Diseases

Disease and Pathogen	Mode of Transmission	Pathogenesis	Clinical Signs	Diagnostics	Treatments
Feline leukemia Feline leukemia virus (FeLV)	Direct: contact with saliva, nasal secretions Iatrogenic transmission though blood transfusion or contaminated needles	Virus replicates in oropharyngeal lymphoid tissue, then spreads to the spleen, thymus, lymph nodes, and bone marrow Patients may become latent carriers	Anorexia Weight loss Fever Generalized lymphadenopathy Signs of severe anemia Evidence of immunosuppression: gingivitis, chronic viral respiratory disease, etc. Evidence of lymphoma	FeLV antigen testing (ELISA and IFA) on blood, bone marrow	Maintain good husbandry and nutritional health Keep animal indoors Semiannual physical examinations, preventive medicine, and routine laboratory work to monitor for anemia Routine dental prophylaxis Antiviral therapy Immunomodulators Blood transfusion Chemotherapy (for lymphoma)
Feline immunodeficiency Feline immunodeficiency virus (FIV)	Direct: inoculation of saliva through bite wounds Transplacental Iatrogenic transmission though blood transfusion	Virus replicates in the salivary glands and lymphoid tissue Patients may become latent carriers	Weight loss Generalized lymphadenopathy Fever Anterior uveitis Evidence of immunosuppression: gingivitis, chronic viral respiratory disease, etc. Evidence of lymphoma	FIV antibody testing (ELISA and Western blot) on blood	Maintain good husbandry and nutritional health Keep indoors Semiannual physical examinations, preventive medicine, and routine laboratory work Routine dental prophylaxis Antiviral therapy Immunomodulators Treatment of secondary disease
Feline infectious peritonitis (FIP) Feline coronavirus (FCoV)	Direct: ingestion of feces (fecal-oral) Indirect: contaminated fomites	Virus replicates in the intestinal tract, a portion with mutated and infected macrophages, thus disseminating throughout the body and causing the clinical disease	*Effusive Form* • Ascites • Pleural effusion • Weight loss • Fever • Anorexia *Noneffusive Form* • Uveitis • CNS signs • Signs of organ failure as granulomas form in the liver, spleen, kidneys, and GI tract	History and clinical signs Serum globulin and albumin concentrations Cytologic examination and analysis of effusions Antigen detection in effusive fluid Tissue biopsy	Thoracocentesis or abdominocentesis Corticosteroids to reduce immune overreaction Immunomodulators
Canine distemper Canine distemper virus (CDV)	Direct: inhalation of airborne virus Direct: contact with urine, feces, mucosal secretions	Infection starts in lymphatic system of the respiratory tract and spreads to the GI and urogenital tracts, and to CNS and optic nerves. Progression of clinical signs often follows progression of infection	Nasal discharge Ocular discharge Cough Fever Diarrhea Anorexia Lethargy Hyperkeratosis of foot pads, nasal planum CNS signs: • Seizures • Head tilt • Ataxia • Paralysis	Clinical signs Antibody titers Virus isolation	Treat dehydration Antibiotics Anticonvulsants Antipyretics Analgesics Anti-inflammatories

TABLE 18.16	Polysystemic Contagious Diseases—cont'd				
Disease and Pathogen	**Mode of Transmission**	**Pathogenesis**	**Clinical Signs**	**Diagnostics**	**Treatments**
Leptospirosis *Leptospira* spp.	Direct: contact with urine Indirect: contaminated fomites *Note:* Cattle and wildlife are reservoirs	Bacterial infection ensues in multiple tissues, particularly liver and kidneys	Anorexia Fever Joint pain Vomiting Diarrhea Evidence of hemorrhage Evidence of hepatitis Evidence of kidney disease Evidence of leptospiral pulmonary hemorrhage syndrome (LPHS)	History and clinical signs Serology/PCR	Antibiotics Treat dehydration Treat kidney disease Treat liver disease

CNS, Central nervous system; *ELISA,* enzyme-linked immunosorbent assay; *GI,* gastrointestinal; *IFA,* indirect fluorescent antibody test; *PCR,* polymerase chain reaction.

TABLE 18.17	Contagious Diseases of the Nervous System and Skin				
Disease and Pathogen	**Mode of Transmission**	**Pathogenesis**	**Clinical Signs**	**Diagnostics**	**Treatments**
Rabies Rabies virus (RV)	Direct: inoculation of saliva into skin, usually through a bite wound *Note:* Reservoir is usually wildlife	The virus travels from peripheral nerves to spinal cord and brain, and then from brain to salivary glands via peripheral nerves Rapid progression of neurologic signs ensues	Apprehension Nervousness Hyperexcitability Aggression Seizures Paralysis Hypersalivation Inability to swallow	Postmortem virus isolation in brain tissue	No therapeutic protocols for infected patients Infection is lethal
Ringworm (dermatophytosis) *Microsporum* spp. and *Trichophyton* spp.	Direct: contact with skin, hair, claws Indirect: contaminated fomites	Dermatophytes infect growing hairs, penetrating the hair shaft and hair follicle and causing a local inflammatory response	Alopecia Erythema Crusting, scaly skin Hyperpigmentation Folliculitis	Dermatophyte test medium culture Direct microscopic evaluation of hair or skin scraping	Topical antifungals: • Ointments • Bath/dip Oral antifungals

TABLE 18.18	Vector-Borne Pathogens				
Disease and Pathogen	**Vector**	**Pathogenesis**	**Clinical Signs**	**Diagnostics**	**Treatments**
Lyme disease *Borrelia burgdorferi*	*Ixodes* spp. tick	Bacterial infection and subsequent inflammation of various tissues, including skin, joint capsule, lymph nodes, kidney, liver, and heart	Fever Anorexia Lameness Swollen joints Lymphadenopathy Signs of kidney failure	History and clinical signs Serology Analysis of joint effusion	Antibiotics Treatment for specific organ damage
Rocky Mountain spotted fever *Rickettsia rickettsii*	*Dermacentor* spp. tick	Rickettsial infection of the vascular endothelium, causing vasculitis and secondary thrombocytopenia	Fever Depression Cough/dyspnea Vomiting/diarrhea Evidence of hemorrhage CNS signs Shock	History and clinical signs Laboratory data Serology/PCR Isolation of pathogen in body fluids and tissue	Antibiotics Fluid therapy Treatments aimed at managing organ-specific damage

Continued

TABLE 18.18 Vector-Borne Pathogens—cont'd

Disease and Pathogen	Vector	Pathogenesis	Clinical Signs	Diagnostics	Treatments
Canine ehrlichiosis *Ehrlichia* spp.	*Rhipicephalus* spp. tick	Rickettsial infection of the vascular endothelium, causing vasculitis and the appearance of macrophages which disseminate throughout the body, particularly to the liver and spleen	Fever Depression Lymphadenopathy Splenomegaly Hepatomegaly Evidence of hemorrhage Lameness, swollen joints	History and clinical signs Laboratory data Serology/PCR Isolation of pathogen in body fluids and tissue	Antibiotics Fluid therapy Blood transfusion Treatments aimed at managing organ-specific damage

CNS, Central nervous system; *PCR*, polymerase chain reaction.

TABLE 18.19 Selection of Small Animal Zoonoses

Disease/ Pathogen	Portal of Exit	Portal of Entry	Patient Presentation	Manifestation in Humans	Prevention in Clinical Setting
Rabies	Saliva	Skin: through bite wound Skin: open wound or abrasion	See Table 18.17.	Fever Lethargy Central nervous system (CNS) signs, including paresis and seizures	Barrier protection when handling alive or deceased patients Wash hands
Plague: *Yersinia pestis*	Respiratory secretions Pus from lymph nodes *Note:* Shared vector = Rodent fleas	Inhalation Mucous membranes Abraded skin	Cough Enlarged tonsils, mandibular and cervical lymph nodes, often draining pus	Fever Headache Swollen, draining lymph nodes	Barrier nursing protocol Wash hands Disinfect surfaces
Cat-scratch fever: *Bartonella* spp.	Flea feces *Note:* Shared vector = Cat fleas	Skin: inoculation through cat scratch or bite	May be asymptomatic Direct correlation with clinical signs still under investigation Associated with gingivitis, uveitis, fever, lymphadenopathy	Lymphadenopathy Fever Signs of infection at scratch site	Avoid being scratched by cat (good restraint, no rough play, wear protective gloves when handling fractious cats) Cat-associated wounds should be washed immediately with soap and water
Ringworm	Hairs	Skin	See Table 18.17	Pruritic, raised, red, circular skin lesions	Barrier nursing protocol Wash hands
Bacterial enteritis: *Campylobacter, Salmonella*	Feces	Oral	Diarrhea	Diarrhea Headache Joint and muscle aches	Barrier nursing protocol for all patients with diarrhea Wash hands Disinfect surfaces Follow personal safety protocol when performing fecal analysis Wash hands
Toxoplasmosis: *Toxoplasma gondii*	Aerosolized spores from dried (old) feces	Oral	Fever Diarrhea Uveitis Ascites	Fever Lethargy Lymphadenopathy Infection of fetus: CNS damage, abortion, stillbirth	Barrier nursing protocol Follow personal safety protocol when performing fecal analysis Wash hands
Leptospirosis	Urine	Mucous membranes Abraded skin	See Table 18.16.	Fever Rash Meningitis Hemorrhage Liver disease Kidney disease	Barrier nursing protocol Wash hands Disinfect surfaces Follow personal safety protocol when performing urinalysis

References

1. Acierno MJ, Brown S, Coleman AE, et al. ACVIM consensus statement: Guidelines for the identification, evaluation, and management of systemic hypertension in dogs and cats. *J Vet Intern Med*. 2018;32(6):1803–1822. https://onlinelibrary.wiley.com/doi/10.1111/jvim.15331.
2. Garden OA, Kidd L, Mexas AM, et al. ACVIM consensus statement on the diagnosis of immune-mediated hemolytic anemia in dogs and cats. *J Vet Intern Med*. 2019;33(2):313–334. https://onlinelibrary.wiley.com/doi/10.1111/jvim.15441.

Recommended Readings

Ballantyne H. *Veterinary Nursing Care Plans*. Boca Raton, FL: CRC Press; 2018.

Brooks HB. *General Pathology for Veterinary Nurses*. Oxford, UK: Wiley-Blackwell; 2010.

Cheville NF. *Introduction to Veterinary Pathology*. 3rd ed. Ames, IA: Blackwell; 2006.

Ettinger SJ, Feldman EC, Cote E. *Textbook of Veterinary Internal Medicine*. 8th ed. St. Louis, MO: Elsevier; 2017.

Merrill L. *Small Animal Internal Medicine for Veterinary Technicians and Nurses*. Ames, IA: Wiley-Blackwell; 2012.

Moore F. Principles of barrier nursing in the veterinary hospital. *Vet Nurse*. 2011;2:258.

Nelson RW, Couto CG. *Small Animal Internal Medicine*. 6th ed. St. Louis, MO: Mosby; 2019.

Norsworthy GD, Grace SF, Crystal MA, et al. *The Feline Patient*. 4th ed. Ames, IA: Wiley-Blackwell; 2011.

Orpet H. The nursing process. In: Orpet H, Welsh P, eds. *Handbook of Veterinary Nursing*. 2nd ed. Oxford, UK: Wiley-Blackwell; 2011.

The Merck Veterinary Manual. 11th ed. White House Station, NJ: Merck & Co; 2016.

Wilkinson JM. *Nursing Process and Critical Thinking*. 5th ed. Upper Saddle River, NJ: Pearson; 2012.

Withrow SJ, Vail DM. *Withrow and MacEwen's Small Animal Clinical Oncology*. 6th ed. St. Louis, MO: Saunders; 2019.

Websites

American College of Veterinary Internal Medicine (ACVIM). *Small Animal Consensus Statement on Leptospirosis: Diagnosis, Epidemiology, Treatment, and Prevention*; 2010. https://onlinelibrary.wiley.com/doi/full/10.1111/j.1939-1676.2010.0654.x.

International Renal Interest Society (IRIS): http://www.iris-kidney.com/.

The Cornell Feline Health Center: https://www.vet.cornell.edu/departments-centers-and-institutes/cornell-feline-health-center.

The Ohio State University College of Veterinary Medicine: The Indoor Pet Initiative: http://indoorpet.osu.edu/.

The American Animal Hospital Association (AAHA) and the American Association of Feline Practitioners (AAFP) have many evidence-based guidelines for small animal patients. The current guidelines are at https://www.aaha.org/ Guidelines (top menu bar) and https://catvets.com/guidelines/practice-guidelines.

The authors strongly recommend the following:

American Animal Hospital Association (AAHA). *Canine Life Stage Guidelines*; 2022.

American Animal Hospital Association (AAHA). *Diabetes Management Guidelines for Dogs and Cats*; 2018.

American Animal Hospital Association (AAHA). *Infection Control, Prevention, and Biosecurity Guidelines*; 2018.

American Animal Hospital Association (AAHA). *Oncology Guidelines for Dogs and Cats*; 2016.

American Animal Hospital Association (AAHA). *Selected Endocrinopathies of Dogs and Cats Guidelines*; 2023.

American Association of Feline Practitioners (AAFP). *Feline Retrovirus Management*; 2020.

American Association of Feline Practitioners (AAFP). *Guidelines for the Management of Feline Hyperthyroidism*; 2016.

American Association of Feline Practitioners (AAFP). *Zoonoses Guidelines*; 2019.

American Association of Feline Practitioners (AAFP) and American Animal Hospital Association (AAHA). *Feline Life Stage Guidelines*; 2021.

19

Large Animal Medical Nursing

MAXON M. GRAHAM AND HOLLY LEBEAU

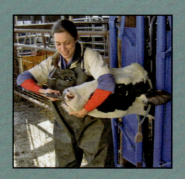

CHAPTER OUTLINE

LEARNING OBJECTIVES

When you have completed this chapter, you will be able to:

1. Pronounce, define, and spell all key terms in the chapter.
2. Explain the importance of a thorough physical examination and medical record for large animal patients.
3. List and describe the most common diseases and conditions of the horse for the gastrointestinal, musculoskeletal, respiratory, hemolymphatic, cardiovascular, neurologic, ophthalmologic, dermatologic, endocrine, and urinary systems, including the causes and pathogenesis of each.
4. Discuss the care of the hospitalized equine patient, including biosecurity, patient monitoring, supportive care, and laboratory diagnostics.
5. List and describe the most common diseases and conditions of ruminants for the digestive, respiratory, reproductive/mammary gland, metabolic, hemolymphatic, cardiovascular, nervous, ophthalmologic, musculoskeletal, dermatologic, and urinary systems, including special care and conditions of the neonate.
6. List and describe the most common diseases and conditions of swine for the gastrointestinal, respiratory, reproductive, nervous, and musculoskeletal systems, including abnormal behaviors.
7. List and describe the common diseases and conditions of camelids, including special care and conditions of the neonate.

KEY TERMS

Agammaglobulinemic
Antitoxin
Colostrum
Colostrometer
Dystocia
Endotoxemia
Epistaxis
Failure of passive transfer (FTP)
Farrowing
Fecal transfaunation
Gangrenous mastitis
Gastrointestinal parasite
Glucose absorption test
Hepatic lipidosis
Hirsutism
Hypoglycemia
Hypoxic ischemic encephalopathy (HIE)

Keratoconjunctivitis
Ketosis
Lymphosarcoma
Myositis
Omphalophlebitis
Pericarditis
Persistent infection (PI)
Polioencephalomalacia
Pregnancy toxemia
Proprioceptive
Pseudopregnancy
Septicemia
Serous
Social hierarchy
Stranguria
Toxoid
Urolithiasis

Introduction

Whether a large animal patient is treated in the field or in a hospital, proper nursing care is vital to its recovery. The veterinary technician or nurse must therefore be familiar with handling and care of large animals and with the medical conditions that affect each species. Most large animal species are prey animals that naturally congregate into herds for protection, and when they are removed from the safety of their herd, it is more likely that they may be spooked or act defensively. This can create a potentially dangerous situation for veterinary personnel and animal handlers. The behavior of any animal can change quickly, and large animals can be dangerous, given their size, weight, and strength.

There are basic handling skills that large animal veterinary technicians/nurses must know and master. (Refer to Chapter 6, "Restraint and Handling of Animals," for additional information on these skills.) Although many veterinary technicians and nurses have some previous experience working with large animals, it may not fully prepare them for working with nervous large animals or those in pain. These cases can challenge even the most experienced handlers. Proper mentorship and training are essential for every large animal practice to ensure the safety of all patients and personnel. In addition, patience, calmness, and planning can go a long way toward avoiding unnecessary stress being placed on the patient.

A complete patient assessment is critical, not only to gain information about vital parameters and potential problems, but also to provide information about the large animal patient's demeanor, habits, and responses. If an animal is not experiencing an immediate medical emergency, it should be allowed a brief time to acclimate to its new environment. Owners and trainers provide valuable insight into their animals' normal behaviors, and the technician can make observations about the patient while gathering information from the owner.

Equine Nursing

Physical Examination

Upon presentation, the patient's history and presenting complaints should be gathered from the owner or the trainer by the veterinary nurse/technician. The horse should be secured in the examination room or stall so that the physical examination can be completed. To avoid self-injury and panic in horses, they are never tied in a clinical setting. Typically, a handler or a veterinary technician will handle the horse during the initial physical examination. Knowing the patient's normal behaviors and vital signs (temperature, pulse rate, and respiratory rate [TPR]) helps staff identify abnormalities to enable early detection of problems and early intervention by veterinary personnel. (Refer to Chapter 7, "History and Physical Examination.")

Be aware that all components of a complete physical examination are important and should be performed. Gathering only TPR data is not an adequate evaluation of a hospitalized patient. Assessing a patient's behavior and attitude and monitoring catheters, bandages, and patient comfort are also very important. A proficient veterinary technician/nurse notes all changes in patient status in the medical record and verbally reports it to the staff on the next shift. In this way, the veterinary nursing team can work seamlessly across shift changes and can respond promptly to changes in patient status. In addition, making thorough observations of patients enables the team to know if a horse is progressing well or not responding to treatment. Regular and thorough patient evaluations also allow the team to recognize when a new problem occurs. Refer to Table 19.1 for normal vital signs in horses.

PUT INTO PRACTICE

Becoming adept at collecting a patient history and performing a thorough physical exam on your large animal patients can help identify issues that may otherwise be missed.

Common Diseases and Conditions of Horses

Care of the Neonate

Foals are born after approximately 330–362 days of gestation. A foal should stand within 1 hour of birth and should nurse within 2 hours. On physical examination, a neonatal foal should be bright, alert, and responsive. Neonatal TPR values are different than adult values: T 99–102°F; P = 80 to 100 beats per minute (bpm); and

TABLE 19.1	Normal Vital Signs in Adult Horses and Foals		
	Adult Horse	Foals (Birth–24 Hours)	Foals (2 Days–Weanling)
Pulse rate	28–44 beats per minute (bpm)	80–100 bpm	40–60 bpm
Respiration rate	8–20 bpm	20–40 bpm	20–40 bpm
Temperature	99.0°F–101.5°F	99.0°F –102°F	99.0°F–102°F
Mucous membranes	Pink, moist	Pink, moist	Pink, moist
Capillary refill time	<2 seconds	<2 seconds	<2 seconds

R = 20–40 breaths per minute. Note that measurement of vitals is not always accurate in foals, who may struggle and attempt to run around, making heart rate and respiration higher than at rest. A healthy foal spends its time nursing every 15 to 30 minutes, sleeping, and moving around. A normal foal should jump up when someone enters the stall and should run behind the mare and begin to nurse. The umbilicus should be dipped in chlorhexidine at birth and monitored for several days. The foal should receive colostrum within the first hours of life. To ensure passive transfer of immunity, a SNAP test is performed at 24 hours. If immunoglobulin G (IgG) levels are low (<800 mg/dL), plasma is given, because foals depend on these antibodies to protect against infection. Neonates that have failure of passive transfer (FPT) are at high risk of systemic inflammatory response syndrome (SIRS), sepsis, corneal ulcers, meconium impaction, diarrhea, and septic arthritis.

Bacteria can enter the foal's body through the umbilical stump, gastrointestinal (GI) system, and respiratory system. Foals may be compromised at birth, particularly if the mare had a difficult birth (dystocia). Other risk factors include gestational age, size, in utero infection, and birthing process. If the foal displays any signs of *hypoxia* (lack of oxygen) or *ischemia* (lack of blood flow), or if it is unable to get up and nurse within 1 or 2 hours, immediate medical attention must be given.

Because of the around-the-clock care and intensive nursing that foals require, many hospitals obtain extra help from paid workers, veterinary medicine and veterinary technician students, and volunteers to help cope with increased hospital demand during peak foaling seasons. The addition of a trained foal team is valuable to keep things running smoothly and relieve overworked veterinary staff (Fig. 19.1).

Hypoxic ischemic encephalopathy (HIE), commonly referred to as "dummy foal" or "equine maladjustment syndrome," is a medical emergency. HIE is believed to result from oxygen deprivation during the birthing process and can vary in severity, depending on the age of the fetus, length of oxygen deprivation, and severity of hypoxia. Dummy foals often seem normal after birth but develop progressive symptoms of HIE, including failure to recognize the mare; inability to stand, walk, or nurse; vocalization; and seizures. Affected foals are basically helpless and require supportive therapy, fluids, oxygen, around-the-clock nursing, antibiotics to prevent infection, and often plasma transfusion, because they often do not receive colostrum. They can harm themselves and others by flailing around and are particularly susceptible to ocular trauma. If supportive therapy is provided early and no severe secondary complications arise, dummy foals can typically recover, with approximately 80% developing into normal adults.

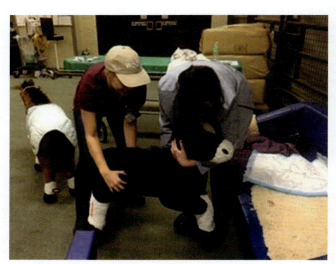

• **Fig. 19.1** Foal team going through training drills to prepare for foaling season.

Diseases of the Gastrointestinal System

The most common signs of GI disease in the adult horse include colic, weight loss, anorexia, diarrhea, and fever. Diagnostic assessment of GI disease may include hematology and serum chemistry, oral examination, rectal examination, abdominocentesis, ultrasonography, radiography, *gastroscopy* (endoscopic examination of the stomach), and fecal diagnostic testing.

Colic

For a thorough discussion of equine colic, refer to the "Gastrointestinal Tract" section in Chapter 25 (Emergency and Critical Care Nursing) and the "Gastrointestinal Tract Surgery" section in Chapter 34 (Large Animal Surgical Nursing). It is important to know that many colics may be resolved medically with fluid replacement and pain management. Recognizing early and slight colic signs is important to correct problems before they persist or worsen.

Enterocolitis

When a horse's GI system is disturbed, microbiome imbalance can result. Many factors, including stress, colic, antibiotic and nonsteroidal anti-inflammatory drug (NSAID) use, and viral or bacterial infections, can cause intestinal inflammation (Table 19.2). Horses with colitis present with potentially severe diarrhea, which can lead to life-threatening hypovolemia, shock, endotoxemia, electrolyte loss, and acid-base imbalance. In addition to diarrhea, clinical signs of colitis include depression, inappetence, abdominal

TABLE 19.2	Common Causes of Enterocolitis in the Adult Horse			
Disease/Etiologic Agent	**Pathogenesis**	**Clinical Signs**	**Diagnosis**	**Treatment**
Infectious				
Salmonellosis/ *Salmonella* spp.	• Bacterial infection caused by exposure to contaminated environment, feed, water, or animals that are actively shedding the bacteria • Risk factors—stress; history of surgery, transportation, or change in feed; concurrent disease, particularly colic; treatment with antibiotics	• Diarrhea • Depression • Anorexia • Colic • Tachycardia • Injected mucous membranes (MMs) and prolonged capillary refill time (CRT)	• Fecal culture • Fecal polymerase chain reaction (PCR) analysis	• Appropriate symptomatic treatment • Isolate horses until five consecutive negative fecal samples are obtained
Clostridiosis/*Clostridium perfringens*, *Clostridium difficile* (clostridial diarrhea)	• Anaerobic bacteria that produce toxins, resulting in profound inflammation and secretion from the GI tract • Overgrowth of *C. difficile* is the most common cause of antibiotic-associated diarrhea	• Diarrhea • Depression • Anorexia • Colic • Tachycardia • Injected MMs • Prolonged CRT	• Fecal PCR analysis or enzyme-linked immunosorbent assay (ELISA) for toxins • Fecal culture	• Appropriate symptomatic treatment • Metronidazole • Isolate horses
Potomac horse fever/*Neorickettsia risticii* (equine monocytic ehrlichiosis)	• Bacterial infection caused by ingestion of infected freshwater insects	• Diarrhea • Depression • Anorexia • Colic • Tachycardia • Injected MMs • Prolonged CRT • Laminitis	• Serology • Whole blood PCR analysis • Response to oxytetracycline	• Appropriate symptomatic treatment • Oxytetracycline
Larval cyathostomiasis/ small *Strongyle* infection	• Re-emergence of encysted larvae from large colon disrupts mucosal barrier, resulting in fluid and protein loss • Most common in horses younger than 6 years of age that have not developed immunity	• Diarrhea • Depression • Anorexia • Colic • Tachycardia • Injected MMs • Prolonged CRT • Weight loss • Ventral edema	• Fecal flotation • Intestinal biopsy	• Appropriate symptomatic treatment • Fenbendazole 10 mg/kg for 5 days or moxidectin
Coronavirus	• Fecal-oral transmission • Most common in cold months	• Fever • Anorexia • Diarrhea *uncommon* • Mild colic	• Fecal PCR analysis	• Anti-inflammatories • Supportive care
Toxic				
Right dorsal colitis/ nonsteroidal anti-inflammatory drug (NSAID) toxicity	• Inhibition of normal gastrointestinal (GI) mucosal barrier, resulting in ulceration • Decreased blood flow can cause kidney damage • Sensitive horses (ponies) can develop toxicity at recommended doses	• Oral ulceration • Anorexia • Lethargy • Weight loss • Colic • Ventral edema • Injected MMs	• History of NSAID use • Total solids— hypoproteinemia • Abdominal ultrasonography— thickening of the right dorsal colon • Gastroscopy—gastric ulcers • Abnormal urinalysis	• Symptomatic treatment • Colloid therapy— hypoproteinemia • Low-bulk, easily digested diet • Antiulcer medications • Sucralfate • Misoprostol

Continued

TABLE 19.2	Common Causes of Enterocolitis in the Adult Horse—cont'd			
Disease/Etiologic Agent	**Pathogenesis**	**Clinical Signs**	**Diagnosis**	**Treatment**
Blister beetle toxicity/ cantharidin	• Ingestion of cantharid, found in blister beetles, irritates the GI and urinary tracts • Exposure occurs after ingestion of hay contaminated by beetles	• Diarrhea • Depression • Colic/anorexia • Tachycardia • Injected MMs • Prolonged CRT • Hematuria	• Chemistry profile— hypocalcemia and hypomagnesemia • Fecal/urine analysis— hyposthenuria and detection of toxin in GI contents or urine	• Symptomatic interventions • Administer mineral oil, activated charcoal, calcium, and magnesium
Antibiotic administration	• Use of some antibiotics alters normal GI flora allowing proliferation of pathogenic organisms in GI tract	• Diarrhea • Depression • Anorexia • Colic • Tachycardia • Injected MMs • Prolonged CRT	• History of antibiotic use • Test for *C. difficile*, *C. perfringens*, and Salmonella	• Appropriate symptomatic treatment • Stop antibiotic administration • Isolate horses

pain, tachycardia (increased heart rate), injected (brick-red) mucous membranes (Fig. 19.2), and prolonged capillary refill time (CRT). The most common life-threatening causes of colitis include infections by *Salmonella* spp., *Clostridium* spp., and *Neorickettsia risticii*. Horses with colitis should be considered contagious and maintained under an isolation protocol. The approach to treatment of horses with colitis is consistent, regardless of the cause. Intravenous (IV) fluid therapy is crucial to support the cardiovascular system, replace fluid losses, and correct electrolyte and acid-base imbalances. Colloid therapy (plasma, hetastarch, dextran) may be necessary because of protein loss, which can lead to peripheral edema as fluid leaks from blood vessels into surrounding tissue. Complications of colitis include laminitis, cardiovascular collapse, cardiac arrhythmias, and thrombophlebitis.

> **TECHNICIAN NOTE**
>
> Equine diarrhea can result in environmental contamination. Be sure to keep the patient's stall clean, wiping feces from the walls, feed and water buckets, and fluid lines. Keep the horse clean and dry, because skin irritation can occur quickly. Wrapping the tail in a rectal sleeve to prevent soiling, cleaning the perineal area, and applying a topical barrier cream several times a day can help to prevent skin breakdown. Always wear proper personal protective equipment (PPE) and change gloves often.

Fecal Transfaunation

Little research has been conducted on the equine microbiome, although its significance in disease management has become evident. It is known that a healthy gut contains good bacterial populations that aid in digestion and that those populations can be altered by disease and illness, prolonging sickness. Repopulation of the gut with healthy flora from another horse, or **fecal transfaunation**, can significantly improve recovery from chronic GI conditions. During fecal transfaunation, the feces of a healthy horse are mixed with water and the fluid strained off. The fluid is then administered into the stomach of a sick horse via a nasogastric (NG) tube so that good bacteria can pass through the stomach and colonize the hindgut. It is critical that the donor horse is healthy and receives negative culture results for harmful organisms, such as *Salmonella* and *Clostridium* species.

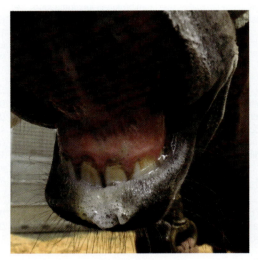

• **Fig. 19.2** Injected mucous membranes in a horse, with toxic line noted above teeth and excessive salivation or dysphagia.

Endotoxemia

Endotoxin, which is a cell wall component of gram-negative bacteria, can enter the bloodstream via compromised tissue and cause significant illness. Endotoxemia can occur secondary to enterocolitis when the GI microbiome is altered and endotoxin-producing bacteria have proliferated. Clinical signs associated with endotoxemia include fever, tachycardia, hyperemic mucous membranes, leukopenia, laminitis, and depression. Endotoxemia may also occur in cases of retained placenta, *metritis* (uterine infection), pneumonia, peritonitis, and large wounds. Horses are extremely sensitive to the effects of endotoxin, and aggressive treatment, which may include surgical excision of compromised intestine, uterine lavage, and drainage of pleural or peritoneal fluid, is required. Early recognition and treatment are critical to a positive outcome, and technicians should monitor at-risk patients closely for any signs of endotoxemia.

Gastric and Colonic Ulceration

Gastric ulceration in horses can have a variety of causes and is common, especially in young horses. Predisposing factors include stress, a high-grain diet, exercise, and NSAIDs. Signs of gastric ulcers include *bruxism* (grinding of teeth), anorexia, weight loss, and abdominal pain after eating. Ulcerations can occur in either the glandular or nonglandular mucosa of the stomach and in the hindgut. Gastric ulcers in the squamous mucosa are thought to be directly related to exposure to the natural gastric acids produced in the stomach. In the glandular region of the stomach, a disruption in blood flow and breakdown of prostaglandins are thought to cause ulcers.

Gastric ulcers can be definitively diagnosed with endoscopy. Hyperkeratosis, which is yellowing and thickening of the mucosa, is often seen in horses that have some degree of irritation. Hyperemia is seen as a reddening of the nonglandular surface. Equine gastric ulcer syndrome (EGUS) is typically graded on a scale of 1 to 4, based on ulcer severity. There are many treatments and compounds on the market to prevent and treat gastric ulcer disease, but the proton pump inhibitor omeprazole is the most successful one. Sucralfate may also be given to coat the stomach walls and lessen pain. Changes in horse management go a long way to prevent ulcers. For example, horses that are worked more than 5 days a week and those that are stalled and do not have access to turn-out have a much higher incidence of ulcers. Management changes, such as providing small, frequent meals; having unlimited access to fresh hay and water; turn-out; reducing workload; and providing companions may all help lower the risk of ulcer.

Potomac Horse Fever

Potomac horse fever (PHF), caused by *Neorickettsia risticii*, produces diarrhea, fever, abortion, and laminitis. This pathogen is acquired through ingestion of mayflies, caddisflies, or snails; therefore cases are most often seen near fresh water. Geographically, clinical disease is observed predominantly in the states east of the Mississippi River and in California. Diagnosis of PHF is based on serum testing for antibodies or polymerase chain reaction (PCR) analysis of whole blood samples. *N. risticii* is very sensitive to treatment with oxytetracycline, and a favorable response to treatment is supportive of the diagnosis. Inactivated bacterin vaccines are commercially available. Although the vaccine is not effective in preventing infection, it may minimize clinical signs, and horses living in the affected areas can be vaccinated. Vaccination should precede the months of peak disease incidence (June through October).

Choke

Choke refers to obstruction of the esophagus, typically by grain or hay. Choke is often caused by dry feed pellets, grains, or processed hay cubes. Horses that rush through eating, compete for food in a pasture situation, have previously choked, or have chronic dental disease are at higher risk. Choke can present much like colic, with clinical signs including anxiety, stretching the neck out, gagging, excessive salivation, and rolling. Feed material may be seen coming from the horse's mouth and nostrils. Choke is considered a medical emergency, and the horse should be evaluated as soon as possible. If the cause is not obvious, the obstruction can be visualized via an endoscopic examination. Clearing of obstruction is achieved through manipulation and hydropulsion by using an NG tube. Heavy sedation is critical to keep the horse relaxed and its head lowered to prevent aspiration of feed and water. Antibiotic therapy is usually started to treat and prevent aspiration pneumonia, which is a common complication of choke, and clearing the obstruction.

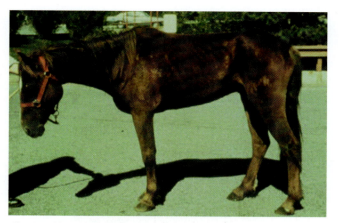

• **Fig. 19.3** Horse in poor body condition caused by chronic weight loss.

> **TECHNICIAN NOTE**
>
> Horses that have been sedated for a procedure should not be given anything to eat until sedation wears off. In a clinical setting, this is a common cause of choke.

Chronic Weight Loss

Horses that present with chronic weight loss, anorexia, lethargy, frequent, intermittent diarrhea, and general dullness can present a clinical challenge (Fig. 19.3). Endoparasites and GI ulcers are among the most common causes and, once they are ruled out, a thorough diagnostic GI workup is critical to reach a diagnosis and prescribe a treatment plan. Ultrasonography of the abdomen may reveal surface abnormalities of the intestines or loops of dilated small intestine, which usually indicate inflammation in the gut. Complete blood count (CBC) and chemistry can identify abnormalities such as inflammation, infection, anemia, and organ dysfunction. Rectal palpation and rectal biopsy may be helpful to diagnose such conditions as neoplasia and irritable bowel syndrome (IBS). Some horses have malabsorption disease that may be caused by a variety of conditions; a **glucose absorption test** may be helpful in determining whether a horse is properly absorbing nutrients. Based on the diagnosis, a horse's treatment plan may include probiotics, corticosteroids to decrease inflammation, diet change, and antibiotics. Horses with chronic weight loss often have a poor long-term prognosis.

Diseases of the Musculoskeletal System

Laminitis

Laminitis ("founder") can be chronic or acute and can affect horses of any breed, age, or discipline. In laminitis, the laminae, which are interdigitations connecting the hoof wall to the sensitive corium underneath, become inflamed and, in severe cases, may eventually begin to pull apart, compromising the structure of the hoof. Many factors seem to increase a horse's risk for laminitis, including stress, illness, endotoxemia, pituitary pars intermedia dysfunction (PPID), equine metabolic syndrome, and corticosteroid administration. Affected horses suffer from severe foot pain and will not want to move or pick up the leg opposite the affected hoof. Because the forefeet are most often affected, horses often shift their weight to the hind feet. Some horses may lie down more than usual to remove excess stress and pain. Recurrent hoof abscesses are common, and rotation and sinking of P3

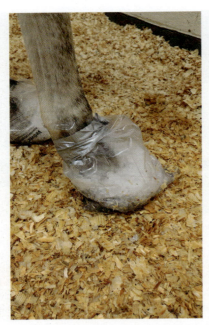

• **Fig. 19.4** Ice bags have been applied to horse's feet to treat laminitis.

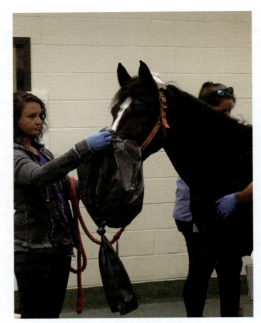

• **Fig. 19.5** A large trash bag is used as a rebreathing bag during a respiratory evaluation.

("coffin bone") is possible. This sequela is extremely painful and associated with a poor prognosis, and cases that reach this point require humane euthanasia. Early monitoring and intervention are key to controlling pain and inflammation and preventing permanent damage. Checking digital pulses and heat in the hoof is an important component of the equine physical examination to detect changes consistent with laminitis. Radiographs of the hoof are taken if inflammation is suspected. Many treatments are available, including NSAIDs, bedding on deep shavings or sand, ice bags placed on affected feet, and vasoconstrictive medications to decrease blood flow to the foot. Empty 5-L fluid bags are handy for soaking hoof abscesses and providing ice for horses being treated for laminitis (Fig. 19.4). Bags can be placed over the hoof, ice added, and the top secured with tape. Caution should be exercised, especially if applying the bags to the hind limbs, because many horses will reject the idea by kicking.

Many supportive shoes, such as NANRICs and Soft-Ride boots, are available, or the use of hoof support packing or foam may provide relief. The long-term use and prognosis of the horse will depend on whether the pain and inflammation can be adequately managed.

Diseases of the Respiratory System

The normal respiratory rate in an adult horse is 8 to 20 breaths per minute. Horses with respiratory disease may display *tachypnea* (increased respiratory rate), *dyspnea* (increased effort), cough (with or without activity), unilateral or bilateral nasal discharge, decreased performance, fever, and *lymphadenopathy* (enlarged lymph nodes). It is often difficult to hear lung sounds under normal conditions in an adult horse in normal body condition. To amplify lung sounds and to encourage the horse to breathe deeper, a rebreathing bag, such as a large, thick trash bag (Fig. 19.5), is placed over the horse's nostrils. Caution should be used, because this procedure can often scare the horse. Some nurses/technicians find it helpful to place a muzzle over the nostrils and then the rebreathing bag over it. It is important that someone monitors

the bag and that the horse is not biting on it or sucking it into its nostrils as its respiration increases. Lung sounds should be auscultated on both sides of the horse, noting harshness, crackles, wheezes, and decreased air flow. Many horses will cough during the examination and take longer to recover. The technician should make sure that the horse is given a break when needed to prevent anxiety and panic.

Diagnostic tests that can be used to assess the upper airway include endoscopy, radiography, computed tomography (CT), and magnetic resonance imaging (MRI). Diagnostic tests performed to assess the lower airway include bronchoscopy, bronchoalveolar lavage (BAL), transtracheal wash (TTW), ultrasonography, radiology, and pulmonary function testing. (Refer to Chapter 17, "Diagnostic Sampling and Treatment Techniques," for more information on performing a TTW). Blood analysis can help determine whether respiratory disease has an infectious or inflammatory cause. Table 19.3 summarizes equine diseases of the respiratory tract.

Bacterial Pneumonia and Pleuropneumonia

Bacterial pneumonia occurs as a result of aspiration of bacteria that normally inhabit the oral cavity and the upper respiratory tract. Horses of all ages can be affected, although young horses are predisposed. Colonization of the lungs by opportunistic bacteria occurs when natural defense mechanisms are compromised or overwhelmed by large numbers of bacteria. Long-distance transportation is a risk factor for the development of bacterial pneumonia, because clearance of debris and bacteria from the trachea is decreased when horses are trailered. Dysphagia and aspiration of feed material because of esophageal obstruction ("choke") can result in bacterial pneumonia. When bacterial infection spreads from lung tissue to the pleural space, called *pleuropneumonia*, pleural effusion can occur.

Clinical signs of pneumonia include exercise intolerance, fever, tachypnea, cough, bilateral mucopurulent nasal discharge, inappetence, and *pleurodynia* (chest pain). Rebreathing examination may reveal crackles and/or wheezes over affected areas and a tracheal

TABLE 19.3   Common Equine Respiratory Diseases

Disease/Etiologic Agent	Pathogenesis	Clinical Findings	Diagnosis	Treatment
Infectious				
Equine influenza	• Contagious viral respiratory disease • Virus transmitted via aerosolization by coughing • Incubation period: 2–3 days • Duration of illness: 3–4 days	• Fever • Cough • Depression • Nasal discharge	• Not typically performed: • Polymerase chain reaction (PCR) analysis • Serology • Virus isolation	• No specific antiviral therapy • Nonsteroidal anti-inflammatories • Rest for at least 3 weeks • Isolate horses
Equine herpesvirus-1 (EHV-1, rhinopneumonitis), and equine herpesvirus-4 (EHV-4)	• EHV-1 and EHV-4 cause respiratory disease • EHV-1 also causes abortion and neonatal neurologic disease • Transmitted via respiratory secretions and fomites • Incubation period: 2–10 days • Duration of illness: 4–5 days	• Fever • Cough • Depression • Nasal discharge • Typically more mild signs than influenza	• Not typically performed: • PCR • Serology • Virus isolation	• No specific antiviral therapy for respiratory cases • Nonsteroidal anti-inflammatory • Rest for at least 3 weeks • Isolate horses
Equine viral arteritis	• Contagious; causes respiratory disease, limb swelling, conjunctivitis, and abortion • Stallions infected after puberty develop persistent infection and infect mares during breeding	• Often asymptomatic • Fever • Anorexia • Serous nasal discharge • Coughing • Limb edema • Abortion	• Serology	• No specific antiviral therapy for respiratory cases • Nonsteroidal anti-inflammatories • Isolate horses
Strangles/*Streptococcus equi* subsp. *equi*	• Contagious bacterial disease • Spread via nasal secretions • Causes • Swelling and abscesses of the submandibular and retropharyngeal lymph nodes • Recovered horses remain contagious for 6 weeks after recovery from clinical disease • Asymptomatic carriers	• Fever • Depression • Anorexia • Painful swellings under the mandible • Purulent nasal discharge • Guttural pouch empyema • Airway obstruction caused by swollen lymph nodes	• Culture or PCR analysis of guttural pouch or nasopharyngeal wash	• Supportive care (anti-inflammatories, fluids) until abscesses have ruptured • Penicillin after rupture of abscesses • Tracheostomy if severe airway obstruction
Bacterial pneumonia	• Colonization of lungs by opportunistic bacteria as a result of compromise of natural defense mechanisms • Risk factors—long-term transportation, dysphagia, aspiration caused by esophageal obstruction (choke)	• Exercise intolerance • Fever • Tachypnea • Cough • Mucopurulent nasal discharge • Anorexia • Chest pain	• Hematology—increased white blood cell count and fibrinogen • Transtracheal wash (TTW) cytology culture and sensitivity • Thoracic imaging	• Broad-spectrum antibiotics based on culture and sensitivity of TTW samples • Nonsteroidal anti-inflammatories • Antiendotoxin therapies
Inflammatory				
Heaves/recurrent airway obstruction (RAO)	• Allergic airway disease of older horses • Airway inflammation, bronchoconstriction, and mucus production	• Cough • Nasal discharge • Flared nostrils • Tachypnea • Dyspnea • Wheezing	• Hematology: normal • Bronchoalveolar lavage (BAL) or TTW cytology • Thoracic radiography	• Environmental management • Systemic or inhaled corticosteroids • Systemic or inhaled bronchodilators

Continued

considered in horses with positive test results and consistent clinical signs. Treatment with IV oxytetracycline or oral doxycycline for at least 1 month is typically required.

Piroplasmosis

Piroplasmosis is a bloodborne disease caused by the parasite *Babesia caballi* or *Theileria equi*. Infection is transmitted via ticks; sharing improperly cleaned needles, surgical, or tattoo equipment; and blood transfusions. Clinical signs include fever, anemia, jaundice, weight loss, ventral edema, and increased respiration. The spleen may also be enlarged. Infected horses are carriers for life and can pass the disease to other horses via blood and often are euthanized. Many racetracks and horse associations require proof of a negative test result.

Diseases of the Cardiovascular System

Horses with cardiac disease are often asymptomatic. Auscultation of a heart murmur will require further examination of the cardiovascular system. When clinical signs do occur, they may include exercise intolerance, tachycardia, weakness, *syncope* (fainting), and respiratory crackles on auscultation. Cardiac disease is diagnosed via auscultation, electrocardiography (ECG) to measure the electrical activity of the heart, echocardiography, or cardiac ultrasonography.

Second-Degree Atrioventricular Block

Second-degree atrioventricular (AV) block is a common arrhythmia in horses, especially fit, athletic animals. Arrhythmia occurs as the result of altered conduction through the AV node, resulting in contracture of the atria without the ventricles. This can occur because of high vagal tone, electrolyte imbalances, and the effects of medications, such as α^2-agonists (xylazine, detomidine). The regularly irregular rhythm, often described as "dropped beats," is often no cause for concern, because regular rhythm will resume with exercise. If arrhythmia is not resolved with exercise, then further diagnostics should be performed.

Atrial Fibrillation

Atrial fibrillation is the most common clinically relevant arrhythmia in horses. Horses are predisposed because of the large size of their atria and their high vagal tone. Clinical signs include exercise intolerance or poor performance. Auscultation of horses with atrial fibrillation reveals an irregularly irregular rhythm. Although most horses with atrial fibrillation do not have underlying heart disease, if heart disease is present, the prognosis is poor. Therefore a complete cardiac workup, including echocardiography, is warranted.

If no underlying issues are found, conversion can be achieved using quinidine via NG tube or oral tablets. Electrical conversion under anesthesia can be accomplished by placing electrodes into the heart with ultrasound guidance.

Diseases of the Neurologic System

Clinical manifestation of neurologic disease depends on which nervous structures are affected. Cerebral (forebrain) diseases may produce altered mentation, altered states of consciousness, head pressing (Fig. 19.6), and seizures. Brainstem lesions can lead to incoordination of limbs and altered breathing patterns. Conditions affecting the brainstem may also damage the cranial nerves, which control the muscles of facial expression, facial sensation,

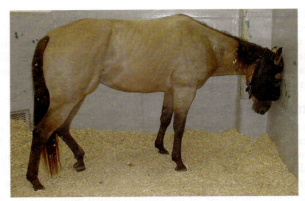

• **Fig. 19.6** Horse head pressing as a sign of cerebral dysfunction.

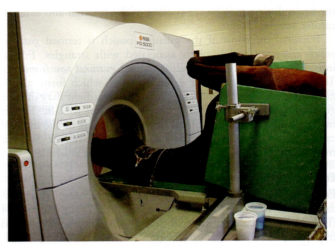

• **Fig. 19.7** Horse undergoing a computed tomography (CT) scan.

mastication (chewing), swallowing, balance, vision, taste, and ocular position. Diagnostic aids for the evaluation of horses with cerebral or brainstem dysfunction include cerebrospinal fluid (CSF) analysis, skull radiography, and CT (Fig. 19.7) or MRI. Damage to the spinal cord causes spinal ataxia (incoordination of the limbs without abnormalities of the brain and brainstem), which may progress to dog sitting and recumbency (Fig. 19.8). Muscle atrophy resulting from a lower motor neuron disorder can indicate a spinal cord disorder. Diagnostic aids to diagnose spinal cord diseases include neurologic examination, cervical radiographic examination, myelography examination, and CSF analysis.

Rabies

Rabies is a zoonotic infection that is universally fatal. Horses usually acquire the infection by a bite wound from a wild animal. Skunks, foxes, raccoons, and bats are the most common reservoirs in North America. Clinical signs are highly variable but often begin as fever, hind limb ataxia, and *hyperesthesia* (hyperresponsiveness to touch). Neurologic signs rapidly progress to involve the brain and the brainstem. The duration of neurologic signs before death is relatively short, ranging from 3 to 10 days. Death is imminent, but euthanasia is usually elected to protect human caretakers.

No accurate antemortem test for rabies is available; it is important to be cautious when handling horses with suspected rabies. The diagnosis of rabies is confirmed with fluorescent antibody staining of brain tissue. People handling potentially rabid horses

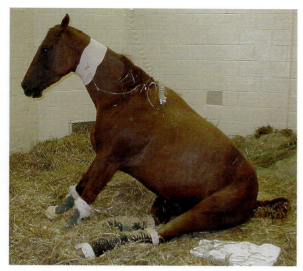

• **Fig. 19.8** Horse in dog-sitting position as a result of a spinal cord dysfunction.

should avoid contact with saliva; should wear gloves, protective eyewear, and disposable outerwear; should wash hands thoroughly; and should avoid contact with CSF. A list of individuals who have had contact with the potentially rabid horse must be kept, and they must be informed of the result of the test (generally within 24–48 hours). Postexposure rabies vaccination should be administered to humans exposed to rabid animals. Individuals with occupational exposure to livestock and wildlife should receive a prophylactic rabies vaccination series.

Horses should be vaccinated against rabies on an annual basis. Vaccinated horses that have been exposed to a rabid animal should be revaccinated promptly and observed for 90 days. Unvaccinated horses with known exposure to rabies should be observed for 6 months and should not be vaccinated.

Viral Equine Encephalitis

Four main types of viral equine encephalitis are known: eastern, western, Venezuelan, and West Nile. The viral equine encephalitides produce rapidly progressive, highly fatal neurologic disease in horses. Mosquitoes transmit the infection; therefore disease incidence is seasonal in most geographic regions. Clinical signs of eastern, western, and Venezuelan encephalitis are practically indistinguishable and include profound depression, fever, ataxia, head pressing, dementia, and multiple cranial nerve abnormalities. Clinical signs of West Nile encephalitis include weakness, ataxia, muscle fasciculations, and cranial nerve deficits (e.g., droopy lip). *Hyperesthesia* (extreme sensitivity to touch) around the head and neck is a common clinical sign. The mortality rate is extremely high with eastern equine encephalitis (75%–100%); moderate with Venezuelan encephalitis (40%–80%); and lower with western encephalitis (30%–50%) and West Nile encephalitis (36%–44%). Treatment consists of supportive care to provide hydration, nutrition, and a clean, dry environment. The prognosis is poor with eastern equine encephalitis and guarded with western, Venezuelan, and West Nile encephalitides. Diagnosis is confirmed by serologic testing (a high titer or a fourfold increase in antibodies to eastern, western, and Venezuelan viruses identified by complement fixation, neutralization, or hemagglutination inhibition assays, or a positive immunoglobulin M (IgM) capture ELISA for West Nile and Venezuelan viruses). Fluorescent antibody or virus

isolation in brain tissue is used to make a diagnosis from postmortem samples.

Vaccines for eastern, western, and West Nile equine encephalitis are highly efficacious, and clinical disease in vaccinated horses is rare. Horses in the United States should be vaccinated against eastern and western equine and West Nile encephalomyelitis viruses before the mosquito season in the spring. Horses living in the southern states with a year-round mosquito season should be vaccinated two to three times per year. Broodmares should receive a booster of their vaccination in the 10th month of gestation (only killed virus vaccines should be used in pregnant animals) to ensure adequate colostral antibody protection for the foal. Vaccination against Venezuelan equine encephalomyelitis is not routinely recommended, because the disease has not been reported recently in the United States and does not currently pose a threat to the US horse population, except for that near the Mexican border.

Equine Protozoal Myelitis

Equine protozoal myelitis (EPM) is a common cause of neurologic disease in horses. Horses are dead-end, aberrant hosts of the protozoan parasites. *Sarcocystis neurona* is the most common protozoan parasite that causes spinal cord disease in horses; opossums are the primary hosts of this parasite, and horses are likely infected via fecal-oral transmission. Birds are secondary hosts and do not appear to be infectious for horses. Clinical signs of EPM are directly referable to the location of the organism in the CNS. Therefore EPM should be considered in any horse demonstrating neurologic signs. Most horses with EPM demonstrate clinical signs such as ataxia, weakness, and muscle atrophy because of spinal cord damage; however, some horses may be asymptomatic. Other signs, such as cranial nerve deficits, may occur. Diagnosis is confirmed by identification of antibodies to the organism in CSF. Treatment of EPM consists of administration of antiprotozoal drugs; treatments approved by the US Food and Drug Administration (FDA) include ponazuril and diclazuril.

Herpes

EHV can produce respiratory disease, abortion, and neonatal and neurologic diseases in horses. EHV is very contagious and spreads from nasal secretions on feed buckets and water troughs and on the clothing and shoes of caretakers. For this reason, horses with neurologic symptoms should be isolated until EHV is ruled out. The neurologic form is characterized by ascending paralysis, with the hind limbs more severely affected compared with the forelimbs. Horses often demonstrate urinary incontinence, poor tail tone, and penile prolapse. Horses are often febrile early in the course of the disease, but the fever may have resolved by the time of examination. Diagnosis is confirmed with PCR testing of whole blood for the neurologic form of the infection. Administration of the antiviral medication valacyclovir may promote recovery and decrease nasal shedding if administered early in the disease process. Recumbency caused by weakness and incoordination in the hind limbs can occur in severe cases and indicates a poor prognosis. Recovery in surviving horses can be prolonged (2 to 3 months), and horses may not return to completely normal neurologic function. Affected horses are often euthanized. Cases are reportable to the state veterinarian.

Wobbler Syndrome

Cervical vertebral malformation is a manifestation of developmental orthopedic disease characterized by compression of the cervical spinal cord by malformed or unstable cervical vertebrae. Males are affected four times more frequently than females, and Thoroughbreds appear to be predisposed. Clinical signs of symmetric incoordination usually begin between 6 months and 3 years of age. The hind limbs usually are more severely affected compared with the forelimbs. The likelihood of disease is determined by evaluation of plain film cervical radiographs, and the diagnosis is confirmed with myelographic examination. Surgical stabilization improves the neurologic status of some patients. Type 2 wobbler syndrome affects older horses that experience cervical compression due to arthritic changes.

Botulism

Botulism is a rapidly progressive, often fatal neurologic disease in horses characterized by profound weakness, muscle fasciculations, and *dysphagia* (inability to swallow). The causal organism, *Clostridium botulinum*, produces a neurotoxin that may gain entry to the body by colonizing the intestinal tract (in foals), infected wounds, or contaminated feedstuff. Colonization of the intestinal tract in foals occurs in certain geographic regions of the United States, especially in Pennsylvania, Ohio, and Kentucky. This is a preventable disease, and it is imperative to vaccinate horses against botulism in endemic areas. The initial series is administered monthly for 3 months and subsequently once yearly. The vaccine is effective, and unvaccinated horses can die quickly after an infection.

Tetanus

Tetanus is a highly fatal neurologic disease in horses characterized by a stiff, stilted gait; hyperexcitability; seizure; and coma. The causative organism, *Clostridium tetani*, is commonly present in the environment and invades wounds or cuts. Tetanus **toxoid** (inactivated) is a safe and efficacious vaccine for preventing clinical disease. Healthy horses without risk factors should be vaccinated annually against tetanus. Unvaccinated horses with a high risk for tetanus (wounds, subsolar abscess, surgery) should receive tetanus **antitoxin** in addition to tetanus toxoid to provide immediate protection against the disease. Tetanus antitoxin is associated with fatal serum hepatitis; its administration should be limited to animals at high risk for the disease.

Ophthalmologic Diseases

A thorough ophthalmic examination is required to diagnose any ocular condition. If the horse requires sedation for the examination, a quick assessment, including menace testing, tracking ability, and pupillary light response (PLR), should be performed prior to sedation. The examiner should always wear gloves, because infectious agents, such as *Pseudomonas*, often complicate eye infections. Horses have incredibly strong eyelids, and a peripheral nerve block to the auricular palpebral branch may be necessary. Once the eyelid is blocked, the examiner may use a thumb and index finger to open the eyelid. By pushing down near the medical canthus, the third eyelid can be seen. One should look for any defects and drainage coming from this area, because it is a common spot for foreign bodies to accumulate. The Schirmer tear test must be performed before any medication is applied to the corneal surface. Local anesthetic drops are applied to numb the cornea, and then ocular pressure is measured with tonometry. The pupils are dilated by using a mydriatic, such as tropicamide, for examination of the retina, fundus, lens, and posterior chamber. Last, fluorescein stain can be used to detect corneal ulceration or defects.

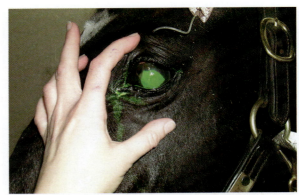

• **Fig. 19.9** Patient with corneal ulceration stained with fluorescein. (Courtesy Dr. Amy Bentz.)

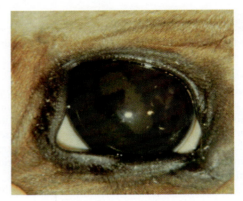

• **Fig. 19.10** Hyphema in the eye of a horse.

Equine Recurrent Uveitis

Equine recurrent uveitis ("moon blindness") is the most common cause of blindness in horses. It is an immune-mediated condition, and many factors (heredity, parasites, leptospirosis) have been implicated in its occurrence; however, the inciting cause is often unknown. Affected horses experience episodes of intraocular inflammation characterized by swelling of the eyelids, corneal edema, and *hypopyon* (inflammatory cellular exudate in the anterior chamber). Over time, the episodes become more frequent and severe and produce permanent ocular damage, including retinal degeneration, cataracts, and *synechiae* (adhesions of the iris to the lens or to the anterior chamber). One or both eyes may be affected. Recurrent uveitis cannot be cured but often can be controlled with long-term anti-inflammatory therapy. Acute episodes are treated with ophthalmic preparations containing atropine and corticosteroids if no corneal ulceration is noted. Systemic anti-inflammatory therapy (e.g., flunixin meglumine) is beneficial. Horses with end-stage uveitis are blind and have small, collapsed ocular globes (*phthisis bulbi*). If a corneal ulcer is present, antimicrobials and NSAIDs are used. Once the ulcer completely resolves, a topical steroid may be used. These cases require diligent observation and long-term treatment.

Corneal Ulceration

Corneal ulceration commonly results from ocular trauma. Fluorescein stain is used to detect corneal abrasions, because it adheres to abnormal cornea. Defects in the corneal surface will stain an apple-green color (Fig. 19.9). Trauma may cause injury that extends into the anterior chamber, causing such signs as hyphema (Fig. 19.10). Corneal ulceration in most horses responds readily without complications to the administration of ophthalmic antibacterial ointment (bacitracin, neomycin, polymyxin B). In some instances, the ulcer is colonized by a fungus (e.g., *Pseudomonas* or *Aspergillus* spp.). These organisms produce collagenase, which destroys the cornea and creates a "melting" corneal ulcer. These ulcers are rapidly progressive, and the eye is prone to rupture. Frequent antimicrobial dosage regimens may require the placement of a subpalpebral lavage system to allow frequent medication administration for a painful eye. Aggressive topical antimicrobial therapy may be successful, but suturing a conjunctival pedicle flap to provide blood supply to the affected area may be necessary to save the globe in some instances. Deep melting corneal ulcers often heal with a fibrous scar that may impair vision in the future.

> **TECHNICIAN NOTE**
>
> Ocular conditions can cause the eye to become extremely itchy, causing the horse to rub it. If a subpalpebral lavage system is in place, it is helpful to apply an eye mask to prevent the horse from damaging the eye and the line.

Diseases of the Skin

Skin diseases are diagnosed using methods that include culture, cytology, histopathology, and allergy testing. Samples are commonly collected using skin scraping, fine-needle aspiration (FNA), and punch biopsy.

Ringworm

Equine dermatophytosis (ringworm) is a fungal infection of the superficial layer of skin. Fungi commonly involved include *Trichophyton* and *Microsporum* spp. Transmission of fungal infection occurs by direct contact between affected animals. Animals younger than 4 years of age are most likely to be affected. Infected areas of skin have a bull's-eye appearance, with circular patches of hair loss and a circle of inflammation at the periphery of the lesion. Diagnosis is confirmed by fungal culture on a commercially available dermatophyte culture medium. Although infection is usually self-limiting, application of topical antifungal drugs will speed recovery.

Rain Rot

Dermatophilosis ("rain scald," "rain rot") is a common bacterial infection caused by *Dermatophilus congolensis* that produces crusting lesions. The crusts can be pulled out with a tuft of hair, and the remaining lesion is a glistening, yellow crater. The organisms readily colonize wet, macerated skin; therefore the disease is common in winter and spring. An impression smear of the tuft should be stained with Wright stain. Organisms are identified as a double chain of cocci with a "railroad track" appearance. The organisms usually are easily cultured and form an applesauce-like colony on specialized growth medium. Affected horses should be bathed with an iodine-based or chlorhexidine shampoo and placed in a dry environment. Administration of penicillin will speed up recovery in severely afflicted horses.

Culicoides Hypersensitivity

Culicoides hypersensitivity is a syndrome characterized by mane and tail rubbing, whereby affected horses develop an allergic pruritic skin condition secondary to the bite of *Culicoides* flies. Body regions typically affected include the face, ears, mane, withers, rump, base of the tail, and ventral abdomen. Dermatitis usually begins as a seasonal condition, but its severity and duration increase as the horse ages. Pruritus usually is noted during the fly season but will vary in duration, depending on the geographic location. The condition is diagnosed by correlating the time of year with physical evidence of self-mutilation, especially in the mane and tail areas. Intradermal skin testing can be useful in confirming the diagnosis. Treatment involves reduced insect exposure and concomitant use of anti-inflammatory medication. Because *Culicoides* breeds in stagnant waters, affected horses should be moved away from ponds, lakes, or irrigation canals. Water troughs and barrels should be cleaned frequently, and the water kept fresh to prevent their use as breeding sites by the flies. Because *Culicoides* feed primarily at dusk, night, and dawn, horses should be kept stabled during these times. Stabling is most effective if the stall is lined with a fine-mesh screen. Stall fans are helpful to reduce exposure, because *Culicoides* cannot fly well in brisk breezes. Application of insecticides and repellents is a necessary part of disease control. The most effective products are those containing pyrethrins with synergists and repellents. Frequent bathing not only decreases scale and crust formation but also seems to decrease pruritus. Corticosteroid therapy is often necessary in these cases to control pruritus.

Sarcodes

Equine sarcoid, a benign, locally invasive tumor of skin, is the most common tumor in horses. These tumors may produce raised, hairless lesions with a corrugated surface that often bleed when traumatized, known as *fibroblastic sarcoids*, or a flattened form known, as *verrucous sarcoids*. The exact cause of sarcoidosis is unknown, but a viral agent is suspected. Surgical resection, cryotherapy (i.e., freezing), laser therapy, immunotherapy (with intralesional mycobacterial cell wall extract), radiotherapy (with iridium-191), and chemotherapy (with intralesional cisplatin) are accepted treatment modalities, with variable rates of success. It is difficult to predict the response to a given treatment modality, and combination therapy is often necessary.

Malignant Skin Masses

Squamous cell carcinomas (SCCs) are neoplastic masses caused by exposure to ultraviolet (UV) light. SCC are usually found in horses with pink, nonpigmented skin and may appear anywhere on the horse, although they are most common near the eyes, on the prepuce in male horses, and on the vulva in mares. Diagnosis is made through biopsy and histopathology. If detected while the tumor is small, resection and cryotherapy can be effective, with or without the use of chemotherapy agents.

Melanomas are typically found on gray horses with black-pigmented skin. Melanomas appear as black masses in hairless areas, such as under the tail, around the anus, or in the sheath of males. Most melanomas in horses are benign but can grow large enough to interfere with normal function, particularly those around the anus, which can interfere with defecation. A vaccine that stimulates the immune system to mount a response against malignant melanocytes is available.

Pigeon Fever

Infection caused by *Corynebacterium pseudotuberculosis* causes three disease manifestations: external abscesses, internal infection, and ulcerative lymphangitis (limb infection). The most common form causes external abscesses in the pectoral region of the horse, leading to swelling that resembles a pigeon's breast, and hence the term *pigeon fever*. Often found in hot, dry climates in late summer to early fall, the pathogen enters the skin through wounds or fly bites. Treatment consists of hot compresses until abscesses can be drained. Once opened, flushing with dilute Betadine daily, disinfecting, and maintaining biosecurity are key. NSAIDs may be used to control pain. The pathogen can spread quickly, making fly control and isolation necessary.

Diseases of the Endocrine System

Pituitary Pars Intermedia Dysfunction (Equine Cushing Disease)

PPID is caused by abnormally elevated hormone levels in blood, particularly cortisol, and is the most common disease condition in horses older than 15 years of age. PPID was formerly referred to as *equine Cushing disease*; however, it is associated with enlargement of the middle lobe of the pituitary gland (pars intermedia) specifically, and this characteristic differentiates it from the human form. PPID causes a variety of clinical signs, including a long, curly haircoat that does not shed seasonally (*hirsutism*); polyuria and polydipsia; laminitis; muscle and weight loss; and chronic infections.

PPID is most often diagnosed with a dexamethasone suppression test or resting plasma adrenocorticotropic hormone (ACTH) levels. The preferred treatment for PPID is oral pergolide. Treatment does not cure the disease but manages the symptoms and is a lifelong commitment. Supportive care, such as clipping long hair in the summer months and regular deworming, hoof care, and dental care, is critical to maintaining a good quality of life for the horse.

Diseases of the Urinary System

Urinary tract disease is relatively uncommon in horses compared with other species. Diagnostic investigation of renal disease may include hematology, serum chemistry, urinalysis, rectal examination (the left kidney can be palpated per rectum), ultrasonography, and *cystoscopy* (endoscopic examination of the bladder and urethra).

Acute Renal Failure

Acute renal failure in horses is most often the result of exposure to toxins. Aminoglycoside antibiotics (gentamicin, amikacin); oxytetracycline; polymyxin B, an antibiotic used in the treatment of endotoxemia; and NSAIDs are commonly implicated. Hypovolemia exacerbates renal damage caused by these drugs. Excretion of hemoglobin, a breakdown product of red blood cells (RBCs), and myoglobin, a breakdown product of muscle, by the kidneys (hemoglobinuria and myoglobinuria) can also result in acute renal failure, because these pigments damage the tubules in the kidneys. Hemoglobinuria is secondary to hemolytic anemia, and myoglobinuria is secondary to rhabdomyolysis. Signs of acute renal failure include *oliguria* (decreased urination), anorexia, and changes in urine concentration. Serum chemistry testing reveals increased blood urea nitrogen (BUN) and creatinine levels. Electrolyte abnormalities may also be present. Urinalysis should be performed (see the "Urinalysis" section). The mainstay of treatment for acute renal failure is administration of IV fluids for diuresis. Frequent monitoring of renal values is necessary to determine response to and duration of fluid therapy. Urine output should be closely monitored.

Polyuria/Polydipsia

Horses normally drink between 4% and 6% of their body weight in water daily. Polydipsia in horses is defined as drinking greater than 10% of their body weight in water daily. Horses normally excrete 1% to 3% of their body weight in urine, because most water is lost via feces. *Polyuria* is defined as excretion of urine greater than 5% of body weight daily.

Polyuria/polydipsia (PU/PD) can result from physiologic causes, including lactation, heat, exercise, diarrhea, and glucocorticoid administration. PU/PD is a common sign of equine PPID in older horses (see Chapter 36, "Geriatric and Hospice Care"). PU/PD can also result from psychogenic excessive water drinking (a behavioral problem), diabetes, or chronic renal failure. A water deprivation test may be performed to differentiate the causes.

Care of the Hospitalized Equine Patient

In the hospital setting, veterinary technicians are an integral part of caring for hospitalized equine patients and responsible for patient monitoring, administration of medications, general daily care of horses, and supervision of lay technical support. This section provides an overview of the daily management of equine patients in the hospital setting. Table 19.4 describes some technician evaluations and interventions that may be encountered when treating equine patients. Refer to Case Presentation 19.1, which demonstrates use of the veterinary technician practice model.

Biosecurity

Horses with contagious diseases should be hospitalized in isolation facilities. The most common diseases that require an isolation protocol are colitis (salmonellosis), strangles (*S. equi equi* infection), and the neurologic form of EHV-1. Personnel wear disposable gloves, boots, and body suits while attending isolation cases and discard the PPE when exiting the isolation area. A disinfectant foot dip should be used when entering and exiting each stall. Horses in isolation should not be walked in areas where other horses are allowed to graze. Waste from the stall should be disposed of in a restricted area, and dedicated equipment should be used to clean the stall. If possible, personnel attending isolation cases should work only with these cases to avoid cross contamination. See the American Association of Equine Practitioners (AAEP) Biosecurity Guidelines for more information on isolation protocols (see "Recommended Websites" at the end of the chapter).

Outside of isolation areas, continued biosecurity should be enforced in the entire clinic. Clean gloves should be donned for handling each patient and manure or stall debris frequently removed from aisles and common spaces. Counters and surfaces should be wiped with disinfectant wipes several times daily to remove infectious pathogens. Hospitals may want to invest in a disinfectant fogger to decontaminate common areas, stalls, and treatment rooms. Surveillance programs are helpful to monitor the risk of nosocomial infections, such as *Salmonella* spp.

Patient Monitoring

The level of patient monitoring required for a hospitalized horse depends on the severity and nature of the disease. Horses with infectious diseases require frequent patient monitoring (e.g., every 4 to 6 hours). Any critically ill patient needs intensive care and monitoring and will likely require IV fluid administration. Such patients will be monitored frequently for signs of discomfort, heart rate, respiratory rate, hydration, CRT, abdominal pain, respiratory distress, shock, laminitis, and GI motility. *Tachycardia* (increased heart rate) is indicative of pain. A rate of 60 bpm or greater indicates serious pain in an adult horse.

TABLE 19.4   Selection of Technician Evaluations and Interventions Applicable to the Equine Patient

Technician Evaluation and Definition	Potential Physiologic Consequences	Clinical Findings	Technician Interventions
Anorexia— complete or partial loss of appetite	• Poor immune function • Decreased wound healing • Dehydration • Electrolyte imbalances • Hypoalbuminemia • Hepatic lipidosis (particularly in animals with concurrent illness or pregnancy) • Cachexia • Hypoglycemia • Seizures • Death	• Loss of appetite for longer than 2 days • Prolonged diminished appetite • Increased total bilirubin • Increased liver values (hepatic lipidosis)	• Administer veterinarian-prescribed treatment for primary disease and antacids • Encourage patient to eat on its own: • Novel, odoriferous foods • Coax/socialization • Enteral feeding via nasogastric tube • Parenteral supplementation of dextrose, amino acids, and lipids
Dehydration—loss of total body water	• Decreased renal perfusion • Electrolyte imbalance	• Tacky/dry mucous membranes • Skin tenting • Increased packed cell volume (PCV) and total protein (TP) • Increased renal values (creatinine, blood urea nitrogen [BUN])	• Administer fluid therapy per veterinarian's order • Monitor fluid intake and urine output
Hypovolemia—loss of intravascular fluid	• Decreased perfusion of kidneys, heart, and brain • Shock	• Dry mucous membranes • Pale to white mucous membranes • Prolonged capillary refill time (CRT) • Tachycardia • Weak pulses • Hemorrhage • Increased PCV and TP • Normal or decreased PCV and decreased TP (blood loss) • Decreased jugular fill • Increased lactate	• Administer fluid therapy per veterinarian's orders • Administer blood transfusion per veterinarian's orders • Monitor for signs of transfusion reaction: • Increased heart rate, temperature, or respiratory rate from baseline • Hives
Endotoxemia—group of clinical signs caused by endotoxin in bloodstream	• Hypovolemia • Shock • Systemic inflammation • Coagulopathies • Laminitis • Gastrointestinal (GI) hypomotility	• Fever • Tachycardia • Hyperemic mucous membranes • Leukopenia • Laminitis • Depression	• Administer veterinarian-prescribed treatments
Pain	• GI hypomotility • Hyperthermia • Anorexia • Weight loss • Depression • Decreased milk production • Recumbency	• Pawing, rolling, looking at flank • Tachycardia • Tachypnea • Decreased locomotion • Decreased response to human interaction • Postural changes	• Administer veterinarian-prescribed analgesics • Monitor for breakthrough pain • Monitor for signs of adverse reaction to pain meds: • Decreased GI motility resulting in decreased fecal output and borborygmi and/or colic (opioids, α^2-agonists) • Increased renal values and/or decreased protein (nonsteroidal anti-inflammatory drugs [NSAIDs]) • Provide comfortable environment: • Deep bedding • Pad feet for laminitis

Continued

TABLE 19.4	Selection of Technician Evaluations and Interventions Applicable to the Equine Patient—cont'd		
Technician Evaluation and Definition	Potential Physiologic Consequences	Clinical Findings	Technician Interventions
Hypoxia—decreased oxygenation	• Death	• Cyanotic mucous membranes • Dyspnea • Tachypnea • Altered mentation • Decreased oxygen saturation • Altered arterial blood gases (ABGs)	• Oxygen therapy • Monitor vitals, watch for changes in respiration • Monitor oxygen saturation and ABGs • Administer veterinarian-prescribed treatments for primary disease
Recumbency—inability to stand	• Pneumonia • Pressure sores • Colic • Urinary tract infection	• Recumbency	• Keep in sternal position if possible • Change position at least every 6 hours • Sling if possible • Deep bedding or pad, head bumper, leg wraps • Give soft feed, mineral oil to keep feces soft • Evacuate rectum twice daily if needed • Place indwelling urinary catheter or catheterize periodically to drain bladder

Patient monitoring forms are designed to identify trends in physical signs. Patient treatment forms coordinate treatment periods when several individuals may be responsible for administering medications. Treatment sheets and monitoring forms may be combined for low-maintenance, elective patients. However, for intensive care patients, monitoring should be more detailed, and many hospitals use a flow sheet, either physical or electronic. It is important to recognize that monitoring and treatment forms are a permanent part of the medical record, which represents a legal document or record of all events during hospitalization.

Supportive Care

Supportive care of hospitalized equine patients can be intensive and involves supporting the patient during the healing period.

PUT INTO PRACTICE

Honing your nursing skills helps you give the best care to your patients and provides your clients with the comfort of knowing you are taking care of their animals. Medication administration, proper feeding, and hygiene care are imperative to the healing of patients.

Medication Administration

Hospitalized horses often must receive oral medications. This can be challenging with horses that are head shy. The technician should go slow, approach the horse's shoulder, and spend a few minutes rubbing the horse with the syringe. The horse can be desensitized by administering a treat, such as molasses or applesauce, through a dose syringe several times. Ensuring that there is enough room so that the horse does not feel claustrophobic can be helpful, because lack of space can make the horse more anxious.

Horses that require frequent injections may become needle shy. A local anesthetic gel can be used to numb the skin before injection. If multiple injections are required and the horse's medical condition does not preclude sedatives, an injectable or oral gel sedative (e.g., detomidine gel) may be administered to facilitate medication.

Intravenous Catheter Care

IV catheters are placed for repeated administration of medications or continuous fluid infusion (Fig. 19.11). It is important to determine ahead of time, if possible, whether the patient will need a short-term or a long-term catheter so that the appropriate type is placed. IV catheters should be flushed with heparinized saline every 6 hours and the catheter site monitored for heat, swelling, and pain. Infection at the catheter site may occur in the subcutaneous tissue or in the vein (i.e., septic thrombophlebitis). Septic thrombophlebitis can be life-threatening in horses and is more likely to occur in horses with endotoxemia, systemic infection, and those being treated with parenteral nutrition.

Feeding

Most hospitalized horses are not on their normal feeding schedule. A patient's diet should be kept as normal as possible. If an animal is anorexic, offering a variety of grass, feeds, and hay may be helpful to provide energy for the body to heal. It must be ensured that horses that are unwilling to move around are offered food and water every few hours. Horses that are dysphagic benefit from enteral nutrition, consisting of a commercial formula or blended pelleted feed. Enteral nutrition can be provided via a small-bore NG feeding tube. Parenteral (IV) nutrition, consisting of IV dextrose, amino acids, and/or a lipid, can be used in horses that cannot tolerate sufficient enteral feeding to meet caloric requirements. Catheter care is critical when parenteral nutrition is provided because of the risk for septic thrombophlebitis. A dedicated line and strict aseptic technique are recommended.

CASE PRESENTATION 19.1

Nursing Care Plan: Bacterial Pneumonia

Signalment: Patches, a 5-year-old Paint gelding
Chief complaint: Owner reports that Patches has had a decreased appetite for 2 days and has been coughing.
Pertinent history: Patches was shipped last week from Oklahoma to Florida. Patches was vaccinated routinely 2 months ago. The owner reports no previous health problems.
Physical examination:
  Body weight—1100 pounds
  Body condition score—5/5
  Temperature—103.5°F
  Heart rate—48 beats per minute (bpm), sinus rhythm; synchronous and strong pulses
  Respiration—28 breaths per minute; wheezes dorsally, quiet ventrally
  Mucous membranes—pink and slightly tacky
  Capillary refill time (CRT)—2 to 3 seconds
  Skin turgor—slightly decreased
  Ears, eyes, and nose—serous discharge both nostrils
  Gastrointestinal system—borborygmi: within normal limits
  Musculoskeletal system—normal
Problem list: Fever, decreased lung sounds in ventral quadrant, history of cough, tachypnea, mild dehydration
Initial diagnostic plan: Lower respiratory disease is suspected based on thoracic auscultation, cough, and tachypnea. A rebreathing examination is performed to further assess the lungs. Crackles are auscultated cranioventrally and wheezes dorsally. The patient coughs during the examination and has a prolonged recovery. Complete blood count (CBC) and serum chemistry are run and reveal leukocytosis and hyperfibrinogenemia (inflammatory leukography) and increased packed cell volume (PCV) and total protein (TP). Based on these findings, an infectious cause of lower respiratory disease is suspected. The history of the patient shipping over a long distance makes bacterial pneumonia likely. Thoracic radiography is performed and reveals an alveolar pattern in the cranioventral lung fields. A transtracheal wash (TTW) is performed to obtain a sample for culture and sensitivity to guide antibiotic therapy and for cytologic examination to confirm infection.
Medical diagnosis (by veterinarian): Pleuropneumonia

Treatment Plan (by Veterinarian)

Treatment	Rationale
Potassium penicillin intravenous (IV) every 6 hours (q6h) Gentamicin IV q24h Metronidazole PO q12h	Broad-spectrum antibiotics are warranted pending culture and sensitivity results from TTW, which will allow selective therapy.
Flunixin IV q12h	Decrease inflammation and relieve fever.
IV fluids	Correct dehydration.

Technician evaluations: Altered ventilation; hypovolemia; hyperthermia; abnormal eating behavior; exercise intolerance; risk of altered gas diffusion; risk of sepsis and endotoxemia

Nursing Care Plan
1. Altered Ventilation

Technician Intervention	Rationale
• Monitor respiratory rate and effort.	• Animals with compromised lung function caused by infection may have elevated respiratory rates and increased respiratory effort.
• Monitor mucous membrane color.	
• Auscultate the thorax for abnormal lung sounds.	• Intensity and quality of abnormal lung sounds may indicate severity of pulmonary disease.
• Monitor nasal discharge: describe quantity, quality, and color.	• Blue discoloration of mucous membranes is indicative of compromised gas diffusion and low levels of circulating oxygen (hypoxia).
	• Nasal discharge is an abnormal finding and should be monitored.
• Monitor heart rate and signs of discomfort.	• Heart rate may increase when the patient experiences pain. Pleural pain is common in horses with bacterial pneumonia and pleuritis.
	• Heart rate may also increase as a compensatory mechanism to improve oxygenation of tissues if the patient is hypoxic.
• Improve air quality.	• Dust may aggravate the respiratory system, because normal clearance mechanisms are compromised.
• Decrease dust in environment.	
• Feed low-dust hay and grain.	
• Remove horse from barn when stalls are being cleaned.	• Administration of oxygen increases oxygen saturation in blood.
• If condition worsens and patient becomes hypoxic, consider giving nebulized nasal oxygen.	

Comfort Care

Good hygiene, mental stimulation, and comfort measures can go a long way toward maintaining a patient's quality of life during hospitalization. Attention should be given to mentally stimulating patients, when appropriate, to prevent depression. Bedding should be clean and adequate, and the patient should be kept clean and dry to prevent skin scald resulting from irritation by urine and feces. Brushing, scratching, and petting go a long way to keep patients comfortable. Rinsing out the mouth of a horse that is on medications or not drinking may be comforting to the horse. If consent is given by the veterinarian and it is safe to do so, the horse may be taken out to graze or walked around.

Hospitalized horses tend to be happier if they can see other animals. If appropriate, housing horses in stalls that face other horses may be helpful. In most clinical settings, the side walls of the stalls are solid to prevent disease spread; this may make horses feel claustrophobic and can cause vocalizing, pawing, and even rearing. If an adjacent stall with a horse is not available, such as in isolation cases,

CASE PRESENTATION 19.1—cont'd

2. Hypovolemia

Technician Intervention
- Place jugular catheter.
- Administer IV fluids, per doctor's orders.
- Maintain catheter.
- Check for patency and thrombosis.
- Heparinize catheter.
- Monitor hydration status via packed cell volume (PCV)/total protein (TP).
- Monitor pulse rate, quality, and intensity.
- Monitor CRT.

Rationale
- IV fluids correct hypovolemia caused by dehydration by increasing the liquid portion of blood.
- Increased blood volume increases perfusion of kidneys and helps prevent damage caused by use of aminoglycoside (gentamicin) and the nonsteroidal anti-inflammatory drug (NSAID) flunixin.
- Blood pressure decreases with dehydration because blood volume is reduced. Pulses become weaker as blood pressure drops.
- Whenever a patient is on IV fluids, it is important to regularly monitor the patient's hydration status, so clinicians are sure that the patient is not being overhydrated or underhydrated.
- Heart rate may increase as the body compensates for decreased tissue perfusion during hypovolemia.
- CRT is slowed during hypovolemia, because blood pressure is reduced and perfusion of gum tissue is reduced.

3. Hyperthermia

Technician Intervention
- Administer flunixin IV q12h per veterinarian's order.
- Monitor body temperature regularly.

Rationale
- Flunixin meglumine is an NSAID that decreases inflammation and reduces fever.
- The veterinary technician monitors temperature to determine whether treatment is effective in reducing fever.
- Infection can worsen if antibiotic therapy is not effective, and body temperature may rise if infection spreads to bloodstream (sepsis).

Technician Intervention
- Monitor for signs of endotoxemia

Rationale
- Gram-negative organisms are a cause of bacterial pneumonia.

4. Abnormal Eating Behavior

Technician Intervention
- Treat primary disease
- Administer antibiotics as per order:
  - Potassium penicillin IV q6h
  - Gentamicin IV q24h
  - Metronidazole PO q12h
- Encourage patient to eat by feeding novel, odoriferous feeds:
  - Offer food by hand if effective
  - Allow to graze if possible
- Feed low-dust hay and grain

- Monitor GI function:
  - Auscultate all four quadrants of the abdomen and record manure production and manure quality
  - Monitor for signs of abdominal pain

Rationale
- Appetite will likely improve with resolution of fever and infection.

- Providing appetizing foods and encouragement increases the likelihood that the patient will eat. Patients need energy for immunologic health.

- Dust may aggravate the respiratory system, because normal clearance mechanisms are compromised.

- Peristalsis can be altered when patients are stall-bound and inactive.

- Illness, such as sepsis, can cause ileus (decreased GI motility).

5. Exercise Intolerance

Technician Intervention
- Hand-walk patient, if possible.
- Allow access to grass.

Rationale
- Activity and pasture improve peristaltic activity.

---

placing a mannequin horse nearby or even a stuffed animal will sometimes help calm an anxious horse (Fig. 19.12).

Recumbency

Recumbent horses are particularly challenging to manage effectively in a hospital setting. Neurologic and musculoskeletal diseases are the most common problems resulting in recumbency in horses. Recumbent horses and foals quickly develop *pressure sores (decubitus ulcers)* over the pelvis (tuber coxae), elbows, and head if not effectively managed (Fig. 19.13). Bedding soaked with manure and urine must be removed frequently, because skin irritation and sores may develop. Pressure sores can rapidly become deep and may infect underlying bony structures. Muscle damage can occur as the result of pressure and decreased circulation. In addition, recumbent horses may have decreased intestinal motility and may fail to void urine. Therefore soft feed, such as fresh grass or feed made into mashes, should be offered to recumbent horses to facilitate fecal evacuation and prevent impaction. Eyes should be checked for corneal ulcers and an ophthalmic lubricant used to prevent them. Horses unable to defecate should have feces manually removed twice daily. Placement of an indwelling urinary catheter or periodic catheterization of the urinary bladder is often necessary when managing recumbent patients. Recumbent horses should be deeply bedded on straw, placed on a padded mat, or

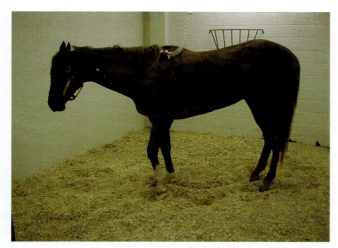

• **Fig. 19.11** Horse with an intravenous (IV) catheter placed and receiving IV fluids.

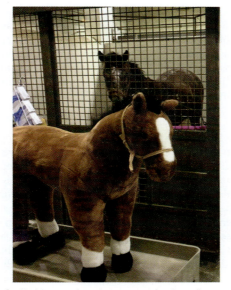

• **Fig. 19.12** Stuffed horse placed near a patient's stall to provide "companionship."

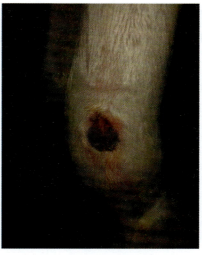

• **Fig. 19.13** Pressure sores in a recumbent horse.

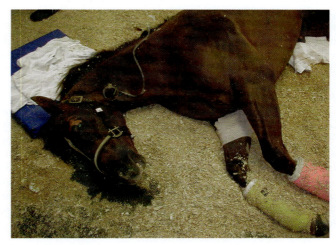

• **Fig. 19.14** Padding is crucial to prevent recumbent horses from injuries. This horse has shifted its head off the provided pad. Note the abrasion above its left eye.

placed on a mattress to prevent the development of pressure sores (Fig. 19.14). The position of the horse should be changed every 6 hours; multiple attendants are required to move an recumbent adult horse. A sling can be used only on horses that can partially support their own weight but are not able to stand on their own. Recumbent adult horses can rarely be managed for longer than 1 or 2 weeks without the development of life-threatening complications (pneumonia, urinary tract infection, colic, pressure sores).

Oxygen and Tracheostomy Monitoring

If the horse has low oxygen levels or is in respiratory distress, oxygen can be administered through a nasal cannula taped to the nostril. The oxygen line can become tangled or kinked if not watched closely. A temporary tracheostomy can provide relief to horses suffering respiratory distress from upper airway obstruction or edema of the head and neck. Tracheostomy tubes must be strictly maintained to keep them clean and patent. Tubes should be removed and cleaned twice a day and kept free of foreign material. Animals with a tracheostomy tube should be given hay and feed on the ground and water kept low so that aspiration does not

occur. Applying a small amount of petroleum jelly below the site will prevent skin irritation from exudate and make cleaning easier.

Plasma and Blood Transfusions

Blood transfusions may be administered to severely anemic patients or those that have lost a significant volume of blood. Horses have eight different blood types, and there is often not adequate time to determine the patient's blood type, so many hospitals have a universal blood donor (AaQq) from which they can collect blood at their facility. Care should be taken to ensure that the donors are healthy, screened frequently for disease, and have not had blood collected from them within the past month. Up to 6 L of blood may be taken from a donor horse, but fluid losses must be replaced and the donor monitored closely after collection. When transfusing a patient, a filtered administration set must be used, and the recipient must be monitored closely for signs of transfusion reaction. (Refer to Chapter 24, "Fluid Therapy and Transfusion Medicine.")

Integrative Medicine

Integrative medicine entails the use of alternative therapies such as acupuncture, chiropractic care, massage, and laser therapy. Complementary therapies may be used alone or in conjunction with traditional therapy and can be particularly helpful in patients that have kidney or liver disease and have limited medication options. (Refer to Chapter 23, "Rehabilitation and Alternative Medical Nursing.")

Laboratory Diagnostics

Clinicopathological testing provides vital information for the veterinarian to identify an impairment of an organ system, confirm a clinical diagnosis, assess patient response to therapy, and formulate a prognosis. The normal values of many clinicopathologic tests vary among species. In addition, species-specific characteristics are associated with diseases and the significance of abnormal findings. This section concentrates solely on equine-specific alterations in clinicopathologic values in health and disease. (Refer to Chapter 11, "Hematology and Cytology," and Chapter 12, "Clinical Chemistry, Serology, and Urinalysis.")

Hematology

CBC provides information pertaining to RBC count, RBC morphology, total WBC count, WBC differential (including neutrophils, lymphocytes, eosinophils, and monocytes), and WBC morphology. RBCs are most easily estimated by using packed cell volume (PCV). The normal range of PCV depends on the breed but generally is between 32% and 45%. Hot-blooded breeds (Thoroughbreds, Arabians, Quarter Horses) have higher resting RBC counts compared with ponies and draft horses. Low PCV (<30%) is indicative of anemia. Horses have a large muscular spleen that normally contains up to one-third of the circulating RBC volume. With excitement and exercise, PCV can increase by as much as 50% secondary to splenic contraction. Therefore resting PCV is highly variable and must be serially evaluated in excitable patients. In addition, splenic response to massive hemorrhage precludes use of PCV to estimate the magnitude of blood loss for at least 24 hours. Total protein levels will decrease and lactate levels will increase in horses with acute blood loss.

Evaluation of the total and differential WBC count is important to identify the presence of infection. In most instances, bacterial infection will manifest as an increase in WBC count (leukocytosis) characterized by an increase in the number of mature neutrophils (mature neutrophilia). Endotoxemia (described above) causes margination and sequestration of WBCs, resulting in a profoundly low WBC count (leukopenia) characterized by low neutrophil count (neutropenia) and immature band neutrophils (left shift). Fibrinogen is a coagulation factor and an acute-phase protein produced by the liver in response to inflammation. Fibrinogen concentrations remain increased until infection has resolved. Serum amyloid A, another acute-phase protein, can be measured with a stallside test to detect inflammation.

Serum Chemistry

A serum chemistry panel provides specific information pertaining to the liver, kidneys, muscles, and serum electrolyte concentrations. In horses, serum normally has a yellow tint as a result of increased bilirubin levels, because horses do not have gallbladders. Serum bilirubin concentrations will increase dramatically if feed is withheld for longer than 24 hours because of a normal physiologic response; this does not indicate liver disease. Most species develop low serum albumin levels with chronic liver disease because of decreased production; however, in horses, production of albumin is maintained, even with marked impairment of liver function. Reliable indicators of liver dysfunction in horses include high serum gamma-glutamyl transferase activity, high serum sorbitol dehydrogenase activity, high serum bile

acid concentrations, low BUN concentrations, and increased ammonia levels.

In most species, renal failure produces low serum calcium and high serum phosphorus concentrations. Horses are obligate calcium excreters, and chronic renal failure often produces a marked increase in the serum calcium concentration. Reliable indicators of renal failure in horses include high serum creatinine and BUN and electrolyte abnormalities, including low sodium and chloride and high potassium and calcium levels. The large equine colon exchanges vast quantities of electrolytes and fluids daily. Horses with colonic inflammation may develop marked electrolyte abnormalities before diarrhea occurs. Low serum sodium, chloride, and potassium levels in horses with abdominal pain or depression often indicate loss of electrolytes into the lumen of the colon and impending diarrhea.

Serum creatine phosphokinase (CK) is an indicator of muscle damage in all species. Horses have large muscle mass in comparison with ruminants and small animals. Moderate increases in serum CK levels (two to four times the normal) readily occur in horses after prolonged transport, prolonged recumbency, exercise in an unconditioned horse, or rolling because of abdominal pain. Moderate increases do not usually indicate primary muscle disease. Horses with primary muscle disease, such as exertional rhabdomyolysis (tying-up, azoturia, Monday morning sickness), have increases in serum CK activity of up to 200 times normal values. Aspartate aminotransferase is an enzyme found in muscle tissue and liver tissue; increases are expected when primary muscle disease or liver disease is present.

Lactate

Lactate, or lactic acid, is produced by cells undergoing anaerobic metabolism as a result of lack of oxygen. Lactate levels in blood therefore increase (hyperlactatemia) in conditions of decreased oxygen delivery to tissues. This most commonly occurs as a result of hypovolemia. In horses, severe hypovolemia is seen with colic and diarrhea. Lactate levels in venous blood can provide an objective measurement of the magnitude of hypovolemia and can help monitor response to fluid therapy. In adult horses, normal lactate levels are lower than 1.5 mmol/L. Other causes of increased blood lactate levels include anemia, cardiac disease, and respiratory disease.

In cases of colic, comparison of the lactate level in peripheral blood with an abdominal fluid sample obtained via abdominocentesis can be useful in determining the viability of the intestine. Colic in which the blood supply to the intestine is compromised, such as a large colon volvulus or a strangulating small intestinal lesion, results in local production of lactate by the ischemic bowel. In such cases, the lactate level in the abdominal fluid will be higher than that in peripheral blood.

Blood Gas Analysis

Blood gas analysis provides information on oxygen and carbon dioxide content, pH, base deficit, and bicarbonate levels in the sample. Arterial samples are indicated to evaluate patients with respiratory disease; venous samples are indicated in patients with diseases affecting metabolic acid-base status, such as diarrhea and kidney disease. (See Chapter 17, "Diagnostic Sampling and Treatment Techniques," for a discussion of sampling techniques for arterial blood gases [ABGs].)

Urinalysis

Urinalysis is essential for evaluation of primary renal disease. (Refer to Chapter 17.) Normal equine urine is usually alkaline (pH 7–9), contains many calcium carbonate crystals, and usually produces a false-positive reaction for protein on urine dipsticks.

Horses have many mucous glands located within the renal pelvis; therefore normal equine urine may appear thick and mucoid. Red urine is abnormal and results from the presence of frank blood (primary urinary tract disease), hemoglobin (hemolytic anemia), or myoglobin (myositis). Differentiation of these sources of red urine requires special testing of urine and serum samples. Urine specific gravity and urinary electrolyte excretion ratios should be obtained to investigate primary renal function. Urine specific gravity indicates the ability of the kidney to concentrate urine; normal values in resting horses should be greater than 1.030. Urinary electrolyte excretion ratios indicate the ability of the kidney to conserve electrolytes. Identification of WBCs and numerous bacteria indicates urinary tract infection. Protein (proteinuria), glucose (glycosuria), and casts in urine indicate renal disease.

Evaluation of Body Fluids

Evaluation of cerebrospinal, synovial (joint), and abdominal cavity fluids provides important information pertaining to inflammation, infection, or neoplasia within that body cavity. These body fluids can be analyzed for total protein, total cell count, differential cell count, and bacterial culture and to identify specific infectious diseases.

Some neurologic diseases in horses require CSF analysis for diagnosis. Because some neurologic diseases, such as rabies, have zoonotic potential, CSF must be collected and handled with caution (e.g., protective eyewear or face shields, laboratory coats, and gloves) to prevent exposure to the infectious agent. CSF can be collected, with the animal under sedation, from the lumbosacral space or in anesthetized horses from the atlanto-occipital space. (See Chapter 17.) Normal nucleated cell counts are less than 5 cells per microliter (predominantly lymphocytes). The normal total protein concentration is variable, depending on the laboratory, but usually is less than 80 mg/dL (higher than in other species). Abnormalities in protein and cell counts can identify an inflammatory, infectious, or neoplastic process, but the results of CSF analyses are often nonspecific. Antibodies to the agents of several equine neurologic diseases (EPM, herpes myeloencephalopathy, equine encephalomyelitis) can be detected in CSF and provide specific information regarding the cause of neurologic signs. Complications associated with a CSF tap include iatrogenic (operator-induced) spinal cord trauma and the introduction of bacteria into the CNS.

Abdominal pain, an abnormal rectal examination, abdominal distention, and fever of unknown origin are indications for abdominocentesis in horses. (See Chapter 17 for more information on sampling techniques.) Normal abdominal fluid is straw-yellow colored and clear, has a total protein of less than 2.5 mg/dL, and has a normal total nucleated cell count of less than 5000/mL (50% neutrophils). Analysis of abdominal fluid can reveal devitalized bowel in horses with acute abdominal pain (colic), abdominal abscesses, tumors in horses with a mass in the abdomen identified via rectal palpation or abdominal ultrasonography, and a ruptured bladder in foals with abdominal distention. Complications of abdominocentesis include traumatic bowel rupture, intra-abdominal hemorrhage from trauma to the spleen, and iatrogenic septic peritonitis.

Bacterial Culture and Susceptibility Testing

The veterinary technician often plays an important role in bacteriologic testing of specimens collected from patients with infectious disease. Specimens (blood, joint fluid, abdominal fluid, feces, urine, wound exudate, infected bone, etc.) are frequently collected for culture from horses with infectious disease. Following proper procedures during collection and transport of these specimens to the laboratory for culture and susceptibility testing improves the chances of growing the causative organism. Specific guidelines must be followed for the collection and transport of different types of specimens. For example, blood is usually placed in a special enhancement medium immediately after collection for transport to the laboratory. Special methods are used for the collection and transport of samples submitted for aerobic and anaerobic culture. Identifying the causative agent in an infectious process and determining the in vitro susceptibility pattern to antibiotics are often critical in choosing the appropriate antibiotic regimen. Fecal samples are often submitted for *Salmonella* spp. or *Clostridium* spp. cultures from horses with diarrhea. Three to five fecal samples for *Salmonella* spp. culture should be submitted at least 24 hours apart. If culture results are negative for these samples, the horses are not shedding *Salmonella* organisms. Fecal samples may be tested for *Clostridium* toxins and *Clostridium* spp. culture; samples should be submitted daily for three consecutive days. Fecal samples may be submitted for other diagnostic tests, such as ELISA for rotavirus, or PCR for *Salmonella* or *Clostridium*.

Polymerase Chain Reaction Testing

PCR testing is a laboratory technique that identifies and amplifies a specific segment of genetic material (DNA or RNA) from bacteria, viruses, or animals. Because DNA samples are unique, this technique allows very sensitive and specific diagnostic testing for bacterial and viral pathogens and for inheritable genetic diseases. The sample tested depends on which test is being performed. For example, PCR is the diagnostic test of choice for the neurologic form of EHV-1. Because the virus circulates within the WBCs, the sample of choice is whole blood. PCR detects a DNA sequence that is unique to the neurologic form of EHV-1 and differentiates it from respiratory forms. PCR is also useful in the diagnosis of PHF by detecting *N. risticii* in whole blood samples, salmonellosis and clostridiosis by identifying specific species of the bacteria in fecal samples, and strangles by identifying *Streptococcus equi* subsp. *equi* in samples from the guttural pouch.

PCR testing can be used to diagnose genetic disorders by identifying the segment of DNA specific to the disease. PCR is used for the diagnosis of several inherited disorders, including hyperkalemic periodic paralysis, polysaccharide storage myopathy, glycogen branching enzyme deficiency, malignant hyperthermia, and hereditary equine regional dermal asthenia. For example, hyperkalemic periodic paralysis is caused by a point mutation (a single nucleotide difference in the DNA sequence) in the sodium channels of muscle cells. PCR analysis of blood or hair samples from the patient allows diagnosis of the disease. Because PCR allows detection of animals that are carriers of a genetic defect, it can be used to screen animals before breeding to eliminate the risk of passing on the disorder.

> **TECHNICIAN NOTE**
>
> Because horses do not have gallbladders, they have a high serum bilirubin level, and their normal serum appears yellow compared with other species. Serum bilirubin concentrations increase dramatically if feed is withheld for longer than 24 hours. This condition, which is called *fasting hyperbilirubinemia*, is a normal physiologic response in horses and does not indicate liver disease.

Summary

Although being an equine veterinary technician can be stressful and overwhelming, it can also be rewarding. It is important to remember to focus on the end goal: a healthy patient. Technicians/

nurses act as the veterinarian's eyes and their patients' advocates, so they must be always aware of their patients' status and can provide updates to the veterinarian as needed. The number of duties related to caring for critically ill horses can be overwhelming, but patient care comes first, whether it is holding a water bucket so that a horse with laminitis can drink, advocating for pain control for a patient in discomfort, or cleaning a horse to lessen the risk of infection. To provide excellent care, technicians must take excellent care of themselves. Although patients always come first when working on the clock, taking time for oneself when the shift is over by doing enjoyable things and focusing on relationships with family and friends are critical to prevent burnout and compassion fatigue.

Food Animal Nursing

Fewer veterinarians are choosing food animal practice as a career, and practice owners have been finding it increasingly difficult to hire veterinary associates. For these individuals, optimizing the use of veterinary technicians/nurses is of great importance. A technician who can confidently and effectively perform the required tasks to assist the practice can improve productivity and revenue by being able to help meet client and patient needs. Veterinarians must focus on tasks that by law, they alone are allowed to perform (surgery, diagnosis, prognosis, and prescribing treatments); however, they can delegate nursing and support care tasks to veterinary technicians/nurses. Veterinary technicians perform numerous tasks in a modern food animal practice, including laboratory procedures, diagnostic tests, diagnostic imaging (Fig. 19.15), anesthesia, preparation of pharmacologic and biological agents, and administration of medications or other treatments. They carry out orders given by the veterinarian to assess and monitor hospitalized patients and complete medication and treatment plans. When assisting at the herd level, veterinary technicians/nurses can take responsibility for ration development, body condition scoring (BCS), and health maintenance visits for herds and flocks. Veterinary technicians can perform necropsies, including recording findings, taking photographs, and collecting tissue specimens for further review by the attending veterinarian. A perceptive, educated, and knowledgeable technician who can anticipate and prepare for the needs of the food animal patient and those of the producer and veterinarian is an invaluable asset to a food animal medical team.

> ### TECHNICIAN NOTE
> Capitalizing on veterinary technician skills in food animal practice can help meet client and patient needs and can improve the practice's productivity, efficiency, and revenue.

When working with large animals, safety should be the primary concern. Gates, ropes, fences, and chutes are helpful for moving and restraining these animals. It is important for veterinary technicians/nurses to become familiar with the different types of chutes and equipment used to be as efficient as possible. Proper footwear and clothing are also important for protection around these animals. Knowledge of the behavior of the species the technician will be working with is crucial. The technician should pay attention to the surroundings and always have an escape route planned. Gathering and handling animals as calmly as possible will promote a calm working environment that is less stressful for the animals and veterinary team. By building trust and implementing low-stress handling techniques, more forceful methods, such as cattle prodding, can potentially be avoided.

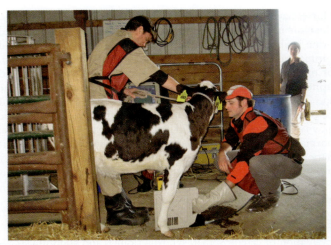

• **Fig. 19.15** Veterinary technicians and nurses in food animal practice may assist with a variety of procedures.

Biosecurity is of utmost importance in a farm/facility or clinical setting. All equipment should be cleaned and disinfected between uses, patients, and farms. Disposable gloves and rubber boots are essential to avoid cross contamination among herds and farms. When new animals are brought to a facility, they should be isolated for a minimum of 30 days before being introduced to the herd to prevent transmission of infectious diseases to established herd members.

> ### PUT INTO PRACTICE
> Implementation of appropriate biosecurity will help your food animal clients know that you understand their concerns and appreciate the importance of keeping their animal safe.

Being able to properly identify patients is another important necessity for food animal technicians. Identifying patients while treating a herd of 50 Black Angus, for example, can be difficult, because they all look the same. Many farmers use ear tags, tattoos, or brands to help identify individual animals within a herd. In cattle, the left ear is used for the farmer's tattoo or tag with a specific identifying number for each animal. The right ear is reserved for regulatory governmental identification, such as a vaccine tattoo, vaccine tag, or other form of permanent identification if there is no visible brand. In goats and sheep, the left ear is used for farm identification, and the right ear holds a scrapie tag for federal identification. In commercial pigs, an ear notching system is used for identification (Fig. 19.16). Notches on the left ear represent the pig's birth number within a breeding season to a particular sow. Notches in the right ear represent the litter number, which signifies the order in which a specific litter was born on that farm. Becoming familiar with this technique can be very useful when working with a herd of pigs to provide treatment or to choose the correct one for a procedure.

Common Diseases and Conditions of Ruminants

Care of the Neonate and Neonatal Diseases
Lambs and Kids

Does and ewes should have a health check and be vaccinated annually with *Clostridium perfringens* type C and D toxoid and *C. tetani* toxoid at least 1 month prior to parturition to ensure the best

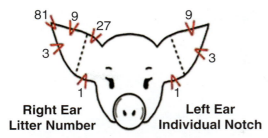

• **Fig. 19.16** Diagram of ear notching system used to identify pigs.

chances for a successful lambing or kidding season. By providing booster doses to the dams before lambing or kidding, the number of colostral antibodies for the neonate will be increased. Small ruminants are born with immature immune systems and rely on colostral antibodies for protection from diseases. Once weaned, these animals will be given their primary vaccination series for these diseases, usually around 2 to 3 months of age.

Sheep are gregarious animals and stay together as a group, even during lambing; this may result in lamb "stealing" by late-pregnant ewes. Therefore lambing in individual pens helps prevent this. A strong ewe-lamb bond is a key component for healthy, happy lambs. The licking of amniotic fluid from the lamb by the ewe clears the lamb's airway, stimulates breathing, and allows the ewe to identify that lamb as her own. Intervention provided during or right after parturition by the owner or the veterinarian might confuse the ewe as to whether the lamb is hers. Ewes can identify their own lamb(s) after only a few hours of contact, whereas lambs require several days before they can identify their mothers. Treatment of the lamb for **hypoglycemia**, chilling, or illness should be provided in the lambing pen, if possible, because separation of the lamb for longer than 1 hour may result in rejection of the lamb by the ewe.

The first week of life, especially the first 48 hours, is the most critical time for lambs and kids. Hypothermia and hypoglycemia are two major problems during this time, when as much as 50% of neonate mortality can occur. Lambs and kids are born with minimal body fat stores; therefore hypoglycemia can develop if newborns do not ingest colostrum (high in fat) within the first 12 to 24 hours. Hypoglycemic kids and lambs rapidly become weak, may not be able to stand and nurse and, if not monitored closely, may become recumbent quickly. The dam's udder should be checked immediately after parturition to ensure that it is producing milk and that mastitis is not present. Ewes tend to have a thick wax plug that blocks the end of the teat before initial nursing. Occasionally, the lamb is unable to remove the plug when it begins to nurse, which results in unsuccessful nursing. Lambs and kids should be examined for congenital problems that might affect nursing, such as cleft palate.

Hypothermia and hypoglycemia usually can be prevented with good management practices. Pens should be built to prevent drafts and may even be designed with a supplemental heat source (heat lamp) for lambs. Securing a corner of the pen and providing a heat source in that area attracts lambs away from the ewe so they may rest safely away from possible accidental trauma caused by the dam. It is helpful to have frozen sheep or goat colostrum on hand. Cow colostrum may also be used, but a small percentage of lambs may develop neonatal isoerythrolysis-type syndrome around 10 days after ingesting cow colostrum. Commercial lamb and kid milk replacers are available for orphan rearing or to supplement neonates of ewes that are poor producers of milk. Lambs and kids

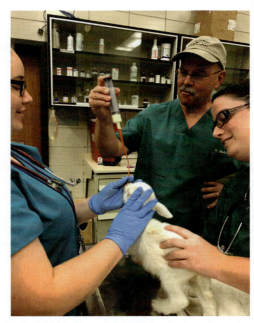

• **Fig. 19.17** Goat kid being administered colostrum through a stomach tube.

need to be fed 10% to 15% of their body weight daily, divided into three to four feedings, during the first few days after birth (Fig. 19.17). Later, twice-daily feeding is adequate. They should be offered hay and starter grain early, but milk should be the major energy source until they are at least 6 weeks old. If a lamb or kid is hypoglycemic and hypothermic, it is best to rewarm the animal before providing any oral therapy. During a hypothermic crisis, the lower esophageal sphincter relaxes, and milk or oral supplements may be regurgitated, potentially resulting in aspiration. Rewarming when the core body temperature is low is best achieved by immersing the neonate in warm water (100°F to 105°F) while taking care to support the head. Veterinary technicians may be instrumental in herd or flock management during the kidding or lambing period. This is when they can use their expertise on bottle feeding neonates and help owners avoid aspiration pneumonia in neonates by choosing properly sized nipples and bottles.

> **TECHNICIAN NOTE**
>
> The key to successful rearing of lambs and kids is identifying the weak and small ones that may get pushed away from the udder by their bigger siblings. It is of utmost importance to keep the neonates warm, dry, and fed.

Enterotoxemia

Enterotoxemia is caused by *C. perfringens*. It is recognized worldwide as a common, frequently fatal disease of young sheep and goats that involve such signs as severe enterocolitis, sudden death, diarrhea in goats, and neurologic signs in lambs. Although outbreaks have occurred in situations where feeding practices were consistent, sudden feed changes, such as accidental exposure to grain, turn-out to lush pasture, feeding bran or molasses mash to animals that have recently given birth and are lactating, and feeding bakery goods, have been associated with enterotoxemia epidemics. In ruminant species, it is believed that *C. perfringens* type D organisms normally reside in the intestines, but sudden ingestion of readily fermentable, carbohydrate-rich feed serves as fuel for rapid proliferation of the organism. Death of the animal is caused by damage to vital neurons, generalized toxemia, and shock. Clinically, lambs show lethargy, overt neurologic signs, minimal diarrhea, and death, as opposed to kids, which show more prominent diarrhea and colic and fewer neurologic signs, followed by death.

Treatment of enterotoxemia consists of IV fluids, *C. perfringens* type C and D antitoxin, anti-inflammatories, and antibiotics. Rations containing high-carbohydrate feeds should be adjusted immediately.

> ### TECHNICIAN NOTE
> Small ruminants are considered highly susceptible to enterotoxemia and should be vaccinated every 6 months.

Coccidiosis

Coccidiosis is a condition commonly found in goats 3 weeks to 5 months old who may or may not have diarrhea. It is caused by a species-specific protozoan parasite (*Eimeria* spp.) that is a normal environmental contaminant. Adult goats are rarely affected; however, it commonly occurs in kids and lambs that are confined and/or stressed at weaning time. Coccidiosis may be subclinical or clinical, but appetite loss and failure to gain weight occur in both situations. Diarrhea, which is the most common clinical sign, can severely debilitate young kids. Dehydration, bloody stool, and death can occur in the worst cases within 24 hours. A veterinary technician can do a microscopic fecal examination to identify the organism and assist the producers in basic sanitary husbandry practices by providing clean bedding and fresh hay and water daily. A coccidiostat, such as amprolium or sulfadimethoxine, is most effective in the early stages of infection.

Endoparasites

Endoparasitism is a severe problem for small ruminants. Although sheep and goats differ in terms of feeding behavior (i.e., sheep graze and goats browse), they can be infected by the same internal parasites. Typical internal parasites include *Haemonchus contortus*, *Ostertagia ostertagi*, and *Trichostrongylus* spp. The most important parasite of small ruminants in North America is *H. contortus*, also known as the *barber pole worm*, aptly named for the spiraling of blood-filled intestines around the white-colored ovary and the uterus. These parasites have developed multidrug resistance after years of indiscriminate anthelmintic administration. As a result, parasite control is a major problem in small ruminant flocks and herds. This is most common in southeastern United States, where the climate is hot and humid most of the year, making this the perfect environment for these parasites. Another parasite that has become more prevalent in goats is the liver fluke, *Fasciola hepatica*. It takes only two to three flukes to do enough damage in a goat's liver to cause anorexia, lethargy, and sudden death.

Severe parasitism results in anemia, pale mucous membranes, subcutaneous edema ("bottle jaw") caused by hypoproteinemia, unthriftiness with poor fleece or wool, and weight loss. Feces may be soft, but diarrhea is rarely observed. Sudden death may occur among animals that have a severe, acute parasite infection. At times, producers will need the veterinary team to advise them regarding husbandry techniques for their herds or flocks. The FAMACHA (FAffa MAlan CHArt) scoring system is a method used to help producers determine the level of anemia present and whether animals should be dewormed. It uses a laminated card with a range of colors that is compared with the color of the lower

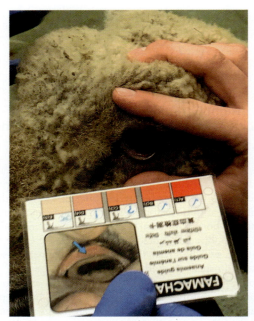

• **Fig. 19.18** FAMACHA (FAffa MAlan CHArt) scoring system used to determine whether deworming is necessary.

conjunctiva of the goat/sheep to determine the degree of possible parasitic load based on a scale of 1 to 5, with 1 being the best and 5 the worst. This scale, along with PCV assessment and fecal examination, is the best way to determine whether the animals require only deworming or blood transfusion therapy (Fig. 19.18).

In severe cases, immediate administration of an effective anthelmintic (dewormer) is recommended. Available dewormers include cydectin, ivermectin, albendazole, and levamisole. Fecal flotation and McMaster fecal egg count can be performed before anthelmintic administration and can be repeated 10 to 14 days after treatment to determine the therapeutic effectiveness of the dewormer. A greater than 90% reduction in fecal egg count per gram of feces indicates that the dewormer is working. Blood transfusions may be required in animals with PCVs of less than 10%. Animals should be kept in a quiet, confined environment and given good-quality forage with high protein content and easy access to water. Prevention of severe parasitism includes pasture rotation, strategic deworming protocols using effective anthelmintics, and selective culling of animals with a heavy parasite burden.

Calves

Dystocia, or difficulty during the birthing process, is common in cattle (Fig. 19.19), and food animal veterinarians often assist cows and heifers during this time. Calves that are delivered via forced fetal extraction or cesarean section are frequently compromised, even if parturition is successful. While the veterinarian attends to the dam, especially in the case of a cesarean section, the veterinary technician can provide intensive care to the neonate. The most important first steps are to place the newborn calf in sternal recumbency and ensure that it is breathing. All mucus should be cleared from the nose, mouth, and upper airway. The calf may be briefly hung upside down with its head off the ground to allow drainage of these fluids, and then the calf should be replaced in the sternal recumbency position. A piece of straw or hay may be used to tickle the nose and stimulate respiration. Additionally, placement of digital pressure on or a small-gauge needle into the nasal

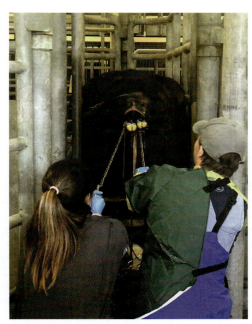

• **Fig. 19.19** A veterinary technician assists a veterinarian deliver a calf from a cow experiencing dystocia.

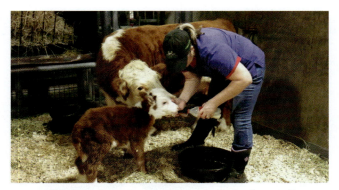

• **Fig. 19.20** A veterinary technician bottle feeding a calf.

septum is often a successful respiratory stimulus. For difficult cases, doxapram hydrochloride, a respiratory stimulant, may be injected under the tongue to induce respiration. If these techniques fail, artificial respiration can be provided by mouth-to-nose resuscitation or by raising and lowering the upper forelimb while simultaneously pressing and releasing the rib cage. Once the calf is breathing, it should be vigorously rubbed dry with a towel, and the umbilical cord should be dipped in iodine or chlorhexidine solution. Care should be taken not to completely remove all afterbirth, because it encourages the cow to smell and lick the calf to foster the cow-calf bond. A well-trained technician will ensure that the calf stays warm, has stood within 30 minutes of birth, and has a suckle reflex.

Colostrum ingestion soon after birth is critically important for neonatal survival and prevention of infectious diseases. The placenta in cattle and other ruminants prevents in utero transfer of immunoglobulins (antibodies) from the dam to the fetus. As a result, these species are essentially **agammaglobulinemic** at birth and rely on ingestion and absorption of colostrum antibodies and nonantibody immune factors to protect newborns from infection during the first few months of life. Transfer of immunity can be compromised by colostrum deficiencies, ingestion failure, or absorption failure. If the cow is weak or rejects the calf, the cow should be restrained, and the colostrum should be milked from the udder and given to the calf via a bottle or an orogastric gravity feeder (Fig. 19.20). It is crucial that the calf receives a full dose of colostrum at 10% of its body weight within the first 4 to 6 hours of life for optimal immunity.

The cow's colostrum may be deficient in immunoglobulins because of age, past diseases, vaccination status, and so on. It is possible to test the colostrum's IgG levels on the farm and in the clinic using a **colostrometer**. If the cow is not lactating sufficiently for the calf to get colostrum and no frozen bovine colostrum is available, a colostrum replacer can be purchased. Once the calf has nursed or colostrum has been administered, the calf's serum is evaluated to determine whether the colostrum has delivered adequate maternal antibodies to the calf.

Several laboratory tests are available for direct or indirect detection of FPT of maternal antibodies, including sodium sulfite precipitation, zinc sulfate turbidity, and serum total solids (STS) analysis. The sodium sulfite test and STS are considered the least expensive tests for routine use and can be run on the farm with the help of a knowledgeable technician. STS can be measured by using a handheld refractometer. STS concentration greater than 5.5 g/dL, in the absence of dehydration, is indicative of successful passive transfer. Primarily, STS testing is useful for monitoring the overall success of a farm's colostrum feeding program. Veterinary technicians can play a valuable role in monitoring a farm's colostrum feeding program by collecting blood samples once weekly from newborn calves (1–7 days old) and analyzing each calf's STS concentration.

Partial or total FPT can make a calf susceptible to a variety of diseases. If a calf fails to acquire passive transfer of immunity, then a plasma transfusion should be given to boost immunity and help prevent any future diseases. Any immunosuppression early in life can predispose the calf to developing an umbilical infection (**omphalophlebitis**), which can manifest as any combination of the following problems: **septicemia**, septic arthritis, anterior uveitis, meningitis, vegetative endocarditis, pneumonia, and diarrhea. These calves should be treated immediately with broad-spectrum antimicrobial agents; supportive therapy, such as with fluids with dextrose and electrolytes; and bottle feeding if they are too weak to stand and nurse. If omphalophlebitis is present and does not respond to antimicrobial therapy, surgical removal of infected umbilical remnants should be considered, if the patient is a good surgical candidate. Septic arthritis should be treated with broad-spectrum systemic antibiotics and IV regional antibiotic perfusion, joint lavage (Fig. 19.21), or arthrotomy.

Calf Scours

Diarrhea, or scours, which is a common problem among young dairy and beef calves, is associated with multiple infectious and noninfectious causes. Viral causes include rotavirus, coronavirus, and bovine viral diarrhea virus (BVDV). Bacterial enteritis may result if the calf is infected by *Escherichia coli*, *Salmonella* spp., *Clostridium* spp., or protozoal pathogens, such as coccidia or *Cryptosporidium*. In addition, a variety of management-related issues, including poor nutrition and improper sanitation, may cause or contribute to the development of diarrhea. Regardless of cause, calves often experience watery diarrhea, which rapidly leads to severe dehydration, metabolic acidosis, hypoglycemia, shock, and hypothermia. Treatment is aimed at rapid replacement of lost fluids and correction of acidosis and electrolyte abnormalities. On farms where calf diarrhea is a persistent problem, it is important to ensure adequate

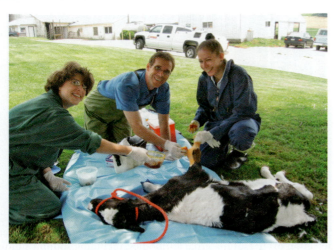

• **Fig. 19.21** Delicate procedures may be performed in the field with the assistance of veterinary technicians.

colostrum feeding, and it may be necessary to vaccinate cows and heifers before calving. Sick, weak calves should be started on warm, balanced IV fluids supplemented with dextrose and bicarbonate. Oral electrolyte solutions may be administered to replace lost fluids, but it is important that the calf's normal milk or milk replacer feedings also be offered. When adding oral electrolytes, they should be given in between milk feedings, not at the same time. Bottle or tube feeding may be necessary during this time.

Some kind of skin protectant, such as vitamin A&D ointment, petroleum jelly, or diaper rash cream, should be used on the calf's perineum and down the legs, where the diarrhea can cause scald, resulting in the calf losing its hair. Bedding should be kept clean and dry.

Diseases of the Digestive System

Several diseases of the GI system are considered an emergency and require rapid assessment by a veterinary technician so that it can be addressed by a veterinarian. Quick recognition of the problem is more likely to have a positive outcome. Other GI diseases are more chronic and can affect the productivity of the animal. A summary of common infectious and noninfectious diseases of adult ruminants is included in Table 19.5.

Rumen dysfunction can be devastating to a ruminant and often requires rumen fluid analysis to determine a cause. Evaluation of a rumen fluid sample includes assessment of color, consistency, odor, pH, microscopic examination, rumen chloride, and redox potential. Testing must be done within 300 minutes of collection or immediately to avoid fluid degradation. The normal color of rumen fluid is olive or brownish green. Grain overload results in fluid that is milky gray, whereas prolonged stasis or decomposition in the rumen changes the fluid color to dark green or black. The consistency of normal rumen fluid is slightly viscous, and salivary contamination increases viscosity. The odor of normal rumen fluid is aromatic and strong, but it develops an acidic smell with grain overload and a putrid odor with stasis and decomposition.

The pH of rumen fluid is normally 6.5 to 6.8 (5.5–6.5 with high-grain diets). Rumen fluid pH of less than 5.5 is suggestive of grain overload. Microscopic examination is performed to assess the types of bacteria present and protozoal activity. In healthy animals, gram-negative bacteria predominate in the rumen. The rumen chloride concentration is normally less than 25 mEq/L but

may be elevated in cases of ileus or obstruction. The redox potential test uses new methylene blue (NMB) to evaluate anaerobic fermentation. To perform the test, 1 mL of 0.03% NMB is mixed with 20 mL rumen fluid (the control sample is untreated rumen fluid). If active the rumen microflora reduces NMB, and the mixture returns to the color of rumen fluid. This usually takes about 3 minutes (1–3 minutes if on a grain diet; 3–6 minutes if on a hay diet). If an animal is inappetent and has poor rumen fluid quality, a rumen transfaunation (Fig. 19.22) can be performed to replace the nutrients that the sick animal is lacking. (Refer to Chapter 25, "Emergency and Critical Care Nursing.")

Pharyngeal Trauma and Abscessation

Improper use of a balling gun, long-dose syringe, speculum, paste dewormer gun, or rigid stomach tube may penetrate the pharynx and cause pharyngeal trauma. Less commonly, a foreign object, such as a stick or wire, may penetrate the pharynx. This may lead to cellulitis, abscess, or hematoma formation. Clinical signs include anorexia, salivation, malodorous breath, extension of the head and neck, feed coming from the nares, and mild bloat. In more severe cases, dysphagia, coughing, and aspiration pneumonia may occur. Careful oral examination of the pharynx is often diagnostic. Gloves should always be worn during palpation of the mouth or the pharynx in cattle because of the risk of rabies. Endoscopy and radiography can be of great benefit in diagnosing the site of the lesion, the extent of the cellulitis, and the presence of a foreign body.

Treatment requires aggressive use of antimicrobial drugs for 10 to 14 days. Anti-inflammatories may help reduce inflammation in the early stages of disease. Supportive therapy is also important, especially if the animal is unable to eat or drink. Feed and water may be administered with a soft stomach tube or via a temporary rumenostomy. The patient's mouth may need to be rinsed and the cud/feedstuff to be manually extracted to allow the lesion to heal until the patient has the ability to swallow and clear the mouth on its own. It is critical that the animal's head is adequately restrained to prevent excessive movement and subsequent injury (Fig. 19.23). The veterinary technician plays an important role in educating food animal producers on the proper use of this equipment.

> **TECHNICIAN NOTE**
>
> Pharyngeal trauma in cattle can be prevented by careful use of oral dosing equipment.

Rumen Indigestion

In ruminants, the term *indigestion* refers to the disruption of normal reticulorumen function; this condition is very common and is self-limiting. It results from a rapid feed change or introduction of feed materials that quickly change the rumen environment. Moldy or overheated feeds are typically implicated. Clinical signs include acute anorexia, reduced rumen motility, and potentially malodorous diarrhea. Diagnosis is usually based on history and clinical signs. Rumen fluid analysis may be useful in confirming the diagnosis. Rumen transfaunation is the single best way to restore normal rumen function, along with oral fluids and probiotics to supplement treatment.

> **TECHNICIAN NOTE**
>
> Indigestion is a very common disease in ruminants and is usually self-limiting.

TABLE 19.5 Common Medically Managed Gastrointestinal Conditions of Ruminants

Disease/Etiologic Agent	Species Affected	Pathogenesis	Clinical Signs	Diagnosis	Treatment
Infectious					
Actinomycosis (lumpy jaw)/*Actinomyces bovis*	Bovine	• Normal bacterial flora of ruminant mouth • Entry via mouth wounds • Infection results in osteomyelitis of the mandible or maxilla	• Hard, immovable bony mass on mandible or maxilla • Inability to masticate • Subsequent anorexia and weight loss	• Oral examination • Radiography • Isolation of organism from infected tissues	• Sodium iodide and antibiotics • Surgical debridement • Anti-inflammatories
Actinobacillosis (wooden tongue)/*Actinobacillus lignieresii*	Bovine, ovine	• Normal bacterial flora of ruminant mouth • Entry via mouth wounds	• Cattle—tongue is hard, with diffuse nodular swellings • Sheep—swellings around lips and face • Excessive salivation • Inability to masticate • Subsequent anorexia and weight loss	• Oral examination • Biopsy and isolation of the organism	• Sodium iodide and antibiotics • Anti-inflammatories
Winter dysentery/coronavirus	Bovine	• Fecal-oral transmission	• Explosive diarrhea • Mild depression • Partial anorexia	• Fecal samples for laboratory diagnostics	• Supportive treatments • Usually spontaneous recovery within a week
Bovine viral diarrhea/bovine viral diarrhea virus (BVDV)	Bovine	• Natural exposure to the virus • Persistently infected animals may have mucosal disease if they are exposed to a cytopathic strain of virus	• Fever • Weight loss • Diarrhea • Mucosal ulceration • Blunted oral papillae • Highly variable clinical presentation	• Physical examination • Identification of virus in blood by laboratory testing • Serology (acute and convalescent)	• Supportive fluid therapy • Prophylactic antibiotics
Parasitism	Bovine, caprine, ovine	• Ingestion of infective larvae	• Chronic diarrhea • Weight loss • Unthriftiness • Pale mucous membranes	• Fecal float	• Anthelmintics
Johne disease/*Mycobacterium paratuberculosis*	Bovine, caprine, ovine	• Oral ingestion during perinatal period • In utero transmission	• Cattle: chronic diarrhea • Weight loss	• Fecal samples for laboratory diagnostics • Serology	• None • Prevention important
Salmonellosis	Bovine, caprine, ovine	• Fecal-oral transmission	• Severe diarrhea, which may include blood or mucus • Fever • Anorexia	• Fecal samples for laboratory diagnostics	• Supportive fluid therapy • Anti-inflammatories • Prophylactic antibiotics
Enterotoxemia/*Clostridium perfringens* types C and D	Bovine, caprine, ovine	• Normal inhabitant of GI tract • Sudden diet change—increased carbohydrates • Rapid overgrowth and subsequent toxin production	• Sudden death • Hemorrhagic diarrhea • Fever • Glycosuria	• Fecal samples for laboratory diagnostics	• Antibiotics • Supportive fluid therapy • Anti-inflammatories • Antitoxin • Prevention with vaccine

Continued

TABLE 19.5 **Common Medically Managed Gastrointestinal Conditions of Ruminants—cont'd**

Disease/Etiologic Agent	Species Affected	Pathogenesis	Clinical Signs	Diagnosis	Treatment
Noninfectious					
Pharyngeal abscessation	Bovine	• Trauma associated with improper oral administration of treatments	• Pharyngeal swelling • Anorexia • Excessive salivation • Malodorous breath • Extension of head and neck • Mild bloat • Fever	• Careful digital palpation of the pharynx per os • Endoscopy • Radiography	• Antibiotics • Anti-inflammatories • Supportive therapy if animal cannot eat or drink
Rumen indigestion	Bovine, caprine, ovine	• Rapid feed changes • Moldy or spoiled feeds • Change in rumen environment	• Acute anorexia • Decreased rumen motility • Malodorous diarrhea	• History • Physical examination • Rumen fluid analysis	• Transfaunation • Supportive fluid therapy
Grain overload (carbohydrate engorgement, lactic acidosis)	Bovine, caprine, ovine	• Excessive intake of carbohydrates • Increased volatile fatty acids (VFAs) and lactic acid • Decreased rumen pH and motility • Increased rumen osmolarity leading to severe dehydration	• Depression • Anorexia • Bloat • Diarrhea • Dehydration • Incoordination • Recumbency • Death	• History • Physical examination • Rumen fluid analysis	• Lavage rumen or rumenotomy surgery • Oral antacids • Antibiotics • Supportive fluid therapy • Anti-inflammatories
Rumen tympany (bloat)	Bovine, caprine, ovine	• Free gas bloat: obstruction of eructation • Frothy bloat: consumption of legumes or grains leading to stable rumen froth	• Severe abdominal distention • Dyspnea • Depression • Anxiety	• History • Physical examination • Passage of orogastric tube	• Passage of orogastric tube • Oral administration of detergent • Supportive fluid therapy • Anti-inflammatories
Traumatic reticuloperitonitis (hardware disease)	Bovine	• Indiscriminate eating habits leading to accidental ingestion of sharp foreign body • Penetration of reticulum and subsequent peritonitis	• Fever • Anorexia • Reluctance to rise or move • Cranial abdominal pain • Kyphosis	• Radiography • Ultrasonography • Blood work (complete blood work [CBC], plasma fibrinogen) • Abdominocentesis	• Oral magnet • Antibiotics • Surgical intervention to remove foreign body

Grain Overload (Carbohydrate Engorgement, Lactic Acidosis)

Grain overload in ruminants results from consumption of excessive amounts of high-carbohydrate feed and subsequent production of large quantities of lactic acid in the rumen. Excess carbohydrate ingestion leads to lower rumen pH and decreases rumen motility. *Streptococcus bovis* organisms then proliferate and produce large amounts of lactic acid, which further lowers rumen pH (4.0–5.0). Additionally, *Lactobacillus* spp. are acid resistant, and this allows them to proliferate and produce more lactic acid. This creates characteristic "splashy rumen" sounds and leads to severe dehydration and metabolic acidosis. If affected animals are not treated early, severe metabolic acidosis may develop, leading to shock and acute death. Animals that do not die of acute acidosis may develop secondary problems, such as rumenitis, liver abscess, laminitis, and/or **polioencephalomalacia**.

Ruminants with grain overload rapidly develop clinical signs of depression, anorexia, bloat, diarrhea, dehydration, incoordination, and recumbency, leading to death. The diagnosis is based on a history of sudden exposure to large amounts of grain, typical clinical signs, and a rumen pH of less than 5.0. Rumen fluid analysis can confirm the diagnosis.

Medical treatment involves rapid removal of rumen contents. In cattle, this may be achieved through lavage of the rumen with

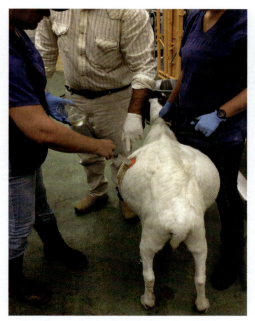

• **Fig. 19.22** This goat has a rumen cannula, through which rumen material can be collected for transfaunation.

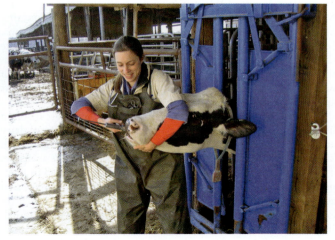

• **Fig. 19.23** This veterinary technician is demonstrating proper restraint of a cow's head during administration of medicine using a balling gun.

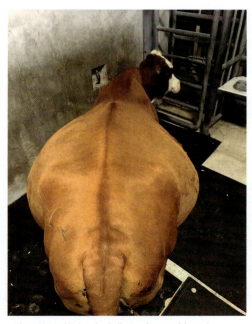

• **Fig. 19.24** Abdominal distension, or bloat, in a cow.

a large-bore stomach tube or by performing rumenotomy surgery. In small ruminants, rumen lavage is not possible with a large-bore tube, and rumenotomy is required. In addition, animals are given oral antacids, antibiotics, anti-inflammatories when rehydrated, and thiamine, all of which help prevent liver abscess, polioencephalomalacia, and laminitis. In more severe cases, IV fluids with sodium bicarbonate should be administered to correct dehydration and acidosis. Whether an animal is treated medically or surgically, rumen transfaunation is often helpful to re-establish normal rumen microflora and improve appetite.

TECHNICIAN NOTE

Grain overload is an emergency and may lead to death if rapid patient assessment and treatment are not provided.

Rumen Tympany (Bloat)

Gas production is a normal occurrence during rumen fermentation, and healthy animals are capable of eructating the gas that the rumen produces. However, in some cases, abnormal distention of the rumen with gas may occur, resulting in bloat (Fig. 19.24). Bloat is described as free gas bloat or frothy bloat, depending on the cause. Free gas bloat results from failure to eructate normally and may be associated with esophageal foreign bodies (choke); motor function abnormalities of the rumen, such as vagal indigestion; body position (lateral recumbency); hypocalcemia; or pharyngitis. Frothy bloat occurs when large quantities of legumes or certain grains are ingested, resulting in development of froth in the rumen that blocks eructation. Clinical signs of bloat include distention of the left paralumbar fossa, discomfort, dyspnea with open-mouth breathing, anorexia, salivation, anxiety, depression, and sudden death.

Treatment of free gas bloat involves passing an orogastric tube. If hypocalcemia is the underlying problem, administration of calcium is therapeutic. Forced exercise stimulates rumen motility and eructation. If an animal is critically bloated and passing a stomach tube is too stressful, an emergency procedure called *rumen trocarization* should be performed.

Frothy bloat requires different treatment, because the froth must first be dissipated before gas can be expelled from the rumen. To reduce surface tension of the froth, several products may be used, including poloxalene, household detergent, mineral oil, or dioctyl sodium sulfosuccinate. Once the frothy bloat becomes a free gas bloat, it can be eructated or relieved via an orogastric tube.

Traumatic Reticuloperitonitis

Traumatic reticuloperitonitis (TRP), or hardware disease, results from penetration of the reticulum by a foreign body and is one of the most common GI problems affecting the forestomach compartments of mature dairy cattle. Their indiscriminate eating habits can lead to accidental ingestion of foreign materials, which settle in the reticulum. Foreign bodies ingested by cattle, such as

wires and nails, are usually ferromagnetic. Following ingestion of a foreign body, four outcomes are possible:
- Attachment of the object to a magnet without further disease problems
- Penetration of the reticular wall with acute inflammation and mild clinical disease if no penetration into the peritoneal cavity occurs
- Perforation of the reticular wall into the peritoneal cavity with acute localized TRP
- Migration of the foreign body with penetration into the peritoneal or thoracic cavity and resulting abscessation (thoracic, reticular, hepatic), vagal indigestion, pericarditis, myocarditis, or other secondary problems.

Acute cases of TRP result in anorexia, a sharp decrease in milk production, reluctance to rise or move, cranial abdominal pain, and kyphosis. Uncomplicated cases may improve in 3 to 5 days, but progression of the severity of signs may indicate failure to contain localized peritonitis or extension of the infection to other organs. A heart rate greater than 90 bpm or a high fever generally indicates more severe disease, such as diffuse peritonitis or pericarditis. A heart rate less than 60 bpm is suggestive of vagal indigestion. Cranioventral abdominal radiography or ultrasonography can offer valuable assistance in the diagnosis of TRP.

Medical treatment of TRP is often successful and is geared toward treating reticulitis and/or peritonitis using systemic broad-spectrum antimicrobials and preventing further perforation of the reticulum by oral administration of a magnet. Even if a foreign body has perforated the reticular wall, a magnet may return the foreign body to the lumen. Surgical intervention may be necessary if TRP fails to respond to medical treatment.

> ### TECHNICIAN NOTE
>
> Traumatic reticuloperitonitis (TRP), or hardware disease, is caused by cattle ingesting sharp metallic objects such as wire. Such sharp objects can perforate the wall of the reticulum, causing peritonitis and liver and reticular abscesses, and can perforate the pericardium, causing pericarditis.

Salmonellosis

Salmonellosis typically manifests as acute diarrhea, but in rare cases, individuals become chronically infected and have recurring bouts of diarrhea with or without fever, anorexia, and dehydration. Severe acute cases may progress to endotoxemia, shock, and subsequent death. Animals that survive may continue to carry and shed the organism, posing a threat to other animals. Submission of multiple fecal samples for culture is necessary to establish a diagnosis. Because of multidrug-resistant strains, the use of antibiotics for the treatment of salmonellosis is controversial. Treatments include anti-inflammatories; fluid therapy, particularly in young animals with septicemia and/or endotoxemia; and potentially antibiotics, depending on the condition of the animal and the strain isolated.

Bovine Viral Diarrhea Virus

Bovine viral diarrhea (BVD) is a viral disease caused by the Bovine Viral Diarrhea Virus (BVDV), is a highly contagious viral disease affecting all ages of cattle; however, most cases are seen in cattle 6 months to 2 years of age. Clinical signs of BVD are sudden onset of fever, depression, oral and GI ulcers and erosions, and diarrhea (sometimes with blood and mucus). BVD also plays an important role in respiratory diseases in cattle by causing immunosuppression and susceptibility to secondary bacterial pathogens. The

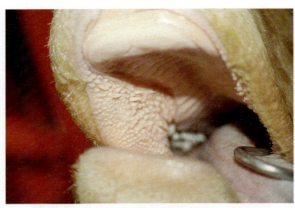

• **Fig. 19.25** Blunted oral papillae seen in a calf with chronic bovine viral diarrhea, or mucosal disease.

disease may progress rapidly through a group of animals. Exposure of pregnant cattle to the noncytopathic strain of BVDV between days 30 and 120 of gestation may result in abortion or an infected fetus which has persistent infection (PI) and becomes immunotolerant to the virus. These calves may look normal at birth, but later in life, will be stunted and unthrifty with diarrhea or pneumonia when exposed to cytopathic strains of BVDV; this results in mucosal disease (MD) in these calves. Clinical signs of BVD-MD include weight loss, anorexia, crusty eyes or muzzle, blunting of oral papillae (Fig. 19.25), and chronic coronary band lesions. MD has a nearly 100% mortality rate. Diagnosis of BVD is made through physical examination, identification of characteristic necropsy findings, virus isolation from tissues or the buffy coat of whole blood samples, and serology (paired samples 2 to 4 weeks apart are most helpful).

No treatment for BVD is available, but antimicrobials are often used to prevent secondary bacterial infection. Vaccination of dairy and beef animals is important to prevent the disease, and both killed virus vaccines and modified live virus vaccines are available. The use of modified live virus vaccines should be avoided in pregnant cows, calves, nursing pregnant cows, and immunosuppressed animals. Use of the modified live virus vaccine in a calf calves experiencing chronic BVD may result in the death of the animal. Incorrect use of vaccines can be financially devastating to farmers, so education is key in the use and timing of vaccination.

> ### TECHNICIAN NOTE
>
> Bovine viral diarrhea (BVD) may cause gastroenteritis, respiratory tract disease, immunosuppression, abortion, in utero infection, and birth defects in cattle.

Johne Disease (Mycobacterium Paratuberculosis Infection)
Cattle

Johne disease is a worldwide animal health issue affecting ruminants. It is characterized by chronic diarrhea and weight loss in cattle and is caused by *Mycobacterium paratuberculosis*, a slow-growing organism (Case Presentation 19.2). The bacterium is transmitted from infected cows to their calves via the fecal-oral route, with calves younger than 6 months being most susceptible to infection. Although infection occurs early in life, clinical signs do not usually develop in cattle until the animal is at least 2 years of age (Fig. 19.26). Diagnosis can be difficult because of the long incubation period and subclinical "shedders," but it should be

CASE PRESENTATION 19.2

Chronic Weight Loss and Diarrhea

A 4-year-old cross-bred beef cow with a 4-month history of weight loss and diarrhea was presented. The cow had been treated with LA200 (Liquamycin; Zoetis, Parsippany, NJ) every other day for three treatments, and she had been dewormed twice with Ivomec Plus (ivermectin and clorsulon; Boehringer Ingelheim Animal Health, Duluth, GA) at monthly intervals beginning 3 months before the cow was seen, with no response.

Clinical findings included emaciation (body condition score of 2 out of 9), submandibular edema, diarrhea, and good appetite. Differentials for chronic weight loss and diarrhea included Johne disease, **gastrointestinal parasites**, chronic salmonellosis, chronic renal disease, chronic liver disease, chronic bovine viral diarrhea, and bovine leukosis virus. Clinical findings, chronicity of the disease, and failure to respond to conventional treatments made Johne disease likely.

A rectal mucosal biopsy was taken, and acid-fast organisms were found within the rectal mucosal cells. The cow was humanely euthanized, and gross and histopathologic findings resulted in a definitive diagnosis of Johne disease. The owner was counseled to cull this cow's offspring, and the attending veterinary technician provided education to the client concerning the impact of the disease on the herd.

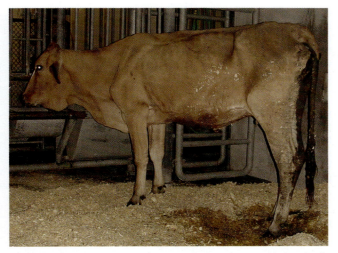

• **Fig. 19.26** Severe emaciation, intermandibular edema, and chronic diarrhea in a cow with Johne disease (caused by *Mycobacterium paratuberculosis*).

high on the differential diagnosis list based on the history, clinical signs, and lack of response to conventional treatments such as antimicrobial and anthelmintic therapy.

Johne disease is a terminal disease for which no effective treatment is available. Control programs in cattle have been outlined for producers who wish to eliminate the disease from their herd. These programs involve the use of repeated serologic testing, fecal cultures, culling of positive or clinically ill animals, and maintenance of separate disease-free and infected herds. It is very important to identify the "shedders" of the group. Veterinary technicians/nurses can educate producers on methods to control the disease and to cull positive or critically ill animals from their herds.

Small Ruminants

Johne disease in small ruminants is a chronic wasting disease. It is not always accompanied by diarrhea, as in cattle. It also is not only infectious to the young but also to adults, which can develop

clinical signs after exposure. Infection from an infected dam can occur in utero or through nursing, or can occur via the fecal-oral route. Agar gel immunodiffusion (AGID) on serum is an accurate diagnostic test, and producers should routinely have this test performed on new animals before they are added to the herd. If Johne disease is found in an animal, it should be culled from the herd.

Diseases of the Respiratory System

There are many pathogens that cause respiratory diseases in ruminants (Table 19.6). Respiratory diseases are very common and can be controlled with a well-designed vaccination protocol. Animals that are stressed as a result of overcrowding, transportation, handling, and poor ventilation are predisposed to infection. Many multivalent vaccines are available and protect against both viral and bacterial respiratory pathogens. Veterinary technicians may play an important role in ensuring appropriate administration of these vaccines on farms.

Bovine Respiratory Disease Syndrome

Bovine respiratory disease syndrome (BRDS; "shipping fever") affects cattle of all ages, but particularly beef calves during the first 45 days in the feedlot and dairy calves younger than 6 months of age. The syndrome is caused by a complex interaction of respiratory viruses, bacteria, and stress.

Generally, a number of viruses, including infectious bovine rhinotracheitis (IBR), BVD, parainfluenza virus (PI3), bovine respiratory syncytial virus, and coronavirus, may cause primary pneumonia or may predispose cattle to secondary bacterial infection by pathogens such as *Pasteurella multocida*, *Mannheimia haemolytica*, and *Histophilus somni*. Each of these bacterial pathogens may also cause respiratory diseases in susceptible animals.

Cattle with BRDS experience depression, causing them to stand with their heads lowered; anorexia; fever (104°F to 107°F); mucopurulent ocular and nasal discharge; cough; and dyspnea. Morbidity and mortality within a group may be quite high, depending on the immune status of the group and the pathogens involved. The diagnosis of BRDS is based on a history of the cattle undergoing stress, clinical signs consistent with pneumonia, and the presence of bronchopneumonia observed on necropsy. Samples from a transtracheal aspirate can be submitted for cytologic examination, bacterial and viral isolation, and antimicrobial sensitivity.

For BRDS treatment of cattle to be successful, early diagnosis and institution of appropriate antimicrobial therapy are important. Individual sick animals should be isolated from the rest of the group and treated with broad-spectrum antimicrobial therapy for at least 5 days. Antimicrobial agents typically used for the treatment of shipping fever include ceftiofur, florfenicol, tilmicosin, tulathromycin, tetracycline, and enrofloxacin. When large numbers of animals are ill, antimicrobial agents may be added to the water or feed to simplify treatment. In addition, fresh water, hay, and adequate shelter should be provided. Preconditioning (castration, dehorning, deworming, and vaccination) of calves before weaning and vaccination before transport from stocker to feeder operations could also decrease stress on cattle during these transitions and may prevent the development or lessen the severity of disease.

TECHNICIAN NOTE

Bovine respiratory disease syndrome (BRDS), which affects primarily feedlot calves and dairy calves younger than 6 months of age, is caused by a complex interaction of respiratory viruses, bacteria, and stress.

TABLE
19.6 **Common Respiratory Pathogens of Ruminants**

Disease/Etiologic Agent	Species Affected	Pathogenesis	Clinical Signs	Diagnosis	Treatment
Bacterial Pathogens					
Pasteurella multocida	Bovine, caprine, ovine	• Normal inhabitant of upper respiratory tract • Stress or concurrent viral infection leads to pneumonia	• Fever • Dyspnea • Cough • Nasal discharge • Ocular discharge	• History • Clinical signs • Transtracheal aspiration for bacterial isolation	• Antibiotics • Anti-inflammatories
Mannheimia haemolytica	Bovine, caprine, ovine	• Normal inhabitant of upper respiratory tract • Stress or concurrent viral infection leads to pneumonia	• Fever • Dyspnea • Cough • Nasal discharge • Ocular discharge	• History • Clinical signs • Transtracheal aspiration for bacterial isolation	• Antibiotics • Anti-inflammatories
Histophilus somnus	Bovine	• Stress or concurrent viral infection leads to pneumonia	• Fever • Dyspnea • Cough • Nasal discharge • Neurologic signs	• History • Clinical signs • Transtracheal aspiration for bacterial isolation	• Antibiotics • Anti-inflammatories
Mycoplasma bovis	Bovine	• Ubiquitous in the environment on some farms	• Variety of clinical syndromes • Relatively mild respiratory signs—mild cough, low fever • Otitis media in calves—head tilt	• History • Clinical signs • Transtracheal aspiration for bacterial isolation	• Antibiotics • Anti-inflammatories
Viral Pathogens					
Infectious bovine rhinotracheitis (IBR)/bovine herpes virus-1	Bovine	• Recent herd additions • Stress • Inhalation	• High fever • Dyspnea • Nasal discharge • Cough • White mucosal plaques • Abortion • Conjunctivitis	• Physical examination and identification of characteristic plaques • Serology (acute and convalescent)	• Prophylactic antibiotics • Anti-inflammatories • Prevention—vaccination
Parainfluenza virus (PI3)	Bovine, caprine, ovine	• Exposure to the virus • Stress	• Fever • Coughing • Nasal discharge • Ocular discharge	• Isolation of virus • Serology (acute and convalescent)	• Prophylactic antibiotics • Anti-inflammatories • Prevention—vaccination
Bovine viral diarrhea/bovine viral diarrhea virus (BVDV)	Bovine	• Natural exposure to the virus • Recent herd additions • Stress	• High fever • Depression • Mucosal lesions • Diarrhea	• Physical examination • Serology (acute and convalescent)	• Prophylactic antibiotics • Anti-inflammatories • Prevention—vaccination
Respiratory syncytial virus (RSV)	Bovine, caprine, ovine	• Spread via infected respiratory secretions	• Subcutaneous emphysema • High fever • Coughing • Dyspnea • Nasal discharge	• Physical examination • Serology (acute and convalescent)	• Prophylactic antibiotics • Anti-inflammatories • Prevention—vaccination
Coronavirus	Bovine	• Natural exposure to the virus	• Fever • Coughing • Nasal discharge • Ocular discharge	• Nasal swab for identification of virus • Serology (acute and convalescent)	• Prophylactic antibiotics • Anti-inflammatories

Aspiration Pneumonia

Force-feeding via a bottle or careless tube feeding in neonates can result in aspiration pneumonia. Inhalation of fluid when passing an NG tube or the presence of a large hole in the nipple of the bottle when a sick animal is too weak to swallow properly can cause aspiration of the contents into the lungs. Clinical signs include coughing, respiratory distress, and pyrexia. Crackles and wheezes may be heard upon auscultation of the lungs. If caught early, antimicrobial and anti-inflammatory treatment is sometimes successful. Care should also be taken to check for a cleft palate if suspected.

Ovine Progressive Pneumonia

Ovine progressive pneumonia (OPP) manifests as progressive respiratory failure but also causes mastitis ("hard bag"), neurologic signs, and arthritis. It can be transmitted to the young that nurse from an infected dam. The pulmonary form is predominant in the United States, and clinical signs include exercise intolerance, open-mouth breathing, exaggerated expiratory effort, and an occasional dry cough. In the later stages of the disease, weight loss occurs despite a good appetite. The disease causes an interstitial pneumonia, and affected animals usually die within 3 to 8 months of onset of clinical signs. Diagnosis is based on clinical signs, necropsy, and serology testing.

Diseases of the Reproductive System/Mammary Gland

Diseases of the reproductive system and the mammary gland are extremely common in ruminants, especially dairy animals. Veterinary technicians may be involved in programs designed to monitor or control these diseases. For example, veterinary technicians may collect aseptic milk samples for culture and then may perform the required laboratory procedures to identify common mastitis pathogens. These procedures provide veterinarians and food animal producers with valuable information that can aid in the treatment of clinical cases and the design of control strategies on a farm.

Mastitis

Cattle

Inflammation of the mammary glands is called *mastitis*. The mammary glands are functionally and anatomically separate glands, and it is possible for only one quarter to be affected. This condition is caused by invasion of a variety of pathogens through the streak canal of the teat. Economically, mastitis is one of the most important diseases in the dairy industry, and it is the single most common disease syndrome in adult dairy cows. Severe environmental contamination of the teats, injury to the streak canal, or improperly functioning milking machine equipment may predispose the udder to infection.

Mastitis may be categorized in several different ways. First, mastitis is either subclinical or clinical. *Subclinical mastitis* refers to an infection of the mammary gland, resulting in elevation in somatic cell count but no clinical change in milk. *Clinical mastitis* refers to an infection resulting in elevated somatic cell count and a clinical change in milk from the affected quarter. Second, mastitis can be subdivided into two broad but overlapping categories based on the source of the infection: contagious and environmental. Contagious mastitis, such as that caused by *Streptococcus agalactiae* and *Staphylococcus aureus*, is spread from an infected mammary gland to a healthy one via contaminated milking equipment, through nursing calves, or by the milker's hands. Environmental

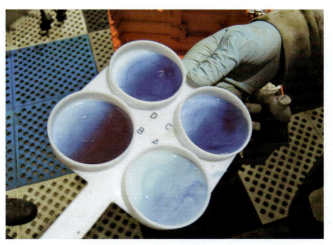

• **Fig. 19.27** Subclinical mastitis in dairy cattle is often identified by using the California mastitis test (CMT). Testing involves stripping milk from each quarter into a corresponding well of the CMT paddle, seen in this photo. A reagent is then mixed with the milk, and the degree of coagulation of the mixture is recorded.

mastitis results when bacteria, such as *E. coli* and *Klebsiella pneumoniae*, from the cow's environment gain access to the mammary gland and cause infection. Clinical mastitis is diagnosed by clinical examination of the milk and udder, but diagnosis of subclinical mastitis relies primarily on use of the California mastitis test (CMT) (Fig. 19.27). (For more information on the CMT and instructions for completing the test, refer to Chapter 17, "Diagnostic Sampling and Treatment Techniques.") Mastitis produces a wide range of abnormal secretions, from milk with flakes or clots to purulent material or blood. Aseptic collection of a milk sample for culture often provides important information on the cause of mastitis and may guide treatment decisions, depending on the pathogen. Cows with toxic mastitis are suffering from endotoxemia and usually have a watery or serous secretion from the affected gland. Gangrenous mastitis causes gangrene of the gland, with a distinct blue line of demarcation separating normal and affected tissues. Secretions from affected glands are watery, gangrenous portions are cold to the touch, and these portions of the gland will eventually slough off. Toxic and gangrenous mastitis may cause death.

Depending on the causative agent, mastitis can be successfully treated if recognized early. Treatment of mastitis involves the use of appropriate antimicrobial therapy—systemic and/or intramammary. Cows with toxic mastitis usually require intensive treatment with anti-inflammatories, IV or oral fluids, and supplemental calcium. Only antibiotics approved for use in dairy cows should be administered for the treatment of mastitis. In addition, antibiotic milk withdrawal times must be closely monitored. The veterinary technician should be familiar with these approved drugs and withdrawal times and can serve as an important resource for education of the dairy farmer.

Prevention of mastitis is of paramount importance in the dairy industry. Control may be achieved by the implementation of the five-point plan for mastitis control, which includes the following:
- Maintenance of hygiene by performing premilking and postmilking teat dipping and keeping cows clean and dry between milkings
- Use of proper milking procedures with well-functioning equipment when milking

- Dry cow treatment of every quarter of every cow and development of a veterinary-prescribed therapeutic plan for clinical cases
- Culling of affected cows as necessary, based on economics
- Maintaining good records on each cow in terms of production, reproduction, milk quality, and clinical mastitis

TECHNICIAN NOTE

Preventing mastitis is of great economic importance, and control may be achieved by ensuring proper hygiene, use of proper milking procedures, appropriate dry cow treatment, culling of affected cows, and maintaining good records.

Small Ruminants

Mastitis in sheep and goats can be caused by a variety of bacteria, including coliforms, *Staphylococcus* spp., *Pseudomonas* spp., *Streptococcus* spp., *and P. haemolytica*. "Blue bag mastitis," caused by *S. aureus* or *P. haemolytica*, is of great concern to sheep and goat producers. *S. aureus* is associated with the gangrenous form of mastitis and may be severe enough to cause death of the animal. Treatment of mastitis in sheep and goats is like that provided for cattle. Be aware that consecutive mastitis episodes can change the conformation of an udder or cause it to become nonfunctional.

Additionally, OPP can result in mastitis in sheep. With this disease, the ewe's udder and milk will appear normal; however, the udder will feel firm when palpated as a result of the presence of fibrous connective tissue that occurs with OPP. Development of fibrous tissue in the udder results in markedly decreased milk production.

TECHNICIAN NOTE

Infection with *Staphylococcus aureus*, likely associated with the gangrenous form of mastitis in sheep and goats ("blue bag mastitis"), may progress rapidly, resulting in the death of the animal.

Retained Placenta (Fetal Membranes)

Retained placenta is a common postpartum disease affecting dairy cattle. After calving, the placenta usually is passed within 2 to 4 hours and is considered retained if it has not been expelled in 12 hours. The cause is unknown, but it is more likely to occur after the birth of twins, after abortion during the last half of pregnancy, and in cases of dystocia. This is not as critical in ruminants as it is in mares. Deficiencies of selenium and vitamins A and E have been suggested to cause an increased incidence of retained placenta.

Manual removal of the placenta should be avoided, because this may result in endometrial damage and infection, with prolonged uterine involution and delayed breeding. Although uterine infusion is controversial, most veterinarians agree that cows with signs of systemic illness resulting from retained placenta should receive systemic antibiotic therapy. Oxytocin can also be used to help the cow or doe in involution of the uterus and expulsion of the retained placental membranes.

Metritis

Postpartum uterine infection, or metritis, is common in dairy cattle and is less common in beef cattle and small ruminants. Uterine infection in ruminants is associated with retained placenta, dystocia, delivery of twins, and unbalanced prepartum diets. The organism most associated with bovine metritis is *Arcanobacterium pyogenes*.

Diagnosis of metritis in cattle is based primarily on findings from physical examination and rectal palpation with the detection of abnormal uterine discharge. Cows with septic metritis usually have fever, anorexia, depression, and decreased milk production. Treatment of metritis involves systemic antibiotic therapy and use of anti-inflammatories. If a dairy farm is experiencing high levels of metritis, it may be important to review dry cow nutrition and evaluate the farm's calving management.

Pseudopregnancy

Pseudopregnancy is a pathologic condition that is more common in dairy goats and that may develop in does with or without exposure to a buck. The condition is characterized by accumulation of fluid in the uterus and one or more corpora lutea on the ovaries. Adult goats seem to be more prone than yearlings to this condition. Out-of-season breeding or delaying breeding until after the first or second estrous cycle during the fall breeding season appears to cause a higher incidence of pseudopregnancy. The doe may exhibit udder development, increased abdominal size, and behavioral signs of pregnancy. Treatment involves the use of luteolytic products, such as Prostaglandin F2α. Successful lysis results in uterine evacuation of fluid.

Metabolic Disorders

Periparturient Hypocalcemia (Milk Fever)

Milk fever is a common, nonfebrile metabolic disease affecting periparturient dairy cows and is the result of acute hypocalcemia, usually occurring within 48 hours of calving. This disease rarely occurs in first-calf heifers, and the incidence of the condition increases with the age and milk production of the cow. The hypocalcemia results from feeding dry cows a high-calcium diet, which causes lack of response by the parathyroid gland and a decrease in vitamin D levels. As a result, the cow is slow to mobilize calcium reserves from bone when there is a sudden demand for calcium at the beginning of lactation.

Cows with hypocalcemia develop muscle tremors, weakness, and a staggering gait, eventually leading to recumbency. Affected cows have a dry nose, rumen atony with bloat, and little to no urine or feces production. Unless treated quickly, the cow may die because of the effects of low serum calcium. Cows in the early stages of milk fever (before recumbency) often respond to the administration of oral calcium. For recumbent cows, slow administration of IV calcium gluconate is the treatment of choice. Cows often respond rapidly to calcium therapy and will begin to lacrimate, eructate, urinate, and defecate during treatment. Additional calcium gluconate should be administered subcutaneously for more prolonged calcium supplementation.

Prevention of milk fever is achieved by providing a well-balanced, low-calcium diet during the dry period. It is important to keep dry cows separate from the rest of the herd so that they can be fed appropriately.

TECHNICIAN NOTE

Milk fever is a common metabolic problem resulting from a severe decline in serum calcium levels in periparturient dairy cows.

Ketosis

Ketosis is usually seen in high-producing dairy cows during the first few months of lactation if they are unable to meet the energy demands of lactation. To provide energy for milk production, the cow begins to mobilize fat, the breakdown of which results in the formation of ketone bodies that accumulate in the blood. Ketosis in dairy cows may result from a primary negative energy balance or may be secondary to a disease process that causes anorexia, such as abomasal displacement, mastitis, or metritis.

Ketones have a characteristic odor that can be detected on the cow's breath; they may be detected in the milk, urine, and blood of affected cows by using a variety of cow-side diagnostic tests. Ketosis usually responds to the administration of energy sources, such as IV glucose or oral propylene glycol. It is important to determine the cause of ketosis and to correct the underlying problem. The cow's ration should be examined to ensure it contains adequate digestible energy to meet requirements for maintenance and lactation. Feed should be offered free choice and in a place easily accessible to the cow.

Pregnancy Toxemia

Pregnancy toxemia is a metabolic disease that commonly affects pregnant ewes and does during late gestation with multiple fetuses. Clinical signs can occur in pregnant animals that are overconditioned, thin, or in normal body condition. This is most often (most commonly) seen in ewes and does that are carrying multiple fetuses. Clinical cases usually follow a period of negative energy balance, resulting in hypoglycemia, increased fat catabolism, and ketosis in susceptible animals.

A diagnosis of pregnancy toxemia should be considered whenever late-pregnant ewes or does appear weak or recumbent. Clinical signs include anorexia, hypoglycemia, ketonemia, ketonuria, weakness, depression, incoordination, mental dullness, and impaired vision, followed by recumbency and death. Urine or blood ketones can easily be checked by using commercially available portable meters. Recumbency is generally indicative of a poor prognosis. Treatment often includes IV dextrose, propylene glycol, B vitamins, and supplemental calcium. In addition, corticosteroids may be used to promote gluconeogenesis, increase appetite, induce parturition or abortion, and assist in lung maturation in the fetus. Furthermore, it is critical to evaluate the remaining herd/flock for evidence of disease and to prevent additional cases. Preventive measures include slowly increasing the grain ration to provide additional energy weeks before parturition, deworming pregnant ewes, and reducing stress.

BCS of ewes or does 4 to 6 weeks before the expected date of parturition allows detection of problems and subsequent time for correction. Late-pregnancy BCSs should increase to a 3 to 3.5 level at parturition. Palpation of the lumbar epaxial musculature is a rapid and relatively simple means of evaluating the BCS in sheep (Box 19.1). Although goats distribute fat deposits in a slightly different manner compared with sheep, this BCS system can also be used in goats to estimate body condition.

Diseases of the Hemolymphatic System

Lymphosarcoma

Lymphosarcoma is the most common neoplastic disease of cattle and is most likely to occur in cattle at 2 to 6 years of age. The adult form of lymphosarcoma is associated with bovine leukosis virus (BLV). Malignant tumors may develop in the lymph nodes, lymph tissue behind the eye or around the spinal cord, abomasum, heart, kidneys, uterus, or other organs; therefore clinical signs may vary greatly, depending on one or more of the organs or systems involved. A positive titer to BLV only suggests exposure to the virus but does not confirm neoplastic disease. No treatment or vaccine is available. Because the virus is spread by infected

---

• BOX 19.1 Body Condition Scores for Sheep

0 = Absence of lumbar musculature and subcutaneous fat, leaving a profound depression between tips of dorsal and transverse spinous processes

1 = Moderate concavity between dorsal and transverse spinous processes

2 = Mild concavity between dorsal and transverse spinous processes

3 = No depression (straight line) between dorsal and transverse spinous processes

4 = Slight bulging (convexity) between dorsal and transverse spinous processes

5 = Profound convexity between dorsal and transverse spinous processes (cannot palpate spinous processes)

---

lymphocytes, every effort should be made to prevent the transfer of blood between infected and noninfected animals (i.e., changing needles and disinfecting surgical instruments between animals).

> **TECHNICIAN NOTE**
>
> Malignant lymphosarcoma tumors associated with bovine leukosis virus (BLV) may develop in peripheral or deep lymph nodes, in lymph tissue behind the eye, or around the spinal cord, abomasum, heart, kidneys, uterus, or other organs; therefore clinical signs may vary greatly, depending on the organs or systems involved.

Caseous Lymphadenitis

Caseous lymphadenitis (CL) is a disease in which abscesses develop in the lymph nodes of small ruminants and is a major cause of sheep meat being condemned. This highly contagious disease is caused by *C. pseudotuberculosis*. The disease is readily spread from animal to animal via contact with contaminated purulent material. The bacterium usually gains entry through broken skin but may also invade intact skin or enter the body via inhalation or ingestion. Then it infects the lymphatic system, where the characteristic abscesses develop. In goats, external abscesses tend to form, whereas in sheep, internal abscesses develop. The disease can become endemic in a herd or a flock and is difficult to eradicate because of its poor response to therapeutics and its ability to persist in the environment for long periods (up to 8 months in soil).

Abscessed lymph nodes have a thick capsule and central cores of dry, green-white caseous material that may displace remnants of lymphoid tissue peripherally. The presence of external abscesses is highly suggestive of CL, but culture is needed to confirm the diagnosis. Weight loss may be observed in cases of chronic, generalized infection.

In general, aggressive culling is recommended in herds or flocks with CL outbreaks, because affected animals serve as reservoirs of infection. Kids and lambs should be separated from infected adults at birth and raised on pasteurized goat or cow colostrum and milk. Treatment techniques include surgical removal of unopened abscesses; lancing, draining, and flushing of opened abscesses; long-term antimicrobial therapy (4–6 weeks); and intra-abscess formalin or antimicrobial injection.

> **TECHNICIAN NOTE**
>
> Caseous lymphadenitis, a highly contagious disease caused by *Corynebacterium pseudotuberculosis*, is the most common cause of lymph node abscesses in small ruminants. Affected animals should be culled immediately to avoid the risk of others becoming infected.

Copper Toxicity

Sheep are more prone than goats to the development of copper toxicity. Sheep absorb copper from the diet in proportion to the amount offered, rather than according to the body's need. Copper accumulates in the liver, causing liver damage that precedes the onset of clinical signs. Usually, stress caused by shipping, handling, traveling to shows, and feed changes will trigger the sudden release of copper from the liver, causing an acute hemolytic crisis. Sources of copper that have been responsible for toxicity in sheep include trace mineralized salt, cattle mineral blocks, horse feed, copper oxide wire particles, and copper sulfate foot baths. Clinical signs include depression, anorexia, weakness, hemoglobinuria, anemia, and icterus.

Although the prognosis is typically poor, therapy with D-penicillamine and ammonium molybdate helps eliminate stored copper. Additional treatments may include diuresis with IV fluids, oxygen therapy, and potentially a blood transfusion. Even if the affected lambs live through the acute hemolytic crisis, significant, irreversible renal damage often results from hemoglobinuria, causing death or necessitating humane euthanasia. "Gun metal gray" kidneys are the indicative sign seen on necropsy.

Anthrax

Bacillus anthracis is the causative agent of this acute disease, which results in sudden death in both animals and humans. Anthrax is endemic in many areas of the southern United States. As a zoonotic disease, humans can easily contract it, and it is important to not perform a necropsy on any animal suspected to have died of anthrax. If anthrax is strongly suspected as the cause of death, the area federal veterinarian should be notified immediately. Anthrax-contaminated carcasses should be buried in lime or incinerated. A live virus vaccine is available, and its use should be considered in high-risk areas. The organism is sensitive to penicillin but, in most cases, treatment cannot be initiated quickly enough to save the animal. In recent years, anthrax has become an important issue in the context of bioterrorism.

> **TECHNICIAN NOTE**
>
> Anaplasmosis, anthrax, clostridial disease, lightning strikes, and bloat are causes of sudden death in cattle.

Anaplasmosis

Anaplasmosis, caused by the intraerythrocytic organism *Anaplasma marginale*, is primarily a disease of adult cattle. It is transmitted via the blood of infected animals. Ticks, biting flies, and reusing infected needles on multiple animals can spread the disease. RBCs infected by the organism are removed from blood by the liver and spleen and subsequently destroyed, resulting in severe anemia. Associated clinical signs include pale mucous membranes, icterus, weakness, and depression or aggressive behavior resulting from anoxia to the brain. Anaplasmosis often causes sudden death without obvious clinical signs, and it must be differentiated from other causes of sudden death, such as anthrax, clostridial disease, bloat, and lightning strikes. The organism is sensitive to tetracycline, so this drug is used for the treatment and prevention of the disease. Other preventive measures include cleaning and disinfecting equipment, such as tattoo kits, ear tags, or any other device that may have blood contamination, and using new needles for each injection. No commercial vaccine is currently available for the prevention of anaplasmosis.

Diseases of the Cardiovascular System

Vegetative or Valvular Endocarditis

Vegetative or ulcerative lesions may develop on the heart valves of cattle, specifically the right AV valve, because of a chronic bacterial infection from other sites. The term *vegetative* comes from the cauliflower-like plaques that form on valves. Treatment is not often successful because of inadequate penetration of lesions by antibiotics and irreversible damage to valves. Penicillin given at high levels for long periods has yielded the best results; however, it is expensive, and relapse is possible.

Pericarditis

Pericarditis is inflammation of the pericardial membrane surrounding the heart. In cattle, it is usually caused by traumatic pericarditis, an extension of traumatic reticuloperitonitis. Pericarditis develops after penetration of the pericardial sac by a metallic foreign body. It results in a mixed bacterial infection that causes severe local inflammation and deposition of fibrinous exudates, leading to a friction rub. Effusion then develops, creating splashing sounds around the heart, especially if the fluid is mixed with gas. Fluid accumulation compromises heart function and can lead to heart failure. Clinical signs include fever, kyphosis, abduction of the elbows, shallow abdominal respirations, and characteristic heart sounds on auscultation. Signs of heart failure occur late in the course of the disease, and death usually results from toxemia or heart failure. Treatment is difficult and requires long-term use of antibiotics and supportive therapies.

> **TECHNICIAN NOTE**
>
> Pericarditis in cattle usually is caused by penetration of the pericardial sac by an ingested metallic foreign body.

Brisket Disease (Mountain Sickness)

Brisket disease occurs in cattle when they are moved to high altitudes and pulmonary hypertension develops because of increased workload on the heart. Right-sided congestive heart failure often results and leads to edema in the brisket region. Additional clinical signs include cyanosis, muffled heart sounds, and dyspnea when resting. Affected cattle can recover if they are moved to a lower altitude, but there may be residual effects on the heart.

Diseases of the Nervous System

Many disorders, from infectious to nutritional, affect the nervous systems of ruminants. Table 19.7 summarizes valuable information about the most encountered neurologic disorders in these species.

Rabies

Rabies is a zoonotic, fatal viral neurologic disease that is most often transmitted by the bite of an infected wild animal, with skunks, raccoons, and foxes being the greatest threat to domestic livestock. There are two forms of rabies: the *furious form*, in which the affected animal demonstrates hyperexcitability, fear, or rage; and the *dumb form*, in which extreme depression, paresis, or paralysis manifests (Fig. 19.28). Definitive diagnosis of rabies is made by examination of the suspected animal's brain on necropsy. Several vaccines are available for use in ruminants. Rabies poses a serious human health concern; therefore proper PPE is required when handling animals suspected of having rabies.

TABLE 19.7   Common Neurologic Diseases of Ruminants

Disease/Etiologic Agent	Species Affected	Pathogenesis	Clinical Signs	Diagnosis	Treatment
Bacterial Pathogens					
Listeriosis/*Listeria monocytogenes*	Bovine, caprine, ovine	• Widely distributed in environment • Ingestion of contaminated feed • Organism invades the host through breaks in mucosa	• Depression • Circling • Head tilt • Facial desensitization and asymmetry • Ataxia • Nystagmus • Dysphagia • Recumbency • Death	• Neurologic examination • Cytologic evaluation of cerebrospinal fluid (CSF) • Isolation of organism • Necropsy	• High doses of antibiotics • Anti-inflammatories • Supportive care (fluids, transfaunation, reduce musculoskeletal injury)
Tetanus/*Clostridium tetani*	Bovine, caprine, ovine	• Infection of deep wounds by spores • Toxin produced during bacterial growth	• Stiff gait • Sawhorse stance • Erect ears • Lockjaw • Recumbency • Death	• History • Clinical signs	• Antitoxin • Antibiotics • Anti-inflammatories • Supportive care (same as for listeriosis)
Thromboembolic meningoencephalitis (TEME)/*Histophilus somni*	Bovine	• Inoculation of respiratory/ genital mucous membranes • Blood clot formation with infection/ bacteremia	• Respiratory signs may precede neurologic signs • Recumbency • Blindness • Cranial nerve deficits • Stargazing (opisthotonus) • Retinal hemorrhage • Death	• History • Identification of clinical signs • Isolation of causative organism from infected tissues • Necropsy	• High doses of antibiotics • Anti-inflammatories • Supportive care (fluids, transfaunation, reduce musculoskeletal injury)
Viral Pathogens					
Rabies	Bovine, caprine, ovine	• Inoculation with contaminated saliva • Migration of virus through peripheral nervous system to central nervous system (CNS) • Zoonotic	• Paralytic form more common than furious form in ruminants • Depression • Dullness • Recumbency • Ataxia • Vocalization • Excessive salivation	• History • Clinical signs • Necropsy	• No treatment • Prevention— annual vaccination
Caprine arthritis encephalitis (CAE)	Caprine	• Ingestion of contaminated colostrum • Close or direct contact with infected animals • Recent herd additions	• Locomotor deficits • Progressive weakness and paralysis • Cranial nerve deficits • Weight loss • Arthritis • Respiratory disease	• Serology • Polymerase chain reaction (PCR) on whole blood	• No treatment • Prevention: • Heat-treat colostrum • Feed colostrum from negative does • Conduct periodic serologic testing of herd and cull or separate positive animals

Continued

TABLE 19.7	Common Neurologic Diseases of Ruminants—cont'd				
Disease/Etiologic Agent	Species Affected	Pathogenesis	Clinical Signs	Diagnosis	Treatment
Parasitic Pathogens					
Meningeal worm/*Parelaphostrongylus tenuis*	Caprine, ovine	• Ingestion of snail or slug with infective larvae • Close proximity to white-tailed deer population	• Ataxia • Weakness • Recumbency • Tetraplegia • Cranial nerve deficits	• History • Clinical signs • CSF analysis is suggestive • Necropsy	• High doses of anthelmintics • Anti-inflammatories • Supportive care (transfaunation, fluids, reduce musculoskeletal injury)
Metabolic					
Polioencephalomalacia	Bovine, caprine, ovine	• Rumen insult leading to decreased thiamine, producing rumen microflora • Increased sulfur consumption in diet or water	• Depression • Anorexia • Blindness • Dorsomedial strabismus • Ataxia • Head pressing • Recumbency • Stargazing (opisthotonus) • Nystagmus	• Clinical signs • Thiamine level determination • Necropsy • Cerebral cortex fluorescence under ultraviolet (UV) light	• Thiamine • Anti-inflammatories • Supportive care (transfaunation, reduce musculoskeletal injury)
Nervous ketosis	Bovine	• Severe ketosis leading to central nervous system signs	• Excessive licking or chewing • Excitement • Hypersensitive • Ataxia	• Clinical signs • Large quantity of ketones detected in urine or blood	• Treatment of ketosis, including dextrose and propylene glycol • Anti-inflammatories

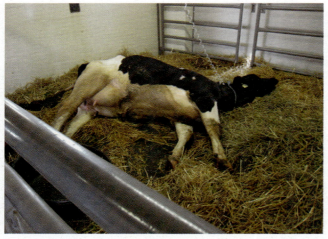

• **Fig. 19.28** Although rabies in cattle is rare, any animal that presents with abnormal clinical neurologic signs (e.g., pharyngeal paralysis, opisthotonus, head pressing) should be suspected to have rabies, and extreme care should be taken to prevent human exposure. (Courtesy Dr. Amy Johnson.)

Scrapie

Scrapie is a transmissible spongiform encephalopathy caused by a prion protein that manifests primarily as weight loss in animals 2 to 5 years of age. Other clinical signs include pruritus with wool loss, ataxia, fine muscle tremors of the face, head pressing, abnormal gait, and disorientation. Scratching of the sheep's back usually will elicit nibbling or licking of the lips. An antemortem diagnosis may be attempted by performing biopsy of the lymphoid tissue of the third eyelid, submandibular lymph node, and rectal mucosa. Postmortem confirmation can be achieved by histopathologic or immunohistochemical examination of the brain. Scrapie is a reportable disease, and there is no known treatment. A scrapie eradication program is currently in place in the United States, and veterinary technicians/nurses play a significant role in this regulatory work.

Tetanus

Tetanus is caused by spores of the bacterium *C. tetani* that produce several potent neurotoxins that are responsible for the typical clinical signs. The disease commonly occurs after spores are introduced through puncture wounds or surgical procedures, such as castration, tail docking, and dehorning. Animals with tetanus develop progressive muscle tetany characterized by a "sawhorse" stance with stiff, erect ears; rigid extension of the limbs (Fig. 19.29); and prolapse of the third eyelid. Affected animals are hyperresponsive to external stimuli such as loud noises. Death usually results from respiratory failure or aspiration pneumonia in bloated animals.

Treatment involves removal of toxin-producing bacteria by debriding and disinfecting wounds or surgery sites. In addition, high doses of penicillin and tetanus antitoxin should be administered. Affected animals should be kept in a quiet environment and provided supportive care.

Tetanus can be prevented by administering tetanus toxoid at least one month before parturition. Vaccination of kids and lambs

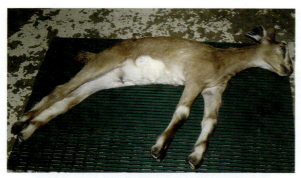

• **Fig. 19.29** Severe extensor rigidity ("sawhorse" position) in a kid with tetanus.

should be initiated by age 6 to 8 weeks. Tetanus toxoid and/or antitoxin should be given to small ruminants any time surgery is performed or an injury occurs.

> **TECHNICIAN NOTE**
>
> Small ruminants are extremely susceptible to tetanus; therefore tetanus toxoid and/or antitoxin should be given to small ruminants any time surgery is performed or injury occurs.

Polioencephalomalacia (Polio)

Polioencephalomalacia is a CNS disease, which results from underlying thiamine deficiency. This disease may occur after sudden ration changes or secondary to grain overload or excessive sulfur consumption. Polio causes neurologic signs that include blindness, ataxia, depression, opisthotonos ("stargazing"), convulsions, coma, and death (Fig. 19.30). Early in the course of the disease, affected animals respond well to treatment with thiamine (10 mg/kg) given every 3 to 6 hours for 3 to 5 days; however, the longer the animal is affected, the longer the recovery takes.

Listeriosis

Listeria monocytogenes is responsible for three different clinical syndromes in ruminants: septicemia, abortion, and neurologic disease. Neurologic involvement is most common in small ruminants and produces fever, anorexia, depression, **proprioceptive** deficits, head tilt, circling, and recumbency. Cranial nerve dysfunction causes unilateral drooping of the ear, eyelid, nose, and lips, with excessive salivation. Although ingestion of contaminated corn silage is frequently blamed, consumption of any rotting, contaminated vegetation can lead to infection.

The organism is sensitive to tetracycline and penicillin, but treatment of listeriosis often is unrewarding. Supportive care with anti-inflammatories and IV fluids is important for a successful outcome (Fig. 19.31). No vaccine is available for protection against this disease. The organism has zoonotic potential and poses a serious risk to human health when contaminated milk, milk products, or meat enters the human food supply. Veterinary technicians/nurses can play an important role in helping producers avoid feed contamination.

Caprine Arthritis Encephalitis

Caprine arthritis encephalitis (CAE) is a multisystemic condition that most often affects dairy goats and causes nonresponsive arthritis (usually in carpi) in adults and acute leukoencephalomyelitis in young goats. It may also cause chronic pneumonia (interstitial), chronic encephalomyelitis, chronic weight loss, and mastitis. The

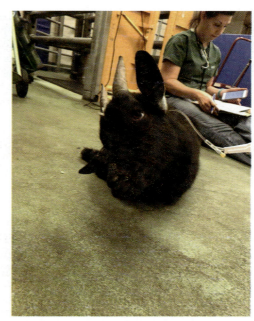

• **Fig. 19.30** A goat with polioencephalomalacia exhibiting torticollis.

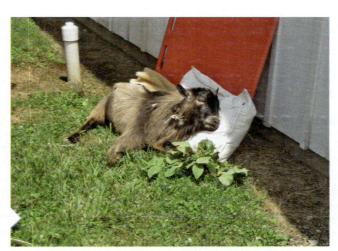

• **Fig. 19.31** Goats diagnosed with listeriosis must be provided with supportive care over an extended period. (Courtesy Dr. Amy Johnson.)

arthritic form is seldom seen before age 1 to 2 years. There is no known treatment for CAE. Transmission occurs primarily through infected colostrum and the milk of infected dams. Positive serology and PCR analysis are used to diagnose CAE; however, only about 15% of seropositive goats ever develop clinical disease. Control and prevention consist of periodic serology testing and aggressive culling of animals that test positive, separating kids from CAE-positive dams at birth, providing colostrum to kids from CAE-negative does, and heat treating colostrum before feeding.

Diseases of the Musculoskeletal System

Lameness in ruminants is most often caused by lesions or problems in the foot. Upper leg problems, such as anterior cruciate ligament rupture, coxofemoral (hip) luxation, fractures, and arthritis, account for remaining cases of lameness. When foot problems occur, they most often are seen in the claws (hooves) that bear the most weight, that is, the front medial and hind lateral claws. It is important to assess all foot problems early because, if not properly treated, many conditions can quickly lead to osteomyelitis and/or septic arthritis. Regardless of the cause of lameness, it can lead to loss of production, including decreased milk production, weight loss, delayed breeding or anestrus, and culling. Intensive housing and feeding of large groups of animals have led to increased incidences of lameness.

TECHNICIAN NOTE

Lameness is commonly encountered in ruminants and most often is caused by lesions or problems in the foot.

Interdigital Necrobacillosis

Cattle

Interdigital necrobacillosis, or foot rot, is an infection of the interdigital skin and underlying tissues. In cattle, it is caused by *Fusobacterium necrophorum*. Infection results in an ulcerated, foul-smelling area between the claws. Swelling may be apparent above the coronary band and, in severe cases, cellulitis up to the carpus or hock may occur. The disease is particularly prevalent when ruminants are kept in wet, muddy conditions. If left untreated, foot rot can invade deeper tissues of the foot, causing septic arthritis, osteomyelitis, and chronic lameness.

Treatment for foot rot can be successful with aggressive topical treatment and systemic antibiotics, such as tetracycline or ceftiofur. In some cases, it may be necessary to keep the animal in a dry stall or debride necrotic tissue and bandage the foot with antimicrobial agents to promote healing. Preventive measures, such as foot baths, are commonly employed on farms.

Small Ruminants

Lameness in multiple animals in a herd or flock usually is caused by contagious foot rot caused by *Dichelobacter nodosus* and *F. necrophorum*. Initial signs occur 10 to 20 days after exposure and include inflammation of interdigital skin, followed by slight undermining of the sole at the heels, which progresses to involve the sole and wall. Some sheep are resistant to infection; some improve, with spontaneous resolution of infection; and others become chronic carriers of the disease. The usual source of bacteria is chronic carrier sheep or previously contaminated surfaces.

Successful treatment involves thorough inspection of all animals and trimming and treatment of all affected animals. Animals should be divided into affected and unaffected groups and placed on clean pastures after treatment. Foot baths are useful for treatment after trimming and may contain copper sulfate or zinc sulfate. Zinc sulfate may be the best choice, because it is less irritating. Copper sulfate poisoning poses a threat if sheep are allowed to drink the foot bath water. Once a treatment program has been initiated, all sheep should be checked weekly, their claws (hooves) trimmed, if needed, and their feet placed in a foot bath. Oxytetracycline is sometimes administered subcutaneously to help decrease healing time. Segregation of infected sheep and goats and culling of chronic carriers are essential for successful foot rot control.

Hoof Wall Deformities and Defects That Can Cause Lameness

There are a number of hoof deformities and defects that can cause lameness in ruminants. White line disease occurs when the sole separates from the hoof wall, allowing dirt and feces to pack into the weakened area, which can lead to foot abscesses. Vertical wall

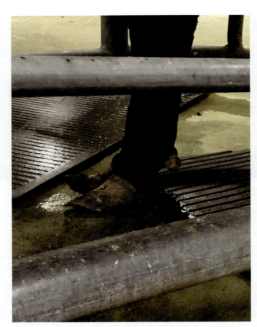

• **Fig. 19.32** Abnormal hoof growth in a goat with a corkscrew claw.

fissures, or cracks, are more common in beef cattle. Dietary deficiencies can lead to microscopic cracks in the hoof wall that can progressively worsen to larger cracks. Horizontal wall grooves ("hardship grooves") can develop when stresses, such as diseases, cause disruption in hoof wall growth. Lesions can be deep and can extend to the sensitive corium, causing lameness. Corkscrew claw is an undesirable, inheritable trait that causes misalignment of the second and third phalanges within the digit and faster growth of the medial and caudal hoof walls, giving the hoof a corkscrew appearance (Fig. 19.32).

Laminitis

Laminitis, or founder, causes diffuse inflammation of the dermis layers of the hoof and involves all parts of the dermis in the cow—not only the sensitive lamina (corium) but also the support system of the third phalanx. Acute laminitis may result from sudden excessive grain ingestion or may occur secondary to other diseases during the postparturient period. Chronic laminitis is more often associated with constant feeding of high-grain diets, as occurs commonly in high-producing dairy cows, feedlot cattle, and show cattle.

Clinical signs include stiffness, pain, reluctance to walk, and difficulty rising. Affected animals spend a lot of time lying down; when they do stand, they may stand with their backs arched, forelimbs crossed, or kneeling on the forelimbs in an attempt to redistribute body weight because of the pain. Acute cases of laminitis are treated by correcting any existing underlying problems and by administering anti-inflammatories. Laminitis often leads to serious sequelae, including sole ulcers, white line disease, abnormal hoof growth with horizontal or vertical hoof wall cracks, underrun heel and sole, and even osteomyelitis or septic arthritis. Frequent hoof trimming helps prevent all these problems.

TECHNICIAN NOTE

Acute laminitis may be caused by sudden excessive grain ingestion or may occur secondary to other diseases during the postparturient period.

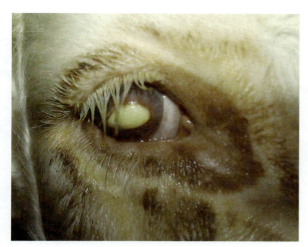

• **Fig. 19.33** A large central corneal ulcer in a bull with infectious bovine keratoconjunctivitis (pinkeye).

Ophthalmologic Diseases

Infectious Keratoconjunctivitis (Pinkeye)

Cattle

Infectious bovine **keratoconjunctivitis**, or bovine pinkeye, is an infectious and contagious ocular disease of cattle caused by *Moraxella bovis* and is characterized by conjunctivitis and corneal ulceration (Fig. 19.33). Flies can serve as vectors of the pathogen and can quickly spread it among animals in a herd. UV light and mechanical irritants, such as dust and weeds, may disrupt the corneal epithelium, making it more susceptible to infection. Initial clinical signs include lacrimation, blepharospasm, and photophobia. If ulceration becomes deep, the cornea may rupture, resulting in vision loss.

Individual treatment of pinkeye usually involves subconjunctival injection of penicillin. Eye patches may be applied to affected eyes to decrease photophobia and protect the eye from flies. More severe cases may require surgery, such as a third eyelid flap or *tarsorrhaphy* (suturing the lids closed) to protect deeper ulcers as they heal. In the case of herd outbreaks, it may be impractical to treat each animal with local therapy, so systemic antibiotics, such as long-acting tetracycline, can be administered to the herd in drinking water.

Small Ruminants

Pinkeye usually is caused by *Chlamydia psittaci* in sheep and *Mycoplasma conjunctivae* in goats, although either organism can cause pinkeye in both species. Carrier animals and apparently uninfected animals in a herd or flock serve as an important source of infection. Both organisms may persist for months in ocular tissue and are spread by contact with infected ocular secretions. Clinical signs, regardless of the cause, include conjunctival hyperemia, ocular discharge, light sensitivity, blepharospasm, corneal edema, and vascularization of the cornea. Severe cases may result in corneal ulceration or corneal abscessation. Both infections are self-limiting, and recovery can be expected in a few weeks; however, systemic and/or topical treatment with tetracycline is recommended to prevent the spread of infection and the development of severe eye lesions leading to loss of sight.

> **TECHNICIAN NOTE**
>
> Pinkeye, or infectious keratoconjunctivitis, is usually caused by *Moraxella bovis* in cattle, *Chlamydia psittaci* in sheep, and *Mycoplasma conjunctivae* in goats. It can cause corneal ulceration, sometimes leading to vision loss.

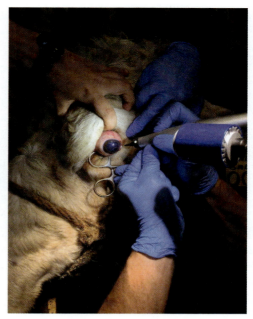

• **Fig. 19.34** Enucleation procedure in a cow.

Ocular Squamous Cell Carcinoma

SCC is the most common ocular neoplasm among white-faced animals that lack pigmentation of the skin surrounding the eye, with Hereford cattle being the most susceptible breed. UV light exposure causes SCC, which often begins as a hyperplastic plaque that progresses to a papilloma or an invasive carcinoma. Lesions appear most commonly on the lateral limbus of the eye, followed by the nasal limbus, the third eyelid, lacrimal caruncle, and the medial canthus. Diagnosis is based on appearance and cytology. Numerous treatments are available, including cryotherapy and surgical excision; however, more extensive lesions may require enucleation (Fig. 19.34).

Diseases of the Urinary System

Pyelonephritis

Pyelonephritis, caused most by *Corynebacterium renale* or *E. coli*, is an ascending urinary tract infection that often affects females because of their short, wide urethra. This infection occurs more often in the periparturient period, when animals are more stressed and the urogenital tract is more susceptible to the entry of bacteria.

Clinical findings include hematuria, pyuria, straining (**stranguria**), frequent urination (*pollakiuria*), and discomfort during urination. Affected animals may have a fluctuating fever, a variable appetite, and decreased milk production. In cattle, if the left kidney is affected, rectal palpation may reveal an enlarged, fluctuant, painful kidney.

Treatment is often unrewarding but may be attempted with high doses of penicillin given over long periods. In valuable animals that have only one kidney affected, nephrectomy may be indicated.

Urolithiasis

Urolithiasis is a common disease of small ruminants that can be life-threatening. Pets and young, castrated male animals fed a high-grain diet and high-calcium forage (e.g., alfalfa, clover) are more likely to develop urinary calculi (uroliths).

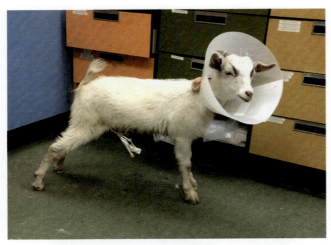

• **Fig. 19.35** Urolithiasis is common in small ruminants. This castrated male goat has undergone a surgical procedure to relieve urinary obstruction.

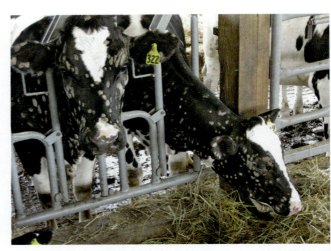

• **Fig. 19.36** This picture depicts extensive lesions associated with dermatophytosis in cattle.

Clinical signs, such as anorexia, weakness, or depression, may be nonspecific. Other signs include dysuria, stranguria with dribbling of urine, vocalization, tail flagging, abdominal distention, and bruxism indicative of discomfort. Clients often misinterpret urinary straining as constipation, and patients are often presented with this complaint. Common locations for obstruction include the urethral process—an appendage at the distal end of the penis—and the urethra at the level of the distal sigmoid flexure.

This condition is an emergency because of the possibility of rupture of the bladder or the urethra. Treatment involves relieving the urinary tract obstruction (Fig. 19.35). Excision of the urethral process under sedation might initially relieve the obstruction but, typically, this is only a temporary solution. The urethra can be flushed to dislodge any other calculi, but these cases frequently require surgery for complete removal of the obstruction. (See Chapter 34, "Large Animal Surgical Nursing.") Because of multiple electrolyte abnormalities that result from urinary obstruction and the risk of cystitis or ascending infection, animals are treated with appropriate fluid and electrolytes, broad-spectrum antimicrobials, and anti-inflammatories.

Prevention of this disease is multifaceted. Urine output should be increased by adding salt to the ration to stimulate water consumption. Ammonium chloride (200–400 mg/kg) can be added to the ration to acidify the urine, helping increase the solubility of uroliths. Certain feeds, such as grain and high-calcium forage, should be reduced significantly or eliminated from the diet.

Diseases of the Skin

Cutaneous Papillomas (Warts)

Cutaneous papillomas are benign neoplasia caused by papillomavirus that appear as tan, white, or gray protruding masses with a dry, horny surface in young cattle. Small warts may be crushed or surgically removed to stimulate development of natural immunity and to hasten healing. Because warts are usually self-limiting, no treatment may be necessary. However, in long-standing, severe, or nonresponsive cases, the immune status of the patient must be considered.

Dermatophytosis (Ringworm)

Trichophyton verrucosum is a fungus that causes ringworm in cattle and is most likely to occur in calves housed in crowded conditions

during the winter. Multiple circular lesions develop, particularly around the head and neck (Fig. 19.36), and typically resolve on their own in 2 to 3 months, if left untreated. If treatment is desired, especially in the case of show animals, topical agents, such as iodine, bleach (1:10 in water), chlorhexidine, or 5% lime sulfur, may be useful. Fungal spores can remain viable in a dry environment for years, so grooming equipment and barns can remain infective.

Contagious Ecthyma (Orf)

Contagious ecthyma (sore mouth, orf) is a common viral disease of small ruminants caused by a poxvirus that produces crusty, proliferative lesions around the mouths and noses of lambs and kids, and similar lesions on the teats and udders of ewes and does (Fig. 19.37). The infection is self-limiting and resolves in 3 to 6 weeks. This is a viral disease, and there is no known treatment; however, antimicrobials may be given to prevent secondary bacterial infections. Supportive therapy may be administered to those lambs and kids that are in too much pain to be able to nurse. The virus is zoonotic (transmissible to humans), so care should be taken when handling infected animals (gloves should be worn), or the veterinary staff should receive the live virus vaccine (gloves should still be worn).

> **TECHNICIAN NOTE**
>
> Contagious ecthyma (sore mouth, orf), a common viral disease of small ruminants, is zoonotic, so care should be taken when handling infected animals.

Common Diseases and Conditions of Swine

Care of the Neonate

Farrowing is the act of a sow giving birth to piglets. It is important to have the farrowing pen or house clean, free from drafts, and warm in preparation for the arrival of a new litter of piglets. Neonatal pigs have few fat stores and require supplemental heat during the first few weeks of life to prevent life-threatening hypothermia. During the first week, the temperature should be 92°F to 95°F (33.3°C–35°C), then gradually lowered over the second and third week to 85°F (31.7°C). The temperature should be closely

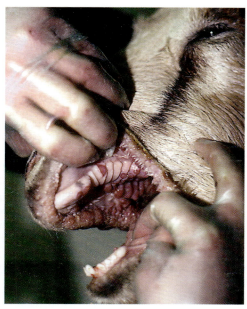

• **Fig. 19.37** Ulcerative and proliferative lesions in and around the mouth of this doe are caused by contagious ecthyma, or orf.

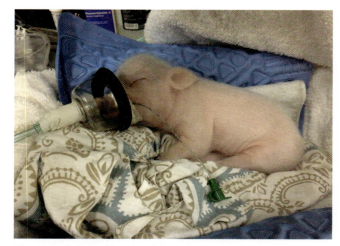

• **Fig. 19.38** A hypoglycemic piglet being treated with a heating pad, enteral nutrition, and supplemental oxygen.

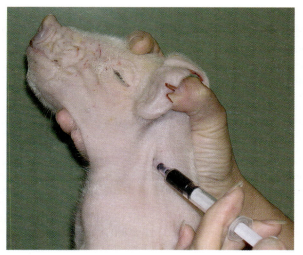

• **Fig. 19.39** Piglets raised in confinement require iron dextran supplementation by age 3 days.

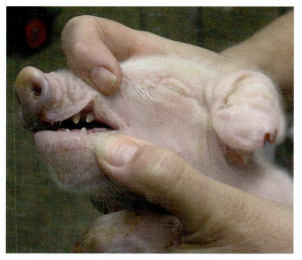

• **Fig. 19.40** Needle teeth in neonatal pigs should be clipped to prevent bite injuries to the dam and littermates.

monitored for the sow and for the neonates; sows prefer cooler temperatures (60°F–65°F) to remain comfortable. Monitoring the activity of the pigs will give insight into their comfort level—if the piglets are too cool, they will pile on top of each other, and if they are too hot, they will move as far as they can get from the heat source.

There should be enough room for the sow to rest comfortably without lying on her piglets. Piglets are not born with maternal immunity, so colostrum intake after birth is important. Adequate nutrition is also important, because hypoglycemia can develop quickly in the undernourished piglet and can lead to death (Fig. 19.38). If the piglets appear hungry, the sow should be examined for mastitis or metritis, which can cause *hypogalactia* (low milk production) or *agalactia* (absence of milk production). Hypoglycemia may lead to a weakened piglet that is susceptible to various diseases or being crushed by the dam when she lies down. Frequent observation of the sow or gilt and of the piglets will help the producer determine whether the nursing behavior is normal. Hypoglycemia in piglets may be treated with 5 to 10 mL of 5% dextrose injected intraperitoneally by using aseptic technique. Pigs that are rejected or orphaned or are not receiving adequate nutrition from the mother may be given supplementation with a milk replacer designed for pigs. Young pigs quickly learn to drink from shallow pans and therefore do not usually require bottle feeding. These piglets can also be offered prestarter feed at an early age.

Processing piglets is less stressful to them when they are a few days old, but it is tedious work. The technician should make sure that all the equipment needed is on hand to make the process go as efficiently as possible. Iron dextran injections at 3 days of age (Fig. 19.39) are necessary for piglets that are not raised on dirt, because they have low iron reserves and can develop anemia. Clipping needle teeth prevents injury to the dam's udder and to other piglets in the litter (Fig. 19.40). Castration and tail docking (Fig. 19.41) are done to reduce the chances of tail biting, which can result in ascending infection of the spinal cord or a spinal abscess. During processing, ear notching is also performed for permanent identification.

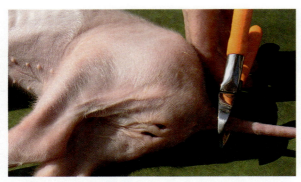

• **Fig. 19.41** Tail docking is often performed at several days of age to prevent tail biting in pigs kept in confinement. Also note the recent castration incisions.

> **TECHNICIAN NOTE**
>
> Prevention of hypothermia and hypoglycemia in the neonatal period is important for successful pig rearing.

Multisystemic Diseases

Erysipelas

Erysipelas ("diamond skin disease") is caused by the bacterium *Erysipelothrix rhusiopathiae*, which is found in dirt or in areas with heavy fecal contamination, and it enters the body through lymphoid tissue, such as the tonsils, or through breaks in the skin. It affects pigs older than 12 weeks of age. Up to 50% of healthy swine may carry and shed the organism. Septicemia quickly develops after infection, and the organisms tend to localize in the skin, heart, and joints. Infection causes high fever and may produce the characteristic diamond-shaped skin lesions. This form often results in death if not recognized early. The treatment of choice for the acute form is penicillin, but nothing is effective for treatment of the chronic form. Immunization against erysipelas is effective and inexpensive, and should be provided at weaning and repeated every 6 months. Erysipelas is zoonotic, and PPE must be worn when handling infected pigs.

Pseudorabies Virus (Aujeszky Disease, Mad Itch)

Pseudorabies is caused by pseudorabies virus (PrV), a contagious herpesvirus. Swine are the natural host for the virus, and although other species are affected by the virus, most are dead-end hosts. Mortality in young pigs is high because of the development of neurologic signs and, in some cases, vomiting and diarrhea. Weanling and growing pigs exhibit fever; pneumonia; a dry, nonproductive cough; and flulike signs. Infection in adults may cause reproductive problems, including early embryonic death, abortion, or stillbirths in pregnant sows or gilts. Serologic tests (e.g., ELISA) are used to screen herds for PrV. No treatment for PrV is known, and vaccination for the disease is closely regulated by state officials. A pseudorabies eradication program is currently in place in the United States, and there have been no closed commercial production herds infected with PrV since 2003. However, the population of feral pigs and those raised outside may still be infected sporadically.

> **TECHNICIAN NOTE**
>
> Pseudorabies virus (PrV) is responsible for the development of neurologic signs in neonatal pigs, flulike signs in growing pigs, and embryonic death, abortion, or stillbirth in pregnant sows or gilts.

Porcine Reproductive and Respiratory Syndrome

Infection with porcine reproductive and respiratory syndrome (PRRS) is prevalent in swine herds in the United States. The virus enters the body through the respiratory tract, resulting in pneumonia. Viremia follows, and the virus may cross the placenta to infect embryos or fetuses. General clinical signs include fever, lethargy, inappetence, and cyanosis of the ears, vulva, tail, abdomen, and snout ("blue ear disease"). The respiratory syndrome manifests as labored breathing with increased secondary respiratory infection, increased postweaning mortality, and decreased rate of gain and feed efficiency. The reproductive syndrome includes abortion, stillbirth, fetal mummies, and the birth of weak piglets. Diagnosis is based on clinical findings, histopathologic examination, virus isolation, immunofluorescence, and/or PCR. No treatment for PRRS is known, but antimicrobials may be administered in the event of secondary bacterial infection. PRRS is an economically devastating disease, and cases must be reported to local authorities. A modified live virus vaccine is available. Control measures vary, depending on the current herd status and the goals of the producer.

Diseases of the Gastrointestinal System

Diarrhea in young pigs from birth to 26 weeks can lead to intensive management, so prevention is critical to avoid outbreaks that can significantly decrease the population.

Diarrhea in Neonatal and Nursery Pigs

Common causative agents of diarrhea in neonatal pigs include enterotoxigenic *E. coli* (ETEC), rotavirus, and coronavirus, and by transmissible gastroenteritis (TGE).

Regardless of the cause of diarrhea in young pigs, good nursing care is important for their survival. Free-choice oral electrolyte solutions should be provided in shallow pans. Antimicrobials may be used if the risk of secondary bacterial infection is present. Additionally, it is important to keep the piglets warm, at least at 90°F (32.2°C), to prevent loss of energy and rapid wasting.

Diarrhea in Grower and Finisher Pigs

Swine dysentery, salmonellosis, proliferative enteropathy (ileitis), and whipworms are common causes of diarrhea in growing and finishing swine. Most treatment is aimed at prevention of these diseases with good sanitation, use of "all-in, all-out" pig facilities, segregated early weaning, and stress reduction. Table 19.8 lists the common infectious causes of diarrhea in grower and finisher pigs.

Diseases of the Respiratory System

Common causes of respiratory disease in swine are *Mycoplasma* pneumonia, PRRS, swine influenza, and *Pasteurella* pneumonia (Table 19.9). Respiratory infection can significantly affect the growth and overall health performance of a pig. Clinical signs typically include coughing, "thumping" or shallow rapid breathing, depression, and weight loss. Prevention of disease is the goal, but antimicrobials can be used to eliminate the causative agents or the secondary pathogens when disease occurs.

Diseases of the Reproductive System

Reproduction and adequate financial return are the goals of any commercial swine operation. The typical length of gestation for swine is 114 days, or 3 months, 3 weeks, 3 days. Subsequently, it

TABLE 19.8	Common Infectious Causes of Diarrhea in Grower and Finisher Pigs			
Disease/Etiologic Agent	**Pathogenesis**	**Clinical Signs**	**Diagnosis**	**Treatment**

Swine dysentery/*Brachyspira hyodysenteriae*	• Fecal-oral route	• Colitis
		• Diarrhea
		• Emaciation
		• Dehydration
			• Isolation and identification of bacteria in colon
			• Fluorescent antibody test on fecal smears
				• Antibiotics sensitive to the organism
				• Prevention:
				  • Maintain a closed herd
				  • Cull affected animals
				  • Segregated early weaning

Salmonellosis	• Sow to piglet via placenta
	• Ingestion of contaminated feed or water
	• Stress caused by overcrowding can increase shedding of organism
		• Enterocolitis leading to profuse watery diarrhea
		• Dehydration
		• Emaciation
		• Septicemia leading to pneumonia or hepatitis
			• Isolation of causative agent via culture or polymerase chain reaction (PCR) assay	• Supportive care (oral fluids, anti-inflammatories)
				• Antibiotics may decrease severity of disease but use with caution because of multiple resistant strains
				• Prevention:
				  • Isolate or cull affected animals
				  • Practice good hygiene in pens, feeding areas, and water sources
				  • Enforce strict biosecurity protocols
				  • Decrease overcrowding of pens
				  • Improve pig comfort

Proliferative enteropathy (ileitis)/*Lawsonia intracellularis*	• Fecal-oral route
	• Feces can be transmitted on boots and rodents
		• Intermittent diarrhea
		• Hemorrhagic diarrhea in older pigs
		• Anorexia
		• Weight loss
		• Melena
		• Anemia
			• Isolation of bacteria from feces via PCR assay
			• Necropsy:
			  • Thickened ileum
			  • Silver staining techniques will show presence of intracellular bacteria
				• Antibiotics
				• Prevention:
				  • Vaccinate young pigs
				  • Segregated early weaning
				  • All-in, all-out facilities
				  • Good sanitation

Whipworms/*Trichuris suis*	• Fecal-oral route	• Anorexia
		• Mucoid to bloody diarrhea
		• Dehydration
		• Death
			• Fecal float
			• Necropsy:
			  • Adult worms in cecum
				• Anthelmintics
				• Prevention:
				  • Good sanitation

is important to optimize the number of piglets weaned per sow throughout the animal's lifetime. Several infectious agents are responsible for poor reproductive efficiency in swine, including PRRS, porcine parvovirus (PPV), brucellosis, and leptospirosis.

Porcine Parvovirus

PPV is present in nearly 100% of swine herds worldwide and is a common cause of infectious infertility. The virus can infect a male or a nonpregnant female and be eliminated with no clinical signs. If a female becomes infected in the first 30 days of pregnancy, the virus crosses the placenta and infects rapidly dividing fetal cells, causing fetal death and resorption. If infected between 30 and 70 days of gestation, the fetus is killed and mummified, and if infected after 70 days of gestation, the fetus builds an immune response and survives to term, although it may be born weak or

dead. The only clinical signs of PPV include reproductive problems in pregnant sows or gilts. Mummies of different sizes, still-births, and live pigs may be present in the same litter. Vaccines are available, but immunity lasts for only 4 to 6 months, so vaccination must be repeated before each breeding.

Leptospirosis

Leptospira pomona and *Leptospira bratislava* are the primary serovars adapted to swine, although other serovars may incidentally infect pigs. Bacteria are shed through the urine and reproductive discharge of infected animals and enter susceptible animals through the mucous membranes or broken skin. Once infection occurs, bacteremia develops, and the organism localizes and multiplies in the kidney. In pregnant females, the virus may cross the placenta and infect and kill the fetuses. Aborted, weak, and

TABLE 19.9   Common Infectious Causes of Respiratory Disease in Pigs

Disease/Etiologic Agent	Pathogenesis	Clinical Signs	Diagnosis	Treatment

Atrophic rhinitis (AR)/*Bordetella bronchiseptica*, *Pasteurella multocida*	• Sow-to-piglet and pig-to-pig contact via nasopharyngeal route
	• Chronic, progressive disease causing nasal turbinate atrophy
	• Environmental factors—high ammonia levels, stress, concurrent disease, suboptimal nutrition can contribute to lesions
		• Early signs:
		  • Sneezing
		  • Mucopurulent nasal discharge
		• Later signs:
		  • Twisted or shortened snouts
		  • Excessive tearing
		  • Epistaxis
		  • Decreased growth rate
		  • Decreased feed efficiency
			• Necropsy:
			  • Degree of nasal atrophy by cross sectioning the snout at level of second premolar
				• Antibiotics
				• Prevention:
				  • Prefarrowing vaccines
				  • All-in, all-out farrowing units
				  • Improved ventilation
				  • Eradication by depopulation and repopulation with AR-negative animals

Swine influenza	• Pig-to-pig contact via nasopharyngeal route
	• Zoonotic
		• Fever
		• Conjunctivitis
		• Rhinitis
		• Nasal discharge
		• Sneezing
		• Coughing
		• Weight loss
			• Virus isolation from nasal or pharyngeal swabs
			• Necropsy:
			  • Virus isolation from trachea or lung tissues
				• Supportive care
				• Antibiotics for secondary infection
				• Prevention:
				  • Vaccination
				  • Good biosecurity protocols

Mycoplasma pneumoniae/*Mycoplasma hyopneumoniae*	• Pig-to-pig contact via nasopharyngeal route
	• Aerosol transmission
	• Most common cause of chronic pneumonia in swine
		• Dry, nonproductive cough
		• Fever
		• Decreased appetite
		• Dyspnea
			• Isolation of organism from nasal swabs
			• Serology
				• Antibiotics
				• Prevention:
				  • Provide adequate ventilation
				  • Avoid overcrowding
				  • Segregated early weaning
				  • All-in, all-out facilities
				  • Vaccination reduces lesions and improves weight gain

Pleuropneumonia /*Actinobacillus pleuropneumoniae*	• Pig-to-pig contact via nasopharyngeal route
	• Aerosol transmission
		• Per-acute:
		  • Death
		• Acute:
		  • High fever
		  • Dyspnea
		  • Coughing
		• Chronic:
		  • Intermittent cough
		  • Reduced appetite
		  • Decreased weight gains
			• Isolation of organism from nasal swabs
			• Serology
			• Necropsy:
			  • Characteristic firm, well-demarcated abscesses associated with pericarditis and pleuritis
				• Antibiotics
				• Prevention:
				  • Monitor herds with serology and cull positive animals
				  • Quarantine replacement animals before introduction to the herd
				  • Metaphylactic antibiotics
				  • Provide adequate ventilation
				  • Avoid overcrowding
				  • Segregated early weaning
				  • All-in, all-out facilities
				  • Vaccination reduces lesions and improves weight gain

Pasteurella pneumonia/*Pasteurella multocida*	• Normal inhabitant of upper respiratory tract • Stress or concurrent infection leads to pneumonia	• Fever • Dyspnea • Moist, productive cough • Anorexia	• Isolation of organism • Serology • Necropsy: • Bronchopneumonia	• Treat primary disease • Antibiotics • Anti-inflammatories

stillborn fetuses may be the only obvious clinical signs. Diagnosis is reached through demonstration of high antibody titers in the dam (interpreted considering vaccination status) or in fetal fluids, culture of the organism, or dark-field microscopy of urine or fetal fluids. Treatment may include tetracycline given in the feed or administration of parenteral tetracycline. Many monovalent and multivalent vaccines are available for the protection of breeding stock; however, the immunity is short-lived, so the animals should be vaccinated every 6 months at breeding. Because this is a zoonotic disease, suspect animals and their samples should be handled with care and PPE used.

> **TECHNICIAN NOTE**
>
> Diseases responsible for abortion and reproductive failure in swine include pseudorabies virus (PrV) infection, brucellosis, porcine reproductive and respiratory syndrome (PRRS), porcine parvovirus (PPV) infection, and leptospirosis.

Diseases of the Nervous System

Salt Toxicity

Salt toxicity, also known as *sodium ion toxicosis* or *water deprivation*, occurs in commercial and pet swine as a result of excessive sodium consumption such as eating dog food, inadequate water intake, or possibly both. Hyperosmolarity develops in the CNS and, when the pig does consume water, osmotic pressure draws fluid into the brain, causing cerebral edema. Affected pigs show signs 36 to 48 hours after fluid deprivation, including restlessness, pruritus, constipation, and thirst, followed by depression, blindness, convulsions, and death. Salt toxicity is a well-recognized entity in commercial swine, but descriptions of medical treatment of affected animals are limited, because it usually is not economically feasible to treat individual commercial pigs. Successful treatment of pet pigs has been reported and consists of slow rehydration with fluids that gradually return sodium to a normal level.

Diseases of the Musculoskeletal System

Porcine Stress Syndrome

Porcine stress syndrome (PSS) is also known as *malignant hyperthermia*. Susceptibility to PSS is caused by a single autosomal recessive gene. However, this defective gene is also closely associated with desirable characteristics such as good feed conversion and high-percent lean meat. The gene for PSS has been identified in almost every breed of swine but is especially prevalent in the Pietrain breed. Stress, halothane, and other anesthetics may precipitate the occurrence of PSS. Severity of clinical signs is related to degree of stress. Signs include muscle and tail tremors, dyspnea, alternating blanched and reddened areas of skin, elevated body temperature (hyperthermia), cyanosis, muscle rigidity, and death. Once clinical signs develop, the affected animal may be treated by removing the stress, applying external cooling, and administering dantrolene sodium, if available. Pigs should be carefully monitored during herd health exams to prevent undue stress to the herd due to overexcitement.

> **TECHNICIAN NOTE**
>
> Porcine stress syndrome (PSS), or malignant hyperthermia, is a genetic disease that results in muscle tremors, hyperthermia, and death. Herd stress during herd health exams may precipitate the development of PSS.

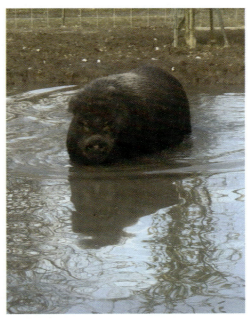

• **Fig. 19.42** Pigs are sensitive to heat and will wallow in mud for better thermoregulation.

Behavioral Disorders

The pig's normal response to fear includes vocalization and attempts to escape, so use of earplugs is critical when working with swine. Pigs are naturally curious and spend a great deal of time exploring their environment. They will use their snouts to investigate and root to forage on grass and dirt. Pigs have poor eyesight and therefore are reluctant to venture into areas with unusual odors and changes in light; however, they have a keen sense of smell. Once familiar with their surroundings, the rooting may lead to destructive behavior. Pigs are sensitive to heat and as a result will wallow in mud for thermoregulation (Fig. 19.42). Additionally, swine maintain clean sleeping and feeding areas.

Swine have a strong social hierarchy that is established through aggressive behavior. This begins as early as the neonatal period, when teat order is established. Then again at weaning, because of commingling of pigs, this hierarchy is re-established. This reordering usually occurs within 12 to 24 hours, with the dominant pig establishing its position first. In established hierarchies, the dominant pig assumes the recumbent position, and its belly is nuzzled by subordinates, possibly as an allogrooming ritual. The sow will also lie down on its side for piglets to nurse when rubbed on her belly. This behavior can be used to encourage a pig in the clinic to lie down on its side with little resistance so that minor examinations can be performed (Fig. 19.43).

Abnormal behavior is likely to develop because of stressful living conditions or during weaning, or with poor ventilation, overcrowding, or an imbalanced diet. Problematic behaviors, such as poor defecation habits, soiling the sleeping and feeding areas, extreme aggression, tail biting, ear biting, and flank biting, indicate environmental or managerial deficiencies. These behaviors can be controlled by providing adequate space and diversions, such as toys (e.g., bowling balls, inner tubes) for pigs to play with inside the pen.

Mature boars have well-developed tusks that they use for slashing, and they will bite each other as part of normal aggressive behavior.

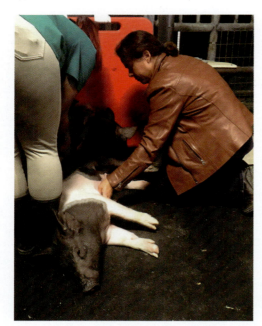

• **Fig. 19.43** This pig is being rubbed on its belly to encourage it to lie calmly for a physical examination.

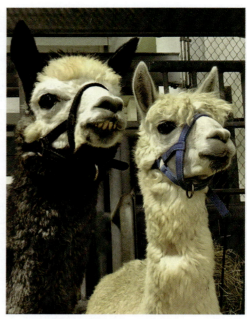

• **Fig. 19.44** South American camelids.

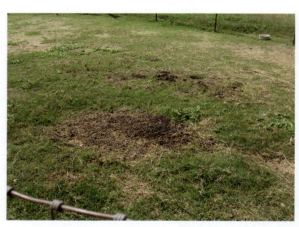

• **Fig. 19.45** South American camelids have pelleted feces and use communal dung piles for defecation.

Aggression toward piglets (hysteria) or savaging of baby pigs usually is exhibited by gilts. Possible causes of hysteria include stress resulting from the inability of the gilt to make a "nest," human in terference during farrowing, and, perhaps, genetic predisposition. Piglets can be removed at birth and reintroduced once parturition is complete, because initiation of nursing often calms the gilt.

Common Diseases and Conditions of Camelids

In general, camelids may be classified as Old World and New World camelids. Old World camelids include dromedary, or one-humped, camels, and bactrian, or two-humped, camels. New World camelids, also called *South American camelids* (SACs), include llamas, alpacas, guanacos, and vicuñas (Fig. 19.44).

SACs originated from the South American Andes; thus they are accustomed to dry, cooler climates and high altitudes. Their life span is 15 to 20 years. Camelids have a complex, three-compartment stomach, with digestion similar to that of ruminants. They will also regurgitate and rechew their food, but they are better equipped to extract energy from poor-quality forage compared with other ruminants. Llamas tend to browse, whereas alpacas prefer to graze. SACs have pelleted feces and use communal dung piles (Fig. 19.45). Llamas are typically used for meat, leather, and fiber, and as pack animals. Alpacas are known for their superior fiber, but they are also used as a source of meat and leather. Two breeds of alpacas—the Huacaya and the Suri—have gained popularity in the United States. The Huacaya breed is the most common; its fiber is crimped and shorter than that of the Suri. The Suri has a haircoat that hangs from the body in ringlets.

Llamas and alpacas are herd animals and therefore need to live with at least one other llama or alpaca. Gelded male llamas or adult female llamas can be used as guardians of sheep, goats, alpacas, cattle, and miniature horses.

TECHNICIAN NOTE

Llamas and alpacas are herd animals and therefore need to live with at least one other llama or alpaca. Gelded male llamas or adult female llamas can be used as guardians of sheep, goats, alpacas, cattle, and miniature horses.

Health Maintenance

Veterinary technicians/nurses can play an important role in helping producers maintain camelid herd health by using veterinary-supervised protocols. Technicians can set up vaccine and deworming protocols, along with hoof trimming and dental care.

Camelids should be routinely vaccinated for *C. perfringens* types C and D and tetanus when they are 2 to 3 weeks of age, again at 6 and 12 months, and annually after that. Other vaccines that are available include those against rabies, equine rhinovirus infection, West Nile virus infection, leptospirosis, and other diseases, depending on herd location and endemic areas.

Internal and external parasite control is necessary and can be effective when customizing the protocol to specific farms.

Camelids are susceptible to many of the same parasites as those that affect sheep and goats, such as *H. contortus*, or barber pole worm. Parasitism can cause anemia and decrease herd numbers if not controlled or if animals are crowded in a small area. Overcrowding can also be a concern in situations where these species are intermingled. Routine fecal examinations, along with pasture rotation and feeding hay and grain off of the ground, are necessary to keep infections to a minimum.

The incisors of a camelid can get overgrown at times and may need filing down. Canine teeth ("fighting teeth") are well developed in intact males and may also need to be blunted or filed down to prevent lacerations to the throat and limbs of others in the herd.

The camelid has two digits on each foot, and the plantar surface has a soft, cornified pad. There is a nail on each toe that may require occasional trimming (Fig. 19.46).

The BCS system in camelids uses a 10-point scale, with 1 indicating emaciation, 5 indicating a desirable BCS, and 10 indicating severe obesity. BCS cannot be determined with a hands-off approach, especially when the camelid has its full fiber. Technicians must put their hands on these animals to determine the accurate score with confidence.

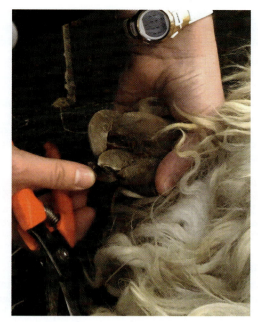

• **Fig. 19.46** Nail trimming is important to prevent overgrowth.

> ### TECHNICIAN NOTE
>
> Veterinary technicians play a vital role in camelid herd health management by establishing management programs, such as vaccination, parasite control, dental examinations, foot trimming, and body condition scoring (BCS).

Care of the Neonate and Neonatal Diseases

Neonatal camelids are referred to as *crias* (Fig. 19.47). The newborn alpaca cria should weigh at least 12 lb at birth, and the normal llama cria should weigh greater than 15 lb. The neonate is covered with an epidermal membrane that is attached to the mucocutaneous junctions, the coronary bands, and the umbilicus, which will flake off shortly after birth. Crias are born with open eyelids and erupted incisors. A veterinary technician can aid in the delivery and management of neonatal crias, providing similar care as that for other food animal species.

Newborns should be closely observed for several hours after birth to ensure that standing and active nursing occurs within the first hour. As with other neonates, the newborn cria should be examined thoroughly, the umbilicus dipped in disinfectant, and the cria weighed daily. The newborn should be alert and should have clear eyes and erect ears. Typically, body temperature is 100°F to 102°F (37.8°C–38.9°C); heart rate 70 to 100 bpm; and respiratory rate 20 to 30 breaths per minute. Comparisons with values for the adult camelid are provided in Box 19.2.

The technician should ensure that the dam has adequate colostrum for passive transfer of maternal antibodies. However, if this is not the case, cow, goat, or sheep colostrum can be substituted. The newborn cria should receive 20% of its body weight in colostrum in four to six feedings during the first 24 hours after birth. If the cria will not nurse, orogastric intubation should be performed to make certain that the cria receives adequate colostral immunity. If colostrum is not available, IV plasma transfusion is strongly recommended. Passive transfer can be evaluated by assessing serum total solid levels and sodium sulfite turbidity. These tests are most beneficial in crias that are 36 hours to 7 days of age.

Orphaned crias may be bottle fed a kid or lamb milk replacer or whole cow's milk and should receive 10% to 15% of their body

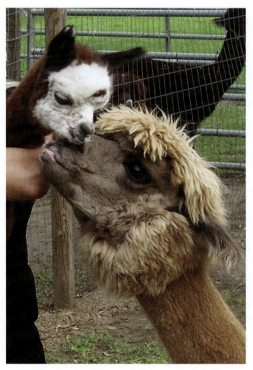

• **Fig. 19.47** The neonatal camelid is referred to as a *cria*. The dam and the cria form strong family bonds. (Courtesy Ms. Vida Palmer.)

weight in milk per day. Initially, this amount can be divided into four to six feedings per day, but feedings can be reduced gradually to two to four feedings per day.

Crias that are considered "at risk" include premature crias, those born to mothers with dystocia, newborns with congenital defects, crias that suffer excessive umbilical bleeding, crias born to the same mating that experienced problems in previous years, and crias that develop FPT. At-risk crias often show abnormalities in vital signs, labored respirations, weakness, depression, failure to nurse, failure

• **BOX 19.2** **Normal TPR Parameters for an Adult Camelid at Rest**

Temperature (T): 99°F to 102.5°F
Pulse rate (P): 60 to 90 beats per minute (bpm)
Respiration rate (R): 10 to 30 breaths per minute

to stand, and straining with failure to pass meconium. Meconium should be passed within 18 to 24 hours after birth; if the cria is straining, a warm soapy water enema can be administered.

TECHNICIAN NOTE

Typically, the temperature, pulse rate, and respiration rate (TPR) of a normal cria are as follows: T = 100°F to 102°F (37.8°C–38.9°C); P = 70 to 100 bpm; and R = 20 to 30 breaths per minute.

Premature Crias

In alpacas and llamas, considerable variation in the duration of gestation has been noted (330–360 days), with some pregnancies lasting longer than 1 year. Therefore trying to predict whether a cria is premature goes beyond duration of gestation. Low birth weight may be the most obvious sign, but there are other signs, such as weakness and inability to stand or hold the head up to nurse. Affected crias have excessive laxity of tendons and ligaments and may walk on their fetlocks; they have nonerect or curled ears because of immature aural cartilage (Fig. 19.48), the haircoat is especially silky, and the rubbery covering of the toe persists for 1 to 2 days (it disappears in 6–12 hours in full-term crias). The incisors are not erupted in premature crias, and the mucous membranes may be dark red because of decreased oxygenation resulting from poor development of the lungs. Prematurity is life-threatening and requires immediate and intensive therapy.

Once prematurity has been diagnosed, the cria should be provided supplemental heat and oxygen. Warmed transfusion of camelid plasma can be administered if the dam cannot supply colostrum. After plasma transfusion, IV fluids with dextrose can be given to meet any existing fluid deficits and to prevent hypoglycemia. A common sign of hypoglycemia in crias is the inability to lift the head to nurse. Premature crias are susceptible to infection, so administration of broad-spectrum antibiotics is usually initiated. If the cria is strong enough to nurse, it should be fed milk at the rate of 10% to 15% of its body weight divided into four feedings a day. If the cria is incapable of nursing, tube feeding via an orogastric tube may be necessary (a stallion urinary catheter works well). Intensive care is continued until the cria matures appropriately or is capable of survival without additional support. Maturity is evidenced by eruption of the incisors and straightening of the ears. Any angular limb deformities may be addressed by application of light support splints; these deformities often improve upon maturity.

TECHNICIAN NOTE

Prematurity in crias can be life-threatening. Most premature crias are incapable of nursing, so it is suggested that a warm transfusion of camelid plasma be administered.

Diseases of the Digestive System

Diarrhea is an important cause of morbidity in neonatal camelids. The most common pathogens causing diarrhea in neonates are

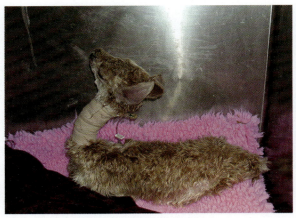

• **Fig. 19.48** Premature crias often have nonerect or curled ears as a result of immature cartilage in the ears.

E. coli, *C. perfringens* (types A, C, and D), coronavirus, *Cryptosporidium* spp., *Giardia* spp., and coccidia. If diarrhea is not treated effectively, it may lead to the development of chronic diarrhea, which may ultimately result in chronic renal failure.

TECHNICIAN NOTE

Diarrhea is an important cause of morbidity in neonatal camelids; if not treated effectively, it may lead to the development of chronic diarrhea, which may ultimately result in chronic renal failure.

Metabolic Conditions

Hepatic Lipidosis

Middle-aged, pregnant, or lactating female camelids are most likely to develop hepatic lipidosis (fatty liver disease), when there is severe anorexia or weight loss within a short amount of time. A negative energy balance results, initiating excessive fat accumulation in the liver cells. This syndrome has been well defined in cats, cows, sheep, goats, ponies, and humans. Unfortunately, in camelids, this disease nearly always has a fatal outcome if it is not recognized early and treated aggressively.

Any animal that is inappetent for an increased amount of time because of stress caused by hot weather, relocation, lactation, or parturition can develop this condition. Offering a variety of appetizing feeds, such as grass clippings or blackberry leaves, can help stimulate feed intake and increase the energy available. Injections of B vitamins can be beneficial for appetite stimulation. If more aggressive oral supplementation is required, a liquid gruel with alfalfa meal, electrolytes, propylene glycol, calcium propionate, and other energy sources can be administered via an orogastric tube. Transfaunation with rumen fluid from cattle, sheep, or goats can be used to repopulate the microbial fauna and restimulate fermentation.

In more severe cases, intensive supportive care and dietary management, including total parenteral nutrition, may be required. The prognosis is always guarded in severe cases of hepatic lipidosis, even with aggressive nutritional support. Close monitoring of feed intake in sick animals is essential to prevent death.

TECHNICIAN NOTE

Anorexia is a hallmark of initiating hepatic lipidosis; therefore therapy must be focused on increasing energy intake immediately.

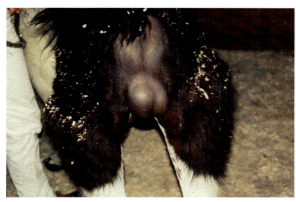

• **Fig. 19.49** Scrotal swelling is a sign of heat stress in intact male camelids. (Courtesy Dr. David Pugh.)

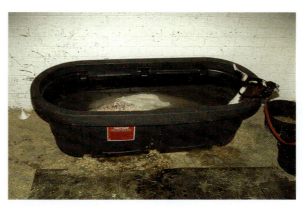

• **Fig. 19.50** Camelids that are recumbent as a result of heat stress may benefit from the use of water flotation tanks. (Courtesy Dr. Christine Navarre.)

Heat Stress

Alpacas and llamas originated from the Andes Mountains of South America, where high heat and humidity are not as common as in many areas of the United States; therefore it is not easy for these animals to adapt to hot, humid conditions. Heat stress must be prevented, because it can lead to severe illness and death.

During the warmer months of the year, trees can provide shade to keep camelids from getting too hot. Barns and shelters with fans and clean, fresh water in different places provide the ideal conditions for camelids to relax and stay cool during the heat of the day. Even an air-conditioned room or area of the barn can help keep animals cool or can be saved as a place to move animals that begin to show signs of heat stress.

Shearing is another important way to help llamas and alpacas keep cool. The fibers trap heat close to the animal's body, and shearing helps the animal lose body heat more effectively through evaporation. If possible, shearing from head to toe (leaving about 1–3 inches of fiber on the body) is most effective, but barrel cuts (e.g., abdomen and thorax only) also help.

> **TECHNICIAN NOTE**
>
> Providing plenty of fresh water, shade, air movement, and small pools will help keep camelids cool and will prevent heat stress; shearing may also be necessary.

It is important to know when llamas and alpacas are most in danger of heat stress. Signs to watch for include nasal flaring, open-mouth breathing, tachypnea, dyspnea, drooling, depression or dullness, anorexia, scrotal swelling in intact males (Fig. 19.49), weakness, trembling, rectal temperature greater than 104°F (40°C), heart rate greater than 90 bpm, and respiratory rate greater than 40 breaths per minute.

Treatment of llamas and alpacas with heat stress should first consist of cooling the animal down by using water or alcohol. Additional cooling with a fan, air conditioner, or water flotation tank are especially useful (Fig. 19.50). The most important aspect of heat stress treatment is prevention.

Diseases of the Nervous System

Meningeal Worm (Parelaphostrongylus Tenuis)

One parasite that is of great importance to llama and alpaca producers is the meningeal worm, *Parelaphostrongylus tenuis*. Llamas and alpacas and other animals, such as domestic small ruminants,

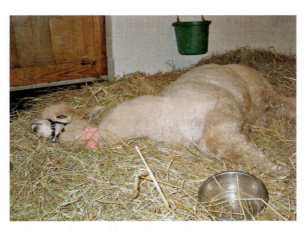

• **Fig. 19.51** Llama with neurologic disease.

are aberrant hosts of this parasite, and the white-tailed deer is the normal host. This parasite does not cause clinical disease in white-tailed deer; it causes high morbidity and mortality in camelids such as alpacas and llamas. *P. tenuis* larvae migrate through the spinal cord, causing neurologic deficits such as ataxia, stiffness, and paralysis (Fig. 19.51). Additionally, gradual weight loss, depression, and death can occur, and neurologic signs generally begin in the hind limbs and progress to the forelimbs. The course of disease may be acute to chronic, ranging from ataxia that lasts months to years or death within days.

> **TECHNICIAN NOTE**
>
> *Parelaphostrongylus tenuis* larvae migrate through the spinal cord of aberrant hosts, such as llamas and alpacas, causing neurologic deficits that may be acute or chronic in nature.

A dewormer such as ivermectin is used for the treatment of meningeal worm infection. Anti-inflammatories are important to reduce inflammation associated with aberrant spinal cord migration and to prevent further clinical signs. Dexamethasone should not be administered to pregnant females, because this drug may induce abortion. Supportive care, including slings, physical therapy, and hydrotherapy, will aid in recovery, especially if the animal is recumbent (Fig. 19.52). The prognosis for survival depends on the severity of clinical signs. The animal that is recumbent has a poorer prognosis. Many animals suffer permanent neurologic

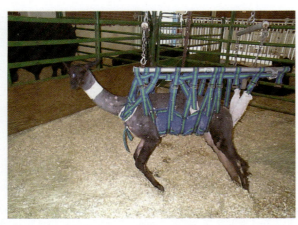

• **Fig. 19.52** Camelids that are unable to stand may benefit from the use of slings and physical therapy. (Courtesy Dr. Christine Navarre.)

deficits but may remain productive members of the herd for breeding and as pets.

TECHNICIAN NOTE

The prognosis for survival from meningeal worm infection depends on how severe the clinical signs are. A poor prognosis is indicated if the animal is recumbent.

Acknowledgments

The authors and publisher wish to acknowledge Jonathan R.O. Garber, Matthew L. Stock, Amy Bentz, Laura Javsicas, Darla Garon, and Danielle Vallotton for their previous contributions to this chapter.

Recommended Readings

Anderson DE, Rings DM. *Current Veterinary Therapy—Food Animal Practice.* 5th ed. St. Louis, MO: Saunders; 2009.

Constable PD, Hinchcliff KW, Done SH, Gruenberg W. *Veterinary Medicine: A Textbook of the Diseases of Cattle, Horses, Sheep, Pigs and Goats.* 11th ed. New York, NY: Saunders; 2017.

Cowart RP. *An Outline of Swine Diseases.* 2nd ed. Ames, IA: Iowa State University, Blackwell Science; 2001.

Divers TJ, Peek SE. *Rebhun's Diseases of Dairy Cattle.* 3rd ed. St. Louis, MO: Saunders; 2018.

Evans CN. *Alpaca Field Manual.* 2nd ed. Manhattan, KS: Able Publishing and Ag Press; 2005.

Fowler ME. *Medicine and Surgery of South American Camelids.* 3rd ed. Ames, IA: Wiley-Blackwell Publishing; 2010.

Fubini SL, Ducharme NC. *Farm Animal Surgery.* 2nd ed. St. Louis, MO: Saunders; 2016.

Holtgrew-Bohling. *Large Animal Clinical Procedures for Veterinary Technicians.* St. Louis, MO: Mosby; 2019.

Orsini JA, Divers TJ. *Manual of Equine Emergencies.* 3rd ed. St. Louis, MO: Saunders; 2009.

Pugh DG, Baird N, Edmondson M, Passler T. *Sheep, Goat, and Cervid Medicine.* 3rd ed. St. Louis, MO: Elsevier; 2020.

Reed S, Bailey W, Sellon D, eds. *Equine Internal Medicine.* 4th ed. St. Louis, MO: Saunders; 2017.

Robinson NE, Sprayberry KA, eds. *Current Therapy in Equine Medicine.* 7th ed. Philadelphia, PA: Saunders; 2014.

Scott PR. *Sheep Medicine.* 2nd ed. London, UK: CRC Press; 2015.

Smith BP, Van Metre DC, Pusterla N. *Large Animal Internal Medicine.* 6th ed. St. Louis, MO: Mosby; 2019.

Smith GW. Bovine neonatology. *Vet Clin North Am Food Anim Pract.* 2009;25:xi.

Smith MC, Sherman DM. *Goat Medicine.* 2nd ed. Ames, IA: Wiley-Blackwell Publishing; 2009.

Van Amstel S, Shearer J. *Manual for Treatment and Control of Lameness in Cattle.* Ames, IA: Blackwell Publishing; 2006.

Zimmerman JJ, et al., ed. *Diseases of Swine.* 11th ed. Ames, IA: Wiley-Blackwell Publishing; 2019.

Recommended Websites

American Association of Equine Practitioners: *Vaccination guidelines.* Available at: https://aaep.org/guidelines/vaccination-guidelines (accessed on July 30, 2024).

American Association of Equine Practitioners: *Infectious disease control.* Available at: https://aaep.org/guidelines/infectious-disease-control (accessed on July 30, 2024).

20
Veterinary Oncology

BETH OVERLEY ADAMSON AND SAMANTHA MORAUX

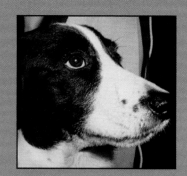

CHAPTER OUTLINE

LEARNING OBJECTIVES

When you have completed this chapter, you will be able to:

1. Pronounce, define, and spell all key terms in this chapter.
2. Discuss the pathogenesis of cancer, including the following:
   - Define oncology and explain mechanisms by which tumors cause clinical signs.
   - Differentiate between malignant and benign tumors.
   - List the classifications of tumors by tissue origin and provide examples of each.
   - Describe the difference between staging and grading and explain how each can be used to make treatment decisions.
3. Discuss the epidemiology of cancer, including the following:
   - List and describe common tumor types.
4. List clinical warning signs that can be associated with cancer.
5. Describe general staging diagnostics for patients with cancer, including the following:
   - Describe what is involved in an initial database for a patient.
   - Discuss how imaging can be used to evaluate a patient.
   - Describe the difference between cytology and histology and list the advantages and limitations of each.
6. Discuss the process of staging cancer.
7. Describe therapeutic options in veterinary oncology, including surgery, radiation, chemotherapy, and palliative and comfort care; discuss safety concerns and side effects related to administration and use of both oral and IV chemotherapy, along with ways to address such concerns and ways to reduce risks of side effects.
8. Discuss complementary, alternative, and integrative therapy and explain why oncologists usually reject alternative medicine but embrace complementary and integrative therapies.
9. List and discuss the common tumors of horses and cattle.

KEY TERMS

Acute radiation toxicity
Adjuvant therapy
Carcinogen
Carcinomas
Chemotherapy
Complementary medicine
Cytotoxic
Definitive treatment
Hemangiosarcoma
Integrative medicine
Lymphoma

Mast cell tumor
Metastasis
Metronomic therapy
Mutagen
Myelosuppression
Nadir
Neoplasm
Neutropenia
Oral tumors
Osteosarcoma
Palliative care

Paraneoplastic syndrome
Teratogen
Tumor grade

Tumor stage
Vesicants

Introduction

Oncology is the study of cancer. There are over 100 different types of cancers, and each type includes several subtypes, with each having its own clinical course and outcome. Patients with some types of cancer have positive long-term outcomes with appropriate therapy. However, some types of cancer are aggressive and have a poor outcome despite treatment. Cancer is a common but complex disease process. It is estimated that 165 million dogs and cats in the United States are at risk of cancer, and approximately 8 million dogs and cats are diagnosed with cancer each year. In one necropsy study, 24% of all dogs had died as a result of cancer; in another study, 45% of dogs older than 10 years of age had died as a result of the disease. It is therefore important for veterinarians and veterinary technicians to understand how to care for and manage patients with cancer.

The words *cancer* and *chemotherapy* evoke strong emotions in clients and conjure images of illness, disfigurement, and death. Many owners fear treatment risks and do not understand that the primary goal of cancer treatment in veterinary medicine is to improve quality of life, not diminish it. Pet owners who seek advice and treatment love their pets as family members, and they expect the same level of professionalism and care for their pet that they expect for themselves. Therefore it is imperative that veterinary personnel know how to discuss, diagnose, and treat cancer in pets.

This chapter focuses on cancer in dogs and cats. In addition, information about the most common types of cancer in horses and cattle is included at the end of the chapter.

Pathogenesis of Cancer

Cancer is a disease in which abnormal cells fail to die. These cells proliferate unchecked, invade normal tissues, and spread to other sites. The terms *tumor*, *neoplasm*, and *mass* characterize discrete clusters of abnormal cells that can be either malignant or benign. Malignant tumors invade local tissues and can *metastasize* (spread) to other parts of the body through blood and lymphatic vessels. Benign tumors may grow large, but they do not spread to distant parts of the body. Both benign and malignant tumors can cause clinical signs, because both can impinge on surrounding tissues and hamper normal system function. One example of a benign tumor is *meningioma*. Although it is benign, it can cause severe neurologic dysfunction, because it localizes in the brain and the spinal cord. Malignant tumors often invade adjacent tissues and can cause severe tissue destruction, inflammation, and necrosis.

Cellular biologists have identified eight fundamental characteristics of cancer cells (Box 20.1). In normal tissues, cells are regulated by a molecular check-and-balance system that controls both cell division and cell death. When abnormal cells arise in the body, molecular mechanisms activate to eliminate these cells by a process called "programmed cell death," or apoptosis. Apoptosis plays a crucial role in developing and maintaining a healthy body.

Cancer arises when apoptosis is interrupted and when molecular signals for cell growth and proliferation continue unchecked. Because the body's regulatory check-and-balance systems are both redundant and complex, cancer development requires a series of molecular modifications that promote cellular proliferation

> ### • BOX 20.1   Fundamental Characteristics of Cancer Cells
>
> 1. They stimulate their own growth.
> 2. They are insensitive to inhibitory signals that would stop their growth.
> 3. They evade their own programmed cell death (apoptosis).
> 4. They have the ability to multiply indefinitely.
> 5. They stimulate the growth of blood vessels that supply increased nutrition to themselves.
> 6. They invade local tissues and can spread to distant sites.
> 7. They follow abnormal metabolic pathways.
> 8. They evade the body's immune defenses.

and growth and/or inhibit apoptosis. These modifications often include mutations in the parts of the deoxyribonucleic acid (DNA) that code for tumor suppressor genes or *proto-oncogenes* (cancer-promoting genes), and nonmutational change of DNA can also promote cancer development. Occasionally, genetic mutations are inherited and present at birth (called *germ line mutations*). More often, mutations occur during somatic cell division and accumulate over time. Such mutations can arise from exposure to *carcinogens* (cancer-causing agents) and to mutagens (e.g., radiation or ultraviolet [UV] light), which can cause mutations (changes in genes) in DNA that may promote tumor development. Local invasion of normal tissues and metastasis to other sites involves complex molecular processes that include abnormal cell-to-cell adhesion, interruption of apoptosis, overexpression or mutation of growth factor receptors, formation of new blood vessels (angiogenesis), and evasion of immune system surveillance.

Malignant tumors cause pain and disability in many ways. They can grow large and invade and destroy normal tissues. They can cause inflammation and become more easily infected compared with healthy tissue. They often bleed readily and can cause pain locally from invasion into muscles, joints, bones, and nerves. They can spread to other sites in the body, such as the lungs, lymph nodes, bone marrow, and liver. A patient with cancer may therefore present with symptoms of pain from both the primary lesion and the growths at secondary sites. Finally, tumors can cause *paraneoplastic syndromes*. These are systemic effects that occur not as a consequence of the physical presence of cancer cells but as a consequence of humoral mediators secreted by certain tumor types. These secreted molecules cause adverse systemic changes, such as *hypercalcemia* (high calcium levels in blood), hypertension, or low blood glucose. The most common paraneoplastic syndrome seen in veterinary medicine is hypercalcemia, which can arise with certain tumor types, such as lymphoma, anal sac carcinoma, squamous cell carcinoma (SCC), and multiple myeloma. Refer to Box 20.2 for a list of paraneoplastic effects.

> ### TECHNICIAN NOTE
>
> Both malignant and benign tumors may grow large locally and cause discomfort. Unlike benign tumor cells, malignant cells are invasive and destroy surrounding tissue. In addition, they can spread by the lymphatic and hematogenous routes to other parts of the body. This is a process known as *metastasis*.

• BOX 20.2 **Paraneoplastic Syndromes**

Some cancers secrete humoral mediators that cause systemic derangements not associated with the local presence of tumor cells. These derangements are called *paraneoplastic syndromes*. Below are examples of paraneoplastic syndromes and some of the cancers that cause them.

Hypoglycemia
Hepatic tumors
Insulinoma
Leiomyoma and leiomyosarcoma

Hypercalcemia
Lymphoma (cats and dogs)
Apocrine gland adenocarcinoma of the anal sac (dogs)
Squamous cell carcinoma (cats)
Thymoma
Multiple myeloma
Parathyroid tumors

Erythrocytosis
Renal carcinoma

Disseminated Intravascular Coagulation
Hemangiosarcoma
Thyroid carcinoma
Mammary carcinoma

Anemia
Lymphoma
Histiocytic sarcoma
Sertoli cell tumor

Hyperproteinemia
Multiple myeloma
Lymphoma
Leukemia

Fever
Lymphoma
Leukemia

Cachexia
Multiple tumors

Neutrophilia
Multiple carcinomas and sarcomas

Hypertrophic Osteopathy
Primary and secondary pulmonary neoplasia

Classification, Staging, and Grading

In addition to being classified as "benign" or "malignant," tumors are further categorized by tissue of origin. Carcinomas, for example, arise from epithelial tissues, such as the skin, mucous membranes, and glandular structures. They usually appear as discrete masses and spread primarily through lymphatic vessels, and can also spread via blood vessels. Sarcomas arise from mesenchymal tissues, such as bone, cartilage, and other connective tissues. They spread most commonly through the bloodstream alone.

The terms *sarcoma* and *carcinoma* refer to two large groups of tumors whose names are further modified by appending a descriptor and/or prefix to these terms. For example, *osteosarcoma* is a sarcoma that arises from bone. *Leiomyosarcoma* is a sarcoma of smooth muscle tissue, and *liposarcoma* is a sarcoma of fat cells. The suffix *-oma* is used to describe tumors. A *lipoma* (versus a liposarcoma) is a benign tumor of fat cells. An *adenoma* (versus adenocarcinoma) is a benign tumor of glandular tissue. Some exceptions include *lymphoma* (sometimes called *lymphosarcoma*), which is a malignant tumor of lymph cells, and *melanoma,* which is a term that describes both benign and malignant tumors. *Insulinomas* can also be malignant, whereas *fibromas* are always benign.

> ### TECHNICIAN NOTE
> Carcinomas arise from epithelial tissue and primarily spread via lymphatic vessels and less commonly through blood vessels, whereas sarcomas arise from mesenchymal (connective) tissue and spread primarily through the bloodstream alone.

Additional methods used to classify tumors include tumor staging and grading. *Tumor stage* indicates how large a tumor is and how far it has spread in the body. Stage is determined by using diagnostic tests, such as caliper measurements, abdominal ultrasonography, thoracic radiography, computed tomography (CT), blood work, urinalysis, magnetic resonance imaging (MRI), and lymph node cytology or biopsy. In contrast, the tumor type and *tumor grade* are determined by an anatomic pathologist, who examines the microscopic appearance of the tumor. Tumor grading systems score tumors on the basis of certain factors, such as mitotic activity, vascular or lymphatic invasion, cellular appearance, and nuclear characteristics. Grade can have prognostic value, and higher-grade tumors are expected to behave more aggressively compared with lower-grade ones. A low-grade mast cell tumor, for example, has a low risk of spread and has the potential to be cured with surgery, and a high-grade mast cell tumor is expected to progress rapidly and spread to other sites. Both tumor stage and grade help the veterinarian formulate a patient's prognosis and treatment plan.

Epidemiology of Cancer

Cancer is a common disease seen in veterinary patients. It is most often diagnosed in middle-aged to older animals, but it can develop in patients of any age. Large-scale surveys from the Morris Animal Foundation have shown cancer to be one of the leading causes of disease-related death in small animal species. It has also been shown that both veterinarians and pet owners consider cancer to be one of their greatest health concerns. Certain dog breeds have a higher incidence of acquiring specific types of cancers compared with other breeds. Some of the more common cancers in veterinary patients include mammary carcinoma, lymphoma, mast cell tumor, soft tissue sarcoma, osteosarcoma, hemangiosarcoma, melanoma, and SCC.

> ### TECHNICIAN NOTE
> Each dog breed has its own unique phenotype and cancer susceptibility risk. Spontaneous cancers in dogs mirror those in humans. Canine and human cancers often share common clinical presentations, pathology, treatment responses, and molecular underpinnings. The National Cancer Institute (https://ccrod.cancer.gov/confluence/display/CCRCOPWeb/Home) takes the One Health Initiative (http://www.cdc.gov/1health/index.html) approach to study canine cancer, aiming to improve the welfare and treatment of human and canine patients alike.

Common Tumor Types

Lymphoma

Lymphoma is a cancer of immune system cells, in which malignant lymphocytes clonally proliferate in lymph tissues throughout

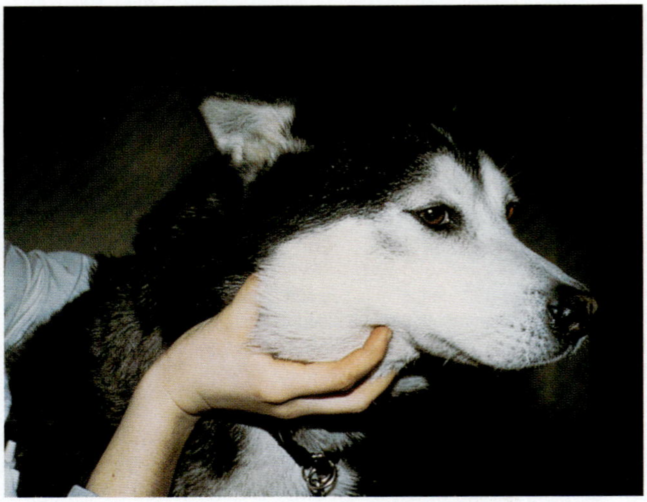

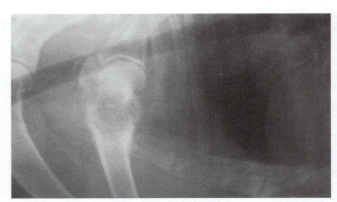

• **Fig. 20.2** Radiograph of a lytic lesion caused by osteosarcoma in the proximal humerus of a dog.

• **Fig. 20.1** Dog with marked enlargement of lymph nodes caused by lymphoma.

the body. In dogs, the most common clinical presentation is multiple, markedly enlarged lymph nodes, which is most commonly seen in middle-aged dogs, but can be seen in younger dogs also (Fig. 20.1). The most common feline presentation is a subacute to chronic history of weight loss and possible vomiting, decreased appetite, and diarrhea in a 12- to 14-year-old cat. A mass or diffuse intestinal thickening may be noted on physical examination. Lymphoma is a heterogeneous disease with a variety of subtypes, each with its own clinical course.

Mast Cell Tumor

Mast cell tumors are the most common malignant skin tumors of dogs. These tumors can mimic the appearances of others and exhibit variable behavior. If diagnosed and treated early, the outcome is usually good. In cats, mast cell tumors most often arise on the face, and some patients develop multiple tumors. Mast cells are immune system cells filled with cytoplasmic granules, which contain chemical mediators, such as histamine, heparin, serotonin, proteoglycans, and proteases. These molecules can be released during degranulation into the body and can cause swelling and inflammation, increased blood vessel permeability, coagulation disorder, and stomach irritation and ulceration. Caution should be taken when manipulating or aspirating larger mast cell tumors. Pretreatment with an antihistamine, such as diphenhydramine, should be considered before biopsy or fine-needle aspiration (FNA) performed on vulnerable tissues. In addition, some types of narcotics, such as morphine, can cause mast cell tumor activation and histamine release, which may result in severe hypotension. Therefore the use of certain narcotics should be avoided in patients with mast cell tumors.

> **TECHNICIAN NOTE**
>
> Avoid the use of morphine in patients with confirmed or suspected mast cell tumors, because morphine can cause mast cell tumor degranulation and histamine release.

Osteosarcoma

This disease occurs most commonly in middle-aged large breed dogs. It primarily affects the bones of the appendicular skeleton (Fig. 20.2). Patients usually present with lameness.

Anti-inflammatories are often tried initially and may help, but the tumor eventually progresses, and lameness returns or persists. A mass may not always be present at the first visit. Therefore radiography should be recommended at the patient's first visit, and owners should be instructed to return in 1 to 2 weeks if pain medications and rest have not resolved the lameness.

Oral Tumors

The most common malignant oral tumor in dogs is melanoma (Fig. 20.3). In cats, it is SCC. These tumors primarily affect older animals. SCC commonly develops under the tongue in cats; therefore a thorough oral examination is important for patients that exhibit trouble eating, oral bleeding, or halitosis. In addition, loose teeth in cats that have no evidence of dental disease may be related to underlying SCC.

Hemangiosarcoma

This tumor occurs most commonly in larger breed, middle- to older-aged dogs. It can arise in many organs, but the most common are the heart, liver, and spleen. The most common presentation in a dog is acute collapse and abdominal swelling. These dogs often present as emergency cases, with pale gums, poor or snappy pulse, distended abdomen, and extreme lethargy. Abdominal radiography or ultrasonography likely will reveal abdominal effusion and possibly a mass. Unfortunately, benign splenic lesions can present in the same way, and the only way to confirm hemangiosarcoma is through tissue biopsy. However, staging diagnostics may show metastases in the lungs, heart, or other locations, and these findings would support the diagnosis of a highly aggressive malignancy, such as hemangiosarcoma.

Other Sarcomas

This large group comprises tumors arising from the mesenchymal (connective) tissues of the body. They often arise in the dermis as firm, invasive, and often nonmovable masses. In cats, they have been noted to arise from injection site locations. Aspirate cytology may help with diagnosis in some, but these tumors exfoliate cells less avidly compared with carcinomas or round cell tumors. Early detection and treatment are key, because these tumors are highly invasive, and major surgery is needed to reduce the risk of tumor recurrence.

> **TECHNICIAN NOTE**
>
> Some tumors, especially those of bone and of the mouth, can be extremely painful. It is imperative to educate clients on the signs of tumors, such as pain and discomfort. Pain medications may be prescribed to reduce pain and to enhance the patient's quality of life.

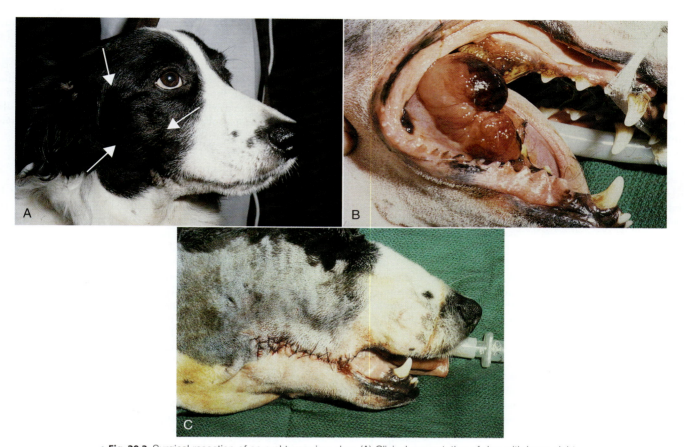

• **Fig. 20.3** Surgical resection of an oral tumor in a dog. (A) Clinical presentation of dog with large, right-sided facial swelling *(inside arrows)*. (B) Before surgery, a portion of the mass is visible via the oral cavity. (C) The same animal immediately after surgical resection and reconstruction.

Carcinomas

Carcinomas are tumors of epithelial tissues and arise from many sites. The more common ones seen in veterinary medicine are mammary carcinomas (primarily in late spayed [after second estrus] or intact females), urothelial carcinomas (e.g., transitional cell carcinoma of the bladder), anal sac carcinomas in dogs, and SCC in cats.

Clinical Signs

In general, clinical signs associated with cancer(s) are nonspecific, but cancer should be considered in patients that exhibit one or more of the following signs:
- Swellings that persist or grow
- Nonhealing wounds
- Weight loss
- Loss of appetite
- Bleeding or discharge from orifices
- Reluctance to exercise or lethargy
- Persistent lameness or stiffness
- Difficulty breathing, urinating, or defecating

When a patient presents with a mass, the diagnostic process begins with a careful clinical history and thorough physical examination. The history should include the presenting complaint (duration, frequency, and progression); available test results; results of treatments for other health issues; current medications; nutrition; and recent travel history. A mass should be measured, and its location and size documented in the record before aspiration of the mass. This is particularly important for mast cell tumors, because they can swell significantly after aspiration. Photos of hard-to-measure masses are useful. All other masses should be noted, measured, and recorded as well.

Diagnostics

Two of the most important factors for long-term treatment success are early detection and appropriate treatment. A "watch and wait" approach is not advised, and diagnostic recommendations should be documented in the veterinary record. If an owner declines diagnostic testing, monitoring recommendations should be made. Owners should be advised to return if the lesion changes (ulcerates, grows and shrinks, causes itching, or swells) and persists. Also, the owner should return if new lesions arise or if lameness or a wound does not resolve in 2 weeks.

Initial Database

The standard of care for animal patients with cancer undergoing treatment includes a complete blood count (CBC), a serum chemistry profile, and urinalysis. These tests provide a general health screen, may help characterize the tumor, and can help identify paraneoplastic syndrome. Other diagnostics are recommended on the basis of tumor type and often include three-view thoracic radiography, lymph node cytology, and/or abdominal ultrasonography.

When performing diagnostics, great care should be taken to use proper technique to ensure accurate results. For example, thrombocytopenia can be an indicator of a poor outcome in some patients and can be a reason to delay treatment. Improper venipuncture technique can lead to an inaccurate result that can affect patient treatment plans. A manual blood smear should be performed to assess cell morphology and to confirm that proper technique was used during blood collection and handling. (Refer to Chapter 11 for information on blood smear preparation.)

TECHNICIAN NOTE

Initial evaluation of oncology patients includes a complete blood count (CBC), accompanied by blood smear examination, a serum chemistry profile, and urinalysis. Other common staging diagnostics include three-view thoracic radiography, abdominal ultrasonography, lymph node palpation, and cytology.

Urinalysis should be obtained, ideally via cystocentesis, at the time blood is collected for serum chemistry evaluation. Thoracic radiography should include three well-positioned views that include the entire chest, including the part that overlaps the cranial abdominal structures.

When performing diagnostic tests, it is imperative to understand tumor behavior and to use proper technique. Mast cell tumors, for example, rarely spread to the thorax. Therefore nodal sampling and abdominal ultrasonography are more important diagnostics for this particular type of cancer. Sloppy or improper biopsy or aspiration techniques may yield inaccurate results and seed tumor cells at additional sites. FNA of a transitional cell carcinoma of the bladder, for example, can seed cancer cells along the needle tract. Therefore cystocentesis would not be the first recommended diagnostic for a confirmed or suspected bladder tumor. In patients under treatment, blood samples ideally should be obtained through venipuncture of the jugular vein rather than the peripheral veins. Peripheral veins may be used in future treatment and ideally should not be compromised.

TECHNICIAN NOTE

When performing diagnostic tests, it is imperative to use proper technique and to have complete understanding of specific tumor biology and behavior to obtain appropriate samples without causing further complications. Cancer-contaminated needles should never be reused and should be immediately disposed of in biohazard waste containers. All samples should be properly and immediately labeled and processed to avoid labeling errors and misdiagnosis. Proper technique should be used to obtain diagnostic-quality radiographs to avoid a missed diagnosis or a delay in diagnosis or treatment.

Imaging

Comprehensive radiography of the thorax is most commonly used for initial evaluation of the presence or absence of metastatic disease. Specialty hospitals may additionally recommend thoracic CT, depending on the type of tumor and its location. It is the imaging modality used for planning radiation therapy, because it is more likely to detect very small lesions compared with other imaging modalities. Before performing expensive, invasive, or risky treatments, it is important to properly stage a patient's cancer, particularly if metastasis is likely. Patients undergoing CT must be either anesthetized or sedated, which can increase risk to an unhealthy patient. In addition, CT is not widely available and can be more expensive than radiography. Therefore CT is not recommended for every case, and initial survey radiography is recommended to detect obvious lesions.

For abdominal imaging, ultrasonography is currently the diagnostic method of choice in veterinary medicine. Abdominal ultrasonography is noninvasive and allows better visualization of organs compared with radiography. Ultrasonography can also guide percutaneous collection of biopsy samples and body cavity effusions.

Cytology and Histology

Histologic examination of the primary tumor is performed by an anatomic pathologist to confirm the diagnosis of cancer. The procedure requires a sample of tumor tissue obtained through either incisional or excisional biopsy. Excisional biopsy attempts to remove the entire tumor and a margin of normal tissue, whereas incisional biopsy procures only part of a tumor. Incisional biopsy may be used before definitive treatment for larger tumors located in complicated locations. Neoplastic tissues and/or associated lymph nodes are collected and preserved in a fixative, such as formalin. Samples are submitted to a pathology laboratory for processing and interpretation by an anatomic pathologist. FNA is another helpful sampling technique. It may be performed concurrently with biopsy or it may be performed independently. Cytology samples obtained through FNA are stained with the modified Wright-Giemsa stain and are submitted to a laboratory service for interpretation by a clinical pathologist. Technicians should be careful not to expose cytology slides to formalin, because partial fixation of cells can alter cell morphology. Some slides can be stained in-house with the Diff-Quik or similar stain and then evaluated immediately by the clinician. Cytology does not usually require anesthesia or sedation and allows for more rapid assessment and identification of cancer cells, if present in the sample. However, biopsy is often still needed to confirm the diagnosis and the tumor grade. Cytology-based diagnoses correlate strongly with biopsy-based diagnoses, but not necessarily vice versa. Some tumor types, such as sarcomas, are poorly exfoliative, which means the absence of cancer cells in a cytology sample does not always rule out cancer.

Cytology is recommended at the start of a workup for most cutaneous lesions. It rarely requires sedation and is often performed by using a 22-gauge needle, 6- to 10-mL syringe, and multiple slides (Fig. 20.4). The needle is inserted into the lesion of interest, and a sample is obtained either by "coring" the sample with a poking motion under the skin or by using light suction with a 10-mL syringe attached to the needle. Cells in the needle hub are sprayed onto slides using the syringe, and another slide is then used to carefully spread the cells on the first slide. Slides are then stained for microscopic evaluation (Fig. 20.5).

Staging

The histologic appearance of the tumor and its grade can help determine which staging tests need to be performed. The process of staging cancer considers the following four aspects of an oncologic disease:

1. The location and type of the tumor
2. The tumor size and its borders
3. The involvement of regional lymph nodes
4. The presence or absence of metastasis and the number of tumors

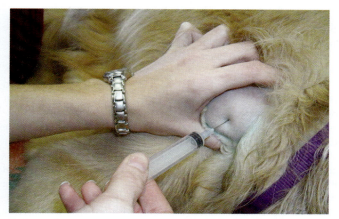

• **Fig. 20.4** Proper technique is important to obtain a diagnostic cytology sample.

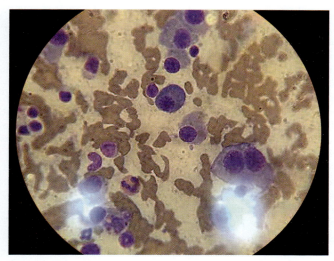

• **Fig. 20.5** Results from fine-needle aspiration. Before submission to an outside laboratory, cytology should be evaluated in-house to confirm that adequate cells are present in the aspirate.

Carefully staging a tumor is essential for planning an appropriate and effective course of treatment. Diagnostic imaging for most cancers usually includes a three-view series of thoracic radiography or thoracic CT. The primary exception is a mast cell tumor, which rarely spreads to the chest. Although thoracic CT is more sensitive than radiography and therefore more likely to detect smaller and more subtle lesions, radiography is always recommended first. If metastatic disease is readily apparent on radiographs, it may not be necessary to perform the more expensive CT, because many owners elect euthanasia or decline treatment at that point. In general, diagnostic tests used for staging cancer should be performed before treatment. However, treatment may be carried out as soon as a diagnosis is made but before staging if a patient is suffering in extremis and there is no other way to alleviate its suffering. For example, a dog with advanced stage lymphoma may have trouble breathing and swallowing as a result of extremely enlarged retropharyngeal lymph nodes. In this case, the dog may benefit from the immediate use of steroids. Treatment, in this case, may quickly alleviate suffering until a definitive diagnosis can be made.

Therapeutic Options

The primary goal of treatment in veterinary oncology is to maintain good quality of life for the patient. The secondary goal is to prolong the patient's life. This approach is different from that in human medicine, where life extension can take precedence over quality of life, particularly during treatment.

Cancer treatment is most successful when cancer is diagnosed and treated early. Therefore thorough physical examination and routine health screening are of utmost importance. The veterinary technician plays an important role by taking a careful history; assessing the patient; and bringing new findings, such as a second mass, to the attention of the veterinarian. New masses should be measured, recorded, and aspirated and the data included as part of the patient record.

Surgery

Surgery is the cancer treatment most likely to provide a positive long-term result; however, it is not recommended for all tumor types. Surgery is best used to treat solitary masses that have not metastasized beyond the primary site and to treat associated regional disease, such as affected lymph nodes. Surgery will not improve survival for most patients with distant metastases; therefore surgery is not recommended in these cases unless it is used to alleviate patient suffering. Surgery can be curative in the case of some small, low-grade tumors. Generally, solitary tumors that are less than 2 cm in diameter and have been completely excised offer the best long-term outcome with surgery. Surgery may also be used in combination with other treatments. Adjuvant chemotherapy (*adjuvant therapy* is treatment given in addition to the primary treatment) is recommended after surgery for high-grade tumors that are likely to metastasize in the future. Adjuvant radiation is often recommended after surgery for locally invasive tumor types, such as larger sarcomas that are hard to completely remove with surgery alone.

Treatment can vary, depending on the stage, grade, location, and type of tumor. Therefore it is best to obtain a diagnosis and perform recommended staging diagnostics before surgical removal of a tumor.

Radiation

Radiation treatment uses high-energy waves to kill cancer cells and shrink tumors. Most often, the radiation used comes from an external mechanical source that targets a beam of high-energy rays on the diseased tissue (this is called *external beam radiation* or *teletherapy*). In veterinary medicine, rarely does radiation come from radioactive material placed within the body (*brachytherapy*). With external beam radiation, the patient is not radioactive after treatment, and the machines delivering such treatment are in facilities designed to protect personnel from treatment effects.

Radiation causes damage to DNA both directly and indirectly, because it forms highly charged particles (called *free radicals*) that damage DNA. Cells with damaged DNA usually stop dividing and die. Radiation can be given as the primary form of treatment, but more often, it is used in addition to other treatments, such as radiation after a surgery when complete tumor removal is not achieved.

Radiation treatment can be used with curative or palliative intent. In the case of a curative intent, radiation is usually given in combination with other treatments. Curative radiation is usually delivered in several small fractions over the course of a month. Palliative radiation is used to reduce pain associated with the presence of a tumor and to improve the patient's quality of life. Palliative radiation treatment involves the administration of larger, less frequent fractions of radiation to the tumor site. In veterinary medicine, palliative radiation is commonly used to treat painful bone tumors, such as osteosarcomas, that cannot be surgically removed.

Radiation does not specifically target cancer cells. It also affects normal cells located within the radiation field. Radiation of normal tissues can cause side effects such as *acute radiation toxicity*, which occurs during treatment but disappears within weeks after treatment. The most common acute side effects include skin reactions, such as hair loss or moist dermatitis, which occur toward the middle to end of the treatment period (Fig. 20.6). Topical medications can be used to minimize discomfort. In addition, the pet owner needs to make sure that the patient is not causing self-trauma to the site through licking or biting. Severe reactions occur in less than 5% of cases. Hair loss also occurs in the radiation field. To minimize the risk of radiation exposure to normal cells, patients are sedated or anesthetized during each radiation treatment. Thus the risks of sedation must be considered when treatment recommendations are made.

TECHNICIAN NOTE

After radiation therapy, the skin within the radiation field may be subject to depigmentation, hyperpigmentation, leukotrichia (white hair), or alopecia. These effects do not cause any harm or discomfort to the animal. Some animals develop moist dermatitis in the mid- and final stages of treatment. Side effects can be minimized with the use of anti-inflammatory agents and with devices that prevent self-trauma.

Chemotherapy

Technically, *chemotherapy* is the use of pharmaceuticals to treat cancer. Traditionally, chemotherapy has been thought of as a small

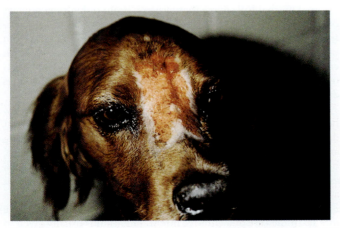

• **Fig. 20.6** Moist dermatitis in a dog receiving radiotherapy for treatment of a nasal tumor.

group of drugs that stop cell proliferation and kill cancer cells by altering tumor cell DNA. Practically, treatment involves a diverse array of therapies that include steroids, nonsteroidal anti-inflammatory drugs (NSAIDs), *metronomic therapies*, traditional chemotherapy, hormonal therapy, immunotherapy, and targeted therapies.

Chemotherapy can be given with injectable or oral drugs and traditionally has been administered periodically, with intermittent tissue recovery times between doses. In contrast, metronomic therapy may be given daily at much smaller doses and does not require recovery periods. Traditional chemotherapy drugs usually directly affect the DNA of both tumor and normal cells. Other treatments affect the metabolism of tumor cells or inhibit the formation of blood vessels in tumors. Some newer treatments inhibit signaling pathways involved in the promotion of cell growth and proliferation. Still others affect covalent bonding within the DNA molecule which, in turn, alters gene expression and the regulation of cellular activities. Finally, much focus has been placed on the development of treatments that modulate the patient's immune system so that it can recognize and attack tumor cells. Table 20.1 provides a list of chemotherapeutic agents used in veterinary medicine.

Most traditional chemotherapy agents target metabolically active, rapidly dividing cells. These agents, however, are not specific to cancer cells; normal cells that are also metabolically active and rapidly dividing will be affected by these treatments as well. Such normal tissues include epithelial cells that line the gastrointestinal (GI) tract, bone marrow–derived cells (e.g., neutrophils), and the cells in hair follicles. Traditional side effects from treatment therefore include vomiting, diarrhea, inappetence, and hair loss (in certain breeds) (Fig. 20.7). Chemotherapy-associated *neutropenia*, although temporary, can also increase the risk for infections at various time points during the course of treatment. Decreases in platelet counts occur and, although they rarely cause problems, it is important to know that treatment will affect the platelet count. Low platelet counts can be one reason for delaying of a prescribed treatment.

Chemotherapy is used in different ways, depending on the patient's condition and the tumor type. It can be administered before **definitive treatment** (called neoadjuvant chemotherapy) to shrink a tumor so that subsequent surgery and radiation can completely eradicate the primary tumor. This is occasionally recommended, for example, for large mast cell tumors. Chemotherapy is also used in addition to surgery or radiation (as adjuvant therapy) to prevent or delay metastasis of high-grade tumors. In systemic tumors that are highly sensitive to chemotherapy, such as lymphoma, leukemia, or multiple myeloma, chemotherapy is used as the primary treatment. Treatment protocols may involve the use of multiple drugs given either concurrently or sequentially for a set period, often over several months.

It is important to know that chemotherapy is not recommended in the treatment of every type of cancer. Lower-grade, slow-growing tumors and certain resistant tumor types are less likely to respond to traditional chemotherapy. It is also important to know that different types of tumors respond differently to various treatments. A particular protocol, for example, is not equally effective on all tumor types or on all patients.

TECHNICIAN NOTE

Chemotherapy is not recommended for every oncology patient. Different drugs are used to treat different tumor types. Drugs with different side effect risks and different mechanisms of action are often combined in a single treatment protocol to optimize effectiveness and, at the same time, minimize risk. The side effects of treatment can be reduced by using medications, such as antinausea medication, prophylactically. When severe side effects occur, the dosage of chemotherapy is either lowered for subsequent treatments or a substitute drug is used.

TABLE 20.1   Chemotherapy Drugs

Chemotherapy	Type of Chemotherapy	What Does It Treat?	Pet Owner Education	Excreted via	Nadir	Is It a Vesicant?
Asparaginase (L-Asparaginase (Elspar)	*Escherichia coli* antineoplastic	• Lymphoid malignancies	• Possible acute tumor lysis syndrome • Anaphylactoid reactions • Vomiting • Diarrhea • Dyspnea • Hypotension • Collapse	• Extracellular spaces	None	No
Carboplatin (Paraplatin)	Platinum antineoplastic	• Squamous cell carcinoma • Ovarian carcinoma • Mediastinal carcinoma • Pleural adenocarcinoma • Nasal carcinoma • Thyroid adenocarcinoma • Melanoma	• Caution with hepatic and renal disease • Not compatible with live or killed annual vaccines • Vomiting • Diarrhea • Anorexia • Lethargy • Bone marrow suppression • Avoid touching urine for several days after treatment	• Liver • Kidney • Skin • Tumor tissue • Excreted in urine over several days after treatment	• Dogs: neutrophils 14 days; thrombocytes 14 days • Cats: neutrophils 17–21 days	Yes
Chlorambucil (Leukeran)	Antineoplastic (immunosuppressant)	• Lymphocytic leukemia • Multiple myeloma • Polycythemia vera • Macroglobulinemia • Ovarian adenocarcinoma (immunosuppressant) • Glomerulonephritis • Inflammatory bowel disease • Immune-mediated skin disease	• Vomiting • Diarrhea • Anorexia • Nausea • Lethargy • Proper handling oral formulation	• Liver	• Complete blood count (CBC) recommended at 0, 1, 2, 4, 8, and 12 weeks, and then every 3–6 months thereafter	No
Cisplatin (Platinol-AQ)	Antineoplastic	• Squamous cell carcinoma • Transitional cell carcinoma • Ovarian carcinoma • Mediastinal carcinomas • Osteosarcoma • Pleural adenocarcinoma • Nasal carcinoma • Thyroid adenocarcinoma • Palliative control of neoplastic pulmonary effusions after intracavitary administration	• Never use in cats • Nephrotoxic • In dogs, nausea and vomiting within 6 hours post-administration • Thrombocytopenia • Ototoxicity • Diarrhea • Seizures • Anaphylactoid reaction • Hyperuricemia • Increased hepatic enzymes • Lethargy • Anorexia	• Liver • Intestines • Kidneys	• 7–10 days	Yes

Continued

TABLE 20.1   Chemotherapy Drugs—cont'd

Chemotherapy	Type of Chemotherapy	What Does It Treat?	Pet Owner Education	Excreted via	Nadir	Is It a Vesicant?
Cyclophosphamide (Cytoxan, Neosar)	Antineoplastic immunosuppressive	• Lymphoma • Leukemia • Carcinoma • Sarcoma (immunosuppressant) • Systemic lupus erythematosus, idiopathic thrombocytopenic purpura, immune-mediated hemolytic anemia	• Sterile hemorrhagic cystitis • Myelosuppression • Anorexia • Vomiting • Diarrhea • Lethargy • Alopecia • Proper handling of oral formulation	• Liver • Urine	• 4–12 hours • Possibly 72 hours	Yes
Cytarabine Cytosine arabinoside (Cytosar-U)	Parenteral antineoplastic	• Lymphoreticular neoplasms • Leukemia	• Myelosuppression • Anorexia • Vomiting • Diarrhea • Lethargy • Conjunctivitis • Oral ulceration • Neurotoxicity • Hepatotoxicity • Proper administration of subcutaneous injections	• Liver • Kidneys • Intestinal mucosa and granulocytes	• 5–7 days	Yes
Dacarbazine (DTIC-Dome)	Parenteral antineoplastic	• Relapsed lymphoma • Soft tissue sarcoma • Melanoma	• Anorexia • Vomiting • Diarrhea • Lethargy • Hepatotoxicity • Serious toxicity risk (bloody vomiting or diarrhea, abnormal bleeding, bruising, urination, depression, infection, shortness of breath, etc.).	• Liver • Kidneys	• 7–10 days	Yes
Doxorubicin HCL Adriamycin (Doxil)	Antibiotic antineoplastic	• Lymphoma • Carcinoma • Leukemia • Sarcoma	• Anaphylactoid reactions • Cardiotoxic • Anorexia • Vomiting • Diarrhea • Lethargy • Alopecia • Caution in *MDR1*-allele mutations • Myelosuppression • Discolored (reddish-orange) urine 1–2 days • Renal toxic in cats	• Bone Marrow • Kidneys • Urine	• 7–10 days	Yes
Fluorouracil (5-FU) (Adrucil)	Antineoplastic agent	• Canine mammary carcinoma • Dermal squamous cell carcinoma • Gastrointestinal tract tumors	• Never use in cats • Anorexia • Vomiting • Diarrhea • Lethargy	• Tumor cells • Intestinal mucosa • Liver • Bone marrow • Urine	• 9–14 days	Yes

Drug	Classification	Indications	Side Effects	Affected Organs/Route	Nadir	
Gemcitabine HCL (Gemzar)	Antineoplastic agent	• Radiosensitizer for nonresectable tumors • Pancreatic carcinoma (humans) • Small cell lung carcinoma (humans) • Lymphoma (humans) • Bladder and soft tissue sarcoma (humans)	• Anorexia • Vomiting • Diarrhea • Lethargy • Myelosuppression • Limited experience "investigational" treatment	• Urine	• 3–7 days	Yes
Lomustine (CeeNu)	Antineoplastic	• Central nervous system neoplasm • Lymphoma • Mast cell tumor	• Myelosuppression • Anemia • Thrombocytopenia • Alopecia • Elevated liver enzymes (icteric) • Metabolites in urine up to 24 hours after dose; use proper personal protective equipment (PPE) • Caution in live vaccines • Proper handling of oral formulation	• Liver • Urine (up to 24 hours after a dose)	• 7–10 days	No
Mechlorethamine HCL (Mustargen)	Antineoplastic	• Lymphoreticular neoplasms • Peritoneal effusions	• Anorexia • Vomiting • Diarrhea • Lethargy • Myelosuppression • Ototoxicity • Hepatotoxicity • Caution with live vaccines	• Urine	• 7–10 days	Yes
Melphalan (Alkeran)	Alkylating agent Antineoplastic	• Ovarian carcinoma • Lymphoreticular neoplasm • Osteosarcoma • Mammary or pulmonary neoplasm	• Thrombocytopenia • Vomiting • Diarrhea • Anorexia • Lethargy • Myelosuppression • Proper handling of oral formulation	• Bone Marrow • Kidneys • Urine	• CBC recommended every week for 2 weeks and monthly thereafter	No
Mitoxantrone HCL (Novantrone)	Antineoplastic	• Lymphoma • Mammary Adenocarcinoma • Squamous cell carcinoma • Renal adenocarcinoma • Fibroid sarcoma • Thyroid or Transitional cell carcinoma • Hemangiopericytoma	• Anorexia • Vomiting • Diarrhea • Lethargy • Myelosuppression • Caution with live vaccines • Blue-green colored urine after treatment	• Liver • Heart • Thyroid • Red blood cells • Urine	• 10 days	Yes

Continued

TABLE 20.1 Chemotherapy Drugs—cont'd

Chemotherapy	Type of Chemotherapy	What Does It Treat?	Pet Owner Education	Excreted via	Nadir	Is It a Vesicant?
Vinblastine (Velban)	Vinca alkaloid Antineoplastic	• Lymphoma • Carcinoma • Mastocytoma • Splenic tumors • Canine mast cell tumors	• Anorexia • Vomiting • Diarrhea • Lethargy • Myelosuppression • Caution in *MDR1* patients • Severe toxicity possible (depression, abnormal bleeding [bloody diarrhea], and/or bruising)	• Bile • Feces • Urine (small amounts)	• 4–9 days	Yes
Vincristine (Oncovin)	Vinca alkaloid Antineoplastic	• Lymphoid and hematopoietic neoplasms (immunosuppressant) • Immune-mediated thrombocytopenia	• Anorexia • Vomiting • Diarrhea • Lethargy • Myelosuppression • May cause constipation in cats • Caution in *MDR1* patients	• Bile • Feces • Urine (small amounts)	• 4–9 days	Yes

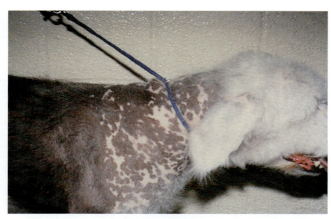

• **Fig. 20.7** Hair loss caused by chemotherapy in an Old English Sheep-dog.

Safe Handling Practices

Environmental contamination and occupational exposure to hazardous drugs are an ongoing concern. Recently, the US Pharmacopeia Convention created USP General Health Chapter <800>, which includes regulations for safe handling of hazardous substances. USP<800> became effective on November 1st, 2023 (after delay due to the coronavirus pandemic), for all health care personnel (in human or veterinary medicine) who receive, store, prepare, administer, transport, or otherwise come in contact with hazardous drugs. Hazardous drugs include not only antineoplastics (e.g., chemotherapy agents) but also other classes of drugs, such as antipsychotics, antibiotics, and benzodiazepines. Examples of hazardous agents are methimazole, spironolactone, paroxetine, warfarin, fluconazole, cyclosporine, and azathioprine. The National Institute for Occupational Safety and Health (NIOSH) List of Antineoplastic and Other Hazardous Drugs safety sheet provides a reference of known hazardous substances. USP is not a regulatory agency, and therefore enforcement of USP<800> is the responsibility of regulatory veterinary boards. Regardless, this USP chapter's recommendations increase the risk of liability for practices that do not comply.

Exposure to chemotherapeutic agents can occur from improper handling of the drug, contaminated packaging, and patient waste. It can occur directly via inhalation of an aerosolized drug, percutaneous absorption, and accidental ingestion. Chronic exposure can cause health problems in hospital personnel, and many chemotherapy agents are well-known *teratogens*, *mutagens*, and *carcinogens*. Special care to minimize exposure should be taken by all personnel, especially immunocompromised individuals and those who are pregnant, nursing, or trying to conceive.

The use of personal protective equipment (PPE) and disciplined adherence to recommended safety guidelines can significantly reduce the risk of exposure to *cytotoxic* and chemotherapeutic agents. PPE should be worn when working with any chemotherapeutic drug and should include gowns, hair covers, shoe covers, chemotherapy-specific gloves, eye protection, and respiratory protection. All respiratory protection should be fitted to each individual. Gowns should have long sleeves with tight-fitting cuffs and should tie in the back. Gowns should be coated with polyethylene or other laminate material to offer the best protection. Personnel should be double-gloved, using chemotherapy-specific gloves, and must meet the American Society for Testing and Materials

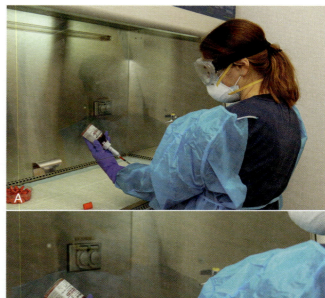

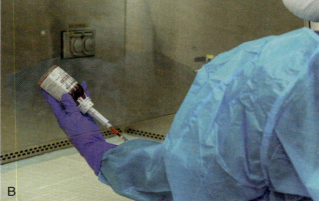

• **Fig. 20.8** (A, B) When drawing up chemotherapeutic agents, it is important to use personal protective equipment (PPE) and a ventilated class II or III laminar flow biological safety cabinet with high-efficiency particulate air (HEPA) filtration. This helps ensure the safety of veterinary personnel and reduces environmental contamination. (Courtesy Moraux Photography.)

(ASTM) standard D6978 or its successor. When double gloving, the first layer of gloves should be under the cuff of the gown, and the second layer should be over the cuff to ensure a proper protective barrier.

When chemotherapy agents are prepared, a ventilated class II or III laminar flow (vertical) biological safety cabinet (BSC) with high-efficiency particulate air (HEPA) filtration should be used (Fig. 20.8A and B). Syringes should be labeled, and chemotherapeutic drugs and saline should be drawn up in a closed system transfer device (CSTD) appropriate for safe administration (Fig. 20.9A and B). Examples of CSTDs are EQUASHIELD and BD PhaSeal. CSTDs were invented to prevent exposure of personnel to drugs, reduce surface contamination, and eliminate direct human uptake via aerosolization or ingestion. In addition, syringes filled with chemotherapeutic agents should be transported to the administration site in a sealed plastic bag (Fig. 20.10). Personnel should never apply makeup, use lip balms, chew gum, smoke, eat, or drink in a room where chemotherapy is administered as these actions increase the likelihood of exposure.

USP<800> has established definitions of primary and secondary Containment Primary Engineering Control (C-PEC) for drug containment and preparation. The primary C-PEC is the room that houses the BSC in which the hazardous drugs are stored and unpackaged. The secondary C-PEC is the outer room that contains the inner room containing the BSC (Fig. 20.11). All injectable chemotherapy agents must be prepared inside a BSC that provides

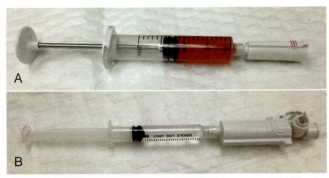

• **Fig. 20.9** (A) Use of closed system transfer devices (CSTDs), as seen here, reduces the risk of aerosolization and accidental splatter of chemotherapeutic agents. (B) Normal saline should be used to flush catheters, rather than heparin, which can precipitate chemotherapeutic agents. (Courtesy Dr. Joanna Bassert.)

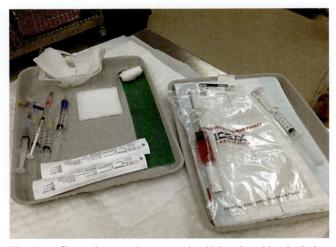

• **Fig. 20.10** Chemotherapeutic agents should be placed in plastic bags before being transported within the veterinary hospital.

International Organization for Standardization (ISO) Class 5 or better. The BSC should be externally vented and should be located in a room that is also externally vented. The room should be maintained at a pressure negative to the pressure of surrounding areas. This includes being away from any drains and water sources. The room must have a minimum of 12 air changes per hour. When antineoplastics are received, they should be segregated from other medications and opened in an area that has immediate access to a spill kit. Full PPE should be worn during unpacking and storing of all antineoplastics.

Safety documentation should be made available to the entire staff, because the risk of exposure to hazardous drugs is always present. The staff should have access to key documents that appropriately communicate information about the hazards. This includes but is not limited to the following:

- Labels on containers of all hazardous drugs
- Safety data sheets (SDSs) for all hazardous chemicals
- List of all hazardous drugs located in the practice setting
- Signs posted before entrances to any areas where hazardous drugs are handled

Appropriate training is also important to those handling hazardous drugs. Every employee should be trained on drug specifics, including proper use of PPE, proper use and cleaning procedures

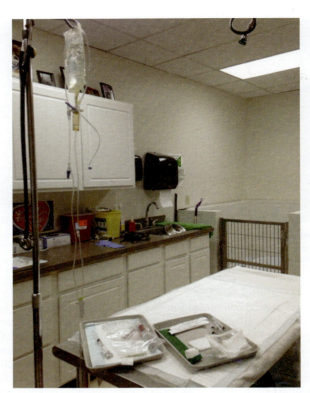

• **Fig. 20.11** A dedicated, quiet room with low traffic flow should be used for the administration of chemotherapy. Ventilation should be turned on during the administration process. (Courtesy Dr. Joanna Bassert.)

of a BSC, spill management, proper disposal of hazardous drugs and contaminated materials, and response to known or suspected exposure to hazardous drugs. The veterinary technician should also understand and be able to relay information about risk of exposure and safety techniques to clients when their pets are taking any type of hazardous drugs. All staff with reproductive capability must confirm in writing that they understand the risks of handling hazardous drugs. It is up to the individual veterinary technician to ensure that safety measures are being implemented by the hospital and report all violations if anyone's safety is at risk.

Administration

Consideration of a patient's temperament is vital to the safe administration of chemotherapy. If a patient is extremely aggressive, sedation may be required to ensure safety to both oncology department personnel and the patient. Inappropriate administration of chemotherapy can cause severe illness, pain, or even patient death. It is imperative that the patient be properly restrained and that specific treatment administration protocols are followed. Veterinary technicians should be knowledgeable about each of the chemotherapeutic drugs being administered. Doses should be triple-checked to avoid overdose as miscalculation may result in serious illness or possibly death. In addition, the correct identity of the patient, the drug, route of administration, and blood work should also be checked before the administration of chemotherapy.

Some chemotherapy agents, called *vesicants*, cause severe tissue irritation, blistering, and sloughing of skin and tissue if they are accidentally administered outside the vein (extravasated). Box 20.3 lists commonly known vesicants and their risks. Extravasation can be extremely serious and potentially life-threatening (Fig. 20.12). It should be reported and treated immediately because

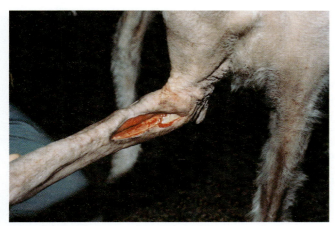

• **Fig. 20.12** Tissue necrosis and sloughing caused by extravasation of a vesicant in a dog.

most problems can be self-limiting with proper management (Table 20.2).

The type of catheter to be placed depends on the type of chemotherapy agent being administered and the patient's temperament. If a large amount of the agent is being administered and the patient is unruly, a butterfly catheter should *not* be used (Fig. 20.13). This is particularly true if the chemotherapeutic agent being administered is a vesicant. In this case, a secured, longer indwelling catheter would be more appropriate to prevent extravasation of the drug. Chemotherapy should be administered only though a clean stick catheter, with the injection site previously prepped using aseptic technique. Intravenous catheters should be flushed before and after administration with sterile saline and not with heparinized saline, because heparin is known to precipitate chemotherapeutic agents. After removal of the catheter, the area around the injection site should be checked for any signs of extravasation, and a bandage should be placed at the site of administration.

Traditionally, chemotherapy is given at the highest possible dose (the maximum tolerated dose) for relatively short periods, with intervals of recovery when no chemotherapy is given. Both normal and abnormal cells are affected by chemotherapeutic agents. The death of normal cells, particularly those that are rapidly dividing, gives rise to side effects. Traditional chemotherapy permits periods of rest between treatments to allow the side effects to recede. Metronomic dosing or therapy is a more recent approach to the administration of chemotherapy. Low doses of oral medications are given daily at home over a long period. Dose intensity is maintained through dose frequency, and this treatment strategy is not appropriate for every patient or tumor. Although it lowers the risk of side effects for patients, it does increase the risk of exposure of clients to chemotherapeutic drugs.

Decontamination and Waste Disposal

A chemotherapy spill kit should be easily accessible, and staff members should be educated in the proper use of spill kits (Box 20.4). If chemotherapy contaminates any part of the PPE, the affected part should be removed immediately, placed in a sealed bag, and disposed of in a hazardous waste container. Linens that come in contact with a chemotherapy agent should be placed in a sealed bag and should be washed immediately and separately from other linens. If there is direct skin contact, the area should be thoroughly cleaned with soap and warm, running water. The skin should not be abraded by scrubbing. A rash may appear and, if it persists for more than an hour, consultation with a medical physician is recommended. If the eye is contaminated, it should be thoroughly rinsed at an eyewash station or with large amounts of water or saline for at least 15 minutes. All liquid environmental spills should be wiped down with an absorbent pad that is then sealed in a bag and disposed of in hazardous waste containers. The affected area should be cleaned multiple times by using a soap or bleach solution and clean water. Broken pieces of a chemotherapy vial should be swept up and placed in a chemotherapy waste container so that it can be disposed of properly. All exposed items should be sealed in a labeled bag and disposed of in hazardous waste containers.

Chemotherapy wastes should be disposed of in leak-proof containers clearly labeled as chemotherapy waste. Similarly, sharps used to administer chemotherapy agents should be disposed of in leak-proof plastic containers intended only for chemotherapy waste. Any linen soiled by contaminated waste, such as feces, urine, saliva, blood, or vomitus, should be washed separately from hospital laundry from other areas. All contaminated laundry should be clearly labeled and should be washed twice, preferably with hot water and bleach, before being returned to the hospital. Proper PPE should be used when handling soiled linens.

> **TECHNICIAN NOTE**
>
> Dogs being treated with chemotherapy should be allowed to urinate only in low-traffic areas. Ideally, the areas would be exposed to plenty of sunlight. Soiled litter from cats receiving chemotherapy should be disposed of in a chemotherapy waste receptacle. All veterinary technicians should wash their hands immediately after handling any patient waste.

Side Effects and Adverse Reactions

Each chemotherapy agent may have its own unique side effects and risks. However, the most common side effects include lethargy, decreased appetite, vomiting, and diarrhea. Most side effects are mild to moderate and self-limiting. However, a small percentage (approximately 5%) of patients may suffer unexpectedly severe toxicity and require hospitalization and supportive care. Patients with comorbid states, such as renal disease or liver disease, may be at increased risk. In addition, certain breeds of dogs are genetically predisposed to have severe reactions to certain chemotherapeutic agents. Many of these dogs are herding breeds or crossed with herding breeds. These dogs have a mutation in the multidrug

From Henry CJ, Higginbotham ML. *Cancer Management in Small Animal Practice*. St. Louis, MO: Saunders; 2010.

TABLE 20.2　Specific Treatments for Extravasated Vesicant Chemotherapeutic Agents

Drug	Antidote	Local Care	Comments
Carboplatin	None	Apply dry cold compress for 20–30 minutes at a time, 4 times a day for the first 24–48 hours following extravasation	
Doxorubicin (Adriamycin)	Dexrazoxane Inject 5–10 times the patient's doxorubicin dose IV over 45 minutes as a separate intravenous infusion within 3 hours of extravasation. Repeat doses at 24 and 48 hours recommended.	Wide surgical resection and debridement may be required	Dimethyl sulfoxide, cold, hydrocortisone shown not effective; immediate pain followed by erythema, edema within hours; ulceration, necrosis within 1–3 weeks
Mechlorethamine (Mustargen)	Isotonic sodium thiosulfate *immediately*	Apply dry cold compresses for 20–30 minutes at a time, 4 times a day for the first 24–48 hours following extravasation	Immediate pain/phlebitis; use 2 mL antidote for every 1 mg drug extravasated with 25-gauge needle or smaller
Vinblastine (Velban)	Hyaluronidase	Apply dry warm compresses for 20–30 minutes at a time, 4 times a day for the first 24–48 hours following extravasation	Inject 1 mL per 1 mL of extravasated fluid subcutaneously at extravasation site. Immediate pain, slow-healing ulcers
Vincristine (Oncovin)	Hyaluronidase	Apply dry warm compresses for 20–30 minutes at a time, 4 times a day for the first 24–48 hours following extravasation	Inject 1 mL per 1 mL of extravasated fluid subcutaneously at extravasation site. Immediate pain, slow-healing ulcers
Vinorelbine (Navelbine)	Hyaluronidase	Apply dry warm compresses for 20–30 minutes at a time, 4 times a day for the first 24-48 hours following extravasation	Inject 1 mL per 1 mL of extravasated fluid subcutaneously at extravasation site. Immediate pain, slow-healing ulcers

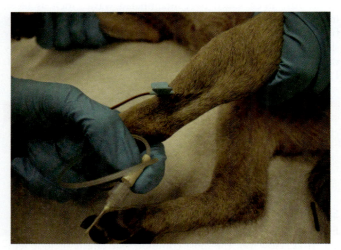

• **Fig. 20.13** A butterfly catheter should not be used to administer a vesicant in an unruly dog. (Courtesy Dr. Joanna Bassert.)

• **BOX 20.4　Chemotherapy Spill Kit**

Chemotherapy spill kits are commercially available, or you can make one yourself with the following contents:
1. Chemotherapy nonspill, heavy-duty, sealable waste-disposable bags
2. Hazardous waste labels
3. Absorbent, plastic-backed chemotherapy diapers
4. Chemotherapy-resistant gown (back closure)
5. Latex gloves or chemotherapy-specific gloves
6. Splash goggles
7. Face masks (respirators are ideal)
8. Disposable dustpan
9. Chemotherapy sharps container
10. Chemotherapy spill sign

TECHNICIAN NOTE

Certain breeds of dogs are genetically predisposed to have severe reactions to chemotherapeutic agents. A complete list of potentially susceptible breeds can be found at http://vcpl.vetmed.wsu.edu/affected-breeds. Many of these dogs are white footed, and the rhyme "four white feet, don't treat" may help oncology personnel remember to test for *MDR1* mutation before treating these dogs.

resistance gene (*MDR1* or *ABCB1*), which results in increased sensitivity to certain medications, including select chemotherapeutic agents (Table 20.3). The rhyme "four white feet, don't treat" is a useful cue for oncology personnel to consider whether *MDR1* mutation testing should be performed before initiating treatment with certain drugs.

The Veterinary Cooperative Oncology Group has produced a scale to standardize the reporting of adverse events. Generally,

TABLE 20.3	"Four White Feet, Don't Treat" Dog Breeds Likely to Carry *MDR1* Mutation	
Breed of Dog	**Frequency**	
Australian Shepherd	50%	
Australian Shepherd, mini	50%	
Border Collie	<5%	
Collie	70%	
English Shepherd	15%	
German Shepherd	10%	
Herding breed (cross)	10%	
Long-Haired Whippet	65%	
McNab	30%	
Mixed breed	5%	
Old English Sheepdog	5%	
Shetland Sheepdog	15%	
Silken Windhound	30%	

Modified from Withrow SJ, Vail DM, Page R. *Small Animal Clinical Oncology.* 5th ed. St. Louis, MO: Saunders; 2013.

• BOX 20.5 Adverse Event Classifications

Grade 1: Mild or asymptomatic effects only. Intervention is not indicated.
Grade 2: Moderate to mild effects. Outpatient intervention is needed.
Grade 3: Medically significant but non–life-threatening. Hospitalization is needed.
Grade 4: Life-threatening. Urgent intervention and intensive care is needed.
Grade 5: Death.

grades 1 or 2 toxicity are considered reasonable. Grades 3 or higher are not acceptable. Box 20.5 provides a condensed, practical version of the consensus report. The side effects of chemotherapy include vomiting, diarrhea, and decreased appetite. Additional side effects that may occur with chemotherapy treatment are discussed below.

Anaphylaxis

Anaphylaxis is a serious and life-threatening allergic reaction that may include difficulty breathing, hypersalivation, increased heart rate and blood pressure, vomiting, abdominal pain, diarrhea, hyperemic mucous membranes with increased capillary refill time, and swelling of the face, tongue, or throat. Pretreatment with diphenhydramine is recommended, because some chemotherapeutic agents can cause anaphylaxis or mast cell degranulation.

Acute Tumor Lysis Syndrome

Acute tumor lysis syndrome (ATLS) is an uncommon syndrome of metabolic derangements that can occur when tumor cells rapidly die within a short period. Animals with advanced lymphoma or leukemia and those with underlying renal disease are at higher risk of developing ATLS, and it is most common after the first dose of treatment. Clinical signs can occur within a few hours to several days after treatment

and may include severe depression, anorexia, vomiting, diarrhea, and rapid decline. Blood work will show significant hyperphosphatemia, possible hypocalcemia, and hyperkalemia. Other findings may include acute renal failure, collapse, and cardiac arrhythmias. ATLS is usually fatal unless immediate treatment is given.

Neutropenia

Neutrophils are the most abundant type of white blood cells, and they are an important part of the innate immune system. Neutrophils have a short half-life and a rapid turnover; therefore they are the cell line most adversely affected by cytotoxic chemotherapy. Typically, the nadir of the neutrophil count occurs approximately 5 to 7 days after the administration of chemotherapy. At this point, if the neutrophils have fallen to less than 1000 cells/µL, the patient is at significant risk for infection. CBC and temperature measurement are recommended at the anticipated nadir to measure the neutrophil count and assess the patient's status. Some patients with a particularly poor prognosis may become hypotensive and hypothermic. If neutrophil counts are too low, future treatments will be delayed. Antibiotics may be prescribed. If a patient is febrile and depressed, hospitalization for systemic treatment and supportive care may be needed.

TECHNICIAN NOTE

Disciplined use of the Oncology Patient Management Checklist (Box 20.6) ensures that patients receive consistently excellent medical care. Use of this tool will reduce the risk of chemotherapy-related mistakes.

Client Education

After chemotherapy administration, it is important to educate the pet owner about the type of chemotherapy received and potential side effects. In addition, drug hazard periods should be described so that the client avoids direct contact with the patient's urine, feces, and vomitus during this period. Clients should be instructed to walk their pet in a sunny, low-traffic area where children do not play. If owners see any feces, urine, or vomitus, they should wear gloves to remove the waste and then wash their hands thoroughly with warm, soapy water. Cat owners should wear gloves and change the litter box frequently, and litter should be replaced weekly after the box has been scrubbed with hot, soapy water. It is not necessary for other cats in the household to use a different litter box, because the risk of exposure to chemotherapeutic agents is small. Table 20.4 lists the hazardous elimination periods of chemotherapeutic drugs in dogs, and Table 20.5 lists elimination periods in humans.

All pet owners should be informed of the potential chemotherapy side effects and the usual timing of such side effects. All efforts should be made to reduce side effects, and these efforts include client education and the prescription of prophylactic medications, such as antiemetics. Owners should be instructed to return for evaluation when the patient's neutrophil count will be at the lowest (**nadir**) so that it can be determined whether antibiotic therapy or supportive care is needed for patient safety. Sepsis can be caused by flora in the patient's own GI tract; however, owners should be instructed to keep their pets away from unknown areas, kennels, unvaccinated animals, and young puppies, particularly during these nadir times.

Oncology Patient Management Checklist

The safety of patients and clients and of veterinary personnel is a high priority. Box 20.6 provides a checklist of questions that

• BOX 20.6 Patient Management Checklist for Veterinary Technicians in Oncology

The following checklist ensures that consistently excellent care is provided to every cancer patient:

Patient Check
- Do we have the right patient?
- Is the patient's weight correct?
- How is the patient feeling?
- Has the doctor preformed a physical examination?
- Did we perform diagnostics (blood work, ultrasonography, radiography)?
- Does the diagnostic work support treatment?
- Does this patient have any pre-existing issues that may interfere with chemotherapy?
- Do we have the pet owner's consent before treatment?
- Are the owners aware of the type of drug being administered and the potential side effects?
- Is the patient due for chemotherapy today?

Drugs
- Is the chemotherapy that the doctor ordered correct for this patient type and cancer type?
- Did we triple-check the dose (in milligrams and in milliliters)?

Pharmacy
- Do we need pretreatment?
- Is PPE required to draw up and administer the chemotherapy?
- Did we draw up the correct chemotherapeutic agent?
- Did we draw up the proper amount?
- Is the syringe properly labeled?

Setup
- Do we have a closed system setup prepared?
- Do we have the proper setup with a disposable, plastic-backed absorbent pad?
- Will this be a treatment that requires fluids?
- Do we have proper flushes and bandages for after treatment (nonheparinized 0.9% sodium chloride [NaCl] flush only)?

During Administration
- How is the patient?
- Is a muzzle needed?

- Is sedation needed?
- Is the staff wearing proper PPE?
- How is the chemotherapeutic agent administered?
- Have we selected a proper administration route?
- Is this drug a vesicant?
- What are the potential side effects of this drug?
- Are we aware of the emergency protocols in place for the drug we are administering?
- Did we use proper aseptic technique during administration?
- Was the drug administered properly?
  - A subcutaneous medication went subcutaneously and did not leak out.
  - There was no blood return on an intramuscular injection, and it did not go subcutaneously.
  - An intravenous injection was given with a clean stick, and the drug was not extravasated.
- Is the patient comfortable during administration?
- Are we filling out the treatment sheet properly and maintaining proper medical records?
- Has all of the remaining chemotherapeutic drug been disposed of correctly
- Have we thoroughly disinfected the chemotherapy administration area?

After Administration
- Have we reviewed side effects with the pet owner again?
- Have we discussed post-treatment concerns?
- Have we discussed the possible nadir of the drug with the pet owner?
- Have we discussed chemotherapy drug exposure risks with the pet owner?
- Does the pet owner have medications to provide supportive care at home or do the owners need prescription refills? (for example, antinausea medications or antidiarrheal medications)
- Have we discussed the future treatment plan? For example, when is blood work due or when is the next treatment scheduled?
- Do we need to schedule any additional diagnostics for the next visit?
- Did the owners receive a copy of their discharge instructions?
- Did we answer all of the owner's questions?
- Are the owners satisfied with the care we are providing to their pet?

TABLE 20.4 Documented Hazardous Period for Dogs (Not Studied in Cats)

Name of Drug	Documented Hazardous Period
Cyclophosphamide (Cytoxan)	1 day
Doxorubicin (Adriamycin)	7+ days
Vinblastine (Velban)	7 days
Vincristine (Oncovin)	3 days

TABLE 20.5 Documented Hazardous Period in Humans

Name of Drug	Documented Hazardous Period
Carboplatin (Paraplatin)	5 days
Cytarabine (Cytosar-U)	3 days
Lomustine (CCNU)	3 days
Mitoxantrone (Novantrone)	7 days

---

help guide efficient management of oncology cases. By regularly reviewing these questions, excellent care of oncology patients and their owners can be ensured.

Palliative Treatment

"*Palliative care*" is often used synonymously with "comfort care." The goal of palliative care is to improve the quality of life of a patient. Palliative care targets symptoms associated with a disease but is not intended to cure a disease or prolong the patient's life. Palliative treatments alleviate pain, lethargy, loss of appetite, nausea, constipation, diarrhea, and fatigue. Medications, such as anti-inflammatory agents, analgesics, appetite stimulants, antinausea medications, and antacids, along with nutritional support, are central to palliative care. In cases of cancer, sometimes the only way to alleviate patient suffering is to

TABLE 20.6 Supportive Care and Pain Management Treatments

Anorexia	Diarrhea	Nausea or Vomiting	Pain	Antacids	NSAIDs
Capromorelin	Bland diet	Maropitant citrate	Amantadine	Famotidine	Deracoxib
Cyproheptadine	Canned pumpkin	Metoclopramide	Buprenorphine	Omeprazole	Carprofen
Mirtazapine	Loperamide	Ondansetron	Gabapentin		Robenacoxib
Prednisone	Metronidazole	Anzemet	Tramadol		Piroxicam
	Rx Clay		Tylenol 3/4		Firocoxib
	Probiotics				

NSAIDs, Nonsteroidal anti-inflammatory drugs.

treat the tumor. Therefore in oncology, management with radiation, surgery, and chemotherapy can also be used for palliative care in certain instances, although the goal of treatment is to improve the patient's quality of life with less regard for prolongation of life. One example is the use of radiation to diminish the pain caused by an unresectable bone tumor. Table 20.6 lists commonly used palliative treatments.

Complementary, Alternative, and Integrative Medicine

Complementary medicine uses nonstandard treatments in combination *with* standard therapy. Alternative medicine, however, uses nonstandard treatments *in place of* standard therapy. *Integrative medicine* is a newer term for an approach to treatment that makes use of complementary, holistic, and conventional treatments in a rational, evidence-based way. The oncologist's main goal in using additional therapies is to improve patient welfare and maximize quality of life.

Many, if not most, oncologists are receptive to the integration of complementary therapies into their practice, but most reject alternative medicine. Alternative treatments are not considered interchangeable with "standard of care" treatments and are considered experimental at best. Standard therapies become standard after clinical trials have been performed and evaluated in the peer-reviewed literature. These trials assess a treatment's safety and dosing (phase I studies), use (phase II studies), and effectiveness (phase III and IV studies). An alternative treatment tested in the same way and found to be superior to standard treatments becomes the new standard of care. Products with unsupported claims of treatment success, particularly for treatments without side effects, should raise suspicion. Nevertheless, many pet owners seek out commercially advertised treatments, such as vitamins, herbs, and homeopathic medicine. When taking a case history, it is important for veterinary technicians to ask owners specifically about the use of these products. The oncologist can then be made aware of them and can discuss the potential benefits and risks of such treatments with the owner. Untested treatments may increase risk of side effects because of toxic drug interactions or lack of quality control in the manufacture of supplements. However, some supplements have shown to be safe and potentially effective. These are discussed in the section below.

Examples of Integrative Therapies

Yunnan Baiyao
Yunnan Baiyao is an herbal supplement that has been used for generations in China and is used to stop bleeding. In oncology, it can be used in patients with intractable epistaxis or hematuria or in patients with bleeding tumors, such as hemangiosarcoma.

I'm-Yunity
I'm-Yunity is a compound derived from the mushroom *Coriolus versicolor*. The active compound, polysaccharopeptide, may have antitumor properties, as indicated by laboratory studies. A veterinary clinical trial to evaluate the role of I'm-Yunity in the treatment of canine hemangiosarcoma is currently under way.

Rx Clay
Rx Clay, also known as *hydrated aluminosilicate clay*, is a mineral that aids in maintaining normal stool consistency and frequency. It is used to treat chemotherapy-associated diarrhea.

Acupuncture
Acupuncture uses needles inserted at specific points in the body to stimulate chemicals in the brain to aid in healing and to promote organ function. Acupuncture does not treat cancer but may help with pain management and improve the patient's quality of life.

Nutritional Management
The owners of animals with cancer are often concerned about nutrition and frequently ask about home-cooked diets. Most recipes for home-cooked diets are not nutritionally balanced to meet the long-term feeding needs of pets. If home feeding is desired, consultation with a board-certified nutritionist should always be recommended, because studies have indicated that most diets found on the Internet or even in books on cancer are not nutritionally balanced. Most high-quality commercial diets are approved by the Association of American Feed Control Officials, and only these should be recommended. Among these, diets high in proteins and omega-3 fatty acids and low in carbohydrates are recommended. Prescription diets targeted toward patients diagnosed with cancer are becoming more readily available commercially. These diets are made with high-quality protein, include digestive support, and are made to be very palatable to encourage appetite. Raw meat diets are never recommended, because they increase the risk of serious infection from

foodborne pathogens such as *Salmonella* and have no proven cancer-fighting effects in veterinary patients. Changes in diet should be introduced gradually, particularly if a high-fat diet is being implemented.

Cachexia refers to metabolic derangement seen mostly in human patients with advanced cancer. It is less commonly seen in veterinary medicine, because most patients are humanely euthanized before advanced wasting occurs. The syndrome involves muscle wasting and loss of the body's fat stores in spite of the patient consuming appropriate amounts of food. Use of antinausea medication, nutritional management, and appetite stimulants can be tried in these patients.

Diarrhea is a common chemotherapy side effect. For a patient with diarrhea, a bland diet of a 50:50 mixture of boiled beef or chicken (no fat, skin, or bones) with plain, steamed rice can be recommended on a temporary basis. Veterinary probiotics or the addition of one to two tablespoons of canned pumpkin to the diet can also help with loose stools. Owners of cats should be made aware that all felines are obligate carnivores and should never be fed a vegetarian diet or one that is deficient in taurine. In addition, cat owners should be informed that anorexia, even for short periods, can cause hepatic lipidosis and significantly compromise the patient's well-being and care. Patient weight and body condition score should be recorded at every visit, and changes should be monitored and noted.

Quality of Life

One of the principal goals of veterinary oncology is to maintain a good quality of life for each patient. A specialized scale has been developed to assess oncology patients' quality of life (Table 20.7). On a 70-point scale, the best quality of life is indicated by a score of 70 and the worst by a score of 1. The scale is applied to seven different aspects of a patient's life: pain, appetite, hydration, self-care, attitude, mobility, and the general assessment of "good versus bad" days. An overall score of 35 or higher is considered acceptable.

Cancer in Horses

Dermal and subcutaneous tumors are common in horses and can occur in both haired and hairless regions of the skin. Cutaneous tumors are often found on eyelids, ears, lips, muzzles, the perianal area, and external genitalia. Any nodular or ulcerated lesion should be noted and monitored. Lesions that persist despite treatment, double in size over the period of 1 month, or grow beyond 2 cm in diameter should be evaluated. Although tumors can be aspirated and cytologically evaluated, the most thorough way to evaluate integumentary tumors is to perform biopsy and histopathologic analysis. Culture may be warranted as part of the routine diagnostic workup, because infections of the skin can also present as nodules or as ulcerated wounds.

Fibromas

Although this is an uncommon tumor of dermal and subcutaneous tissues, it is one of the most common tumors in the frog of a horse's foot. This is considered a benign lesion and is therefore unlikely to spread to other sites. Treatment involves surgical removal, and the expected outcome with surgical excision is good.

TABLE 20.7	Quality of Life (HHHHHMM Scale)	
Score	**Criterion**	
0–10	**HURT:** Is there adequate pain control (including breathing ability)?	
0–10	**HUNGER:** Is the pet eating enough? Does the pet require hand feeding or a feeding tube?	
0–10	**HYDRATION:** Is the pet dehydrated? Does it need subcutaneous fluids?	
0–10	**HYGIENE:** Pet needs to be brushed and cleaned, especially after elimination.	
0–10	**HAPPINESS:** Does the pet express joy/interest? Does it respond to its environment? Does the pet show signs of boredom/loneliness/anxiety/fear?	
0–10	**MOBILITY:** Can the pet get up without assistance? Does the pet want to go for a walk? Is the pet experiencing seizures or stumbling?	
0–10	**MORE GOOD THAN BAD:** When bad days start to outnumber good days, the quality of life becomes compromised, and euthanasia needs to be considered.	
Total	**A total of 35 points is considered an acceptable quality-of-life score.**	

From Villalobos A. *Canine and Feline Geriatric Oncology: Honoring the Human-Animal Bond.* Hoboken, NJ: John Wiley; 2007.

Melanoma and Melanocytoma

Melanocytic tumors are cutaneous tumors derived from melanocytes. These tumors usually appear on hairless regions of dark-skinned gray horses. These horses can develop multiple lesions at one site. Melanomas can be benign or malignant. The tumors most commonly develop in middle-aged to older horses and can be found under the tail, around the eye, on the lips or muzzle, and on the external genitalia. Melanocytic tumors are usually pigmented. Treatment includes surgical removal, the administration of medical agents (e.g., cisplatin/carboplatin and cimetidine), radiation therapy, and use of the canine melanoma vaccine ONCEPT.

Squamous Cell Carcinoma

SCC is the second most common tumor of the horse and the most common tumor of the eyelid and external genitalia. SCC is believed to be solar induced, being more common in horses that live in sunny areas. Other factors, such as chronic irritation, may also lead to the development of these lesions. SCC occurs most commonly in middle-aged to older horses and occurs most often in areas of unpigmented or lightly haired skin, such as the skin on the eyelids and the muzzle or around the anus and the external genitalia. Lesions of the eyelids present as raised bumps or weeping, red wounds. These tumors are locally invasive and usually require surgical removal for treatment. If extensive, surgery may include enucleation of the globe.

Sarcoid

Sarcoid is the most common type of skin tumor in horses. They are locally invasive but rarely metastasize. They can be difficult to remove and may invade deeper tissue layers and bone. They are often found in haired skin and take on different presentations (occult, verrucous, nodular, and fibroblastic). Although the etiology is unknown, association with exposure to bovine papillomavirus has been hypothesized. Treatment options include surgical excision, cryotherapy, immunotherapy, and intralesional injections of chemotherapeutic agents, such as cisplatin, carboplatin, or 5-fluorouracil. Radiotherapy has also been used for refractory cases.

Cancer in Cattle

SCC is relatively more common in cattle and can result in significant economic losses for the producer and pain in the affected animals. These tumors are associated with prolonged exposure to the sun and are therefore more commonly seen in open-range cattle that have little to no access to shade. It also tends to occur in nonpigmented regions of the skin, such as the skin on the face, around the eyes, and on the ears in Herefords (see Chapter 34). Middle-aged and older animals are more likely to be affected compared with younger ones. Treatment options include excisional surgery or cryosurgery; cattle that are diagnosed with SCC are often culled.

Recommended Readings

American Veterinary Medical Association. *Senior Pet Care (FAQ)*; 2015. 2015. Available at: https://www.avma.org/resources-tools/pet-owners/petcare/senior-pets.

Bronson RT. Variation in age at death of dogs of different sexes and breeds. *Am J Vet Res*. 1982;43:2057–2059.

Cornell University. *New York State Veterinary Diagnostic Laboratory Animal Health Diagnostic Center Samples for Hematology*; 2015. Available at: https://ahdc.vet.cornell.edu/sects/clinpath/sample/test/hema.cfm.

Veterinary Diagnostics Institute. *Canine Health & Cancer Screen*; 2014. 2015. Available at: http://vdilab.com/page.php?id=85.

Veterinary Cooperative Oncology Group. *Veterinary Cooperative Oncology Group—Common Terminology Criteria for Adverse Events (Vcog-Ctcae) Following Chemotherapy or Biological Antineoplastic Therapy in Dogs And Cats, v1.1*; 2011. Available at: Veterinary Cooperative Oncology Group-Common Terminology Criteria for Adverse Events (VCOG-CTCAE v2) following investigational therapy in dogs and cats - PubMed (nih.gov).

Washington State University. *College of Veterinary Clinical Pharmacology Lab*; 2014. 2015. Available at: http://vcpl.vetmed.wsu.edu/.

Withrow SJ, Vail DM, Page RL, et al. *Withrow and MacEwen's Small Animal Clinical Oncology*. 5th ed. St. Louis, MO: Elsevier; 2012.

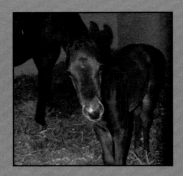

CHAPTER OUTLINE

LEARNING OBJECTIVES

When you have completed this chapter, you will be able to:

1. Pronounce, define, and spell all key terms in this chapter.
2. Define the neonatal period for puppies and kittens, obtain an accurate and thorough clinical history for all littermates and parents, and describe the procedure for physical examination of a neonate, including equipment needed and potential abnormalities.
3. Explain the timeline of normal development in neonatal puppies and kittens.
4. Do the following regarding performance of diagnostic procedures and routine maintenance in neonatal puppies and kittens:
   • Discuss how to perform diagnostic procedures on a neonatal puppy or a kitten.
   • Discuss appropriate times to administer medical treatments to neonatal puppies and kittens and explain proper nutrition, preventive medicine, and behavior to the owner.
5. Do the following regarding common concerns and disorders in puppies and kittens:
   • Explain common concerns of neonatal puppies and kittens, such as hypothermia, dehydration, hypoglycemia, malnutrition, fading puppy or kitten syndrome, and neonatal isoerythrolysis in kittens.
   • Discuss proper care of an orphaned neonatal puppy or kitten and common complications involved with orphaned neonates.
6. Do the following regarding the perinatal period and the high-risk mare:
   • Differentiate between normal and abnormal perinatal periods in the mare and explain how to care for a high-risk mare.

   • Identify the stages of labor in a mare and describe how to treat any complications that may arise at each stage.
7. Describe the normal development of a neonatal foal that occurs during the first 24 hours after birth and identify normal vital signs and behavior.
8. Do the following regarding care of the sick foal:
   • List the signs of a critically ill foal, including symptoms of prematurity and dysmaturity and classic early clinical signs of disease.
   • Identify common sites and procedures for venous and arterial blood collection and the appropriate needles, syringes, and restraint techniques to be used in the neonatal foal.
   • Identify parameters that should be monitored in the hospitalized foal and describe complications that may arise during hospitalization.
   • Describe proper nursing care for the foal to prevent contamination, including washing of hands and injection sites, changing of intravenous (IV) fluid lines, and maintenance of IV and jugular catheters.
   • Explain appropriate physical therapy for the recumbent foal, the necessity for keeping it in the sternal position and for frequent changes in recumbency, and the proper restraint techniques that can be used for the ambulatory foal.
9. Explain alternative methods that can be used to ensure that nutritional needs are met if a foal is unable to nurse from the mare.

KEY TERMS

Congenital
Dehydration
Foal
Genetic
Hypoglycemia

Hypothermia
Mare
Neonatal period
Urachus

Introduction

Human medicine is rich with volumes of books containing tables, graphs, and guidelines, such as "Denver scores," that detail normal and abnormal development of babies and are readily available to clinicians for assessment of human pediatric patients. In contrast, veterinary medicine is challenged by diversity among species and breeds of animals and by the far broader ranges of what constitutes "normal" and "abnormal." In relative terms, veterinary personnel must rely on far fewer reference resources, and this makes empirical experience and the observations of breeders and the foster community critically important. Because the development of body systems continues well after birth, young animals are particularly vulnerable to age-related problems. A thorough history and physical examination are important for detecting developmental complications and illnesses. This chapter addresses normal neonatal development and the most common reasons for illness in the puppy, the kitten, and the **foal**.

Neonatology of Puppies and Kittens

Definition

During the **neonatal period**, which is the first 4 weeks of life, puppies and kittens fully depend on their mothers for nutrition, warmth, care, and overall survival. The first 14 days compose the most critical period, followed by weeks four through eight, when weaning occurs. This is especially true in the foster environment. The discussion in this section pertains to puppies and kittens in a highly vulnerable time of their lives.

History

The history should include the number of ill animals, the method by which they were raised, including use of a milk replacer, their normal environment, the behavior of each puppy or kitten within the litter, body weight curves, duration and types of clinical signs, and medications given. The history of the queen or the bitch should include vaccination status, nutrition, medications or supplements given during pregnancy, problems during pregnancy or birth, and whether the disorder has been seen in previous litters or relatives. Clients should be encouraged to bring the whole litter so that the patient can be compared with its littermates as well as to ensure others in the litter are not affected. The mother should also be brought in at the same time.

> **TECHNICIAN NOTE**
>
> Because of the unusual or nonspecific clinical signs associated with ill puppies and kittens, it is important to obtain a comprehensive history of not only the patient but also of littermates, parents, and, if possible, other relatives.

Physical Examination

Physical examination of the neonate and the juvenile patient can be challenging. If more than one neonate is being examined, it is important to properly identify everyone, for example, by drawing pictures of unique markings or by using different-colored collars or identification bands for those individuals that are similar in appearance. The use of a permanent marker on the inside of the pinna will offer a semi-permanent form of identification, especially in feline neonates due their smaller size. This aids in identification as it can be difficult to keep siblings with similar colors and patterns with minimal unique markings easily identified. While convenient, it is not recommended to use animal ID bands around the neck of a neonate because of the possibility of asphyxiation and their lower mandible or limbs becoming caught in the band, causing emotional distress and physical trauma. Physical examinations in neonates should be performed as thoroughly as in adult animals, but there are some specific differences that deserve particular attention.

Typically, kittens weigh 90–110 g at birth; however, it should be noted that the smaller and pedigree feline and canine breeds (toy or teacup) will have a significantly lower birth weight. For example, a feline pedigree breed, the Singapura, normally weighs 50–60 g at birth, and their adult weight is typically 4 pounds. Maine Coon kittens can weigh >110 g at birth—they are considered a giant feline breed, and intact males can grow to 25–30 pounds. There is no one "normal" weight for all kittens and puppies as their breed affects what "their" normal is. It is not uncommon for premature kittens weighing less than 40 g at birth to survive with aggressive nursing care.

A pediatric stethoscope with a 2-cm bell and a digital thermometer that allows rapid body temperature measurement without causing great discomfort are helpful tools. Because the neonate can have a body temperature lower than 94°F (34.4°C), a digital thermometer, which can measure temperatures as low as 85°F (29.4°C), is necessary. In the feline neonate, it is important to use a thin tipped oral human thermometer as rectal thermometers may be too wide for their anus to accommodate, causing injury. It is not necessary to take daily CORE body temperatures on a neonate *unless the kitten presents as ill or compromised*. Neonates cannot regulate their body temperatures and should therefore be placed on a warm, clean surface for examination. Feline neonates in particular have a high body to surface area. Keeping them warm is key as hypothermia can be caused in minutes depending on the temperature of the environment and the surface they are lying on. It is important to have the neonate arrive in a warm carrier with either the mother, siblings, or an artificial thermal source provided for warmth and emotional comfort. To evaluate a neonate's hydration status, their urine color, instead of skin turgor, is evaluated (Fig. 21.1). Kittens lack skin turgor in their first 6 weeks of life and their high body water–low body fat

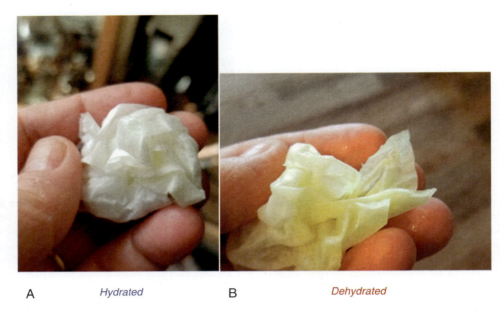

A *Hydrated*   B *Dehydrated*

• **Fig. 21.1** (A) Clear urine indicates adequate hydration in a neonate. (B) Yellow urine indicates dehydration.

ratio makes determining dehydration by skin turgor unreliable. The neonate will have clear to pale yellow urine if adequately hydrated. The neonate is born with hair that covers most of the body, except the ventral abdominal skin. Lack of hair or a sparse hair coat anywhere else may indicate a **genetic** abnormality of the skin or a premature birth (Fig. 21.2). Typically, the forelimbs and muzzle will be hairless with a sheen present on the skin, making them appear "gummy" or "rubbery" (Fig. 21.3). The neonate normally has hairless, dark-pink ventral abdominal skin. Bluish and dark-red discolorations (dusky abdomen) are indicative of distress (i.e., cyanosis, omphalitis, and sepsis) (Fig. 21.4). Other than urine and feces, a discharge from any orifice is abnormal. The head is specifically examined for open fontanels, cleft palate, bulging eyes from behind closed eyelids (neonatal ophthalmia), and abnormal formation of the nose and external ears. Flattening or malformations of the chest are noted and are suggestive of pectus excavatum (Fig. 21.5). Neonatal puppies are mildly pudgy, and neonatal kittens are generally on the lean side. Neither of them should ever be bloated, which would be a sign of distress. The abdomen and the **urachus** are specially examined for defects of the abdominal wall or a persistent urachus. The umbilicus should be thoroughly examined for any redness surrounding the cord and/or discharge. The cord should be trimmed back to as small as safely possible to prevent umbilical trauma from blankets, the queen/dam during cleaning, or siblings in the litter. The genitals and the anus are visually checked for patency, along with stimulating them for urination and defecation. Make any notation of genital mutilation from sibling genital suckling in the litter. The tail is examined for muscle tone, length, curliness, and kinks. Abnormalities in tone, leakage of urine and feces, or inability to eliminate with stimulation may indicate neurologic problems such as abnormal innervation of the distal pelvis. Other skeletal abnormalities, such as ulnar hypoplasia (Fig. 21.6), "swimmer's legs" (Fig. 21.7), and twisted leg/tendon contracture (Fig. 21.8A–D) should be noted and, if possible, treated immediately with rehabilitative exercises or taping/hobbling of the limbs to correct the issue.

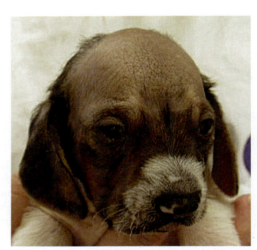

• **Fig. 21.2** Two-week-old abnormal puppy displaying hairlessness and cloudy, slightly crusty eyes.

If hospitalized, neonates should be kept in an incubator away from other patients to prevent any cross contamination and potential passage of diseases they do not have current immunity against. It is important to fulfill the emotional needs of neonates in the hospital by gentle handling; grooming with a new, clean toothbrush; and providing fresh, warm meals to prevent further illnesses. It is highly advisable that the care of neonates is assigned to team members who are not working with other ill patients that day.

TECHNICIAN NOTE

Neonatal puppies and kittens should be examined in a clean room free of contamination from previous patients. Freshly washed, clean towels and blankets should be available for the patient to be examined upon as their body temperature can be compromised. Examination gloves should be worn to minimize the spread of infectious agents to neonates with immature immune systems.

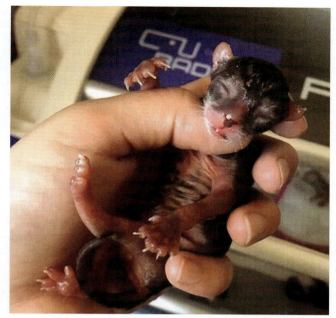

• **Fig. 21.3** Typically, the forelimbs and muzzle will be hairless with a sheen present on the skin, making them appear "gummy" or "rubbery." (Courtesy Tara Hatch.)

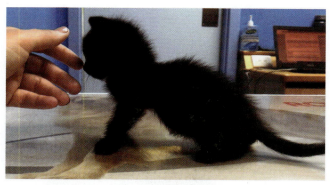

• **Fig. 21.5** Example of pectus excavatum. (Courtesy Tara Hatch.)

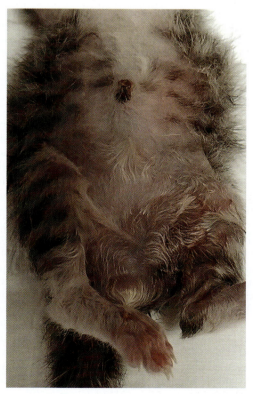

• **Fig. 21.4** Advanced omphalitis and sepsis in a neonatal kitten. The neonate normally has hairless, dark-pink ventral abdominal skin. Bluish and dark-red discolorations (dusky abdomen) are indicative of distress. (Courtesy Ellen Carozza.)

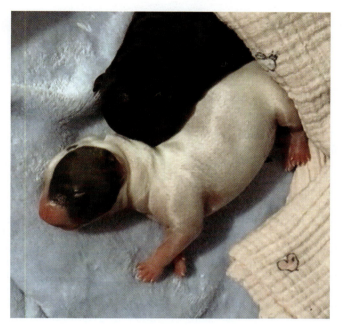

• **Fig. 21.6** Example of ulnar hypoplasia. (Courtesy Tara Hatch.)

Normal Development

During the first week of life, newborn kittens and puppies sleep through most of the day (80%) and nurse vigorously for a short time every 2 to 4 hours. The only motor skills present are crawling, suckling, purring, and distress vocalization. The feline neonate can exhibit stress responses such as hissing as early as a few days old when handled by unfamiliar hands. Neonates only respond to stimuli, such as odor, touch, and pain. The queen or the bitch initiates urination and defecation in the neonate by licking the urogenital area. By the age of 3 days, kittens and puppies should be able to lift their heads, and by 1 week, they can crawl in a coordinated manner. Puppies and kittens are unable to maintain their body temperatures during the first 2 weeks of life, and a low body temperature at birth (94.5°F–97.3°F [34.5°C–36.3°C]) rises to 94.7°F to 100.1°F (34.8°C–38.3°C) during the first week of life. Heart and respiratory rates may be irregular at birth (pulse [P] = 160–200 beats/minute [bpm] in the puppy and greater than 200 beats per minute (bpm) in the kitten; respiration

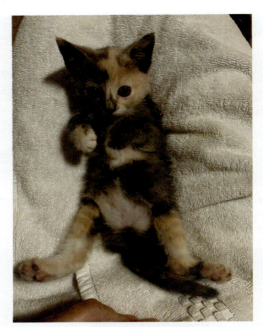

• **Fig. 21.7** Example of "swimmer's legs" (Courtesy Raven Farina.)

[R] = 10–20 breaths per minute), and respiration has no abdominal component. During the first week, the respiratory and heart rates of neonates increase (P = 200–220 bpm; R = 16–35 breaths per minute). The umbilical cord dries during the first day of life and falls off within 3 to 7 days. Any wet umbilicus should be evaluated for trauma and disinfected with a tincture of iodine to help prevent infection. The flexor tone present at birth switches over to extensor tone after the fourth day of life in puppies, and specific neurologic reflexes are present (Box 21.1). Male kittens are born with descended testicles that move in and out of the scrotum freely until age 5 to 7 months. However, owing to the free testicular movement, the scrotum can easily be confused for female genitalia as the tissue folds in upon itself, appearing as labia. Female kittens' urogenital folds along the vulva (Fig. 21.9A–D), likewise, can be interpreted wrongfully as testicles. Knowing the visual cues ensures a more accurate sexing the first time.

If differentiation is difficult, apply some warm water on a cotton ball and dampen the area to look for a vaginal slit or prepuce. Rare cases of hypodiasis (Fig. 21.10), a congenital defect seen in males where the urethra is not located at the tip of the penis, can cause difficulty in sexing the kitten. In many cases, the penis curves and can cause urination issues as the cat ages, along with retained testicles. While many of these cats retain their testicles, any that do eventually descend may present along the sides of the prepuce as opposed to below the anus and above the prepuce in normally developed cats. In dogs, the testicles do not descend until age 6 to 8 weeks.

During the second week of life, kittens and puppies begin to crawl, and the body temperature slowly rises toward normal adult levels. Kittens and puppies will have doubled their birth weight by 7–10 and 10–12 days, respectively. The healthy neonatal kitten should gain 10–30 g per day depending on the breed, whereas the healthy neonatal puppy should gain 5% to 10% of weight daily. It is important to note that any significant daily gains in excess of 30 g per day can indicate an increase in water weight, not body mass. Therefore it is important to track daily trends to catch any

signs or illnesses early, before it is too late to treat. Kittens begin to open their eyes at age 7 to 12 days, and the external ear canals open at age 14 to 16 days. The cornea is slightly cloudy as a result of increased water content, and all neonates are born with grayish/blue eyes. By 7 weeks of age, their permanent eye color will begin to emerge. Kitten eye color can range through shades of green, copper, and blue, and sometimes lilac is seen in Asian breeds. Heterochromia (odd-eyed) is typically seen in white-coated cats (Fig. 21.11). By age 3 weeks, puppies and kittens are able to stand and have good postural reflexes. Refer to Box 21.2 for details about the development of specific organ systems.

Congenital abnormalities are common, especially in feline colonies and when canine and feline breeders mate animals with genetics too closely related. Some common genetic abnormalities presented are orofacial deformities such as cleft lip/palate and atresia ani (anal deformities). Atresia ani is a severe and potentially life-threatening defect in neonates and is graded in four categories, ranging from mild to severe. Polydactyly is a common skeletal abnormality in felines (Fig. 21.12), in which they are born with an abnormal number of digits on each paw, while syndactyly, in which the kitten is born with fused digits (Fig. 21.13), is less common. In extreme skeletal anomalies in both species, limbs and digits that are not fully developed can be present and may or may not affect the quality of life of the neonate as it ages.

TECHNICIAN NOTE

The sex of kittens can be determined at birth by evaluating their anatomy; however, it may take a keen eye in some cases. Males may or may not have a distinct scrotum with a rounded prepuce, whereas females will have a vertical slot. If, owing to the presence of fur, there is a discrepancy on determining the sex visually, one can use some water or saline on a cotton ball to wet the fur down for a more accurate determination. Not all congenital defects warrant euthanasia. Each animal should be evaluated for quality of life, which includes their ability to eat, drink, eliminate, and ambulate without assistance.

Diagnostics

Blood can be easily obtained from the jugular vein in neonates; however, no greater than 10% of the circulating volume should be drawn over the course of a week. If the neonate is ill, no greater than 5% of the circulating volume should be drawn. In the feline neonate, a U-100 insulin syringe can be used easily for small sampling without compromising the integrity of the sample for diagnostic results and helps prevent venous trauma. For hospitalized neonates, it is worthwhile posting a chart next to the patient on which every veterinary technician can record the amount of blood drawn to prevent the patient from becoming anemic. Extra precautions should be considered for the already anemic pediatric patient as sampling can cause the animal to become further compromised. Utilizing laboratory diagnostics that request the smallest sample possible can help prevent further blood loss/waste. The technician can calculate blood volume by using the calculation: Total blood volume in cats = 66 mL/kg × body weight (BW; kg). Because of the small amount of sample drawn at any given time, a collection tube of appropriate size should be used to ensure that the anticoagulant does not dilute the sample and result in false laboratory data. The use of avian blood collection tubes may prove beneficial for neonatal patients. It is a common phenomenon in felines to see mildly elevated metabolic "normals" compared with their adult counterparts.

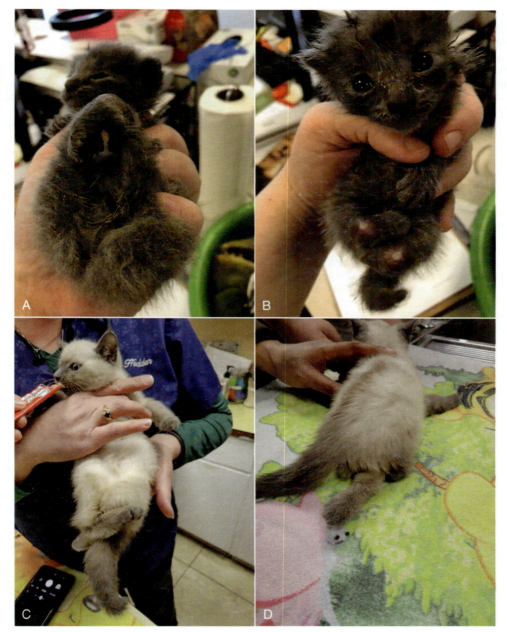

• **Fig. 21.8** (A–D) Examples of twisted leg/tendon contracture. (A, B Courtesy Nicole-Elaine Farrell; C, D Courtesy Tara Trillo.)

To obtain urine samples from the neonate, simply stimulate them to urinate by gently rubbing the genital area with a moistened cotton ball. Alternatively, the bladder can be carefully expressed. Cystocentesis should be performed by skilled staff only, employing the assistance of ultrasonography and using a 25-gauge needle. The bladder will be located against the abdominal wall. Obtaining a blind sample is possible; however, the likelihood of injuring other organs is more probable due to the lack of abdominal fat.

Imaging techniques include radiography and ultrasonography. An ultrasound examination is best performed using a 7.5-MHz transducer, and neonates generally tolerate this imaging technique better than radiography. For optimal contrast, whole-body radiography should not be performed; the technician should rather focus on the area of interest. Radiography of the neonate is best reserved for thoracic studies. If possible, a normal littermate should be radiographed for comparison. In the feline neonate, full body radiographs may be necessary due to their size and the inability to collimate the radiograph beam to a smaller area of less than 2 inches. Digital dental radiographs can be utilized to perform diagnostic quality images on limbs and feet with detail.

Parasitology

Although parasites are a common issue with pediatrics, gastro-intestinal (GI) distress may not be parasite related but bacterial or viral in nature or owing to dietary indiscretion. Performing routine fecal flotation may not provide accurate results due to

- *Suckling reflex:* Should be present at birth; puppy or kitten will try to suck or chew on a finger.
- *Pressing reflex:* Should be present at birth; puppy or kitten will press its head against a bowed hand.
- *Flexor tone:* Present until age 3 to 4 days; when a puppy or kitten is held by the head, it will "roll up" and adduct its hind limbs.
- *Extensor tone:* After age 4 days, a puppy or kitten held by its head will stretch its back and hind limbs.
- *Lumbar reflex:* Forcefully rubbing a healthy puppy or kitten in the lumbar region will result in vocalization and great activity.
- *Extensor reflex:* Patient is placed in dorsal recumbency, and the toe of a hind limb is pinched. If the puppy or kitten is younger than 3 weeks of age, it will adduct the other hind limb. *Note:* This is normal!
- *Magnus reflex:* Patient is placed in dorsal recumbency, and its head is bent toward one side. Before age 3 weeks, it will stretch its legs on this side and bend the legs on the other side.
- *Tonic neck reflexes:* Patient is held by the thorax, and its neck is bent toward one side; it should stretch the limbs on this side. The head is bent dorsally; the forelimbs should be stretched and the hind limbs adducted. Present until 3 weeks of age.
- *Hopping reflex:* Already present at age 2 to 4 days.
- *Anogenital reflex:* If patient's anogenital region is stimulated with a moist cloth or cotton, it should urinate or defecate. Present until age 3 to 4 weeks.
- *Palpebral and corneal reflexes:* Should be present as soon as the eyes are open.
- *Menace reflex:* Can be present as early as age 2 weeks but usually not until age 10 to 14 weeks.

the small fecal sampling. Preparing a saline wet mount as well as performing a stained fecal cytology will allow for more accurate results in determining a cause for diarrhea.

The technician needs to be familiar with the common parasite life cycles as most neonates will not be positive for parasitic worm infections until at least 2 weeks of age. They are more prone to protozoan, viral, and bacterial infections in a dirty environment or if a queen is already infected, passing it to her kittens during cleaning or by them lying on her dirty fur. *Campylobacter* and *Clostridium* infections are not only common but can be contagious between littermates.

Fly egg infestations in puppies and kittens can cause serious internal larval infestations and should not be confused with tapeworm infections, particularly in the first 2 to 3 weeks of life, due to the *Dipylidium* (tapeworm) lifecycle. Flies will typically lay eggs on any open orifice, as well as the umbilicus, and within 48 hours hatch into larvae that will feed upon the moist tissues. They do not need dead tissue to feed. Not only is this painful to the neonate, it can also cause serious internal damage resulting in death. Although an extralabel use, the drug nitenpyram has been shown to be safe at a smaller dosage for the neonate than the adult and quite effective in destroying infection by fly larva and fleas in as little as 30 minutes.

Flea infestations are not only common in neonates but are also life-threatening for many. Regardless of the animal's age, they should be bathed in warm water using a mild dish soap such as Dawn blue dish soap. Using a flea comb or clean mascara wand, the fleas can be easily combed out and drowned by dipping the comb or wand into a cup of Dawn-infused water. Take the precaution of putting a ring of soap around the neonate's neck to prevent fleas running up to the face and ears. Although an off-label use, many clinicians will treat the neonate afterwards with a topical flea preventative to prevent reinfestation. The environment should be kept clean, and kittens should be monitored for future *Dipylidium* infections due to the fleas.

Routine Maintenance

Healthy neonatal puppies and kittens born to healthy mothers with good maternal instincts require almost no care during the first weeks of life. If neonates were delivered via cesarean section, the umbilical remnant should be treated with tincture of iodine (1%), and the neonates should be encouraged to nurse as quickly as possible to ensure colostrum uptake when recovered from anesthesia. Monitoring the interaction between the mother and her offspring is extremely important at all times after a cesarean section, especially during nursing interactions and when traveling to home, because this is the time the mother may harm the neonates. It is not uncommon for a stressed queen or bitch to kill and consume their offspring because of confusion and stress. If nursing cannot occur for various reasons and there is little to no risk of blood type incompatibility, blood samples for plasma or serum can be obtained from the bitch or queen and given orally to their offspring in the first 24 hours of life to help them develop immunity. The only difference between plasma and serum is that plasma hosts clotting factors that may also be beneficial to the offspring. Giving intraperitoneal (IP) injections is not recommended as there is the possibly of harming internal organs. The plasma or serum should be warmed to body temperature before administration.

Beginning at 2 weeks of life, kittens and puppies should be dewormed with at least three doses of pyrantel pamoate (4.54 mg/kg orally) at 2-week intervals to eliminate roundworms. Vaccinations are categorized into CORE and NON-CORE vaccinations for both species. Starting any vaccination series is not recommended until 4 weeks of age due to the potential for cerebellar hypoplasia in the growing neonate. CORE vaccinations for the feline pediatric recommended by the American Association of Feline Practitioners and the American Animal Hospital Association are those for feline viral rhinotracheitis, calicivirus, panleukopenia (FVRCP),

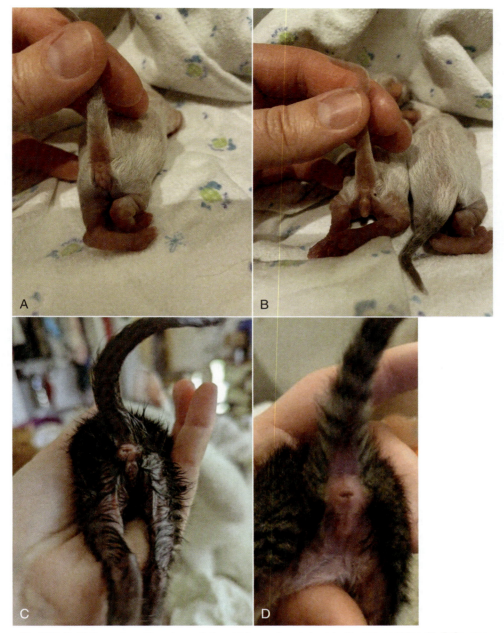

• **Fig. 21.9** (A–D) Examples of female genitalia, which may be confused with male testicles. (A, B Courtesy Karin Lathin; C Courtesy Lana M. Corbo; D Courtesy Meisha Gustafon.)

feline leukemia, and rabies. Vaccinations after the pediatric series are completed and those for future immunity are lifestyle dependent.

Common Concerns and Disorders in Puppies and Kittens

Neonatal illnesses that require immediate attention are listed in Box 21.3.

Hypothermia

Hypothermia is a serious problem in neonates. A neonate is considered hypothermic if its body temperature drops below

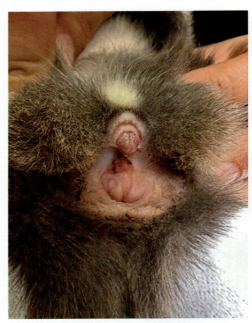

• **Fig. 21.10** Example of Hypodiaasis, a congenital defect in males. In cases of Hypodiasis, a congenital defect in males where the urethra is not located at the tip of the penis, can cause difficulty in sexing the kitten. In many cases the penis curves and can cause some urination issues as the cat is older as well as testicles remaining undescended. If testicles do descend, they typically will present along the sides of the prepuce vs. above. (Courtesy of Dr. Victoria Liberman.)

94°F (34.4°C) at birth, below 96°F (35.6°C) at 1 to 3 days of age, or below 99°F (37.2°C) at 1 week of age. Clinical signs in a chilled neonate with body temperature above 88°F (31.1°C) include restlessness, continuous crying, red mucous membranes, and skin that is cool to the touch. In many cases, lethargy and a stuporous mentality may also be present, particularly in kittens. However, muscle tone is still good, respiratory rate is greater than 40 breaths per minute, and heart rate is greater than 200 bpm. When body temperatures fall into the range of 78°F to 85°F (25.5°C–29.4°C), the neonate appears lethargic and uncoordinated but responsive. Thickened saliva or moisture is seen around the corners of the lips, heart rate drops to less than 50 bpm, and respiratory rate is between 20 and 25 breaths per minute. Typically, a cardiac arrhythmia is also noted in neonates that are failing. No abdominal sounds are heard, and metabolism is impaired, resulting in hypoglycemia (see later discussion in this chapter). With body temperature below 70°F (21.1°C), the neonate would appear to be comatose or presumed dead. At times these kittens may begin agonal breathing, which can be misinterpreted as normal deep breaths. Hypoxia also contributes significantly to hypothermia. Therefore the neonate should be provided with proper ventilation or oxygen administration whenever possible.

Treatment consists of slowly (approximately 2°F/hour) reheating the patient by providing appropriate ambient temperature and humidity. It is essential that the temperature be monitored carefully, because the neonate cannot escape if the temperature is too warm, and thermal burns may occur. Supplying warm air and oxygen in a veterinary neonatal incubator such as the Rcom, a circulating air avian brooder, or a veterinary oxygen cage is optimal for rewarming the hypothermic neonate. Warm intravenous (IV) fluids can also be given but at no more than 2°F (1.1°C) above body temperature.

Warmed lactated Ringer solution (LRS) with 50% dextrose can be administered orally to a hypothermic neonate. This will slowly warm them while supporting the glycogen stores of the liver and helping prevent GI collapse. However, food, including formula, should not be given orally until the patient exhibits audible gut sounds and is appropriately rewarmed, because the hypothermic neonate also suffers from GI stasis. When hypothermic neonates are tube fed, the milk replacer may be regurgitated and aspirated, resulting in pneumonia, or the stomach contents will clot and ferment, leading to bloat. A downward spiral can form and ultimately results in circulatory collapse and death.

Rapid rewarming will result in heat shock, with increased respiratory rate and effort. Eventually, the patient will become cyanotic and can develop diarrhea and seizures. Raising the neonatal body temperature by more than 4°F (2.2°C) within an hour usually has fatal consequences as a result of delayed organ failure.

TECHNICIAN NOTE

Hypothermia in the neonate is a serious problem. Gut motility can slow and even stop with decreasing body temperature, ultimately causing ileus. Feeding a hypothermic neonate can cause milk replacer to be regurgitated and aspirated, resulting in pneumonia, or the stomach contents may ferment, leading to bloat. Use clear, warm liquids only until thermoregulation is present. Once normal body temperature is reached, tube feeding is the safest way to feed the critical neonate (Figs. 21.14A–D and 21.15). Bottle or syringe feeding should not be attempted in the absence of a strong suckle response.

Dehydration

Any disease process or imbalance of fluids or electrolytes will quickly lead to **dehydration** in the neonate. Tacky to dry mucous membranes indicate 5% to 7% dehydration. At 10% dehydration, the mucous membranes are dry, and in a neonate that is at least 4 weeks of age, a decrease in skin elasticity is noticeable. In the feline neonate, shallowing of the face and eye sockets is more apparent when dehydrated.

Fluid requirements are high in neonates, but total volumes that can be given are low. All fluids should be warmed to 98°F to 99°F (36.6°C–36.7°C) before administration unless the neonate is substantially colder. Boluses can be given at 3.3 mL per 100 g of the neonate's weight over 5 to 10 minutes. The maintenance dose is 6 mL/kg per hour. To this, 50% of the deficit is added over 6 hours (deficit = BW × % dehydrated). It is often easiest to place a short 23- or 25-gauge catheter into the jugular vein for fluid administration. Another option is intraosseous (IO) fluid delivery; the bone is soft enough that a 20-, 22-, or 24-gauge needle, depending on the species, can be placed into the proximal tibia or the proximal femur, with fluids given at the same rate as IV fluids. It is important that each bone not be punctured more than once because fluid will leak out if there is another hole present. Administering fluids at a constant rate is best accomplished by using a syringe pump or a pediatric drip set (60 drops/mL). If IV or IO access is not available, fluids are given by the oral (PO) route with a feeding tube if not able to suckle. Subcutaneous (SC) fluids are not recommended in the neonate, especially if they are hypovolemic, because the absorption rate is much slower as a result of vasoconstriction. If recommended, SC fluids should be limited to neonatal patients with euvolemia and mild dehydration of <5% to prevent fluid overload and abscess formation in the area of administration.

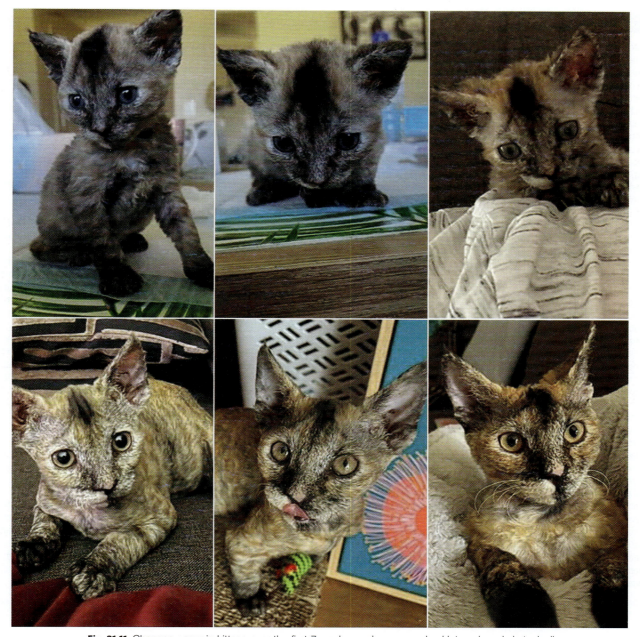

• **Fig. 21.11** Changes occur in kittens over the first 7 weeks, such as eye color. Heterochromia is typically seen in white-coated cats. (Courtesy Jessica Broadhead.)

TECHNICIAN NOTE

Dehydration occurs very quickly in neonates, because their fluid requirements are much greater than those of adults and because they are less able to conserve fluids. Therefore fluid replacement therapy is a key element in nursing a neonate back to health. It is important to use an intravenous catheter (IVC) that fits the vein and the patient, not the largest IVC that can be placed with force, especially in the feline patient, as this may be the only opportunity to place an IVC in the neonate. Once the animal is better hydrated, a larger catheter can be utilized when homeostasis has occurred. The feline neonate should have catheters of smaller sizes (24–26-gauge) applied to prevent phlebitis and bone fractures.

Hypoglycemia

A variety of clinical signs may occur in a neonate with **hypoglycemia** (serum glucose <30 mg/dL in the canine and <50 mg/dL in the feline), including tremors, crying, irritability, increased appetite, dullness, head pressing into corners, isolating themselves from the rest of the litter, lethargy, coma, stupor, and seizures. In hand-reared cases, many feline neonates will paddle their feet in frustration when offered food or fight the caregiver and push away at the bottle when becoming hypoglycemic. This should be addressed immediately before it progresses to a more serious stage of hypoglycemia.

- *Heart:* At birth, the right and left ventricles have approximately the same mass, changing to an ultimate adult ratio of 1:2 to 1:3 throughout puberty and changing in cardiac axis and shape. During this time, the canine heart changes from an ellipsoid shape at birth to a more globoid shape in adulthood. At age 1 month, puppies and kittens still have lower blood pressure, stroke volume, and resistance in the peripheral vasculature compared with adults, but they have higher heart rate, cardiac output, and central venous pressure. Responses to cardiovascular drugs during the first weeks of life are less intense than in adults. Development of the heart has been well studied in the dog, and it has been shown that normal adult values of the parameters are reached by age 7 months. It is important to keep these differences in mind when evaluating chest radiographs, electrocardiograms, and echocardiograms.

- *Immune system:* Virtually no antibodies are transferred in utero to canine and feline fetuses, and they are born immunologically immature. Puppies and kittens are dependent on the colostral transfer of antibodies (passive immunity) for postnatal protection against infectious diseases. In puppies and kittens, colostrum needs to be ingested within the first 24 and 16 hours of life, respectively, whereby mainly immunoglobulin G (IgG) and IgA are absorbed. Thereafter the gut seems to be closed for further absorption. Depending on the type of maternally derived antibodies, these may last from 6 to 16 weeks after birth. Relative to the size of the puppy, the greatest size of the thymus is noted at birth, but its absolute size will be greatest at puberty, after which it begins to atrophy. Although the thymus and the immune system are thought to be mature by age 3 to 4 months, puppies and kittens have the ability to produce functional IgM shortly before birth. Lymph node structure is normal at birth, but few lymphocytes are present; these increase in number during the first months of life. Lymph nodes should be palpable at birth, with facial nodes easier to palpate because of their increased reactivity.

- *Liver:* Drugs that require hepatic metabolism should be carefully administered to neonatal patients, because the liver does not reach full metabolic capacity until well after the neonatal period. Neonatal albumin and plasma protein levels are significantly lower than in adults. Dosages of drugs that are bound to albumin or plasma proteins must be adjusted accordingly. The liver is the site of the production of most coagulation factors. Because of its immaturity, many coagulopathies may be exacerbated during the neonatal age. Because growing requires rapid bone turnover, serum concentrations of alkaline phosphatase (ALP) are often elevated, but they should never be increased more than twofold to threefold in healthy, growing animals. Serum ALP and gamma glutamyl transferase (GGT) are not reliable indicators of liver disease during the first 2 weeks of life, because both are present in colostrum and are absorbed through the gut, increasing ALP and GGT levels greatly in the neonate. Lack of an increase in ALP and GGT in a puppy younger than 2 weeks can be used as an indicator of not having received colostrum.

- *Kidney:* The neonate is particularly susceptible to dehydration, because water makes up 82% of body weight, and water turnover is about twice that of an adult. Because of the neonate's limited ability to conserve fluid and the immaturity of the kidney, fluid requirements are high at 13 to 22 mL/100 g body weight per day. Nephrons are not completely formed until the third week of life, and the glomerular filtration rate increases from 21% at birth to 53% by age 8 weeks. Whereas tubular secretion generally is thought to be mature by age 8 weeks, some reports indicate that it takes 6 months for tubular function to be complete. Either way, this explains the low urine specific gravity until age 8 weeks (1.006–1.017), increased concentrations of amino acids and proteins, and glycosuria—a common finding in neonates up to 2 weeks of age. Given the immaturity of renal function, medications that affect kidney development should be avoided, and dosages of those that are excreted through the kidney must be adjusted to the patient's age.

- *Thyroid:* Serum thyroid hormones differ between puppies and kittens and their adult counterparts and differ significantly with time during the first 12 weeks of life. Therefore it is critical to know the exact age of puppies or kittens and to not use the standard reference range for adult normal dogs or cats, respectively. Lack of thyroid hormones in the neonate leads to much more serious disease than in the adult because of involvement of the thyroid in development. Clinical signs in affected puppies and kittens may be as mild as apathy and failure to thrive or as severe as joint and bone abnormalities, complete dullness, extremely stunted growth and, in cats, constipation. Serum thyroid hormones should be determined at the slightest suspicion of hypothyroidism because the earlier treatment is initiated, the better the outcome. Therapy is performed as in adults, but thyroid levels should be checked frequently in young patients and results compared with normal values for the corresponding age group.

- *Gastrointestinal (GI) system:* The neonate is born with a sterile GI system, which will develop its own flora to assist digestion during the first few days of life. GI peristalsis is weaker (slower), intestinal blood flow is reduced, and gastric fluid has a higher pH. Medication, changes in the environment, or disease will cause upset to this yet-fragile system, and this is most commonly apparent in the form of diarrhea. The most common causes of diarrhea in the orphaned neonate are overfeeding and inappropriate dilutions of milk replacer.

Treatment consists of giving dextrose slowly by the IV or IO route at 0.5 to 1 g/kg as part of a 5% to 10% dextrose solution in normal saline. Care should be taken when giving 5% dextrose mixed with LRS, because the mixture will become hypertonic, and volume replacement will have to be monitored carefully. Higher concentrations of IV dextrose should be avoided, because its irritant nature can cause phlebitis. Dextrose can be given at higher concentrations directly to the oral mucous membrane if the neonate is not dehydrated or hypothermic (1–2 mL of a 5%–15% dextrose solution). Because they may cause tissue damage, dextrose solutions should never be given by the SC route. After treatment, blood glucose levels should be monitored for the development of hyperglycemia. Oral routes of sugar solutions are well tolerated and can allow for quick recovery while IV or IO access is being obtained. Although high fructose corn syrup (HFCS) tends to be utilized in practice, it is also a hypertonic solution. Neonates that are significantly compromised should not have concentrated HFCS administered on the gumline or under the tongue; it should be diluted slightly so it is no longer a thick syrup and given one to two drops under the tongue or along the maxillary gumline. The patient should be kept at a downward angle of 5–10 degrees until it is responsive and swallowing to minimize the risk of aspiration of the sugar solution. Oral sugar solutions should be given every 10 to 15 minutes until the patient is responsive and eating/drinking on their own.

TECHNICIAN NOTE

Hypoglycemia is one of the most common causes of seizures and sudden comatose episodes in neonatal puppies and kittens. Stuporous mentality, sudden aggression, and coma are also common signs of hypoglycemia in the neonatal kitten.

Neonatal Isoerythrolysis in Kittens

Cats with blood type A have low titers of naturally occurring antibodies against blood type B red blood cells (RBCs). Therefore type

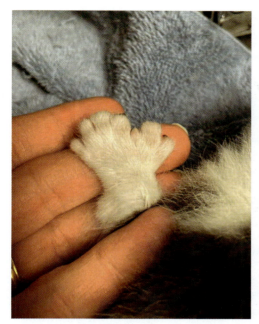

• **Fig. 21.12** Example of polydactyly in cats. (Courtesy Denise Breda Cunningham.)

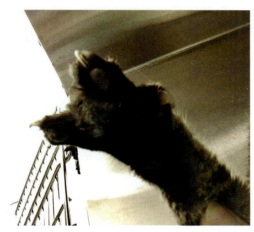

• **Fig. 21.13** Example of syndactyly in cats. (Courtesy Olivia G. Ripca.)

• **BOX 21.3** **Neonatal Illnesses That Need Immediate Attention**

- Hypothermia
- Dehydration
- Hypoglycemia
- Neonatal isoerythrolysis
- Malnutrition

B kittens born to type A queens do not show any clinical signs of incompatibility reactions after ingestion of colostrum containing alloantibodies. However, all type B cats have high titers of naturally occurring antibodies against type A RBCs. This may lead to incompatibility reactions when type A kittens receive colostral antibodies from a type B queen. Clinical signs are variable and

range from jaundice, red/orange urine, and death within the first 2 days of life to no signs at all (which is rare). In some cases, the tail tip becomes necrotic and falls off at 10 to 14 days of life. Other symptoms seen are sudden limb edema that subsides after several days of aggressive nursing care. In some cases, the neonate may lose a digit or two due to necrosis. Kittens at risk for neonatal isoerythrolysis (NI) must be removed from their queens only during the first day of life.

Malnutrition

Regular feeding leads to good hydration in the neonate. Three feedings per day are not enough for the neonate; not only is this inadequate for the appropriate amount of nutrition, daily caloric needs, and fluid requirements for the neonate, it also does not meet their emotional needs. Ideally, the neonate should be fed every 2 to 4 hours, depending on age and demands. The use of a species-specific commercial milk replacer with a formulation that comes closest to the mother's milk should be used, because many milk replacers easily cover the daily caloric requirements of both puppies and kittens (Table 21.1), yet the ratios of protein, fat, and carbohydrate requirements are vastly different between the species. Before and after each meal, the neonate should be encouraged to urinate and defecate as they will consume more food. Neonates are weighed at least twice daily on a suitable scale until weaned to ensure proper weight gain. Weekly weight monitoring is recommended to continue after weaning until the neonate is adopted. Stimulating the neonate with a clean toothbrush along their head and body replicates allogrooming during nursing and can help prevent and ease emotional distress as nursing is not just an act of nourishment but is also for comfort. Feline and canine neonates should be fed in a sternal position, and they should be in control of how much milk they draw from the bottle. It is important NOT to have any large lumps or formula clots in the bottle as it can clog the nipple. Not only does this cause frustration in the neonate, but it can also cause aspiration pneumonia if the clot passes through the nipple and a rush of liquid of a volume they cannot swallow safely should enter the neonate's mouth. The neonate should be able to accommodate 4 mL of liquid volume per 100 g of bodyweight; however, it is important to monitor the neonate for bloating.

Bottle babies should have their own bottle and nipple system clearly marked with their identification. Wildlife nipples such as the Miracle Nipple tend to fit the feline neonate's mouth better than many of the commercial bottles available for use, especially for smaller feline breeds or premature neonates. The kitten should be fed with the same nipple and bottle until it is weaned or the nipple is worn out.

Tube feeding is necessary if a neonate will not nurse from a bottle, does not have a strong suckle reflex, or is not gaining the expected weight because of illness or malformations. However, a neonate should never be milk replacer via tube if its body temperature is lower than normal for its age, for reasons described previously. Feeding warmed LRS with dextrose would be appropriate in this scenario. Nasogastric (NG) tubes with premarked measurements (Fig. 21.14A) make superior feeding tubes; however, if one is not available, a red rubber catheter can be used. To tube feed, first the distance from the tip of the neonate's nose to the last rib should be measured (see Fig. 21.14A and B). With a felt-tip pen or a piece of tape, a mark is made at 75% of this distance on a feeding tube, measuring from the distal end of the feeding tube. The syringe with the milk replacer is connected to the tube and primed with the liquid being fed to remove

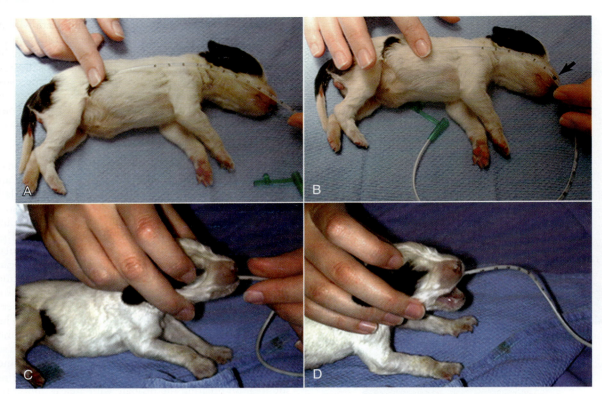

• **Fig. 21.14** (A–D) Tube feeding. (A) Measure from the tip of the nose to the last rib. (B) Make a mark at 75% of length *(arrow)*. (C) Gently insert tube to the mark. (D) Check for negative pressure and give milk slowly.

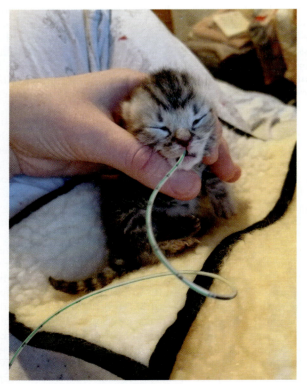

• **Fig. 21.15** Example of proper feeding tube placement in kitten. (Courtesy Laura Davies.)

air bubbles. Then this length of a clean and dry feeding tube is inserted gently into the left side of the mouth of the neonate while holding them upright. No force is needed, because most neonates will swallow the feeding tube easily. A crying neonate proves that the feeding tube is, in fact, in the esophagus and not in the lungs. Negative pressure also indicates that the feeding tube is in the lower esophagus and not in the lungs. The size of the neonate being tube fed will dictate the size of tube to be used. Small kitten neonates may only tolerate a 3.5-French (Fr) tube, but a larger tube size such as a 5.0 or 8.0 Fr can be used as the neonate grows.

> **TECHNICIAN NOTE**
>
> Tube feeding is a safe and efficient method of supplementing neonates, especially when more than one neonate needs to be fed. The risk of aspiration is less with this method than with syringe or bottle feeding. The downside of tube feeding is that it lacks the emotional connection the neonate needs with nursing alone. It is important to handle, groom, and provide additional comfort to tube-fed neonates.

The Critical Neonate

The critical neonate is characterized by anorexia, lethargy, emaciation, birth defects, and death. Kittens or puppies may be stillborn or born small, weak, and unable to nurse, resulting in dehydration, hypothermia, hypoglycemia, and death within the first few days of life. Other neonates appear healthy during the first weeks of life but become weak, depressed, and anorexic, or die of malabsorption at the time of weaning.

TABLE 21.1   Overview of Requirements and Milk Comparison

Age	Puppies, kcal/100 g per day	Kittens, kcal/100 g per day	Fluids for Both, mL/100 g
Week 1	13–15	<38 at birth; 28 thereafter	18 mL average
Week 2	15–20	28	Range, 13–22
Week 3	20	27	Same
Week 4	≥20	25	Same

	Bitch's Milk	Queen's Milk	Cow's Milk‡	Goat's Milk‡
Fluid content	77	79	88	87
Fat, %	9.5	8.5	3.5	4.1
Protein, %	7.5	7.5	3.3	3.6
Lactose, %	3.4	4.0	5.0	4.7
Calcium*	0.24	0.18	0.12	0.13
Phosphorus*	0.18	0.16	0.10	0.16
ME†, kcal/100 mL milk	146	121	70	69

*g/100 mL.

†Metabolizable energy.

‡When mixing cow's or goat's milk as a milk replacer for neonates, be aware that to meet the fat or protein requirements, the lactose concentrations will be far too high and will cause diarrhea. Commercial milk replacers are a better choice.

Causes of neonatal death include poor management with inadequate educational resources, malnutrition, inappropriate environmental conditions, congenital and genetic defects, infection and, at times, human error. Management and environmental problems can be easily detected by obtaining a detailed history or inspecting the facility. Nutritional deficiency can be caused by an inadequate diet for the mother or the neonate. It is important to document the animal's vitals daily and to notify the clinician immediately so that medical care can be initiated if any "abnormals" are noted. Animals in foster care should be cared for by properly trained individuals who can provide the level of nursing care required for the case to succeed. Many times, despite our efforts, the neonate will succumb to its illness.

Treatment involves aggressive supportive care for the sickly neonate and removal of causative factors. If causes are not immediately apparent, necropsy of neonates that have died is recommended.

TECHNICIAN NOTE

"Fading puppy syndrome" and "fading kitten syndrome" are not recognized syndromes or diagnoses of death, and these cases should not be termed as such. They will have failed to thrive for specific reasons, whether from infectious disease, parasites, congenital defects, environmental causes, nutritional indiscretion, or trauma. "Critical neonate" is not a diagnosis but rather, a clinical description, and requires further workup to identify the cause.

Orphan Care

Kittens or puppies may need to be hand-raised because of maternal death or abandonment, lack of milk, maternal aggression, large litter size, malformation, or trauma. Materials needed include warm and clean bedding, milk bottles with a variety of different rubber nipples, feeding tubes, syringes, a gram scale, cotton balls, hand sanitizers, and fur clippers; it may be necessary to isolate the orphan from other animals. Orphaned kittens or puppies from different litters should not be introduced to each other until after a quarantine period of 3 to 5 days to prevent disease transmission. If different litters are mixed immediately, there is a higher probability of disease transmission and higher mortality rate. Each orphan must be weighed twice daily, and records should be kept. Losses should be monitored closely as they are an early indication of fluid loss or illness. Ambient temperature of 84°F to 90°F (29°C) and 90°F to 95°F (32°C–35°C) for canine and feline neonates, respectively, and humidity of 55% to 60% should be provided during the first week of life, if possible, especially if using an incubator as their microenvironment. During the second week, ambient temperature can be lowered to 79°F to 84°F (26.1°C–29.0°C), and to 73.4°F to 79°F (23°C–26.1°C) during the third week. The neonate must be kept warm and always hydrated. Proper nutrition or supplementation and clean and dry housing should be provided. After feeding, the orphan must be stimulated to urinate and defecate.

Overfeeding with milk replacers often results in diarrhea and bloating that can cause death due to the inability to digest soured food in the stomach, while underfeeding leads to dehydration, malnutrition, and lack of weight gain and can ultimately lead to death in many cases if not corrected quickly. Homemade formulas are often deficient in growth factors, amino acids, and other nutrients essential for growth. Commercial milk replacers should be carefully evaluated, and homemade milk replacers should be made under the guidance of a veterinarian and, ideally, a board-certified veterinary nutritionist. Currently, the liquid veterinary formula Feline EmerAid HDN is an acceptable diet for the neonate in practice if no kitten formula is available for use. Because of

Considerations When Administering Medication to the Pediatric Patient

- Higher total body water (up to 82% of body weight)
- Less fat
- Less muscle mass
- Muscle not well vascularized
- Lower plasma protein concentration
- Higher gastric pH
- Weaker/slower gastrointestinal peristalsis
- Lower intestinal blood flow
- Better intestinal absorption of proteins
- Intestinal flora not fully developed
- Blood—brain barrier not fully developed
- Liver—some enzymes need up to 4 months to develop
- Kidney—glomerular filtration developed by 3 to 4 weeks; tubular secretion developed by 6 months

differences in physiology, many medications will not be absorbed and metabolized at the same rate as in adults. Box 21.4 outlines the main physiologic differences between neonates and adults that should be considered when administering medications.

TECHNICIAN NOTE

Goat's milk alone is not an appropriate substitute for the feline or canine neonate for any period longer than 24 hours. There are commercial domestic pet formulas available made with goat's milk with the proper nutrition ratios added. Ideally, the dams milk should be utilized, even if only partly in addition to species-specific commercially provided formula.

TECHNICIAN NOTE

Weight loss, or lack of weight gain, is the first indication that a neonate is not doing well. Therefore proper identification and accurate twice-daily weight recordings for each orphan will help ensure that a problem is identified before it is too late for treatment.

Neonatology of Foals

The term *neonate* encompasses foals from birth to 1 month of age, with *perinatal* referring to the short period just before and after birth. The neonate foal is a complex unit of multiple immature systems that must rapidly adapt to life outside of the uterus, combined with a naïve immune system vulnerable to outside insult. This section focuses on two critical areas: the perinatal period and the neonatal period. Because of this, subtle yet life-threatening changes can occur rapidly. Normal foal development and potential diseases of neonatal foals that require intensive care will be discussed.

The Perinatal Period and the High-Risk Mare

Most **mares** have routine pregnancies and deliver healthy foals. The mare's health is an important aspect to consider before the breeding process ever takes place to better ensure a healthy foal. Age, nutrition, medical conditions, and previous foaling history are all important factors to consider prior to breeding, because some mares develop problems during late-term pregnancy and require treatment. These mares, referred to as *high-risk mares*,

often exhibit early warning signs that indicate a problem with the pregnancy.

The normal gestational period in the mare is approximately 340 days; however, the gestational period is quite variable among mares (320–400 days) and even between sequential pregnancies in the same mare. Once the mare has been bred via natural or artificial means, sequential pregnancy checks via rectal examination and transrectal ultrasonography should be performed at 15, 30, and 90 days to confirm pregnancy, address twin pregnancies, and evaluate the amniotic and allantoic fluids. Mares at high risk for any reason should be monitored closely throughout pregnancy to quickly recognize and address such concerns as premature development of the udder, vaginal discharge, or lactation (dripping or streaming milk) as early as possible.

TECHNICIAN NOTE

Unless delivery is imminent, the mare should *not* have milk dripping or streaming from her udder. Premature lactation occurs for three reasons:
1. Twins are present.
2. Placentitis has developed.
3. The owner has miscalculated the delivery date.

Methods used to monitor high-risk mares include video monitoring and telemetry to monitor the heart rates of the mare and the foal. Management of these mares involves treating the primary problem in the mare, maintaining the pregnancy, and supporting the fetus. Assessment of the mare includes a thorough physical examination, baseline bloodwork (complete blood count [CBC]/serum chemistry), rectal palpation, and vaginal examination (with discretion).

Placentitis is a leading high-risk complication in the mare and usually involves an ascending infection via the cervical star. Vaginal discharge, premature udder development, and lactation are the most prominent clinical signs. Transrectal and transabdominal ultrasonography are used to assess the uteroplacental thickness and attachment, echogenicity and depth of fetal fluids, fetal heart rate, fetal aortic diameter, and fetal activity. The fetal cardiac pulse can be monitored transrectally once the fetus moves into an anterior presentation and the head and neck move into view at 180 days' gestation or later. The fetal cardiac pulse has been shown to directly correlate with the fetal heart rate. The fetal heart rate and fetal activity decrease in late gestation; however, prolonged tachycardia, bradycardia, or arrhythmias can be indicative of fetal compromise. Treatment of placentitis includes broad-spectrum antimicrobial therapy that achieves therapeutic levels across the placenta, nonsteroidal anti-inflammatory drugs (NSAIDS; most commonly flunixin meglumine), and progestin (i.e., altrenogest) to suppress premature delivery. Nasal oxygen supplementation to the mare may increase oxygen to the foal but is not always readily available. Many mares respond quickly to treatment, and clinical signs, such as premature udder development and lactation, resolve. Left untreated, most affected mares will deliver premature foals with a poor prognosis for survival. High-risk mares may be referred to a veterinary hospital for attended foaling and immediate access to medical intervention as needed.

Many mares exhibit classic preparturition physical changes, including increased udder enlargement ("bagging up"); pelvic ligament relaxation over the tail head; and vulvar softening and elongation. Typically, mares produce prefoaling secretions that accumulate or "wax up" on the teats. However, some mares, especially primiparous mares that have not previously foaled, may show few to no clinical signs or very rapid changes immediately prior to foaling. Other mares may routinely exhibit signs 2 to 3 weeks before delivery. Colostral calcium content rises near parturition. Calcium carbonate ($CaCO_3$) levels can be measured via diagnostic laboratory tests, commercial kits, and simple hard-water test kits. Typically, mares with a less than 200 parts per million (ppm) $CaCO_3$ content will not foal within 24 hours. A more precise indicator of imminent parturition is a significant drop in colostral pH less than 7 (6.5 or lower) on the day of parturition. Mares with a prolonged decrease in milk pH often deliver dysmature or critically ill foals. There is also a high correlation between the pH and electrolyte concentrations in milk, with an elevation in calcium, magnesium, and potassium concentrations and a drop in sodium and chloride concentrations within 1 to 2 days before foaling. Milk from most mares exhibits an inversion in the ratio of the concentration of sodium and potassium. Despite the different methods that are available, the best approach for determining when a mare will foal is to have well-trained staff monitor the mare's behavior 24 hours a day and note any changes.

Prefoaling mares often have a significant drop in body temperature on the day of parturition, so daily monitoring of rectal temperature may be useful. Significant behavior changes, including aggression, docility, restlessness, vocalization, and decreased appetite, may be observed in mares close to parturition. Another key note to remember is that many mares tend to foal late at night or very early in the morning.

Normal parturition has three distinct stages. At the onset of stage 1 labor, the mare should be left alone but be closely monitored, because she can stop labor if she feels threatened and resume later. The mare often becomes restless, paces, flank watches, may bite and/or kick at her sides and abdomen, and frequently postures to urinate or defecate. At this time, the foal's forebody is beginning to rotate up into the dorsosacral position, pushing the head and extended forelimbs into the pelvic canal. Stage 1 labor often lasts 1 to 2 hours or longer and ends when the chorioallantois membrane ruptures (water breaks), releasing allantoic fluid. If sweating is observed along the mare's shoulders, foaling should occur within 30 minutes. For veterinary technicians, this time is crucial. It is best to notify the veterinarian, stay near the mare, ensure that all necessary equipment is available, and wrap the mare's tail with brown gauze to keep it clean. Box 21.5 lists equipment needed to manage high-risk foaling.

Stage 2 labor progresses rapidly as oxytocin is released, stimulating vigorous uterine and abdominal contractions, and the foal moves into the pelvic canal. Most mares deliver a foal while in lateral recumbency but may get up and down several times to assist in the rotation and positioning of the foal. The foal is delivered rapidly, often within 10 to 15 minutes after rupture of the chorioallantois membrane. The umbilical cord (comprising two umbilical arteries, vein, and urachus) should be left intact until the mare breaks it upon standing. It is an extreme emergency if the foal is not delivered within 30 minutes. If the foal's nose is protruding from the vulva, an endotracheal tube can be placed in the foal's trachea and breaths delivered via an Ambu Bag to supply oxygen while preparing for a cesarean section. A prolonged duration of stage 2 labor directly affects the survival of the foal and sometimes that of the mare as well.

Stage 3 labor involves expulsion of the fetal membranes (placenta), usually within 3 to 4 hours. The placenta is considered retained if it is not delivered within 6 hours. Some mares may exhibit mild discomfort or colic signs that may be alleviated with a dose of an NSAID such as flunixin meglumine. The placenta

should be examined and weighed (normal weight is ≈11% of foal's BW) to ensure that it is intact and has been completely expelled. After foaling, the mare should exhibit immediate interest in the foal, demonstrated by nickering (vocalization) and cleaning/stimulating the foal. A mare and foal should be left undisturbed immediately after delivery to allow for proper bonding. This is a crucial time between mare and foal, especially in primiparous mares. Intervention should only occur if the foal is in distress, in danger from the mare, or unable to stand and nurse within a reasonable period. The mare will be thirsty and will need fresh, clean water. Additional bedding should be added to the stall, because it will be slippery from fetal fluids. Postpartum complications of the mare may include mild colic, large colon volvulus, uterine artery hemorrhage, retained placenta, peritonitis, endotoxemia, and laminitis. Depending on the problem, the foal may be able to stay with the mare or may need to be removed and raised as an orphan (called a "bucket baby") or "grafted" onto a nurse mare.

TECHNICIAN NOTE

High-risk mares should have an attended foaling at a veterinary hospital to ensure optimal survival of the mare and the foal. Foaling equipment should be kept close to the mare's stall for easy access. Once stage 2 labor has started, sweating is often noted around the mare's shoulders, and normally, the mare will deliver the foal within 30 minutes.

The Neonatal Period: The Normal Foal

Postfoaling events should occur rapidly, with very specific milestones. Foals are born with hypoxemia and hypercapnia, stimulating spontaneous breathing within seconds of delivery. A normal foal will right itself into a sternal position within 2 to 3 minutes and have the suckle reflex within 5 to 10 minutes, demonstrated by an extended, curled tongue and sucking of air, especially when stimulated (i.e., rubbing the nose). The foal should attempt to rise within 30 minutes, stand within 1 hour, and successfully nurse within 2 hours of birth. The neonatal foal has very limited stores of glycogen and endogenous fat that are used up quickly after birth, making it imperative that a foal stand and nurse within 1 to 2 hours after birth. The ingestion of good-quality colostrum is not only important for its transfer of protective immunoglobulins but also provides up to 50% more energy compared with milk. Once

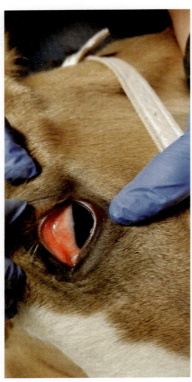

• **Fig. 21.16** Examination of a foal's eye. A neonate foal's eyes should be inspected for white sclera and large, round pupils.

it stands, a foal will demonstrate a base-wide stance and ambulate with a hypermetric (exaggerated) gait.

Every neonate should receive a complete physical examination within 8 to 24 hours of birth. A healthy neonatal foal will be bright, responsive, and reactive, and will stay close by the mare's side or flank. During the first week of life, foals nurse often and play/sleep within close proximity (3–15 feet) of the mare. The foal's nursing and swallowing behavior should be observed. If the mare has an engorged udder or is streaming milk or the foal has evidence of dried milk on its face, this indicates a sick foal that is not nursing adequately.

Normal vital parameters include a rectal temperature of 99°F to 102°F, a heart rate of 80 to 120 bpm, and a respiration rate of 30 to 40 breaths per minute, with slight abdominal effort. The oral mucous membranes should be pink and moist, with a capillary refill time (CRT) of less than 2 seconds. The nostrils should be clean and dry. The eyes should be clear with white sclera, and neonates younger than 1 day of age have eyes with large, round pupils that gradually become smaller and more oval, like those of an adult horse (Fig. 21.16). Foals often have a slower pupillary light response compared with an adult and do not demonstrate the menace response; this is a learned response developed over the first 2 weeks of life.

Upon auscultation, the heart should have a strong beat with a regular rhythm and a synchronous pulse (palpate the facial, brachial, and metatarsal arteries). A holosystolic (machinery) flow murmur may be present and is normal if the foal is otherwise healthy. This murmur normally resolves within a day or two but can persist longer. The lungs should be clear on auscultation, although a healthy foal may have transient, slightly harsh airway sounds. Respiratory rate, effort, and pattern should also be used to assess respiratory function. The thorax should be palpated and

assessed for the presence of rib fractures, which can occur during parturition. Gastrointestinal (GI) motility or borborygmi (peristaltic activity) is assessed with bilateral auscultation of the abdomen within four quadrants and is generally classified as normal, increased, decreased, or absent in each quadrant. The umbilical remnant should be small and dry on palpation. The umbilicus and inguinal area should be palpated for evidence of hernias within the body wall.

The musculoskeletal system is evaluated by observing the gait and movement of the foal. A hypermetric gait in all four limbs is normal in neonate foals. Foals may exhibit mild flexor tendon laxity at birth that often self-corrects with exercise and time. The joints of all four limbs should feel tight on palpation, with no evidence of heat or effusion. Healthy foals are excitable and easily stimulated. It is normal for foals to respond to visual, auditory, and tactile stimuli with exaggerated, jerky movements, especially around the head. This behavior of head "bobbing" becomes extremely apparent during restraint; it is also normal for a healthy foal to struggle, fall limp in the handler's arms, and then react explosively when stimulated.

Routine Neonatal Therapy

Routine care for all foals includes monitoring the foal's attitude, appetite, urination, and fecal production. The umbilical remnant is a potential entry site for bacteria (i.e., *Staphylococcus* spp.); therefore once the foal is standing, the remnant should be treated with a 0.5% solution of 2% chlorhexidine solution three or four times over the first 24 hours. Meconium or "first feces" is the black, tarlike fecal material that is passed within a few hours after birth; some foals may require an enema to assist with initial defecation. Warm, mild soapy water solutions of about 200 to 400 mL may be administered gently by gravity flow via a well-lubricated enema kit catheter or tubing. Foals normally urinate within 6 to 10 hours, with colts (males) tending to urinate sooner than fillies (females). Adequately hydrated foals will urinate often, and urine should be clear with a low specific gravity (1.001–1.015). A normal foal nurses frequently (five to eight times) every hour between periods of sleep and activity, consuming approximately 150 mL/kg or more of colostrum and milk within the first 24 hours.

Foals are born with a completely naïve immune system, dependent on the protective antibodies obtained through the ingestion of colostrum. Colostrum is a thick, sticky, yellow-colored fluid produced by the mare during the last few weeks of gestation. Good-quality colostrum provides immunoglobulins (including immunoglobulin G [IgG]), nutrients, vitamins, B-lymphocytes, and growth factors that aid in the development of the foal's immature immune system and GI tract. Vaccination of the mare 4 to 6 weeks prior to foaling increases the concentration of vital immunoglobulins in the colostrum. Colostrum quality can be evaluated prior to the foal nursing with a Brix refractometer and/or colostrometer. Colostrum with a Brix reading of 20% to 30% or higher is considered good. A colostrometer measures the specific gravity of colostrum. The greater the antibody density, the higher the specific gravity (1.08–1.09 is considered acceptable).

Colostral antibodies are best absorbed within the first 6 to 8 hours of life, when special cells allow the large immunoglobulins to transfer out of the intestinal lumen to the bloodstream via the lymphatic system. After 24 hours, these large protein molecules are no longer able to pass through. An average 45-kg foal should ingest 2 to 4 liters of colostrum. All foals should have their IgG measured approximately 12 hours after birth to determine whether adequate immunity has occurred. Failure of passive transfer (FPT) occurs when a foal does not ingest an adequate amount of colostrum within the first 12 to 24 hours of life or if the colostrum is of poor quality. Foals must be monitored closely to identify subtle changes as FPT is associated with increased risk of infection or sepsis. A simple, commercial point-of-care test (enzyme-linked immunosorbent assay [ELISA]: SNAP Foal IgG ELISA; IDEXX Inc., Westbrook, ME) can be used to obtain quick, reliable assessment of passive immunity transfer. IgG levels of 800 mg/dL or greater indicate adequate transfer, whereas levels 200 mg/dL or less indicate FPT. This can be addressed with oral administration of good-quality colostrum via nasogastric intubation within approximately 12 hours of birth or by IV administration of plasma. Plasma is obtained from hyperimmunized donors and contains high levels of IgG and must be administered via a filtered blood IV set. One liter of plasma can raise the serum IgG level 50 to 200 mg/dL in a 45-kg foal.

> **TECHNICIAN NOTE**
>
> A neonatal foal needs to be monitored closely for appropriate developmental milestones. The immunoglobulin G (IgG) level in the foal should be measured within 12 hours of birth to ensure that passive transfer of maternal antibodies has occurred.

Laboratory Evaluation

In addition to a physical examination, a newborn foal's examination should include basic bloodwork with an IgG assessment, a CBC, and a serum chemistry evaluation. Normal parameters vary significantly between neonate foals and adult horses. In general, foals have a higher packed cell volume (PCV) and hemoglobin (Hb) concentration for the first 24 hours before gradually decreasing. The total white blood cell (WBC) in neonates is like adults, except neonate foals will have a greater than 2:1 ratio of neutrophils to lymphocytes. Neutropenia with band cells (premature neutrophils) is indicative of an ongoing infection or septicemia. Thrombocyte (platelet) values are similar between foals and adults. In general, fibrinogen levels in the neonate should not exceed 400 mg/dL. The ingestion and absorption of colostrum directly correlates to the globulin levels in the newborn foal; therefore before ingestion of colostral immunoglobulins (IgG), the total plasma protein concentration in foals is considerably lower than in adult horses (5.2–8.0 mg/dL). Some serum chemistry values are in the higher range in foals than in adult horses, whereas others remain similar. Elevated bilirubin and mild icterus may be observed in the neonate. Severe icterus or an increased plasma concentration of conjugated bilirubin could indicate NI, septicemia, or placental dysfunction in the mare. Kidney function in neonates is like that in adult horses, with serum creatinine and blood urea nitrogen (BUN) on the high side of the normal range. An elevated creatinine during the first 48 hours of life may indicate placental dysfunction in the mare. Prerenal azotemia (elevated creatinine and urea) can be seen with dehydration and hypovolemia. The liver enzymes, including gamma glutamyl transferase (GGT), sorbitol dehydrogenase, and alanine transaminase, will all be elevated. Glucose is also consistently elevated in healthy foals as a result of constant nursing. A key point to remember: the trend of serial laboratory results, rather than any single value at a given point, is more indicative of the direction of a disease process.

The Neonatal Period: The Sick Foal

By default, any gestational abnormality displayed in the mare (i.e., twins, placentitis) automatically places the foal into a higher risk category for disease. Postpartum factors, such as FPT or any abnormal behavior observed in the foal, are also high risk concerns. If foals are compromised for any reason, they are more likely to develop bacteremia (bacterial infection in the bloodstream) and sepsis. Three main sites of entry for bacteria are the GI tract, the respiratory tract, and the umbilicus. Initially, foals may appear normal but deteriorate rapidly within 24 to 48 hours. The neonate's lack or loss of affinity for the mare (manifesting as aimless wandering) is often the first clinical sign observed and may be an early indication of neonatal maladjustment syndrome (NMS) or dummy foal syndrome, which requires immediate veterinary intervention. Other early indicators of disease or abnormalities prompting evaluation include lethargy, fever, decreased appetite, decreased suckle reflex, and increased recumbency. All foals should be monitored for normal mentation, nursing, defecation, urination, and activity during the first week of life.

Premature foals are the result of gestational abnormalities in the mare. In general, foals are considered premature if delivered before 320 days' gestation. Characteristic signs of prematurity include small body size, low birth weight, a dome-shaped forehead, floppy ears, silky hair coat, entropion, flexor laxity, angular limb deformities, decreased muscle tone, generalized weakness, and inability to rise without assistance. Radiography may further validate prematurity by identifying incomplete ossification of cuboidal bones in the carpus and the tarsus. These foals require strict, confined management until ossification occurs to prevent severe nonreparative joint damage. Premature foals require intensive supportive care because they are prone to multiple simultaneous body system dysfunctions or disease processes. Dysmature foals are those that are delivered at full-term gestational age but present with similar characteristics of premature foals. Post-term foals are carried for an extended period past full term and become increasingly abnormal the longer they are in utero. These foals have "outgrown" the placenta and tend to present with a normal to large body frame, emaciation, long hair coat, weak suckle, flexor contracture, and fully erupted incisors.

> **TECHNICIAN NOTE**
>
> Early indicators of disease or abnormalities in the foal prompting evaluation include lethargy, fever, decreased appetite, decreased suckle reflex, and increased recumbency. Foals can become critically ill quickly and can rapidly deteriorate, so they need to be monitored closely for normal mentation, appetite, activity, urination, and defecation, especially in the first week of life.

Admitting the Critically Ill Foal

Regardless of the initial cause for concern in a foal, early detection and immediate, aggressive intervention, including hospitalization, are often required for a positive outcome (Box 21.6). When possible, critically ill foals should be referred to a hospital with adequate facilities and staff experienced with the intensive supportive care that neonate foals require. Upon admission to the hospital, critically ill foals require a competent team approach for diagnostic evaluation, stabilization, and ongoing care. Often, these foals arrive weak or recumbent, requiring proper foal handling knowledge. If it is necessary to carry a foal, the handler needs to place one arm around the front of the chest and the other arm behind the haunches and then lift and carry the foal. It is easy to displace fractured ribs or rupture the bladder by improperly lifting a foal from under the thorax and the abdomen. The foal should be placed in semisternal recumbency on a padded bed separate from the mare (if possible), quickly assessed, and stabilized.

• BOX 21.6 Common Diseases of Neonatal Foals

- *Neonatal encephalopathy:* "Dummy foal" or neonatal maladjustment syndrome, which results in abnormal behavior, poor nursing ability, and weakness and is associated with other problems, such as sepsis, neonatal gastroenteropathy, and neonatal nephropathy
- *Neonatal gastroenteropathy:* Abnormal gastrointestinal (GI) tract motility and absorption leading to intolerance of enteral nutrition, such as reflux noted after feeding
- *Neonatal nephropathy:* Renal insufficiency that may resolve or may be too severe for recovery
- *Neonatal isoerythrolysis:* Acute, severe anemia caused by destruction of the foal's red blood cells because of maternal antibodies causing an incompatibility reaction
- *Sepsis or septic shock:* Acute, severe bacterial infection causing multiorgan dysfunction, including poor perfusion of the limbs, cardiovascular collapse, and metabolic derangements, such as profound hypoglycemia
- *Meconium retention:* Meconium is retained in the colon, and the foal will display abdominal discomfort, such as tail flagging and rolling
- *Colitis:* Development of acute diarrhea, often caused by an infectious organism, such as rotavirus, *Salmonella* spp., or *Clostridium* spp., requiring immediate treatment in an isolated stall
- *Patent urachus:* Foal's urachus not closed and leaks urine
- *Ruptured bladder:* Foal's urinary bladder or associated structures (e.g., ureters) developing a tear, with urine leaking into the abdomen
- *Septic arthritis or septic physitis:* Development of an infected joint or growth plate
- *Failure of passive transfer (FPT):* Foal not receiving maternal antibodies from the mare's colostrum within 24 hours of age
- *Musculoskeletal abnormalities (e.g., flexural deformities, angular limb deformities):* Tendon contracture, or valgus or varus problems causing deviated limbs
- *Prematurity:* Foal born before 320 days' gestational age and exhibiting typical signs, such as low birth weight, soft hair coat, floppy ears, domed head, and incomplete ossification of cuboidal bones
- *Dysmaturity:* Very large foal born at greater-than-expected gestational age (e.g., 400 days), with long hair coat and erupted incisors; often has limb deformities
- *Entropion:* Lower eyelid rolling inward to the cornea, causing corneal abrasion or ulceration

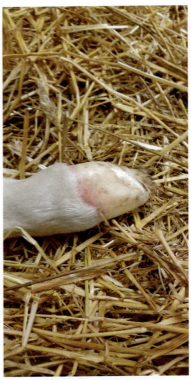

• **Fig. 21.17** Hyperemic coronary band of a septic neonatal foal.

Initial assessment of a critically ill foal often reveals signs of hypothermia, hypoglycemia, dehydration, sepsis, and hypovolemia. Clinical vital parameters and a quick examination should be obtained to facilitate immediate stabilization of the foal. Findings may include obtunded mentation; a low rectal temperature (<99°F); tachycardic (>150 bpm) or bradycardic (<60 bpm) heart rate; and/or tachypneic (>60 bpm), decreased (<20 bpm), or dyspneic respiration rate with abdominal effort. The mucus membranes may be cyanotic, hyperemic, or tacky, with a prolonged CRT of greater than 2 seconds. Ulcerations, petechiae, cyanosis, hyperemia, or icterus may also be seen elsewhere (eyes, ears, nostrils, vulva, and urethra). The eyes may appear sunken, with miotic pupils, and exhibit entropion (rolling in of the lower eyelids), uveitis, hypopyon, hyphema, or cataracts. Upon auscultation of the heart, detection of a murmur in a compromised foal may indicate an underlying abnormality that can result in pulmonary hypertension and hypoxemia. Abnormal crackles and wheezes auscultated in the lungs may present bilaterally or unilaterally. Sounds may be decreased or absent as a result of atelectasis (partial collapse of alveoli, causing decreased air movement) in recumbent foals. Edema or crepitus over the thorax may indicate rib fractures, which often occur near the heart at the costochondral junction of ribs three to eight and can be confirmed with ultrasonography. GI motility may be present, hypermotile, hypomotile, or absent. The presence of abdominal distension indicates enteritis or colitis, obstruction, torsion, or uroperitoneum (ruptured bladder or urachus). If the foal has mild colic, it will often flag its tail when defecating. The foal may roll onto its back and fold its front legs over the chest to indicate abdominal pain. Meconium retention (impaction) is a common cause of colic signs in the neonate foal and requires medical and sometimes surgical intervention. A thorough examination of the umbilicus (for heat, pain, edema, moisture, patency, or mucopurulent discharge) is necessary, because it is a common source of infection or omphalitis in the neonate. Any feces or lack thereof should be noted and specimens collected. Palpation of all four limbs, particularly the joints, is essential, because infections can occur rapidly as a primary infection or secondary to a previous or ongoing infection elsewhere in the foal. Cold distal limbs with poor digital pulse quality are indicative of poor cardiovascular perfusion and sepsis. Sepsis may also be indicated by hyperemic discoloration of the coronary band of the hoof wall (Fig. 21.17). Table 21.2 lists important considerations for evaluating the critically ill foal.

A well-organized team will simultaneously initiate stabilization of the critical foal during the initial examination, including oxygen therapy, stallside diagnostics, IV catheterization, and fluid therapy. As a degree of peripartum hypoxemia may be present, oxygen administration is beneficial to all critical foals. However, it is ideal to aseptically obtain an arterial blood gas (ABG) sample via the medial brachial artery or the lateral great metatarsal artery before administration of oxygen. The ABG sample should be obtained by using a specialized 1-mL blood gas syringe, with the plunger pulled back to 0.5 mL to allow arterial blood to fill the syringe. An ABG analysis provides accurate measurement of

TABLE 21.2 Key Physical Assessments and Self-Guiding Questions Regarding a Neonatal Foal

Physical Assessment	What to Check	Nursing Assessment Questions
Mentation and walking	• Observe the foal for signs of dullness, depression, and reluctance to move.	• Is the foal quiet and depressed or reluctant to move?
• Body condition and hair coat	• Evaluate the foal's size and body condition; many foals are about 100 pounds (45 kg). • Foals should have an adequate body condition and a soft hair coat. • If possible, it is ideal to weigh the foal every day for the first few weeks.	• Is the foal smaller or larger than expected? • Does the foal have adequate body condition? • Is the foal thin with a silky or overlong hair coat?
• Vital signs	• Assess temperature, pulse, and respiration.	• Does the foal have a fever or hypothermia? • Is the foal's heart rate increased or decreased? • Is respiratory rate increased or decreased?
• Hydration status and cardiorespiratory system	• Assess the following: • Mucous membrane color and quality • Capillary refill time (CRT) and jugular vein refill time • Pulse quality • Thoracic auscultation to assess heart rate and rhythm and detect heart murmurs or to assess pulmonary sounds • Assess whether the foal's respiratory rate and effort are within normal limits • Assess whether periods of apnea are occurring (greater than 20 seconds of breath holding)	• Are the foal's oral mucous membranes pink and moist with CRT greater than 2 seconds, or dark purple, injected, and icteric, with petechiae? • Are the foal's heart rate and rhythm consistent and within normal limits? • Are pulses strong or weak? • Does the foal have stable blood pressure? • Are nasal discharge, coughing, or other abnormalities noted on thoracic auscultation of the respiratory system?
• Abdomen, urination, and defecation	• Check for signs of abdominal pain, such as pawing or rolling • Auscultate both sides of the abdomen • Note whether the foal is urinating and defecating and how often, and if the foal strains, flags its tail, or has diarrhea or skin scalding	• Is the foal comfortable or painful? • Are borborygmi or abdominal distention present? • Do you see any urine or fecal material from the foal? • Is the external umbilical remnant small and dry or moist and large?
• Integument and eyes	• Check for decubitus ulcers, urine and/or fecal scalding, linear dermal necrosis over hocks, generalized edema, presence of entropion, corneal ulceration, hyphema, miotic pupils, injected or icteric sclerae	• Do the foal's jugular veins at the site of catheter placement have any signs of swelling or thickening? • Is the foal clean and dry? • Are the foal's eyes open and comfortable, or do they appear closed and painful?
• Metabolic derangements	• Check whether the foal's glucose levels are within normal limits	Is the foal hypoglycemic or hyperglycemic?
• Musculoskeletal assessment	• Check for joint swelling (effusion), acute lameness, joint contracture, incomplete ossification of cuboidal bones, and tendon and ligament laxity	• Is the foal walking comfortably, or does it appear lame and reluctant to move?

peripheral oxygenation. Oxygen therapy may be administered via the flow-by method, a nasal cannula or, if necessary, endotracheal intubation. A nasal cannula should be used for prolonged oxygen therapy. The cannula is inserted in the nasal passage to a point just below the level of the medial canthus of the eye and is secured to a neonate halter or the foal's muzzle. Humidified oxygen may be supplied at a flow rate of 5 to 10 L/min.

A peripheral vein, such as the cephalic or saphenous vein, may be used to obtain blood for diagnostic samples, leaving the jugular veins for venous catheterization. In addition to the ABG analysis, PCV, total protein (TP), lactate, blood glucose, and IgG (if the foal is at least 12 hours old), should be assessed quickly. Enough venous blood should be collected for a CBC, serum chemistries, electrolytes, and fibrinogen levels.

The jugular vein is most often used for venous catheterization and requires strict aseptic technique, because catheter sites are primary portals of iatrogenic infection. Catheter placement is easiest to perform in a sedated foal. Once sedated, the foal is placed in lateral recumbency and properly restrained by three assistants, using bony areas such as joints to avoid soft tissue trauma. Placing a rolled towel under the neck will improve visualization and stabilization of the jugular vein, especially in a dehydrated foal. The catheter site should be clipped and aseptically prepared with chlorhexidine scrub solution and alcohol with a bleb of local anesthetic (lidocaine or mepivacaine) injected SC at the catheter insertion site. A 16-gauge or 14-gauge, 3.5-inch or 5.5-inch long, over-the-wire (OTW), long-term, nonreactive polyurethane catheter (i.e., Milacath; Mila International, Inc., Florence, KY) is the standard of care for use in all foals. These catheters come in single, double, or triple lumen, with or without an integrated extension set allowing venous access for blood collection, fluid therapy, and partial or total parental nutrition. Blood for anaerobic and aerobic culture can be obtained aseptically via the catheter before antibiotic therapy is initiated. A needleless port or injection cap is placed on the end of the extension set, the line is flushed with heparinized saline, and the catheter is secured with suture. The catheter site is covered with sterile gauze sponges and wrapped with Elastikon or ExpandDover elastic tape (Johnson & Johnson Elastikon Tape).

Shock fluid therapy at a short-term rate of 20 mL/kg per hour can begin immediately by using isotonic fluids, such as LRS, PlasmaLyte, Normosol-R, or Hartmann solution, to stabilize dehydration or hypovolemia. Foals with hypoglycemia (normal is 80–160 mg/dL) can be administered 1% to 10% (20–200 mL of 50% dextrose/1 L of fluid) dextrose solutions as a continuous rate infusion (CRI). Bolus administration of dextrose solutions should be avoided, because it can exacerbate neurologic signs and result in rebound hypoglycemia. Blood glucose levels require careful monitoring as hyperglycemia is also detrimental to the neonatal foal. The normal maintenance fluid requirement in the neonate foal is 90 mL/kg per 24 hours.

Hypothermia should be addressed with gradual warming blankets, warm fluid bags, heat lamps, or forced-air warming units (Bair Hugger; 3M Inc., St. Paul, MN). A compromised foal has difficulty with thermoregulation and can overheat quickly, resulting in hyperthermia. Hyperthermia affects ventilation and pulmonary function, increases caloric requirements, and may induce seizure activity.

Indirect blood pressure is easily obtained with a properly sized cuff positioned correctly at the base of the foal's tail (obtain at least three readings for average blood pressure). Blood pressure should be monitored closely because hypotension is one of the first indications that a foal is not responding to treatment. The use of antibiotic therapy will be determined after CBC and serum chemistry results are obtained. Once the foal has been stabilized, further diagnostics, such as radiography and ultrasonography, may be used to further evaluate the foal's status to determine immediate and long-term care in the hospital.

TECHNICIAN NOTE

Once a neonatal foal is admitted to a veterinary hospital, blood pressure should be monitored closely, because hypotension is one of the first signs that the foal is not responding to treatment.

Over the course of hospitalization, the foal may require additional treatment, including maintenance of fluids, nutritional support, blood pressure support, treatment for orthopedic conditions, and a ventilator. The best outcome for a neonatal foal occurs with early detection of disease on the farm, followed by rapid intervention before the foal becomes critically ill. See Case Presentation 21.1.

TECHNICIAN NOTE

A critically ill neonatal foal should be evaluated and treated quickly by a veterinary team at a referral hospital for an optimal outcome.

Monitoring and Nursing Care

Vigilant 24-hour monitoring and nursing care provided by trained intensive care team members is the most important factor for hospitalized critically ill foals. Subtle changes in behavior or clinical parameters signifying improvement or deterioration in the foal's condition occur rapidly. Identifying and addressing these changes quickly can have a significant impact on the successful outcome of the foal. Some complications of hospitalized foals include resistant nosocomial infections, multiple sites of infection, corneal ulcers, decubital ulcers, and malnutrition. Positive or negative trends in clinical parameters can be identified readily on flow sheets. Complete physical examinations should be performed multiple times daily, paying particular attention to catheter sites, joints, umbilicus, and lung fields.

The hallmarks of nursing care for the foal include strict attention to asepsis and attention to detail. Gloves should always be worn when directly handling the neonate, administering medications, changing fluids or IV lines, and so on. Vigilant monitoring of catheter sites is required. If heat, pain, swelling, or "ropiness" is observed, catheters should be removed immediately to prevent thrombosis of the vein. Catheters should be flushed with heparinized saline every 6 hours if IV fluids are not being administered, and saline should be flushed between administrations of multiple medications to prevent precipitate formation. Needles and syringes should not be reused, injection caps should be changed daily, and accidently disconnected lines should be considered contaminated and replaced. The interval for catheter replacement depends on the type of catheter used and the status of the vein. Skin injection sites should be clean and dry, with intramuscular injections limited to the semimembranosus region of the hind limb. Foals should be kept clean, dry, and warm; recumbent foals are susceptible to fecal and urine dermatitis and scalding. Continual replacement of bedding, diapers, and other absorbent pads is required to prevent this from occurring. Separate caretakers for each foal is ideal; however, if it is necessary to care for multiple foals, the technician should wash hands, change gloves, use separate equipment, and treat the least critical patient first to avoid cross contamination.

A recumbent foal requires constant attention and needs to be maintained in sternal recumbency and turned every 2 hours to facilitate adequate lung perfusion, minimize atelectasis, and prevent decubitus ulcers (bed sores) that occur over the bony structures of the elbows, hips, and hocks. Sternal recumbency can be accomplished with the use of pads, pillows, or bean bags (Fig. 21.18). Recumbent or weak foals should be encouraged or stimulated to stand, ambulate, and nurse. Physical therapy, consisting of complete passive range of mobility in all four limbs, is beneficial in recumbent, nonambulatory foals. Two persons may be required to safely and correctly stand or turn over large foals, taking care to never grab the foal around the abdomen or thorax or roll the foal over on its back to change recumbency. The tail may be used to assist a foal to stand; however, the tail should not be used to lift the

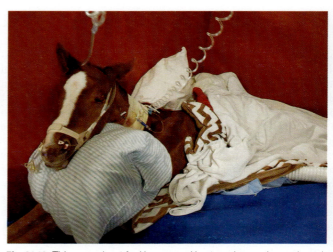

• **Fig. 21.18** This recumbent foal is propped in sternal recumbency by using pillows and padding.

CASE PRESENTATION 21.1

Septicemia in a Neonatal Foal

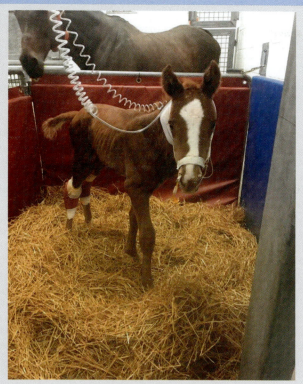

• **Fig. 21.A** The foal is maintained in a foal stall, but permitted to nurse every 2 hours. Foal improvement demonstrated with standing, walking, and beginning to nurse.

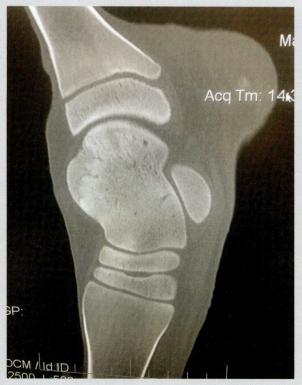

• **Fig. 21.B** Radiograph of the foal's tarsus, showing severe osteomyelitis. Multifocal osteomyelitis lesions of right carpal bone, right distal radius, bilateral tarsal bones, and bilateral tibiae.

A large, 1-day-old Thoroughbred colt presented with signs of colic and suspected sepsis. The foal reportedly stood to nurse approximately 2 hours after birth but was then up and down the remainder of the night, exhibiting signs of colic. The referring veterinarian noted that the foal was ambulatory but weak and dehydrated. Abdominal ultrasonography revealed a distended stomach and hypomotile loops of small intestine. A nasogastric tube was passed with extreme difficulty because of gastric distension; no reflux was obtained. Bloodwork indicated leukopenia, elevated lactate, and greater than 800 mg/dL of immunoglobulin G (IgG). The foal was treated with intravenous (IV) fluids, hyperimmune plasma, ceftiofur, metronidazole, ceftazidime, and flunixin meglumine prior to referral.

Upon admission to a specialty hospital, the colt was able to stand with assistance but was very dull in mentation. Vital parameters included rectal temperature 94.0°F; heart rate 72 beats per minute (bpm); respiratory rate 40 breaths per minute; tacky, pink mucous membranes; and capillary refill time (CRT) less than 2 seconds. The foal was sedated with diazepam, and an IV catheter was aseptically placed in the left jugular vein. Blood was drawn, and samples for complete blood count (CBC), serum biochemistry, and blood culture were submitted. Results indicated severe leukopenia ($1.5 \times 10^3/\mu L$) with neutrophilic toxic changes, including Döhle bodies; hyperlactemia (91.1 mg/dL); hypoglycemia (38 mg/dL); and mild azotemia (BUN 35 mg/dL; creatinine 2.44 mg/dL). Abdominal ultrasonography confirmed the presence of a markedly distended stomach and distended, amotile loops of small intestine. The foal received a 1-L bolus of LRS and a 1-L bolus LRS + 5% dextrose, then was placed on a CRI of LRS + 5% dextrose solution at maintenance rate (90 mL/kg per hour). The foal was also placed on prokinetic CRIs of lidocaine and metoclopramide. Antibiotic and anti-inflammatory therapy were initiated with ceftiofur and flunixin meglumine. Tentative diagnoses at this time were colic as a result of enteritis/ileus, sepsis, and neonatal ischemic encephalopathy. The owners were advised of the poor prognosis, but they elected to continue treatment.

The next day, the foal was transferred to the equine internal medicine service, where an indwelling nasogastric feeding tube was placed to drain gastric reflux, a nasal cannula was placed to provide oxygen therapy, and an indwelling urinary catheter was placed to drain an enlarged bladder. Antibiotic therapy was adjusted to include amikacin and metronidazole, and ceftiofur was increased in frequency to four times daily. Ongoing medical therapy included sucralfate to protect the gastric mucosa, flunixin meglumine, IV fluids (LRS); lidocaine to stimulate gastric motility; and Clinimix 5/20 (dextrose and amino acids). CRI was initiated at 25% of the foal's caloric needs. The foal was assisted to stand every 2 hours with recumbency change, and pads were used to maintain the foal in sternal recumbency to prevent atelectasis.

The foal gradually improved over a week of hospitalization and began to stand, walk, and nurse while still receiving adequate nutritional supplementation (Fig. 21.A). After a week of hospitalization, the foal was bright, alert, and responsive and moved freely about the stall, nursing frequently. Although the foal exhibited laxity in all four limbs, no lameness was observed. No heat or effusion was palpated within joints or distal limbs. The foal continued to be maintained on IV antibiotic therapy, gastroprotectants, probiotics, and flunixin meglumine.

Approximately 10 days after admission, the foal was evaluated for continued tendon laxity and palpable effusion in both tarsi and the right carpus, although no lameness was noted. Full-series radiography was performed on both carpi and tarsi joints, at which time there was no obvious evidence of bony changes. The foal was anesthetized stallside, and an arthrocentesis was performed on the right carpus and both tarsocrural joints. Cloudy, cellular joint fluid consistent with sepsis was obtained for fluid analysis and aerobic culture. Approximately 500 mL of LRS was lavaged through the right carpus, and all joints were injected with amikacin. A full-limb bandage was placed on the right forelimb, and both hocks were bandaged. The white blood cell (WBC) counts in all submitted samples was elevated. Each day, the foal was placed under general anesthesia to perform regional limb perfusions and copious joint lavages. The foal was confined to a heavily straw-bedded foal cage to limit activity, yet was allowed to nurse every 2 hours. A multidrug-resistant *Escherichia coli* strain was isolated from the

Continued

foal from recumbency, as fractures can occur. Ambulatory foals are generally restrained with one arm around the chest and one around the hindquarters or by grasping the base of the tail (using the "less is best" theory). If necessary, a single person can easily lay a neonate foal down using the "foal folding" technique. This requires the handler to stand at the foal's side and simultaneously fold the head/neck and the hindquarters (by grasping the base of the tail) in toward each other, allowing the foal to slide down the front of the handler's body to the ground. The recumbent foal can then be properly restrained in lateral recumbency, with the same handler applying pressure directly behind the ears, a second handler restraining the forelimbs between their own legs, and a third person restraining the hind limbs in the same manner.

Neonatal Foal Nutrition

A healthy foal will consume about 15% of its BW on day one, and up to 25% to 30% of its body weight daily, gaining 2 to 4 lb/day over the first month of life. While the foal is in the hospital, every attempt should be made to encourage it to nurse from the mare to meet its caloric requirements; however, this may not be an option in a critically ill foal. Foals that are unable to nurse but which maintain a good suckle reflex may be fed milk from a pan/bucket or bottle (least desirable). Medical complications, such as aspiration pneumonia, and long-term behavioral dysfunction without appropriate development of social skills gained from being raised by the mare, are concerns. A small-diameter indwelling nasogastric feeding tube can be placed in weak foals to allow for enteral feeding every 2 hours (foals are able to nurse around these tubes). Correct feeding tube placement can be difficult, because their small diameter makes them difficult to palpate in the esophagus. Radiographic confirmation may be used to position the feeding tube; the radiopaque stylet and tip of the feeding tube should be visualized caudal to the diaphragm. Because feeding tubes can be dislodged inadvertently by the foal, tube placement should be verified before each feeding. If the foal is not nursing, mares in the hospital with a sick foal should be milked out every 2 hours to stimulate continued milk production. The mare's udder and the caretaker's hands should be clean. Fresh mare's milk is the ideal source of enteral nutrition in a foal and is easily digestible; however, frozen mares' milk or foal replacers (high salt content) may be used. Cow's milk must be diluted, or 2% milk with 50% dextrose (20 g/L) may be used. Goat's milk is palatable but may cause metabolic abnormalities. Complications, such as diarrhea,

constipation, colic, and dehydration, can occur when substituting fresh mare's milk. All utensils used in feeding foals should be thoroughly cleaned and disinfected before and after use, because the GI tract is a potential portal for infection. Once reconstituted, milk replacers should be kept refrigerated and should be discarded after 2 hours at room temperature.

If possible, a hospitalized foal should be weighed daily. Although the resting energy requirement in a sick neonate is approximately one-third (50 kcal/kg per day) of the requirements of a healthy foal, the GI tract often is compromised and cannot tolerate enteral feeding. It is best to start the foal out on small volumes of milk (about 1%–5% of the body weight) given up to every 2 hours and increased as tolerated by the foal. Foals should be standing or placed in sternal recumbency during and for 30 minutes after receiving enteral feeding to prevent regurgitation and aspiration. Discontinue enteral feeding if regurgitation, abdominal distention, colic, or severe diarrhea occurs. Critically ill neonates may require IV parenteral nutritional supplementation for sufficient energy intake, because it prevents catabolism. Dextrose-containing solutions can be used for short durations of about 24 to 48 hours at a starting rate of 4 to 8 mg/kg per minute. Constant rate infusion pumps should be used when administering dextrose solutions, and strict monitoring of blood glucose is required. Critically ill foals sometimes do not tolerate even low rates of dextrose solutions, necessitating exogenous insulin therapy for regulation. After 24 to 48 hours, if enteral feeding is absent or continues to decrease, parenteral solutions with added amino acids might be warranted. Commercial premixed products are available. The initial parenteral flow rate should be one-quarter of the end target rate, increasing every 4 to 6 hours as the foal tolerates, dependent on blood glucose levels. Total parenteral nutrition comprises glucose, amino acids, and lipids, which is readily used by foals as an energy source. However, lipids are also a perfect medium for bacterial growth and require strict aseptic technique during administration. The use of multilumen catheters and regular changing of IV lines and injection ports decreases contamination risk.

> **TECHNICIAN NOTE**
>
> Fresh mare's milk is the ideal source of oral nutrition for foals and is easily digestible. When available, mare's milk should be used to feed healthy and critically ill neonatal foals. Milk replacers formulated for foals can also be used, but they often have a high salt content and can be difficult for neonatal foals to digest.

Summary

Working with compromised neonatal foals is extremely challenging and requires time, effort and skill. However,

sometimes, despite a veterinary medical team's best efforts, a foal dies or is ultimately euthanized. This can be disheartening to the veterinary nurses and doctors who worked hard to save the foal's life. Nevertheless, many foals do survive, despite poor odds, and this is due, in great part, to the tireless efforts of dedicated veterinary personnel. It is this level of caring and dedication that moves the profession of veterinary technology forward.

Recommended Readings

Neonatology of Puppies and Kittens
Casal ML. Feline paediatrics. In: Raw ME, Parkinson TJ, eds. *The Veterinary Annual*. London, UK; 1995:210.

Davidson AP. Approaches to reducing neonatal mortality in dogs. In: Concannon PW, England III G, Verstegen J, Linde Forsberg C, eds. *Recent Advances in Small Animal Reproduction*. Ithaca, NY: International Veterinary Information Service; 2003.

Gunn-Moore D. *Small Animal Neonatology: They Look Normal When They are Born and Then They Die*. Prague: Czech Republic; 2006. WSAVA Proceedings.

Hotson-Moore P, Hughes A. *BSAVA Manual of Practical Animal Care*. Wiley; 2007.

Little SE. *The Cat: Clinical Medicine and Management*. St. Louis: Elsevier Saunders; 2012.

Lopate C. *Management of Pregnant and Neonatal Dogs, Cats, and Exotic Pets*. Wiley-Blackwell; 2012.

Margolis CA, Casal ML. Neonatal Resuscitation. In: Drobatz KJ, Hopper K, Rozanski E, Silverstein DC, eds. *Textbook of Small Animal Emergency Medicine*. Wiley-Blackwell; 2018.

Neonatology of the Foal
Bucca S, Carli A, Fogarty UMG. How to assess equine fetal viability by transrectal ultrasound evaluation of fetal peripheral pulses. Orlando, FL: *AAEP Proceedings*; 2007:335–338.

Cannisso IF, Ball BA, Trodesson MH, Silva ESM, Davolli GM. Decreasing pH of mammary gland secretions is associated with parturition and is correlated with electrolyte concentrations in pre-foaling mares. *Vet Rec*. 2013;173(9):218.

Cassino IF. Update on placentitis in mares: Diagnosis and treatment. Extracted from Canisso IF, Ball BA, Erol E, Squires EL, Trodesson M. Comprehensive review on equine placentitis. In: Las Vegas, NV: *AAEP Proceeding*; 2015.

Chapman AC. *Nursing Care for Neonatal Foals*. Online Proceedings: ACVIM; VIN; 2008.

McKenzie III HC, Geor RJ. How to provide nutritional support of sick neonatal foals. *AAEP Proc*. 2007;53:202–208.

Paradis MR. *Normal Foal Nutrition*. In: Anaheim, CA: AAEP Proceedings; 2012:399-401.

Reef VB, Vaala WE, Worth LT, et al. Ultrasonic assessment of fetal well-being during late gestation: Development of an equine biophysical profile. *Equine Vet J*. 1996;28:200–208.

Stoneham SJ. *Assessing the Newborn Foal, Equine Neonatology*. A Caseload Approach; 2006:1–11. Chapter 1.

Wilkins PA. *High-Risk Pregnancy, Equine Neonatology*. A Caseload Approach; 2006:13–29. Chapter 2.

22

Care of Birds, Reptiles, and Small Mammals

LORELEI D'AVOLIO

CHAPTER OUTLINE

LEARNING OBJECTIVES

When you have completed this chapter, you will be able to:

1. Define and spell all key terms in this chapter.
2. Do the following regarding the intake process and examination of birds:
   - Collect an accurate and thorough clinical history for an avian patient and explain proper capture and restraint techniques for an effective and timely examination with minimal stress to the patient.
   - Discuss proper nutrition and husbandry of pet birds.
   - Discuss the physical examination process.
3. Explain sample collections and diagnostic procedures commonly used in birds and describe proper anesthetic techniques.
4. Describe the common routes for administering medication to birds, gavage, hand-feeding, and grooming.
5. Discuss avian nutrition.
6. Manage the hospitalized avian patient.
7. List the materials needed to properly treat and handle reptiles in the veterinary hospital with regard to zoonotic diseases, transmission, and prevention of *Salmonella* and understanding of the information needed for an accurate and thorough clinical history of a reptile patient.
8. Describe sample collections and diagnostic procedures commonly used in reptiles.

9. Understand anesthesia and intubation recommendations for the chelonian, snake, and lizard.
10. Describe husbandry requirements for the reptilian patient, including nutrition, temperature, humidity, lighting, and substrate requirements.
11. Explain the proper care of ferrets, including handling, grooming, phlebotomy, anesthesia, nursing management, and nutritional requirements.
12. Discuss the common presenting complaints of ferrets.
13. Explain the proper care of rabbits, including housing, nutritional requirements, anesthetic techniques, and intravenous access.
14. Describe some common presenting complaints in pet rabbits.
15. Explain the proper care of rodents, including antibiotic therapy, anesthetic techniques, antiparasitic agents, and nutritional requirements, specifically for guinea pigs, hamsters, gerbils, rats, and chinchillas.
16. Describe the proper care of hedgehogs and sugar gliders, including husbandry requirements, dietary requirements, and common disease conditions.

KEY TERMS

Apteric
Chelonian
Cloaca
Conjunctivitis
Crepuscular
Crop
Dysbiosis
Ecdysis
Giardia

Gram stain
Heterophils
Molting
Palpebral edema
Poikilothermic
Precocious
Preferred optimal temperature zone
Scutes

Introduction

Exotic pet ownership in the United States is increasing and consequently, more owners are willing to pay for specialized health care for these unique animals. This chapter will discuss nondomestic pet species, with particular attention paid to individual requirements of birds, reptiles, and commonly kept small mammals. It is important to note that approximately 85% of the presenting disease problems of companion exotic animals result from pet owners' lack of knowledge of basic nutrition and husbandry for that particular species. With so much misinformation available online now, it is imperative that the veterinary community, including veterinary technicians, take the lead in serving as the information resource for owners of companion exotic species. With proper education of pet owners, all species covered in this chapter will have a greater chance of living fulfilled and healthy lives.

Birds

Birds should be transported in a pet carrier made of durable fabric or plastic that a parrot cannot destroy, with a sturdy perch and locks to prevent accidental escape. Owners can be creative: a shoe box with holes and the lid secured with rubber bands could be appropriate for a parakeet, and small dog/cat crates can be used for transporting larger parrots. Owners should bring photos of the enclosure at home to give a more accurate visual description of cage size, hygiene, and cage furniture/enrichment. Owners should also bring fresh samples of droppings from the cage for evaluation and samples of the food offered to the birds, any supplements used, and any medications the birds may currently be taking.

> **TECHNICIAN NOTE**
> Owners should be advised to take photos of the enclosure at home and bring droppings from the cage to allow the medical team to visually evaluate them.

Taking the Clinical History

Obtaining a proper history from pet bird owners is a critical part of the health examination and something many technicians do when starting appointments for the veterinarian. The following is a suggested list of questions to ask bird owners either on a history form they can fill out or in an interview during the visit:
- *Signalment* (includes species, gender, and age).
- *Origin:* Where was the bird obtained? How long has it been owned by the current owner?

- *Environment:* What are the dimensions, construction, and design of the cage? What is the design and composition of the water and food bowls, substrate, and perches? Where is the bird kept (indoors or outdoors)? In what room of the house is it kept (e.g., kitchen or garage, where potential toxins may be located)? Are insecticides, household cleaners, air fresheners, or other chemicals used around the house in the vicinity of the cage?
- *Enrichment/Exercise:* Is the bird allowed out of the cage and, if so, for how long? Are the wings clipped? If not, is the bird allowed to fly freely, and how well is it supervised? If the bird does not fly, what other forms of exercise does it get? What kind of foraging and enrichment opportunities are available to the bird?
- *Diet/Appetite:* What foods are offered to the bird (e.g., commercially formulated diet, seed, fruits, vegetables, grain)? Of the foods offered, what does the bird actually eat (e.g., 50% pellets, 30% fruit, 10% nuts, 10% vegetables). How often and how much is the bird fed? Are vitamins and minerals added to the food? How often is the water changed?
- *Feces:* Questions regarding the consistency, color, odor, and number of droppings per day are all important. Have feces been previously submitted for parasite evaluation?
- *Other pets:* Are there other birds in the same cage or in the household? Does the owner maintain a quarantine policy? Are there other, potentially predatorial, animals in the home? If so, how do the owners keep the bird safe?
- *Sleep patterns:* Is the bird cage covered at night? If so, for how many hours?
- *Molting cycle:* When did the bird go through its last general molt? Are any abnormalities evident in the feather coat or feather growth?
- *Behavior:* What is the overall attitude and behavior of the bird? Does it have a chosen "mate" in the home? Is it social with a variety of people? Have behavior-related problems been reported in the past (e.g., feather destruction, overvocalizations, extreme aggression, etc.)?
- Previous medical history
- Presenting complaint

The Physical Examination Process

Capture and restraint are usually necessary for an examination but can be very stressful for the birds and the veterinary staff. Birds that are aggressively captured and restrained can develop serious phobias or other unwanted behaviors, and this should be avoided.

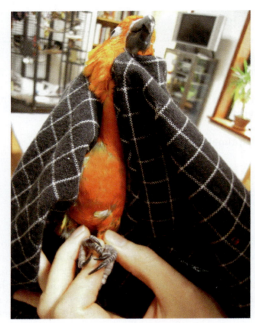

• **Fig. 22.1** Once the bird is held in a towel, technicians must be careful to restrain the head safely while taking care not to compress the chest.

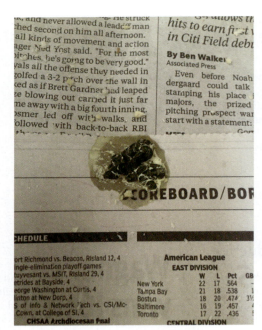

• **Fig. 22.2** Normal psittacine stool, with solid feces, white urates, and liquid urine.

Good technique for capture and restraint takes practice, and these procedures should be performed calmly and gently. A small towel can be presented, along with food treats and soft words to calm the bird. The towel should be placed gently around the bird's wings and head, with care being taken not to damage the eyes. Birds should not be chased around the examination room, snatched quickly from a carrier, or yanked or pulled from a cage. Some birds that experience more anxiety than others may benefit from anxiolytic agents, such as midazolam (2 mg/kg intranasally), to prevent a severe stress response. Midazolam can easily be reversed with flumazenil at the end of the visit.

Birds do not have a diaphragm, and their chest must be able to expand and contract to allow them to breathe. Once in the towel, technicians must be careful to restrain the head, wings, and feet safely while not compressing the chest (Fig. 22.1). Once the examination has been completed, positive reinforcement, provided by communicating gently with the bird, offering food rewards, or preening, will aid in transitioning the bird back to the owner or to the transport carrier.

Sample Collections and Procedures Commonly Used in Birds

Fecal Analysis

Avian droppings have three components: (1) feces, which are generally brown to green and formed like normal stool; (2) uric acid, which is how avian kidneys convert and excrete ammonia, and is generally white and pasty; and (3) urine, which is the liquid part (Fig. 22.2). Technicians should become familiar with the appearance of normal stool to determine the difference between polyuria (excessive urine output) and diarrhea (unformed or liquid changes in the fecal part of the dropping). Fecal parasites may be detected on fresh smears with saline and a coverslip. This is the best method of checking for protozoa such as *Giardia,* which can cause gastrointestinal problems. Fecal flotation will allow parasite ova (e.g., ascarids, *Capillaria* spp.) to float to the slide surface.

Fecal sedimentation is an important procedure for the diagnosis of flukes, which may be seen in wild avian species, including raptors. Fecal specimens that are **Gram stained** may provide information regarding the microbial flora (e.g., bacteria or fungi) of the patient's digestive tract by selectively staining different kinds of microbiota with different colors. Most pet bird species have predominantly gram-positive organisms, which appear pink with the Gram stain, inhabiting the digestive system. Gram-negative bacteria will stain purple. This test can also be helpful in diagnosing candidiasis, *Clostridium perfringens* infection, or avian gastric yeast *Macrorhabdus* sp. (Fig. 22.3).

TECHNICIAN NOTE

Most pet bird species have predominantly gram-positive organisms inhabiting the digestive system.

Cloacal Swab

A cloacal swab is often performed on avian species to obtain samples for polymerase chain reaction (PCR) analysis. The DNA samples are used to test for infectious diseases, such as *Chlamydia psittaci* or polyomavirus infection. Cloacal swabs are also used to obtain samples for microbial culture or viral isolation. Swabs should gently be inserted through the vent, which is the entrance into the **cloaca**. The cloaca is the common chamber where urine, urates, feces, eggs, and semen terminate before being pushed out through the vent. Microculturettes should be used to avoid causing trauma to this delicate tissue.

Crop Sampling

The **crop** is an outpouching of the esophagus located above a bird's sternum, where food is stored before digestion (Fig. 22.4). Samples may be taken directly with a sterile swab or by using a tube to flush and remove sterile saline from the crop. When obtaining samples, a beak speculum must be used to prop open the beak (Fig. 22.5) to prevent the patient from biting/breaking the

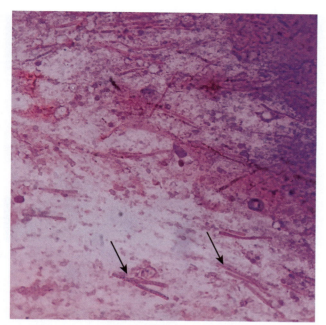

• **Fig. 22.3** Avian gastric yeast *(black arrows)* can be found on a gram-stained fecal smear under 100× oil immersion.

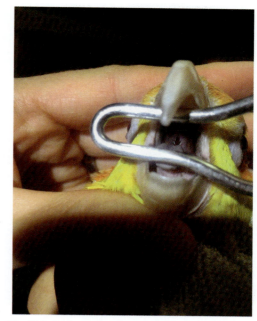

• **Fig. 22.5** Oral examination with a metal beak speculum.

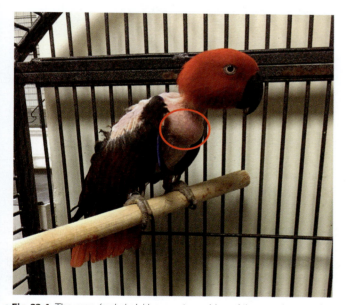

• **Fig. 22.4** The crop *(red circle)* is an outpouching of the esophagus where food is stored prior to digestion.

culturette and swallowing the tip or damaging their beak on the tube. The culturette or sampling tube should be placed through the bird's oral cavity into the crop. Tubes should be made of soft, durable rubber or stainless steel with a ball tip to protect the delicate lining of the crop from getting ripped by rough or pointed edges. An important tip is to always use a tube that has a diameter larger than the glottis to prevent accidentally placing the tube into the trachea. Sterile saline is flushed into the crop, agitated, and then aspirated back though the tube. The saline can then be used to perform a direct microscopic examination, in which a wet mount technique is used to evaluate the sample for protozoan parasites (e.g., *Trichomonas* spp.), avian gastric yeast, and *Candida albicans*. Slides may be prepared for cytologic examination with Diff-Quik

or Wright stain and then examined to look for inflammatory cells, such as **heterophils**, which are analogous to neutrophils and are the most abundant granulocytes in avian, reptile, and some small mammalian species. Culturette samples may be submitted for culture and sensitivity.

> **TECHNICIAN NOTE**
>
> An important tip is to always use a tube that has a diameter larger than the glottis for feeding or performing a crop wash to avoid accidentally placing the tube into the trachea.

Hematology/Phlebotomy

Hematology is an important part of the diagnostic evaluation of avian patients. Common venipuncture sites include the right jugular vein, basilic vein, and the medial metatarsal vein. Each location of blood collection has its own advantages and disadvantages; the veterinarian and the technician will often choose their own sites of preference, but the right jugular vein is the recommended site for most, if not all, pet bird species. A blood sample should never be obtained from a clipped claw "toenail." This is painful for the patient and often causes lameness for several days after the procedure. It also may result in poor blood flow, low yield, and invalid or contaminated results.

The right jugular vein is large and is easily found in most birds on the right dorsolateral aspect of the neck (Fig. 22.6). However, it is highly mobile and therefore can be difficult to stabilize. In most birds, the right jugular vein is located in an *apteric* (normal area of skin where feathers do not grow) tract lateral to the trachea. With practice and proper restraint, avian jugular venipuncture becomes an easy procedure to perform.

> **TECHNICIAN NOTE**
>
> The right jugular vein is the recommended site for venipuncture in most, if not all, companion avian species.

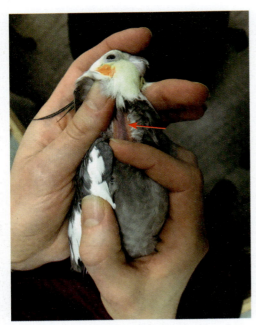

• **Fig. 22.6** The apteric area and right jugular vein *(red arrow)*.

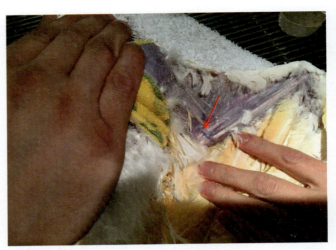

• **Fig. 22.7** The basilic vein *(red arrow)*. Ventral view of humerus, radius, and ulna.

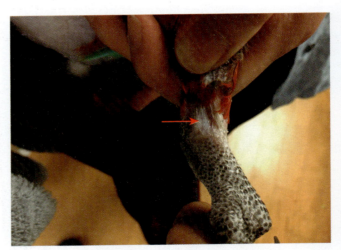

• **Fig. 22.8** The medial metatarsal vein *(red arrow)*.

The basilic vein is accessible and easy to visualize (Fig. 22.7) in birds weighing greater than 300 g; however, when the needle is removed from this vein, it is common for a large hematoma to form. Technicians should apply pressure to the site for at least 1 minute after the needle has been removed to prevent or reduce hematoma formation. In larger parrot species and other birds, the basilic vein is a good choice for placement of intravenous (IV) catheters, particularly after the bird is anesthetized. Securing this catheter can, however, be challenging, and practicing bandaging techniques by using the wing feathers and a figure-of-eight bandage to tape in the catheter properly is recommended.

The medial metatarsal vein (Fig. 22.8) is another option for psittacine patients weighing greater than 300 g. Similar to the basilic vein, this site can be prone to bleeding and hematoma formation. In larger birds weighing greater than 400 g, the medial metatarsal vein is also a good choice for placement of IV catheters, which are easier to secure in this location.

Safe sample collection volumes from birds should never be greater than 1% of the bird's body weight. Technicians should take into account the potential for hematoma formation before sampling avian patients (e.g., a 45-g lovebird can tolerate blood loss of 0.45 mL, and assuming a small hematoma may form, the technician should only take 0.3 mL). The goal should always be to take the minimum amount required to fulfill the testing needs. Most tests will not require more than 1 mL of blood, and using a 1 mL syringe is sufficient. As a general rule, 29-gauge needles should be used for birds weighing less than 50 g, 27-gauge needles for birds weighing 50 to 150 g, and 25-gauge needles for birds weighing greater than 150 g. This will help minimize perivascular bleeding and hematoma formation, which can be life-threatening in small avian patients.

TECHNICIAN NOTE

Safe blood collection volumes from birds should never be greater than 1% of the bird's body weight.

Radiography

Orthogonal images include the ventrodorsal (VD) and lateral views (Figs. 22.9 and 22.10) of the whole body and are standard for avian patients. Technique charts must be developed by using the equipment available and will vary depending on machine technology; however, digital radiology has significantly simplified the process for achieving high-quality images in birds. Because good positioning and absence of motion are important for high-quality radiographs, it is generally recommended that most avian patients be sedated or anesthetized, except those with medical conditions that prevent safe sedation. Proper positioning is essential for diagnostic evaluation. For the VD view, it is critical that the keel bone and spine be aligned and for the lateral view that the hip bones overlie each other.

Other, more sophisticated diagnostic procedures include computed tomography (CT), rigid endoscopy, coelomic ultrasonography, biopsy, cytologic collection, and bone marrow aspiration. The technician's role for most of these procedures may include preparing equipment and tools, securing the animal with good restraint, providing diligent anesthesia monitoring, and obtaining images and samples.

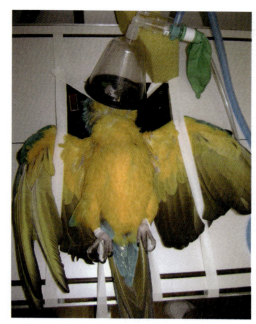

• **Fig. 22.9** Ventrodorsal positioning for radiography.

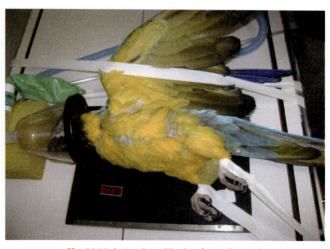

• **Fig. 22.10** Lateral positioning for radiography.

Anesthesia and Analgesia

Before any patient is anesthetized for a procedure that may produce pain, proper analgesia should be considered. Studies show that some birds have a predominant number of kappa receptors, whereas mammals have predominantly mu receptors. This means that many complete mu agonists commonly used in mammalian medicine may not be effective in birds, and evidence-based studies support this. Analgesics that work on kappa receptors, such as butorphanol (which has partial kappa agonist activity) in combination with nonsteroidal anti-inflammatory drugs (NSAIDs) and neuropathic pain blockers (e.g., gabapentin), have been shown to be the most effective analgesics currently available for birds.

Using a mask or induction box without premedicating with sedation to induce anesthesia in birds causes severe stress and should be avoided. Sedation should be used prior to induction and will decrease catecholamine release, which can complicate anesthesia. Anxiolytic agents, such as midazolam, and analgesics/sedatives, such as butorphanol or alfaxalone, will not only prevent

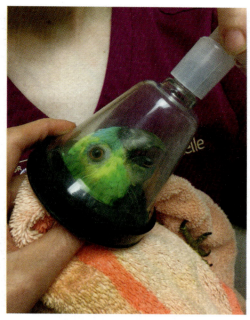

• **Fig. 22.11** Mask induction of a macaw.

stress, but also decrease the minimum anesthetic concentration (MAC) for gas anesthesia or even replace the need to use gas anesthesia, depending on the procedure. Sedatives such as telazol, dexmedetomidine, or acepromazine, used for other species, are not recommended for use in birds because of concerns about profound cardiac suppressive effects.

Isoflurane and sevoflurane gas with oxygen are both used for induction and maintenance of anesthesia for most common procedures in birds. Sevoflurane has a slightly higher MAC but a lower blood gas partition coefficient, which means higher concentration is required, but induction and recovery are faster. Due to the lower tidal volume of small birds, use of a non rebreathing anesthesia circuit such as a Jackson-Rees circuit with a 0.25- to 0.5-L reservoir bag is best.

Once sedated, a mask or induction chamber may be used to induce the patient and prepare for intubation (Fig. 22.11). For gas induction, it is recommended that the patient be preoxygenated with 100% oxygen for 3 to 5 minutes before adding the anesthetic gas. At 4% to 5% flow of isoflurane or 7% to 8% of sevoflurane, rapid induction occurs in most avian patients, and they are ready for intubation in less than 1 minute; subsequently, the rate should be lowered to 1% to 4%, depending on their response and the anesthetic used.

For intubation, a noncuffed tube is used in birds, because their trachea is made of completely closed cartilaginous rings, and pressure from a cuff could cause pressure necrosis of the mucosal layer, leading to a stricture. A cotton swab can be used to push down the tongue to expose the glottis (Fig. 22.12), and a properly sized tube will easily slide into the trachea. Once intubated, a gag should be placed in the beak to prevent the bird from breaking the tube during recovery.

TECHNICIAN NOTE

For intubation, a noncuffed tube is used in birds because their trachea is made of completely closed cartilaginous rings, and pressure from a cuff could cause severe pressure necrosis of the mucosal layer.

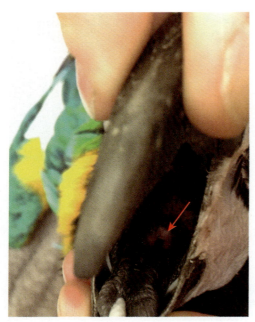

• **Fig. 22.12** A cotton swab presses down the tongue to visualize the glottis *(red arrow)*.

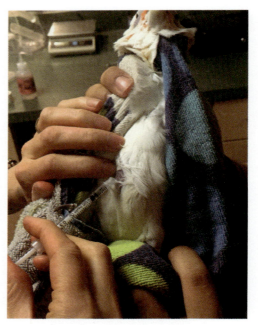

• **Fig. 22.13** Intramuscular injection.

Thorough anesthesia monitoring should take place, similar to the monitoring in other animals under general anesthesia. Monitoring devices for anesthetized birds include electrocardiography (ECG), peripheral capillary oxygen saturation (SpO_2) evaluation, mainstream capnography, Doppler ultrasonography, and indirect blood pressure monitoring. Average temperatures for birds are 99°F to 105°F. Technicians should be aware that placing temperature probes in the crop and cloaca does not provide an accurate measurement but does give estimates and can show trends and changes.

Intravenous (IV) or intraosseous (IO) fluids should be administered via constant rate infusion or syringe pump. IV sites will be based on patient size and include the medial metatarsal vein, basilic vein, or jugular vein. IO sites include the proximal tibiotarsus or distal ulna. Technicians should be prepared to ventilate birds manually or mechanically as needed and have all emergency drugs calculated and drawn up before administration of anesthetic drugs in the event they are required and need to be quickly administered via the IV or IO route.

Administration of Medication to Birds

Administration of drugs in food or water is an unreliable way to provide medications to birds. Medications will not reach adequate therapeutic levels because of inconsistent intake, particularly if the birds are sick and the food or water has a bitter taste. Administration of tablets to birds (particularly parrots) is likewise difficult and unreliable. With the advancement of veterinary compounding pharmacies, many medications can be formulated into oral suspensions that are flavored to enhance palatability. Although this does require instructing owners how to properly restrain their birds, which can be challenging, this is the best option for administering oral medications. Intramuscular (IM) injection of medication in birds should be given in the large pectoral muscle mass on either side of the keel bone (Fig. 22.13) with a small-gauge needle recommended, as 25-gauge or smaller. IV drugs can be administered via the jugular, basilic, or medial metatarsal vein.

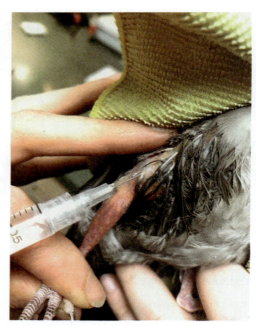

• **Fig. 22.14** Subcutaneous injection in the inguinal area.

These IV sites may only be accessible for one-time use because of hematoma formation unless an IV catheter is placed. IO catheters can be used to administer fluids and medications in the same way as IV support. Subcutaneous (SC) fluid therapy or medications should be provided in the apteric areas of the inguinal regions (Fig. 22.14). It is important that technicians can visualize the fluid bolus under the skin while administering SC fluids. If fluids are accidentally given through the SC tissue and into the body cavity or air sac, the avian patient could be at risk of drowning. Caution should also be taken to determine if certain medications are dangerous when given via the SC or IM route. For example, enrofloxacin has a high pH and can cause pain and tissue damage when given IM.

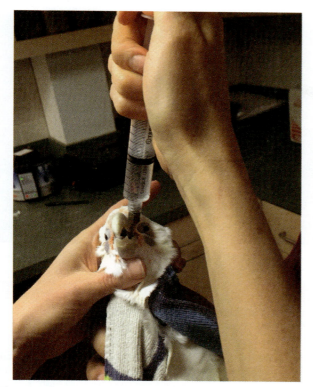

• **Fig. 22.15** Gavage tube technique for fluids, medication, or liquid food.

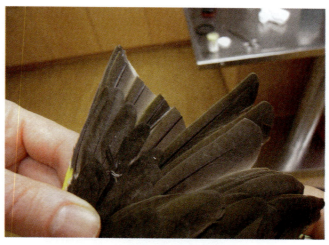

• **Fig. 22.16** Proper wing trimming.

> ### TECHNICIAN NOTE
> Intramuscular (IM) injection of drugs is recommended in the large pectoral muscle mass of birds.

Gavage and Hand-Feeding

Passing a tube into the crop of the psittacine bird is an important technique to learn in order to obtain diagnostic samples and also because gavage feeding is often necessary to administer medications and/or nutritional supplementation (Fig. 22.15). Formula options, such as Lafeber's Omnivore Critical Care Formula (Lafeber Co., Cornell, IL—currently referred to as EmerAid), can be chosen on the basis of a bird's nutritional requirements. Food that is administered by using a feeding tube should have a temperature between 99°F and 101°F. If the temperature is too low, motility can be slowed and ileus can occur. If the temperature is too high, thermal burns in the crop can result. These injuries can be prevented by careful preparation and temperature monitoring of food by the attending technician.

The glottis of the bird is located at the base of the tongue and is easy to visualize. A soft, round-tip feeding tube may be passed into the crop by passing it over the glottis into the esophagus and the crop. The tube can be easily palpated at the level of the thoracic inlet to ensure proper placement. While gavage feeding, technicians should watch the back of the bird's mouth to ensure that formula does not begin to accumulate. If the crop is overfilled, the bird may start to aspirate. If this happens, the bird should be immediately placed down, as it has a better chance of clearing its airway by itself compared with the technician or the veterinarian trying to do it by using cotton-tipped applicators.

When hand-feeding baby birds, a commercially available avian baby formula, such as Kaytee Exact (Exact, Kaytee Inc., Chilton, WI) is generally recommended. Baby birds often do not require

gavage feeding, because a feeding response can be elicited when the corners of their beaks are stimulated. Carefully putting a long-tipped syringe in the corner of the mouth and aiming at a point behind the glottis should stimulate a baby bird to bob its head, facilitating the formula to be fed as the bird swallows. Baby birds should be weighed one or two times per day to chart weight gain. It is essential that a gram scale that weighs in at least 1-g increments be used for all avian patients. The crop should be monitored for appropriate emptying as delayed emptying is a sign of illness.

> ### TECHNICIAN NOTE
> It is essential that a gram scale that weighs in at least 1-g increments be used for all avian and exotic animal patients; no substitutions are acceptable.

Grooming of Birds

Grooming procedures that veterinary technicians often perform include nail trimming, beak trimming, and clipping wing feathers, each with pros and cons that technicians should be familiar with. Allowing birds to fly provides them with vital exercise and can prevent serious psychological damage. Technicians should educate clients about the importance and the dangers of flight (escape through open doors or windows; accidents with ceiling fans, boiling water, etc.). If there is no option but to trim a bird's wings (e.g., if the bird is taken outside without a harness), wing trimming can be an acceptable practice to ensure its safety. Fig. 22.16 illustrates one technique for clipping the flight feathers of pet birds. Both wings should be clipped evenly and symmetrically to ensure stability. No more than 10 primary flight feathers need to be trimmed at the length of the primary coverts, and heavy-bodied birds, such as African gray parrots, usually only require the distal four or five feathers trimmed to prevent flight. If only one wing is clipped, the bird cannot control its flight and will become prone to injury. Owners who insist on wing trimming should be reminded that feathers will grow back unpredictably and the birds could fly unexpectedly at any time, requiring owners to be cautious in situations that are potentially dangerous for the birds.

Toenails can be trimmed in a few different ways in pet birds. Very long nails can be clipped with human nail trimmers or by electrocautery, and then a Dremel motor tool (Dremel, Inc., Racine, WI) can be used to buff the sharp corners. Chemical

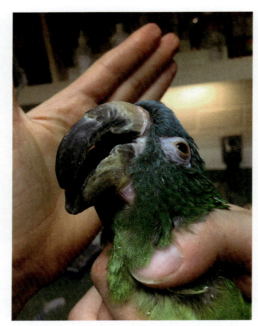

• **Fig. 22.17** A severely overgrown, diseased beak.

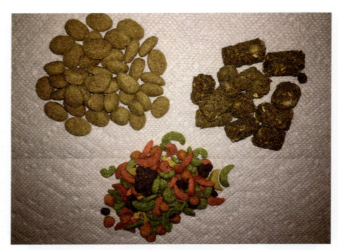

• **Fig. 22.18** Examples of commercially available pelleted diets.

cautery (silver nitrate sticks or styptic powder) should be available in case bleeding occurs during trimming. Technicians should alert owners that birds with newly trimmed nails may be clumsy and could have difficulty holding on to certain surfaces.

Beak trimming may be indicated in certain instances. Sometimes, the keratin layers are thicker than normal, and using a Dremel tool to smooth the top layer can provide cosmetically pleasing results for the owners. But trimming of the shape or length of the beak should only be done when medically required. An overgrown beak is often mistakenly thought to result from lack of things to chew or grind on; in fact, it is usually a sign of trauma, infection, or metabolic disturbance (Fig. 22.17). Clipping or grinding a parrot's beak can cause changes in the occlusal surface and may result in permanent malocclusion; only technicians trained in proper shaping should perform the procedure.

Avian Nutrition

Pet birds originate from a vast variety of geographic regions with unique vegetation, weather patterns, and seasonal changes. They evolved over millions of years to eat the foods indigenous to that locale; thus each species of bird has different nutritional needs, and no one particular diet available can meet the requirements of all birds. In the past, all-seed diets or seed diets supplemented with fruits and vegetables were recommended as the correct diet for companion avian species. This outdated recommendation has led to nutritionally induced diseases and the premature death of innumerable pet birds. Fortunately the development and general acceptance of commercially made pelleted diets, which are combined with nutritious whole foods, have reduced the occurrence of many nutrition-related illnesses, such as vitamin A deficiency.

Seed diets are deficient in certain nutrients, such as specific amino acids, vitamins (particularly vitamin A), trace minerals, and macrominerals (e.g., calcium and sodium), and are high in fat. In addition, seeds are not the primary or natural diet of most companion avian species. Of the few birds that do consume seeds in the wild (budgerigars and cockatiels), it is important to recognize that the seeds they consume are alive, sprouting, and growing, and that these birds naturally consume a wide variety of seeds. Commercial pet seed mixes are limited in variety, dried, processed with colors and additives, and often sit on pet store or warehouse shelves for weeks to months, which further diminishes their nutritional potency.

Fruits and vegetables sold for human consumption can be a valuable addition to the diet of pet birds. However, many fruits and vegetables are deficient in protein, vitamins, and minerals, and birds may select food items on the basis of water and sugar content, texture, color, and taste rather than their nutrient content. This can cause overeating of high-calorie, low-nutrient food, resulting in obesity. Good options for fruits are vitamin A–rich sources, such as papaya or mango, and low glycemic index fruits, such as berries. Good options for vegetables are broccoli, winter squashes, string beans, or sweet potatoes. Technicians should remind owners that birds will selectively eat less nutritious items (apples, grapes, bananas), and they should consider eliminating them from the daily available options.

The major benefits of commercially prepared pelleted diets are nutrient balance and convenience (Fig. 22.18). Owners should be warned that birds accustomed to eating seeds may be reluctant to try new foods. The conversion process could take time as the new foods are gradually introduced. Owners should monitor the consistency and quality of the droppings, looking for signs such as dark brown or black feces, which indicate the bird may not be eating enough. Owners should be advised to weigh the bird to ensure it is not losing too much weight and should be encouraged to try several brands of pellets until the right one for the bird is identified.

Table 22.1 presents a recommended psittacine diet. Currently, it is recommended that a commercial pelleted diet be provided

TABLE 22.1   **Recommended Psittacine Diet**

Food Group	What It Supplies	What It Lacks
Cereals and whole grains (commercial pelleted diets are primarily cereal and grain based, with vitamin and mineral supplementation added), 40%–50%	Protein, fat, B vitamins, fiber	Vitamins A, D, and K, calcium (unless using commercial pellets, which are supplemented)
Vegetables (e.g., dark-green leafy, winter squash, sweet potato, broccoli), 20%–30%	Vitamins A and K, fiber, carbohydrates ± calcium	Proteins, fats, vitamin D_3
Fruit (e.g., papaya, pomegranates, berries), approximately 15%–20%	Sugars, simple carbohydrates, antioxidants, vitamin A and C	Proteins, minerals
Meats/insects/fish, approximately 5%	Protein, fat, calcium, omega fatty acids	Fiber, vitamins, antioxidants

to companion avian species. Supplementation with a high-quality seed mixture, raw nuts, vegetables, and to a lesser extent, fruits completes the diversified diet. Birds can also safely share healthy human meals with their owners. Sharing cooked eggs, legumes, whole grains, and even lean meats or fish can be fun and healthy for pet birds when these items are not fed to excess. It is very important that owners know that avocado is toxic to birds and therefore should never be offered. "Junk food" (pizza, chips, cookies) have dangerously high levels of sugar, salt, and fat, which can be harmful to psittacines.

TECHNICIAN NOTE

It is very important that owners know that avocado is toxic to birds and therefore should never be offered to them.

Technicians should also educate owners about the importance of foraging. In the wild, birds spend much of their time flying many miles to find food sources. They have to crack nuts, peel fruits, and scavenge for insects in tree barks. Owners should be encouraged to provide opportunities to their birds in captivity to mimic some of these behaviors. Instead of just leaving a dish or two filled with food, the bird could be provided with challenges that it must overcome to obtain its meals or treats. Opening lids, tearing apart paper towels with food inside, or using the many commercially available foraging toys is a great way to keep captive birds active and stimulated. This can contribute to exercise opportunities and good mental health.

Technicians should be prepared to educate owners about ways to alter diets when pet birds become reproductively active. The calcium and protein requirements of the hen will increase as she generates eggs and feeds her chicks. These requirements will vary by species and additions to the diet, such as eggshells, cuttlebone, and live insects, may be appropriate. The addition of ultraviolet B (UVB) radiation may also assist with vitamin D synthesis and consequent calcium absorption (see the section on "Reptiles" for more information on UVB radiation).

The addition of high-quality vitamin and mineral supplements is controversial. Birds (and all animals) should ideally obtain their nutrition from healthy foods rather than from supplements. Oversupplementing could cause serious problems, such as vitamin D toxicosis, which can damage the kidneys. Birds that are eating a diet based on commercial pellets should not be supplemented with multivitamins. In instances where supplementation is recommended by a veterinarian, the supplement should be sprinkled on the food, not added to water, because many nutritional elements are denatured after a few hours, and because vitamins may taint the water with abnormal color or flavor, which can discourage the bird from drinking.

Insoluble grit (e.g., quartz, silica) is stored in the bird's ventriculus (gizzard) to mechanically break down food. This should only be offered to birds (e.g., doves) that do not hull their seeds. Oversupplementation of insoluble mineral grit may lead to gastrointestinal (GI) disease. Soluble grit (e.g., oyster shell, cuttlebone, mineral block) is completely digested and serves as a source of minerals (e.g., calcium, phosphorus). Birds that are resistant to eating pelleted diets or that are reproductively active may require additional calcium in their diet, and soluble grit is a good option.

TECHNICIAN NOTE

Insoluble grit (e.g., quartz, silica) is stored in the ventriculus (gizzard) to mechanically break down food. This should only be offered to birds (e.g., doves) that do not hull their seeds. Soluble grit (oyster shell, cuttlebone, or mineral block) is completely digested to obtain minerals.

Although feeding a well-balanced food diet is essential, it is easy to overlook the single most important dietary component: water. Because birds have no sweat glands, water intake plays an important role in thermoregulation. Breeding females may require increased amounts of water for egg production and for heat regulation while incubating eggs. Fresh, preferably filtered water should be available at all times. Many birds enjoy dunking pellets or food in their water, or take baths in their water dishes. These are positive behaviors; however, owners should be encouraged to change the water more frequently in these instances.

TECHNICIAN NOTE

Because birds have no sweat glands, water intake plays an important role in thermoregulation.

Managing the Hospitalized Avian Patient

Maintaining a proper hospital environment for birds is a vital component to successful case management. When possible, birds should be housed in a room separate from predatorial species. Fear and stress can further compromise a bird's fragile immune system, and sights and sounds of barking dogs or loudly vocalizing cats can significantly contribute to a bird's stress level. If this is not possible, using visual barriers, such as cage covers, is recommended. Additionally, birds that are suspected to have infectious diseases, such as *C. psittaci* infection, should be kept in separate rooms isolated from other birds. Standard cage banks with Plexiglass cage fronts or incubator units are helpful to prevent aerosolized pathogens from spreading. These units are also much easier to disinfect compared with wire cages. Large parrots do well in standard dog/cat cages or crates with perches, food, and water dishes. Any perches or cage furniture should be either disposable or easy to sanitize.

Sick birds have difficulty maintaining and regulating body temperature, as do birds with poor feather coats. Therefore these birds should be kept warm but not hot. Temperatures between 80°F and 90°F are best. The bird should be observed for signs of heat stress, which include panting, extended wings, and depression. An environmentally controlled cage or incubator should be available for avian patients in intensive care. Ceramic heat-emitting devices can be used to provide radiant heat if incubators are not available.

Chlamydia psittaci Infection

C. psittaci infection was historically considered the most likely differential diagnosis in sick parrots because of poor quarantine conditions and overcrowding. Prevalence of this infection has decreased with the ban on importation of parrots into the United States; however, it is still of significant concern. Clinical signs in birds can be nonspecific but may include upper respiratory infections, bright green stool or diarrhea, and vomiting. Psittacosis, which is caused by *C. psittaci*, is a zoonotic disease transmissible to humans. Birds suspected of infection with *Chlamydia* should be isolated, gloves and masks should be used to protect hospital personnel, and the feces of sick birds should be disposed of properly after thorough cleaning of the cage and bagging of disposable substrate. Transmission occurs primarily through inhalation of the infectious elementary body and can cause severe respiratory infection in humans.

> **TECHNICIAN NOTE**
>
> *Chlamydia psittaci* can be transmitted to humans, making psittacosis a zoonotic concern. Transmission occurs primarily through inhalation of the infectious elementary body and can cause severe respiratory infection in humans.

Reptiles

Although the pet reptile population does not match pet dog and cat populations, statistics show that the popularity of the reptile pet is increasing as is the need for high-quality veterinary care. The diversity of reptile species maintained in captivity requires education of owners about the health, nutritional, and environmental management of these pets. In many cases, it is the responsibility of the technician to not only handle and collect diagnostic samples but also educate owners about their captive reptile. It is therefore vital that technicians educate themselves on the husbandry needs of the most common reptiles seen in captivity.

Once a veterinary hospital decides to treat reptile species, a few pieces of specialized equipment are needed to provide an adequate hospital environment. Required medical equipment includes a gram scale, an incubator designated specifically for reptiles to prevent disease transmission to other species (Fig. 22.19), a rubber mouth speculum to facilitate oral examinations without damaging delicate teeth, snake sexing probes for gender determination, and rigid and nonrigid feeding tubes. Reptile housing equipment

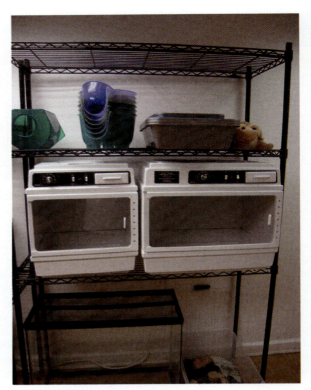

• **Fig. 22.19** Reptile incubators are necessary for proper hospital care.

must be adaptable to the different species that may be hospitalized. Examples of hospital caging and equipment include aquatic tanks with water heaters, tanks/vivariums with secure ventilated tops, UVB lighting (fluorescent light tubes or mercury vapor bulbs), heat bulbs or ceramic heat emitters, under-tank heat pads, humidifiers and misters, water filters, basking areas, and hide boxes.

> **TECHNICIAN NOTE**
>
> In many cases, it is the responsibility of the technician to not only handle and collect diagnostic samples but also educate owners about their captive reptile.

Taking the Clinical History

The following is a list of questions to ask clients regarding reptile patients:

- *Signalment:* What is the species, age, and gender of the patient?
- *Origin:* Do the owners know whether the reptile was captive bred or wild caught?
- *Environment:* Cage design, construction materials, substrates, perches, branches, hide boxes, water sources, temperature, humidity, photoperiod and exposure to direct sunlight or artificial UVB radiation and lighting, type of heat source, and the temperature gradient should be evaluated. For aquatic species, questions pertaining to water quality, filter systems used, sources of water, and frequency of water changes are important.
- *Food:* How often is food offered? How much is consumed? Are supplements used? Are insects gut loaded (fed nutritious meals before consumption)? Is food presented alive or dead?

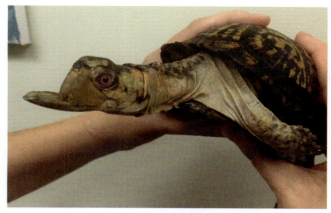

• **Fig. 22.20** A box turtle with a severely overgrown beak.

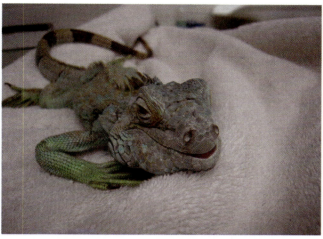

• **Fig. 22.21** Iguana with nutritional secondary hyperparathyroidism.

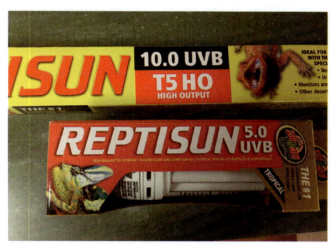

• **Fig. 22.22** Examples of ultraviolet B lights.

- *Drinking water:* How often is the water cleaned or changed? How is it offered to the animal (drippers, misters, soaking bowls, pools, etc.)?
- *Feces:* How often does the animal defecate? What is the color and consistency of the stool? Has the owner previously submitted a fecal sample for a parasite evaluation?
- *Cagemates:* Are there other reptiles in the collection? If so, what species are they? Are they housed in the same enclosure? Does the owner maintain a quarantine policy?
- *Behavior:* What is the attitude and behavior of the patient, and have any recent changes been noted?
- **Ecdysis** *(Shedding):* How often does ecdysis occur and when was the last period of ecdysis?
- *Previous medical history:* Has the animal been ill previously? Have other animals in the collection ever been ill or died?

Reptile Nutrition and UVB Radiation

Dietary requirements vary significantly from species to species, and improper feeding is a significant causative factor in many reptile disease processes. Technicians working with reptiles should become well versed in the dietary requirements of commonly seen species and be prepared to recommend high-quality reptile supplements, such as Repashy Superfoods (Specialty Pet Diets and Supplements, Oceanside, CA). There are several excellent supplements available, and the veterinarian will guide owners in this choice.

Vitamin A deficiency is commonly diagnosed in reptiles and usually manifests as an overgrown beak (*chelonians*; turtles and tortoises) (Fig. 22.20), stomatitis, dysecdysis, *palpebral edema* (inflammation of the eyelid), and *conjunctivitis* (inflammation of the conjunctival tissue around the eye). Prevention includes feeding vitamin A–rich foods, such as carrots, dark leafy greens, bell peppers, and cantaloupe, to species that consume vegetables and fruits, and feeding gut-loaded insects with vitamin A–rich foods to insectivores. Additionally, powdered multivitamins should be regularly sprinkled on food (Reptivite Reptile Vitamins; Zoomed, San Luis Obisbo, CA).

Nutritional secondary hyperparathyroidism (NSHP) is the most common of the metabolic bone diseases that are prevalent in captive reptiles. It is caused by low calcium intake, low vitamin D_3 intake (or lack of access to UVB radiation), or excessive phosphorus intake (e.g., through feeding of animal protein to herbivores) (Fig. 22.21). Like humans, reptiles require vitamin

D_3 (cholecalciferol) to absorb ingested calcium. The only way to synthesize vitamin D_3 is by exposing the skin to UVB radiation at 280- to 315-nanometer (nm) wavelengths. Exposing the animal to UVB radiation, either naturally or artificially plus feeding appropriate calcium-rich diets will help prevent NSHP. Direct unfiltered sunlight or artificial lighting with UVB bulbs is needed; UVB radiation will not pass through window glass or terrarium plastic. Many types of light bulbs are marketed as "full spectrum" or "reptile lights" but actually do not provide UVB radiation. Technicians should verify that clients have purchased lights that produce UVB radiation (Fig. 22.22) by asking about cost (UVB bulbs are significantly more expensive than regular "reptile" lights) and proper "UVB" labeling on the bulb. Additionally, these bulbs lose UVB potency in approximately 6 months, even if the visual light is still functional. Clients should be advised to purchase new bulbs every 6 months or have their bulbs tested with a UVB meter (Solarmeter, Glenside, PA.). The required amount and intensity of UVB radiation vary by species.

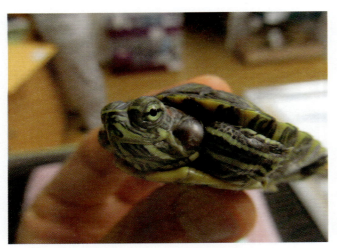

• **Fig. 22.23** Aural abscess in a red-eared slider.

- 85% vegetables, such as collards, radishes, turnip greens, dandelions, kale, cabbage, bok choy, broccoli, cauliflower, and summer and winter squash
- 10% fruits, such as grapes, papayas, pears, peaches, plums, dates, melons, strawberries, raspberries, mangoes, and tomatoes
- 5% high-protein foods (based on species), such as commercially formulated, species-specific; pellets; cereals; mice; eggs; and insects

[a]*This is a basic guide; there are many different species of chelonians with varied requirements that should be considered.*

Chelonians (Turtles, Terrapins, and Tortoises)

Chelonians are diurnal (awake during the day) and should have UVB radiation available for several hours. This will assist with shell formation and stimulate appetite and normal basking behaviors. Multivitamins containing vitamin D should be used cautiously and based on species and UVB exposure, because oversupplementation of vitamin D is dangerous. Chelonians living outside in direct sunlight may never need a vitamin D supplement, whereas indoor chelonians receiving an uncertain amount of UVB radiation should be supplemented regularly. Calcium supplementation, however, should be offered three to five times a week, regardless of UVB exposure.

Vitamin A deficiency is common in chelonians. Clinical signs include respiratory infection, edematous conjunctivitis, urogenital tract obstruction, and aural abscesses (Fig. 22.23). Hypovitaminosis A can be prevented by providing a proper diet that supplies beta carotene, which is found in such foods as earthworms, small fish, and orange or yellow vegetables, and by adding a vitamin supplement.

Land tortoises are primarily herbivorous but occasionally scavenge insects and small rodents. In captivity, diets should be composed primarily of vegetables (dark leafy greens, squash, legumes), some fruits (papaya, berries), and limited quantities of high-protein foods (Box 22.1). A variety of commercially available chelonian foods that are based on species can be used in conjunction with fresh food items. Successful care of captive tortoises relies heavily on varying the diet with proper vitamin and mineral supplementation. A shallow water dish should be provided to allow consumption and soaking, and should be changed daily or more often if soiled, because chelonians tend to defecate in water.

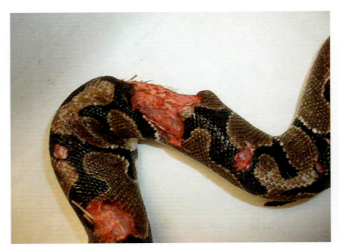

• **Fig. 22.24** This snake has sustained multiple injuries after being attacked by a live rat.

Aquatic turtles need a variety of foods to achieve a balanced diet. Much of the diet should be composed of whole animals, such as earthworms, goldfish, or guppies. Insects, such as crickets, mealworms, and grasshoppers, are also acceptable options. Feeding meats, such as hamburger, deli meats, or shellfish, is not recommended. Vegetables, such as dark leafy greens, carrots, bell peppers, cabbage, or romaine lettuce, should be offered regularly. Commercial diets are available in floating stick or pellet forms, but supplementing these diets with natural foods as described is important both for nutrition and animal enrichment. It should be noted that aquatic turtles will instinctively feed only if they are in water.

TECHNICIAN NOTE

Successful care of captive tortoises relies heavily on varying the diet.

Snakes

Snakes are strict carnivores. They eat a variety of prey items based on species and size, including rabbits, rats, mice, gerbils, chickens, and lizards. The size of the prey item fed should be about the same diameter as the snake's body and about one-eighth of the animal's length. Feeding frozen or freshly killed rodents is strongly recommended to prevent injury caused by live prey bites (Fig. 22.24). Most species of snake feed once every 1 to 2 weeks, but the frequency of feeding depends on the age and signalment of the snake. Clients should be encouraged to keep records of eating and defecating patterns as a means of monitoring health trends in their pet. Enclosures should be kept at the proper **preferred optimal temperature zone** (POTZ) for that species, particularly to aid in digestion. Water should be supplied on a daily basis for drinking, soaking, and to increase humidity in the environment.

The incidence of nutritional deficiency in the captive snake is rare, because most snakes are fed whole prey, which are nutritionally complete; therefore use of supplements is not required. Because of this, snakes do not typically require the amount of UVB radiation required by other reptiles; however, the current recommendation is to offer low-level UVB exposure during the day, with locations for the snake to hide.

Lizards

Captive lizards can be herbivores, insectivores, omnivores, or carnivores. Herbivorous lizards, such as iguanas, require a varied diet, with vitamin and mineral supplementation to ensure adequate nutritional balance. Recommended diets for herbivores include chard, mustard greens, and herbs, along with protein-rich sources, such as collards, turnip greens, kale, bok choy, and broccoli with leaves. Vegetables, including green beans, okra, carrots, and squash, are also healthy options. Fruit can be used as treats and can include small amounts of berries or melons. A variety of commercially available herbivorous lizard foods are appropriate to use in conjunction with fresh food items. It is important to note that certain vegetables, such as spinach, soybeans, and beet greens, contain oxalic acid that binds calcium and other trace minerals, inhibiting absorption, and should therefore be avoided. Herbivores should never be fed meat-based protein sources, such as commercial dog and cat food, because this will ultimately cause renal disease and death.

Insectivorous lizards, such as chameleons, need to consume a variety of insects. Good options include phoenix worms/soldier fly larvae, silkworms, superworms, dubia cockroaches, and crickets properly gut loaded with healthy, vitamin-rich vegetables. Mealworms and waxworms, although more readily available at most pet stores, have an inverse calcium-to-phosphorus ratio and should not make up a large part of a lizard's diet. Insects should be dusted with calcium supplements three to five times per week and with a multivitamin one to two times per week.

Omnivorous lizards, such as bearded dragons, require a variety of invertebrate or vertebrate prey, vitamin and mineral supplementation, and fresh vegetables. A variety of commercially available omnivorous lizard foods are appropriate to use; however, it is considered vital that these reptiles also eat fresh produce and insects, both to ensure nutritional balance and to provide enrichment for the animal. It is currently recommended that juvenile species be fed a higher insect-driven diet with insects, as described above for insectivores. As the lizard grows, vegetables, as described above for herbivores, should be increased. An adult omnivorous lizard should be encouraged to eat approximately 70% vegetables and 30% insects; however, this will vary by species.

Carnivorous lizards, such as monitor lizards, eat a diet similar to that of snakes, but their diet can be more varied. In addition to rodents, they enjoy eggs, chicks, fish, insects, and other forms of whole prey. It is recommended that prekilled frozen prey items be fed instead of live.

Most lizards, such as savannah monitors, are diurnal and require day feedings plus time to bask in UVB radiation; however, some, such as leopard geckos, are nocturnal. Nocturnal reptiles require night feedings and a lower output of UVB radiation during the day while they hide. Regardless of the light cycle of a species, it is currently recommended that all reptiles be offered some form of UVB radiation during the day, whether they are hiding or basking.

Water should be provided in a bowl for bathing and drinking for all reptiles, even the desert species. The water source should be changed daily or more often if soiled. It should be noted that some lizards (e.g., chameleons) will drink water only if it is in the form of droplets on plant leaves, similar to dew. Therefore it is important to spray or mist the animal's enclosure several times a day. In addition, most lizards should be sprayed with water or bathed/soaked daily to prevent dysecdysis associated with low humidity.

> **TECHNICIAN NOTE**
> Feeding commercial dog food or cat food to herbivorous lizards will cause renal disease and death; these should be avoided.

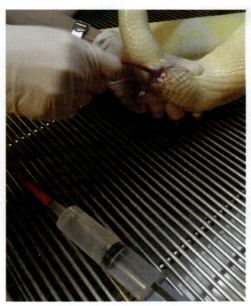

• **Fig. 22.25** Colonic wash.

Sample Collection and Diagnostic Procedures

Diagnostic approaches for reptiles are similar to those for other small animal species. Technicians who have the proper sampling equipment and the desire to succeed can master any of the procedures discussed in this section.

Fecal Sampling

Fecal material can be very useful in diagnosing parasite infestations, bacterial infections, and the presence of blood in the GI tract. A fresh sample should be examined under a wet mount for protozoan parasites. Other tests include flotation, sedimentation, and culture and sensitivity. Technicians may wish to review Chapter 13, "Parasitology," regarding these procedures. If a fecal sample is not available at the time of examination, a warm water bath often will stimulate a reptile to defecate. If this is not productive, specimens may be collected by performing a colonic wash. This is done by passing a lubricated rubber tube or catheter through the cloaca into the colon (Fig. 22.25). Sterile saline is administered through a syringe, and a typical flush or enema is performed. The recommended volume of saline for a colonic wash is 1% or less of the animal's weight.

Stomach Lavage

A stomach wash is used to examine the upper GI tract, especially for identification of *Cryptosporidium* (a common protozoan parasite found in many reptile species). This procedure is well tolerated by most reptiles and is quick and easy to execute. A lubricated soft rubber catheter is advanced through the mouth into the stomach, which lies in the midcranial body area. Sterile isotonic saline is administered through a syringe inserted into the catheter, and a simple flush is performed after the stomach is agitated through external palpation. Samples obtained are used for direct microscopic examination for parasites, to prepare slides for cytologic examination, or for culture and sensitivity.

Urine Sampling

Many, but not all, reptiles have urinary bladders. However, all reptiles do have a cloaca into which the reproductive, GI, and

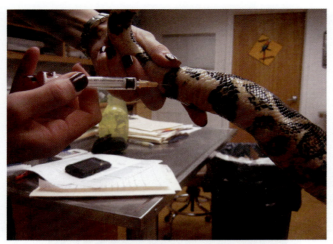

• **Fig. 22.26** Phlebotomy from the coccygeal vein of a snake.

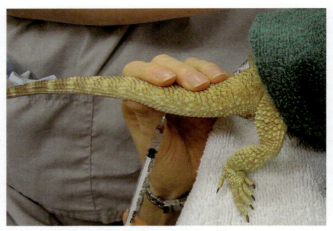

• **Fig. 22.27** Phlebotomy from the caudal tail vein of a bearded dragon.

urinary tract contents drain before the excretions exit the body. Urine samples collected from voids on a countertop or tabletop have a high likelihood of being contaminated after excretion from the cloaca. Accurate urinalysis may be performed on fresh urine samples obtained via cystocentesis in reptiles with bladders. Cystocentesis may be performed on turtles by advancing a needle cranial to the hindlimb.

> ### TECHNICIAN NOTE
> Many, but not all, reptiles have urinary bladders, but all reptiles have a cloaca where the excretions from the urinary, gastrointestinal, and reproductive tracts combine and pass through before exiting. Therefore voided urinary samples are likely to be contaminated.

Skin Sampling

Clinical dermatologic diseases are common in reptilian species, often resulting from poor humidity (too much or too little, depending on the species), unsanitary water (aquatic species), or nutritional deficiencies. Skin specimens may be cultured for bacterial and fungal organisms, scraped for cytologic evaluation, or biopsied for histopathology. Samples for dermatologic analysis may be taken by using sterile cotton-tipped culturettes or by aseptically collecting pieces of affected skin, scales, or dermal *scutes* (the individual pieces covering bone that make up the carapace, or the dorsal aspect of the shell).

Phlebotomy

As with birds, it is important to take only the required amount of blood for tests and no greater than 1% of the reptile's body weight. Technicians should have all collection tubes and sampling equipment ready before the actual blood draw to prevent clotting. Blood collection sites in snakes include the caudal or coccygeal vein of the tail (Fig. 22.26), the ventral abdominal vein, the palatine vessels, or through cardiocentesis. Cardiocentesis should not be performed on snakes weighing less than 200 g. For lizards, the caudal tail vein is the most accessible site (Fig. 22.27); however, blood may also be collected from the ventral abdominal vein. In chelonians, jugular veins are easily used for venipuncture sites (Fig. 22.28) as long as the head can be retracted safely from the shell. Other sites include the subcarapacial sinus (Fig. 22.29), the caudal tail vein, or the brachial plexus. The site chosen will depend on the

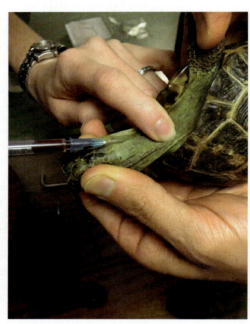

• **Fig. 22.28** Phlebotomy of the jugular vein in a Russian tortoise.

size of the reptile and the experience of the technician. Clipping of nails or toes should never be considered for blood collection.

Radiography

For many species, radiographs may be taken on nonsedated animals by restraining them in plastic boxes or acrylic tubes. It is important to remember to take at least two views: (1) a VD or a dorsoventral (DV) view, and (2) a lateral view, preferably by using the lateral beam technique. For turtles, a third view (anteroposterior [AP] view) should be taken, also by using the lateral beam (Fig. 22.30). Contrast studies may be done by gavage feeding or orally administering barium sulfate; however, GI transit times are long, and it may take up to 1 week to complete a GI barium study on some species. Ultrasonography can be used in all reptilian species. Using copious ultrasound gel will facilitate visualization through scales and thick skin. When available, computed tomography (CT) is a valuable diagnostic tool, especially in large chelonians (Fig. 22.31).

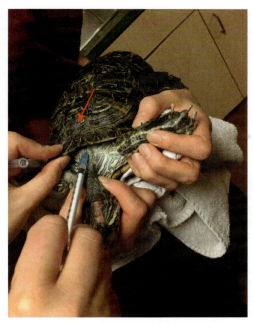

• **Fig. 22.29** Phlebotomy from the subcarapacial sinus in a red-eared slider, with a red arrow indicating where the sinus lies beneath the carapace.

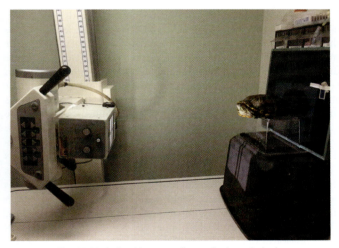

• **Fig. 22.30** Lateral beam radiography in a chelonian.

Anesthesia and Analgesia

Because of the lack of pharmacokinetic studies on anesthetic agents in reptiles, it is very important to remember that many of the drug dosages used by clinicians have been developed on the basis of anecdotal experience. A current exotic animal formulary with proper species-specific recommendations is mandatory (see the "Recommended Reading" list). Evaluating pain in reptiles can be challenging because of their stoic appearance, but technicians should be aware of the ways pain manifests in reptiles and be able to discuss proper analgesic protocols with other veterinary staff. Combinations of sedatives and analgesics work synergistically and are safe and effective to use in the same manner that they are used in mammals. They include alpha$_2$ agonists (e.g., dexmedetomidine), pure mu-opioids (e.g., hydromorphone), benzodiazepines (e.g., midazolam), local anesthetics (e.g., lidocaine), neuroactive steroids (e.g., alfaxalone), and others. Multimodal analgesia and

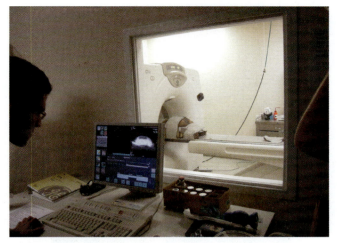

• **Fig. 22.31** Computed tomography scan of a sulcata tortoise.

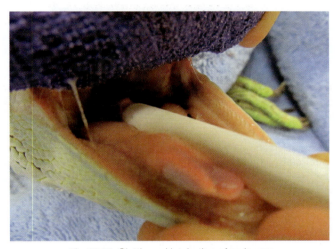

• **Fig. 22.32** Glottis and intubation of an iguana.

anesthesia provide much greater analgesia and the desired sedative effects compared with an induction agent used alone.

Induction through use of a gas anesthetic agent is not recommended in reptiles because of their ability and propensity to not breathe for long periods. Propofol is a popular choice as an induction agent because of ease of IV access in the caudal tail or the jugular vein of many reptiles; however, technicians must be aware of the common side effects, including apnea and cardiovascular depression. Because of the unique metabolism of many reptiles, drug clearance is prolonged; therefore drugs with reversible antagonistic agents may be preferable.

Isoflurane or sevoflurane are the inhalant anesthetic agents of choice for reptiles, and intubation with assisted ventilation is mandatory for all anesthetized reptiles for adequate anesthetic control and outcome. In herbivores, the glottis is located in the back of the oral cavity at the base of a sticky, fleshy tongue (Fig. 22.32). Carnivores tend to have a rostrally located glottis (Fig. 22.33), and the glottis of omnivores is located in between the location of the glottis in that of the carnivore and that of the herbivore. As with birds, many reptiles have complete cartilaginous rings; therefore uncuffed endotracheal tubes should be used. Use of positive-pressure ventilation at four to six breaths per minute based on species, size, and estimated tidal volume is recommended throughout the procedure.

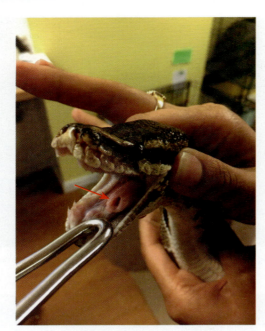

• **Fig. 22.33** Glottis (*red arrow*) of a snake.

Anesthesia should be monitored as in nonreptile species. SpO_2, capnography, and ECG are all valuable monitoring tools; however, these tools are not designed for animals, such as reptiles with a three-chambered heart or nucleated red blood cells. Technicians should not interpret the readings literally but should instead be monitoring trends throughout the anesthetic procedure to be aware of changes in that particular animal. Doppler ultrasonography for monitoring heart rate and an ambient thermometer to measure temperature should be used during every anesthetic procedure. All poikilotherms should be kept at their POTZ, which is the temperature at which individual species will thrive, before, during, and after a procedure to ensure the proper effect and metabolism of the anesthetic agent. Controlling the POTZ is done by manipulating the ambient temperature with heat devices such as forced hot air or radiant heat sources. One important difference between reptiles and mammals is that the stimulus to breathe in reptiles is low oxygen saturation, whereas in mammals, it is increased carbon dioxide concentration. Therefore technicians should be careful to ensure that during recovery, reptiles are ventilated properly with room air rather than with 100% oxygen until completely awake.

Husbandry and Treatments in the Hospital

Reptiles require a controlled microenvironment both at home and in the hospital. Temperature and humidity are important, because these animals are **poikilothermic** (they depend on their environment for regulation of their body temperature). A temperature gradient should be provided by using a thermostat at each end of the enclosure, resulting in a cooler end and a warmer end based on the POTZ for that species. This allows the animal to somewhat self-regulate their temperature comfortably, similar to behavior exhibited in a wild environment. For most species, temperature should not exceed 32°C (90°F) or dip below 24°C (75°F). Humidity is the other important environmental consideration that is determined by species-specific requirements. In general, most captive reptile species respond well to humidity ranges of 50% to 70%. The technician must remember that rainforest species usually require higher humidity, whereas desert species do better in lower humidity ranges.

For many species, a variety of aquaria are sufficient for short-term hospitalization. Any substrate used should be easily cleaned and disinfected or disposable, such as newspaper. Hide boxes or areas of seclusion should be provided for all reptiles, with perches for arboreal species such as iguanas and some snakes. Water sources should always be available, regardless of animals being "desert" species, and changed daily or more often if soiled. UVB radiation as described above should be used.

Gavage feeding in snakes, chelonians, and some lizards is an important technique that the veterinary technician should learn. A tube should be premeasured for the distance from the oral cavity to the stomach, well lubricated, and passed gently into the stomach. Once the tube has been placed properly, liquid food, water, or medication can be injected slowly through the tube into the stomach. For patients that are anorexic, gavage feeding of commercial critical care supplements as suggested by the clinician, such as Carnivore, Omnivore, or Herbivore Critical Care (Oxbow Animal Health, Omaha, NE), can be used.

Reptiles have a renal portal system that routes blood from the caudal third of the body through a capillary network into the kidneys before sending it to the general circulation. Because of this, injections should be administered to reptiles in the cranial half of the animal's body, especially if the drug is nephrotoxic (Fig. 22.34). IM injection sites are primarily the epaxial muscles and the muscles of the forelimbs. Oral medications are easily given either per os or through gavage feeding as previously described. Liquid suspensions are preferred over tablets, which are difficult to administer and not consistently absorbed.

IV catheters can be placed but are challenging because of the thick skin and scales of reptiles. In most species, a surgical cut-down procedure is required to visualize a vein for catheterization (Fig. 22.35). Large species of lizards have cephalic veins and abdominal veins that can accommodate a catheter. Jugular vein catheters often can be placed in chelonians without a cut-down procedure if the head can be restrained to facilitate placement. Snakes require a cut-down of their jugular vein for IV access. A good option for lizards and chelonians is to place IO catheters. IO catheters can be placed in the distal femur or proximal tibia of lizards (Fig. 22.36), or the distal humerus or carapace/plastron bridge in chelonians. Local anesthetics and analgesics should be used prior to IO catheter placement.

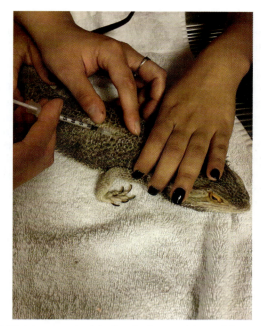

• **Fig. 22.34** Intramuscular injection in the cranial epaxial muscles of a bearded dragon.

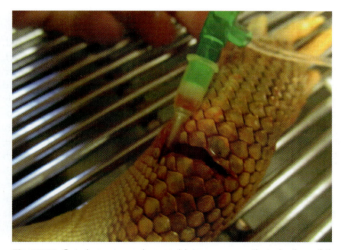

• **Fig. 22.35** Cut-down procedure and intravenous catheterization of the cephalic vein in an iguana.

Salmonella spp.

Salmonella spp. are considered part of the normal GI flora of all reptiles and are often shed when reptiles are immunosuppressed. If humans are infected, they can develop severe GI disease. To reduce exposure to this infectious and zoonotic bacterium, reptiles should be maintained in good health and without undue stress. Individuals handling reptiles should practice excellent hygiene and should always wash their hands afterward.

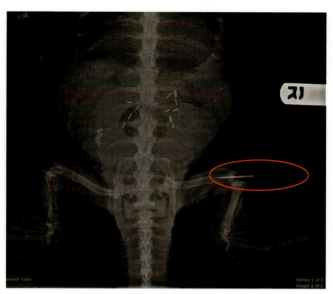

• **Fig. 22.36** Radiograph of an intraosseous catheter *(red circle)* in the proximal tibia of a tegu.

PUT INTO PRACTICE

When interacting with clients and reptiles, remember actions speak louder than words; do not handle reptiles in ways that may expose you to *Salmonella,* such as holding near the face, kissing, or nuzzling the animal.

Small Mammals

Ferrets

Handling and Grooming

Although ferrets are usually not aggressive, they may nip or bite when nervous. However, when scruffed by the nape of the neck, ferrets become very docile, almost immobilized, and most grooming procedures are thus facilitated. Ferret nails are sharp and owners often request nail trimming. Ferrets do not have retractable claws, but they do have a vascular "quick" delineation that can be used as a landmark to trim. If bleeding occurs, silver nitrate sticks or styptic powder can be used for cautery. Ferrets also tend to have wax buildup in their ears, and technicians will need to clean them. Standard mammalian otic solutions are safe to use with fine-tipped cotton swabs to clean the delicate folds. *Otodectes cynotis* (ear mites) are common in ferrets, and technicians should be aware of the difference between ear mite infestation and normal wax buildup. In general, ferrets do not require baths. Owners should be educated that ferrets have a musky odor that routine bathing will not eliminate.

Phlebotomy

Common locations for collecting blood samples include the jugular vein or cranial vena cava for large samples and the cephalic or lateral saphenous for small samples. The ferret's thick skin and SC fat make visualization of the jugular vein difficult, and the cranial vena cava may be preferred for easier sampling. Positioning requires either a firm scruff of the neck by the assistant or restraint of the head and neck by the phlebotomist (Fig. 22.37). With experience, it is possible to obtain a blood sample with the use of restraint alone, without sedation. However, sedatives may

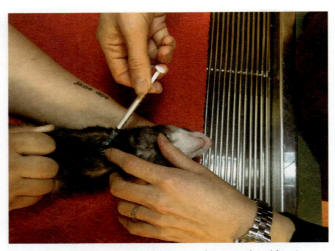

• **Fig. 22.37** Vena cava phlebotomy of an unsedated ferret.

be preferred for safe, stress-free phlebotomy in instances where the ferret is very active or nervous. It is vital that the ferret is not able to move or pull away during vena cava phlebotomy because of the risk of lacerating the vein.

TECHNICIAN NOTE

The ferret's thick skin and subcutaneous fat make visualization of the jugular vein difficult. For drawing adequate blood samples the cranial vena cava may be preferred.

Anesthesia and Analgesia

Current protocols for ferret anesthesia and pain management are similar to those for cats. Multimodal combinations of premedication, induction, maintenance, and postanesthetic agents are key. These combinations should include NSAIDs, alpha$_2$ adrenergic agonists and their reversal agents, opioids, benzodiazepines, dissociative agents, inhalants, and local anesthetics, which will vary based on the procedure. For longer procedures, ferrets should be intubated with a cuffed endotracheal tube, using a technique similar to that used for cats. To prevent hypoglycemia, ferrets should not be fasted for longer than 3 to 4 hours before anesthesia. Because they have a short GI transit time, even with this short fasting, they usually do not vomit as a result of anesthetic or analgesic use.

Hospitalization Care

Ferrets are notorious for disliking oral medications. Using palatable treats such as Nutrical (Vetroquinol Global, Forth Worth, TX), dairy products, and sweets to mask the bitter taste of medications can help. Flavored compounded medications are much easier to administer compared with pills.

Parenteral administration techniques are similar to those used in cats; however, ferrets generally need firm scruffing of the neck, as described previously, to be able to tolerate injections. SC injections can be administered between the shoulder blades and IM injections can be given in the epaxial, gluteal, or the thigh muscles. IV catheterization is possible in the cephalic or jugular veins; however, active ferrets may need sedation to be able to tolerate this procedure.

Ferrets defecate frequently and when nervous, and patients often readily produce fecal samples during an examination if allowed to explore the floor of the examination room. A small, lubricated feline fecal loop will also provide a sufficient sample for test evaluation.

Ferrets will be less stressed in the hospital if given an enclosure with soft bedding to wrap themselves and hide in. They generally like hammocks, fleece blankets, or even pillowcases. Food and water should be made available at all times unless instructed otherwise by the veterinarian. Ferrets do not necessarily become litter trained, but they do routinely choose to use the corners of rooms or enclosures to urinate and defecate. Offering litter or bedding in those areas or a corner litter box may make cleaning easier. Their normal body temperature is between 99°F and 104°F, and supplemental heat or cooling should be used as needed to help maintain their temperature in this range.

Nutrition

Ferrets are strict carnivores, with dietary requirements of roughly 30% protein and 25% fat with very low fiber. Feeding whole prey diets of chicks, mice, and rats can be used; however, there are several commercially available, ferret-specific diets that will provide the proper nutrition for these animals. Technicians should assist clients in finding a product that contains the highest quantity of animal protein rather than soy or pea as the primary ingredients, because grain and legume proteins have been associated with urinary stones in ferrets. Small quantities of fruit or cooked meat can be offered as treats. Fresh water should be provided on a daily basis, preferably in a bowl rather than in a water bottle.

General Information and Common Presentations

In the United States, the vast majority of captive ferrets are spayed, neutered, and descented before reaching the pet trade. However, technicians should be aware of a potentially fatal clinical problem of the intact female ferret. Female ferrets are induced ovulators and occasionally will not cycle out of estrus unless bred or artificially stimulated. These animals become severely anemic and thrombocytopenic because of the toxic effects of estrogen on bone marrow. Signs of estrogen toxicity are vulvar swelling and discharge, lethargy, and anorexia. Estrogen toxicity is best managed through prevention by educating the client. Female ferrets not intended for breeding should be spayed before their first estrus cycle. Ferrets that have been spayed or neutered by a breeding facility at an early age will have tattooed dots on the surface of the ear pinna (Fig. 22.38). Regardless of descenting, ferrets retain a musky odor.

TECHNICIAN NOTE

Ferrets that have been spayed or neutered and descented by a breeding facility at an early age will have one or two tattooed dots on the surface of the ear pinna.

Hyperadrenocorticism is a common problem in pet ferrets, resulting from hypertrophy of the adrenal gland. Clinical signs include hair loss, pruritus, an enlarged vulva in females (Fig. 22.39), and stranguria in males. It is theorized that causes include the environment (most ferrets in the United States live inside and are not exposed to UV light), breeding practices/genetics, diet, and early sterilization. These theories are based on the fact that in other countries, ferrets live outside, are left intact or sterilized later in life, eat more animal protein, and have a dramatically lower rate of hyperadrenocorticism compared with those in the United States. Treatment options include gonadotropin-releasing hormone (GnRH) agonists, such as leuprolide acetate or deslorelin

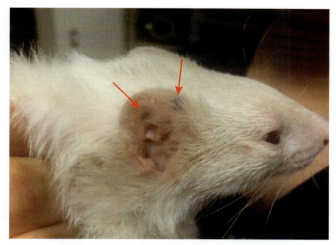

• **Fig. 22.38** Tattoos on the pinna of a ferret indicating that it has been altered/descented.

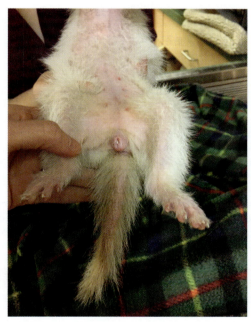

• **Fig. 22.39** Hair loss and an enlarged vulva, common in female ferrets with adrenal disease.

implants, which stop the production of sex hormones and thus alleviate the symptoms of hyperadrenocorticism. These drugs do not cure the disease, however, and need to be continued for the life of the ferret. Performing an adrenalectomy can be curative if the adrenal glands can be completely removed. It is hypothesized that not sterilizing ferrets at least until 6 months of age may decrease the risk of adrenal disease.

Ferrets are susceptible to human influenza, and clients should be counseled that any members of the family with influenza should not handle the ferret. Human influenza in a ferret must be differentiated from canine distemper and bacterial pneumonia, to which ferrets are also susceptible. All exhibited signs are similar to those of human respiratory disease, such as nasal and ocular discharge, coughing, and sneezing. However, canine distemper is far more dangerous than influenza and has a very high mortality rate. Canine distemper also manifests symptoms of

chin, lip, and anal lesions in the ferret, something not seen in influenza cases.

Parasites that present problems for dogs and cats are also a problem for ferrets. Heartworm prevention is required in animals that are exposed to mosquitoes. Fleas commonly plague ferrets, even if the ferrets are maintained within a household setting, and can spread intestinal parasites. Ferrets are also often infested by ear mites at breeding facilities and pet stores. Currently, there are commercial flea treatments formulated specially for ferrets. According to the American Heartworm Society, there is no approved drug therapy to treat heartworm infection in ferrets. Heartworm prevention is accomplished through extralabel monthly usage of imidacloprid/moxidectin topically.

Ferrets are fond of chewing, preferring soft rubbery objects, and should be watched closely for foreign body ingestion. A ferret, particularly a young kit that is vomiting, anorexic, and lethargic, should be suspected of having a GI obstruction. Toys for ferrets should be limited to objects that they cannot break or ingest, or "ferret tubes" that they can crawl into to play.

There are many fairly common neoplastic diseases in ferrets, including insulinoma, lymphoma, and fibrosarcoma. If a ferret is depressed or moribund, a blood glucose test should be performed, because hypoglycemia is a common concurrent result of these diseases.

Ferrets are one of the few exotic species that are regularly vaccinated. Only canine distemper and rabies vaccines are recommended. It is unlikely that an indoor ferret will be exposed to rabies virus, but some jurisdictions require it, and the IMRAB 3 rabies vaccine (Boehringer Ingelheim Pharmaceuticals, Inc., Ridgefield, CT) will protect the ferret in the event of exposure and will support its quarantine if a human is bitten. Ferrets are highly susceptible to vaccine reactions. Signs of a vaccine reaction include swelling and redness at the vaccination site, drooling, vomiting, rapid breathing, and increased body temperature. Ferrets that receive vaccines should be monitored for at least 20 minutes after the procedure is completed.

Rabbits

The rabbit is not a rodent but rather, is a lagomorph of the family Leporidae. Rabbits are *crepuscular* (most active at dusk and dawn) and come in many breeds and sizes, ranging from the Flemish Giant (6–7.5 kg) to Dutch and miniature breeds (1–2 kg). It is a common misconception that rabbits make good "caged" pets, similar to a guinea pig or hamster. Rabbits are dynamic, curious animals that require a lot of exercise, play, companionship, and enrichment to be healthy and content. If proper husbandry practices are maintained, a pet rabbit should live 8 to 10 years. Restraining and handling rabbits must be done carefully. They have extremely powerful hind legs and will kick violently when scared or when their hind area is not supported. The force of this

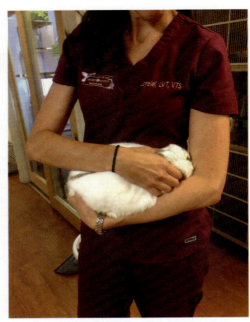

• **Fig. 22.40** Proper rabbit handling.

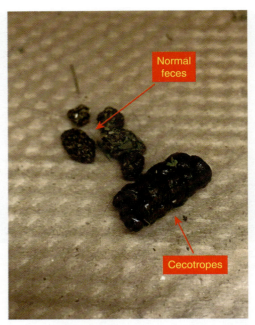

Normal feces

Cecotropes

• **Fig. 22.41** A rabbit cecotrope.

often luxates the lumbar vertebrae; this is a mortal injury. Rabbits should be held securely, with their bodies gently restrained like a "football" (Fig. 22.40) or wrapped safely in a towel.

Nutrition

Rabbits are herbivores, using hindgut fermentation in a large cecum to digest the high-fiber diet they require. The cecum is an outpouching of the intestines at the junction of the small and large intestines where unique bacteria, fungi, and protozoa symbiotically use the difficult-to-digest grasses the rabbit needs. Large amounts of fiber and water are needed for the cecum to function properly, and foods that are high in sugar or carbohydrates can damage the delicate flora and cause serious intestinal problems.

The recommended pet rabbit diet should be composed primarily (80%–90%) of a variety of grass hays, such as timothy, orchard, or oat hay. Legume hay, such as alfalfa, is lower in fiber and higher in protein and calcium compared with grass hay and should be fed in small amounts to adult rabbits. Hay should be available ad libitum and with a variety of options for both flavor/texture enrichment and to provide a more complete nutritional balance. A grass-based pellet, such as Oxbow Animal Health's variety of rabbit foods (Oxbow Animal Health, Omaha, NE), can be used in moderation as a supplement but should not be fed at more than a quarter cup per kilogram of body weight per day. Overfeeding of pellets can not only cause obesity but also distract the rabbit from eating proper amounts of hay, which is vital for dental and GI health. All commercial feed should have a mill date of manufacture clearly printed on the bag; it is recommended to purchase feed within 90 days of production to ensure that vitamins, such as vitamin E, do not oxidize, rendering them inert. Technicians should be diligent in encouraging clients not to feed rabbit food that has seeds, dried fruits, or colored treats mixed in. These additives contain sugars and starches that can disrupt the flora of the cecum and are highly caloric and may contribute to obesity.

Fresh greens or other vegetables can be healthy additions to the rabbit diet in moderation. Greens, such as kale, green lettuces,

carrot tops, and herbs, can be fed at a rate of approximately two cups per kilogram of body weight per day, as long as the rabbit does not develop diarrhea. Tiny pieces of carrots, banana, or other sugary treats should only be fed strictly in moderation.

Although most mammals typically excrete approximately 2% of ingested calcium in their urine, rabbits excrete up to 60%. Because of this, rabbit urine can range from being clear yellow to chalky white to appearing as a "sludge" because of the formation of calcium crystals or calculi in the urinary tract. It is recommended that high-calcium vegetables and hay (broccoli, spinach, alfalfa hay) be fed only in limited quantities to prevent this.

> **TECHNICIAN NOTE**
> The recommended pet rabbit diet should be composed primarily (80%–90%) of a variety of grass hays, such as timothy, orchard, or oat hay.

Another important component of a rabbit's diet is the ingestion of cecotropes or "night feces." These feces are completely different compared with the typical dry, hard pellets that rabbits pass all day. They are small, clumped together, and mucus covered in comparison to normal rabbit feces (Fig. 22.41). Cecotropes are generated in the cecum and are consumed directly from the anus, generally in the crepuscular hours. They contain vital nutrients, such as vitamins B and K, beneficial bacteria, fatty acids, and significant amounts of fiber. It is vital that rabbits are able to consume these and, if deprived, they will ultimately suffer various forms of malnutrition. Obesity, spinal arthritis, or other problems can cause a rabbit to not be able to ingest cecotropes. When owners complain that they see cecotropes left in the litter, technicians should know that this is a potential sign of illness and should call for a veterinary visit.

The rabbit's bacterial flora is important for technicians to be aware of, because many antibiotics will destroy vital cecal bacteria, allowing harmful bacteria such as *Clostridium difficile* to increase excessively. This can be deadly for rabbits. Antibiotics that are considered toxic to rabbits include clindamycin, lincomycin, erythromycin, ampicillin, cephalosporins, and amoxicillin/clavulanic acid.

Anesthesia and Analgesia

Unlike ferrets, rabbits have a very slow GI transit time and should not have food withheld longer than 1 to 2 hours before anesthesia. Herbivores should always have food in their GI tract to maintain function and, because many rabbits do not eat immediately after anesthesia, fasting them can have dangerous consequences, including GI stasis. Additionally, rabbits are not capable of emesis, so emptying the stomach before surgery is not important. Technicians should be aware that many rabbits naturally produce atropine esterase, which inactivates atropine, so glycopyrrolate may be a better option for rabbits suffering from bradycardia or hypersalivation.

> **TECHNICIAN NOTE**
>
> Technicians should be aware that many rabbits naturally produce atropine esterase, which inactivates atropine.

Injectable anesthetic agents include combinations of dissociative agents (e.g., ketamine), alpha$_2$ adrenergic agonists (e.g., dexmedetomidine), benzodiazepines (e.g., midazolam), and the neuroactive steroid alfaxalone. Isoflurane or sevoflurane are the inhalation anesthetic agents of choice. Intubating rabbits can be difficult because of their deep oral cavity and small oropharyngeal opening. In average-sized rabbits, it is almost impossible to visualize the tracheal opening. With practice, however, technicians can master the technique of blind intubation, or they can use a rigid endoscope for ease of visualization and assistance with placement. When available, the supraglottic airway device, V-gel (Docsinnovent, Hemel Hempstead, UK), can be used to provide airway support in lieu of true intubation.

As a prey species, rabbits are particularly sensitive to the effects of pain and stress, and a good plan for analgesia is critical. Adrenergic responses caused by stress can dramatically slow GI tract transit time, which can cause life-threatening ileus in rabbits. Signs of pain may include a hunched posture, teeth grinding, or sensitivity to certain parts of the body. Similar to dogs and cats, there are many resources for a Rabbit Grimace Scale to help technicians recognize and quantify the level of discomfort a rabbit may be in. Rabbits tolerate analgesics well, and proper pain management should include combinations of local analgesics, NSAIDs, and narcotics, such as partial and complete mu-agonists and antagonists.

Intravenous Access

The marginal ear vein can be used for placing IV catheters and giving injections, and the central artery can be used for arterial sampling. Although these sites can be convenient and fast in a laboratory setting, complications include lack of proper blood volume and sloughing or necrosis of the ear as a result of damage by IV drug injections or damage to blood supply. This is not acceptable in clinical practice. For pet medicine, the safer phlebotomy sites are the lateral saphenous and jugular veins. With proper, safe restraint, these veins are easily accessible and yield appropriate blood volumes. The cephalic vein is difficult, because it tends not to provide adequate volumes of blood; however, it is the placement site of choice for IV catheterization. Placement may require sedation in an active rabbit; however, the techniques are similar to those used in any other small mammal (Fig. 22.42).

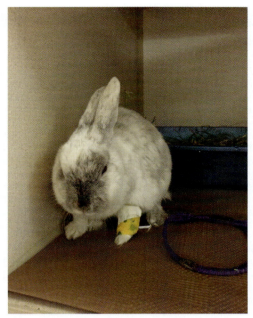

• **Fig. 22.42** Rabbit with an intravenous catheter in the cephalic vein.

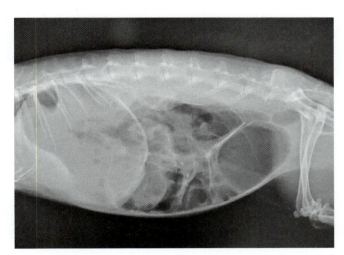

• **Fig. 22.43** Lateral radiograph typical for a rabbit suffering from gastrointestinal stasis; the stomach is bloated and the intestines and cecum are full of gas.

> **TECHNICIAN NOTE**
>
> For pet rabbit medicine, the best phlebotomy sites are the lateral saphenous and jugular veins.

Common Presentations

The most common ailment in pet rabbits is anorexia, which often leads to gastric stasis and intestinal ileus, and is often referred to as *GI stasis syndrome*. There are many possible causes for this situation. A rabbit with anorexia should be examined for dental malocclusion, trichobezoars (hairballs) causing a gastric outflow obstruction, dehydration, trauma/pain, dietary problems (e.g., lack of fiber), and stress. All of these problems, as well as others discussed below, can cause secondary GI stasis, which is often more dangerous than the primary problem. GI stasis is extremely

CASE PRESENTATION 22.1

Gastric Stasis

Clover, a 2-year-old mixed-breed male lop rabbit (lagomorph), presented to the veterinary hospital with a 4-day history of decreased appetite, 24 hours of complete anorexia, and what the owners describe as "constipation," or not passing any stool. Clover was adopted from a rabbit rescue 1 year prior. He lives primarily in a hutch approximately 3 feet long by 4 feet wide, which is located in the bedroom of the owners' 8-year-old daughter. Clover is permitted to play outside of the hutch for 1 or 2 hours every day. His diet consists of ad libitum commercial rabbit seed and pellet mix of an unknown brand, a daily handful of timothy hay, and a carrot or small bit of lettuce a few days a week. His favorite treats are pieces of cereal, pieces of peanut butter and jelly sandwich, and apple slices, which are given almost every day. The owners suspect that their child has been giving him more treats recently. Water is offered from a sipper bottle and changed when the level becomes low. The owners are not giving Clover any supplements. They observe that he has been shedding more over the past few weeks but have not been able to brush him because of his dislike of being combed. The owners say he seems depressed and has been sitting quietly in the litter box for the past 12 hours, rejecting even his favorite foods.

On physical examination, Clover is found to be quiet, alert, and approximately 10% dehydrated. He has signs of discomfort on abdominal palpation and is grinding his teeth intermittently throughout the examination. His temperature is 98.8°F, and he is slightly tachypneic and tachycardic. He weighs 2.2 kg and has a body condition score of 4/5. His oral examination reveals sharp enamel points on the lingual aspect of the right and left lower molars. Blood is collected from the lateral saphenous vein, and the only abnormalities are an increased packed cell volume (PCV) (53%), creatine phosphokinase (CPK) (950 U/L), alkaline phosphatase (49 units/L), and alanine aminotransferase (70 units/L). Abdominal radiography shows marked gaseous dilation of the stomach, intestines, and cecum, with potential foreign body presence in the stomach. Based on the history, physical examination, and diagnostic findings, a diagnosis of gastric stasis with ileus, often referred to as *gastrointestinal (GI) stasis syndrome*, is confirmed.

GI stasis is common in pet rabbits and is often characterized by anorexia, decreased to no fecal production, and a distended stomach filled with food material and hair (ingested during grooming). Rabbits eating high-carbohydrate, low-fiber diets with little opportunity for exercise may develop decreased GI motility, increasing the likelihood of stasis and ileus. Changes in gastric motility and function may result in GI fluid loss and subsequent inability to excrete the hair out of the stomach, resulting in the formation of a gastric trichobezoar (hairball). Occasionally changes in GI motility result in the accumulation of gastric ingesta only, without formation of a trichobezoar. Other potential causes for GI stasis include any possible reason for anorexia in rabbits, such as dental disease, stress, pain, or chronic inflammatory disease. Rabbits may groom excessively during heavy shedding periods, during the prepartum period, or as a result of flea and mite infestation. Lack of exercise also leads to obesity and a slower GI transit time. It is believed that the cause of Clover's stasis is poor nutrition and husbandry, and that the overgrown points on the teeth are secondary to a lack of fibrous chewing material. Additionally, Clover has been shedding more heavily and ingesting an increased amount of hair.

Clover's treatment plan starts with pain management to help alleviate the discomfort of the dilated GI tract. Buprenorphine 0.05 mg/kg subcutaneously twice daily (SC BID) and meloxicam 1 mg/kg SC BID are administered for the 3-day duration of his hospital stay. A 24-g intravenous (IV) catheter is placed in his left cephalic vein, and 150 mL/kg per day IV Normasol (Normasol, Hospira, Inc., Lake Forest, IL) is administered for 48 hours, followed by 100 mL subcutaneously twice daily until discharge. The prokinetic agents metoclopramide (0.5 mg/kg IV BID) and cisapride (1 mg/kg) orally twice daily (PO BID) are administered to aid motility. Clover is sedated with ketamine 5mg/kg intramuscularly (IM) and dexmedetomidine 0.15mg/kg IM, and anesthesia is induced with isoflurane via a face mask. The sharp points of his mandibular molars are filed with a high-speed hand drill until the teeth are smooth and even. Dexmedetomidine is reversed with atipamezole. Clover recovers uneventfully in a heated cage. Eight hours later, Clover's temperature has increased to normal (101.8°F) and he seems to be in less pain (tooth grinding has ceased and the abdomen is not as tense); however, he has still not defecated. He is syringe fed Herbivore Critical Care Formula (Oxbow Company, Murdock, NB) at a rate of 50 mL/kg per day and encouraged to hop around safe spaces in the hospital for exercise and increased motility.

By day 3 of hospitalization and supportive care, Clover has started producing small fecal pellets and is eating on his own. The most important part of his recovery includes client education about making the necessary changes to prevent this situation from happening again. They are instructed to increase Clover's diet to predominantly (80%) high-fiber grass hay, which could include a combination of timothy, oat, brome, orchard, or other grass hay. They are also told to switch to a rabbit pellet that is made from grass hays and does not have seeds, oats, or any dried fruits, only pellets. They are instructed that they should only feed a quarter cup of pellets per kilogram of body weight daily. Fresh vegetables are to be limited to dark-green leafy vegetables or herbs, such as kale, carrot tops, chard, and parsley. Low glycemic index fruits, such as cantaloupe or blueberries, may be given in only very tiny amounts a few times a week. Giving human foods, such as cereal and bread, should be avoided. It is therefore also recommended that they move Clover's enclosure outside of the child's bedroom for an adult to monitor dietary intake. The clients are advised to use a large, heavy crock as a water bowl (with daily changes) instead of the sipper bottle to encourage Clover to drink more water. It is also recommended that Clover be placed in a much larger enclosure and allowed more time out of it, at least 3 to 4 hours a day, for exercise. Veterinary technicians also demonstrate various ways to safely restrain and brush Clover to remove excess hair, particularly during heavy shedding periods.

Clover's owners are very receptive to the recommendations for changes in husbandry. They return for a follow-up examination 2 weeks later, and Clover is doing very well. He is eating mostly hay and enjoying the new vegetables. His fecal production is normal, and his teeth are aligned perfectly. The owners claim that he also seems much more active as a result of the new diet and exercise opportunities. It is anticipated that as long as they continue this proper regimen, he should have no relapses and will continue to enjoy excellent health.

painful because of gas buildup (Fig. 22.43) and can be life-threatening, as illustrated in Case Presentation 22.1. Prevention of these problems is the best way to avoid stasis.

Rabbits have aradicular (having no root) hypsodont (having long crowns) elodont (continuously growing) dentition. They require tremendous amounts of fibrous material (e.g., hay) to chew, which keeps the occlusal surfaces worn properly. In the face of improper diet (inadequate amounts of hay) and poor breeding practices (breeding for small-sized rabbits with petite faces), malocclusion often occurs, leading to elongated or diseased incisors (Fig. 22.44) and sharp enamel points on molars. Rabbits with these conditions present with drooling, anorexia, a malodorous oral cavity, and oral pain. Most tooth-trimming procedures are done with the patient under general anesthesia and require rabbit-specific dental instruments to properly examine and safely trim the affected teeth. Positioning devices, drills, oral specula, and other unique instruments are required (Figs. 22.45 and 22.46). If malocclusions are left untreated, jaw abscesses, osteomyelitis,

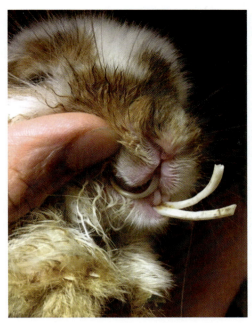

• **Fig. 22.44** Diseased incisor teeth of a rabbit.

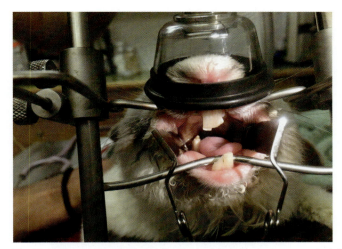

• **Fig. 22.46** An anesthetized rabbit with dental malocclusion on a dental restraint device.

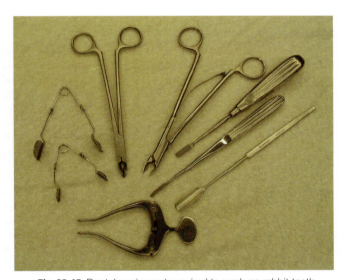

• **Fig. 22.45** Dental equipment required to work on rabbit teeth.

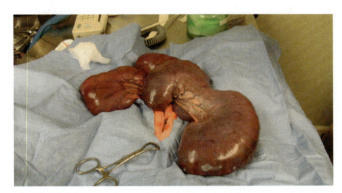

• **Fig. 22.47** Adenocarcinoma in a rabbit undergoing an ovariohysterectomy.

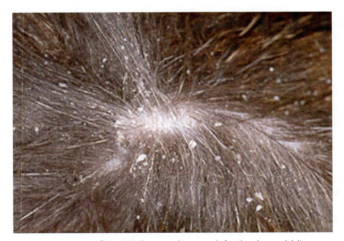

• **Fig. 22.48** *Cheyletiella parasitovorax* infection in a rabbit.

and sinusitis can all develop, potentially leading to severe illness, secondary GI stasis, and death.

Intact female rabbits have a high likelihood (up to 80%) of developing uterine adenocarcinoma or other reproductive system diseases (Fig. 22.47). Signs can include bloody discharge (often mistaken for bloody urine), painful abdomen, and anorexia. Preventive spaying should be recommended for all female rabbits, both to reduce this common presentation and to avoid unplanned pregnancies.

Skin problems can be caused by bacterial dermatitis, parasites (e.g., ear mites [*Psoroptes cuniculi*], fur mites [*Cheyletiella parasitovorax*]) (Fig. 22.48), or dermatophytes. Fungal organisms that have been noted to cause dermatopathy in rabbits include *Microsporum gypseum* and *Trichophyton mentagrophytes*. Flea prevention and control measures are needed for outdoor rabbits; however, technicians should be aware that fipronil (Boehringer Ingelheim Pharmaceuticals, Inc., Ridgefield, CT) is highly toxic to rabbits. Ulcerative foot lesions, or pododermatitis (Fig. 22.49), on the ventral surface of the rear hocks is usually caused by poor husbandry practices, such as use of wire-bottomed caging, or result from obesity and lack of exercise.

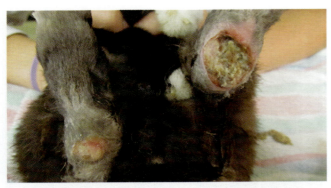

• **Fig. 22.49** Pododermatitis lesions on the hocks of a rabbit.

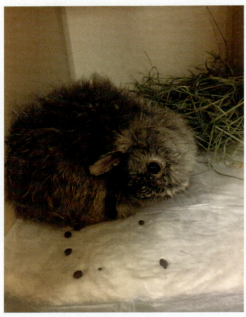

• **Fig. 22.50** Head tilt in a rabbit, commonly seen with *Encephalitozoon cuniculi* infection.

Encephalitozoon cuniculi is a microsporidial intracellular protozoan parasite that can cause neurologic changes ranging from mild ataxia and a slight head tilt (Fig. 22.50) to severe torticollis. It can also cause damage to the eyes, kidneys, and heart. This is a very common problem in breeding facilities, and rabbits often harbor the parasite in spore form, which can erupt and cause symptoms years after initial exposure. *E. cuniculi* is spread through urine, and good hygiene and quarantine are the best preventive measures.

Heat stress/stroke is common when adequate cooling is not provided in warm temperatures. Rabbits should have access to cool stone or tiles, ample fresh water, and cool hiding areas when the temperature is higher than 80°F.

Diarrhea is very dangerous in rabbits, causing life-threatening dehydration. Causes include intestinal parasites, such as coccidiosis (*Eimeria* spp.), colibacillosis, *Clostridium* infection, mucoid enteropathy, or ingestion of contraindicated antibiotics.

Pasteurella multocida infection is another common problem in rabbits. Clinical signs include nasal discharge, abscesses, conjunctivitis, and respiratory distress.

Rodents

Rodent species commonly seen in the veterinary hospital include guinea pigs, hamsters, gerbils, rats, and chinchillas. Although all of these animals are rodents, each species has particular anatomic characteristics, dietary requirements, and diseases. Blood collection in most rodent species can be accomplished by using the anterior vena cava or the jugular vein while the patient is sedated.

Antibiotic Therapy

Similar to rabbits, guinea pigs and chinchillas experience toxic and often fatal reactions to antibiotics such as penicillin, bacitracin, erythromycin, ampicillin, lincomycin, gentamicin, clindamycin, and vancomycin. They cause severe intestinal microbial imbalance (*dysbiosis*), causing intestinal ileus. Antibiotics that are considered safe include enrofloxacin, ciprofloxacin, chloramphenicol, oxytetracycline, and trimethoprim-sulfadiazine. Hamsters, gerbils, and rats, however, tolerate most antibiotics well. An exotic animal formulary is essential in an exotic animal practice to obtain specific information and dosages.

> **TECHNICIAN NOTE**
>
> Blood collection in most rodent species can be accomplished by using the anterior vena cava or the jugular vein while the patient is sedated.

Anesthesia and Analgesia

Safely anesthetizing rodents can be challenging for a few reasons. Intubation can be almost impossible in guinea pigs and chinchillas because of the palatal ostium. This is a tiny opening between the anterior and posterior oropharynx that makes visualization of the glottis impossible, and passing a tube blindly can damage the surrounding tissue. Other smaller rodents (mice, rats, and hamsters) are too small to intubate in a clinical setting. IV catheterization in these species is also difficult because of size and often requires an IO catheter.

In chinchillas and guinea pigs, combinations of ketamine, dexmedetomidine, alfaxalone, and benzodiazepines are injectable sedative/anesthetic agents that may be used to decrease anxiety and achieve a smooth induction. Once sedated, these animals can have an IV or IO catheter placed, and general anesthesia can be easily induced and maintained with isoflurane or sevoflurane. Because most of the smaller rodents are not intubated and IV catheters are not used, it is considered safer to use only an anxiolytic drug, such as midazolam, with a narcotic prior to gas induction to avoid complications that may occur with other sedatives and tranquilizers. Gas induction alone by box or mask is very stressful for all rodents and should be avoided. Once the rodent is sedated, it is fastest for the patient and safest for the veterinary staff to use the smallest induction chamber available (Fig. 22.51).

Local analgesics, narcotics, and NSAIDs are all safe and effective for use at proper dosages in pet rodents, and the dosages are significantly higher than those for dogs and cats. Rodents tolerate partial and full mu-opioids well and, like rabbits, cannot vomit. Use of analgesics is important to prevent pain that can cause rodents to chew incision sites, increase catecholamine release, and result in the animal becoming anorexic. In guinea pigs and chinchillas, these responses can cause GI stasis syndrome, similar to that of rabbits.

While a rodent is under anesthesia, monitoring equipment should be used, as with any other patient. A Doppler flow device

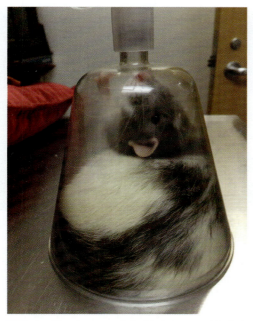

• **Fig. 22.51** A rat in a large mask that is being used for induction.

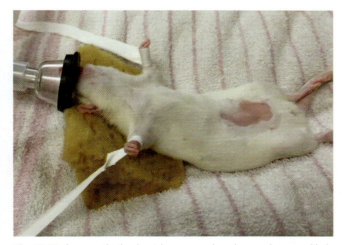

• **Fig. 22.52** An anesthetized rat in proper dorsal recumbency with her head and chest elevated above the level of her abdomen to allow easier respiration.

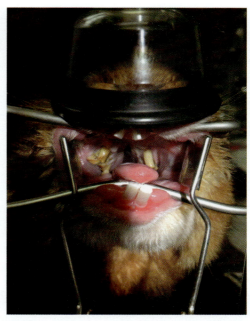

• **Fig. 22.53** Guinea pig on a dental restraint device with severely overgrown cheek teeth.

should be placed over the heart to monitor heart rate and rhythm. SpO₂, cardiac function (use of ECG with atraumatic clamps), temperature, and respiration rate should all be constantly monitored during anesthesia. These small animals become cold quickly and should be kept on heat support. Because most are not intubated and because they have very small thoracic cavities, it is recommended that rodents be positioned with the head and neck elevated to minimize pressure on the lungs and to maximize respiration (Fig. 22.52).

Antiparasitic Agents

Rodents often have lice when purchased. Ivermectin and selamectin (Revolution; Zoetis Inc., Florham Park, NJ) can be used to treat ectoparasites. Common intestinal parasites include coccidia and pinworms, which are safely treated with various anthelmintic drugs. See Chapter 13 for additional information on parasitology.

Guinea Pigs

The cavy, or guinea pig, has a long gestation (64 days), which leads to the birth of large, **precocious** young (relatively developed, mature, and mobile at birth). Although the female has only two mammary glands, she can successfully raise litters of three or more offspring. The most common guinea pig species kept as pets are the English or American, Abyssinian, and Peruvian long-hair types.

Guinea pigs should have access to monitored exercise time outside of an enclosure, and spacious, well-ventilated, plastic-bottomed wire enclosures should be used to house them. Soft padded substrate, such as fleece, towels, or bath mats, should line the bottom to protect feet and absorb urine. Guinea pigs do not require a particulate matter substrate; however, if the owners prefer it, a soft recycled paper product is recommended. Wood chips should be avoided because of artificial toxic odors and the sharp, pointed edges of the chips that can damage the delicate feet, mouth, and eyes of guinea pigs. Enclosures should always have a hiding spot for these shy animals and a variety of toys, such as balls, hay chew toys, and tubes for enrichment.

Like rabbits, guinea pigs have aradicular hypsodont elodont dentition, which may become maloccluded and overgrown without proper fibrous hay to chew (Fig. 22.53). Trauma, which can occur if the animal is dropped, can crack the incisors, also causing irregular growth. Molar spurs and malocclusions can cause severe pain and infection, resulting in anorexia and GI stasis/ileus, as in the rabbit. Lack of adequate hay to chew and grind is the main cause of overgrown teeth in guinea pigs.

At age 7 or 8 months, the pubic symphysis in female guinea pigs becomes fused. Pregnancy after this time is likely to result in a nondeliverable dystocia. If the sow is experiencing dystocia, retrieval of the young by cesarean section is often the only option to save her and the babies. Signs include vaginal bleeding, straining, and extreme lethargy. Cystic ovaries and other reproductive diseases are very common in intact female guinea pigs. Signs of

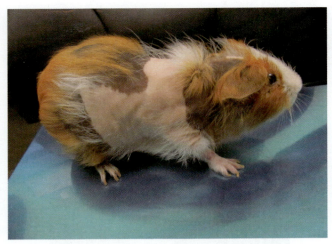

• **Fig. 22.54** Guinea pig with cystic ovaries, displaying bilateral hair loss before ovariohysterectomy.

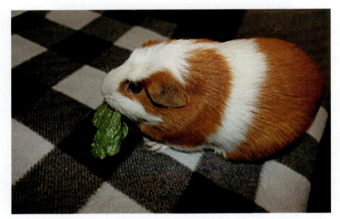

• **Fig. 22.55** Guinea pig after ovariohysterectomy, with resolved cystic ovaries and fur regrowth.

bilateral hair loss, vaginal bleeding, and weight loss often indicate a reproductive disease, and ovariohysterectomy is generally curative (Figs. 22.54 and 22.55).

Footpad dermatitis (bumblefoot) resulting in ulcers may develop in animals placed in wire-bottomed cages. Guinea pigs tend to be sedentary, and an overweight animal placed on metal grates is susceptible to development of sores. If left untreated, these wounds can advance to severe infection and osteomyelitis.

Nutrition

Guinea pigs are herbivores, but their digestion differs slightly from that in rabbits. Guinea pigs do not produce cecotropes; however, they do have coprophagous behavior (eating of feces). The recommended diet is similar to that for rabbits and should include ad libitum grass hay, such as timothy or orchard hay, plus a grass-based, commercial guinea pig pellet with select green leafy vegetables. A high-fiber/hay-based diet will reduce the incidence of ileus and overgrown teeth. Urinary calculi are common in pet guinea pigs (Fig. 22.56) as a result of high dietary calcium intake, such as with excessive alfalfa hay or calcium-rich vegetables. As in rabbits, avoiding high-calcium foods will prevent the formation of kidney and bladder stones.

Like humans, guinea pigs lack the enzyme L-gulonolactone oxidase, which is necessary to produce ascorbic acid (vitamin C).

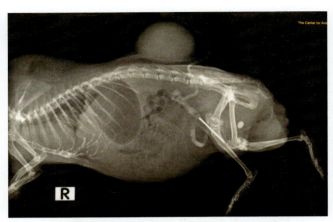

• **Fig. 22.56** Radiograph of a urolith in a guinea pig; an intraosseous catheter has been placed in the proximal tibia.

Therefore guinea pigs require ascorbic acid supplementation of 10 mg/kg per day. Many guinea pig pellets contain vitamin C; however, better options include offering vitamin C–rich foods, such as kale, parsley, and peppers. Use of vitamin C in the water is discouraged, both because it is not stable for very long in water and because it can impart an unpalatable flavor and discourage hydration. Clinical signs of vitamin C deficiency include alopecia, anorexia, and poor wound healing, along with eventual periodontal disease and temporomandibular joint inflammation.

Fresh water is essential for guinea pigs and should be provided daily. Water consumption prevents dehydration, ileus, and bladder stone formation. Heavy, shallow crocks instead of sipper bottles offer the best opportunity for guinea pigs to drink adequate amounts.

> **TECHNICIAN NOTE**
>
> Like humans, guinea pigs lack the enzyme L-gulonolactone oxidase, which is necessary to produce vitamin C, so they require a dietary ascorbic acid supplement.

Hamsters

The golden hamster is native to Syria and comes in many color varieties. Teddy Bear and Chinese Dwarf hamsters are also popular in the pet trade. Unique anatomical features include cheek pouches that extend along the head and neck to the proximal dorsum of the back, used to store and move food (Fig. 22.57), and noticeable sebaceous glands that appear as dark brown patches of skin on each side of the caudal lateral abdominal region; these are used to mark territory and in mating rituals.

Hamsters live for 18 to 24 months, have a gestation length of 16 days, and produce, on average, five offspring. If disturbed by human presence, the female may cannibalize her litter or hide them in her cheek pouches, which can cause suffocation. Hamsters tend to fight brutally and therefore should be housed alone. Males can be identified by their greater anogenital distance and pair of large scrotal sacs.

> **TECHNICIAN NOTE**
>
> If disturbed by human presence, the female may cannibalize her litter or hide them in her cheek pouches, which can cause suffocation.

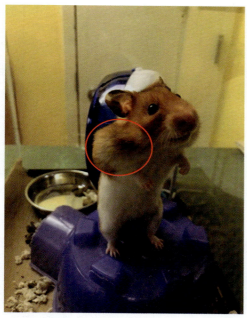

• **Fig. 22.57** A hamster with full cheek pouches *(red circle)*.

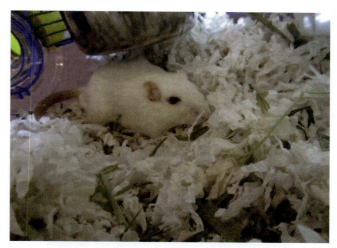

• **Fig. 22.58** A gerbil with appropriate digging substrate.

Hamsters are nocturnal and have a tendency to bite, especially when awakened. Many hamsters are purchased as pets for children, but owners should be warned about their nature and taught how to handle them with caution. Hamsters that are dropped or accidentally flung after they bite can sustain life-threatening traumatic injuries. Hamsters should be picked up by cupping the hands under their bodies and restrained gently with hand towels. Scruffing at the nape can be an effective way to restrain them; however, they are prone to eye proptosis during scruffing, so attention should be paid to the eyes if using this restraint.

Hamsters have hypsodontic elodont incisors and, unlike guinea pigs and rabbits, anelodont premolars and molars (they do not continuously grow). They are good at chewing through plastic cage material, which often results in escape. Cages should be well-ventilated, high-quality hard plastic or glass enclosures. Hamsters love to dig, bury, and hide in deep particulate substrate. Aromatic shavings, such as cedar or pine, may cause ocular and respiratory irritation and should therefore be avoided. Recycled paper products are safer and more comfortable for use as substrate. Sipper bottles work well for dispensing water, and vessels made of nonchewable material should be used as food bowls. Hamsters are very active at night and require an exercise wheel to accommodate the animal's active physical nature.

Hamsters are omnivorous. A commercially made pelleted hamster diet is preferred over a seed-based product, which can lead to obesity and malnutrition. Treats, including small amounts of seed, fruits, vegetables, and healthy human foods, may be given to hamsters, but the base diet should consist of a pelleted hamster product.

Wet tail is a general term used to refer to diarrhea in the hamster. This potentially life-threatening problem is most often caused by bacterial infection and dysbiosis but can also be caused by intestinal parasites or viral infection. Other common illnesses in hamsters include trauma, dermatitis (fungal, parasitic, or bacterial), cheek pouch impactions, reproductive disease (mostly females), and various kinds of tumors.

Gerbils

The Mongolian gerbil, which is native to Mongolia and northeastern China, is a popular pet. It is an active burrowing animal adapted to the desert environment (Fig. 22.58). The gerbil has a life span of 3.5 years and a gestation duration of 25 days. Litter sizes average five offspring. Gerbils have dentition and dietary requirements similar to the hamster. They are friendly rodents and may be housed in commercially available hamster enclosures to prevent escape. They tend to be more active during the day compared with hamsters and also enjoy digging, running on a wheel, and taking dust or sand baths. Gender is determined by measuring the urogenital distance, which is much longer in the male than in the female. Female gerbils tend not to cannibalize their young or fight with other adults. In fact, males assist with care of the young. It is recommended that gerbils be kept in pairs, ensuring they are spayed or neutered to avoid large numbers of births.

Gerbils have long tails and are prone to "tail slip," which occurs when the fur and skin from the tail comes off when they are inappropriately picked up by the tail. This can result in the need for tail amputation. Restraint should be similar to that of a hamster.

Certain gerbil lines are prone to epileptiform seizures. Stress caused by handling, change of environment, or a weakened immune system can induce these seizures; however, they do not typically cause severe or permanent harm.

Rats

Despite the stigma, rats are clean, intelligent animals that can be trained and make great pets. Rats seldom bite, but caution must be used in stressful situations or around food. Rats may live up to 3 years. Commercial rodent cages can be obtained for proper housing. The substrate should be similar to that provided for other rodents, although they do not tend to dig or burrow as much as gerbils and hamsters do; therefore deep particulate substrate is not necessary. Rats should have hiding areas and plenty of enrichment to stimulate them, such as running wheels, climbing ropes, and foraging toys. They are very social animals and should be housed in pairs or groups. Rats are omnivores, and several excellent formulated rat pellets are available. Treats (e.g., vegetables, fruit, healthy human foods) may be provided in small, regulated quantities. Rats, like gerbils and hamsters, have hypsodontic elodont incisors and benefit from wood chew toys.

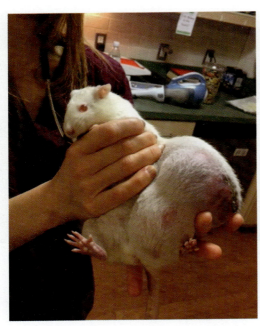

• **Fig. 22.59** A rat with a very large mammary tumor.

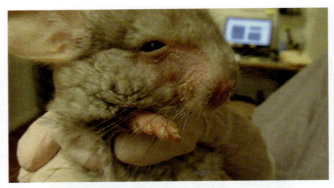

• **Fig. 22.60** A chinchilla with *Trichophyton mentagrophytes*.

TECHNICIAN NOTE

Rats seldom bite, but caution must be used in stressful situations or around food.

Rats are highly susceptible to neoplasia, particularly mammary gland tumors (Fig. 22.59). These tumors are believed to be driven by excess estrogen that is produced when pituitary gland tumors stimulate estrogen release from the ovaries. Performing an ovariohysterectomy of rats younger than 6 months of age decreases the incidence of mammary tumors. *Mycoplasma* spp. respiratory infections are commonly diagnosed and may appear clinically as dyspnea with signs of nasal discharge. Enrofloxacin and doxycycline have been used to effectively treat *Mycoplasma* spp. infections in rats; however, most infections are recurrent. Rats that are ill or under stress can develop ocular and nasal discharge called *chromodacryorrhea*, which is tinged red as a result of the pigment from harderian gland secretions. Owners often mistake this pigment as blood.

Chinchillas

Chinchillas are native to the Andes mountains in South America and have become fairly common pet rodents, known for their very soft fur. These rodents have a shy disposition and do well living with at least one other chinchilla. They are sexually mature at 6 to 8 months of age and have a long gestation period of 111 days. They have one to three offspring that are born precocious, with full hair coats, open eyes, and teeth. Chinchillas can live up to 20 years.

Chinchillas are nocturnal, and enclosures should have hiding areas for them to rest during the day. They have very delicate feet that can be damaged in traditional rodent wheels; however, wheels designed with flat surfaces, specifically for chinchillas, are ideal for providing exercise at night.

Like rabbits and guinea pigs, all of a chinchilla's teeth are hypsodont and elodont, and they require large amounts of hay and roughage to keep their teeth filed. Chewing material, such as

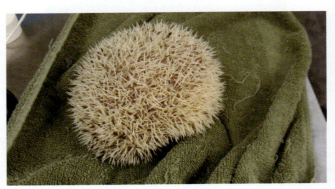

• **Fig. 22.61** A hedgehog that has tucked into itself, making a defensive ball.

sticks, bark, and deer antlers, make great toys and help keep teeth filed. Grass- or hay-based pellets can be given in small amounts to supplement ad libitum hay. An important component of their care is providing them with formulated chinchilla dust to bathe in several times a week. This natural behavior helps absorb oil and dirt to keep their dense fur healthy. Dust should be provided in a box or tray, and water baths should never be given.

Chinchillas are nervous animals that do not readily enjoy demonstrations of human affection. When scared, they will try to escape, and females often defend themselves by spraying urine and barking/chirping, but they rarely bite. Proper restraint is accomplished by grasping the body and supporting the rear area. If their tail is grasped, it is very easy to accidentally fracture or pull the skin or fur off, as with a gerbil. Common problems include traumatic injuries, GI stasis, dental disease, and malocclusion. Chinchillas are also commonly seen after purchase as juveniles to be suffering from *Trichophyton mentagrophytes* (ringworm) infection (Fig. 22.60) and giardiasis.

Hedgehogs

The African hedgehog is a shy nocturnal animal that likes to hide, stay in dark quiet areas, and burrow. Hedgehogs may be housed similarly to rodents in a 20-gallon (or larger) enclosure lined with absorbable paper bedding. Although hedgehogs spend most of the day hiding, they are very active at night. Hiding huts, running wheels (made for hedgehogs, not rodents), and soaking/swimming receptacles are vital for providing comfort and physical enrichment.

- 3 teaspoon (tsp) commercially available hedgehog diet, such as Mazuri Insectivore Diet (Mazuri Exotic Animal Nutrition, St. Louis, MO), fed per manufacturer's directions
- 1 tsp fruit and vegetable mix
- Four to eight live insects that have been gut loaded, such as dubia roaches, phoenix worms, superworms, or crickets.

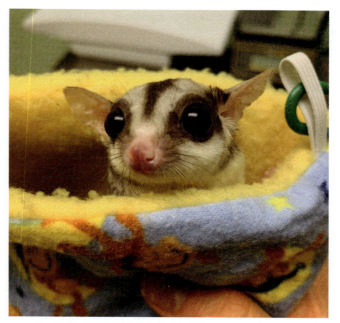

• **Fig. 22.63** A sugar glider being held safely in a fleece pouch.

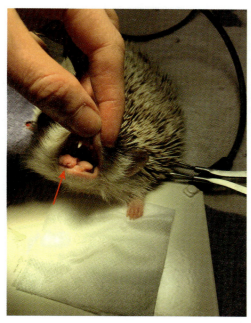

• **Fig. 22.62** A sedated hedgehog with an oral mass *(red arrow)*.

The life span of hedgehogs is 3 to 5 years. Biannual physical examinations are recommended for teeth cleaning, nail trimming, and tumor checks. One feature of hedgehog medicine is that most hedgehog patients must be sedated or anesthetized, even for a simple examination. Their spines are very sharp, so caution must be taken during handling; gloves may be necessary, particularly before anesthesia is administered (Fig. 22.61). Hedgehogs are not rodents or porcupines, and they rely on an insectivore-omnivore diet (Box 22.2).

Blood collection is performed while the animal is anesthetized, and collection sites include the cranial vena cava and the jugular vein. Diseases commonly diagnosed in hedgehogs are neoplasia (particularly in the oral cavity) (Fig. 22.62), obesity, otitis externa, dermatitis, external parasites, and respiratory disease.

Sugar Gliders

Sugar gliders are nocturnal marsupials that are native to Australia (Fig. 22.63). Like hedgehogs, they are unusual pets with unique qualities that should be considered carefully by a potential owner before a purchase is made. They are very social animals and should not be made to live alone. Without companionship, sugar gliders often develop undesirable psychological behaviors, such as genital self-mutilation.

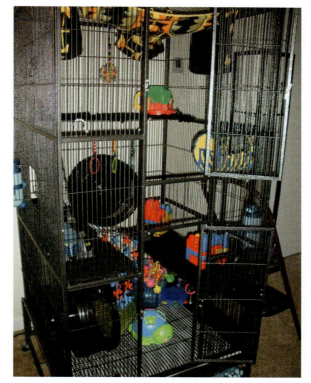

• **Fig. 22.64** An appropriate sugar glider enclosure.

Sugar gliders are arboreal, and housing should be a tall wire enclosure (Fig. 22.64) with branches and places to hide, such as a bird nesting box. The wire mesh should have spacing no larger than one square inch to prevent escape. The bottom tray should be lined with shredded paper or pelleted paper products for easy cleaning and optimal absorption of urine, food, and water.

Blood collection is best performed using the cranial vena cava or jugular vein while the animals is anesthetized. Giving benzodiazepines prior to anesthesia will decrease stress and is recommended over gas induction alone. Restraint of sugar gliders is similar to that of a small bird, using caution around the mouth. Needle-sharp incisors can cause a painful injury if they bite.

Despite their name, sugar gliders should not consume large amounts of sugar or fruit. In the wild, they eat eucalyptus gum, sap, insects, nectar, eggs, and small animals. This diet is difficult to replicate in captivity. Commercial pelleted glider diets, such as Mazuri Insectivore Diet (Mazuri Exotic Animal Nutrition, St. Louis, MO), supplemented by small amounts of insects, fruits, and vegetables, are appropriate. Malnutrition and hypocalcemia are common conditions diagnosed in sugar gliders, and proper supplementation is mandatory. Overfeeding of high-sugar foods can cause obesity in captive sugar gliders.

Acknowledgments

The author and the publisher wish to acknowledge the contributions of Thomas N. Tully, Jr., to previous editions of this chapter.

Recommended Readings

Altman RB, Clubb SL, Dorrestein GM, et al. *Avian Medicine and Surgery*. St. Louis, MO: Saunders; 1997.

Carpenter JW. *Exotic Animal Formulary*. 6th ed. St. Louis, MO: Saunders; 2022.

Campbell TW. *Avian and Exotic Animal Hematology and Cytology*. 5th ed. Ames, IA: Wiley-Blackwell; 2022.

Harrison GJ, Harrison LR, Ritchie BW. *Avian Medicine: Principles and Application*. Lake Worth, FL: Wingers Publishing; 1994.

Speer Brian. *Current Therapy in Avian Medicine and Surgery*. St. Louis, MO: Saunders; 2015.

Longley LA. *Anesthesia of Exotic Pets*. St. Louis, MO: Saunders; 2008.

Mader D. *Reptile and Amphibian Medicine and Surgery*. 3rd ed. St. Louis, MO: Saunders; 2019.

Meyer J, Donnelly TM. *Clinical Veterinary Advisor: Birds and Exotic Pets*. St. Louis, MO: Saunders; 2013.

O'Malley B. *Clinical Anatomy and Physiology of Exotic Species: Structure and Function of Mammals, Birds, Reptiles and Amphibians*. Germany: Saunders; 2005.

Quesenberry K, Carpenter JW. *Ferrets, Rabbits, and Rodents: Clinical Medicine and Surgery*. 4th ed. St. Louis, MO: Saunders; 2020.

Tully TN, Dorrestein GM, Jones AK. *Handbook of Avian Medicine*. 2nd ed. St. Louis, MO: Saunders; 2009.

23

Rehabilitation and Integrative Medical Nursing

LEILANI ALVAREZ AND DEANA CAPPUCCI

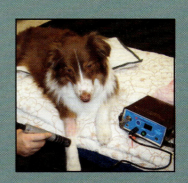

CHAPTER OUTLINE

LEARNING OBJECTIVES

When you have completed this chapter, you will be able to:

1. Pronounce, define, and spell all key terms in this chapter.
2. List the common indications for veterinary rehabilitation.
3. Understand the principles and implementation of therapeutic exercise and manual therapies.
4. Compare and contrast the therapeutic modalities used in veterinary rehabilitation, including electrical- and magnet-based therapies, light- and sound-based therapies, and superficial thermal therapies.
5. List supportive and assistive devices commonly used for animal patients.
6. List commonly used nutraceuticals and chondroprotectants and describe their therapeutic uses.
7. Explain the principles and techniques of acupuncture and describe the role of the veterinary technician in acupuncture therapy.
8. Describe how veterinary spinal manipulative therapy can benefit animal patients and explain the role of the veterinary technician.
9. Describe the role of veterinary herbal medicine.

KEY TERMS

Acupuncture
Cryotherapy
Extracorporeal shockwave
Goniometer
Gulick
Hydrotherapy
Intervertebral disk disease
Low-level laser therapy
Massage
Myotherapy

Neuromuscular electrical stimulation
Nutraceutical
Passive range of motion
Rehabilitation
Therapeutic ultrasonography
Thermotherapy
Transcutaneous electrical nerve stimulation
Veterinary physical rehabilitation
Veterinary spinal manipulative therapy

Introduction

Integrative medicine is a growing field of veterinary medicine. It is a group of diverse medical and health care systems, practices, and products that are not presently considered part of conventional medicine. Integrative medicine utilizes complementary modalities *in conjunction with* conventional medicine, whereas alternative medicine is used *instead of* conventional medicine.

This chapter offers an overview of the integrative modalities most commonly used in veterinary practice today. The following therapies will be discussed: acupuncture, veterinary spinal manipulative therapy, herbal medicine, and nutraceuticals. Case reports will illustrate the principles and practice of various therapies. For additional information, refer to the section "Recommended Reading and Resources" at the end of this chapter.

Physical Rehabilitation

Physical rehabilitation is the newest recognized specialty by the American Veterinary Medical Association (AVMA). The human equivalent, physical therapy, has been in existence since World War I. Equine rehabilitation began in the 1960s, and canine rehabilitation began in the mid-1980s. In 1997, certification programs in both canine and equine rehabilitation were established. The term *physical therapy* is a protected term in the United States, and the term *physiotherapy* is a protected term in Canada, the United Kingdom, and some states in the United States; these terms can only be used exclusively by trained physical therapists. In the veterinary field, terms *rehabilitation* or *veterinary physical rehabilitation* are used. In 2010, the AVMA approved the College of Veterinary Sports Medicine and Rehabilitation (ACVSMR) as a specialty in veterinary medicine, and in 2017, the National Association of Veterinary Technicians (NAVTA) recognized the Academy of Physical Rehabilitation Veterinary Technicians (APRVT) as one of the newest veterinary technician specialties.

Rehabilitation can be defined as relief of pain and restoration of mobility and function. The term *physical therapy* (or *physiotherapy*) is more specific, referring mainly to the physical aspects of a disability or disorder, whereas *rehabilitation* is a broader term that may encompass lifestyle management and physical intervention. Rehabilitation, by nature, is a team effort. Patients do best when a collaborative effort is made by the primary veterinarian, the specialist (surgeon, neurologist, or other), the rehabilitation team, and the patient's owner. The rehabilitation team may consist of a veterinarian (board certified in rehabilitation or certified through an approved course), a physical therapist (certified through an approved veterinary course), and one or several veterinary technicians and/or physical therapy assistants. All team members must be dynamic in their roles and responsibilities. Good communication and feedback are essential to a successful rehabilitation program.

TECHNICIAN NOTE

The role of the veterinary technician in a rehabilitation program is often extensive. Training and certification programs are available for technicians. In many rehabilitation practices, the veterinary technician is the primary caregiver, performing all exercise-based and assistive therapies and most manual and modality-based treatments.

Before implementing a rehabilitation protocol, it is imperative for the veterinarian to fully evaluate each patient and determine their overall health to ensure that the therapies performed

---

• BOX 23.1   **Common Problems of Physical Dysfunction**

Pain
Inflammation (swelling, heat)
Reduced range of motion
Hypermobility
Muscle atrophy
Muscle tightness
Muscle spasm and trigger points
Fibrosis and scarring
Abnormal gait (lameness, pacing)
Neurologic dysfunction (placing reaction deficits)
Ataxia
Weakness
Exercise intolerance

---

during a rehabilitation session are appropriate for the patient. In rehabilitation, treatment is based on a problem list of dysfunctions (Box 23.1). These are often grouped into primary and secondary, or compensatory, problems. Rehabilitation therapy should be tailored to the individual patient, not the disease, according to the animal's signalment, condition, and other concurrent conditions. An assessment of a patient for rehabilitation therapy starts with a complete physical examination, orthopedic examination, neurologic examination, and rehabilitation examination. There are multiple components to a rehabilitation examination: gait analysis, goniometry, strength testing, muscle mass measurement, and a thorough assessment of myofascial tissues. Gait analysis is important in determining lameness, whether it is done subjectively by watching the patient walk and trot or objectively by force plate analysis or pressure sensitive walkway. A **goniometer** is used to measure the range of motion (ROM, both flexion and extension) of all distal joints, including the carpus, elbow, shoulder, tarsus, stifle, and hip (Fig. 23.1). A **Gulick** is used for indirect muscle mass measurement, which can be performed on the limbs to determine muscle atrophy, and around the abdomen to determine weight loss (Fig. 23.2). Strength testing is measured by lifting one limb at a time and determining if a patient can hold that position in neutral or on elevated ground without compensation. Strength is measured on a scale of 0–5. Normal strength (5/5) is noted if the patient can hold a single limb down for 15 sec while the contralateral limb is elevated at tarsal height. Fair strength (3/5) is noted if the patient can hold a single limb down on neutral ground without compensation while the contralateral limb is elevated. Lower grades of strength (<3/5) are considered poor or trace strength due to compensation in ability to weight bear on neutral ground.

It is imperative to examine the entire patient and compare the values of the unaffected limb with those of the affected limb. It is also important to repeat the measurements at a desired recheck examination to determine the effectiveness of the rehabilitation therapy. The goals of therapy must be established with a corresponding timeline, and the individual goals of the owners should also be discussed with them. Once the evaluation is performed and the goals are determined, a rehabilitation program can be prescribed. It should be kept in mind that the program might change, because the patient may exceed or be unable to meet the goals of the original plan.

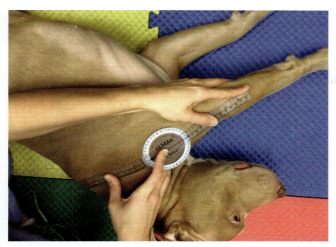

• **Fig. 23.1** Goniometer measurement of the shoulder joint in a dog.

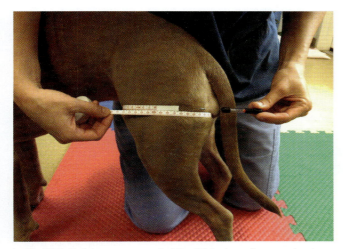

• **Fig. 23.2** Gulick measurement of the thigh circumference of a dog.

TECHNICIAN NOTE

Depending on the state or provincial regulations and individual hospital protocols, all or some of the evaluation may be done by a veterinarian or a physical therapist. It is important for any technician involved in rehabilitation practice to have a thorough knowledge of the evaluation process. While some states may allow for a veterinary technician or assistant to perform a rehabilitation evaluation, the authors do not support this and would rather recommend that veterinary technicians always work alongside a veterinarian who is highly trained in rehabilitation.

The first thing to consider when starting rehabilitation therapy is pain management. If the patient is in too much pain, it will be reluctant to perform certain tasks. A multimodal approach to pain management is highly recommended, because pain control can be achieved in a variety of ways and tailored to the individual patient. A multimodal approach may include pharmaceuticals, such as NSAIDs and opioids, nutraceuticals, and chondroprotectants; acupuncture; manual therapy; and therapeutic modalities. The modalities discussed in this section include the following: exercise-based therapy (therapeutic exercises, hydrotherapy, and land treadmill); manual therapy (passive ROM and massage); electrical-based therapy (neuromuscular stimulation, pulsed electromagnetic field therapy); light- and sound-based therapy

(low-level laser therapy, **therapeutic ultrasonography**, and extra-corporeal shockwave); superficial thermal agents (heat and cryotherapy); and assistive devices.

One of the goals of rehabilitation is to restore function within the damaged tissue. To understand how to rehabilitate the injured tissue, the technician first needs to understand tissue healing and its response to disuse. There are three phases of healing: inflammatory, reparative, and remodeling. The inflammatory phase involves an acute vascular response followed by infiltration of cell mediators that typically lasts 2 to 5 days (or sometimes longer if there is infection or other compromises). Hemostasis is formed by creating a hematoma, or a fibrous plug. The formation of the fibrin plugs initiate chemotaxis, or cell signaling. Neutrophils are the first cells to appear, and their function is wound debridement and phagocytosis of microorganisms to minimize potential infection. Macrophages appear a few days later, leading into the reparative phase through angiogenesis and fibroplasia for scar tissue formation. The reparative phase, also known as the *proliferative phase*, is characterized by the influx of epithelial cells or fibroblasts, which are the primary cells that make up scar tissue. This phase typically lasts 2 weeks (or longer if tissue is compromised) after the initial injury, preparing the cell matrix to increase tensile strength. The remodeling, or maturation, phase is the final aspect of wound healing in which the collagen fibers create cross-link patterns to maintain stable scar tissue formation. The stronger the collagen deposition and cross-link formation, the more adequate is the resulting tensile strength of the tissue. Tensile strength can continue to increase over the course of 1 year or longer.

Bone healing occurs through primary or secondary healing. Primary healing, or direct bone healing, occurs when there is direct formation of bone across the fracture line, which creates reabsorption canals that lie parallel to the long axis of the bone. Osteoblasts move through this canal to prepare to lay down new bone formation. Secondary healing, or indirect bone healing, occurs when there is a large gap formation between fragments, and a callus is formed. The callus size is related to the amount of instability at the fracture site. Wolff's law states that bone will be remodeled according to the appropriate stress forces applied and reabsorbed where no force is delivered. This concept means that applying weight-bearing forces through the healing phase results in the formation of stronger bone. When bone is immobilized, it is reabsorbed, with most bone loss occurring closest to bone marrow, resulting in weakened bone. Studies have indicated that weight bearing and controlled rehabilitation contribute to better bone healing and return of tensile strength.

Tendon healing depends on whether the tendon is covered by a vascular paratenon or a synovial sheath. Paratenon-covered tendons rely on fibroblasts and capillaries from surrounding tissues to invade the injured tendon to promote healing. Synovial-sheathed tendons rely on intrinsic blood supply and infiltration of the inflammatory phase to initiate the healing response. Immobilization for synovial-sheathed tendons is critical at this initial phase to allow for adequate healing. After the inflammatory phase, collagen deposition continues initially as type III but refigures into stronger formation of type I as the repair and remodeling phase continues. Collagen deposition requires a minimum of up to 28 days for appropriate fiber alignment and can take up to 4 months. The goal of tendon repair is to minimize adhesion formation to facilitate return to maximum function. Early controlled passive movement may be initiated within the first 3 weeks of repair to allow proper alignment of collagen fibers; however, end ROM should be avoided until the remodeling phase is complete to avoid excessive gap formation.

Muscle injury results in damage to myofibrils caused by contusions, ruptures, ischemia, or strains. Muscle healing proceeds from the initial inflammatory phase, resulting in hemostasis, followed by repair with scar tissue formation. Immobilization for a minimum of 2 to 3 weeks is important to protect repair and prevent remobilization stress, which could prolong the healing process. After the reparative phase, controlled movement at the site of injury can help align and orient muscle fibers. If the motion is too excessive, the gap widening expands and the muscle will heal with more fibrous tissue. Scar tissue within the muscle is undesirable because of the potential for injury recurrence and a decrease in approximately 50% muscle contractile strength. Immobilization of a muscle can lead to disuse atrophy and can happen rapidly within the first week of immobilization, increasing over time. Controlled mobility is important for muscle fiber recruitment and for the prevention of atrophy.

Clinical Indications

The goals of rehabilitation are to decrease pain and restore, maintain, and promote optimal function, fitness, wellness, and quality of life, because these factors relate to movement disorders and general health. That said, most animals that are seen in the clinic can benefit from rehabilitation. The most common indications for rehabilitation include osteoarthritis; orthopedic conditions (dysplasia, fractures, cruciate ligament tears, meniscal tears, patellar luxation, tendinopathies); neurologic conditions (intervertebral disk disease, fibrocartilaginous embolism, wobbler syndrome, polyneuropathy); strengthening for athletic performance; and weight management. Box 23.2 lists the most common conditions treated in rehabilitation facilities.

Exercise-Based Therapy

Exercise is essential to any rehabilitation program. Intensity level and duration are dependent on the patient's level of function. For seniors and geriatric patients that have arthritis or are neurologically weak, exercise needs to be very gentle and may be performed with a great deal of assistance. Sessions would be short and frequent (three or four 5- to 10-minute sessions over the day). For an athletic animal almost at the stage of returning to competition, exercise can be very rigorous and demanding (two to three 20- to 30-minute sessions per day, with cardio, strength, and sport-specific activity intermixed). As a rule, it is best to start out conservatively to prevent the patient from an initial setback. By assessing the response to initial sessions, the therapist can better tailor a program that challenges the patient without causing excessive fatigue or pain.

Therapeutic Exercises

Therapeutic exercises are used to improve strength, balance, and coordination. Various exercises can be used to build muscle strength, increase weight bearing, improve stamina and endurance, and retrain muscles. Specific exercises are based on the individual patient's needs and clinical condition. Examples of therapeutic exercises and their purposes are provided in Table 23.1

PUT INTO PRACTICE

It often behooves the technician working with physical rehabilitation therapy to be in shape themselves. Give yourself permission to go to the gym and strengthen those muscles. Your patients will reap the rewards.

• BOX 23.2   **Common Conditions Treated at Rehabilitation Facilities**

Musculoskeletal
Osteoarthritis
Developmental orthopedic disease (hip dysplasia, elbow dysplasia, osteochondritis dissecans)
Joint injuries
Sprains, strains, muscle tears
Muscle contractures
Tendonitis and bursitis
Cranial cruciate ligament injuries (partial or full tears)
Joint replacement
Fracture repair
Arthrodesis
Amputation

Neurologic
Intervertebral disk disease
Fibrocartilaginous embolism
Peripheral neuropathy
Degenerative myelopathy
Cervical spondylomyelopathy
Degenerative lumbosacral stenosis

Other
Weight management
Wound healing
Athletic conditioning

TABLE 23.1   **Therapeutic Exercises**

Exercise	Type	Use
Sit to stand	Strengthening	Pelvic limbs
Walking on a hill	Endurance	Incline: pelvic limbs Decline: thoracic limbs
Zigzag/weave	Proprioception Coordination	Whole body
Backward walking	Strengthening	Pelvic limb
Balance board	Balance Proprioception	Limbs on the board
Balance board	Strengthening	Limbs not on the board
Play bow	Strengthening	Thoracic limb
Cavaletti poles	Proprioception	Gait training
Sit up and wave	Strengthening	Core, thoracic limbs

Strengthening exercises can target specific muscle groups, such as hamstrings and gluteals. They are used when atrophy is present or when increased strength in specific areas is desired. Some exercises target a broader range of muscles, such as the abdominal or paraspinal muscles (Fig. 23.3). These are core-strengthening exercises and are appropriate at some level for every patient undergoing rehabilitation. Core muscles are not only abdominal and back muscles but also include the muscles that connect the limb to the trunk (for example, shoulder and hip flexor muscles are important core stabilizers). Stretching exercises

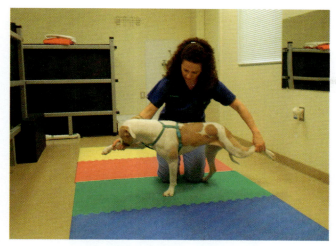

• **Fig. 23.3** Two-leg standing exercise.

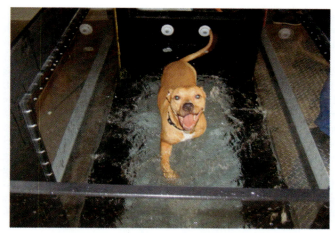

• **Fig. 23.5** A dog walking on the underwater treadmill.

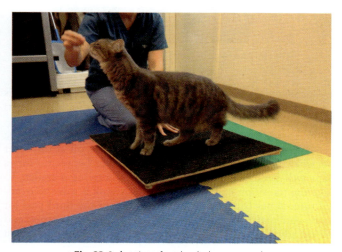

• **Fig. 23.4** A cat performing balance exercise.

can also be targeted to a specific muscle or group of muscles and can be active or passive.

Proprioception exercises help a patient develop better body awareness. Balance exercises improve overall stability (Fig. 23.4). Both types of exercise not only help patients that are weak and ataxic, but they also help improve athletic performance when seconds count. These exercises are also crucial for rehabilitation of a patient with an injured joint, because ligaments contain proprioceptive fibers, which often are damaged by joint injury.

Endurance exercises focus on the cardiovascular system and are whole-body exercises. They may include walking, jogging, and swimming. Walking is the cornerstone of rehabilitation and is recommended for all patients. It is important that the animal be on a leash while walking, starting with about 5 minutes and gradually working up to 30 to 45 minutes (to be increased by 5 minutes per week, if tolerated). Hills or stairs can be added to encourage more weight bearing (uphill or up the stairs for pelvic limb strengthening, and downhill or down the stairs for thoracic limb strengthening). Neuromuscular re-education exercises involve posture and gait corrections that vary in the degree of therapist assistance needed. The weaker the muscle or the more abnormal the gait pattern, the higher the level of assistance needed. Generally, the patient is required to do as much as physically possible, and the therapist assists as needed in attaining the correct posture and gait.

An exercise plan is generally developed by the senior veterinarian or the physical therapist. The rehabilitation technician helps the patient perform the exercises, modifying them according to patient response. Technicians may also be responsible for teaching clients how to help their animals perform the exercises at home.

Hydrotherapy

Hydrotherapy involves the use of water to promote physical activity (Fig. 23.5). It takes advantage of the physical properties of water, such as temperature, buoyancy, and hydrostatic pressure, for therapeutic purposes. The buoyancy of water decreases stress on the joints. The hydrostatic pressure of water reduces edema. The viscosity and surface tension of water improve strengthening and proprioception.

Walking on an underwater treadmill in warm water provides the benefits of increased joint ROM, improved muscle flexibility and mobility, enhanced circulation, and facilitation of front-to-rear and side-to-side balance. Because it can relieve pain and increase muscle strength while putting decreased weight on the joints, this activity is extremely beneficial in the treatment of osteoarthritis. It is also an invaluable tool when working with patients with neurologic deficits, because many patients can take steps in water before they can perform voluntary motion on land. Swimming, without an underwater treadmill, also provides many of these benefits, especially for elbow and carpal ROM. However, dogs most commonly swim with stronger thoracic limb strokes, so this may not be the best treatment if the goal is to strengthen the pelvic limbs.

For companion animals, massage, stretching, and exercises can also be done in water before, during, or after swimming or walking on the underwater treadmill. It is generally more difficult and even dangerous to be in a hydrotherapy tank with horses, so massage and stretching are generally done on land.

> **TECHNICIAN NOTE**
>
> Athletic dogs and horses can benefit from underwater treadmill and swimming for conditioning and for improving athletic performance.

Dynamic variables in the aquatic environment include buoyancy, resistance, flexion and extension of the limbs, speed, and patterning. Buoyancy can be enhanced with the use of a life vest, which makes swimming easier. Resistance can be increased with the use of jets. To maximize flexion, balloons or water wings can be used, or the water level can be lowered to just above the joint that is desired to maximize flexion. When the depth of water is changed, resistance, buoyancy, and flexion/extension are affected. The deeper the water, the greater the buoyancy and the easier the movement for the patient. The maximum strengthening occurs when the water level is at the stifle, as this water depth allows 85% of normal weight bearing (91% of weight bearing occurs at the level of the tarsus and 38% at the level of the greater trochanter). Altering treadmill speed will affect the speed of the patient, thereby changing the intensity of the workout. *Patterning* can be defined as teaching the body to act in a certain way without conscious thought (a human example would be riding a bicycle or skiing). With animals, proper gait can be achieved by moving their limbs or stimulating their limbs to move in a certain pattern (walk, trot, or pace).

Although the veterinarian determines the variables associated with hydrotherapy, the technician plays a very important role. In addition to keeping detailed records of each session, the technician stays in the pool or hydrotherapy tank with the canine patient, facilitates correct motion, monitors the patient, and provides massage, stretching, or exercises as needed. If the patient has fecal incontinence, before it gets into the pool, the technician can use a cotton swab to rectally stimulate the patient to defecate outside of the pool. When the patient is done with the pool, the technician may towel dry and/or blow dry the patient. Technicians should also be responsible for pool care (testing the water and adding any chemicals that may be needed). For equine patients, training the horse to safely enter and exit the treadmill (whether an in-ground system or a tank system is used), while monitoring and adjusting the variables and holding the lead would be responsibilities of the technician.

> **TECHNICIAN NOTE**
>
> Although the veterinarian determines the variables associated with hydrotherapy, the technician plays a very important role. In addition to keeping detailed records of each session, the technician stays in the pool or hydrotherapy tank with the canine patient, facilitates correct motion, monitors the patient, and provides massage, stretching, or exercises as needed.

Land Treadmill

Land treadmills are used for increasing strength and endurance and for re-educating on front-to-back balance and normal foot placement (Fig. 23.6). Walking either just uphill or just downhill can alter habitual compensation after an injury. By walking uphill, a patient with nonclinical hip dysplasia can strengthen the muscles around the hip, decreasing laxity and delaying the onset of clinical signs. After surgery, when a patient places a limb laterally, the patient will often place it back in normal position when walking on a treadmill, especially if the treadmill is set at an angle that decreases weight on that limb. Although treadmills re-create the same motion as walking on land, fewer muscles are used, because the belt movement reduces the body's need for self-propulsion. Therefore the benefits of the treadmill are maximized when the treadmill is set to uphill or downhill motion. Land treadmills can also be used for a wide variety of other exercises that can intermix with other equipment, such as physioballs, to add additional challenge or target specific muscles. For example, to target pelvic limb lateral stabilizers, the patient can balance the forelimbs on a

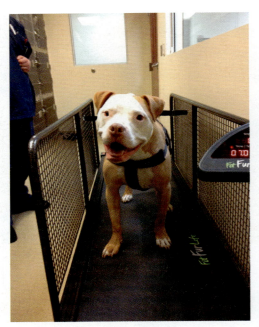

• **Fig. 23.6** A dog walking on the land treadmill.

physioball and the hindlimbs sidestep as the belt is running. This is an excellent exercise to strengthen lateral hindlimb stabilizers and an excellent core and proprioceptive exercise.

The goal of teaching patients to use the treadmill is to have them be comfortable getting on at one end and off at the other end when done and enjoying the workout in between. Horses adapt well because this movement is like entering a trailer. To make the transition easier, the patient can walk across the treadmill three times (sitting and then standing on the third pass for canine patients). On the fourth pass, the treadmill is started and quickly advanced to a normal pace with no hesitation between steps. Starting the treadmill too slowly will cause awkwardness and therefore should be avoided. It is important to ensure that patients look in a forward direction to avoid habitual sidewinding.

> **TECHNICIAN NOTE**
>
> The technician's role is to teach the patient to use the treadmill without fear, to monitor the patient for gait changes and weariness while on the treadmill, and to record the time, speed, angle, and progress of the patient.

Manual Therapies

Massage

Massage is defined as systematic manipulation of the soft tissues of the body for the purpose of obtaining or maintaining health. Massage has been performed for thousands of years. More than 70 types of human massage techniques are known, many of which can be applied to animals.

> **TECHNICIAN NOTE**
>
> The technician, if properly trained, can play a key role in massage therapy. Most massage certification courses are available to technicians, allowing them to be the primary massage therapists for animal patients. Training schools are listed at the end of this chapter.

Types of Massage

Shiatsu is a Japanese form of massage that means "finger pressure." Shiatsu practitioners use finger pressure at specific points in the body (correlating with acupuncture points) to promote circulation and stimulate the nervous system.

In trigger point massage, or **myotherapy**, the therapist feels for taut bands or knots that have a point of maximal tenderness. Pressure on these points can cause local pain, referred pain, and muscle spasms. The manual technique for deactivating a trigger point is ischemic compression. When direct pressure is applied over the point, the tissue becomes ischemic (blood is pushed out of the tissue) and when the pressure is removed, the tissue becomes hyperemic (blood quickly infiltrates the tissue). This often relieves the tension, band, or knot, and thus the pain. This pressure is usually held for 8 to 15 seconds, and if a spasm is felt during application of pressure, pressure should be maintained until the muscle stops firing.

Sports massage can be classified into event massage and maintenance massage. Event massage (related to a massage done on an athlete before, during, or after competing) can be further categorized into pre-event, interevent, and postevent massage. The goal of pre-event massage is to get the animal relaxed and ready for the event. Interevent massage keeps the patient tuned up and ready for the next event, and postevent massage flushes out metabolic waste and reduces muscle spasms and soreness. The goal of maintenance massage is to prevent injury and expedite the healing of injured tissue.

Swedish massage is the most used massage technique. Studies have shown that massage is beneficial for reducing stress, enhancing blood and lymph circulation, decreasing pain, promoting sleep, reducing swelling, enhancing relaxation, and increasing the oxygen capacity of blood.

Massage Techniques

Effleurage is the most common stroke used for animals. It is a gliding stroke that follows the contour of the body. Hand over hand, thumb over thumb, and one hand on either side of the body are the most common variations. It is repeated several times at the beginning and at the end of the massage to evaluate the tissue and enhance blood flow (warm it up and then aid in flushing lactic acid). Animals usually prefer these strokes to flow with the direction of the hair. Although effleurage is often thought of as a light stroke, deeper strokes are used to lengthen muscles and assist with stretching.

Pétrissage, or kneading, consists of rhythmic lifting, squeezing, and releasing tissue. It helps remove metabolic waste and promotes circulation. The hands form a "C" shape and can be alternated in a circular motion, can "roll" the skin, or can spread up and out to help widen or broaden the muscle.

Friction is the manipulation of tissue performed to promote circulation. It is commonly used over tendons when tendonitis is present, over trigger points, and over joint capsules with excessive fibrous tissue. It is also used to break up skin adhesions and scar tissue (wait 3 to 4 weeks after injury or surgery before applying this technique). When friction is applied to deep tissue, one finger or thumb is placed on the skin and either rubs the skin or is attached to the skin and rubs the tissue underneath. This can be done longitudinally (with muscle fibers), across fibers (perpendicular to the muscle fibers), circularly, diagonally, or in a "J" pattern.

Tapotement is a tapping motion of the hands or fingers. When done for a short time, it stimulates nerve endings (pre-event sports massage or for toning of atrophied muscles). When done for a longer time, it has a more sedative effect. *Coupage*, which is used to loosen phlegm congestion in the lungs, is a form of tapotement. The hands are cupped, and strokes start at the caudal aspect of the ribs and move forward. Proper positioning using wedges or pillows can help maximize the effectiveness of coupage. This stroke may be continued for 5 to 10 minutes on each side.

Vibration is rapid shaking or slower rocking of the tissue. The speed of vibration affects the outcome: faster vibrations are stimulatory, whereas slower speeds are inhibitory. Vibration differs from tapotement in that the therapist's hands do not leave the patient's skin. It can aid in relaxing muscles and reducing trigger point activity and, when used over a joint capsule in the proper position, it can act as joint mobilization.

TECHNICIAN NOTE

Effleurage is a very effective massage technique most commonly used in animals. It is a gliding stroke that follows the contour of the body. It is often used to open or close a massage session as it can be calming to the patient and helps to flush toxins.

The duration of a small animal massage is usually 30 minutes; for a large animal, it is approximately 1 hour. A sequence is the arrangement of massage strokes.

A typical example of a sequence would be as follows:

- Start with effleurage on the face and head.
- Continue down the back and sides.
- Use petrissage over the paraspinal muscles (including kneading, circles, or strokes going with or perpendicular to the muscle fibers).
- Apply ischemic compression on trigger points, if found.
- Move on to one side of the neck.
- Carry on down the thoracic limb.
- Perform effleurage with strokes running from the toes to the heart to flush toxins.
- Continue by using skin rolls along the body wall.
- Apply the same techniques used in the thoracic limb to treat the pelvic limb.
- Gently flip the patient over if the patient is a canine or walk around to the other side if it is an equine.
- Repeat the techniques on the other side.
- Finish up with a final effleurage.

Signs of relaxation include sighing, yawning, licking the lips, hanging the head (equine), burping, and flatulence. Signs that the pressure is too great include increased respiratory rate, opening of eyes (if previously closed), fidgeting, incessant licking (canine), or swishing of the tail (equine).

Massage Contraindications

Areas of the body called *endangerment sites* should be avoided because they are too delicate to withstand massage. These areas include the throat, eyeballs, the brachial plexus, the abdomen (deep, near the aorta), and the area over the kidneys, among others. Other contraindications for massage include areas around infected lesions, open wounds, acute injury, inflammation, or hemorrhage, and the period after a recent high fever. Caution should be considered when performing massage close to a suspected neoplasm and should never be performed directly over a neoplasm. Precautions should be taken when massaging a patient with heart disease or over an area with a neoplasm.

Passive Range of Motion

Passive range of motion (PROM) is the use of stretching to prevent loss of normal ROM, return normal ROM if absent, increase

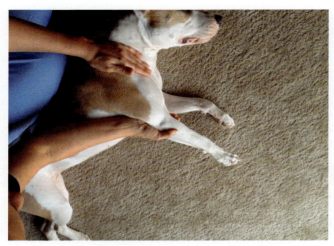

• **Fig. 23.7** Passive range of motion on the shoulder of a dog.

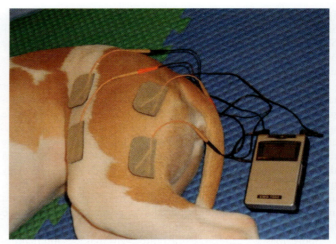

• **Fig. 23.8** Neuromuscular electrical nerve stimulation being performed on the quadriceps and biceps femoris muscles of a dog.

cartilage nutrition in the joint, and stimulate cartilage regeneration (Fig. 23.7). Most of the nutrition received by chondrocytes comes from the capillary-rich synovial capsule, which then bathes the cartilage via the synovial fluid. If the joint is stationary, joint fluid is not circulated, and less nutrition is available to the chondrocytes.

Rules of PROM include the following:

- It should never be painful.
- If the patient is lying in lateral recumbency, keep the worked limb parallel to the ground to prevent torquing of joints.
- Hold the joint flexed for 10 to 20 seconds, hold it in extension for 10 to 20 seconds, and then repeat these 3 to 10 times.
- Massage the muscles that are being stretched.
- Guide the limb but do not pull it.
- Do not hyperextend the carpus or tarsus, because permanent tendon or ligament damage may occur. These joints are flexed and relaxed unless a contracture issue involves these joints.

The technician can take an active role in PROM, performing this modality under a veterinarian's direction. This can be done successfully in equine and canine patients and other species with appropriate training.

Electrical-Based Therapies

Neuromuscular Stimulation

Neuromuscular electrical stimulation (NMES) is the application of electrical current to elicit a muscle contraction (Fig. 23.8). The main purpose of NMES in rehabilitation is to attain muscle strengthening. Clinical indications include reducing disuse atrophy (after surgery or an injury), reversing muscle atrophy (in a patient that is not using a limb after surgery or an injury), and strengthening selected muscles (neuromuscular re-education). Although NMES is an effective treatment, it is not without risk. Refer to Box 23.3 for a list of contraindications to NMES stimulation being used.

A voluntary muscle contraction first recruits the small-diameter, slow-twitch, type I fatigue-resistant fibers. Constant tension of the muscle is maintained by asynchronous recruitment of those fibers—some are relaxing as others are contracting. An electrically induced muscle contraction first recruits large-diameter, fast-twitch type II fibers because of their low threshold for electrical excitation. These fibers tend to be recruited simultaneously and, as they fatigue, tension in the muscle begins to decrease. With continued NMES therapy, properties of fast-twitch type II muscle

• **BOX 23.3** **Contraindications for Neuromuscular Electrical Stimulation**

Over the heart or cardiac pacemakers
Seizure disorders
Over areas of peripheral vascular disease or thrombophlebitis
Over areas of decreased pain or temperature sensation
Over areas of infection
Over neoplasms
Over the carotid sinus
Any time active motion is contraindicated

fibers begin to resemble those of slow-twitch type I muscle fibers and decrease the fatigability of the muscle.

In treating a patient, pads are placed over the motor point of the muscle (the area in which the least electricity is needed to produce a contraction—usually where a nerve enters the muscle) and over a distal point (usually just proximal to the musculotendinous junction) on the muscle. If a solid contraction cannot be created, the proximal pad should be rearranged to make sure it is truly over the motor point.

Treatment parameters usually are determined by the attending veterinarian or the physical therapist and include frequency (pulses per second, measured in hertz); pulse duration (measured in microseconds); intensity, duty cycle (contraction time versus relaxation time); ramp (time to full contraction); and treatment time. Waveform or current type (versus direct current) may be determined by the type of machine used.

The technician's role in NMES is to shave and clean the skin with alcohol, apply gel, attach the pads, and use the NMES machine to obtain a strong yet pain-free contraction. The patient should be monitored throughout the session, because pads sometimes migrate, causing reduced effectiveness or even discomfort if placed incorrectly. Finally, the session should be recorded in the patient's record, with details of all the treatment variables described previously and any unusual reactions noted. Knowledge of anatomy is essential for performing this task. Muscles and muscle groups that are routinely stimulated include triceps muscles, paraspinal muscles, gluteal muscles, biceps femoris muscles, quadriceps muscles, and cranial tibial muscles. Thoracic limb flexor muscles, thoracic limb extensor muscles, deltoid muscles, and gastrocnemius muscles also may be stimulated.

Transcutaneous electrical nerve stimulation (TENS) is the use of electric current to stimulate the nerves to release endogenous opioids and thus relieve pain and muscle spasm. TENS units most frequently use frequencies of 75 to 100 Hz for pain relief. The disadvantage of using TENS units is that the pain often returns relatively quickly.

Interferential therapy can be used with one frequency in one direction and another in a perpendicular direction and where they are superimposed, summation is followed by cancellation of the current. It can also be used with two pads on one side for topical treatment or muscle stimulation. This therapy is most effective in treating deep, aching, and chronic pain, but it can also be used for acute pain and electroanalgesia. The pads should be placed directly across the painful region (e.g., when treating a painful stifle, the pads can be placed on the medial and lateral aspect of the knee directly across from each other).

Most units have attached leads that are placed on either side of the area to be treated or, in the case of interferential therapy, on all four sides. Before the leads are attached, the treatment area typically is shaved and cleaned with alcohol to remove hair and dead skin. Reusable or carbon pads are attached to the unit's leads with gel to increase conductivity. The frequency is set, and the amplitude is adjusted so the patient can feel a sensation but has no pain.

> **TECHNICIAN NOTE**
>
> The technician's role in TENS is to administer and record the treatment. This includes shaving the treatment area if needed, applying gel and pads, and setting the machine to the proper frequency and intensity.

Pulsed Electromagnetic Field Therapy

All atoms produce electromagnetic fields, and every organ in the body has its own unique bioelectromagnetic field. All cells in the body communicate via electromagnetic fields, and tissues are very sensitive to changes in electromagnetic activity. Pulsed electromagnetic field therapy (PEMF) has been used therapeutically for over a century. Modern PEMF was reborn in the 1930s when diathermy machines were adapted to not emit heat. In the late 1970s, low-powered PEMF devices were approved by the US Food and Drug Administration (FDA) for human use. In the 1990s, new PEMF devices were manufactured to be portable and target soft tissues for the reduction of swelling, inflammation, and edema. Studies of these newer targeted PEMF devices have demonstrated efficacy in improving wound, nerve, and bone healing and for reducing pain. Two prospective canine studies on postoperative hemilaminectomies demonstrated efficacy of PEMF (Assisi Loop) in reduction of pain. Specifically, dogs receiving sham therapy were almost twice as likely to receive opioids after hospital discharge compared with dogs receiving PEMF therapy. PEMF devices are easy to use (Fig. 23.9) and penetrate bandages, making this a useful modality for patients that are recovering postoperatively. PEMF is also relatively safe, with the primary contraindication being cardiac arrhythmias or patients with a pacemaker, because the electrical signal may cause interference.

Light- and Sound-Based Therapies

Photobiomodulation

Photobiomodulation (also known as laser therapy or low-level laser therapy [LLLT]) is the stimulation of tissue with light to achieve a therapeutic effect (Fig. 23.10). *Laser* stands for "light

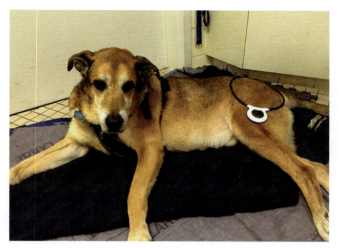

• **Fig. 23.9** A pulsed electromagnetic field therapy (PEMF) device known as the Assisi loop is applied to the targeted tissue (hip) for treatment. The device is manually turned on and treatment will configure for 15 minutes.

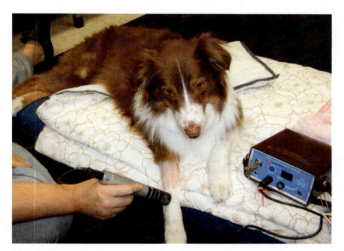

• **Fig. 23.10** Low-level laser therapy is being performed on the carpus of a dog.

amplification by stimulated emission of radiation." It is a form of phototherapy that uses a nonionizing form of light in the visible and infrared spectrum. This light, in the form of photons, stimulates endogenous chromophores to elicit a photochemical response. Common chromophores are hemoglobin, melanin, water, and cytochrome c oxidase, which is the second to last enzyme within the mitochondrial respiratory chain. It is within this enzyme that the regenerative properties of laser occur. Activation of cytochrome c oxidase forms intracellular signaling of adenosine triphosphate (ATP) molecules, reactive oxygen species, and nitrous oxide. ATP is important for many of the biochemical processes within the cell. It not only gives energy to cells but also controls carrier ions for sodium/potassium ion (NA+/K+) pumps and calcium ion (Ca+) pumps, which are important for cell function. ATP is also responsible for the release of growth factors, which trigger cellular proliferation and is important for cell repair and tissue healing. Reactive oxygen species are produced by oxygen metabolism and, at low concentrations, can stimulate cell proliferation, nerve cell regeneration, cytokine modulation, growth factors, and other inflammatory mediators to activate cell healing. Activation of nitrous oxide regulates circulation and acts as a neurotransmitter, which causes vasodilation, reduces edema, improves lymph drainage, reduces pain, and promotes angiogenesis. Laser also stimulates proliferation of fibroblasts and new epithelial cells, which help wound healing, and stimulates collagen production, which is essential for tissue repair. Laser reduces proinflammatory cytokines and tissue necrosis factor-alpha, interleukin-1, and prostaglandin E2. Laser helps decrease pain by inhibiting A-delta and C nerve fibers, thus decreasing the nociception threshold and reducing nerve conduction velocity. Laser also decreases pain by releasing beta-endorphins and serotonin. According to the mechanism of action, three main therapeutic effects are created with LLLT: decreased pain, decreased inflammation, and improved tissue healing.

The power of the laser is the rate at which the energy is emitted over time and is measured in watts (W) or milliwatts (mW) 1 W=1 J/sec. For example, a 1-W laser can deliver 60 J/min. Wavelength determines the depth of penetration to the targeted tissue in which the chromophores will absorb the light. Wavelengths in the range of 600 to 700 nm are often used for superficial tissue, whereas wavelengths of 780 to 950 nm penetrate deeper tissue. The energy density (or energy fluence, commonly referred to as *dose of light*) is the amount of energy being emitted per surface area measured as joules per square centimeter (J/cm^2). The deeper the targeted tissue, the greater the energy required for the desired physiologic response. The total amount of joules is the energy emitted over time and is usually referred to as *dosage*. To determine the dosage, measure the surface area (cm^2) and multiply by the J/cm^2. For example, would multiply the dose (4 J/cm^2) by the treatment area (50 cm^2) to calculate the total amount of energy to be delivered to that treatment area (200 total J).

The most common indications for LLLT include treating pain associated with degenerative joint disease, **intervertebral disk disease**, surgical procedures, and soft tissue injuries. It is also used to stimulate healing of wounds and ulcers, stimulate acupuncture points, treat trigger points, reduce edema, and reduce inflammation associated with stomatitis, gingivitis, and cystitis.

> **TECHNICIAN NOTE**
>
> The technician's role in low-level laser therapy (LLLT) is to deliver treatment according to the veterinarian's directions.

Therapeutic Ultrasound

Therapeutic ultrasound is the use of sound waves to treat tissue (Fig. 23.11). This modality works by increasing collagen extensibility, increasing blood flow, decreasing pain and muscle spasms, increasing enzyme activity, accelerating wound healing by modulating the inflammatory process, and enhancing transdermal delivery of certain medications (phonophoresis). Refer to Box 23.4 for a list of clinical applications for therapeutic ultrasonography.

Therapeutic ultrasound has both thermal and nonthermal effects. Variables that determine the amount of heat produced by the sound wave include frequency, intensity, duty cycle, duration of exposure, and size and type of the tissue to be treated. At a frequency of 1 megahertz (MHz), the depth of penetration is 4 to 5 cm, whereas at a frequency of 3 MHz, penetration depth is only 1 to 2 cm. The proximity of the bone and the thickness of the tissue determine the frequency that is used. Intensity determines whether thermal or nonthermal effects will be seen. Intensities over 1 watt by square centimeters (W/cm^2) produce thermal effects that increase circulation and help reduce joint contractures. Intensities less than 1 W/cm^2 produce nonthermal effects that

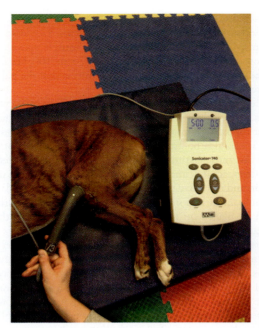

• **Fig. 23.11** Therapeutic ultrasound being performed on the patellar tendon of a dog.

> • **BOX 23.4** **Clinical Applications of Therapeutic Ultrasound**
>
> *Joint contracture and scar tissue:* heats and stretches to improve range of motion
> *Tendonitis and bursitis:* increases blood flow and decreases pain
> *Pain and muscle spasm:* increases pain threshold and reduces muscle spindle activity
> *Wound healing:* used at low intensity 2 weeks after injury

enhance wound healing. The duty cycle is the fraction of time that the sound wave is emitted during a pulse period. In a continuous mode, intensity is constant and can be destructive to tissue but may be beneficial for stretching scar tissue. In a pulsed mode, most commonly 20% or 50%, the wave is interrupted in an on/off pattern. Pulsed ultrasound is used to enhance healing and eliminate swelling. Time is determined by the size of the area being treated and by the size of the ultrasound probe (sound head). Generally, an area twice the size of the sound head is treated for 5 minutes. As sound increases the temperature in the tissue, it is important to continuously move the sound head. If it is held stationary, burns of the skin, muscle, or periosteum may result.

> **TECHNICIAN NOTE**
>
> The technician's role in therapeutic ultrasound is to shave the treatment area, clean the area with alcohol, apply coupling gel, and administer ultrasound treatment under the veterinarian's direction. Treatment is also charted after the therapy session; charting includes details on areas treated, duration, duty cycle, frequency, intensity, and response to treatment. Passive stretching of muscles immediately following treatment is recommended.

Extracorporeal Shockwave

Extracorporeal shockwave therapy consists of high-energy, focused sound waves that deliver energy to a specific focal point in the body. These sound waves dissipate mechanical energy into tissues, which initiates biological responses at the cellular level. It increases expression of cytokines and growth factors; leads to decreased inflammation, neovascularization, and cellular proliferation; increases serotonin activity in the dorsal horn; and promotes descending inhibition of pain signals. It speeds wound healing; speeds bone, tendon, and ligament healing; and decreases pain. It is important to note there are different types of focused shockwave therapy (electrohydraulic, electromagnetic, and piezoelectric), and machines are not equal in efficacy. In veterinary medicine, evidence in focused shockwave only exists for electrohydraulic therapy. Nonfocused shockwave therapy (radial shockwave) has demonstrated evidence in the treatment of osteoarthritis in animals. Electrohydraulic shockwave has supporting evidence as a positive treatment of osteoarthritis, tendinopathies, wounds, lumbosacral disease, and nonhealing fractures.

Focused extracorporeal shockwave therapy produces a loud sound, and certain electrohydraulic machines with deep penetration may cause an uncomfortable sensation that would necessitate sedation for the procedure. Newer electrohydraulic devices offer nonsedated options for treating patients, and piezoelectric shockwave is also safely tolerated without sedation. Nonsedated extracorporeal shockwave is most utilized in veterinary rehabilitation. The treatment itself is relatively short (3–5 minutes) and well tolerated. Earplugs (in the form of cotton balls or earmuffs) may help to decrease reactivity for noise-sensitive animals.

In dogs, electrohydraulic extracorporeal shockwave therapy has been shown to speed healing of osteotomies after tibial plateau leveling osteotomy (TPLO) 14 days faster and lead to a full recovery compared with no treatment. It has also been shown to significantly reduce patellar desmitis in TPLO cases. In elbow osteoarthritis cases, there was a 4.5% increase in peak vertical force after shockwave therapy compared with a decrease of 2.6% with no treatment. In cases of shoulder lameness (caused by instability, calcification, and/or inflammatory tendinopathies of the shoulder), 88% of dogs treated with shockwave therapy showed improvement. Recent research has also demonstrated efficacy for electrohydraulic shockwave therapy in the treatment of canine lumbosacral disease.

> **TECHNICIAN NOTE**
>
> Extracorporeal shockwave therapy produces a loud sound and uncomfortable sensation caused by the pressure wave. Historically, patients required sedation for treatment; however, new advances in shockwave equipment provide a less intense sensation that most patients tolerate without sedation.

Superficial Thermal Therapy

Cold and heat therapies affect physiologic changes in the body. Cold and heat therapies can be extremely beneficial for the patient undergoing rehabilitation and these therapies are easy and simple to implement in every practice.

Cryotherapy is the application of cold to the body to decrease pain and inflammation. It causes vasoconstriction, which reduces postoperative bleeding and bruising (when the cooling agent is removed, a rebound vasodilatation occurs—red coloration may be seen in the skin), slows nerve conduction (thereby decreasing pain), and decreases enzyme activity (thereby decreasing inflammation). The larger the animal, the longer it takes to cool the deep tissue. Studies have demonstrated that cooling packs should be applied for 10–20 min to reach appropriate temperature at the target tissue. Small dogs may need only 10 minutes, while larger breeds (and especially dogs with heavy coats) may need 15–20 minutes.

After surgery, cold can be applied by filling a disposable paper cup three-quarters full of water and freezing it. The paper is unraveled, and gauze can be placed at the incision to prevent water from contaminating the incision. Commercial cool packs are easy to keep in the freezer. A mixture of alcohol and water in a reusable zipper freezer bag at a ratio of 1:2 stays cold and malleable, although double bagging is recommended to prevent cold leaks. If the patient has been shaved or is short coated, wrapping the alcohol bag in a towel may be required. Machines made for cooling can either spray liquid nitrogen on the affected area or use a flowing ice bath in conjunction with compression to decrease swelling and pain. Studies in canine postoperative cruciate surgery have demonstrated that the combination of cold and compression simultaneously is superior for decreasing pain, swelling, lameness and improving ROM compared with no therapy or cold therapy alone. In large animals, running a cold hose over an injury is also effective. Therapeutic ice boots are available for equine extremities.

Thermotherapy is the application of heat to the body to reduce pain. Heat increases circulation, increases muscle contractility, increases the ability of collagen to stretch, and decreases pain. The recommended method is wet/moist heat. A hand towel for small areas or a bath towel for larger areas may be folded into thirds and rolled (to be unrolled around a joint) or accordion-folded (to be placed over a flat surface). The towel is held under warm to hot running water and then applied to the area. If it is not possible to keep a hand on the towel because it is too hot, it is also too hot for the patient. A big, thick towel or plastic wrap may be placed over the wet towel to contain the heat.

Heat can be applied for 10 to 15 minutes over areas of chronic arthritis, before exercises to warm up muscles and joints, or if an area is cold to the touch on examination (signifying a chronic condition with decreased blood perfusion). Sweat wraps can be used on equine extremities and commonly contain dimethyl sulfoxide, nitrofurazone, or dexamethasone, surrounded by plastic and a quilted wrap. This is thought to decrease inflammation and swelling.

Contraindications

Cryotherapy and thermotherapy should not be applied over areas that do not have appropriate sensation or perfusion, because tissue damage may occur.

Assistive Devices

Some patients cannot reach the previous level of function or do not achieve an acceptable level of function or comfort without an assistive device. These devices include harnesses, slings, and protective devices, ranging from simple ones, such as boots and nail covers, to complex custom orthotics, prosthetics, and wheelchairs. Not only do these devices help the patient recover or adapt physically, but they also benefit many patients by providing the emotional lift gained from increased mobility and independence. Assistive devices also benefit the caregivers by allowing the pet to move more independently, thereby lessening the physical burden from lifting or assisting the patient.

Harnesses and Slings

Harnesses and slings are often used in canine patients when full independence is expected to return shortly. They allow clients and therapists to assist the dogs via weight and balance support without injuring themselves in the process. Some slings are simple, with a fabric support that slides under the abdomen, and some harnesses are fully adjustable, with support for both thoracic and pelvic limbs. Large animals that need weight-bearing and balance assistance can benefit from a harness and sling system attached to a ceiling beam. Although stall confinement is necessary for these patients, the benefits of being upright reduce complications that may occur when a horse or cow is recumbent. Because of their large size and body weight, pressure sores and life-threatening gastrointestinal stasis can develop rapidly in large animal patients that must endure prolonged recumbency.

> **TECHNICIAN NOTE**
>
> The more complex the harness, the more instruction the owners will need on how to apply, fit, and adjust the harness to their pet and on how to use it properly on a regular basis.

Protective Devices

Paws and nails may be traumatized when patients are unable to lift their feet properly because of paresis or paralysis; instead, they may knuckle and drag their paws. Nail caps can be applied to protect nails from wear if enough nail is present at the base to allow proper attachment of the cap. Nail caps are helpful when knuckling is present, because they allow the foot to maintain direct contact with the ground. There are also rubber nail grips that can be applied to nails to improve traction as the weight-bearing aspect of the nail contacts the ground. This can be useful, particularly for mild paresis or for dogs with temporary weakness. Proper application of the nail grips is key for successful use. Replacement is typically needed every 2 to 4 weeks. The hair around the paws and on the palmar/plantar surfaces should be adequately groomed to prevent slipping, which could lead to injury. Boots can be helpful in protecting not only the nails but also the entire paw. Although boots reduce tactile ground contact, they can be useful to prevent the dorsum of the foot from becoming traumatized by the patient. Boots can be heavy and durable or light and disposable.

For large animals, boots are used to assist recovery from hoof injuries and are available in a variety of configurations. Some are fastened by straps and levers and are removable (these are beneficial when medication needs to be applied); others are more like a glue-on shoe and are semipermanent.

Clients should also be educated on navigating the home environment by providing traction surfaces such as yoga mats or carpet runners in high-traffic areas of the home.

> **TECHNICIAN NOTE**
>
> The technician can be trained specifically to apply nail grips, which should be checked routinely during rehabilitation visits to ensure there are no signs of nailbed infections or other complications. If nail grips have been lost, the technician should replace them.

Braces, Orthotics, and Prosthetics

Sometimes patients cannot bear their full weight on a weak or injured limb. Commercially available braces and wraps may provide light to moderate support for recovery while strengthening exercises are carried out. These braces are commonly available for the carpus and the tarsus in dogs and for the hock and the fetlock in horses. Neoprene braces are available for stifles, shoulders, and

elbows in dogs. When a patient requires rigid support or needs support in a joint that is not commonly braced, such as the stifle, a custom orthotic is indicated. An orthotic device may be used not only to provide support but also to limit or protect ROM. Orthotics are commonly used in horses suffering from traumatic injury, typically on the lower limb, and in dogs suffering from a cranial cruciate ligament tear. Prosthetics are used to replace a part of the limb that is missing or requires amputation. A custom fit is necessary to prevent pain and ensure correct balance and stability.

It is important that the introduction of assistive devices be progressive and positive. Complications resulting from use of assistive devices include skin irritation and ulceration, chewing, breakdown and wear, and lack of acceptance by the patient. Formal rehabilitation to facilitate acclimation to the device, careful monitoring, and excellent client education increase the likelihood of success.

> **TECHNICIAN NOTE**
>
> The technician may be involved in cast molding the affected limb so that a model limb can be generated by the orthotist or the prosthetist.

Wheelchairs

Wheelchairs allow a paretic patient freedom of movement and a means of performing regular exercise. If properly introduced to a patient, they are not only accepted but are fully enjoyed by both the patient and the client. Although they offer greater freedom of movement for the patient, wheelchairs can tip or become stuck on surrounding obstacles; therefore supervision is important. Initially, they should be used for very short (5- to 10-minute) periods to allow the patient to adjust. Some dogs using wheelchairs may have difficulty eliminating, but most learn and adapt with time.

Wheelchairs range from fully adjustable aluminum frames with two wheels, a neoprene seat, and a harness to complex four-wheeled "quad" carts with head and neck support. It is important that each wheelchair or cart be properly fitted for the individual patient's balance and comfort. If the balance is not appropriate, it may be difficult or uncomfortable for the patient to move in the apparatus. Case Presentation 23.1 demonstrates the benefit of using wheelchairs in patients with paresis or paralysis.

> **TECHNICIAN NOTE**
>
> Sometimes it takes 30 to 45 minutes to adjust an assistive cart to fit properly, introduce the patient to walking confidently, and teach the client the basics of cart care and troubleshooting.

Acupuncture

Definition and Mechanisms of Action

Acupuncture is defined as the stimulation of a specific point (acupuncture point) on the body by using a specific method, which results in a physiologic effect. These physiologic effects include both systemic and local effects as acupuncture stimulates both the central and peripheral nervous systems. Some of the systemic effects include the release of endogenous substances such as beta-endorphins, dynorphins, enkephalins, serotonin, and various hormones. Acupuncture can also improve blood flow; release somatotropin in chronic pain; and modulate thyroid function, among other functions. The local effects of acupuncture include

CASE PRESENTATION 23.1

Using an Assistive Device for a Quadriplegic Patient

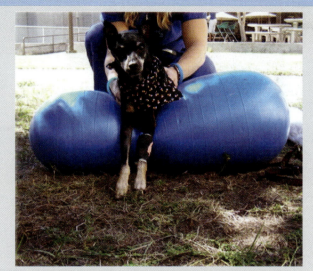

• **Fig 23.A** Patient being balanced on peanut-shaped exercise ball.

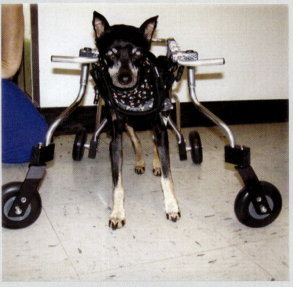

• **Fig 23.B** Patient in quad cart.

A 13-year-old castrated male Miniature Pinscher was presented to an emergency clinic in an acutely quadriplegic state. Initial examination revealed lack of motor response in all four limbs and presence of deep pain perception. Myelography confirmed type I intervertebral disk disease with compression of the spinal cord at C3 and C4. A ventral slot procedure was performed on the day of presentation to relieve spinal cord compression. After surgery, the patient was still quadriplegic and had significant neck pain. Therapy started 5 days after ventral slot surgery and consisted of the following:

Weeks 1 to 2: Passive range of motion, massage, low-level laser therapy, and acupuncture

Weeks 3 to 6: Continued therapy as weeks 1 to 2 and added balance on a peanut-shaped exercise ball (Fig. 23.A), underwater treadmill, and assisted walking in a quad cart (Fig. 23.B)

Weeks 7 to 12: Continued therapy as weeks 1 to 6 and added assisted standing, assisted walking, assisted sitting to standing, and weight-shifting exercises

Weeks 13 to 17: Added assisted walking on a land treadmill and progressed to unassisted walking

Progress and outcome: Three weeks into therapy, the patient was able to walk in a quad cart; however, he was still unable to stand without assistance. Over the next 7 weeks, he slowly regained the ability to stand with minimal assistance. After 16 weeks of therapy, the patient had progressed to being able to stand and walk without assistance.

---

muscle relaxation and spasm relief; release of bradykinin, which leads to vasodilation; and production of local prostaglandins, leading to smooth muscle relaxation.

Acupuncture Points

Research shows that most acupuncture points are located in areas on the skin that have decreased electrical resistance or increased electrical conductivity. In addition, it has been found that acupuncture points are closely associated with free nerve endings, veins, lymphatics, and an aggregation of mast cells. There are about 150 to 200 acupuncture points in animals. The majority of acupuncture points correspond to motor points. The motor point is the point in a muscle which, when electrical stimulation is

applied, will produce a maximal contraction with minimal intensity of stimulation. Motor points are located in areas where nerves enter muscles. For instance, SI-9 is located at the junction of the deltoid muscle and triceps brachii and is supplied by axillary and radial nerves.

Methods of Stimulation

Acupuncture points can be stimulated by various means, including acupressure, dry needle, electroacupuncture, aqua-acupuncture, moxibustion, gold implantation, pneumoacupuncture, and laser acupuncture. *Acupressure* is applying firm digital pressure to an acupuncture point for a specific length of time (Fig. 23.12). This is the least invasive type of stimulation and can be performed by

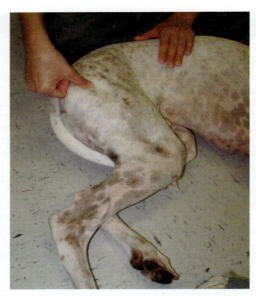

• **Fig. 23.12** Acupressure being performed on a dog with hip pain.

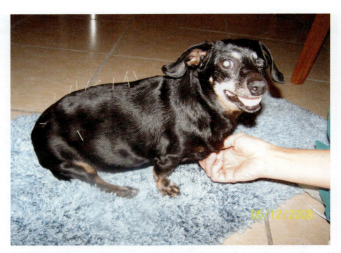

• **Fig. 23.13** Dry needle acupuncture is being performed on a dog with epilepsy.

veterinary technicians and pet owners. Dry needling is the insertion of a sterile filiform needle into an acupuncture point to elicit a response (Fig. 23.13). These needles are typically left in place for 15 to 30 minutes. *Dry needling* is the most common technique in veterinary medicine. *Electroacupuncture* involves applying electrical current to the dry needles to increase the therapeutic response (Fig. 23.14). This modality is preferred, because the frequency and amplitude can be adjusted, and a stronger stimulation can be induced compared with the use of a dry needle alone. Low-frequency (1–40 hertz [Hz]) electroacupuncture predominantly stimulates A-delta fibers and releases beta-endorphins and met-enkephalins. High-frequency (80–120 Hz) electroacupuncture predominantly stimulates C fibers and releases dynorphins. Very-high–frequency (200 Hz) electroacupuncture predominantly stimulates serotonergic fibers and releases serotonin and epinephrine. *Aqua-acupuncture* is the injection of a sterile liquid (i.e., saline, vitamin B_{12}, lidocaine, Adequan, etc.) into an acupuncture point (Fig. 23.15). This causes prolonged stimulation of the acupuncture point until the liquid is absorbed, and it has the added benefit of the medicinal properties of the substance used. *Moxibustion* is the use of a Chinese herb called *Artemisia vulgaris*, which is rolled into a cigar shape and burned just above the acupuncture point without touching the skin (Fig. 23.16)). This is a warming technique that is therapeutic for older patients with chronic pain. *Gold implantation* is the injection of sterile pieces of gold, whether in a bead or wire form, into acupuncture points for permanent implantation. Gold implantation provides long-term stimulation for chronic conditions. *Pneumoacupuncture* is the injection of air under the skin in the subcutaneous space to produce pressure by air and stimulate the acupuncture points, nerves, and muscles. Pneumoacupuncture is used solely for muscle atrophy. *Laser acupuncture* is the use of LLLT to emit light to penetrate the tissues and stimulate acupuncture points.

Clinical Indications

Acupuncture can be used to treat a variety of diseases as a sole treatment or in conjunction with conventional medicine and/or surgery. Treatable conditions include but are not limited to pain and lameness; musculoskeletal, neurologic, and dermatologic disorders;

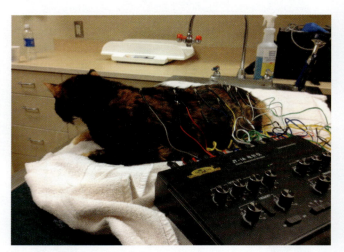

• **Fig. 23.14** Electroacupuncture being performed on a cat with back pain.

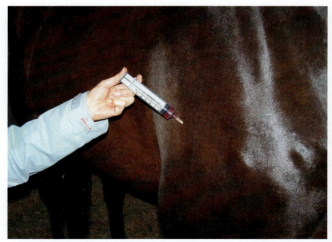

• **Fig. 23.15** Aqua-acupuncture with vitamin B_{12} being performed on a horse with shoulder pain.

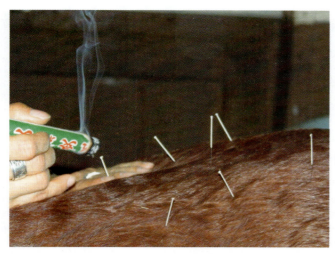

• **Fig. 23.16** Moxibustion being performed on a horse with osteoarthritis.

behavioral disorders; and gastrointestinal problems. Acupuncture may also improve quality of life in geriatric patients and in those with cancer or chronic disease. Case Presentation 23.2 depicts an example of the use of acupuncture to decrease lumbosacral pain.

Cautions and Contraindications

Although acupuncture is typically considered a safe and minimally invasive modality, there are some conditions that warrant caution or contraindication. For example, caution must be exercised when treating a weak, debilitated, or obtunded patient. Generally, fewer needles and less stimulation are used. Inserting needles directly into skin lesions, ulcers, scar tissue, the umbilicus, tumors, or masses is contraindicated. Specific acupuncture points around the abdomen and lumbar area are to be avoided in pregnancy. Electroacupuncture wire leads should not be connected through or across a known or suspected tumor or mass. Electroacupuncture should not be used in patients with a history of seizures, pacemaker use, or severe arrhythmia.

> ### TECHNICIAN NOTE
>
> At the end of the treatment, the technician should carefully remove the acupuncture needles and dispose of them in a sharps container. If resistance is felt when the needle is removed, tapping around the needle, rolling it back and forth, or gently holding down the skin on either side of the needle while pulling the needle gently will ease it from the tissue. If electroacupuncture is to be performed, the technician should set the frequency according to the veterinarian's direction and then set the intensity according to the patient's tolerance.

Veterinary Spinal Manipulative Therapy

Veterinary spinal manipulative therapy (VSMT) is like chiropractic in humans. It is used to manually restore reduced motion in the spine and limbs, thereby improving patient mobility, comfort and, in many cases, nervous system function.

Pathophysiology

A *subluxation* or a *vertebral subluxation complex* (VSC) involves an abnormal relationship between two adjacent vertebrae. This involves an anatomically complex area known as the *motor unit*, consisting of muscles, ligaments, connective tissue, a spinal nerve

CASE PRESENTATION 23.2

Acupuncture for Lumbosacral Pain Reduction

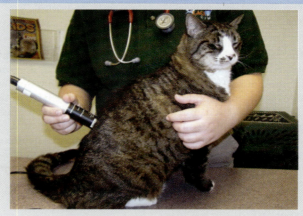

• **Fig. 23.A** Patient receiving laser therapy.

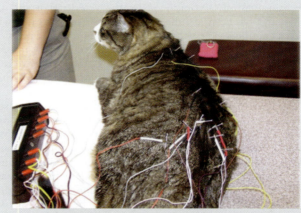

• **Fig. 23.B** Patient receiving electroacupuncture.

A 12-year-old castrated male domestic short hair cat was presented by his owner for recent changes in behavior and activity. The owner reported that the cat had not been jumping onto furniture and counters in the past 6 months, although this used to be normal behavior for him. The cat also exhibited a general decrease in activity. He had been spending more time sleeping and hiding and less time interacting with the other cats in the household. Diagnostic testing revealed degenerative lumbosacral stenosis, which was causing the patient chronic pain and discomfort. The prescribed treatment plan included low-level laser therapy, electroacupuncture, and walking on the land treadmill. For the first 2 weeks of treatment, the cat received low-level laser therapy (Fig. 23.A) and electroacupuncture (Fig. 23.B) along the back and lumbosacral junction twice a week. At the 2-week recheck, the owner reported that the cat had started seeking attention more often and seemed more social with the other cats in the house. The examination during this visit revealed that the pain level had been reduced, so walking on the land treadmill was added to the treatment protocol. Weekly treatments thereafter consisted of low-level laser therapy along the back and lumbosacral junction, followed by 15 to 20 minutes of walking on the land treadmill, and ending with electroacupuncture. After 1 month of therapy, this patient became more active at home and returned to jumping on furniture and counters. The pain level was significantly reduced for the remainder of the cat's life with ongoing weekly therapy.

and other smaller nerves, blood vessels, lymphatics, and cerebrospinal fluid. The hallmark or "triad" of signs that occurs with a subluxation includes altered mobility, pain on palpation, and abnormal tension in the surrounding paraspinal muscles.

The causes of chiropractic subluxation can vary from overt trauma to minute repetitive stress to the area, such as abnormal spinal movement secondary to thoracic limb lameness. Clinical signs range from mild discomfort to reduced reflexes to serious organ dysfunction. By determining where abnormal motion occurs and correcting reduced motion in the spine, normal biomechanics can be restored to the body and the normal neurologic pathways reset, thus aiding proper nervous system function. Restoration of full motion to limb joints can be equally important in maintaining spinal health.

Treatment

Once examination is completed by the veterinarian and the problem area has been identified, the patient can be treated with VSMT. Often, it is easiest to treat patients in a standing position. However, sometimes the sitting or sternal recumbent position may work better for small animal patients. Cats are easier to treat while they are lying on the treatment table than when they are forced to stand.

The veterinarian will check the motion between two spinal segments by applying pressure that is aligned with the way the joint surface glides. If reduced mobility is found in a given area, the veterinarian takes the motion as far as it will go and applies a short, quick motion in the plane of normal motion of the joint. Sometimes a popping noise (like cracking of a knuckle) will accompany the adjustment, although this is more common in humans than in animals. The adjustment should generally be painless for the patient, although sometimes a problem area may present some temporary mild discomfort. If a seriously painful area is found, the veterinarian will likely avoid treating that area altogether, at least until further diagnostics have been performed. It is important to keep the patient relaxed and to make the treatment a positive experience (for both the patient and the client); therefore all problem areas may not be corrected in a single visit. Immediately after treatment, the technician may be asked to massage the patient or walk the animal for several minutes to help it "hold" the adjustment. Afterward, some period of rest or reduced exercise is usually recommended, and massage and stretching may also be recommended. After treatment, the veterinarian will instruct the client on aftercare and follow-up visits and will provide additional recommendations.

Restraint is particularly important for first-time patients, because they may be nervous or frightened. Restraint can be simple, such as gentle petting, soothing words, or a food distraction. Often, a patient may have to be repositioned so that the veterinarian is in the best position to perform the necessary adjustment. Most patients accept and even enjoy the treatment, and only gentle physical restraint is necessary. It may, however, be necessary to use more rigorous methods of restraint, depending on the situation. Some canine or feline patients may need to be muzzled. Some horses may require twitching or hobbling, especially if they are not used to being routinely handled. If necessary, cattle may be restrained in a chute.

Herbal Medicine

The term *herbal medicine* refers to the practice of using plant materials (including flowers, stems, leaves, bark, seeds, and roots) to treat patients. Herbal medicine is the most ancient known medicine and the foundation of modern medicine. Herbal medicine is divided into three branches based on its country of origin: Chinese, Western, and Ayurvedic. Chinese herbs can be used in the form of single herbs or, more commonly, in a herbal formula. A herbal formula is a combination of two or more single herbs that work synergistically to create a therapeutic effect. Western herbal medicine can be traced back to the ancient Greeks and Native Americans and typically uses single herbs. Ayurvedic herbal medicine originated in India and is believed to predate Chinese herbal medicine. Ayurvedic herbs are typically used in a formula of two or more herbs, like Chinese herbs. Tables 23.2–23.4 list the commonly used herbs.

Many herbs are safe at many times the therapeutic dose, but others have a low margin of safety. Many medicinal herbs have not been proven safe for use in pregnancy, and some are toxic to cats. This is important to remember, because many clients equate herbs with complete safety. They need to be educated on the proper use of herbs and on their side effects, just as they should be with any prescribed medication.

The technician should become familiar with herbal pharmacy, just as they are familiar with pharmaceuticals. Information about the medicinal use of herbs can be found in the *Materia Medica*, which is similar to a drug formulary. If working in a practice with a veterinarian who uses therapeutic herbs, the veterinary technician should be familiar with commonly used preparations and should be able to properly prepare and dispense them. As with all practices, veterinary technicians are responsible for client education and for reviewing home care instructions with the pet owner.

Nutraceuticals (Also Known as Supplements)

Nutraceuticals are naturally occurring and biologically active products that can be supplemented in a patient's diet to provide a health benefit. Many types of nutraceuticals are available to treat a variety of conditions. Because these are not considered pharmaceutical drugs, the FDA does not regulate them. A brief discussion of the most common supplements used for the treatment of osteoarthritis (Table 23.5) is provided next.

TABLE 23.2 Commonly Used Chinese Herbal Medicines

Chinese Name	Common Name	Scientific Name	Clinical Indications
Sheng jiang	Ginger	*Zingiber officinale*	Nausea
Huang lian	Coptis	*Coptis japonica*	Inflammation
Sheng di huang	Rehmannia	*Rehmannia glutinosa*	Kidney support
Chi shao	Red peony	*Paeonia rubra*	Pain
Wu rong	Maitake	*Grifola frondosa*	Immune system support
Yunnan baiyao	(Proprietary blend)		Hemorrhage

TABLE 23.3 Commonly Used Western Herbal Medicines

Common Name	Scientific Name	Active Components	Clinical Indications
Aloe	*Aloe vera*	Gel layer of leaf	Skin irritation, burns (topical)
Cranberry	*Vaccinium macrocarpon*	Fruit	Urinary tract infection
Dandelion	*Taraxacum officinale*	Root (whole plant)	Diuretic
Echinacea	*Echinacea purpurea*	Whole plant	Immune support
Ginkgo	*Ginkgo biloba*	Leaves	Promotes mental alertness
Hawthorn	*Crataegus laevigata*	Leaves, berries, blossoms	Supports heart function
Milk thistle	*Silybum marianum*	Seeds, fruit, leaves	Liver support, detoxification
Slippery elm	*Ulmus fulva*	Bark	Soothes the gastrointestinal tract
Valerian	*Valerian officinalis*	Root	Anxiety, sleep disorders

TABLE 23.4 Commonly Used Ayurvedic Herbal Medicines

Common Name	Scientific Name	Clinical Indications
Ashwagandha	*Withania somnifera*	Fatigue, skin disease
Boswellia	*Boswellia serrata*	Arthritis (anti-inflammatory)
Cinnamon	*Cinnamomum zeylanicum*	Digestive disorders
Licorice	*Glycyrrhiza glabra*	Soothes urinary and gastrointestinal tracts
Shatavari	*Asparagus racemosus*	Bladder infection
Turmeric	*Curcuma longa*	Arthritis, liver support

Glucosamine and Chondroitin

Glucosamine inhibits enzymes that are responsible for cartilage degradation and decreases the production of inflammatory mediators. Chondroitin stimulates the production of glycosaminoglycans, inhibits degradative enzymes, enhances production of hyaluronic acid, and prevents degeneration of type II collagen within articular cartilage. While in vitro data is promising for glucosamine and chondroitin sulfate, prospective studies show mixed evidence for efficacy. The most recent systematic reviews in veterinary medicine concluded that glucosamine/chondroitin has poor evidence and should no longer be recommended for the treatment of osteoarthritis in dogs or cats. Evidence is also lacking in horses.

Omega-3 Fatty Acids

Omega-3 fatty acids (i.e., eicosapentaenoic acid [EPA] and docosahexaenoic acid [DHA]) decrease pain and lameness, improve weight bearing, and can decrease the need for nonsteroidal anti-inflammatory drugs (NSAIDs) in dogs with osteoarthritis. In addition, they have been shown to have beneficial effects in

TABLE 23.5	Commonly Used Nutraceuticals		
Supplement	**Primary Target Area(s)**	**Functions**	**Route of Administration**
Glucosamine	Joints	Lubricates joints, protects cartilage, decreases inflammation	Oral
Chondroitin	Joints	Lubricates joints, protects cartilage, inhibits joint degradation	Oral
Omega-3 fatty acids	Joints, skin, heart	Decreases joint pain, inhibits inflammation	Oral
Perna canaliculus	Joints	Decreases joint pain and inflammation	Oral
Polysulfated glycosaminoglycans	Joints	Decreases joint pain and inflammation, protects cartilage	Intramuscular, subcutaneous, or intra-articular
Hyaluronic acid	Joints	Decreases joint pain and inflammation	Intra-articular or oral

the treatment of cardiovascular disease and dermatologic disorders. Omega-3 fatty acids have the highest level of evidence for supplements that benefit the treatment of canine osteoarthritis. Omega-3 fatty acids are available in therapeutic joint diets, in gel capsules, or in liquid oil form for oral administration.

Perna Canaliculus

Perna canaliculus, the New Zealand green-lipped mussel, is composed of omega-3 polyunsaturated fatty acids, a variety of carotenoids, and other bioactive compounds. It has anti-inflammatory and antiarthritic effects. It has been shown to alleviate the symptoms of degenerative joint disease and arthritis in cats and chronic orthopedic pain in dogs. In horses, it decreases the severity of lameness and joint pain and provides improved joint flexion in limbs with lameness attributed to osteoarthritis.

Polysulfated Glycosaminoglycans

Polysulfated glycosaminoglycans are semisynthetic products derived from bovine trachea that stimulate collagen synthesis, inhibit collagen breakdown, and decrease pain and inflammation in joints. They are typically delivered via intramuscular or subcutaneous injection in canine patients and intra-articular injection in equine patients.

Hyaluronic Acid

Intra-articular injection of hyaluronic acid decreases pain and inflammation and stimulates endogenous production of hyaluronic acid in horses with joint disease. Hyaluronic acid is commonly combined with a steroid, such as triamcinolone, for its anti-inflammatory properties.

If an intra-articular injection is going to be administered, the technician should perform a thorough surgical preparation of the affected joint before the veterinarian administers the injection. In most cases, the patient will need to be sedated and should be properly and safely restrained by the technician during the procedure. Hyaluronic acid is also available in oral forms as a chew or capsule.

TECHNICIAN NOTE

Technicians should be familiar with the various nutraceuticals and supplements available to treat osteoarthritis.

Summary

Rehabilitation therapy and integrative medicine encompass a vast array of techniques and therapies. This chapter offers an overview of some of the more common modalities and is not a comprehensive guide to rehabilitation or integrative medicine. Many of the individual subjects discussed in this chapter have their own texts and are taught in courses lasting months to years. The veterinary technician may become skilled in many of these modalities and can serve as an excellent source of information for clients regarding other treatments, such as acupuncture and VSMT. As clients experience the benefits of physical therapy and integrative medicine in their own health care, they are increasingly interested in pursuing the same care for their pets. As the demand for complementary veterinary medicine and rehabilitation grows, more veterinarians are pursuing advanced certification and are seeking veterinary technicians with training and experience in these areas.

Acknowledgments

The author and publisher wish to acknowledge the contributions of Laurie McCauley, Christine Jurek, and Carolina Medina to previous editions of this chapter.

Recommended Reading and Resources

Books

Bockstahler B, Levine D, Millis D. *Essential Facts of Physiotherapy in Dogs and Cats. Rehabilitation and Pain Management.* Babenhausen, Germany: BE Vet Verlag; 2004.

Duerr F. *Canine Lameness.* Hoboken, NY: John Wiley; 2020.

Gaynor JS, Muir WW. *Handbook of Veterinary Pain Management.* 3rd ed. St. Louis, MO: Elsevier Inc; 2015.

Goldberg ME, Tomlinson J. *Physical Rehabilitation for Veterinary Technicians and Nurses.* Hoboken, NJ: John Wiley; 2018.

Millis D, Levine D. *Canine Rehabilitation and Physical Therapy.* 2nd ed. Philadelphia, PA: Elsevier Inc; 2014.

Reigel R, Godbold J. *Laser Therapy in Veterinary Medicine, Photobiomodulation.* Ames, IA: John Wiley; 2017.

Salvo S. *Massage Therapy Principles and Practice.* 5th ed. St. Louis, MO: Saunders; 2005.

Schreiber M. Sports massage for the equine athlete, Equissage, Round Hill, VA. Available at: http://www.equissage.com/.

Whalen-Shaw P. Canine massage: An instructional guide, Integrated Touch Therapy, Circleville, OH. Available at: http://www.integrated-touchtherapy.com/.

Xie H. *Traditional Chinese Veterinary Medicine. Fundamental Principles (Volume 1).* Reddick, FL: Jing Tang; 2005.

Zink C, Van Dyke J. *Canine Sports Medicine and Rehabilitation.* 2nd ed. Hoboken, NJ: Wiley-Blackwell; 2018.

Journals

Alvarez LX, McCue J, Lam NK, et al. Effect of targeted pulsed electromagnetic field therapy on canine postoperative hemilaminectomy: A double-blind, randomized, placebo-controlled clinical trial. *J Am Anim Hosp Assoc.* 2019;55:83–91.

Barbeau-Grégoire M, Otis C, Cournoyer A, et al. A 2022 systematic review and meta-analysis of enriched therapeutic diets and nutraceuticals in canine and feline osteoarthritis. *Int J Mol Sci.* 2022;23(18):10384.

Crook T, McGowan C, Pead M. Effect of passive stretching on the range of motion of osteoarthritic joints in 10 Labrador Retrievers. *Vet Rec.* 2007;160:545–547.

Draper WE, Schubert TA, Clemmons RM, et al. Low-level laser therapy reduces time to ambulation in dogs after hemilaminectomy: a preliminary study. *J Small Anim Pract.* 2012;53(8):465–469.

Drygas KA, McClure SR, Goring RL, et al. Effect of cold compression therapy on postoperative pain, swelling, range of motion, and lameness after tibial plateau leveling osteotomy in dogs. *JAVMA.* 2011;238:1284–1291.

Duerr F, Elam L. Small animal orthopedic medicine. *Vet Clin Small Anim.* 2022;52(4):841–1068.

Gallagher A, Cross AR, Sepulveda G. The effect of shock wave therapy on patellar ligament desmitis after tibial plateau leveling osteotomy. *Vet Surg.* 2012;41:482–485.

Groppetti D, Pecile AM, Sacerdote P, et al. Effectiveness of electroacupuncture analgesia compared with opioid administration in a dog model: A pilot study. *Br J Anaesth.* 2011;107(4):612–618.

Haussler KK. Back Problems. Chiropractic evaluation and management. *Vet Clin North Am Equine Pract.* 1999;15(1):195.

Kathmann I, Cizinauskas S, Doherr MG, et al. Daily controlled physiotherapy increases survival time in dogs with suspected degenerative myelopathy. *J Vet Intern Med.* 2006;20:927–932.

Monk M, Preston C, McGowan C. Effects of early intensive postoperative physiotherapy on limb function after tibial plateau leveling osteotomy in dogs with deficiency of the cranial cruciate ligament. *Am J Vet Res.* 2006;67:529–536.

Sems A, Dimeff R, Ianotti JP. Extracorporeal shockwave therapy in the treatment of chronic tendinopathies. *J Am Acad Orthop Surg.* 2006;14:195–204.

Vandeweerd JM, Coisnon C, Clegg P, et al. Systematic review of efficacy of nutraceuticals to alleviate clinical signs of osteoarthritis. *J Vet Inter Med.* 2012;26(3):448–456.

Zidan N, Fenn J, Griffith E, et al. The effect of electromagnetic fields on post-operative pain and locomotor recovery in dogs with acute, severe thoracolumbar intervertebral disc extrusion: A randomized placebo-controlled, prospective clinical trial. *J Neurotrauma.* 2018;35(15):1726–1736.

Professional Organizations

Academy of Physical Rehabilitation Veterinary Technicians: www.aprvt.com
American Academy of Veterinary Acupuncture: www.aava.org
American Association of Rehabilitation Veterinarians: www.rehabvets.org
American Association of Traditional Chinese Veterinary Medicine: http://www.aatcvm.org
American College of Veterinary Sports Medicine and Rehabilitation: www.vsmr.org
American Holistic Veterinary Medical Association: www.ahvma.org
American Physical Therapy Association: www.apta.org
American Veterinary Chiropractic Association: www.animalchiropractic.org
International Association of Veterinary Rehabilitation and Physio Therapy: www.iavrpt.org
International Veterinary Academy of Pain Management: https://ivapm.org

Massage Schools

Equissage: www.equissage.com
Healing Oasis: www.thehealingoasis.com
Integrated Touch Therapy, Inc: www.integratedtouchtherapy.com

Rehabilitation Certification Training

Canine Rehabilitation Institute, Inc: www.caninerehabinstitute.com
Healing Oasis, Healing Oasis: www.thehealingoasis.com
University of Tennessee: https://www.utvetrehab.com/canine-rehab-ccvp/
North Carolina State University, Northeast Seminars: https://www.ncsuvetce.com/canine-rehab-ccat

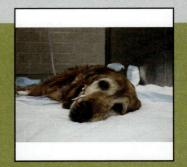

24

Fluid Therapy and Transfusion Medicine

COURTNEY BEITER, EDWARD COOPER, OLIVIA M. HOLT WILLIAMS, AND
MARGARET MUDGE

CHAPTER OUTLINE

LEARNING OBJECTIVES

When you have completed this chapter, you will be able to:

1. Recognize, define, and apply all key terms in the chapter.
2. Explain the indications for fluid therapy and describe the body fluid compartments, including movement of fluids between these compartments.
3. Compare and contrast crystalloid and colloid fluids, and describe the uses for and characteristics of each.
4. Do the following regarding the administration of fluids and fluid therapy additives:
   - Discuss the objectives of each phase of fluid therapy and the specific products and administration rates used during each phase.
   - Compare and contrast the indications for and techniques used to administer fluids by the intravenous, subcutaneous, intraosseous, and enteral routes.
   - Explain the indications for and techniques used to administer potassium chloride, dextrose, and sodium bicarbonate.
5. Do the following regarding monitoring and complications of fluid therapy:

- Describe the methods used to monitor the effectiveness of fluid therapy.
- Discuss common complications of fluid therapy, including appropriate interventions.
6. Do the following regarding transfusion medicine:
   - Describe the indications for blood, plasma, and blood component transfusion.
   - Discuss the selection and care of blood donors.
   - Explain pretransfusion testing, including blood typing, antibody screening, and cross matching.
7. Do the following regarding collection techniques, blood products, and product administration:
   - Describe the techniques used to collect blood from dogs, cats, and horses.
   - List blood products, including the indications for and benefits provided by each.
   - Describe the technique used to administer blood products to a patient, including calculation of administration rates.
   - Discuss patient monitoring during blood transfusions and recognition and management of transfusion reactions.

KEY TERMS

Agglutination
Anaphylaxis
Anemia
Blood type
Coagulopathy
Colloid
Cross match
Crystalloid fluid
Dehydration
Fluid resuscitation
Hemolysis

Hypersensitivity
Hypertonic
Hypotonic
Hypovolemia
Isotonic
Maintenance rate
Oncotic pressure
Packed cell volume
Replacement fluid rate
Transfusion reaction

Introduction

Fluid therapy is an extremely important aspect of patient care, especially in the setting of emergent and critical illnesses. The optimal fluid type, the amount to be given, and the route of administration can vary considerably, depending on the patient's clinical picture. Despite extensive research, no single approach to fluid administration has been proven to consistently offer a clear advantage. Furthermore, fluids are not without potential risks and complications. Consequently, formulating a fluid therapy plan (that addresses what type, how much, and how fast to give fluids) can offer considerable challenge. Very simply stated, the key is to give the adequate amount of an appropriate fluid as dictated by the patient's clinical condition and to not give too much. Although it would be desirable to have one formula and fluid type that suits all patients, one size most certainly does not fit all. Thus to develop and implement an appropriate fluid therapy plan, it is important to understand the body fluid compartments and the characteristics of different fluid types, consider the rates and routes of administration, monitor the effectiveness of achieving fluid therapy goals, and recognize potential complications. The first part of this chapter provides a systematic approach to fluid therapy that is intended to guide these decisions in the treatment of large and small animals.

Along with effective fluid therapy, blood product transfusions can be a lifesaving or life-prolonging component of treatment, and veterinary technicians and nurses play an integral role in the collection, processing, and administration of blood and blood products. The technician should be able to recognize severe hemorrhage and life-threatening anemia and should be aware of available blood products. In many practices, the veterinary technician is responsible for collection of blood from donor animals and for separation and storage of blood components. Proper blood product administration and monitoring are also important responsibilities, because blood transfusion is not without risks and adverse effects. The second part of this chapter provides information on indications for blood transfusion, pretransfusion testing, blood donor selection and blood collection, processing of blood components, blood product storage, transfusion administration, and transfusion reactions.

Fluid Therapy

Indications for Fluid Therapy

The decision to initiate fluid therapy is based on various clinical and practical considerations. Generally, fluids are used to replace those which have been lost or to keep up with the basic physiologic need for water when the patient cannot do so for itself. Some related indications, among others, are provided in Box 24.1.

Body Fluid Compartments

To understand the effects of different fluid types after they are administered, a general understanding of body fluid compartments is extremely important. The body is made up of approximately 60% water (referred to as *total body water [TBW]*). TBW is spread across the intracellular fluid (ICF) and extracellular fluid (ECF) spaces (Fig. 24.1). The primary barrier between these spaces is the cell membrane. ECF is further divided into interstitial (ISF) and intravascular (IVF) fluid spaces. The primary barrier between these spaces is the endothelial surface layer (ESL), which is comprised of the vascular endothelium and the glycocalyx (a glycoprotein and glycolipid layer covering the endothelial surface) (Fig. 24.2). Relative to differences in these compartmental distributions, the circulating blood volume for different species can be variable, ranging from as little as 40 mL/kg for cats to 100 mL/kg for alpacas. Box 24.2 lists normal circulating blood volumes for various species.

TECHNICIAN NOTE

Relative to differences in these compartmental distributions, the circulating blood volume for different species can be variable, ranging from as little as 40 mL/kg for cats to 100 mL/kg for alpacas (see Box 24.2).

These fluid compartments are important to consider because of differences in barrier permeability to assorted substances provided in intravenous (IV) fluids (water, electrolytes, colloids, etc.). For example, water can move across all barriers (ESL and cell membrane)

• BOX 24.1 Clinical Indications for Fluid Therapy

- Maintaining hydration
- Replacing fluid deficit (dehydration)
- Replacing ongoing losses
- Treating decreased oncotic pressure
- Treating hypovolemia
- Treating shock states
- Improving/increasing urine production
- Correcting acid-base balance or electrolyte disorders
- Maintaining intravenous access and delivering other medications

entirely based on concentration gradient. Therefore the volume of distribution for water is the TBW. Electrolytes, however, can move freely across the ESL but cannot move across the cell membrane unless actively transported, so they will distribute throughout the ECF based on relative proportions of ISF and IVF. In other words, when an electrolyte solution is administered, approximately one-fourth will remain in the vascular space and three-fourths will move into the interstitium. Large molecules, such as colloids, do not readily move across the vascular endothelium and so are *relatively* confined to the vascular space. This means that IV administration of colloids will result primarily in expansion of the vascular volume, at least in the immediate sense. Furthermore, colloids may have the ability to move fluid from the interstitium into the vascular space by increasing the **oncotic pressure** of blood.

Types of Intravenous Fluids

IV fluids are typically classified based on their composition and physiochemical properties. Two main categories are crystalloids and colloids.

Crystalloids

Crystalloid solutions contain various electrolytes in water and are further characterized because of their osmolality compared with the osmolality of blood (Table 24.1).

Hypotonic fluids have an osmolality less than that of blood (normal plasma osmolality is approximately 280–310 mOsm/L)

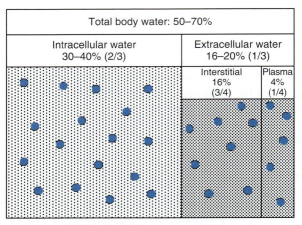

• **Fig. 24.1** Diagram of body fluid compartments.

Total body water: 50–70%		
Intracellular water 30–40% (2/3)	Extracellular water 16–20% (1/3)	
	Interstitial 16% (3/4)	Plasma 4% (1/4)

• BOX 24.2 Circulating Blood Volume for Various Species

• Cats	40–60 mL/kg
• Small ruminants	75 mL/kg
• Horses	80 mL/kg
• Dogs	80–90 mL/kg
• Alpacas	100 mL/kg

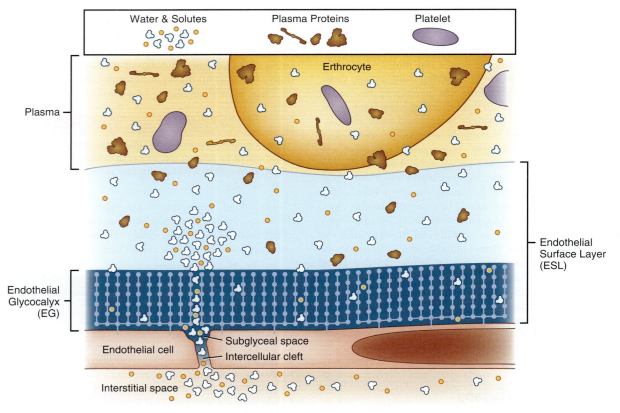

• **Fig. 24.2** Endothelial surface layer.

TABLE 24.1	Assorted Crystalloid Solutions and Electrolyte Compositions						
Fluid	Sodium (Na)	Potassium (K)	Chloride (Cl)	Calcium (Ca)	Magnesium (Mg)	Osmolality, mOsm/kg	Sodium Bicarbonate Precursors
Dextrose 5% in water (D$_5$W)	0	0	0	0	0	287	0
0.45% Sodium chloride (NaCl)	77	0	77	0	0	154	0
0.9% NaCl	154	0	154	0	0	308	0
Lactated Ringer solution	130	4	109	3	0	278	28 lactate
Plasmalyte 148/A	140	5	98	0	3	294	27 acetate
Normosol R	140	5	98	0	3	294	23 gluconate
3% NaCl	513	0	513	0	0	1026	0
7% NaCl	1198	0	1198	0	0	2396	0

All values in mEq/L unless otherwise indicated.

and provide water in greater proportion than electrolytes. Examples of hypotonic fluids include dextrose 5% in water (D$_5$W); 0.45% sodium chloride (NaCl); and "maintenance" fluids, such as Normosol M and Plasmalyte 56. Hypotonic fluids may be used to replace a free water deficit and to treat hypernatremia (high blood sodium). Given the decreased tolerance for sodium load in neonates and patients with heart disease and kidney disease, hypotonic fluids may be more ideally suited to replace deficits or maintain hydration in these patients. It should be emphasized that these fluids should never be used in fluid resuscitation (administered rapidly as a bolus), because they are ineffective for expanding vascular volume and could cause overly rapid changes in blood osmolality.

TECHNICIAN NOTE

Given the decreased tolerance for sodium load in neonates and patients with heart and kidney disease, hypotonic fluids may be more ideally suited to replace deficits or maintain hydration in these patients.

Isotonic crystalloids have an osmolality approximately equal to that of blood and provide water in equal proportion to electrolytes. Examples of isotonic crystalloids include 0.9% NaCl (normal saline [NS]) and balanced electrolyte solutions (BESs), such as Plasmalyte 148, Normosol R, and lactated Ringer solution (LRS). Because these fluids have applications in resuscitation, rehydration, and replacement of ongoing losses, they are, by far, the most used crystalloids. As previously indicated, IV administration of an isotonic crystalloid will result in rapid redistribution to the interstitial space so that as little as 25% to 35% (or less) will remain in the vascular space after 20 to 30 minutes.

In addition to providing water and electrolytes, isotonic crystalloids can affect acid-base balance. Because of its relatively high chloride content, 0.9% NaCl has acidifying effects, and BESs contain sodium bicarbonate precursors and have alkalinizing effects. This might make NS the ideal choice for the vomiting patient with hypochloremic metabolic alkalosis, or BES may be the ideal choice for a patient with severe acidemia. Isotonic crystalloids are not without potential adverse effects, especially if given in very large quantities. For example, these fluids have the potential to

cause tissue edema and create acid-base disturbances. In addition, currently there is concern that the high chloride content of 0.9% NaCl may cause acute kidney injury and increase the need for renal replacement therapy in human patients.

Hypertonic crystalloids have an osmolality greater than that of blood and provide electrolytes in greater proportion than water. Examples of hypertonic fluids include 3% and 7% hypertonic NaCl. It is important to note that 23% NaCl solutions are available but must be diluted to a concentration no greater than 7.5% to avoid osmotic injury. The high osmolality of hypertonic saline will cause a shift of fluid from the interstitium to the intravascular space, promoting rapid expansion of vascular volume to aid in resuscitation. However, because electrolytes readily redistribute across the endothelium, the effects are transient, lasting only 20 to 30 minutes. Another therapeutic application of hypertonic saline is treatment of head trauma or traumatic brain injury. The osmotic effects of this fluid help draw fluid out of the cerebral interstitium, thereby decreasing intracranial pressure and simultaneously increasing blood volume and blood pressure. Hypertonic saline should not be administered any faster than 0.5 to 1 mL/kg per minute, because rapid volume expansion can trigger reflex bradycardia.

See Fig. 24.3 for a summary of suggested uses of the various types of crystalloids.

Colloids

Colloid solutions contain high–molecular-weight molecules suspended in an isotonic crystalloid. As was previously discussed, these larger molecules tend to remain within the vascular space through prohibition by the ESL, thereby conferring oncotic pressure (the portion of total osmotic pressure contributed by colloids). Colloids can be classified as natural (e.g., plasma or albumin solutions) or synthetic (e.g., hydroxyethyl starch suspended in crystalloid solution). Given their tendency to initially remain within the vascular space and provide relatively efficient and more prolonged volume expansion, colloids are well suited for use in resuscitation. In addition, they can be used to provide oncotic support for patients with hypoproteinemia. Synthetic colloids have been associated with the potential to cause coagulopathy. However, this has not been shown to be associated with increased risk of

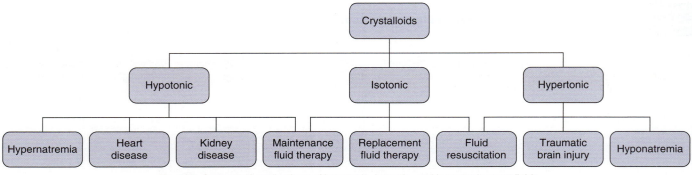

• **Fig. 24.3** Suggested applications of hypotonic, isotonic, and hypertonic crystalloids.

bleeding or need for transfusion. More recently, considerable concern has been raised regarding the potential for renal injury caused by hydroxyethyl starch solutions. In critically ill human patients, increased risk of acute kidney injury and the need for renal replacement therapy have been documented, resulting in significantly reduced use of synthetic colloids in human medicine and in veterinary medicine. Studies investigating the impact on veterinary patients have shown mixed results, with some showing no impact and others demonstrating concern regarding accumulation of synthetic colloid in the kidneys and potential injury. As such, these solutions should be used with caution for ongoing long-term infusions, especially in patients with or at risk for kidney injury/disease. If available, natural colloids (e.g., plasma) may be a better option for providing oncotic support.

> **TECHNICIAN NOTE**
>
> Given the tendency to remain within the vascular space and provide relatively efficient and prolonged volume expansion, colloids are well suited for use in resuscitation.

Specifics of Fluid Administration

Phases of Fluid Therapy

Resuscitation Phase. Fluid resuscitation is aimed at restoration of vascular volume to reverse **hypovolemia** and/or a shock state. Typically, the amount administered during resuscitation is determined based on the amount of vascular volume lost and the relative efficiency with which fluid expands the intravascular space (Table 24.2). These volumes are determined based on the assumption that patients in hypovolemic shock have lost approximately 30% of their blood volume (25–30 mL/kg in dogs and horses; 12–18 mL/kg in cats) and dividing that volume by the efficiency (increase in vascular volume for 1 mL of fluid administered). The "ideal" fluid for resuscitation has not been determined, as it may vary depending on the patient's clinical needs. In some circumstances, it might not be just one fluid type that is indicated, and a mixed resuscitation (using different types of fluids) might be warranted. By combining the beneficial effects (e.g., profound expansion from hypertonic saline, prolonged effects of colloids), total doses of each fluid can be reduced and the side effects thus diminished.

The "classic" volumes determined as "shock doses" for these different fluids are meant to serve as a guideline. Fluid administration should be titrated to effect based on clinical response. In the traditional approach to fluid resuscitation, this is typically achieved by giving some fraction of the shock dose over some period (e.g.,

one-fourth over 15 minutes). However, there is some evidence to suggest that this traditional approach, with rapid administration of large volumes, may not be ideal in some patients. For example, in patients with uncontrolled bleeding, there is potential to exacerbate blood loss with rapid volume expansion and increasing perfusing pressure. Furthermore, it may be that rapid administration is actually less effective, because there is disruption of the glycocalyx, and a greater portion of the volume may move out of the vascular space. This has led to the notion that a more cautious and gradual (revised) approach to fluid resuscitation may be indicated, with smaller volumes administered over a similar or longer period (so a "slowless" rather than a bolus), for example, giving 10 mL/kg of an isotonic crystalloid over 20 to 30 minutes rather than the "classic" 20 to 30 mL/kg given over 15 to 20 minutes (see Table 24.2).

> **TECHNICIAN NOTE**
>
> Volumes determined as "shock doses" for different fluids are meant to serve as guidelines. Fluid administration should be titrated to effect based on clinical response.

In either of these approaches, after each bolus or "slowless" administration, the patient should be reassessed for improvement in perfusion parameters. It is important that blood pressure is not used as the sole means of determining the need for fluid resuscitation or response to therapy. Generally, arterial blood pressure is highly preserved and therefore decreases only in advanced stages as the patient decompensates. Along these lines, it is also the first parameter to normalize, even though hypovolemic shock may continue. Therefore changes in heart rate (HR), capillary refill time (CRT), mucous membrane color, mentation, warmth of distal extremities, and so on are more useful in helping to guide therapy (see the section "Monitoring Fluid Therapy"). If perfusion parameters have not improved with the initial bolus, it should be repeated. If a full "shock dose" has been administered, but the patient is not yet stable, investigation should be conducted into the sources of ongoing loss or causes of shock unrelated to hypovolemia (cardiogenic, vasodilatory, etc.), and other interventions may be necessary (vasopressors, inotropes, etc.).

In large animals that require immediate resuscitation, it is difficult to deliver "shock doses" of isotonic **crystalloid fluids** or colloids within 10 to 15 minutes. Instead, hypertonic saline can be delivered quickly because of the small volume required and can be followed by isotonic crystalloids. Placement of a second jugular catheter can be helpful in delivering the large volumes needed, and high-volume oscillating pumps can be used to increase the speed of fluid delivery. However, high delivery pressures may cause

Fluid Resuscitation Guidelines

TABLE
24.2

Fluid	Efficiency	Total Shock Dose (mL/kg)		Initial Bolus, mL/kg (classic) Initial Slowless, mL/kg (revised)
Isotonic crystalloid	0.25–0.33	Dog/Horse	80–90	20–30 10–15
		Cat	40–60	10–15 5–10
Hypertonic crystalloid	4-6	Dog	3–6	3–6 N/A
		Cat/Horse	2–4	2–4 N/A
Colloid	1–1.5	Dog	20–30	5 2–3
		Cat/Horse	10–15	3–4 1–2

Efficiency reflects the increase in vascular volume for each milliliter administered. Bolus given over 15 to 20 minutes in the classic approach, 20 to 30 minutes in the revised approach.

damage to the jugular veins, so this method should be used only when necessary.

Replacement Phase. Once resuscitation has been achieved (or in cases in which it was not necessary), the next phase of fluid therapy is *replacement*. Replacement fluid therapy involves correction of dehydration, replacement of ongoing losses, and provision of maintenance fluid requirements. It is generally assumed that fluid losses are isotonic in nature (vomiting, diarrhea, blood loss, etc.); therefore an isotonic crystalloid is most commonly used during replacement.

TECHNICIAN NOTE

Replacement fluid rate = Dehydration + Ongoing losses + Maintenance

To determine the contribution of dehydration to the replacement rate, the fluid deficit should be calculated by multiplying the patient's body weight (BW) in kilograms by the estimated percent dehydration expressed as a decimal (see Chapter 25 regarding assessment of hydration). For example, a 30-kg dog with 8% dehydration would have a fluid deficit of 2.4 L (30 × 0.08). The length of time over which the deficit will be replaced must then be determined. Depending on the clinical situation, replacement over 4 to 24 hours may be acceptable, with chronic loss replaced more slowly. For those that replace fluids more slowly (12–24 hours), the argument is made that rapid rehydration will result in expansion of the vascular volume with loss through the kidneys and ineffective rehydration. There should be further consideration for feline and neonatal patients and for those with cardiac or kidney disease, because these patients are particularly associated with decreased fluid tolerance, and thus slower rehydration is recommended. Once the time frame for replacement is determined, the fluid deficit is divided by the number of hours over which fluids will be administered. (See the Case Presentations in this chapter for examples of calculations.)

Provision for ongoing loss is determined by quantifying or estimating fluid losses over a period and then increasing the fluid administration rate accordingly. Examples of ongoing losses

include vomiting, diarrhea, bleeding, increased insensible losses (panting), and inappropriate urinary losses. It is important to not include appropriate urinary losses (1–2 mL/kg per hour) in a calculation of ongoing losses, because these are accounted for in the maintenance rate. Quantifying water losses can be accomplished by using collection devices (catheters, drains, etc.) or by weighing fluids (e.g., vomit, diarrhea, urine) collected in absorbable pads. This is achieved by weighing the soiled pads and subtracting the weight of the pads themselves. Then every gram of weight measured is equal to 1 mL of fluid loss. If it is not possible to measure losses because they are on the floor or outdoors, volumes can be estimated. In either case, the volume of losses that occur over a given period (e.g., 4–8 hours) should be divided by the number of hours over which they occurred, and the resulting rate (in mL/hour) added to the fluid administration rate for the next period. (See the Case Presentations for examples of calculations.) It is important to also consider that increasing fluid rates could serve to drive ongoing losses (especially urinary or gastrointestinal [GI] losses). If escalation of fluid rate to match losses results in progressively increased diarrhea, urine production, and so on, then fluids should be decreased and those losses no longer replaced.

The maintenance rate is meant to supply the basic physiologic need for water lost through urine, the GI system, and insensible losses (as from the respiratory tract). Various guidelines have been used to determine the daily maintenance fluid requirement (expressed in milliliters per day [mL/day]), including the formulas 30*Body weight (kg) + 70, 40 to 60 mL/kg per day, and 2 to 4 mL/kg per hour. Although straightforward, these guidelines assume a linear relationship between body weight and daily fluid requirement and do not take into account the impact of body surface area-to-volume ratios on metabolic rate. An allometric scale, as represented by the formula $132 \times$ Body weight $(kg)^{(3/4)}$ for dogs, and the formula $80 \times$ Body weight $(kg)^{(3/4)}$ for cats, may better predict metabolic water requirements for some patients. As shown in Table 24.3, the linear calculations mentioned above tend to underestimate the needs of small patients (especially those weighing <10 kg) and can overestimate the needs of large patients (especially those weighing >30 kg) compared with the allometric

TABLE 24.3	Comparison of Equations for Calculating Maintenance Fluid Rates			
BW, kg	2–4 mL/kg per hour	60 mL/kg per day	30 × BW + 70/day	132 × BW$^{(3/4)}$/day (dog) 80 × BW$^{(3/4)}$/day (cat)
1	2–4	2.5	4.2	5.5 3.3
5	10–20	12.5	9.2	18.4 11.1
10	20–40	25	15.4	30.9 18.7
15	30–60	37.5	21.7	41.9
20	40–80	50	27.9	52.0
30	60–120	75	40.4	70.5
40	80–160	100	52.9	87.5
50	100–200	125	65.4	103.4

Fluid rate based on indicated equation (in mL/hour).
BW, Body weight.

scale. In horses, a maintenance rate of 40 to 60 mL/kg per day is typically used. Larger (draft breed) horses are given maintenance fluids at a lower rate (40 mL/kg per day), and neonates are given maintenance fluids at a higher rate (up to 90–100 mL/kg per day).

TECHNICIAN NOTE

There are several ways to calculate maintenance fluid rates. Linear calculations (e.g., 60 mL/kg per day) tend to underestimate rates in small canine patients (weight <10 kg) and overestimate rates in large patients (weight >30 kg), compared with the allometric scale (132 × Body weight (kg)$^{(3/4)}$ for dogs).

The replacement rate determined by this process should serve as a good starting point, provided it is followed up with periodic reassessment of hydration status and revision of the fluid therapy plan (see the section "Monitoring Fluid Therapy").

Maintenance Phase. Once dehydration has been corrected and there are no longer any ongoing losses, the patient can be moved to the maintenance phase of fluid therapy. Patients that present without dehydration or ongoing losses may start out on a maintenance rate during hospitalization if they are unwilling or unable to drink adequately on their own. Maintenance rates are determined as described previously. Isotonic crystalloids are often used for maintenance fluid therapy. However, these fluids (intended for replacement) provide sodium and chloride in an amount that is more than what is needed for maintenance purposes (because patients normally drink water, not salt solution, to maintain fluid balance). Hypotonic, or "maintenance," crystalloids better match true maintenance requirements but, for reasons of availability and ease, isotonic fluids are most often used. For most patients with normal cardiac and renal functions, the excess electrolyte load is easily handled and excreted by the kidneys, thereby justifying this common practice. For neonatal foals that are not nursing and require only maintenance fluid therapy, a hypotonic solution, such as 0.45% NaCl with 2.5% to 5% dextrose, is preferable to

replacement fluids. (See Case Presentations 24.1–24.3 for examples of fluid rate calculations and fluid administration in two dogs and a horse, respectively.)

Routes of Administration

Several factors should be considered when determining the optimal route for fluid administration. These factors include the nature of the disease process, the stability of the patient, the magnitude of the fluid deficit and ongoing losses, the characteristics of the fluid loss, the decision of whether to treat the animal as an inpatient or an outpatient, the expected length of the hospital stay (if needed), the equipment and technical expertise required, and the ultimate goal of fluid therapy for that patient. Possible routes of administration in small animals include IV (central or peripheral), subcutaneous (SC), intraosseous (IO), and oral (PO); in large animals, routes of administration include the IV route and the enteral route via a nasogastric tube.

Intravenous Route. The IV route offers several advantages, especially for acutely and/or critically ill patients (those requiring urgent or immediate attention). The IV route allows the ability to administer fluids rapidly for volume expansion. In addition, multiple different fluid types can be given intravenously, including hypotonic, isotonic, hypertonic crystalloids, colloids, and blood products. Because of the ability to rapidly titrate fluid administration, the IV route is preferred for fluid resuscitation, intraoperative fluid therapy, use in anesthetized patients, replacement of significant dehydration and ongoing losses, and use in critically ill patients in general.

TECHNICIAN NOTE

Because of the ability to rapidly titrate fluid administration, the IV route is preferred for fluid resuscitation, intraoperative fluid therapy, use in anesthetized patients, replacement of significant dehydration and ongoing losses, and use in critically ill patients in general.

CASE PRESENTATION 24.1

Fluid Rate Calculations and Fluid Administration in a Dog

A 5-kg castrated male mixed-breed dog was presented with a history of severe vomiting, bloody diarrhea, lethargy, and anorexia over the previous 2 days. On the initial physical examination, heart rate (HR) was 200 beats per minute (bpm), pulses were weak, the mucous membranes were pale, capillary refill time (CRT) was 4 seconds, and the patient was found to be depressed. Systolic arterial blood pressure as measured with a Doppler monitor was 60 mm Hg (normal, 110–140 mm Hg). Dehydration was estimated to be 10%. Blood glucose was also found to be 48 mg/dL.

Resuscitation Phase

Plasmalyte was started intravenously at a rate of 10 mL/kg (50 mL total) over 20 minutes. In addition, 0.5 g/dL of dextrose (2.5 g, or 5 mL diluted to 10 mL with sterile water) was administered over 3 to 5 minutes. The patient was then reassessed. Systolic arterial blood pressure increased to 100 mm Hg, HR was 180 bpm, CRT was 3 seconds, and a slight improvement in mentation was evident, along with an increase in pulse quality.

Because the physical parameters improved but were not normal, a repeat bolus of 50 mL (10 mL/kg) Plasmalyte was administered intravenously over 30 minutes. A second reassessment revealed further improvement as evidenced by systolic arterial blood pressure of 120 mm Hg, HR of 140 bpm, CRT of 2 seconds, and increased responsiveness. Blood glucose was reassessed and found to be 115 mg/dL. At this point, the resuscitation phase was complete.

Replacement Phase

Because dehydration was determined to be 10% on presentation, 0.5 L (500 mL) of fluid (0.1 × 5 kg) was needed to correct the fluid deficit. However, given that 100 mL of fluid had already been administered, this left 400 mL of fluid deficit. The attending veterinarian elected to replace this deficit over 12 hours at an administration rate of 33 mL/hour (400 mL/12 hour).

The maintenance rate for this patient was calculated as 18 mL/hour ([132 × 5$^{(3/4)}$] ÷ 24), so replacement fluids were started at a rate of 51 mL/hour (33 mL/hour + 18 mL/hour), which was rounded to 50 mL/hour. It was also decided that 2.5% dextrose would be add to the 1-L fluid bag. This was accomplished by adding 50 mL of 50% (0.5 g/mL) dextrose to 1 L of Plasmalyte. At this rate, during the first 4 hours, the patient was estimated to have had 120 mL in ongoing losses from vomiting and diarrhea (30 mL/hour). Therefore the fluid rate for the next 4 hours was increased to 80 mL/hour (50 mL/hour + 30 mL/hour) to replace this loss.

During this time, estimated ongoing losses decreased to 60 mL (15 mL/hour), so the maintenance rate for the subsequent 4 hours was adjusted to 65 mL/hour (50 mL/hour + 15 mL/hour) to reflect this decrease. After 12 hours, it was believed the patient was rehydrated, although fluid loss resulting from vomiting and diarrhea continued. For the next 36 hours, the fluid rate was adjusted to include only maintenance fluid rate and ongoing losses. With resolution of ongoing fluid loss, the replacement phase was complete.

Maintenance Phase

At the onset of the maintenance phase, the fluid administration rate was reduced to the maintenance rate of 18 mL/hour. Shortly thereafter, the patient started to eat and drink. The maintenance rate was gradually reduced and then discontinued, at which point the maintenance phase was complete.

CASE PRESENTATION 24.2

Fluid Rate Calculations and Restrictive Fluid Administration in a Bleeding Dog

A 30-kg spayed female, Labrador Retriever was presented after she was hit by a car 30 to 45 minutes earlier. On initial physical examination, heart rate (HR) was 160 beats per minute (bpm), femoral pulses were moderate, the mucous membranes were pale pink, capillary refill time (CRT) was 3 seconds, hydration was normal, and the patient was found to be depressed but ambulatory. Systolic arterial blood pressure as measured with a Doppler monitor was 70 mm Hg. Quick trauma ultrasonography (focused assessment with sonography for trauma [FAST] examination) revealed a moderate amount of echogenic fluid, suspected to be hemorrhage.

Resuscitation Phase

Because of concerns about active bleeding and taking a restrictive approach to fluid resuscitation, Plasmalyte was started intravenously at a rate of 10 mL/kg (300 mL total) over 30 minutes. The patient was then reassessed. Systolic arterial blood pressure increased to 100 mm Hg, HR was 150 bpm, CRT was 3 seconds, and a slight improvement in mentation was evident, along with an increase in pulse quality. Although some signs of compensation persisted, further fluid boluses were not administered in order to limit the potential of exacerbating bleeding.

Replacement Phase

Maintenance for this patient was determined to be 70 mL/hour ([132 × 30$^{(3/4)}$] ÷ 24). Because there was no indication of dehydration in this patient, replacement of deficit did not need to be accounted for. However, because decreased circulating volume was anticipated and with potential ongoing loss of fluid (hemorrhage), it was decided that the patient would be placed on 2× maintenance (140 mL/hour) with continued close monitoring of vital signs and blood pressure. Over the next 6 hours, the patient's blood pressure remained at 100 to 110 mm Hg, HR decreased to 120 to 130 bpm, and the remainder of the vital signs stabilized. The administration rate was then reduced to a maintenance rate (70 mL/hour).

correction of dehydration, a peripheral vessel, such as the cephalic or saphenous vein can be used. In horses, the jugular vein can be used.

If a catheter is placed in a critically ill patient, such as one that may need serial blood sampling or constant rate infusions of multiple medications, a central line may be of benefit. Central line (multilumen) catheters are also useful when medications that may not be compatible are simultaneously administered, because these catheters have multiple lumens through which medications can be administered (Fig. 24.4). Usually, this is done through the jugular vein, but central line catheters can be placed in the lateral or medial saphenous vein and advanced into the caudal vena cava (peripherally inserted central catheter, or PICC).

Care should be taken by using aseptic technique when placing an IV catheter. This is especially true for central venous catheters. The catheter site should be clipped and enough hair removed from the area to ensure that there will be no contamination from the surrounding fur. A surgical scrub, such as chlorhexidine, should be used to clean the site by starting in the center and gradually moving outward until the gauze is clean. The site can then be wiped clean with alcohol or Zephiran (Sanofi-Aventis, Bridgewater, NJ) solution. Proper restraint is key for catheter placement. The holder should occlude the vessel above the patient's elbow for catheters being placed in the cephalic vein and above the stifle for catheters being placed in the medial or lateral saphenous vein. If a catheter is being placed into the jugular vein, the vessel should be occluded at the thoracic inlet. Ultrasonographic guidance may be needed when placing lateral thoracic

Multiple sites are available for IV catheter placement, including cephalic, medial, and lateral saphenous, dorsal pedal (in dogs and cats), lateral thoracic (in horses), and jugular veins. One should take into consideration the reason for IV catheter placement when choosing a vein to use. If a catheter is placed for routine fluid therapy or for

CASE PRESENTATION 24.3

Fluid Rate Calculations and Fluid Administration in a Horse

A 500-kg Quarter Horse gelding was presented with a 48-hour history of diarrhea, inappetence, and lethargy. On initial physical examination, the heart rate (HR) was 70 beats per minute (bpm) and pulses were weak, the mucous membranes were congested and dark pink, capillary refill time (CRT) was 4 seconds, and the patient was observed to be depressed. Dehydration was estimated to be 10%.

Resuscitation Phase

Lactated Ringer solution (LRS) was administered intravenously at a rate of 20 mL/kg (10 L total) over 20 to 30 minutes. The patient was then reassessed, and it was found that HR was 40 bpm, CRT was 2 seconds, and the patient was responsive and had urinated. At this point, the resuscitation phase was complete.

Replacement Phase

Because dehydration was determined to be 10% on presentation, 50 L (0.1 × 500 kg) was needed to correct the fluid deficit. However, given that 10 L of fluid had already been administered, this left 40 L of fluid deficit. The attending veterinarian elected to replace this deficit over 18 hours at an administration rate of 2.2 L/hour (40 L/18 hours).

The maintenance rate for this patient was calculated as 1.25 L/hour (500 kg × 60 mL/kg per day ÷ 24). Therefore replacement fluids were started at a rate of approximately 3.5 L/hour (2.2 L/hour + 1.25 L/hour). During the first hour, the patient continued to have watery diarrhea, with estimated losses of 1 L/hour. The maintenance rate was increased to 2.25 L/hour (1.25 L/hour + 1 L/hour) to replace this loss, increasing the replacement fluid rate to 4.55 L/hour (2.2 L/hour + 2.25 L/hour). The patient was reassessed every 4 hours, and packed cell volume (PCV) and total protein (TP) were checked every 6 hours during ongoing large fluid loss.

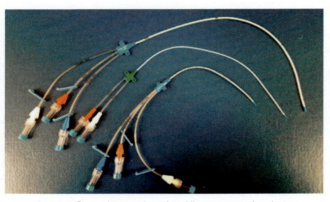

• **Fig. 24.4** Several examples of multilumen central catheters.

catheters in horses. Once placed, the catheter should be secured by using tape when it is placed in a peripheral vessel. Central line catheters should be sutured in place to ensure that they do not slip or back out of the vein. All catheters should then be wrapped to help keep the insertion site clean and the catheter more secure.

All catheters should be closely monitored daily for the development of any complications. For peripheral venous catheters, this includes checking the patient's foot for swelling or the presence of phlebitis and flushing the catheter to check for patency. The catheter tape and wrap should be monitored for excessive tightness or slipping. Any concerns should be addressed immediately. If a patient's foot is swollen, the catheter tape or wrap may need

to be loosened or replaced. If the catheter is no longer patent when flushed or if evidence of phlebitis (pain or irritation when the catheter is flushed) is found, the catheter should be removed and replaced (possibly in a new location). All catheters should be closely monitored for signs of infection, including swelling, irritation of or discharge from the catheter site, and fever. If a patient acquires a fever of unknown origin while in the hospital, any IV catheters should be removed and replaced in a different vein as a precaution.

Central venous catheters should always be unwrapped at least once a day. The site should be cleaned by using a surgical scrub, wiped with an alcohol or Zephiran (Sanofi-Aventis, Bridgewater, NJ) solution, and then rewrapped with bandage material. In adult horses that remain standing, the catheter can be wrapped or left unwrapped at the clinician's discretion. Gloves (sterile or nonsterile) should always be worn when central venous catheters are handled so that the possibility of introducing infection can be minimized. Patients with jugular vein catheters should be monitored closely for facial swelling, which can result from the bandage being placed too tightly or from jugular vein thromboses.

IV fluids are administered one of two ways: (1) by using a gravity-fed system and (2) by using a fluid pump. With a gravity-fed system, fluids are kept elevated above the patient and flow into the body by gravity. The fluid rate is manually adjusted by opening or closing the roller clamp on the administration set. The rate is largely dependent on the patient's position and therefore should be closely monitored to avoid fluid overload or insufficient flow. For smaller patients, a Buretrol device (Baxter, Deerfield, IL) can be placed between the fluid bag and the administration set to decrease the risk of fluid overload. The Buretrol device holds a maximum of 150 mL and can be clamped off just below the fluid bag so that no more than 150 mL can be administered unless it is refilled. It is extremely important to properly calculate the fluid rate based on the delivery rate of the drip set (the number of drops/mL) to avoid fluid overload or insufficient flow. To perform the fluid rate calculation, one will need to know the desired fluid infusion rate and the size of the drip set to be used (typically 10 drops/mL or 60 drops/mL for small animal patients) (See Box 24.3 for sample calculations.) However, when using a drip set, it is important to remember that any major change in position of the patient or the fluid bag will affect the rate. When it is necessary to deliver fast rates in resuscitation, it may be useful to apply a pressure bag that can allow administration of 1 L in 15 minutes or less.

Whenever possible, a fluid pump should be used to administer IV fluids, because this will help ensure accuracy of fluid administration. The type used most often is a volumetric pump (Fig. 24.5), which can be programmed to deliver any volume of fluid over a set amount of time. However, most of these units have a maximum infusion rate of 1 L/hour, and so a straight drip set ± pressure bag is needed for higher rates. In addition, administration of fluids at very low rates (especially <2 mL/hour) may be more accurately achieved through use of a syringe pump (Fig. 24.6). For large animals, large volumes of IV fluids are often required and are usually delivered by gravity. An example of a large animal fluid administration setup is shown in Fig. 24.7.

Calculation for Fluid Drips Sets

Example #1: The prescribed fluid infusion rate is 100 mL/hour, and the drip set has a delivery rating of 10 drops/mL.

$$\frac{\frac{100 \text{ mL}}{h} \times 1\,h}{60 \text{ min}} = \frac{\frac{1.66 \text{ mL}}{\text{min}} \times 1 \text{ min}}{60 \text{ s}}$$

$$\frac{\frac{0.02 \text{ mL}}{s} \times 10 \text{ drops}}{\text{mL}}$$

$$\frac{0.2 \text{ drops}}{s} = \frac{1 \text{ drop}}{5 \text{ s}}$$

where h is hours, min is minutes, and s is seconds.
In this example, the drip rate would be 1 drop every 5 seconds.

Example #2: The prescribed fluid infusion rate is 20 mL/hour, and the drip set has a delivery rating of 60 drops/mL.

$$\frac{\frac{20 \text{ mL}}{h} \times 1\,h}{60 \text{ min}} = \frac{\frac{0.33 \text{ mL}}{\text{min}} \times 1 \text{ min}}{60 \text{ s}}$$

$$\frac{\frac{0.0055 L}{s} \times 60 \text{ drops}}{\text{mL}}$$

$$\frac{0.33 \text{ drops}}{s} = \frac{1 \text{ drop}}{3 \text{ s}}$$

where h is hours, min is minutes, and s is seconds.
In this example, the drip rate would be 1 drop every 3 seconds.

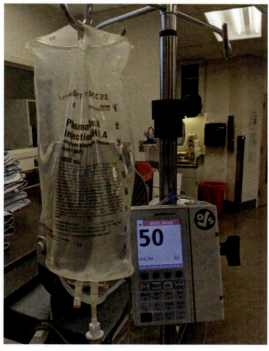

• **Fig. 24.5** A volumetric fluid pump.

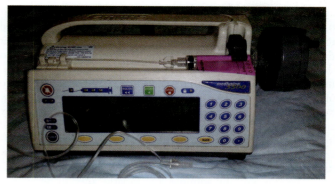

• **Fig. 24.6** Example of a syringe pump.

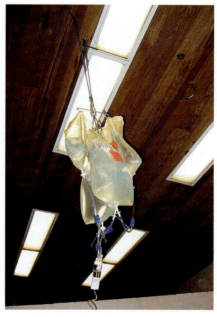

• **Fig. 24.7** A total of 20 L of crystalloid fluids can be administered to large animal patients by using transfer sets and a large-bore coil administration set. The coiled extension and swivel hanger allow the horse to move freely in the stall while intravenous (IV) fluids are administered.

Subcutaneous Route. The subcutaneous (SC or SQ) route can be used to administer large volumes of fluid for slow absorption over time and gradual fluid replacement. This route can be used to reverse mild-to-moderate dehydration or to prevent the development of dehydration in patients that are not eating or drinking. SC fluids can also be helpful in patients that need fluids but cannot be hospitalized or require intermittent fluid therapy that the client can provide at home (e.g., patients with renal failure). This route of administration should not be chosen for patients with severe dehydration or significant electrolyte imbalances that need to be corrected. SC fluids certainly should not be used in patients that are hypovolemic or hypotensive, because volume expansion will not be rapid enough, and the peripheral vasoconstriction associated with shock will result in significantly impaired absorption of fluid from the SC space.

TECHNICIAN NOTE

The subcutaneous (SC) route of administration should not be chosen for patients with severe compromise from dehydration, hypotension, or significant electrolyte imbalance.

TECHNICIAN NOTE

When using a drip set, it is important to remember that any major change in position of the patient or the fluid bag will affect the rate of administration!

Subcutaneously administered fluids should be isotonic (LRS or 0.9% NaCl) and should have an osmolality approximately equal to that of ECF. Dextrose solutions with concentration greater than 2.5% should not be given subcutaneously, because skin sloughing and abscess formation may occur. The volume of SC fluid to be administered can be calculated at approximately 30 to 60 mL/kg per day (or approximately one-half to full maintenance rate). SC fluids usually are absorbed in 6 to 8 hours, so the dose can be divided accordingly (typically, no more than 20–30 mL/kg at a time). The total volume should be divided to be administered in as many different spots as possible to avoid causing any discomfort to the patient. Although useful in small animals, SC fluids are not typically administered to large animals because of the large volume of fluids needed and the lack of adequate SC space in these patients.

SC fluid administration is relatively safe and easy and can be done at home when appropriate. However, complications may occur. SC administration of Plasmalyte 148 can cause discomfort because of the acidic pH (less likely with Plasmalyte A, which has been balanced to a pH of 7.4). Owners should be instructed to use a new needle each time fluid is administered; otherwise, pathogens might be introduced and abscess formation could occur. Pressure necrosis is possible if too much fluid is administered into one spot. Despite the relatively slow absorption of SC fluids, it is possible to cause fluid overload in a patient with underlying heart disease.

Intraosseous Route. The intraosseous (IO) route (or intermedullary route) offers an alternative when IV access is not possible, as in neonatal patients or small-sized or young patients with cardiovascular collapse. Bone marrow does not collapse in patients with hypovolemia, and so in some patients this space may be easier to access than a vein. This route provides rapid dispersion of fluids through bone marrow and medullary venous channels, and thus essentially has the same effect as IV administration. The same dosage calculations used for IV resuscitation and replacement can be used when fluids are given by the IO route. In addition, any medication that is given intravenously is safe to administer intraosseously. Because IO catheters can be difficult to maintain, they are best used for the short term. Once the patient has been resuscitated, an IV catheter should be placed.

TECHNICIAN NOTE

Dosage calculations used for intravenous (IV) resuscitation and replacement can also be used when fluids are administered through an intraosseous (IO) catheter.

Various sites, including the tibial tuberosity, the trochanteric fossa of the femur, the wing of the ilium, and the greater tubercle of the humerus, can be used for IO catheterization. To prevent pain during needle placement, the periosteum should be anesthetized by using a 1% lidocaine solution before catheterization is attempted. Many different types of needles can be used, depending on the patient and the availability of supplies. Options include bone marrow needles, spinal needles, commercial IO needles, and hypodermic needles. The insertion site should be aseptically clipped and prepared to avoid introducing pathogens and causing osteomyelitis. Aspiration of bone marrow using radiography can help confirm proper placement. Potential complications of IO catheter placement include infection at the insertion site and development of osteomyelitis.

Enteral Route. Enteral fluids are often used in large animal patients, particularly equids. Enteral fluids may be indicated for various reasons, such as when treating a large colon impaction; they may be used simultaneously with IV fluids and may include osmotic agents. Enteral fluids can also be a cost-effective way to maintain hydration status, because they are delivered via a nasogastric tube and do not require the use of costly fluids, fluid lines, and catheters. Enteral fluids may be administered at scheduled intervals (usually every 2–4 hours), or they can be given as a constant rate infusion. Deciding between these two methods of administration may ultimately depend on the intensive care unit (ICU) staff and how well the patient tolerates nasogastric intubation. When enteral fluids are delivered as a constant rate infusion, the nasogastric tube should be placed and secured to the halter with tape. A "Christmas tree" adaptor is then placed on the end of the nasogastric tube, and a carboy containing fluids and an administration set are then connected to the adaptor. The carboy is raised above the patient and fluid is administered by gravity. For the average adult 500-kg horse, a rate of 1 L/hour should be used for maintenance. When enteral fluids are being administered at scheduled intervals, boluses no greater than 8 L at a time should be given to the average adult 500-kg horse.

Enteral fluids can also be used for at-home management of small animal patients with nasogastric tubes (in hospital), or with esophagostomy or gastrostomy feeding tubes in place at home. For some patients (e.g., those with chronic kidney disease), this may be preferable and better tolerated compared with intermittent SC fluid administration. Giving enteral water provides a more physiologic source of hydration and does not carry the sodium burden of isotonic crystalloids (which may not be well tolerated in kidney disease or heart disease).

TECHNICIAN NOTE

Enteral fluids are not to be used for patients in shock—they should be used only in patients with a normally functioning gastrointestinal (GI) tract.

Fluid Additives

Potassium

Patients may present with hypokalemia or may develop hypokalemia in the hospital for a variety of reasons. Hypokalemia can be seen with GI losses, such as vomiting or diarrhea, and with urinary losses. Specific causes include chronic renal failure, postobstructive diuresis, dialysis, hyperadrenocorticism (Cushing disease), diabetic ketoacidosis, and primary hyperaldosteronism. Some medications, such as loop diuretics, thiazide diuretics, amphotericin B, and penicillin, can also cause hypokalemia.

Signs of hypokalemia vary, depending on the severity of the condition. Some patients have no clinical signs. Patients with serum potassium values lower than 3.0 mEq/L may exhibit certain signs, such as polyuria/polydipsia (PU/PD), decreased ability to concentrate urine, and muscle weakness. Patients may exhibit cardiovascular signs, including the development of ventricular and supraventricular arrhythmias. When serum potassium is less than 2.0 mEq/L, patients are at risk for severe muscle weakness and even respiratory paralysis.

Patients with hypokalemia should be placed on IV potassium supplementation. This can be done by using potassium chloride (KCl; 2 mEq/mL) or potassium phosphates (K+; 4.4 mEq/mL). To avoid adverse cardiac effects, potassium should not be administered intravenously at a rate faster than 0.5 mEq/kg per hour (potassium maximum). See Table 24.4 for guidelines regarding potassium supplementation.

TABLE 24.4	Guidelines for Routine Intravenous Supplementation of Potassium in Dogs and Cats			
Patient Serum K Levels (mEq/L)	Suggested K Supplementation (mEq/L)	Resulting K Concentration (mEq/mL)	Equivalent K CRI Rate (mEq/kg per hour)	
3.5–5	20	0.02	0.1	
3–3.4	30	0.03	0.2	
2.5–2.9	40	0.04	0.3	
2–2.4	60	0.06	0.4	
<2	80	0.08	0.5	

TECHNICIAN NOTE

To avoid adverse cardiac effects, potassium should not be administered intravenously at a rate faster than 0.5 mEq/kg per hour (potassium maximum).

Dextrose

Patients can present with hypoglycemia or can become hypoglycemic for a variety of reasons, including neonatal or juvenile hypoglycemia, starvation, hepatic insufficiency, hypoadrenocorticism (Addison disease), insulin overdose, sepsis, insulinoma, non–islet cell tumors, pregnancy, and "hunting dog hypoglycemia." Hypoglycemia should be suspected and blood glucose checked in patients that show clinical signs, such as weakness, seizures, ataxia, collapse, stupor, or muscle tremors. Once a patient is found to be hypoglycemic, treatment should be started immediately. Dextrose (50% or 0.5 g/mL) can be administered slowly at a dose of 0.5 to 1 mL/kg intravenously. It is recommended that dextrose be diluted 1:1 (to a 25% solution) to avoid phlebitis, which may occur with administration of 50% dextrose. If hypoglycemia does not resolve, an additional bolus can be given. The patient should then be placed on IV fluids containing dextrose. If indicated, a balanced electrolyte solution can be used, and dextrose can be added to make a concentration of 2.5% to 10%. To avoid osmotic injury and phlebitis, hypertonic solutions (those containing greater than 5% dextrose) should be administered only via a central vein. To make a dextrose-containing solution, the desired concentration (%) is multiplied by the desired volume (in milliliters) and divided by stock concentration of dextrose (typically 50%). Therefore to create a 2.5% solution in 1 L of fluid, 50 mL (2.5% × 1000 mL ÷ 50% = 50 mL) is added.

Sodium Bicarbonate

Sodium bicarbonate can be administered for the treatment of metabolic acidosis; however, its use is controversial and depends largely on the nature and severity of the disturbance. In most cases of metabolic acidosis (e.g., lactic acidosis, diabetic ketoacidosis, renal failure), direct treatment of the underlying cause is recommended, because sodium bicarbonate provides only temporary improvement in acid-base balance. For example, in patients with diabetic ketoacidosis, resolution of acidosis is often achieved with fluid and insulin therapy alone. Poor tissue perfusion and lactic acidosis in animals in shock should be addressed with volume restoration and shock reversal, not with administration of sodium bicarbonate. Furthermore, administration of sodium bicarbonate has not been shown to result in improved outcomes in patients with metabolic acidosis.

• BOX 24.4 Calculations for Sodium Bicarbonate Deficit and Isotonic Sodium Bicarbonate

Total Sodium Bicarbonate Deficit

$$\text{Base deficit} \times 0.3 \times \text{Body weight (kg)} = \text{Deficit in mEq}$$

In cases of acute metabolic acidosis, administer one-third of the calculated dose rapidly (over 5–10 minutes), with the rest administered over the next 12 to 24 hours.

Preparing Isotonic Sodium Bicarbonate (typically used in foals and calves)

Remove 150 mL of water from a 1-L bag of sterile water and then add 150 mL 8.4% (1 mEq/mL) sodium bicarbonate ($NaHCO_3$), or remove 250 mL of water from a 1-L bag of sterile water and then add 250 mL 5% (0.595 mEq/mL) $NaHCO_3$. Both dilutions will result in a final concentration of 150 mEq/L.

Because severe acidemia (pH <7.1) can lead to life-threatening cardiovascular complications, sodium bicarbonate should be used only in extreme cases in which the pH is less than 7.1 and when other directed therapy is not available or has not served to successfully restore acid-base balance. Isotonic sodium bicarbonate is most often used to treat metabolic acidosis with bicarbonate losses in large animals with severe diarrhea. If sodium bicarbonate therapy is indicated, the dosage can be calculated as shown in Box 24.4.

TECHNICIAN NOTE

Sodium bicarbonate should be used only in extreme cases in which the pH is less than 7.1 and directed therapy is unavailable or has not served to restore acid-base balance.

Sodium bicarbonate can also be administered to patients with hyperkalemia, because it helps promote a shift of potassium ions (K^+) into cells in exchange for hydrogen ions (H^+). Because of the potential for adverse effects, its use is reserved for cases with severe hyperkalemia (K^+ >10 mEq/L). For this purpose, sodium bicarbonate can be administered intravenously at a dose of 1 to 2 mEq/kg over 5 to 10 minutes.

Finally, oral sodium bicarbonate supplementation may be indicated for large animal patients with chronic metabolic acidosis (e.g., those with diarrhea).

Several potential adverse effects are associated with sodium bicarbonate administration. It is extremely important to note that sodium bicarbonate should never be administered to a patient with respiratory acidosis (hypoventilation or high partial pressure of carbon dioxide [$PaCO_2$]), because sodium bicarbonate is rapidly converted to carbon dioxide (CO_2) and so could worsen this condition. Administration of sodium bicarbonate can also result in paradoxical central nervous system (CNS) acidosis. This means that acidosis in the brain actually worsens despite improvement in peripheral acid-base balance. Finally, administration of oral sodium bicarbonate may cause gum ulcers in some patients. Therefore care should always be taken to wipe excess sodium bicarbonate from around the mouth.

Monitoring Fluid Therapy

Resuscitation Phase

As was previously stated, the primary goal of the resuscitation phase is to restore vascular volume and tissue perfusion. Monitoring fluid therapy during this phase is geared toward assessing cardiovascular stability, blood volume, and perfusion parameters (including HR, pulse quality, CRT, mucous membrane color, warmth of distal extremities, and mentation). (See Chapter 25, "Emergency and Critical Care Nursing," for a more detailed description of these parameters.)

Tissue perfusion and cardiovascular stability can also be monitored by measuring arterial blood pressure. Complete discussion of blood pressure monitoring is beyond the scope of this chapter, but it is important to note that it is a relatively insensitive marker for blood flow. The compensatory response is aimed at sustaining blood pressure, even though perfusion to some tissues may be impaired. In other words, low blood pressure is bad, but normal blood pressure does not mean that everything is normal. When fluid therapy is monitored and resuscitation is gauged, it is very important to assess perfusion parameters and other data in conjunction with blood pressure. Under most circumstances, efforts should be made to normalize and maintain systolic blood pressure between 110 and 140 mm Hg (or mean blood pressure between 80 and 100 mm Hg).

One potential exception to using these blood pressure guidelines is fluid therapy in the face of ongoing hemorrhage (e.g., hemoabdomen) when aggressive fluid therapy may result in exacerbation of bleeding and worsening of the clinical condition. With that in mind, targeting a lower "minimally acceptable" blood pressure (90–100 mm Hg systolic, 60–70 mm Hg mean) as part of a more restrictive approach to fluid resuscitation may be beneficial in these cases.

TECHNICIAN NOTE

When fluid therapy is monitored and resuscitation is gauged, it is very important to assess perfusion parameters and other data in conjunction with blood pressure.

Measurement of blood lactate levels has also received a great deal of attention as a potential guide to fluid therapy. Lactate, a byproduct of anerobic metabolism, accumulates when tissues do not receive enough oxygen. Successful fluid resuscitation should result in significant reduction in elevated lactate levels (normal blood levels should be <2 mmol/L). However, some causes of hyperlactemia are unrelated to perfusion, as other factors can affect lactate production and clearance; this can sometimes limit the usefulness of blood lactate levels as a guide to fluid therapy.

Replacement Phase

As was previously mentioned, assessment of hydration status is an important component of determining replacement fluid rates. As such, frequent monitoring of hydration is an equally important component of determining when the replacement phase should end. What follows is a brief overview of the key components of assessment of hydration and response to replacement fluid therapy. (For a complete review of hydration assessment, refer to Chapter 25.)

Hydration status and response to replacement fluid therapy can be monitored in various ways, including aspects of physical exam and laboratory data (Box 24.5). Unfortunately, numerous other factors can potentially affect these parameters and can obscure the assessment of dehydration or rehydration. For example, skin turgor tends to be less accurate in obese or geriatric patients. Panting dogs typically have dry mucous membranes regardless of hydration status, and kidney disease will impair the usefulness of specific gravity of urine. For small animal patients,

---

• BOX 24.5   Hydration Parameters

Physical examination
    Skin turgor
    Tackiness of mucous membranes
    Sunken eyes
    Cardiovascular compromise
    Body weight
Laboratory data
    Packed cell volume/total protein (PCV/TP)
    Urine output
    Urine specific gravity
    Hypernatremia (free water loss)

---

frequent monitoring of body weight can be an effective way to track changes in hydration and body water. Generally, a change in body water is the major reason for a short-term change in body weight (over the course of 1 day or less). A notable exception would be the occurrence of a surgical procedure, such as limb amputation or splenectomy. In patients that have not had a short-term change in body weight related to surgery, a change in body weight of 1 kg signifies a change in body water content of 1 L. Weighing a patient at least one or two times per day or more often in some cases can be helpful in determining whether a fluid deficit has been corrected or if the patient is becoming overhydrated. For example, a 20-kg dog believed to be 5% dehydrated (which corresponds to a 1-L fluid deficit) should weigh 21 kg after correction of the deficit. Changes in body weight are not as reliable in large animal patients, because GI ingesta and fluid retention could also have a significant impact on weight, resulting in a heavier reliance on parameters such as physical exam and packed cell volume (PCV) and total protein (TP).

TECHNICIAN NOTE

For small animal patients, frequent monitoring of body weight can be an effective way to track changes in hydration and body water. This is less reliable in large animal species.

Complications of Fluid Therapy

Although fluid therapy is often a cornerstone of treatment, it is important to realize that it does not come without complications, such as the risk of administering an excessive quantity of fluids, causing volume overload and/or a positive fluid balance. Most patients with normal heart and kidney functions can tolerate a large volume of fluids, but compromised patients, especially cats and neonates, are at greater risk. One of the most significant concerns is the development of pulmonary edema from left-sided volume overload of the heart. Because of this, respiratory rate (RR) and pattern should be closely monitored in patients receiving fluids. If the RR increases by greater than 20%, if respiratory effort increases, or if the patient develops pulmonary crackles, fluids should be discontinued and the veterinarian contacted immediately. Patients with volume overload can also develop cavitary effusion (effusions into a body cavity) or peripheral edema (Fig. 24.8). The development of positive fluid balance has been associated with worse outcomes in both human and veterinary patients, particularly in the ICU setting. As such, there should be caution regarding the total volume of fluid administered, particularly if signs of positive fluid balance have developed.

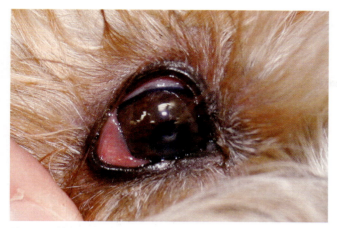

• **Fig. 24.8** Note the swollen, edematous conjunctiva associated with overhydration. Conjunctival edema is called *chemosis*.

Certain types of fluids can result in coagulation abnormalities. Synthetic colloids, such as hetastarch, have been implicated in causing prolonged coagulation times and impaired platelet function. This effect may be reduced with some synthetic colloids (e.g., VetStarch; Abbott Inc., Abbot Park, IL) but may still be a concern. In addition, administration of large volumes of fluid, especially in the face of major blood loss, can result in a dilution coagulopathy. This involves a decrease in coagulation factors and platelets when blood is replaced by fluids that do not contain these components. As previously mentioned, synthetic colloids have also been associated with acute kidney injury in humans.

Although fluid therapy is often used to treat electrolyte and acid-base disturbances, it can also be responsible for causing these problems. For instance, patients can develop major changes in both sodium and chloride levels in blood, depending on the type of fluid given; significant fluid-induced diuresis can be associated with the development of hypokalemia unless the patient is supplemented appropriately; and certain fluid types (e.g., 0.9% NaCl) are acidifying, whereas some others (e.g., Plasmalyte, LRS) are alkalinizing.

Transfusion Medicine

Indications for Blood and Plasma Transfusion

Indications for blood transfusion include acute hemorrhage, chronic anemia, and hemolytic anemia. Causes of acute hemorrhage include trauma, surgical bleeding, coagulopathy, and intracavitary bleeding. Physical examination findings, such as pale mucous membranes, delayed CRT, tachycardia, tachypnea, and lethargy and/or dull mentation, may indicate a need for blood transfusion, especially when blood loss is estimated to be greater than 30% of blood volume. Acute blood loss can result in hypovolemic shock, in addition to loss of red blood cell (RBC) mass, leading to the assessment parameters that may include cold extremities, hypotension, and increased blood lactate concentrations. Additional findings in horses include sweating and colic. It is important to remember that PCV can still be within normal reference ranges during severe, acute hemorrhage, but PCV and TP will decrease as body fluid redistributes over the first 12 hours after hemorrhage (or more rapidly if IV fluid resuscitation is administered). TP will decrease before PCV decreases substantially, especially in horses and dogs, because splenic contraction sustains the

PCV. Blood transfusion is likely necessary if PCV drops to less than 20% to 25% during an acute bleeding episode, although the decision should still be based on the full clinical picture. In cases of acute hemorrhage, whole blood or packed red blood cells (PRBCs) and plasma, often in conjunction with crystalloids or colloids, are used to restore oxygen-carrying capacity and circulating volume.

> **TECHNICIAN NOTE**
>
> Blood transfusion is likely to be necessary if **packed cell volume** (PCV) drops to less than 20% to 25% during an acute bleeding episode, although the decision should be based on the full clinical picture.

In patients with chronic or hemolytic anemia, PCV and TP can be more useful indicators of the need for blood transfusion. No universally accepted threshold has been established in veterinary medicine regarding an absolute transfusion trigger. For example, in more chronic cases, the tolerance of anemia may allow patients to have minimal clinical signs down to a PCV of less than 12% to 15%. However, once the previously mentioned physical examination findings have developed (tachycardia, tachypnea, and lethargy), the patient likely needs a blood transfusion. Patients with PCV above this level may need a transfusion if they have a concurrent disease, such as a respiratory condition or sepsis. Because animals with hemolytic or chronic anemia are normovolemic, PRBCs are indicated for transfusion, although whole blood may also be used. For both acute and chronic anemia, blood transfusion will at least temporarily boost the oxygen-carrying capacity of blood, but it is also essential to diagnose and treat the underlying cause of the anemia.

Platelet transfusions are indicated for patients with severe thrombocytopenia and life-threatening hemorrhage and/or a need for surgical intervention. In the presence of life-threatening bleeding or necessary surgical procedure, a platelet count of 10,000/μL in a cat or 20,000/μL in a dog may indicate the need for a platelet transfusion. However, platelet transfusions may be less beneficial for patients with immune-mediated thrombocytopenia, because transfused platelets will be rapidly destroyed and so are reserved for emergency treatment in extreme circumstances.

Plasma transfusions are indicated for treatment of coagulopathy, hypoalbuminemia, and failure of passive transfer (FPT) of immunity (in large-animal neonates). Fresh plasma and fresh frozen plasma contain clotting factors (I, II, V, VII, VIII, IX, X, XI, XII), anticoagulant proteins (antithrombin, protein C, protein S), and immunoglobulins. Plasma can also be used for colloid support, particularly when TP is less than 4.0 g/dL or albumin is less than 2.0 g/dL. However, a very large volume of plasma is needed to significantly raise blood albumin levels. In large-animal neonates (e.g., foals, crias, and calves) with FPT of immunity (from the colostrum), hyperimmune plasma is used to increase the serum immunoglobulin concentration. Immunoglobulin G (IgG) concentration less than 800 mg/dL in foals or TP concentration less than 5.5 g/dL in calves is an indication for plasma transfusion if the animal is older than 12 hours of age as they are no longer able to absorb colostrum. Box 24.6 lists commercial sources of fresh frozen equine plasma. In animals with von Willebrand disease, cryoprecipitate may be used, because it contains more concentrated von Willebrand factor (in addition to factor VIII, fibrinogen, factor XIII, and fibronectin). Cryoprecipitate typically would be administered to a patient with known deficiency needing to

TABLE 24.5　**Blood Donor Recommendations**

Donor Species	Minimum Weight	Minimum PCV	TP
Canine	25 kg	45%	Within reference range
Feline	5 kg	35%	Within reference range
Equine	450 kg	35%	≥6.0 g/dL

PCV, Packed cell volume; *TP*, total protein.

undergo a surgical procedure or experiencing life-threatening bleeding associated with primary hemostatic dysfunction.

TECHNICIAN NOTE

Plasma transfusions are indicated for treatment of coagulopathy, hypoalbuminemia, and failure of passive transfer (FPT) of immunity (in large-animal neonates).

Blood Donors

Healthy animals with a good temperament and adequate PCV and body weight may be selected as blood donors. Recommended body weight, PCV, and TP for blood donors are shown in Table 24.5. Some referral hospitals will choose to use in-house donors; others may collect and bank blood from "volunteer" donors or client-owned animals. Blood products are also commercially available and can be stored on site. All donors should be current on vaccinations and free of parasites at the time of donation. A thorough physical examination, complete blood count, and chemistry profile should be performed on animals being considered as blood donors.

Canine and feline donors should be between 1 and 7 years of age and should have good jugular vein access. Feline donors should be housed indoors only. Donor animals should not be on medication, except those used for prevention of heartworms, fleas, or ticks, and should be tested for blood-borne infectious diseases. Canine donors should test negative for heartworm antigen, babesiosis, leishmaniasis, ehrlichiosis, anaplasmosis, neorickettsiosis, and brucellosis. Feline blood donors should test negative for feline leukemia virus, feline immunodeficiency virus, hemoplasmosis, and bartonellosis. Equine donors should test negative for equine infectious anemia and ideally also for equine viral arteritis, glanders, dourine, piroplasmosis, brucellosis, equine hepacivirus, equine parvovirus, and equine pergivirus. They should also be vaccinated for rhinopneumonitis, tetanus, Eastern and Western encephalitis, rabies, and West Nile virus. Additional testing may be needed, depending on the travel or exposure history of the donor animal. PCV should be determined for all donor animals before each blood collection.

Pretransfusion Testing

Blood Typing

Blood typing should be performed in animals to be used as blood donors, and any stored blood products should be clearly labeled with donor information and blood type. Horses have 8 major blood systems and 34 blood factors within 7 of these systems. As a result of the vast numbers of blood systems and factors, no true "universal" equine blood type is known. The ideal donor horse is Aa and Qa negative, because these blood types appear to be the most immunogenic and have been commonly associated with

neonatal isoerythrolysis. A horse of the same breed is more likely to have a similar blood type, so choosing a donor of the same breed may increase the likelihood of having a compatible donor. It would be preferable to determine the blood type of the horse that will receive the transfusion so that the best blood match can be selected. However, blood must be sent to an equine blood typing laboratory, so this is not a practical method of selecting a donor horse in an emergency. A rapid equine blood typing method identifies Ca antigens (Alvedia, Limonest, France); however, there is not a stallside test for Aa or Qa antigens. Cattle have greater than 70 recognized blood group factors, but factor J is the only one for which naturally occurring antibodies have been identified. Donor cattle should be negative for factor J.

Numerous dog erythrocyte antigens (DEAs) have been identified for canine patients. Among these, DEA 1.1, 1.2, and 7 have been shown to be the most immunogenic and therefore the most important in canine transfusion medicine. The presence of circulating anti-DEA 1.1 antibody in a recipient will cause **agglutination** and **hemolysis** if DEA 1.1–positive blood is transfused. Rapid blood typing cards (Fig. 24.9A) or immune chromatographic test kits (see Fig. 24.9B) can be used to detect DEA 1.1.

Some testing laboratories and blood banks can provide extensive canine blood typing for several other erythrocyte antigens. Currently, typing is available for DEA 1.1, 1.2, 3, 4, 5, and 7. When blood banks test for all these antigens, the universal donor is one that is positive for only the DEA 4 antigen (because this antigen occurs in 98% of dogs) and negative for all other DEAs. Ideally, only these dogs would be included in the blood donor program; however, only 15% of the population falls under this category. To broaden the donor pool, dogs that are positive for DEA 1.1 may be used as donors for DEA 1.1–positive recipients.

In any case, dogs do not typically have naturally occurring antibodies; therefore a major transfusion reaction is less likely after a first transfusion of RBCs. However, once exposed to a foreign DEA, a canine patient will become sensitized. It is recommended that blood types of all donors and recipients be identified before transfusion (for at least DEA 1.1) so that type-specific blood can be administered.

TECHNICIAN NOTE

Among the dog erythrocyte antigens (DEAs), DEA 1.1, 1.2, and 7 have been shown to be the most immunogenic and therefore the most important in canine transfusion medicine.

The blood group system in cats consists of blood types A, B, and AB. A is the most common blood type, especially for Domestic Shorthair and Domestic Longhair breeds (which represent 95%–99% of cats in the United States). Type B is far less common

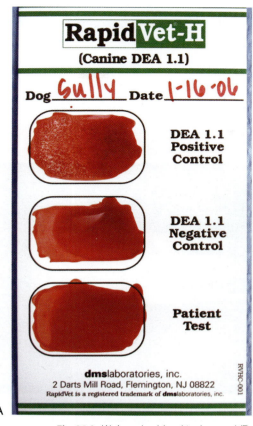
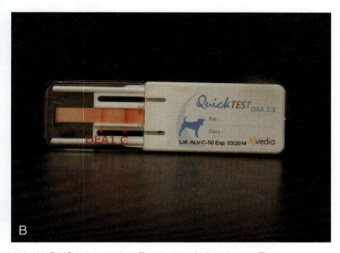

• **Fig. 24.9** (A) A canine blood typing card (Rapid Vet-H; DMS Laboratories, Flemington, NJ) is shown. The patient sample does not agglutinate, indicating that the pet is dog erythrocyte antigen (DEA) 1.1 negative. (B) An immune chromatographic method of blood typing (Quick Test; Alvedia, Lyon, France) is also demonstrated. Binding of red cells to antibody on the strip forms a red line and indicates blood type.

but is seen with greater frequency in some breeds (e.g., 40%–50% of Devon Rex and British Shorthair; 10%–20% of Abyssinian, Persian, Himalayan, and Sphinx). Feline blood typing cards are commercially available and involve a standard agglutination reaction with antitype antibodies (Fig. 24.10A) or immune chromatographic test kits (see Fig. 24.10B).

Unlike dogs, cats have naturally occurring circulating alloantibodies (antibodies to antigens of another cat) to the blood type they do not have. In other words, type B cats have high levels of anti–A antibodies, so transfusion of type A blood into a type B cat could result in a severe, potentially fatal hemolytic transfusion reaction. If type B blood is transfused into a type A cat, the lifespan of the transfused cells will be significantly reduced but, overall, the transfusion reaction will not be nearly as severe (anti–B antibodies are weaker by comparison). Type AB cats can receive blood from a donor with any blood type. Because of the risk for transfusion reaction, no universal donor is known, and blood typing should be performed in all cats before transfusion. If typing cards are not available, a **cross match** (see the section "Cross Matching") can be used to help determine whether patients are compatible.

In addition to A and B antigens, evidence indicates the presence of another erythrocyte antigen that can result in acute hemolytic reaction. Circulating alloantibodies against this antigen (called *Mik antigen*) have been detected. Currently, no way to directly test for the presence of Mik antigen is known, so a cross match is advisable even if the cat has not been previously transfused. There

is some evidence that suggests no difference in the outcome or lifespan of transfused RBCs in cats, whether cross matching is performed or not. As such, the strength of the recommendation to perform blood typing in all cats has diminished.

Antibody Screen

Donor animals should ideally be screened yearly for alloantibodies. Antibody screens are most often performed in mares that may be at risk of having anti-RBC antibodies to the foal's blood type (leading to neonatal isoerythrolysis if the foal ingests colostrum).

In horses and dogs, an initial emergency transfusion may be given without pretesting, because the likelihood of naturally occurring RBC antibodies is low. It is important to check for a history of previous transfusion or foaling (horses), because the likelihood of sensitization to RBC antigens is high in these cases. Development of RBC antibodies occurs 3 to 7 days after transfusion, so it is imperative that cross matching be performed before any subsequent transfusions.

Cross Matching

Cross matching is a readily available diagnostic procedure that can be performed on site. Major cross matching detects agglutination reactions between the donor's RBCs and the recipient's plasma. Minor cross-matching detects agglutination reactions between the donor's plasma and the recipient's RBCs. Equine cross matching results may be difficult to interpret because of normal rouleaux

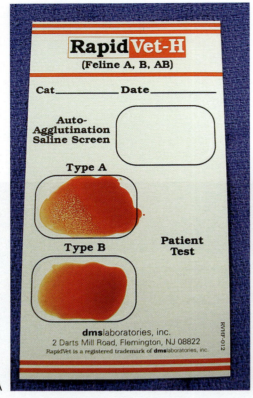

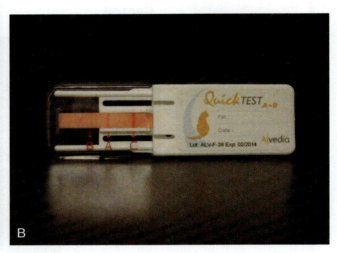

• **Fig. 24.10** (A) A feline blood typing card (Rapid Vet-H; DMS Laboratories, Flemington, NJ) is shown. Note the agglutination that indicates this cat is blood type A. (B) An immune chromatographic method of blood typing (Quick Test; Alvedia, Lyon, France) is also demonstrated. Binding of red blood cells to antibody on the strip forms a red line and indicates blood type.

formation (stacking) of equine RBCs; rouleaux should disperse when a small amount of saline is mixed with blood, whereas agglutination will not disperse. Cross matching results can also be difficult to interpret in animals with immune-mediated hemolytic anemia because of the autoagglutination of patient RBCs. The exact procedure for performing cross-matching is described in numerous texts.

TECHNICIAN NOTE

Major cross matching detects agglutination reactions between the donor's red blood cells (RBCs) and the recipient's plasma. Minor cross matching detects agglutination reactions between the donor's plasma and the recipient's RBCs.

Routine cross matching evaluates agglutination reactions but does not test for hemolytic reactions. Rabbit serum can be used for hemolytic testing, but this is not routinely performed as part of cross matching. Cross matching also does not necessarily predict the lifespan of the transfused RBCs or the development of antibodies to transfused RBCs, and transfusion reactions have been reported even when cross matching shows compatibility. However, the risk of transfusion reaction is significantly increased if a patient is given incompatible blood.

Blood Collection

The recommended maximum blood donation for dogs is 15% to 20% of blood volume or approximately 13 to 17 mL/kg.

Commercially available blood bags have a standard unit volume of 450 mL, so donor animals should be at least 25 kg if they are to donate 1 unit of blood. Commercially available 450-mL collection bags have a 16-gauge needle attached to the collection line. The donor is usually restrained in lateral recumbency. After clipping and sterile preparation of the jugular area, the needle is inserted into the jugular vein. Specific step-by-step instructions for blood collection in dogs are provided in Procedure 24.1, and similar procedures can be found elsewhere for cats and horses.

The recommended maximum blood donation for cats is 11 to 15 mL/kg, and the standard blood volume collected is 50 to 70 mL. Cats usually need to be sedated or anesthetized for the blood collection procedure. Blood collection in cats is performed by using an 18- to 19-gauge needle or a butterfly catheter attached to a syringe or a collection bag containing anticoagulant. The ratio of anticoagulant solution to blood should be 1:7. Pediatric (75-mL) transfer packs are commercially available and are good options for storage of feline blood.

The recommended maximum blood donation for horses is 20% of blood volume or approximately 16 mL/kg body weight. Donor horses should be weighed and should have PCV and TP measured before blood collection. Ideally, PCV should be greater than 35%. Blood is collected from the jugular vein, and both jugular veins may be used if a large volume of blood is needed immediately (Fig. 24.11). Vacuum canisters may be used to speed the collection process, but glass bottles with vacuum are not recommended, because glass inactivates platelets and can damage RBCs. Commercially available 450-mL blood collection bags may be used in horses, as can 2-L and 4-L bags with sodium citrate anticoagulant.

PROCEDURE 24.1

Protocol for Canine Whole Blood Collection

1. Perform a predonation physical examination, including body weight measurement and blood chemistry.
2. Assess TPR.
3. Evaluate jugular vein quality and location.
4. Place the donor on the examination table in the lateral recumbent or sternal position. Make the animal as comfortable as possible.
5. Shave a 1-inch square area of skin over the jugular vein.
6. Perform a standard three-pass sterile prep on the phlebotomy site.
7. Place a collection bag on a gram scale and set the scale to zero.
8. Clamp the collection line 3 to 4 inches distal to the needle by using a plastic hemostat to avoid damage to the collection line.
9. Have an assistant apply pressure to the jugular vein at the thoracic inlet to allow for distention and clear identification of the vessel.
10. Remove the needle cap. Insert the needle, bevel side up, into the jugular vein.
11. Release the clamp from the collection line.
12. Collect 405 g to 480 g of whole blood, carefully rocking the blood bag back and forth to mix blood and anticoagulant (each time an additional 50–75 mL has been collected).
13. Have the assistant release pressure over the vein.
14. Clamp the collection line with plastic hemostats.
15. Apply a 4 × 4–inch gauze sponge against the phlebotomy site.
16. Remove and cap the needle while holding pressure on the phlebotomy site with the sponge.
17. Wrap the phlebotomy site with 4-inch–wide Vetrap. Gauze and wrap should be left in place for 30 minutes to avoid bruising or hematoma formation.
18. Apply a hemiclip to the collection line or heat seal the collection line at least 2 inches above the bag to imprint a unique identifying line number on the bag.
19. Carefully agitate the collection bag to thoroughly mix blood and anticoagulant.
20. Label the collection bag with donor identification, date, time, and amount collected.
21. Record the donation in the donor record, including the donor's weight and TPR, and the blood chemistry, PCV, and TP results. Make sure to note the vessel and patient position used and any problems encountered during the donation process.

PCV, Packed cell volume; *TP*, total protein; *TPR*, temperature, pulse, and respiration.
From Lucas RL, Lentz KD, Hale AS. Collection and preparation of blood products. *Clin Tech Small Anim Pract.* 2004;19:55.

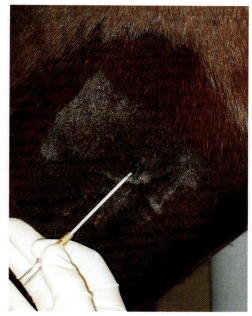

• **Fig. 24.11** A 14-gauge, 2-inch intravenous (IV) catheter is directed toward the horse's head to optimize blood flow during collection.

Collections can also be made by addition of anticoagulant to an empty sterile collection bag.

For all species, the maximum blood collection volume should be calculated based on *lean* body weight. During blood collection from any animal, the donor's HR, RR, mucous membrane color, and attitude should be monitored. Volume replacement with 20 to 40 mL/kg of an IV crystalloid fluid is recommended when 20% of the blood volume is collected. For smaller collection volumes that are tolerated with no clinical signs of hypovolemia, the donor does not require IV fluids. All donors should have access to fresh water and food after blood collection.

Several anticoagulant options may be used for blood collection. If blood will be transfused immediately, the anticoagulant sodium citrate is acceptable, but it will not support RBC metabolism during storage. If blood is going to be stored, citrate-phosphate-dextrose or citrate-phosphate-dextrose-adenine should be used. When shed or cavitary blood is collected for autologous

transfusion, it may be collected into a blood bag with a reduced amount of anticoagulant and then filtered before administration. Recommendations for the ratio of anticoagulant to free blood range from 1:7 to 1:20. Commercially available devices are also available to collect, wash, and filter free (shed or cavitary) blood (Cell Saver, Haemonetics, Boston, MA).

To achieve optimal RBC viability during storage, blood bags should be weighed to ensure adequate fill (blood to anticoagulant ratio). Sterility is very important during the collection and processing of blood for storage, because bacterial contamination and growth may cause a significant transfusion reaction. To minimize bacterial contamination, a closed collection system should be used and a tube sealer should be used to seal the collection tubing, which can be sealed in several increments for later testing or cross matching.

Whole blood and PRBCs are refrigerated at 33.8°F (1°C) to 42.8°F (6°C), ideally in a dedicated blood bank refrigerator with an alarm system that signals temperature breaches. Donor name, date of collection, blood type, and intended recipient (if known) should be clearly indicated on each blood bag. Blood from different species should be stored in separate refrigerators or at least on separate shelves, with clear labeling (Fig. 24.12).

Blood Products

Whole blood can be given directly or can be processed to make PRBCs and plasma. To separate the components, blood is centrifuged (at 39.2°F [4°C]) at a relative centrifugal force of 5000 × g for 5 minutes. Plasma is transferred to a satellite bag by using a plasma extractor, and an additive solution is mixed with the PRBCs. Plasma that is used within 8 hours of collection is labeled fresh plasma. Plasma that is placed in a freezer within 8 hours of collection and is less than 1 year old is fresh frozen plasma (FFP). FFP is stored at temperatures less than or equal to 0°F (–18°C). FFP should be used within 1 year of freezing to ensure optimal clotting factor activity, although there is evidence

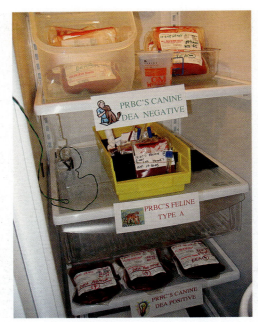

• **Fig. 24.12** This refrigerator has been converted into a dedicated blood bank refrigerator. A temperature monitor is provided, and the shelves are clearly labeled.

to suggest adequate activity beyond a year. If plasma is thawed but not needed, it can be refrozen within 1 hour of thawing and will maintain coagulation factor activity. Plasma that is frozen longer than 8 hours after collection or FFP that is older than 1 year of age is considered frozen plasma. Labile clotting factors (factors V and VIII) will be decreased in frozen plasma compared with FFP, although levels are still likely to be clinically efficacious.

Equine hyperimmune plasma is a US Department of Agriculture (USDA)–regulated product, and the shelf life for immunoglobulin efficacy is 2 to 3 years. Ideally, equine hyperimmune plasma ideally is collected by plasmapheresis to minimize any RBC contamination. In horses, up to 20 mL/kg of plasma can be collected every 30 days.

TECHNICIAN NOTE

Plasma that is used within 8 hours of collection is fresh plasma. Plasma that is placed in a freezer within 8 hours of collection and is less than 1 year old is considered to be fresh frozen plasma (FFP).

Canine PRBCs have been shown to have a shelf life of 20 days when stored in citrate-phosphate-dextrose-adenine-1 and 35 days when stored in an additive solution, such as Nutricel (ProNature Laboratories, Canterbury, NSW, Australia). In horses, washed RBCs are needed in cases of neonatal isoerythrolysis. The mare is the ideal blood donor for the foal; however, the mare's plasma contains antibodies directed against the foal's RBCs. A technique of centrifugation—removal of plasma supernatant and washing with saline three times—is used to prepare washed RBCs.

Other blood products that can be processed from whole blood include cryoprecipitate, cryo-poor plasma (or cryosupernatant), platelet-rich plasma, and platelet concentrate. Cryoprecipitate has a shelf life of 1 year. Platelet concentrate must be stored at room temperature and should be used within 5 to 7 days.

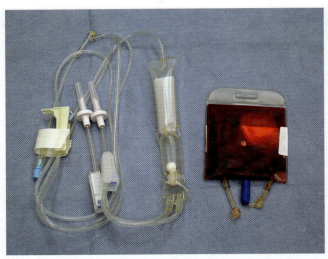

• **Fig. 24.13** Commercially available blood administration set with in-line filter to prevent inadvertent infusion of clots.

Blood Product Administration

Refrigerated blood can be transfused directly, because warming may cause deterioration of RBCs. In hypothermic patients or in those receiving large volumes of blood, it should be warmed at least to room temperature (71.6°F [22°C]) but no warmer than body temperature (98.6°F [37°C]). Blood products are administered using a commercial blood delivery set with an in-line filter (Fig. 24.13). Standard filters have a pore size of 170 to 260 µm, and the filter and administration set should be changed after administration of 2 to 4 units of blood. Blood should not be given concurrently with hypertonic or hypotonic solutions. It should also not be given with calcium-containing solutions (e.g., LRS), because the calcium in the fluids can overwhelm the citrate anticoagulant, resulting in activation of the coagulation cascade.

TECHNICIAN NOTE

Blood should not be given concurrently with hypertonic or hypotonic solutions and should not be given with calcium-containing solutions (e.g., lactated Ringer solution [LRS]).

Determination of Volume and Rate

Blood products should initially be given slowly so that the animal can be monitored closely for signs of transfusion reaction, and the transfusion can be stopped if needed. Approximately 0.3 mL/kg is given over the first 20 to 30 minutes, after which the rate can then be increased if needed. The rate of transfusion will depend on the patient's volume status and can be as high as 20 to 40 mL/kg per hour if volume resuscitation is needed. It is not recommended to exceed 2 to 4 mL/kg per hour in patients with significant cardiac disease. The transfusion should be completed within 4 hours to prevent bacterial growth and ensure platelet functionality (in the case of fresh whole blood). In other words, blood products should be administered as quickly as needed but as slowly as the situation will allow.

The total volume of blood to be transfused can be calculated on the basis of estimated blood loss (for acute blood loss) or PCV (for chronic or normovolemic anemia). See Box 24.7 for specific guidelines and Case Presentation 24.4 for a clinical example. An estimate of the patient's blood volume is needed to determine the

• BOX 24.7   Calculation for Blood Transfusion Volume for Chronic or Normovolemic Anemia

$$\text{Blood transfusion volume (mL)} = \frac{\text{Wt (kg)} \times \text{Blood volume}\left(\frac{\text{mL}}{\text{kg}}\right) \times \left[\left(\text{Desired PCV} - \text{Actual PCV}\right)\right]}{\left[\text{Donor PCV}\right]}$$

PCV, *Packed cell volume.*

CASE PRESENTATION 24.4

Equine Blood Transfusion

History and Signalment
A 4-year-old Friesian mare (600 kg) was presented to the hospital with acute onset of lethargy and pale mucous membranes. No treatments had been administered before admission to the referral hospital.

Initial Examination
On presentation, the mare appeared lethargic and mildly anxious. The heart rate (HR) was 88 beats per minute (bpm; normal, 28–40 bpm), respiratory rate (RR) was 36 breaths per minute (normal, 8–18 breaths per minute), and temperature was 99.0°F (normal, 98.5–100.5°F). The mucous membranes were very pale and slightly tacky, and the extremities were cold. Basic blood work showed packed cell volume (PCV) of 18% (normal, 28%–40%), total protein (TP) of 5.5 g/dL (normal, 5.5–7.5 g/dL), and blood lactate of 15 mmol/L (normal, <2 mmol/L). Abdominal ultrasonography showed a large amount of free fluid and a large mass in the right side of the abdomen. Rectal examination confirmed the right abdominal mass (possible ovary), and pain was associated with palpation. An abdominocentesis was performed. The sample was red and had a PCV of 14% and TP of 5.8 g/dL (results similar to those on the peripheral blood sample taken on admission). Cytologic examination confirmed that it was consistent with peripheral blood, but there was no evidence of neoplasia or infection. Preliminary diagnosis was intra-abdominal hemorrhage and shock secondary to blood loss from the mass.

Fluid Therapy and Transfusion Plan
The mare was housed in the intensive care unit (ICU) and was started on lactated Ringer solution (LRS) at a rate of 10 mL/kg per hour. In the meantime, 8 L of whole blood was collected from a donor horse into citrated bags and transfused immediately.

On the basis of the signs of shock, blood loss was estimated to be at least 30%.

$$\text{Total blood volume} = 600\,\text{kg} \times 0.08 = 48\,\text{L}$$

$$30\% \text{ of } 48\,\text{L} = 14.4\,\text{L blood lost}$$

Four hours after transfusion, blood work was repeated. The mare's PCV was 12%, TP was 4.1 g/dL, lactate was 6.0 mmol/L, and HR remained high (80 bpm). Because the mare did not show adequate clinical improvement, a second transfusion was indicated. Two other donor horses were cross matched but were found to be incompatible on both major and minor matches. Because these horses did not match, the owner elected to bring in a related Friesian horse to obtain donor blood. An additional 8 L of whole blood was transfused over 2 hours. After the second transfusion, PCV increased to 14%, TP increased to 6.0 g/dL, lactate was <2 mmol/L, and HR decreased to 54 bpm.

transfusion volume (see earlier in this chapter). Once blood loss and blood volume have been estimated and PCV of the donor animal (or PCV of the stored blood) is known, the desired volume for transfusion can be calculated.

In general, the goal should be to replace 25% to 50% of the blood lost in acute hemorrhage and/or target an increase in PCV of approximately 10%, with the goal of reversing the clinical signs that prompted transfusion in the first place. A useful guideline in dogs is that 2 mL/kg of whole blood or 1 to 1.5 mL/kg of PRBCs will raise PCV by 1%.

> ### TECHNICIAN NOTE
> A useful guideline for red blood cell (RBC) transfusion in dogs is that 2 mL/kg of whole blood or 1 to 1.5 mL/kg of packed red blood cells (PRBCs) will raise packed cell volume (PCV) by 1%.

Before FFP is administered, the plasma should be thawed in a water bath at 86°F (30°C) to 98.6°F (37°C). Generally, the amount of plasma required to correct a coagulation abnormality is approximately 10 to 15 mL/kg in dogs and 5 to 8 mL/kg in cats. Although this can serve as a guideline, coagulation times (activated partial thromboplastin time [APTT] and prothrombin time [PT]) ideally would be assessed after the transfusion is completed to ensure the values have normalized.

In adult horses, plasma usually is given in 1-L increments "to effect" to treat coagulopathy. "To effect" means that treatment is continued until the desired effect is achieved. In neonatal foals with FPT of immunity, hyperimmune plasma is given at a dose of approximately 20 to 40 mL/kg. IgG concentration should be rechecked after transfusion of hyperimmune plasma in these patients.

Monitoring and Transfusion Reactions
The recipient's HR, temperature, RR, and attitude should be monitored every 15 minutes during the first hour of a transfusion, with particular attention given during the first 15 minutes. Transfusion reactions from acute allergic (type I) hypersensitivity can include erythema, urticaria, pruritus, or anaphylaxis. In horses, sweating and piloerection and muscle fasciculation may be components of an allergic reaction. In canine and feline patients, these reactions tend to be more severe when plasma-containing blood products are used. If an allergic reaction is suspected, the transfusion should be stopped immediately (if severe) or slowed (if mild). Most allergic reactions will resolve on their own; however, some will require administration of antihistamines (or, rarely, corticosteroids), and severe anaphylactic reactions may require administration of epinephrine (although the incidence of this appears to be very low).

Acute hemolytic transfusion reactions typically occur during or within hours of transfusion. This reaction occurs when there is incompatibility between donor and recipient blood, resulting in rapid destruction of transfused RBCs (e.g., when type A blood is administered to a type B cat). This process typically occurs when preexisting antibodies are present and is classified as cytotoxic (type II) hypersensitivity. Clinical signs include hemoglobinemia, hemoglobinuria, and progressive anemia or lack of increase in

PCV. In addition, the highly inflammatory nature of this reaction can lead to signs of systemic inflammatory response, disseminated intravascular coagulation, shock, cardiovascular collapse, and death. Severity of signs is directly related to the volume of transfused blood. When acute hemolytic transfusion reactions occur, the transfusion should be stopped immediately, and supportive care initiated.

Delayed hemolytic transfusion reactions can occur longer than 24 hours after transfusion and can result in RBC lysis. Hemolysis of donor blood may occur before transfusion as the result of improper handling. Improper storage, excessive warming of the blood, administration with hypertonic solution, and use of peristaltic pumps are examples of improper handling that can lead to RBC destruction.

Nonhemolytic immune reactions, such as fever, may also occur with blood or plasma transfusion and are the most common reactions seen in veterinary patients. Fever is thought to be caused by donor leukocytes and accumulation of pyrogenic cytokines over time. Therefore older units of blood products are more likely to cause this response. Decreasing the rate of infusion is typically all that is needed to treat nonhemolytic immune reactions. Another potential immunologic response is transfusion-related acute lung injury (TRALI). This reaction occurs when leukocyte antibodies from the donor interact with recipient leukocytes, triggering an inflammatory response and leading to the development of protein-rich edema fluid in the lungs. Clinical signs include an increase in RR and respiratory effort, development of pulmonary crackles and dyspnea, and fever. No direct therapy is available (diuretics are not beneficial); rather, intervention is largely supportive (supplemental oxygen or mechanical ventilation). Available evidence suggests that this rarely occurs in veterinary medicine.

Perhaps the most significant nonimmune acute reaction is transfusion-associated circulatory overload (TACO). This can occur with large or rapidly delivered volumes of blood products, especially in patients with normal blood volume (e.g., those with immune-mediated hemolytic anemia or chronic anemia). Cats and patients with cardiac disease are particularly at risk. Clinical signs typically are related to pulmonary congestion and include increased RR and effort, development of pulmonary crackles, and dyspnea. These signs can be very difficult to distinguish from TRALI, although the clinical circumstances may help (e.g., a large volume administered to a small patient would support TACO). If a patient develops TACO, the transfusion should be slowed or discontinued, supplemental oxygen provided, and possibly, a single dose of furosemide administered. Other potential complications of blood transfusion include transmission of infectious disease, bacterial contamination, citrate toxicity (leading to ionized hypocalcemia and hypomagnesemia), and hypothermia associated with high-volume transfusions.

In horses, the incidence of adverse reactions with plasma is 10%, and the incidence of adverse reactions with whole blood transfusion has been reported to be 16%. The incidence of transfusion reactions in dogs has been reported to be approximately 10% to 15%. In cats, the incidence of reactions to red cell transfusion has been reported to be approximately 5% to 10% when type-specific blood is given. No reports have described plasma transfusion in cats.

It is important to assess the response to transfusion. Physical examination, PCV, blood lactate, and oxygen extraction are among the parameters that should be monitored. It is important to remember that with acute or ongoing hemorrhage, PCV may not increase after transfusion. The primary goal of blood transfusion is to improve oxygen delivery to the tissues, so all of the information from physical examination and laboratory data should be considered before an additional transfusion is performed.

Recommended Readings

Bracker KE, Drelich S. Transfusion reactions. *Compend Emerg Med.* 2005;27.

Cooper ES, Guillaumin J, Her J, et al. *Small Animal Fluid Therapy.* Boston, MA: CABI; 2023.

Crabtree NE, Epstein KL. Current concepts in fluid therapy in horses. *Front Vet Sci.* 2021;29(8):658774.

Davis H, Jensen T, Johnson A, et al. 2013 AAHA/AAFP fluid therapy guidelines for dogs and cats. *J Am Anim Hosp Assoc.* 2013;49(3):149.

DiBartola SP. *Fluid, Electrolyte, and Acid-base Disorders in Small Animal Practice.* St. Louis, MO: Elsevier; 2011.

Fielding CL, Magdesian KG. *Equine Fluid Therapy.* Ames, IA: Wiley Blackwell; 2015.

Finfer S, Myburgh J, Bellomo R. Intravenous fluid therapy in critically ill adults. *Nephrology.* 2018;14:541.

Kuo KW, McMichael M. Small animal transfusion medicine. *Vet Clin North Am Small Anim Pract.* 2020;50(6):1203.

Lucas RL, Lentz KD, Hale AS. Collection and preparation of blood products. *Clin Tech Small Anim Pract.* 2004;19:55.

Mudge MC. Acute hemorrhage and blood transfusions in horses. *Vet Clin Equine.* 2014;30:427.

Muir WW, Ueyama Y, Noel-Morgan J, et al. A systematic review of the quality of IV fluid therapy in veterinary medicine. *Front Vet Sci.* 2017;4:127.

Odunayo A, Nash KJ, Davidow EB, et al. Association of Veterinary Hematology and Transfusion Medicine (AVHTM) transfusion reaction small animal consensus statement (TRACS). Part 3: Diagnosis and treatment. *J Vet Emerg Crit Care.* 2021;31(2):189.

Radcliffe RM, Bookbinder LC, Liu SY, et al. Collection and administration of blood products in horses: Transfusion indications, material, methods, complications, donor selection, and blood testing. *J Vet Emerg Crit Care.* 2022;32(S1):108–122.

Rudloff E, Hopper K. Crystalloid and colloid compositions and their impact. *Front Vet Sci.* 2021;8:639848. https://doi.org/10.3389/fvets.2021.639848.

Zaremba R, Brooks A, Thomovsky E. Transfusion medicine: an update on antigens, antibodies and serological testing in dogs and cats. *Top Companion Anim Med.* 2019;34:36.

Zarychanski R, Abou-Setta AM, Turgeon AF, et al. Association of hydroxyethyl starch administration with mortality and acute kidney injury in critically ill patients requiring volume resuscitation: a systematic review and meta-analysis. *JAMA.* 2013;309:678.

25

Emergency and Critical Care Nursing

ANDREA M. STEELE, DARCY ADIN, AND JARRED WILLIAMS

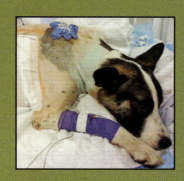

CHAPTER OUTLINE

LEARNING OBJECTIVES

When you have completed this chapter, you will be able to:

1. Pronounce, define, and spell all key terms in this chapter.
2. Triage a patient over the phone and upon arrival at the veterinary hospital.
3. Do the following regarding emergency and critical care assessment, initial diagnostics, and first aid:
   - Assess hydration and recognize hypovolemia in critical care patients.
   - Identify the diagnostic tests most commonly used in emergency and critical care settings.
   - Explain the principles of basic first aid.
   - Identify the ideal location for an emergency care station and/or resuscitation area and explain how to set up and stock a crash cart.
4. Compare and contrast the different types of shock, explain how each is treated, and identify and explain advanced emergency techniques most commonly performed on small animals.
5. Discuss disorders of the respiratory system seen in critically ill small animal patients.
6. Do the following regarding cardiopulmonary resuscitation:
   - List the common causes of cardiopulmonary arrest and explain the principles of cardiopulmonary resuscitation (CPR).
   - Describe the principles of basic and advanced life support in small animals and care of the postarrest patient.
7. Describe methods used to monitor critically ill patients and the principles of effective patient monitoring.
8. Identify key aspects of recumbent patient care.
9. List common small animal emergencies and discuss appropriate patient stabilization and treatment.
10. Do the following regarding canine and feline electrocardiography:
    - List the indications for and discuss the principles of electrocardiography.

- Explain the processes used to acquire, analyze, and interpret an electrocardiogram.
- Identify and explain the significance of common cardiac arrhythmias.

11. Describe initial management, assessment, diagnostic, and treatment procedures for common equine emergencies.
12. Describe initial management, assessment, diagnostic, and treatment procedures for common food animal emergencies.

KEY TERMS

Abdominocentesis
Acidosis
Arrhythmia
Asystole
Atrial fibrillation
Atrial premature complexes
Azotemia
Borborygmi
Capillary refill time
Cardiopulmonary resuscitation
Chest tube
Choke
Colic
Defibrillation
Disseminated intravascular coagulation
Down animals
Dystocia
Electrocardiography
Endometrial
Eructation
Fetatome
Fetotomy
Hyperventilation
Hypovolemia
Hypoxemia
Hypoxia
Ileus
Ischemia
Mastitis

Metritis
Multiple organ dysfunction syndrome (MODS)
Pneumothorax
Pulse oximeter
Regional nerve block
Reperfusion injury
Rumen tympany
Rumenostomy
Sepsis
Syncope
Systemic inflammatory response syndrome (SIRS)
Tachycardia
Tachypnea
Thoracocentesis
Thromboembolism
Tracheostomy
Tracheotomy
Traffic flow
Transfaunation
Triage
Tube cystostomy
Tympany
Urethal process
Urethrostomy
Urolithiasis
Uterine prolapse
Uterine torsion
Ventricular premature complexes
Ventricular tachycardia

Introduction

This chapter reviews many topics that a well-educated critical care veterinary technician or nurse must understand to provide exemplary care to critical patients, such as triage to determine whether a condition is truly an emergency warranting immediate treatment.

Basic trauma stabilization, patient assessment and monitoring, and care of the critical patient are important aspects of the critical care technician's responsibility. This chapter includes how to approach common emergencies in dogs, cats, horses, and food animals, as well as proper techniques for performing abdominocentesis, thoracocentesis, and placement of thoracostomy tubes. Use of electrocardiography (ECG) for detection and treatment of common arrhythmias is also discussed.

Emergency and Critical Care Nursing: Small Animal

Triage

Telephone Triage

Frequently, the first contact veterinary professionals have with owners whose animals are critically ill is via the telephone. Thus

it is crucially important that the veterinary technician can quickly differentiate patients with life-threatening injuries or illnesses from patients that can wait until their family veterinarian is available. An established system for asking pertinent questions can aid the technician in determining how to advise clients over the phone and ensure that important information is obtained.

Initially, the person answering the phone should obtain a name and a phone number so that the caller can be contacted if the call is disconnected. Next, the veterinary technician should determine whether the animal is in a life-threatening situation, such as respiratory compromise or severe bleeding. If such a situation is evident, the caller should be referred to the closest veterinary facility for immediate attention. Other situations that may require immediate care include toxin exposure, acute changes in neurologic status, and excessive heat or cold exposure.

It is important to remember that the person on the other end of the phone may be distraught and likely does not understand medical language. Speak in simple terms with nonleading questions but do not delay transport in obvious critical situations.

If allowed by the state and veterinary practice, first aid advice may be provided but should be limited to simple tasks, such as compressing a bleeding wound. Do not get into more involved tasks that could result in the owner been bitten and injured or those that may take too much time. In situations where the patient may be in pain, advise the owner to be cautious, because the animal may bite. Although it is important to provide and obtain time-sensitive information over the phone, transport of an animal that is critically ill, injured, or exposed to a toxin should not be delayed just to obtain routine historical information.

It is important to convey some financial information to the owner, and this is often done in the form of an emergency estimate. The value will vary by location, clinic, and possible condition being quoted; however, it is usually a basic fee that will include the emergency examination, allocate some money for quick diagnostics (such as point-of-care blood work) or stabilization (IV catheter, fluids, pain medications), and allow for an assessment to be made to provide the owner with a more detailed estimate once the doctor has made a plan. Many clinics would use a range of $500–$1000, depending on the situation. It is important that the owner is aware that there is an expectation of financial compensation so they are not caught unprepared.

In-Hospital Triage

When an emergent patient arrives, assessment and triage are most often performed by a veterinary technician or nurse. **Triage** is a process for sorting ill or injured animals into groups based on their need for or likely benefit from immediate medical treatment. It is a method of "prioritizing" patients and is used when several emergency cases are present at the same time. It is one of the most important aspects of emergency medicine and requires time and practice to become truly skilled.

Several triage scales have been suggested for veterinary emergencies and provide a simple framework for veterinary technicians and veterinarians to quickly assess, categorize, and initiate treatment of veterinary emergencies. Commonly used triage scales include the Animal Trauma Triage Score (Drobatz, 1994), and the Veterinary Triage List (Rhuys, 2012).

Initial triage should include a brief history, a quick physical examination, and targeted discussion with the owners about resuscitation status and initial treatment, if necessary.

TECHNICIAN NOTE

Animals assessed as unstable, potentially infectious, or disturbing to other clients because of the nature of their illness should be immediately taken to the clinic's treatment or holding area.

The initial task is to perform a primary survey, which will give brief information on the most important aspects of the patient's condition. The primary survey can be used to perform a brief, targeted examination based on the ABCs:

A: Airway/Attitude
B: Breathing, Bleeding
C: Cardiovascular, Circulation

The primary survey does not require the veterinary technician to measure respiratory rate (RR) or heart rate (HR) but only to assess whether it is abnormal (fast or slow) or normal. A more thorough, detailed examination and vital parameter assessment will be done in the treatment phase.

The primary survey can be further broken down into three *actions:* LOOK, LISTEN, and FEEL. All the ABCs can be assessed by using these actions, and many will occur simultaneously, beginning with the approach to the patient. In triage, every moment counts, and the veterinary technician must become skilled in acquiring many details at once. The primary survey begins as you *look* at the patient from a distance, then approach and finally touch the patient. Keep in mind that if a patient "fails" any of the assessments along the way, the primary survey must be aborted, and emergency treatment initiated.

From a distance, and without moving, *look* at the patient:

Airway: Is the patient breathing? If not, the primary survey is aborted, and emergency treatment is initiated. If the patient is breathing, *look* and assess the quality of the respiration. What is the respiratory pattern like? Is it regular or irregular? Shallow or very deep? Is there increased effort (abdominal component)? Is the rate normal or abnormal? *Listen* (still from a distance) to the patient's breathing. Can you hear respiratory sounds associated with inspiration or expiration?

Attitude: Is the patient bright, alert, and responsive; quiet, alert, and responsive; or nonresponsive? Is it interacting with its owner or other people/pets in the room?

Bleeding: Is there visible bleeding? Is the bleeding arterial (pulsating, copious)? Is it compressible?

PUT INTO PRACTICE

Proficiency with the LOOK, LISTEN, and FEEL technique may help you pick up on subtle nuances with your patients. Assessing your patient from a distance really allows the patient to let their guard down so you can really see them for how they are feeling in that moment.

From a distance, very important information has been quickly obtained. The technician may be able to determine how emergent the patient's condition is or whether further information may be required. If further information is necessary, the patient must be approached. Approaching the patient should evoke some response in a healthy animal. For example, a dog may wag its tail, sniff the air, stand up to greet you, or may move into a protective position in front of its owner (even very ill dogs may still do this). Cats in carriers can be difficult to observe, and you may need to ask the owner to move the cage to a more visible position. Observe the cat's ear position, pupil size, and its general demeanor. It may exhibit fear, interest, or disinterest, or may be nonresponsive. Again, these cues or responses are used in assessment of the triage scale.

After approaching the patient, LOOK, LISTEN, and FEEL can be used to finish the primary survey:

LOOK: Note the response of the patient to your approach, presence, and touch. Look at the mucous membranes and note the color (normal pink, cyanotic, injected pink, red, muddy, brown), check the **capillary refill time** (≤2 seconds is generally considered normal), and assess if the mucous membranes feel dry, tacky, or moist.

LISTEN: Quickly auscultate the heart, lungs, and trachea. Does the heart sound regular? Is there a murmur? Are there increased lung sounds? Auscultate the trachea to localize abnormal sounds (large airways versus small airways and parenchyma).

FEEL: Assess pulse rate (strong, weak, bounding, snappy), and, while auscultating, determine whether a pulse deficit is present. Do the mucous membranes and limbs feel warm, cool, or hot to the touch?

TECHNICIAN NOTE

Remember, at *any* point during the primary survey, the assessment can be discontinued and emergency treatment initiated as necessary.

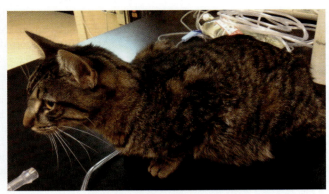

• **Fig. 25.1** A cat exhibiting classic orthopnea. Note the extended head and neck, and the "perched position" with the elbows abducted to avoid placing pressure on the sternum.

The remainder of the initial examination is completed once it is determined that the patient does not require emergency treatment or after stabilization has occurred. At this time, a more thorough secondary examination is conducted to identify other, non-life—threatening problems.

Respiratory System

As the patient is approached, its RR, effort, and pattern should be observed. An increased RR (**tachypnea**) may reflect decreased oxygen in blood (**hypoxemia**), thoracic trauma, or shock, or may be related to a nonrespiratory source, such as pain, stress, increased body temperature, traumatic brain injury, or metabolic **acidosis**. A decreased RR (*bradypnea*) is commonly associated with exposure to toxins or elevated intracranial pressure. The effort involved in breathing may provide clues as to the origin of the problem. For instance, inspiratory dyspnea results in long, slow inspirations with short exhalations and can indicate an extrathoracic airway obstruction, such as laryngeal paralysis, or swelling associated with an acute hypersensitivity reaction. In contrast, expiratory dyspnea with increased abdominal effort on expiration often develops if an intrathoracic airway obstruction, such as a mass compressing the airway or an inhaled foreign body, is present. The term *labored breathing* is often used to describe breathing that is prolonged and deep. Fast, short, and shallow breaths are the hallmark of a restrictive breathing pattern and reflect impaired ability to expand the lungs, as with rib fractures, pleural space disease (pleural effusion, **pneumothorax**, or tumors), or late in diseases of the lung tissue. *Orthopnea* is the term used to describe the condition of maintaining a specific posture to ease breathing. This occurs when dyspnea is so severe that the patient is "air hungry" and does everything it can to keep the airway open. Veterinary patients with orthopnea will extend the neck and stand or crouch with the elbows slightly away from the sides (Fig. 25.1). They become extremely distressed, combative, or aggressive when placed in any other position.

> ### TECHNICIAN NOTE
>
> If in doubt about a patient's respiratory status, *always* administer supplemental oxygen until further assessment can be completed.

The next part of assessing the respiratory system is the hands-on examination. First, the color of the mucous membranes is quickly checked. Any patient whose mucous membranes are blue, purple, or dusky needs supplemental oxygen immediately. Similarly, patients with brick red, brown, or injected (mottled pink, purple, or red) mucous membranes warrant a closer look because these colors could indicate dangerous conditions such as carbon monoxide (CO) poisoning, heatstroke, or **sepsis**, which require immediate intervention. Icteric (yellow) mucous membranes indicate high levels of bilirubin and may be because of liver dysfunction or red blood cell destruction. White mucous membranes could indicate a life-threatening condition such as internal hemorrhage and shock or a chronic anemia, and it is vitally important to differentiate between the conditions.

The final component of the respiratory section of the initial triage examination is thoracic auscultation. Decreased or dull lung sounds can indicate a diaphragmatic hernia, severe pulmonary contusions, pneumothorax (if decreased dorsally), or pleural effusion (if decreased ventrally). Increased or harsh bronchovesicular sounds or crackles can indicate pulmonary edema or contusions. **Borborygmi** in the thorax might indicate a diaphragmatic hernia but can also be referred from the abdomen. Any absence of lung sounds warrants further investigation in the treatment area.

Cardiovascular System

The initial triage examination of the cardiovascular system involves assessment of mentation (because decreased mentation can indicate shock), HR and rhythm, pulse quality, capillary refill time (CRT), extremity temperature, and mucous membrane color and temperature. HR and rhythm should be assessed by digital palpation of the pulse and thoracic auscultation with a stethoscope. An abnormally fast HR, called **tachycardia**, can indicate compensation for a shock state, **hypoxia**, pain, anemia, anxiety, or any combination thereof. An inappropriately slow HR, termed *bradycardia,* can indicate a life-threatening arrhythmia or, in animals with urethral obstruction, an extremely elevated potassium level. An important species difference to note is that cats in shock are often bradycardic. If arrhythmia is detected, electrocardiography (ECG) should be performed.

> ### TECHNICIAN NOTE
>
> Cats in shock often present with bradycardia rather than with tachycardia (as is seen in dogs).

Pulse quality can provide a great deal of information about the patient's cardiovascular state. *Pulse pressure* is the difference between systolic and diastolic pressures, and *pulse quality* is a description of how quickly pulse pressure changes and how long each pulse lasts. In a weak or thready pulse, the pulse pressure is lower than normal and typically occurs in conjunction with tachycardia. It can indicate hypotension, hypovolemia, or decompensated shock. A pulse that is "snappy" has a very large pulse pressure with an extremely rapid rise and fall. This type of pulse often occurs with anemia, patent ductus arteriosus, or severe aortic regurgitation. Generally, if you are unable to palpate the dorsal metatarsal arterial pulse in a dog, the mean arterial pressure (MAP) is likely less than 80 mmHg. If you cannot palpate a femoral pulse in a dog or a cat, the MAP is likely less than 60 mmHg. In either case, pulse palpation should never be a substitute for an accurate blood pressure measurement, although it can be used in the primary survey to determine if the patient is stable.

While assessing mucous membrane color, it is crucial to also check the CRT. A normal CRT is 1 to 2 seconds. Prolonged CRT may indicate the patient needs intravenous (IV) fluids or other interventions. A shortened CRT is most associated with the hyperdynamic stage of sepsis and may not reflect increased perfusion to the tissues.

Neurologic System

The focus of the initial triage neurologic examination is to determine whether evidence of traumatic brain injury (TBI) is present. Findings that support TBI include abrupt changes in mentation; changes in pupil size, symmetry, and responsiveness; altered gait or posture; altered proprioception; and evidence of trauma to the head. Any of these findings should trigger immediate intervention or a more thorough neurologic evaluation.

Mentation can be categorized as normal, dull/depressed, obtunded/delirious, stuporous, or comatose. A normal animal is alert and interactive with its environment. A dull or depressed animal is interactive with its environment but is not bright and eager to interact. An obtunded or delirious animal reacts appropriately to stimuli but at a lower level or slower pace than normal. A stuporous animal is completely disconnected from the environment and reacts only to noxious (painful or prolonged) stimuli. A comatose animal is completely disconnected from the environment and does not react to any stimulus at all.

> ### TECHNICIAN NOTE
>
> Elevated carbon dioxide (CO_2) levels can be extremely dangerous for a patient with increased intracranial pressure and traumatic brain injury (TBI). Frequently reassess breathing in any patient with symptoms of TBI.

Evaluating the pupils can provide insight into the extent and location of brain injury in traumatized or acutely ill patients. Unresponsive, large "fixed and dilated" (mydriatic) pupils can indicate an irreversible midbrain lesion. Unresponsive midrange pupils are suggestive of a lesion in the medulla. Anisocoria (asymmetry in pupil size) may indicate an acute cerebral injury (e.g., blood clot, hemorrhage, or brain injury) or Horner syndrome, in which the nerves controlling the pupil are affected, but the brain is not injured. In some animals, anisocoria is normal and may not reflect any disease process.

Once overall mentation and pupils have been evaluated, the animal's posture should be more closely evaluated. Three classic postures are related to neurologic injury: decerebrate posture, decerebellate posture, and Schiff-Sherrington posture. Decerebrate posture is characterized by extreme rigidity of all four limbs. It may involve *opisthotonos* (arching of the neck and back) and indicates a complete disconnect between the forebrain and the brainstem. It is often accompanied by a stuporous to comatose mentation and carries a grave prognosis. Decerebellate posture signifies severe injury to the cerebellum. Typically, the animal presents with rigid forelimbs and flexed hind limbs, although rigidity may be noted in all four limbs. The main difference between this posture and decerebrate posture is that decerebellate animals will have normal mentation. Schiff-Sherrington posture can mimic decerebrate or decerebellate posture. Typically, when the animal is on its side, the forelimbs are rigid, and the hind limbs are flaccid. However, the animal has a normal mentation and often can ambulate when picked up and placed on its feet. The Schiff-Sherrington posture is associated with a T3–L3 spinal cord lesion.

Completing the Initial Triage Examination

Once initial assessment of the respiratory, cardiovascular, and neurologic systems has been completed, a quick abdominal palpation to check for pain, tympany, or a fluid wave is conducted.

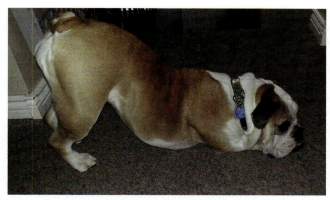

• **Fig. 25.2** A dog displaying a classic "praying posture" commonly observed with abdominal pain. (Courtesy Alison Downie, RVT, VTS [SAIIM].)

> • **BOX 25.1** **Assessment of Dehydration Based on Physical Examination Findings**
>
> Less than 5% dehydration: not clinically detectable
> 5% dehydration: mild mucous membrane dryness
> 7% dehydration: mild loss of skin turgor, dry mucous membranes, possible mild tachycardia
> 10% dehydration: pronounced loss of skin turgor, dry mucous membranes, tachycardia, weak pulses, sunken eyes
> Greater than 10% dehydration: severe loss of skin turgor, sunken eyes, shock, coma, death

Individual organs are not assessed during triage. If significant pain is detected, this may indicate a problem that requires surgery or a disease such as pancreatitis. Animals with severe abdominal pain often adopt a posture with an arched back and hind limbs moved backward; others repeatedly stretch into a "praying" posture, with the forelimbs down and stretched in front of them while they remain standing with the hind limbs in the normal position (Fig. 25.2). Tympany raises concerns that an intestinal structure is gas filled, such as the stomach in a gastric dilatation-volvulus (GDV) or a loop of small intestine with complete obstruction. A fluid wave could indicate hemorrhage from an internal organ, fluid buildup from inflammation or heart failure, or other diseases.

> ### TECHNICIAN NOTE
>
> Appropriate pain control is always important when treating a critically ill or injured patient.

Assessment of Hydration and Hypovolemia

Part of the initial assessment of every patient presented on an emergency basis is hydration status. Common causes of dehydration in veterinary patients include vomiting, diarrhea, excessive panting, polyuria, or decreased water intake. Unfortunately, precise methods to quantify dehydration are not available, although several subjective measures may be used (Box 25.1).

The earliest detectable signs of dehydration are tacky or dry mucous membranes. This is typically assessed in the oral cavity. CRT is normal until severe dehydration develops, leading to shock. Lack of skin turgor is checked by tenting the skin of the animal. With moderate to severe dehydration, agitation and restlessness can be seen, with progression to apathy and a comatose state. Body weight can be used to provide an objective measure of dehydration if the normal weight for the animal is known for comparison.

Common laboratory abnormalities in dehydrated animals include hemoconcentration, azotemia, hypernatremia, and elevated albumin. If azotemia is noted, urine specific gravity should be checked. If it is greater than 1.050, azotemia can be considered prerenal (i.e., resulting from decreased renal blood flow) and secondary to dehydration in most cases. Isosthenuria (urine specific gravity: 1.012–1.018 in dogs, 1.012–1.022 in cats) in the face of dehydration and azotemia suggests that renal disease is present.

During patient assessment, it is important to differentiate a dehydrated animal from a hypovolemic animal. Hypovolemia is loss of intravascular volume and commonly occurs with shock, trauma, hemorrhage, or profuse vomiting and diarrhea. Animals with hypovolemia tend to present with tachycardia and prolonged CRT. Because hypovolemia is an acute process, skin turgor may be normal. In severe cases, hypovolemic shock can be recognized by the presence of tachycardia, weak pulses, hypotension, and prolonged CRT. Hypovolemic shock is a true emergency that should be addressed immediately.

TECHNICIAN NOTE

Differentiating dehydration from hypovolemia is very important. Hypovolemic shock is a true emergency and must be addressed immediately.

Treatments for hypovolemia are aimed at restoring the blood volume quickly and include IV catheterization, administration of IV fluids, and possibly blood transfusions for hemorrhaging patients. Identification of the source of hypovolemia is important. Additional tests, such as radiography or ultrasonography, may be needed to identify the cause, and emergency surgery may be required for stabilization.

In contrast, treatment for dehydration involves replacement of the fluid deficit over several hours. If the patient has severe hypernatremia, rehydration should be even more gradual, possibly over 48 to 72 hours, to allow for fluid to shift from the intravascular to interstitial space. During rehydration, patients should be monitored for ongoing fluid loss, such as through vomiting, diarrhea, or polyuria, and fluid therapy plans adjusted accordingly (see Chapter 24).

Initial Diagnostics

The initial treatment area should be equipped to perform limited, high-yield diagnostics. These diagnostics are performed after the initial triage examination to determine the overall stability of the patient. These initial diagnostics include packed cell volume (PCV), total protein (TP), blood glucose, blood gas analysis, blood pressure, pulse oximetry (Fig. 25.3), ECG, and point-of-care ultrasound (POCUS) of the thorax and abdomen to determine whether free fluid or air is present in the abdomen or thorax. Blood gases (venous or arterial), electrolytes, and lactate are also very useful point-of-care analyses. An animal with high PCV and TP may be very dehydrated, whereas a low PCV may indicate red blood cell (RBC) loss or destruction. The color of serum can also lend clues to the underlying disease process. Icteric or hemolytic serum could indicate extravascular or intravascular hemolysis.

Blood gas analysis provides information about the acid-base and respiratory status of the patient. Normal blood pH for veterinary patients is 7.4. If the pH is low, there is a buildup of acid in

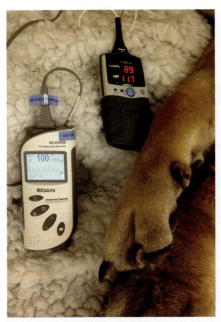

• **Fig. 25.3** A pulse oximeter provides a convenient means of monitoring oxygenation in critical or anesthetized animals. There are several factors that can cause the pulse oximeter to give unreliable readings. It is important that the patient is monitored by other means to ensure safety. In this picture, two pulse oximeters are giving very different readings on the same patient: on the left, 100% and on the right, 87%. Both gave an accurate heart rate of 117 beats per minute. The one on the right gave the more accurate values, and the patient required intervention.

the system, such as with diabetic ketoacidosis. If the pH is high, there is excess base or loss of acid, as occurs with severe vomiting. An elevated carbon dioxide (CO_2) level indicates an upper airway obstruction or hypoventilation. A decreased CO_2 level indicates hyperventilation, which can be related to hypoxemia, pain, stress, anxiety, or hyperthermia, or it can occur as compensation for a metabolic acidosis. The partial pressure of oxygen in arterial blood (PaO_2) can be used to assess pulmonary function on arterial samples. A normal patient will have a PaO_2 of 80 to 100 mmHg when breathing room air. It is concerning when a patient's PaO_2 falls below 70 mmHg. If a patient cannot maintain a PaO_2 above 70 mmHg with supplemental oxygen, mechanical ventilation is warranted. Many blood gas analyzers also provide a blood lactate level. A lactate level above 2 mg/dL can indicate poor perfusion and should lead to further evaluation of the patient's fluid status.

The ability to monitor blood pressure is crucial for proper stabilization and management of a critically ill animal. The most common methods are indirect Doppler measurement, oscillometric measurement, and direct arterial catheterization. Normal arterial blood pressure values for dogs and cats are in the range of 100 to 140 mmHg (systolic), 60 to 80 mmHg (diastolic), and 70 to 100 mmHg (mean). Reasonable initial reference points for blood pressure comparison vary by species and breed (in dogs).

Pulse oximetry is a key part of determining a patient's overall stability. The pulse oximeter is an instrument that determines the percent saturation of hemoglobin with oxygen. Normal animals have a pulse oximetry reading between 95% and 100%. Readings less than 92% indicate extreme disease and should be addressed immediately with supplemental oxygen. Remember that a pulse oximeter requires pulsatile blood flow to function, so if the patient's perfusion is poor or if the mucous membranes are highly pigmented, you might not be able to obtain a reading. Hemoglobin bound to CO registers as saturated on pulse oximetry, so pulse oximetry is not reliable in cases of smoke inhalation or CO poisoning.

> **TECHNICIAN NOTE**
>
> The initial treatment area should be equipped for packed cell volume/total protein (PCV/TP), blood glucose, blood pressure, pulse oximetry, and electrocardiography (ECG) monitoring. Blood gas analysis and ultrasonography capabilities are also helpful.

ECG is useful for monitoring the stability of a patient and response to treatment. Specific ECG rhythms and appropriate treatments are discussed later in this chapter. POCUS is used to quickly assess body cavities for the presence of fluid. Four sites in the abdomen (the subxiphoid area, around each kidney, and at the bladder) are imaged on abdominal POCUS. The heart is imaged from both sides, and each half of the thorax is imaged dorsally and ventrally during thoracic POCUS examination. If any fluid or free air is detected, a sample can be obtained by thoracocentesis or abdominocentesis.

The Secondary Survey

During the secondary survey, a more detailed physical examination is conducted, and non-life—threatening problems are addressed. The spine should be gently palpated. Any step defects or points of tenderness may indicate a spinal problem, such as luxation, fracture, or intervertebral disk herniation. Diffuse spinal pain may indicate problems, such as meningitis. A complete neurologic examination can help the clinician determine whether a concurrent neurologic deficit is present and requires further treatment and evaluation.

The head should be examined for additional signs of trauma not detected on the initial examination. The eyes are evaluated for scleral hemorrhage, corneal ulceration, lacerations, or development of anisocoria. It is important to recheck the pupils during the secondary examination as increased intracranial pressure can develop quickly. It is also imperative to perform a full cranial nerve examination and look in the oral cavity for broken teeth, bleeding, or swelling. The ears are examined for the presence of fluid or foreign material.

Wounds should be clipped, thoroughly cleaned and flushed with sterile saline, and bandaged. Each limb is carefully palpated for pain, swelling, lacerations, or malformations. A splint should be applied to stabilize any fracture or joint instability. Additional pain control and/or sedatives should be provided, if necessary, to properly clean wounds and apply bandages or splints. Throughout the initial stabilization, diagnostics, and secondary treatment phases, fluid therapy should be provided as discussed in Chapter 24.

The Emergency Care Station and Resuscitation Area

Patient treatment areas should be easily accessible (out of the main hospital traffic flow), clean, and well stocked. IV catheters, IV fluids, fluid pumps, administration sets, and needles and syringes should be available in the emergency area. An oxygen source, suction apparatus, and a crash cart must be in close proximity. It is important that the treatment area has functional clippers with working blades, surgical scrub, and tape to secure catheters. In addition, an easily readable **cardiopulmonary resuscitation** (CPR) flow chart should be prominently displayed (Fig. 25.4).

Crash Cart

The place where emergency drugs and supplies are kept is referred to as the *crash cart*. Depending on the size and focus of a clinic, the crash cart may range from a tackle box to a full, rolling cart with attached defibrillator. The crash cart must contain emergency medications, needles, syringes, a laryngoscope, various endotracheal (ET) tubes, and a bag-valve-mask resuscitator, commonly referred to as an *Ambubag*. Larger carts should also contain instrument packs for such procedures as **tracheostomy** or open-chest CPR.

> **TECHNICIAN NOTE**
>
> At a minimum, all items in the emergency crash cart must be inspected once a month for proper function and drug expiration. After inspection or use, the crash cart should be restocked.

Red rubber or polyvinyl chloride (PVC) catheters of various sizes have multiple uses in the treatment and resuscitation areas. In situations where the upper airway is completely obstructed, disrupted, or otherwise inaccessible to orotracheal intubation, a large-bore IV catheter placed percutaneously into the trachea will allow administration of oxygen while emergency tracheostomy materials are being prepared.

Shock and Systemic Inflammatory Response Syndrome

Shock is a complex syndrome resulting from altered blood flow or impaired oxygen delivery to tissues. If shock is left untreated, it may lead to death or serious complications. Prompt recognition of shock and appropriate treatment are crucial for patient survival. Early stages of shock are easily overlooked because of various compensatory mechanisms that are meant to preserve blood flow and oxygen delivery. Patients with early or compensated shock present depressed or anxious and are often tachycardic and tachypneic. Pulse quality can be normal, decreased, or increased. As shock progresses and cardiac output decreases, more severe alterations occur, including severe tachycardia, altered mental status, hypotension, pale mucous membranes, and weak pulses. The terminal stages of shock involve massive vasodilation, hypotension, and cardiac arrest.

Shock can be caused by numerous underlying conditions, leading to variable physical examination findings. The type of shock most commonly seen in cats and dogs is *hypovolemic shock*, which is the result of decreased intravascular fluid volume. Common predisposing events include trauma, hemorrhage, and severe vomiting or diarrhea. Patients in hypovolemic shock may have delayed CRT, weak pulses, pale mucous membranes, and altered mentation. Treatment is aimed at restoring intravascular volume. Treatment with IV fluids or a blood transfusion may be indicated. *Distributive shock* occurs from maldistribution of blood flow from inappropriate vasodilation leading to pooling of blood in the capillaries. This type of shock is seen with anaphylaxis, sepsis, heatstroke, and envenomation. Fluid therapy is essential in the treatment of distributive shock. Treatment often includes vasopressors to restore normal vascular tone. Weak or bounding pulses and pink mucous membranes are generally seen. *Obstructive shock* occurs when venous return to the heart is impaired.

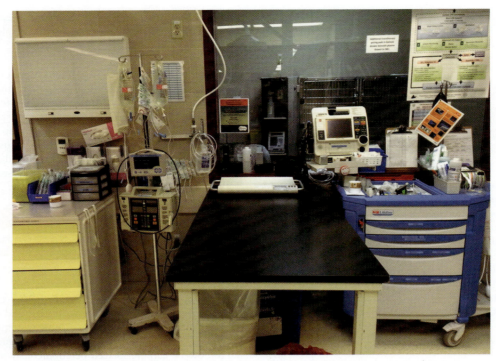

• **Fig. 25.4** An effective emergency area is easily accessible and is spacious enough to contain an array of emergency supplies.

In veterinary medicine, this type of shock can occur with GDV (when the distended stomach impairs venous return from the abdomen) or pericardial tamponade (when increased intrapericardial pressure causes collapse of the right atrium). Obstructive shock is best treated by addressing the underlying cause. *Cardiogenic shock* occurs secondary to problems in the heart itself. Patients will have weak pulses, hypotension, and pale mucous membranes. Other signs of cardiac failure, such as cold extremities, pulmonary edema, or ascites, and a heart murmur, are often present. Fluids are contraindicated in cardiogenic shock. Treatment relies on improving heart function. Diuretics are needed to resolve pulmonary edema.

Septic shock occurs after a severe infectious insult, such as pneumonia, parvovirus, gastric or intestinal perforation, or an infected bite wound. Septic shock can also occur as a sequela to severe tissue damage, such as after heatstroke or pancreatitis. Translocation of bacteria from the gastrointestinal (GI) tract into the bloodstream transports them to damaged organs. This can occur during any form of shock and is difficult to treat as altered blood flow may impair antibiotic delivery to the damaged organ. The inflammatory response associated with sepsis causes increased vasodilation, so septic animals often present with bright red mucous membranes (Fig. 25.5) and bounding pulses. Sometimes generalized erythema occurs, and fever is often present. As septic shock progresses, hypotension worsens, and the patient becomes pale, with weaker pulses. Therapy for septic shock involves treating the source of infection and providing fluid therapy and broad-spectrum antibiotics.

TECHNICIAN NOTE

Animals that present with septic shock often have bounding pulses, bright red mucous membranes, and fever.

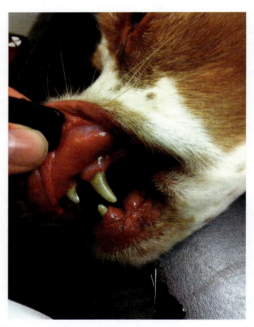

• **Fig. 25.5** Hyperemic (injected) mucous membranes are seen in this dog suffering from sepsis secondary to an acute abdomen.

During shock, an inflammatory response develops, even if no infection is present. Normally, an inflammatory response is restricted to discrete areas of infection or damage. However, shock results in widespread tissue hypoxia and damage, and the inflammation can progress from a local response to a systemic response (Box 25.2). This widespread inflammatory phenomenon is called *systemic inflammatory response syndrome (SIRS)*.

• BOX 25.2 **Common Causes of Systemic Inflammatory Response Syndrome (SIRS)**

Trauma
Surgery
Shock
Cardiopulmonary arrest (CPA) and cardiopulmonary resuscitation (CPR)
Pancreatitis
Heatstroke
Envenomation
Immune-mediated disease
Neoplasia—solitary tumor or metastatic disease
Infection (sepsis)

• BOX 25.3 **Definition of Systemic Inflammatory Response Syndrome (SIRS)**

To meet the SIRS criteria, dogs must meet two or more of the following, and cats must meet three or more:

1. *Heart rate (HR):* Tachycardia (>120–150 beats per minute [bpm] in dogs and 200–225 in cats), although some cats may have bradycardia (HR <140 bpm)
2. *Respiratory rate (RR):* Increased (most sources cite RR >40 bpm and/or $PaCO_2$ <30 mm Hg)
3. *Body temperature:* Increased (>103°F [39.4°C]–104.0°F [40°C]) or decreased (<99.0°F [37.2°C]–100.4°F [38°C])
4. *Leukogram:* Leukopenia (<5000 WBCs/μL) or leukocytosis (>18,000–20,000 WBCs/μL) or left shift (>5%–10% bands)

SIRS results in widespread vasodilation, leading to hypotension, tachycardia, tachypnea, fever and, often, marked increases or decreases in white blood cell count (Box 25.3). During SIRS, inflammatory mediators are released into the circulation; this causes recruitment and activation of white blood cells (WBCs) and platelets (PLTs). Activated WBCs cause additional tissue damage and inflammatory response throughout the body. As the endothelial lining of blood vessels and organs becomes damaged, PLTs are activated, and the clotting cascade is initiated. Microscopic clotting occludes capillaries, causing greater impairment of blood flow to organs and worsening the inflammatory response. As PLTs and clotting factors are consumed by inappropriate clotting, normal physiologic clotting mechanisms fail, and spontaneous bleeding can occur. This pattern of concurrent thrombosis and bleeding is called *disseminated intravascular coagulation* (DIC) and is among the most serious complications of shock. Despite treatment, DIC is often fatal. Another challenging complication of shock and sepsis is **multiple organ dysfunction syndrome (MODS)**. As the SIRS response progresses to microvascular clotting, organ failure may occur. Without timely and aggressive intervention, MODS can lead to permanent organ failure and death. Organs affected by MODS can include the kidneys, liver, lungs, brain, and heart. Treatment is focused on maintaining blood flow with fluid therapy, vasopressors, antibiotic therapy, transfusions of blood components, and mechanical ventilation. The prognosis for SIRS that has progressed to DIC and MODS is poor.

TECHNICIAN NOTE

Systemic inflammatory response syndrome (SIRS) is a secondary effect of shock and causes widespread inflammation. It can lead to disseminated intravascular coagulation (DIC), which is among the most serious complications of shock and is often fatal.

Advanced Emergency Techniques

Abdominocentesis

Abdominocentesis is primarily diagnostic but can also be therapeutic. With the animal in left lateral recumbency, the ventral abdomen is clipped and aseptically prepared around the umbilicus. With sterile gloves worn, the clinician places a 20- or 22-gauge needle or an over-the-needle catheter in the four quadrants around the umbilicus (Fig. 25.6). The needle or catheter is gently and slowly advanced through the skin and abdominal musculature until the tip "pops" into the peritoneal cavity. The

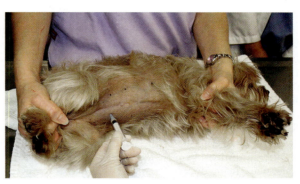

• Fig. 25.6 Abdominocentesis is performed by gently inserting a needle into the abdomen at four locations around the umbilicus until a sample of effusion is obtained.

needle is slowly advanced, or the catheter slid off the stylet. Each needle should be left in place while the others are being inserted. Once fluid is seen, no additional needles need to be placed. Fluid samples should always be collected in red-top and purple-top tubes for analysis. At other times, no fluid is obtained, and ultrasound-guided abdominocentesis or diagnostic peritoneal lavage should be considered. If the fluid obtained is hemorrhagic, it should be observed for clotting. If the fluid develops a clot, it is fresh blood rather than free fluid from within the abdomen. Alternatively, if ultrasonography is available, POCUS can help identify pockets of fluid, and the operator can sample the fluid under ultrasound guidance.

Thoracocentesis

Thoracocentesis is both diagnostic and therapeutic. The lateral thorax is clipped and aseptically prepared on one or both sides. If ultrasonography is available, POCUS is performed to identify fluid or air location. Supplies are gathered: a needle, butterfly or IV catheter, collection tubing, a three-way stopcock or centesis valve, and a syringe of appropriate size. By using sterile technique, the needle or catheter is blindly inserted at the seventh to ninth intercostal spaces or at the space indicated by ultrasonography. If pneumothorax is suspected, the needle or catheter should be inserted in the dorsal third of the thorax. For pleural effusion, the needle or catheter should be in the ventral third of the thorax. The needle or catheter should always be advanced off the cranial aspect of the rib and into the pleural space, and needles or butterfly catheters should be directed with the bevel side facing the lungs and the sharp tip parallel to the chest wall. The collection tubing and three-way stopcock are quickly attached to the needle or catheter, and suction gently applied with the syringe.

Thoracic Drain Placement

Placing a tube in the thoracic cavity is necessary if large amounts of air or fluid are present. A thoracic drain (**chest tube**) should be placed if more than two thoracocenteses are needed within a few hours. Chest tubes are commercially available both as large-bore rigid tubes and as Seldinger (guidewire) placed, flexible, fenestrated catheters.

To prepare for thoracic drain placement, the skin is clipped and aseptically prepared on the affected side(s). The seventh, eighth, or ninth intercostal space is identified at the junction of the upper one-third and the lower two-thirds of the thorax. This will be the entry point for the thoracic drain. The length from the insertion site to the desired tip location is measured and noted. Although tunneling is usually preferred to reduce the risk of a pneumothorax around the insertion site, Seldinger catheters tend to kink if tunneled too much.

A lidocaine bleb is injected at the insertion site and allowed to sit for approximately 5 minutes. A permanent marker can be used to identify the rib space above the point of entry to avoid contaminating the prepared skin. Sterile gloves are donned, and a small procedure drape is used to cover the site.

The introducer catheter (an over-the-needle catheter included in the Seldinger kit) is introduced perpendicular to the skin between the two ribs and at the site of the lidocaine. Once in the pleural space (often a distinct "pop" is felt), the catheter is advanced off the stylet while being directed cranially. The stylet is removed, and a gloved finger is used to cover the catheter hub while the coiled guidewire is removed from the kit. The guidewire has a soft J-bend in the end, which will prevent damage to lung tissue, and has markings every 10 cm. The "J" is pulled back into the introducer coil to straighten it, and the tip is placed into the introducer catheter and advanced as far as desired, depending on the patient's size. Adapter wings are included in the kit for use when less than 20 cm will be placed in the chest; however, this type of drain must be inserted a minimum of 10 cm, because there are multiple fenestrations on the first 10 cm of the tube. Once at the desired depth, the guidewire is left in place and kept stable so that it does not move, and the coiled wire cover and introducer catheter are removed so that only the wire remains in the chest. Finally, the soft chest tube is fed onto the end of the wire and advanced to the chest wall. By using two hands to firmly hold onto the wire and chest tube hub, the tip of the chest tube is pushed through the chest wall and into the pleural space. As soon as it begins to easily advance into the chest, the chest tube is redirected cranioventrally and advanced to the predetermined point. Once the chest tube is at the desired depth, the guidewire is removed. Immediately, a three-way stopcock is attached to prevent air from entering the chest. A Chinese finger trap suture is used to hold the tube in place, and the chest is bandaged. Once the tube is in place and secured, fluid or air are removed from the chest by gentle suction. The chest tube and lines should then be carefully attached to the bandage around the patient's thorax and labeled (Fig. 25.7).

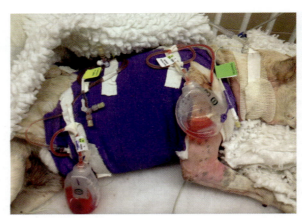

• **Fig. 25.7** This trauma patient has a thoracic drain, multiple Jackson-Pratt drains, and a feeding tube. It is important to keep all tubes neat, tidy, and well labeled to avoid errors.

Respiratory System Support and Oxygen Therapy

Disorders of the respiratory system are common in critically ill animals. These patients can suffer from structural problems, such as brachycephalic syndrome or collapsing trachea; problems with the lung tissue, such as pneumonia, hemorrhage, edema, or cancer; or even extrapulmonary problems, such as fractured ribs. Assessment of the patient's respiratory effort and breathing pattern can indicate which portion of the respiratory system is involved. Thoracic percussion can be used to determine whether pleural effusion is present.

TECHNICIAN NOTE

Observing the respiratory pattern and performing careful auscultation can provide clues to the underlying cause of dyspnea.

Mucous membrane color can be a sign of respiratory function. Normal animals have pink mucous membranes, whereas animals with poor respiratory function have pale, gray, or cyanotic mucous membranes. An important caveat when noting "pink" mucous membranes is that there are varying shades of pink, from bright pink to pink with purple or blue undertones. It is important not to assume that "pink" is always normal, because it requires a significant amount of deoxyhemoglobin (<5 g/dL) to appear cyanotic (blue).

Animals with respiratory difficulty or distress *(dyspnea)* should be handled very carefully. Common procedures, such as restraint, examination, IV catheter placement, and radiography, can cause an animal with dyspnea to decompensate to cardiac arrest; these procedures should be avoided, if possible, until the patient is less distressed. Oxygen support to conscious animals is provided by nasal cannulas or catheters, flow-by, face mask, and oxygen cage or oxygen hood (Figs. 25.8 and 25.9). Animals with dyspnea benefit from sedation before handling or procedures; however, careful monitoring is important, because certain drugs can interfere with respiration, and the patient may require intubation. If pleural effusion or pneumothorax is suspected, thoracocentesis is indicated to allow the lungs to inflate properly. The technique for thoracocentesis is described in Chapter 17. Performing thoracocentesis before thoracic radiography is helpful, because it allows expansion of the lungs, making radiographic identification of tumors and lesions much easier.

TECHNICIAN NOTE

In animals with severe dyspnea, handling should be minimized and stressful procedures, such as radiography, should be postponed until the animal's condition is more stable or the animal has been placed under gentle sedation.

Pulse oximetry and arterial blood gas (ABG) measurement provide valuable information about a patient's respiratory status. Pulse oximeters come with a cliplike probe, which is designed to attach to a vascular, poorly haired area such as the tongue, lip, ear flap, or toe webbing. Some models come with a rectal probe and cover, which can be used in recumbent and anesthetized animals in place of the conventional probe.

The pulse oximeter measures only the percent of hemoglobin molecules that are saturated with oxygen. It does not reflect the

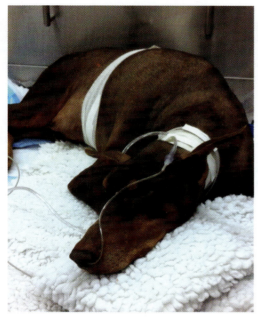

• **Fig. 25.8** This dog is receiving supplemental oxygen through a nasal catheter.

oxygen diffused in blood, or PaO_2. As long as pulmonary function is normal, even animals with severe anemia can have normal pulse oximetry readings, because although they have severely decreased hemoglobin levels, saturation of remaining hemoglobin molecules may be normal.

If the pulse oximeter displays an abnormal reading, immediate evaluation of the patient is warranted. HR, pulse quality, mucous membrane color, and RR and effort should be noted. Common causes of machine error include poor perfusion to the probe site, hypothermia, interference from hair or oral pigmentation, and patient movement. Depending on the patient's status, an ABG analysis may be performed to evaluate the blood oxygen content.

Capnography, which is a noninvasive means of measuring CO_2 levels, can also provide information about respiratory system function. End-tidal carbon dioxide ($ETCO_2$) levels reflect the amount of CO_2 present in expired air at the end of exhalation and, because CO_2 readily crosses from the bloodstream to the alveolus, should accurately reflect blood CO_2 levels. Increased $ETCO_2$ readings may indicate that the patient is hypoventilating or is rebreathing CO_2 in an anesthesia circuit with exhausted soda lime. Decreased $ETCO_2$ readings may indicate that the patient is hyperventilating or has decreased cardiac output.

ABG monitoring provides information about respiratory function. Arterial blood samples are obtained from the dorsal metatarsal artery or the femoral artery. To obtain an arterial blood sample, the fur in the area is clipped, and alcohol is used to clean the site. The pulse is palpated with a finger, and the other hand gently guides the needle into the artery. Specialized arterial draw syringes are often used as they are vented and fill on their own. The angle used for arteriopuncture is steep, and the syringe is often nearly perpendicular to the artery (Fig. 25.10).

Mechanical ventilation is a means of providing long-term intensive respiratory support to critically ill dogs and cats. Many referral veterinary practices have specialized critical care ventilators, which allow for fine alterations in breathing support and oxygen delivery. Short-term mechanical ventilation can be accomplished by using a standard anesthesia ventilator. Ideally, the ventilator is used to deliver oxygen mixed with room air, and the patient is anesthetized with IV medications during ventilation (Fig. 25.11).

Typical continuous monitoring of a ventilator patient includes an arterial catheterization, direct blood pressure monitoring,

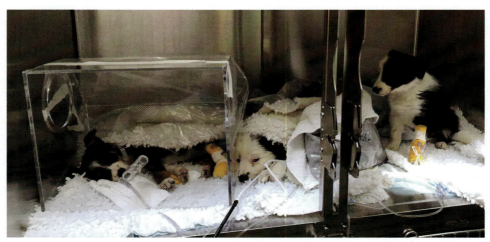

• **Fig. 25.9** An oxygen hood allows these young puppies to stay in the same cage together, even though only one is oxygen dependent.

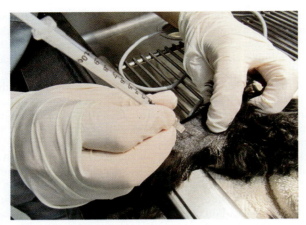

• **Fig. 25.10** Proper technique for obtaining an arterial blood gas sample from the dorsal metatarsal artery.

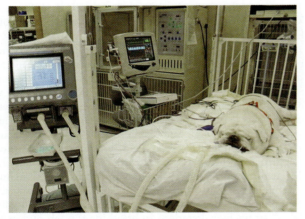

• **Fig. 25.11** Patients on mechanical ventilation require intensive, around-the-clock nursing care and monitoring.

$ETCO_2$ monitoring, pulse oximetry, temperature monitoring, and placement of a central line and an indwelling urinary catheter. Nursing care of the ventilator patient is a highly labor-intensive process. Every 4 to 6 hours, administration of an eye lubricant, swabbing of the oral cavity to remove secretions, inspection of all catheters, inspection and maintenance of the ET or tracheostomy tube, passive range-of-motion exercises, and repositioning to prevent pressure ulcers should be performed. Patients are at risk for pressure ulcers and peripheral edema, especially of the face and limbs, after 24 hours of recumbency. In some cases, the tongue can become severely edematous, requiring continued ventilation or tracheostomy. Pneumonia, a common complication during mechanical ventilation, can lead to sepsis and organ failure.

TECHNICIAN NOTE

Patients undergoing mechanical ventilation require extensive monitoring and intensive nursing care.

Cardiopulmonary Arrest

Cardiopulmonary arrest (CPA) involves cessation of spontaneous respirations and lack of a perfusing heart rhythm. In veterinary medicine, CPA most often occurs as the terminal event in a chronic disease process. However, previously healthy animals can experience CPA after trauma, critical illness, or anesthesia complications. CPR involves resuscitative efforts employed after CPA occurs.

Identifying patients at high risk for CPA is essential, because time is crucial for successful CPR. These patients present with underlying cardiac disorders, respiratory disease, severe trauma, or shock. Other patients at risk for CPA include those with acid-base and electrolyte disorders, seizures, anemia, or increased vagal stimulation (vagal tone), and those under general anesthesia. Some animals will have respiratory arrest before a full CPA. In these cases, the animal stops breathing, but the heart continues to beat for a short time before complete CPA occurs. Identifying these patients as soon as possible after respiratory arrest is crucial for survival. Other indications that a patient may suffer a CPA include sudden tachycardia or bradycardia, pallor, changes in pulse strength, increased RR or effort, and even acute agitation or depression.

TECHNICIAN NOTE

The first step in the resuscitation effort is to alert other team members to the crisis and move the patient to a centralized area where the crash cart and oxygen are accessible.

Cardiopulmonary Resuscitation

When CPA is suspected, the patient should be briefly assessed by quickly evaluating respiration (absence is sufficient cause to start CPR), ensuring the airway is clear, and calling for help, which should take no longer than 10 to 15 seconds. At this point, resuscitative measures must begin immediately. Resuscitation is commonly classified as basic life support (chest compressions and ventilation) or advanced life support (medications, **defibrillation**, and open-chest procedures).

Basic Life Support

Once CPA is suspected to have occurred, first responders should immediately start chest compressions, because delaying compressions is worse than performing them on an animal not in CPA (according to Reassessment Campaign on Veterinary Resuscitation [RECOVER] Initiative Guidelines). Once initiated, chest compressions should be continued in 2-minute cycles. As additional staff members arrive, the airway is secured by placement of an ET tube, and breaths are delivered at 10 breaths per minute using a bag-valve-mask resuscitator or rebreathing bag and anesthetic circuit. Oxygen is generally indicated at this point, although CPR can be performed successfully without oxygen.

The RECOVER Initiative, the first evidence-based guidelines for veterinary CPR, identifies properly administered chest compressions as one of the most important features of successful CPR. Posture, technique, and proper compression point are key.

In cats and small dogs (weighing less than 5–7 kg), the animal is placed in lateral recumbency, and the caregiver's hand encircles the ventral chest. Compressions are performed directly over the heart. The caregiver should be very careful to use the whole hand, not just the fingertips, to administer compressions (Fig. 25.12). Alternatively, a two-handed technique may be used with caution, taking into consideration that the patient is small and that the chest wall is generally very compliant. It is easy to overdo compressions on such small patients.

In larger dogs, positioning and technique for delivering chest compressions depend on patient size and conformation (keel,

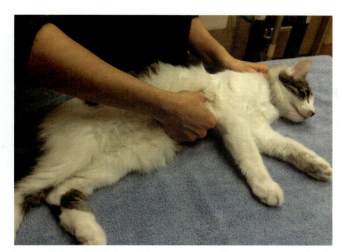

• **Fig. 25.12** One-handed technique for cardiopulmonary resuscitation in a cat or small dog.

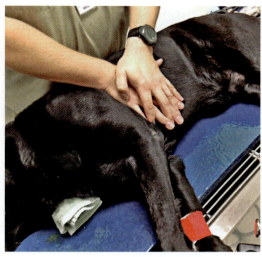

• **Fig. 25.13** Proper hand placement for cardiopulmonary resuscitation in a medium- to large-sized dog using the cardiac pump technique.

round, or flat chested), and a two-handed technique is used, with two different possible positions and three compression points. Proper compressions using the two-handed technique are administered with interlocked hands and straight arms in line with the shoulders to the heels of the hands. The heel of the hand will be over the compression point. During compressions, the arms remain straight, and the force of compression comes from the core by bending at the waist. Using an adjustable height table or a footstool or placing the patient on the floor will help the technician to stay in the proper position.

In "keel-chested" dogs, such as Greyhounds, which have a deep, narrow thoracic cavity, the cardiac pump technique is used to compress the heart directly at approximately the fifth intercostal space, with the dog in lateral recumbency.

In "round-chested" dogs, which have a chest with a similar width and depth, the thoracic pump technique is used, and compressions are applied to the widest part of the chest (approximately the seventh intercostal space, midway between spine and the sternum), with the dog in lateral recumbency (Fig. 25.13). With this technique, the heart is not directly compressed, and blood flow is dependent on changes in intrathoracic pressure that occur with each compression and recoil. When the chest is compressed, blood is forced out of the heart, and venous return to the right atrium occurs when pressure is released. To generate adequate pressure to cause passive blood flow, each thoracic compression should compress the thoracic wall by 30% to 50%. Compressors must imagine "lifting off" the chest wall to allow for complete chest recoil. This becomes more difficult as fatigue sets in and is one of the reasons compression cycles should be limited to 2 minutes.

Regardless of the technique used, successful CPR depends on performing quality chest compressions. In cats and dogs, a rate of 100 to 120 compressions per minute is recommended. At the moment that compressors are changing, a quick 10- to 15-second assessment of the patient is key to determining whether there is return of spontaneous circulation (ROSC). Compressions should not be stopped until the full 2-minute cycle is complete, at which point a quick assessment is made, and a new compressor steps in for 2 minutes.

Monitoring the effectiveness of chest compressions is best accomplished with the use of an $ETCO_2$ monitor. In CPA, $ETCO_2$ is zero, because no pulmonary blood flow is occurring. As chest compressions restore perfusion, $ETCO_2$ should rise and ideally reach 15 mm Hg or higher. A sudden increase in $ETCO_2$ may indicate ROSC.

> **TECHNICIAN NOTE**
>
> Pulse palpation and mucous membrane color are not reliable indicators of adequate chest compressions. End-tidal carbon dioxide ($ETCO_2$) measurements above 10 to 15 mm Hg are more dependable indicators of successful compressions.

Interposed abdominal compressions are used to enhance venous return to the heart during CPR. With this technique, the abdomen is compressed during the recoil phase of chest compression. Increased abdominal pressure can facilitate blood flow toward the heart. Complications of interposed abdominal compressions include organ contusions (especially of the liver) and hemoabdomen.

> **TECHNICIAN NOTE**
>
> Care should be taken to minimize any interruptions in chest compression, even for intubation and catheter placement.

In some cases, closed-chest compressions are not adequate to generate blood flow during CPR. A quick decision by the clinician to perform open-chest CPR is vital to the animal's survival. Some clinicians also elect to perform open-chest CPR on giant-breed dogs or on patients that have suffered a witnessed traumatic or anesthetic arrest. Open-chest CPR involves making an incision in the left fifth intercostal space, freeing the heart from its attachments, and directly massaging the heart from apex to base, mimicking normal contraction. If desired, the descending aorta can also be gently occluded by another team member's hand. This promotes preferential delivery of blood to the brain and the heart. The decision to pursue open-chest CPR should be made early in the resuscitation attempt—ideally immediately or after the first or second cycle of resuscitation—to maximize the chances of success.

Once CPA is identified and chest compressions are under way, the animal's airway must be secured. ET intubation should be performed in the position that the animal is in (usually lateral recumbency) to avoid lifting the head and affecting blood flow to

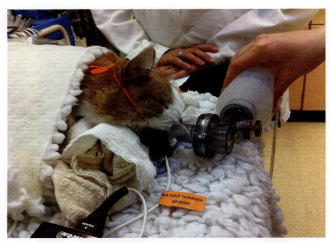

• **Fig. 25.14** A bag resuscitator is being used to ventilate a cat experiencing respiratory arrest.

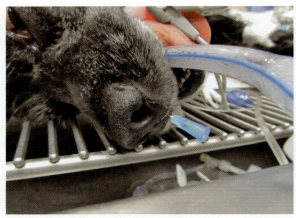

• **Fig. 25.15** A needle inserted at the Governor Vessel 26 (GV 26) acupuncture point.

the brain. It is imperative that the veterinary technician practice this technique in advance of an arrest on routine surgeries such as spays and neuters to become comfortable and competent. A laryngoscope *must* be used, and the tube *must* be visualized while going into the trachea. Any delay by esophageal intubation will reduce the chances of survival. Once the tube has been placed, it should be secured with a gauze tie and the patient connected to an oxygen source. Assisted breathing is initiated immediately. A bag resuscitator is a portable, easy-to-use device that connects to oxygen (Fig. 25.14). An anesthesia machine can also be used to deliver 100% oxygen to the animal during CPR, with breaths provided by using the rebreathing bag. If a pressure manometer is present, a target of 20 cm water (H_2O) for each breath is appropriate. Regardless of the patient's size, 10 respirations per minute should be administered, with 1-second inspirations and 5-second expirations.

> ### TECHNICIAN NOTE
> Excessive ventilation of the patient during cardiopulmonary resuscitation (CPR) causes cerebral vasoconstriction and decreased blood flow to the brain.

Acupuncture is a complementary technique that may be helpful in stimulating respiration when other measures have failed. The acupuncture point Governing Vessel 26, which is located at the nasal philtrum at the level of the ventral edge of the nares, can be stimulated (Fig. 25.15). A 25-gauge needle is applied to the bone at this point and is twirled to stimulate respiratory centers in the brainstem.

Advanced Life Support

If the patient is still in CPA after the first cycle, advanced life support techniques, which include medications or defibrillation, are often employed. Several drugs are available to assist in CPR, and the team must properly interpret an electrocardiogram to determine which is indicated. Four main arrest rhythms in dogs and cats are easily identifiable on ECG and are broken into two categories: (1) **asystole**, or pulseless electrical activity (PEA); and (2) pulseless **ventricular tachycardia**, or ventricular fibrillation. Asystole ("flatline") is complete cessation of all mechanical and electrical activity in the heart. PEA occurs when the electrical system of the heart is functioning (as evidenced by complexes on ECG), but no mechanical heartbeat occurs in response to electrical stimulation.

The appearance of this rhythm can be diverse, but it often mimics a ventricular arrhythmia, with wide, bizarre QRS complexes. While pulseless, many monitors will mistake the complexes and provide an HR. A defining feature for PEA is that the rate would be less than 200 beats per minute (bpm) and often far less. Asystole and PEA are commonly treated with low-dose epinephrine or vasopressin given every *other* BLS cycle (every 4 minutes). Atropine may be considered every other cycle as well. Ventricular fibrillation (VF) is highly disorganized contractile activity of the heart. It is often preceded by rapid pulseless ventricular tachycardia (PVT). If the monitor provides an HR, it would be greater than 200 bpm. The treatment of choice for these arrest rhythms is defibrillation. After the first 2-minute cycle of CPR or as soon as VF or PVT are diagnosed by ECG, an electrical defibrillator is used to attempt conversion back to a perfusing rhythm by stopping the heart and allowing the autonomic heart rhythm to restart effective contractions. Immediately after the shock is administered, another team member resumes chest compressions and completes the 2-minute cycle of CPR. If defibrillation is not successful and the patient remains in a shockable rhythm, it can be repeated at a 50% higher setting during the next CPR cycle. The defibrillator should be used only by trained personnel.

Alcohol should never be used near defibrillator paddles because of fire risk. The recommended initial dose depends on the defibrillator type: biphasic defibrillators use 2 to 4 joules per kilogram (J/kg) and monophasic (most older models) 4 to 6 J/kg. Initially, a setting at the lower end of this range is used. RECOVER guidelines suggest a 50% dose increase after an unsuccessful shock. Open-chest defibrillation requires specific paddles and a modified dose of electricity (0.2–0.4 J/kg).

In certain cases, additional medications may be indicated during the CPR attempt. See Table 25.1 for a list of common CPR drugs and their indications. The IV route is preferred for drug administration during CPR. If a catheter was not placed before CPA, one is placed as the patient is being intubated. Animals have very poor blood pressure during CPR, so a cutdown may be needed to secure venous access. An intraosseous (IO) catheter may be placed manually in small or young patients, or by using an IO drill in adult patients, to deliver medications during CPR. When drugs are administered via intraosseous access or through a peripheral vein, follow with an adequate volume of flush to ensure the medication reaches the heart and lungs. Sometimes, IV or IO access cannot be achieved during CPR. In these situations, certain

TABLE 25.1 Drugs Dosages Commonly Used During Cardiopulmonary Resuscitation

Drug Name	CPR Dose	Indications	Adverse Effects
Epinephrine	0.01–0.1 mg/kg IV (1 mL/10 kg)	Asystole, PEA. Used at low dose (0.01 mg/kg) every 4 mins. High dose (0.1 mg/kg) can be considered in prolonged CPR	Arrhythmias, hypertension
Atropine	0.04 mg/kg IV	Bradyarrhythmias, vagally mediated arrests, AV block	Arrhythmias, tachycardia, decreased GI motility
Vasopressin	0.8 mU/kg IV (0.4 mL/10 kg)	Asystole, PEA. Can be used in place of second dose of epinephrine	Arrhythmias, hypertension

AV, Atrioventricular; CPR, cardiopulmonary resuscitation; GI, gastrointestinal; IV, intravenous; PEA, pulseless electrical activity.

drugs can be administered through the ET tube. While there is little evidence to support intratracheal (IT) use, RECOVER guidelines recommend diluting the drug and delivering though a long catheter (such as a urinary catheter) that is longer than the ET tube. Generally, the dose used is twice the IV dose. Drugs that are caustic to the lungs (magnesium, bicarbonate, etc.) should never be administered through an ET tube. Drug uptake by the pulmonary circulation is impaired by some conditions, such as pulmonary edema, which may negate use of the IT route. Intracardiac injection of emergency drugs is not recommended because of the risk of damage to the heart muscle or laceration of the coronary arteries.

TECHNICIAN NOTE

Drugs that are safe to administer through an endotracheal (ET) tube are easily remembered by the acronym NAVEL (naloxone, atropine, vasopressin, epinephrine, lidocaine).

If the patient has experienced CPA from hypovolemic or hemorrhagic shock, fluid boluses should be given during the CPR attempt to restore vascular volume. Small crystalloid boluses of 10 to 15 mL/kg can be given at the start of CPR. A blood transfusion may also be given during CPR if indicated. It is important to remember that excessive fluid administration is detrimental, because it predisposes the animal to fluid overload.

During CPR, numerous activities occur. A designated team member must record the dose and route of all drugs administered (with times) and details of defibrillation attempts and circumstances that led to the patient's CPA. This ensures the medical record remains as complete as possible. RECOVER provides information and an extensive CPR Record that can be downloaded for free at https://recoverinitiative.org/cpr-guidelines/.

Finally, it is important to educate owners about realistic expectations when CPA occurs in their pets. In hospitalized animals, death often occurs as the result of a chronic or overwhelming disease. The odds of surviving until hospital discharge are very poor in these patients, with up to 82% undergoing another CPA within 12 hours. Dogs and cats undergoing CPA from trauma or anesthesia complications have greater chances of survival, but the overall survival rate for all causes of witnessed in-hospital CPA is 4% to 9%. If interventions are performed while the animal is in respiratory arrest only, approximately 30% of dogs and 58% of cats are expected to survive. Given these grim statistics, it is reasonable to discuss CPR with owners of critically ill animals upon admission and to determine their wishes should the pet experience CPA. "Do not resuscitate" orders can be written if the owner and the clinician agree that this is the best strategy for the patient.

Care of the Postarrest Patient

After a successful CPR attempt, the patient will require intense nursing care and monitoring. For the patient to have the best chances of survival, treatment should be focused on resolving the underlying cause of CPA (if possible) and anticipating and treating the systemic effects of CPA and resuscitation.

After resuscitation, the cardiovascular system is subjected to the effects of local ischemia and reperfusion injury of the heart muscle. Cardiac function is further compromised by the effects of inflammatory mediators and other substances released by peripheral tissues as reperfusion occurs throughout the body. Even the medications used during the CPR attempt itself, such as epinephrine and atropine, can contribute to ongoing cardiac stress by potentiating reperfusion injury and increasing the oxygen demands of an already stressed heart. In the postarrest period, patients often develop severe arrhythmias and systemic hypotension, which predispose them to another episode of CPA. Continuous ECG and blood pressure monitoring are imperative in the postarrest patient. These animals generally require treatment with antiarrhythmic medications and medications given to support cardiac contractility and blood pressure.

The respiratory system is very fragile after CPA and CPR. Often, these patients have underlying respiratory disease, making the lungs especially vulnerable to ongoing injury. After CPR, the patient is at risk for pulmonary edema, atelectasis, pulmonary thromboembolism, and acute respiratory distress syndrome, as well as for injuries resulting from the CPR attempt itself. The force used to generate adequate chest compressions can inadvertently result in pulmonary contusion, hemorrhage, or even rib fractures. During CPR, 100% oxygen is administered, and most patients require ongoing oxygen support for hours to days after an arrest. Mechanical ventilation is often needed in the immediate postarrest period.

The GI tract is subjected to severe insult during CPA. Hypoxia and hypotension lead to microscopic breakdown of the GI mucosal barrier, and this causes translocation of intestinal bacteria into the systemic circulation, potentially causing sepsis.

Acute kidney injury is also common after CPA. The kidneys have protective mechanisms to prevent extreme alterations in perfusion. These are overridden in severe shock and cardiac arrest, leaving the kidney vulnerable to hypotension and hypoxia. Electrolytes, kidney parameters, and urine output should be monitored closely in the postarrest period. Changes in urine output (polyuria or oliguria) can reflect significant renal injury, even if blood work values are normal. Careful monitoring of "in-and-out" fluid is essential for maintaining fluid balance in the postarrest patient.

The central nervous system (CNS) is also dramatically affected by CPA. Similar to the kidneys, the brain normally has autoregulatory mechanisms to ensure a constant supply of oxygen and nutrients while avoiding intracranial hypertension and fluid overload. When these mechanisms are lost during CPA, hypoxic brain injury occurs rapidly. After CPR, the brain is highly susceptible to reperfusion injury, which manifests as cerebral edema. Alterations in mental state and nerve function are common in the postarrest period. Initially, evaluation of neurologic function is performed at least hourly and includes evaluation of pupillary light response, pupil size and symmetry, spontaneous respiratory efforts, response to stimulus, and motor responses. Common neurologic abnormalities in the postarrest period include coma, stupor, anisocoria, miosis, altered pupillary light response, and decreased or absent corneal reflex. A positive prognostic indicator is recovery of these basic reflexes. Dilated or midrange nonresponsive pupils can signify a severe brainstem injury and carry a worse prognosis than anisocoria or miosis. Other poor prognostic indicators include failure to resume spontaneous ventilation, seizures, and loss of the ability to regulate basic body functions such as temperature and HR. After CPA, cortical blindness is very common. If the animal recovers, it often will regain vision, although permanent blindness is possible.

Blood glucose concentrations should also be monitored closely in the postarrest period. Patients commonly develop hyperglycemia as a result of stress as well as exposure to exogenous catecholamines such as epinephrine. Hyperglycemia can be detrimental to neurologic function and should be avoided. Some patients will develop hypoglycemia as a result of sepsis and reperfusion.

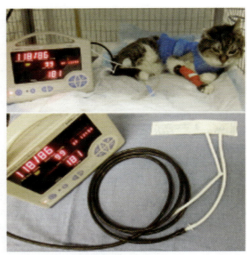

• **Fig. 25.16** An oscillometric blood pressure monitor. Note that this patient's arterial pressures are as follows: systolic, 118 mmHg; diastolic, 86 mmHg; mean, 99 mmHg.

TECHNICIAN NOTE

After successful cardiopulmonary resuscitation (CPR), patients should receive frequent neurologic assessments and should be monitored for the development of organ failure.

Many drugs are used to support the patient in the immediate postarrest period. Lidocaine is an antiarrhythmic medication used to treat rapid or unstable ventricular tachycardias. It is commonly given as a bolus, which may convert the patient's heart back to a normal sinus rhythm. Lidocaine can then be administered as a constant rate infusion (CRI) to control ventricular arrhythmias. When used as a CRI, lidocaine also provides systemic analgesia.

Mannitol is an osmotic diuretic that is used to decrease cerebral edema in the postarrest patient. Like lidocaine, mannitol has free radical scavenging properties that may be useful following reperfusion. Because of its diuretic properties, mannitol should be used judiciously in patients with existing renal failure, and fluid balance should be monitored closely.

Dopamine is a synthetic catecholamine administered as a CRI. This medication improves blood pressure by causing peripheral vasoconstriction. A related drug, dobutamine, increases cardiac output by enhancing cardiac contractility. Both medications can cause tachycardia and arrhythmias, so ECG and blood pressure monitoring are essential when they are used. Ideally, a central line is used for administration; however, use of a dedicated peripheral IV catheter is also acceptable.

Vasopressin may be administered as a CRI in hypotensive patients to improve blood pressure. This drug has the advantage of working well in an acidic environment. Cardiac arrhythmias can occur, so continuous ECG monitoring is needed.

Furosemide is a loop diuretic that is used occasionally in the postarrest period. Its diuretic effects increase urine output and cause volume contraction. Furosemide can help resolve cardiogenic pulmonary edema or fluid overload but should not be used in patients that are hypovolemic.

A positive outcome depends on anticipating and being prepared to handle the common complications of CPA. These animals often require around-the-clock care and monitoring to minimize the chances of another arrest event. The prognosis for survival and return to function after CPA is guarded to poor, and most survivors require several days of intensive care.

Patient Monitoring

Arterial Blood Pressure Monitoring

During each cardiac cycle, blood pressure varies from a maximum (systolic pressure) to a minimum (diastolic pressure). MAP is the average pressure over the course of the cardiac cycle. Blood pressure is generally expressed as a fraction (systolic/diastolic). Normal systolic pressures range from 80 to 140 mm Hg and diastolic pressures from 50 to 80 mm Hg. This reflects a MAP of 70 to 100 mm Hg. Maintaining adequate MAP is especially important in the brain and the kidneys, because these organs are highly sensitive to alterations in blood pressure.

Indirect or noninvasive blood pressure monitoring is used most often in veterinary practices with a Doppler or oscillometric device (Fig. 25.16). Oscillometric devices are often paired with other monitoring equipment in the same machine, such as ECG, pulse oximetry, and CO_2 monitors, or can be standalone. They calculate the systolic and diastolic pressures after measuring the MAP. Often, these machines can be set to automatically measure and record blood pressure at preset intervals, which makes them especially useful during anesthesia or in the intensive care unit.

Doppler blood pressure monitoring relies on an auditory signal to determine the arterial blood pressure (Fig. 25.17). For this technique, hair is clipped over an appropriate artery, and ultrasound gel is applied to enhance sound transmission. The Doppler crystal is positioned directly over the artery and is maneuvered until a clear pulse is heard. A blood pressure cuff of appropriate size is placed proximal to the transducer, and a sphygmomanometer is used to inflate the cuff until the pulse sound disappears. The cuff is then slowly deflated until the pulse is heard again. The point

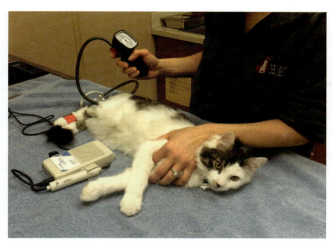

• **Fig. 25.17** Obtaining a Doppler blood pressure measurement in a cat.

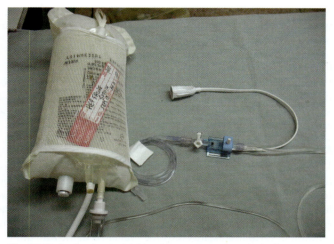

• **Fig. 25.18** A direct arterial blood pressure setup, including pressure transducer, rigid tubing, and pressure bag with heparinized saline.

where the pulse becomes audible again is the systolic pressure. This technique cannot be used to reliably assess diastolic or MAP in animals. Because the Doppler measurement must be taken manually, this technique is subject to operator variability.

> ### TECHNICIAN NOTE
> The blood pressure cuff width should be approximately 40% of the circumference of the limb at the site of cuff placement.

Direct or invasive blood pressure measurement is the gold standard for blood pressure monitoring. This technique requires catheterization of an artery and the use of specialized monitoring equipment. The most common sites for arterial catheter placement are the dorsal metatarsal and femoral arteries, although the tail artery can also be used. The femoral artery should be catheterized only in anesthetized or recumbent patients because of the risk for hemorrhage if the catheter is dislodged. Unlike veins, arteries cannot usually be visualized under the skin, and catheter placement is accomplished by digital palpation of the artery. Before the arterial catheter is placed, the fur is clipped, and the site is prepped with surgical scrub and wiped with alcohol. Sterile gloves should be worn during placement of arterial catheters. Arterial puncture often results in vasospasm, which can make threading the catheter challenging. Pausing for a few seconds after getting a flash of arterial blood in the catheter will allow the spasm to subside. The catheter should be slowly advanced and then securely taped in place. To monitor blood pressure, the arterial catheter is connected to a pressure transducer (Fig. 25.18), which generates a waveform on the electronic monitor (Fig. 25.19). These monitors will display systolic, diastolic, and mean blood pressures. It is important to keep the transducer at the level of the atrium to obtain the most accurate measurements. *No medications should ever be given through an arterial catheter.* To prevent blood clots from forming on the catheter tip, arterial catheters should be flushed every 2 hours.

> ### TECHNICIAN NOTE
> Arterial catheters should be labeled clearly to prevent accidental intra-arterial administration of medications. Never administer medications through an arterial catheter.

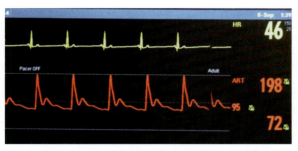

• **Fig. 25.19** An arterial blood pressure waveform on a multiparameter monitor.

Care of the Recumbent Patient

Airway and Endotracheal or Tracheostomy Tube Care

Airway care of the recumbent patient includes humidification, sterile suctioning as needed, repositioning of the ET tube, and changing the ET tube as needed. Repositioning the ET tube is important to prevent pressure damage to the tracheal endothelium. Humidification prevents desiccation of the sol layer and the mucosa, which preserves mucociliary clearance. Suctioning ensures removal of airway secretions that may clog the ET tube. Patients with a tracheostomy tube will also require care of the stoma, keeping it clean at all times. In both cases, hand hygiene is very important prior to handling any airway tubing to help reduce the risk of pneumonia.

Patient Comfort

Patient comfort is an important component of caring for the recumbent pet. Appropriate bedding is absorbent, easily cleaned or changed, and provides adequate padding to prevent the development of decubitus ulcers. Personal toys and blankets can reassure pets when they are in an unfamiliar environment. Many recumbent patients are in a fair amount of discomfort or pain, and maintaining appropriate pain control is vital for their return to function. Recumbent patients that require mechanical ventilation have additional considerations. Mechanical ventilation is most effective when the patient is anesthetized to a depth that allows complete control of its ventilatory process and reduces the stress associated with the patient's awareness of being intubated. These patients will need frequent changing of sides to avoid positional discomfort and help maintain skin integrity. The technician should always be monitoring for any redness over bony prominences as the start of a possible decubitus ulcer.

Intravenous Catheter Monitoring and Care

IV catheters should be monitored for patency, evidence of infection (heat, redness, swelling or pain), and phlebitis at least once a day. If IV fluids are not continuously administered though the catheter, it must be flushed regularly.

Nutrition and Hydration

Many recumbent patients do not eat appropriately because of their medical condition. Adequate enteral or parenteral nutrition (enteral route is always preferred) is important to support metabolism, albumin production, immune function, and GI integrity, and to prevent catabolism and complications such as refeeding syndrome. Hydration status must be evaluated daily, with adjustment of fluid therapy as needed.

Ocular Care

Proper ocular care, including periodic examinations and frequent application of sterile eye lubricant, is important to prevent ophthalmic complications such as corneal ulcer development. Applying fluorescein stain to the corneas daily will reveal potential ulcers at the earliest stage possible, allowing for appropriate treatment.

Oral Care

Keeping the oral mucosa moist using glycerin-based oral solutions and preventing pressure sores on the tongue are important nursing care items for comatose or anesthetized patients. Cleaning the oropharynx with dilute chlorhexidine solution or saline and suctioning debris help prevent pulmonary aspiration during repositioning of the tracheostomy or ET tube and decrease bacterial growth.

Range of Motion

Performing range-of-motion exercises at least four times a day will help decrease peripheral edema and will prevent contracture and atrophy of muscles from prolonged recumbency.

Urinary Catheter Placement and Care

Urinary catheters are important for keeping the patient clean, reducing the risk of urine scalding, and monitoring urine output and specific gravity. They also allow changes in urine appearance (i.e., color, clarity, and odor) to be monitored. Using aseptic technique for placing, using a closed urine collection system, avoiding catheter disconnections, and avoiding retrograde flow of urine from the bag into the bladder are just several strategies to reduce catheter-related urinary tract infection.

Standards of Care and Emergency Protocols

Common Emergencies

Respiratory Distress

The mainstay of treatment for animals in respiratory distress is to minimize stress. Oxygen supplementation must be provided immediately, and these patients often benefit from sedation. Butorphanol has minimal effect on the cardiovascular system and is considered safe for most patients at a dose of 0.2 mg/kg (0.1 mg/lb), as ordered by the veterinarian. The patient should then be placed immediately into an oxygen cage if available or provided with flow-by oxygen. If thoracic auscultation suggests pneumothorax or pleural effusion, thoracocentesis should be performed. Animals with suspected heart failure should receive furosemide, and cats with suspected asthma should receive two puffs from an albuterol inhaler. The IV catheter can wait until the patient is more stable and the sedation can take effect. After the patient has been stabilized, additional diagnostics can be performed. If the patient is at risk of respiratory failure, a rapid-sequence induction and intubation to take control of airway and breathing should be performed.

> **TECHNICIAN NOTE**
>
> Animals in respiratory distress, especially cats, can die as a result of even small amounts of stress. Oxygen, sedation, and time should be used to decrease their stress enough to allow safe handling.

Trauma

For the traumatically injured patient, an appropriate triage examination is performed, and all life-threatening injuries addressed immediately. IV access must be established as early as possible. Analgesia should be initiated early in the treatment protocol. During the secondary examination, all non-life—threatening problems should be addressed. It is important to operate under the presumption that pulmonary contusions and TBI have occurred and to treat the patient accordingly. Oxygen should be provided and the whole body positioned at a 30-degree angle so the head is elevated until these conditions are ruled out. The trauma patient should be reassessed continuously during the initial stabilization period and then a minimum of once every 3 to 5 minutes until the patient's condition is completely stable. See Case Presentation 25.1 for an example of emergency management of a trauma patient.

Acute Abdomen

The term *acute abdomen* refers to sudden onset of abdominal pain that is often severe and of unknown cause. When assessing a patient that presents with an acute abdomen, it is important to obtain a complete history from the owner (Box 25.4). Patients with a history of collapse with pale mucous membranes should be closely monitored for intermittent abdominal hemorrhage. Many causes of diarrhea are infectious, and some can be zoonotic, so it is important to wear gloves and practice infection control when handling these patients.

Gastric Dilatation-Volvulus

Patients with GDV present with acute signs ranging from agitation and repeated retching to lateral recumbency and shock. Abdominal distention is often a feature of this condition; however, dogs with a very long thorax may not display the classic abdominal distention, because the stomach remains within the thoracic cage. Initial stabilization requires placement of large-bore IV catheters in the forelimbs, rapid fluid administration, and possible decompression of the stomach by trocarisation or orogastric intubation. Radiographic confirmation of GDV should lead straight to surgery.

Urethral Obstruction

Upon presentation, animals with complete urethral obstruction may strain to urinate, or they may be stuporous from hypovolemic shock and hyperkalemia. If a patient suspected of urethral obstruction presents with bradycardia, it should be immediately evaluated for hyperkalemia. Calcium gluconate should be administered (0.5–1 mL/kg or 0.25–0.5 mL/lb) if hyperkalemia

CASE PRESENTATION 25.1

Emergency Management of a Canine Trauma Patient

Freddy, a 3-year-old neutered male Australian Cattle Dog mix, was presented to the emergency clinic after being hit by a train while out on a walk. Freddy was off leash and when the owner (who was wearing headphones) realized a train was coming, Freddy did not return immediately and paused on the tracks, where he was struck. Freddy attempted to get out of the way at the last moment, but his left hind leg was caught by the train and traumatically amputated. The owner immediately picked Freddy up, ran back to the vehicle, and presented Freddy to the emergency room (ER) within 15 minutes of the incident.

Freddy was triaged by the veterinary technician on duty and immediately taken to the emergency treatment area. The primary survey was brief, because Freddy had suffered significant blood loss. He was quiet but responsive, his gums were pale, and his limbs were cool. In the emergency area, one veterinary technician applied pressure to the amputation site, which continued to bleed (without pulsing), while another worked on gaining intravenous (IV) access and initial blood work. Flow-by oxygen was provided, and initial vital signs and diagnostics were obtained with the following results:

Heart rate (HR): 180 beats per minute (bpm), with weak pulses
Respiratory rate (RR): 60 respirations per minute (rpm)
Temperature: 38°C (100.4°F)
Mucous membranes: Pale, with capillary refill time (CRT) >2 seconds
Blood pressure (BP): 110/45 mm Hg; mean arterial pressure (MAP) 68 mm Hg
Peripheral capillary oxygen saturation (SpO$_2$): 93% on room air, 98% on
      oxygen
Electrocardiography (ECG): Sinus tachycardia
Packed cell volume (PCV): 42%
Total solids (TS): 4.8 g/dL
Venous blood gas: Respiratory alkalosis (likely caused by hyperventilation)
Electrolytes: Within normal ranges
Lactate: 5.2 mmol/L
Complete blood count (CBC): No significant abnormalities
Biochemical profile: No significant abnormalities

The veterinarian diagnosed Freddy as being in hypovolemic shock and, once cephalic IV access was obtained, a dose of hydromorphone and a 10-mL/kg bolus of Plasma-Lyte A were administered. Reassessment followed:

HR: 120 bpm, with fair pulses
RR: 36 rpm
Mucous membranes: Visibly pinker, with CRT <2 sec
BP: 120/65 mm Hg; MAP 78 mm Hg

The bleeding from the amputation site decreased significantly, and the artery was retracted and sealed (see figure).

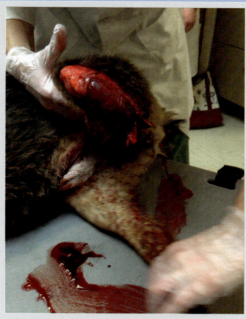

Traumatic amputation of the hind limb following a collision with a train.

Repeat PCV/TS an hour after initial presentation (28%/3.6 g/dL) showed that Freddy had lost a significant amount of blood but did not require a transfusion, because he was clinically stable and otherwise young and healthy.

Overall pleased with Freddy's initial response to treatment, the veterinarian ordered Freddy to be put on twice maintenance fluids, a fentanyl constant rate infusion (CRI) to address ongoing pain, and intravenous (IV) cefazolin every 8 hours (q8hr). Radiographs of Freddy's left hind limb and pelvis revealed his tibia and fibula were completely transected and crushed.

Freddy was taken to surgery for a complete hind limb amputation, and he did very well under anesthesia. His recovery was uneventful, and he continued to improve on maintenance fluids and fentanyl CRI over the next 24 hours. After his CRI was discontinued, hydromorphone was given as needed for pain. A "to go home" analgesia plan of gabapentin and meloxicam (after confirming normal renal values) was started. Freddy was discharged the next day and subsequently made a full recovery.

• BOX 25.4   Relevant Information When Assessing a Patient With an Acute Abdomen

- Is the patient vomiting? If so, describe the character of the vomitus.
- Is the patient having diarrhea? If so, include a description.
- Have periodic episodes of pale mucous membranes and collapse been reported?
- Is vaginal or preputial discharge present?
- For male patients: Is the patient intact? If so, have both testicles descended?

---

is confirmed. Once the calcium gluconate has been administered, additional measures, such as fluid therapy, dextrose administration, and possibly insulin, should be initiated. Appropriate sedation and urethral deobstruction should be performed to stabilize the patient.

Toxin Exposure

Information about toxin exposure including specific toxins, decontamination techniques, and treatments are discussed in Chapter 26, "Toxicology."

Canine and Feline Electrocardiography

ECG is a diagnostic tool that records electrical impulses generated by the specialized conduction system of the heart during each heartbeat. It is the test of choice for rhythm assessment and may provide information regarding cardiac chamber sizes.

Principles of Electrocardiography

The surface ECG records electrical activity of the heart using leads that consist of positive (+) and negative (–) electrodes attached to the skin. A wavefront of depolarization traveling toward a (+)

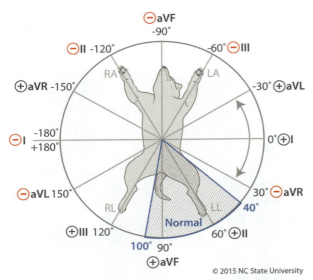

• **Fig. 25.20** The frontal plane hexaxial lead system consists of leads I, II, III, aVR, aVL, and aVF. The leads are 30 degrees apart, and each lead consists of a positive and a negative electrode. The normal mean electrical axis of 40 to 100 degrees is shaded. (Figure created by Alice MacGregor Harvey, medical illustrator, MA.)

electrode is recorded as a positive deflection on the ECG (above the baseline), whereas a wavefront traveling away from a (+) electrode is recorded as a negative deflection (below the baseline). Multiple leads (I, II, III, aVR, aVL, and aVF) are used to obtain different views of cardiac depolarization in the frontal plane (Fig. 25.20).

Leads I, II, and III are bipolar leads that record electrical activity between a (+) and (−) electrode in different locations (Fig. 25.21). Lead I is recorded with the (+) electrode on the left arm or forelimb (LA) and the (−) electrode on the right arm (RA) or forelimb. Lead II is recorded with the (+) electrode on the left hind limb (LL) and the (−) electrode on the RA. Lead III is recorded with the (+) electrode on the LL and the (−) electrode on the LA. Leads aVR, aVL, and aVF are augmented unipolar leads that record the electrical activity between a (+) electrode and the summation of the forces from the other two electrodes. These leads record half the voltage of the bipolar limb leads, and the ECG machines augment their signal to make them comparable in size with leads I, II, and III. Lead aVR is recorded with the (+) electrode on the RA and the reference (−) electrode as the combined average of the LA and the LL. Lead aVL is recorded with the (+) electrode on the LA and the reference (−) electrode as the combined average of the RA and the LL. Lead aVF is recorded with the (+) electrode on the LL and the reference (−) electrode as the combined average of the RA and LA.

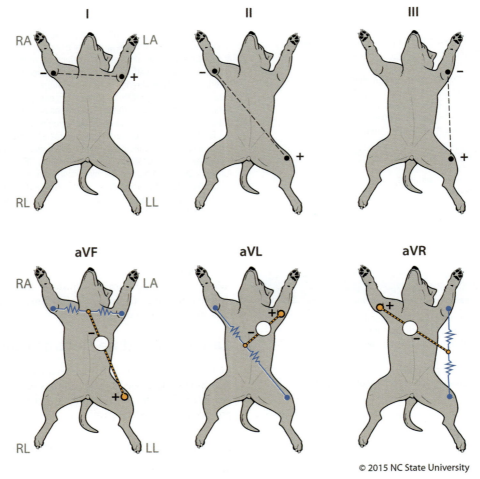

• **Fig. 25.21** Electrode placement is depicted for the generation of bipolar limb leads (I, II, III) and unipolar augmented leads (aVR, aVL, aVF). (Figure created by Alice MacGregor Harvey, medical illustrator, MA.)

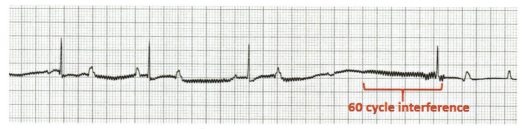

• **Fig. 25.22** Lead II ECG demonstrating 60-cycle electrical interference, which occurs when the leads detect the 60-hertz (Hz) signal created by electrical 110-volt alternating current (AC).

Acquisition of the Electrocardiogram

ECG should be performed in a quiet environment, with the patient in right lateral recumbency on a pad. Nearby electrical equipment should be unplugged to reduce 60-cycle electrical interference (Fig. 25.22). The limbs should be perpendicular to the body and the electrodes placed just below the elbow and stifle using alligator clips or adhesive patches. Alcohol or conductive gel applied to the electrodes enhances conduction of electrical activity. The electrodes on many ECG machines are color coded and often labeled using human anatomic terms (RA = right arm; LA = left arm; RL = right leg; LL = left leg). Respiratory artifact may be minimized by placing the electrodes more distally on the limb. The electrocardiogram is recorded at a paper speed of 50 mm/second or 25 mm/second and voltage (sensitivity) of 10 millimeters per millivolt (mm/mV).

> ### TECHNICIAN NOTE
>
> To perform electrocardiography (ECG), the white electrode (RA) is placed on the right forelimb, the black electrode (LA) is placed on the left forelimb, and the red electrode (LL) is placed on the left hind limb. The green electrode (RL) is the ground and is placed on the right hind limb (Fig. 25.23).

> ### PUT INTO PRACTICE
>
> Proficiency in acquiring a diagnostic ECG takes time and practice. Listening to normal patient hearts and completing ECG on many patients will help you to increase your skills in recognizing abnormal sounds and performing diagnostic ECGs.

Basic Cardiac Conduction and Electrocardiography Waveforms

The specialized cardiac conduction system is composed of the sinoatrial (SA) node, the atrioventricular (AV) node, the bundle of His, left and right bundle branches, and Purkinje fibers (Fig. 25.24). Pacemaker cells in the SA node initiate an impulse that propagates quickly through the atrial myocardium causing atrial depolarization (corresponding to the P wave on ECG). The impulse is conducted more slowly through the AV node to allow complete atrial depolarization to occur before ventricular depolarization. Conduction through the AV node corresponds to the PR interval on ECG. After conduction through the AV node, the impulse conduction velocity increases dramatically, traversing the bundle of His, left and right bundle branches, and Purkinje fibers to cause coordinated, nearly simultaneous left and right ventricular depolarization corresponding to the QRS complex on ECG. Ventricular repolarization follows depolarization and corresponds to the T wave on ECG (Fig. 25.25A).

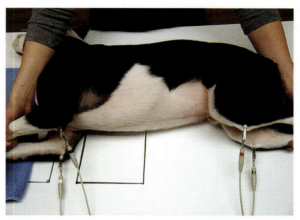

• **Fig. 25.23** Example of correct positioning and lead placement for electrocardiography recording. The dog is in right lateral recumbency and the limbs are perpendicular to the body. The white electrode is on the right forelimb, the black electrode is on the left forelimb, the green electrode is on the right hind limb, and the red electrode is on the left hind limb.

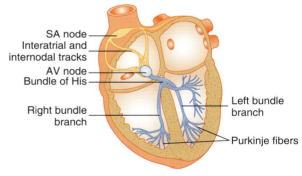

• **Fig. 25.24** The cardiac conduction system. (From Thomas J, Lerche P. *Anesthesia and Analgesia for Veterinary Technicians.* 4th ed. St. Louis, MO: Mosby; 2011.)

Indications for Electrocardiography

The most common reason for the use of ECG is to investigate arrhythmia. Physical examination abnormalities that should prompt ECG evaluation include an irregular rhythm, bradycardia, or tachycardia. Arrhythmias are commonly present in patients with advanced cardiac disease but may also be caused by drugs (e.g., digoxin, albuterol); toxins (e.g., Bufo toad toxicosis); myocarditis; and systemic diseases, such as electrolyte abnormalities (especially potassium and calcium); thyroid disease; abdominal neoplasia (especially splenic and adrenal); GDV; trauma; sepsis;

and shock. ECG should always be performed on patients with a history of syncope (fainting) or episodic weakness, because these conditions are commonly caused by cardiac arrhythmias, some of which are life-threatening.

Because routine ECG only records the cardiac rhythm for a small portion of the day (typically 1 to 5 minutes), it is possible that an intermittent arrhythmia will not be detected. If a rhythm disturbance is clinically suspected despite a normal ECG, longer monitoring is necessary. A Holter monitor digitally records the ECG measurement of a patient over a 24- or 48-hour period and is used to diagnose suspected arrhythmia or to further characterize the frequency and severity of arrhythmias detected by routine ECG (Fig. 25.26). Holter monitor findings can help guide treatment and diagnostic plans and can rule in or rule out an arrhythmic cause of syncope if collapse occurs during the recording. Holter monitoring is also used to document adequate suppression of arrhythmia after treatment with antiarrhythmic medication. The cardiac rhythm of hospitalized patients can be continuously monitored by using an anesthesia ECG machine or telemetry, which transmits the ECG signal to a monitor, thus avoiding wire placement on the patient.

ECG waveforms may also provide information to suggest cardiac chamber enlargement; however, ECG is more specific than sensitive for this purpose. The finding of a chamber enlargement pattern on ECG strongly supports its presence; however, normal waveform measurements do not rule out chamber enlargement. Echocardiography is much more sensitive for cardiac chamber enlargement detection compared with ECG.

ECG can also reveal abnormal results in other clinical situations, such as electrolyte abnormalities (e.g., absent P waves and tented T waves in hyperkalemia; Fig. 25.27), drug toxicities (e.g., QT prolongation; Fig. 25.28), and pericardial effusion (small QRS complexes; sinus tachycardia; and *electrical alternans*, which is an alternating height of the QRS complexes; Fig. 25.29). ECG recording should be monitored during anesthesia and during pericardiocentesis to screen for arrhythmias and HR abnormalities that could suggest procedural complications, electrolyte abnormalities, or depth of anesthesia.

Electrocardiographic Analysis

The ECG should be evaluated in a systematic manner, analyzing four basic features: HR, rhythm, measurement of waveforms and intervals, and mean electrical axis (MEA). The standard ECG paper has a grid of 1-mm boxes. The paper is further subdivided

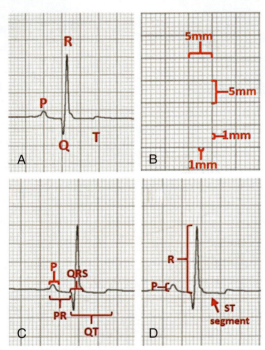

• **Fig. 25.25** Paper speed 50 mm/second, sensitivity 10 mm/mV. (A) A sinus beat with labeled P-QRS-T waves. Note the lack of an obvious S wave. It is not uncommon for Q waves or S waves to be absent in normal QRS complexes. (B) Standardized electrocardiography (ECG) paper. Each thin line represents 1 mm, and each thick line represents 5 mm, both vertically and horizontally. (C) Demonstration of the proper measurement for P wave width, QRS width, PR interval, and QT duration. (D) Demonstration of the proper measurement for P wave and R wave height. The ST segment should not significantly deviate from the baseline.

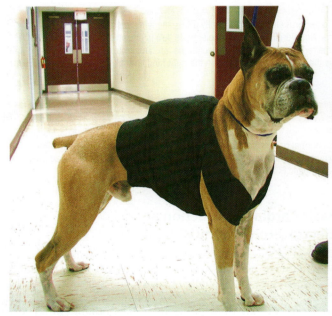

• **FIGURE 25.26** A Boxer dog wearing a 24-hour Holter monitor.

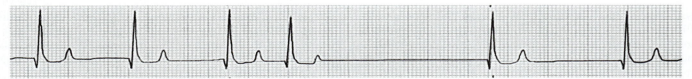

• **Fig. 25.27** Lead II electrocardiogram from a dog with atrial standstill resulting from hyperkalemia. Note the flat baseline, absence of P waves, supraventricular-appearing QRS complexes, and tented T waves. The average heart rate is slow (50 beats per minute). Paper speed is 25 mm/second.

every 5 mm by thicker and darker lines, creating a grid of 5-mm boxes (Fig. 25.25B). Vertical measurements of waveforms represent the strength of the electrical impulse expressed in millivolts, and horizontal measurements of waveforms represent time expressed in seconds. Standard calibration is 10 mm/mV, making each vertical 1-mm box equivalent to 0.1 mV and each 5-mm box 0.5 mV. Paper speed is typically recorded at 50 mm/second or 25 mm/second, making each horizontal 1-mm box 0.02 second or 0.04 second, respectively, and each 5-mm box 0.1 second or 0.2 second, respectively.

HR can be calculated as an average or an instantaneous HR. Average HR is useful when the rhythm is irregular, and instantaneous HR is useful when the rhythm is regular or when calculating the instantaneous rate of a premature beat. Average HR is determined by counting the number of QRS complexes in a predetermined time period and multiplying the number of complexes by a factor (20 when 3-second period is used, 10 when a 6-second period is used) to calculate the number of beats per minute. A 3-second period will equal 150 mm at 50 mm/second and 75 mm at 25 mm/second. In contrast, instantaneous HR is calculated using only two heartbeats by counting the number of millimeters between two R waves and dividing this number into 3000 when the paper speed is 50 mm/second (3000 mm occurs during 1 minute at 50 mm/second) or into 1500 when the paper speed is 25 mm/second (1500 mm occurs in 1 minute at 25 mm/second).

After calculating HR, the rhythm should be identified. Asking the following questions in a stepwise manner can help fully evaluate the rhythm:

1. *Is the rhythm regular or irregular?* If irregularity is present, it should be noted whether there is a pattern to the irregularity (i.e., *regularly irregular* or *irregularly irregular*). This will aid in determining whether an arrhythmia is present (e.g., an irregularly irregular rhythm might indicate premature beats or atrial fibrillation) or if the rhythm is of sinus origin (e.g., a regularly irregular rhythm is consistent with respiratory sinus arrhythmia).

2. *Are P waves present and, if so, is there a P wave, for every QRS and a QRS for every P wave, with a consistent PR interval?* A "yes" supports sinus rhythm, whereas a "no" could indicate an arrhythmia.

3. *Are the QRS complexes supraventricular or ventricular in appearance?* Supraventricular complexes arise from above the ventricles (sinus node, atria, or AV node), so they utilize the normal, rapidly conducting pathways in the ventricle and are therefore narrow and upright in leads I, II, III, and aVF. They should have an associated P wave; however, depending on the site of impulse formation (e.g., sinus or atrial tissue or junctional), the P wave could be visible or might be buried within the QRS complex. Ventricular origin complexes appear wide and bizarre compared with normal beats, because they arise from the ventricular muscle and do not utilize the normal conduction system. They may be positive or negative in leads I, II, III, and aVF, and they are not associated with P waves. A general rule for this determination is the "90% rule"; if the QRS complexes appear greater than 90% like a normal QRS complex, they are probably of supraventricular origin, and if they are less than 90% like a normal QRS, they are probably of ventricular origin.

4. *Are premature beats present and, if so, are they supraventricular or ventricular in origin?* The answers to these questions should lead to the correct rhythm diagnosis on most electrocardiograms.

Each sinus beat waveform and interval on ECG should be identified and the amplitude and width measured in lead II to evaluate for chamber enlargement patterns or conduction delays (Figs. 25.25C and D). Normal canine and feline waveform and interval measurements are available in Table 25.2. The P wave documents atrial depolarization; therefore measurement abnormalities may indicate atrial enlargement. The width is measured from the beginning to the end of the P wave, and the height is measured from the baseline to the top of the P wave. A tall P wave (P-pulmonale) is consistent with right atrial enlargement (Fig. 25.30A), and a wide P wave (P-mitral) suggests left atrial enlargement (Fig. 25.30B). The PR interval is measured from the beginning of the P wave to the beginning of the QRS complex (or the R wave if no Q wave is present) and is mainly affected by conduction time through the AV node. Prolongation of the PR interval can occur because of increased vagal tone or structural AV nodal disease and is called *first-degree AV block* (Fig. 25.31). The QRS complex indicates

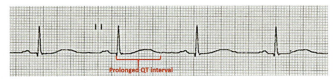

• **Fig. 25.28** Lead II electrocardiogram showing sinus rhythm with a long QT interval of 0.32 seconds. Paper speed is 50 mm/second.

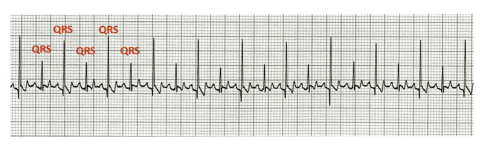

• **Fig. 25.29** Lead II electrocardiogram showing sinus rhythm with electrical alternans in a dog with pericardial effusion. Note the changing QRS morphology (especially R wave height) on an every-other-beat basis. Paper speed is 25 mm/second.

TABLE 25.2	Normal Canine and Feline Waveform and Interval Measurements	
	Canine	**Feline**
Heart rate, bpm	Puppy: 70–220	120–240
	Toy breed: 70–180	
	Standard: 70–180	
	Giant breed: 60–140	
Rhythm	Sinus rhythm	Sinus rhythm
	Sinus arrhythmia	
	Wandering pacemaker	
P wave		
Height	Max: 0.4 mV	Max: 0.2 mV
Width	Max: 0.04 seconds (giant breed, 0.05 seconds)	Max: 0.04 seconds
PR interval	0.06–0.13 seconds	0.05–0.09 seconds
R wave height	Small breed: 2.5 mV	Max: 0.9 mV
	Large breed: 3.0 mV	
QRS width	Small breed: 0.05 seconds	Max: 0.04 seconds
	Large breed: 0.06 seconds	
ST segment		
Depression	No more than 0.2 mV	None
Elevation	No more than 0.15 mV	None
QT interval	0.15–0.25 seconds	0.12–0.18 seconds
Electrical axis	+40 to +100 degrees	0 to +160 degrees

Bpm, Beats per minute; *mV,* millivolts.

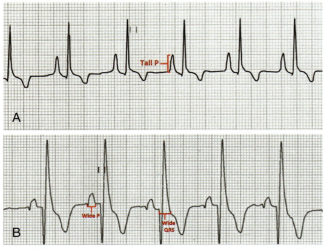

• **Fig. 25.30** Lead II electrocardiograms showing sinus rhythm. Paper speed is 50 mm/second and sensitivity is 10 mm/mV. (A) P-pulmonale is present as evidenced by a tall P wave (0.6 mV), suggesting right atrial enlargement. (B) P-mitrale is present as evidenced by a wide P wave (0.06 seconds), suggesting left atrial enlargement. The QRS complex is wide (0.07 seconds), suggesting left ventricular enlargement.

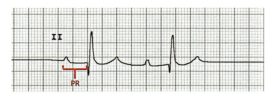

• **Fig. 25.31** Lead II electrocardiogram showing sinus rhythm with a prolonged PR interval of 0.16 seconds, indicating first-degree atrioventricular block. Note that the P wave is still related to the QRS complex and the rhythm is sinus. Paper speed is 50 mm/second.

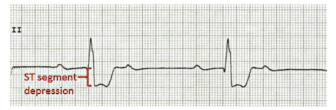

• **Fig. 25.32** Lead II electrocardiogram showing sinus rhythm with an ST segment depression of 0.7 mV indicating regional myocardial ischemia. The ST segment should be no lower or higher than 0.2 mV compared with the baseline. Paper speed is 50 mm/second and sensitivity is 10 mm/mV.

ventricular depolarization and can therefore reveal abnormalities of ventricular size or activation. QRS width is measured from the beginning of the Q wave (or the R wave if there is no Q wave) to the end of the S wave, and R wave height is measured from the baseline to the top of the R wave. A tall R wave in lead II suggests left ventricular enlargement, and a deep S wave suggests right ventricular enlargement. A wide QRS complex may indicate ventricular enlargement, bundle branch block, or a ventricular ectopic beat, and the specific diagnosis will depend on other ECG findings (e.g., whether P waves are associated or not) (Fig. 25.30B).

The ST segment indicates the time from ventricular depolarization to repolarization and should normally be at baseline level, because it is a period of electrical quiescence. Regional myocardial ischemia can cause elevation or depression of the ST segment (Fig. 25.32).

The T wave is associated with ventricular repolarization and can be positive, negative, or biphasic. T wave abnormalities are uncommon in dogs and cats except for tall, tented T waves, which are a hallmark finding of hyperkalemia (Fig. 25.27).

The QT interval represents the summation of ventricular depolarization and repolarization and varies inversely with HR. It is measured from the beginning of the QRS complex to the end

of the T wave. Interpretation of the QT interval is challenging because of the complex effects of the changing HR with sinus arrhythmia on QT duration. There are numerous causes of QT prolongation, such as medications (e.g., some antiarrhythmics, antibiotics, and antipsychotics), electrolyte abnormalities, and genetic abnormalities and, when it is significant, it can predispose to dangerous arrhythmia formation.

The MEA is the net direction of all potentials involved in ventricular depolarization and is typically discussed only in reference to the QRS complex. Because the left ventricle has the greatest mass, the normal MEA is directed toward the left ventricle. If right ventricular hypertrophy or right bundle branch block is present, the

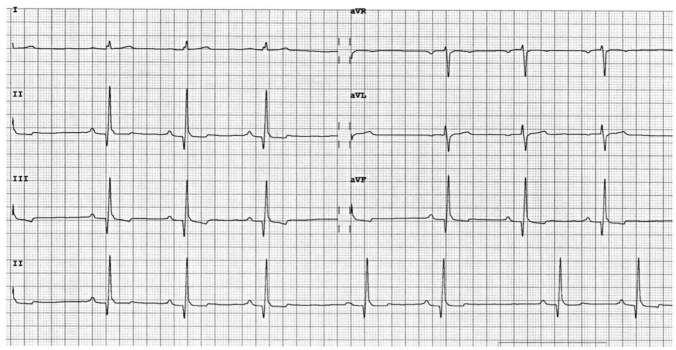

• **Fig. 25.33** This is a 6-lead electrocardiogram with a lead II rhythm strip at the bottom. The paper speed is 50 mm/second, and sensitivity is 10 mm/mV. The rhythm is sinus with a heart rate of 100 beats per minute. The six leads can be used to demonstrate determination of the mean electrical axis (MEA), as described in the "Electrocardiographic Analysis" section. Lead II has the tallest R wave (1.8 mV from baseline to R wave peak); therefore the positive pole of lead II (+60 degrees) is the MEA, which is normal for a dog. The R wave height in lead aVF is also tall (1.6 mV), so the MEA is directed somewhere between the positive pole of lead II (+60) and lead aVF (+90), both of which are normal in the dog. Fig. 25.31 is used for reference.

MEA can shift to the right. The simplest method to estimate MEA is to find the lead with the tallest R wave in a standard six-lead system (remembering that the R wave is always a positive waveform). The positive pole of this lead roughly equates to the MEA, because the net impulse direction is toward this positive pole (Fig. 25.33).

Cardiac Arrhythmias

An *arrhythmia* is a disturbance in the rate, regularity, or site of cardiac impulse formation. Arrhythmias that originate above the AV node are classified as supraventricular arrhythmias, whereas arrhythmias that originate below the AV node are ventricular arrhythmias. Arrhythmias can also be categorized on the basis of HR. Those with a slow HR are termed *bradyarrhythmias*, and those with a fast HR are termed *tachyarrhythmias*.

Normal Rhythms
Normal Sinus Rhythm
Sinus rhythm refers to normal rhythm in dogs and cats in which each beat is initiated by SA nodal discharge. It is characterized by a regular rhythm, normal HR, and consistent association between P waves and QRS complexes (Fig. 25.33).

Sinus Arrhythmia
Sinus arrhythmia (Fig. 25.34) is a normal rhythm in dogs that is usually associated with high vagal tone and/or with breathing (e.g., respiratory sinus arrhythmia). When associated with breathing, HR increases with inhalation and decreases with exhalation.

It is a *regularly irregular* rhythm (patterned) and is commonly associated with a wandering pacemaker, which is characterized by taller P waves when HR increases and smaller P waves when HR decreases. Sinus arrhythmia is not a normal finding in a cat and when it occurs, it can indicate excessive vagal tone caused by underlying CNS, respiratory, or GI disease.

Sinus Bradycardia
Sinus bradycardia refers to regular rhythm that originates from the SA node but is slower than normal. It is often a physiologic response to high vagal tone, drugs (e.g., anesthetics, calcium channel blockers, beta blockers), or systemic disease (hypothermia or hypothyroidism). Specific therapy is not warranted unless the patient is symptomatic (e.g., weakness or collapse); however, addressing the primary cause is indicated (e.g., reducing drug doses, warming, treating hypothyroidism). Atropine can be administered to abolish vagal tone if the patient is bradycardic or to demonstrate a vagal origin to the rhythm.

Sinus Tachycardia
Sinus tachycardia refers to regular rhythm that originates from the SA node but is faster than the normal HR. It typically occurs as a normal physiologic response to high sympathetic tone caused by pain, excitement, stress, anxiety, or drugs (e.g., atropine, methylxanthines, catecholamines), or as a response to fever, shock, hemorrhage, hyperthyroidism, anemia, hypoxia, or congestive heart failure. Specific therapy typically is not warranted; however, the underlying cause of sinus tachycardia should be addressed.

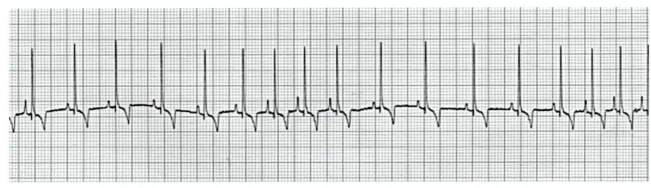

• **Fig. 25.34** Lead II electrocardiogram showing a sinus arrhythmia at an average rate of 125 beats per minute (bpm). Note the patterned appearance to the slowing and acceleration of the rhythm. Also note the wandering pacemaker, which is evidenced by increased P height when the heart rate is faster and decreased P height when the heart rate is slower. Wandering pacemaker is a normal finding that often accompanies sinus arrhythmia. Paper speed is 25 mm/second and sensitivity is 10 mm/mV.

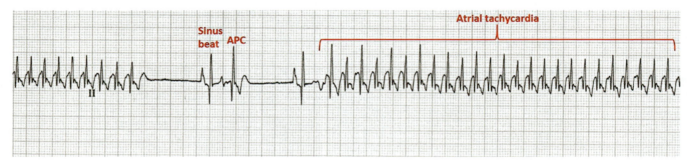

• **Fig. 25.35** Lead II electrocardiogram showing an atrial premature complex (APC) following a sinus beat and a run of atrial tachycardia following another sinus beat. The premature atrial beats appear about 90% like the normal sinus beats and are preceded by a negative ectopic P wave, therefore having characteristics of an APC. The atrial tachycardia is rapid (300 beats per minute). Paper speed is 25 mm/second.

Disturbances of Supraventricular Impulse Formation

Atrial Premature Complexes

Atrial premature complexes (APCs) (Fig. 25.35) are abnormal impulses originating from the atrial myocardium instead of the SA node. On an electrocardiogram, an APC appears as a premature QRS complex nearly identical in shape to the normal sinus QRS complex. Each APC is associated with a P wave that occurs earlier than normal. This premature P wave can have an abnormal appearance and might be superimposed on the previous T wave. APCs are commonly associated with atrial enlargement secondary to structural cardiac disease, but other causes include atrial neoplasia, hyperthyroidism, and hypoxia. Therapy is usually not indicated for single APCs; however, Holter monitoring can be performed to determine whether atrial tachycardia is occurring at other times during the day that might prompt treatment.

TECHNICIAN NOTE

Atrial premature complexes (APCs) are differentiated from ventricular premature complexes (VPCs) by QRS shape and by the presence or absence of a P wave. APCs have a premature but normally shaped QRS and are associated with a P wave, whereas VPCs have an abnormal, "wide and bizarre" QRS and are not associated with a P wave.

Atrial Tachycardia

Atrial tachycardia (Fig. 25.35) is defined as four or more APCs in succession and often has a sudden onset and termination. The QRS complexes appear normal, and P waves are typically present but are buried in the previous T wave or ST segment, making them sometimes difficult to identify. Atrial tachycardia is usually a regular rhythm with HR in excess of 200 to 300 bpm. Underlying etiologies are like those of APCs; however, unlike single APCs, therapy with antiarrhythmic medications is indicated, especially if the patient experiences weakness, hypotension, or collapse. Junctional tachycardia is like atrial tachycardia; however, because the ectopic rhythm starts in the AV nodal region, P waves can occur before, during, or after the QRS complex. The term *supraventricular tachycardia* (SVT) is commonly used to describe both atrial and junctional tachycardias, because sometimes they are indistinguishable on surface ECG.

Atrial Flutter

Atrial flutter (Fig. 25.36) is a rapid rhythm with supraventricular QRS complexes and saw-toothed flutter waves instead of P waves. Flutter waves are similar in appearance to wide P waves but without a return to an isoelectric baseline between them. The HR in atrial flutter can be regular or irregular (but in multiples of a common denominator), depending on how many impulses are

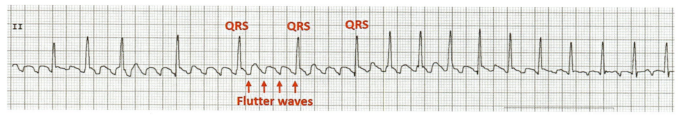

• **Fig. 25.36** Lead II electrocardiogram showing atrial flutter. Negative flutter waves are very rapid and, because the AV node cannot conduct this rapidly, the heart rate is variable, from 150 beats per minute (bpm) to 300 bpm. Paper speed is 50 mm/second.

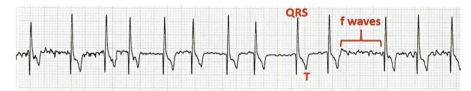

• **Fig. 25.37** Lead II electrocardiogram showing atrial fibrillation with an average rate of 130 beats per minute after treatment with medication to slow the rate. The rhythm is irregularly irregular and supraventricular in morphology, and no discernable P waves are present. The baseline shows fibrillation (f) waves. The paper speed is 25 mm/second.

conducted to the ventricles through the AV node. This rhythm often occurs secondary to severe left atrial enlargement and commonly degenerates into **atrial fibrillation**. Drug therapy typically is warranted, although pharmacologic or electrical cardioversion to sinus rhythm can be attempted.

Atrial Fibrillation

Atrial fibrillation (Fig. 25.37) is a rapid, *irregularly irregular* rhythm with supraventricular morphology QRS complexes, no identifiable P waves, and the presence of fibrillatory waves (f waves). It is often caused by severe left atrial enlargement secondary to underlying structural cardiac disease (e.g., advanced degenerative valve disease, dilated cardiomyopathy). The sudden onset of this rapid arrhythmia and loss of atrial contraction can cause collapse or precipitate congestive heart failure in dogs with underlying heart disease. Less commonly, atrial fibrillation occurs in giant-breed dogs with structurally normal hearts (referred to as *lone atrial fibrillation*) or as the result of high vagal tone. Atrial fibrillation is rare in cats because of their small size. Therapy with medications to slow the ventricular response rate is indicated when HR with atrial fibrillation is high. Slowing the rate allows for improved filling of the ventricles and improved cardiac output. If no underlying cardiac disease is present, electrical or pharmacologic conversion to sinus rhythm can be considered.

Disturbances of Ventricular Impulse Formation

Ventricular Premature Complexes

Ventricular premature complexes (Fig. 25.38) are abnormal beats originating from the ventricular myocardium. The typical appearance is a wide and bizarre QRS complex that can be positive or negative, indicating that QRS originated from outside the normal conduction system. There is no association with P waves, and QRS occurs earlier than normal. VPCs may occur as single, monomorphic beats (all abnormal QRS complexes are identical) or as polymorphic beats (abnormal QRS complexes differ in appearance). The appearance of two sequential VPCs is called a *couplet*, and that of three VPCs in a row is called a *triplet*. A rhythm in which every other

beat is a VPC is called *bigeminy*, and one in which every third beat is a VPC is called *trigeminy*. There are many causes of VPCs, including structural cardiac disease, arrhythmogenic right ventricular cardiomyopathy, GDV, splenic disease (neoplasia, hematoma), trauma, sepsis, drugs/toxins (e.g., digoxin, digitalis glycosides), electrolyte abnormalities, hyperthyroidism, and excessive catecholamines. Single, monomorphic VPCs are typically not treated; however, 24-hour Holter monitoring is indicated to screen for more serious arrhythmias throughout the day that would indicate need for treatment.

Ventricular Tachycardia

Ventricular tachycardia (Fig. 25.39) is a run of four or more VPCs in succession at a rapid rate (>180 bpm). Ventricular tachycardia can be sustained (>30 seconds) or nonsustained (< 30 seconds) and monomorphic or polymorphic. Rapid ventricular tachycardia requires emergency treatment with lidocaine to suppress the arrhythmia because of the high risk of sudden death. Other factors that indicate a need for treatment include associated clinical signs of weakness, hypotension, or collapse; the presence of underlying structural disease; R-on-T phenomenon; and breeds of known risk for sudden death, such as Boxers and Doberman Pinschers.

TECHNICIAN NOTE

R-on-T phenomenon (see Fig. 25.39) occurs when the QRS of the ventricular premature complex (VPC) falls on the T wave of the preceding beat. The downslope of the T wave is considered a vulnerable period when ventricular fibrillation can be initiated with a stimulus. R-on-T phenomenon typically occurs with very rapid ventricular tachycardia rates and indicates the need for antiarrhythmic treatment, such as with lidocaine, in the emergency setting.

Accelerated idioventricular rhythm (AIVR) (Fig. 25.40) is a ventricular rhythm with a relatively normal rate (typically between 60 and 160 bpm) that competes with the normal sinus rhythm. AIVR is often caused by extracardiac disease (e.g., vehicular trauma, splenic masses, GDV) that affects the heart through

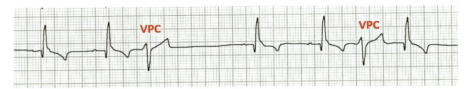

• **Fig. 25.38** Lead II electrocardiogram showing ventricular premature complexes (VPCs) in a trigeminal pattern. The VPCs are wide and bizarre compared with sinus beats and are not preceded by a P wave. Paper speed is 50 mm/second.

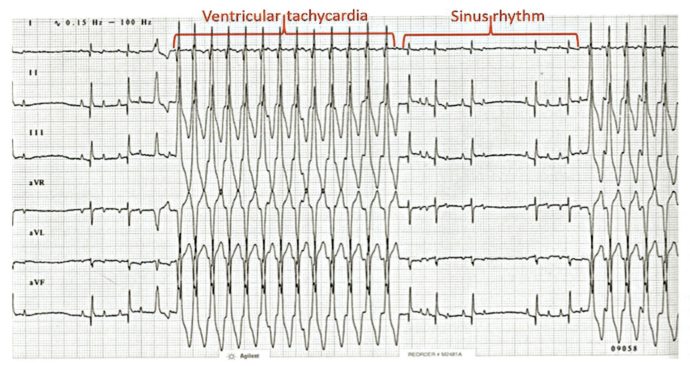

• **Fig. 25.39** Six-lead electrocardiogram showing paroxysmal (bursts) monomorphic ventricular tachycardia (VT). The VT is rapid (300 beats per minute) and shows R-on-T phenomenon, indicating that this is a dangerous rhythm requiring treatment. Paper speed is 25 mm/second.

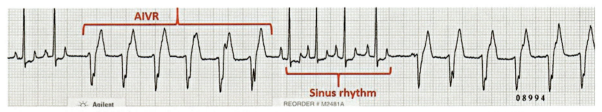

• **Fig. 25.40** Lead II electrocardiogram showing intermittent accelerated idioventricular rhythm (AIVR). AIVR is a ventricular rhythm that occurs at a rate similar to the sinus rate (slower than ventricular tachycardia), thereby competing with the sinus rhythm. Paper speed is 25 mm/second.

perfusion deficits or depressant factors. Antiarrhythmic therapy is rarely indicated for AIVR, because the overall rate is similar to the sinus rate, and R-on-T phenomenon does not typically occur at rates between 60 and 160 bpm. The underlying etiology should be addressed, which can help resolve the AIVR.

Ventricular Fibrillation

Ventricular fibrillation (Fig. 25.41) is a life-threatening rhythm characterized by chaotic, irregular waves resulting from lack of organized ventricular activity. On ECG, no P-QRS-T complexes are present, and only irregular oscillations of varying size are noted. ECG lead attachment should be verified, and electrical defibrillation should be performed immediately to restore sinus rhythm.

Ventricular Asystole

Ventricular asystole is the absence of any ventricular activity and appears as a flat baseline on ECG. Immediate therapy to restore a rhythm should be instituted (e.g., with epinephrine).

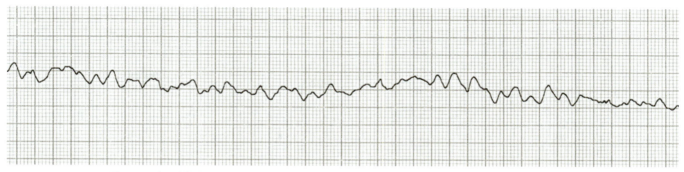

• **Fig. 25.41** Lead II electrocardiogram showing ventricular fibrillation. No P-QRS-T complexes are visible, and the baseline shows chaotic oscillations of fibrillation.

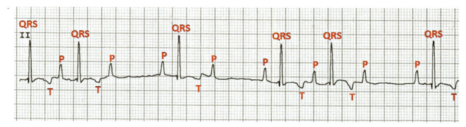

• **Fig. 25.42** Lead II electrocardiogram showing second-degree atrioventricular block. The second, fourth, and seventh P waves are not conducted to a QRS complex, while the remaining P waves are associated with QRS complexes. Paper speed 50 mm/second.

Disturbances of Impulse Conduction

Atrial Standstill

Atrial standstill (see Fig. 25.27) is a rhythm in which atrial depolarization does not occur when the SA node discharges. It is characterized by lack of P waves, a flat baseline, supraventricular morphology QRS complexes, and bradycardia. The most common cause of atrial standstill is hyperkalemia associated with systemic disease, because high extracellular potassium concentration impairs the ability of the atrial myocardium to conduct an impulse. Prominent tented T waves are also noted with hyperkalemia. The sinus node continues to control the rhythm through the interatrial tracts without atrial myocardial depolarization (and therefore without P waves) until hyperkalemia is very severe, which is called a *sinoventricular rhythm.* Treatment is directed at restoring normokalaemia.

Atrial standstill that occurs with normal serum potassium concentration is usually a result of replacement fibrosis of the atrial muscle and is called *persistent atrial standstill* (or *silent atrium*). Because the sinus node cannot conduct impulses to the atria or the AV node, the AV node supports heart rhythm with a junctional escape rhythm at 40 to 60 bpm. Underlying etiologies of persistent atrial standstill include atrial myocarditis or genetic predispositions (e.g., English Springer Spaniels appear predisposed). Pacemaker implantation is necessary to treat atrial standstill not caused by electrolyte disturbances.

First-Degree Atrioventricular Block

First-degree AV block (see Fig. 25.31) occurs when conduction through the AV node is delayed, causing a prolonged PR interval on ECG. Sinus rhythm is maintained, and HR is normal. First-degree AV block can be caused by elevated vagal tone, AV nodal fibrosis, or medications. Direct therapy is not indicated, because the rate and the rhythm are normal.

Second-Degree Atrioventricular Block

Second-degree AV block (Fig. 25.42) is a rhythm characterized by intermittent disruption of AV nodal conduction. On an ECG tracing, some P waves are followed by QRS complexes, while others are not. Second-degree AV block is further subdivided into Mobitz type I and Mobitz type II second-degree AV block. Mobitz type I (Wenckebach periodicity) is caused by high vagal tone and is characterized by progressive prolongation of the PR interval until AV nodal conduction is blocked. Mobitz type II is considered more serious and is characterized by a consistent PR interval before AV block.

Third-Degree Atrioventricular Block

Third-degree AV block (complete heart block) (Fig. 25.43) occurs when there is no conduction of sinus impulses through the AV node and the rhythm is maintained by an escape rhythm. Complete heart block usually occurs as the result of degeneration and fibrosis of the AV node; however, drugs (e.g., digoxin or beta blocker toxicity), infiltrative myocardial disease, and myocarditis are other possible causes. ECG shows complete dissociation of the P waves and QRS complexes, and HR is very low (30–60 bpm). Atropine responsiveness is typically lacking, and pacemaker implantation is indicated to resolve the bradycardia. There is some risk of sudden death with untreated third-degree AV block.

Bundle Branch Block

Bundle branch block is a conduction disturbance that occurs when the cardiac impulse is blocked at the level of the left or right bundle branch but is conducted normally through the opposite bundle branch. The rhythm is sinus, so P waves are present and temporally related to the widened QRS complex. The ventricle with the bundle branch block must be depolarized through cell-to-cell conduction after the normally depolarized ventricle.

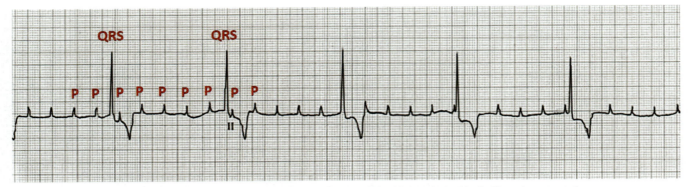

• **Fig. 25.43** Lead II electrocardiogram showing third-degree atrioventricular block. There is no association of the P waves with the QRS complexes (the PR interval is not constant, indicating the P waves are dissociated from the QRS). The underlying ventricular rate is slow (35 beats per minute), consistent with a ventricular escape rhythm. Paper speed is 25 mm/second.

Cell-to-cell conduction is a slower process, so the QRS is wider than normal and terminally directed toward the ventricle with the bundle branch block. ECG appearance of both types of bundle branch block is a wide QRS complex with associated P waves; however, with a left bundle branch block pattern, QRS is positive in leads I, II, III, and aVF with a normal MEA (Fig. 25.44A), and with a right bundle branch block pattern, QRS is negative (deep S waves) in leads I, II, III, and aVF with a right axis shift (Fig. 25.44B). Right bundle branch block can be associated with underlying right ventricular disease or can be an incidental finding not associated with detectable cardiac disease. Left bundle branch block is commonly associated with severe left ventricular disease. Direct treatment for either bundle branch block is not indicated, because the rhythm is still sinus.

TECHNICIAN NOTE

Bundle branch block and ventricular premature complex (VPC) both have wide QRS complexes, but a sinus beat with a bundle branch block has an associated P wave, whereas a VPC does not have an associated P wave.

Disturbances of Impulse Formation and Conduction

Sick Sinus Syndrome

Sick sinus syndrome is a disease of the conduction system characterized by abnormal sinus impulse formation and conduction causing a combination of arrhythmias (sinus arrest, sinus bradycardia, atrial tachycardia), AV nodal conduction block, and intermittent failure of escape beats (Fig. 25.45). Because both rapid and slow rhythms often coexist, the term "bradycardia-tachycardia syndrome" has been coined. The underlying cause is unknown; however, some breeds are overrepresented (older female Miniature Schnauzers, Cocker Spaniels, West Highland White Terriers, and Dachshunds). Clinical signs are related to weakness and episodic collapse. Atropine testing will determine whether there is a vagal influence that could suggest potential benefit from medications that increase HR (e.g., theophylline, hyoscyamine); however, most patients that have symptoms of sick sinus syndrome require pacemaker implantation to prevent syncope.

Escape Beats and Escape Rhythms

Junctional escape beats occur when the AV node acts as a subsidiary pacemaker if a sinus impulse is not generated or conducted. ECG appearance of a junctional escape beat is a narrow,

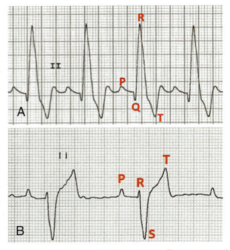

• **Fig. 25.44** Lead II electrocardiogram strips. Paper speed is 50 mm/second; sensitivity is 10 mm/mV. (A) Sinus rhythm with a left bundle branch block. The Q wave is narrow and followed by a very wide R wave as a result of cell-to-cell depolarization toward the (+) pole of lead II (toward the left ventricle). (B) Sinus rhythm with a right bundle branch block. The R wave is narrow and followed by a very wide S wave as a result of cell-to-cell depolarization away from the (+) pole of lead II (toward the right ventricle).

supraventricular morphology QRS complex that occurs after a pause of greater than 1 second, with a negative or retrograde P wave occurring before, on, or after the QRS complex (Fig. 25.45). *Ventricular escape beats* occur when the bundle of His and Purkinje fibers act as subsidiary pacemakers in the event that a sinus or junctional impulse is not generated or conducted. A ventricular escape beat appears as a wide and bizarre QRS complex without a P wave that occurs after a pause of approximately 2 seconds (it is different from a VPC, because it is not premature). Prolonged failure of higher pacemaker sites will result in "rescue" of the heart rhythm by an escape rhythm (successive escape beats). The intrinsic rate of junctional escape rhythms is 40 to 60 bpm, whereas the rate of ventricular escape rhythms is 30 to 40 bpm (Fig. 25.43). Escape rhythms should not be suppressed with antiarrhythmic medications, because this can result in asystole and death.

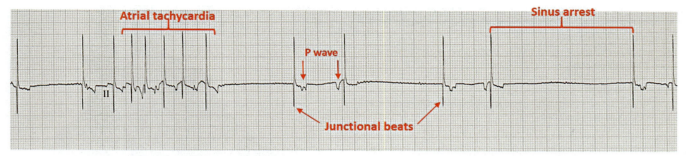

• **Fig. 25.45** Lead II electrocardiogram showing characteristics of sick sinus syndrome. Atrial tachycardia is present, and the ectopic P waves are visible in the preceding T wave. Sinus arrest is present (pause greater than two heartbeat intervals). Ectopic but nonpremature atrial complexes are present, as indicated by the prominent negative P waves. Junctional escape beats occur after a pause of about 1.5 seconds, and the P waves associated with retrograde atrial conduction from these beats can be noted in the ST segment. Paper speed is 25 mm/second.

TECHNICIAN NOTE

An atropine response test can be performed by administering atropine 0.04 mg/kg subcutaneously and rechecking the electrocardiography (ECG) reading in 30 minutes. Abolition of pauses and atrioventricular (AV) nodal block with a heart rate (HR) above 150 beats per minute (bpm) indicates that elevated vagal tone is the cause of the bradyarrhythmia (termed a full atropine response). An inadequate response indicates the presence of conduction disease. Dogs with bradyarrhythmia that are not atropine responsive should not be anesthetized without pacemaker support, because anesthesia can suppress escape rhythms and increase the risk of anesthesia complications or death.

Emergency and Critical Care Nursing: Equine

In equine practice, emergencies make up a large portion of the caseload. The most common emergencies are directly related to the GI system (e.g., colic), the respiratory system (e.g., respiratory distress), and the musculoskeletal system (e.g., fractures, wounds). When emergencies occur, there are two potential waves of action: field response and referral. The field veterinary team is on the front line of triage, action, and care. For emergencies to be treated efficiently and effectively, the veterinary staff needs to be organized, prepared, and thoughtful.

Gastrointestinal Tract

One of the most common emergencies in equine practice is colic. The term *colic* refers to any condition that causes abdominal pain. Horses exhibiting signs of colic in the field can be broadly divided into two categories: those that will resolve with minimal or no treatment and those that will not. The former group encompasses the vast majority of cases. The recommendation is for all patients with colic to receive professional medical attention, but many patients will improve before a veterinarian arrives. In cases that improve, it is impossible to determine the exact cause of the discomfort, although it is believed that gas accumulation within the bowel or spasmodic colic (cramping of the GI tract) is the most common cause. A large percentage of patients will respond to administration of analgesics (e.g., flunixin meglumine), hand walking, sedation with xylazine or detomidine, and laxatives (e.g., mineral oil) given through a nasogastric tube. When there is no response to this level of treatment, patients require more intensive treatment (medical or surgical) to correct the condition. It is important to remember that GI pain that is unresponsive to

treatment is a potentially life-threatening condition; therefore early recognition and referral to a tertiary medical center capable of aggressive therapy is essential for the survival of these patients.

For the veterinary hospital staff to be successful in dealing with these emergencies, team members must be prepared with proper supplies and technical support. When setting up for an emergency, the veterinary technician or nurse should envision the events that may transpire. However, it is common for an emergency to be encountered in routine practice; therefore a minimum colic setup should consist of the supplies listed in Box 25.5.

General Physical Examination

Once the doors of the trailer are opened after arrival of the patient to the hospital, an immediate visual assessment of pain and the severity of the condition should commence. It is important for veterinary team members to assume control and ensure safety of the environment while maintaining their own safety. Once unloaded from the trailer, the patient should be moved to the designated examination area. The examiner needs a thermometer, a stethoscope, and a keen sense of observation to perform a thorough physical examination.

The typical colic examination should include assessment of pain, attitude, temperature, pulse, respiration, mucous membrane color, CRT, and GI motility. The degree of pain can be related to the severity of GI disease.

TECHNICIAN NOTE

Horses that are stoic can be very difficult to assess accurately, because the level of pain they exhibit may not reflect the severity of their disease.

Mild pain is recognized by pawing, stretching out—with or without attempts to urinate, curling the upper lip ("flehmen response"), or standing quietly without any desire to move or eat. Horses frequently respond to light sedation or mild exercise such as walking. Those with moderate pain can exhibit similar signs, but usually in combination with an elevated HR (>50 bpm). They may attempt to repeatedly lie down and stand up, and even occasionally roll while recumbent. Horses with moderate pain often remain comfortable for only short periods (<1 hour) or not at all, despite sedation. Severe abdominal pain manifests as a violent attempt by the animal to throw itself to the ground, inability to stand for short periods, constant rolling while down, and banging of the side of the head on the ground. Sedation may have no

Nasogastric (NG) Intubation
NG tube, two or more buckets, pump, towels, elastic or nonelastic adhesive tape, and 3-mL syringe case

Standard Blood Work
20-gauge needle, 12-mL syringe, and purple (ethylenediaminetetraacetic acid [EDTA]), red-top, and blue-top tubes

Sedation
Xylazine, detomidine, butorphanol, romifidine, and acepromazine

Intravenous (IV) Catheterization
14-gauge × 5¼-inch catheter or smaller (based on patient size), short extension with injection port, suture, normal saline flush, clippers, chlorhexidine or povidone-iodine scrub, 3 mL mepivacaine, examination gloves, and sterile gloves

Ultrasonography
Ultrasound machine, 70% isopropyl alcohol, ultrasound gel, and clippers

Rectal Examination
Palpation sleeve, water-soluble lubricant, towels, hyoscine butylbromide (if requested by the attending veterinarian), and lidocaine in a syringe with a long extension tubing connected (if requested by the attending veterinarian)

Abdominocentesis
Clippers, chlorhexidine or povidone-iodine scrub, 3 mL mepivacaine, examination gloves, sterile gloves, 18-gauge × 1.5-inch needles, teat cannula, metal bitch catheter, Tuohy needle, sterile 4 × 4-gauge sponges, #15 scalpel blade, purple-top tube with the EDTA shaken out, and red-top tube

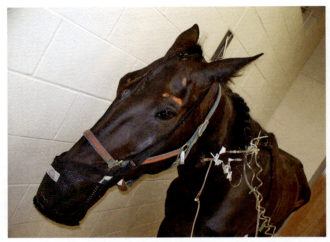

• **Fig. 25.46** Patients with colic can present with external trauma from pain. Note the periorbital swelling and abrasions.

effect, despite the type or amount. A history of severe pain before arrival is often confirmed by the presence of abrasions over the head, face, eyes, and bony prominences of the body (Fig. 25.46), as well as a large amount of dirt, hay, or mud in the haircoat.

TECHNICIAN NOTE
Abdominal distention can be difficult to assess in a large horse; therefore it is always important to question the owner regarding the horse's normal abdominal contour.

GI motility can be estimated by auscultation of the abdomen with a stethoscope, beginning in the paralumbar fossa and proceeding along the caudal edge of the costal margin toward the xiphoid on both sides of the abdomen. Sounds typically heard may be the result of increased intestinal motility ("borborygmi"). Normal increased intestinal motility is perceived as prolonged fluid rushing that occurs every 2 to 4 minutes. In addition, high-pitched tinkling sounds can be auscultated in the right paralumbar fossa every 2 to 4 minutes and are routinely associated with cecal motility. The complete absence of GI sounds in a patient with colic is always a significant finding. When GI sounds are documented in the record, it is common practice to record the auscultation by abdominal quadrant (upper right, upper left, lower right, and lower left) and by intensity of the sounds (absent, decreased, normal, or increased). Frequently, a very large volume of gas accumulates in the lumen of the bowel, severely stretching the walls of the large bowel and the cecum. To detect this accumulation, simultaneous auscultation and percussion of the abdomen is necessary. This is achieved by percussing or "flicking" the area of

the flank circumferentially around the head of the stethoscope and listening for a characteristic "ping."

TECHNICIAN NOTE
Various medications can alter heart rate (HR), respiratory rate (RR), attitude, degree of pain, and gastrointestinal (GI) motility; therefore it is always beneficial to assess these parameters before administration of medications.

Many colic workups include submission of blood for a complete blood count (CBC), biochemical profile, PCV, TP, lactate, and fibrinogen; therefore the necessary blood tubes should be available. After the physical examination and blood work, the complete colic workup may include the procedures described in detail next.

Nasogastric Intubation
Passage of a nasogastric tube is an extremely important and common procedure that may be performed by a veterinarian or an experienced veterinary technician. Horses will not typically vomit, and therefore excessive accumulation of gas or fluid within the stomach can lead to rupture if the gas or fluid is not removed. When very full, an engorged stomach can be the cause of pain, and removal of this fluid or gas can lead to temporary or permanent pain resolution. Usually, reflux of fluid or gas out of the nasogastric tube indicates that the horse is unable to pass fluid or air through the GI tract in an oral-to-aboral direction. Typically, the reason for this is a small intestinal functional disorder (ileus) or mechanical obstruction causing the ingesta to back up into the stomach, causing severe distention and pain. Excess fluid that is removed is termed *gastric reflux*, and the amount should be noted.

TECHNICIAN NOTE
Because of the severe consequences of gastric rupture, nasogastric intubation should be performed in all patients examined for abdominal pain.

Nasogastric tubes are available in a variety of sizes and materials (Table 25.3). In general, the size of the patient determines the size of the tube and, in very small horses, such as American Miniatures and foals, a stallion catheter can be used. To perform the procedure, the patient may need to be restrained with a twitch,

| TABLE 25.3 | Relative Sizes of Nasogastric Tubes Used in Equine Patients of Different Sizes | | |

TABLE 25.3 Relative Sizes of Nasogastric Tubes Used in Equine Patients of Different Sizes

Patient Size	OD, inches	ID, inches	Length, feet
Miniature horse	¼(6.4 mm)	⅛(3.2 mm)	5
Foal	⅜(9.5 mm)	¼(6.4 mm)	10
Yearling	⁷⁄₁₆(11 mm)	¼(6.4 mm)	12
Small horse	½(12.7 mm)	⁵⁄₁₆(7.9 mm)	12
Large horse	⅝(15.9 mm)	⅜(9.5 mm)	12
Extra-large horse	¾(19.1 mm)	½(12.7 mm)	10

ID, Inner diameter; *OD*, outer diameter.

sedated, or both. The smooth end of the tube is lubricated with water or a water-soluble lubricant and is passed through the nose, ventral meatus, and pharynx until the epiglottis is reached. Before it can be advanced farther, it must be ensured that the horse has swallowed to promote movement of the tube down the esophagus and into the stomach. Waiting for this to happen requires patience on the part of the operator. Once the tube is in the stomach, fluid or air may be readily evacuated, or it may be necessary to pump in 1 to 2 liters of water to create a siphon effect that will promote emptying. Evacuation of stomach contents in this fashion should continue until the stomach is sufficiently empty. The total amount of water that was introduced to create the siphon should be subtracted from the total amount of gastric reflux; the result is considered the net amount of reflux and should be recorded. If no reflux is obtained, introduction of various therapeutic agents (e.g., mineral oil, water, electrolytes) may be indicated. The normal stomach contents are light green to yellow, may be foamy, have minimal odor, and usually are less than 2 L in volume. If greater than 2 L of reflux is obtained, the tube may be left in place and secured for future attempts at fluid retrieval.

TECHNICIAN NOTE

Epistaxis (nosebleed) is a common occurrence after removal or passage of a nasogastric tube. This is rarely a serious complication and generally resolves within minutes.

Abdominal Palpation per Rectum

It can be very difficult to identify the cause of colic based on the physical examination and nasogastric intubation alone; therefore rectal palpation is performed by a veterinarian to identify what section of the GI tract, if any, is responsible for colic signs. Major questions to answer during a rectal examination include the following: (1) Are the normally palpable structures in the correct location? (2) Is an abnormal amount of gas distention noted? (3) Is the small intestine distended and palpable? (4) Is a palpable impaction present in the colon, cecum, or ileum? (5) Are any masses present in the abdominal cavity or in surrounding organs? (6) Is the bowel located in the inguinal rings?

Rectal tears are, by far, the most serious complication of rectal examination, and they can be life-threatening. To minimize the risk for this complication, the horse should be restrained, ideally in a standing stock whenever possible and sedated and/or twitched whenever necessary. A plastic rectal sleeve is used to protect the veterinarian's arm from fecal contamination, and copious amounts of water-soluble lubricant are essential. For horses that strain, hyoscine butyl bromide can be administered intravenously, or 2% lidocaine can be administered intrarectally or, less frequently, by caudal epidural injection to relax the GI tract. Upon completion of the examination, it is important to examine the sleeve for evidence of blood.

TECHNICIAN NOTE

Rectal examination of a patient with colic should be performed only by a veterinarian and on a horse that is adequately restrained.

Abdominal Ultrasonography

Because of the size of the horse, it is impossible to evaluate the entire abdomen by rectal palpation. Therefore when it is available, transabdominal ultrasonography can be a valuable tool for performing a more thorough evaluation. It may be necessary to clip long or thick hair to obtain an acceptable image; however, efforts should first be made to obtain an image by saturating the hair and skin with isopropyl alcohol. The best images are obtained with probes that are 2.5 to 10 megahertz (MHz) in frequency.

Common abnormalities that can be identified by transabdominal ultrasonography include distention of the small and large intestines, increased wall thickness of GI viscera, and abnormal motility of specific portions of the GI tract. Transabdominal ultrasonography can also be used to assess the appearance of the kidneys, liver, spleen, and reproductive tract and to determine the amount and appearance of abdominal fluid. It is important to remember that thoracic problems can lead to signs of colic; therefore the chest should also be examined for abnormalities, such as diaphragmatic hernia, pneumonia, pleural fluid, or neoplasia.

Abdominocentesis

An *abdominocentesis*, or a "belly tap," evaluates the abdominal fluid, which bathes the GI tract, and is a very important method of assessing the health of the bowel. The abdominal cavity should be a sterile environment, although this can change in the presence of devitalized or ruptured bowel. Therefore it is essential to maintain aseptic technique when performing a belly tap. A 10 × 10-cm area of the most dependent part of the abdomen, usually centered 3 to 5 cm caudal to the xiphoid and 3 to 5 cm to the right of the midline, is clipped. The area is cleaned with an initial surgical prep, followed by a sterile surgical prep, and is then blocked with 2 to 5 mL of 2% lidocaine infused into the skin and subcutaneous tissues at the intended site for centesis. A variety of instruments, such as needles and teat cannulas, may be used to collect abdominal fluid. Once the abdomen has been entered, the fluid should be allowed to drip into purple-top (ethylenediaminetetraacetic acid [EDTA]) and red-top tubes. The fluid is examined visually for color and clarity. Additional information may be obtained by measuring TP, glucose, and lactate and by submitting a sample to the laboratory for cell count, cytologic examination, Gram staining, and culture. Normal peritoneal fluid values are listed in Table 25.4.

Abdominal Radiography

Although not a standard diagnostic procedure for most colic examinations, radiography can be valuable for diagnosing a few specific conditions. Generally, images of the abdomen reveal

<table>
<tr><td colspan="3">**TABLE 25.4**   **Normal Peritoneal Fluid Values**</td></tr>
<tr><td>**Gross Appearance**</td><td>**Cellularity**</td><td>**Molecular Components**</td></tr>
<tr><td>Clear or straw/ yellow colored</td><td>WBC ≤5000 cells/μL ≈50% neutrophils</td><td>TP ≤2.5 g/dL Lactate ≤ 2.0 mmol/ dL Glucose >50 mg/ dL OR <50 mg/ dL difference from blood glucose pH >7.3</td></tr>
</table>

dL, Deciliter; *μL,* microliter; *mmol,* millimole; *TP,* total protein; *WBC,* white blood cell.

low detail because of the large size of a horse's abdomen and the limited ability of the equipment to produce enough radiation to create highly detailed images. It is important to remember that images of the abdomen require a lot of radiation, so personnel should be fully protected to minimize exposure. Radiography is most useful for identifying enteroliths (stones within the GI tract) and sand accumulation, for examining foals and small horses such as American Miniature Horses (in which a rectal examination is not possible), and for performing contrast studies to identify gastric emptying delay.

Specific Conditions

The goal of the examination and diagnostic testing is to decide on a diagnosis and formulate an effective therapeutic plan. Unfortunately, an absolute diagnosis is not always possible after a workup; however, appropriate management of the condition is necessary. To help formulate a plan in the absence of a diagnosis, it is important to have an idea of common conditions affecting each part of the GI tract. Box 25.6 lists common conditions that affect each section of bowel. It is important to remember that each condition may be associated, to some degree, with the region of the country the horse is in, the age and breed of the horse, the diet and function of the horse (broodmare, racehorse, etc.), and its medical history.

Abdominal Exploration

After examination and workup, surgical intervention may be necessary. When a preoperative diagnosis is accurate, abdominal exploratory surgery is undertaken for therapeutic purposes; however, most colic surgeries are the final and most invasive diagnostic step and are also therapeutic. When this occurs, it is important to remain efficient, because the patient will require preoperative preparation to minimize anesthetic time and to increase the likelihood of a positive outcome. In all cases, an IV catheter should be placed, through which perioperative antibiotics, fluids, anti-inflammatories, sedatives, and anesthetic induction drugs can be administered.

TECHNICIAN NOTE

The most common reason for surgical intervention in the patient with colic is continual pain despite sedation.

If it is safe to do so, the ventral abdomen should be clipped from the xiphoid to the inguinal region and from flank to flank,

---

• BOX 25.6   **Common Conditions of the Gastrointestinal Tract**

- Esophagus
  - Obstruction (choke)
- Stomach
  - Impaction
  - Ulceration
  - Neoplasia
- Small intestine
  - Intraluminal obstruction
    - Ascarid impaction
    - Intussusception
    - Ileal impaction
  - Extraluminal obstruction
    - Lipoma
    - Herniation
    - Epiploic foramen entrapment
    - Scrotal hernia
    - Umbilical hernia
    - Mesenteric rent
    - Congenital abnormality
    - Diaphragmatic hernia
- Volvulus
- Ileus
  - Duodenitis/proximal jejunitis
- Large intestine
  - Intraluminal obstruction
    - Cecal impaction
    - Large colon impaction
    - Small colon impaction
    - Cecocolic intussusception
    - Enterolithiasis
  - Extraluminal obstruction
    - Large colon displacement
    - Large colon volvulus
- Ileus
  - Right dorsal colitis
  - Salmonellosis

---

and an initial surgical prep should be performed to remove all gross contamination. The hooves should be picked out and debris removed. Once the patient is anesthetized, a final touchup of the clipping and another initial scrub can be performed. When the patient is in the final location for surgery, a final surgical prep should be performed, using chlorhexidine or povidone-iodine scrub. See Case Presentation 25.2 for an example of emergency management of a horse with colic.

Respiratory Tract

The primary purpose of the respiratory tract is delivery of oxygen to tissues and cells and elimination of carbon dioxide. Failure of oxygen exchange can lead to respiratory distress, which is an emergency. Most commonly, but not exclusively, respiratory emergencies present as the result of an inability of oxygen to diffuse across the alveoli because of lung disease (e.g., pneumonia), inability of the lungs to expand enough to take in sufficient oxygen (e.g., because of pneumothorax), or inability of oxygen to reach the lungs (e.g., because of upper airway obstruction or bronchoconstriction). It is important to remember that a horse can present with respiratory distress or, to a lesser degree, tachypnea if it is unable to deliver oxygen to the tissues (e.g., because of anemia).

CASE PRESENTATION 25.2

Emergency Management of an Equine Patient With Colic

History and Signalment

A 14-year-old Thoroughbred gelding was presented with a 2-hour history of signs of colic. A feed change to coastal Bermuda hay was made 3 days prior to the onset of signs of colic. No significant findings were identified by the referring veterinarian, and the horse was referred for further workup because of persistent signs of colic. Before referral, the horse received 150 mg of xylazine and 500 mg of flunixin meglumine intravenously and had a nasogastric tube passed to evaluate stomach contents and volume. No nasogastric reflux was obtained.

Initial Physical Examination

Upon presentation, the horse was found to be colicky, which included signs of stretching out and wanting to lie down. His jugular refill and pulse quality were normal. His temperature was 100°F/37.8°C (normal 98.5°F [36.9°C] to 100.5°F [38.1°C]), pulse rate was 52 beats per minute (bpm) (normal 28–40 bpm), respiratory rate was 12 bpm (normal 8–18 bpm), and breath sounds were present in all lung fields. Mucous membranes were pink and moist, and capillary refill time (CRT) was 2 seconds. Weight was estimated to be approximately 1000 lb (454 kg). Gastrointestinal sounds were absent. The horse's ears and extremities were warm to the touch. After the physical examination, 150 mg of xylazine was given intravenously.

Diagnostic Workup

Results of complete blood count (CBC) and chemistry profile revealed a mildly elevated packed cell volume (PCV) (42%; normal 28%–40%), mildly elevated total protein (TP) (7.7 g/dL; normal 5.5–7.5 g/dL), normal total white blood cell count (WBC) (7900 cells/μL; normal 4700–10,600 cell/μL) with normal differential, normal creatinine (1.4 mg/dL; normal 0.3–1.8 mg/dL), and mildly elevated lactate (2.1 mmol/L; normal <2.5 mmol/L).

A nasogastric tube was passed, and 4 liters of net reflux were obtained. Upon transrectal palpation, multiple loops of distended small intestine were felt. Transabdominal ultrasonography revealed multiple loops of a motile, distended small intestine, with a normal wall thickness of 3 to 4 mm. A pocket of peritoneal fluid was observed, and abdominocentesis was performed to evaluate the fluid. The fluid was cloudy and straw colored (pale yellow), with a normal total WBC (1300 cells/μL; normal <5000 cells/μL), elevated TP (3.1 mg/dL; normal<2.5 mg/dL), and normal lactate (1.6 mmol/L; normal <2.5 mmol/L).

Therapeutic Intervention

Upon completion of the physical examination and colic-related diagnostics, an intravenous (IV) catheter was placed in the left jugular vein. The presumptive diagnosis was a nonstrangulating obstruction of the small intestine. Medical management was attempted, but the colic persisted despite sedation. Therefore surgical exploration was recommended and accepted by the owner. The horse was given a preoperative dose of antibiotics (IV potassium penicillin and gentamicin). The horse was then sedated, anesthetized, and placed in dorsal recumbency for a ventral midline laparotomy. The ventral abdomen was aseptically prepared and draped in routine fashion. Upon exploration of the abdomen, an ileal impaction was identified and pushed into the cecum. The jejunum oral to the impaction was distended and fluid filled. This fluid was decompressed into the cecum. Evaluation of the remainder of the abdomen revealed no other abnormalities. The horse recovered from anesthesia without incident. Over the next 24 hours, the patient produced approximately 2 L/hour of reflux, which was removed via an indwelling nasogastric tube. The patient was maintained on maintenance IV fluids, and all lost fluid was replaced parenterally. The patient continued to receive potassium penicillin and gentamicin, as well as flunixin meglumine intravenously, for 5 days. Postoperatively, after 48 hours, water was introduced, followed by a gradual increase in food on days three to five. By day six, the patient was on free-choice timothy hay, and all medications were discontinued.

Outcome

The horse was discharged 7 days after admission, and the owners were instructed to keep him on stall rest, with hand walking/grazing for 1 month, followed by another month of small paddock turnout. Two months following surgery, the patient resumed normal pasture turnout and returned to exercise after 3 months. This case illustrates how a rapid, efficient, and coordinated response to this life-threatening emergency by an organized, prepared, and thoughtful veterinary team in the field and at the referral hospital resulted in a positive outcome for both the patient and its owner.

When a patient presents with respiratory distress, it is important to quickly identify the cause. The most efficient way to do this is to divide respiratory emergencies into two broad categories: upper airway and lower airway emergencies.

Upper respiratory tract emergencies are among the most common types of respiratory emergencies. They are almost always the result of obstruction of airflow to the lungs and typically present with severe distress, anxiety, and a loud noise on inspiration (inspiratory stridor). In contrast, conditions of the lower respiratory tract are usually caused by lung disease (pneumonia or asthma) or failure to inflate the lungs (caused by pneumothorax). Pneumonia is characterized by the presence of abnormal lung sounds, including crackles and wheezes, and asthma is characterized by rapid, shallow breaths, expiratory stridor, and abnormal lung sounds. Pneumothorax is often secondary to external trauma to the chest cavity that allows influx of air into the pleural space, which collapses the lung and prevents re-expansion. A patient with this condition will present with rapid, shallow breathing and expiratory stridor; however, lung sounds will be absent. It is important to remember that severe pneumonia can lead to pleuropneumonia, and severe external trauma can lead to thoracic bleeding. Both conditions can cause accumulation of fluid in the chest cavity and can present like a pneumothorax.

> ### TECHNICIAN NOTE
> The mediastinum of the horse is incomplete, so a pneumothorax can be bilateral; however, in many horses, the mediastinum becomes imperforate, and the pneumothorax is unilateral. Consequently, it is important to evaluate both sides of the chest and to never assume that the condition is unilateral.

General Physical Examination

A respiratory emergency is readily identifiable, even at a distance from the patient, because the most common signs of respiratory distress include an increased RR (tachypnea), flaring of the nostrils, exaggerated thoracic or abdominal movements, inspiratory or expiratory noise (stridor), and blue to pale blue coloration of the mucous membranes (cyanosis). Affected horses are frequently anxious, panicky, weak, depressed, sick, or reluctant to move the body or chest because of pain. Horses in severe respiratory distress, especially that resulting from upper airway obstruction, may be so anxious or hypoxic or in so much pain that they may be uncontrollable, unpredictable, and at risk for sudden death. Therefore it is essential that the veterinarian and the veterinary technician secure the environment and maintain the safety of clients, staff, themselves, and, whenever possible, the patient.

Oxygen is vital to life, and the absence of it, even for brief moments, can be devastating. Therefore the respiratory examination should be conducted with great efficiency and careful preparation. For all respiratory emergencies, oxygen, supplies for a temporary tracheotomy, and an IV catheter should be prepared and ready. If the patient is in severe respiratory distress because of an upper airway obstruction, a temporary tracheotomy should be performed immediately before the physical examination. Once the patient's condition is stable, a thorough physical examination should be performed. Auscultation of the lungs and trachea is extremely important for differentiating between upper and lower airway disease and for characterizing the severity of the disease. Examination of mucous membranes for color is very important, because cyanotic (blue) membranes provide a tremendous amount of insight into the degree of hypoxia. As with any physical examination of a horse, evaluation of HR, temperature, and GI sounds is very important.

Once an airway has been secured and the physical examination is complete, it is important to perform diagnostics to find and correct the cause of the distress. It is important to remember that the patient may be systemically unstable and may need oxygen therapy during the diagnostic procedures, or more time may be needed to stabilize the patient before diagnostic tests are performed. If the patient has been stabilized and is amenable to testing, the diagnostics described next are the most common and valuable tests for finding the source of the disease.

Thoracic Ultrasonography

Ultrasonography is a noninvasive method of evaluating the thoracic cavity. When transthoracic ultrasonography is performed, it is important to saturate the patient's hair with isopropyl alcohol or to clip the hair and apply gel to obtain an acceptable image. The best images are obtained with probes that are 2.5 to 10 MHz in frequency. Thoracic ultrasonography can be used to evaluate the amount and appearance of the pleural fluid, the serosal surface of the lungs, and, in diseased lungs that are not properly aerated, the deeper parenchyma. Common abnormalities that can be identified include pneumonia, pleuropneumonia, lung abscesses and tumors, and the presence of fluid or air in the pleural space.

> **TECHNICIAN NOTE**
>
> It is important to remember that thoracic problems can lead to signs of colic as well as respiratory distress. Therefore patients with colic should have a thoracic ultrasound examination performed to rule out diaphragmatic hernia, pneumothorax, and pleuropneumonia.

Radiography

Radiography of the head and neck can help identify pharyngeal swelling, tracheal swelling or compression, foreign bodies, or guttural pouch abnormalities leading to an upper airway obstruction (Fig. 25.47). Thoracic radiography is excellent for identifying a collapsed lung, pleural fluid, pneumonia, equine asthma, abscesses, neoplasia, and pulmonary edema.

Upper and Lower Airway Endoscopy

Endoscopic evaluation of the upper airway is an invaluable diagnostic tool when an upper airway obstruction is suspected. The nasal meatus, pharynx, and guttural pouches can be visualized for evidence of swelling, mass-occupying lesions (neoplasia, abscesses, etc.), and foreign bodies. This is also an excellent opportunity to identify the size of the opening to the trachea and to assess whether a tracheotomy tube should be placed in patients that are not yet in

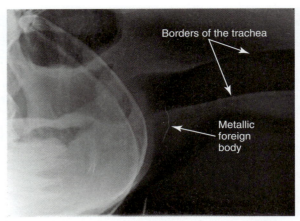

• **Fig. 25.47** Radiography can be an excellent method for identifying upper airway foreign bodies. Note the linear metallic foreign body located in the proximal trachea.

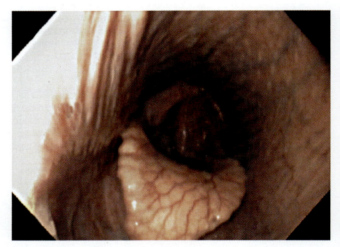

• **Fig. 25.48** Patients in respiratory distress can present with an upper airway obstruction. Note the marked decrease in the size of the opening of the trachea.

respiratory distress but are certainly in danger (Fig. 25.48). After a complete examination of the pharynx and the upper airway has been performed, the endoscope can be moved into the trachea to the bifurcation of the bronchi. This area should be evaluated for swelling or thickening, which can occur with severe asthma or bronchitis. As the endoscope is slowly removed, the trachea can be evaluated for swelling or compression, increased or abnormal secretions or discharge, and laceration of the tracheal mucosa.

Thoracocentesis

Horses with lower airway conditions that limit expansion of the lungs, such as pneumothorax or pleural effusion, need the pleural space reduced to its normal volume. This can be done through a procedure known as *thoracocentesis*, or "chest tap." This is a potentially life-saving procedure in which the pleural cavity is entered with a needle, catheter, teat cannula, or large chest tube. As with abdominocentesis, thoracocentesis must be performed aseptically. The location for thoracocentesis is very important and is based on the need to remove pleural fluid or air.

For removal of pleural fluid, ultrasound guidance is most helpful to identify an area of the thorax that has a large amount of effusion (typically, a ventral, dependent area). With the horse properly

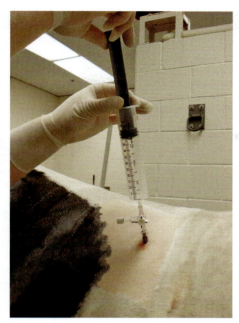

• **Fig. 25.49** Example of a teat cannula, a three-way stopcock, and syringe evacuation of air from a pneumothorax.

sedated and restrained, the area in which the centesis will be performed should be clipped and aseptically prepared. The skin, subcutaneous tissue, and intercostal muscle should be blocked with 10 to 20 mL of mepivacaine. The vein-artery-nerve complex is located along the caudal aspect of each rib; therefore a stab incision into the skin should be made with a #10 or a #15 scalpel blade along the cranial aspect of the rib. The desired instrument should then be placed through the stab incision and intercostal muscle and into the pleural space. For removal of air from the pleural space, this procedure is identical, except that the incision generally is made dorsally between the 12th and 15th ribs (because air rises to this location).

Temporary evacuation of fluid or air can be accomplished using the teat cannula, IV catheter, or needle. Because of the risk of introducing air into the chest cavity, evacuation should be performed with a three-way stopcock and syringe with active suction for correction of a pneumothorax, or with a one-way valve (i.e., Heimlich valve) for removal of pleural effusion (Fig. 25.49).

TECHNICIAN NOTE

If pneumothorax is the result of a laceration of the thoracic wall, the wound should be repaired or sealed before and along with evacuation of the air to restore negative intrathoracic pressure.

If it is necessary for fluid to be evacuated continuously or over a prolonged time, a chest tube can be placed and sutured into position with a one-way valve secured in place. As would be expected, patients should be monitored very closely for respiratory distress because of possible recurrence of pleural effusion or pneumothorax. Patients with indwelling chest tubes should have these tubes regularly checked to ensure patency and to confirm that the valve is in place and functional.

Transtracheal Wash

If a diagnosis of pneumonia is made, it may be necessary to obtain a bacterial culture and cytologic preparation of respiratory secretions before antimicrobial therapy is started. This is best performed with a transtracheal wash (TTW). To perform a TTW, the skin over the cranial one-third of the trachea should be clipped and aseptically prepared. A site located in the middle of this clipped area, directly on midline and between the tracheal rings, should be identified. The skin and subcutaneous tissue at this site should be anesthetized with 3 to 5 mL of mepivacaine, and a stab incision made through the skin with a #15 blade. A sharp trocar with a sleeve is placed into the trachea between two cartilaginous rings, and the trocar is removed. A TTW tube is passed through the sleeve and down into the trachea. Approximately 20 to 30 mL of sterile saline is injected into the tube and allowed to flow into the trachea. This fluid is then collected via the tubing with a new syringe, and the sample is submitted for cytologic examination and culture. The tube is then removed, and a small amount of antimicrobial can be injected into the sleeve and subcutaneous opening as the sleeve is removed.

Oxygen Administration

Oxygen supplementation can be beneficial for patients suffering from any respiratory tract disease that leads to a decrease in blood oxygen content. Blood oxygen is most accurately determined by measuring PaO_2 through blood gas analysis. Patients with a PaO_2 of less than 100 mmHg should receive oxygen supplementation, although in patients with a PaO_2 less than 60 mmHg, the need is especially critical. When a blood gas analysis is not readily available, HR, RR, mucous membrane color, and lactate concentration can be evaluated. In patients in which oxygen intake by the lungs is adequate, but delivery to or uptake by the tissues is inadequate (e.g., anemia), oxygen supplementation will have only a very modest benefit, because the oxygen-carrying capacity of RBCs is likely fully saturated.

To supplement a patient with oxygen, three items are needed: (1) an oxygen source, (2) a method of measuring and regulating the amount to be given, and (3) a means of oxygen delivery. The rate of oxygen flows a patient needs is dependent on its size and the degree of hypoxia. Adults may need at least 15 L/minute for effective therapy; smaller patients, such as foals and American Miniature Horses, may require as little as 5 L/minute.

It is important to remember that the oxygen that comes out of the tank is dry, unlike the ambient oxygen we breathe. Therefore to avoid drying out respiratory mucous membranes, a bubble humidifier is attached to the oxygen delivery tubing (Fig. 25.50).

Unless anesthetized, oxygen typically is delivered passively via a nasal cannula with multiple small fenestrations. The tip of the cannula is positioned in the nasopharynx and secured to the halter or is sutured to the skin of the nostrils by placing adhesive tape in a "butterfly pattern" over the cannula and suturing the tape to the skin. To determine the approximate distance to the nasopharynx, the cannula is measured from the opening of the nares to the medial canthus of the eye. Oxygen delivery tubing is then used to connect the oxygen source at the bubble humidifier to the nasal cannula. This tubing usually is long, and it is typically hung from a position above the stall, such as a fluid hook.

Tracheotomy

A temporary tracheotomy is essential for relieving respiratory distress caused by an upper airway obstruction. This procedure is frequently life-saving, and it is one that all veterinary professionals must be familiar with. When it is performed on the standing and awake patient, sedation and restraint should be used, *if possible*, without compromising the patient. The most used and desirable location for the tracheotomy is along the ventral midline of the neck, where the trachea can be clearly identified and isolated under the skin and

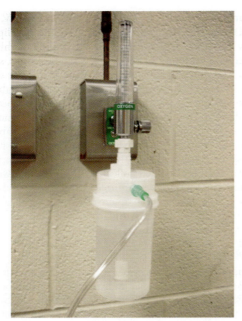

• **Fig. 25.50** Oxygen source, flow meter, bubble humidifier, and outflow tubing.

subcutaneous tissue, typically between the cranial and middle third of the neck. If time permits, this area should be clipped, aseptically prepared, and infiltrated with 10 to 20 mL of lidocaine or mepivacaine.

It must always be remembered that horses in severe respiratory distress can be unpredictable and dangerous. When such situations arise, a tracheotomy may have to be performed without clipping, aseptic preparation, local analgesia, sedation, or even much restraint. An exit strategy should always be maintained, the number of people near the patient should be minimized, and personnel should proceed with caution, speed, and efficiency.

> **TECHNICIAN NOTE**
>
> A tracheotomy is a life-saving procedure that should be familiar to all veterinarians and technicians.

The choice of a tracheotomy tube may vary considerably from patient to patient and is based on personal preference. Several different sizes and styles of silicone or stainless steel tubes are available. The size of the tube is dictated by the size of the patient, but generally, the largest possible tube that will not cause damage to the tracheal rings should be placed. Indwelling tracheotomy tubes can induce production of a variable amount of mucus and discharge that can clog the tube, causing recurrence of respiratory distress if the tube is not regularly cleaned and maintained. Therefore close attention to tube maintenance is paramount. The tube should be cleaned as necessary (which may be as frequently as two to four times a day) and should remain in place until the source of the upper airway obstruction has been resolved. Once the condition has resolved, the tube can be removed, and the tracheotomy incision left to heal by secondary intention.

Musculoskeletal System

Musculoskeletal injuries, such as fractures, lacerations, infections (of the joint, soft tissue, or foot), and luxation, are common emergencies in equine medicine. Because of the size and temperament

> • **BOX 25.7** **Guidelines for Fracture Stabilization**
>
> 1. Stabilize the patient and control hemorrhage.
> 2. Relieve pain and anxiety.
> 3. Control wound infection.
> 4. Prevent neurovascular trauma.
> 5. Prevent trauma to muscle and skin adjacent to fracture site.
> 6. Minimize trauma to fractured bone ends.

of horses, these injuries, especially fractures, can be severe and life-threatening. When these injuries are identified, immediate veterinary attention to the injury is essential for maximizing the chance of a positive outcome. Diagnosing an orthopedic injury, although not always easy, is typically straightforward in an emergent situation. This fact is especially true when the injury involves the *distal limb*, which is defined as any area below the carpus or the tarsus, because of the minimal amount of soft tissue covering this area. In general, the extent of the procedures necessary to diagnose most injuries is limited to physical examination, radiography, ultrasonography, and arthrocentesis.

Fractures

Like many acute and severe injuries in horses, bone fractures can cause great distress and pain. It is always important to perform a general assessment of the horse first to ensure that it is stable and to control the environment. Controlling the environment usually means calming the horse, often with sedation, and minimizing the number of people involved and at risk. It is important to remember that it may be very difficult to adequately sedate a horse that has a large sympathetic surge (e.g., a racehorse). It is also important to remember that it is possible to oversedate this type of patient and worsen the injury, owing to increased weight bearing. Therefore an experienced and conscientious team is important for managing equine fractures. Once the horse and the environment have been secured, a swift and accurate assessment of the injured limb should commence. Accurate identification of the region of injury should lead to one of two scenarios. If radiography equipment is readily available and can be used without having to move the horse, radiographs can be taken to accurately evaluate the injury before transport. If this is not the case, the limb should be stabilized based on the region of suspected injury. Goals of stabilization should be to decrease pain, minimize or eliminate further injury, minimize damage to soft tissues and vasculature, minimize swelling, and enable some degree of weight bearing. Box 25.7 outlines important steps in the first aid of a fracture. The next sections detail recommended fracture stabilization techniques for achieving these goals.

> **TECHNICIAN NOTE**
>
> Appropriate fracture stabilization and immediate medical attention are the most important ways to maximize the likelihood of a successful outcome.

Distal Forelimb Fracture

This region includes the distal metacarpus, proximal and middle phalanges, and sesamoid bones. The goal of stabilizing this area is to align the bony column and protect the soft tissues of the fetlock and the pastern from excessive compression. A bandage of moderate thickness is applied from the coronary band to the proximal metacarpus. A rigid splint (PVC, wood, etc.) is then secured to the dorsal aspect of the limb with nonelastic tape and is extended all the way to the ground to include the foot. A commercially

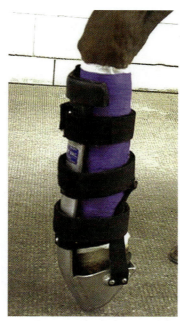

• **Fig. 25.51** Kimzey Leg Saver splint applied to the distal limb of a horse with a fracture.

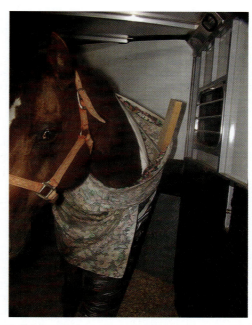

• **Fig. 25.52** Full-limb Robert Jones bandage with a caudal and lateral splint extending to the withers for transport of a patient with a suspected distal radial fracture.

available splint called the *Kimzey Leg Saver* (Kimzey, Inc., Woodland, CA) is an acceptable alternative (Fig. 25.51). This form of external coaptation is acceptable for fracture of the bones as well as for luxation of the fetlock joint, laceration of the flexor tendons, and disruption of the suspensory apparatus because of fracture through both proximal sesamoid bones.

Distal to Mid-forelimb Fracture

This region includes the mid- to proximal metacarpus and carpus. The goal of stabilizing this area is to align the bony column and prevent the lower limb from moving. A bandage is applied from the coronary band to the highest point of the elbow. This bandage can be a modified Robert Jones bandage, which is composed of multiple layers of sheet cotton or similar material compressed by gauze. A caudal splint, extending from the ground to the point of the elbow, is secured with nonelastic tape. A second splint is secured laterally, again from the ground to the point of the elbow. This form of external coaptation is commonly used for mid- to proximal metacarpal fractures.

Mid-forelimb Fracture

This region includes the radius and the elbow. The goal of stabilization is to realign the bony column and prevent movement of the radius in any direction, especially abduction. Bandaging and stabilization are the same as those described previously for fractures of the mid- to proximal metacarpus, except that the lateral splint should be long enough to traverse from the ground, across the shoulder joint, and to the proximal margin of the scapula. The most proximal portion of this splint should be secured by wrapping bandage material around the neck and chest, between the forelimbs, over the withers, and under the girth in a "figure-of-eight" pattern (Fig. 25.52). This form of external coaptation is commonly used for radial fractures.

Elbow Fracture

If the patient can extend, plant, and move the limb, splint stabilization is not necessary. With some olecranon fractures, the triceps

apparatus is disrupted, and the patient is unable to extend and fix the leg. In these cases, the goal of stabilization is to lock or fix the carpus in extension. A bandage of medium thickness is applied from the coronary band to the highest point of the elbow, and a caudal splint extending from the ground to the point of the elbow is secured with nonelastic tape.

Proximal Forelimb Fracture

This region includes the humerus and the scapula. It has a large amount of muscle mass and cannot be properly stabilized, so no attempt at stabilization should be made. The only exception is the case of a distal humeral fracture in which the triceps apparatus has been compromised. In these scenarios, a light bandage with caudal splint can be applied to lock the carpus in extension.

Distal Hind Limb Fracture

The distal hind limb can be stabilized as per the previously described distal forelimb fracture, except that the rigid splint is applied along the plantar aspect of the limb. A Kimzey Leg Saver is an acceptable alternative.

Distal to Mid-Hind Limb Fracture

This region includes the mid- to proximal metatarsus. Fractures in this region are treated as described for the forelimb, except that a moderate bandage is placed, and a plantar splint is applied up to the point of the calcaneus (proximal extent of tarsus).

Mid-Hind Limb Fracture

This region includes the tarsus, tibia, and stifle. The goal of stabilization is to realign the bony column and prevent collapse and movement of the bones. A modified Robert Jones bandage is placed from the coronary band to the stifle. A lateral splint extending from the ground to the hip is secured with nonelastic tape. The most proximal end of the splint is secured by wrapping bandage material over the hip, between the hind limbs, under the flank, and over the lumbar spine in a "figure-of-eight" pattern. This form of external coaptation is commonly used for tibial fractures.

Proximal Hind Limb Fracture

This region includes the femur and the pelvis. Because the area is heavily muscled, further stabilization is not possible and is contraindicated, because it could further increase trauma to the fracture site.

Soft Tissue Injury

All other musculoskeletal injuries commonly seen in the horse involve the soft tissues in some fashion. These injuries are usually visible (e.g., lacerations); however, their extent can be misleading because punctures, abscesses, or tendon injuries may also be present. The remainder of this section discusses common soft tissue injuries encountered as emergencies.

Wounds

Lacerations and punctures can occur on any part of the body but are most frequent on the distal limb. These injuries usually result from contact with loose metal, wire, wood, or other horses. Because of the minimal soft tissue covering of the distal limb, minor skin wounds can become life-threatening events when joints, tendon sheaths, or vessels are involved; therefore all wounds should be evaluated with the idea that the injury could be worse than it appears. Initial triage and evaluation of soft tissue injuries can have a profound influence on the prognosis of the patient.

General Examination

Initial examination should include a general assessment of the patient, with particular attention to blood loss. The vein-artery-nerve complex of the distal limb is very superficial and is commonly involved. Blood loss can be very difficult or impossible to accurately quantify; therefore HR, RR, mucous membrane color, PCV, TP, and lactate levels are important factors to evaluate. If ongoing hemorrhage is occurring, it is vital that an attempt is made to slow or stop it. When advising the owner over the phone or when working in the field with limited supplies available, ordinary materials, such as towels wrapped tightly over the wound and secured with duct tape, can be effective. It is likely that a bandage of this type will become soaked quickly with blood; however, leaving it in place may allow a clot to form and may slow the hemorrhage (although the clot may be unstable). If the limb is still bleeding upon presentation to the veterinary medical staff, hemostatic forceps (Kelly or mosquito) may be used to isolate and ligate the vessel. Following hemostasis, the physical examination, and stabilization of the patient, a more thorough evaluation of the limb should be performed. A description of this evaluation is provided in Chapter 27.

The size of the area clipped depends on the location of the wound. If a synovial structure (joint or tendon sheath) is clearly not involved, only the wound needs to be clipped. If there is any possibility that the wound (a laceration or puncture) could involve a joint or tendon sheath, the area should be clipped widely and circumferentially.

Arthrocentesis

For injuries suspected of synovial involvement, a site away from the wound that allows needle access to the suspected joint or sheath should be identified and aseptically prepared. The introduction of a needle into a joint is called *arthrocentesis*, or "joint tap." This procedure should be performed by a veterinarian, because many possible sites are unique to each synovial structure. Depending on

TABLE 25.5	Normal Synovial Fluid Values	
Gross Appearance	Cellularity	Molecular Components
Clear or straw/ yellow colored, viscous	WBC ≤500 cells/μL ≈10% neutrophils	TP ≤2.5 g/dL Lactate ≤2.0 mmol/dL Glucose >50 mg/ dL OR <50 mg/ dL difference from blood glucose pH >7.3

dL, Deciliter; *μL,* microliter; *mmol,* millimole; *TP,* total protein; *WBC,* white blood cell.

the structure that is to be entered, an 18- or 20-gauge, 1.5-inch needle is introduced under sterile conditions after the skin overlying the tap site is aseptically prepared. Once the structure has been entered, a small volume of synovial fluid should be obtained (1–3 mL), evaluated for color and viscosity, and placed into a purple-top (EDTA) tube for cytologic examination and lactate, glucose, and TP evaluation. Normal values for joint fluid are listed in Table 25.5. Extra fluid can be obtained for bacterial culture; however, this infrequently yields bacterial growth and is not commonly useful.

> **TECHNICIAN NOTE**
>
> When arthrocentesis is performed, the needle should *never* be introduced through a wound. A site distant from the wound should *always* be used to assess the integrity and involvement of a synovial structure. Synovial structures are easily contaminated and may become infected.

After the synovial fluid sample is obtained, sterile isotonic fluids should be injected into the synovial structure, and an assistant should evaluate the wound for evidence of leakage of saline from the synovial structure; this would indicate communication of the wound with the joint or tendon sheath. If the synovial structure distends with saline and nothing exits the wound, it is likely (but not guaranteed) that the structure is not involved. Excess fluid should be evacuated, and a small amount of antibiotic may be injected into the joint before the needle is removed. If it is determined that the synovial structure is involved, the owner should be informed that a more aggressive approach may be necessary that would involve lavage of the joint and prolonged use of antibiotics (regionally and/or systemically). These cases are often associated with a potentially worse prognosis and increased cost. If it was clear that the synovial structure was not involved, the workup should focus on the wound.

Wound Management

Once the surrounding skin has been clipped and evaluated, the wound can be cleaned and managed as described in Chapter 27.

> **TECHNICIAN NOTE**
>
> Wounds, especially deep ones, should not be lavaged with saline under pressure until it has been ensured that a synovial structure is not involved.

Radiography

Radiographic evaluation of the wound provides the best assessment of bony structure involvement. More specifically, radiography can be used to detect early hairline fractures, fractures of the small bones (e.g., splint bones), or foreign bodies (e.g., metal or gravel), and to evaluate the risk of developing a bone sequestrum.

TECHNICIAN NOTE

A *sequestrum* is a nonviable segment of bone that acts as a foreign body and frequently prevents full wound healing until it is removed.

Ultrasonography

Ultrasonography is helpful for evaluating the structure of tendons and ligaments and for identifying foreign bodies without mineral content (e.g., glass, wood, other organic matter). Portable ultrasonography machines are sufficiently powerful to be used in the field for evaluation of most distal limb injuries.

Wound Closure

The decision of how to treat a wound is usually multifactorial and considers the anticipated future use of the patient, the level of financial commitment by the owner, and the extent of the injury. If a synovial structure is involved, recommended therapy may include surgery under general anesthesia and joint lavage with or without arthroscopic evaluation. When the wound clearly does not involve a synovial structure, management may involve suturing the laceration. This requires the use of standing sedation or general anesthesia.

In most situations, a general pack of instruments that includes a scalpel handle, hemostatic forceps (mosquito and Kelly), thumb forceps (Brown-Adson and rat-tooth), needle drivers (Mayo-Hegar or Olsen-Hegar), and scissors (Mayo and Metzenbaum) is sufficient for suturing a laceration. A selection of Penrose drains of varying sizes is useful to ensure proper drainage when necessary. Preoperative and postoperative care generally consists of administration of antibiotics, anti-inflammatories, analgesics, and prophylactic tetanus toxoid if the vaccination history is unknown or if the tetanus vaccine was given more than 4 to 6 months before the injury occurred.

Emergency and Critical Care Nursing: Food Animal

It is not uncommon for owners to place high economic or sentimental value on farm animals; therefore many farm animal owners are willing to seek emergency veterinary care whenever necessary. Emergency treatment requires prompt action, as well as safety considerations on the part of the owner, the veterinarian, and the veterinary support staff.

TECHNICIAN NOTE

The veterinary technician or nurse must be familiar with the emergency condition and the procedure at hand and should be able to anticipate the veterinarian's next step.

Patient Restraint and Safety

Emergency situations are not an excuse to compromise the safety of the veterinary team, the owner, or the patient. Because of their large size, many farm animal patients pose a unique set of challenges compared with other domesticated animals. This increases the level of danger when handling even the mildest-mannered patients.

Considerations for Drug Use in Food-Producing Animals

Certain regulations apply to the use of specific pharmaceuticals in food-producing animals that do not apply to the use of these drugs in non-food—producing species. Some drugs are prohibited from being used in an extra-label manner, and many others are strictly forbidden in food-producing animals. Refer to Chapter 28 ("Pharmacology and Pharmacy") for more information about these regulations, particularly Table 28.12 for a list of drugs that are prohibited from use in food-producing animals. The *entire* veterinary team should be aware of these drug regulations, and attention should be paid to withdrawal times to avoid drug residues in meat and milk. The Food Animal Residue Avoidance Databank (www.farad.org) should be consulted regarding current drug regulations and withholding times.

Gastrointestinal System
General Physical Examination

Before providing emergency treatment, the veterinarian will perform a thorough physical examination of the patient, which is critical for making an accurate diagnosis and for initiating appropriate treatment. The physical examination should include measurement of HR and RR, assessment of body temperature, and evaluation of lung and heart sounds. One of the most important aspects of the physical examination regarding the gastrointestinal tract is auscultation and percussion of the lateral abdominal wall to listen for hyperresonant sounds, which are referred to as *pings*. Pings represent gas pockets within the viscera and can be a sign of displaced abdominal viscera.

Most veterinarians perform rectal palpation as part of a routine physical examination, because it is useful for assessing caudal abdominal structures, including the uterus, cecum, small intestines, caudal sac of the rumen, and left kidney in cattle. A large, distended abomasum can be palpated rectally in some cases. The veterinarian should be provided with an arm-length plastic rectal sleeve and copious amounts of lubricant. If the veterinarian is palpating several cows, a new, clean sleeve/lubricant should be used for each cow.

Ancillary Diagnostics

Other diagnostic tests that can be very useful for assessment of abdominal disease include abdominal ultrasonography, abdominocentesis, abdominal radiography, and blood work. If the veterinarian wishes to perform other diagnostics, the veterinary technical staff should be familiar with these procedures and the necessary equipment.

Emergency Intervention

The veterinary team must be prepared to act quickly to stabilize the patient and prepare for emergency surgery. If severely compromised, the cow should have a jugular IV catheter placed and should be started on IV fluids. Classic biochemical abnormalities which occur alongside GI disease include hypokalemia, hypochloremia, and metabolic alkalosis. Administration of a nonalkalinizing balanced electrolyte solution (lactated Ringer solution) is best. If the cow is in hypovolemic shock, a liter of hypertonic saline (7% sodium chloride [NaCl]) can be administered intravenously to quickly increase the circulating blood volume. (*Note:* The effect of hypertonic saline is temporary because it is a crystalloid and will eventually leave the vascular space.) Hypertonic saline must always be followed with additional IV fluids or oral fluids to avoid hypernatremia.

Among the most acute and life-threatening bovine abdominal emergencies are volvulus of the abomasum or cecum. Intestinal obstruction can result from a volvulus of some or all intestinal structures. A volvulus is especially serious, because vascular supply is compromised.

Abomasal ulcers can result in focal or diffuse peritonitis. The rumen produces large amounts of gas, predisposing ruminants to rumen tympany ("bloat") if there is failure to expel this gas. Bloat can be life-threatening if it leads to respiratory compromise. Vagal indigestion is a multifactorial condition that results in dysfunction of the forestomachs and abomasum that can also lead to profound ruminal and abdominal distention.

TECHNICIAN NOTE

Volvulus of the abomasum and of the cecum are among the most acute and life-threatening conditions of the bovine abdomen.

Abdominal surgery to correct an abomasal volvulus, a cecal volvulus, or another GI abnormality is typically performed in the right flank (paralumbar fossa) with the animal standing. The right side of the cow is clipped and aseptically prepared. The prepped area should extend from the tuber coxae (point of the hip) cranially to the 12th intercostal space and from dorsal midline (spine) ventrally to the flank fold (Fig. 25.53). The surgical site is desensitized by performing a local or regional nerve block (paravertebral nerve block, inverted-L block, or line block). A final surgical prep is done, and the cow should be moved to the operating room or to the area prepared for sterile abdominal surgery.

TECHNICIAN NOTE

Abdominal surgery to correct an abomasal volvulus, a cecal volvulus, or another gastrointestinal (GI) abnormality is typically performed in the right flank region (paralumbar fossa), with the animal standing.

The necessary equipment will vary, depending on the surgeon's preference. A list of common surgical equipment for performing abdominal surgery in cattle is provided in Box 25.8.

Specific Gastrointestinal Conditions
Diarrhea
Diarrhea is a nonobstructive GI problem that can result in profound dehydration, low protein, and hypovolemic shock within hours of onset. Young animals are especially vulnerable to the sequelae of diarrhea, which can result from dietary, parasitic, bacterial, or viral causes; successful treatment depends on an accurate diagnosis. If significantly dehydrated, patients should have a jugular catheter placed for administration of IV fluids. Animals that are suffering from hypovolemic shock may benefit from an IV bolus of hypertonic saline. Oral fluids and electrolytes, especially bicarbonate-containing fluids, may also help restore hydration.

Parasitism
Most farm animals will have a low level of GI parasites, which is not usually considered an emergency; however, overload can result in malabsorption, diarrhea, and dehydration. Some parasites, for example, *Haemonchus contortus*, are avid blood feeders and can cause profound anemia. These problems are especially common in small ruminants (sheep and goats) and camelids. The presenting complaint is usually weakness and weight loss, and this condition can be fatal if not treated. Mucous membrane color (lower eyelid

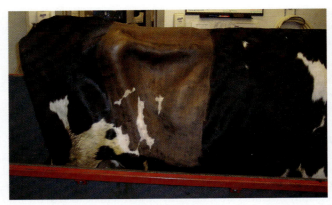

• **Fig. 25.53** Cow prepared for right flank surgery. Abdominal surgery in cattle is commonly performed in the right paralumbar fossa. The surgical prep should extend from the tuber coxae cranially to the 12th intercostal space and from the dorsal midline ventrally to the flank fold.

• **BOX 25.8** **Surgical Equipment for Abdominal Surgery in Cattle**

- Large drape
- Towel clamps (quantity = 10)
- Hemostats (quantity = 10 Kelly, 5 mosquito)
- Scalpel
- Mayo scissors
- 4 × 4 gauze sponges
- Basin with warmed isotonic saline
- Sterile palpation sleeves
- Suture and needles
- Suction and decompression set

or vulva in females) should be assessed as a part of the physical examination, and PCV/TP should be performed. A blood transfusion may be necessary to stabilize these patients. Owners can be educated to monitor mucous membrane color so that treatment can be administered before anemia becomes life-threatening. Use of FAMACHA cards is helpful for recognizing various stages of anemia.

Emergencies Involving the Rumen
Ruminal Tympany
In ruminal tympany ("bloat"), excessive gas accumulates within the rumen. Affected animals have abdominal distension prominent on the upper left side. Microbes that live in the rumen normally produce a large amount of gas, which should be expelled periodically through the esophagus (eructation). Bloat is caused by an inability to properly expel this gas. One type of bloat termed *frothy bloat* occurs when a foamlike substance forms within the rumen and cannot be expelled like normal gas. *Free gas bloat* occurs when a physical blockage (choke) or decrease in rumen motility prevents eructation.

Bloat is life-threatening when the distended rumen pushes cranially on the diaphragm, inhibiting normal respirations. Emergency decompression is necessary in these cases. In cases of free gas bloat, an esophageal tube is usually sufficient to relieve excessive gas accumulation. Frothy ruminal contents do not pass well through a tube, and pharmacologic therapy may be necessary to break down the foam. Poloxalene (50 g orally for cattle weighing ≥500 kg), a surfactant, can be used to relieve frothy bloat by breaking the surface tension of the foam.

Rumenostomy

Surgical decompression of the rumen may be necessary. **Rumenostomy**, a surgical procedure creating a permanent hole in the rumen, is performed in the left flank (paralumbar fossa region), providing a permanent escape for gas in animals that chronically bloat.

As a last resort, rumen trocars (Fig. 25.54) are available to puncture the rumen and allow the gas to escape. These devices are inserted through the left flank into the rumen. Most devices have a tapered, threaded shaft that holds the rumen onto the trocar to prevent the rumen from slipping off the device and away from the body wall. Use of these devices is discouraged by the author, because leakage of rumen contents invariably results in peritonitis. However, in certain instances of respiratory depression, it may be a life-saving procedure.

Solid ingesta may need to be removed from the rumen in cases of grain overload or toxin ingestion. Standard-size esophageal tubes are easily plugged with rumen contents and are not effective for removing solid ingesta. A Kingman tube, a large-bore esophageal tube, can be used for removal of ingesta, liquid, and gas from the rumen (Fig. 25.55). To pass a Kingman tube, the patient's head must be securely restrained. A mouth gag that is designed to be used with the Kingman tube is placed in the mouth and securely tied around the head. A thin layer of lubricant or mineral oil can be applied to the tube to aid in passage. With the head extended, the tube is passed through the center hole of the mouth gag until the pharyngeal area is reached. Gentle pressure should be exerted on the tube until the tube passes the pharyngeal region and begins to go down the esophagus. The tube will encounter resistance before entering the rumen; slightly withdrawing the tube, rotating it 90 degrees, and advancing the tube may facilitate its passage. To assist in recovery of rumen contents, the cow's head and the end of the tube should be held low. Filling the tube with water and allowing the water to drain will create a siphon, which may aid in draining rumen contents. Flushing the tube with water can also overcome blockage of the tube by fibrous rumen material. If the Kingman tube is not sufficient for emptying rumen contents, a rumenotomy may be indicated.

Choke

Choke (esophageal obstruction) is usually caused by swallowing a foreign body. Clinical signs include gagging, retching, and excessive drooling. Animals can still breathe, but the condition can be very frightening to watch as the animal retches for long periods without relief. If the animal cannot eructate and expel gas produced in the rumen, severe bloat can result. In cattle, choke is often caused by swallowing apples or hedge apples (Fig. 25.56). In camelids, choke is commonly caused by rapid consumption of pelleted feed material. A palpable ball of feed material or a foreign body may be felt over the cervical esophagus but may not be palpable if the obstruction is at the thoracic inlet. The choke often resolves spontaneously, but veterinary intervention may be necessary to relieve the obstruction. If an obstructive ball of feed material can be palpated, the area should be gently massaged to facilitate breakup of the mass. If massage is unsuccessful or a large foreign body is present, the mass should be moved into the rumen or first stomach compartment by using an esophageal tube. Appropriate tube size varies by animal, but the esophagus is very distensible, and a typical large animal nasogastric tube works well for most adults. Adult cattle usually require a more rigid tube than is needed for sheep and goats. Coating the tube with some obstetric lube or mineral oil may aid in passage and decrease esophageal or pharyngeal trauma. Animals can be panicked and may require sedation for safe passage of an esophageal tube.

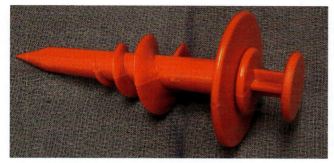

• **Fig. 25.54** Rumen trocar used to relieve severe bloat in cattle. The main risk with the use of this device is leakage of rumen fluid around the trocar, which will cause peritonitis. Therefore use of this device is discouraged except in emergency situations.

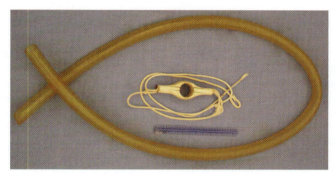

• **Fig. 25.55** Kingman tube with mouth gag. This tube is used to remove ingesta, liquid, and gas from the rumen of cattle with severe rumen distention. (*Note:* for size comparison, the ruler is 30 cm in length.)

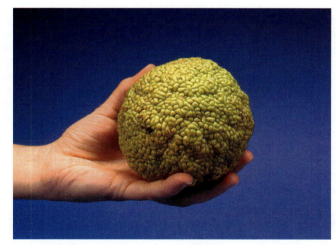

• **Fig. 25.56** Photo of a hedge apple. These firm fruits frequently cause esophageal obstruction (choke) when swallowed by cattle. (Courtesy Dr. Bruce Hull, Columbus, Ohio.)

Rumen Fluid Analysis and Transfaunation

Analysis of rumen contents may be necessary. Parameters include measurement of rumen pH, a methylene blue reduction test, and microscopic examination of ruminal fluid. pH should be measured with a pH meter or with pH paper (normal pH ≈7). Animals that are accustomed to high-grain diets may have a rumen pH as low as 5.5. The methylene blue reduction test is used to determine microbial function. A 0.5 mL of 0.03% methylene blue is added to 9.5 mL of strained ruminal fluid to make a total of 10 mL in a clear glass tube. A second tube of ruminal fluid serves as a color control. Methylene blue will color ruminal contents blue; healthy ruminal flora will reduce methylene blue to a colorless solution, and the rumen fluid will resume its normal color within 5 minutes. Delayed return to normal color indicates decreased rumen flora activity.

> **TECHNICIAN NOTE**
>
> Normal rumen pH should be approximately 7.

A drop of ruminal fluid should be placed on a microscope slide and viewed under low power (×10 objective). Many motile protozoa should be seen per low-power field. It is normal to see organisms of different sizes, and they should appear active. If the slide or the rumen contents are allowed to cool, the protozoa will appear less active. Successful rumen fluid analysis should be carried out as soon as possible after collection and not subjected to variants in temperature.

Transfaunation is the transfer of ruminal microbes from one individual to another and may be beneficial if a patient's ruminal contents are abnormal. The purpose of a transfaunation is to enhance rumen function by repopulating the rumen with healthy rumen microbes. Rumen transfaunation can be performed in any ruminant species, because rumen flora is similar across species (e.g., bovine rumen contents can be given to a goat or sheep). Ruminal fluid typically is collected from a rumen-cannulated cow (Fig. 25.57). Rumen fluid is separated from the fibrous ruminal contents (multiple methods of separation exist). The liquid portion is used for transfaunation, and the fibrous material is discarded or replaced back into the donor rumen. Rumen fluid can be filtered with cheesecloth to remove small fibrous material that may clog the pump and tube during administration (Fig. 25.58). A device that filters the rumen fluid can be inserted through the rumen cannula so the rumen fluid will be filtered as it is being pumped out of the donor cow, making collection a one-step process (Fig. 25.59). Rumen fluid is administered via an esophageal tube like the one used for administration of oral fluids. It is important to administer rumen fluid while it is still warm, because cooling of the fluid may kill rumen microflora.

> **TECHNICIAN NOTE**
>
> Once collected, rumen fluid should be used as soon as possible, because the microorganisms will become less effective with time.

Respiratory System

Respiratory Distress

Respiratory distress can be life-threatening and is a frightening experience for both the animal and the owner. Animals may act aggressively or become delirious. Safety precautions should always be followed to avoid placing the veterinarian, veterinary staff, owner, or patient in unnecessary danger. A thorough physical examination should be performed to make a diagnosis but may be abbreviated until the animal is stabilized.

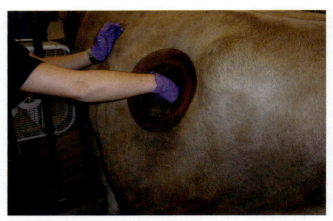

• **Fig. 25.57** Collection of rumen contents from a rumen-cannulated cow.

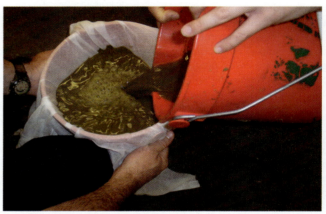

• **Fig. 25.58** Rumen fluid being strained with cheesecloth to remove particulate matter before it is pumped through an esophageal tube.

If the patient is in respiratory distress, stabilization should be a higher priority than the physical examination. The veterinary team should be prepared to administer oxygen, if necessary, which can be accomplished via nasal cannula, face mask, or endotracheal (ET) tube. The equipment necessary to achieve safe and effective oxygen delivery should be readily available.

> **TECHNICIAN NOTE**
>
> When dealing with patients in respiratory distress, the veterinary team should be prepared to administer oxygen if necessary. Stabilization takes priority over the initial exam.

Tracheostomy

If a patient is presented with an upper airway obstruction, a tracheostomy can be performed to help the animal breathe under adequate restraint. To optimize restraint and expose the neck for the procedure, the head can be cross tied with two halters, one coming off either side of the head. An approximately 10- × 10-cm area should be prepared for aseptic surgery. This area should be centered on ventral midline over the palpable trachea at the junction of the cranial third and the middle third of the trachea (Fig. 25.60). Adult cattle can accommodate tubes with a 10- to 20-mm internal diameter (ID). Calves and small ruminants will require 5- to 10-mm ID tubes. Young lambs, kids, and crias may require smaller sizes.

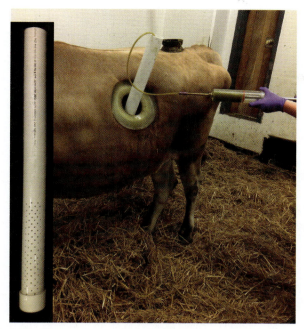

• **Fig. 25.59** The one-step method of collecting rumen fluid. A 2-inch piece of PVC pipe, perforated at the bottom, is inserted through the rumen cannula. The small perforations allow rumen fluid to accumulate in the pipe while preventing larger particulate matter from entering the tube. Flexible tubing is passed into this pipe, and rumen fluid is aspirated with a large syringe attached to the end. The inset shows the perforated pipe used for the one-step method of collection.

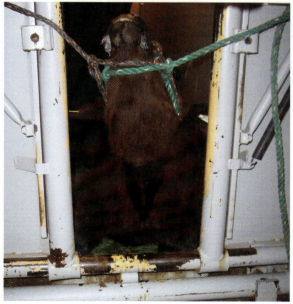

• **Fig. 25.60** Calf positioned for a tracheostomy. Two halters are placed on the head, one coming off of either side to keep the head and neck elevated and straight. The mid-to-cranial cervical region is prepped for surgery.

> **TECHNICIAN NOTE**
>
> If the technician is unsure which tracheostomy tube would be best for the specific application, multiple tubes should be prepared.

Musculoskeletal Injuries

Orthopedic Emergencies and Downer Animals

Orthopedic problems can be extremely problematic in large animals. Fractures and other musculoskeletal problems can be more difficult to repair because of increased forces applied to the fixation. Physical therapy and rehabilitation can be labor intensive, time consuming, and dangerous. Animals that cannot stand or ambulate are at great risk for secondary problems such as sores, pneumonia from recumbency atelectasis, and muscle damage resulting from compression. This discussion will be limited to orthopedic emergencies in cattle.

> **TECHNICIAN NOTE**
>
> Animals that cannot stand or ambulate are at great risk for secondary problems such as sores, pneumonia from recumbency atelectasis, and muscle damage resulting from compression.

Fractures and Joint Luxation

Animals with traumatic injuries must be evaluated for life-threatening issues before addressing any orthopedic problem. Unstable fractures should be stabilized to prevent additional damage to the bone or neurovascular structures. Distal fractures (metacarpus, radius, metatarsus, or tibia) should be stabilized immediately with a splint or heavy bandage to confer stability. Proximal fractures (humerus or femur) are not easily stabilized with splints but typically have enough surrounding muscle that they are inherently more stable than distal fractures. In smaller patients, slings may afford some support for proximal fractures.

Joint luxation should receive prompt veterinary care. Joint luxation that is presented, diagnosed, and treated within a few hours after injury has a good chance of successful resolution, and many of these luxations can be corrected by closed (nonsurgical) techniques. This is especially true with shoulder and hip luxation. After several hours, muscle contracture around the limb and debris accumulating within the joint increase the difficulty of reducing the joint luxation, necessitating surgical reduction.

> **TECHNICIAN NOTE**
>
> The prognosis for successful treatment of joint luxation depends on how rapidly it is treated.

Life-threatening problems should be corrected before the joint luxation is treated. Radiography may be useful for assessing the luxation and formulating a treatment plan. Traction is often needed in cases of joint luxation or displaced fracture in large animals.

Down Animals

Animals that cannot stand are referred to as ***down animals***, or "downers." Causes include sepsis and shock; metabolic causes, such as hypocalcemia and hypokalemia; orthopedic problems, such as fractures, dislocations, and ligament tears; neoplasia, such as tumors caused by bovine leukosis virus; and neurologic diseases. In many cases, the cause remains unknown, but it is important to make an accurate diagnosis so that the underlying disease process can be treated appropriately. Regardless of the reason the patient is down, secondary skin, muscle, and nerve damage can result, making supportive and physical therapy a mainstay of treatment.

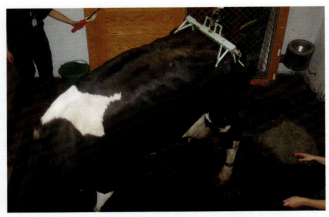

• **Fig. 25.61** Cow being lifted in hip lifters. The hip lifters are clamped down around the wings of the ileum, and a hook connected to a hoist is attached to the center of the device is used to lift the hind end of the cow.

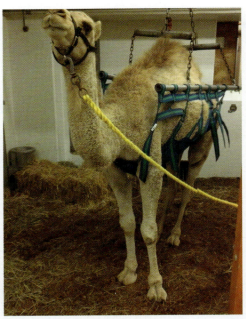

• **Fig. 25.62** Dromedary camel assisted to stand by a sling. The sling is suspended by a hoist from the ceiling.

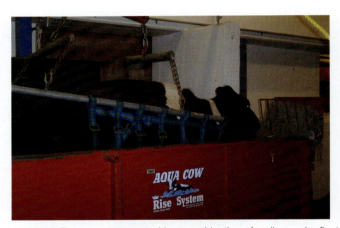

• **Fig. 25.63** Down cow supported in a combination of a sling and a float tank. Although each method of support is designed to work independently, the sling offers a level of protection against the cow going down and drowning in the float tank. The sling is actually supporting very little of the cow's weight, because the animal is being supported by the water.

Exceptions may be made for certain orthopedic and neurologic situations but, ideally, down animals should be assisted to stand. Several devices can be used to help down cattle stand. A hip lifter is an apparatus that is clamped tightly over the wings of the ileum. A hook in the center of the device allows attachment of a hoist (Fig. 25.61). Hip lifters are lightweight and easy to apply and use; however, the animal may slip out of the device, and these devices only lift the rear end of the animal. Animals that cannot bear weight on their front will tip forward. Prolonged use of hip lifters can result in skin sores and musculoskeletal trauma over the hip area. Slings (Fig. 25.62) lift animals more evenly (front and back). Once the animals are standing, slings do a better job of distributing the weight; however, they are designed only to assist an animal to stand, and animals that are completely unable or unwilling to stand will develop complications from prolonged use of slings. Slings are more difficult to apply; it usually takes a team of several experienced people to properly fit a large cow into a sling. Hydrofloatation (Fig. 25.63) is another option for assisting down cows to stand and is the best option for supporting cattle for long periods. Hydrofloatation of cattle requires specialized float tanks and a team of experienced personnel. Hydrofloatation causes the least trauma and is likely to produce the most favorable outcome. It does, however, carry some unique risks, including drowning of the animal, hypothermia, and infection if submerged in dirty water. Ideally, water should be changed often to prevent infections.

TECHNICIAN NOTE

Hydrofloatation is an option for assisting down cows to stand; it is the best option for supporting cattle for long periods. Water changes will help in preventing subsequent infections during usage of float tanks.

Dog/Wild Animal Attacks

Camelids, sheep, and goats are frequent targets of animal attacks (particularly dog attacks). Frequently, the owner's dog is the attacker. Owners should be informed that the attack is likely to occur again if precautions are not taken. If an unknown animal is responsible for the attack, greater concern is raised about infectious diseases, such as rabies. Although rabies is not common in camelids, sheep, and goats, it can occur in these species. Attacks can occur anywhere on the body but commonly occur around the head, neck, or extremities; serious life-threatening injury can result and may require emergency therapy.

If severe blood loss has occurred, the animal may need a blood transfusion. The color of the mucous membranes should be noted, and PCV/TP should be measured as part of the examination; blood donors or homologous blood should be available. If the animal is still bleeding, hemostasis should be of primary concern. Animals may be in shock after the attack because of the traumatic event or because of blood loss. An IV catheter should be placed in the jugular vein for administration of fluids (for shock) or blood, if needed. Neck wounds may directly involve the jugular vein, or resulting cellulitis may make jugular catheterization difficult. In these cases, other peripheral vessels may be used for catheterization.

Although puncture wounds may look superficial, they usually involve deeper structures; this trauma often is not directly obvious. Bite wounds are always contaminated. The depth of these wounds should be explored with a narrow sterile probe. Tissue with questionable viability may be left undebrided until it is known that it is not viable. Other equipment and supplies that should be made available include sterile normal saline for lavage and a 20-mL syringe. A 10- to 12-French (Fr) red rubber catheter is also useful for lavage of deep wounds. Animals may remain panicked and not easily restrained after an animal attack, and sedation may be needed to treat their wounds appropriately. Animal attacks should be considered emergencies and may have fatal consequences.

Dystocia and Obstetric Emergencies

Obstetric emergencies must be dealt with in a prompt manner to ensure the health of the dam and the fetus. **Dystocia** (difficult birth) represents most obstetric emergencies. Management of these cases often requires two or more people. A trained assistant or technician is of utmost importance to the veterinarian and should be knowledgeable of the art of fetal extraction. Often, veterinary technicians will play a lead role in fetal extraction, because they possesses physical traits that the veterinarian may be lacking. For instance, for managing bovine dystocia, good upper body strength and long arms are an advantage, but for managing dystocia in small ruminants, camelids, and pigs, small hands are invaluable. Veterinary technicians should learn each veterinarian's particular style of obstetric management, because many techniques are available and every veterinarian has their personal preferences.

Dystocia Box and Equipment

A dystocia kit is useful to keep all needed obstetric equipment in one centralized location. Ideally, the kit should be mobile so that it can be moved quickly to the patient (Fig. 25.64). Suggested contents of a farm animal dystocia kit are listed in Box 25.9.

Some veterinarians prefer to use sterile sleeves to perform vaginal examinations; others prefer to scrub their hands and arms carefully before examining the cow. In addition to protecting the uterine environment, sleeves protect the arms of the veterinarian. If the veterinarian prefers to use sterile sleeves, these should be available, along with sterile lubricant. Certain lubricants can be very toxic if introduced into the abdominal cavity. For this reason, some lubricants are not recommended if a cesarean section (C-section) is a possibility or if uterine trauma is extensive.

Sterile obstetric chains should be available for assisting in vaginal extraction of calves. Proper placement of obstetric chains should be ensured to prevent injury to the calf. The chain should be wrapped around the calf's leg proximal to the fetlock, and a half-hitch should be placed below the fetlock. A calf jack is a winch that is used to apply traction on obstetric chains; it can be very useful in helping to extract a large fetus, especially when help is limited. The operator must be very careful that too much force is not applied or trauma to the fetus or dam may result.

TECHNICIAN NOTE

Sterile obstetric chains should be available for assisting in vaginal extraction of calves. Each chain should be accompanied by at least two handles so that the assistant can help with the delivery.

A **fetatome** is a device that uses obstetric wire to perform a **fetotomy** (cutting a dead fetus into smaller parts that can be extracted more easily). Operation of a fetatome requires two people—one to place the fetatome and hold it in position, and an assistant to make the cut.

A Krey hook is a device that can be used to grab fetal parts when a fetotomy is performed. It is designed such that when

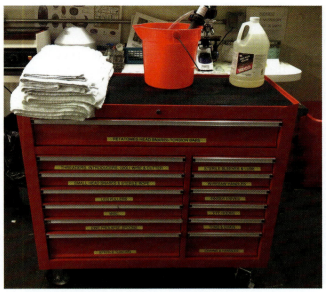

• **Fig. 25.64** Dystocia kit. Toolbox is used to contain all of the commonly used equipment for management of bovine dystocia. Drawers are labeled so that the equipment is organized and easy to find in an emergency. The box is on wheels so that it is easily moved around the clinic. Inventory of the equipment in the box should be routinely made so that the box is stocked with all of the needed supplies at all times.

• BOX 25.9	Suggested Items to Be Included in a Farm Animal Dystocia Kit

- Obstetric chains
- Chain handles
- Head snare
- Eye hooks
- Krey hook
- Finger knife
- Sterile water-based lubricant
- Bucket
- Pump
- Soft tube
- Fetatome
- Obstetric wire
- Wire introducer
- Wire passer
- Wire cutters
- Calf jack
- Soft rope (clothesline)

traction is applied, it clamps more forcefully onto the fetus. Eye hooks can also be used in cattle to attach directly under the medial canthus of the eyes to help apply traction to the head. Because of the orbital anatomy of cattle, they can be applied to live calves without causing severe trauma. A finger knife is a useful tool for making cuts in a fetus while protecting maternal tissues.

A bucket, a pump, lubricant, and a uterine lavage tube are useful to pump water and lubricant into a contracting uterus to distend and lubricate the birth canal.

Examination

Every case of dystocia should begin with a thorough examination. Vaginal and rectal examinations should be performed on animals in dystocia. A rectal examination can allow the veterinarian to feel the outside of the uterus and may be useful for diagnosis of **uterine torsion**. Most other information can be obtained by performing a vaginal examination.

The perineal area should be prepped before the vaginal examination. The perineal scrub is not intended to achieve asepsis but to decrease uterine and vaginal contamination so that manure and dirt are not carried into the vagina. This reduces the incidence of metritis and reduces the risk for abdominal contamination if a C-section is performed. If a rectal examination is performed, the perineal area is not cleaned until after it has been completed. Some veterinarians prefer to begin by cleaning out the rectum so that the cow does not defecate on the clean field. The tail should be tied out of the way to prevent contamination of the area once it has been cleaned.

Epidural Anesthesia

Epidural anesthesia can be useful; however, if vaginal delivery is to be performed, the dam will no longer be able to assist in the delivery process. Also, overzealous administration of epidural anesthesia can cause the animal to become recumbent.

> **TECHNICIAN NOTE**
>
> Epidural anesthesia can be useful for reducing the pain associated with vaginal manipulation and for decreasing the force of uterine contractions so that vaginal manipulation of the fetus can be accomplished.

Vaginal Delivery

In most cases, vaginal delivery affords advantages over C-section, including faster delivery of the fetus, faster recovery of the dam, and fewer postparturient complications. Vaginal delivery can be successfully performed with the fetus presented head first or hind limbs first. If the fetus is presented in anterior presentation (forelimbs first), the head and both forelimbs must be extended into the pelvis of the dam. If the fetus is delivered in posterior presentation (hind limbs first), both hind limbs are extended and presented in the birth canal. If the fetus is in posterior presentation and the hind limbs are retained so that the rump of the fetus is presented first, the presentation is termed a *breech presentation.* Breech fetuses must be repositioned before successful vaginal delivery can be performed.

> **TECHNICIAN NOTE**
>
> Vaginal delivery can be successfully performed with the fetus presented head first or hind limbs first.

Cesarean Section

The incision for a C-section may be made in the flank, on the ventral midline, or paramedian. Adequate restraint is important for any animal undergoing C-section. A headgate-and-chute system with a removable side panel is preferred for standing C-sections. C-sections can be performed in small ruminants that are awake and standing; however, because of increased difficulty in keeping the animal restrained, the surgeon will often elect to place these animals in right lateral recumbency. In cattle, the tail is tied to prevent contamination of the surgical site. An epidural is recommended to keep the cow from straining during the procedure but, as noted previously, too much local anesthetic can cause the cow to become weak and recumbent during the procedure.

Before surgery is performed, the appropriate area should be clipped and aseptically prepared. Most commonly, C-sections in ruminants are performed on the left flank with the animal awake.

> • **BOX 25.10** **Equipment for Bovine Cesarean Section**
>
> - Surgery pack
>   - Towel clamps (quantity = 10)
>   - Hemostats (10 Kelly, 5 mosquito)
>   - Mayo scissors
>   - Needle holders
>   - 2 scalpels
>   - 4 × 4 gauze sponges
>   - Uterine forceps
> - Drapes
> - Suture with needles (surgeon's choice)
>   - Uterus (absorbable)
>   - Body wall (absorbable)
>   - Skin (nonabsorbable)
> - Obstetric chains
> - Sterile sleeves
> - Basin with sterile saline

A liberal area should be prepared from caudal to the tuber coxae (the point of the hip) to the 12th intercostal space and from the dorsal midline to the flank fold to decrease the risk for abdominal contamination during surgery. Regional nerve blocks, such as proximal or distal paravertebral nerve blocks, are preferable over line blocks.

Before the C-section, the surgeon's table should be set up with the equipment listed in Box 25.10.

In cattle, assistance commonly is required to extract the calf. The assistant need not scrub but should wear a sterile gown and gloves. The assistant usually assumes the role of neonatologist after extraction of the calf and therefore should be well versed in care of the neonate.

> **TECHNICIAN NOTE**
>
> When a cesarean section (C-section) is performed in cattle, assistance is almost always required to extract the calf.

Uterine Torsion

Uterine torsion, a condition in which the gravid uterus twists in relation to the maternal pelvis, is a cause of dystocia in cattle and camelids and may be corrected by rolling the animal. Rolling a cow to correct uterine torsion usually requires multiple personnel. The direction of the torsion is important to know, because this will influence the direction in which the animal will need to be rolled. The uterus must be immobilized while the animal is rolled. In cattle, this is accomplished by the "plank-in-the-flank" method. The cow is cast onto the desired side with a long rope. Other ropes are used to tie the limbs together. A long 2- × 12-inch board is placed in the flank directly in front of the tuber coxae. An assistant (usually the largest person in the group) stands on the plank near the flank end. The cow is slowly rolled in the desired direction, while the assistant bounces up and down on the board. The cow then is palpated and rolled again if necessary. For severe twists, multiple rolls may be necessary to fully correct the torsion. A detorsion rod can also be used to untwist the uterus of a cow. This method requires the presence of an open cervix and the possibility to pass the rod and a hand into the uterus. The calf's limbs are secured to the rod, and the rod is used to flip the calf and the uterus.

Camelids can also suffer from uterine torsion, and similar principles apply. Conservative therapy for correction involves rolling the llama or the alpaca. Typically, an assistant will palpate the uterus through the abdomen and will stabilize the uterus while the animal is rolled. Surgical correction is another option for uterine torsion in cases refractory to conservative management and in animals that have had a previous torsion. If a torsion is severe (>180 degrees), the animal may show signs of toxic shock or hemorrhage after correction. Signs may include pale mucous membranes, tachycardia, tachypnea, recumbency, seizures, and death. The veterinary team should watch carefully for these clinical signs after a torsion is corrected.

Small Ruminant Dystocia

The same principles apply to dystocia in small ruminants. In these cases, the most common limiting factor for vaginal manipulation is the size of the veterinarian's hands. Assistants who have smaller hands are frequently called upon to manipulate the fetus vaginally. It must be remembered that the uterus of small ruminants is more easily ruptured than the uterus of cattle. Therefore care must be taken when vaginal manipulation is performed.

Uterine Prolapse

Uterine prolapse occurs when the uterus folds inside out through the cervix and the vulvar lips. Sequelae of uterine prolapse include uterine trauma with potential tearing of the uterine wall and damage to the uterus because of restriction of blood supply (ischemia). If the weight of the uterus applies too much traction on the vasculature of the uterus, the uterine artery can rupture, causing fatal hemorrhage.

> **TECHNICIAN NOTE**
> Caution must be used if a cow with a uterine prolapse is transported over a long distance in a trailer before correction.

The external environment can be detrimental to the **endometrial** (inner uterine) lining. A drape or a large plastic bag makes a good surface for protecting the uterus against further contamination and trauma during correction. Before correction of the prolapse, the endometrial surface should be gently cleansed. Warm water or saline is sufficient, because antiseptic solutions have the potential for causing chemical damage to the endometrial surface. An epidural should be administered to the cow to decrease straining and to allow the uterus to be replaced with less force. Elevation of the uterus above the vulva can help with reduction. After the uterus has been replaced, the veterinarian typically will perform another procedure, such as a Buhner suture, to keep the uterus from prolapsing again.

Toxic Metritis and Toxic Mastitis

Cattle with severe metritis and mastitis can develop endotoxemia from absorption of endotoxins. These animals may present with signs of toxic shock (tachycardia and tachypnea), with weakness or neurologic deficits, or they may be down. A CBC and biochemistry profile should be performed so that therapy can be specifically tailored to the patient's needs. Cattle may require IV fluid support, and hypertonic saline may be used to help restore circulating blood volume. If the animal is down on presentation, supportive therapy should be provided to prevent nerve and muscle damage.

Urolithiasis in Small Ruminants

Urethral obstruction caused by urolithiasis (urinary calculi or stones) is common in ruminants, especially sheep and goats, and is seen almost exclusively in males. Factors predisposing to development of obstructive urolithiasis include early castration, high-grain diets (high phosphorus), legume forages, and dehydration.

> **TECHNICIAN NOTE**
> Formation of most stones is associated with ingestion of high-phosphorus diets, such as those high in concentrates (grain).

Complete urethral obstruction from urolithiasis is the most common presentation. Failure to treat these animals in a timely fashion can result in bladder rupture, urethral rupture, or death. Several treatment options exist. The best option will depend on use of the animal; the age of the animal; concurrent problems, such as urethral rupture, bladder rupture, or severe metabolic derangements; and the veterinarian's experience and preferences. See Case Presentation 25.3 for an example of emergency management of urethral obstruction caused by urolithiasis.

History and Physical Examination

The veterinarian can usually diagnose urethral obstruction with a good history and physical examination. The owner should be questioned about the animal's presenting signs, the duration of the problem, when the animal was last observed to urinate, the quality of the urination (full stream versus dribbling), access to water, any drugs or other treatments administered, and dietary history.

These animals are usually in pain; additional restraint may be necessary to perform a physical examination. Acepromazine is preferred over xylazine for sedation, because xylazine has diuretic properties and can increase urine production. Acepromazine has vasodilatory properties, so caution must be employed in animals that appear to be in shock. The veterinarian may wish to perform a rectal examination to palpate the penis and the urethra, so supplies needed for a rectal examination should be available. Ultrasonography can be a very useful diagnostic tool to evaluate the size of the bladder and the presence of any free fluid (urine) within the abdomen. A 5.5-MHz convex probe is ideal for transabdominal ultrasonography. If the animal has formed radiopaque stones, radiography may be useful to determine the quantity and location of the stones (Fig. 25.65). However, many urinary calculi (e.g., struvite stones) are not radiopaque and will not be visible on survey radiographs. Therefore the absence of visible stones on radiographs does not rule out a diagnosis of urolithiasis. In cases of chronic obstruction, metabolic derangements are common, with potentially fatal consequences, so a biochemistry profile is useful under these circumstances. Electrolytes that can contribute to metabolic abnormalities (sodium, chloride, and potassium) should be measured. Measuring blood urea nitrogen and creatinine is useful in assessing the severity of azotemia.

> **TECHNICIAN NOTE**
> The absence of visible stones on radiographs does not rule out a diagnosis of urolithiasis.

Treatment

Severe metabolic derangements should be addressed before the obstruction is relieved. This is especially important if the animal is to undergo general anesthesia. Although somewhat counterintuitive, obstructed animals generally will benefit from IV fluid therapy before the obstruction is resolved. An IV catheter should be placed in the jugular vein. For most small ruminant patients,

CASE PRESENTATION 25.3

Emergency Management of Urethral Obstruction

Brutus, a 4-year-old neutered male American Pygmy goat, was presented to the clinic with a history of constipation. He was fed grain and given "treats" at home. The goat was straining to defecate, was not eating, and was uncomfortable for 3 days before admission. The owner administered three enemas (one a day since the signs started) and offered a mild laxative with his daily grain, but Brutus refused to eat it.

Upon physical examination, Brutus was found to be uncomfortable and straining to defecate. Digital rectal examination revealed no feces in the rectum, but the urethra was palpated ventrally to the rectum and was found to be pulsating. The prepuce was dry, and a few crystals were found on the hair of the prepuce. The owners were questioned about the last time the goat was observed to urinate; they indicated that this had occurred about 4 days earlier.

A presumptive diagnosis of obstructive urolithiasis was made, and abdominal ultrasonography was performed. The bladder measured approximately 10 cm, but no free fluid was found in the abdomen. The technician placed an intravenous (IV) catheter in the jugular vein and drew blood for a biochemistry profile; 0.9% saline was started at maintenance rate before laboratory results were received. The profile revealed severe azotemia with blood urea nitrogen and creatinine of 105 mg/dL and 8 mg/dL, respectively. Potassium was 6.9 mEq/L (high). The veterinarian ordered dextrose to be added to the fluids to help lower blood potassium.

After 60 minutes on the new fluid regimen (0.9% sodium chloride with 5% dextrose at 1.5 times the maintenance rate), the goat was taken to surgery for tube cystostomy. The goat was anesthetized and was maintained under general anesthesia with isoflurane. Multiple uroliths (stones) were cleaned from the bladder, and a 20-French (20-Fr) Foley catheter was placed through the abdominal wall into the bladder. Surgery, anesthesia, and recovery were uneventful.

After surgery, Brutus was fed free-choice hay but no grain. He was given ammonium chloride to acidify his urine and dissolve any stones in the urethra. Seven days after surgery, the tube was clamped off, and the goat was observed to urinate through his urethra. The clamp was left on the tube for 24 hours, and after a night of successful urinations with the tube clamped, the bulb of the tube was deflated and the tube was pulled.

The owners were told that urolithiasis is a common problem in male goats, especially in those that receive grain in their diets, and that most straining in male goats is caused by urinary blockage, not constipation. They were advised to feed no grain at all and were told that good-quality grass hay serves as a sufficient diet for pet goats. They were also advised to monitor the goat closely at home for urination, because recurrence may occur.

The owners changed Brutus's diet as recommended and stopped feeding grain entirely. They reported that Brutus was doing well after surgery and discharge from the clinic, and they were very pleased with the service provided by the veterinary team.

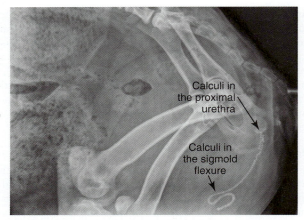

• **Fig. 25.65** Radiograph of a male goat with multiple urinary calculi. Calculi line the proximal urethra, including the sigmoid flexure.

a 16-gauge, 3.5-inch catheter works well. Hyperkalemia (high potassium) is a common electrolyte abnormality in obstructed animals and may lead to fatal cardiac arrhythmias, so potassium-containing fluids are avoided. Normal strength saline (0.9% NaCl) is the ideal fluid, because affected animals are frequently deficient in sodium and chloride. Sodium bicarbonate and dextrose can also be given intravenously to help drive potassium into the cells, thus decreasing blood potassium levels.

Treatment objectives for patients with obstructive urolithiasis are to (1) stabilize the patient, (2) allow urinary drainage, (3) achieve diuresis and waste removal, and (4) restore patency to the urinary tract.

The most common place for calculi to lodge and cause an obstruction in goats is the **urethral process**, a small, curved extension of the urethra located at the distal end of the penis. If the urethral process can be visualized, it can be amputated. The most difficult part of this procedure is exteriorization of the penis. Acepromazine at a dose of 0.05 mg/kg given intravenously will allow the animal to relax and will make it more tolerant of penile exteriorization. The goat should be positioned on its rump, with its hind limbs pulled forward toward its head. This positioning will facilitate penile exteriorization. One person should hold the goat in this position while another attempts to retract the prepuce. Once the penis is visualized, a third person should roll a gauze square into a strip and wrap it around the shaft of the penis just proximal to the glans penis. The gauze strip should be twisted firmly around the penis to keep it from retracting back into the prepuce. If the gauze is wrapped around preputial tissue, the penis will retract through the prepuce and will be lost. **Urethrostomy** is a process that involves creating an opening in the urethra proximal to the obstruction. Urethrostomy can be performed rapidly and typically does not require general anesthesia. Sedation, epidural anesthesia, or a local nerve block is usually sufficient. The procedure may be performed with the animal standing, but positioning the animal on a table with the hind limbs hanging over the edge or elevating the rear quarters of the animal with the limbs spread apart may facilitate the procedure. The procedure can be performed in the perineal region (referred to as *perineal urethrostomy*), or it can be performed in a more ventral location. For urethrostomy, the area from the tail head (dorsal margin) to the area of the scrotum (ventral margin) and laterally from one thigh to the other should be clipped and prepped for surgery. The penis will be exteriorized in this location and the urethra opened to provide urine drainage. Complications include hemorrhage from the penile stump and stricture of the urethra at the surgery site. This is a quick procedure, but it often is not associated with a good long-term outcome because of the possibility of stricture. It is also not an option for breeding animals.

TECHNICIAN NOTE

Urethrostomy is a process that involves creating an opening in the urethra proximal to an obstruction. Urethrostomy can be performed rapidly and may not require general anesthesia.

A **tube cystostomy** involves placement of a Foley catheter in the bladder to provide temporary diversion of urine while urinary stones

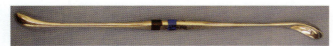

• **Fig. 25.66** Bladder spoon. This double-ended spoon is used during a cystotomy procedure to clean the bladder of uroliths.

are dissolved or passed. This procedure involves a ventral abdominal approach. The catheter can be placed with a percutaneous technique under ultrasound guidance, or it can be placed with the animal under general anesthesia. The technique varies, depending on economics, patient status, available equipment, and surgeon preference. For surgical placement, the following equipment should be prepared: a general surgery pack, a basin and sterile saline, a bulb syringe for lavage of the open bladder and the abdomen, equipment to provide sterile suction, a bladder spoon for removing uroliths from the bladder (Fig. 25.66), electrocautery, and a Foley catheter. The appropriate size of the Foley catheter varies, depending on the patient, but catheters smaller than 16-Fr are not recommended, because they are easily plugged with blood clots or calculi. The Foley catheter is left in place for about 1 week to allow urine to drain. During this time, the animal is medically managed to dissolve the stones and to relax the urethra. The tube is then occluded, and the patient is observed to confirm passage of urine through the urethra. If the patient can urinate successfully, the tube is removed. This procedure is associated with a better long-term outcome compared with urethrostomy and is the recommended procedure for breeding animals.

> **TECHNICIAN NOTE**
>
> Foley catheters smaller than 16-French (16-Fr) are not recommended for urethrostomy, because they are easily plugged with blood clots or calculi.

Many cases of urolithiasis can be prevented by management changes on the farm—most importantly, dietary changes. Urine acidifiers like ammonium chloride can be fed to help dissolve phosphatic calculi that form preferentially in alkaline urine. It is very important to always have adequate fresh water available, because dehydration can predispose to stone formation. A salt and mineral block will increase thirst and water intake.

> **TECHNICIAN NOTE**
>
> Prevention is a very important aspect of urolithiasis management. The most important recommendation for owners of pet male goats and sheep is to feed *no* grain.

Acknowledgment

The authors and publisher wish to acknowledge Kirk Ryan, Lee Ann Eddleman, Charles T. McCauley Ann Peruski, Michelle Goodnight, Grace VanHoy, and Andrew Niehaus for their contributions to previous editions of this textbook.

Recommended Readings

Anderson DE, Rings M. *Current Veterinary Therapy: Food Animal Practice*. 5th ed. St. Louis, MO: Saunders; 2009.

Auer JA, Stick JA. *Equine Surgery*. 5th ed. St. Louis, MO: Elsevier; 2019.

Ford RB, Mazzaferro EM, eds. *Kirk and Bistner's Handbook of Veterinary Procedures and Emergency Treatment*. 9th ed. St. Louis MO: Elsevier; 2012.

Fowler ME. *Medicine and Surgery of Camelids*. 3rd ed. Ames, IA: Wiley-Blackwell; 2010.

Fubini SL, Ducharme NG, eds. *Farm Animal Surgery*. 2nd ed. St. Louis MO: Elsevier; 2017.

Mason DE, Ainsworth DM, Robertson JT. Respiratory emergencies in the adult horse. *Vet Clin North Am Equine Pract*. 1994;10:685.

Mudge MC, Bramlage LR. Field fracture management. *Vet Clin North Am Equine Pract*. 2007;23:117.

Orsini JA, Divers T, eds. *Equine Emergencies: Treatment and Procedures*. 4th ed. Philadelphia, PA: Saunders; 2014.

Peterson ME, Talcott PA, eds. *Small Animal Toxicology*. 3rd ed. St. Louis, MO: Saunders; 2013.

Silverstein D, Hopper K. *Small Animal Critical Care Medicine*. St. Louis, MO: Elsevier; 2015.

Smith BP, Van Metre DC, Pusterla N, eds. *Large Animal Internal Medicine*. 6th ed. St. Louis, MO: Mosby; 2019.

Theoret CL, Schumacher J, eds. *Equine Wound Management*. 3rd ed. Ames, IA: Wiley-Blackwell; 2016.

Recommended Websites

Academy of Veterinary Emergency and Critical Care Technicians and Nurses. Available at, www.avecctn.org.

Food Animal Residue Avoidance Databank. Available at: www.farad.org.

26
Toxicology

KARA RICHMOND AND TINA WISMER

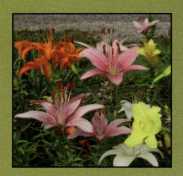

CHAPTER OUTLINE

LEARNING OBJECTIVES

When you have completed this chapter, you will be able to:

1. Pronounce, spell, and define all the key terms in this chapter.
2. Assess and stabilize a patient presenting with a toxicologic emergency.
3. Use appropriate decontamination techniques for ocular, dermal, and oral toxin exposure to prevent absorption and/or remove the toxin from the body.
4. Provide supportive care to a patient being treated for toxicosis.
5. Do the following regarding common household hazards, including dangerous food items, household cleaning agents, and miscellaneous household items:
   * Identify the toxic component of the item or product.
   * Describe clinical signs expected with toxicosis.
   * Describe specific decontamination techniques used to prevent absorption and/or remove the toxin from the body.
6. Do the following regarding dangerous plants, including *Rhododendron* species, cardiac glycoside–containing plants, castor

beans, cycad palms, lilies, and insoluble calcium oxalate crystal–containing plants:
   * Identify the toxic component of the item or product.
   * Describe clinical signs expected with toxicosis.
   * Describe specific decontamination techniques used to prevent absorption and/or remove the toxin from the body.
7. Do the following regarding pesticides, including ant and roach baits, flea/tick products, methomyl, molluscicides, and rodenticides:
   * Identify the toxic component of the item or product.
   * Describe clinical signs expected with toxicosis.
   * Describe specific decontamination techniques used to prevent absorption and/or remove the toxin from the body.
8. Do the following regarding antifreeze products, including methanol, propylene glycol, and ethylene glycol:
   * Identify the toxic component of the item or product.

- • Describe clinical signs expected with toxicosis.
- • Describe specific decontamination techniques used to prevent absorption and/or remove the toxin from the body.
9. Do the following regarding human medications, including acetaminophen, nonsteroidal anti-inflammatory drugs, aspirin, pseudoephedrine, amphetamines, isoniazid, calcipotriene, and 5-fluorouracil:
   - • Identify the toxic component of the item or product.
   - • Describe clinical signs expected with toxicosis.

- • Describe specific decontamination techniques used to prevent absorption and/or remove the toxin from the body.
10. Do the following regarding drugs of abuse, including marijuana, cocaine, ethanol, and methamphetamine:
    - • Identify the toxic component of the item or product.
    - • Describe clinical signs expected with toxicosis.
    - • Describe specific decontamination techniques used to prevent absorption and/or remove the toxin from the body.

KEY TERMS

Acids
Adsorbent
Alkali
Anticoagulant
Antiemetics
Cathartics
Cationic detergents
Corrosive
Decontamination

Emetic
Enterohepatic recirculation
Gastric lavage
Hydrocarbon
Metabolic acidosis
Nonsteroidal anti-inflammatory drugs
Toxicosis
Toxin

Introduction

Animals have a natural curiosity, and many are adept at accessing areas where toxic substances, such as baits, cleaners, chemicals, and medications, are stored. Pets may also chew through child-resistant bottles or heavy plastic containers. Some products, such as flavored medications or pest control baits, may be particularly attractive to pets. Prevention of poisoning by "pet proofing" the home environment is the only safe choice. The veterinary technician can educate pet owners on ways to make their homes "poison safe." However, if a pet has been exposed to a toxicant, prompt action is needed to prevent potentially life-threatening problems.

Toxicity is dependent on the substance, the exposure dose and the species, breed, age, and size of the animal. Different species of animals may be more sensitive to certain **toxins** (e.g., cats and acetaminophen). Pediatric, geriatric, and pregnant patients can present their own challenges. Both the very young and the very old can have decreased kidney and liver functions, making them more susceptible to toxicants. Proper and prompt treatment of poisonings, including stabilization and **decontamination**, is essential.

Assessing the condition of the pet, stabilizing the animal, preventing absorption of the toxicant, controlling clinical signs, and instituting ancillary measures are critical areas in which veterinary technicians play a key role.

Managing Poison Emergencies

Every veterinary practice must be prepared for the emergency management of poisoned patients. Often, the first instinct of an animal owner whose pet has been exposed to a potential poison is to call a veterinary practice. Veterinary technicians should be equipped to recognize what constitutes a toxicologic emergency, give basic first aid advice, and provide clear directions to the

appropriate veterinary hospital if needed. The following questions should be asked to evaluate the situation:

1. What is the current clinical status of the animal? Severe clinical signs necessitate immediate veterinary assistance (bleeding, unconsciousness, dyspnea, seizures).
2. What was the animal exposed to and through what route (oral, ocular, dermal)?
3. How much of the toxin was the animal exposed to (weight, volume, or quantity)?
4. When did the exposure occur?
5. How old is the animal and how much does it weigh?
6. Is the animal male or female? If female, is she lactating or pregnant?
7. Does the animal have any history of health problems?
8. Is the animal currently on any medications?
9. Has the animal had any recent surgeries?
10. Has the owner taken any steps to treat the animal?
11. Are there any other animals that may have been exposed?

PUT INTO PRACTICE

Creating a list of questions to be posted by the phone can help when a client calls with a possible poisoned pet. Having these questions posted makes remaining calm and supportive during the phone call much easier for all staff.

This information can be helpful to prepare for the office visit. After reviewing this information with the staff veterinarian, basic first aid advice or at-home decontamination recommendations may be given and/or the client told to bring the animal directly into the hospital. In the case of large animals, a farm call may be needed. While waiting for the client's arrival, the veterinary technician can prepare the necessary equipment and medications and can help investigate the toxicant by scanning a reference in the practice library or by consulting with veterinary toxicology specialists at the American Society for the Prevention of Cruelty to Animals (ASPCA) Animal Poison Control Center (888-426-4435).

In cases where symptomatic animals are presented and the owner suspects poisoning, history taking is similar but needs to be broader. In this case, the following questions should be included:

1. Where does the animal live (indoors, outdoors, fenced area, or is it allowed to roam)?
2. Are there any medications, dewormers, insecticides, rodenticides, or plants in the animal's environment?
3. When did the owner last notice the animal being normal?

Assessment of the Patient's Condition

Initial management of a potential toxicosis starts with assessing the present condition of the pet. The assessment should be performed quickly and include the following: assessment of respiratory rate, capillary refill time (CRT), mucous membrane color, heart rate (HR), and core body temperature. Examination of a pet that is unconscious, in shock, seizing, or in cardiovascular or respiratory distress must be conducted simultaneously with stabilization measures. With stable animals, the technician should obtain a comprehensive history of the pet and the exposure and perform a thorough physical examination.

Stabilization of Vital Functions

The general rule of toxicology is to "treat the patient, not the poison." The ABCs (airway, breathing, circulation) should be addressed before attempting any type of decontamination. A patent airway should be established, and artificial respiration given if the animal is dyspneic or cyanotic. The cardiovascular system should be monitored closely, and any cardiovascular abnormalities should be corrected. Placement of an indwelling intravenous (IV) catheter may be necessary for the administration of medications and IV fluids.

Decontamination

Decontamination is performed to prevent absorption of toxicants. Information gained from the history is crucial when dealing with toxicosis and often affects the way the animal is treated. Clinical signs and time frame will determine whether decontamination is needed and whether it will be helpful. Some toxicants can cause clinical signs quickly, whereas others can have a delayed onset of signs. Depending on the situation, certain methods of decontamination are more beneficial than others. The patient's age, weight, and previous medical history can also affect the method of decontamination.

External Exposure

Ocular Exposure

With any ocular exposure, the eyes should be flushed repeatedly with tepid water or saline solution for a minimum of 20 to 30 minutes. Eye flushing should begin as soon as possible and is often done by the pet owner. Ocular exposure to corrosive agents should be considered an emergency. The eyes should be examined for corneal damage and monitored closely for excessive redness, lacrimation, or pain. Follow-up examinations may be needed to establish the level of corneal damage.

Dermal Exposure

For dermal exposures, the animal should be bathed in a mild liquid dishwashing detergent. Baths may need to be repeated to completely remove oily toxicants. The animal should be rinsed well with warm water and thoroughly towel dried to prevent chilling. The technician or owner performing the bath should wear proper personal protective equipment (PPE; i.e., rubber gloves, apron, and eye and respiratory protection) to protect themselves from toxin exposure.

When dealing with sticky substances (e.g., gum, glue traps, tar, etc.), the use of chemical solvents should be avoided, because they may cause dermal irritation or burns. To remove sticky substances from mammals, a small amount of vegetable oil, mineral oil, mayonnaise, or peanut butter should be worked through the rest of the substance until it breaks down into "gummy balls." Afterward, the animal should be washed with liquid dishwashing detergent as described above. For birds, the same instructions apply, but mineral oil should not be used, because it is very difficult to remove from feathers.

Oral Ingestion

Dilution

Dilution with milk or water is recommended in cases of corrosive or irritant ingestion. A dosage of 1 to 3 mL/lb body weight is suggested. For exotic animals, juicy fruits or vegetables can be used in place of milk.

Emesis

Emesis (induction of vomiting) can be performed in some cases of toxin ingestion. The patient's species, length of time since ingestion, previous and current medical conditions, and the type of poison can affect the decision to induce emesis. Dogs, cats, pigs, and ferrets can vomit. Emesis is contraindicated in rodents, rabbits, birds, horses, and ruminants. Emesis is more likely to be productive if the animal is fed a small, moist meal before vomiting is induced. Time since ingestion is important, because some medications may be quickly absorbed (10–15 minutes), whereas chocolate can stay in the stomach for up to 8 hours.

Any animal that has a previous history of cardiovascular abnormalities, poorly controlled epilepsy, or recent abdominal surgery or is severely debilitated is not a candidate for emesis induction. Emesis should not be induced in any animal that is severely depressed or in a coma (risk of aspiration), is hyperactive (this could trigger a seizure), or has already vomited.

Another factor affecting the decision to induce emesis is the nature of the substance ingested. Emesis is contraindicated for corrosive materials, such as cationic detergents, acids, and alkalis, because of re-exposure and injury of the esophageal tissues to the corrosive material. Dilution with milk or water in combination with gastrointestinal (GI) protectants is recommended in cases of ingestion of corrosive substances.

Emesis is also contraindicated with hydrocarbon (petroleum distillate) ingestion; the main concern is the risk of aspiration. Many of these products are light and easily inhaled into the lungs. See Table 26.1 for examples of hydrocarbon-containing products.

TABLE 26.1	Hydrocarbon Classes With Examples of Common Substances
Petroleum distillates	Diesel fuel
	Gasoline
	Naphtha (lighter fluid)
	Stoddard solvent
	Mineral spirits
	Mineral oil
	Kerosene (number 1 fuel oil)[a]
	Jet fuel
	Fuel oil
	Lubricating oils (motor oil, grease)
	Petroleum jelly/petrolatum jelly
	Paraffin wax
	Asphalt
Other aliphatic hydrocarbons (alkanes, alkenes, alkynes)	Butane
	Ethane
	Hexane
	Methane
	Propane
Aromatic hydrocarbons	Benzene
	Toluene
	Xylene
Selected terpenes	Turpentine
	Pine oil (pine oil cleaner)
Chlorinated (halogenated) hydrocarbons	Carbon tetrachloride
	Chlorinated hydrocarbon insecticides
	Chloroform
	Methyl chloride
	Methylene chloride
	Tetrachloroethylene
	Trichloroethane
	Vinyl chloride
	Trichloroethylene
Other hydrocarbons	Automatic transmission fluid
	Coal pitch and coal tar pitch volatiles
	Naphthalene
	Machining fluids
	Waste oils

[a]*Note:* Kerosene is often called *paraffin* in the United Kingdom and other countries. This confusion is thought to be responsible for some poisoning accidents in humans, particularly in children.

A 3% hydrogen peroxide solution has been shown to be an effective emetic for dogs, ferrets, and pigs. The mechanism of action of hydrogen peroxide is the release of oxygen and mild irritation to the gastric mucosa. The dosage for hydrogen peroxide is one teaspoon (5 mL) per 5 lb of body weight and should not exceed a total dose of three tablespoons (45 mL). Typically, vomiting occurs within 15 or 20 minutes if there is food in the stomach and the peroxide is fresh. If vomiting does not occur, peroxide administration can be repeated one additional time. Cats have an increased risk of developing hemorrhagic gastroenteritis after hydrogen peroxide administration, so it is not recommended in this species. More concentrated hydrogen peroxide products, such as food-grade hydrogen peroxide or hair products, should not be used. These higher concentrations can cause severe GI hemorrhage.

Apomorphine hydrochloride is a centrally acting emetic agent for dogs. It acts by stimulating the vomiting center or chemoreceptor trigger zone (CRTZ). Apomorphine is available as an injectable solution and as a capsule of powder for administration into the conjunctival sac. The sedation that may develop can be reversed with naloxone. Another centrally acting emetic agent for dogs is ropinirole (Clevor, Vetoquinal, Fort Worth, TX, United States) eye drops. It also works by stimulating the CRTZ.

The cat vomiting center is different than dogs, and apomorphine and ropinirole will not work. Alpha$_2$ adrenergic agonists (xylazine, dexmedetomidine) can be used to induce emesis in cats. Severe central nervous system (CNS) depression can be reversed with either yohimbine or atipamezole.

Salt or salt water should never be used as an emetic. Salt is not an effective agent, and there have been cases of sodium toxicosis reported because of its use as an emetic. Animals also do not vomit in response to sticking a finger down the throat, and both the animal and the owner can be injured in this process.

Animals should be monitored during the emesis process. Ingestion of vomitus by the animal or another animal in the household is counterproductive. Emesis should be induced on a hard surface, where the vomitus can be examined. Animals generally vomit only 40% to 60% of their stomach contents. If the toxin is not seen in the vomitus, it cannot be assumed that it came back up.

TECHNICIAN NOTE

Always advise owners of the correct amount of hydrogen peroxide to give to their animal. One teaspoon (5 mL) per 5 lb of body weight is the recommended dose, with a maximum dose of three tablespoons (45 mL).

Activated Charcoal

Activated charcoal is an adsorbent (a substance that attracts other materials or particles to its surface) that can bind to toxins, thereby preventing their absorption into the bloodstream. By adsorbing the toxicant, activated charcoal facilitates its excretion via the feces. It is administered orally when an animal ingests a toxin or if enterohepatic recirculation of metabolized toxicants can occur. The recommended dose of activated charcoal for most species of animals is 1 to 2 g/kg body weight. Repeated doses of activated charcoal may be indicated when enterohepatic recirculation occurs. Activated charcoal can be given orally with a large syringe or with a stomach tube. In symptomatic or uncooperative animals, anesthesia may be needed. A cuffed endotracheal tube should always be used in the sedated or clinically depressed animal to prevent aspiration.

Activated charcoal is contraindicated in animals that have ingested caustic materials. These materials are not absorbed systemically, and the charcoal may make it more difficult to see oral and esophageal burns. Other chemicals that are not effectively adsorbed by activated charcoal include ethanol, methanol, fertilizer, fluoride, petroleum distillates, heavy metals, iodides, nitrates, nitrites, sodium chloride (NaCl), and chlorate. Risks of charcoal administration include aspiration and hypernatremia secondary to fluid shifts into the GI tract.

Cathartics

Cathartics decrease GI transit time. Cathartics are used to enhance elimination of the activated charcoal and adsorbed toxicant complex, and so are often administered along with activated charcoal. Cathartics can be added to solutions of activated charcoal or given separately. Contraindications for using cathartics include diarrhea and dehydration.

Enemas

Enemas are helpful when elimination of toxicants from the lower GI tract is desired. The general technique is to use plain warm water or soapy warm water. Premixed phosphate enema solutions for humans are contraindicated in small animals because of the potential electrolyte and/or acid–base imbalances they may cause. Enemas are not performed in birds because of the risk of introducing fecal bacteria into the oviduct.

Gastric Lavage

Gastric lavage is a method of gently pumping the stomach contents out of the animal. Gastric lavage should not be performed in cases of caustic or petroleum distillate ingestion and should always be performed with the animal under general anesthesia with a cuffed endotracheal tube in place to protect the airway and prevent aspiration. The procedure involves inserting a fenestrated lavage tube into the stomach to the level of the xiphoid cartilage. The stomach should then be lavaged repeatedly with physiologic-temperature water until the fluid drawn out of the stomach is clear in color. It is important not to use greater than 10 mL/kg in rabbits because of the risk of stomach rupture.

> **TECHNICIAN NOTE**
> Using body-temperature water for gastric lavage can help decrease the risk of hypothermia.

Enterogastric Lavage

Enterogastric lavage, also known as the "through-and-through lavage," may be necessary when potentially lethal oral ingestion has occurred. After a gastric lavage, the stomach tube is left in place. An enema is performed to eliminate large pieces of fecal matter from the colon and upper large intestines. The distal end of the enema tube is attached to a water source, and body-temperature water is slowly allowed to fill the tube and enter the intestinal tract in a retrograde manner. Water is allowed to flow until the water and fecal material flow out through the stomach tube. This process is continued until the color of the fluid passing out of the stomach tube is clear.

Supportive Care

Veterinary technicians and nurses play a critical role during decontamination by routinely evaluating vital signs and any parameters likely to be affected by the toxicant. Hydration, CRT, HR, blood pressure, and temperature should be closely monitored.

Blood samples may be needed to perform a complete blood count, chemistry panels, or clotting profiles to monitor the effects of the poison on different body systems. Blood, vomitus, and urine may also be collected to check for toxins. Samples collected should always be kept properly labeled, especially if legal action is a possibility. Samples can always be discarded later if not needed.

Ancillary measures, such as nutritional support, are key components for complete recovery for the pet. Anorectic cats and ferrets are at risk for developing hepatic lipidosis and hypoglycemia; therefore it is extremely important to maintain nutritional requirements. A pharyngostomy tube may be necessary to provide adequate nutrition to the animal.

Good nursing care should be continued until the pet completely recovers. The amount of time that supportive care is needed will vary with the toxicant ingested. Some toxins are eliminated from the body within minutes or hours, whereas others can take days or even years (as with lead) to be eliminated.

> **TECHNICIAN NOTE**
> Assessment, stabilization, history taking, and decontamination are critical areas in which veterinary technicians and nurses play a key role.

Household Hazards

Dangerous Food Items

Some types of food that are safe for humans can be dangerously toxic to pets. Pet owners are often tempted to give table scraps to their pets as a special treat, and pets may also encounter potentially dangerous food in trash cans or dumps. If a pet is exposed to a dangerous food item, prompt action will be needed to prevent a potentially life-threatening problem.

Moldy Food

Moldy food may contain tremorgenic mycotoxins, such as penitrem A and roquefortine C. Tremorgenic mycotoxins are neurotoxins produced by molds and can induce muscle tremors, ataxia, and convulsions that can last for several days. The severity of signs can range from mild to severe. Diagnosis of tremorgenic mycotoxins involves sample analysis of the moldy food or the stomach contents by an accredited veterinary diagnostic laboratory. Treatment goals after tremorgenic mycotoxin ingestion include minimizing absorption through decontamination procedures such as emesis, lavage, and potential administration of activated charcoal; controlling tremors with methocarbamol; and providing supportive care. With early and aggressive treatment, the prognosis is good.

> **TECHNICIAN NOTE**
> Tremorgenic mycotoxins produced by molds on food are relatively common and possibly underdiagnosed as a cause of tremors and seizures in animals.

Chocolate

Chocolate contains theobromine and caffeine, which are methylxanthine stimulants. Depending on the dose, methylxanthines can cause vomiting, polyuria, polydipsia, diarrhea, hyperactivity, increased HR, tremors, seizures, and potentially death. The amount of methylxanthines present in chocolate varies with the type of chocolate (Table 26.2). Generally, the darker and more

TABLE 26.2	Methylxanthine Content of Various Types of Chocolate	
Type of Chocolate	Methylxanthines (mg/oz)	
White chocolate	1.1	
Milk chocolate	65	
Semisweet (dark) chocolate	165	
Baking chocolate	400	

bitter the chocolate, the more toxic it likely is. Unsweetened baking chocolate contains almost seven times more theobromine compared with the same amount of milk chocolate, and white chocolate (a combination of cocoa butter, sugar, butterfat, milk solids, and flavorings without cocoa beans) contains negligible amounts of methylxanthines.

TECHNICIAN NOTE

The darker and more bitter the chocolate, the more toxic it is.

Although theobromine and caffeine have a lethal dose 50 (LD_{50}; dose that will be lethal to 50% of patients) of 100 to 200 mg/kg, signs of toxicity can be seen well below this dose. Gastrointestinal signs begin at doses greater than 20 mg/kg, cardiovascular effects are seen at doses above 40 mg/kg, and neurologic effects are seen at doses exceeding 60 mg/kg. Early treatment, including emesis, cardiovascular monitoring, and supportive care, is extremely helpful with chocolate poisoning. Activated charcoal is only recommended when used with IV fluids to prevent the development of hypernatremia (fluid shifts). In addition, fluid diuresis may help enhance elimination. Caffeine can be resorbed by the bladder wall, which may result in extended duration of clinical signs. Veterinary staff should take extra steps to keep the patient's bladder empty, either through catheterization or frequent walking. Acepromazine works well to control methylxanthine-induced agitation, and beta blockers can be used to control tachycardia. See Case Presentation 26.1 for discussion of a case of chocolate toxicosis.

Onions

Onions and other members of the *Allium* family can be harmful to all animals. Other members of this genus include garlic, leeks, shallots, and chives. Pieces of onion, onion powder, or even cooked onion can cause damage to the red blood cells (RBCs), which could result in anemia. The primary toxic principle is

CASE PRESENTATION 26.1

Chocolate Toxicosis

As one of the veterinary technicians on duty, you answer a phone call from a client who tells you that her Whippet got into the kitchen and ingested some chocolate. To determine whether the dog needs medical attention or if the owner can watch the dog at home, more information must be gathered. The *who*, *what*, and *when* of this situation are all important unknowns that must be determined.

Through thorough questioning, you can find out that the 27-pound healthy male castrated dog (*who*) ate 4 to 5 oz of solid dark chocolate (*what*) approximately 2 hours ago (*when*). The dog is still asymptomatic at this point in the conversation.

To determine whether this amount could be toxic for the dog, some simple calculations must be performed. Dark chocolate contains 165 mg of methylxanthines per ounce. Using the worst-case scenario of ingestion of 5 oz of dark chocolate, you figure that the dog ingested a maximum of 825 mg of methylxanthines (5 oz × 165 mg/oz). Converting the dog's weight to kilograms (27 lb × 1 kg/2.2 lb), you find that he weighs 12.27 kg. By dividing the maximum dose ingested by the dog's weight (825 mg ÷ 12.27 kg), you calculate that the dog has ingested up to a dose of 67.2 mg/kg of methylxanthines. Doses greater than 60 mg/kg are known to cause vomiting, diarrhea, agitation, tachycardia, tremors, and potentially seizures.

You inform the owner that emesis should be induced to eliminate the potentially toxic dose of chocolate. The owner has no hydrogen peroxide at home and so is advised to bring the dog into your clinic. Upon arrival, a quick physical examination reveals a heart rate of 160 beats per minute, a respiratory rate of 24 breaths per minute, and a temperature of 102.1°F. The mucous membranes are moist and pink, and capillary refill time is 1 second. The dog is bright, alert, and responsive, and paces around the examination room while you are speaking with the owner. After taking the dog to the treatment area, apomorphine is administered via the conjunctival sac. Within 5 minutes, the dog produces a large amount of brown liquid vomitus with chocolate chunks (Fig. 26A).

Upon estimating the amount of chocolate ingested and the amount obtained on emesis, it appears that at least two-thirds of the chocolate have been recovered. This would leave a maximum of approximately 275 mg (22.5 mg/kg) of methylxanthines in the dog's gastrointestinal

tract. At doses over 20 mg/kg vomiting and diarrhea may still occur, but cardiac or neurologic signs are not expected. At this point, the dog may be monitored in the clinic or at home. Luckily for this patient, the prompt action of the owner and the preparedness of the veterinary staff changed this potentially life-threatening situation to one with only minor consequences.

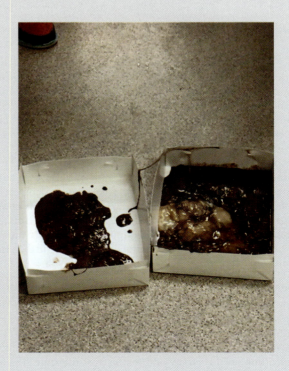

n-propyl disulfide, which causes oxidative damage to erythrocytes, resulting in hemolysis. Toxicoses from fresh, dried, or powdered plant material have been reported in dogs and cats. Cats are at higher risk because of the higher number of free sulfhydryl groups on their hemoglobin (eight vs. four for dogs and two for humans).

In one study, dogs given an extract equivalent to 5 g whole garlic/kg body weight once daily for 7 days developed decreased RBC count, decreased packed cell volume (PCV), and decreased hemoglobin concentration. Even chronic feeding of commercial baby food containing onion powder has been reported to cause toxicity in cats. For acute exposures, decontamination should occur at doses greater than 10 g/kg of garlic or 15 g/kg of onion per dog and greater than 1 g/kg of garlic or 5 g/kg of onion in cats.

Clinical signs associated with onion poisoning include hemolytic anemia, hemoglobinuria, vomiting, weakness, and pallor. Decontamination includes inducing emesis within 2 hours of ingestion. Administration of activated charcoal should be considered with large exposures to garlic or onion powder. Afterward, the animal should be monitored for the development of hemolysis, azotemia, and/or hematuria. These signs may not be seen for 3 to 7 days after exposure. Whole blood transfusions should be considered with critical patients, and fluid diuresis is recommended in patients with hemoglobinuria. In addition, supportive care should be administered until the patient recovers fully.

Macadamia Nuts

Ingestion of macadamia nuts may cause problems in dogs. Clinical signs include weakness, depression, vomiting, ataxia, tremors, and hyperthermia. The toxic principle is unknown. The lowest dose reported to cause clinical effects is 2.4 g/kg. In most cases, dogs develop clinical signs within the first 12 hours after ingestion. Treatment includes decontamination procedures, such as induction of emesis, and supportive care. The prognosis in most cases is extremely good, and dogs return to normal within 24 to 48 hours.

> **TECHNICIAN NOTE**
>
> Macadamia nut toxicosis often causes hindlimb paresis in dogs.

Yeast Bread Dough

Ingestion of uncooked yeast bread dough can be life-threatening to dogs. Production of ethanol and carbon dioxide during the rising process results in intoxication and bloating. Signs may include severe abdominal pain, bloating, vomiting, ataxia, and depression. In cases of recent ingestion in asymptomatic dogs, emesis could be induced. Administration of cold water or ice cubes by mouth or via a stomach tube will slow the rising process. Because ethanol can cause **metabolic acidosis**, it is important to monitor the acid-base balance and correct this with sodium bicarbonate if indicated. As large amounts of ethanol can cause coma, respiratory depression, hypothermia, and hypotension, the vital signs of symptomatic animals must be monitored closely. See the "Ethanol" section for further treatment information.

Grapes and Raisins

Grapes, raisins, and Zante currants (all *Vitis* spp.) have been shown to cause kidney failure in some dogs when eaten. The exact mechanism for kidney failure is not known, but the toxin is tartaric acid. The concentration of tartaric acid in grapes/raisins varies depending on the variety and maturity of the fruit. This may

account for the fact that some dogs do not develop signs. Cooking raisins has been anecdotally observed to be less toxic than fresh fruit (ASPCA Animal Poison Center Database: unpublished data, 2002–2021). Processed products, such as wine, jam, and juice, are detartrated and do not cause renal toxicity. With recent ingestion, induction of vomiting is recommended. This should be followed by IV fluid diuresis for 48 hours. During this time, the patient should be monitored for azotemia by performing periodic blood analysis. Activated charcoal is not recommended due to possible complications and lack of published studies showing it to be effective. Dogs have also been reported to have developed acute kidney injury after ingestion of tamarinds and cream of tartar, both of which are high in tartaric acid.

Xylitol

Xylitol is a sugar alcohol that is found in many "sugar-free" human food items (gum, candy, baked goods, peanut butter), and it may also be found in certain dental products, chewable medications, cough drops, and other products. Xylitol is used as a sugar substitute and has plaque-blocking properties. Xylitol toxicosis has been well documented in dogs and causes severe hypoglycemia secondary to the release of insulin. There have also been reports of liver failure and secondary coagulopathy from an unknown mechanism. Hypoglycemic symptoms of xylitol poisoning in dogs can occur soon after ingestion (baked goods, candy) or up to 8 hours later (gum) and include weakness, depression, ataxia, and vomiting. Biochemical analysis may show increased liver enzymes (alanine transaminase, aspartate transaminase) and/or liver failure within 24 hours after xylitol ingestion.

Ingestion of xylitol doses over 100 mg/kg by a dog can cause hypoglycemia. Emesis should be induced with recent ingestion if the patient is asymptomatic. After decontamination, the dog's blood glucose should be monitored frequently for hypoglycemia. During the monitoring period, the animal should have access to food and be encouraged to eat. If hypoglycemia is noted, IV dextrose should be used. If the dose is greater than 400 to 500 mg/kg, liver enzymes should be monitored and liver protectants started.

> **TECHNICIAN NOTE**
>
> Always consider xylitol toxicity if an animal has eaten a chewable or sugar-free medication.

Household Cleaning Agents

Acids

Hydrochloric acid, sulfuric acid, nitric acid, phosphoric acid, oxalic acid, and sodium bisulfate are all examples of household acids. Common sources include toilet bowl cleaners, drain openers, metal cleaners, antirust compounds, gun barrel cleaners, automobile battery fluid, and pool sanitizers. Acids are corrosives that have a low pH and can produce severe chemical burns on contact with tissue. The severity of tissue damage produced is directly related to the concentration and contact time with the acid. Acid burns are initially painful, and animals will typically only ingest small amounts. Concentrated acids, if ingested, may produce severe burns in the GI tract. Most cases of acid exposure result in gagging, hypersalivation, vomiting, and pain. In cases of ingestion of corrosive agents, vomiting should not be induced. The initial treatment should be oral dilution with a few laps of milk or water. The patient should be monitored and treated by a veterinarian for oral or esophageal burns if needed. These animals may need pain control, antibiotics, and nutritional support. For dermal exposure, flush the area with water and treat any burns as needed.

Alkalis

Alkalis (alkaline or basic chemicals) are found in drain openers, oven cleaners, bathroom and household cleaners, radiator cleaning agents, hair relaxers, alkaline batteries, electric dishwasher soaps, some oven cleaner pads, and cement. Lesions from alkalis are typically deeper and more penetrating than those caused by acidic compounds as they are initially nonpainful. The ability of alkalis to generate corrosive injury depends on concentration, pH, viscosity, amount ingested, and duration of contact with tissue. The full extent of the burns can be delayed for several hours. Clinical signs and treatment are the same as for acids. Animals exposed to alkalis can present with very high body temperatures secondary to the release of inflammatory compounds in the body.

> **TECHNICIAN NOTE**
> Both acids and alkalis cause burns; however, alkali burns often take several hours to fully develop, therefore possibly being deeper and more penetrating.

Bleach

Household bleaches typically contain less than 5% sodium hypochlorite, and household mildew removers contain up to 5% calcium hypochlorite. Nonchlorine or colorfast bleach may contain sodium peroxide, sodium perborates, or enzymatic detergents. Household bleaches are mild-to-moderate mucosal irritants. Bathing and dilution are the cornerstones of treatment. Nonchlorine bleaches can cause vomiting, which may be hemorrhagic in some cases.

Detergents

Detergents are nonsoap surfactants in combination with inorganic ingredients, such as phosphates, silicates, or carbonates. Detergents are classified according to their charge in solution as nonionic, anionic, or cationic surfactants.

Anionic and nonionic detergents are found in shampoos, dishwashing detergents, laundry detergents, and electric dishwashing detergents. Anionic and nonionic detergents are irritants, and their toxicity is generally limited to cutaneous, ocular, oral, or GI irritation. Dilution and a period of NPO (nothing by mouth) usually suffice as therapy.

Cationic detergents can be found in fabric softeners, some liquid potpourri oils, germicides, disinfectants, and sanitizers. Cationic detergents are rapidly absorbed and may produce severe local and systemic toxicity. Oral ulcerations, hyperthermia, stomatitis, and pharyngitis can be seen. The lesions are very similar to acid and alkali burns and are treated the same way.

Miscellaneous Household Items

Zinc

Sources of zinc include galvanized hardware, such as wire, screws, bolts and nuts, and US pennies. Pennies minted since 1983 contain 99.2% zinc and 0.8% copper. Ingestion of only one penny has the potential to cause zinc poisoning. Zinc is ionized in the acidic environment of the stomach, thus allowing for absorption into the bloodstream, where oxidative damage to the RBCs occurs. Clinical signs of zinc toxicosis may include hemolytic anemia, hemoglobinuria, weakness, renal failure, and death.

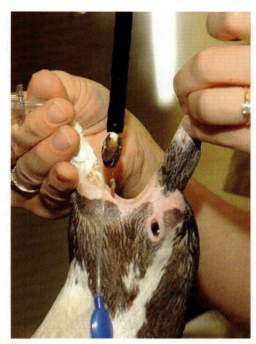

• **Fig. 26.1** Coins are removed via endoscopy from a penguin under general anesthesia.

Radiography of the abdomen may reveal the presence of metallic objects in the GI tract. Serum zinc levels may be submitted by using whole blood collected in royal blue–top vacutainers and then spun down to minimize contamination with exogenous zinc. Blood zinc levels greater than 10 parts per million (ppm) are considered diagnostic of zinc toxicosis in avia and mammals.

It is imperative to remove the source(s) of zinc from the GI tract via endoscopy (Fig. 26.1) or surgery. The use of chelators is generally not necessary, as zinc levels drop quickly after removal of the zinc object. Some pets may need a blood transfusion before or after surgery. IV fluids will help protect the kidneys from the free hemoglobin.

> **TECHNICIAN NOTE**
> When surgically removing metallic objects, follow-up radiography should always be performed before closing to ensure that all metallic items have been successfully removed from the digestive tract.

Lead

Sources of lead include paint, toys, drapery weights, linoleum, automotive batteries, plumbing materials, galvanized wire, solder, stained glass, fishing sinkers, lead shot, foil from champagne bottles, and improperly glazed bowls. Lead must be in an acidic environment to be absorbed into the bloodstream (stomach, synovial joint). Lead embedded in muscle tissue, such as lead pellets, may not be a problem. Young animals have increased lead absorption abilities compared with adults.

Lead affects multiple body systems, including GI, renal, CNS, and hematopoietic. Lead increases the fragility of the RBCs, leading to anemia and capillary damage. It can also cause segmental demyelination of neurons and necrosis of the renal tubular epithelium, GI tract mucosa, and liver parenchyma. Clinical signs seen with lead poisoning are often nonspecific and may include lethargy, weakness, anorexia, regurgitation, vomiting, diarrhea, polyuria, ataxia, circling, and convulsions. Lead is one of the only toxins that will cause intermittent seizures.

Radiography may reveal evidence of metallic objects. Blood levels of lead can confirm lead toxicoses. Lead levels below 0.35 ppm in dogs and 0.5 ppm in birds are rarely associated with clinical signs. Basophilic stippling and nucleated RBCs may also be seen with lead poisoning.

Removal of lead particles via bulk diet therapy, endoscopy, or surgery is recommended. Succimer and calcium ethylenediaminetetraacetic acid (Ca EDTA), both considered effective chelating agents, can be administered if symptomatic. In addition, good supportive care, including seizure control, is recommended until full recovery. If the source of lead is from the household, it should be recommended that any children in the house also be tested for lead.

Nicotine

Tobacco products contain varying amounts of nicotine, with cigarettes containing 13 to 30 mg and cigars containing 15 to 40 mg. Nicotine can also be found in gums, patches, and liquid forms for use in electronic cigarettes or as an insecticide. Signs often develop quickly (usually within 15–45 minutes) and include excitation, tachycardia, tachypnea, salivation, vomiting, and diarrhea. Muscle weakness, twitching, depression, bradycardia, shallow respiration, collapse, coma, and cardiac arrest can follow the initial period of excitation. Death occurs because of respiratory paralysis. With recent ingestion in asymptomatic animals, emesis can be induced (not with liquid nicotine products). Activated charcoal is most effective when given within 1 hour of the exposure but is rarely recommended. Patients should be monitored closely and treated symptomatically. Artificial respiration would be indicated in patients with respiratory paralysis.

> **TECHNICIAN NOTE**
>
> Some nicotine gums also contain xylitol, which can cause hypoglycemia and liver failure.

Silica Gel Packets

Silica gel is used as a desiccant and often comes in paper packets or plastic cylinders. It is used to absorb moisture in leather, medication, and food. It is also used as the base of some types of cat litter. Silica is considered "chemically and biologically inert." However, with ingestion, it is possible to see signs of GI upset, such as nausea, vomiting, and inappetence, although only mild signs occur with ingestion of small amounts. Instances of foreign body obstructions are possible but rarely seen. The risk for an obstruction depends on the amount of material ingested in comparison with the patient's weight.

Toilet Tank Drop-In Tablets

Toilet tank "drop-in" tablets typically contain corrosive agents (alkali or cationic detergents). Corrosive effects can be seen if the actual tablet is chewed or swallowed. When a tank "drop-in" cleaning product is used in a toilet, the actual concentration of the cleaner is low in the toilet bowl water. Drinking toilet bowl water containing diluted cleaner only causes gastric irritation. Common signs seen with toilet bowl water ingestion include mild vomiting and nausea.

Glow-in-the-dark Products

Dibutyl phthalate, also known as *n-butyl phthalate*, is a liquid found in various glow-in-the-dark products commonly sold at fairs, carnivals, and novelty stores. Almost all pets that bite into glow-in-the-dark jewelry will drool or foam at the mouth excessively in response to the bitter taste of the liquid. The pet can be offered milk or treats to remove the bitter taste. Any glowing liquid must be washed off or signs will recur when the animal grooms itself.

Batteries

Flashlights, remote controls, toys, watches, hearing aids, and other battery-operated items pose a risk of battery exposure. When batteries are chewed by animals and the alkaline contents are released, chemical burns can penetrate deeply into local tissue. In addition, swallowing battery casings may result in GI obstruction. Button batteries can become lodged in the esophagus and can generate an electric current that can cause significant tissue damage and perforation of the esophagus. Treatment of battery exposure is the same as for exposure to any alkaline product and includes observation and treatment of burns incurred (see discussion under "Alkalis"). Radiography is often used to determine the location of the battery when the casing is missing or a button battery was swallowed. Intact batteries can be removed through induction of emesis, bulking of the diet, or endoscopy. If the casing is punctured, it may need to be surgically removed.

Ice/Snow Melts

The most common ingredients in ice melts are NaCl, potassium chloride, calcium chloride, magnesium chloride, calcium carbonate, and calcium magnesium acetate. Electrolyte imbalances and oral and GI irritation are possible after ingestion of large amounts of ice melts, salt, or rock salt. Pet-safe ice melts containing urea are considered safe for dogs and cats but not for ruminants. In case of dermal exposure, dermal decontamination of the pet should be performed. Close attention should be paid to removal of the crystals lodged between paw pads. Dermal irritation is possible with prolonged skin contact.

Dangerous Plants

Plant exposures are a common occurrence among various animals, including exotics, small animals, horses, and livestock. Exposures can occur with ornamental plants, house plants, and naturally occurring wild plants. Toxicity varies greatly depending on the species of the plant and the type of animal affected. For example, true lilies (*Lilium* spp.) can cause kidney failure in feline species, but generally only cause mild GI symptoms in canines. It is also important to ask the owner if any herbicides, pesticides, or fertilizers have been used on or around the plant to determine whether there is additional risk from these chemicals.

Precise identification of a plant can sometimes be difficult. Identifying the Latin name is the best way to evaluate the plant's toxic potential. If the Latin name is unknown, taking the plant to a garden center or researching on the Internet are possible ways to identify the plant.

> **TECHNICIAN NOTE**
>
> Animals may ignore certain plants for years before deciding on a particular day to eat them.

Rhododendron Species

Members of the *Rhododendron* family, including azalea and rhododendron, contain grayanotoxanes, which can lead to cardiovascular dysfunction. Clinical signs include vomiting, diarrhea, abdominal pain, weakness, depression, cardiac arrhythmias, hypotension, shock, cardiopulmonary arrest, pulmonary edema, dyspnea, CNS depression, and seizures. Signs generally occur within 4 to 12 hours of ingestion and may persist for several days. Severe poisoning has been reported in ruminants and horses, whereas dogs and cats mainly have GI signs. Veterinary treatment and observation is always recommended.

Cardiac Glycoside–Containing Plants

Hundreds of cardiac glycosides have been identified in various plants, including oleander (*Nerium oleander*), lily of the valley (*Convallaria majalis*) (Fig. 26.2), and foxglove (*Digitalis purpurea*) (Fig. 26.3). In most cases, all parts of the plant are toxic, and even small amounts can cause significant clinical signs. Clinical signs generally develop within several hours of ingestion, and signs may persist for several days after removal of plant material from the GI tract. Clinical signs include vomiting, diarrhea, and cardiac arrhythmias. Veterinary treatment and observation are recommended.

See Table 26.3 for a list of other cardiotoxic plants.

Castor Beans

Castor beans (*Ricinus communis*) contain ricin, a water-soluble toxin found in all parts of the castor bean plant but in the highest concentration in the seeds. Oil extracted from the seeds (castor oil) is used medicinally and is nontoxic. Ingestion of one seed is potentially lethal, and veterinary treatment is always recommended. There is no antidote, so supportive care is necessary. If the seeds are swallowed whole (not chewed), the ricin will not be released and clinical signs will not occur.

Cycad Palms

Cycad or sago palms (*Cycas, Zamia*) are found naturally in the sandy soils of tropical to subtropical climates but may also be grown as houseplants in more temperate climates (Fig. 26.4). Most parts of the plant are toxic, but the seeds contain a higher concentration of cycasin and are most often associated with toxicosis in small animals. Ingestion of one or more seeds has resulted in liver failure and death in dogs. Livestock and horses can develop neurologic signs after eating the foliage. Treatment is symptomatic and supportive. Early decontamination is critical to prevent liver damage.

See Table 26.4 for a list of other hepatotoxic plants.

> **TECHNICIAN NOTE**
> Cycad palms may be sold without warning labels as houseplants.

Lilies

Easter lilies (*Lilium longiflorum*), tiger lilies (*Lilium tigrinum*), rubrum or Japanese lilies (*Lilium speciosum* and *Lilium lancifolium*), and various day lilies (*Hemerocallis* spp.) (Fig. 26.5) can

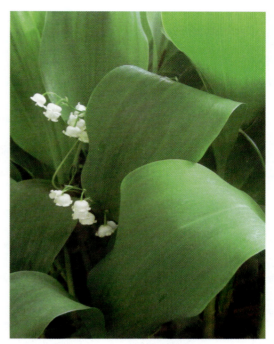

• **Fig. 26.2** *Convallaria majalis*, or lily of the valley. (Courtesy Laura Stern.)

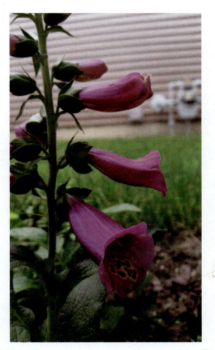

• **Fig. 26.3** *Digitalis purpurea*, or foxglove. (Courtesy MaryEllen Malysiak.)

cause acute renal failure and death in cats. The toxic principle is unknown. Even minor exposures (a few bites of a leaf, ingestion of pollen, etc.) may result in toxicosis. In felines, all exposures to lilies should be considered potentially life-threatening.

Affected cats often vomit within a few hours of exposure to lilies, but the vomiting quickly subsides and the cats may appear normal. Elevations in kidney values can occur as early as 12 to 18 hours after ingestion. Within 24 to 72 hours of ingestion, renal failure develops and is accompanied by vomiting, depression,

TABLE 26.3	Cardiotoxic Plants	
Common Name	**Latin Name**	**Comments**
Milkweed	*Asclepias* spp.	Cardiac glycosides—arrhythmias, hyperkalemia, death; others are neurotoxic
Yew	*Taxus* spp.	Arrhythmias, death
Avocado	*Persea americana*	Myocardial degeneration in rabbits, goats, caged birds; sterile mastitis
Cotton	*Gossypium* spp.	Gossypol in pigment glands
White snakeroot	*Ageratina altissima*	Myocardial necrosis in horses
Monkshood	*Aconitum* spp.	Bradycardia, hypotension, death
Larkspur	*Delphinium* spp.	Sudden death

TABLE 26.4	Hepatotoxic Plants	
Common Name	**Latin Name**	**Comments**
Cocklebur	*Xanthium strumarium*	New growth is most toxic
Ragwort Rattlebox Comfrey	*Senecio* spp. *Crotalaria* spp. *Symphytum* spp.	Pyrrolizidine alkaloids—chronic liver damage in grazing animals Can also cause dermatitis (photosensitization)
Blue-green algae	*Microcystis* spp., *Oscillatoria* spp., *Nodularia* spp.	Liver necrosis (can also cause neurologic signs)
Lantana	*Lantana* spp.	Cholestasis, bile duct proliferation, liver failure in grazing animals
Mushrooms	*Amanita* spp. *Galerina* spp. *Lepiota* spp.	Vomiting, liver failure, death
Blue panicum, kleingrass Puncture vine Bunchgrass Agave	*Panicum* spp. *Tribulus terrestris* *Nolina* spp. *Agave lecheguilla*	Formation of crystals in the bile ducts, secondary photosensitization in grazing animals

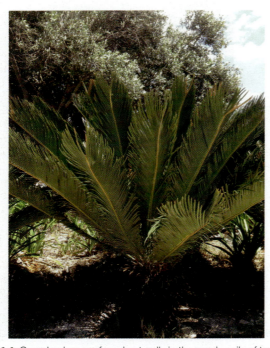

• **Fig. 26.4** Cycad palms are found naturally in the sandy soils of tropical to subtropical climates but may be used as houseplants in more temperate climates. (Courtesy Tina Wismer.)

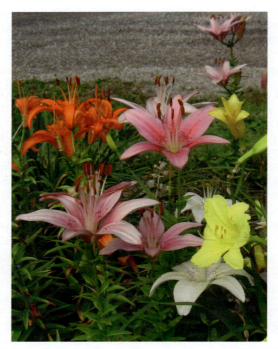

• **Fig. 26.5** A collection of *Lilium* and *Hemerocallis* spp. Acute renal failure and death can occur in cats that consume various lilies. (Courtesy Laura Stern.)

anorexia, and dehydration. Death generally occurs within 3 to 6 days of ingestion.

Veterinary treatment is always recommended for cats that have ingested lilies. Early decontamination by a veterinarian (emesis, oral administration of activated charcoal, and administration of a cathartic) in combination with IV fluid therapy has been shown to effectively prevent lily-induced kidney failure. Wash off any pollen from the coat. Delaying treatment beyond 18 hours frequently results in death or euthanasia as a result of severe kidney failure. Dialysis can be of help in some severely affected animals.

See Table 26.5 for a list of other nephrotoxic plants.

Insoluble Calcium Oxalate–Containing Plants

Philodendron species, calla lily (*Zantedeschia* spp.), elephant ears (*Caladium* spp.), dumb cane (*Dieffenbachia* spp.), peace lily (*Spathiphyllum* spp.), pothos (*Epipremnum* spp.), and many other varieties of plants contain insoluble calcium oxalate crystals. Chewing of the plant material can cause needle like raphide crystals to be expelled into the oral cavity and can result in painful oropharyngeal edema. Clinical signs associated with these plants include oral irritation; intense burning and irritation of the mouth, lips, and tongue; excessive drooling; vomiting; and difficulty swallowing. Airway compromise from tissue swelling could be life-threatening, although severe effects are a rare occurrence. Dilution with milk can help reduce the severity of the clinical signs.

There is a wide variety of common plants that can be poisonous to animals if ingested, but they cannot all be covered in this chapter. Tables 26.6 to 26.9 include lists of plants that can cause medical problems in various species.

TECHNICAL NOTE
Most common houseplants contain insoluble calcium oxalate crystals.

Pesticides

Ant and Roach Baits

Ant and roach baits may be referred to as *hotels, disks, stations, traps,* or *baits.* The baits usually contain inert ingredients, such as peanut butter, breadcrumbs, sugar, and vegetable or animal oils, in addition to the insecticide. Insecticides commonly used in these baits are fipronil, indoxacarb, avermectin, boric acid, and hydramethylnon. These insecticides have a wide margin of safety (therapeutic index) and are present in small quantities within the baits,

TABLE 26.5   Nephrotoxic Plants

Common Name	Latin Name	Comments
Sorghum	*Sorghum* spp.	Ataxia, cystitis in horses
Grapes/raisins	*Vitis* spp.	Renal failure in dogs
Oak	*Quercus* spp.	Gallotanins in grazing animals
Pigweed	*Amaranthus* spp.	Perirenal edema, renal failure
Shamrock Sorrel, dock Rhubarb	*Oxalis* spp. *Rumex* spp. *Rheum* spp.	Soluble calcium oxalate crystals form in the kidney; ruminants can eat enough to cause hypocalcemia

TABLE 26.6   Neurotoxic Plants

Common Name	Latin Name	Comments
Water hemlock	*Cicuta maculate*	Seizures, death
Sorghum	*Sorghum* spp.	Ataxia, cystitis in horses
Milkweed	*Asclepias* spp.	Seizures (others are cardiotoxic)
Blue-green algae	*Anabaena flos-aquae*	Seizures, salivation, vomiting, diarrhea; others are hepatotoxic
White snakeroot	*Ageratina altissima*	Tremors, ataxia in ruminants (milk sickness)
Marijuana	*Cannabis sativa*	Ataxia, sedation, occasionally agitation, urinary incontinence (dogs)
Yellow jessamine	*Gelsemium sempervirens*	Muscle weakness, seizures, death
Yesterday, today, and tomorrow	*Brunfelsia* spp.	Tremors (can last for weeks), seizures
Dallis grass Perennial ryegrass Bermuda grass Phalaris grass	*Paspalum* spp. *Lilium perenne* *Cynodon dactylon* *Phalaris* spp.	Fungal infection of plant causes grass staggers, tremors in grazing animals
Horsetail Brakenfern	*Equisetum* spp. *Pteridium aquilinum*	Ataxia, paresis secondary to thiamine deficiency (horses); anemia, bladder, and GI tumors in ruminants
Locoweed	*Astragalus* spp. *Oxytropis* spp.	Ataxia

TABLE 26.7   Plants Causing Reproductive Adverse Effects

Common Name	Latin Name	Comments
Ponderosa pine Monterey cypress Common juniper	*Pinus ponderosa* *Cupressus macrocarpa* *Juniperus communis*	Abortion (isocupressic acid) in cattle
False hellebore	*Veratrum californicum*	Cycloptic lambs if ingested on day 14 of pregnancy
Tobacco Poison hemlock Lupine	*Nicotana* spp. *Conium maculatum* *Lupinus* spp.	Neuromuscular blocking resulting in limb deformities
Fescue	*Festuca* spp.	Infected with fungus, prolonged gestation, abortion, dystocia, agalactia in horses

TABLE 26.8   Plants Causing Dermal Lesions

Common Name	Latin Name	Comments
St. John's wort Buckwheat	*Hypericum* spp. *Fagopyrum* spp.	Dermatitis, photosensitization (helianthrones) in grazing animals
Giant hogweed Queen Anne's lace Spring parsley Dutchman's breeches	*Heracleum mantegazzianum* *Amni majus* *Cymopterus* spp. *Thamnosma* spp.	Dermatitis, photosensitization (furcoumarins [psoralens]) in grazing animals
Hairy vetch	*Vicia villosa*	Granulomatous dermatitis in cattle

TABLE 26.9   Plants Causing Miscellaneous Effects

Common Name	Latin Name	Comments
Black walnut	*Juglans nigra*	Laminitis in horses
White and yellow sweet clover	*Melilotus* spp.	Fungal growth can produce dicoumarol (anticoagulant); bleeding in cattle
Red maple	*Acer rubrum*	Hemolysis in horses
Poinsettia	*Euphorbia pulcherrima*	Gastrointestinal upset (toxicity has been exaggerated)
Tulips Daffodils	*Tulipa* spp. *Narcissus* spp.	Gastroenteritis; bulbs are the most toxic part
Apple Cherry	*Malus* spp. *Prunus* spp.	Seeds, bark, and leaves contain cyanide; problems most commonly seen in grazing animals
Hops	*Humulus lupulus*	Severe hyperthermia and death in dogs

TABLE 26.10   Insecticides Commonly Used as Topical or Oral Flea/Tick Control

Family of Insecticides	Insecticide	Adverse Effects
Pyrethrins	Etofenprox Permethrin Phenothrin	Wide margin of safety with low concentrations Taste reactions (drooling) if ingested Paw and ear flicking (cats) Dermal paresthesia with concentrated products Tremors in cats with concentrated products (especially permethrin)
Insect growth regulators	Pyriproxyfen, methoprene	Mild gastrointestinal upset if ingested
Avermectins	Ivermectin Moxidectin Selemectin	Ataxia, tremors, lethargy if ingested
Nitroguanide	Dinotefuran	Drooling, vomiting if ingested Application site irritation
Tetracyclic macrolide	Spinetoram, spinosad	Vomiting, ataxia
Oxadiazine	Indoxacarb	Vomiting, ataxia
Phenylpyrazole	Fipronil	Drooling if ingested; application site irritation; seizures and death in rabbits
Neonicotinoid	Imidacloprid Nitenpyram	Drooling, vomiting if ingested Can see hyperactivity as fleas die with nitenpyram
Isoxazoline-substituted benzamide	Fluralaner, afoxolaner Sarolaner	Vomiting, diarrhea, lethargy Can rarely see tremors, ataxia, and seizures even at therapeutic doses
Chitin synthesis inhibitor	Lufenuron	Mild gastrointestinal upset

making them a hazard of low toxicity to dogs and cats. If ingested, the plastic or metal container can act as a foreign body, causing additional problems. Outdoor ant baits used to treat yards come in granular or spray form. Dogs are more sensitive to bifenthrin than other pyrethroids, and bifenthrin-containing insecticides can cause tremors and fasciculations. Symptoms are typically seen within 4 to 8 hours. Treatment includes decontamination, fluids, and supportive care to manage tremors.

Flea/Tick Products

Oral flea preventatives and topical spot-on products are commonly used due to their effectiveness and ease of administration. Some products prevent flea egg development, and others kill adult fleas and ticks. These products have replaced most of the sprays, shampoos, dips, and collars that were commonly used in the past. Approved insecticides have a wide margin of safety when used appropriately; however, all insecticides have the potential for adverse effects. Common adverse effects seen with appropriately used products are generally mild. Table 26.10 documents the commonly used topical spot-on and oral flea and tick products and their adverse effects.

In cases where the pet develops a dermal reaction, mild redness at the application site, hair loss, paresthesia, and behavior changes may be seen. Paresthesia can be caused by topically applied concentrated pyrethrins. Owners may think that the animal is experiencing a tingling sensation at the application site. If these symptoms are seen, the animal should be bathed in a mild liquid dishwashing detergent and towel dried to prevent chilling. Fractious animals may need to be sedated by a veterinarian for the procedure. Examination by a veterinarian may be needed if the skin continues to be red or painful.

Ingestion of topical insecticides or sprays may result in a taste reaction, especially in cats. Dogs and cats are unable to get rid of bitter taste by spitting, so when they have a bad taste in the mouth, they tend to drool. Giving the animal a tasty treat, such as a few laps of milk, water, or tuna juice, will help dilute the bad taste and stop the drooling.

Cats have been shown to be extremely sensitive to concentrated permethrin. Currently, there are multiple brands of permethrin spot-on products available over the counter as topical flea control labeled "for dogs only." The packaging of these products often has multiple warnings against use in cats; however, inappropriate application of concentrated permethrin products still occurs frequently and can result in muscle tremors and seizures in cats. Problems can even occur in cats that groom or closely interact with dogs, including sharing common sleeping areas, in the first 24 hours after application of concentrated permethrin.

The first step for treating symptomatic cats exposed to permethrin compounds involves controlling muscle tremors with methocarbamol. Choices for seizure control include diazepam, propofol, barbiturates, or inhalant anesthetics. After stabilization, the entire body of the cat should be bathed using a mild liquid dishwashing detergent. Supportive care, such as thermoregulation, fluid therapy to maintain hydration, and nutritional support, should be provided as needed until full recovery. Some cats may experience symptoms for up to 3 days.

> **TECHNICIAN NOTE**
>
> Always read and follow label directions when using flea and tick products. Many products that are safe for use in dogs are extremely toxic to cats.

Methomyl

Methomyl is a highly toxic carbamate insecticide that can be found in fly baits. Carbamate insecticides competitively inhibit acetylcholine esterase, causing parasympathetic effects. Clinical signs include SLUDDE (salivation, lacrimation, urinary incontinence, diarrhea, dyspnea, and emesis) syndrome, bradycardia or tachycardia, and seizures. Immediate veterinary treatment is required, because signs can occur within minutes of methomyl ingestion. The antidote of choice is the anticholinergic atropine.

Molluscicides

Metaldehyde was commonly found in snail or slug bait and is highly toxic; fortunately, its use is becoming rarer. The onset of clinical signs is typically seen within 30 minutes to 3 hours of ingestion and include increased HR, panting, drooling, ataxia, hyperthermia, tremors, and seizures. In some cases, liver and kidney failure may occur within 2 to 3 days of exposure. Veterinary treatment and observation are always required, and many of these animals will require gastric lavage to remove the bait from the digestive tract and methocarbamol to stop the tremors.

Sodium feredetate and ferric phosphate are the newer iron-based types of molluscicides that cause direct caustic or irritant effects on the intestinal mucosa. Vomiting, lethargy, and diarrhea (often bloody) occur within 0.5 to 6 hours. Treatment includes limiting absorption with magnesium hydroxide, protecting the GI mucosa, and chelation if needed to remove excess iron from blood.

Rodenticides

There are multiple types of rat or mouse baits available commercially, but the most common are **anticoagulants**, bromethalin, and cholecalciferol. Other pesticides, such as strychnine and zinc phosphide, may be used to control wild rodent populations.

Anticoagulants

Anticoagulant rodenticides (Table 26.11) act by competitive inhibition of vitamin K epoxide reductase, thus halting the recycling of vitamin K. Vitamin K is an important component in the production of blood-clotting factors; thus toxicity with anticoagulant rodenticides interferes with hemostasis. Clinical signs of anticoagulant poisoning may not be observed for 3 to 7 days after ingestion and include hemorrhage, pale mucous membranes, weakness, exercise intolerance, lameness, dyspnea, coughing, and swollen joints. Often, the animal is not taken to a veterinarian until the clinical signs become severe.

Animals that are seen ingesting the bait can be made to vomit. If induction of emesis is unsuccessful, vitamin K_1 should be started. Animals with clinical signs should be stabilized immediately. Transfusions with whole blood, fresh plasma, or fresh-frozen plasma may be necessary to replace clotting factors. Oral vitamin K_1 is an antidote for anticoagulants and should be given with a fatty meal to enhance absorption. Length of treatment will depend on the exact bait ingested but is often 30 days or longer.

> **TECHNICIAN NOTE**
>
> Rodents often move rodenticide-containing baits from the protective boxes, which allows pets access to them. Clients should be made aware of this.

Bromethalin

Bromethalin causes uncoupling of oxidative phosphorylation in the CNS, leading to cerebral edema and neurologic signs. Depending on the dose, clinical signs of bromethalin toxicosis can occur any time from 8 to 96 hours after exposure and include muscle tremors, seizures, hyperexcitability, forelimb extensor rigidity, ataxia, CNS depression, loss of vocalization, paresis, paralysis, and death. Cats are more sensitive to bromethalin compared with

TABLE 26.11	Anticoagulant Rodenticides
Brodifacoum	Bromadiolone
Chlorophacinone	Difenacoum
Difethialone	Diphacinone
Pindone	Warfarin

dogs. Guinea pigs are not affected by bromethalin, because they cannot make the toxic metabolite (desmethylbromethalin).

Aggressive decontamination is most important with bromethalin ingestion. Repeated doses of activated charcoal (every 8–12 hours) may be needed. If activated charcoal is given, sodium levels should be monitored for hypernatremia. The prognosis is poor for animals showing severe signs. A definitive diagnosis of bromethalin toxicosis can only be made at postmortem examination.

Cholecalciferol

Cholecalciferol (vitamin D_3) increases intestinal absorption of calcium, stimulates bone resorption, and enhances kidney reabsorption of calcium. This causes a serum calcium increase, leading to soft tissue mineralization, kidney failure, and death. Clinical signs usually have a delayed onset, occurring 18 to 36 hours after ingestion. The most common signs seen with cholecalciferol toxicosis include vomiting, diarrhea, inappetence, depression, polyuria, and polydipsia.

Decontamination is important with cholecalciferol ingestion. Administration of repeated doses of activated charcoal or cholestyramine is recommended, along with monitoring of serum calcium, phosphorus, creatinine, and blood urea nitrogen. Elevations in calcium are treated with IV fluid therapy (0.9% NaCl), prednisone, and furosemide. Pamidronate is the preferred treatment for persistent hypercalcemia. The goal is to prevent soft tissue calcification, because this cannot be reversed. Symptomatic patients may need to be treated for weeks.

Zinc Phosphide

Zinc phosphide is a rodenticide used in mole and gopher baits and is highly toxic. After ingestion, phosphide is converted to phosphine gas by stomach acid. The released phosphine gas causes severe respiratory distress. Clinical signs are seen soon after ingestion, typically within 15 minutes to 4 hours. Zinc phosphide causes vomiting, dyspnea, and seizures. Death occurs because of respiratory failure. These animals should be seen immediately by a veterinarian. Affected animals should be made to vomit outside or in another well-ventilated area away from other patients. Phosphine gas exposures are also dangerous to humans and smells like rotten fish. If people in the area can smell it, they should contact a human poison control center.

> **TECHNICIAN NOTE**
> If any of the staff members experience a headache or shortness of breath while managing a zinc phosphide case, they should seek medical attention.

Antifreeze Products

Ethylene Glycol

Ethylene glycol (EG) is the most dangerous type of antifreeze. Most commercial antifreeze products contain between 95% and 97% EG. The minimum lethal dose of undiluted EG antifreeze is 4.4 to 6.6 mL/kg in dogs and 1.4 mL/kg in cats. EG can cause drunkenness, metabolic acidosis, acute renal tubular necrosis, and death. The clinical signs will change as the parent compound (an alcohol) is metabolized. Peak blood levels of EG are reached within 1 to 4 hours after ingestion. In most cases of EG poisoning, vomiting is seen within the first few hours and signs of depression, ataxia, weakness, tachypnea, polyuria, and polydipsia within 1 to 6 hours. By 18 to 36 hours, acute renal failure develops.

> **TECHNICIAN NOTE**
> Ethylene glycol (EG) is the most dangerous form of antifreeze and causes acute renal failure.

Commercial EG test kits are available for cage side veterinary use. Most are accurate from 30 minutes up to 12 hours after ingestion. The test kit insert should be consulted and directions followed carefully. The blood sample should be obtained before giving any treatment, as both activated charcoal and some injectable medications can cause a false-positive result. Do not use alcohol to wet down the fur for the blood draw, as this can also affect results.

Induction of emesis is only helpful in cases of very recent ingestion. The goal of treatment of EG toxicosis is to slow down or block its metabolism. Fomepizole or ethanol is used to block the production of toxic EG metabolites. Fluid diuresis and correction of acidosis with sodium bicarbonate are also important components of therapy. Treatment must be started as soon as possible, because once renal values have increased, the prognosis is poor.

Methanol

Methanol (also known as *methyl alcohol* or *wood alcohol*) is commonly found in windshield washer fluid and varies in concentration from 20% to 100% (20%–30% is most common). Methanol's metabolite, formaldehyde, is rapidly oxidized by aldehyde dehydrogenase to formic acid, which can cause metabolic acidosis, seizures, and retinal toxicity (blindness) in primates but not other species. With small exposures in nonprimates, only mild gastric upset is seen. Larger exposures can cause sedation and ataxia. In the case of ingestion of a large amount, the animal should be monitored and treated for acidosis.

Propylene Glycol

Propylene glycol is the main ingredient in "safer" forms of engine antifreeze or coolants. It is typically used in boats and RVs, and to winterize waterlines. Propylene glycol is approximately three times less toxic to dogs compared with EG; however, in toxic quantities, acidosis, liver damage, and renal insufficiency could occur. Clinical signs of propylene glycol toxicosis include CNS depression, weakness, ataxia, and seizures. With ingestion of large amounts, diuresis and supportive care, such as treatment for acidosis, should be provided.

Human Medications

It should be noted that any medication can be dangerous to an animal, depending on the dose and frequency. Human medications that are potentially dangerous to animals are discussed below. All require veterinary consultation, treatment, and monitoring.

Acetaminophen

Acetaminophen is a synthetic nonopiate derivative of *p*-aminophenol that is often used as an analgesic. In dogs, it can be used therapeutically at a dose of 10 mg/kg every 12 hours. Clinical signs of liver injury can be seen in dogs at 100 mg/kg and methemoglobinemia at 200 mg/kg. In cats, 10 mg/kg has produced signs of toxicity. Cats are more sensitive to acetaminophen, because they are deficient in the enzyme glucuronidase that detoxifies acetaminophen. Clinical signs include depression, weakness, tachypnea, dyspnea, vomiting, methemoglobinemia, hypothermia, facial or paw edema, hepatic necrosis, and death. The antidote is acetylcysteine, which can decrease mortality and morbidity.

> **TECHNICIAN NOTE**
>
> Cats are more sensitive to acetaminophen compared with dogs; a dose of 10 mg/kg can cause toxicity in cats, whereas 100 mg/kg is the toxic dose for dogs.

Nonsteroidal Anti-inflammatory Drugs

Nonsteroidal anti-inflammatory drugs (NSAIDs) include over-the-counter medications, such as ibuprofen and naproxen; prescription products, such as diclofenac and indomethacin; and veterinary medications, such as carprofen and deracoxib. These drugs, which have anti-inflammatory, antipyretic, and analgesic properties, can cause vomiting, stomach ulcers, and acute renal failure in animals. At high doses, ibuprofen and phenylbutazone can also have CNS effects, such as seizures, ataxia, and coma. Cats are considered more sensitive than dogs, because cats have a limited glucuronyl-conjugating capacity to metabolize NSAIDs.

The primary goal of treatment is to prevent or treat gastric ulceration, renal failure, and CNS effects. IV fluids, antiemetics, and GI protectants are the mainstays of therapy. Length of treatment will vary depending on the substance ingested. The prognosis is good if the animal is treated promptly and appropriately.

Aspirin

Aspirin can be used therapeutically in both dogs and cats but must be used cautiously in cats because of their inability to rapidly metabolize and excrete salicylates. Symptoms of acute aspirin overdose in dogs and cats include depression, vomiting, stomach ulcers, anorexia, hyperthermia, acidosis, and liver injury. Vomiting can be seen, even at therapeutic doses. Treatment consists of fluids, antiemetics, and GI protectants. Salicylates can also be found in teething ointments, Pepto-Bismol, and wart removers.

Pseudoephedrine and Amphetamines

Pseudoephedrine is a stimulant found in cold and flu medications as a nasal decongestant. It is similar in structure to amphetamines. Many medications to treat attention deficit/hyperactivity disorder are also amphetamines. They can cause increased blood pressure, tachycardia, ataxia, mydriasis, hyperactivity, tremors, and seizures. Acepromazine, beta blockers, and fluids are important parts of treatment. Diazepam is contraindicated because it can increase agitation and dysphoria.

> **TECHNICIAN NOTE**
>
> Many medications to treat attention deficit/hyperactivity disorder are amphetamines and are commonly ingested by household pets.

Isoniazid

Isoniazid is a medication used to treat tuberculosis. Overdoses produce life-threatening signs of seizures, acidosis, and coma. Pyridoxine (vitamin B_6) is a direct antagonist of isoniazid. Dogs are very sensitive, as they have a reduced ability to metabolize this medication.

Calcipotriene

Calcipotriene is a synthetic derivative of vitamin D_3. It is used as a topical ointment to treat psoriasis in humans. An overdose of calcipotriene can cause hypercalcemia, which can result in kidney failure, cardiac failure, and possibly death. Treatment is the same as for cholecalciferol rodenticides (see "Cholecalciferol").

5-Fluorouracil

5-Fluorouracil (5-FU) is a topical anticancer cream. It is used in humans to treat solar and actinic keratoses and some superficial skin tumors. 5-FU, like other anticancer agents, attacks rapidly dividing cells, such as bone marrow stem cells and the epithelial layer of the intestinal crypts. Early effects seen with 5-FU exposure in dogs include seizures, tremors, vomiting, and ataxia. Cardiac arrhythmias, respiratory distress, and hemorrhagic gastroenteritis are also seen. Clinical signs develop within 1 hour, and death often occurs within 6 to 16 hours after exposure. In those that survive the initial effects, it is possible to see bone marrow suppression with evidence of neutropenia 4 to 20 days after exposure.

Recreational Drugs

Marijuana

Marijuana can go by many different names, such as *flower*, *pot*, *grass*, *Mary Jane*, and *weed*. More concentrated forms can be called hash, wax, rosin, oil, and dabs. As a fresh plant, marijuana is not considered toxic, but toxicity increases when the plant is damaged by heating, drying, smoking, or aging. Marijuana can be found in three basic forms: (1) as a dried herb (composed of top leaves and buds); (2) rosin (hash or hashish); and (3) a sticky liquid (hash oil). These forms can be used to make edible products, such as cookies or brownies. Through selective breeding, the potency of marijuana has been increased over the years, making it more dangerous to animals.

In dogs, the onset of clinical signs generally occurs about 30 to 90 minutes after ingestion. Symptoms may last for up to 72 hours. Initial signs can include nervousness and disorientation, which can progress to depression (which may last up to 18–36 hours). Mydriasis, hypothermia, nystagmus, urinary incontinence, and ataxia have also been seen. Marijuana exposure is rarely fatal, although death can occur in severe cases. Decontamination by emesis may be attempted, but because of the antiemetic properties of cannabis, it may not be effective. Activated charcoal with a cathartic can be given if the pet is asymptomatic. Supportive care should include fluids, thermoregulation, assisted respiration if needed, and diazepam if agitation is seen. Lipid therapy has been anecdotally helpful in comatose patients. If baked goods were involved, the risk of chocolate toxicosis must also be considered. Some edible products may also contain xylitol as a sugar substitute. Urine drug tests are commonly false-negative, as dogs make different metabolites than people.

> **TECHNICIAN NOTE**
>
> An animal with ataxia that exhibits dribbling of urine should be considered intoxicated by marijuana until proven otherwise.

Cocaine

Cocaine is a natural alkaloid derived from the coca plant (*Erythroxylon coca*). It is a potent CNS stimulant with sympathomimetic effects. Street cocaine is often adulterated and can come in a variety of concentrations. Street names for cocaine include *crack*, *rock*, *snow*, *blow*, *nose candy*, and *speedball* (cocaine and heroin). Cocaine can be detected in plasma, stomach contents, and urine. When absorbed orally, cocaine can be detected in plasma within 30 minutes. Because cocaine is better absorbed in the small intestine than in the stomach, peak levels are slightly delayed to between 50 and 90 minutes after ingestion.

Initially, dogs present with signs of serotonin syndrome and stimulatory signs. Serotonin syndrome is a spectrum of clinic signs caused by increased CNS serotonergic activity and increased serotonin levels. Cardiovascular, nervous, GI, metabolic, and respiratory systems are affected. Symptoms can range from lethargy and sedation to CNS excitement, hyperactivity, hyperthermia, tachypnea, tachycardia, erratic behavior, and possibly seizures. Other possible signs of cocaine are vomiting, hypersalivation, tachycardia, hypertension, and hyperthermia. Dogs may later become depressed and comatose. Death may result from hyperthermia, cardiac arrest, or respiratory arrest. Because of the quick onset of symptoms, emesis should only be induced within 15 minutes of ingestion, because the patient can deteriorate rapidly. An alternative is gastric lavage under anesthesia followed by administration of activated charcoal. HR, heart rhythm, blood pressure, and electrolyte level should be monitored throughout treatment. Diazepam can be used to control tremors and seizures, naloxone to inhibit cocaine-induced agitation, and cyproheptadine to treat serotonin syndrome. For life-threatening tachyarrhythmias, a beta blocker, such as propranolol, can be used.

Ethanol

In published reports, the lowest reported LD of ethanol poisoning was 5.5 mL/kg in a dog and 6 mL/kg in a cat. See Table 26.12 for average alcohol concentrations found in commonly ingested alcohol products (200 proof = 100% ethanol). Depending on the amount of alcohol ingested, clinical signs of ethanol poisoning can include vomiting, ataxia, CNS depression, hypotension, hypothermia, arrhythmias, respiratory depression, and coma. Treatment is generally symptomatic and supportive. Fluid diuresis and respiratory support are used on an as-needed basis while monitoring temperature and cardiac function. Aspiration is a concern, as ethanol affects the closing of the epiglottis during vomiting. With treatment and monitoring, the prognosis is good.

Methamphetamine

Methamphetamines are stimulants. For clinical signs and treatment of methamphetamine exposure, refer to the "Pseudoephedrine and Amphetamine" section. Clinical signs occur quickly after ingestion.

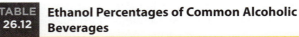

TABLE 26.12 Ethanol Percentages of Common Alcoholic Beverages

Type of Drink	Percentage of Ethanol
Beer	4%
Craft beer	4%–>10%
Wine	10%
Vodka	40%
Whiskey	43%
Grain alcohol (Everclear)	95%

Acknowledgments

The authors would like to thank Jill A. Richardson and Mary Ellen Malysiak for their previous work on this chapter.

Recommended Readings

Burrows GE, Tyrl RJ. *Toxic Plants of North America*. 2nd ed. Ames, IA: Wiley-Blackwell; 2013.

Cortinovis C, Caloni F. Household food items toxic to dogs and cats. *Front Vet Sci*. 2016;3:26.

Dunayer EK, Gwaltney-Brant SM. Acute hepatic failure and coagulopathy associated with xylitol ingestion in eight dogs. *J Am Vet Med Assoc*. 2006;229(7):1113–1117.

Hooser SB, Khan SA. Common toxicologic issues in small animals: an update. *Vet Clin North Am Small Anim Pract*. 2018;48(6):899–1118.

Lee KW, Yamato O, Tajima M, et al. Hematologic changes associated with the appearance of eccentrocytes after intragastric administration of garlic extract to dogs. *Am J Vet Res*. 2000;61:1446–1450.

Means C. Bread dough toxicosis in dogs. *J Vet Emerg Crit Care*. 2003;13(1):39–41.

Meola SD, Tearney CC, Haas SA, et al. Evaluation of trends in marijuana toxicosis in dogs living in a state with legalized medical marijuana: 125 dogs (2005–2010). *J Vet Emerg Crit Care*. 2012;22(6):690–696.

Peterson ME, Talcott PA. *Small Animal Toxicology*. 3rd ed. St. Louis, MO: Elsevier; 2013.

Schell MM. Tremorgenic mycotoxin intoxication. *Vet Med*. 2000;95(4):283–286.

Simmons DM. Onion breath. *Vet Technician*. 2001;22(8):424–427.

Slater MR, Gwaltney-Brant S. Exposure circumstances and outcomes of 48 households with 57 cats exposed to toxic lily species. *J Am Anim Hosp Assoc*. 2011;47(6):386–390.

Wegenast CA, Meadows ID, Anderson RE, et al. Acute kidney injury in dogs following ingestion of cream of tartar and tamarinds and the connection to tartaric acid as the proposed toxic principle in grapes and raisins. *J Vet Emerg Crit Care*. 2022;32(6):812–816.

27

Wound Management and Bandaging

ERIN SCOTT, JOSEPH LOZIER, AND JARRED WILLIAMS

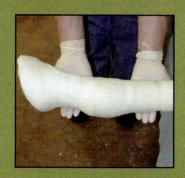

CHAPTER OUTLINE

LEARNING OBJECTIVES

When you have completed this chapter, you will be able to:

1. Pronounce, define, and spell all key terms in the chapter.
2. Identify the phases of wound healing and describe patient, wound, and treatment factors that adversely affect wound healing.
3. Do the following regarding wound management in the small animal:
   - Describe the objectives and principles of immediate wound care, including wound lavage.
   - Describe the goals and methods of wound debridement.
   - Differentiate among primary, delayed primary, and secondary wound closure and among primary-, second-, and third-intention healing.
   - Compare methods of managing wound drainage and wound infection.
   - Explain the nature and appearance of abrasions, lacerations, degloving injuries, penetrating wounds, burns, decubitus ulcers, and pressure sores and discuss the methods used to treat each.
4. Identify the principles of bandaging and discuss the purpose of the primary, secondary, and tertiary layers of a bandage, including the specific materials used for each.
5. Discuss the uses for and characteristics of the following external coaptation methods in small animals and their application technique:

   - Robert Jones bandage and modified Robert Jones bandage
   - Casts and splints
   - Ehmer, 90/90 flexion, Velpeau, and carpal flexion sling, hobbles
   - Bandages for the head, chest, abdomen, tail, and areas that are difficult to bandage, such as the pelvis and the axilla
6. Explain aftercare of bandages, splints, casts, and slings, including complications that may occur.
7. Discuss the principles of equine wound care, including treatment of exuberant granulation tissue.
8. Do the following regarding application of bandages, splints, and casts in horses:
   - Discuss uses for, characteristics of, and the technique used to place a lower limb wound bandage or a support bandage on an equine limb.
   - Discuss uses for and characteristics of equine casts and splints, and techniques used to place a cast or a splint on an equine limb.
   - Describe the technique used to remove a cast.
9. Discuss uses for and characteristics of bandages, splints, and casts used for cattle and describe technique used to place a claw block and a modified Thomas splint on a ruminant limb.

KEY TERMS

Abrasions
Active drain
Carpal flexion sling
Collagen

Contralateral
Cytotoxic
Dead space
Debridement

Decubitus ulcers
Degloving injury
Dehiscence
Dermis
Ehmer sling
Eschar
Epidermis
Epithelialization
External coaptation
Extracellular matrix
Exuberant granulation tissue
Fibroblasts
First-degree burn
Fourth-degree burn
Granulation tissue
Hypertonic
Inflammatory phase
Inguinal
Isotonic
Lacerations
Lag phase
Maturation phase
Modified Robert Jones bandage

Modified Thomas splint
Moist wound healing
Myofibroblast
Negative-pressure wound therapy
Nonadherent dressing
Nonocclusive
Occlusive
Passive drain
Penetrating wounds
Primary closure
Primary-intention wound healing
Proliferative phase
Re-epithelialization
Robert Jones bandage
Second-degree burn
Second-intention wound healing
Secondary closure
Semiocclusive
Spica splint
Third-degree burn
Third-intention wound healing
Velpeau sling

Wound Healing

Phases of Wound Healing

The skin forms an important protective barrier against insults from the environment. When injured, either by trauma or by a purposeful insult such as a surgical incision, the physiologic phases of wound healing begin. Wound healing is a continuous process that starts at the moment of injury and lasts up to months thereafter. It can be divided into three phases—inflammatory, proliferative, and maturation—which are distinct in their characteristics but overlap in the timeline of healing (Box 27.1). These phases are best observed in a wound left to heal by second-intention healing (Fig. 27.1).

• BOX 27.1 | **Phases of Wound Healing**

Inflammatory (Lag)
- Begins immediately and lasts 3 to 5 days
- Characterized by formation of a blood clot within the wound, release of growth factors, and recruitment of macrophages and neutrophils to clean up the wound and modulate healing
- Wound at its weakest during this phase

Proliferative
- Begins after 2 to 3 days
- Characterized by invasion of fibroblasts, formation of granulation tissue, deposition of collagen, epithelialization across healthy granulation tissue, and wound contraction by myofibroblasts
- Wound strength increases considerably during this phase

Maturation
- Begins after about 3 weeks and lasts weeks to months
- Collagen fibers remodel and align, and a final gain in wound strength occurs

---

The **inflammatory phase** begins immediately. As the injury occurs, blood is released into the wound via injured blood vessels. Platelets aggregate and form a fibrin clot within the wound, which aids in control of bleeding and stabilizes the wound edges. The clot also allows growth factors to be released as part of the clotting cascade. Within a few hours, wound macrophages and neutrophils are recruited and modulate wound healing by releasing more growth factors. They also help remove bacteria and cellular debris from the wound. Wound exudate is the combination of white blood cells and fluid leaked from blood vessels and lymphatics. The inflammatory phase lasts for 3 to 5 days and is often called the *lag phase*, because wound strength is at its lowest during this phase and **dehiscence** is most likely. Dehiscence is a partial or total separation of previously approximated wound edges from surgical or primary closure. This time frame may be extended up to 10 days in animals that are at risk of slower healing times due to existing comorbidities.

TECHNICIAN NOTE

During the inflammatory phase of wound healing (the first 3–5 days) wound strength is minimal and dehiscence may occur.

The **proliferative phase**, or the repair phase, begins 3 to 5 days after injury and continues for 2 to 4 weeks, depending on the wound type and size. It is marked by **fibroblasts** and endothelial cells entering the wound. Growth factors released into the wound stimulate cell proliferation and recruitment, and production of an **extracellular matrix** (ECM). As cells migrate into the wound, new vessels are formed by angiogenesis to supply oxygen and nutrients to newly forming tissue. **Granulation tissue** creates a surface for **re-epithelialization** and is a source of fibroblasts, **myofibroblasts**, endothelial cells, inflammatory cells, and new blood vessels, all connected by the ECM. Healthy

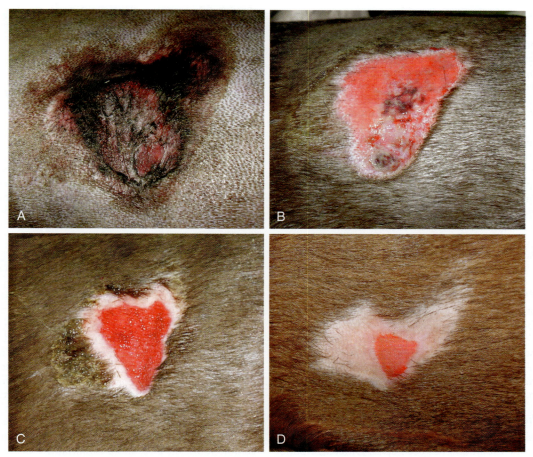

• **Fig. 27.1** Phases of wound healing. (A) The inflammatory phase. Contamination and nonviable tissue have to be eliminated. (B) Beginning of the proliferative phase. Granulation tissue begins to cover the wound. (C) Wound contraction. Epithelial cells begin to migrate across the wound. (D) Epithelialization is well advanced; once complete, the maturation phase will begin.

granulation tissue is pink to reddish in appearance because of an abundance of capillaries; poor quality granulation tissue is pale from a lack of appropriate blood supply. Fibroblasts begin to deposit **collagen** into the wound, thus increasing wound strength. Once the wound bed is covered by granulation tissue, fibroblasts decrease in number and are replaced by collagen-rich tissue. Epithelial cells can now migrate across healthy granulation tissue to re-establish a barrier between the wound and the environment. **Epithelialization** usually begins 4 to 5 days after the injury. Starting at the wound edges, cells advance in a single layer across the wound until they meet in the middle. New epithelial cells are formed at the wound margins to replace keratinocytes and supply more cells for migration, thereby thickening the epithelial layer. If a scab is present, epithelialization occurs underneath it, and the scab will eventually fall off. A **moist wound healing** environment enhances cell migration and cleanup, and is preferred over allowing a wound/scab to dry out. Once the wound is covered by keratinocytes, a new basement membrane is formed, and cells begin to differentiate to re-epithelialize skin. New epithelium tends to be friable and to bleed easily. Wound contraction of the full-thickness skin edges occurs as the result of contraction of myofibroblasts within the granulation tissue. It helps to reduce the size of the wound, sometimes considerably. Contraction begins about 1 week after injury and can last for several weeks.

The final phase of wound healing is the **maturation phase**, which begins approximately 3 weeks after injury and continues for weeks to months and sometimes years. It is characterized by remodeling and realignment of collagen fibers along tension lines. During this phase, the wound tissue gains the most strength, although it will only regain 80% of its original strength.

A surgically closed wound with direct apposition of wound edges can heal by **primary wound healing**. The wound will still undergo the three different phases of wound healing; however, in the proliferative phase, granulation tissue does not form, because no defect is present between wound edges. Epithelialization begins after a few days and crosses the incision directly. Because of poor wound strength during the inflammatory (lag) phase, apposition depends entirely on surgical closure during this time. This is why dehiscence is usually seen within the first 3 to 5 days after surgery. Thereafter, wound strength gradually increases, taking the tension off the sutures or staples.

Factors Influencing Wound Healing

Wound healing is influenced by many factors, such as patient health, wound classification, and concurrent treatment. It is important to consider these factors, because they can considerably delay the phases of wound healing or predispose the patient to infection.

Patient Factors

Although aging is not a disease, older animals often have concurrent health problems that may alter their healing capabilities. Endocrinopathies have several effects on wounds. Cushing disease and hypothyroidism delay wound healing, diabetes mellitus alters tissue perfusion and release of oxygen, and hyperglycemia interferes with defense against infection. Chronic viral infections, such as feline leukemia virus (FELV) and feline immunodeficiency virus (FIV), can also delay healing and predispose the animal to opportunistic infections. Orthopedic or neurologic problems may lead to periods of prolonged recumbency, with increased pressure on certain body parts causing decubitus ulcers and poor wound healing. Poor nutritional status, such as emaciation, or diseases that cause low protein and albumin levels (e.g., certain liver diseases, protein-losing nephropathy/enteropathy) will delay wound healing and alter wound strength. Conversely, obesity is associated with increased risk of wound infection and dehiscence, because decreased vascularization of fatty tissue leads to a decreased capacity for healing.

Concurrent Treatment Factors

Oncologic radiation therapy can lead to tissue fibrosis and vascular scarring, both of which negatively affect wound healing. Certain types of chemotherapy can suppress bone marrow function and decrease resistance to infection, thereby contributing to wound healing difficulties. Corticosteroids, especially when used long term, decrease the body's inflammatory response, increase the risk for infection, and delay all phases of wound healing.

Wound Classification

Wounds are classified based on their degree of contamination and/or the length of time the wound has been open. Different wound classes have different timelines for and probabilities of successful healing.

- *Clean wounds:* Atraumatic and surgically created under aseptic conditions.
- *Clean contaminated wounds:* Created by controlled surgical entry into contaminated areas, such as the gastrointestinal (GI) tract, respiratory tract, or urogenital tract. The contamination is typically minimal and easily removed.
- *Contaminated wounds:* Recent traumatic wound with bacterial contamination resulting from contamination by pavement, soil, or saliva from a bite, also major contamination by bacteria from the GI or urogenital tract during surgical procedures.
- *Dirty wounds:* Older wound with obvious infection. Contains more than 10^5 bacterial organisms per gram of tissue; could be caused by abscess of bite wound, puncture wound from contaminated foreign material, or necrotic tissue.

TECHNICIAN NOTE

Infection stops the progression of wound healing, and corticosteroid usage delays all phases of wound healing.

Small-Animal Wound Management

Wound Management

Many animals present with wounds after experiencing trauma, such as a vehicular accident or a bite by another animal. Stabilization of the patient must take precedence over any definitive wound care. A temporary clean bandage should be applied

---

• BOX 27.2   Steps in Proper Wound Management

1. Prevent further contamination
2. Remove foreign debris and contamination
3. Debride nonviable tissue
4. Manage wound drainage
5. Protect the wound through the inflammatory and proliferative phases
6. Select appropriate wound closure

---

quickly to protect the wound until it can be properly managed. Once stabilized, the animal can receive appropriate wound care (Box 27.2). If open fractures are present, care must be taken to avoid contaminating deeper tissues by pushing bone back underneath the skin.

Immediate Wound Care

The first objective must be to prevent further contamination of the wound. Gloves must be worn when handling open wounds and a sterile bandage should be placed when appropriate. The wound can be covered with moist sterile gauze or with sterile water-soluble lubricant, such as K-Y Jelly (Johnson & Johnson Medical, Arlington, TX). As the hair around the wound is clipped, hair falling into the wound is caught by the sterile lube and can be flushed out after clipping. The surrounding skin should then be gently cleaned with an antiseptic, such as chlorhexidine or povidone-iodine scrub, but care must be taken to avoid getting the antiseptic in the wound, because it is **cytotoxic** to wound cells. The wound is then lavaged with a warm **isotonic** crystalloid fluid (preferably lactated Ringer solution [LRS]) to remove the water-soluble lubricant and, more importantly, any foreign and loose necrotic debris. Fluid bags punctured over 24 hours previously should not be used because of the risk of bacterial contamination. Wound lavage pressure between 7 lb and 8 lb per square inch (psi) is the ideal pressure to achieve debris removal without damaging tissues. To achieve this, a 1-L bag of body-temperature LRS is placed inside a pressure bag, which is inflated to 300 mm Hg of pressure. It is connected via an extension set to an 18-gauge 2-inch over-the-needle catheter (with the stylet removed). This allows the sterile tip of the catheter to be used to lavage the subcutaneous space, if dead space is present (Fig. 27.2). This method is preferable to the syringe and three-way stopcock method, because the high pressure delivered by the syringe system can easily damage tissues. However, if no pressure bag is available, this method can be employed if only gentle pressure is applied to the syringe. Sterile saline bottles with holes or needles in the top consistently fail to reach pressure levels needed to effectively clean debris from the wound and should not be used. The volume of irrigation solution used will vary, depending on wound size and the degree of contamination.

TECHNICIAN NOTE

A 1-L bag of warm lactated Ringer solution (LRS) within a compression bag pressurized to 300 mm Hg produces the correct amount of pressure for wound flushing, regardless of the size of the needle or catheter used.

In highly contaminated wounds, such as those containing road debris or soil, tap water can be used initially instead of sterile isotonic fluids because in such cases, the main benefit comes from the volume, rather than the type, of fluid used. A dilute antiseptic

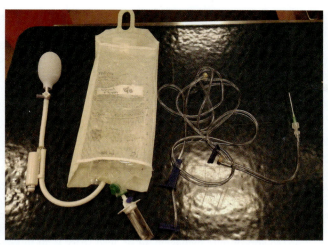

• **Fig. 27.2** Setup of a wound lavage system with the use of a 1-L bag of lactated Ringer solution inside a pressure bag connected via a primary extension set to an 18-gauge catheter with the stylet removed. The tip of the catheter should always be kept sterile.

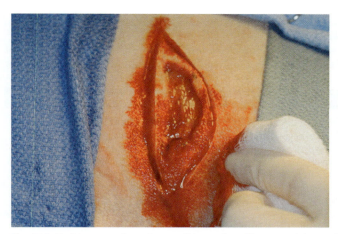

• **Fig. 27.3** En bloc resection of a small laceration. The wound is small enough and has loose surrounding skin to allow primary closure of the newly created fresh wound.

• BOX 27.3 Types of Wound Debridement

Staged Surgical Debridement
Obviously compromised tissue is removed, and tissue of questionable health is preserved and removed at a later stage if needed. Used for larger wounds with substantial trauma.

En Bloc Excision
If surrounding skin allows, small wounds can be excised completely and closed primarily.

Mechanical
An adherent primary bandage layer is used to nonselectively debride heavily contaminated wounds. Use only in the inflammatory phase.

Biological
Maggots can be used to ingest necrotic tissue. Used for chronic wounds with poor tissue health.

---

can be added to the lavage fluid, but the cytotoxic potential must be kept in mind. Common mixtures include a 0.05% dilution of chlorhexidine solution (1 part 2% chlorhexidine to 40 parts sterile water) and a 0.1% dilution of povidone-iodine solution (1 part 10% povidone-iodine solution to 100 parts sterile saline), although, because of povidone-iodine's cytotoxic potential, chlorhexidine is generally preferred.

> **TECHNICIAN NOTE**
>
> In heavily contaminated wounds, the volume of the flushing fluid is more important than its sterility, and thus tap water may be used initially.

Wound Debridement

The goal of **debridement** is removal of obviously contaminated, devitalized, or necrotic tissue and elimination of foreign debris from the wound (Box 27.3). Surgical debridement should always be performed by using aseptic techniques, including wearing sterile gloves, a sterile gown, caps, masks, and sterile drapes. If the wound is extensive or complex, an open fracture is present,

or abdominal or thoracic penetration is suspected, debridement should be performed in the surgical suite with the patient under general anesthesia. If the patient is too unstable to undergo general anesthesia, epidurals and local blocks can be used to facilitate patient comfort during debridement. Obviously necrotic tissues should be excised, but those with questionable viability should be reassessed later by using staged debridement, which allows for better preservation of viable tissues, especially on distal limb wounds. Smaller wounds may be debrided *en bloc* (as one unit) and closed primarily (Fig. 27.3). Mechanical debridement with the use of an adherent primary bandage layer, such as a wet-to-dry bandage, can be performed for initial management of highly contaminated wounds. A wet-to-dry bandage causes nonselective debridement; although it is effective, it causes several undesirable side effects (see the section "Principles of Bandaging"). Specific maggot species can also be used to selectively debride dead tissue by ingesting necrotic and liquefied tissue.

Wound Closure

Surgically created wounds can be closed by direct apposition and will heal by **primary-intention wound healing** across the incision (Box 27.4). Clean traumatic lacerations may also undergo **primary closure** after wound lavage. Small wounds with contamination can be excised en bloc and closed primarily. Wounds with a questionable degree of contamination or excess drainage may require a 2- to 3-day period of open wound management before they undergo delayed primary closure (Fig. 27.4). This short period of open wound management facilitates elimination of contamination and improves wound health. To be considered *primary closure*, wound closure has to occur before granulation tissue has formed.

> **TECHNICIAN NOTE**
>
> Mildly contaminated wounds that are otherwise amenable to primary closure can be managed for 2 to 3 days before closing. This method of wound management is known as *delayed primary closure*.

Wounds requiring a longer period of open wound care, such as heavily contaminated wounds, can undergo **secondary closure**. These wounds are allowed to form a healthy bed of granulation tissue, which is then folded onto itself with closure of the skin.

This type of healing is also referred to as *third-intention wound healing*.

Second-intention wound healing refers to the process of healing by contraction and epithelialization, and is indicated for heavily contaminated wounds for which delayed closure or en bloc excision is not possible. Except for surgical debridement, surgical closure is not performed. This form of wound healing is often employed in areas with little skin (e.g., the distal limbs). The newly epithelialized wound is often friable and easily traumatized. Second-intention healing in the distal limb can produce contraction over joints, muscles, or tendons, creating impaired function, and may not be desirable.

• BOX 27.4   Methods of Wound Closure

Primary Closure With Primary-Intention Wound Healing

Surgical apposition of wound edges with sutures or staples. Can be performed in fresh, clean wounds with little loss of soft tissue, such as surgically created wounds. Primary-intention wound healing occurs. Epithelialization begins within 1 to 2 days, because cells can cross over the incision. Granulation tissue is not needed. En bloc debridement can convert a small, contaminated wound into a clean wound, which then can be closed primarily.

Delayed Primary Closure

Appropriate for wounds older than 6 to 8 hours, with some contamination and questionable ability to heal with primary closure. The wound is treated as an open wound for 2 or 3 days to allow drainage and elimination of infection, and then the wound is surgically closed primarily. Closure occurs before granulation tissue appears.

Secondary Closure

Appropriate for wounds older than 6 to 8 hours, for infected necrotic wounds, and for failed primary wound closure. The wound is allowed to form healthy granulation tissue and then is closed by apposition of granulation surfaces or by excision of granulation tissue and primary closure. This is also known as *third-intention wound healing*.

Second-Intention Wound Healing

Appropriate for wounds older than 6 to 8 hours or for infected, necrotic wounds. The wound is allowed to heal by granulation tissue formation and epithelialization. Disadvantages of this type of healing are the length of time required for complete healing, the cost associated with prolonged treatment, the fragility of the newly epithelialized wound, loss of function as a result of excessive scarring or contraction, and poor cosmetic results.

Wound Drainage

Dead space is created when soft tissue planes are disrupted by surgery (e.g., removal of a mass, removal of fluid) or trauma (e.g., bite wounds, penetrating wounds), and is often accompanied by fluid or blood accumulation. Excessive fluid accumulation can further separate tissue planes and can delay or prevent normal wound healing. Furthermore, fluid accumulation increases the risk of infection, so appropriate management of dead space is an important consideration in wound management and healing. If a significant amount of dead space exists or if wound exudate is expected, passive or active wound drains may be used in conjunction with wound closure. The location of the wound and the amount of drainage will dictate which type of drain can be used.

Passive drains, such as the Penrose drain, function by allowing fluid to flow along the drain surface as the result of capillary action. These drains must exit in a dependent location so that fluid can gravitate toward the exit skin incision. If exudate builds up or a scab forms on the end of the drain, a warm-water soak and gentle scrubbing will remove it. If needed, twice-daily flushing with sterile saline can be used to maintain patency. Because the goal of the drain is to remove fluid and exudate away from the wound, a bandage should not be used. These drains are kept in place for 3 to 5 days before removal and subsequent skin closure.

Active drains, commonly referred to as *closed suction drains*, work by creating a vacuum within the wound and allowing wound fluid to be removed via a rigid fenestrated

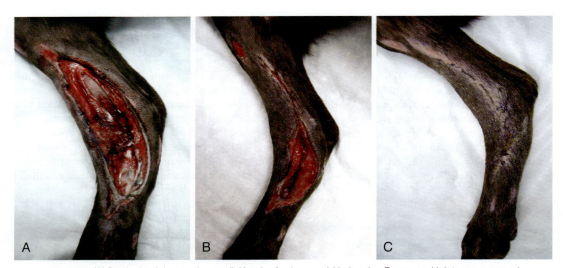

• **Fig. 27.4** (A) Degloving injury to the medial hock of a 1-year-old Labrador. Bones and joints are exposed. The wound has been surgically debrided where safe. After placement of an occlusive nonadherent dressing for 2 days, delayed primary closure of the most proximal part of the wound was performed. (B) Day 6: The proximal incision is healing by primary intention and the distal wound is developing healthy granulation tissue. Secondary closure of the distal part of the wound is performed by apposing the skin edges over healthy granulation tissue. (C) Day 18: Both aspects of the wound have healed completely. Delayed primary and secondary closure significantly reduced the wound management period compared with second-intention wound healing.

drain into an external collection container. This fluid can then be measured and collected for cytology analysis or culture and sensitivity. Although more expensive than passive drains, closed suction drains play an important role in the management of more extensive wounds and those with a large amount of drainage. Drains are removed when the amount of wound fluid decreases (usually after 3–5 days), because the simple presence of a drain will stimulate some fluid production. Normal fluid production of an invasive drain will be 1 to 2 mL/kg/day.

Negative-pressure wound therapy (NPWT) refers to the controlled application of a vacuum to a wound and can be used in situations where normal drains cannot be used, such as distal limb wounds, wounds with extensive dead space and a large amount of expected fluid production, or before use of skin flaps and grafts. Benefits of NPWT include increased vascularization, improved granulation tissue formation, and reduction in wound size.

Wound Infection

A wound is considered infected when the bacterial count is greater than 100,000 (10^5) organisms per gram of tissue. Signs of a wound or incisional infection include swelling, heat, and redness of surrounding tissues.

TECHNICIAN NOTE

Signs of a wound or incisional infection include swelling, heat, and redness of surrounding tissues. Wound drainage itself is not a sign of infection.

Healthy wounds may exude clear serosanguinous fluid. Discharge from infected wounds can be copious and of varying consistency, color, and odor. With severe infection, systemic signs such as lethargy, fever, pain associated with the wound, and changes in appetite and drinking may occur. The use of antimicrobials depend on the severity of infection, the type of organism, the condition of the wound, and the general health of the patient (see the section "Factors Influencing Wound Healing"). If the overall wound status is favorable (good blood supply, superficial infection, minimal foreign body contamination), antimicrobials may not be needed, because local wound defenses can often eliminate infection. Wounds with healthy granulation tissue are inherently resistant to infection and do not require antimicrobial use. If the infection involves deeper tissues and is well established, oral antimicrobials are appropriate for stable patients; however, if the infection is severe and/or the patient is immunocompromised, intravenous drug administration is indicated. Antibiotics are often chosen empirically based on efficacy against common skin pathogens, such as *Staphylococcus* and *Streptococcus* spp. Signs of infection should resolve within 2 to 3 days of treatment. If the infection persists, a resistant organism is present in the wound, and microbial culture and susceptibility testing are recommended to appropriately target antimicrobial therapy. The use of topical antimicrobial drugs, such as silver sulfadiazine (Silvazine; Smith & Nephew, Fort Washington, PA), is often not effective against deep tissue infection, because these agents cannot reach deeper parts of the wound. However, they may be effective in eliminating superficial infection without the use of systemic antimicrobials. Other topical agents, such as aloe vera, honey, and sugar, can be used to treat wound infection and are incorporated as the primary layer within a bandage (see the section "Principles of Bandaging").

Types of Wounds

Abrasions and Lacerations

Abrasions are partial-thickness dermal wounds that are common in animals that sustain vehicular accident–related injuries. Because of the preservation of parts of the **dermis**, these wounds heal well by re-epithelialization. Maintaining a moist wound environment will speed epithelialization and is preferred over allowing the wound to dry out and scab over.

Lacerations are produced by tearing of skin and deeper tissues. Tissues are relatively sharply incised, and trauma to the surrounding area is minimal. Fresh lacerations with minimal contamination can be lavaged, debrided, and closed primarily. If small enough, the older lacerations can be excised en bloc and closed primarily. Secondary closure may be performed if the wound is heavily contaminated.

Degloving Injuries

A **degloving injury** occurs when a large section of skin is torn off from the underlying tissue, like removal of a glove. Degloving injuries are common in dogs that jump off or fall out of a moving vehicle and are dragged along the pavement. These injuries can lead to severe tissue loss, usually involving the distal limbs. Bone abrasion and joint exposure are common. These wounds often require weeks to months of wound care. Because of the nature of the injury, degloving wounds tend to be heavily contaminated with foreign debris and have varying amounts of devitalized tissue. Aggressive wound lavage and wound debridement precede granulation tissue formation. Because of lack of loose skin for wound contraction, large defects require skin grafting.

Penetrating Wounds

Penetrating wounds encompass a wide range of injuries, including wounds from bites, bullets, arrows, sticks, and antlers. Bite wounds are the most common type of penetrating wound in veterinary patients. Penetrating wounds can be challenging to assess, because they often cause extensive injury to deeper tissues that is not immediately apparent on inspection of the skin. Because of the elastic nature of skin, surface wounds may look small, but underlying structures may be severely damaged. Any penetrating wounds that may involve abdominal or thoracic wall penetration should be sealed with sterile gauze and a sterile adhesive occlusive film such as Ioban (3M, Maplewood, MN) until surgical exploration is possible. Along with having tissues crushed and lacerated, bite victims are often shaken violently, which adds to separation of tissues and creation of dead space. Penetrating wounds should always be considered contaminated. Penetrating objects should only be removed under sterile surgical conditions in case the object is occluding a lacerated blood vessel. Management of these wounds includes exploration, lavage, and debridement. The type of closure depends on the ability to remove contaminated and damaged tissue. Drains are commonly used in penetrating wounds with extensive dead space.

TECHNICIAN NOTE

Penetrating wounds can be challenging to assess, because they often cause extensive injury to deeper tissues that is not apparent on inspection of the skin.

Burns

Burns are classified based on how deeply into the tissues the injury reaches and how large the affected area is. Although burns can be caused by accidental or deliberate injury in the animal's environment (burns caused by house fires, hot car engines, electrocution, scalding by hot liquid, heating pads/blankets, etc.), they are more often caused by accidental inappropriate use of heating blankets and lamps, hair dryers, or poorly grounded electrocautery units in a veterinary facility. **First-degree burns** are superficial and are confined to the outermost layer of the skin (**epidermis**). Affected skin is reddened and painful but re-epithelializes within 1 week with topical wound management. **Second-degree burns** are the result of full-thickness epidermal and partial-thickness dermal injury. The epidermis can appear yellow-white, black, or charred and may slough and leak plasma. The area can be painful or nonpainful to the touch, and hair follicles can be spared or destroyed. The full extent of the damage may not be known until several days after the injury (often called "declaring" itself). Second-degree burns, if not severe, will heal by epithelialization with minimal scarring in 10 to 21 days. Severe second-degree burns may require surgical intervention, and systemic effects are possible. **Third-degree burns** are full-thickness injuries of the epidermis and deep-layer dermis, characterized by a thick, leathery, black layer of dead tissue called *eschar*, and are insensitive to touch. Treatment requires extensive surgical interventions, with eschar removal, wound debridement, and application of skin grafts and flaps if second-intention healing is not possible. Life-threatening systemic effects, such as sepsis and multiple organ failure, are likely. **Fourth-degree burns** involve tissue extending beyond the dermis, including muscle, tendon, and bone. Surgical intervention is required to prevent scarring that restricts movement. Animals with fourth-degree burns are critically ill and require intensive care to survive.

Many animals that present to a veterinary facility with burn wounds will require acute stabilization for shock, including fluid replacement and pain management, before a wound treatment plan can be initiated, although a quick, nonstick, sterile dressing should be applied to any open wound during stabilization. Additional long-term management may require nutritional support and blood product transfusion(s) in severe cases.

> **TECHNICIAN NOTE**
>
> Burns can range in severity from minor to those requiring life-saving stabilization before wound treatment can be initiated. Wound treatment for severe burns can last weeks to months and require intensive hospitalization and treatment.

Burn Treatment

First- and shallow second-degree burns can be managed much like a wound fit for second-intention healing. The focus for minor burn healing also involves debridement, infection prevention, and healing bed hydration. Additionally, burns produce a large amount of exudate, which will need to be absorbed by the bandage material. Several options exist for this primary and secondary layer, which is covered more in depth in the later section, "Principles of Bandaging."

In the past several years, several new treatment options have been proposed for burns in veterinary patients. Part of the challenge of treating patients with severe burns comes from the length of time for healing and increased risk of complications during that time. If these novel interventions can decrease the length of time to healing, patient mortality will decrease.

Platelet-Rich Plasma

Platelet-rich plasma is obtained by drawing blood from the patient, which is then spun down to isolate the platelets and then applied directly to the wound. In this way, the process of platelet degranulation, which includes growth factors, induces cellular proliferation, mitosis, chemotaxis, matrix formation, collagen synthesis, and angiogenesis, and is theorized to decrease the healing time frame. This process would be especially useful in severe second- and third-degree burns as well as patients with diabetes mellitus, all of which decrease useful blood flow to the site.

Tilapia Skin Grafts

Tilapia grafts are used successfully in cases where a standard skin graft technique has failed or is not an option, or where appropriate follow-up care cannot be provided, such as in large, dangerous wild animals. When properly prepared, tilapia skin retains its high amounts of omega-3s and collagen. The grafts provide additional pain relief, may decrease healing times, and decrease the number of bandage changes required.

Decubitus Ulcers and Pressure Sores

Decubitus ulcers develop over bony prominences as the result of skin compression on hard surfaces during long periods of recumbency. Patients with orthopedic and neurologic problems, extremely obese animals, and large- and giant-breed dogs with little soft tissue coverage over these bony prominences are at particular risk. The most common location for a decubitus ulcer is the elbow (lateral or caudal surface of the olecranon). These ulcers can be frustrating to treat, so efforts must be focused on prevention. Animals that are prone to such ulcers must be housed on soft, clean, and dry surfaces and may benefit from commercially available pressure-relieving sleeves. Surgical closure usually fails if the wound continues to be exposed to surface pressure. Advanced reconstructive surgery is required in large ulcers that have failed to respond to conservative treatment.

Inappropriate or prolonged periods of bandaging (especially with a splint or a cast) can lead to pressure necrosis of the skin, particularly over the olecranon, the calcaneus, and the bony prominences of the feet. As with decubitus ulcers, the best treatment for bandage-associated pressure sores is prevention. Susceptible areas must not be padded more (because more padding will cause increased pressure during compression) but must be protected with the use of doughnut-shaped bandage material, such as a rolled-up stockinette or cast padding. Reddening of the skin with hair loss is an early sign of excessive pressure. White, purple, or black discoloration indicates severe damage to the dermis, which usually leads to sloughing and an open wound. Most pressure sores are treated by second-intention healing after the splint or the cast has been modified or removed.

Principles of Bandaging

Bandages are applied for two main reasons: (1) management of soft tissue wounds, and (2) stabilization of bone and joint injuries. Additionally, postoperative bandages help decrease hemorrhage and edema, eliminate dead space, increase patient comfort, and protect the wound from damage caused by the patient or the environment (Box 27.5).

Most bandages consist of three distinct layers: (1) the primary layer, which is in direct contact with the wound; (2) the secondary layer; and (3) the tertiary layer (see Table 27.1 for a list of bandage materials, including their uses and functions). The primary layer is most important for wound protection and healing because it directly influences the wound environment.

BOX 27.5 Functions of a Bandage

Soft Tissue Wounds

- Protects the wound from the environment and from the patient
- Aids in debridement of the wound surface
- Manages exudate
- Creates an environment for wound healing
- Provides hemostasis
- Decreases hematoma/seroma formation
- Provides support and comfort
- Delivers topical agents

Orthopedic Injuries

- Stabilizes fractures or joints
- Maintains splints or casts in position
- Restricts motion
- Prevents weight bearing
- Protects soft tissues from further injury
- Decreases swelling

It may be adherent or nonadherent and may be **nonocclusive, semiocclusive,** or **occlusive.** The type of primary layer depends on the phase of wound healing and the amount of exudate present. The secondary layer absorbs and holds exudate (if present) and provides some immobilization and support. If a large amount of exudate is produced, as would happen with a burn or highly infected wound, the secondary layer must be thicker to allow absorption of fluid into the bandage without causing strike-through into the tertiary layer. The tertiary layer is the protective outer layer that keeps the other layers in place and determines the amount of pressure and support applied. This final layer must not be occlusive, or moisture will accumulate within the bandage.

TECHNICIAN NOTE

Most bandages consist of three layers. The primary layer contacts the wound, the secondary layer provides structure and padding, and the tertiary layer holds and protects the other two.

TABLE 27.1 Examples of Primary, Secondary, and Tertiary Bandage Layers

Bandage Layer	Use and Function	Product Examples
Primary		
Adherent	Nonselective debridement	Sterile wide-mesh gauze
Hypertonic/hyperosmolar	Draws fluid and debris away from the wound; antimicrobial effect because of hypertonicity and low water content within the wound; some enhanced wound healing; use on highly exudative, contaminated, and infected wounds	Hypertonic sodium chloride dressing (20%) (e.g., CURASALT[a]), granulated sugar, honey
Nonadherent semiocclusive	*Moderately to highly exudative wounds* Maintains a moist wound environment, draws fluid and debris away from the wound	*Hydrophilic* Variety of hydrogels (e.g., Curagel[a]) and hydrocolloids (e.g., Ultec Hydrocolloid Dressing[a]), absorptive foam (e.g., Hydrosorb Plus Foam[a]) *Nonhydrophilic* Polyurethane film (e.g., Bioclusive[b])
Nonadherent occlusive	*Minimally exudative wounds* Maintains a moist wound environment, promotes epithelialization, protects new epithelium	*Hydrophilic* Variety of hydrogels (e.g., NU-GEL[b]) and hydrocolloids (e.g., Tegaderm Hydrocolloid[c]) *Nonhydrophilic* Tegaderm Transparent Dressing[c]
Nonadherent nonocclusive	Covers surgical incisions, protects recently epithelialized surfaces	Teflon pads (e.g., Telfa pads[a]), petrolatum-impregnated gauze (e.g., Adaptic[b])
Secondary		
Padding	Absorbs exudate, provides support	Cast padding,[c] rolled cotton[b]
Tertiary		
Conforming gauze	Conforms and holds secondary layer	Kling[b]
Nonocclusive elastic bandage	Holds and protects secondary layer	Vetrap[d]
Nonocclusive elastic adhesive tape	Holds and protects secondary layer	Elastikon[b]

[a]Kendall/Covidien, Mansfield, MA.
[b]Johnson & Johnson Medical, Arlington, TX.
[c]3M Skin and Wound Care, St. Paul, MN.
[d]3M Animal Care Products, St. Paul, MN.

Adherent Primary Layer

A wet-to-dry bandage uses an adherent primary layer for nonselective debridement. It must be used only in the inflammatory and debridement stages of heavily contaminated wounds. To apply a wet-to-dry bandage, moist sterile gauze is placed onto the wound bed and is then covered by a relatively thick, absorptive secondary layer. Moisture on the wound surface helps dilute exudate and debris, which then are wicked into the dry secondary layer. As the gauze dries, it adheres to the wound bed, and mechanical debridement occurs when the dried gauze is pulled away from the wound. Although such debridement is effective, it is nonselective and will remove not only diseased tissue but also healthy tissue, such as new granulation tissue, thereby delaying the healing process. Wet-to-dry bandages must be changed at least once per day and more often if fluid strike-through of the tertiary layer occurs, because bacteria from the environment can penetrate the bandage and contaminate the wound. In addition, this technique often causes bleeding and pain when the gauze is removed, necessitating proper analgesia or sedation. Because of these undesirable consequences and studies showing that the body's own phagocytic processes are very effective when given a moist healing environment, the wet-to-dry bandage has largely been replaced by a nonadherent primary layer.

Nonadherent Primary Layer

This type of primary layer is in direct contact with the wound bed but does not firmly adhere to it. A nonadherent primary layer is used once granulation tissue has formed or epithelialization has begun to protect and promote second-intention wound healing. A semiocclusive nonadherent primary layer is permeable to air and fluid, and allows exudate to be absorbed by the secondary layer. An occlusive nonadherent primary layer is impermeable to air and retains moisture. Such materials as hydrogels and hydrocolloids can be used as semiocclusive or occlusive primary layers. Moisture-retaining primary layers provide many benefits during wound healing, such as maintaining a warm and moist environment, aiding in selective debridement, and improving epithelialization; therefore they are the primary layer of choice.

TECHNICIAN NOTE

Moisture-retaining primary layers provide many benefits, including improved epithelialization, and are the preferred primary layer for most wounds.

A great variety of nonadherent primary layers are available for the veterinary patient. Highly absorptive primary layers, such as **hypertonic** saline or calcium alginates, may be required for highly exudative wounds. Some materials, such as hydrogels, hydrocolloids, and polyurethane film or foam, allow absorption of wound fluid while creating a moist wound healing environment. They are best used on wounds with minimal exudate and can be applied throughout the inflammatory and repair phases. This type of layer is much less painful when changed and allows longer intervals between bandage changes once the wound is in the proliferative phase. The moist wound healing environment enhances cell activity and improves granulation tissue formation and epithelialization. A lower infection rate is seen with moist wound healing; however, bacteria may be trapped underneath the occlusive layer if it is not applied correctly and changed at appropriate intervals. Petrolatum-impregnated sterile gauze is an example of a nonadherent nonocclusive layer commonly used in the proliferative phase. Teflon pads are nonadherent and are frequently used to cover surgical incisions and epithelialized skin. Case Presentation 27.1 illustrates the principles of bandage material selection for management of an open wound.

Sugar, Honey, and Silver

Sugar and honey are frequently incorporated into the primary layer of a bandage, because they assist debridement, possess antimicrobial activity, and provide a moist wound healing environment. Sugar assists in wound healing by creating a hyperosmolar environment that draws macrophages into the wound, thereby accelerating sloughing of devitalized tissue. Sugar is useful for debriding large wounds, degloving or shearing injuries, or infected wounds. After debridement and lavage, the area is patted dry with a sterile towel and the sugar applied in a thick layer. Sterile towels or lap sponges are then used as the primary layer, with a thick, absorbent secondary layer. Because fluid wicking dilutes the sugar, frequent bandage changes are required.

Manuka honey or medicinal honey can be used during the debridement phase, over infected granulation tissue, or for burns. It is similar to sugar in that it creates a hypertonic environment but has the added benefit of providing a rich energy source for wound cells, and its acidity and hydrogen peroxide levels lend antibacterial properties. After lavage and debridement, honey-soaked gauze is applied as a primary layer, with a thick, absorbent secondary layer. As with sugar, the bandage needs to be replaced at least once per day.

One percent silver sulfadiazine (SSD) cream has been a mainstay of burn treatment for decades. There are currently many silver-impregnated products (compounded creams, meshes, etc.) on the market today. There have been many studies comparing these novel products to SSD cream in terms of effectiveness and patient comfort.

Bandage, Cast, Splint, and Sling Application in Small Animals

A variety of bandages, splints, casts, and slings are available for use in cats and dogs—each with its own indications regarding when and where it should be used. Distal limb bandages are often applied to protect wounds and to stabilize bone or joint injuries. Splints, casts, and slings are used to provide further stability to orthopedic injuries or to prevent weight bearing. Only injuries below the elbow or stifle joint can be effectively immobilized; even with splints or casts, movement of joints and bones is possible. For other body parts, bandages need to be modified. Proper sedation or anesthesia greatly facilitates the application of any bandage. In nonsedated animals, proper restraint is paramount to avoid movement during bandage application.

Distal Limb Bandages

The **Robert Jones bandage** can be used to temporarily immobilize limbs distal to the elbow or stifle joint. This bandage relies on an extremely thick secondary layer, such as cast padding or cotton, which is tightly compressed to cause uniform compression of the distal limb (Fig. 27.5A–C). Because of the large amount of bandage material necessary and the resultant cumbersome bandage, the traditional Robert Jones bandage is not often used in small animals.

The **modified Robert Jones bandage** is the most commonly applied distal limb bandage in small animals (Fig. 27.6A–F). It uses a much thinner secondary layer and often is referred to as a *soft-padded bandage*. Because less padding

CASE PRESENTATION 27.1

Management of a Degloving Injury

A 2-year-old intact male German Shepherd Dog sustained a degloving injury of the medial aspect of the left hind foot after jumping out of a moving car. Three days later, the dog was presented at the clinic with a large full-thickness skin wound involving the dorsomedial aspect of the metatarsi (Fig. 27A), with visible foreign body contamination and areas of nonviable tissue.

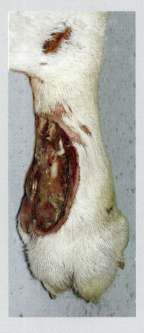

Parts of metatarsal bones #2 and #3 were exposed. The wound was lavaged with copious amounts of fluid, and some tissue was carefully surgically debrided. A wet-to-dry bandage was applied for additional nonselective debridement. After placement of sterile saline-soaked sponges into the wound (Fig. 27B),

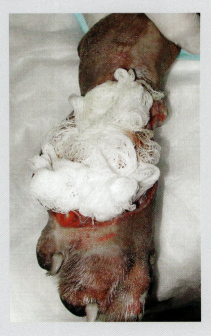

several dry sponges were placed over the wet sponges (Fig. 27C), followed by a thick absorptive secondary layer of cast padding (Fig. 27D). Elastic gauze and an outer protective layer were applied. Bandage changes were performed daily. Wet-to-dry bandages were discontinued on day 3 as the wound required no further aggressive debridement (Fig. 27E).

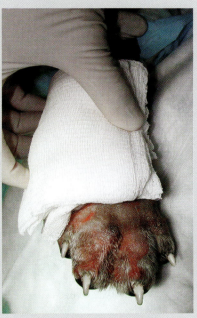

Hydrogel, a nonadherent semiocclusive primary layer, was applied (Curagel; Kendall/Covidien, Mansfield, MA) and was changed every 2 to 3 days. On day 14, healthy granulation tissue covered the wound bed except the metatarsal bones (Fig. 27F). On day 21, previously exposed metatarsal bones were covered with granulation tissue and some wound contraction had occurred (Fig. 27G).

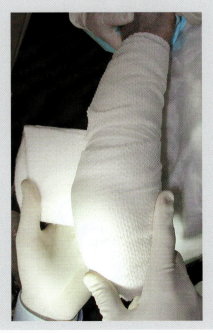

Continued

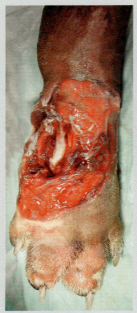

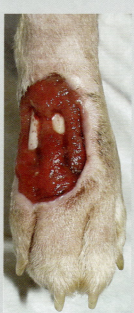

was present (Fig. 27H); epithelialization was noted at the wound edges and continued to cover 50% of the remaining wound by day 42 (Fig. 27I). The primary layer was switched to a Teflon pad (Telfa pad; Kendall/Covidien, Mansfield, MA), and bandage changes were reduced to every 4 to 5 days. Epithelialization was complete by day 60. (Fig. 27J).

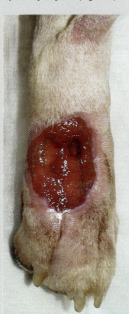

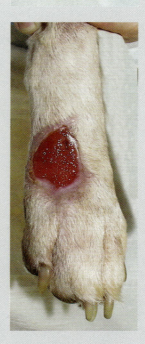

The primary layer was switched to petrolatum-impregnated gauze (Adaptic; Johnson & Johnson Medical, Arlington, TX), covered by a few dry gauze sponges to help absorb wound fluid. Bandage changes were made every 2 to 3 days. By day 36, wound size had been reduced by greater than 60% because of wound contraction, and healthy granulation tissue

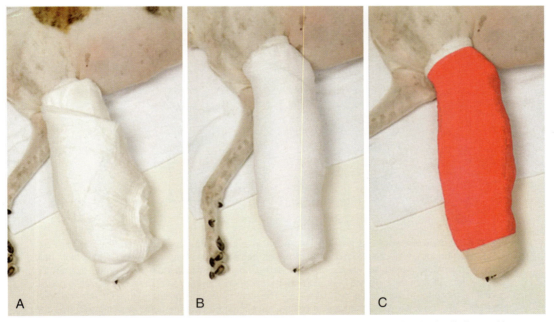

• **Fig. 27.5** Robert Jones bandage. (A) Large amounts of rolled cotton are applied to the forelimb, reaching above the elbow. (B) The thick layer of rolled cotton is evenly compressed with elastic gauze to provide stabilization of the fracture beneath. (C) A tertiary protective layer has been applied, and the distal part of the bandage has been reinforced with elastic adhesive tape. Note how the toenails of the middle two toes are still visible for assessment of swelling.

is used, the tertiary layer must not be overly tight or pressure necrosis may occur. Splints and casts can easily be incorporated into the bandage. The tips of the toes or toenails are often excluded from bandaging to allow for daily inspection. Care must be taken to avoid leaving too much toe exposed, because this will lead to compromised blood flow and swelling.

TECHNICIAN NOTE

The modified Robert Jones bandage is the most commonly applied distal limb bandage in small-animal medicine.

The appropriate primary layer is first selected. If slippage of the bandage is a concern, small strips of adhesive tape can be applied

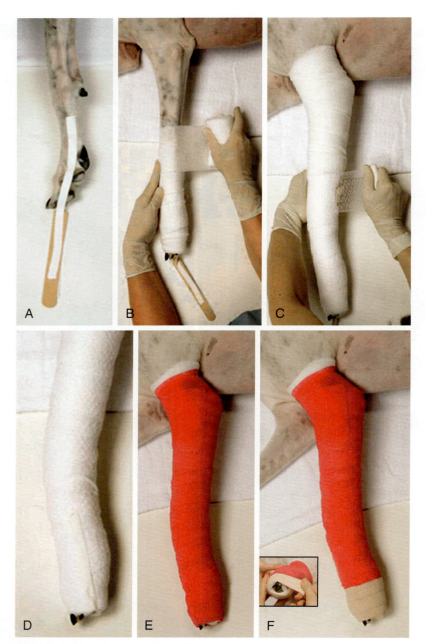

• **Fig. 27.6** Modified Robert Jones bandage. (A) Two thin strips of adhesive tape are placed to form stirrups. (B) Cast padding is applied from distal to proximal, with each pass overlapping about 50%. Note how the tips of the middle toenails are visible. To avoid chafing, none of the subsequent layers must contact the skin. (C) After sufficient padding has been applied, the secondary layer is compressed with elastic gauze. Gauze is evenly applied from distal to proximal. (D) The stirrups are now pulled up to adhere to the outer gauze layer. (E) The outer protective layer is placed. Care must be taken to avoid applying this layer too tightly. Note how a thin rim of cotton is visible at the proximal extend of the bandage. (F) Strips of nonocclusive elastic tape are used to reinforce the distal end of the bandage for walking. Note how the middle two toes can easily be assessed for swelling.

to the lateral and medial aspects of the foot before bandaging as stirrups. For prolonged bandaging, the portion of adhesive tape on the foot itself can be left for several bandage changes while new thin strips of tape are applied on top of it to form new stirrups. Oftentimes, stirrups are not needed and should not serve as a substitute for proper bandaging technique. If necessary, small strips of cotton can be placed between the toes to decrease abrasions from toenails rubbing against skin or sprinkled with

moisture-control powder, such as Gold Bond (Sanofi Consumer Healthcare, Bridgewater, NJ) to help absorb moisture. "Doughnuts" (doughnut-shaped pads) made of soft, nonabrasive material can be placed over bony protuberances or compromised tissue to decrease pressure on these areas. The secondary layer consists of cast padding. The thickness of the secondary layer depends on the amount of exudate (if present) and compression desired. Cast padding is unrolled smoothly without folds or wrinkles, starting at

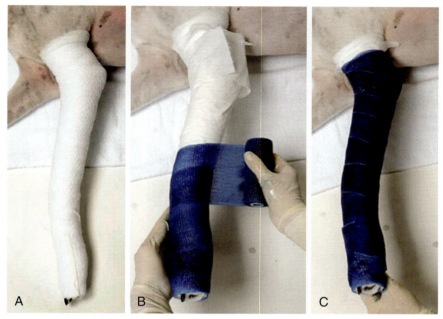

• **Fig. 27.7** Forelimb cast. (A) Casts and splints are applied over a modified Robert Jones bandage before the outer protective layer is applied. This bandage must not be too thick so as to prevent loosening of material underneath and rubbing of the cast or splint. (B) A thin layer of toilet paper or paper towels is applied over the elastic gauze to prevent the casting material from adhering to it. The fiberglass tape is applied from distal to proximal, with up to 50% overlap. Care must be taken to prevent indentations with fingers or creases, folds, and wrinkles, because these can cause pressure points on the skin. (C) Several layers of fiberglass tape are applied, taking care to avoid having casting material touch the skin. This material is allowed to harden, is possibly bivalved, and then is covered by a protective layer.

the level of the toenails and proceeding proximally. Starting at the bottom should help decrease edema in the lower limb. Padding should be 50% overlapped as the material is unrolled. To avoid placing a secondary layer that is too thin and will slip easily, at least three to four layers of cast padding are applied. If the elbow or stifle joint is to be included, cast padding must be applied as far proximal to the elbow or stifle as possible to avoid slipping over these high-motion joints. Larger dogs require a surprising amount of cast padding to thicken the secondary layer enough to avoid collapse of the bandage by slippage. Once the desired thickness of padding has been applied, elastic gauze or Kling (Johnson & Johnson Medical, Arlington, TX) is used to compress the secondary layer. This gauze is applied distally, moving proximally with 50% overlap and even compression. If a splint or a cast is used, it is applied at this point and is held in place by another layer of elastic gauze or Kling. Finally, the outer protective layer is applied from distal to proximal. This layer must not touch skin directly, because it can cause abrasions. Unlike large animals, cats and dogs do not tolerate excessive tightness of a bandage; therefore the tertiary layer must not be too tight. If properly applied, this bandage will not need to be taped to the limb at the proximal extent. Tape can be used over the foot to provide greater resistance against wear, or Elastikon may be used to help with traction.

Casts and Splints

Casts and splints are used to provide stability for joint injuries or fractures, for temporary support until surgery, as a means of definitive treatment, or as an adjunct after surgical stabilization. They are incorporated into a modified Robert Jones bandage between the elastic gauze layer and the outer protective layer and must only be used for injuries below the elbow or stifle joint, because they cannot effectively immobilize injuries above those joints.

TECHNICIAN NOTE

Distal limb bandages are not appropriate for fractures above the elbow or the stifle, because they cannot effectively immobilize injuries above those joints.

Casts encircle the entire limb. Fiberglass casting tape is the preferred material, because it produces a lightweight yet very rigid cast (Fig. 27.7A–C). A modified Robert Jones bandage is placed over the distal limb, except for the outer protective layer. The bandage must not be too thick to avoid the cast loosening, and it must have an even surface free of wrinkles or creases. The technician should wear gloves and immerse the fiberglass casting tape in water to activate the setting; excess water is then shaken out. A layer of toilet paper applied to the bandage before casting tape application will prevent undesirable adhesion of the tape to the bandage. The tape is then unrolled evenly over the soft-padded bandage from distal to proximal, avoiding folds, wrinkles, or indentations, because these can cause pressure necrosis underneath. The casting material must not contact skin at the ends of the bandage. While the casting tape is overlapped by 30% to 50%, two to three layers are applied to the limb. Once hardened, a protective outer layer

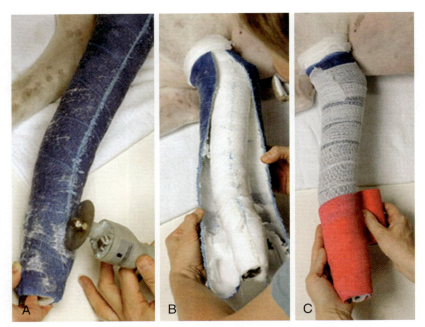

• **Fig. 27.8** Bivalving a forelimb cast. (A) An oscillating saw is used to cut the cast on both sides and create halves. This saw will not injure the patient. (B) The bivalved cast is removed. The layer of toilet paper between the casting material and the elastic gauze prevented the two layers from adhering. (C) The bivalved cast is reapplied to the bandaged limb. Elastic gauze is used to firmly hold both halves together. The tertiary layer is applied.

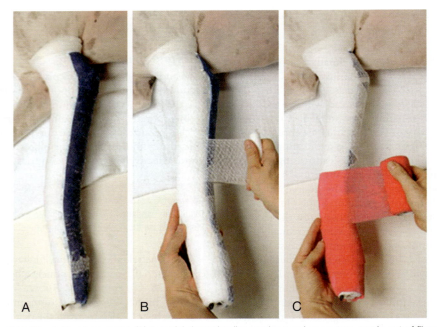

• **Fig. 27.9** Caudal forelimb splint. (A) A prefabricated splint can be used or custom-made out of fiberglass tape. Splints are generally applied to the caudal surface of the forelimb and the lateral surface of the pelvic limb over a modified Robert Jones bandage. (B) Elastic gauze is used to secure the splint to the bandage. (C) A protective outer layer is placed, and the foot is reinforced with elastic tape.

can be applied to prevent excessive soiling of the cast. Casts are often bivalved (cut on both sides) with an oscillating cast saw to create halves, which then are kept together by elastic gauze or tape and the outer protective layer (Fig. 27.8A–C). Although bivalving a cast weakens its stability, it allows for fast removal of the cast in an emergency and is generally recommended.

A variety of prefabricated splints made of plastic or aluminum are available (lateral and spoon splints). Alternatively, fiberglass casting tape or thermoplastic material can be used to make custom splints (Fig. 27.9A–C). Using fiberglass tape allows great flexibility, because it can be applied in any fashion desired. Most forelimb splints are applied to the caudal limb surface, and hind limb splints are applied laterally unless only the metatarsi and the foot are splinted, in which case a caudal splint is used.

The original indication for the Schroeder-Thomas splint was to immobilize distal femoral fractures that otherwise could not be bandaged. This splint suspends the limb in a rigid metal frame fashioned to match the outline of the leg. This splint is not used to treat fractures as it causes muscle contracture with permanent loss of limb function.

A spica splint maintains the forelimb or the pelvic limb in extension through application of a soft-padded bandage and addition of a strong lateral support splint that curves over the shoulder or pelvis. This type of splint is most used in the forelimb after elbow luxation reduction when the elbow must be kept in extension and overall mobility of the affected limb must be reduced. Prolonged immobilization must be avoided to prevent muscle contracture and joint damage.

Slings

An Ehmer sling is a non–weight-bearing sling applied to the pelvic limb to protect the hip joint after injury. It is used primarily after closed reduction of craniodorsal hip luxation and selectively after surgery associated with the coxofemoral joint. In principle, a properly applied Ehmer sling will internally rotate and abduct the femur, thereby forcing the femoral head into the acetabulum and maintaining reduction. Broad elastic tape is used to make a "figure-of-eight" loop around the stifle and hock while both joints are held in flexion and the hock is externally rotated (Fig. 27.10A–F). On rare occasions, the tape is wrapped around the abdomen to further reduce movement at the hip joint. If only the limb is encircled, care must be taken to apply adhesive tape as far proximally on the femur as the flank fold will allow to prevent slippage of the sling over the cranial aspect of the stifle joint. Most patients develop skin irritations around the flank fold and inguinal area due to the tape; unless severe, these may be treated conservatively for the duration of sling application. The limb must be inspected daily, because the sling can lead to significant swelling of the foot. If this occurs the sling must be altered or removed. To prevent muscle and joint contracture, non–weight-bearing slings should not be maintained for longer than 2 to 3 weeks.

> **TECHNICIAN NOTE**
> To prevent muscle and joint contracture, non–weight-bearing slings should not be maintained for longer than 2 to 3 weeks.

The 90/90 flexion sling is a non–weight-bearing sling, which consists of a simple loop of adhesive tape wrapped around the stifle and hock while both joints are held at about 90 degrees of flexion. After repair of distal femoral fractures in puppies, use of this sling is critical to prevent quadriceps tie-down or contracture by keeping the affected muscles stretched. The sling is applied immediately after repair and is maintained for 2 to 3 days until postoperative pain and swelling have decreased.

The Velpeau sling is a non–weight-bearing sling for the forelimb and is used to immobilize all joints of the affected leg. It is mainly applied after reduction of medial shoulder joint luxation or after reconstruction of tenuous fractures. The entire forelimb is flexed and brought up against the thoracic wall, and a soft-padded bandage is applied to keep it in place (Fig. 27.11A–D). Care must be taken to not impair breathing, because this bandage encircles the chest.

A carpal flexion sling is a simple, non–weight-bearing forelimb sling that is applied with the carpus in flexion (Fig. 27.12A–F). It prevents weight bearing but allows movement of the elbow and shoulder joint. It can also be used to relieve tension on the carpal flexor tendons after injury or surgical repair. If used for an inappropriate length of time, contracture of the carpal flexor tendons may occur.

Hobbles prevent abduction of the pelvic limbs and are used after reduction of ventral hip luxation. They can be applied at the level of the stifle joints or at the metatarsi (Fig. 27.13). Because of the vast amount of hip mobility in cats and dogs, hobbles may not protect entirely against reluxation, and patients must be supported with an abdominal sling and be kept on nonslip flooring.

Bandages for Other Locations

A tie-over bandage can be applied to locations on the body where traditional limb bandages cannot be used or would be impractical, for example, the axillary and inguinal areas or around the pelvis. This type of bandage uses suture loops that encircle the wound edges and are used as anchor points for bandage material. The wound is covered with appropriate primary and secondary layers. A protective tertiary layer, such as a paper drape cut to size, is used to cover the bandage. The layers are then held in place by strands of large suture or umbilical tape that crisscross over the bandage from one suture loop to another (Fig. 27.14A–D). When a tie-over bandage is changed, the skin suture loops are maintained while the umbilical tape is cut for removal of the bandage.

Adhesive drapes can be used instead of tie-over skin sutures to hold the primary and secondary bandage layers in place. The adhesive drape will also act as the outer protective layer. Adhesive drapes are useful for wounds on relatively flat surfaces, such as the chest or abdominal wall.

Three-layer soft-padded bandages that encircle a body part are usually used for the head, chest, abdomen, and tail. Instead of a tertiary layer, such as Vetrap, elastic materials, such as stockinette, can be used to hold the primary and secondary layers in place. Head bandages are often applied to the ear after injury or surgery to absorb wound drainage, to provide compression against dead space, or to protect the ear from injury caused by head shaking. The affected pinna may be incorporated into the bandage, so when the bandage is cut and removed, great care is required to avoid accidentally cutting into the ear (Fig. 27.15A–F). A head bandage is often applied immediately after surgery while the animal is still under general anesthesia. These animals must be closely monitored during the recovery period for potential respiratory compromise as a result of airway compression by a tight bandage. Other complications include corneal abrasions if the bandage is placed too close to the eye.

Bandages around the chest are often applied in a "figure-of-eight" pattern around the forelimbs to prevent slippage (Fig. 27.16). Care must be taken to avoid restricting respiratory function by applying the bandage too tightly. Figure-of-eight bandages can be difficult to place around the caudal abdomen or pelvis (especially in male dogs) so as to allow urination and defecation. Soiling of the bandage is common and necessitates changes.

Tail bandages often require a small strip of adhesive tape applied to the skin at the proximal end to keep the bandage from slipping off (Fig. 27.17A–D). Syringe casing or other additional protection can be added to the tip of the tail if needed.

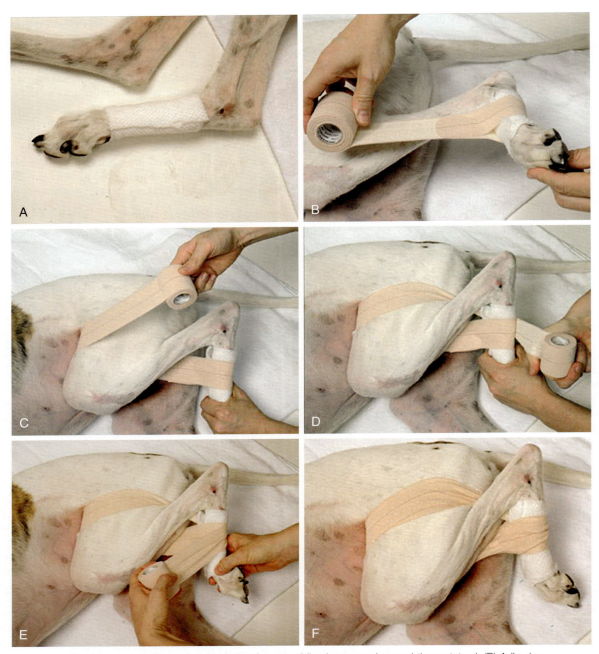

• **Fig. 27.10** Ehmer sling. (A) A thin layer of cast padding is wrapped around the metatarsi. (B) Adhesive tape is applied around the metatarsi and is taped back onto itself to prevent constriction of soft tissues. (C) With the hock and the stifle held in full flexion, the tape is passed medially and then cranially around the thigh as far proximally as possible. This prevents slippage of the tape over the stifle joint. (D) The tape is then passed caudally over the lateral thigh and looped back medially around the hock. (E) If necessary, the tape is passed one more time in the same manner. (F) The Ehmer sling is primarily non–weight-bearing. When properly placed, it results (in principle) in internal rotation and abduction of the femur.

TECHNICIAN NOTE

Head bandages can cause life-threatening respiratory compromise, especially when placed while the patient is still under general anesthesia. Thus patients must be closely monitored during the recovery period.

Aftercare for Bandages, Splints, Casts, and Slings

The length of time that a bandage should be kept on depends on the underlying condition. Prolonged immobilization leads to muscle atrophy, contracture of soft tissues, and joint changes; therefore any type of bandage should be removed as soon as possible. Bandage changes are required on a regular basis, because complications occurring under the bandage are not obvious to the observer. Wound bandages may have to be changed up to three times a day if exudate is copious. Once healthy granulation tissue has formed or the wound is in the epithelialization phase, bandage changes can be decreased to every 2 to 3 days. When there is no wound (e.g., closed fractures, joint injuries), bandages should be

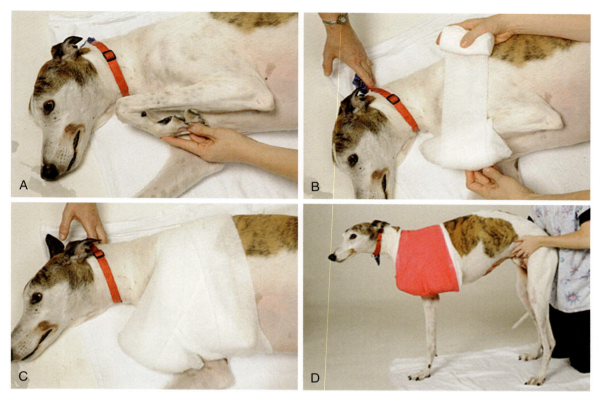

• **Fig. 27.11** Velpeau sling. (A) The entire forelimb is bandaged in flexion. (B) A soft-padded bandage is applied, beginning with the carpus held in flexion. (C) The secondary layer is continued over and around the chest. (D) Elastic gauze and a tertiary layer complete the Velpeau sling. This sling prevents weight bearing on the forelimb.

changed once a week to allow assessment of the limb for bandage-associated complications.

It is important to severely limit exercise to short bathroom walks on a leash until the bandage is removed; activity will increase the risks for shifting of bandage material, development of chafing and sores, and complications during healing.

Monitoring of distal limb bandages includes daily inspection of the toes for swelling (indicated by increased distance between the toe-nails) or decreased viability (decreased warmth or abnormal color). The bandage must be kept dry and clean and must be protected when the animal goes outside. Plastic bags, reclosable plastic bags, empty IV fluid bags, or commercial booties can be used as water-proof coverings; however, they must only be kept in place for short periods to prevent moisture accumulation and subsequent soft tis-sue maceration. Most cats and dogs require an Elizabethan collar to protect the bandage from being chewed or licked. A bandage, splint, cast, or sling that is inappropriately tight or that has slipped may impair blood flow, leading to swelling and possible tissue necrosis. Foul odor from the bandage or a sudden behavior change in the ani-mal, such as increased lameness or biting at the limb, are indications that bandage complications are occurring. Good client education regarding bandage care requirements and possible bandage-associ-ated complications is paramount in the care of the animal.

Large-Animal Wound Management

Wound Care in Horses

Wound management in horses starts with basic wound care and is no different from that provided for small companion animals. However, the size and nature of the animal and the location of the injury may dictate the approach to wound care. The initial care includes clipping hair from around the wound, cleansing and debriding, and preparing the wound for closure (if applicable).

Preparing the Wound

Initial treatment of the wound includes using clippers to remove hair from around the edges of the wound. Methods used to lavage a wound are like those described for small animals. It is impor-tant that lavage is performed under pressure, because this will dislodge debris and bacteria from the wound. A water hose with moderate pressure is good to remove large amounts of dirt and debris; however, caution should be used with a spray nozzle and strong pressure, as this system could drive dirt and bacteria into the tissue.

Local Versus General Anesthesia

One important step in treating a wound in any horse is providing appropriate restraint. If the wound is to be closed, tranquilization or general anesthesia may be needed. If tranquilization is used, local or regional anesthesia is also necessary for debridement and closure of the wound. Local infiltration is performed by injecting a local anesthetic (mepivacaine or lidocaine) approximately 1 cm from the wound edge subcutaneously around the entire wound (Fig. 27.18). If possible, a ring block or a nerve block (e.g., a pal-mar nerve block) can be performed to anesthetize the portion of the limb distal to the block (Fig. 27.19). If a wound is to be sutured, the same considerations for wound closure in small com-panion animals apply to large animals.

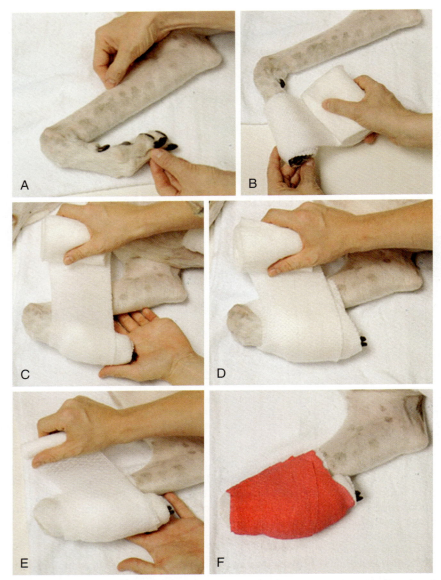

• **Fig. 27.12** Carpal flexion sling. (A–D) The carpus is bandaged in flexion. The soft-padded bandage begins around the foot, then continues over the distal forelimb with the carpus in flexion. (E and F) Elastic gauze and a protective outer layer are applied. This sling prevents weight bearing on the forelimb while allowing movement of the shoulder and elbow.

Exuberant Granulation Tissue in Open Wounds

Open wounds on the distal aspect of the limb of the horse are notorious for developing exuberant granulation tissue, commonly referred to as "proud flesh" (Fig. 27.20). Various measures, including limb immobilization (as with a cast), wound bandaging, cryotherapy, electrocautery, and application of topical corticosteroids, can be undertaken to maintain appropriate granulation tissue during healing. Surgical excision appears to be the best method of removing and controlling exuberant granulation tissue (Fig. 27.21). Regardless of the decision to close a wound or allow healing by second intention, bandaging should be part of the wound care provided.

Bandage, Splint, and Cast Application Techniques for Horses

Bandages and casts serve many purposes and are named based on the location they cover and the purpose that they serve. Various materials are available for use in a bandage or cast, but the most important aspect for selection is their proper application and function. Development of good bandaging and cast-application skills is important in ensuring proper function of the bandage or cast. Application and purposes of different types of bandages and casts used in horses are discussed.

Bandages

Lower Limb Wound Bandage

A lower limb wound bandage covers a wound on a limb distal to the carpus or tarsus. After the wound has been cleaned, a topical antimicrobial preparation may be applied. A nonadherent dressing is then placed directly over the wound. The wound dressing is secured to the limb with *rolled conforming gauze*, which is wrapped around the limb with light pressure, with overlapping and with minimal wrinkles to prevent formation of pressure lines. It is wrapped approximately 2 to 4 cm proximal and distal to the wound edges (Fig. 27.22).

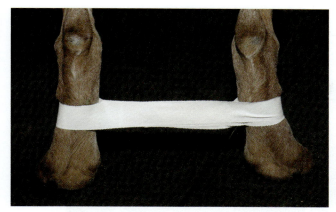

• **Fig. 27.13** Hobbles. A strip of adhesive tape is applied around the metatarsal bones of both pelvic limbs. The tape must not be too tight to avoid swelling and constriction of blood flow to the foot. The width of the hobbles should not be greater than the width of the animal's pelvis. Hobbles are used to prevent abduction of the hip joints after ventral coxofemoral luxation.

The *padded layer* is applied next. Sheets cut from a cotton combine roll, rolled cotton, layered cotton sheets, quilted leg wraps, or a military field bandage can be used (Fig. 27.23). The padded layer is secured to the limb with a roll of conforming gauze. Pressure is applied during wrapping to compress and conform the padding to the limb. The *outer shell* of the bandage is finished with elastic wrap (Vetrap bandage tape; 3M Animal Care Products, St. Paul, MN; or an Ace bandage), adhesive elastic tape (Elastikon; Johnson & Johnson Medical, Arlington, TX), or a flannel track wrap. If an Ace bandage or track wrap is used, it is secured with white tape cut into strips or placed around the bandage in a "barber pole" fashion (Fig. 27.24). Elastikon is placed around the top and bottom of the bandage, with half of the tape sticking to the wrap and half to the skin, to prevent slippage and to keep debris (e.g., bedding shavings) from getting inside the bandage (Fig. 27.25A–D).

Lower Limb Support Bandage

A lower limb support bandage is used to provide support for soft tissues (e.g., ligaments, tendons) of the limb **contralateral** to the injured leg, which is bearing more weight because of decreased weight-bearing ability on the injured limb. The bandage also minimizes static limb edema in a confined, inactive horse. A support bandage is placed on the lower limb in the manner previously described for the lower limb wound bandage, except that the underlying wound dressing and inner conforming gauze layer are not used. It is unnecessary to place wide adhesive elastic tape around the top and bottom. Typically a reusable cotton wrap will suffice.

Splint Application

A splint is rigid material added to a limb bandage to reinforce immobilization of a particular part of a limb. Various materials, including wooden slats, metal bars, low-temperature thermoplastic material, and casting material, can be used as reinforcement. However, the material most commonly used is PVC (polyvinylchloride) pipe because of its light weight and strength. A 10-cm–diameter pipe split into thirds is ideal. It can be bent to conform to the fetlock angulation by heating along the area to be angled. The length and width of the splint vary, depending on the size of the limb and the area splinted. According to the amount of immobilization required, splints can be placed the full length of the forelimb or from just below the carpus or tarsus all the way to the ground surface. In most situations, they are placed on the flexor surface (back) of the limb. Splints are used in such situations as extensor or flexor tendon lacerations and flexure deformities in foals or for needed limb support (as in radial nerve paresis).

A support bandage is placed on the limb first. It should be long enough to cover the limb above and below the ends of the splint. This is very important, because it will prevent the development of pressure sores. Once the bandage is in place, the splint is secured to the limb with adhesive tape (Fig. 27.26). Splints should be reset frequently (at least once per day), particularly in foals. Because of advances in limb splinting for large animals, specially designed splints are now available (DynaSplint; DynaSplint Systems, Inc., Severna Park, MD).

> **TECHNICIAN NOTE**
> A bandage should cover the limb well above and below the ends of a splint to prevent pressure sores.

Cast Application

A cast is the **external coaptation** most frequently used to manage various orthopedic injuries or problems when maximum support and immobilization are required. Casts are commonly used for lower limb problems; however, full-limb application is sometimes indicated in large animals. Distal limb casts can be efficiently placed with the animal under general anesthesia or in the standing sedated patient; however, full-limb application is preferably performed with the animal under general anesthesia, as it is more difficult to place in the standing patient. Indications for use of a cast include lower limb fractures, tendon lacerations, support of the lower limb during anesthetic induction or recovery for orthopedic surgery, heel bulb lacerations, and luxation of the tarsus, fetlock, or pastern. A cast may also be used as an adjunct to internal fixation.

For optimal effectiveness in immobilization, a cast must immobilize the joint proximal and distal to the injury. Full-limb casts must extend up to the elbow or stifle as far as possible. The most frequently used material today is fiberglass (e.g., Delta-Lite; Johnson & Johnson Medical, Arlington, TX). It is appealing because it is lightweight, strong, and relatively easy to apply. However, some veterinarians prefer to use an initial layer of traditional plaster of Paris under the fiberglass. Plaster conforms well to the contour of the limb, reducing the risk of pressure sores. A limb cast must be applied properly or serious problems, such as pressure necrosis, can occur. It is important to remember that applying excessive padding under a cast can result in compression of the padding and loosening of the cast, leading to the development of cast sores.

> **TECHNICIAN NOTE**
> Excessive padding under a cast can result in compression of the padding and loosening of the cast, leading to the development of cast sores.

All necessary materials should be collected before the procedure is begun (Fig. 27.27A–B). Proper application of a cast is essential, especially if it is to remain on the limb for a prolonged period (4–6 weeks).

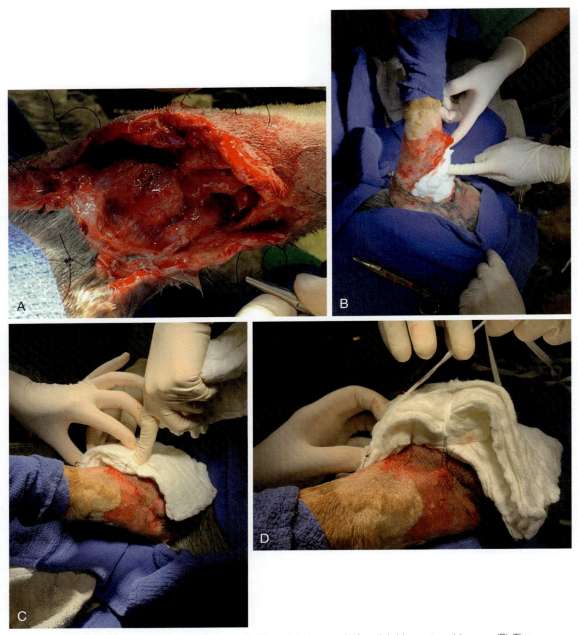

• **Fig. 27.14** Open wound management. (A) The original wound after debridement and lavage. (B) The application of a nonadherent primary layer using appropriate sterile technique. (C) Application of a secondary moisture-wicking layer. (D) Application of a tie-over bandage using laparotomy sponges to protect the primary and secondary layers and provide extra moisture wicking.

Preparation of the Foot

When applying a cast to the animal under general anesthesia, it is preferable to position the horse in lateral recumbency so that the limb to which the cast will be applied is uppermost. Debris is cleaned from the sole, the horseshoe is removed, and the hoof is trimmed. The limb is placed in an extended position perpendicular to the body. Effective support of the limb is essential to maintain it in alignment. Some veterinarians use a wire looped through holes drilled in the hoof to improve traction (Fig. 27.28A–C).

Preparation of the Limb Before Cast Application

The skin that will be covered by the cast must be clean and dry. It can be powdered with talcum or boric acid to help keep the area under the cast dry. If a wound or surgical site is present, a three-layer bandage consisting of a nonadherent dressing, conforming gauze, and adherent elastic tape is used to cover it. The limb is then covered with a double layer of stockinette (Figs. 27.29 and 27.30). Any wrinkles are smoothed out, and towel clamps may be used to secure the stockinette above the area to which the cast will be applied (Fig. 27.31). A strip of orthopedic felt (5–7 cm wide) is placed around the limb at the most proximal limit of the cast. This is held in place with 1-inch white tape (Fig. 27.32). A second piece of felt can be placed along the palmar/plantar aspect of the fetlock, over the sesamoid bones. When a full-limb cast is used, a doughnut pad cut from orthopedic felt is placed over the accessory carpal bone of the forelimb. A thin strip of orthopedic felt is

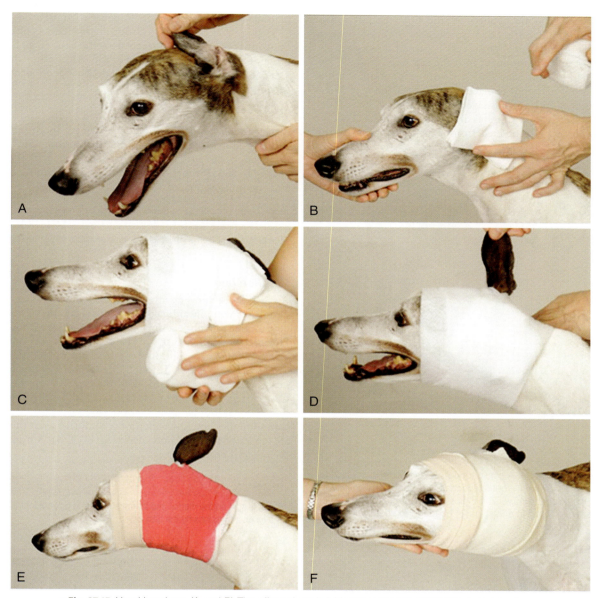

• **Fig. 27.15** Head bandage. (A and B) The affected ear is laid across the top of the head, and a primary layer can be applied if indicated. (C and D) Cast padding is applied, with the unaffected ear spared. If desired, elastic gauze can be used to cover the padding; however, care must be taken to not tighten the bandage too much. (E and F) The tertiary layer can consist of such material as Vetrap or the more elastic stockinette. Both are held in place by a strip of elastic tape.

placed over the gastrocnemius tendon and the point of the hock of the hind limb to prevent the development of pressure sores.

A roll of support foam can be applied next. It is applied over the stockinette, and its purpose is to provide padding under a cast to reduce the development of pressure sores (Fig. 27.33).

Application of the Cast Material

Gloves should be worn when casting material is applied. Initially, some veterinarians may apply two layers of 3-inch plaster material. Application of the cast material is usually started at the proximal or distal aspect of the limb. Approximately 1 cm of orthopedic felt is left exposed above the top of the cast to prevent formation of a sore.

To begin, the fiberglass material is held in a bucket of clean water until it is thoroughly wet, and the excess water is shaken

out. The warmer the water, the faster the curing process of the resin, resulting in premature hardening of the fiberglass cast material. The cast material is overlapped by one-third to one-half of its width as it is applied. As the fiberglass casting material is worked toward the foot, the traction wires (if being used) are cut, and an assistant supports the limb (Fig. 27.34).

TECHNICIAN NOTE

It is important to ensure that the initial layer of casting material applied to the limb is without wrinkles or finger imprints, which may create pressure sores.

More pressure is applied to the succeeding layers of fiberglass. This will allow them to laminate better and improves cast strength. Generally, five to six layers (four to five rolls) of 4- or

5-inch fiberglass tape are applied. At the time the last roll of cast material is applied, the excess stockinette is cut off, leaving approximately 4 cm. This 4-cm excess is turned down over the top of the cast and incorporated into the last layer (Fig. 27.35). A wedge block (made of wood, plastic, rubber, or another roll of fiberglass casting material) is placed underneath the heel and is also incorporated with the last layers (Fig. 27.36). A heel wedge allows the horse to walk more easily while wearing a cast. The bottom of the cast is protected from wear by capping it with

hard acrylic (e.g., Technovit; Jorgensen Laboratories, Loveland, CO) (Fig. 27.37). Finally, elastic adhesive tape is placed around the top of the cast and attached to the skin (Fig. 27.38), or a piece of stockinette is pulled over the top and taped to the cast and the limb above it to prevent debris (wood shavings) from getting under the cast.

Stall confinement is mandatory after cast application, and the patient must be monitored daily. Indications for cast change or removal include breakage, increased lameness, swelling above the cast, and exudate coming out of the top or through the cast. Reaction and tolerance to the cast vary among horses. If there is any doubt, the cast should be removed and the limb evaluated.

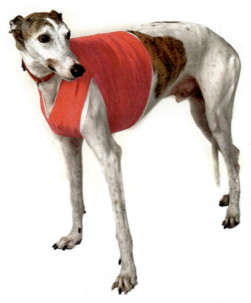

• **Fig. 27.16** Chest bandage. A soft-padded bandage with cast padding, elastic gauze, and a protective outer layer has been placed by crisscrossing between the two forelimbs. This helps keep the bandage in place. Care must be taken to avoid applying this bandage too tightly to prevent respiratory compromise.

TECHNICIAN NOTE

The presence of flies on the cast is a good indicator of the development of cast sores.

Cast Removal

A cast is best removed with the animal standing. If cast removal is performed with the animal under general anesthesia, the limb may be reinjured when the animal is trying to recover from anesthesia. However, if another cast is to be applied, general anesthesia can be used. The cast is split on the medial and lateral surfaces with a cast saw (Fig. 27.39A). Through this approach, potential injury to flexor and extensor tendons with the cast saw can be prevented. Cast cutters are made to oscillate, so it is best to push into the cast material, not along it, because this will reduce the chance of lacerating the skin. Once the cast is completely, cut the two halves are separated with cast spreaders (Fig. 27.39B). A support wrap is then placed on the limb.

TECHNICIAN NOTE

A cast is split on the medial and lateral surfaces to prevent injury to the flexor and extensor tendons by the cast saw.

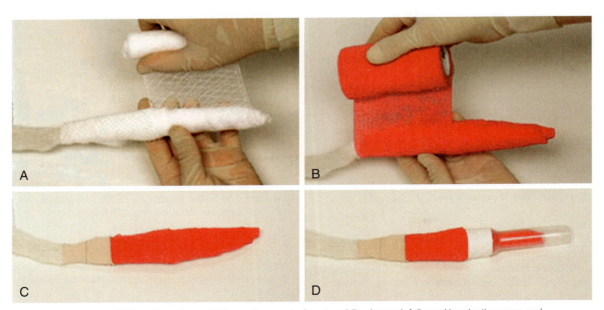

• **Fig. 27.17** Tail bandage. (A and B) A small amount of cast padding is used, followed by elastic gauze and a tertiary layer. (C) Adhesive tape at the proximal end helps to prevent slippage of the bandage. (D) A rigid covering (e.g., syringe casing) can be added to the tip of the tail to provide further protection.

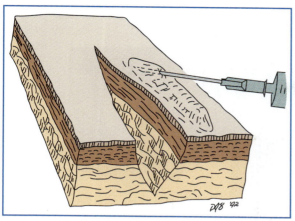

• **Fig. 27.18** Proper technique for infiltration of a wound edge with a local anesthetic. The needle should enter through the skin at the point of the last injection.

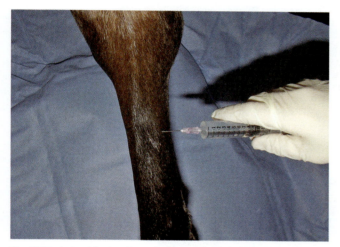

• **Fig. 27.19** A ring block using a local anesthetic is infiltrated subcutaneously around the limb of a horse to triage a distal limb wound.

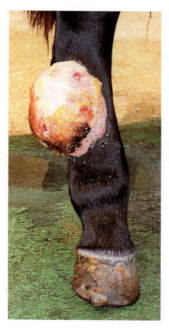

• **Fig. 27.20** Exuberant granulation tissue on the metatarsus of a horse.

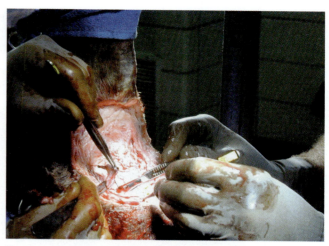

• **Fig. 27.21** Exuberant granulation tissue being excised from the dorsum of a horse's tarsus.

Bandage, Splint, and Cast Application Techniques for Cattle

Similar principles of limb bandaging and cast application apply to cattle. Most casts, bandages, and splints are applied in cattle as described in the horse. Bandages and casts are tolerated remarkably well by cattle, making them excellent candidates for therapy for many wounds and fractures. Placing the animal in lateral recumbency is preferred for procedures involving external coaptation, because cattle often are often not amenable to cast or bandage application and removal in the standing position. Achieving recumbency can be accomplished by using chemical sedation, a hydraulic tilt chute or table, or casting with rope techniques, often in combination with sedation.

Sores caused by the cast rubbing against the skin are a common complication and can be avoided with proper cast padding. It is important to ensure that pressure points, such as the accessory carpal bone and the very top of the cast, are adequately padded. Unlike in the horse, it is necessary to use padding between the claws and underneath the dewclaws in ruminants (Fig. 27.40). Velpeau and Ehmer slings, as described for small animals, can be implemented effectively in small ruminants and camelids.

Application of a Claw Block

Cattle have two weight-bearing digits on each foot, which is an advantage in the management of lameness confined to one digit. A wooden or rubber block (available in different shapes or sizes) can be glued to the sound digit, elevating the foot and thereby alleviating pressure on the affected digit (Fig. 27.41).

Debris must be removed and the claw trimmed and kept dry to provide effective bonding of adhesive to the claw. The block is bonded to the surface of the claw with acrylic cement such as Technovit (Jorgensen Laboratories, Loveland, CO) or polyurethane hoof cement (Vettec; Vettec Hoof Care Products, Oxnard, CA) (Fig. 27.42).

Modified Thomas Splint

Modified Thomas splints are often used in farm animals along with casts for external support to provide traction and to maintain alignment of the limb. They can be used for any long-bone fracture distal to the elbow and the stifle but are especially useful for radius and tibia fractures, as these bones cannot be adequately stabilized with a

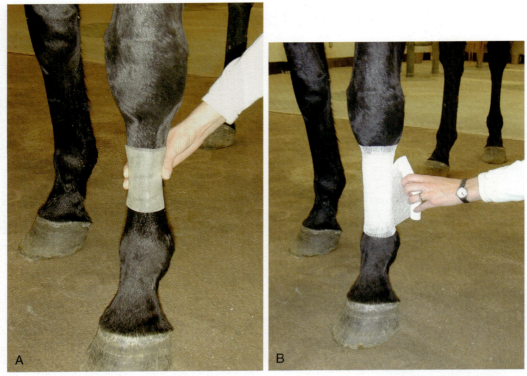

• **Fig. 27.22** Application of wound dressing to the distal region of the limb of a horse. (A) A nonadherent dressing is applied directly over the wound. (B) Conforming gauze is applied to hold the nonadherent dressing over the wound.

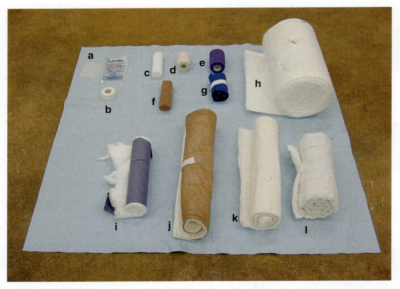

• **Fig. 27.23** Various materials can be used in a leg bandage for large animals: nonadherent wound dressing *(a)*, white tape *(b)*, white roll gauze *(c)*, Elastikon (Johnson & Johnson Medical, Arlington, TX) *(d)*, Vetrap bandage tape (3M Animal Care Products, St. Paul, MN) *(e)*, brown gauze *(f)*, track wrap *(g)*, combine cotton roll *(h)*, rolled cotton *(i)*, military field bandage *(j)*, layered cotton sheets *(k)*, and quilted leg wraps *(l)*.

plain cast alone. They are also useful in long oblique or comminuted fractures in which a plain cast will not provide enough support. The splint essentially acts as a crutch, with a hoop placed in the axillary or inguinal region and two support bars that run parallel to the limb cranially and caudally, linking the hoop to a footplate distally. With this design, as the patient bears weight, it is distributed between the hoop and footplate, largely bypassing the limb and unstable area. Although this technique can be very useful in ruminants of all sizes, complications are common and include pressure sores in the inguinal/axillary region and malunion or nonunion of the fracture.

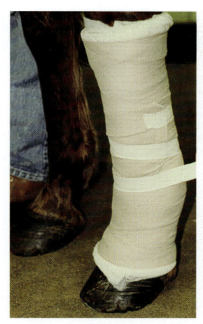

• **Fig. 27.24** If white medical tape is used to secure the outer layer of the bandage on a horse's limb, it is secured in a "barber pole" fashion to reduce the chance of a tourniquet effect.

The splint may be made of steel conduit, steel rod, or aluminum rod, depending on the size of the patient. A template using flexible tubing can be used to size the ring that will encircle the proximal part of the limb (Fig. 27.43). The ring can be bent by using a conduit bender or around a support beam or something similar to bend an aluminum rod for smaller patients (Fig. 27.44). The ring should not impinge on any bony prominences and is padded with cotton (Fig. 27.45) to reduce pressure sores in the axillary or inguinal region. Covering the padding with a water-impervious tape (duct tape) can reduce sores created by damp, fabric-based tape rubbing against the skin.

> ### TECHNICIAN NOTE
> Covering the padding with a smooth, water-impervious tape (duct tape) can reduce sores created by damp, fabric-based tape rubbing against the skin.

Support bars connect to the ring and extend distally (Fig. 27.46). Supports should bend away (lateral) from the flat plane of the ring to allow the ventral part of the ring to fit into the axillary or inguinal region (Fig. 27.47). A metal rod bent into a flat U-shape and attached to the extension with tape can serve as a footplate (Fig. 27.48A and B). Alternatively, sophisticated splints for larger ruminants may have an adjustable footplate. Wire secures the hoof to the splint through holes in the hoof wall (Fig. 27.49A and B). Traction is placed on the limb as the splint is applied. Excessive traction must be avoided, because too much pressure in the axillary or inguinal region can interfere with venous drainage or distract the fracture fragments.

> ### TECHNICIAN NOTE
> It is important to avoid applying excess traction when the hoof is secured to a modified Thomas splint, because this will create too much pressure in the axillary or inguinal region, and the pressure can interfere with venous drainage or distract the fracture fragments.

Once the splint is in position, the limb and splint are covered with cast material (Fig. 27.50). Casting tape is applied first to the limb alone and then used to incorporate the casted limb into the frame (Fig.27.51A and B). The cast material should be applied as proximally as possible (Fig. 27.52). The bottom of the splint can be protected from wear by application of acrylic hoof-bonding material (Fig. 27.53). A calf with a completed modified Thomas splint is shown in Fig. 27.54.

Acknowledgments

The authors and publisher wish to acknowledge the previous contributions of Giselle Hosgood, Bianca Hettlich, Harry Markwell, and Andrew Niehaus.

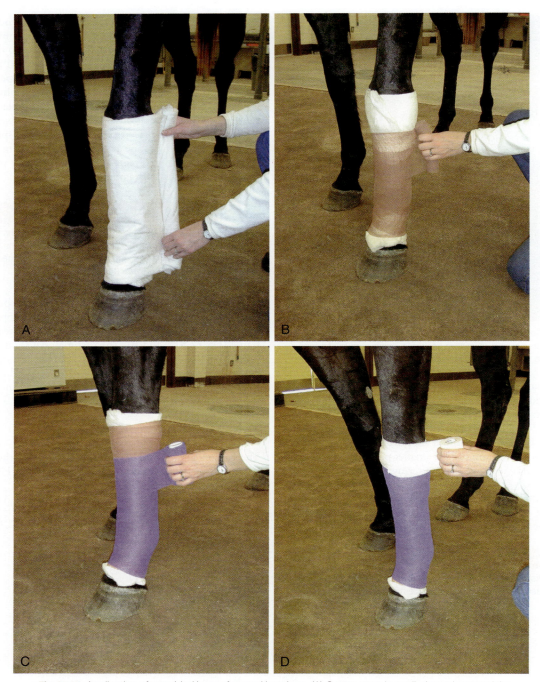

• **Fig. 27.25** Application of a padded layer of wound bandage. (A) Cotton wrap is applied snugly around the limb. (B) Conforming gauze is used to secure the padded layer to the limb. (C) Vetrap bandage tape (3M Animal Care Products, St. Paul, MN) is applied as the outer shell of the bandage. (D) Wide adhesive tape is used to provide a seal between the skin and the bandage.

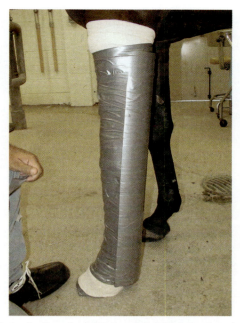

• **Fig. 27.26** Application of a full-limb splint. A thick bandage is placed on the limb. The splint (polyvinylchloride [PVC] pipe) is positioned along the flexor surface and is secured to the bandage with duct tape.

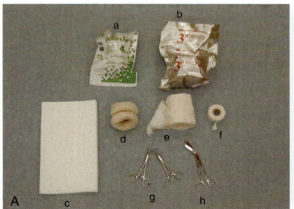

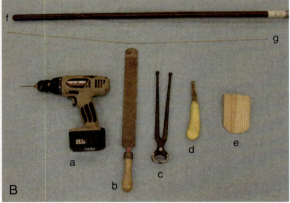

• **Fig. 27.27** Materials needed to apply a limb cast to a large animal. (A) Cast material *(a)*, support foam *(b)*, orthopedic felt *(c)*, orthopedic stockinette (3-inch) *(d)*, cast padding *(e)*, white tape (1-inch) *(f)*, towel clamps *(g)*, and bandage scissors *(h)*. (B) One-eighth–inch drill bit and hand drill *(a)*, hoof rasp *(b)*, shoe pullers *(c)*, hoof knife *(d)*, wooden wedge block *(e)*, broom handle *(f)*, and wire (approximately 30 cm) *(g)*.

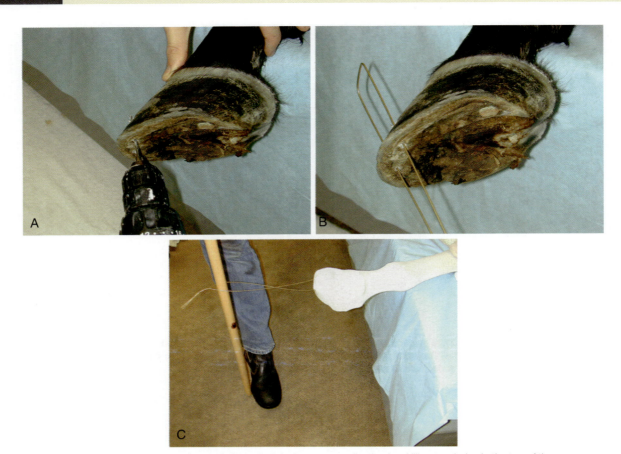

• **Fig. 27.28** Traction can be applied to a limb before cast application by drilling two holes in the toe of the hoof (A) and threading a loop of wire through the holes (B) with a broomstick placed in the loop to apply traction (C).

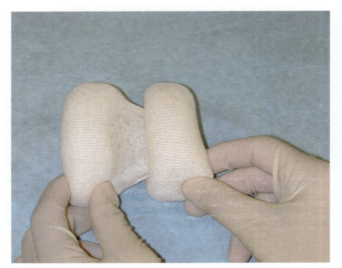

• **Fig. 27.29** Orthopedic stockinette used under a cast is prerolled. One end is rolled outward and the other end is rolled inward until both ends meet at the midpoint of the stockinette.

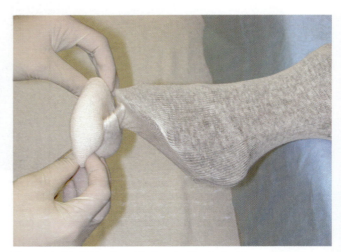

• **Fig. 27.30** A twist is placed in the stockinette just beneath the toe, and the inward roll is unrolled up the leg.

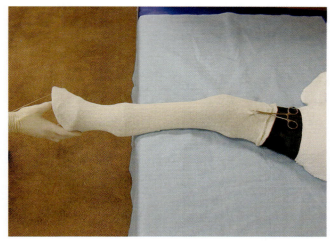

• **Fig. 27.31** Before cast material is applied, the orthopedic stockinette is secured with towel clamps to the medial and lateral aspects of the limb above the area to which the cast will be applied.

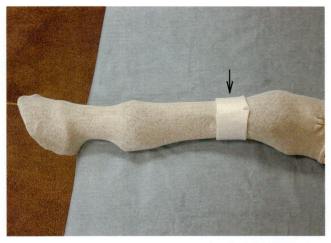

• **Fig. 27.32** A strip of orthopedic felt (5–7 cm wide) *(arrow)* is placed around the limb at the most proximal limit of the cast. The ends are held in place with 1-inch white tape.

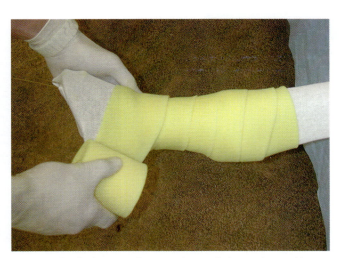

• **Fig. 27.33** A roll of support foam can be applied over the stockinette to provide padding under the cast to prevent the formation of pressure sores.

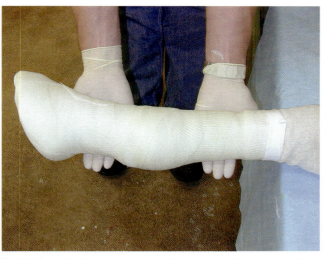

• **Fig. 27.34** As the fiberglass cast material is applied, an assistant holds the limb out by resting it on the palms of the hands under the metacarpus or metatarsus region. This method prevents finger impressions in the uncured cast material.

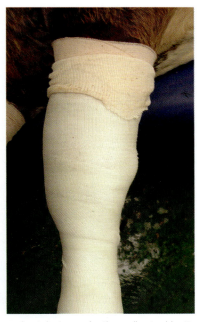

• **Fig. 27.35** Approximately 4 cm of orthopedic stockinette left exposed on top of a cast is pulled down over the cast top and incorporated into the last layers of the cast.

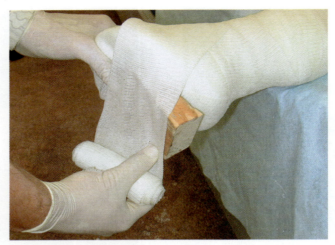

• **Fig. 27.36** A wooden wedge block is placed underneath the heel and incorporated with the final layers of cast material.

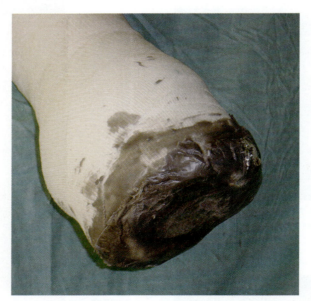

• **Fig. 27.37** The bottom of the cast is protected from wear by capping it with hard acrylic. (From Technovit; Jorgensen Laboratories, Loveland, CO.)

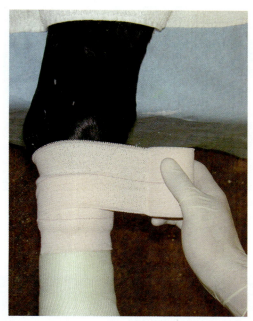

• **Fig. 27.38** Elastic adhesive tape is placed on top of the cast to form a seal between the skin and the cast and prevent debris from getting inside the cast.

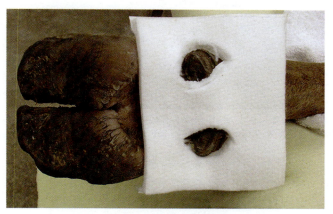

• **Fig. 27.40** A piece of orthopedic felt with holes cut out can be placed between the dewclaws to reduce motion under a cast and to help prevent the development of pressure sores.

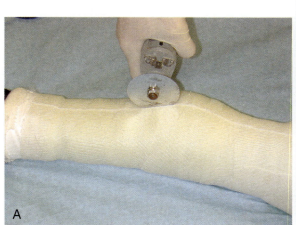

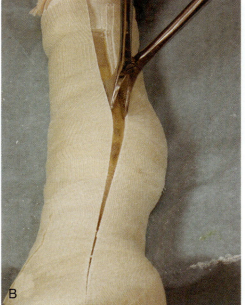

• **Fig. 27.39** Removal of a limb cast from a horse. (A) With a Stryker saw, the cast is split on the medial and lateral surface, and the cut is continued under the foot. (B) Once the cast is completely cut, the halves are separated with cast spreaders.

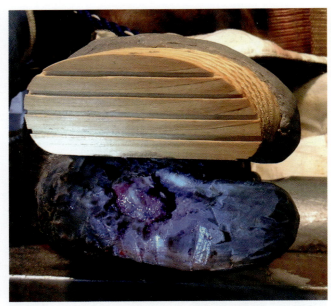

• **Fig. 27.41** A claw block made from wood. Grooves are cut on both sides of the block to improve traction and bonding.

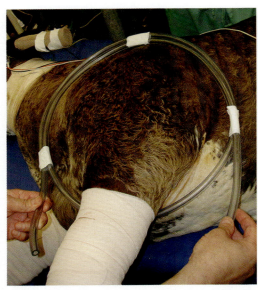

• **Fig. 27.43** A template, devised from a nasogastric tube or other similar flexible tubing, is used to construct the metal ring of a modified Thomas splint that will encircle the proximal part of the leg.

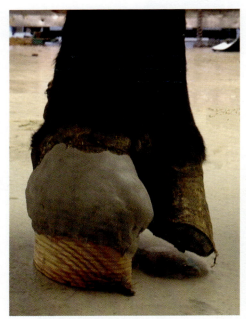

• **Fig. 27.42** A wooden block is cemented to the sound digit with polymethyl methacrylate. The cow stands on the hoof block (viewed from the dorsal aspect of the foot), which prevents the affected digit from bearing weight.

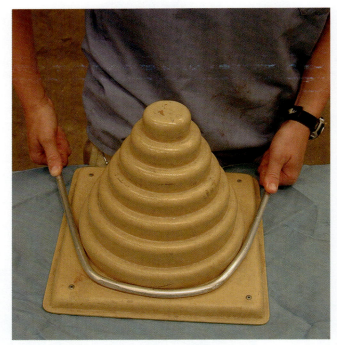

• **Fig. 27.44** A ¼-inch aluminum rod is bent to construct a modified Thomas splint.

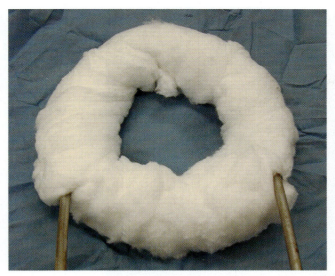

• **Fig. 27.45** A metal rod is bent into a ring to construct the proximal part of a modified Thomas splint. Once the ring is constructed, it is padded with cotton.

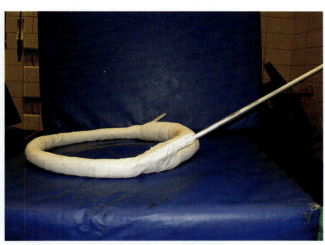

• **Fig. 27.47** Construction of a modified Thomas splint. Supports come off the ring at an angle to allow the ring to properly fit under the axillary or inguinal region.

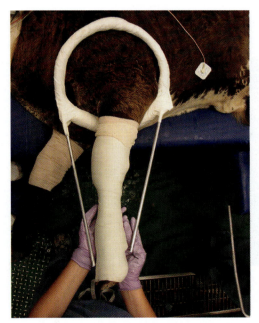

• **Fig. 27.46** Construction of a modified Thomas splint. Supports of the splint come off the edge of the ring and are positioned cranial and caudal to the limb.

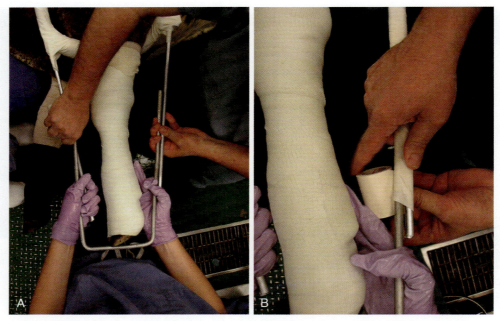

• **Fig. 27.48** The footplate in this design of a modified Thomas splint is constructed from a piece of metal rod that is bent into a flat "U" shape (A), positioned under the foot, and connected to the ends of the supports of the splint with a combination of twisted wire loops and lots of tape (B).

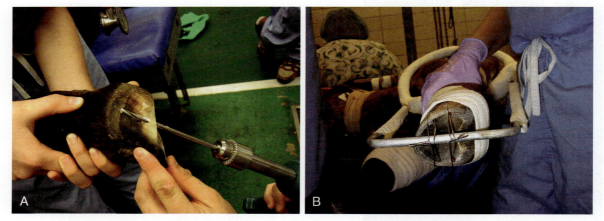

• **Fig. 27.49** Holes are drilled into the hoof walls near the toes (A) and are wired to the bottom of the splint (B) when a modified Thomas splint is applied.

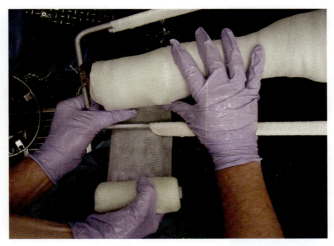

• **Fig. 27.50** The limb and the modified Thomas splint are covered with layers of cast material to stabilize the limb.

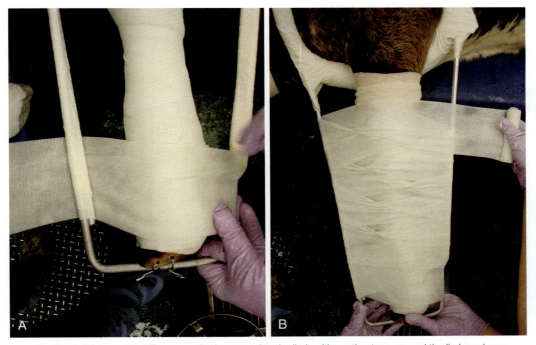

• **Fig. 27.51** (A) A modified Thomas splint is secured to the limb with casting tape around the limb and supports of the splint. (B) The casting tape is twisted 180 degrees with each passage of the material.

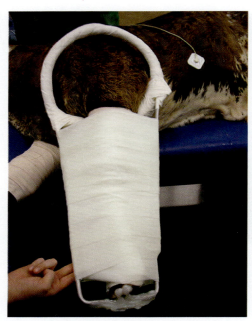

• **Fig. 27.52** The cast material is placed as proximally as possible when a modified Thomas splint is applied.

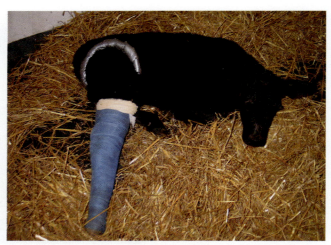

• **Fig. 27.54** Young calf with a distal tibial fracture managed with a Thomas splint covered with fiberglass casting tape. The splint frame was constructed with an aluminum rod.

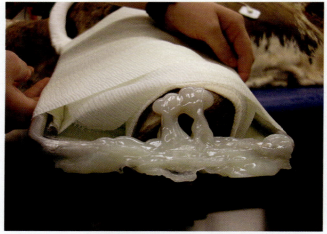

• **Fig. 27.53** The bottom of a modified Thomas splint is protected from wear by applying a polyurethane hoof-bonding material.

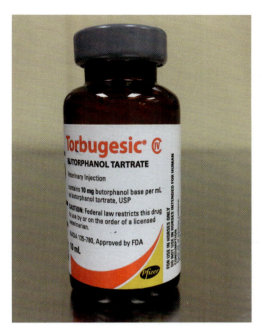

• **Fig. 28.1** Label on a bottle of butorphanol. Note the large "C" containing the Roman numeral "IV" to the right of the trade name (Torbugesic), indicating that this is a schedule IV-controlled substance.

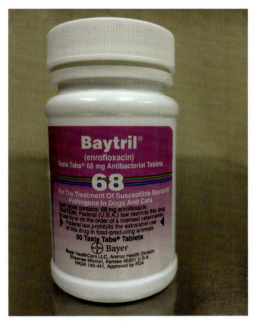

• **Fig. 28.2** Label on a bottle of medication. Note the trade name (Baytril) and the generic name (enrofloxacin) of the drug.

Drug Nomenclature

Drugs can be identified by many different names. The *chemical name* of a drug describes its chemical structure and is determined during the development of the drug compound. During development, a drug's **generic name**, which officially identifies it and is used by all manufacturers, will also be established by the developing company and the FDA. When a particular manufacturer produces and markets a drug, they will assign it a **trade name**, or *brand name*. Because multiple manufacturers may produce the same drug, one generically named drug may be known by multiple trade names. For example, the generic drug methimazole, used to treat hyperthyroidism, is manufactured under the trade names Tapazole and Felimazole. The trade name can be identified by the ® (registered) or ™ (trademark) symbol after it and is often capitalized. On a drug label, the generic name is typically listed after the trade name and is usually not capitalized. Fig. 28.2 shows an example of a drug bottle with both generic and trade names displayed.

Systemic Approach to Drug Classification

In the sections below, drugs commonly used in veterinary patients will be presented based on the primary diseases or conditions they are used to treat, organized according to the body system. Drugs in this chapter are identified by their generic name only.

Antimicrobial Drugs

Antimicrobials, a large class of drugs, include antibacterial and antifungal compounds that are used to kill or inhibit the growth of microorganisms.

Antibacterial Drugs

The term *antibacterial* is used in reference to substances that kill or inhibit the growth of bacteria. Antibacterial drugs, also commonly called *antibiotics*, are classified according to their MOA, their spectrum of activity (gram-positive, gram-negative, or anaerobic organisms), and whether they are **bactericidal** (kill bacteria) or **bacteriostatic** (inhibit bacterial replication).

The goal of antibacterial therapy is to assist the body's natural defenses in the elimination of bacterial pathogens while minimizing the risk of toxicity to the patient. Important factors to consider in the effort to maximize the **efficacy** of antibacterial therapy include: (1) establishing a preliminary or definitive diagnosis, including identification of the primary site or organ system affected, and (2) collecting appropriate samples for bacterial culture and sensitivity testing. Antibacterial therapy is often started while waiting for bacterial culture and sensitivity testing results and is based on the most likely infecting organism, the antimicrobial's spectrum of activity, the site of infection, and the risk for toxicity. This method of choosing a specific antibacterial based on observation and experience is called *empirical antibacterial therapy*.

Table 28.2 provides a summary of the classes of antibacterial agents most used in veterinary patients, including information on MOA, the spectrum of activity, and clinically important side effects. The most common side effects associated with all classes of antibacterial drugs are vomiting and diarrhea, which can occur for two reasons: (1) antibacterial compounds affect not only the targeted bacterial pathogen but also the normal gastrointestinal (GI) microflora, causing bacterial imbalance in the microbiome; and (2) some antibacterial drugs directly irritate the stomach. For example, the oral antimicrobial amoxicillin/clavulanic acid commonly causes anorexia and vomiting in cats.

> **TECHNICIAN NOTE**
>
> Antibacterial therapy is based on the bacterial pathogen identified, the site of infection, and the drug's spectrum of activity and MOA. Appropriate samples should be collected for bacterial culture and sensitivity; however, empirical antibacterial therapy is often initiated while waiting for results.

TABLE 28.2	Classes of Antibacterial Agents Commonly Used in Veterinary Patients[a]		
Class	Examples	Primary Spectrum of Activity	Side Effects and Notes Regarding Use
Penicillins MOA: interfere with the development of bacterial cell wall (bactericidal)	Penicillins: narrow spectrum • Penicillin G • Penicillin V	• Gram-positive aerobes • Obligate anaerobes	• Diarrhea • Hypersensitivity reactions
	Penicillins: aminopenicillins • Ampicillin • Amoxicillin		
	Penicillins: potentiated aminopenicillins • Amoxicillin + clavulanate • Ampicillin + sulbactam	• Also effective against beta-lactamase–producing *Staphylococcus* • Gram-negative aerobes	
Cephalosporins MOA: interfere with the development of bacterial cell wall (bactericidal)	Cephalosporins: first generation • Cefazolin • Cephalexin • Cefadroxil	• Gram-positive aerobes • Penicillinase-producing *Staphylococcus*	• Diarrhea • Vomiting, anorexia • Hypersensitivity reactions
	Cephalosporins: second generation • Cefotetan • Cefoxitin	• More gram-negative efficacy than first generation but slightly less gram-positive efficacy	
	Cephalosporins: third generation • Cefotaxime • Cefpodoxime • Ceftiofur • Ceftriaxone • Cefovecin	• Even more gram-negative efficacy, with significantly less gram-positive efficacy • Beta-lactamase resistant	
	Cephalosporins: fourth generation • Cefepime	• Have a broader spectrum of activity than the third generation • Effective against *Pseudomonas aeruginosa* and certain Enterobacteriaceae species	
Aminoglycosides MOA: inhibit bacterial ribosomal protein production (bactericidal)	Gentamicin Amikacin Neomycin Tobramycin	• Gram-negative aerobes	• Kidney toxicity • Otic toxicity • Avoid use in dehydrated patients • Poor GI absorption, mainly administered parenterally
Sulfonamides MOA: inhibit bacterial production of folic acid (unpotentiated sulfonamides: bacteriostatic; potentiated sulfonamides: bactericidal)	Sulfonamides • Sulfadiazine • Sulfamethoxazole • Sulfadimethoxine Potentiated sulfonamides • Sulfadiazine + trimethoprim • Sulfamethoxazole + trimethoprim • Sulfadimethoxine + ormetoprim	• Gram-positive aerobes • Gram-negative aerobes • Some protozoa	• Diarrhea • Bone marrow suppression • Hypersensitivity reactions in dogs involving joints, bone marrow, skin, liver, and dry eye • Teratogenic
Fluoroquinolones MOA: disrupts bacterial DNA supercoiling and storage (bactericidal)	Enrofloxacin Orbifloxacin Marbofloxacin Ciprofloxacin Pradofloxacin	• Gram-negative aerobes • *Brucella* • *Chlamydia* • *Mycobacterium* • *Mycoplasma* • *Rickettsia*	• Diarrhea • Young animals—cartilage damage • Cats—blindness at high doses • Seizures (in patients with a history of seizures) • Should not be used during pregnancy • Ciprofloxacin contraindicated in horses

TABLE 28.2	Classes of Antibacterial Agents Commonly Used in Veterinary Patients[a]—cont'd		
Class	**Examples**	**Primary Spectrum of Activity**	**Side Effects and Notes Regarding Use**
Amphenicols MOA: bind to ribosomes and inhibit bacterial protein synthesis (bacteriostatic at standard doses)	Chloramphenicol Florfenicol	• Gram-positive aerobes • Gram-negative aerobes • Obligate anaerobes • *Rickettsia* • *Chlamydia* • *Mycoplasma*	• Diarrhea • Bone marrow suppression • Gloves to be worn when handling tablets to avoid accidental absorption • Chloramphenicol use is illegal in food-producing animals • Florfenicol approved for use in cattle
Macrolides MOA: inhibit bacterial protein synthesis (bacteriostatic)	Erythromycin Clarithromycin Tilmicosin Azithromycin Tylosin Tulathromycin	• Gram-positive aerobes • Obligate anaerobes • Penicillinase-producing *Staphylococcus* • *Mycoplasma*	• Diarrhea • Erythromycin and tylosin may cause fatal diarrhea in horses
Lincosamides MOA: inhibit bacterial protein synthesis (bacteriostatic at lower concentrations, bactericidal at higher concentrations)	Clindamycin Lincomycin Pirlimycin	• Gram-positive aerobes • Obligate anaerobes • *Mycoplasma*	• Diarrhea • Contraindicated in horses
Tetracyclines MOA: bind to bacterial ribosomes and inhibit protein synthesis (bacteriostatic)	Tetracycline Oxytetracycline Doxycycline Minocycline	• Gram-positive aerobes • *Chlamydia* • *Rickettsia* • *Borrelia* • *Mycoplasma*	• Diarrhea • Esophageal strictures in cats • Decreased oral absorption when given with calcium- and iron-containing products, antacids, and sucralfate • Binds to the enamel of developing teeth in neonates, causing yellow discoloration • Doxycycline (intravenous) contraindicated in horses
Nitroimidazoles MOA: disrupt bacterial synthesis of DNA and nucleic acids (bactericidal/protozoacidal)	Metronidazole Ronidazole	• Obligate anaerobes • Protozoa	• Neurotoxicity (dose-related) • Use illegal in food-producing animals
Carbapenems MOA: interfere with the development of bacterial cell wall (bactericidal; bacteriostatic against some bacteria)	Imipenem Meropenem	• Broad spectrum against gram-positive and negative aerobes and anaerobes • Multidrug-resistant bacteria	• Diarrhea • Vomiting/anorexia • Hypersensitivity reactions • Seizures (associated with rapid infusion)

[a]Including spectrum of activity, MOA, and clinically important side effects.

Antifungal Drugs

Fungal infection can arise from a variety of fungal organisms (e.g., *Blastomyces, Histoplasma, Cryptococcus, Coccidioides, Aspergillus*); yeasts (e.g., *Candida, Malassezia*); and dermatophytes (e.g., *Microsporum* spp., *Trichophyton* spp.). Skin and ear infections are generally treated with topical antifungals, such as clotrimazole and nystatin, whereas disseminated infections are treated with systemic antifungals, including amphotericin B, ketoconazole, fluconazole, and itraconazole.

Antifungals are selectively toxic to fungal organisms as they bind to or inhibit the synthesis of ergosterol in the cell membrane, leading to cell death. Side effects associated with antifungal therapy occur when the antifungal drug targets the major sterol in mammalian cell membrane cholesterol (a substance similar to ergosterol). Systemic fungal infection often necessitates weeks to months of antifungal treatment. For the duration of therapy, each patient must be monitored closely for drug side effects, including decreased appetite, anorexia, and vomiting. Routine liver

TABLE 28.3   Common Antiparasitics Used in Treatment of Endoparasites in Veterinary Species

Drug	Mechanism of Action	Target Species	Activity	Side Effects and Other Comments
Benzimidazoles: Fenbendazole Albendazole Oxibendazole Febantel Oxfendazole	Bind parasitic beta-tubulin	Cattle Goats Sheep Horses Poultry Pigs Dogs Cats	Nematodes Lungworms Cestodes *Giardia*	Wide margin of safety Teratogenic
Tetrahydropyrimidines: Pyrantel pamoate Pyrantel tartrate Morantel tartrate	Agonist at parasitic nicotinic acetylcholine receptors	Sheep Cattle Swine Horses Dogs Cats	Nematodes	Use not recommended in horses intended for food consumption
Praziquantel	Alter parasite intracellular calcium concentration, causing detachment and digestion by the host	Dogs Cats Cattle Sheep Goats Pigs Horses	Cestodes Trematodes	Wide margin of safety Vomiting at high doses (dogs)
Epsiprantel	Alter parasite intracellular calcium concentration, causing detachment and digestion by the host	Dogs Cats	Cestodes	Wide safety margin
Avermectins: Ivermectin Doramectin Selamectin *Milbemycins:* Milbemycin oxime Moxidectin	Agonist at invertebrate glutamate-gated chloride channels, causing flaccid paralysis	Cattle Sheep Horses Swine Dogs Cats	Nematodes Arthropods	Genetic predisposition for central nervous system toxicity in Collies and related herding breeds Restricted use in lactating dairy cows (except some topical formulations)
Sulfadimethoxine	Prevent parasite production of folic acid, preventing replication	Dogs	*Coccidia* *Toxoplasma*	Many side effects, including crystalluria, hypersensitivity reactions, keratoconjunctivitis sicca, bone marrow suppression, and polyarthritis
Metronidazole	Antiprotozoal activity is poorly understood	Dogs Cats	*Giardia* *Balantidium coli*	Use in food-producing animals prohibited
Melarsomine	Arsenical compound, exact mechanism unknown	Dogs	Adult heartworms	Must be administered intramuscularly Treatment contraindicated in severe cases of heartworm disease Toxic to cats

and kidney function monitoring is recommended during treatment with systemic antifungal therapy because of the potential for significant organ toxicity in association with specific antifungal therapies.

Antiparasitic Drugs

Endoparasitic Drugs

Endoparasites include nematodes (roundworms [including stomach worms], hookworms, whipworms, lungworms, and heartworms); cestodes (tapeworms); trematodes (flukes); and protozoa (*Giardia, Coccidia*). Available antiparasitic drugs target different classes of parasites by using a variety of MOAs, and antiparasitic compounds that are often used in combination to broaden their spectrum of activity. Table 28.3 summarizes the more common antiparasitic drugs used to treat endoparasite infection in veterinary patients, including target species, antiparasitic activity, and side effects.

Widely used macrocyclic lactones (avermectins [ivermectin, doramectin, and selamectin] and milbemycins [milbemycin oxime and moxidectin]) are considered broad-spectrum antiparasitic agents with activity against various nematodes and arthropods. In dogs, macrocyclic lactones are commonly used as heartworm preventive agents or, in some cases, as part of a multidrug treatment protocol for heartworm disease (see Case Presentation 28.1), whereas in ruminants, horses, and pigs, they are used primarily to treat GI nematodes and arthropod infestations.

CASE PRESENTATION 28.1

Multimodal Treatment for Heartworm Disease

Harley, a 4-year-old, 16-kg male Shepherd mix was adopted from a local shelter to be used in a veterinary technology training program. Upon arrival at the school, a heartworm antigen test revealed that Harley was positive for heartworm disease. A thorough physical examination and observation showed no obvious clinical signs of heartworm disease, such as coughing, exercise intolerance, or abnormal lung sounds. After analysis of a blood smear confirmed the presence of microfilaria and thoracic radiographs showed mild enlargement of the pulmonary vasculature, Harley's case of heartworm disease was graded as mild to moderate in severity. The American Heartworm Society's website (see "Recommended Readings") was consulted for the most current heartworm treatment protocol before initiation of treatment.

The next day, glucocorticoid therapy was started to decrease inflammation caused by the presence of the heartworms and to reduce the risk of pulmonary thromboembolism throughout treatment. A tapered dose of prednisone at 10 mg two times daily for 7 days, followed by 10 mg once a day for 7 days, then 10 mg every other day for 14 days was prescribed. Doxycycline was also started at 200 mg two times daily for 28 days to reduce the obligate bacterial species *Wolbachia* that *Dirofilaria immitis* harbor, which is thought to contribute to pulmonary inflammation. On the first day of treatment (and on days 30, 60, and 90), an ivermectin-based heartworm-preventive therapy was administered to eliminate larval stages that may not be susceptible to the adulticide that will be used. Harley's exercise was restricted, eliminating running and vigorous play, to reduce the risk of pulmonary embolism.

On day 60, along with the ivermectin-based heartworm-preventive therapy, the adulticide melarsomine 25 mg/mL at a dose of 2.5 mg/kg (40 mg/ 1.6 mL) was injected into the left epaxial muscle two inches from the spinous process of the fourth lumbar vertebra. A 1.5-inch, 22-gauge needle was used to ensure intramuscular administration. Prednisone therapy was started again at the same tapered dosing schedule that was used previously, and Harley's activity level was restricted to cage rest and leash walks only.

On day 90 of treatment, a second melarsomine injection (40 mg/1.6 mL) was administered into the right epaxial muscle, followed by a third injection 24 hours later (day 91) into the left epaxial muscle. After the third melarsomine injection, prednisone administration was started again at 10 mg two times daily for 7 days, followed by 10 mg once daily for 7 days, then 10 mg every other day for 14 days. Strict exercise restriction continued for an additional 6 weeks, and Harley was closely monitored for signs of thromboembolism (coughing, gagging, pulmonary congestion). Thirty days after the last melarsomine injection (day 121), a blood smear was examined to look for the presence of microfilaria. None were found. Year-round heartworm prevention was established with an ivermectin product, and a heartworm antigen test was to be performed 6 months from the date of completion of treatment and then yearly thereafter.

Harley's case is an example of multimodal treatment of heartworm disease. Treatment not only consisted of an adulticide to kill off the adult heartworms and ivermectin to eliminate larval stages but also an anti-inflammatory (prednisone) to minimize the inflammation associated with heartworm presence and doxycycline to reduce the number of *Wolbachia* was also administered. Exercise restriction, although difficult for many clients to implement, was an integral part of treatment, as pulmonary embolism caused by dying and dead worms is a constant threat during heartworm treatment. Remember that the only exit route for these dead worms is through the phagocytic action of the white blood cells. This multidrug treatment protocol has been proven to better minimize inflammation and organ damage compared with adulticide therapy alone. The drugs used in the treatment eliminated Harley's heartworm infection and allowed him to live a long, healthy life.

Macrocyclic lactones are highly lipophilic drugs with wide tissue distribution and a prolonged effect. In food-producing animals, a significant portion of the drug is eliminated through the mammary glands, restricting the use of macrocyclic lactones (except for some of the topical formulations) in lactating dairy cows. Each of the macrocyclic lactones used in food-producing animals (cattle and sheep) requires a withdrawal period after administration.

The limited use of macrocyclic lactones in dogs is likely caused by increased sensitivity in some breeds (Collies and other herding breeds) to the higher doses of macrocyclic lactones needed to treat GI nematode or arthropod infection. The sensitivity of Collies to macrocyclic lactones is associated with genetic alteration of the gene coding for the important drug efflux pump, P-glycoprotein. Dogs with the P-glycoprotein mutation are at increased risk for central nervous system (CNS) toxicity when macrocyclic lactones (e.g., ivermectin) are used at higher concentrations.

Ectoparasitic Drugs

Ectoparasites include insects (e.g., flies, lice, fleas) and ascarines (e.g., ticks, mites). Strategies for ectoparasite control include preventing host-parasite interaction through the use of contact insecticides, such as organophosphates and pyrethrums (pyrethrin or pyrethroids), or controlling ectoparasitic infestation with insecticide or adulticide therapy. The most common means of drug delivery for ectoparasite control is topical application, although oral control options are available.

Ectoparasiticides have a variety of MOAs and include those that function as repellents, others that target the parasite's nervous system, and still others that target the growth and development of the parasite. Toxicity is a risk associated with ectoparasiticide use, and signs of toxicity must be closely monitored during use. Table 28.4 compares the MOA of the ectoparasiticides commonly used in veterinary patients and clinical signs associated with toxicity.

With the development of safe and effective ectoparasiticides that preferentially target the nervous system of invertebrates or their growth and development, the use of more toxic products (e.g., pyrethrums in cats, organophosphates, and carbamates) have become relatively infrequent in veterinary medicine.

Endocrine Drugs

Thyroid Supplementation and Antithyroid Drugs

Thyroid hormones are produced by the thyroid gland and are essential throughout the body for normal growth, organ function, and metabolism. Thyroid hormones are used by multiple body systems; therefore alterations in normal thyroid hormone concentrations result in a diverse set of clinical signs. The prevalence of thyroid disease in veterinary patients varies, depending on the species. *Hypothyroidism*, a condition associated with low circulating thyroid hormone concentrations, is a relatively common disease in dogs and horses and is treated with levothyroxine (L-thyroxine, $[T_4]$).

High thyroid hormone concentration, or *hyperthyroidism*, is the endocrine disease most diagnosed in cats and is commonly treated with methimazole or with the administration of radioactive iodine.

TECHNICIAN NOTE

Serum thyroid concentrations are measured 4 to 6 hours after dosing (peak drug concentration) to assess response to L-thyroxine therapy. Once hypothyroidism is controlled, routine monitoring of serum thyroid levels every 6 to 12 months is recommended.

TABLE 28.4 Ectoparasiticides Commonly Used in Veterinary Patients

Ectoparasiticide	Mechanism of Action	Target Host	Target Parasite	Clinical Signs of Toxicity
Contact Insecticides				
Pyrethrin Pyrethroids (synthetic pyrethrin) Permethrin Flumethrin Deltamethrin Cyphenothrin	Target voltage-gated sodium channels of the axonal cell membrane	Cattle Swine Dogs	Mosquitoes Ticks Fleas Mites	Hyperexcitability, tremors, salivation, weakness Not safe for use in cats
Dinotefuran (neonicotinoid)	Inhibit nicotinoid acetylcholine receptors	Dogs Cats	Fleas Ticks Flies Lice Mosquitoes	Canine products should not be used in cats
Lime sulfur	Forms pentathionic acid and hydrogen sulfide after application	Dogs Cats Horses	Mites Lice	Skin irritation
Agents That Target Parasite's Nervous System				
Amitraz	Monoamine oxidase inhibitor	Dogs Cattle Swine	Ticks Lice Mites	CNS depression via alpha-adrenergic agonist activity in mammals
Avermectins	Target invertebrate glutamate-gated chloride channels Cross reactivity with mammal GABA and glycine-gated chloride channels	Cattle Swine Dogs Cats	Lice Mites Flies Grubs Ticks	CNS depression Ataxia Some dog breeds (Collies and related herding breeds) are susceptible to CNS toxicity
Imidacloprid (neonicotinoids)	Competitive inhibition of invertebrate nicotinic acetylcholine receptors	Dogs Cats	Fleas (larvae, adults)	Tremors
Nitenpyram (neonicotinoids)	Competitive inhibition of invertebrate nicotinic acetylcholine receptors	Dogs Cats	Fleas	Well tolerated
Fipronil	Noncompetitive blockade of chloride ions through GABA and invertebrate glutamate-gated chloride channels	Dogs Cats	Fleas Ticks	Hyperactivity Convulsions
Isoxazolines: Afoxolaner Fluralaner Lotilaner Sarolaner	Noncompetitive blockade of chloride ions through invertebrate GABA-gated chloride channels	Dogs Cats	Fleas Ticks Mites	Well tolerated
Spinosad Spinetoram	Activation of invertebrate acetylcholine receptors	Dogs Cats	Fleas	Vomiting Diarrhea Anorexia
Agents That Target Parasite's Growth and Development (Insect Growth Regulators)				
Pyriproxyfen Methoprene	Juvenile hormone analogs (maintain insect development in immature egg or larval stages)	Dogs Cats Cattle	Fleas Flies Mosquitoes	Well tolerated
Lufenuron Diflubenzuron	Insect development inhibitors (inhibit chitin synthesis and deposition, interfering with the development of insect's exoskeleton)	Dogs Cats Horses	Fleas Flies	Tissue reactions to injectable lufenuron

CNS, Central nervous system; *GABA*, gamma-aminobutyric acid.

TABLE 28.5 Differences Among Types of Insulin Currently Available

Type	Source	Activity, U/mL	Syringe	Action Profile	Onset, hours	Duration, hours	Target Species	Route
Regular insulin	Human recombinant	100	U-100	Fast	0.5	2–5	Dog Cat	IV IM SQ
NPH	Human recombinant	100	U-100	Intermediate	2–4	12–24	Dog Cat	SQ
Glargine	Synthetic analog	100	U-100	Long	4–6	12–24	Cat	SQ
PZI	Porcine zinc suspension	40	U-40	Long	4–6	8–12	Dogs and cats	SQ
PZIR[a]	Human recombinant	40	U-40	Long	4–6	10–12	Cat	SQ

[a]Approved by the US Food and Drug Administration for use in cats.

IM, Intramuscular; *IV,* intravenous; *NPH,* neutral protamine Hagedorn; *PZI,* protamine zinc insulin; *PZIR,* protamine zinc insulin recombinant; *SQ,* subcutaneous.

Drugs to Treat Adrenal Disease

Diseases of the adrenal gland occur as a result of *hyperadrenocorticism* (an increase in function) or *hypoadrenocorticism* (a decrease in function). Hyperadrenocorticism, also called *Cushing disease,* is caused by the excessive production of cortisol by the adrenal gland and occurs in both dogs and horses.

Medical therapy with mitotane or trilostane is used most for the treatment of hyperadrenocorticism. Both mitotane and trilostane decrease the production of cortisol but through different mechanisms. Mitotane is directly cytotoxic to the *adrenal cortex* (the region of the adrenal gland that produces cortisol), whereas trilostane reversibly inhibits the enzymatic conversion of steroid hormones to cortisol. The goal of either therapy is to decrease the cortisol levels and resolve the clinical signs of hyperadrenocorticism (i.e., increased eating and drinking, panting, and weight gain).

Hypoadrenocorticism, also called *Addison disease,* refers to decreased production of the steroid hormones cortisol (a glucocorticoid) and aldosterone (a mineralocorticoid) by the adrenal gland. Hypoadrenocorticism can be a spontaneous disease (most commonly in dogs) or can occur in association with treatment for hyperadrenocorticism. Hypoadrenocorticism can be treated with fludrocortisone or with prednisone and deoxycorticosterone pivalate (DOCP).

Fludrocortisone is a synthetic steroid hormone that has both mineralocorticoid (aldosterone) and glucocorticoid (cortisol) activity, so it can be used alone. As an alternative, DOCP can be used, but it provides only mineralocorticoid activity; therefore concurrent therapy with a glucocorticoid (prednisone) is required.

> ### TECHNICIAN NOTE
> If a patient with hyperadrenocorticism treated with mitotane or trilostane develops signs of hypoadrenocorticism, the animal must be evaluated immediately, because hypoadrenocorticism can be a life-threatening disease.

Insulin

Diabetes mellitus (DM) is a disease of impaired carbohydrate, protein, and fat metabolism associated with insulin deficiency or resistance. Insulin is a hormone produced in the beta cells of the pancreas and is responsible for the cellular uptake of glucose. Patients with insulin deficiency require injections of supplemental insulin, whereas those with insulin-resistant DM are treated with diet and activity modification.

Insulin is made up of a series of linked amino acids (AAs) specific to each species but with little variation. Because insulin is well conserved across species, available therapeutic insulin products may be animal derived (porcine or bovine); human derived genetically engineered (human recombinant); or synthetic. In clinical practice, the source of insulin can be best matched to the species to be treated based on AA sequence similarities.

Other differences between insulin products include their *biological activity* (or ability to decrease blood glucose) and the action of insulin. The biological activity of insulin is expressed as units of activity per milliliter (units/mL). The activity determined for each type of insulin corresponds to the type of syringe needed to administer the appropriate dose (insulin with a bioactivity of 40 units/mL requires a U-40 insulin syringe, and insulin with a bioactivity of 100 units/mL requires a U-100 insulin syringe). The actions of the currently available insulin products are characterized by their speed of onset and anticipated duration of action. Insulin types are subdivided into fast, intermediate, and long-acting insulin. Table 28.5 summarizes the differences among currently available types of insulin.

Insulin therapy needs to be individualized for each patient because of significant species and individual variations in the *action profile* (the clinical response to insulin will vary among patients and within a patient from day to day). Therefore regulation of the insulin level and treatment requires monitoring for clinical signs (i.e., appetite, water consumption, and activity), body weight, and blood glucose levels by using glucose curves and/or serum fructosamine levels.

> ### TECHNICIAN NOTE
> The biological activity of insulin is expressed as units of activity per milliliter (units/mL). The activity determined for each type of insulin corresponds to the type of syringe needed to administer the appropriate dose. Insulin with a bioactivity of 40 units/mL requires a U-40 insulin syringe, and insulin with a bioactivity of 100 units/mL requires a U-100 insulin syringe.

Gastrointestinal Drugs

Therapeutic strategies used in the treatment of GI disease include nonspecific supportive therapies and targeted therapies based on the primary underlying disease process. Diseases affecting different organ systems often present with GI clinical signs (e.g., kidney disease, liver disease). Symptomatic supportive care is often necessary before a definitive diagnosis can be established, at the onset of targeted therapy, or during periods of clinical relapse.

GI drugs include *antiemetics*, which are used to stop or control vomiting, and *emetics*, which can be administered to induce vomiting in the case of toxin ingestion. *Antidiarrheals* are used to control diarrhea, and *laxatives* are used to increase the fluid content of stool and/or increase peristalsis to encourage defecation. *Prokinetics* can also be used to increase peristalsis in cases of constipation or ileus. *Antiulcer drugs* are used to prevent or treat mucosal ulcers in the stomach or intestines. Drugs can also be used to stimulate the appetite in an anorexic patient or supplement digestive enzymes. Table 28.6 lists the common symptomatic and supportive therapies used in the treatment of GI disease.

Cardiovascular Drugs

Heart disease is associated with structural damage to the heart or rhythm disturbances of the heart; it may result from damaged cardiac muscle, valvular disease, pericardial disease, rhythm abnormalities, or altered coronary circulation. Heart disease can progress to congestive heart failure (CHF), resulting in the accumulation of fluid in the lungs, body cavities, and tissues (edema). Treatment of patients with heart disease is dependent on the nature of the primary problem but often involves the use of multiple drugs, including diuretics (to reduce fluid accumulation), inotropic agents (to improve the contractility of cardiac muscle), antihypertensives (to modulate blood pressure), and antiarrhythmics (to control heart rhythm abnormalities).

Diuretics

Diuretics are used to eliminate *edema* (fluid buildup) in cases of CHF. Diuretics are also used for some disease processes that affect the kidney, liver, and GI tract to reduce associated fluid retention. The therapeutic goal of diuretic therapy is to increase sodium and water excretion. Diuretics achieve this goal by inhibiting the reabsorption of sodium at different parts of the nephron or collecting duct during urine formation. The mechanisms employed to inhibit sodium reabsorption may also alter potassium reabsorption or secretion, so potassium levels may be affected. The sites of action, specific actions, and side effects associated with the diuretics commonly used in veterinary patients are summarized in Table 28.7. Of the diuretics listed, furosemide has the most potent diuretic effect and is most commonly prescribed.

> ### TECHNICIAN NOTE
>
> Diuretics eliminate *edema* (fluid buildup in tissues) by altering the reabsorption of sodium with secondary effects on water and potassium levels in the body. Monitoring hydration and electrolyte levels in patients treated with diuretics is essential.

Inotropic Agents

Drugs used to improve the contractility of cardiac muscle fibers are known as *inotropic agents* or *positive inotropes*. The two main inotropic agents used in veterinary patients are digoxin and pimobendan. Digoxin is a naturally derived drug from the plant *Digitalis purpurea*, or common foxglove, that is used in patients with myocardial disease or CHF to improve the ability of the heart to pump blood. Digoxin increases the calcium concentration in cardiac muscle cells, thereby increasing the strength of muscle

contractions. In addition, digoxin inhibits the ongoing activation of the sympathetic nervous system resulting from CHF.

Digoxin has a *narrow therapeutic index* (low ratio between therapeutic plasma levels and toxic plasma levels). Clinical signs associated with toxicity include GI signs (anorexia, vomiting, or diarrhea) and life-threatening arrhythmias, which can be detected by electrocardiography (ECG) monitoring. To evaluate its effectiveness and minimize side effects, therapeutic drug monitoring is recommended. Treatment for digoxin toxicity requires drug withdrawal.

Pimobendan is both a positive inotrope and a balanced vasodilator (combination of venous and arterial dilation) used in the treatment of dogs and cats with CHF. Positive inotropic effects result from its inhibition of the enzyme phosphodiesterase III, found in cardiac muscle cells and blood vessels. Inhibition of phosphodiesterase III increases intracellular calcium levels, which strengthens cardiac muscle contractions and dilates blood vessels. Pimobendan does not increase the risk of cardiac arrhythmias and does not require therapeutic drug monitoring. Overall pimobendan is well tolerated by dogs and cats, although it does produce much higher blood concentrations in cats, with a half-life almost three times longer than in dogs. Reported side effects include low blood pressure, GI upset, anxiety, and kidney failure.

Antihypertensives

Antihypertensives (drugs that lower blood pressure) are used in the treatment of patients with heart failure and other conditions associated with hypertension, including kidney disease, DM, and hyperthyroidism. Antihypertensive drugs dilate blood vessels and are subdivided based on their MOA and the vessels they dilate (veins, arteries, or pulmonary vessels). Table 28.8 summarizes commonly used antihypertensives.

Antiarrhythmics

Antiarrhythmics are used to treat *arrhythmias* (disturbances in heart rhythm), including alterations in heart rate, rhythm, or the site of impulse origin or conduction. Arrhythmias can originate from the atria (referred to as *supraventricular arrhythmias*) or from the ventricles (referred to as *ventricular arrhythmias*). Antiarrhythmics are subdivided into classes I through IV based on their pharmacologic effects on the action potential of cardiac cells. Table 28.9 summarizes commonly used antiarrhythmics based on class, MOA, and side effects.

> ### TECHNICIAN NOTE
>
> Because of the upregulation of beta receptors found in the bronchial smooth muscle, blood vessels, and fat cells, beta-adrenergic blockers require a gradual dose reduction before discontinuation of therapy to prevent the development of fatal arrhythmias. Consequently, clients should be advised to follow instructions carefully as the drug is being withdrawn.

Anticoagulants

Anticoagulants are used to prevent the formation of life-threatening blood clots, or *thrombi*, in patients with cardiovascular disease and other systemic diseases (e.g., protein-losing nephropathy, protein-losing enteropathy, or immune-mediated hemolytic anemia) associated with thrombus formation.

Hypertrophic cardiomyopathy is a condition in cats that commonly causes thrombus formation. Thrombi typically form in the left atrium of the heart and can dislodge and block the aortic bifurcation, causing a saddle thrombus that leads to pelvic limb ischemia.

TABLE 28.6   Common Symptomatic and Supportive Therapies Used in the Treatment of Gastrointestinal Disease

Drug	Mechanism of Action	Side Effects
Antiemetics		
Metoclopramide	Dopamine antagonist Increases gastric emptying	Contraindicated in patients with GI obstruction
Dolasetron Ondansetron	Serotonin receptor antagonist	Arrhythmias
Maropitant citrate	Neurokinin 1 receptor antagonist	Subcutaneous injection is painful when parenteral product is stored and administered at room temperature
Mirtazapine	α_2 receptor antagonist Serotonin receptor antagonist	Sedation Hypotension Tachycardia
Prochlorperazine Chlorpromazine	Dopamine receptor antagonist Histamine receptor antagonist Cholinergic receptor antagonist Adrenergic receptor antagonist	Sedation Hypotension Lowered seizure threshold
Dimenhydrinate Diphenhydramine Meclizine	Histamine receptor antagonist	Sedation
Dronabinol	Affects cannabinoid receptors in the vomiting receptor	Sedation Dizziness Ataxia
Emetics		
Apomorphine	Dopamine receptor agonist	Sedation
Dexmedetomidine	α_2 receptor agonist	Sedation
Ropinirole	Selective dopamine agonist	Transient, mild lethargy Increased heart rate
Xylazine	α_2 receptor agonist	Sedation
Antidiarrheals		
Loperamide Diphenoxylate	Increases segmental contractions Decreases intestinal secretions	Sedation P-glycoprotein substrate—use contraindicated in dogs with P-glycoprotein mutation Constipation
Bismuth subsalicylate Kaolin/pectin	Coats inflamed mucosa Binds bacteria and toxins	Constipation Use contraindicated in cats Some OTC kaolin–containing products contain salicylates—use contraindicated in cats and dogs concurrently treated with steroids or NSAIDs
Probiotics	Re-establish normal GI bacterial flora	The bacteria used are species specific
Laxatives and Emollients		
Lactulose Magnesium sulfate Magnesium hydroxide	Draw water into the colon	Dehydration
Bisacodyl Castor oil	Irritate intestinal mucosa, causing increased peristalsis	Abdominal cramping Diarrhea
Psyllium	Increases fecal bulk Increases peristalsis	Administer with water to avoid esophageal irritation (especially in cats)
Docusate sodium Docusate calcium Docusate potassium	Reduce water absorption from the colon	Abdominal cramping Diarrhea
Petroleum products	Lubricate intestinal tract	

Continued

TABLE 28.6	Common Symptomatic and Supportive Therapies Used in the Treatment of Gastrointestinal Disease—cont'd	
Drug	**Mechanism of Action**	**Side Effects**
Prokinetics		
Cisapride	Serotonin receptor agonist (only available through compounding pharmacies)	Arrhythmias
Metoclopramide Domperidone	Dopamine receptor antagonist	Restlessness, involuntary movement
Antacids and Antiulcer Drugs		
Famotidine Cimetidine Ranitidine	Histamine antagonist	Many drug-drug interactions
Omeprazole Lansoprazole	Proton pump inhibitor	
Sucralfate	Promotes gastric ulcer healing, inactivates pepsin, absorbs bile acids, and increases gastric mucosal prostaglandin synthesis	
Appetite Stimulants		
Capromorelin	Ghrelin receptor agonist	Salivation
Cyproheptadine	Serotonin receptor antagonist	Sedation Dry mouth
Mirtazapine	α_2 receptor antagonist Serotonin receptor antagonist	Sedation Hypotension Tachycardia
Digestive Enzyme Supplements		
Pancrelipase	Supplements deficient digestive enzymes	Abdominal pain Diarrhea Oral irritation

GI, Gastrointestinal; *NSAID*, nonsteroidal anti-inflammatory drug.

TABLE 28.7	Summary of Site of Action, Specific Action, and Side Effects Associated With Diuretics Commonly Used in Veterinary Patients		
Diuretic	**Site of Action**	**Specific Action**	**Side Effects**
Furosemide	Kidney—loop of Henle	Inhibits sodium/potassium/chloride ($Na^+/K^+/2Cl^-$) reabsorption	Hypokalemia Hypochloremia Metabolic alkalosis
Hydrochlorothiazide	Kidney—distal tubule	Inhibits Na^+/Cl^- reabsorption	Hypokalemia
Spironolactone	Kidney—distal tubule Kidney—collecting duct	Inhibits aldosterone	Hyperkalemia (as a result of potassium-sparing effect)

Commonly used anticoagulants include heparin, clopidogrel, and aspirin. Heparin inhibits the conversion of prothrombin to thrombin, interfering with clot formation. Although it can be used to prevent blood clots from enlarging, it cannot dissolve them once they have formed. It can also be used to treat disseminated intravascular coagulation (DIC). Clopidogrel is used to inhibit platelet aggregation to prevent the formation of thrombi. Side effects, such as anorexia and vomiting, can be alleviated by administering oral medication with food. Aspirin may also be used in cats to prevent thrombus formation but should be used cautiously because of its slow metabolism in this species.

Respiratory Drugs

Respiratory disease can interfere with the body's ability to efficiently keep air flowing to and from the lungs, supply tissues with oxygen, and eliminate carbon dioxide waste. Many of the drugs used for respiratory conditions palliatively treat clinical signs to make the patient more comfortable. It is imperative to also identify the primary condition and provide treatment to restore proper respiratory function. Respiratory drugs include *antitussives*, which control coughing; *mucolytics* and *expectorants*, which decrease the thickness of mucous and help the body eliminate it

TABLE 28.8 **Antihypertensives Commonly Used in Veterinary Patients**

Drug	Mechanism of Action	Main Use	Therapeutic Effects	Side Effects and Other Comments
ACE inhibitors Enalapril Benazepril	Inhibit angiotensin-converting enzyme (ACE)	Treatment of CHF, hypertension, and proteinuria	Systemic vasodilation (↓ aldosterone, ↓ blood volume and edema)	Benazepril is eliminated by both the kidneys and liver, so is preferred in patients with kidney disease (vs. enalapril, which is eliminated by the kidneys only)
Angiotensin receptor blocker Telmisartan	Block angiotensin (AT₁) receptors	Treatment of systemic hypertension in cats	Prevents vasoconstriction caused by activation of the renin-angiotensin-aldosterone system, ↓ blood pressure	GI upset Anemia Anorexia Approved for use in cats only
Calcium channel blockers Amlodipine	↓ Calcium movement into vascular smooth muscle cells	Treatment of hypertension	Peripheral vasodilation ↓ Blood pressure	Hypotension
Hydralazine	Alters calcium metabolism of vascular smooth muscle cells	Treatment of CHF and secondary treatment of hypertension	Arteriolar dilation	Hypotension Reflex tachycardia GI upset
Phosphodiesterase V (PDE5) inhibitor Sildenafil	Inhibits PDE5 found in the smooth muscle of pulmonary vasculature	Treatment of pulmonary hypertension	Pulmonary vasodilation	Possible GI upset

CHF, Congestive heart failure; *GI*, gastrointestinal; *PDE5*, phosphodiesterase type 5.

TABLE 28.9 **Antiarrhythmics Commonly Used in Veterinary Patients**

Class	Mechanism of Action	Examples	Clinical Use	Side Effects
I	Blockade of fast sodium channels (slow action potential conduction)	Lidocaine Quinidine Mexiletine Procainamide	Ventricular tachycardia Supraventricular and ventricular tachycardias Atrial fibrillation (horses)	GI, CNS Urticaria, nasal inflammation, GI disturbances Laminitis
II	Beta-adrenergic blockade (prolongation of action potential)	Propranolol Atenolol	Supraventricular tachycardia Ventricular tachycardia	Cardiovascular depression Propranolol avoided in dogs and cats with respiratory disease
III	Potassium channel blockers (prolongation of the refractory period), beta-adrenergic blockade (prolongation of action potential)	Sotalol Amiodarone	Ventricular tachycardia (Boxer ventricular tachycardia and syncope) Ventricular tachycardia and fibrillation	Cardiovascular depression GI, hepatopathy Cardiovascular depression ↑ Liver enzymes thyroid disfunction
IV	Calcium channel blockade (impair impulse propagation)	Diltiazem Amlodipine (for high BP)	Supraventricular tachycardia (atrial fibrillation)	Cardiovascular depression Systematic hypotension may exacerbate CHF

CNS, Central nervous system; *GI*, gastrointestinal.

through coughing; and *decongestants*, which reduce swelling and congestion of the nasal passages. *Bronchodilators* and antihistamines are used to widen the lumen of the lower airways, countering bronchoconstriction. *Respiratory stimulants* directly stimulate the respiratory center of the brain to increase respiration. Table 28.10 describes respiratory drugs commonly used in veterinary medicine, their MOA, and their side effects.

Anticonvulsants

The most used anticonvulsants for long-term control of epileptic seizures in veterinary patients are phenobarbital, potassium bromide (KBr), and levetiracetam. These drugs work by influencing the release of neurotransmitters and by decreasing seizure-associated neuronal activity. Side effects of all three drugs include

TABLE 28.10   Respiratory Drugs Commonly Used in Veterinary Patients

Drug	Mechanism of Action	Side Effects
Antitussives		
Butorphanol Hydrocodone Dextromethorphan	Centrally acting, suppressing the cough center of the brainstem	Sedation
Expectorants		
Guaifenesin (glycerol guaiacolate [GG])	Increase watery secretions from airways, thinning mucus	Mild hypotension Tachycardia
Mucolytics		
Acetylcysteine	Decreases viscosity of respiratory mucus	Vomiting, nausea, rashes, or hives (rare)
Decongestants		
Pseudoephedrine Phenylephrine	Vasoconstriction in swollen nasal passageways, reducing edema	Tachycardia
Bronchodilators		
Aminophylline Theophylline	Interference with calcium release for muscle contraction, forcing relaxation of smooth muscle in airways	CNS stimulation GI upset
Albuterol Terbutaline	Beta$_2$-receptor agonist	Tachycardia
Diphenhydramine Chlorpheniramine	Histamine receptor antagonist	Sedation Dry mouth
Respiratory Stimulants		
Doxapram	Direct stimulation of the medullary respiratory center	Hypertension Arrhythmias Seizures

CNS, Central nervous system; *GI*, gastrointestinal.

dose-dependent sedation and/or ataxia, with possible polydipsia (increased water intake); polyuria (increased urine volume); polyphagia (increased food intake); and weight gain with phenobarbital use.

Phenobarbital is used commonly as a first-line anticonvulsant, except in patients with evidence of hepatotoxicity or an underlying hepatopathy, in which case KBr may be used as a first-line therapy in dogs. If single-drug therapy is ineffective or does not adequately control seizure activity, the second drug (typically KBr) is added because the two drugs will act synergistically (work together to produce an enhanced result). If seizure activity is still not adequately controlled, levetiracetam can be added as a third drug or may be used in place of phenobarbital or KBr if either is not well tolerated.

KBr is not recommended in cats because 40% of cats treated with KBr develop asthmalike symptoms associated with eosinophilic bronchitis. Phenobarbital is the anticonvulsant of choice in cats, with the addition of levetiracetam if necessary. When levetiracetam and phenobarbital are used concurrently, significant drug interactions cause increased clearance and a decreased half-life of levetiracetam, requiring potential dosage adjustments. Clinical use of both phenobarbital and KBr requires therapeutic drug monitoring to ensure appropriate blood levels. Phenobarbital can also cause reversible hepatotoxicity; serial liver enzyme monitoring should be performed during therapy.

Levetiracetam should be administered every 8 hours (TID) to maintain effective serum concentrations. Higher doses may

be needed if administered with phenobarbital. Extended-release (XR) tablets can be administered every 12 hours (BID). No clinical monitoring is required.

Both status epilepticus and *cluster seizures* (several seizures occurring in succession) require immediate treatment. To stop seizure activity, diazepam (a benzodiazepine tranquilizer) is typically administered intravenously in the hospital setting. If IV access is not available, or if the owner wishes to keep the drug at home to be used in the event of an emergency, diazepam may be administered rectally through a red rubber catheter or compounded suppositories. Alternatively levetiracetam may be administered intravenously or subcutaneously (by the owner in the home setting) for treatment of status epilepticus or cluster seizures. The injectable, but not the oral version, can be given rectally.

> **TECHNICIAN NOTE**
>
> Diazepam is often administered intravenously or rectally (by owners at home) to treat patients with status epilepticus or experiencing cluster seizures.

Immunosuppressants

Immune-mediated diseases involve an abnormal immune response against the body's own normal tissues or cells and are treated with immunosuppressive drugs. These drugs target the immune system (primarily lymphocytes) via different MOA and are used, either alone or in combination, to treat a variety of immune-mediated diseases (hemolytic anemia, thrombocytopenia, skin disease, polyarthritis, systemic lupus erythematosus, and many others). The goal when these agents are used is to control the disease without producing significant side effects. This is achieved by stabilizing the underlying disease process by using immunosuppressive doses (generally higher doses) and then by gradually decreasing (or tapering) the amount of each drug, administered at the lowest dose necessary for long-term control of symptoms.

Glucocorticoids are the most commonly used immunosuppressive agents. They are available in a variety of formulations that differ in chemical structure and are classified as short-acting (hydrocortisone), intermediate-acting (prednisone/prednisolone, methylprednisolone, triamcinolone), or long-acting (dexamethasone, betamethasone) glucocorticoids.

Long-acting glucocorticoids are eliminated from the body very slowly. This causes three problems: First, the slow elimination significantly suppresses the production of natural glucocorticoids by the adrenal gland. Second, it prolongs the duration of side effects because once the drug is given, it stays in the body until it is naturally eliminated. Third, the slow rate of elimination makes it difficult to taper the dose effectively. For these reasons, the use of long-acting agents is best avoided. Glucocorticoids are available in oral, injectable, topical, otic, and ophthalmic forms.

Cyclosporine A, azathioprine, tacrolimus, and chlorambucil are other immunosuppressive agents used for those animals that do not respond to glucocorticoids alone or for those experiencing significant side effects. Azathioprine use is not recommended in cats due to its bone marrow suppression effects.

Anti-inflammatory Drugs

Inflammation is the result of tissue injury. During the inflammatory process, phospholipids in cell membranes are broken down by the enzyme phospholipase to arachidonic acid. Arachidonic acid, an essential omega-9 fatty acid, is then broken down by both cyclooxygenase-2 (COX-2) and lipoxygenase, creating *inflammatory mediators*, such as prostaglandins, thromboxanes, and leukotrienes, which are released into the surrounding tissues and blood. It is the action of these inflammatory mediators that cause the well-known signs of inflammation: redness, heat, swelling, and pain. Both glucocorticoids (steroids) and NSAIDs are used to treat inflammation. The concurrent administration of NSAIDs and glucocorticoids is contraindicated because of the significant risk of gastric ulceration and/or gastric or intestinal perforation.

Glucocorticoids are available in many forms (i.e., tablets, suspensions, solutions, and topical forms) and are classified according to their duration of action, as described above. Glucocorticoids reduce inflammation by blocking enzymatic the action of phospholipase. Glucocorticoids are very potent anti-inflammatories, but long-term use or high doses can cause significant side effects, such as immunosuppression, delayed wound healing, polyuria/polydipsia polyphagia, and DM.

NSAIDs mainly reduce inflammation by blocking COX-2, although a few also block lipoxygenase. The most significant side-effect seen with NSAID use is GI upset and gastric ulcer formation because of concurrent inhibition of COX-1, which participates in gastric mucosal protection. COX-2–specific NSAIDs (e.g., deracoxib, firocoxib, robenacoxib, meloxicam, and carprofen) preferentially inhibit COX-2 and, to some extent, spare COX-1 and therefore may be less likely to cause GI side effects. Other significant adverse effects associated with NSAIDs include acute kidney injury, especially in dehydrated or hypovolemic patients,

TABLE 28.11	Common Anti-inflammatory Drugs Used in Veterinary Medicine[a]
Glucocorticoids	**Nonsteroidal Anti-inflammatory Drugs**
Cortisone	Phenylbutazone
Hydrocortisone	Ketoprofen
Dexamethasone	Carprofen
Prednisone	Etodolac
Prednisolone	Flunixin meglumine
Methylprednisolone	Meclofenamic acid
Methylprednisolone acetate	Diclofenac sodium
Prednisolone sodium succinate	Deracoxib
Triamcinolone	Firocoxib
Betamethasone	Robenacoxib
Flumethasone	Meloxicam
Fluocinolone	Tepoxalin
Side Effects	**Side Effects**
Immunosuppression	GI ulceration
Delayed wound healing	Bone marrow suppression
GI ulceration	Bleeding tendency
Abortion	
Polyuria/polydipsia	
Polyphagia/weight gain	
Thinning of the skin	
Muscle wasting	

[a]Including side effects.

and hepatotoxicity in some patients. Common anti-inflammatory drugs used in veterinary medicine are listed in Table 28.11, along with significant side effects.

TECHNICIAN NOTE

The use of glucocorticoids concurrent with nonsteroidal anti-inflammatory drugs (NSAIDs) is contraindicated because of the increased risk of GI bleeding, ulceration, or perforation.

Dietary Supplements/Nutraceuticals

Dietary supplements fall somewhere between the food and drug categories; in some cases only a fine line divides a dietary supplement from a drug. Nutraceuticals, along with vitamins, minerals, and herbs, fall under the category of *dietary supplements*. Nutraceutical products commonly used in veterinary patients include *S*-adenosylmethionine (SAMe), milk thistle, glucosamine, and chondroitin.

A **nutraceutical**, as defined by the North American Veterinary Nutraceutical Council, is a "nondrug substance that is produced in a purified or extracted form and administered orally to provide agents required for normal body structure and function with the intent of improving the health and well-being of animals." Legally nutraceuticals are not considered prescription or OTC medications, and they are dispensed and administered without medical supervision. Although they are readily available to consumers, no efficacy or safety evaluations from the FDA are required before the marketing and sale of nutraceuticals. In addition, the raw materials, manufacturing process, and product stability of nutraceuticals are not evaluated or standardized; therefore product composition may vary, and bioequivalence between products cannot be ensured.

Drug Administration

Different drug dosage forms are available for administration by a variety of routes. Drugs are often injected into different tissues (**parenteral** drug administration) or administered orally (**nonparenteral** drug administration). Oral dosage forms are most commonly used and include tablets (flavored and unflavored), capsules, and oral suspensions. Depending on the drug's stability at a low gastric pH and the preferred site of intestinal absorption, some oral dosage forms are enteric-coated to prevent drug exposure to the low pH of the stomach and to delay absorption until the drug reaches the higher pH of the small intestine. Oral tablets that are enteric-coated should not be split or crushed for administration. The only tablets that should be split or cut are those that are scored by the manufacturer because this ensures that the drug will be evenly distributed between the split fractions.

Injectable products provided as solutions or suspensions are available for administration via subcutaneous (SQ), intramuscular (IM), or intravenous (IV) injection. A few injectable drugs are well absorbed when administered transmucosally because of the ability of the drug to cross the oral mucous membranes in some species. For example, the opioid analgesic buprenorphine is absorbed very well when administered transmucosally to cats. Other commonly used dosage forms include topical preparations, such as creams, lotions, sprays, ophthalmic ointments or solutions, and otic medications.

Additional routes of administration include other injection methods (intraarterial, intraarticular, intraperitoneal, intracardiac, intradermal, epidural, and intraosseous), transdermal administration, intrauterine and intramammary infusions, and inhalation of a vaporized drug, as in inhalation anesthesia.

Dosage Terminology

When a drug is prescribed for a patient, the amount of the drug is typically calculated based on the weight of the animal in kilograms (kg). The **dosage** of the prescribed drug is the expression of the amount of drug per body weight (e.g., milligrams per kilogram [mg/kg]). The drug **dose** is the amount of drug, in units, that will be given with each administration. It is important to communicate to the client the *dosage interval*, or frequency of drug administration (e.g., once a day, three times a day, or every 12 hours) and the duration of the treatment. It is not appropriate to designate the dosage interval using medical abbreviations, such as BID, TID, or QID. The most accurate way to designate dosage intervals is in hours to ensure the medication is given at the correct interval. The complete *dosage regimen* includes the drug dosage, dosage interval, and duration of treatment, as shown in Box 28.2.

When recording drug doses on treatment forms, medical records, or other legal documents the dose must be recorded in units, such as milligrams. Many drugs are available in multiple concentrations, and if recorded as a volume or number of tablets it will not be clear how much drug was actually administered.

Basic Pharmacokinetics

Pharmacokinetics (PK) is the study of drug movement in the body (i.e., absorption, distribution, metabolism, and excretion). Fig. 28.3 provides a schematic diagram that illustrates the steps of pharmacokinetics. Knowledge of a drug's PK is important because it is used to determine appropriate drug doses, dosing regimens, and withdrawal times in food animals. In addition, PK is used

---

• BOX 28.2 **Example of a Complete Dosage Regimen**

Cephalexin 22 mg/kg t.i.d. × 14 d

(Interpretation: Cephalexin is prescribed at 22 milligrams per kilogram of body weight, to be administered three times per day (every 8 hours) for 14 days)

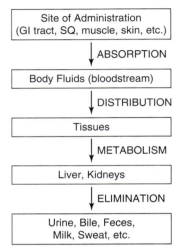

• Fig. 28.3 A schematic diagram used to describe the compartmental movement of drugs in the body.

during drug development to establish effective and safe dosage forms and regimens.

Drug Absorption

Absorption is the movement of a drug from the site of administration (gastrointestinal [GI] tract, muscle, subcutaneous tissues, respiratory tract, or skin) to the circulating blood. Cell membranes are composed of lipids; therefore drug absorption across cell membranes is most effective for drugs that are lipid soluble (or **lipophilic**) and uncharged (or nonionic), such as fluoroquinolones and glucocorticoids. Water-soluble (or **hydrophilic**) drugs are often poorly absorbed and distributed, and therefore require administration by injection (parenteral administration) to achieve effective **therapeutic blood levels** (the blood level at which the drug will have the desired effect).

Bioavailability refers to the fraction of a drug dose that reaches the bloodstream. When administered intravenously, a drug is 100% bioavailable (expressed as a bioavailability of 1). In contrast, only a fraction of a drug administered outside of a vein reaches the bloodstream. Bioavailability is influenced by the dosage form of the drug, the vascularity of the site of administration, the mechanism of absorption, and the metabolism of the drug.

The most common extravascular route of drug administration is the oral route, where the primary site of absorption is the small intestine because of its high surface area and alkaline pH. The intestinal blood vessels that absorb oral drugs lead directly to the liver via the portal vein, causing many drugs to be broken down through liver metabolism before they have a chance to be distributed to tissues. This is termed the **first-pass effect** and explains why some drugs are not effective when administered orally and require parenteral administration. For example, butorphanol (an opioid analgesic that undergoes significant liver metabolism after absorption from the GI tract) is only 20% bioavailable (bioavailability of 0.2) when administered orally, but it is 100% bioavailable when administered intravenously.

> **TECHNICIAN NOTE**
>
> *Bioavailability* refers to the fraction of a drug dose that reaches the bloodstream. When administered intravenously, a drug is 100% bioavailable (expressed as a bioavailability of 1). In contrast, only a fraction of a drug administered outside of a vein reaches the bloodstream for distribution to the cells.

Drug Distribution

Distribution is the movement of an absorbed drug from the blood to various tissues of the body. The drug leaves the vascular space by moving through the fenestrations (pores) of the blood vessel wall.

In addition to the chemical properties of the drug (lipid solubility, pH, and molecular weight), factors that influence the distribution of the drug to tissues include: (1) relative tissue blood flow (because highly perfused tissues achieve higher drug concentrations); (2) degree of protein binding; (3) degree of tissue binding (because a drug with high affinity for tissue binding will tend to concentrate in tissues); and (4) physical anatomic barriers (the blood-brain barrier [BBB], epidural barrier, blood-testis barrier).

After absorption into the bloodstream, a portion of the drug binds to blood proteins, primarily albumin. The "bound" drug is too large to fit through the fenestrations and will not be able to move out into tissues. It is only the "free" or "unbound" portion of the drug that will be distributed. This must be taken into consideration when administering highly protein-bound drugs to patients with hypoproteinemia. If less protein is available for binding, a higher portion of the drug will be distributed to tissues, making adverse side effects or overdose more likely.

The most important physical barrier to drug movement is the BBB. Because of the lack of fenestrations in the capillaries of the brain and the presence of a protective layer of glial cells a barrier is formed, limiting the entry of drugs into the CNS. Another important component of the BBB is the P-glycoprotein pump (a protein that protects the brain from exposure to various drugs and substances by actively pumping them out of the cells). How tissue barriers influence drug distribution can be observed in individuals that have a genetic mutation producing a nonfunctional P-glycoprotein pump (a condition affecting Collies and a few other herding breeds). When given ivermectin (a drug that is normally prevented from entering the CNS by the BBB), dogs carrying the genetic mutation are at increased risk for CNS toxicity because ivermectin is able to enter the brain. Examples of other drugs affected by P-glycoprotein pump functionality include milbemycin, selamectin, moxidectin, vincristine, ketoconazole, loperamide, digoxin, and cyclosporine.

Drug Metabolism

Metabolism (or **biotransformation**) is the chemical modification of a drug to an active, inactive, or toxic metabolite. Metabolism most commonly inactivates or detoxifies drugs or makes them more water soluble for elimination in urine or bile. In contrast, prodrugs (drugs administered in an inactive form) are metabolized to their active form. Examples of prodrugs include

benzodiazepines, enalapril, and codeine. In addition, some drugs, such as acetaminophen and cyclophosphamide, are changed into toxic metabolites.

Drugs are metabolized by enzyme systems. Enzyme systems central to the metabolism of substances are located primarily in the GI tract, liver, and kidney but are also present in other tissues. The liver is considered the major site of drug metabolism in the body. Drug metabolism generally occurs in two steps or phases. Phase I involves the alteration of the drug by *cytochrome P450 (CYP 450) enzymes* found in the liver. Each species and individuals within each species have variable quantities of specific CYP 450 enzymes. These differences cause variations in the metabolism of drugs among patients. During phase II, various enzymes conjugate (i.e., add) a substance to the drug to inactivate it and facilitate its elimination.

> **TECHNICIAN NOTE**
>
> The major site of drug metabolism, or biotransformation, is the liver. The liver contains enzyme systems that chemically alter the drug to facilitate its removal from the body.

Drug Elimination

Elimination is the removal of a drug from the body. Routes available for drug elimination include urine, bile, feces, expired air, milk, sweat, saliva, and tears. Relative to other sites, the kidneys eliminate many drugs and their metabolites from the body. The liver also plays a significant role in drug elimination. Drugs diffuse into liver cells and are incorporated into bile production. Bile is then secreted into the duodenum, with elimination of the drug in feces. Because of the significant role the kidneys and liver play in drug elimination, loss of renal or hepatic function may cause drugs to accumulate in the body. Many drugs must be given at lower doses or avoided altogether in these situations. Pharmacokinetic values that describe drug elimination are clearance and half-life.

Drug clearance (Cl) is the rate at which a drug is removed from an organ or from the body, expressed as the volume of plasma-cleared drug per unit time (mL/minute). It is used to measure the efficiency of drug elimination and to determine the dosage regimen necessary to achieve a stable concentration in blood, called a *steady state*. Steady state is reached when the amount of drug administered equals the amount of drug eliminated.

Half-life ($t_{1/2}$) is the time required for the amount of a drug in the body to decrease by one-half or 50%. With each subsequent half-life after administration, the drug concentration is incrementally lowered by half the level it was at the beginning of that half-life. The half-life of a drug provides an estimate of the duration of its effect and is therefore used to estimate the dosing interval. The time needed to reach steady-state plasma concentration or time for 97% of a drug to be removed from the body is approximately five-times the half-life.

Half-life is also used to establish a withdrawal time for drugs used in food-producing animals. As drugs travel throughout the body, the drugs, or their metabolites, known as *drug residues*, can be present in edible tissues (muscle) or products (milk, eggs). Consumption of animal products containing drug residues can cause allergic reactions or disease in humans and contributes to antibiotic resistance. The withdrawal time is the period after drug administration during which the food products contain an unacceptable amount of drug residue, rendering them unacceptable for harvesting or consumption.

Basic Pharmacodynamics

Pharmacodynamics (PD) is the study of the biochemical and physiologic effects of drugs on the body. Clinically relevant PD parameters include MOA, the relationship between drug concentration and effect, side effects, and adverse reactions.

Mechanism of Action

The mechanism by which a drug causes its desired effect, or MOA, typically requires that the drug has direct physical interaction with cellular components, resulting in an alteration of the cell's normal physiology. Exceptions to this rule are drugs that produce effects based on their physical characteristics alone. Most commonly, the action of a drug involves interaction with a target protein, such as a receptor, within a specific cell type. Receptors are specific proteins on the cell surface that activate a cascade of cellular events when triggered by interaction with a natural substance (endogenous substrate) that is specific to the receptor. Cell receptors are a key component of intracellular communication and cell function. Many pharmacologic compounds (natural and synthetic) are used to activate (act as an **agonist**) or block (act as an **antagonist**) the action of an endogenous substrate at its receptor.

Side Effects and Adverse Drug Reactions

Side effects or adverse reactions are the undesired effects associated with a drug; they are commonly linked to its MOA. Side effects can result from the interaction of a drug with multiple tissue or cell types (other than the target cell or tissue), or from alteration of the patient's physiology and/or drug pharmacokinetics. Clinically important adverse reactions can occur at standard or inappropriate doses, can arise when other drugs are given concurrently resulting in an interaction between two or more drugs, or can occur as the result of altered drug PK (absorption, distribution, metabolism, or elimination). Adverse drug reactions can be subdivided into two types: dose-dependent and idiosyncratic.

Dose-dependent drug reactions are predictable, affect all members of a species, and often affect multiple species. The likelihood of these reactions increases as the drug dose increases. Because these reactions are dose-dependent, **therapeutic drug monitoring** can help prevent them and confirm whether the drug is the cause of a suspected reaction. A dose-dependent drug reaction often responds to dose reduction or to brief drug withdrawal.

Idiosyncratic drug reactions are unpredictable, affect only a small portion of treated animals, and may or may not affect multiple species. These reactions are not dose-dependent, but the risk of a reaction increases with the dose. They do not occur immediately but, rather, after several days of treatment, and are often associated with an immune system response (e.g., fever, antibody production, or T-cell sensitization). Therapeutic drug monitoring does not help identify or avoid these reactions. Treatment requires drug withdrawal and drug avoidance in the sensitized patient. An example would include antibiotic sensitivity to penicillin. These can occur randomly and would require avoidance in the future.

Impact of Disease on Drug Pharmacokinetics

During illness a drug's PK can significantly change, making dosage adjustments necessary. Diseases that most commonly affect drug PK include cardiovascular disease, kidney disease, and liver disease. A decrease in major organ function is seen with age, and this influences drug PK in geriatric patients.

Cardiovascular Disease

Cardiovascular disease alters the distribution of blood flow to tissues through changes in water and sodium balance, and long-term activation of the sympathetic nervous system. More blood is distributed to the brain and the heart, increasing the risk of toxicity to these organs. For example, the risk for arrhythmias and nausea caused by digoxin toxicity is increased in patients with congestive heart failure (CHF).

Alterations in GI, hepatic, and renal blood flow resulting from cardiovascular disease can affect drug absorption, distribution, metabolism, and elimination. For example, the total absorption and absorption rate of the diuretic furosemide is decreased in patients with CHF. In addition, patients with heart disease or CHF are often taking multiple drugs that alter the activity of the sympathetic nervous system, control heart rate and rhythm, and influence electrolyte and fluid balance, increasing the risk of adverse drug events or drug interactions.

Kidney Disease

The kidneys are the major organ involved in drug elimination. Kidney disease or failure can cause decreased drug elimination, increasing plasma drug concentrations and the risk for adverse drug reactions or toxicity. Therefore dose adjustments are recommended for drugs primarily excreted by the kidney (fluoroquinolones, aminoglycosides, enalapril, digoxin, and chloramphenicol in cats). Dose adjustments also may be necessary for drugs associated with increased risk for side effects in these patients (cephalosporins, sulfonamides, tetracycline, furosemide, cimetidine, metoclopramide, and nonsteroidal anti-inflammatory drugs [NSAIDs]). For example, NSAIDs inhibit prostaglandins (PGs), including beneficial PGs that maintain renal blood flow. The resulting decreased blood flow to the kidneys can cause significant problems in a patient with a renal disease that likely already has compromised renal blood flow.

The kidneys also play a significant role in maintaining the body's fluid and electrolyte balance. Increased fluid retention associated with kidney disease can alter the volume of distribution, especially for drugs primarily distributed to the vascular compartment or plasma (penicillins, cephalosporins, and aminoglycosides).

Potential drug interactions in patients with kidney disease are associated with the use of antacids and phosphate binders (drugs often used to help treat the effects of kidney disease), which may reduce the absorption of orally administered antibiotics, including fluoroquinolones, tetracyclines, and sulfonamides.

Liver Disease

The liver is the primary site of drug metabolism. The liver houses the metabolic enzymes that convert lipophilic drugs to more water-soluble metabolites for elimination by the kidneys. Dosage adjustment should be considered in the presence of liver failure for drugs metabolized by the liver, including metronidazole, chloramphenicol, and benzodiazepines.

TECHNICIAN NOTE

Dose adjustments may need to be made for patients with liver or kidney disease, because these are the major organs for drug metabolism and elimination.

Aging and Drug Pharmacokinetics

Normal aging leads to a change in body composition (decreased lean body mass and total body water; increased fatty tissue) and redistribution of blood flow to the brain and heart, in part as a result of decreased cardiac output. This altered distribution of tissues and blood in geriatric patients influences the distribution of drugs. Additional changes in physiology associated with aging include decreased drug absorption from the GI tract, decreased hepatic metabolism, and decreased renal excretion.

Reduced kidney function associated with aging has the most clinically significant impact on drug elimination. Reduced drug elimination through the kidneys results in increased drug plasma concentration when standard doses are given. Therefore drugs excreted primarily by the kidneys often require dosage adjustment to minimize the risk of toxicity in geriatric patients.

Regulatory Pharmacology

Drug Laws and Regulations

State and federal laws regulating drug use in the United States are designed to work in conjunction with each other. Federal laws are the fundamental regulations for drug approval and use, enacted to ensure that available drugs are safe, effective, and prepared in accordance with manufacturing standards. State laws are in place to control the distribution of drugs within the state. For example, state laws oversee individuals authorized to prescribe and dispense drugs, the required record keeping, and the licensing of drug distributors. There are variations in state laws, so each licensed practitioner is required to know the laws in the state where they practice. Veterinarians found to violate federal or state laws regulating the transport, sale, or use of drugs may be subjected to any of the following: warning letters, fines, temporary or permanent loss of state veterinary license, or imprisonment.

Federal regulation of drugs began in the mid-1800s, but it was not until the enactment of the Federal Food, Drug, and Cosmetic (FFD&C) Act in 1938 that manufacturers were required to provide evidence of safety under conditions prescribed on the label. The FFD&C Act also required product labeling to include directions for use, warnings, active ingredients, and shelf life. The

FFD&C Act remains the law regulating the approval, use, safety, and efficacy of drugs, although it has been amended many times to make it more effective. Federal regulating bodies that oversee veterinary products include the FDA, the US Department of Agriculture (USDA), and the Environmental Protection Agency (EPA). The FDA's Center for Veterinary Medicine (CVM) is the governing body that regulates the manufacture and distribution of drugs, food additives, and medical devices used in veterinary species. The CVM oversees regulations regarding approval, safety, efficacy, and postapproval monitoring. The USDA's Animal and Plant Health Inspection Service (APHIS) Center for Veterinary Biologics oversees veterinary biologicals (vaccines, antitoxins, and diagnostics used to prevent, treat, or diagnose animal diseases). The EPA's Pesticide Regulation Division oversees pesticides, including those used on inanimate objects, rodenticides, and insecticides.

The official legal drug compendium for the United States is the US Pharmacopoeia (USP)–National Formulary (NF). The USP is a compilation of all drug substances and products and is focused on providing active ingredients. There are several additional sources available for drug information, including active ingredients, indications, and dosage recommendations. The Compendium of Veterinary Products (CVP) (see "Recommended Readings") is a compilation of information about veterinary drugs and biologicals that is available in print, online, and as a digital application. In addition, drug package inserts are often included with bottles or vials of drugs that are purchased.

TECHNICIAN NOTE

The US Food and Drug Administration (FDA), the US Department of Agriculture (USDA), and the Environmental Protection Agency (EPA) are the federal regulating bodies that oversee veterinary drug products.

Extra-label Drug Use

In 1994, the FFD&C Act was amended to include extra-label drug use by veterinarians, as provided under the Animal Medicinal Drug Use Clarification Act (AMDUCA). Under the AMDUCA, veterinarians can legally use or prescribe certain approved animal and human drugs for the treatment of veterinary species in an extra-label fashion, provided specific conditions are met. Before the AMDUCA was signed, this practice was illegal.

Extra-label drug use is defined as follows: "…actual use or intended use of a drug in an animal in a manner that is not in accordance with the approved labeling. This includes but is not limited to, use in a species not listed in the labeling, use for indications (disease and other conditions) not listed on the labeling, use at dosage levels, frequencies, or routes of administration other than those stated in the labeling, and deviation from labeled withdrawal time based on these different uses." Extra-label drug use enables veterinarians to use their professional judgment in the treatment of veterinary species under certain conditions but requires them to make every effort to initially use an approved drug at an approved dosage. Specific conditions that must be met when an approved drug is used include a valid VCPR, appropriate animal identification, and documentation, such as drug labeling and record keeping. Box 28.3 provides information on the specific criteria that must be met for extra-label drug use in veterinary species and for extra-label use in food-producing animals. Extra-label drug use is prohibited for enhancement of animal production or reproduction, growth promotion, routine disease prevention, alteration of cost of therapy, or as a feed additive. In addition, as

• BOX 28.3   Criteria Used to Determine Extra-label Drug Use in Veterinary Species and as required for Food-producing Animals Under AMDUCA.

1. There is no approved new animal drug that is labeled for such use and that contains the same active ingredient in the required dosage form and concentration, except where a veterinarian finds, within the context of a valid veterinarian-client-patient relationship, that the approved new animal drug is clinically ineffective for its intended use.
2. Before prescribing or dispensing an approved new animal or human drug for extra-label use in food animals, the veterinarian must:
   a. Make a careful diagnosis and evaluation of the conditions for which the drug is to be used.
   b. Establish a substantially extended withdrawal period before marketing of milk, meat, eggs, or other edible products supported by appropriate scientific information, if applicable.
   c. Institute procedures to ensure that the identity of the treated animal or animals is carefully maintained.
   d. Take appropriate measures to ensure that assigned time frames for withdrawal are met and no illegal drug residues occur in any food-producing animal subjected to extra-label treatment.
3. Such use must be accomplished in accordance with an appropriate medical rationale; and
4. If scientific information on the human food safety aspect of the use of the drug in food-producing animals is not available, the veterinarian must take appropriate measures to ensure that the animal and its food products will not enter the human food supply.
5. Extra-label use of an approved human drug in a food-producing animal is not permitted if an animal drug approved for use in food-producing animals can be used in an extra-label manner for the particular use.

stated under AMDUCA, the FDA-CVM may prohibit the extra-label drug use of approved new animal or human drugs under other circumstances. For example, specific drugs or drug classes are prohibited for use in food-producing animals (Table 28.12) because of their potential to adversely affect human health. The extra-label use of a prohibited drug in food-producing animals is considered one of the most serious regulatory violations by the FDA.

TECHNICIAN NOTE

Specific drugs or drug classes are prohibited for use in food-producing animals because of their potential to adversely affect human health. The extra-label use of a prohibited drug in food-producing animals is considered one of the most serious regulatory violations by the US Food and Drug Administration (FDA).

Drug Residues and Withdrawal Times in Food-Producing Animals

The presence of drug residues in edible products derived from food-producing animals (meat, poultry, eggs, and milk) is regulated by the FDA and the EPA to protect the public food supply and environment. Enforcement of these regulations minimizes the effects that food residues have on public health and on the economy. Drugs of concern that are commonly used in veterinary food-producing animals include antimicrobials, pesticides, and herbicides.

The term *drug residue* is defined as the presence of a drug or its metabolite in cells, tissues, organs, or any edible products of an

TABLE 28.12   Drugs Prohibited for Use in Food-producing Animals Under AMDUCA

All Food-Producing Animals	Comments
• Chloramphenicol	• Banned in 1984 because of observed reversible, dose-related bone marrow suppression in many species. Humans may develop an idiosyncratic bone marrow toxicosis that can be fatal.
• Nitroimidazoles	• Include metronidazole, dimetridazole, ipronidazole. Risk for mutagenicity and carcinogenicity.
• Clenbuterol	• Toxicity and death associated with human consumption of edible tissues (liver).
• Nitrofurans	• Include furazolidone and nitrofurazone. Banned in 1991 because of concerns about carcinogenicity and mutagenicity.
• Fluoroquinolones	• Banned in 1997 because of concerns for microbial drug resistance in humans (e.g., *Salmonella* spp.).
• Glycopeptides	• Vancomycin: banned in 1997 because of concerns about microbial drug resistance in humans. Reserved for treatment of methicillin-resistant *Staphylococcus aureus* infection in humans.
• Cephalosporins (not including cephapirin)	• Prohibited in 2012 in cattle, swine, chickens, and turkeys (major species of food-producing animals) because of concern for microbial drug resistance in humans. Prohibited uses include (1) for disease prevention purposes; (2) at unapproved doses, durations, or routes of administration; and (3) if the drug is not approved for that species and production class.
Dairy Cattle	**Comments**
• Sulfonamides	• Prohibited in lactating dairy cows. Concerns of carcinogenicity. *Exception*: Sulfonamides with an approved labeled indication for use in lactating dairy cows (sulfadimethoxine, sulfabromomethazine, sulfamethoxypyridazine).
• Phenylbutazone	• Use prohibited in female dairy cattle 20 months of age or older.
Chickens, Turkeys, and Ducks	**Comments**
• Adamantanes • Neuraminidase inhibitors	• Drugs used for treating or preventing influenza A.

AMDUCA, Animal Medicinal Drug Use Clarification Act.

animal (eggs, milk, etc.). The FDA and the EPA have established tolerances for drugs, pesticides, and other chemicals in tissues of food-producing animals that are used to determine safe drug withdrawal times. The use of drugs in food-producing animals requires the establishment of drug withdrawal times (based on pharmacokinetic data) as a condition for approval. **Withdrawal time** is the period after the last administered drug dose to a food-producing animal during which that animal cannot be slaughtered, and animal products, such as eggs or milk, cannot be used. When a drug is used in an extra-label fashion in food-producing animals, the veterinarian is responsible for making every effort to determine an extended withdrawal time. Useful resources, such as the Food Animal Residue Avoidance Database (FARAD), are available for consultation in determining withdrawal times (see "Recommended Readings").

In addition, as has been mentioned, some approved drugs (for animals and humans) used in veterinary species are prohibited for use (including extra-label use) in food-producing animals because of the significant threat that they pose to human health. Drugs with no approved labeled veterinary indication are considered illegal for use in food-producing animals.

Drug Compounding

Drug compounding is defined as any manipulation of a drug other than that described on the approved drug label. This practice is sometimes necessary to ensure that a particular patient receives an appropriate amount of a drug. Circumstances under which a drug may be compounded include those in which a drug cannot be accurately dosed (e.g., because available tablets cannot be cut into small enough pieces to ensure that the correct amount is given) or will not be accepted (e.g., because the available form has an offensive taste). Drug compounding, however, raises concerns about the development of adverse reactions or treatment failures associated with the loss of the drug's stability, purity, and potency after the alteration of the original dosage form.

The FDA-CVM has recognized the need for drug compounding in veterinary medicine to meet the medical needs of the diverse veterinary patient populations and considers compounding of a drug under the classification "extra-label drug use more effectively." Consequently, under AMDUCA rules, a veterinarian can legally compound an approved animal or human drug for use in a veterinary species.

In addition, the FDA-CVM has developed Compliance Policy Guidelines (CPGs) on compounding drugs for animals (see "Recommended Readings"). CPGs indicate that drug compounding cannot be done from *bulk chemicals* (raw chemical ingredients used to produce the manufactured dosage form). It is also stated under AMDUCA that extra-label drug use is not allowed for bulk drugs. Compounding cannot be used to produce a new animal drug. Compounding bulk drugs and mass marketing of compounded drugs to avoid the FDA drug approval process are illegal practices.

> ### TECHNICIAN NOTE
>
> Although compounded products are not regulated by the US Food and Drug Administration (FDA), compounding must be performed in compliance with regulations stated for extra-label drug use. For example, compounded drugs used in food animals cannot violate regulations on tissue or milk residues. Thus if a product is compounded, the compounder is required to establish and document an expiration date and an appropriate withdrawal time in food-producing animals.

Veterinarians may prescribe compounded drugs through compounding pharmacies, which are commercial businesses that prepare and sell compounded drugs for veterinary patients.

Accreditation of a compounding pharmacy by a compounding accreditation board is obtained at the discretion of the pharmacy. Compounding pharmacies that have undergone accreditation show their willingness to follow compounding recommendations, ensuring as much as possible that their compounding methods are ethical, follow established regulations, and are based on available science.

It is typically not legal to dispense medications previously compounded by a pharmacy as a "prescription" to leave the veterinary practice and be taken home by clients. This means that a clinic cannot legally order a bulk compounded medication and sell it in individual doses for clients to take away. It can only legally be used by the purchaser in the hospital.

The Veterinary Pharmacy

Drug Procurement

Veterinary and human drugs that are FDA approved can be obtained directly from the drug manufacturer or through drug distributors, which provide access to a variety of products through a single source. The CVP provides a comprehensive list of veterinary pharmaceutical companies and their product lines (see "Recommended Readings").

Most veterinary facilities maintain a pharmacy with an inventory of commonly used drugs that are dispensed to clients directly. Veterinarians may also prescribe a human drug that can be obtained at a retail pharmacy. Other sources of veterinary pharmaceutical products available to owners are local feed stores, mail-order suppliers, and internet pharmacies. Online sites can also serve as a source of health care information. Despite the perceived convenience of information and products available on the internet, the information provided may not always be accurate, and products can be of questionable quality. Thus clients must maintain healthy objectivity and a cautious perspective when exploring internet sources.

> ### PUT INTO PRACTICE
>
> Do you remember the First In/First Out Rule? Drugs should be dispensed in the order in which they arrived at pharmacy. Always place new stock behind current stock to avoid wastage.

Regulation of online pharmacies is primarily in the hands of each state's board of pharmacy, although some federal oversight is required. The National Association of Boards of Pharmacy does not have a role in regulating online pharmacies. Hallmarks of a reputable internet pharmacy are that it: (1) requires a valid hard copy or verbal prescription provided directly from the prescriber with a valid VCPR; (2) provides a toll-free telephone number and street address on its website; (3) allows direct contact with its pharmacists for consultation; and (4) is certified as a Verified Internet Pharmacy Practice Site (VIPPS).

VIPPS is a voluntary accreditation program of the National Association of Boards of Pharmacy that provides a VIPPS seal of verification to internet pharmacies that are appropriately licensed and legitimately operated. To attain the VIPPS seal, the online pharmacy is required to undergo and successfully complete a thorough review to ensure compliance with the same state and federal laws and regulations that a traditional retail pharmacy must observe. A VIPPS also provides a mechanism for reporting any errors or inconsistencies made by a VIPPS-certified pharmacy.

Drug Storage and Disposal

The storage recommendation for a drug is established by the drug manufacturer, based on the results of stability studies conducted on the manufactured finished product. To ensure the safety and potency of a drug for the lifetime of the product, storage recommendations must be followed to prevent premature degradation. Storage recommendations for a particular drug product are available in the package insert accompanying the product.

Product expiration dates are provided by the manufacturer to ensure the purity and potency of the final dosage form based on controlled stability studies. The expiration date ensures product purity and potency only if the product is stored in accordance with the manufacturer's recommendations. The FDA requires standard expiration dates (month, day, and year) on all approved drug products. Exceptions to this rule are drugs regulated by the EPA (pesticides, rodenticides, and insecticides), for which no expiration date is included on the manufactured product, but the required shelf life is a minimum of 5 years.

Drug disposal is governed by the Department of Environmental Quality, the EPA, the FDA, and local boards of pharmacy. The disposal of controlled substances is regulated by the DEA. Expired drugs and unused drugs should not be poured down the drain, flushed down the toilet, thrown in the trash, or discarded on the ground. The expired drug should be returned to the manufacturer or the distribution company for credit or should be sent to a reverse distribution company (RDC). An RDC functions as the intermediary between the drug purchaser and the drug vendor. The RDC provides credit to the drug purchaser for a returned drug; when credit is not acceptable, the RDC discards or destroys a returned drug on a cost per pound basis. Approved disposal of a controlled substance is provided only through an RDC. There is a chain of command paperwork trail required to show all handlers from the veterinary clinic to the RDC. This paperwork is kept on file for as long as the clinic exists.

> **TECHNICIAN NOTE**
>
> Expired drugs and unused drugs should not be poured down the drain, flushed down the toilet, thrown in the trash, or discarded in the ground. These practices allow the drug to enter the water stream, increasing the potential exposure of humans and wildlife to the drug. The expired drug should be returned to the manufacturer or the distribution company for credit or should be sent to an RDC.

Prescribing and Dispensing Drugs

Prescription Writing

Correct prescription writing and reading are essential for the accurate dosing and dispensing of drugs. A veterinary prescription is valid only if written or authorized by a licensed veterinarian. Essential elements required by law on a written prescription include: (1) the printed or stamped name, address, and telephone number of the licensed veterinarian; (2) the DEA registration number of the licensed veterinarian (required on all prescriptions for controlled substances); (3) the legal signature of the licensed veterinarian; (4) the drug name, concentration, and quantity (#, the number of pills or milliliters of liquid to be included in the script); (5) directions for use; (6) the full name and address of the client; (7) identification of the animal (name and species); (8) any cautionary statements (e.g., withdrawal times for food animals); and (9)

the number of refills (if applicable). Prescriptions for dispensing controlled substances require two additional components. Not only is the legal signature of the licensed veterinarian required, but the licensed veterinarian's name must also be printed. Also, the number of refills allowed is dictated by the controlled substance being dispensed. No refills are allowed for Schedule II drugs, and refills are limited to five times or 6 months (whichever comes first) for Schedule III and Schedule IV drugs.

Legal prescription writing allows the use of standardized abbreviations. Table 28.13 provides a list of recognized and accepted abbreviations commonly used in prescription writing. An example of a properly written prescription that uses common abbreviations to provide directions for use is shown in Fig. 28.4.

When medications are dispensed that are intended to be taken home with the patient to be administered by the owner, a label must be affixed to the bottle or vial with the following information: (1) the name, address, and phone number of the dispensing veterinary clinic or pharmacy; (2) the name of the client; (3) identification of the animal (name and species); (4) the date dispensed; (5) directions for use; (6) the name, concentration, and quantity of the drug dispensed; (7) the name of the prescribing veterinarian; and (8) if the dispensed drug is a controlled substance, the label must contain the following statement: "Caution: Federal law prohibits the transfer of this drug to any person other than the patient for whom it was prescribed." In addition, any medication that is dispensed for home use must be provided in a child-resistant container, as required by the Poison Prevention Packaging Act, enacted in 1970. Other label requirements include precautions, requirements for refrigeration, and, for suspensions and other liquids, directions to shake well before use. These requirements are often in the form of small adhesive stickers to place on the bottle without obscuring the label.

> **TECHNICIAN NOTE**
>
> The abbreviation "s.i.d." is not a universally accepted abbreviation for "once a day" outside of veterinary medicine; therefore it should not be used in prescription writing. Alternatively the terms "every 24 hours" or "q24hr" should be used.

Drug Calculations

An important aspect of dispensing and administering drugs is calculating the accurate dose, infusion volume, and conversion between units of measure. Correctly calculating the dose is just as essential to a good patient outcome as determining an accurate diagnosis and treatment plan. Some of the most common calculations made by a veterinary technician are outlined in following sections. These include: (1) converting between units of measure, (2) converting the recommended dosage for a patient into the correct drug dose, (3) performing calculations by using percent solutions, and (4) performing calculations needed to successfully deliver a drug by constant rate infusion (CRI).

Converting Between Units of Measure

Conversions are most commonly performed between units of measurement within the metric system, because most drug dosages are expressed as the number of milligrams of drug per unit body weight in kilograms (mg/kg). By using known conversion factors and keeping track of the units carefully, one can readily calculate conversions between units of measure. Box 28.4 contains some common units of conversion. Conversions between metric and

TABLE 28.13   **Latin Abbreviations Commonly Used and Accepted in Prescription Writing**

Latin Abbreviation	Interpretation	Latin Abbreviation	Interpretation
AD	Right ear	mg	Milligrams
AS	Left ear	ml or mL	Milliliter
AU	Both ears	NPO	Nothing by mouth
bid	Two times a day	OD	Right eye
cap	Capsule	OS	Left eye
Cc	Cubic centimeter	OU	Both eyes
g or gm	Gram	PO	Per os (by mouth)
Gr	Grain	prn	As needed
ggt(s)	Drop(s)	q (q × hour)	Every (every × hour)
IC	Intracardiac	qid	Four times a day
IM	Intramuscular	qod	Every other day
IO	Intraosseous	Sig	Directions to client
IP	Intraperitoneal	stat	Immediately
IU	International Units	Sub Q, SQ, SC	Subcutaneous
IV	Intravenous	susp	Suspension
Kg	Kilograms	tid	Three times a day
Lb	Pound	tab	Tablet
m^2	Meter squared	Tbsp, T	Tablespoon (15 mL)
mEq	Milliequivalents	tsp, t	Teaspoon (5 mL)

Rx: Enrofloxacin, 136 mg, # 14; **Sig:** give 1 tab PO q 24 hours

Interpretation: Dispense 14, 136 mg tablets of enrofloxacin with the following directions for use: Give 1 tablet orally every 24 hours.

• **Fig. 28.4** Example of a properly written prescription using common abbreviations to describe directions for use and the correct interpretation of the prescription for accurate filling.

• **BOX 28.4**   **Common Units of Conversion**

Metric System Conversions

1 kilogram (kg) = 1000 grams (g)
1 g = 1000 milligrams (mg)
1 mg = 1000 micrograms (µg or mcg)
1 liter (L) = 1000 milliliters (mL)
100 mL = 1 deciliter (dL)
1 mL = 1000 microliters (µL)
1 cc = 1 mL

Metric-to-English System Conversions

1 kg = 2.2 lb
1 grain (gr) = 64.8 mg

English systems of measure are sometimes necessary, especially in association with body weight (pounds to kilograms and kilograms to pounds), or for dispensing medications that use grains as a unit of measure (e.g., phenobarbital). Sample calculations for converting between units of measure are provided in Box 28.5.

Calculating the Correct Drug Dose

Most often, the veterinarian will prescribe the dose of a drug in milligrams or will indicate the dosage to be administered in milligrams per kilogram of body weight. In either case, depending on the formulation of the drug, the veterinary technician administering the drug will need to calculate the amount of drug to be administered to the patient in milligrams or milliliters (mL). Calculating the dose of an oral drug in milligrams or the dose of an injectable solution in milliliters requires careful unit conversions, knowledge of the patient's weight, and knowledge of the concentration of the drug in either solid or liquid dosage form (Box 28.6).

TECHNICIAN NOTE

The single most important rule in successfully performing drug calculations is to keep track of the units; this often requires writing out the equations and canceling the units.

Using Percent Solutions

The use of injectable drugs with concentration expressed as a percent of the drug in a solution can create much confusion for many technicians and veterinarians alike. The fundamental concept to keep in mind when working with percent solutions is that percent means "per one hundred," and this way of expressing concentration is equivalent to a ratio of parts of the drug per 100 parts of the solution.

• BOX 28.5　Sample Calculations for Conversion of Units of Measure

I.　A dog's body weight was recorded in the medical record in pounds (lb). Convert this dog's weight (95 lb) to kilograms (kg).

$$95\ \text{lb} \times \frac{1\,\text{kg}}{2.2\ \text{lb}} = 43.2\,\text{kg}$$

II.　A cat is prescribed buprenorphine at a dosage of 30 μg/kg for transmucosal administration. The concentration of buprenorphine in the vial is 0.3 mg/mL. Convert the dosage of buprenorphine from μg/kg to mg/kg.

$$\frac{30\,\text{"μg}}{\text{kg}} \times \frac{1\,\text{mg}}{1000\ \text{μg}} = \frac{0.03\,\text{mg}}{\text{kg}}$$

• BOX 28.6　Sample Calculations for Correct Drug Doses

I.　Dr. Smith just diagnosed pneumonia in a 30-kg dog and would like to prescribe doxycycline at a dosage of 5 mg/kg orally every 12 hours. Calculate the dose of doxycycline (in mg) that needs to be administered twice a day.

$$30\ \text{kg} \times \frac{5\,\text{mg}}{\text{kg}} = 150\,\text{mg}$$

II.　You need to administer 30 μg/kg of buprenorphine via the transmucosal route to a cat that weighs 5 kg. Buprenorphine is available as a 0.3-mg/mL solution. Calculate the volume (in mL) of buprenorphine that needs to be administered to this cat.

$$5\ \text{kg} \times \frac{30\,\text{μg}}{\text{kg}} = 150\,\text{μg}$$

$$150\ \text{μg} \times \frac{1\,\text{mg}}{1000\ \text{μg}} \times \frac{1\,\text{mL}}{0.3\ \text{mg}} = 0.5\,\text{mL}$$

Percent solutions can be expressed as volume/volume (vol/vol), meaning the number of milliliters of a drug in 100 mL of solution. For example, a 10% solution (vol/vol) contains 10 mL of the drug in 100 mL of solution. Percent solutions can also be expressed as weight/volume (wt/vol), meaning the number of grams of the drug in 100 mL of solution. For example, a 10% (wt/vol) solution contains 10 g of the drug in a total of 100 mL of solution. Percent solutions can be expressed as weight/weight as well, meaning the number of grams of the drug in 100 g of a mixture. For example, a 10% weight/weight solution contains 10 g of the drug in a total of 100 g of a mixture (Box 28.7).

Constant Rate Infusion

Some drugs are delivered intravenously using CRI, usually expressed in micrograms or milligrams per unit of time. Drugs are delivered via CRI for a variety of reasons. Some drugs, such as fentanyl and dobutamine, are given by CRI, because their half-lives are so short that intermittent bolus dosing is not effective. Other drugs, such as metoclopramide, are more efficacious when given by CRI, because plasma levels can remain fairly constant, rather than fluctuating. CRI is also used when dehydration is severe enough to impair absorption of a drug given subcutaneously or intramuscularly (as may happen when regular insulin is used to treat a patient that has diabetic ketoacidosis and is dehydrated).

• BOX 28.7　Sample Calculations Using Percent Solutions

I.　Convert a 5% solution into mg/mL.

$$5\% = \frac{5\ \text{g}}{100\,\text{mL}} \times \frac{1000\,\text{mg}}{1\ \text{g}} = \frac{50\,\text{mg}}{\text{mL}}$$

II.　You are asked to administer ivermectin to a 1000-lb horse at a dosage of 0.2 mg/kg. Ivermectin is available as a 1% solution.

a.　Convert a 1% solution into mg/mL.

$$1\% = \frac{1\ \text{g}}{100\,\text{mL}} \times \frac{1000\,\text{mg}}{1\ \text{g}} = \frac{10\,\text{mg}}{\text{mL}}$$

b.　Convert the horse's weight into kilograms.

$$1000\ \text{lb} \times \frac{1\,\text{kg}}{2.2\ \text{lb}} = 454.5\,\text{kg}$$

i.　Calculate the dose of ivermectin to be administered to the patient.

$$454.5\ \text{kg} \times \frac{0.2\,\text{mg}}{\text{kg}} = 90.9\,\text{mg}$$

ii.　Calculate the volume of ivermectin to be administered.

$$90.9\ \text{mg} \times \frac{1\,\text{mL}}{10\ \text{mg}} = 9.09\,\text{mL}$$

• BOX 28.8　Sample Calculation of Constant Rate Infusions

• A 30-kg dog was just diagnosed with ventricular tachycardia and requires an immediate IV infusion of lidocaine, which will be administered at a CRI of 50 mcg/kg/minute. Calculate the amount of lidocaine (in milligrams) that needs to be added to a 1000-mL bag of Normosol-R, which is currently running at an infusion rate of 65 mL/hour.

$$\frac{\dfrac{50\,\text{μg}}{\text{kg}\ /\ \text{min}} \times 30\ \text{kg} \times 1000\ \text{mL}}{\dfrac{65\ \text{mL}}{\text{h}} \times \dfrac{1\,\text{h}}{60\ \text{min}}} = 1{,}384{,}615\,\text{μg}$$

$$1384{,}615\ \text{μg} \times \frac{1\,\text{mg}}{1000\ \text{μg}} = 1385\,\text{mg}$$

When CRI is given, an appropriate drug volume must be added to an appropriate volume of base solution (often a bag of IV fluids). The following equation can be used to calculate the amount of drug (in micrograms or milligrams) that should be added to the base solution when CRI is prepared (Box 28.8).

$$M = (D \times W \times V) \div (R)$$

M = Amount of drug (microgram [μg] or mg) to be added to the base solution

D = Dosage (μg/kg per minute or mg/kg per minute)

W = body weight (kg)

V = Volume of base solution (mL)

R = Infusion rate (mL/minute)

> **TECHNICIAN NOTE**
>
> When CRI is calculated, the formula $M = (D \times W \times V) \div (R)$ can be used to calculate the amount of drug (in micrograms or milligrams) to be added to the base solution (often a bag of fluids), where M = amount of drug (μg or mg) to be added to the base solution; D = dosage (μg/kg per minute or mg/kg per minute); W = body weight in kg; V = volume of base solution (mL); and R = infusion rate (mL/minute).

Acknowledgments

The authors and publisher wish to acknowledge the contributions of Marvene Augustus, Sonya Bremer Boss, Katrina Viviano, and Angela Beal to previous editions of this textbook.

Recommended Readings

American Heartworm Society. *Heartworm Guidelines*. Available at: http://www.heartwormsociety.org.

American Veterinary Medical Association. *Best Management Practices for Pharmaceutical Disposal*. Available at: https://www.avma.org/KB/Policies/Pages/Best-Management-Practices-for-Pharmaceutical-Disposal.aspx.

Bill RL. *Clinical Pharmacology and Therapeutics for Veterinary Technicians*. 4th ed. Elsevier: St. Louis, MO.

Compendium of Veterinary Products, DVMetrics-CVP. Available at: https://www.dvmetrics.com/products/cvp-compendium-of-veterinary-products.

Martin-Johnson L. *Applied Pharmacology for Veterinary Technicians*. 6th ed. Saunders: St. Louis, MO.

Occupational and Safety Health Administration. *OSHA Technical Manual: Controlling Occupational Exposure to Hazardous Drugs*, Washington, DC, U.S. Department of Labor, OSHA. Available at: https://www.osha.gov/hazardous-drugs.

Papich M. *Saunders Handbook of Veterinary Drugs: Small and Large Animal*. 4th ed. Saunders: St. Louis, MO.

Plumb D. *Veterinary Drug Handbook*. 9th ed. Wiley-Blackwell: Ames, IA.

Rannazzisi JC, Caverly MW. *Practitioner's Manual—An Informational Outline of the Controlled Substance Act of 1970*. US Department of Justice, Drug Enforcement Administration; 2006. available at: https://www.in.gov/dhs/files/DEA_Practicioner_Manual.pdf.

Romich JA. *Fundamentals of Pharmacology for Veterinary Technicians*. 3rd ed. Cengage Learning: Boston, MA.

US Department of Agriculture. *Food Animal Residue Avoidance Database (FARAD)*. Available at: http://www.farad.org/.

US Food and Drug Administration. *Animal Medicinal Drug Use Clarification Act of 1994 (AMDUCA)*. Available at: https://www.fda.gov/animal-veterinary/guidance-regulations/animal-medicinal-drug-use-clarification-act-1994-amduca.

US Food and Drug Administration, Center for Veterinary Medicine. *Compliance Policy Guides (CPG)*. Available at: https://www.fda.gov/media/74810/download.

29
Pain Management

TASHA McNERNEY

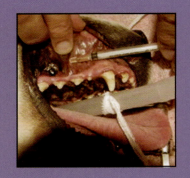

CHAPTER OUTLINE

LEARNING OBJECTIVES

When you have completed this chapter, you will be able to:

1. Pronounce, define, and spell all key terms in the chapter.
2. Explain how the technician can use effective communication, observation, and interpretation skills to advocate for the patient and help provide effective and appropriate analgesia.
3. List common causes and physiologic and behavioral signs of pain in small animals, including the negative effects of untreated pain.
4. Describe the physiologic aspects of pain, including the phases of nociception in mammals; and compare acute, chronic, inflammatory, neuropathic, somatic, and visceral pain; and explain the significance of the "wind-up phenomenon."
5. Do the following regarding the treatment of pain in small animals:
   - Describe the basic principles of effective analgesia protocol design and pain management, including pre-emptive and multimodal analgesia concepts.
   - Compare and contrast agents used to treat pain in small animals, including nonsteroidal anti-inflammatory drugs (NSAIDs), local anesthetics, opioids, and α^2-agonists.
   - List the analgesics commonly given by constant rate infusion (CRI) and perform the calculations required to administer a drug by CRI.
   - List the "adjunctive analgesics" and nonpharmacologic treatment options for pain control and describe the uses and benefits of each.
6. Do the following regarding the treatment of pain in large animals:
   - List causes and signs of pain in large animals and explain why large animals often are undertreated for pain.
   - Compare and contrast agents used to treat pain in large animals, including NSAIDs, opioids, α^2-agonists, and local anesthetics.
   - Discuss the role of joint supplements, chondroprotective agents, miscellaneous agents, alternative and complementary therapy, and good husbandry in the treatment of pain in large animals.
7. Describe analgesic agents and techniques commonly used in horses, cattle, sheep, goats, camelids, and pigs, and explain how economics and drug residues influence the decision to treat pain in food animals.

KEY TERMS

Agonist
Allodynia
Antagonist
Breakthrough pain
Dysphoria
Hyperalgesia
Modulation
Multimodal analgesia

Neurotransmitter
Nociception
Omentopexy
Partial agonist
Pre-emptive analgesia
Transduction
Transmission
Wind-up phenomenon

Introduction

The practice of pain management has become mainstream in veterinary medicine over the past decades. Optimal use of analgesic drugs, combinations, methods of administration, and integrated therapies (e.g., Eastern medicine, rehabilitation, etc.) are continually being improved and developed as more is learned about analgesia and how animals feel and express pain. The search continues for the most objective, scientific methods of measuring and assessing pain in nonverbal patients. Veterinary technicians and nurses continue to play a vital part in pain management, and many veterinarians rely heavily on the ability of the veterinary technician to recognize and report animal pain and use this input to guide decision making. In their roles as patient advocates, human neonatal and pediatric nurses and veterinary nurses give patients a voice and attend to their needs.

The task of advocating for a nonverbal patient can be daunting. Veterinary technicians and nurses are responsible for the quality of patient care and the overall condition of patients but are not free to prescribe or initiate therapy. This shows why a team approach to pain management is best, with the technician and clinician working together to improve patient outcomes. Knowledge of the physiology of pain and the pharmacology of analgesics is essential for good communication between veterinarians and veterinary technicians. Optimally, the veterinarian regards the technician as an integral member of the pain management team. The skilled veterinary technician is a source of vital information who is required to choose and administer appropriate analgesics. They are trusted caretakers of recovering patients. The success of this relationship is extremely important for all hospitalized patients, whether the case is an elective, routine, or emergent one.

The Role of the Veterinary Technician as a Patient Advocate

Communication

Veterinary technicians use critical thinking, observation, and interpretation skills to make important pain management recommendations. Discussing each case directly with the clinician might include the technician's particular concerns and observations about a patient or a general approach to managing different types of pain. Based on the interaction with patients, the veterinary technician may offer suggestions for adjustments in analgesic regimens, changes or additions to drug protocols, and the addition of sedatives if needed.

Veterinary technicians and nurses often complain that their requests for patient analgesia go unheeded. The actual method of communication used plays a large part in achieving a positive outcome. For example, "Can I give Charlie something for pain?" is inadequate to convey the situation and often results in the response, "No." To be effective, technicians must present two sets of information: (1) what the patient is doing that indicates painfulness, and (2) what has already been done that is considered inadequate. For example, "Dr. X, the black Labrador Charlie, who had cruciate repair yesterday, is not doing as well as I would like. Even though his bladder is empty, and I have offered him food and water, he seems restless and has difficulty getting comfortable. He is panting excessively, although his temperature is normal. I checked the bandage, and it does not seem too tight. The record says he received morphine last night at midnight, which allowed

him to sleep for 4 hours, but he has not had any morphine since. Would you like me to repeat the dose to see if it makes him more comfortable?" This approach delivers the necessary information to gain the veterinarian's confidence in the technician's assessment skills and knowledge of the case. The veterinarian is more likely to agree to administer pain medication under these circumstances.

Veterinary technicians and nurses can also be vital to administering pre-emptive medication, which is often overlooked in a busy hospital setting. For example, "I have noticed a difference in the recovery of animals that are given nonsteroidal anti-inflammatory drugs (NSAIDs) before surgery. Would you like me to give an NSAID to this patient now?" This approach also applies to the administration of long-acting opioids, constant rate infusions (CRIs), and the performance of local or regional nerve blocks. Veterinary technicians should provide as much feedback as possible regarding which analgesic protocols are working well and which need to be improved to increase patient comfort.

Patient Assessment

Historically, animal pain has been recognized and treated only in those patients that display overt behavioral signs, such as vocalization. When clinicians wait for signs, patients are forced to prove that they are in pain before they are given analgesics. Dogs and cats instinctively hide pain just as they would in the wild to avoid becoming prey. Once animals display obvious signs of pain, the pain intensity that they are experiencing is likely to be severe. Old or severely debilitated patients may be too ill or weak to display changes in behavior. Patients should never be required to prove they are in pain. A sound approach to pain management favors anticipating the severity and duration of pain likely to occur with any procedure, condition, or surgery. In many cases, animals do "appear" to tolerate pain better than humans. There are several explanations for this. In contrast to the pain detection threshold (the point at which pain nerve fibers are stimulated to send signals), pain tolerance (the greatest intensity of pain voluntarily tolerated) varies widely among species and between individuals within a species. Like humans, animals tolerate pain to a certain point before they show changes in behavior. Awareness that patients may exhibit a wide range of pain tolerance and a broad spectrum of behaviors can improve pain recognition and treatment.

Recently, research in pain management has shifted toward identifying and even predicting known painful events. For example, severe pain is expected with disk herniation, extensive inflammation, medical or surgical fracture repair, limb amputation, declawing, ear canal ablation, and so forth. Moderate pain is expected with cruciate repair, laparotomy, mass removal, castration, dental procedures, and so forth. This approach encourages treatment, without requiring proof of pain, of patients that undergo painful procedures or disease processes. It does not, however, consider the vast variation in pain tolerance among individuals. It seems reasonable to incorporate both concepts to develop a genuinely effective analgesic plan (i.e., receive direction according to what is a painful event and be prepared to provide adequate analgesia for the expected pain level, also to look at the individual and tailor analgesic protocols accordingly).

Veterinary technicians observe patients closely for extended periods and are usually the first to notice status changes. Familiarity with individual patients' personalities and usual reactions to stimuli gives insight into the meaning of behaviors. Experience establishes expectations of how particular patients may react to painful stimuli. This includes differences in expression between dogs and cats and young and old, and variations among certain breeds. For example, Siberian Huskies and Dobermans, breeds known for being more "vocal," are thought to be more "sensitive" to pain or to possess a lower pain threshold compared with other breeds, whereas Greyhounds and Labrador Retrievers remain stoic in the face of pain. The skilled technician armed with a pain scoring system agreed upon within the hospital factors this into the pain assessments.

Companion animals retain survival instincts despite being bred into captivity. These instincts include a drive to hide signs of pain from potential predators to avoid appearing weak compared with the rest of the pack. Much to their detriment, even in a setting without predators, dogs and cats attempt to hide their pain from humans, therefore reaching a high threshold of pain before showing changes in behavior. Conversely, some animals express more pain than expected due to a low pain threshold, which should be managed appropriately.

Signs of Pain

In veterinary medicine, pain is seldom diagnosed based on a single observation or physiologic value. Because pain is an individual, subjective experience, assessment depends on the combination of good examination skills, familiarity with species, breed, and individual behaviors, knowledge of the degree of pain associated with particular surgical procedures or illnesses, and recognition of the signs of stress and pain.

Signs of pain in animals can be categorized as physiologic or behavioral (Table 29.1). Physiologic pain signs may be obvious and include increased heart rate, blood pressure, increased respiratory rate, and vocalization. More subtle behavioral changes, such as general restlessness, decreased appetite, not sleeping, resenting handling, and not assuming a normal position, may be even more significant. Clinical signs of pain in dogs and cats most often reported include tachycardia, increased respiratory rate, restlessness, increased temperature, increased blood pressure, abnormal posturing, inappetence, aggression, frequent movement, facial expression, trembling, depression, and insomnia. Less frequently reported are anxiety; nausea; pupillary enlargement; licking, chewing, and staring at the surgical site or wound; poor mucous membrane color; salivation; decreased carbon dioxide; and head pressing.

Clinical manifestations may differ between species and even among members of the same species. Standing or sitting for long periods and sleeping in an atypical position are considered signs of pain for dogs. For cats, abnormal posture, hiding, and aggression are common signs of pain. Because the signs of pain are so varied and diverse, any abnormal sign in a veterinary patient that cannot be attributed to another cause is suspected of indicating pain.

TECHNICIAN NOTE

Signs of pain vary among animals. Patients should assume normal positions (what you would expect to see at home) while caged in the hospital. Standing for long periods or sleeping in an abnormal position indicates discomfort. Normal posture and behaviors (sleep patterns, eating, drinking, and elimination) are good indications that the patient is comfortable.

All patients should be evaluated for pain upon admission and at regular intervals throughout the hospitalization period. The observer's subjective opinion and physiologic signs can be described by using a pain scale, such as the visual analog scale (VAS). One pain scale option is the Colorado State University

TABLE 29.1 Behavioral Signs of Pain in Dogs and Cats

Posture	Temperament	Vocalization	Locomotion	Other
Dogs				
• Tail between legs • Arched or hunched back • Twisted body to protect pain site • Drooped head • Prolonged sitting position • Tucked abdomen • Lying in flat, extended position	• Aggressive • Clawing • Attacking, biting • Escaping	• Barking • Howling • Moaning • Whimpering	• Reluctance to move • Carrying one leg • Lameness • Unusual gait • Unable to walk • Chewing painful areas	• Unable to perform normal tasks • Attacks other animals or people if pain site is touched (self-trauma) • No interest in food or play
Cats				
• Tucked limbs • Arched or hunched head and neck or back • Tucked abdomen • Lying flat • Slumped body • Drooped head	• Aggressive • Biting • Scratching • Chewing • Attacking • Escaping • Hiding	• Crying • Hissing • Spitting • Moaning • Screaming • Purring	• Reluctance to move • Carrying one leg • Lameness • Unusual gait • Unable to walk • Inactive	• Attacks if pain site is touched • Absence of grooming • Dilated pupils • No interest in food or play

Pain Scale (Fig. 29.1A and B), developed for use in canines and felines. It uses numeric, pictorial, and descriptive assessments to allow the user to derive a "score" for the level of pain the patient may be experiencing.

Veterinary technicians and nurses are educated to recognize pain in animals and are instinctively skillful observers of behavioral changes in patients, noticing the subtlest expressions of potential pain. Most experienced technicians have an innate sense of how painful most procedures, conditions, and surgery are likely to be because of their repeated and prolonged exposure to animals in the recovery phase. However, it is often difficult for even the most experienced veterinary nurse to distinguish between pain and other stress. For example, postoperative patients frequently display aberrant behavior several minutes to hours after surgery. These behaviors may include vocalization, thrashing, rolling, self-mutilation, and tachypnea. When these behaviors are thought to be related to stress other than pain, they are often referred to as **dysphoria**, a general term defining an emotional state characterized by anxiety, depression, or unease. Abnormal postoperative behaviors sometimes are referred to as *emergence delirium*, attributed to residual gas anesthetics. Some animals do, in fact, display this response upon awakening, but anesthetic-related behaviors should resolve within several minutes. Behaviors that persist beyond a few minutes require further investigation and attention. In any case, it can be difficult to distinguish pain, dysphoria, and reaction to narcotics or general anesthetics. Rapid control of the patient using sedation and analgesia is essential, regardless of the cause of pain.

The Science of Pain Management

Is There a Purpose for Pain?

In human medicine, preventing and treating pain are now recognized as essential parts of overall patient management. Pain is

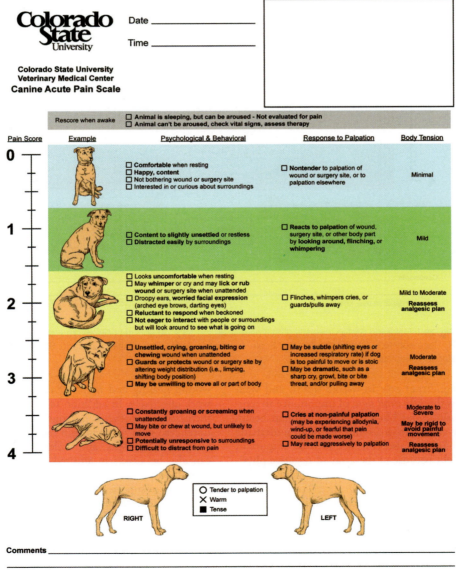

A

© 2006/PW Hellyer, SR Uhrig, NG Robinson

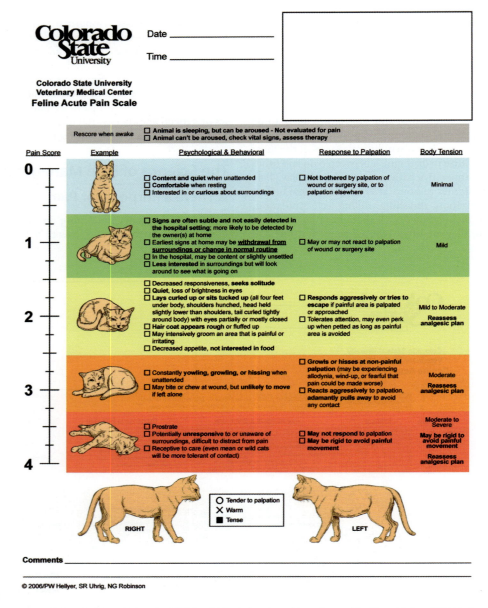

Colorado State University
Veterinary Medical Center
Feline Acute Pain Scale

Date _____

Time _____

Rescore when awake	☐ Animal is sleeping, but can be aroused - Not evaluated for pain ☐ Animal can't be aroused, check vital signs, assess therapy		
Pain Score	**Example**	**Psychological & Behavioral**	**Response to Palpation**	**Body Tension**

0
☐ Content and quiet when unattended
☐ Comfortable when resting
☐ Interested in or curious about surroundings

☐ Not bothered by palpation of wound or surgery site, or to palpation elsewhere

Minimal

1
☐ Signs are often subtle and not easily detected in the hospital setting; more likely to be detected by the owner(s) at home
☐ Earliest signs at home may be withdrawal from surroundings or change in normal routine
☐ In the hospital, may be content or slightly unsettled
☐ Less interested in surroundings but will look around to see what is going on

☐ May or may not react to palpation of wound or surgery site

Mild

2
☐ Decreased responsiveness, seeks solitude
☐ Quiet, loss of brightness in eyes
☐ Lays curled up or sits tucked up (all four feet under body, shoulders hunched, head held slightly lower than shoulders, tail curled tightly around body) with eyes partially or mostly closed
☐ Hair coat appears rough or fluffed up
☐ May intensively groom an area that is painful or irritating
☐ Decreased appetite, not interested in food

☐ Responds aggressively or tries to escape if painful area is palpated or approached
☐ Tolerates attention, may even perk up when petted as long as painful area is avoided

Mild to Moderate

Reassess analgesic plan

3
☐ Constantly yowling, growling, or hissing when unattended
☐ May bite or chew at wound, but unlikely to move if left alone

☐ Growls or hisses at non-painful palpation (may be experiencing allodynia, wind-up, or fearful that pain could be made worse)
☐ Reacts aggressively to palpation, adamantly pulls away to avoid any contact

Moderate

Reassess analgesic plan

4
☐ Prostrate
☐ Potentially unresponsive to or unaware of surroundings, difficult to distract from pain
☐ Receptive to care (even mean or wild cats will be more tolerant of contact)

☐ May not respond to palpation
☐ May be rigid to avoid painful movement

Moderate to Severe

May be rigid to avoid painful movement

Reassess analgesic plan

RIGHT   LEFT

○ Tender to palpation
✕ Warm
■ Tense

Comments _____
_____
_____

© 2006/PW Hellyer, SR Uhrig, NG Robinson

B

• **Fig. 29.1** Colorado State University (CSU) pain scale for dogs (A) and cats (B). (From Hellyer PW, Uhrig SR, Robinson NG. Canine Acute Pain Scale and Feline Acute Pain Scale. Colorado State University Veterinary Medical Center, 2006.)

considered to play a significant role in overall health and well-being and is regarded as the *fifth vital sign*, of importance to temperature, pulse, respiration, and blood pressure. Human health care providers not only view pain as a symptom of an underlying disease or condition, but they also consider pain an important syndrome in its own right because of the array of negative physiologic events attributable to pain, regardless of the patient's underlying disease or condition.

Pain triggers a series of physiologic changes that increase stress. Although the nervous system is the main target of pain transmission and provides the means for the body to react to that information, the body's response to pain signals is not limited to the nervous system. Most, if not all, of the body's major systems are affected by inadequately controlled pain (Box 29.1). For example, increased cortisol levels that accompany pain may interfere with

wound healing and may reduce the immune system's ability to work effectively. In addition to suppressing the immune system, increased sympathetic nervous system activity associated with unrelieved pain may result in increased catabolism and metabolic rate, anorexia, ileus, and atelectasis. The cardiovascular system can also be adversely affected, resulting in increased heart rate and blood pressure, irregular heart rhythms, and coagulopathies. Reducing or suppressing the stress response by managing pain can minimize adverse effects on the entire body. It is obvious that as with humans, animals in pain require more intensive medical care than those in which pain is adequately managed. The standards of the American Animal Hospital Association (AAHA) require pain assessment in every patient, regardless of the presenting complaint. Other requirements include making repeat regular assessments (including pain scoring) throughout hospitalization and

---

> **• BOX 29.1 Negative Effects of Pain in All Mammals**
>
> **Cardiovascular System**
> Arrhythmias
>
> **Gastrointestinal System**
> Nausea, vomiting
>
> **Pulmonary System**
> Tachypnea
> Hypoxemia
> Pulmonary edema
> Pulmonary hypertension
> Respiratory acid-base imbalance
>
> **Renal System**
> Renal hypertension
>
> **Metabolic System**
> Cachexia
> Increased oxygen demand
> Negative nitrogen balance
>
> **Immune Function**
> Hemorrhage
>
> **Sleep Pattern**
> Behavior changes

> **• BOX 29.2 Summary of AAHA Pain Management Standards**
>
> - Pain assessment for every patient, regardless of presenting complaint
> - Assessment recorded in the medical record
> - Use of pre-emptive pain management
> - Appropriate pain management for anticipated level and duration
> - Pain management for *all* surgical procedures
> - Reassessment for pain throughout procedures
> - Medical and chronic pain also treated
> - Written protocols
> - Teaching clients to recognize pain in their pets

anesthesia (unconscious) do not perceive that they are in pain. However, nociception can occur even when an animal is in a state of unconsciousness, as with general anesthesia.

> **TECHNICIAN NOTE**
>
> Without the benefits of analgesia, the nervous system is still activated to process pain signals while patients are under anesthesia, triggering negative physiologic effects even though no pain-related behaviors are seen.

As the anesthesia wears off and consciousness returns, postoperative pain perception occurs. This explains why many patients display pain signs immediately upon waking. Appropriate pain management is designed to interrupt nociception, even if the patient is under general anesthesia, and should be initiated whenever pain is anticipated. Analgesia is recommended before *all* surgical procedures, because it results in a much smoother and comfortable recovery.

Neuropathic Pain and Wind-Up Phenomenon

Pain traditionally has been subdivided into acute and chronic types. *Acute pain* is described as a sharp stabbing sensation and *chronic pain* as dull, persistent throbbing. Chronic and acute pain are two different types of pain experienced by veterinary patients, and each requires a different approach to treatment. Acute pain is sudden and usually occurs because of an injury or trauma. It is characterized by a rapid onset, and it is usually easy to locate the source of the pain, for example, an injury such as a laceration or burn. Acute pain is protective in nature, serving as a warning signal to the body that something is wrong. Acute pain is typically treated with medications such as opioids, NSAIDs, and local anesthetics.

Chronic pain, on the other hand, is pain that persists over a long period of time, typically for weeks or even months. Chronic pain can be caused by a variety of factors, including arthritis, cancer, and nerve damage. Unlike acute pain, chronic pain serves no protective purpose and can significantly impact an animal's quality of life. Chronic pain is often more difficult to treat than acute pain and may require a combination of medications, physical therapy, and other interventions. When it comes to the transmission of pain signals, there are two types of nerve fibers that play a significant role: *A-fibers* and *C-fibers*.

A-fibers are large, myelinated nerve fibers that transmit pain signals rapidly. These fibers are responsible for the sharp, immediate pain associated with acute pain. C-fibers are small, unmyelinated nerve fibers that transmit pain signals more slowly. These fibers are responsible for the dull, persistent pain associated with chronic pain. Different treatment modalities are used to address each type

recording those assessments in the medical record. A full listing of AAHA pain management standards can be found on their website (www.aahanet.org) (Box 29.2).

Physiology of Pain

Nociception and the Pain Pathway

From a physiologic standpoint, pain is processed in the same manner in all mammals. **Nociception**, derived from the Latin word *nocere* ("to injure"), includes three distinct phases: **transduction**, **transmission**, and **modulation**. The pain pathway begins at the site of tissue damage (evidenced by localized redness, heat, and swelling—classic signs of inflammation). Regardless of the cause of inflammation (e.g., injury, tumor, surgical incision), nociceptors, the specialized nerve endings, convert mechanical, chemical, and thermal energy into electrical impulses (transduction) once their threshold is exceeded. If the noxious stimulus is large enough to exceed the nociceptor's threshold, a nerve impulse is generated and transmitted along peripheral nerves to the spinal cord (transmission). The highly specialized nerve fibers carry pain information and are distinct from other nerve fibers that typically carry pleasant or neutral sensations. Once at the spinal cord, a nerve impulse may be projected upward to the thalamus and then to other parts of the brain, or it may be transmitted to a nerve cell located entirely within the central nervous system (CNS) that activates sympathetic reflexes (Fig. 29.2). In this way, the sensation of pain is dampened (modulation).

The fourth phase of the pain pathway is perception. Perception occurs in the conscious brain and is the awareness that "this hurts." Although the terms *pain* and *nociception* are often used interchangeably, they are not synonymous and are differentiated by "consciousness." This means that patients under general

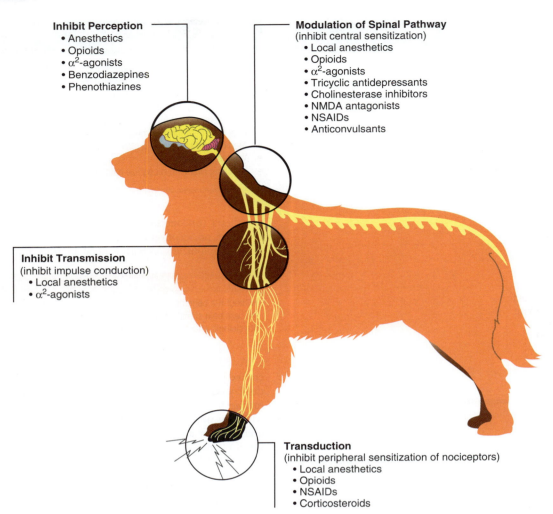

Inhibit Perception
- Anesthetics
- Opioids
- α^2-agonists
- Benzodiazepines
- Phenothiazines

Modulation of Spinal Pathway
(inhibit central sensitization)
- Local anesthetics
- Opioids
- α^2-agonists
- Tricyclic antidepressants
- Cholinesterase inhibitors
- NMDA antagonists
- NSAIDs
- Anticonvulsants

Inhibit Transmission
(inhibit impulse conduction)
- Local anesthetics
- α^2-agonists

Transduction
(inhibit peripheral sensitization of nociceptors)
- Local anesthetics
- Opioids
- NSAIDs
- Corticosteroids

• **Fig. 29.2** Nociception. Sites of analgesic action along the pain pathway. (From Tranquilli WJ, Grimm KA, Lamont LA. *Pain Management for the Small Animal Practitioner.* Jackson, WY: Teton NewMedia; 2004.)

of pain. For acute pain, medications such as opioids, NSAIDs, and local anesthetics can be used to manage pain. For chronic pain, nonopioid analgesics such as gabapentin, amantadine, and tramadol can be used to help manage pain. Additionally, physical therapy, acupuncture, and other complementary therapies can be used to help manage chronic pain in veterinary patients.

Most pain is related to inflammation, but unpleasant sensations may arise directly from the nerves involved in pain transmission. When attributed to nerves, these sensations are generally described as "neuropathic." Therefore it may be more appropriate to classify pain as *inflammatory* (with subsets of acute and chronic) or *neuropathic* (present in the nerves, irrespective of ongoing inflammation). Neuropathic pain is described as a persistent stabbing, aching, burning, itching, or tingling sensation, with or without an observable cause; it can occur along with inflammatory pain or as a separate syndrome. Treating neuropathic pain may allow patients to return to a normal or near-normal state. A commonly used neuropathic pain reliever in human and veterinary medicines is gabapentin (Neurontin) (see the section "Administration of Analgesics and Analgesic Techniques").

An extreme form of neuropathic pain occurs when the CNS is bombarded by persistent pain impulses. This can have a profound effect on the architecture of the nervous system, altering pain processing. When spinal neurons are subjected to repeating or high-intensity nociceptive impulses, these neurons become progressively and increasingly excitable, even after the stimulus is removed. This condition is known as *central sensitization* or the **wind-up phenomenon** and leads to nonresponsive or chronic intractable pain. Wind-up is the culmination of two distinct phases of change in the nervous system. First, the pain-transmitting nerve fiber threshold is reset to a lower level, resulting in **hyperalgesia**, where less and less stimulation is required to initiate pain. In the second phase, nerve fibers that normally carry pleasant or neutral information are recruited and become part of the pain transmission process, a phase termed **allodynia.** It results in the interpretation of normally harmless sensations as pain. The presence of hyperalgesia and allodynia collectively is considered the wind-up phenomenon. This is apparent, for example, in the Dachshund with vertebral disk disease that cries out in pain when any part of its body is touched, or in the Cocker Spaniel with a chronic ear infection that can no longer tolerate normal petting. People suffering from a migraine headache can attest to both an increase in pain sensitivity and normally innocuous sensations (light touch by hand, clothing, wind, etc.) becoming unpleasant. The wind-up phenomenon highlights the need for effective analgesia to treat pain before it begins and at regular intervals once it occurs. The wind-up phenomenon is an important concept in pain management. Most patients experiencing acute pain can be managed by using common analgesics, such as NSAIDs. Patients experiencing wind-up require additional therapy, just as the migraine sufferer would not likely be helped by taking two ibuprofen tablets, even though this approach would be adequate to treat a common headache. A variety of approaches can be used to "unwind" the patient, aimed at resetting neurologic processing so that conventional medications will work again. These approaches are discussed in the section "Administration of Analgesics and Analgesic Techniques."

Treatment of Pain in Small Animals

Environmental and Emotional Care

Pain has both physical and psychological components. Fear and anxiety can exacerbate pain, and vice versa. Attending to an animal's physical and perceived emotional needs can reduce stress and consequently minimize pain levels. Environmental factors may affect the perception of pain in pet animals. The hospitalized patient in unfamiliar surroundings may be comforted by a favorite blanket or toy. If possible, felines should have separate housing, away from barking dogs or the sounds of the treatment room, to minimize stress and anxiety. Veterinary technicians must be adept at "reading" patients, because the emotional needs of individual dogs and cats vary greatly. Environmental care, such as providing a clean cage of appropriate size, extra padding, and careful positioning to reduce pressure on painful areas, is important. Designate the patient's cage as a safe zone so that animals do not associate contact with an unpleasant experience. Any procedure that might be considered noxious should be performed after taking the patient out of the cage if possible. This allows the animal to feel comfortable and safe when in the cage. Nonpharmacologic actions can reduce pain by removing other stressors. However, tending to a patient's comfort needs should not be seen as a substitute for analgesia.

When it comes to animals and veterinary medicine, pain can also have a profound effect on their emotions and well-being. Here is how pain can impact animals emotionally:

- Behavioral changes: Animals in pain may exhibit changes in behavior, such as restlessness, aggression, or withdrawal. They may become less interested in their surroundings, refuse to engage in activities they previously enjoyed, or exhibit signs of fear or anxiety.
- Loss of appetite and reduced activity: Pain can lead to a loss of appetite and decreased activity levels in animals. They may become lethargic or reluctant to move, as certain movements or actions can exacerbate their pain. This decrease in activity can contribute to emotional distress and a sense of malaise.
- Fear and anxiety: Animals experiencing pain may become fearful or anxious, especially when their pain is associated with specific activities, such as veterinary visits or handling. The fear of experiencing pain again can lead to heightened anxiety and avoidance behaviors.
- Aggression or defensive behavior: Animals in pain may display aggression or defensive behavior because of their discomfort. They may snap, growl, or bite when approached or touched, as they perceive these actions as potential threats to their painful areas.
- Altered sleep patterns: Pain can disrupt an animal's sleep patterns, leading to difficulty in getting comfortable and obtaining restful sleep. This sleep disturbance can contribute to increased irritability and further impact their emotional well-being.

It is crucial for veterinary nurses and techs to recognize and address the emotional impact of pain on animals. Proper pain management in veterinary medicine involves not only identifying and treating the underlying cause of pain but also considering the emotional well-being of the animal.

Principles of Administering Analgesia

Improved understanding of the impact of pain on the body is shaping new philosophies in managing patients' pain. Several basic principles are used in the approach to designing analgesic protocols and are particularly important in managing pain effectively.

1. *The best way to treat pain is to prevent it.* This is the concept of **pre-emptive analgesia**. All research in human and veterinary medicine shows that preventing pain is unquestionably the best approach to treatment. It is an easy concept to grasp but not so easy to remember and to implement. That is because it has become common to treat animal pain "on request" (i.e., when we see overt signs of pain), despite the rational knowledge that once the signs are present, it is already too late. The opportunity to manage pain most effectively in that patient has already been missed. Administering pre-emptive analgesics whenever possible appears to be much more effective than using the same agent to treat pain once it occurs. Analgesia given before a noxious stimulus occurs helps reduce postprocedure analgesia requirements, minimizes detrimental effects of pain, improves the handling of patients, and potentially lowers sedation or anesthetic requirements. Reducing pain signaling helps prevent hypersensitization at the spinal cord and neuropathic pain syndromes.

2. *Using drug combinations or a multimodal approach often produces better pain relief compared with single agents.* The physiology of nociception gives rise to the concept of **multimodal analgesia**. Multimodal analgesia takes advantage of the synergistic effects obtained by combining two or more classes of analgesic drugs to alter more than one phase of nociception (transduction, transmission, modulation, and perception). Attacking pain from many angles is more effective than doing so from only one. Because the pain pathway has distinct phases, pain can be interrupted at various points. For example, in addition to pre-emptive NSAIDs (that work on transduction), a local block (that works to block signal transmission) may be performed and opioids administered (they work on modulation and perception, respectively). Using analgesics from these three different classes provides better pain control and confers the added benefit of allowing the use of lower doses of individual agents, thereby reducing overall side effects. Effective analgesia can also reduce the amount of inhalant anesthetic required for a procedure.

3. *Matching analgesics* (based on dosage and duration of action) to the degree of expected surgical pain, rather than to the patient's ability to express pain in a recognizable way, is a more effective way to ensure pain relief.

4. *Maintaining an analgesic plane once pain control is established.* This may include the use of epidurals, CRI, or continued bolus dosing. Patients are weaned off pain treatment as they are transitioned out of the intensive care unit. Regimented treatment (i.e., dosing at regular intervals) is helpful in maintaining an analgesic plane. Otherwise, a "roller coaster effect" occurs, leaving the patient in varying degrees of pain between treatments. Keeping a patient out of pain is always more efficacious than continual efforts to take the patient out of pain.

5. *Adopting the approach of "Don't quit till the pain quits."* This approach includes sending the patient home with pain relief agents. Many professionals agree that most soft tissue procedures, such as spaying or neutering, require 3 to 4 days of postoperative analgesia, whereas orthopedic procedures probably require a supply for 7 to 10 days. Of course, the needs of individual patients may vary, and owners should be advised to request additional analgesia if they perceive their pets to be in pain beyond the anticipated period.

6. Dispelling the pain myth that *pain is beneficial in limiting a recovering animal's activity* is critical to patient care. Although this is one of the most widely held myths about pain, studies demonstrate that animals in pain tend to be restless, change positions frequently, and bite, chew, and/or lick at painful sites, whereas pain-managed animals tend to rest and recover quietly. Besides being morally questionable, allowing animals to remain in pain for the purpose of restraint is not a medically sound policy. The type of pain produced by tissue injury, inflammation, or direct damage to the nervous system is never beneficial. The previously described negative effects of pain far outnumber any benefit, real or imagined. Providing effective analgesia reduces the pain-induced stress response, thereby enhancing patient comfort and recovery.

Administration of Analgesics and Analgesic Techniques

The basic principles of pain management currently applied in practice, as described above, include pre-emptive (preventive) analgesia, multimodal analgesia (using different classes of drugs simultaneously to interrupt the pain pathway at various points), and appropriate follow-up analgesia (postoperative and take-home). Using this strategy, an analgesic plan is designed for each patient to maximize pain control, maintain them on an analgesic plane, and reduce unwanted side effects (Table 29.2).

Choosing the correct analgesic therapy requires an understanding of both the pharmacokinetics of a wide range of drugs and the levels or types of pain associated with various conditions. Typically, five categories of drugs—NSAIDs, local anesthetics, opioids, dissociative, and α^2-agonists—are used in various combinations to inhibit the nociceptive process at more than one site. For this reason, combinations are more effective than single agents. Pain relief, as assessed by the criteria previously described, is the only true measure of successful treatment. More recently, several classes of drugs have been added to the pain management regimen as adjunctive therapy in nonresponsive cases, including *N*-methyl-D-aspartate (NMDA) receptor antagonists (for efficacy against wind-up) and anticonvulsants (for efficacy against neuropathic pain).

Anticipating pain level and duration provides a starting point for analgesic protocols. The initial approach is based on knowledge of the mechanisms of pain, drug dosages and expected duration of treatment, pain assessment, and knowledge of expected levels of pain for injuries, surgery, and diseases (Box 29.3). Patients should be continually evaluated for breakthrough pain that persists beyond the usual treatment protocol or pain that persists beyond the expected period. Categorization of the expected severity (mild, moderate, severe) of pain is used to establish the initial type of analgesia and the duration of treatment. Later dosages can be adjusted according to individual patient responses. For example, mild pain may be manageable with NSAIDs alone or in combination with a weak opioid, whereas moderate pain may require the addition of a stronger opioid. Severe pain might be best approached with

TABLE 29.2	Monitoring Patients Taking Analgesics
Adverse Effect	**Monitoring**
Opioids	
Sedation, low blood pressure, respiratory depression, vomiting	Mentation, blood pressure, respiratory rate, and nature
Local Anesthetics	
None unless given by CRI. Then nausea, vomiting, neurologic signs, and seizures	Observe regularly for muscle tremors and GI upset
NSAIDs	
GI disturbances, GI bleeding, renal disturbances	General observation, hydration status, stool quality, and urine production
α^2-Agonists	
Bradycardia, cardiac arrhythmias, hypertension, peripheral vasoconstriction	Femoral pulse rate and quality, heart rate and rhythm, and blood pressure

CRI, Constant rate infusion; *GI*, gastrointestinal; *NSAIDs*, nonsteroidal anti-inflammatory drugs.

• BOX 29.3 Sound Approach to Developing an Individual Pain Management Protocol

The initial approach should be based on the following questions:
- How painful is the condition, procedure, or surgery expected to be?
- Are there any underlying factors, such as stress, anxiety, fear, or pre-existing chronic pain conditions, that could be causing an increased pain response?
- What is the normal behavior and disposition of the particular breed and for this animal in particular?
- Are there any contraindications to particular drugs or drug classes for this patient's condition?
- Does this animal have a history of drug sensitivities?

an NSAID and a full opioid agonist, or it may require CRI or additional therapies. Local and regional blocks can and should be added to the pain management plan whenever feasible. When specific nerves cannot be identified for blocking, lidocaine can be administered via CRI for excellent systemic analgesia.

> **TECHNICIAN NOTE**
>
> A variety of techniques may be used to administer analgesics. Experienced veterinary technicians and nurses can deliver drugs by the oral, transmucosal, subcutaneous (SQ), intramuscular (IM), intravenous (IV), transcutaneous, and epidural routes and via continuous rate infusion (CRI).

NSAIDs provide analgesia by modifying the inflammatory response. Pharmacologic actions of NSAIDs include analgesia, antipyresis (fever reduction), and control of inflammation. Because they treat the underlying problem (inflammation) and pain is diminished as a result, NSAIDs are considered a therapeutic class of analgesics. Since the time that NSAIDs were approved for use in dogs and introduced into the market, they have been universally accepted as the treatment of choice for osteoarthritis. NSAIDs remain the most widely used analgesics in the treatment of chronic pain. However, they are also extremely effective in reducing acute pain in the perioperative period (around surgery). Recent changes in our understanding of pain in animals and the best ways to manage it and new US Food and Drug Administration (FDA) drug approvals have led to NSAIDs becoming one of the most widely used classes of veterinary analgesics in a variety of situations.

Research shows that pretreatment with NSAIDs greatly reduces intraoperative and postoperative pain resulting from procedures on soft tissues and from orthopedic procedures. Therefore patients undergoing treatments ranging from spaying and neutering to cruciate ligament repair potentially benefit from NSAID administration, especially when given pre-emptively. NSAIDs have been shown to have a synergistic effect when combined with other classes of drugs, such as opioids. NSAIDs have an onset of action of 45 to 60 minutes. The duration of action is typically 24 hours in dogs and varies from 8 to 96 hours in cats. NSAIDs are best suited for treating mild to moderate pain, whether acute or chronic in nature. In addition to controlling postoperative pain, NSAIDs are extremely effective in controlling inflammatory pain associated with traumatic soft tissue injury, ophthalmic conditions, otitis, gingivitis, and pain caused by some cancers. Often, patients with severe acute pain can be weaned to NSAIDs alone as their pain diminishes.

Current FDA-approved veterinary NSAIDs for use in dogs include carprofen (Rimadyl), meloxicam (Metacam), deracoxib (Deramaxx), grapiprant (Galliprant), and firocoxib (Previcox). It should be noted that grapiprant is only approved to control pain and inflammation associated with osteoarthritis. Meloxicam (Metacam) and robenacoxib (Onsior) are approved for use in cats in the United States. Regardless of the use of NSAID, patients should be normotensive (have normal blood pressure), and have normal renal and liver function, no bleeding abnormalities, and no potential for gastric ulceration. Patients that receive NSAIDs preoperatively *must* have blood pressure monitored intraoperatively, and intravenous (IV) access must be maintained for the administration of IV fluids if necessary. Patients that are receiving corticosteroids or aspirin should not be given NSAIDs. Two different NSAIDs should not be administered concurrently. Acetaminophen (commonly known as Tylenol, its brand name) is not a nonsteroidal anti-inflammatory drug. It is an over-the-counter pain reliever for people but does not have much anti-inflammatory activity. Veterinarians will sometimes use acetaminophen to relieve pain in dogs but never in cats. **Acetaminophen is fatal to cats** as they lack certain enzymes that the liver needs to safely break down the drug.

Because of the receptors targeted by NSAIDs, the most reported adverse events in dogs are related to the gastrointestinal (GI) tract and include vomiting, diarrhea, GI bleeding, and GI perforation, whereas in cats, signs are more commonly related to the renal system and include renal failure.

TECHNICIAN NOTE

Meloxicam (Metacam) is approved for a one-time 0.3 mg/kg dose for acute pain in cats; however, this dose is considered unsafe, and most of the adverse effects attributed to meloxicam in cats have occurred because of this overdose. The one-time dose most commonly and safely used is 0.1 mg/kg. Robenacoxib (Onsior) is approved at 1 mg/kg for three doses for acute pain in cats and is a safe and effective dose. Outside the United States (EU, UK, and Canada), both drugs are approved for the treatment of chronic pain in cats at a dose of 0.1 mg/kg on the first day and 0.05 mg/kg every day following. Dosages as low as 0.01–0.03 mg/kg may be effective in some cats and may be safe for some cats with chronic kidney disease. Robenacoxib is approved at the same dose for both acute and chronic pain, with no limit on the duration of therapy for either drug. Acetaminophen (Tylenol) should never be administered to cats as it can be fatal.

Take-home Analgesia with NSAIDs

The availability of NSAIDs has improved outpatient pain management in dogs. These drugs are convenient to administer (once a day, chewable), are relatively inexpensive, and provide long-lasting pain relief compared with other analgesics. The current anecdotal recommendation for dogs from pain management experts is that elective soft tissue procedures, such as spaying or castration, require 3 to 5 days of postoperative treatment with NSAIDs. Orthopedic procedures may require treatment for 7 to 10 days or longer. Of course, each individual animal must be evaluated for the presence of pain that persists beyond the expected time or pain that is of significant intensity and requires additional analgesics. Currently, there are no approved NSAIDs for chronic use in cats. However, carprofen (Rimadyl) has been administered anecdotally to cats off-label at 2 mg/kg every 4 days for chronic inflammatory pain.

Local and Regional Anesthetics

Local anesthetics work by totally disrupting neural transmission of information. Blocking transmission of painful signals is one of the most effective ways of managing pain. Nerve blocks routinely administered by veterinary technicians include canine and feline blocks used in dental treatments and feline declawing. The use of lidocaine as a systemic blocking agent given via CRI is becoming increasingly popular. Recent research has led to the revival of the use of local or regional analgesia. Applying analgesia directly to affected nerve endings can provide excellent pain control while reducing the need for the use of systemic drugs.

Lidocaine, the most widely used local anesthetic, takes effect in 1 to 3 minutes, and its effect lasts for 60 to 90 minutes. Lidocaine's duration can be extended by combination with a 1:200,000 dilution of epinephrine. The addition of epinephrine is commonly used in dentistry blocks. Epinephrine should *never* be used in circumferential limb blocks, such as those used for toe amputations. Other drugs, such as buprenorphine and dexmedetomidine, can be added to local anesthetics to extend their duration of action and increase analgesia. Bupivacaine takes longer to take effect (15 minutes), but its anesthetic and analgesic effects last 6 to 8 hours. Bupivacaine is not effective as a topical analgesic but is an excellent choice for local infiltration. Nocita is a long-acting local anesthetic product that provides extended-release delivery of bupivacaine, providing up to 72 hours of postoperative pain relief. Nocita lasts for up to 72 hours, because the bupivacaine is encapsulated in a liposomal layer that degrades over time and slowly releases bupivacaine for long-lasting local analgesia. Nocita is administered during surgery in the layers of closure and requires special training prior to use.

Blocking agents, such as lidocaine and bupivacaine, are considered safe if correctly administered. Most cases of toxicity in small animals occur as a result of accidental overdose or inadvertent IV administration. Signs of toxicity include seizures, coma, neurotoxicity, and cardiovascular collapse.

TECHNICIAN NOTE

Does the drug name end in *-caine*? If so, it is used for regional analgesia. *-caine* is a suffix used in pharmacology to name local anesthetics. The names of all local anesthetics end with the suffix "-caine," and they block nerve transmission via sodium channels. Differences between individual agents are noted in time to onset and duration of action. Most procedures in small animals are best performed with the use of the longest-acting agent possible (bupivacaine); however, the gold standard and most widely used local anesthetic is lidocaine, owing to its safety and effectiveness.

Routes of Administration

Topical Analgesia. Application of topical analgesia to the surface skin or mucosa can reduce pain associated with minor procedures, such as wound suturing, venipuncture, arterial puncture, nasal cannulation, and urinary catheterization. Solutions of lidocaine, bupivacaine, tetracaine, and epinephrine can be used alone or in various combinations to provide desensitization at the application site. Gauze pads soaked with solutions can be applied directly to the site. Alternatively, several commercially prepared topical anesthetic creams and jellies can be applied as a thick paste. Regardless of the application method selected, 20 to 30 minutes of direct contact time is required to ensure effective analgesia.

Local Infiltration. Injection of lidocaine or bupivacaine into local tissue can reduce pain associated with various painful procedures. This technique is useful for small mass removal, digit amputation, arterial catheter placement, thoracocentesis, abdominocentesis, bone marrow sampling, and so forth. The entry area is infiltrated with small amounts of local anesthetic before tissue penetration. An appropriate waiting time must be observed based on the type of local analgesic used to ensure adequate desensitization of the area, as described earlier.

Circumferential Ring Block. This block is especially effective for use in feline declawing or toe amputations and involves subcutaneous (SQ) injection of bupivacaine or lidocaine. The dosage is 1 mL of 0.5% bupivacaine/10 lb of body weight divided among injection sites. Sterile saline can be added to achieve sufficient coverage in smaller cats. Injections are made just above the carpal bend on the top side of the paw and just above the accessory carpal pad on the underside (Fig. 29.3). The skin is tented horizontally, and the needle is inserted under the skin. As the needle is withdrawn, the drug is injected slowly to leave behind a "line." When this is done on both surfaces, the lines will connect, creating a bracelet or ring block around the limb. This four-injection technique (for two paws) provides a regional nerve block sufficient to eliminate pain for up to 8 hours after surgery. Recently, Nocita gained FDA approval for pain following onychectomy in cats. Nocita is a sterile aqueous suspension of multivesicular liposomes containing bupivacaine. The liposomes are microscopic structures designed to gradually release bupivacaine from the vesicles. This is important as the liposomes do not diffuse readily from where they are deposited, providing up to 72 hours of blocked nerve signal transmission.

RUMM Block

A radial, ulnar, median, and musculocutaneous (RUMM) block is used to block the distal forelimb and is especially useful for procedures involving the carpus or digits. To perform the nerve blocks on the humerus, prepare the two injection sites. First, prep the areas on the inside and outside of the upper limb (humerus) for the injections. Remember to always use proper sterile technique and prioritize the animal's comfort and safety during the procedure.

To block the radial nerve, start by positioning the animal on its side, with the limb you are going to work on facing upwards. Find the spot for the injection by locating the middle and lower parts of the humerus. It is near where the brachialis muscle meets the triceps. To locate the radial nerve, run the thumb along the humeral shaft between the brachialis and triceps to feel the nerve crossing there. Use a 22-gauge needle and insert it from behind, going straight toward the humerus at the level of the nerve. Once the needle touches the bone near the nerve, pull it back slightly, check for any fluids by pulling the plunger (aspirate), and if everything is clear, inject the local anesthetic.

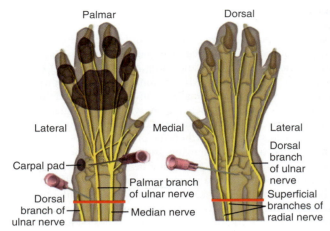

• **Fig. 29.3** Circumferential block for feline declawing. Landmarks are shown, indicating proper site for subcutaneous injection of local anesthetic to provide block of the three major nerves in the feline forelimb.

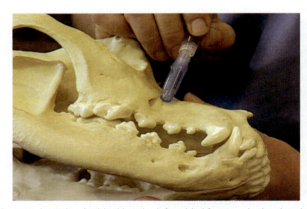

• **Fig. 29.4** Location for blocking the infraorbital foramen in the dog. Infraorbital foramina are the sites for injection to provide nerve block to the entire maxilla. The left and right foramen can be located easily just above the third premolar and about midway up the gum line.

To block the ulnar, median, and musculocutaneous nerves, keep the animal on its side, but this time, have the limb working downward. The ulnar, median, and musculocutaneous nerves are all on the inner side of the humerus. Locate the brachial artery's pulse between the biceps brachialis and the inner part of the triceps, roughly a third of the way up from the elbow. To block the ulnar and median nerves, inject the local anesthetic behind the artery after checking for any fluids in the needle (negative aspiration). For the musculocutaneous nerve, inject the local anesthetic in front of the brachial artery, again after ensuring no fluids are in the needle. Alternatively, a single injection behind the artery can be done to numb all three nerves.

Dental Nerve Blocks

The entire muzzle can be anesthetized by blocking the infraorbital and mandibular foramen. This relatively simple technique is effective for dental extractions, oral mass removal, fracture repair, mandibulectomy, maxillectomy, and nasal biopsy (Fig. 29.4). Lidocaine or bupivacaine can be used. Epinephrine can be added to reduce bleeding by coating the syringe with epinephrine before the local anesthetic is drawn up. The size of the foramen limits the volume of administration. Typically, about 0.5 mL per site is appropriate for a 50-lb dog, whereas about 0.1 mL per site is adequate for cats.

Pleural Space

Interpleural bupivacaine infusion after thoracotomy surgery may have some analgesic benefits. Bupivacaine (1.5–2 mg/kg) is injected via an indwelling chest tube into the pleural space. Analgesia is thought to occur by direct blocking of the intercostal nerves. For maximum coverage, patients are held in sternal recumbency for 5 to 10 minutes after injection and are gently rolled from side to side. Drug absorption through the pleural tissue should be considered.

Epidural Nerve Block

Injection of opioids (preservative-free morphine or fentanyl) and/or local anesthetics (lidocaine, bupivacaine) directly into the epidural space has been used to provide analgesia to the caudal half of the body while minimizing sedative effects. This is a reasonably simple and safe technique. An injection is generally performed at the lumbosacral space between L7 and S1. Epidural catheters can be inserted to allow long-term analgesic administration. Caudal epidurals, also known as sacrococcygeal blocks, are especially useful for felines undergoing urethral obstruction catheterization, canines or felines undergoing tail amputations, anal sac infections or surgeries, and perianal-urethrostomy patients.

Ultrasound-guided Blocks

Ultrasound-guided nerve blocks play a crucial role in veterinary medicine, especially for hind limb surgeries, where specific blocks such as femoral and sciatic nerve blocks are commonly employed. These blocks provide effective pain management and facilitate successful surgical procedures (Fig. 29.5).

Femoral and Sciatic Nerve Block. The femoral nerve block targets the femoral nerve, which supplies sensory innervation to the anterior thigh and motor innervation to the quadriceps muscle group. It is commonly used for surgeries involving the distal hind limb, such as stifle joint procedures or surgeries on the distal limb. Ultrasound imaging allows visualization of the femoral nerve and surrounding structures. After identification, the veterinarian inserts a needle near the nerve under continuous ultrasound guidance. A local anesthetic, such as lidocaine or bupivacaine, is injected to provide regional anesthesia to the femoral nerve, ensuring pain relief during the surgical procedure. The sciatic nerve block targets the sciatic nerve, which is the largest nerve in the hind limb. It provides sensory and motor innervation to the posterior thigh, lower leg, and foot. The sciatic nerve block is commonly used for surgeries involving hock, hind foot, or digit procedures.

Intravenous Analgesia

IV administration of lidocaine via CRI is an effective technique for managing a variety of pain states. At the cardiac dose of 25 to 50 µg/kg per minute, lidocaine provides analgesia for visceral pain (e.g., pancreatitis, parvovirus) and is a beneficial analgesic adjunct in procedures with extensive nerve damage, such as limb amputation. Lidocaine given via CRI can be administered as a sole agent or in conjunction with other analgesics.

> ### TECHNICIAN NOTE
> The addition of analgesics such as buprenorphine to local blocking agents may prolong the duration of postoperative analgesia and sensory blockade without an increase in side effects. In a study evaluating the effect of adding buprenorphine to bupivacaine in an infraorbital nerve block and its effects on the minimum alveolar concentration of isoflurane, the anesthetic requirement for patients that received the combination was less than that for patients that received bupivacaine alone.

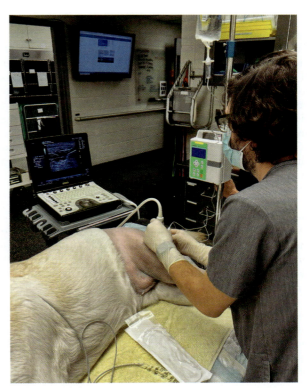

• **Fig. 29.5** Ultrasound-guided nerve block performed by a veterinary technician.

Opioids

Opioids are the most used analgesics in hospitalized patients because of their efficacy, rapid onset of action, and safety. The efficacy of various opioids is determined by the specific receptors in the brain and in the spinal cord that are affected by them. Receptors are classified as mu, kappa, and sigma receptors. Mu receptors are responsible for providing analgesia and feelings of euphoria. Kappa receptors are chiefly responsible for providing sedation. Sigma receptors are less clinically relevant and are thought to be responsible for the adverse effects of opioid administration, such as dysphoria, excitement, restlessness, and anxiety. Opioid drugs are classified as **agonists** (i.e., they stimulate the opioid receptors) or **antagonists** (i.e., they block specific opioid receptors). Also, mixed agonist-antagonist opioids stimulate some receptors while blocking others, and partial agonists cause partial stimulation of receptor sites. In general, pure agonists (working at all receptors) are the most potent of opioids, but they also cause the most severe adverse effects. Mixed agonist-antagonist and partial agonist opioids can provide reasonably good analgesia without many of the deleterious side effects of pure agonists. Side effects may include vomiting, constipation, excitement, respiratory depression, bradycardia, and panting. The type of opioid is chosen based on the degree of analgesia required and the specific needs or limitations of the individual patient. In the United States, the approved pure agonists used most often are morphine, hydromorphone, and fentanyl.

> ### TECHNICIAN NOTE
> Emesis (vomiting) is a common side effect of some opioids, particularly morphine and hydromorphone, and occurs most frequently when used as an intramuscular or subcutaneous premedication rather than as an analgesic in an animal already in pain.

Pure antagonists have the effect of reversing the narcotic properties of agonists. The availability of opioid antagonists makes opioid use extremely safe, because drug effects can be rapidly reversed. Opioids are metabolized by the liver and excreted via the kidneys and should be used with caution in patients with renal or hepatic disease. Opioids are most effective when administered before the onset of pain. As a class, these drugs produce minimal respiratory and cardiac side effects in animals, and any patient experiencing pain is a candidate for opioid analgesia.

Opioids can be administered through numerous routes, including IV, intramuscular (IM), SQ, transcutaneous, epidural, and oral routes, and via CRI. Opioids can be administered concurrently with other analgesics.

Severe Pain

Morphine Sulfate (Pure Opioid Agonist). Morphine is the gold standard for pure opioid agonists. All other drugs in this class are compared with morphine in terms of efficacy, duration of action, and cost. Morphine is commonly used to provide maximal analgesia and sedation. Its relatively low cost and excellent efficacy are the reasons that it is preferred over other opioids in some cases. However, morphine has additional side effects, particularly systemic hypotension and vomiting, which make it less desirable in many instances. Cats are particularly sensitive to morphine; therefore lower doses are used in cats. It is common for cats to experience hyperthermia resulting from the use of morphine. The typical dosage for dogs is 1.0 to 1.5 mg/kg given by the IV route every 4 to 6 hours. The dosage in cats is 0.25 to 1.0 mg/kg given via the SQ or IM route every 4 to 6 hours.

Hydromorphone (Pure Opioid Agonist). Hydromorphone has similar properties to morphine in terms of providing analgesia but appears to have fewer side effects. Specifically, hydromorphone is less likely than morphine to induce vomiting or hypotension. Elevated body temperature has been noted, especially in cats. This hyperthermia is usually self-limiting and transient. The typical dosage in dogs is 0.1 to 0.2 mg/kg given by the SQ or IM route and 0.03 to 0.1 mg/kg by the IV route. The dosage in cats is 0.05 to 0.1 mg/kg given via the SQ or IM route and 0.01 to 0.025 mg/kg by the IV route. The duration of action is 3 to 4 hours.

Fentanyl Citrate (Pure Opioid Agonist). Fentanyl is an extremely potent synthetic opioid with rapid onset but short duration of action when administered via the IV or IM routes. It is most efficaciously used as a CRI due to the short duration of action (approximately 20–30 minutes).

Moderate to Severe Pain

Buprenorphine (Buprenex) (Partial Mu Agonist). Buprenorphine, a partial mu agonist, has an effect of longer duration compared with morphine because of its slow dissociation from receptors, providing analgesia for approximately 6 to 8 hours. Partial agonists avidly bind and partially activate mu receptors. Buprenorphine is recommended for moderate pain in the dog and for moderate to severe pain in the cat given by the IV or IM routes. Additionally, buprenorphine is readily absorbed oral transmucosal (OTM) in felines due to the unique oral pH in this species. Buprenorphine is also absorbed by the OTM route in canines; however, the dosing needs to be adjusted and often increased due to first-pass metabolism. Transmucosal administration can provide analgesia for up to 8 hours from a single appropriate dose. Transmucosal buprenorphine has been the primary analgesic for take-home use in cats. It is extremely easy for owners to administer and provides analgesia of varying duration depending on the dose.

The dose for buprenorphine in dogs and cats is 0.02 to 0.06 mg/kg administered intramuscularly, intravenously, or transmucosal; however, higher doses are required for ongoing pain management. Simbadol (buprenorphine injection) is a higher concentration formulation of buprenorphine labeled specifically for use in cats; it is delivered by the SQ route at a dose of 0.24 mg/kg to provide 24 hours of continuous pain relief. Simbadol can be repeated for up to 3 consecutive days.

Mild Pain

Butorphanol Tartrate (Torbugesic) (Mixed Agonist-Antagonist). Butorphanol is a kappa agonist and a mu antagonist. As a kappa agonist, it is a mild analgesic with marked sedative properties. Whereas the sedative effects of butorphanol may last for 1 to 2 hours or longer, the effect of analgesia lasts only about 45 minutes—an important consideration for managing pain of any greater duration. As a mu antagonist, butorphanol can be used to reverse adverse events thought to be associated with mu opioid agonists, such as hydromorphone. The dosage is 0.2 to 0.8 mg/kg given by the SQ, IM, or IV route.

> ### TECHNICIAN NOTE
> Butorphanol should not be used as the sole analgesic unless mild pain of short duration (<1 hour) is expected.

Opioid Reversal

Naloxone Hydrochloride (Pure Opioid Antagonist). One of the reasons for the safety of opioids is the clinician's ability to rapidly reverse its sedation and adverse side effects. Antagonists work by blocking opioid action at the receptors. Onset of reversal occurs within 1 to 2 minutes of IV administration and can last for 1 to 4 hours. Treatment may be repeated when narcotics with a longer duration are reversed. The typical dosage is 2 µg/kg by the IV route.

Butorphanol Tartrate (Torbugesic) (Mu Antagonist). See the description in the section "Mild Pain."

α^2-Agonists

Xylazine and dexmedetomidine are α^2-agonists that have been widely used in veterinary medicine. Dexmedetomidine is the first premedication labeled for use as a sedative/analgesic in dogs and cats, and is the most potent and selective α^2-agonist available in the United States. α^2-agonists, which are nonnarcotic and nonscheduled (uncontrolled) agents, can be useful as adjuncts in a balanced analgesic protocol. The main effect is to produce significant sedation accompanied by visceral and somatic analgesia. This drug class can be used in a variety of ways as a premedication, for rough recovery rescue, and for ongoing management of in-hospital pain and anxiety. α^2-agonist combinations are also extremely effective in cats for a variety of surgical and nonsurgical procedures.

α^2-agonists inhibit the release of the excitatory **neurotransmitter** norepinephrine to produce analgesia and sedation. α^2-agonists are short-duration analgesics, and their effects can be rapidly reversed with alpha$_2$ antagonists. This characteristic makes these drugs suitable for procedures requiring short-term restraint and analgesia. α^2-agonists may bind to the same receptors as opioids and act synergistically with them. Dosages of other analgesic and anesthetic agents can be significantly reduced if given concurrently with α^2-agonists. α^2-agonists can have profound effects on the cardiovascular and nervous systems, but these adverse events can be minimized by using low dosages. Bradycardia and vomiting are the side effects most seen with α^2-agonists.

> ### TECHNICIAN NOTE
>
> α^2-agonists cause vasoconstriction—like constriction that occurs when a water hose is kinked—and the narrowing of blood vessels causes increased blood pressure or hypertension. Because heart rate normally goes up when blood pressure is low and goes down when blood pressure is high, slowed heart rate is expected. Bradycardia is considered a normal finding when α^2-agonists are used.

Advantages of α^2-Agonists Over Other Sedatives

Other commonly used sedatives (e.g., acepromazine, diazepam) do not provide pain relief. Analgesia achieved with α^2-agonists is of moderate intensity and moderate duration. Even more important, α^2-agonists work synergistically with opioids (e.g., butorphanol or morphine) and increase the duration of pain relief. Other advantages are that the degree of sedation can be "tailored" or "titrated" by using different dosages and/or different drug combinations to provide mild to profound sedation and that α^2-agonists are reversible. Atipamezole is most used to reverse the effects of dexmedetomidine. Atipamezole is the safest of all the reversal agents, because it works almost exclusively by simply displacing dexmedetomidine from the alpha$_2$ receptors so that nerve function can return to normal. After administration of atipamezole, patients usually awaken in about 5 to 10 minutes and can stand or walk within 10 minutes.

α^2-agonists are used in a variety of ways to provide patient comfort: for premedication before surgery, combined with an opioid; as a CRI for extremely anxious hospitalized patients; as an analgesic for short procedures, such as radiography; and as a rescue drug for patients experiencing rough recovery from anesthesia. α^2-agonists are most commonly used in cats in a combination called "kitty magic," which consists of an α^2-agonist, an opioid (most commonly buprenorphine), and ketamine. The addition of ketamine makes the combination a protocol for general anesthesia, rather than just a protocol for sedation. Minor surgical procedures can be performed after the administration of kitty magic, or kitty magic can be administered before a gas anesthetic for more advanced procedures. α^2-agonists can also be administered as a CRI for patients with continual anxiety or pain.

> ### TECHNICIAN NOTE
>
> Like any sedative, α^2-agonists work best when they are administered to an animal that is not overly agitated or anxious. Agitated patients should be placed in a quiet place for 15 minutes after administration to allow the drug to take effect. Handling, loud noises, or any other sudden stimuli may cause a startle reaction, even if the animal is sedated. Caution should be used, especially around the animal's head and neck, to avoid being bitten.

Dexmedetomidine has been extensively used and valued as a "rescue" drug for patients that are experiencing rough recovery after anesthesia. Excitement in recovery (sometimes called *emergence delirium*) is not appropriate, whether it is caused by pain or by residual effects of anesthesia, because both cause tremendous physiologic stress and side effects that include tachycardia (high heart rate); hypertension (high blood pressure); cardiac arrhythmias (abnormal electrical activity of the heart); ventilation abnormalities (e.g., increased respiratory rate [i.e., tachypnea] with

> ### • BOX 29.4 Calculating Constant Rate Infusions
>
> Step 1. Set up the equation based on dosage: µg/kg per minute = µg to add to bag
>
> Step 2. Replace hash marks with times signs: µg × kg × minutes = µg to add to bag
>
> Step 3. Enter known information: dose and weight
>
> Step 4. Solve for hours: fluid bag size ÷ hourly rate = # hours bag will last
>
> Step 5. Solve for minutes: # hours above × 60 minutes/hour
>
> Step 6. Solve equation: µg × kg × minutes = µg to add to bag
>
> Step 7. Convert µg to mg; divide answer by 1000
>
> Step 8. Calculate drug volume and add to bag desired: mg ÷ concentration in mg/mL = mL
>
> A controlled rate infusion pump is required, because the rate of drug delivery must be precisely controlled. This can be a syringe pump, a cassette pump, or a rotary pump.

decreased volume of breaths [i.e., tidal volume]); cortisol release (which impairs proper healing); and a predisposition to GI ileus and ulceration. Dexmedetomidine is an excellent choice (in heart-healthy patients), because it provides both sedation and analgesia. Patients who require repeated rescue doses of dexmedetomidine can be administered the sedative via low-dose CRI for continued sedation and analgesia.

Constant Rate Infusions

CRIs allow continuous low-dose administration of various analgesics. Optimally, a CRI is established before tissue damage occurs (i.e., preoperatively) and is run for 6 to 12 hours postoperatively. CRI analgesia is also effective in the management of hospitalized patients with pre-existing or persistent medical pain. Many agents can be delivered, but this method is most commonly used with local anesthetics (lidocaine), opioids (morphine or fentanyl), NMDA antagonists (ketamine), and α^2-agonists (e.g., dexmedetomidine [Dexdomitor]). These drugs can be used as single agents or in combination with one another. Technicians should be adept at calculations for a CRI (Box 29.4). (For further discussion of CRI calculations, see Chapter 28, "Pharmacology and Pharmacy.")

Drugs Commonly Administered via CRI

The main advantage of giving opioids via a CRI is that it prevents the peaks and valleys typically seen with opioid bolus dosing. A lower dose of opioids can be used in a CRI; this can reduce unwanted side effects, such as dysphoria or panting. As a very cost-effective analgesia plan, morphine given via CRI is useful for managing any severe pain and can be safely combined with ketamine and/or lidocaine. The CRI dose for morphine in dogs is 0.2 to 0.5 mg/kg *slow* IV loading bolus, followed by 0.1 to 0.3 mg/kg per hour CRI.

Fentanyl is a full opioid agonist with properties like those of morphine. The main advantage of fentanyl over morphine is its rapid onset of action and short half-life, which allows for rapid cessation of unwanted side effects. The CRI dose for fentanyl in dogs is 2 to 5 µg/kg IV loading dose, followed by 5 to 20 µg/kg per hour CRI intraoperatively; for cats, the dose is 1 to 2 µg/kg IV loading dose, followed by 5 to 20 µg/kg per hour CRI.

Lidocaine is a local anesthetic that provides excellent systemic analgesia when delivered intravenously. Because it is safe for use in patients with GI disturbances, lidocaine is a good choice for analgesia in patients with gastric dilatation-volvulus, pancreatitis, or similar disorders. Lidocaine seems to also benefit patients undergoing procedures with excessive nerve trauma, such as complicated back surgeries or limb amputations. IV lidocaine is extremely short acting and can be discontinued without residual effect almost immediately. Lidocaine CRI should be discontinued if the patient shows signs of toxicity, including muscle tremors, seizures, nausea, or vomiting. The CRI dose for lidocaine in dogs is 1 to 2 mg/kg IV, followed by 30 to 50 µg/kg per minute. Lidocaine CRI dosages have been reported for cats but typically, lidocaine is not recommended for use in cats because of the potential for severe cardiotoxic effects.

Ketamine at CRI dosing is an NMDA receptor antagonist and, as such, is used to reverse or prevent wind-up phenomenon, which causes stimulation of NMDA receptors in the spinal cord. Wind-up will be most evident in the postoperative period once the patient has regained consciousness. However, ketamine, as an NMDA receptor antagonist given as an intraoperative CRI, binds at these CNS receptors and prevents wind-up. Ketamine should always be given in combination with other analgesics and can be delivered in the same infusion. The CRI dosage for ketamine in dogs and cats is 0.5 mg/kg IV loading bolus, followed by 10 µg/kg per minute CRI during surgery and 2 µg/kg per minute for 24 hours after surgery.

Morphine-Lidocaine-Ketamine Combination

The morphine-lidocaine-ketamine (MLK) infusion combines an opioid (morphine), a local anesthetic (lidocaine), and ketamine to provide optimal analgesia and to treat wind-up. The recipe for MLK is shown in Table 29.3.

Dexmedetomidine

CRI of dexmedetomidine is commonly used in human patients, including children who are agitated in the hospital, resistant to ventilators, or in narcotic withdrawal. Similar success has been reported in veterinary patients, particularly in breeds prone to anxiety. The CRI dose for continued dysphoria, anxiety, or pain in dogs and cats is 1 to 3 µg/kg per hour. Dexmedetomidine (Dexdomitor) can be added to CRI of other drugs, including MLK.

Neuropathic Pain Relievers

Gabapentin (an anticonvulsant) plays an important role in reducing neuropathic pain and central sensitization. Gabapentin is increasingly popular in both human and veterinary medicine as the first choice in patients whose pain does not respond to conventional therapies, especially when nerve involvement or neuropathic pain is suspected. Indications for initiating gabapentin therapy include the following:

- Chronic degenerative conditions, such as osteoarthritis and cancer
- Dermatologic conditions, such as lick granuloma and chronic skin or ear infection
- Persistent biting, licking, chewing, and scratching of body areas
- Resistance to being touched at unaffected body sites
- Limping or obvious signs of pain not associated with current inflammation

A typical starting dose is 10 mg/kg orally two to three times per day in dogs and 5 mg/kg two to three times per day in cats. Patients should be re-evaluated for response frequently, with dose adjustments made every 5 to 7 days until full efficacy is reached. Sleepiness is the side effect most reported at higher doses. Gabapentin should not be stopped abruptly; patients should be weaned

TABLE 29.3	Recipe for Morphine-Lidocaine-Ketamine (MLK)	
Amount of Each Drug Added to a 500-mL Bag of Lactated Ringer Solution	**Rate at Which Each Drug Is Infused, Provided Fluids Are Administered at a Rate of 10 mL/kg Per Hour**
10 mg morphine (0.66 mL)	Morphine 0.2 mg/kg per hour
120 mg lidocaine (6 mL 2%)	Lidocaine 2.5 mg/kg per hour
100 mg ketamine (1 mL)	Ketamine 2 mg/kg per hour

off. *Caution:* Neurontin elixir contains xylitol and can be used in cats but is not recommended for use in dogs.

Nonpharmacologic Treatment Options

When possible, multimodal therapy that includes both pharmacologic and nonpharmacologic modalities should be used to treat pain, whether acute or chronic. Nonpharmacologic options include thermotherapy, massage, therapeutic exercise, aquatic therapy, acupuncture, electrical stimulation, therapeutic ultrasonography, extracorporeal shock wave therapy, and low-level laser, among others. Many of these modalities (e.g., acupuncture) provide direct pain relief; others (e.g., many therapeutic exercises) are associated with pain relief secondary to improved function and strength. (See Chapter 23, "Rehabilitation and Alternative Medical Nursing," for more detailed information about these treatment options.)

Case Presentations 29.1, 29.2, and 29.3 provide examples of analgesic protocols designed to manage pain associated with feline fracture repair, canine ovariohysterectomy with tooth extraction, and surgical repair of a herniated disk in dogs, respectively.

Treatment of Pain in Large Animals

Large animal pain management has many challenges. Although it is not known exactly how many large animal patients receive analgesia in the United States, a survey of Canadian veterinarians has provided some insight into just how few horses, steers, and piglets receive analgesic drugs. According to the survey results, for routine procedures such as castration in patients younger than 6 months, only 0.001% of piglets, 6.9% of beef calves, and 18.7% of dairy calves received pain medication. Analgesia improved slightly in older patients, among which 19.9% of beef calves and 33.2% of dairy calves older than 6 months received some analgesic drugs. In horses, 95.8% of patients received analgesics for castration, and more than 90% of veterinarians used analgesic drugs for other equine surgery, for cesarean section in sows and cows, and for bovine claw amputation and *omentopexy* (suture of the greater omentum to the abdominal wall to induce collateral portal circulation). However, even when analgesia was provided, it was often inadequate. In most cases, a single agent was used to treat levels of pain that would have required multimodal analgesia for adequate pain control, and often, that agent was a drug with a short duration of action.

Identifying and Anticipating Pain

Why is pain in large animals so grossly undertreated? Fortunately, because of the similarities among all animals, we can use our existing knowledge about small animals, combined with knowledge of species-specific treatment and economic perceptions of

CASE PRESENTATION 29.1

Feline Fracture Repair

An 8-lb, 3-year-old spayed female Siamese cat is seen for a distal radius/ulna fracture after an unknown trauma. Surgical repair of the fracture is recommended by the clinician. Pain is expected to be severe immediately after surgery and for 5 to 7 days postoperatively. How would you design an analgesic protocol that provides maximum pre-emptive, multimodal, and take-home analgesia for this cat?

Pre-emptive Pain Management

- Give one dose of nonsteroidal anti-inflammatory drug (NSAID) subcutaneously (SQ) 1 to 2 hours before surgery.
- Administer 0.02 to 0.03 mg/kg buprenorphine combined with 3-5 μg/kg dexmedetomidine intramuscular (IM) with sedation 30 to 45 minutes before anesthesia.
- Perform RUMM block with bupivacaine and allow 15 minutes to onset of action.
- If possible, place Nocita at the time of closure to provide long-lasting local anesthetic.

Postoperative Pain Management

- Administer subsequent doses of buprenorphine transmucosal every 6 to 8 hours or Simbadol (buprenorphine injection) SQ every 24 hours until discharge.

Take-Home Pain Management

- Dispense buprenorphine to be given every 8 hours transmucosal by owners for 3 days, or administer Simbadol SQ every 24 hours, up to three doses.
- Re-evaluate on day four and continue buprenorphine as needed. NSAID may be repeated at this time if deemed necessary.
- Administer gabapentin for 2 to 4 weeks, tapering off to prevent neuropathic pain.

CASE PRESENTATION 29.2

Canine Ovariohysterectomy (Spay) and Tooth Extraction

A 2-year-old Golden Retriever is being spayed, but physical examination reveals a fractured premolar tooth that needs to be removed while the dog is under general anesthesia. What analgesia do you think would be appropriate for these two procedures?

Pre-emptive Pain Management

- Give a nonsteroidal anti-inflammatory drug (NSAID) subcutaneous (SQ) 1 to 2 hours before surgery.
- Administer a premedication combination of a strong opioid, such as hydromorphone, combined with an α²-agonist for sedation and analgesia about 15 minutes before induction.
- Perform an infraorbital nerve block on the affected maxillary side by using approximately 0.5 mL of 0.5% bupivacaine.

Postoperative Pain Management

- Administer additional doses of hydromorphone every 6 hours for 12 to 24 hours or more frequently if dictated by pain scoring systems.
- Can change to buprenorphine for its longer-lasting effects (6 to 8 hours) in the evening if personnel are unavailable to assess during the night.

Take-Home Pain Management

- Continue once-daily NSAIDs for 3 to 5 days postoperatively (longer if indicated).

CASE PRESENTATION 29.3

Surgical Repair of Herniated Disk

A 9-year-old neutered male Dachshund has acute lameness progressing within several hours to inability to walk. Owners report that the dog has been walking "funny" for several weeks. After magnetic resonance imaging (MRI) confirms a herniated disk, surgery is scheduled to be performed immediately. How do you think this dog's pain should be managed before, during, and after surgery?

Before Surgery

- The dog is started on steroids immediately and therefore should *not* receive additional nonsteroidal anti-inflammatory drugs (NSAIDs).
- Fentanyl-lidocaine-ketamine (FLK) continuous rate infusion (CRI) is started to treat existing pain and prevent the wind-up phenomenon.

During Surgery

- Continue FLK infusion throughout the surgery.

Postoperative Pain Management

- FLK infusion is continued for 12 to 24 hours postoperatively.
- Steroids are continued.
- Pain scoring on regular intervals to reassess pain plan.

Take-Home Pain Management

- Send home on once-daily NSAIDs for several weeks.
- After 2 weeks, the dog can walk and does not appear to be in pain but is chewing persistently at his left hind toes. What could be added to treat this assumed nerve pain?
- Gabapentin is added, and the signs resolve in 3 days. Gabapentin is continued for 2 to 4 weeks, tapering off slowly to not cause rebound pain.

veterinarians and producers, to educate our colleagues in large animal veterinary practice. Here are the main reasons why pain in large animals is not adequately addressed:

1. *"Animals don't feel pain."* As in the case of pain in small animals, this perception is false. All mammals have a similar pain pathway, so if a procedure or injury would be painful to humans, it will be painful to other mammals, including large animals.
2. *"Animals don't show pain."* It is instinctual for an animal to not show pain unless it is in so much discomfort that it can no longer hide its distress. It must be remembered that most farm animals are "prey" animals and, in their world, the weakest member of the herd might become a meal for a "predator." It is in their best interests to be stoic. Thus each patient should be treated based on anticipated pain intensity and should not be forced to prove that it is in pain.
3. *"A limited number of analgesic drugs are available for farm animals."* This, also often true, is absolutely no excuse for not treating pain. The analgesic drug classes that are available in small animal medicine (NSAIDs, opioids, local anesthetic agents, α²-agonists, etc.) are also available in large animal medicine. However, it is true that some species differences have been reported in how patients respond to a drug (e.g., horses can get excited after opioid administration) and in how drugs are "handled" in the body (e.g., orally administered drugs may be inactivated in the rumen). However, effective drugs are available for each species; they are discussed in the section "Species-Specific Information" later in the chapter.

4. *"Owners or producers will not pay for analgesia."* This may be true if it is allowed to be true. It is not true of most horse owners, and this is reflected by the large percentage of veterinarians in the Canadian study who reported providing at least some analgesia for their equine patients. However, most farm animals have an absolute economic value (which is generally low), and the value to the producer is in the herd rather than in each individual animal; thus medical care for the individual animal is not a priority, and pain relief falls in this category. However, to counter that argument, many analgesic drugs (e.g., lidocaine) are inexpensive and can be used without significant additional costs. Furthermore, the stress of pain causes decreased food intake, weight loss, decreased milk production, and other side effects, which can be expensive for the producer. (Additional information on this topic is provided in the section "Cattle, Sheep, and Goats" of this chapter.)

In a few instances, pain management in large animal medicine might be slightly ahead of that in small animal medicine. For instance, practitioners of equine medicine are extremely comfortable with the use of NSAIDs for the treatment of acute and chronic musculoskeletal pain and with the use of α^2-agonists to control acute abdominal pain (or colic). Of course, this perceived comfort level with analgesics sometimes stems from factors other than concern about the welfare of the patient. As an example, NSAIDs are administered, because lame horses are not highly functional and certainly will not perform well if they are to be placed in competition. Colic pain is treated because severe GI pain can make horses extremely violent and dangerous to humans. Whatever the reason for administering analgesic agents may be, the benefit to the patient is the same. Veterinarians and veterinary technicians should continue to stress the message that large animals do indeed feel pain and that pain must be treated in all animals (Fig. 29.6).

> ### TECHNICIAN NOTE
>
> All mammals, including large animals, have a similar pain pathway and do experience pain, although they may not show signs of pain. Pain causes deleterious effects (e.g., hypertension, arrhythmias, gastrointestinal [GI] ulceration, ileus, delayed healing) and should be treated based on what the anticipated pain level would be after a painful stimulus—not based on what the patient exhibits.

Identifying pain in large animals can be extremely difficult, because these animals, which evolved in a prey-predator society, are in the "prey" group. This means that they instinctively hide weakness (and pain is a weakness) to survive. However, because the pain pathway is similar in all mammals, the phrase "If it hurts you, it hurts them" is appropriate in determining if a patient might be in pain, whether the patient shows pain or not. Unfortunately, as with small animals, the negative effects of pain (see Box 29.1) happen any time pain occurs and can be detrimental to the patient, including causing delayed healing. Treatment of pain is not just an ethical issue—it is also a medical issue. Species-specific signs of pain are listed in Box 29.5.

Furthermore, because these animals often do not show pain until it is too severe to be hidden, the sequelae of pain may well be advanced by the time it is realized that the patient is in pain. The degree of pain in the patient should be anticipated and analgesia administered based on that expectation rather than based on demonstration of pain.

Treating Pain in Large Animals

All the analgesic drug classes used to treat small animals can be used to treat large animals, but fewer FDA-approved drugs for

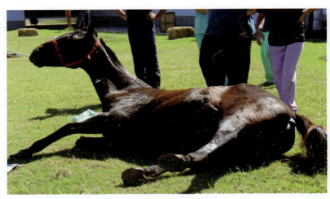

• **Fig. 29.6** Painful horse rolling. Horses occasionally will roll in the pasture, presumably as a way to scratch an itchy back. However, horses that are rolling and thrashing violently and repeatedly are generally in pain, and the source of the pain is almost always the GI tract. This degree of pain requires immediate attention.

• **BOX 29.5** **Signs of Pain in Horses and Farm Animals**

General Signs of Pain
Decreased interest in food or anorexia
Lethargy
Excitement, restlessness
Pawing
Vocalizing (especially cattle)
Bruxism
Reluctance to move
Lying down more frequently or for longer periods than usual
Any abnormal behavior

Additional Signs of Gastrointestinal (GI) Pain
Kicking at or looking at abdomen
Violently trying to roll
Stretching out in abnormal posture (especially horses)
Standing with abdomen "tucked" (especially cattle)
"Dog sitting" (especially foals with GI pain)

Additional Signs of Musculoskeletal Pain
Lameness
Abnormal gait
Positive response to hoof testers or flexion tests

Other Signs of Pain (Horses Only)
Reluctance to be bridled (may be head or tooth pain)
Reluctance to be saddled (may be back pain)
Reluctance to be ridden (may be back pain, lameness, or general pain)

---

large animal species are available and, in general, less is known about the use of these drugs (Box 29.6). However, affordable, effective analgesic drugs are available for all species.

The principles of pain management include use of the following:
1. Pre-emptive analgesia (for surgical pain)
2. Multimodal analgesia (any time pain is moderate to severe)
3. Analgesia of a duration that covers the entire painful period (this applies to both acute and chronic pain)
4. Regardless of which analgesic drugs are chosen for the patient, these principles should be addressed every time an analgesic protocol is formulated. Drug classes that can be used in large animal analgesic protocols are listed in Tables 29.4 and 29.5.

The US Food and Drug Administration (FDA) approval of a drug for use in a particular species is gained only after a rigorous amount of research has proved that the drug is both safe and effective in that species. Thus FDA approval guarantees that the drug has been studied in the target species. However, many "off-label," or non–FDA-approved, drugs are used when no approved drug is available for treatment or when non–FDA-approved drugs may be more effective or safer than approved drugs. FDA-approved drugs may also be used in a non–FDA-approved way (e.g., dexmedetomidine is approved for use in dogs but not as a premedication to anesthesia, yet it is commonly used this way) or at a non–FDA-approved dose (e.g., the dose of xylazine used clinically in horses is generally lower than the FDA-approved dose). Not all of the products mentioned in this chapter are FDA approved, but all are commonly used in veterinary practice, and all can be referenced in the veterinary literature.

PUT INTO PRACTICE

As an advocate for your large animal patients, you can discuss with your veterinarian the need for pre-emptive and postop analgesia for any patient that will be having surgery.

Nonsteroidal Anti-inflammatory Drugs

NSAIDs are an ideal choice for most painful conditions because of their anti-inflammatory and analgesic properties. Thus any time pain is caused by inflammation, NSAIDs can treat the source of pain and the pain itself (Fig. 29.7). NSAIDs are relatively safe, easy to administer, inexpensive, and have a long-lasting effect (12–24 hours). Because of their long duration of action, NSAIDs are ideal for pairing with more potent but short-acting drugs, such as opioids and α²-agonists. Depending on which drug is chosen, NSAIDs can be administered via the IV, IM, SQ, per os (PO), or transdermal route. The most commonly used NSAIDs in large animals are phenylbutazone ("bute") and flunixin meglumine (Banamine), but other NSAIDs are also available (Tables 29.4 and 29.5). In large animals, the primary side effect of NSAID use is GI ulceration.

TECHNICIAN NOTE

The most common side effect associated with nonsteroidal anti-inflammatory drug (NSAID) use in all species is gastrointestinal (GI) upset or ulceration; large animals are more likely to experience ulceration. Patients with GI ulceration tend to stop eating and appear lethargic. Pain may cause animals to stand with their backs "hunched" (especially ruminants) or to stretch out in abnormal postures (especially horses). Adult horses often grind their teeth when they are in pain, and foals may "dog sit" when they have stomach pain. Anorexia, lethargy, and/or abnormal behavior in any patient that is on therapy should prompt immediate evaluation of the patient and assessment for possible drug side effects.

Opioids

Opioids are the most potent class of analgesic drugs and should be used to treat all cases of moderate to severe pain, especially acute pain. The opioid most used in large animals is butorphanol, but morphine, buprenorphine, and fentanyl are also used. Although rare in patients with pain, opioids may cause excitement in horses and pigs without pain. Thus opioids are generally administered with a sedative (e.g., xylazine, romifidine, detomidine) in these species. Cattle, sheep, and goats generally become lightly sedated with opioids but may exhibit behavioral changes such as restlessness and vocalization. Camelids are sensitive to the sedating properties of opioids. Opioids can be administered via the IV, IM, SQ, transdermal, epidural, and intra-articular routes and via CRI. Opioids are used primarily for acute medical or surgical pain. Other than butorphanol, opioid administration in large animals has been uncommon. However, use of morphine is increasing.

α²-Agonists

α²-agonists, such as detomidine, xylazine, and romifidine, are used more commonly in large animals than in small animals. Although these agents are generally considered sedatives, they provide moderate pain relief. α²-agonists are often combined with opioids (primarily butorphanol) for improved sedation and enhanced analgesia in patients that are experiencing acute pain (e.g., patients with colic) and patients that will undergo minor procedures (e.g., wound repair). The dosage of α²-agonists is highly variable among species, because the response to α²-agonists is highly variable. Ataxia secondary to profound sedation is the most common side effect of this class of drugs in large animals. The decrease in heart rate that often follows administration of α²-agonists is rarely a matter of concern, because it is a normal physiologic response to increased blood pressure caused by α²-agonist–mediated vasoconstriction.

TECHNICIAN NOTE

There is a wide variation between species in the sedation dose of α²-agonists. Pigs are most resistant and require high dosages for sedation. Horses are next in sensitivity and require moderately high dosages. Cattle, sheep, and goats are the most sensitive, and all of these species require approximately one-tenth of the equine dose. Dose sensitivity of camelids falls between those of horses and ruminants.

Local Anesthetic Drugs

Local anesthetic drugs are some of the most effective, least expensive, and yet underused analgesic drugs available. Local anesthetic drugs are ideal for pain control in all species, because they block the transmission of painful impulses without causing systemic effects. Lidocaine, bupivacaine, and mepivacaine (or Carbocaine) are used locally in large animals, and lidocaine can be administered intravenously as a CRI. Mepivacaine is often chosen for diagnostic nerve blocks, because it has an intermediate duration of action between lidocaine and bupivacaine (Fig. 29.8). For true analgesia (i.e., blocking nerves to control the pain of laminitis), longer-lasting drugs, such as bupivacaine, should be used. Lidocaine CRI is commonly used to control intraoperative and postoperative pain, especially GI pain in horses.

Miscellaneous Agents

Ketamine

Ketamine is an NMDA receptor antagonist that is given as a CRI to treat the pain of "wind-up" (see the section "Neuropathic Pain and Wind-up Phenomenon"). Ketamine CRIs can be added to multimodal analgesic protocols in patients experiencing pain that is difficult to control. Ketamine CRIs have been shown to be useful in a variety of large animal species, including horses and llamas.

Antispasmodic Agents

Antispasmodic agents (e.g., hyoscine butyl bromide [Buscopan]) are frequently administered as part of a multimodal plan in the initial treatment phases of colic in horses.

TABLE 29.4   Analgesic Drug Dosages for Horses

Drug Class/Drug	Dose (mg/kg unless stated)	Route	Dosing Interval	Comments
NSAIDs				
Phenylbutazone	2–4	PO, IV	q12h	FDA approved for use in horses; reduce dose to 2 mg/kg on second day; used most commonly for musculoskeletal pain
Flunixin meglumine	1	PO, IV, IM	q12h or q24h	FDA approved for use in horses; used most commonly for GI pain and treatment of endotoxemia
Ketoprofen	2–3	IV	q24h	FDA approved for use in horses
Firocoxib	0.1	PO	q24h	FDA approved for use for up to 14 days for control of pain and inflammation associated with equine osteoarthritis
Diclofenac sodium	5-inch ribbon of cream	Topical, over painful joint	q12h	FDA approved for treatment of joint pain and inflammation for up to 10 days
Carprofen	0.7	IV	q24h	Approved for horses in countries other than the United States
Meloxicam	0.6	IV	q12h	Approved for horses in countries other than the United States
Opioids				
Morphine	0.1–0.3	IV	q3–4h	Inject slowly if administered IV; horses may have excitatory response
	0.1–0.2	Epidural	q24h	qs to 10–30 mL with sterile saline
	0.1	Intra-articular	Once, intraoperative	
Butorphanol	0.02–0.1	IM, IV	q2–3h	FDA approved for relief of pain associated with colic at 0.1 mg/kg; ataxia associated with label dose; lower dosages are generally used clinically
	23.7 µg/kg per minute (0.013 mg/kg per hour)	IV	CRI	Loading dose 0.02 mg/kg
Fentanyl	Two of the 100-µg patches/450 kg	Transdermal	Change patches at 48 hours	Can be used without sedation—no excitement noted
Buprenorphine	0.004–0.006	IV, IM, SQ		
Tramadol	2	IV		Analgesic effects unknown
α²-Agonists				
Detomidine	0.01–0.02	IV	q2–4h	FDA approved as a sedative-analgesic
	0.02–0.04	IM		
	0.06	PO		
	0.15–0.3 µg/kg per minute	IV	CRI	Loading dose 6–10 µg/kg; adjust CRI to achieve desired sedation
Romifidine	0.04–0.120	IM, IV	q2–4h	FDA approved as sedative-analgesic and as a preanesthetic
Xylazine	0.5–1.0	IV	q2–4h	FDA approved as a sedative-analgesic
	1.0–2.2	IM		
	0.17	Epidural		Generally added to lidocaine
Medetomidine	0.005–0.007	IV	q2–4h	Loading dose 5 µg/kg
	3–5 µg/kg per hour	IV	CRI	
Local Anesthetic Drugs				
Lidocaine	As needed for tissue infiltration; total dose <5 mg/kg	Tissue		
	50 µg/kg per hour	IV	CRI	Intraoperative or postoperative or for medical pain
	0.35	Epidural		May be combined with morphine or xylazine
	0.35	Intra-articular		

TABLE 29.4 Analgesic Drug Dosages for Horses—cont'd

Drug Class/Drug	Dose (mg/kg unless stated)	Route	Dosing Interval	Comments
Bupivacaine	As needed for tissue infiltration; total dose 2 mg/kg			Longer duration of action than lidocaine; can also be used for epidural and intra-articular administration
Mepivacaine	2–15 mL	Tissue		FDA approved for use in horses; dosages are from label
	5–20 mL	Epidural		
	10–15 mL	Intra-articular		
Joint Supplements and Chondroprotective Agents[a]				
Sodium hyaluronate	10–40 mg/joint	Intra-articular	Every 7 days	
Polysulfated GAGs	250 mg/joint	Intra-articular	Every 7 days	
	500 mg	IM	Every 5 days	
Other Agents				
Ketamine	40 µg/kg per minute	IV	CRI	FDA approved for one-time injection for spasmodic, flatulent, or impaction colic in horses; administer slowly
Antispasmodic agents (hyoscine butylbromide [Buscopan])	0.3	IV	One dose	

[a]Numerous products are included in this category, and two examples are listed here. Use of these products should be governed by proven efficacy.

CRI, Constant rate infusion; *FDA,* US Food and Drug Administration; *GAGs,* glycosaminoglycans; *IM,* intramuscular; *IV,* intravenous; *NSAIDs,* nonsteroidal anti-inflammatory drugs; *PO,* oral; *q2–3h,* every 2 to 3 hours; *q2–4h,* every 2 to 4 hours; *q3–4h,* every 3 to 4 hours; *q12h,* every 12 hours; *q24h,* every 24 hours; *qs,* as sufficient; *SQ,* subcutaneous.

TABLE 29.5 Analgesic Drug Dosages for Farm Animals (Cattle, Sheep, Goats, and Pigs) and Camelids

Drug Class/Drug	Species	Dose (mg/kg unless stated)	Route	Dosing Interval	Comments
NSAIDs					
Phenylbutazone	All	4–6	PO	q24–48h	Prohibited in dairy cattle older than 20 months of age
		2–4	IV		
Flunixin meglumine	All	1	PO, IV, IM	q12–24h	FDA approved in some species; withdrawal times are published
Ketoprofen	All	2–3	PO, IV, IM, SQ	q24h	Widely used because of low cost, but absorption may be erratic
Aspirin	Cattle, sheep, goat	100	PO	q12h	
Carprofen	All	0.7	IV	q24–48h	
Meloxicam	Cattle	0.5 mg/kg	SQ, IV	q24h	
	Pig	0.4 mg/kg	IM	q24h	
Opioids					
Morphine	All	0.05–0.1	IV	q3–4h	Inject slowly if administered intravenously. May cause excitement, especially in pigs
		0.1–0.4	IM		
		0.1	Epidural		Commonly combined with local anesthetic agent
	All	0.1–0.2	Epidural	q6–12h	Dilute with 0.05 mL/kg sterile saline or combine with bupivacaine at 1.5 mg/kg
	All	0.1	Intra-articular	Once, intraoperative	

Continued

| TABLE 29.5 | Analgesic Drug Dosages for Farm Animals (Cattle, Sheep, Goats, and Pigs) and Camelids—cont'd |

Drug Class/Drug	Species	Dose (mg/kg unless stated)	Route	Dosing Interval	Comments
Butorphanol	All	0.01–0.2	IM, IV	q2–3h	Camelids are extremely sensitive to sedative properties
	Pig	0.2 mg/kg	IM, IV	q2–3h	
Fentanyl	Sheep, goat	50 µg/hour	Transdermal	48–72 hours	Dosage is for adult animals of the respective species
	Pig	50 µg/hour			
	Camelid	150–225 µg/hour			
Buprenorphine	Sheep, goat	0.015	IV, IM		Rarely causes sedation or excitement
	Pig	0.01	IV, IM		
	Camelid	0.01	IV, IM		
α²-Agonists[a]					
Detomidine	Cattle, sheep, goat	0.003–0.01	IM, IV	q2–4h	
	Pig	0.1	IM, IV	q2–4h	
Romifidine	Cattle, sheep, goat	0.003–0.005	IM, IV	q2–4h	
	Pig	0.1	IM, IV	q2–4h	
Xylazine	Cattle, sheep, goat	0.1–0.3	IM	q2–4h for all	Alpacas are more resistant than llamas and require a dose of 0.3–0.6 mg/kg by IV or IM route
	Camelid	0.05–0.1	IV		
	Pig	0.2–0.4	IV, IM		
		2.2–4.4	IM		
			Epidural		
Medetomidine	Camelid	0.01–0.03	IV, IM	q2–4h	
	Pig	0.08	IV, IM	q2–4h	
	Sheep, goat	0.004–0.01	IV, IM	q2–4h	
Dexmedetomidine	Camelid	0.005–0.015	IV, IM	q2–4h	
	Sheep, goat	0.002–0.005	IV, IM	q2–4h	
	Pig	0.04	IV, IM	q2–4h	
Local Anesthetic Agents					
Lidocaine	All	As needed for tissue infiltration; total dose, ≤5 mg/kg	Tissue	q1–3h	Goats sensitive to side effects—dose carefully
	All	0.2–0.4	Epidural	q1–3h	
	All	0.1	Intra-articular	q1–3h	
Bupivacaine	All	As needed for tissue infiltration; total dose, ≤2 mg/kg	Tissue	q4–6h	Goats sensitive to side effects—dose carefully; do not give intravenously

[a]α²-agonists cause profound sedation in ruminants and camelids, but pigs are fairly insensitive to α²-agonist–induced sedation.

FDA, US Food and Drug Administration; *IM*, intramuscular; *IV*, intravenous; *NSAIDs*, nonsteroidal anti-inflammatory drugs; *PO*, oral; *q1–3h*, every 1 to 3 hours; *q2–3h*, every 2 to 3 hours; *q2–4h*, every 2 to 4 hours; *q3–4h*, every 3 to 4 hours; *q4–6h*, every 4 to 6 hours; *q6–12h*, every 6 to 12 hours; *q12h*, every 12 hours; *q24h*, every 24 hours; *qs*, as sufficient; *SQ*, subcutaneous.

Joint Supplements and Chondroprotective Agents

Joint supplements and chondroprotective agents, such as nutraceuticals, chondroitin sulfate, hyaluronic acid, and glycosaminoglycans, are used more commonly in horses than in any other species, although they can be used in all the species mentioned in this chapter. These products generally are not truly analgesic agents, but they may help improve joint health, thereby decreasing pain. However, some may have an anti-inflammatory or other effect. These products are appropriate to add to a multimodal protocol (e.g., with NSAIDs) and sometimes are used alone for mild to moderate pain, especially in performance horses that cannot receive other pharmaceuticals because of drug administration

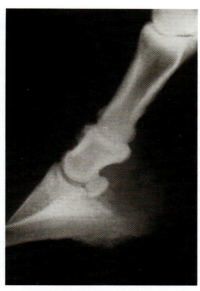

• **Fig. 29.7** Radiograph of the pastern joint of a horse with "high ringbone." This is a slowly progressive disease that causes mild to severe lameness (depending on the degree of the pathologic condition) that will limit the usefulness of the horse. Mild pain generally can be controlled with nonsteroidal anti-inflammatory drugs and light use, but more severe pain requires multimodal therapy.

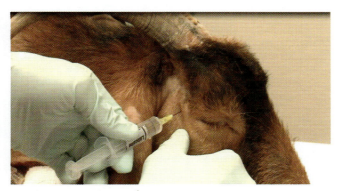

• **Fig. 29.8** Location for blocking the cornual branch of the zygomaticotemporal nerve in preparation for a dehorning procedure in a goat. In addition, the cornual branch of the infratrochlear nerve must also be blocked. It is important to note that both nerves must be blocked in goats, as opposed to cattle, in which only the cornual branch of the zygomaticotemporal nerve supplies the horns.

rules. Many products are included in this category. The choice of which one(s) to use should be based on proven efficacy of the product.

Most nutraceuticals and other feed additives are not regulated by the FDA; thus proof of their efficacy and safety based on research is not required by law. Reports of efficacy generally are anecdotal and are not backed by research. Furthermore, the true content of the product is not regulated, and some products have been shown to have a lower percentage of active ingredients than the percentage listed on the label. This does not mean that these products do not work. However, it means that only products that are shown to be safe and effective and those that come from reputable companies should be used.

Alternative and Complementary Therapy

Alternative and complementary therapy encompass many modalities, including acupuncture, spinal manipulative therapy, massage, low-level laser therapy, extracorporeal shock wave therapy, magnetic therapy, and many others (see Chapter 23, "Rehabilitation and Alternative Medical Nursing" for information on alternative treatment options). However, not all the alternative modalities have scientific credibility, and all treatment modalities should be carefully researched before they are endorsed. These treatments may be used for acute pain, but more commonly, they are added to a multimodal protocol for chronic pain or are used when pharmaceuticals are not allowed (e.g., in performance horses that will be drug tested).

Good Husbandry

Good husbandry and nursing care are always a major part of an effective pain management program. This includes not only attention to comfort, as in small animals, but also attention to species-specific details, such as proper shoeing in horses with foot and limb pain and proper udder care in lactating dairy cattle.

Species-Specific Information

Horses

Horses generally receive better analgesic treatment than is received by other large animals for several reasons:
1. Like dogs and cats, they are more likely to be treated as "companion animals."
2. Horses generally are performance animals, and pain can affect their performance.
3. Horses may become violent and dangerous when in acute pain—especially with GI pain.
4. Unlike cattle and pigs, most horses do not have an absolute economic value; thus the owners are more likely to spend money on care.

A greater number of analgesic agents have been researched in the horse; thus we have more information about how to use these drugs in this species. NSAIDs are the mainstay for both acute and chronic pain, and equine practitioners are often more apt than small animal practitioners to prescribe NSAIDs. Opioids are used with increasing frequency in horses. Morphine is a potent analgesic drug that is used intraoperatively as an IV injection or in the epidural or intra-articular space. Morphine is often used intramuscularly in patients with postoperative pain or in patients with chronic pain. When morphine is used parenterally in the horse, it is often combined with an α2-agonist or acepromazine to reduce the chance of an excitatory response. Butorphanol is the most commonly used opioid in horses; it is routinely combined with an α2-agonist for the treatment of acute pain. Buprenorphine, albeit somewhat expensive in adult horses, has been shown to provide analgesia and has a longer duration of analgesia compared with butorphanol. Fentanyl patches have been used in adult horses and in foals for acute pain; tramadol has been used in a few horses (with mixed success) for the control of chronic pain. Other agents that are routinely used in horses include chondroprotective agents for joint pain and antispasmodic agents for GI pain. Ketamine and lidocaine CRIs are used more and more commonly for treating intraoperative and postoperative pain and medical pain (e.g., nonsurgical colic). Local and regional types of blockades (e.g., epidurals, intra-articular blocks) are fairly standard treatments for pain in horses.

See Case Presentation 29.4 for an example of an analgesic protocol designed to manage pain associated with severe colic in a horse and Case Presentation 29.5 for an example of an analgesic protocol designed to manage pain associated with osteoarthritis in a horse.

TECHNICIAN NOTE

Do not be afraid to use potent opioids (e.g., morphine) in horses, especially for intraoperative and postoperative pain. These drugs are highly effective and inexpensive. However, like cats, horses may exhibit excitement after receiving a potent opioid, so a sedative (e.g., xylazine, romifidine, detomidine) should generally be administered at the same time. Excitement is rare in horses with pain but is common in horses that are not in pain.

Cattle, Sheep, and Goats

Except for animals kept as individual pets, valuable beef herd sires, and high-producing dairy cows, the least likely large animal patients to receive analgesia are food-producing herd animals, such as cattle, sheep, and goats. This is because these animals often have an absolute economic value with a narrow profit margin, and pharmaceutical residue in animal tissues is not generally accepted in the food industry. Some drugs are totally prohibited in this group of patients, whereas other drugs have a withdrawal time that must be considered between drug administration and the time that meat and/or milk can be used.

Drug Residues in Meat and Milk

Because drug residues in the food supply could be harmful to humans, there are strict regulations regarding the use of many pharmaceuticals in food-producing (meat and milk) animals. For instance, the use of phenylbutazone is completely prohibited in dairy cattle 20 months of age or older. However, some forms of flunixin meglumine (but not all brands) are approved for use in cattle and pigs, with withdrawal times of 72 hours for milk, 10 days for meat from cattle, and 12 days for meat from pigs. Because regulations change, people dealing with food-producing animals should routinely update withdrawal information on the drugs they are using. The best source for information is the Food Animal Residue Avoidance Databank at www.farad.org.

Finally, many food-producing animals are ruminants and delivery of an oral drug into the rumen can inactivate the drug, slow absorption, or otherwise alter the drug's action or the patient's response to the drug. Fortunately, most oral drugs that are available to treat pain can be used in ruminants; of course, IV, IM, SQ, transdermal, epidural, intra-articular, and local tissue infusion routes of administration can all be used as well.

TECHNICIAN NOTE

The latest guidelines for withdrawal times of drugs in food-producing animals can be obtained from the Food Animal Residue Avoidance Databank at www.farad.com.

All of the drug classes used in horses can be used in ruminants. The most used NSAIDs are phenylbutazone, flunixin meglumine, and aspirin. α^2-agonists are commonly used for acute pain, but because these species are extremely sensitive to the sedating effect of α^2-agonists, low dosages should be used. Butorphanol is also commonly used for acute pain, and morphine is used occasionally. Fentanyl patches, buprenorphine, and both ketamine and lidocaine CRIs have been used to control pain in small ruminants

---

CASE PRESENTATION 29.4

Severe Colic

Lightning, a 4-year-old Quarter Horse mare, was found 1 hour ago kicking at her abdomen and trying to lie down and roll. She appears to be in extreme pain and is being sent to a surgical referral center for colic surgery. How might the horse be made comfortable for the ride to the referral center?

ANSWER: Multimodal therapy is required for this degree of pain. Potent analgesic drugs that act quickly are the best choice. A combination of an α^2-agonist (xylazine, detomidine, and romifidine are all appropriate) and an opioid (most likely butorphanol) should be administered intravenously.

CASE CONTINUED: At the referral center, the surgeon decides to go to surgery immediately. What analgesic protocol would you expect to be recommended preoperatively and intraoperatively?

ANSWER: Pre-emptive multimodal analgesia is required. Some analgesia is most likely still present from the α^2-agonist–opioid combination; however, more α^2-agonist will be needed for induction of anesthesia, and the opioid will have to be repeated at induction or just before the surgeon makes an incision. IV morphine just before the incision would be an excellent choice, because it is a potent, long-lasting opioid. Although the previously administered butorphanol is an agonist-antagonist opioid and could potentially decrease the effectiveness of the pure opioid agonist morphine, butorphanol has a short duration, and any clinical effects are likely minimal within 1 to 2 hours. An NSAID should be administered if one was not given before arrival at the referral center. Continuous rate infusion (CRI) of lidocaine with or without ketamine could be administered intraoperatively.

CASE CONTINUED: The horse recovered well, but now, 6 hours after surgery, she seems a bit uncomfortable. What can be done postoperatively to control the pain?

ANSWER: Unless the horse is only mildly uncomfortable and would need only one dose of analgesic drugs, CRI is the best choice. Lidocaine, ketamine, or butorphanol (or a combination of two or three of these drugs) can be used. The best choice is probably lidocaine, because it is inexpensive, is not a controlled drug, and causes neither sedation nor excitement (unless overdosed). Ideally, in the attempt to anticipate pain rather than force the patient to show pain, CRI should have been started *before* the horse became uncomfortable. Multimodal analgesia will be required, so the horse should be continued on an NSAID (long duration and anti-inflammatory properties). Flunixin meglumine is the most used NSAID to treat colic pain.

CASE PRESENTATION 29.5

Osteoarthritis

Rajah, an 11-year-old Arabian mare, has been diagnosed with osteoarthritis of the pastern joint ("high ringbone"). The horse has been a competitive endurance horse, but its owner is willing to retire it. However, the owner still wants a "performance" horse, because she would like to do some light trail riding with Rajah. What might the veterinarian recommend to control chronic pain in this horse?

ANSWER: Nonsteroidal anti-inflammatory drugs (NSAIDs) will be the mainstay of treatment, because they will help control both the pain and the inflammation associated with this disease. Phenylbutazone is the most likely choice. Addition of nutraceuticals to the feed, intramuscular (IM) administration of glycosaminoglycans, and injection of hyaluronic acid with or without steroids directly into the joint are all excellent adjuncts to NSAIDs. Proper shoeing will also greatly benefit Rajah. An increased dose of NSAIDs may be needed immediately before and the day after long rides to keep Rajah comfortable and able to enjoy the trail.

Dehorning

Bucky, a 6-year-old Spanish goat, comes to your practice for dehorning. How will you manage his surgical pain?

ANSWER: For multimodal pre-emptive analgesia, sedate Bucky with an α^2-agonist (xylazine, medetomidine, dexmedetomidine, or romifidine would be a good choice) combined with butorphanol. Use bupivacaine to block the nerves to the horn and give one dose of flunixin or ketoprofen intravenously.

Bone Fracture

Willow, an 8-year-old adult female llama, has a fractured tibia and will be undergoing surgery today. How will you handle the pain associated with this surgery?

ANSWER: For pre-emptive multimodal analgesia, administer butorphanol and xylazine (or medetomidine, dexmedetomidine, or romifidine) as a premedication to anesthesia and give a dose of a nonsteroidal anti-inflammatory drug (NSAID) intravenously. Once the patient has been anesthetized, administer an epidural block of morphine and bupivacaine. For pain after the epidural wears off, there are three options: (1) place an epidural catheter (which is *easy* to do in large animals and one of the author's personal preferences for this case) and administer morphine twice daily for 2 to 3 days; (2) place a fentanyl patch for 72 hours of analgesia; or (3) keep Willow on a lidocaine-ketamine CRI (this is probably the least practical, because this patient will not likely be on fluids postoperatively). Whichever method is chosen, it should be combined with intravenous (IV) NSAIDs. Subsequently, the patient should be discharged from the hospital with instructions to the owner to give oral NSAIDs to Willow for 10 to 14 days.

such as sheep and goats; however, caution should be used with lidocaine to avoid overdose.

Analgesic techniques are not as common in adult cattle simply because treatment of pain in this group is not as common. By far the most used analgesic drugs in ruminants are local analgesic agents (primarily lidocaine and bupivacaine); techniques include local field blocks (tissue block at the site of surgery or injury), IV regional blocks, epidurals, paravertebral blocks, and cornual blocks, among others. For a description of these blocks and how to perform them, refer to the chapter "Ruminant and Swine Local and Regional Anesthetic and Analgesic Techniques" in *Lumb and Jones Veterinary Anesthesia and Analgesia* (see "Recommended Readings" in this chapter). See Case Presentation 29.6 for an example of an analgesic protocol designed to manage pain associated with dehorning a goat. Alternative and complementary techniques, such as acupuncture, are also appropriate for analgesia in ruminants.

TECHNICIAN NOTE

Local anesthetic agents are an excellent choice for analgesia in all ruminants. However, keep in mind that sheep and goats are easily overdosed, so drug dosages in these species must be calculated carefully.

Camelids

Camelids (e.g., llamas, alpacas) are more likely to receive analgesic treatment compared with cattle, sheep, and goats (but not as likely as horses), because use generally is constrained neither by an absolute economic value nor by entry into the human food chain. These animals have a GI tract similar to that found in ruminants, with a "third compartment" that functions like a rumen. Thus drug administration issues are the same in camelids as they are in ruminants, in which orally administered drugs may be inactivated. All drugs used in other ruminant species can be used in camelids. NSAIDs are generally the first treatment for both acute and chronic pain. α^2-agonists and butorphanol are used to treat acute pain, but these drugs cause profound sedation in camelids, so they are used only when sedation is appropriate. Other treatment modalities include fentanyl patches, lidocaine CRIs, ketamine CRIs, local or regional blockade, and alternative and complementary therapies, such as acupuncture.

See Case Presentation 29.7 for an example of an analgesic protocol designed to manage pain associated with surgery to repair a bone fracture in a llama.

Pigs

Lack of good pain management in swine practice rivals that in cattle practice, but high-producing boars and sows, along with

BOX 29.7 Summary of Veterinary Technicians' and Nurses' Responsibilities

Veterinary technicians and nurses typically are responsible for the following:
- Assessing patients
- Identifying (or predicting) pain
- Providing nonpharmacologic comfort and care
- Differentiating pain from other stress
- Requesting appropriate analgesia and/or sedation
- Helping to develop appropriate protocols for pain management
- Administering medications, performing analgesic techniques
- Monitoring and treating drug effects
- Assessing patients postoperatively
- Communicating with clients
- Logging controlled substances

pot-bellied pigs kept as pets, may receive more effective pain treatment. Like ruminants, pigs generally have an absolute economic value and are affected by their likely entry into the human food chain. All of the drugs discussed previously for use in other species can be used in pigs.

Summary

Providing effective pain management is not an individual endeavor. It requires a team approach involving everyone who participates in patient care. As true patient advocates, veterinary technicians and nurses constitute a vital force in this effort. A successful technician understands the goals of pain control and the analgesic options. Combining keen observation with good technical skills, the veterinary technician or nurse appropriately assesses pain and then requests and administers analgesics to their patients. Paying attention to environmental and emotional needs and differentiating other stress from pain is part of a technician's daily routine (Box 29.7). Veterinary technicians and nurses have played a vital role in bringing animal pain management to the forefront of veterinary practice. Through continued teaching and vigilant practice, technicians no doubt will be credited in large part with continuing improvements in the practice of veterinary pain management. Much work is still to be done, particularly in the arena of large animal practice. Although it is true that large animals hide pain (often even better than small animals), and some economic constraints and species-specific limitations have been applied in drug use or administration, it is not true that large animals do not feel pain. Pain management is often initiated by veterinary technicians or nurses, because they often spend the most time with patients and are most likely to recognize pain.

Recommended Readings

Bath GF. Management of pain in production animals. *Appl Anim Behav Sci*. 1998;59:147.

Benson GJ, Rollin BE, eds. *The Well-being of Farm Animals: Challenges and Solutions*. Ames, IA: Blackwell Publishing; 2004.

Bockstahler B, Levine D, Millis D. *Essential Facts of Physiotherapy in Dogs and Cats: Rehabilitation and Pain Management*. Höst, Germany: BE VetVerlag; 2004.

Chopra K, Arora V. An intricate relationship between pain and depression: Clinical correlates, coactivation factors and therapeutic targets. *Expert Opin Ther Targets*. 2014;18(2):159–176. https://doi.org/10.15 17/14728222.2014.855720.

Gowan RA, Baral RM, Lingard AE, et al. A retrospective analysis of the effects of meloxicam on the longevity of aged cats with and without overt chronic kidney disease. *J Feline Med Surg*. 2012;14(12):876–881.

Hewson CJ, Dohoo IR, Lemke KA, et al. Canadian veterinarians' use of analgesics in cattle, pigs, and horses in 2004 and 2005. *Can Vet J*. 2007;48:155.

Mama K, Hendrickson D. Pain management and anesthesia. *Vet Clin North Am Eq Pract*. 2002;18(1):xi–xii.

Robenacoxib approval EU: https://eee.ema.europa.eu/en/medicines/veterinary/EPAR/onsior.

Sparkes AH, Heiene R, Lascelles BD, et al. ISFM and AAFP consensus guidelines: Long-term use of NSAIDs in cats. *J Feline Med Surg*. 2010;12(7):521–538.

Tranquilli WJ, Grimm KA, Lamont LA. *Pain Management for the Small Animal Practitioner*. Jackson, WY: Teton NewMedia; 2004.

US Department of Agriculture: Animal Welfare Act and Regulations. Available from https://www.nal.usda.gov/awic/animal-welfare-act. Accessed 23.08.13.

Valverde A, Gunkel CI. Pain management in horses and farm animals. *J Vet Emerg Crit Care*. 2005;15:295.

Valverde A, Sinclair M. Ruminant and swine local and regional anesthetic and analgesic techniques. In: Grimm KA, Lamont LA, Tranquilli WJ, Greene SA, Robertson SA, eds. *Lumb and Jones Veterinary Anesthesia and Analgesia*. 5th ed. Ames, IA: Blackwell Publishing; 2015.

30
Veterinary Anesthesia

PHILLIP LERCHE, ANN B. WEIL, HEATHER CARTER, AND
CARL O'BRIEN

CHAPTER OUTLINE

LEARNING OBJECTIVES

When you have completed this chapter, you will be able to:

1. Pronounce, define, and spell all key terms in the chapter.
2. Differentiate general anesthesia, sedation, tranquilization, neuroleptanalgesia, and local anesthesia; differentiate among the periods of general anesthesia (premedication, induction, maintenance); and list the objectives of anesthesia and techniques used to achieve these objectives, including the concept of balanced anesthesia.
3. Discuss each aspect of patient preparation for anesthesia, including fasting, gathering historical information, physical assessment, stabilization, and physical status classification.
4. Do the following regarding injectable anesthetic agents:
   - Describe the ways anesthetic agents are classified, and differentiate among agonists, partial agonists, agonist-antagonists, and antagonists.
   - Describe the effects, adverse effects, properties, and uses of anticholinergics, phenothiazine and benzodiazepine tranquilizers, alpha$_2$ adrenergic agents, opioids, propofol, alfaxalone, dissociatives, etomidate, and guaifenesin.
5. Explain how vapor pressure, blood-gas partition coefficient, and minimum alveolar concentration influence the way inhalant anesthetics are used and describe the effects, adverse effects, properties, and uses of halogenated inhalant anesthetics.
6. Do the following regarding the use of anesthetic equipment:
   - Discuss the characteristics, uses, and maintenance of endotracheal tubes, laryngoscopes, and anesthesia masks and chambers.
   - Describe the characteristics of an anesthesia machine, including the four general machine systems.
   - Explain how to assemble an anesthesia machine, check for leaks, and set the pop-off valve before use.
   - Describe the structure, function, and use of each component of the carrier gas supply, including compressed gas cylinder, pressure gauge, pressure-reducing valve, flowmeter, and oxygen flush valve.
   - List and calculate the oxygen flow rates used for various species, systems, and periods of the anesthetic procedure.
   - Describe the structure, function, and uses of precision and nonprecision vaporizers.
   - Discuss rebreathing and nonrebreathing systems, and explain the criteria used to choose an appropriate breathing system for any given patient.
   - Describe the structure, function, and use of each component of the breathing system, including unidirectional flow valves, reservoir bag, pop-off valve, carbon dioxide absorber canister, pressure manometer, negative pressure-relief valve, and breathing tubes.
   - Discuss the function and uses of passive and active scavenging systems.
   - Describe the procedures used to maintain anesthesia machines.
7. Do the following regarding endotracheal intubation:
   - Discuss the principles of endotracheal intubation, including the equipment needed to place an endotracheal tube and the criteria used to select and prepare an appropriate endotracheal tube for any given patient.
   - Describe placement of an endotracheal tube in a small animal (SA), horse, adult ruminant, and small ruminant; how to check an endotracheal tube for proper placement; and how to inflate the cuff.
   - Discuss laryngospasm and other complications of intubation, including causes and methods of prevention.
   - Compare and contrast supraglottic airway devices and endotracheal tubes.
8. Do the following regarding anesthetic monitoring:
   - Explain the principles of anesthetic monitoring and how monitoring parameters can be used to identify the classic stages and planes of anesthesia.
   - Identify physical monitoring indicators of circulation, oxygenation, and ventilation.
   - Discuss the methods used to assess vital signs, including normal values, and common causes of abnormal values.
   - Describe methods used to assess reflexes and other monitoring indicators, and explain how they are used to determine anesthetic depth.
   - Discuss the function, setup, and limitations of monitoring equipment used to assess circulation, oxygenation, and ventilation, and interpretation of data generated by these instruments.
9. Do the following regarding SA anesthesia:
   - Describe the sequence of events required to take an SA patient from consciousness to surgical anesthesia and back to consciousness.
   - Describe agents and methods commonly used to induce anesthesia in an SA patient through intramuscular or intravenous injection, mask, or chamber.
   - Describe agents and methods used to maintain anesthesia in an SA patient and considerations for patient positioning, comfort, safety, and recovery.
10. Explain the sequence of events in an anesthetic event in a horse, including ways in which the anesthetic procedure for equines differs from that for an SA patient.
11. Explain the sequence of events in an anesthetic event in a ruminant, including ways in which the anesthetic procedure for ruminants differs from that for an SA patient.
12. List the common problems and emergencies, associated causes, and interventions in relation to anesthesia.

KEY TERMS

Analgesia
Anesthesia
Anesthetic induction
Anesthetic maintenance
Anesthetic protocol
Apnea
Atelectasis
Ayre's T-piece
Bain coaxial circuit
Balanced anesthesia
Barbiturates
Carbon dioxide absorber canister
Cyanosis
Exhalation unidirectional valve
Flowmeter
General anesthesia
Hypercarbia
Hypnotic
Hypotension
Hypothermia
Hypoventilation
Hypovolemia
Hypoxemia
Hypoxia
Line pressure gauge
Local anesthesia
Miosis

Mydriasis
Narcosis
Negative pressure relief valve
Neuroleptanalgesia
Nonrebreathing system
Oxygen cylinder
Oxygen flush valve
Oxygen saturation
Pneumothorax
Pop-off valve
Premedication
Preoxygenation
Pressure manometer
Pressure-reducing valve
Rebreathing system
Reservoir bag
Respiratory minute volume
Sedation
Tachycardia
Tachypnea
Tank pressure gauge
Tidal volume
Tranquilization
Vaporizer inlet port
Vasodilatation
Ventilation
Yoke

Introduction

Anesthesia is a unique discipline for several reasons. First, anesthesia is performed not for its own sake, but to allow veterinary professionals to do things that otherwise would not be possible. For instance, anesthesia enables surgery, dentistry, endoscopy, and other procedures that require patient immobility, unconsciousness, and pain control. It enables treatment, handling, and transport of exotic and feral animals. In some patients, it is necessary to perform certain procedures, such as nail trims, grooming, and radiographic studies, which—although not painful—evoke fear, cause discomfort, and are unwelcome.

Second, the practice of anesthesia involves much more than choosing machine settings, checking reflexes, or watching monitoring devices. It is an extremely complex discipline that involves the use of complex equipment, administration of potentially dangerous drugs, and awareness of an intricate set of monitoring parameters that enable the anesthetist to assess the well-being of the patient.

Also general anesthesia is, by nature, a high-risk procedure. Anesthetic drugs cause adverse physiologic changes in cardiac output, blood pressure, respiratory drive, and central nervous system (CNS) function, which can be dangerous and even life-threatening if not monitored and managed. A solid understanding of what is an expected or "normal" response to the drugs given in a protocol is necessary in order to recognize when the patient response is not normal and requires intervention by the anesthetist. Although a competent anesthetist is never controlled by fear, a healthy respect for the risks of anesthesia must be always maintained to keep the "edge" required for best performance.

Finally, changes in the status of anesthetized patients occur quickly and unexpectedly—often within minutes or even seconds. This urgency demands a high level of awareness and an ability to make critical decisions rapidly and effectively to ensure patient safety. Vigilant patient monitoring is the cornerstone of excellent anesthesia care.

This unique combination of the frequent use, complexity, high risk, and fast pace of veterinary anesthesia tests the knowledge and abilities of even the most experienced veterinary technician or nurse. Therefore the successful practice of anesthesia demands that the technician be prepared, skillful, alert, and attentive.

What Is Anesthesia?

Anesthesia is defined as an absence of sensation that affects the whole body or an isolated part or region of the body. Tranquilization and sedation are, by convention, included in the study of anesthesia because these techniques are frequently used in conjunction with anesthesia. Effects appropriate for each patient vary depending on the procedure, and may include light to heavy sedation, local anesthesia, general anesthesia, muscle relaxation, **analgesia**, or a combination of all these effects.

General anesthesia is characterized by unconsciousness and insensibility to feeling and pain induced by administration of anesthetic agents given alone or in combination. General anesthesia provides an environment in which general surgery or other painful procedures can be performed without the danger of patient movement or injury to personnel. *Induction* of anesthesia is the process that is used to take the patient from a state of consciousness to general anesthesia. *Maintenance* of anesthesia is the process used to keep the patient under general anesthesia until recovery.

In contrast, *local anesthesia* is the loss of sensation in a localized body part or region induced by administration of a drug or other agent without loss of consciousness. Local anesthesia is used for procedures that do not require the patient to be unconscious and for adjunctive pain control. Administration of local anesthetic to remove a skin tumor, a nerve block performed on a horse to localize lameness, and an epidural used to provide analgesia for a patient undergoing an orthopedic procedure are all examples of local anesthesia.

Premedication refers to the administration of an agent or agents before induction of general anesthesia to calm and relax the patient, ease induction and recovery, minimize adverse effects, reduce the amount of the general anesthetic agent needed, provide muscle relaxation, or provide pain control. A variety of tranquilizers, sedatives, anesthetics, and anticholinergics are used alone or in combination for this purpose. Premedication is also referred to as *preanesthesia*.

Sedation is a state of calm or drowsiness; *tranquilization* is a state of relaxation and reduced anxiety. Many tranquilizers also produce some degree of sedation. Consequently, these terms are often used interchangeably, even though they have somewhat different meanings.

Neuroleptanalgesia is a state of profound sedation and analgesia produced by simultaneous administration of an opioid and a tranquilizer. Neuroleptanalgesia is commonly used to perform minor procedures, such as wound treatment or radiography, and is a common premedication plan in an anesthetic protocol.

The objectives of anesthesia are to produce loss of sensation in the whole body or a body part or region, and to provide muscle relaxation, analgesia, and alteration of consciousness appropriate to the procedure. In addition, patient safety must be preserved and adverse effects minimized, with special attention to respiratory and cardiovascular function. This can seldom be achieved with the use of only one drug. This is why concurrent administration of two or more anesthetic drugs is commonplace. The use of drugs with complementary effects, referred to as *balanced anesthesia*, enables the anesthetist to fulfill these diverse objectives. Although many protocols are commonly used, premedication with morphine and dexmedetomidine, anesthetic induction with a ketamine-midazolam mixture, anesthetic maintenance with sevoflurane gas, and administration of a local anesthetic block for pain control constitute one example of balanced anesthesia.

PUT INTO PRACTICE

Anesthesia can be intimidating to a new veterinary nurse/technician. Observe, ask questions, learn from others, and become familiar with all aspects of each case. Breaking the process into steps can help. Start with the machine and learn its function and how to troubleshoot. Study the different pharmaceuticals used and learn your clinic's protocols. Become familiar with each patient's needs and assess them thoroughly prior to the anesthetic event. The more anesthetic cases you do, the more knowledge you will gain.

Patient Preparation

The technician must accurately identify factors that can compromise a patient and must effectively communicate this information to the veterinarian before beginning any anesthetic procedure. Specifically, careful patient preparation is important for the following reasons:

- To minimize the likelihood of preventable complications, such as aspiration of gastrointestinal (GI) contents
- To allow for treatment of any problems that may endanger the patient, such as dehydration, bleeding, organ dysfunction, or organ failure

• BOX 30.1 Physical Findings That Should Be Reported to the Veterinarian

- Dehydration, obesity, or cachexia
- Change in consciousness or any other sign of neurologic disease (e.g., seizures, ataxia, abnormal pupil size, recent behavior change)
- Pale mucous membranes or prolonged capillary refill time (CRT)
- Abnormal mucous membrane color (e.g., cyanosis or icterus)
- Abnormal heart rate (HR) or rhythm, or heart murmur
- Weak or irregular pulse
- Increased respiratory effort or rate
- Abnormal lung sounds, such as wheezes or crackles
- Marked hypothermia or hyperthermia

TABLE 30.1 Fasting Recommendations

Species	Food Withholding Time (hours)	Water Withholding Time (hours)
Dogs and cats	8–12[a]	0–4
Horses	8–12	0–2
Cattle	24–48	8–12
Small ruminants	12–18	8–12
Neonates and pediatric patients (<8 weeks old)	None	None

[a]Note that patients weighing less than 2 kg should be fasted for shorter lengths of time.

- To allow the veterinarian to make anesthetic drug choices based on facts about the patient's condition
- To make the anesthetist aware of potential problems that the patient may experience during the procedure.

Evaluation of the patient is an important part of preanesthetic preparation and it starts with proper patient identification. Further evaluation involves acquisition of a complete patient history, a thorough physical examination, and diagnostic testing with a focus on the nervous, cardiovascular, and pulmonary systems because the health status of these systems is closely associated with the outcome of any anesthetic procedure. The purpose of these procedures is to uncover abnormalities that may impair the patient's ability to compensate, as this may lead to unanticipated complications or may impact the patient's ability to eliminate the anesthetics. See Box 30.1 for a list of physical findings that should be reported to the veterinarian.

Fasting Recommendations

Swallowing reflexes become sluggish, lower esophageal sphincter tone decreases, and patients may experience nausea or vomiting during anesthetic procedures. This combination of factors may allow stomach contents to reflux into the esophagus and the pharynx, resulting in a range of mild to devastating complications, including aspiration of stomach contents into the lungs, postanesthesia esophagitis, and esophageal stricture. Therefore it is vital to observe fasting recommendations before any anesthetic procedure is performed in common domestic species. Fasting recommendations vary widely from practice to practice; however, some guidelines are provided in Table 30.1.

TABLE 30.2 American Society of Anesthesiologists Physical Status Classifications

Classification	Risk	Criteria	Representative Conditions
ASA I	Minimal	Normal, healthy patient	Patients undergoing elective procedures (OHE, castration, or declaw)
ASA II	Low	Patient with mild systemic disease	Neonatal, geriatric, or obese patients Mild dehydration Low-grade heart murmur
ASA III	Moderate	Patient with severe systemic disease	Anemia Moderate dehydration Compensated major organ disease
ASA IV	High	Patient with severe systemic disease that is a constant threat to life	Ruptured bladder Internal hemorrhage Pneumothorax Pyometra
ASA V	Extreme	Moribund patient that is not expected to survive without the operation	Severe head trauma Pulmonary embolus Gastric dilatation-volvulus End-stage major organ failure
ASA VI		A declared brain-dead patient whose organs are being removed for donor purposes	(Note that this classification is not used in veterinary patients)

ASA, American Society of Anesthesiologists; *OHE*, ovariohysterectomy.

TECHNICIAN NOTE

Ensure that fasting instructions have been observed before administering anesthesia to *any* patient.

Patient Stabilization

Abnormalities identified during patient evaluation must be treated before the anesthetic is administered. Patient stabilization includes treatment or correction of dehydration, **hypovolemia**, anemia, cardiac arrhythmias, respiratory compromise, major organ failure, or electrolyte or acid-base imbalance and may involve administration of fluids, blood, oxygen, and pharmaceutical agents, such as antibiotics, analgesics, or a wide variety of other agents. The veterinary technician or nurse will be intimately involved in this stabilization process and must be knowledgeable on the calculation of doses, placing intravenous (IV) catheters, setting fluid administration rates, and administration of drugs, blood, and oxygen, as ordered by the veterinarian.

Physical Status Classification

Information gleaned from patient evaluation is used to determine the physical status classification. This system, developed by the American Society of Anesthesiologists (ASA), is a subjective rating of the patient's condition based on historical, physical, and laboratory findings, and places the patient into one of six classes (Table 30.2). This system is a tool that can be used to guide the anesthetist in appropriate patient management, because anesthetic protocols are often based on physical status classification. This classification is somewhat subjective, so the technician must use best judgment based on the criteria listed. Any surgery that is an emergency, regardless of ASA class, is additionally assigned the letter "E." While a healthy

dog that needs to be anesthetized to remove a stick wedged in its mouth may be ASA class 1E, a horse with colic requiring surgery may be a class 5E.

Anesthetic Plans

General anesthesia is mostly delivered via a balanced anesthesia technique, which requires the use of drugs that provide analgesia, unconsciousness, muscle relaxation, and amnesia. No single agent that adequately provides these characteristics exists, so drugs from multiple pharmacologic classes are used in an anesthetic plan to provide optimal patient care. Agents used in veterinary patients may be classified in one of several ways. They may be grouped according to the route of delivery (topical, oral, injectable, or inhalant) or by primary use (preanesthesia, sedation, induction, or maintenance). Agents may also be grouped into drug classes based on chemistry. Agents in any given class tend to have similar actions, properties, uses, and effects.

Agonists, Partial Agonists, Mixed Agonist-Antagonists, and Antagonists

Drugs work by binding to specific receptors on or inside the cells of target tissues. In the case of many anesthetics, these target tissues are in the central or peripheral nervous system. Most drugs are *agonists* (i.e., they bind to receptors and exert one or more effects). Some drug classes, such as opioids and alpha$_2$ adrenergics, include drugs called *antagonists*, which block or reverse the action of the corresponding agonist. These antagonists are referred to as *reversal agents*. The opioid class includes agents that are classified as partial agonists and those that are classified as mixed agonist-antagonists. *Partial agonists* bind to receptors and exert a partial or milder effect than an agonist, whereas *mixed agonist-antagonists* partially reverse the effects of pure agonists.

Anticholinergics

Although not true anesthetic agents, anticholinergics are used to counteract the effects of parasympathetic nervous system stimulation, such as bradycardia and excess salivation. Although many anesthetics cause these effects to some degree, dissociatives have a notable tendency to cause excess salivation; opioids and alpha$_2$ adrenergic agonists are especially likely to cause bradycardia. Atropine and glycopyrrolate are the most used anticholinergics in veterinary patients.

Anticholinergics have many effects expected to result from a parasympathetic nervous system blockade, including increased heart rate (HR), reduced tear secretions and salivation, reduced gastrointestinal (GI) activity, and dilatation of the pupils, especially in cats. Protective ophthalmic ointment should be applied to all patients undergoing heavy sedation or general anesthesia to prevent corneal dryness, as these processes reduce tear production and distribution.

Many potential adverse effects, including tachycardia, cardiac arrhythmias, bronchodilation, mydriasis, and ileus, are known. Bronchodilation caused by these drugs can increase anatomical dead space, which increases the risk for hypoxemia and hypoventilation. Mydriasis may render the pupillary light reflex unreliable. Anticholinergics may cause thickening of mucus in small airways, especially in cats, which can result in blockage. Routine use of anticholinergics in small-animal (SA) patients is no longer common.

In ruminants, copious salivary secretions become more viscid, pool in the pharynx, and may be aspirated, thus predisposing the patient to airway blockage. Horses may develop colic from GI stasis. Therefore anticholinergics are avoided in these species unless they are necessary to treat bradycardia.

Atropine is a rapid-acting agent that is available in SA strengths (0.4 mg/mL and 0.54 mg/mL) and large-animal (LA) strength (15 mg/mL). Glycopyrrolate (0.2 mg/mL) is like atropine, except that glycopyrrolate has a slower onset and a longer duration. It is less likely to cause tachycardia, cardiac arrhythmias, and ileus, suppressing salivation more effectively. Unlike atropine, it does not cross the placental barrier and will not adversely affect fetuses if used for cesarean section (C-section). It also does not cross the blood-brain barrier and thus has less impact on vision.

> **TECHNICIAN NOTE**
>
> Anticholinergics are used to counteract bradycardia and hypersalivation. The large-animal (LA) concentration of injectable atropine is approximately 30 to 40 times stronger than small-animal (SA) concentrations. Never mix these drugs up.

Tranquilizers and Sedatives

Tranquilizers and sedatives are commonly used to restrain patients for minor procedures, such as grooming, diagnostic imaging, blood draws, nail trims, and wound treatment. They are also used as premedications and to produce analgesia and muscle relaxation. Each drug has unique properties and must be chosen based on desired effects. For instance, dexmedetomidine (an alpha$_2$ adrenergic agonist) produces analgesia and muscle relaxation, whereas acepromazine minimizes vomiting and development of cardiac arrhythmias. Tranquilizers and sedatives may be used in combination or with other anesthetic agents to produce a combination of effects not achieved with one drug.

Phenothiazine Tranquilizers

Phenothiazine tranquilizers are used to calm and sedate patients before general anesthesia and improve the quality of anesthetic induction and recovery by reducing anxiety. The phenothiazine tranquilizer used most for this purpose is acepromazine. It may be used alone or in combination with other agents. An example of such a combination is "BAG" (butorphanol, acepromazine, and glycopyrrolate).

Acepromazine induces mild-to-moderate sedation and has antiemetic and antiarrhythmic properties. Unlike many other agents, it causes little respiratory or cardiac depression. It has a relatively long duration of action and has no direct antagonist.

Acepromazine blocks (antagonizes) alpha$_1$ adrenergic receptors in the sympathetic nervous system, resulting in dose-dependent peripheral vasodilatation. Consequently, the main adverse effect of acepromazine is hypotension, which can lead to cardiovascular collapse if given to hypovolemic patients. Acepromazine also can cause hypothermia or hyperthermia, changes in HR, third eyelid prolapse, and paradoxical excitement or aggression. Adverse effects specific to horses include excitement, sweating, tachypnea, and penile prolapse, which can lead to permanent injury. Many clinicians will not use this drug in breeding stallions.

Acepromazine should be given intramuscularly at least 15 minutes before induction, allowing the patient to remain in a quiet area, because the tranquilizing effect may be overridden by stimulation, especially in excited patients. Note that the commonly used dose of the injectable form of acepromazine is significantly lower than the dose suggested on the label. Use of higher doses will not increase the level of sedation but will worsen hypotension.

When administering acepromazine intravenously it is given slowly, avoiding intra-arterial injection, especially in the horse. Boxers, Greyhounds, giant-breed dogs, Collies, Australian Shepherds, and debilitated, young, or geriatric patients may be sensitive to this drug, whereas Terriers and cats are relatively resistant. Owners must be instructed to use caution when handling patients that have received this drug, because personality changes may occur, resulting in aggression.

> **TECHNICIAN NOTE**
>
> The commonly used dose of acepromazine (about 0.01–0.05 mg/kg in small animals [SAs] with a maximum dose of 2 mg in dogs and 1 mg in cats; 0.01–0.03 mg/kg in horses) is significantly lower than the dose suggested on the label. Higher doses will increase hypotension but not sedation.

Benzodiazepine Tranquilizers

Benzodiazepines are most often used in combination with other agents, such as opioids and dissociatives, to produce a range of effects from sedation to general anesthesia. Benzodiazepines are controlled substances with diazepam, midazolam, and zolazepam commonly used in veterinary patients. Zolazepam is one of the two components in the product Telazol. The other component of this product is tiletamine (see "Dissociatives" for a discussion of this drug). A benzodiazepine antagonist (flumazenil) is available; however, it is seldom used in SAs because of the low incidence of benzodiazepine-related side effects.

The effects of benzodiazepines may last a few hours and include anxiety reduction and mild-to-moderate sedation, although many healthy dogs are resistant to these drugs, and sedation in cats is often unpredictable. Other effects include skeletal muscle relaxation and anticonvulsant activity.

Benzodiazepines are relatively safe and minimally affect the cardiopulmonary system, but they can produce adverse effects that vary among species. Dogs, especially those that are young and healthy, tend to experience CNS excitement, anxiety, and fear, and may become more difficult to control. Aggressive animals may lose inhibition, which prohibits the use of benzodiazepines in these patients. Horses may experience muscle fasciculations, weakness, and mild ataxia.

After intramuscular (IM) injection, diazepam is erratically absorbed and causes pain. It can also cause bradycardia, apnea, hypotension, and pain if given rapidly intravenously due to the propylene glycol vehicle.

Diazepam should not be stored in syringes or IV bags, because it is soluble in plastic and will lose potency. Diazepam is commonly mixed with ketamine (a dissociative anesthetic) in equal volumes and given intravenously to induce general anesthesia in SAs and small ruminants.

Midazolam is more potent than diazepam but can be used with ketamine in place of diazepam for induction of anesthesia. Midazolam is water soluble, compatible with various agents, and is a substitute for diazepam, which is not water soluble and therefore cannot be mixed with other agents except ketamine.

> **TECHNICIAN NOTE**
>
> As a result of incompatibility with most other agents, injectable diazepam can be mixed only with ketamine. When administering diazepam by intravenous (IV) injection, it is given slowly. Diazepam is a painful injection, even when properly given intravenously.

Alpha$_2$ Adrenergic Drugs

Alpha$_2$ adrenergic agonists (α^2-agonists) are sedatives that are used alone or in combination with opioids, dissociatives, and other agents to produce a wide spectrum of effects, from mild sedation to general anesthesia and including analgesia and muscle relaxation. Dexmedetomidine, medetomidine, and xylazine are α^2-agonists most used in SA patients. Xylazine, detomidine, and romifidine are used most in LA patients. Zenalpha is an α^2-agonist/peripheral antagonist combination (medetomidine/vatinoxan) released in 2022 to the US market for use in dogs.

The main therapeutic effects of α^2-agonists are sedation (CNS depression), analgesia, and muscle relaxation; they may cause vomiting in dogs and cats. Cardiovascular effects include initial hypertension, followed by prolonged hypotension. Bradycardia is common and cardiac output is decreased. At high doses, these drugs cause a decrease in both respiratory rate (RR) and depth. In horses xylazine causes lowering of the head and relaxation of the facial muscles, leading to drooping of the ears and lower lip. Relaxation of limb muscles leads to ataxia and a wide-based stance.

α^2-agonists can cause significant bradycardia, reduced cardiac output, hypotension, hypertension (dexmedetomidine) and cardiac arrhythmias, including heart block. They can cause respiratory depression, especially when combined with other agents, and respiratory distress in brachycephalic dogs. Other adverse effects include pain upon IM injection, muscle tremors, changes in body temperature, increased urine production, and hyperglycemia. In dogs, bloating secondary to aerophagia (swallowing of air) may occur, and horses may sweat. Ruminants may experience profound respiratory depression, hypersalivation, bloat, diarrhea, premature delivery, or abortion. Because sedated patients are sensitive to auditory stimuli, horses may kick, SAs may move, and aggressive patients may bite in response to loud noises.

Sedation produced by these drugs can be profound and prolonged, as can cardiovascular depression. Therefore standard doses should only be given to young, healthy patients, and caution should be used in geriatric, diabetic, pregnant, pediatric, or sick patients. Most clinicians do not recommend routine use of anticholinergics with α^2-agonists as this predisposes the patient to further decreases in cardiac output, increases in myocardial work, and development of arrhythmias and hypertension.

Xylazine is used in many domestic and exotic species as one component of anesthetic mixtures and is also used to induce vomiting in cats after ingestion of toxins. Xylazine is available in SA (2%, or 20 mg/mL) and LA (10%, or 100 mg/mL) concentrations. Ruminants are extremely sensitive to this drug, requiring about 10% of the dose used for horses. Swine require a high dose, so xylazine usually is given in combination with other drugs in this species.

Dexmedetomidine is used primarily in SAs and exotic animal species. Compared with xylazine, it is more potent and is less likely to produce side effects. This drug is available in two formulations that differ in concentration. Dexdomitor (0.5 mg/mL) is intended for use in medium- to large-sized dogs and cats, whereas Dexdomitor 0.1 (0.1 mg/mL) is intended for use in dogs weighing less than 20 lb and in cats weighing less than 7 lb to ensure dosing accuracy. The reversal agent atipamezole can be given after either formulation to awaken patients undergoing minor procedures.

Detomidine (Dormosedan) and romifidine (Sedivet) are α^2-agonists used in horses to produce sedation for some procedures, such as dental work, and as a part of anesthetic combinations. Detomidine has a longer duration of action and provides more profound sedative and analgesic activity compared with xylazine. Romifidine generally causes less muscle relaxation and outward sedation signs compared with those produced by xylazine or detomidine. At the time of writing, romifidine is only available in Europe and Canada.

> **TECHNICIAN NOTE**
>
> When giving α^2-agonists, monitor the patient closely for hypotension, cardiac arrhythmias, bradycardia, and abnormal temperatures. Use special caution in geriatric, pediatric, and sick patients. Both large-animal (LA) and small-animal (SA) concentrations of xylazine are available. Do *not* mix these up.

Alpha$_2$ adrenergic antagonists increase HR and blood pressure, and stimulate the CNS. They are used to "wake" patients after sedation or anesthesia and to reverse adverse effects of α^2-agonists. These agents also reverse desirable effects, such as analgesia, and can cause hypotension if administered rapidly IV. Therefore an alternative analgesic must be administered if pain control is warranted. Adverse effects include apprehension caused by rapid arousal, excitement, muscle tremors, and salivation.

Atipamezole (Antisedan) reverses the effects of dexmedetomidine and other α^2-agonists. Dexdomitor is formulated such that an equal volume of the sedative and reversal is used in dogs, whereas Dexdomitor 0.1 is not. The dose in cats is half the volume of the sedative given when Dexdomitor 0.5 mg/mL is used. After the reversal, sudden arousal has been reported in patients heavily sedated with dexmedetomidine, resulting in the occurrence of bites and possibly vomiting or diarrhea. Atipamezole may also be used to reverse detomidine. Dexmedetomidine has a longer duration of action than atipamezole, so reversal shortly after initial administration of dexmedetomidine may need to be repeated.

Alpha$_2$ antagonists may be given intramuscularly in all species. When given intravenously, alpha$_2$ antagonists should be given slowly to effect (see subsection "Induction of Anesthesia" in "Small-animal Anesthesia") to avoid the excitation and aggression that are sometimes seen with rapid reversal. IV use in cats may cause unwanted severe salivation and excitement, and is contraindicated. Thus IV use should be reserved for emergency and critical situations.

50 mg of each drug per milliliter. Once reconstituted, Telazol is stable for 14 days if refrigerated. Telazol is used as an induction agent in healthy dogs and cats, especially if the animals are aggressive. Because it may cause hyperthermia, especially in dogs, body temperature must be closely monitored. Telazol is frequently combined with α^2-agonists and opioids to produce injectable anesthetic combinations in a variety of species.

A mixture of ketamine and diazepam (or midazolam) is commonly used to induce general anesthesia in dogs, cats, and horses. This combination has an onset of about 30 to 90 seconds and provides 5 to 10 minutes of working time. In SAs, the two drugs are mixed in a 1:1 volume ratio and are given at a dosage of about 1 mL of the mixture per 20 lb of body weight intravenously slowly to effect (over 30–90 seconds). Diazepam or midazolam (0.03–0.05 mg/kg) can be added to ketamine (2.2 mg/kg) for induction of anesthesia in horses.

Ketamine–alpha$_2$ adrenergic agonist mixtures are used to provide anesthesia in dogs, cats, horses, and exotic animals. These mixtures cause significant cardiovascular and respiratory depression and must be used cautiously. Other dissociative mixtures include TKX (Telazol-ketamine-xylazine), TKD (Telazol-ketamine-Dexdomitor), TTDex (Telazol-butorphanol-dexmedetomidine), GKX (guaifenesin-ketamine-xylazine) and MKX (midazolam-ketamine-xyalzine).

Ketamine (2 mg/kg) can be added to propofol (2 mg/kg), colloquially referred to as "ketofol," to minimize the cardiovascular side effects of each of the drugs. Respiratory side effects are like those seen with propofol.

> **TECHNICIAN NOTE**
>
> Unlike most other anesthetics, dissociative agents cause normal or increased muscle tone, sensitivity to light and sound, intact reflexes, increased heart rate (HR), and increased blood pressure.

Etomidate

Etomidate is a short-acting, injectable, imidazole-derivative sedative-**hypnotic** used for anesthetic induction in dogs and cats and is not a controlled substance. Etomidate causes minimal changes in cardiovascular and respiratory functions and decreases both intracranial pressure and intraocular pressure. It has a significantly wider therapeutic index compared with propofol. Therefore it is the agent of choice for patients with severe heart disease or shock. Etomidate produces good muscle relaxation but no analgesia.

Although etomidate has a wide margin of safety, adverse effects include vomiting, muscle movements, sneezing, and excitement during induction and recovery. It also suppresses adrenocortical function. Premedication is recommended to reduce these adverse effects. IV injections may be painful and may cause phlebitis; rapid injection or repeat doses can cause hemolysis. Administration through a running IV fluid line will decrease pain and hemolysis. If hemolysis occurs, patients may have hematuria after anesthesia. Etomidate is not in common use because of its relatively higher cost and adverse effects.

Guaifenesin

Guaifenesin, also known as "GG" (glyceryl guaiacolate), is an injectable muscle relaxant and sedative used in combination with other agents for short procedures or to improve the quality of induction and recovery in LAs. Guaifenesin was, at one time,

commonly administered to ruminants and horses to produce muscle relaxation and as one ingredient in combinations called "double drip" (ketamine and GG) and "triple drip" (xylazine, ketamine, and 5% GG, also known as GKX). It is now only available from compounding pharmacies and so is used less often.

Barbiturates

Barbiturates, a class of drugs developed in the early 1900s, were once used extensively for induction and maintenance of general anesthesia in a variety of species. Pentobarbital sodium, a barbiturate used to induce and maintain general anesthesia in laboratory animals by means of intraperitoneal injection, is the only barbiturate-class general anesthetic still in regular use.

Inhalant Anesthetics

Inhalant anesthetics are liquid agents that are vaporized in oxygen and are unique in that they are administered to the patient's lungs via an anesthetic breathing system by endotracheal tube, mask, or chamber. Vapor pressure, blood-gas partition coefficient, and minimum alveolar concentration (MAC) measure the properties of these agents, which influence the way they are used. A basic knowledge of these concepts is therefore necessary in order to use inhalant anesthetics effectively and safely.

Vapor pressure is a measurement of the tendency of a liquid to evaporate. Agents with high vapor pressure evaporate readily, reaching dangerously high concentrations if not regulated, and therefore must be administered using an agent-specific precision vaporizer.

The blood-gas partition coefficient is a measurement of the tendency of an agent to dissolve in blood. It is associated with the speed of induction, recovery, and change in depth of anesthesia, each of which is faster when agents with a low partition coefficient are used and slower when agents with a high partition coefficient are used.

Minimum alveolar concentration (MAC) is the percent concentration of an agent present in the alveoli in the lungs that is required to prevent a response to surgical stimulation in 50% of patients and therefore is a measurement of the potency of an agent. An agent with high MAC is less potent (more of the agent is required to attain surgical anesthesia) compared with an agent with low MAC. Typically, a dial setting of approximately 1.5 times the MAC is required to reach surgical anesthesia in most patients.

Halogenated Anesthetics

These inhalant agents are used in a wide variety of species to induce and maintain general anesthesia. Isoflurane and sevoflurane are the halogenated anesthetics most used in veterinary patients.

Halogenated anesthetics cause CNS depression, hypothermia, respiratory depression, hypotension, and muscle relaxation. Although they cause myocardial depression, cardiac function is maintained close to preanesthetic levels. These agents have little or no analgesic effect postoperatively.

Both isoflurane and sevoflurane have high vapor pressures (240 mm Hg and 160 mm Hg, respectively) and must be administered via a precision vaporizer. Both agents also have low blood-gas partition coefficients (1.46 and 0.68, respectively), resulting in relatively rapid induction, recovery, and changes in depth of anesthesia.

Halogenated anesthetics induce dose-dependent hypotension, which is more prominent with sevoflurane than with isoflurane. They can also cause vomiting, nausea, and ileus in addition to dose-dependent respiratory depression, which can progress to apnea. Although the primary route of excretion for these agents is through the lungs, the amount that is metabolized by the liver and excreted by the kidneys varies from agent to agent. About 2% to 5% of sevoflurane is metabolized, whereas only about 0.2% of isoflurane is metabolized.

Reports have described fire or extreme heat production when sevoflurane is used with desiccated (dry) carbon dioxide (CO_2) absorbent. This problem is more common when low oxygen flow rates are used over a long time. To prevent this complication, the machine should be turned off when not in use, absorbent granules replaced regularly, the use of low oxygen flow avoided for protracted periods, and the temperature of the absorbent canister monitored.

Although isoflurane and sevoflurane are similar, subtle differences have been noted in the way they are used. Because isoflurane is irritating to mucous membranes, patients may struggle and hold their breath during mask or chamber induction. In contrast, sevoflurane is not irritating, making it ideal for anesthetic induction via mask. Some of the chief advantages of sevoflurane are rapid induction, recovery, and changes in anesthetic depth associated with this agent. Safe use therefore requires subtle dial changes and vigilant monitoring on the part of the veterinary anesthetist.

> **TECHNICIAN NOTE**
>
> Although the frequent perception is that sevoflurane is safer than isoflurane, it can cause more hypotension and, because of its more rapid response time, the patient must be monitored even more closely than with isoflurane.

Anesthesia Equipment

Endotracheal Tubes

An endotracheal tube is a device that is placed inside the trachea of an unconscious patient, attached to a breathing circuit, and used to administer oxygen and inhalant anesthetics. Endotracheal tubes increase patient safety because they maintain an open airway; minimize the likelihood of pulmonary aspiration of blood, stomach contents, and other substances; facilitate administration of supplemental oxygen; and allow the anesthetist to ventilate the patient when necessary. Because of these benefits, many veterinarians prefer to place an endotracheal tube in all patients undergoing general anesthesia, even those not receiving inhalant anesthetics.

Endotracheal tubes are available in a variety of sizes, lengths, and types to accommodate the wide size variation of veterinary patients; they may be made of red rubber (Fig. 30.1D), silicone rubber (see Fig. 30.1A), or polyvinyl chloride (see Fig. 30.1C and E). Murphy tubes have a side hole called the *Murphy eye* (Fig. 30.2J) at the beveled end that permits airflow in the event of blockage of the tip. The patient end of a Cole tube is tapered and has no cuff (see Fig. 30.1B). This type is used for small patients and for birds, which do not have an expandable trachea.

An endotracheal tube consists of the following parts: the connector (see Fig. 30.2D) is attached to the breathing circuit of the anesthesia machine or to an Ambu bag. The cuff (see Fig. 30.2H) is a balloonlike part at the beveled patient end (see Fig. 30.2I), which, when inflated, creates a seal between the tube and the tracheal mucosa. This prevents mixing of room air and anesthetic gases, and aspiration of solid materials around the tube. Liquids can sometimes move past the cuff; lubrication of the cuff prior to placement helps to minimize this. In ruminants, the head should be placed in a sloping position, with the mouth lower than the throat to allow drainage, and suction should also be available (see section on ruminant anesthesia below). The cuff is connected by a small tube to the pilot balloon (see Fig. 30.2B) and a valve (see Fig. 30.2A), which is used to inflate the cuff. The pilot balloon allows the anesthetist to monitor cuff inflation.

Although several different scales may be used to measure the diameter of an endotracheal tube, internal diameter (ID) is most common (see Fig. 30.2G). Tubes for dogs and cats range in size from 3 to 14 mm ID. Small ruminants, swine, and foals require tubes between 6 and 18 mm ID. Small exotic animals may require tubes as small as 1 mm ID. Horses and mature cattle require sizes ranging from 16 to 30 mm ID.

Laryngoscopes

Laryngoscopes are used to visualize the larynx while placing endotracheal tubes. A laryngoscope consists of a handle and a blade that is used to depress the base of the tongue, which aids in visualizing the larynx, and it also includes a light source for illuminating the throat (Fig. 30.3). Common blade sizes range from 0 (small) to 5 (large), although longer blades are available for use in swine and some exotics. Miller blades are straight (see Fig. 30.3A and C), and McIntosh blades are curved (see Fig. 30.3B and D). Laryngoscopes are often used in small ruminants, camelids, and swine, and may be helpful in dogs and cats, but they are not used in adult cattle, which are intubated by digital palpation, or in horses, which are intubated blindly.

Supraglottic Airway Devices

A supraglottic airway device (SAD) functions in a similar way to an endotracheal tube but is designed to create a seal around the laryngeal opening without invading the tracheal lumen. Although not in common use, SADs offer an alternative to conventional endotracheal tubes in such species as cats and rabbits, in which endotracheal intubation is challenging and often results in a higher incidence of complications. SADs have several reported advantages, including decreased likelihood of laryngospasm, decreased resistance to breathing, decreased risk of airway trauma during intubation, and no postoperative coughing or other effects related to tracheal irritation. The V-Gel (Millpledge Veterinary, Retford, UK) SAD is available in several sizes for cats and rabbits. To ensure proper placement, the anesthetist must follow the prescribed set of steps as described on the manufacturer's website.

Masks

Masks are cone-shaped devices used to administer oxygen and anesthetic gases to patients that are not intubated (Fig. 30.4). Masks are usually made of plastic or rubber, come in a variety of sizes, and have a rubber gasket designed to create a seal around the patient's muzzle. The smallest mask that comfortably fits the patient should be selected. Masks may be used to induce or maintain anesthesia. They are frequently used to administer anesthetic gases to SA patients, in which intubation is difficult. Masks may also be used to administer oxygen during the preanesthetic and postanesthetic periods. Unlike endotracheal tubes, masks do not

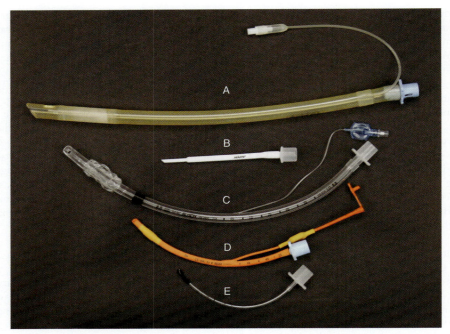

• **Fig. 30.1** Endotracheal tube type, material, and size comparison. (A) Cuffed 11-mm silicone rubber tube. (B) 2.5-mm Cole tube. (C) Cuffed 8-mm polyvinylchloride (PVC) tube. (D) Cuffed 4-mm red rubber tube. (E) Uncuffed 2-mm PVC tube.

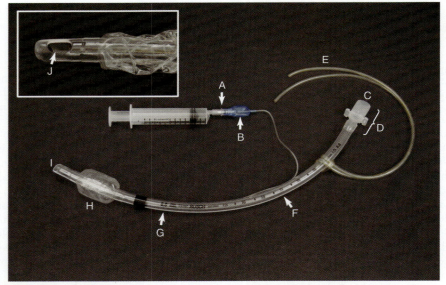

• **Fig. 30.2** Endotracheal tube parts. (A) Valve with syringe attached. (B) Pilot balloon. (C) Patient end. (D) Connector. (E) Tie. (F) Measurement of length from the patient end (cm). (G) Measurement of internal diameter (ID) (mm). (H) Inflated cuff. (I) Patient end. (J) Murphy eye.

maintain an open airway, do not protect against aspiration, and do not afford the ability to ventilate the patient.

Anesthetic Chambers

Anesthetic chambers are solid boxes used to induce general anesthesia in SA patients that are feral, vicious, or intractable, or cannot be handled without undue stress (Fig. 30.5). Chambers are usually clear to allow the anesthetist to observe the patient. They have two ports: one is attached to a fresh gas source, and the other allows waste gas to exit. A common way to set up a chamber is to attach the inhalation tube and the exhalation tube of a semiclosed rebreathing system to each port in place of the Y-piece. Chambers prevent close monitoring of the patient during induction, thus necessitating extreme care when patients are anesthetized by this method.

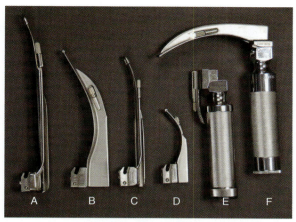

• **Fig. 30.3** Laryngoscope handles and blades. (A) Size 4 Miller blade. (B) Size 4 McIntosh blade. (C) Size 2 Miller blade. (D) Size 1 McIntosh blade. (E) Laryngoscope handle with size 00 Miller blade in unlocked position. (F) Laryngoscope handle with size 3 McIntosh blade in locked position (note that the light turns on when the blade is locked).

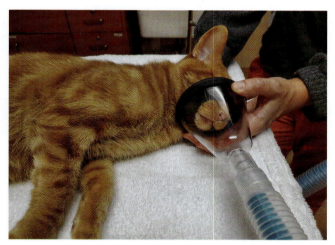

• **Fig. 30.4** Proper anesthetic mask placement on a feline patient. Note the good fit around the patient's muzzle to minimize leakage.

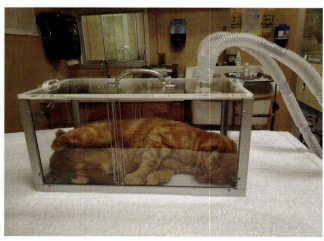

• **Fig. 30.5** Anesthesia chamber attached to the corrugated breathing tubes of a semiclosed rebreathing circuit in place of the Y-piece.

The Anesthesia Machine

Anesthesia machines are used to deliver inhalant anesthetics and oxygen to patients during administration of general anesthesia. These machines are complex and have many specialized and distinct parts that must be properly used and maintained to ensure patient safety. Many different makes and models are in common use, ranging from state-of-the-art machines to those that have been in service for many years, so the veterinary technician may encounter machines of highly varied appearance, size, and age. The basic function and uses are similar, however, and have not changed significantly over the past several decades. For this reason, complete knowledge of anesthesia machine systems and associated equipment, along with a review of the owner's manual, will prepare the technician for operation of any machine that they may encounter.

An anesthesia machine consists of the following general systems:

1. The *carrier gas supply* (Fig. 30.6A) delivers oxygen and other carrier gases to the patient at a controlled flow rate. Compressed gas cylinders, the pressure-reducing valve, the tank and line pressure gauges, the flowmeters, and the oxygen flush valve are part of this system.
2. The *anesthetic vaporizer* (see Fig. 30.6B) vaporizes a precise concentration of liquid inhalant anesthetic and mixes it with carrier gases.
3. The *breathing circuit* (see Fig. 30.6C) delivers the anesthetic and oxygen mixture to the patient via endotracheal tube, mask, or chamber and conveys expired gases away from the patient. Breathing circuits may be classified as rebreathing circuits (see Fig. 30.6) or as nonrebreathing circuits (Fig. 30.7).
4. The *scavenging system* disposes of waste and excess anesthetic gases (Fig. 30.8).

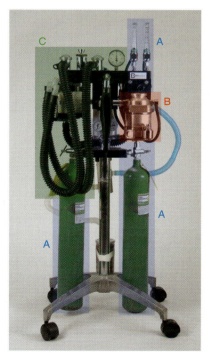

• **Fig. 30.6** Anesthesia machine systems. (A) Carrier gas supply. Note the two size E compressed gas oxygen cylinders beside the "As" at the bottom of this image. (B) Anesthetic vaporizer. (C) Breathing circuit. Note that the scavenging system (see Fig. 30.8) is not visible in this view.

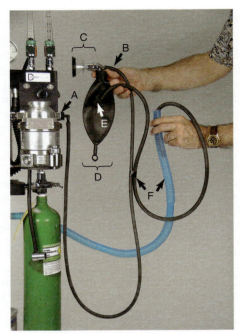

• **Fig. 30.7** Parts of a nonrebreathing circuit. (A) Outlet port of the vaporizer with keyed fitting. (B) Fresh gas inlet. (C) Connector with mask attached. (D) Reservoir bag. (E) Pressure-relief valve. (F) Scavenging hose.

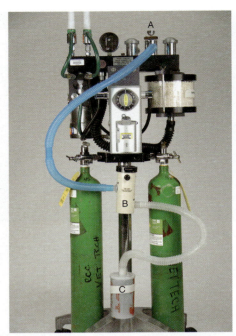

• **Fig. 30.8** Scavenging system. Waste gas exits from the pop-off valve (A) of this rebreathing system (or the discharge hose of a nonrebreathing system), flows through the interface (B), and finally into a charcoal canister (C) or, alternatively, into an outlet pipe in the ceiling or wall.

Preparing the Machine

Box 30.2 highlights the steps required to prepare an anesthesia machine for use.

Machine Assembly

Before using any anesthetic machine all necessary parts, including the vaporizer inlet and outlet port hoses, the reservoir bag, the corrugated breathing tubes, the scavenging system hoses, and any other parts required for the machine that are being used, should be attached.

Checking for Leaks

To check the low-pressure system of a **nonrebreathing system** for leaks, the patient connector and the scavenging hose or pressure-relief valve is occluded. Oxygen is turned on to fill the bag. When the bag is full, the flowmeter is turned off. The system has no leaks if the bag remains inflated for at least 10 seconds.

To check the low-pressure system of a rebreathing system for leaks, the machine is assembled and all connections secured. The pop-off valve is closed completely. The thumb is placed over the Y-piece, and the oxygen flush valve and the oxygen flowmeter are used to fill the reservoir bag until the pressure manometer indicates a pressure of 30 centimeters of water (cm H_2O). The flowmeter is then turned off. No leaks are present if the pressure is maintained for at least 10 seconds. If the pressure begins to drop, the flowmeter may be turned back on just enough to maintain pressure at 30 cm H_2O. If greater than 300 mL/minute is necessary to do so, steps should be taken to locate and repair the leak. The pop-off valve should be opened to release the generated pressure to verify it is working properly.

Setting the Pop-off Valve

When using a semiclosed rebreathing system, the pop-off valve (also referred to as *adjustable pressure-limiting*, or *APL*, *valve*) is

---

• BOX 30.2 Preparing an Anesthesia Machine for Use

1. Check the quantity of carrier gases in the compressed gas cylinders and replace them if needed.
2. Check the level of inhalant anesthetic in the anesthetic vaporizer and refill it if necessary.
3. Select a rebreathing system or a nonrebreathing system based on patient size and requirements.
4. If using a rebreathing system, select an appropriately sized reservoir bag and breathing tubes.
5. Assemble the machine and check the low-pressure system for leaks.
6. Set the pop-off valve.
7. Assemble, turn on, and adjust the scavenging system.

---

adjusted immediately after checking the low-pressure system for leaks. With the Y-piece occluded, oxygen flow is turned back on to the anticipated maximum for that procedure. A general rule of thumb is about 1 to 3 L/minute for patients weighing less than 30 kg, about 3 to 5 L/minute for patients weighing 30 kg or more, and 10 L/minute for LA patients. Then the pop-off valve is opened gradually until the pressure manometer indicates pressure of 1 to 2 cm H_2O.

TECHNICIAN NOTE

It is essential that the anesthetic machine and breathing circuit are assembled correctly and checked for leaks prior to each use, i.e., before every case. To prevent potentially life-threatening complications, it is imperative that the pop-off valve is in the open position prior to commencing anesthesia.

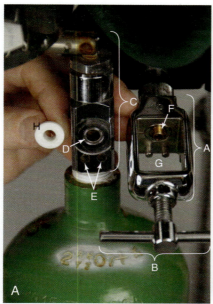
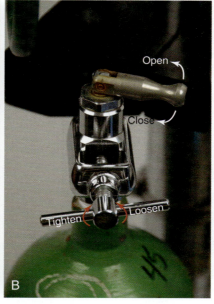

• **Fig. 30.9** (A) *(right image)* Parts of a compressed gas cylinder and yoke. *A*, Yoke. *B*, Wing nut. *C*, Outlet valve. *D*, Valve port. *E*, Pin holes. *F*, Nipple of yoke. *G*, Index pins. *H*, Nylon washer. (B) Opening and closing the outlet valve; loosening and tightening the wing nut.

Carrier Gas Supply

The gases into which the liquid inhalant anesthetic evaporates and that carry the vaporized anesthetic to the patient are referred to as *carrier gases*. Oxygen is the carrier gas used during all anesthetic procedures. Oxygen administration is necessary throughout anesthesia not only to carry the anesthetic but also to compensate for the diminished RR, **tidal volume** (V_T), and available oxygen that most patients experience during anesthesia.

Compressed gas cylinders store carrier gases at high pressure (see Fig. 30.6A). They may be attached to the yoke (Fig. 30.9A) of the anesthesia machine or may be stored in a remote location and connected to the machine via gas lines. An outlet valve is located on the top of all compressed gas cylinders (see Fig. 30.9C). This valve must be opened when the cylinder is in use by turning the valve stem counterclockwise until it is fully open. When opened, gas will flow through the yoke and into the anesthetic machine. The valve is closed by turning it clockwise (see Fig. 30.9, *right side*).

Compressed gas cylinders are usually owned by a supplier that will pick up and refill them as needed. It must be always ensured that at least one spare full tank is available before commencing any anesthetic procedure. If the primary tank runs out, a second tank is thus always available.

Three holes are visible on the face of the outlet valve. The large hole is the valve port, where the gas exits the cylinder (see Fig. 30.9D). This port fits onto the nipple of the yoke (see Fig. 30.9F), with a washer in between (see Fig. 30.9H). The two smaller holes (see Fig. 30.9E) fit onto index pins (see Fig. 30.9G), which hold the cylinder in place. These holes and pins are a specific distance apart for each gas—a feature that prevents a cylinder containing the wrong gas from being attached to the yoke.

When removing a cylinder from the machine, it is important to make sure that the outlet valve is closed and the oxygen is evacuated ("bled off") from the system (see later section on tank pressure gauges for a review of this procedure). The cylinder should be supported, the wing nut loosened (see Fig. 30.9B), and the valve port backed off the yoke. The tank is carefully lowered until the valve clears the yoke. When attaching a full cylinder, first, the valve port is inspected for cleanliness and then a clean, undamaged washer is placed between the valve port and the nipple. The tank is gently raised into place, lining up the valve port and the pin holes with corresponding structures on the yoke. The wing nut is tightened as securely as possible by hand. The valve is opened slowly to listen for leaks. If a leak is present, the holes are rechecked for proper alignment, the wing nut tightened further, or a new washer used.

Compressed gas cylinders may contain different gases. To prevent confusion, oxygen cylinders are color-coded as green (United States) or white (international). These cylinders are available in two sizes, called *E-tanks* (see Fig. 30.6A, *bottom*) and *H-tanks*. E-tanks are stored on the yoke of the anesthesia machine or in a rack. H-tanks are much larger and are stored on a movable cart or chained to the wall and are often used to feed centralized oxygen sources. A centralized oxygen source is one in which the oxygen from an H-tank is piped to outlets at various points around the hospital. These outlets are then connected to anesthesia machines via quick-release connectors.

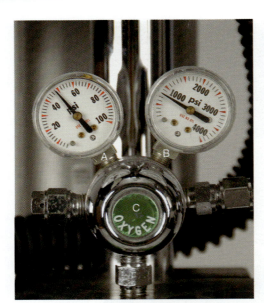

• **Fig. 30.10** (A) Line pressure gauge (registering 48 pounds per square inch [psi]). (B) Tank pressure gauge (registering 800 psi). (C) Pressure-reducing valve.

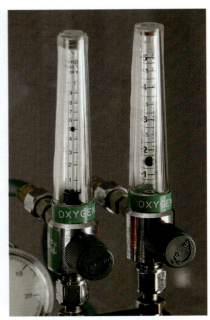

• **Fig. 30.11** Oxygen flowmeters with ball indicators. The flowmeter on the left is adjusted to 0.5 L/minute, and the flowmeter on the right is adjusted to 1.5 L/minute for a total oxygen flow of 2 L/minute.

In some practices, an oxygen concentrator or a bulk oxygen tank is used as a primary oxygen source. An oxygen concentrator is a machine that extracts oxygen from room air, and a bulk oxygen tank contains a large quantity of oxygen in liquid form.

The tank pressure gauge (Fig. 30.10B) indicates the pressure in a compressed gas cylinder. When full, a cylinder contains oxygen at a pressure of approximately 2200 pounds per square inch (psi). As oxygen is used, cylinder pressure gradually decreases. Oxygen cylinders should be changed when the pressure reaches 500 psi or a level at which the tank does not contain enough gas to last the anticipated length of the procedure. It is important to check the pressure before and throughout the anesthetic period to make sure there is enough oxygen to complete the procedure.

The volume of oxygen contained in an E-tank (expressed in liters) can be estimated by multiplying the pressure in psi by a factor of 0.3. A full tank therefore contains about 660 L of oxygen (2200 psi × 0.3 = 660). At a flow rate of 1 L/minute, this will last about 660 minutes, or 11 hours. The volume of oxygen in an H-tank in liters is about three times the pressure in psi. An H-tank with a pressure of 2200 psi therefore contains about 6600 L of oxygen (2200 psi × 3 = 6600, or 110 hours). When a compressed gas cylinder is turned off, the tank pressure gauge will continue to register pressure until the system is evacuated or "bled off." This is accomplished by depressing the oxygen flush valve until the gauge reads 0 psi.

The pressure-reducing valve (see Fig. 30.10C) reduces the pressure of gas exiting the compressed gas cylinder to 40 to 50 psi. This pressure is maintained regardless of the pressure in the cylinder. The line pressure gauge (see Fig. 30.10A) (not present on some machines) indicates pressure in the line connecting the pressure-reducing valve and the flowmeter(s). When the oxygen is turned on, this gauge should read 40 to 50 psi. Both parts function passively and require no action on the part of the machine operator.

The flowmeter (Fig. 30.11) controls the rate at which carrier gas is delivered to the patient and reduces the pressure from 40 to 50 psi to 15 psi. Carrier gas flow rates are expressed in liters per minute. Flowmeters are gas specific and are color coded to match the compressed gas cylinders; that is, green for oxygen in the United States. Some machines, such as the one pictured in Fig. 30.11, have two oxygen flowmeters. The meter on the right is used for flow rates greater than 1 L/minute, and the meter on the left is used for flow rates less than 1 L/minute.

The flowmeter is turned on by turning the dial counterclockwise. All flowmeters have a ball or rotor indicator that rises to a height proportional to the flow of gas. The *center* of a ball indicator or the *top* of a rotor indicator is read. These meters are turned off by turning the dial clockwise just until the ball or rotor drops to zero. Even though the knob can still be turned, it should *not* be turned any further to prevent damage to the valve.

Oxygen flow rates must be carefully chosen to ensure patient safety, produce desired changes in anesthetic depth, and conserve carrier and anesthetic gases. Although in some practices, it is common to use a standard rate of 1 to 2 L/minute for most SA patients, using specific rates will improve patient response, cost savings, and safety. Oxygen flow rates depend on the type of equipment and system used. When a rebreathing system is used, higher rates should be used during induction and recovery, and when changing anesthetic depth. Lower rates may be used during maintenance (Box 30.3 lists recommended oxygen flow rates).

The oxygen flush valve (Fig. 30.12F) delivers pure oxygen at 35 to 75 L/minute directly to the breathing circuit, bypassing the flowmeter and the vaporizer. The oxygen flush valve is used to quickly fill an empty reservoir bag with fresh oxygen but will dilute the concentration of the inhalant anesthetic in the breathing circuit. It is also used to deliver fresh oxygen to a critically ill patient or to flush the inhalant anesthetic out of the circuit during recovery from anesthesia or during a crisis. To flush the circuit, the vaporizer is turned off, the gases forced out of the reservoir bag using gentle hand pressure, and the valve pressed to refill the bag with fresh oxygen. When using this valve, only short bursts should be used to avoid overfilling the bag and damaging the patient's

Oxygen Flow Rates

Oxygen Flow Rates for Small Animals, Foals, Calves, and Small Ruminants

Chamber and Mask Inductions
Chamber induction:
- 5 L/minute

Mask induction: (300 mL/kg per minute or 30 times V_T)
- 1–3 L/minute for patients weighing 10 kg or less
- 3–5 L/minute for patients weighing more than 10 kg

Rebreathing Systems
Semiclosed system after induction, during a change in anesthetic depth, or during recovery:
50–100 mL/kg per minute (approximately 0.5–1 L/10 kg body weight/minute) up to a maximum of 5 L/minute. (This is approximately equal to ¼–½ of the RMV.)
- Approximately 0.5–1 L/10 kg body weight/minute up to a maximum of 5 L/minute

Semiclosed system during maintenance: (20–40 mL/kg per minute)
- Approximately 0.2–0.4 L/10 kg body weight/minute with a minimum of 250 mL/minute regardless of patient size
  Note: The use of a maintenance rate of 0.2 L/10 kg/minute is sometimes referred to as low flow.

Semiclosed system during maintenance with minimal rebreathing: (200–300 mL/kg per minute)
- Approximately 2–3 L/10 kg body weight/minute up to a maximum of 5 L/minute
- Note: At this flow, the machine functions in a manner similar to a nonrebreathing system.

Nonrebreathing Systems (used only for patients weighing 7 kg or less)
Mapleson A (Magill), modified Mapleson A (Lack), and modified Mapleson D (Bain) systems: (100–200 mL/kg per minute. This is equal to approximately 0.75–1.0 times the RMV.)
- Approximately 0.25–1.5 L/minute

Modified Mapleson D systems (Bain) with no rebreathing, Mapleson E systems (Ayre's T-piece), and Mapleson F systems (Jackson-Rees and Norman mask elbow):
(300–400 mL/kg per minute. This is equal to approximately 2–3 times the RMV.)
- Approximately 1–3 L/minute

Oxygen Flow Rates for Large Animals
Rebreathing Systems Note: rebreathing systems are only used in LA patients
Semiclosed system after induction, during a change in anesthetic depth, or during recovery:
Approximately 8–10 L/minute
Semiclosed system during maintenance:
Approximately 3–5 L/minute

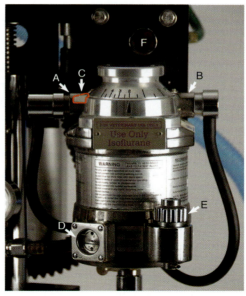

• **Fig. 30.12** Precision anesthetic vaporizer for isoflurane set on 2%. (A) Inlet port with a keyed fitting leading from the flowmeters. (B) Outlet port with a keyed fitting leading to the fresh gas inlet. (C) Safety lock. (D) Indicator window. (E) Fill port. (F) Oxygen flush valve (part of the compressed gas supply).

the agent used (purple for isoflurane, yellow for sevoflurane) (see Fig. 30.12). The vaporizer is turned on by disengaging the safety lock (see Fig. 30.12C) and turning the dial to the desired percent concentration.

> **TECHNICIAN NOTE**
> The level of liquid anesthetic in the vaporizer should be noted before each procedure. To function properly, it must be between the upper and lower lines of the window (see Fig. 30.12D). Refill as needed but always keep the vaporizer at least one-half full. Overfilling a vaporizer will result in anesthetic overdose; underfilling will lead to an inability to keep the patient anesthetized.

Except for some older models, the amount of inhalant anesthetic gas vaporized by a precision vaporizer is independent of variables such as ambient temperature, oxygen flow rate, RR and respiratory depth, and back pressure. This allows precise delivery of high vapor pressure inhalant agents, such as isoflurane and sevoflurane. Precision vaporizers are located out of the breathing circuit because of their high resistance to gas flow and are therefore known as *vaporizer out-of-circle* (Fig. 30.13).

All precision vaporizers will be somewhat affected by very high or very low carrier gas flow rates. Specifically, oxygen flows more than 10 L/minute or lower than 500 mL/minute may affect output. When flows are significantly less than the patient's **respiratory minute volume** (RMV) (200 mL/kg per minute), output will decrease slightly because of a dilution effect by expired gases. Therefore higher dial settings may be needed under these circumstances.

Vaporizer Inlet Port and Outlet Port and the Fresh Gas Inlet
The vaporizer inlet port (see Fig. 30.12A) is the point where oxygen and other carrier gases enter the vaporizer from the flowmeters. The vaporizer outlet port (see Fig. 30.12B) is the point where

lungs because of pressure buildup (a serious complication known as *barotrauma*).

Anesthetic Vaporizers
The anesthetic vaporizer holds liquid inhalant anesthetic and adds controlled amounts of vaporized anesthetic to the carrier gas. Vaporizers may be classified as precision or nonprecision vaporizers.

Precision Vaporizers
The inhalant anesthetics isoflurane and sevoflurane require the use of a precision vaporizer designed and color coded specifically for

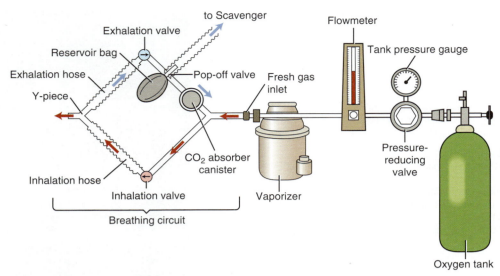

• **Fig. 30.13** Diagram of an anesthetic machine with a rebreathing circuit and vaporizer out-of-circle (VOC). Note that the vaporizer is located outside the breathing circuit.

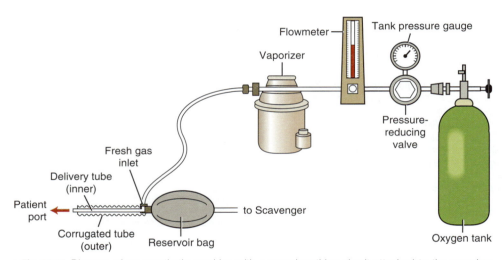

• **Fig. 30.14** Diagram of an anesthetic machine with a nonrebreathing circuit attached to the vaporizer outlet port.

oxygen, inhalant anesthetic, and other carrier gases exit the vaporizer. The point at which these gases enter the breathing circuit is referred to as the *fresh gas inlet*. Vaporizer outlet and inlet ports are connected to hoses with keyed fittings that prevent the operator from inadvertently attaching the wrong hose to the wrong vaporizer port.

Breathing Circuits

Breathing circuits circulate fresh gases to the patient and convey waste gases to the scavenging system. During inhalation and exhalation, the patient's lungs act like bellows to move air through the breathing circuit. Nonrebreathing systems do not resist air movement and are generally used for very small patients, because they minimize the work required to breathe. In contrast, rebreathing systems resist air movement, thus impairing the ability of very small patients to move gases through the circuit.

Use of a nonrebreathing system (Fig. 30.14) is recommended for patients weighing less than 7 kg and required for patients

weighing less than 2.5 to 3 kg. A nonrebreathing circuit is attached to the outlet port of the anesthetic vaporizer in place of the keyed fitting of a rebreathing circuit (see Fig. 30.7A). Fresh oxygen and inhalant anesthetic are delivered to the patient through a fresh gas inlet (see Fig. 30.7B), while exhaled gases pass into the scavenging system (see Fig. 30.7F), often after passing through a reservoir bag (see Fig. 30.7D). These systems flush out expired gases with the use of a relatively high oxygen flow rate (100–400 mL/kg per minute) and consequently do not require a CO_2 absorbent canister or unidirectional valves. Nonrebreathing circuits are available in a variety of configurations in which the position of some parts, including the fresh gas inlet, the reservoir bag, and the scavenger outlet, varies. These circuits are grouped using the Mapleson classification system into classes A through F, based on the position of the parts. The Magill circuit (Mapleson A), the Lack circuit (modified Mapleson A), the **Bain coaxial circuit** (modified Mapleson D), **Ayre's T-piece** (Mapleson E), the Jackson-Rees circuit (Mapleson F), and the Norman mask elbow (Mapleson F) are nonrebreathing circuits in common use.

Nonrebreathing systems have disadvantages. They do not conserve gases, moisture, or body heat, thus increasing the vigilance required to maintain patient body temperature. Waste gas scavenging is more difficult with some systems.

Manual ventilation is more challenging when using a nonrebreathing circuit, because most do not have a pressure manometer or an adjustable pop-off valve. When using a Bain coaxial circuit, these disadvantages can be overcome by using a universal control arm (also referred to as *Bain block*). The *universal control arm* is a device that when attached to a Bain circuit provides a conventional pop-off valve and manometer, increasing the ease and precision with which manual ventilation can be provided.

> **TECHNICIAN NOTE**
>
> After a nonrebreathing circuit is removed, the keyed fitting leading to the fresh gas inlet of a rebreathing circuit may be inadvertently left unattached to the vaporizer outlet port. If this happens, anesthetic gas will discharge into the room instead of discharging into the circuit, resulting in failure to keep the patient anesthetized and exposure of personnel to anesthetic gas. Checking the machine for leaks before each procedure will prevent this error.

Rebreathing systems deliver anesthetic gases to the patient, remove CO_2, and recirculate CO_2-free exhaled gases to the patient. These systems are also called *circle systems*, because the gases move in a modified circular pattern (see Fig. 30.13). Fresh oxygen and inhalant anesthetic enter the breathing circuit through the fresh gas inlet, and excess and waste gases exit the circuit through the pop-off valve. A rebreathing system may be used for patients weighing 2.5 kg or more, provided it is fitted with pediatric breathing tubes when used to anesthetize patients weighing between 2.5 and 7 kg.

Rebreathing systems offer several advantages. They may be operated with lower gas flow rates and therefore are more economical than nonrebreathing systems. They allow waste anesthetic gas to be efficiently and easily scavenged. These systems also minimize body heat and moisture loss, and allow observation and control of patient ventilation. These systems also have some disadvantages. Infectious agents may be transferred from patient to patient via microbe-laden moisture that condenses inside the machine parts and is inhaled by subsequent patients. Because the parts of these systems restrict air movement, they are not intended for use in very small patients (<2.5 kg).

A semiclosed rebreathing system (partial rebreathing system) is a safe, practical, and economical system used in general practice in all patients weighing 2.5 kg or more. When a semiclosed rebreathing system is used, the pop-off valve is left partially open, the oxygen flow rate is higher than the metabolic needs of the patient (>10 mL/kg per minute), and waste gases exit through the pop-off valve.

A closed rebreathing system (total rebreathing system) is identical to the semiclosed system, with two exceptions. The pop-off valve can be nearly or entirely closed, and the oxygen flow rate is just enough to meet the metabolic needs of the patient (5–10 mL/kg per minute). In other words, in this system, approximately the same amount of fresh gas is added to the circuit as the amount the patient consumes. Except for equine and bovine anesthesia, closed systems are infrequently used in practice because of the constant monitoring required, although most veterinary anesthesia texts include a detailed protocol for using these systems.

Rebreathing Circuit Parts

Unidirectional flow valves keep the flow of gases in a rebreathing circuit going one way as the patient breathes. The inhalation

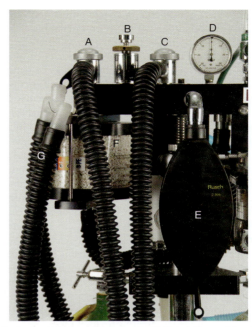

• **Fig. 30.15** Parts of a rebreathing circuit. (A) Exhalation unidirectional flow valve. (B) Pop-off valve. (C) Inhalation unidirectional flow valve. (D) Pressure manometer. (E) 2-L reservoir bag. (F) Carbon dioxide (CO_2) absorbent canister. (G) Small-animal (SA) corrugated breathing tubes.

(inspiratory) valve (Fig. 30.15C) opens to allow gas to flow through the corresponding corrugated breathing tube and into the patient's lungs during inspiration. During expiration, the exhalation (expiratory) valve (see Fig. 30.15A) opens to allow expired gases to flow through the corresponding corrugated breathing tube into the CO_2 absorbent canister. Thus inhalation of expired gases containing CO_2 is prevented.

The reservoir bag (breathing bag) (see Fig. 30.15E) is a storage reservoir for anesthetic gases. It provides compliance in the circuit by holding gases that enter the patient's lungs during inspiration and receives gases breathed out by the patient during expiration. It therefore should deflate during inspiration and inflate during expiration. The reservoir bag allows the anesthetist to visually observe patient respirations and to manually ventilate for the patient when necessary. Reservoir bags are available in a variety of sizes.

The bag should contain enough gas to fill the patient's lungs during inhalation, but it should not be so large as to prevent visualization of respiratory movements. The following rules of thumb can be used when selecting a bag: 500 mL for up to 3 kg; 1 L for 4 to 7 kg; 2 L for 8 to 15 kg; 3 L for 16 to 50 kg; 5 L for 51 to 150 kg. Patients weighing greater than 150 kg or that are intubated with at least an 18-mm endotracheal tube require an LA anesthesia machine that uses 35-L bags.

> **TECHNICIAN NOTE**
>
> Tidal volume (V_T) is the amount of air that passes into or out of the lungs during a normal breath. Normal V_T is about 10 to 15 mL/kg body weight. The size of the reservoir bag ideally should be at least five times the patient's V_T, although this is not always practical or necessary.

When in use, the reservoir bag should be approximately three-fourths full at peak expiration. The amount of gas in the bag is influenced by a variety of factors, including oxygen flow, pop-off valve adjustment, and scavenging system adjustment. Low oxygen flow rates, a fully open pop-off valve, or a maladjusted scavenging system can cause emptying of the bag. This will prevent the patient from filling its lungs with anesthetic gases during inspiration and will impair manual ventilation of the patient. In contrast, high oxygen flow rates, a closed pop-off valve, or a malfunctioning scavenging system may result in an overfilled bag. This may impair the patient's ability to exhale or may cause a buildup of pressure within the lungs and will impair monitoring of respirations by sight.

The pop-off valve (adjustable pressure-limiting valve) (see Fig. 30.15B) allows excess gases to exit the breathing circuit, transfers these waste gases to the scavenging system, and prevents buildup of excess pressure within the circuit. The pop-off valve allows a range of settings from fully closed to fully open to maintain optimal volume in the reservoir bag. When fully open, it releases when gas pressure in the circuit exceeds 0.5 to 1 cm H_2O. As the valve is tightened, more pressure is required for release. When a semi-closed rebreathing system is used, the valve is kept partially open when the patient is spontaneously breathing. It is closed *only* when manual ventilation is provided so that gases may be forced into the patient's lungs with the use of hand pressure. It should be closed only enough to provide the amount of breath required to ventilate the patient. After each breath provided by manual ventilation, it must be opened again to allow escape of gases and to prevent excess pressure in the chest. Excess intrathoracic pressure due to a closed pop-off valve will lead to severe, life-threatening cardiac compromise of the patient due to a rapid and precipitous decrease in cardiac output. Barotrauma may lead to pneumomediastinum and/or rupture of the lung with resultant tension pneumothorax. If any of these occurs and is not recognized and corrected immediately, death of the patient can occur.

The CO_2 absorbent canister (see Fig. 30.15F) is connected to the exhalation valve and receives expired gases. The canister holds absorbent granules, such as calcium hydroxide, which passively remove CO_2 from expired air.

Absorbent granules in the canister must be fresh to prevent the patient from rebreathing toxic levels of CO_2. When saturated, the granules will no longer absorb waste CO_2 and therefore should be changed after 6 to 8 hours of use, when one-third to one-half of the granules become saturated or after 30 days if either of the previous criteria are not met. Fresh absorbent granules can be crushed and are white, but when saturated, they become hard and turn an off-white color that is visibly distinguishable from the original. Most absorbents also contain a pH indicator that will cause a color change to

blue or violet when saturated. The color reaction does not always occur, however, and will dissipate after a few hours if not noted.

The pressure manometer (see Fig. 30.15D) indicates pressure (expressed in cm H_2O) in the breathing circuit and in the patient's lungs. This pressure is influenced primarily by oxygen flow and pop-off valve adjustment. The pressure manometer should read 0 to 2 cm H_2O when the patient is breathing spontaneously. It should read no greater than 20 cm H_2O in SAs or 40 cm of water in LAs when manual or mechanical ventilation is provided unless the chest cavity is open, in which case the pressure can be somewhat higher. Excessive pressure in the circuit can result in dyspnea, lung damage, pneumothorax, and decreased cardiac output. Therefore frequent monitoring of the pressure is critical during any anesthetic procedure.

The negative pressure-relief valve admits room air into the breathing circuit if a vacuum is detected, thus preventing patient asphyxiation. A vacuum may occur if the scavenging system exerts excessive suction, if the oxygen flow is too low, or if the oxygen cylinder is empty.

The corrugated breathing tubes (see Fig. 30.15G) complete the breathing circuit by carrying anesthetic gases to and from the patient. The Y-piece connects the inhalation and exhalation corrugated breathing tubes. Opposite ends of the breathing tubes attach to the unidirectional valves. The remaining port of the Y-piece is then connected to a mask or to an endotracheal tube. LA tubes are 50 mm in diameter and SA tubes (Fig. 30.16A) are 22 mm in diameter. Pediatric tubes (see Fig. 30.16B), which are shorter and smaller than conventional SA tubes, decrease mechanical dead space and are intended for patients weighing between 2.5 and 7 kg.

Dead space is defined as breathing passages and tubes that convey fresh oxygen to the alveoli but in which no gas exchange can occur. Increased dead space decreases the amount of fresh air that reaches the alveoli and is therefore available to the patient. *Mechanical dead space* is produced by the Y-piece, the portion of the endotracheal tube extending beyond the mouth, and anything placed between these structures, such as an apnea sensor or capnograph monitor, whereas *anatomical dead space* includes the mouth, nasal passages, pharynx, trachea, and bronchi. It is to the patient's advantage to decrease dead space as much as possible.

The universal F-circuit (see Fig. 30.16C) is a type of SA breathing tube in which the inhalation tube is located within the exhalation tube. This arrangement is designed to conserve body heat. As cold inspired gases travel through the inner turquoise tube, warm

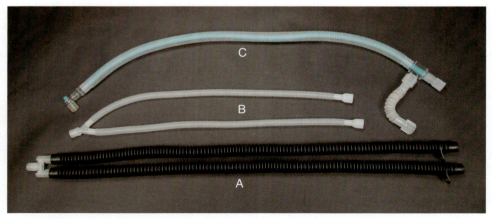

• **Fig. 30.16** Corrugated breathing tubes. (A) Standard 22-mm small-animal (SA) breathing tubes. (B) 15-mm pediatric tubes. (C) Universal F-circuit.

expired gases travel through the outer transparent tube, warming inspired gases.

Scavenging System

The scavenging system is connected to the pop-off valve (see Fig. 30.8A) or another breathing circuit outlet and transfers waste anesthetic gases outside the building through a system of hoses and pipes. Active scavenging systems use a vacuum pump or fan to remove waste gas, whereas passive scavenging systems work by gravitational flow. Active scavenging systems have a vacuum regulator that can be adjusted to prevent inadequate or excessive vacuum. They also have an interface (see Fig. 30.8B), which stores waste anesthetic gases until they can be evacuated and provides positive and negative pressure relief should excess pressure or vacuum develop within the breathing circuit.

All scavenging systems must be checked periodically to ensure that the tubes are not blocked and that the vacuum regulator and interface valves are properly adjusted according to the manufacturer's instructions. Excess vacuum from an active scavenging system will draw all gas out of the breathing circuit. This may lead to asphyxiation and can be recognized by a collapsed reservoir bag. Obstruction of the scavenging system will have the same effect as a closed pop-off valve and is indicated by a full reservoir bag or pressure buildup in the circuit.

An activated charcoal cartridge (see Fig. 30.8C) is attached to the discharge hose of the scavenging system and may be used as an alternative when a conventional scavenging system is not available. Activated charcoal will absorb commonly used halogenated inhalant anesthetics as waste gas is filtered through the cartridge. Activated charcoal cartridges should be weighed before use and must be replaced after 12 hours of use or a weight gain of 50 g.

Maintenance of the Anesthesia Machine

All anesthesia machines require regular maintenance to keep them functioning properly. Much of the maintenance of individual parts can be performed by the anesthetist, but the machine should be inspected and maintained by a repair professional at least once a year to ensure its proper operation.

The tank pressure gauge, line pressure gauge, pressure-reducing valve, flowmeters, oxygen flush valve, pop-off valve, negative pressure-relief valve, and pressure manometer do not require regular maintenance but should be checked by a repair professional for proper function annually or whenever a problem is suspected. Corrugated breathing tubes, reservoir bags, and other detachable rubber parts should be cleaned periodically with a mild disinfectant, such as chlorhexidine, rinsed, dried, inspected for holes or defects, and replaced as necessary.

Unidirectional flow valves should be disassembled, cleaned with 70% isopropyl alcohol or mild disinfectant, air dried, and inspected before reassembly to ensure that neither the valve nor the valve seat is damaged or warped. An incompetent valve will allow rebreathing of expired CO_2—a serious and potentially fatal complication.

> **TECHNICIAN NOTE**
>
> During any anesthetic event, if an elevated inspired carbon dioxide (CO_2) concentration is detected on an end-tidal CO_2 ($ETCO_2$) monitor or is otherwise suspected, check the unidirectional valves to be sure they are opening and closing as the patient breathes. A stuck valve will cause rebreathing of CO_2, a dangerous complication to be corrected immediately.

To change the CO_2 absorbent, the canister should be disassembled, the exhausted granules should be disposed of, the gaskets should be checked for damage, and each part should be cleaned with mild soap and water. The parts should be rinsed, dried, and reassembled. The canister is filled loosely with fresh absorbent granules, leaving at least one-half inch of air space at the top. After reassembly, the canister must be air tight. The CO_2 canister gasket is a frequent place for leakage, so it must be checked carefully for proper alignment after the absorbent is changed.

Principles of Endotracheal Intubation

Placement of an endotracheal tube offers several important advantages. It helps to maintain an open airway and allows inhalant anesthetics and oxygen to be administered precisely. It prevents pulmonary aspiration of stomach contents, blood, fluid, or other debris. It permits careful observation of RR and respiratory depth, and gives the anesthetist the ability to ventilate the patient when needed. The following equipment is required to perform endotracheal intubation:

- Appropriately sized endotracheal tubes
- Hard roll of gauze or IV tubing to secure the tube
- A gauze sponge to grasp the tongue
- A syringe to inflate the cuff (3 mL for cats; 12 mL for dogs and pigs; 20 mL for small-hoof stock, calves, and foals; and 60 mL for adult horses and adult cattle)
- A good examination light
- A laryngoscope with an appropriately sized blade for some species
- A stylet if intubating small ruminants or swine, if using a tube of narrow diameter, or if using any other tube that requires additional support
- Lidocaine to minimize laryngospasm (cats, small ruminants, and swine)

Selecting a Tube

A tube of appropriate diameter and length should be selected. At least three tubes of different sizes should be prepared so that if the first choice does not fit the patient's trachea, other options are always available. The following rules of thumb may be used to select the diameter: most cats require a 3- to 4.5-mm tube. The appropriate size for a dog is based on the patient's body weight. A 9.5- to 10-mm tube is prepared for a patient weighing 20 kg. The size is increased or decreased by approximately 1 mm for each 5-kg body weight less than or greater than 20 kg. In other words, a 7.5- to 8-mm tube is prepared for a 10-kg patient or a 10.5- to 11-mm tube for a 25-kg patient. It must be kept in mind that the usefulness of this rule of thumb depends on a variety of factors, including the patient's body condition and conformation, and the rule may not apply to all patients, particularly brachycephalic breeds and small or obese animals. Hounds will often require a larger-than-expected endotracheal tube.

A 7- to 12-mm tube is prepared for sheep and goats; a 6- to 14-mm tube for swine; a 9- to 16-mm tube for foals; a 9- to 18-mm tube for calves; and a 22- to 30-mm tube for adult horses and cattle.

Next, the appropriate length of tube is determined. The endotracheal tube should ideally extend from the tip of the nose to the thoracic inlet. If the tube is too long, one of two problems may occur. If inserted too far, the beveled end may inadvertently be advanced into only one mainstem bronchus, thus supplying only one lung with oxygen and anesthetic. If inserted cranial to the thoracic inlet, the portion of the tube extending from the mouth will increase mechanical dead space. Either situation will predispose the patient to hypoventilation and hypoxemia. If the tube is too short, it may not be long enough to reach the trachea.

Preparing the Tube

Each tube should be checked for blockages, holes, or other damage. It should be ensured that the connector is securely attached, and the cuff is checked by inflating it. If intact, the cuff should remain inflated after the syringe is detached from the valve. If the tube is soft or narrow, a stylet that does *not* extend beyond the end of the tube is used to stiffen the tube during placement. The tube can be lubricated with a small amount of sterile water-soluble lubricant or with the patient's saliva immediately before placement.

> **TECHNICIAN NOTE**
>
> Before placing an endotracheal tube, check the length, diameter, and cuff. Make sure that the connector is not loose and that the tube is not damaged or blocked with dried mucus.

Successful endotracheal tube placement requires knowledge of the anatomy of the pharynx and the larynx, including the glottis, epiglottis, vocal folds, and soft palate (Fig. 30.17B and C). Proper restraint, positioning, and visualization are also critical for success. The induction agent must be administered until the patient is in a state of readiness for intubation, which is characterized by unconsciousness, lack of voluntary movement, sufficient muscle relaxation to allow the mouth to be held open, and absent pedal and swallowing reflexes.

Intubation Procedures

Intubation Procedure for Small Animals

See Fig. 30.17.
- Place the patient in sternal recumbency.
- An assistant grasps the maxilla behind the canine teeth, extends the neck, and raises the head.
- Grasp the tongue with a gauze sponge and open the mouth fully by firmly pulling the tongue out and down.
- Adjust the light so that you have good illumination of the larynx.
- If necessary, use the tube or laryngoscope to gently displace the soft palate dorsally until the glottis can be visualized (see Fig. 30.17C).
- Gently insert the tube past the vocal folds using a rotating motion. If the tube is too large to pass easily, exchange the tube for one of smaller diameter, but *never force the tube*.
- After the tube is placed, gently transfer the patient to lateral recumbency.
- Check the tube to ensure that it is advanced to an appropriate distance and is oriented to match the natural curve of the trachea.
- Secure the tube with roll gauze or used IV tubing (over the nose for dolichocephalic dogs and behind the head for cats and brachycephalic dogs). Make sure the tie is secure enough not to slip but that it does not compress the tube.
- Connect the tube connector to the breathing circuit.
- Inflate the cuff and check for leaks (see the information for appropriate cuff inflation technique further on in the chapter).

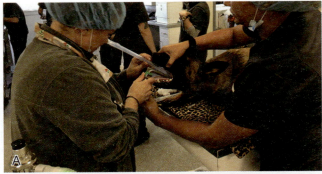
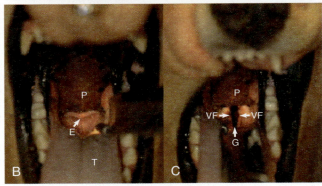

• **Fig. 30.17** (A) Proper position for endotracheal intubation in a small animal. (B) The anatomy of the pharynx and larynx: *P*, palate; *T*, tongue; *E*, epiglottis, which in this view is covering the glottis. (C) In this view, the epiglottis has been displaced ventrally with a laryngoscope. The glottis (*G*) is visible as the dark, oval opening between the vocal folds (*VF*), which move apart when the patient inspires and relax as the patient expires.

- Ensure a patent airway by checking the position of the patient and tube. The neck and tube should assume a gentle natural curve.

Intubation Procedure for Horses

Endotracheal intubation is performed blindly in this species because the larynx is impossible to visualize from the mouth. See Fig. 30.18.
- Extend the patient's head to line up the mouth, oropharynx, and larynx.
- Place a speculum or a mouth gag.
- Advance the tube over the tongue, taking care to stay in the center of the oropharynx so that the molar teeth do not damage the cuff.
- During inspiration, advance the tube *gently*.
- If resistance is encountered, stop and pull the tube back 10 to 15 cm.
- Repeat if unsuccessful, rotating the tube 90 degrees each time.
- Once the tube passes easily into the larynx and trachea, check for correct replacement by feeling for air passing out of the tube on expiration. If the horse is apneic, pressure on the thorax will produce the same effect. It may be helpful to apply gentle pressure externally on the larynx (cricoid pressure) or to flex, then re-extend the head if intubation is unsuccessful after a few attempts.

Intubation Procedure for Adult Cattle

Endotracheal intubation is also performed blindly in adult cattle. See Fig. 30.19.

- Place a speculum or a mouth gag.
- Extend the patient's head and neck.
- Insert your arm into the patient's mouth.
- Palpate and then reflect the epiglottis forward.
- Remove your arm and grasp the endotracheal tube, with the beveled end protected in your palm.
- Guide the tube into the larynx using your hand that is in the patient's mouth while using your other hand to advance the tube into the trachea.

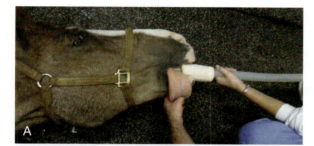

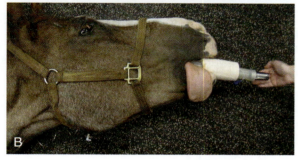

• **Fig. 30.18** Equine intubation. (A) The anesthetist advances the endotracheal tube blindly through a speculum in the mouth and into the larynx with the head extended. (B) The anesthetist feels for movement of air when the horse breathes out to confirm correct placement of the tube in the trachea.

Intubation Procedure for Small Ruminants and Small or Young Cattle

These patients are intubated using a technique like that used for SA patients. The oral cavity is long and narrow in these animals, so visualization of the larynx requires use of a laryngoscope with a long blade, and intubation is facilitated using a stylet.

- Extend the patient's head and neck.
- Hold the mouth open.
- Gently pull the tongue down and out by grasping it with a gauze sponge.
- Insert a stylet that protrudes from the patient end of the endotracheal tube to facilitate intubation.
- Once the larynx is visualized, insert the stylet no more than 2 to 5 cm into the trachea.
- While holding the stylet firmly in position, pass the tube over the stylet into the larynx.

Because of limited space in the mouth, it may be necessary to remove the laryngoscope while passing the endotracheal tube. Goats may develop laryngospasm, so topical lidocaine may be used to desensitize the larynx before intubation. It is imperative to inflate the cuff as soon as a ruminant is intubated to prevent aspiration of regurgitated material or saliva. It is useful to have suction available, to keep the head elevated higher than the rumen to prevent passive regurgitation, and to keep the nose in a downward sloping position (when not otherwise extended during intubation) to reduce the chance of aspiration.

Checking for Proper Placement

An endotracheal tube can easily be misplaced into the esophagus and therefore may appear to be correctly placed when it is not. This will result in an inability to keep the patient anesthetized and put the patient at risk for aspirating and/or developing hypoxemia; therefore confirmation of proper placement is essential. The following techniques may be used to confirm proper placement:

- Revisualize the larynx to confirm successful intubation (dogs, cats, and small ruminants).
- Watch for expansion and contraction of the reservoir bag as the animal breathes.

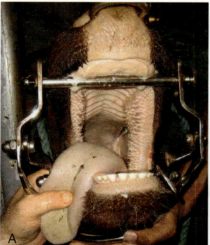 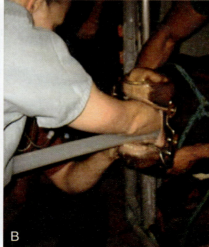 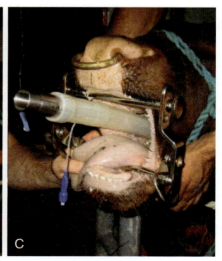

• **Fig. 30.19** Bovine intubation. (A) A mouth gag is placed and the head extended by an assistant. (B) The anesthetist palpates the larynx with their fingers and directs the endotracheal tube into the trachea. (C) With the tube in place, the cuff can be inflated and the mouth gag removed.

- Feel for air movement from the tube connector as the patient exhales.
- Palpate the neck. The only naturally firm structure in the neck is the trachea. If the tube is properly placed, only one firm structure should be palpable. Palpation of two firm structures (the tube and the trachea) indicates placement of the tube inside the esophagus.
- If the patient is able to vocalize (whine or cry), the tube is not in the correct location (this most commonly applies to dogs).
- When using an end-tidal carbon dioxide ($ETCO_2$) monitor, the presence of a normal waveform indicates proper placement.
- Check that the motion of the unidirectional valves coincides with breathing. (*Note:* this is not always a reliable indicator of successful intubation.)

Cuff Inflation

The cuff of the endotracheal tube must be gently inflated until a seal is formed between the trachea and the cuff. This will prevent leakage of anesthetic gases and mixing with room air, which will result in a variety of complications, including contamination of the surgery suite with waste gases and difficulty keeping the patient anesthetized. To inflate the cuff, extend the patient's head to straighten the airway. Attach an air-filled syringe to the valve port. Have an assistant close the pop-off valve and gently compress the reservoir bag. Listen for gas leakage around the tube, which may sound like a soft hiss or gurgling. Slowly inflate the cuff until the leaking just ceases at a pressure of 20 cm H_2O. Avoid overinflation of the cuff, which can result in a variety of mild to serious complications.

Laryngospasm

Laryngospasm is a complication in which the glottis forcibly closes during intubation. This complication is most encountered in cats, swine, and small ruminants. It is extremely difficult to place a tube in a patient experiencing laryngospasm, because the glottis closes as soon as it is touched and cannot be safely forced open. Laryngospasm can lead to **hypoxia** and **cyanosis** in severe cases but it is prevented using one or more of the following strategies:

- Apply 2% injectable lidocaine via a syringe directly to the glottis before placement. Wait 30 to 60 seconds for the lidocaine to take effect before attempting intubation; 0.1 mL is appropriate for cats, whereas 1 to 2 mL can be used in sheep, goats, and pigs. Alternatively, lidocaine gel can be swabbed onto the arytenoid cartilages.
- Make sure that the patient is adequately anesthetized before attempting intubation, because laryngospasm decreases with increasing anesthetic depth.
- Prepare carefully, wait for the glottis to open before attempting placement, and try to insert the tube the first time. Repeat attempts worsen laryngospasm.
- *Do not force the tube.* This can lead to severe and potentially life-threatening complications, including tracheal rupture, pneumothorax, and pneumomediastinum.

Complications of Intubation

Numerous hazards are associated with endotracheal intubation (Box 30.4). Most are associated with tracheal irritation, trauma, or failure to protect the airway. Although the larynx and the trachea of mammals are relatively resilient structures, excessive force will

> **• BOX 30.4** Complications of Endotracheal Intubation
>
> **Cuff Not Inflated/Underinflated**
> - Inability to create a seal between cuff and trachea
> - Difficulty with or inability in keeping the patient anesthetized
> - Aspiration of stomach contents
> - Aspiration of foreign material and fluid during dental cleaning
> - Pollution of the work space with anesthetic gas
>
> **Tube Diameter Too Small**
> - Inability to create a seal between cuff and trachea, leading to the same complications as when cuff is not inflated
> - Small tubes more likely to block with mucus
> - Increased resistance to breathing with increased respiratory effort
>
> **Cuff Overinflated/Tube Diameter Too Large**
> - Necrosis of the tracheal mucosa
> - Possibility of tracheal rupture in extreme situations
>
> **Tube Too Long**
> - If placed past the thoracic inlet, intubation of only one mainstem bronchus, leading to hypoxia and difficulty in keeping the patient anesthetized
> - If extending beyond the mouth, increased mechanical dead space, leading to hypoventilation and hypoxia
>
> **Tube Too Short**
> - Inability to intubate the patient successfully
> - Displacement of the tube from the glottis if the patient's body position is changed
>
> **Overzealous Intubation**
> - Tracheal irritation, leading to tracheitis and postoperative cough
> - Trauma or tracheal rupture, resulting in pneumomediastinum and/or pneumothorax
>
> **Tube Kinked or Obstructed**
> - Dyspnea and hypoxemia
> - Asphyxia and cardiac arrest if not corrected
>
> **Tube Not Removed Before Return to Consciousness**
> - Damage to the tube from chewing
> - Blockage of the airway
> - In extreme situations, a severed portion of the tube can be aspirated or swallowed
>
> **Tube Not Cleaned and Disinfected**
> - Transmission of infectious agents, leading to tracheitis, bronchitis, or pneumonia
> - Blockage of the tube with dried mucus or other foreign material

result in damage, perforation, rupture, or irritation of the delicate mucosa. An endotracheal tube must therefore be chosen, maintained, placed, and monitored with care.

Monitoring the Anesthetized Patient

There is a common misperception that modern anesthetic agents are safe. This belief can lead to the erroneous assumption that careful monitoring is not important, but patient monitoring is, and always has been, one of the cornerstones of the successful practice of anesthesia, because conditions that may lead to serious complications are often subtle and must be recognized and corrected without delay. Serious complications of anesthesia often develop rapidly and, if not prevented, are devastating for the patient, the owner, and the anesthetist. Consequently, the anesthetist must develop the ability to remain vigilant and be prepared to manage periods of urgency and crisis. This requires that the anesthetist be knowledgeable, alert, and watchful for subtle changes in the condition of the patient.

Effective monitoring requires continuous investigation of data from the patient, equipment, and monitoring devices, and effective communication with surgeons and the entire patient care team. This approach promotes safety and efficiency, and reduces boredom or distractions.

During any general anesthetic procedure, the anesthetist must strike a delicate balance between sufficient depth of anesthesia to produce unconsciousness and insensitivity to pain without endangering the life of the patient by compromising cardiovascular and respiratory system function. Monitoring allows the anesthetist to achieve this balance through careful observation and precise regulation of the amount of anesthetic administered.

The American College of Veterinary Anesthesia and Analgesia (ACVAA) has published a set of guidelines for patient monitoring, entitled "Recommendations for Monitoring Anesthetized Veterinary Patients" (available at http://www.acvaa.org/veterinarians/guidelines). These guidelines are designed to improve the level of patient care and to decrease the incidence of anesthetic complications by providing specific recommendations for monitoring, including methods, frequency, and record keeping. Familiarity with these guidelines will help the veterinary anesthetist provide state-of-the-art care for all anesthetized and sedated patients.

> ### TECHNICIAN NOTE
>
> The principles of patient monitoring are as follows:
> - Monitor patients frequently using your hands, eyes, and ears.
> - Always check multiple parameters.
> - Never depend on instrumentation alone.
> - Do not attempt to judge depth of anesthesia on the basis of drug doses or dial settings.

Stages and Planes of Anesthesia

In the early 1900s, a system of stages and planes of general anesthesia was developed to describe patient responses to diethyl ether, an early inhalant anesthetic that is no longer used in clinical practice. Changes in patient behavior, body movements, ocular signs, reflexes, and vital signs in response to the progression from consciousness to deep surgical anesthesia were observed and documented. Under this system, general anesthesia was divided into four stages (I–IV), and stage III was subdivided into four planes (1–4).

Stage I—Period of Voluntary Movement

During this stage, the patient gradually loses consciousness. This stage is usually characterized by fear, excitement, and struggling. HR and RR increase, and the patient may pant, urinate, or defecate. Near the end of stage I, the patient loses its ability to stand and becomes recumbent.

Stage II—Period of Involuntary Movement

During this stage, also known as the *excitement stage*, the patient loses voluntary control and assumes an irregular breathing pattern. It is usually characterized by involuntary reactions in the form of vocalizing, reflex struggling, or paddling. HR is often elevated, pupils are dilated, muscle tone is marked, and reflexes are present.

Stage III—Period of Surgical Anesthesia

During this stage, the patient is unconscious and progresses gradually from light to deep stage III anesthesia. This stage is characterized by progressive muscle relaxation, decreasing HR and RR, and loss of reflexes. The pupils gradually dilate, tear production decreases, and the pupillary light reflex is lost. The increase in HR and RR seen in response to surgical stimulation during light anesthesia is gradually lost. Many anesthetists divide stage III into three planes, corresponding to inadequate, optimal, and excessive depths of anesthesia, which may be referred to as *light stage III anesthesia*, *surgical anesthesia*, and *deep stage III anesthesia*.

Stage IV—Period of Anesthetic Overdose

During this stage, the nervous, cardiovascular, and respiratory systems are extremely depressed. Breathing stops, muscle tone is flaccid, pupils are widely dilated, and all reflexes are absent. The heart stops and death follows quickly unless rapid action is taken.

Principles of Monitoring

Healthy patients (physical status class ASA I) should be monitored at least every 5 minutes during any general anesthetic procedure. Higher risk patients (physical status classes ASA II–V) must be monitored more frequently and, in some cases, continuously. Ultimately, the anesthetist must judge the frequency of monitoring that is appropriate for each patient. An anesthetic record should be used to document monitoring parameters, drug administration, and other information pertinent to the procedure (Fig. 30.20).

At any given time during an anesthetic event, the patient should be somewhere between consciousness and surgical anesthesia. Careful observation of the patient based on expected responses enables the anesthetist to determine the stage and plane the patient is in. For instance, unconsciousness, intact reflexes, eyes in a central position, marked jaw tone, and movement in response to stimulation are all expected responses from a patient in light stage III anesthesia—a point inappropriate to perform surgery. In contrast, absent palpebral, pedal, and swallowing reflexes; moderate jaw tone; eyes in a ventromedial position; and an intact corneal reflex are all expected responses from a patient in surgical anesthesia—an appropriate stage to begin the procedure.

Many factors can influence progression through the stages of anesthesia and interpretation of physical signs. For instance, patients induced using IV agents often pass through stages I and II so quickly that they are minimally noticeable. In contrast, when anesthesia is induced with an inhalant agent, it takes longer to reach surgical anesthesia and the patient may be difficult to control while passing through these stages. Premedication generally decreases the excitement seen during stages I and II and therefore eases passage into surgical anesthesia.

In addition, the anesthetic protocol will influence the interpretation of physical signs. For example, after induction with an $alpha_2$ adrenergic agonist, the patient will often have a much lower HR compared with that after induction with an inhalant agent. A patient may have dilated pupils if given a dissociative agent but, conversely, may have constricted pupils if given an opioid. Consequently, physical signs must be interpreted considering the agents administered.

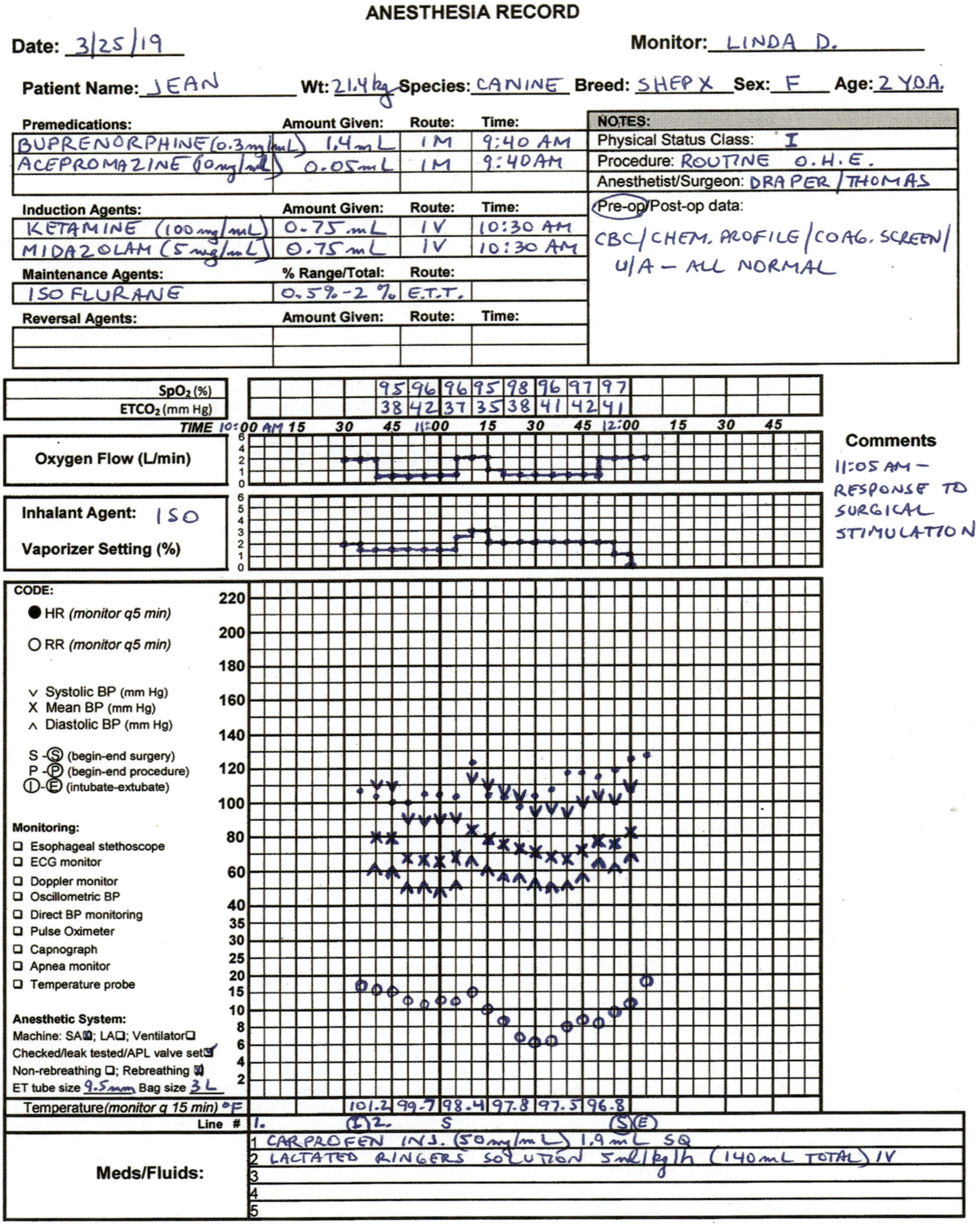

ANESTHESIA RECORD

Date: 3/25/19   **Monitor:** LINDA D.

Patient Name: JEAN   **Wt:** 21.4 kg **Species:** CANINE **Breed:** SHEP X **Sex:** F **Age:** 2 Y.O.A.

Premedications:	Amount Given:	Route:	Time:
BUPRENORPHINE (0.3 mg/mL)	1.4 mL	IM	9:40 AM
ACEPROMAZINE (10 mg/mL)	0.05 mL	IM	9:40 AM

NOTES:
Physical Status Class: I
Procedure: ROUTINE O.H.E.
Anesthetist/Surgeon: DRAPER / THOMAS
Pre-op/Post-op data:
CBC / CHEM. PROFILE / COAG. SCREEN / U/A — ALL NORMAL

Induction Agents:	Amount Given:	Route:	Time:
KETAMINE (100 mg/mL)	0.75 mL	IV	10:30 AM
MIDAZOLAM (5 mg/mL)	0.75 mL	IV	10:30 AM

Maintenance Agents:	% Range/Total:	Route:
ISOFLURANE	0.5% - 2%	E.T.T.

Reversal Agents:	Amount Given:	Route:	Time:

SpO₂ (%)	95 96 96 95 98 96 97 97
ETCO₂ (mm Hg)	38 42 37 35 38 41 42 41

TIME 10:00 AM 15 30 45 11:00 15 30 45 12:00 15 30 45

Oxygen Flow (L/min)

Inhalant Agent: ISO
Vaporizer Setting (%)

Comments
11:05 AM — RESPONSE TO SURGICAL STIMULATION

CODE:
● HR (monitor q5 min)
○ RR (monitor q5 min)
∨ Systolic BP (mm Hg)
X Mean BP (mm Hg)
∧ Diastolic BP (mm Hg)
S - Ⓢ (begin-end surgery)
P - Ⓟ (begin-end procedure)
Ⓘ - Ⓔ (intubate-extubate)

Monitoring:
☐ Esophageal stethoscope
☐ ECG monitor
☐ Doppler monitor
☐ Oscillometric BP
☐ Direct BP monitoring
☐ Pulse Oximeter
☐ Capnograph
☐ Apnea monitor
☐ Temperature probe

Anesthetic System:
Machine: SA☒; LA☐; Ventilator☐
Checked/leak tested/APL valve set ☒
Non-rebreathing ☐; Rebreathing ☒
ET tube size 9.5mm Bag size 3 L

Temperature (monitor q 15 min) °F	101.2 99.7 98.4 97.8 97.5 96.8

Line # 1.   (I) 2.   S   (S)(E)

Meds/Fluids:
1 CARPROFEN INJ. (50 mg/mL) 1.9 mL SQ
2 LACTATED RINGERS SOLUTION 5 mL/kg/h (140 mL TOTAL) IV
3
4
5

• **Fig. 30.20** Anesthesia record. This form is used to document the anesthetic protocol, monitoring parameters, treatments, and other information pertinent to the procedure.

After considering each of these factors, the anesthetist must ultimately answer two questions:

1. Is the patient safe or in danger?
2. Is the depth of anesthesia inadequate, excessive, or appropriate for the procedure being performed?

Monitoring parameters are the physical signs used to answer these questions. They are subdivided into vital signs, reflexes, and other indicators of anesthetic depth. Although all monitoring parameters are evaluated together, some are more useful for answering the first question, whereas others are more useful for answering the second.

Vital Signs

Vital signs are used primarily to evaluate the cardiovascular and pulmonary systems. Vital signs include HR and heart rhythm, RR and respiratory depth, mucous membrane color, capillary refill time (CRT), blood pressure, and temperature. These parameters are used principally to answer the question, "Is the patient safe or in danger?" They are only loosely correlated with the depth of anesthesia. Specifically, patients in lighter planes of anesthesia tend to have higher HR, RR, and blood pressure; pinker mucous membranes; and more rapid CRT, whereas patients in deeper planes experience opposite effects (Table 30.3). However, other factors may change this association. For example, a patient in light stage III anesthesia given an opioid agonist may have a decreased HR. Conversely, a patient in deep stage III anesthesia may have an elevated HR if in shock. Although vital signs are helpful in determining anesthetic depth, other parameters are better suited to this purpose.

The ACVAA's Recommendations for Monitoring Anesthetized Veterinary Patients group vital signs into three classifications: (1) indicators of circulation; (2) indicators of oxygenation; and (3) indicators of ventilation.

Indicators of Circulation

Indicators of circulation include HR and heart rhythm, mucous membrane color and CRT, pulse strength, and blood pressure. HR, measured in beats per minute (bpm), and heart rhythm (Table 30.4) may be monitored by palpation of the chest wall, palpation of the pulse, auscultation, or use of monitoring equipment. HR generally decreases gradually in response to increasing anesthetic depth, because most anesthetic agents are cardiovascular depressants. This effect is extremely variable, however, and is influenced by the specific agents used, blood pressure, pre-existing illness, and other factors. Although bradycardia is caused to some degree by most anesthetic agents, opioids and alpha$_2$ adrenergic agonists are particularly likely to have this effect. Conversely, dissociatives and anticholinergics may cause tachycardia.

During anesthesia, the normal heart rhythm is normal sinus rhythm (NSR) or sinus arrhythmia in dogs and NSR in cats. LAs typically exhibit NSR, but sinus arrhythmia may also be observed. Athletic horses may exhibit first- or second-degree atrioventricular (AV) block. Cardiac arrhythmias can be induced by anesthetic agents, particularly alpha$_2$ adrenergic agonists, anticholinergics, and dissociatives but can also be caused by other conditions, such as hypoxia, gastric dilatation-volvulus, **hypercarbia**, pre-existing heart disease, and trauma.

Mucous membrane color (Table 30.5) is monitored by observing the color of the oral mucous membranes. CRT (see Table 30.5) is the time it takes (in seconds) for normal color to return after

TABLE 30.3 Relationship Between Vital Signs and Anesthetic Depth

Vital Sign	Depth: Too Light	Depth: Surgical Anesthesia	Depth: Too Deep
Heart rate	Usually elevated	Variable	Usually decreased
Respiration rate	Usually elevated	Variable	Usually decreased
Pulses	Strong	Palpable but often less strong	Weak/nonpalpable
Mucous membrane color/ capillary refill time	Normal/normal	Normal but may be somewhat paler/normal	Pale/prolonged

TABLE 30.4 Normal and Abnormal Heart Rate and Rhythm

Species	Normal HR, beats per minute (bpm) (awake/at rest)	Normal HR, bpm (anesthetized)	Report to the Veterinarian If:[a]
Dog[b]	60–180	60–150	Large dogs: <60 or >140; Small dogs: <70 or >160
Cat	120–240	120–180	<100 or >200
Horse	30–45	28–40	<25 or >60
Cattle	60–80	50–80	<40 or >100

[a]In addition to the rates listed, any arrhythmia should be reported to the veterinarian.
[b]Because of the extreme variability of size, large dogs tend to have lower rates, whereas small dogs and puppies have higher rates.
HR, Heart rate.

digital pressure is applied to the gums near the base of a tooth. If oral tissues are pigmented, the tongue, conjunctiva, or mucous membranes of the prepuce or vulva can be used as alternatives.

Pale mucous membranes indicate poor capillary perfusion, vasoconstriction, or anemia resulting from any cause. Prolonged CRT indicates poor capillary perfusion.

Blood pressure can be monitored by indirect measurement (obtained with a Doppler monitor or an oscillometric monitor) or by direct measurement (obtained with an arterial catheter) (see "Monitoring Equipment"). Pulse strength (see Table 30.5), as determined by palpation of a peripheral artery (e.g., the lingual, femoral, carotid, or dorsal pedal artery in SAs, or the facial, auricular, digital, or dorsal pedal artery in LAs), gives the anesthetist a rough but potentially inaccurate indication of blood pressure. A strong pulse is suggestive of normal blood pressure and a weak pulse is suggestive of hypotension; however, a weak pulse can also be a result of vasoconstriction and hypertension. Bounding pulses may be palpated with congenital cardiac abnormalities such

TABLE 30.5	Normal and Abnormal Mucous Membrane Color, Capillary Refill Time, and Pulse Strength		
Vital Sign (all species)	Normal (awake/at rest)	Normal (anesthetized)	Report to the Veterinarian If:
Mucous membrane color	Pink (often described as "bubblegum pink")	Pink (may be somewhat paler than when awake)	Pale or blue
CRT	<2 seconds	<2 seconds	>2 seconds
Pulse strength	Palpable with one pulse closely after each heartbeat	Often somewhat decreased in strength but still palpable	Nonpalpable Irregular Excessively weak

CRT, Capillary refill time.

TABLE 30.6	Normal and Abnormal Respiratory Rate, Effort, and Tidal Volume		
Species	Normal (awake/at rest)	Normal (anesthetized)	Report to the Veterinarian If:
Dog	10–30 (panting is normal)	8–20	<6 or >20
Cat	15–30	8–20	<6 or >20
Horse	8–20	6–12	<6 or >20
Cattle	8–20	6–12, although rapid, shallow breathing is common	<6 or >20
All species	Normal effort and V_T	Normal effort; approximately 25% decrease in V_T	Increased effort; >25% decrease in V_T

V_T, Tidal volume.

as a patent ductus arteriosus and are associated with hypotension under anesthesia. Pulse strength varies widely among individuals, so the anesthetist should assess the pulse as a point of reference before administering an anesthetic.

Indicators of Oxygenation

Pulse oximetry and measurement of dissolved blood oxygen through blood gas analysis are the best indicators of oxygenation. Mucous membrane color, the only physical indicator of oxygenation, will change from pink to cyanotic in severely deoxygenated nonanemic patients, but this does not warn of deoxygenation in sufficient time to permit timely intervention and is not accurate in the presence of anemia. Therefore it is, at best, a very crude indicator of tissue oxygenation.

Indicators of Ventilation

Indicators of ventilation include RR, respiratory effort, V_T, capnography, and blood gas analysis. RR measured in breaths per minute, respiratory effort, and V_T (Table 30.6) are monitored by observing movement of the chest wall, expansion and contraction of the reservoir bag, or movement of unidirectional flow valves or by using monitoring equipment. Auscultation, an important tool for evaluating lung sounds, does not work well for monitoring RR and respiratory depth. It is advisable to observe the patient's respiratory depth and quality while the patient is awake as a point of reference.

Because most anesthetic agents are respiratory system depressants, anesthetized patients often experience a decrease in RR and about a 25% decrease in V_T directly related to anesthetic depth. This hypoventilation can lead to atelectasis, resulting in decreased gas exchange and hypoxemia. This effect is common during anesthesia, particularly in the dependent lung (the one nearest the table). Many clinicians recommend gentle inflation of the lungs by periodic manual ventilation about every 2 to 5 minutes during anesthesia to prevent this complication. This technique is referred to as "bagging" or "sighing" the patient.

In addition to the effects of anesthetic agents, many other potential causes of hypoventilation are known, including postinduction apnea. As the term implies, *postinduction apnea* is a phenomenon

that commonly occurs after anesthetic induction for the following reason: during induction, all patients pass through lighter stages of anesthesia, during which hyperventilation occurs for a period ranging from several seconds to a few minutes. Hyperventilation of sufficient length will cause the patient to expire excessive quantities of CO_2, which results in a decreased concentration of CO_2 in blood. In response to this decreased concentration, the patient hypoventilates or stops breathing until a normal CO_2 level is re-established.

Postinduction apnea can be frightening and dangerous if not understood and must be managed promptly with supportive care. Supportive care involves careful monitoring of other parameters, including oxygen saturation, and periodic manual ventilation about two to four times per minute to maintain adequate oxygen levels until the patient begins to breathe spontaneously. When managing postinduction apnea, excessive ventilation should be avoided so that the normal CO_2 level can be re-established. Use of a capnograph allows precise measurement of CO_2 levels and is a useful tool for managing this problem. The patient must breathe or be ventilated sufficiently to transition from injectable anesthesia to inhalant anesthesia.

During anesthesia, the patient should exhibit normal respiratory effort. Dyspnea indicates a serious patient problem or machine malfunction that must be addressed promptly. Abdominal breathing is a unique breathing pattern associated with dangerously excessive anesthetic depth. It is characterized by a rocking motion of the abdomen and chest because of paralysis of the respiratory muscles, and immediate action must be taken to remedy this.

Body temperature (Table 30.7) should be monitored about every 15 to 30 minutes with a rectal thermometer or probe. Although body temperature can be estimated by touching the skin of the paw or ear, it cannot be accurately determined this way. Hypothermia is experienced by most patients during anesthesia and can lead to bradycardia, prolonged recovery, and predisposition to anesthetic overdose if severe. Hypothermia usually occurs rapidly after induction and is often of a relatively large magnitude.

| TABLE 30.7 | Normal and Abnormal Body Temperatures | | | |

Species	Normal (awake/at rest)	Normal (anesthetized)	Report to the Veterinarian If:
Dog and cat	37.8°C–39.2°C (100°F–102.5°F)	Variably decreased	>39.7°C (103.5°F) or <36.1°C (97°F)
Horse	37.2°C–38°C (99°F–100.5°F)	Variably decreased	>38.6°C (101.5°F) or <36.1°C (97°F)
Cattle	37.8°C–39.2°C (100°F–102.5°F)	Variably decreased	>39.7°C (103.5°F) or <36.1°C (97°F)

| TABLE 30.8 | Interpretation of Reflexes and Other Indicators of Depth of Anesthesia | | | |

Indicator	Inadequate Depth	Surgical Anesthesia	Excessive Depth
Palpebral reflex	Present	Decreased or absent[a]	Absent
Swallowing reflex	May be present	Absent	Absent
Pedal reflex	Present	Absent	Absent
Corneal reflex[b]	Present	Present	Absent
Muscle tone	Marked	Moderate	Flaccid
Eyeball position	Usually central	Usually ventromedial	Central
Pupil size	Constricted	Gradually larger	Widely dilated
PLR	Present	Gradually nonresponsive	Absent
Lacrimal secretions	Present	Gradually decreased	Absent
Nystagmus[c] (horses)	Fast	Slow or absent	Absent
Response to surgical stimulation	Marked increase in HR, RR, or V_T	Mild or no increase in HR No increase in RR or V_T	No increase in HR, RR, or V_T

[a]Absent when halogenated inhalant agents are used (small animals); may be sluggish when other agents are used to maintain anesthesia or in large animals.

[b]The corneal reflex is not reliable in small animals.

[c]Nystagmus may also be caused by severe hypoxia or hypercarbia in horses.

HR, Heart rate; PLR, pupillary light reflex; RR, respiratory rate; V_T, tidal volume.

Therefore the following steps should be taken to reduce heat loss during all anesthetic procedures:

- Do not allow the patient's body to contact stainless steel.
- Place a heat-retaining surface under the patient, such as a warm-water circulating blanket, a blanket, a towel, or lamb's wool.
- During preparation of the surgery site, avoid the use of alcohol as a rinsing agent and avoid wetting the hair excessively.
- Avoid excessively low ambient temperatures in the surgical suite.

In malignant hyperthermia (MH), a complication of general anesthesia, body temperature progressively rises to dangerous levels. MH is caused by a genetic defect in muscle metabolism and occurs in the presence of some anesthetic drugs, such as halogenated inhalant anesthetics and neuromuscular blockers. It is most common in pigs but has also been reported in other species. MH is a medical emergency that must be promptly recognized, reported, and treated. Early signs include muscle rigidity, skin that is red and hot to the touch, and excessive production of CO_2, which leads to exhaustion of the CO_2 absorbent and elevated CO_2 levels on the capnograph.

Reflexes and Other Indicators of Depth of Anesthesia

Reflexes are involuntary protective responses to stimuli (e.g., blink reflex when lightly touching an animal's eyeball). Reflexes and other indicators of anesthetic depth are used to answer the question, "Is the anesthetic depth inadequate, excessive, or appropriate for the procedure being performed?" See Table 30.8.

The palpebral reflex is induced by gently tapping the skin at the medial or lateral canthus of the eye with a finger. This reflex is present when anesthesia is too light, progressively diminishes with increasing depth, and is generally absent in surgical anesthesia in SAs, but it should still be present in horses and ruminants until they are in a moderately deep plane of anesthesia.

The swallowing reflex is a normal reflex that occurs in response to the presence of saliva or food in the pharynx. It is detected by watching the throat for swallowing motions. The swallowing reflex is generally present when anesthetic depth is inadequate but is absent in surgical and deeper stages of anesthesia and therefore is used to determine whether anesthesia is too light.

The pedal reflex is the withdrawal of a limb in response to a painful stimulus. To induce this reflex, a limb is placed in a relaxed position and a toe vigorously pinched. Withdrawal of the limb indicates inadequate depth of anesthesia.

The corneal reflex is induced by placing a drop of sterile artificial tears on the cornea. When the reflex is present, the eyeball will retract slightly within the orbit. In lighter planes of anesthesia, a blink response may also occur. This response is difficult to interpret when the eyes are in a ventromedial position and is not reliable in SAs, but it should be present during all planes of surgical anesthesia in LAs and therefore helps determine whether anesthetic depth in an LA patient is excessive.

Muscle tone is most frequently determined in SAs by assessing jaw tone. The jaws are opened with the fingers and resistance is assessed. Muscle tone is high when the depth of anesthesia is inadequate, gradually diminishes with increasing depth, and is described by using the terms *marked*, *moderate*, *loose*, and *flaccid*. Muscle tone may be assessed by observing the size of the anal opening, which will be closed at lighter planes and progressively more open at deeper planes. Geriatric animals may have a "stiff" jaw that is related to arthritis and not an inappropriately light plane of anesthesia. Jaw tone is highly individualized to the patient.

Eye position and pupil size are also useful in determining anesthetic depth. Eye position is central (straight forward) in light anesthesia, gradually shifts to a ventromedial position (toward the chin), and finally shifts back to a central position in deep anesthesia. In most patients, ventromedial deviation is common during surgical anesthesia. In some horses, eye position may change from ventromedial to central and back again. This is usually indicative of surgical anesthesia. The presence of nystagmus (rapid involuntary movements of the eye) usually indicates a light plane of anesthesia in any patient.

Response to Surgical Stimulation

When stimulated by cutting or manipulation of viscera, HR, RR, V_T, or blood pressure may increase. A sudden, marked increase in any of these parameters indicates inadequate depth of anesthesia. Mild changes in HR may occur, however, even in surgical anesthesia. It is important to realize that the appropriate depth for each patient may vary somewhat depending on the degree of surgical stimulation and pain associated with the procedure.

Monitoring Equipment

Use of monitoring equipment is a valuable addition to physical assessment but should never be performed alone. The main advantages of such equipment are that it gives early warning of impending problems before serious consequences develop, and it allows measurement of certain physical parameters, such as blood pressure, oxygen saturation, or expired CO_2, which is not possible with physical assessment. Monitoring equipment allows the anesthetist to assess the patient more precisely than would otherwise be possible. For instance, a pulse oximeter can detect hypoxemia long before cyanosis is visible. A capnograph can accurately and rapidly warn of inadequate or excessive ventilation, and an oscillometric monitor can detect subtle changes in blood pressure before a change in pulse strength is evident. In this section, use of this equipment is reviewed. However, use of touch, sight, and smell are also appropriate to be used by anesthetists on their patients.

Mechanical Indicators of Circulation

The *esophageal stethoscope* (Fig. 30.21) is a device designed to amplify the sound of the heartbeat so that the anesthetist can monitor the heart from a distance. Although this device is not capable of determining heart rhythm, the anesthetist can be alerted to a possible arrhythmia by noting changes in HR, irregularity, or interruption in heart sounds. Esophageal stethoscopes are inexpensive and are easy to operate and maintain.

Parts include esophageal catheters of various sizes, a sensor, and a base unit, which amplifies and converts heart sounds into an audible electronic signal. To use the esophageal stethoscope, the closed end of an appropriately sized catheter is lubricated and inserted into the esophagus to the level of the heart (about the fifth rib). The free end is attached to the electronic base via the sensor, and the position of the catheter and the volume are adjusted until the signal is audible.

The base should be cleaned as needed and batteries must be changed periodically. Catheters should be washed with a disinfectant and dried after use. Immersing the catheter or introducing water inside the catheter should be avoided.

The *electrocardiography (ECG) monitor* is used to monitor HR and heart rhythm. Electrodes are attached to specific locations on the patient's skin, and electrical activity of the heart and HR are displayed on a screen in real time. These monitors generally require little care. When using the ECG monitor, it is important to realize that it is possible for the heart to stop beating and for electrical activity to continue for a time after the heart has stopped. The technician should never depend on this monitor alone as a guarantee of patient safety but also utilize a stethoscope and pulse assessment by feel during surgery.

The *Doppler ultrasound monitor* (Fig. 30.22) is a device that detects the flow of blood through small arteries and converts this motion into an audible signal. Blood flow is converted to a continuous sound like that of a heart murmur. Parts include an electronic base unit that processes the signal and a probe that emits and receives ultrasound waves. The hair overlying a small artery must be clipped and the skin cleaned and covered with a generous amount of ultrasound gel. The probe is positioned over the artery, adjusted until an audible signal is detected, and then taped in place.

Placement of a Doppler ultrasound probe requires patience and finesse. It must be oriented parallel to and precisely over the artery, and must make firm but not excessive contact. Subtle differences in position of only 1 or 2 mm can make the difference between success and failure in acquiring a signal.

Doppler ultrasound probes are delicate and expensive, and must be handled carefully. They should be cleaned by wiping gently with a gauze sponge. Gentle cleaning with tap water is acceptable, but the probe must not be immersed, scrubbed, or autoclaved.

In SA patients, Doppler ultrasound probes may be placed on the ventral surface of a paw proximal to the metacarpal or metatarsal pad, on the ventral surface of the tail base, on the dorsomedial surface of the hock, or on the medial surface of the thigh in patients weighing less than 5 kg (10 lb). In LA patients, the ventral

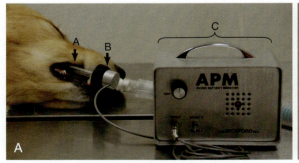
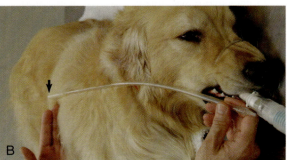

• **Fig. 30.21** (A) Esophageal stethoscope. *A,* Catheter. *B,* Sensor. *C,* Base unit. (B) Measurement of the catheter to the level of the fifth rib or the caudal border of the scapula *(arrow).*

tail is the most frequently used site. Fig. 30.23 shows common locations for placement of the probe.

When used with the sphygmomanometer, the Doppler monitor can also be used to determine blood pressure (see Fig. 30.23, *top left*). A properly fitted cuff is placed on the forelimb, metatarsus, or tail base, with the cuff balloon centered over the artery. The width of the cuff should be 30% to 50% of the circumference of the extremity (Fig. 30.24, *inset*). After establishing a good Doppler signal, the cuff is inflated until the artery is occluded (the signal

can no longer be heard). The pressure is gradually decreased until the audible signal can be heard again. This represents the systolic pressure. These instruments tend to consistently underestimate systolic blood pressure in cats but are fairly accurate in dogs. All indirect blood pressure measurements are subject to many inaccuracies, however, and must be interpreted considering other signs. Table 30.9 provides normal blood pressure values during anesthesia.

The *oscillometric blood pressure monitor* (see Fig. 30.24) is a device that is used to measure blood pressure and HR. Parts include a blood pressure cuff and a computerized base unit that inflates and deflates the cuff and analyzes signals received by the cuff.

A cuff is placed around a limb or a tail with the balloon centered over an artery, and the unit is turned on. The cuff is inflated and deflated automatically by the machine. The unit detects oscillations within the cuff bladder caused by pulsations of the arteries. Because of the changes in intracuff pressure, systolic, mean, and diastolic pressures are calculated. The cuff can be placed around the forelimb, metatarsus, metacarpus, or tail of SA and LA patients. Fig. 30.25 shows examples of locations for cuff placement. For proper operation, the cuff should be at the same horizontal plane as the heart. This device is more accurate in SA patients weighing more than 7 kg; however, this method of determining blood pressure has shown to be inaccurate in LA patients.

Mechanical Indicators of Oxygenation

The *pulse oximeter* (Fig. 30.26) is a device that is designed to detect changes in the oxygen saturation of hemoglobin. Red and infrared wavelength light is passed through or reflected from a tissue bed, detected by a sensor, and analyzed. The sensor is sensitive to blood pulsation in the arteries, so it also determines HR. The machine determines the percent oxygen saturation ($\%SpO_2$) by calculating the difference between levels of oxygenated and

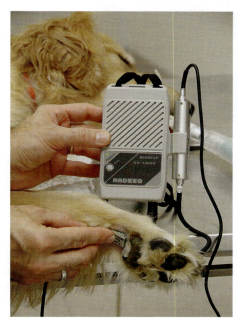

• **Fig. 30.22** Doppler monitor: base unit with the probe positioned over the ventral surface of the metacarpus proximal to the metacarpal pad.

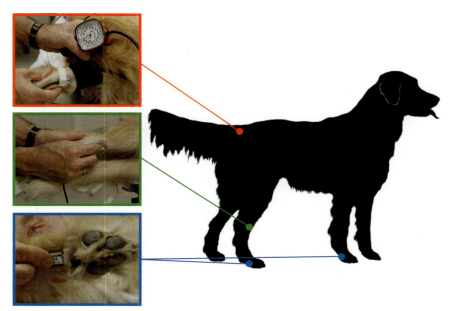

• **Fig. 30.23** Locations for Doppler ultrasound probe placement. *Red*, Determination of systolic blood pressure with the use of a sphygmomanometer, with the cuff placed around the tail base and the probe placed on the ventral surface of the tail distal to the cuff. *Green*, Probe over the dorsomedial surface of the hock. *Blue*, Probe proximal to the metatarsal pad or the metacarpal pad.

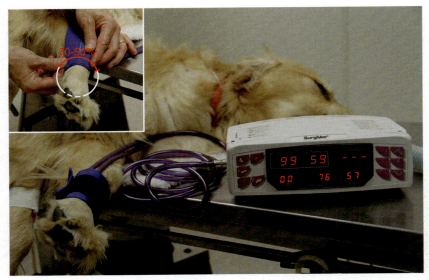

• **Fig. 30.24** Oscillometric blood pressure (BP) monitor with a cuff placed on the metacarpus. The following measurements are indicated—systolic BP: 99 mm Hg; diastolic BP: 59 mm Hg; mean arterial pressure (MAP): 76 mm Hg; heart rate (HR): 57 beats per minute (bpm). *Inset*, An appropriately sized blood pressure cuff should be selected, the width of which should be 30% to 50% of the circumference of the extremity.

TABLE 30.9	Normal Blood Pressure Values During Anesthesia	
Blood Pressure Value (mm Hg)	**Small Animal**	**Equine**
Systolic	100–160	>80
Mean	60–90	60–90
Diastolic	50–70	>50
Minimum acceptable mean during anesthesia	60	70
Hypertension	Systolic >160	Systolic >140

deoxygenated hemoglobin. Both HR and oxygen saturation are digitally displayed.

Normally, when breathing pure oxygen, hemoglobin in the lungs is at least 97% saturated with oxygen. Therefore during oxygen administration, oxygen saturation should be greater than 95%. Saturation between 90% and 95% indicates desaturation and signals the need to determine a cause. Saturation of less than 90% indicates hypoxemia that requires treatment. Saturation of less than 85% for longer than 30 seconds is a medical emergency.

Parts include a computerized base unit and a variety of probes. Pulse oximeter probes are classified as transmission or reflective. Transmission probes are constructed in a clamplike configuration. One of the jaws houses a light source, and the other houses a sensor that detects the transmitted light. Transmission probes must be applied over a nonpigmented tissue bed that is thin enough to allow light transmission, such as the tongue, lip, ear, flank fold, prepuce, vulva, digital web, nasal septum, or foot of SA patients. Although these probes can function through a thin haircoat, excessive hair will prevent operation. The lingual probe and the

"C" probe are examples of transmission probes. Fig. 30.27 shows examples of probe types and placement.

Reflective probes are often long and narrow. The light source and the sensor are located next to each other on one side of the probe. These probes are covered with a protective sleeve and placed inside a hollow organ, such as the esophagus or the rectum, with the side housing the light source and sensor in contact with a tissue bed. When a reflective probe is placed in the rectum, care must be taken to digitally displace the feces from the wall of the rectum and place the correct side of the probe against the tissue. A reflective probe may also be taped against the ventral surface of the tail (see Fig. 30.27).

Pulse oximeter probes can be frustrating to work with, because of the high incidence of signal loss. When this happens, values will no longer appear on the display, the numbers will be incorrect, or an alarm may sound, and the probe must be readjusted or moved to a different location. Probe function is adversely affected by many factors, including tissue pigmentation, motion, excessive pressure, orientation in relation to ambient light, and patient conditions such as anemia, icterus, vasoconstriction, or edema. Box 30.5 presents suggestions for troubleshooting signal loss.

Pulse oximeters require little maintenance but must be handled with care. Probes should be cleaned with alcohol or another mild disinfectant but must not be immersed, scrubbed, or autoclaved. (See Case Presentation 30.1 for an example of the use of a pulse oximeter to monitor oxygenation.)

Mechanical Indicators of Ventilation

The *capnograph*, also known as an end-tidal CO_2 monitor (Fig. 30.28), is a device that measures the level of CO_2 present in inspired and expired air. Parts include a computerized base unit and a fitting that is placed between the endotracheal tube connector and the breathing circuit.

The capnograph enables the anesthetist to estimate the partial pressure of CO_2 in the patient's bloodstream and is one of the best indicators of adequate respiration. Because CO_2 is produced at the tissue level, carried by the vascular system, and eliminated by the

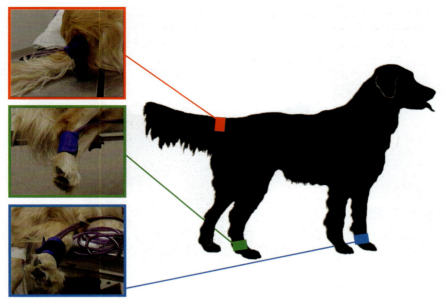

• **Fig. 30.25** Locations for placement of a blood pressure cuff. *Red*, Base of the tail. *Green*, Metatarsus. *Blue*, Metacarpus.

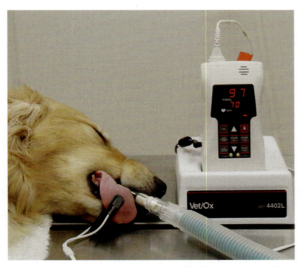

• **Fig. 30.26** Pulse oximeter with transmission lingual probe. The upper number (97) represents the percent oxygen saturation (%SpO$_2$). The lower number (70) represents heart rate (HR) in beats per minute (bpm).

lungs, abnormal readings may be caused by diseases of the lungs, cardiovascular system, or tissues, and by equipment malfunction.

In normal animals, during inspiration, the level should be 0 mm Hg. At the end of expiration, the level should rise to 35 to 45 mm Hg when the patient is awake and to 40 to 55 mm Hg when anesthetized. This increase during anesthesia occurs as the result of the respiratory depression that accompanies general anesthesia. Any change in the configuration of the curve can indicate a problem and should be explored.

End-tidal CO_2 as measured by a capnometer may not correlate as closely to arterial CO_2 levels in LA species, particularly in the presence of severe atelectasis or imbalance between ventilation and perfusion of the lungs. Arterial blood gas analysis is often indicated in these instances.

Interpretation of capnograph tracings is complex and is beyond the scope of this chapter. The student is encouraged to explore the recommended readings for additional information.

Small-animal Anesthesia

A successful anesthetic procedure requires not only careful preparation but also a good understanding of the sequence of events involved in taking a patient from consciousness to surgical anesthesia and back to consciousness. Procedure 30.1 summarizes these events when an SA patient is induced with injectable agents and maintained with an inhalant agent.

Selecting a Protocol

An anesthetic protocol is a list of premedication and anesthetics for a particular patient, including dosages, routes, and order of administration. Anesthetic protocols are commonly selected by the attending veterinarian according to their training and clinical experience. A suitable protocol takes into account patient signalment, pre-existing problems, physical status class, and the procedure to be performed.

After the protocol is known, all drug dosages, oxygen flow rates, and fluid administration rates are calculated and checked *carefully*, because most anesthetic agents have narrow therapeutic indices and overdosing can easily occur. All protocols should be approved by the attending veterinarian prior to use.

TECHNICIAN NOTE

The volume (in milliliters) of each injectable anesthetic drug to be given must be calculated with extreme care. The general formula for most injectable anesthetics is as follows:

Volume (mL) = Drug dosage (mg or µg/kg or lb body weight)
× Patient body weight (kg or lb) ÷ Drug concentration (mg or µg/mL)

Note: When this calculation is performed, drug dosage and body weight units must be the same (kg or lb), as must drug dosage and drug concentration units (mg or µg).

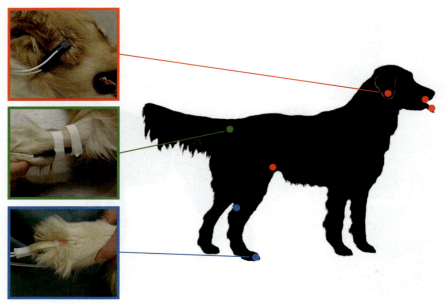

• **Fig. 30.27** Examples of pulse oximeter probes and locations for placement. *Red,* Transmission probe on the ear flap. Additional red dots show alternate placement locations for this probe (tongue, lip, and flank fold). *Green,* Reflective probe taped to the ventral surface of the tail base. *Blue,* "C"-probe (a transmission probe) on the toe web. The other blue dot shows an alternative placement location for this probe (the skin fold between the Achilles tendon and the tibia).

• BOX 30.5   Suggestions for Troubleshooting Pulse Oximeter Signal Loss

Transmission Probes
- Make sure the patient is safe by assessing vital signs.
- Remove and replace the probe.
- If the tongue is dry, wet it.
- Ensure that the pressure placed on the tissue by the probe is not excessive or inadequate.
- When possible, the jaw with the sensor should be oriented toward the ceiling to avoid interference from ambient light.
- Choose a different area that is not pigmented, covered with excessive hair, icteric, or edematous.
- If the area is heavily haired, clip the hair, and gently cleanse the area.

Reflective Probes
- Ensure the patient is safe by assessing vital signs.
- Ensure the side with the light source and sensor is oriented toward the tissue.
- Check for adequate tissue contact.
- When the probe is placed in the rectum, ensure that feces are not between the probe and the tissue.

Patients with ASA III to ASA V physical status classification require use of modified protocols based on the patient's primary condition (Table 30.10). Management of these cases can be challenging and requires customization of the anesthetic protocol by the attending veterinarian.

Equipment Preparation

During typical induction of anesthesia, anesthetic agents are administered; the patient becomes unconscious and recumbent; the endotracheal tube is placed, secured, cuffed, and attached to the machine; the anesthetic gas level is adjusted; the patient is positioned and monitored; and adjustments are made as needed—all within the first few minutes of the procedure. Because these events follow one another so rapidly, the technician has little to no time to leave the patient to locate necessary equipment. Therefore all equipment must be carefully gathered, checked, and organized before the procedure is begun.

The Preanesthetic Period

The preanesthetic period is the time before induction of general anesthesia. During this period, a physical assessment is performed, patient history and results of laboratory tests are reviewed, the patient is stabilized, an IV catheter is placed, and fluid administration is started. Premedication, including tranquilizers, α^2-agonists, opioids, dissociatives, anticholinergics, or a combination of these, are administered to calm and prepare the patient for anesthetic induction. Premedications are chosen to produce a specific set of desired effects, such as sedation, analgesia, and muscle relaxation. Most are given intramuscularly, although some may be administered intravenously. After IM injection, the patient is placed in a quiet but observable location for about 15 to 20 minutes for the agents to take effect before proceeding; otherwise, the patient may partially override the beneficial effects. Prior to induction, providing oxygen by mask or cannula for 5 to 10 minutes will allow the lungs to fill with an increased percentage of oxygen. A tightly fitting mask can increase the oxygen concentration in the lungs to close to 100%. This is called *preoxygenation*, and it increases body oxygen storage and tolerance to apnea. Although preoxygenation is useful, it is often not well tolerated in many patients, so it is often reserved for more compromised individuals.

CASE PRESENTATION 30.1

Anesthesia of a Canine

Cocoa, a 2-year-old 15.2-kg female Spaniel mix, was anesthetized in preparation for a routine ovariohysterectomy (OHE). Based on preanesthetic assessment, she was classified as a physical status class ASA I patient. Cocoa was premedicated with 0.1 mg/kg acepromazine given by intramuscular (IM) injection 15 minutes before anesthesia was induced with a mixture of 5 mg/kg ketamine and 0.25 mg/kg diazepam given by intravenous (IV) injection. After reaching surgical anesthesia, she was maintained with isoflurane at 2.5% and oxygen at a rate of 0.5 L/minute. Pulse oximetry was used to monitor Cocoa via a transmission probe placed on the tongue. After surgical preparation, she was transferred to the operating room. For the first 10 minutes of surgery, Cocoa's oxygen saturation (SpO$_2$) was in the range of 96% to 99%. Then, over a 3-minute period, SpO$_2$ gradually fell to 92%, although heart rate (HR; 85 beats per minute [bpm]), respiratory rate (RR; 8 breaths per minute), mucous membrane color, and refill remained normal.

The normal SpO$_2$ for patients breathing oxygen is 95% or greater. Low SpO$_2$ can be caused by many factors, including pre-existing disease, pulmonary edema, loss of signal, airway blockage, lack of adequate oxygen flow, and respiratory depression. When faced with this situation, the veterinary technician must rapidly determine whether the decrease is real or an artifact and then, if real, must explore possible causes and correct the problem without delay.

The technician determined that the patient was in no immediate danger based on assessment of the other vital signs. Pre-existing disease was deemed unlikely, as indicated by this patient's medical history. The technician rapidly checked the airway, checked the oxygen supply, turned the oxygen up to 3 L/minute, and ruled out pulmonary edema based on normal lung sounds. Because pulse oximeter probe signals are frequently lost due to excess probe pressure, drying of the tissue, patient movement, interference from ambient light, and other factors, the technician removed the probe, rewetted Cocoa's tongue, and replaced the probe, with careful attention to location, orientation, and pressure.

Despite these measures, SpO$_2$ remained between 90% and 93%. Although RR was normal, careful observation revealed a V$_T$ estimated to be less than 50% of normal. Manual ventilation was initiated with a maximum inspiratory pressure of 20 cm of water. After the first breath, SpO$_2$ rapidly returned to 96%. Intermittent positive pressure breaths were given about every 30 seconds for the first 2 minutes and then about every 5 minutes for the duration of the procedure. Oxygen saturation remained in the normal range. This case illustrates the importance of careful observation of respiratory depth during anesthesia which, in this patient, was insufficient to maintain an adequate oxygen level.

Induction of Anesthesia

During induction of anesthesia, the patient is taken from consciousness to unconsciousness. Agents commonly used for anesthetic induction in SAs include a mixture of ketamine and diazepam, propofol, alfaxalone, neuroleptanalgesics, and inhalant anesthetics. Except for inhalant anesthetics, these agents are most often given intravenously.

Intravenous Induction

To induce general anesthesia by the IV route, the calculated volume is drawn up and administered *to effect* until the patient can be intubated, or until the patient is at an adequate plane of anesthesia for completion of the planned procedure. The term "to effect" means that the drug is administered gradually in increments until the desired stage of anesthesia is reached. The entire calculated dose may or may not be given.

Immediately after giving the patient an initial dose, HR and RR are checked to ensure the patient is stable and breathing. Muzzles and other restraint devices are removed. It is important to make sure the patient has passed through stage II and that anesthetic depth is adequate to allow intubation. While the drug is given, there must be interplay between administration of the drug and monitoring of the patient. After giving the initial dose, the vital signs, pedal reflex, palpebral reflex, and jaw tone are rapidly checked; more drug may be given if needed, and the values are rechecked. If the patient is in light anesthesia and needs more drug or starts to wake up while being intubated, a much smaller amount is given to effect (about one-fifth to one-tenth of the original volume) until the patient is in an adequate plane of anesthesia. Although all are given to effect, different induction agents should be given at slightly different rates as described below.

Propofol

Propofol is given "to effect," with approximately one-fourth of the total calculated dose given every 30 seconds until the patient is at an adequate depth for endotracheal intubation. The drug is administered rapidly enough to take the patient through stage II and into stage III.

Ketamine-Diazepam or Ketamine-Midazolam

These agents should be given slowly to effect over 60 to 120 seconds.

Alfaxalone

Alfaxalone should be given at a rate of one-fourth the calculated dose every 15 seconds to effect.

Intramuscular Induction

To induce anesthesia by using the IM route, the entire calculated volume is drawn up and administered. In general, the dosage for IM injection is about two to three times the corresponding IV dosage. When given intramuscularly, anesthetic agents have a slower onset and a longer duration than when given intravenously. Typically, induction takes 5 to 20 minutes. After the peak effect, if the anesthetic depth is inadequate, additional injectable drug is given intramuscularly or intravenously, or an inhalant agent is administered through a mask until intubation. Note that some drugs, such as propofol and etomidate, *must not* be given intramuscularly.

Mask Induction

Mask induction requires the use of a rapid-acting inhalant anesthetic, such as isoflurane or sevoflurane. Once induction has been completed, an endotracheal tube can be placed to maintain anesthesia for the duration of the procedure. Mask induction is a special challenge for several reasons. Many patients struggle, necessitating skillful restraint (enough to prevent operator and patient injury but not so much as to restrict chest excursions or the airway). It is more challenging to monitor mucous membrane color and refill, and ocular indicators of anesthetic depth, because the mask partially obscures the eyes and the muzzle; however, the patient should be monitored carefully

To induce anesthesia by using a mask, a well-fitted mask is attached to the breathing circuit and held over the patient's muzzle. Pure oxygen is administered for 2 to 3 minutes at the recommended rate, and then the vaporizer is turned on to 0.5% to 1% for about 30 seconds to allow the patient to become accustomed

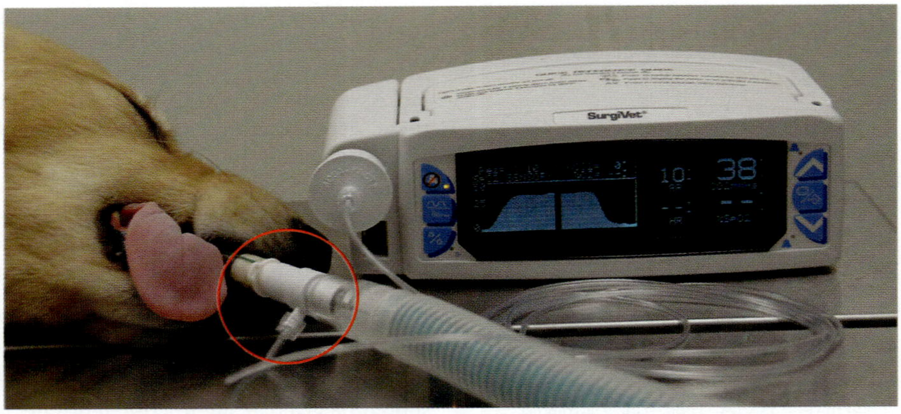

• **Fig. 30.28** Capnograph registering an end-tidal carbon dioxide ($ETCO_2$) level of 38 mm Hg and a respiratory rate (RR) of 10 breaths per minute (bpm) *(upper right)*. The spacer *(circled)* is located between the breathing circuit and the endotracheal tube connector. The graph indicates carbon dioxide (CO_2) levels throughout the respiratory cycle which, in normal awake patients, is 35 to 45 mm Hg during expiration and 0 mm Hg during inspiration.

PROCEDURE 30.1

Sequence of Events for a Small-Animal Anesthetic Procedure[a]

1. Assess, prepare, and weigh the patient (see the section on "Patient Preparation" in this chapter).
2. Determine the protocol (anesthetic agents, including dosages, routes, and sequence of administration).
3. Calculate the volume of each agent to be given, including fluid administration rates (preanesthetic, induction, maintenance, and analgesic agents).
4. Calculate the oxygen flow rates (see Box 30.3).
5. Prepare equipment required to administer drugs (scales, syringes, needles, agents, reversal agents, emergency cart, controlled substance log).
6. Prepare fluid administration equipment (clippers, antiseptic scrub, intravenous [IV] catheters, tape, saline flush, catheter cap, administration extension set, fluids).
7. Prepare equipment for endotracheal intubation (see the section on "Principles of Endotracheal Intubation" in this chapter).
8. Prepare monitoring equipment, including anesthesia record, stethoscope, monitors, and probes (see the section on "Monitoring the Anesthetized Patient" in this chapter).
9. Assemble and test the anesthetic machine (see the section on "Anesthesia Equipment" in this chapter).
10. Administer premedications intramuscularly approximately 15 to 20 minutes before or intravenously approximately 5 to 10 minutes before anesthetic induction.
11. Place an IV catheter, attach the fluid administration set, and begin fluid administration.

12. Administer the induction agent.
13. Check the patient's readiness for intubation.
14. Place and secure the endotracheal tube (see the section on "Principles of Endotracheal Intubation" in this chapter).
15. Turn on the oxygen and connect the endotracheal tube to the breathing circuit.
16. Check the patient's vital signs.
17. Turn on the inhalant anesthetic to the appropriate level.
18. Determine the patient's anesthetic depth and commence regular monitoring.
19. Position and secure the patient for the procedure, paying attention to padding, maintenance of an open airway, unrestricted blood flow, and unrestricted chest excursions.
20. Attach monitoring devices.
21. Continue to monitor and adjust anesthetic and oxygen levels as needed until completion of the procedure.
22. Prepare the patient for recovery.
23. Discontinue the anesthetic and extubate the patient at the appropriate time (i.e., return of swallowing reflex).
24. Remove monitoring equipment, IV catheters, and any other equipment no longer needed.
25. Prepare the patient for continued hospitalization or discharge by applying bandages, administering medications, and performing any other procedures ordered by the veterinarian.

[a]Induction with an IV agent and maintenance with an inhalant agent.

to the smell of the gas. The setting is increased to 3% to 5% if using isoflurane and 4% to 6% with sevoflurane. Some clinicians recommend a gradual increase over several minutes, allowing the patient time to become accustomed to the gas. Other anesthetists increase the vaporizer setting immediately, especially if the patient is difficult to handle when using the gradual method. If the patient struggles, it is important to monitor carefully for cyanosis or other problems and be ready to act quickly if the patient becomes compromised. As soon as the patient is in lateral recumbency, readiness for intubation should be assessed and the anesthetic level

adjusted. Mask induction generally is *not* appropriate for brachycephalic breeds.

Chamber Induction

Chamber induction may be used only for patients small enough to fit comfortably into the chamber. This technique is commonly used in place of a mask for SA patients that are aggressive or difficult to handle. Once induction has been achieved, an endotracheal tube can be placed to maintain anesthesia for the duration of the procedure.

TABLE 30.10 Recommendations for Physical Status Class ASA III to ASA V Small-animal Patients

Primary Condition	Example Protocols and Other Considerations	Avoid These Agents/Circumstances
Cardiac disease	Premedicate with opioids and benzodiazepines Etomidate, propofol, or alfaxalone induction Ketamine/diazepam induction may be acceptable if cardiac disease is mild Maintain with isoflurane or sevoflurane Maintain blood pressure in normal range	Acepromazine in patients with congestive heart failure α^2-agonists Mask/chamber induction (as a result of stress) Ketamine/Telazol
Liver disease	No premedication or use opioids if needed Preoxygenation before induction Propofol, alfaxalone, or etomidate induction if mild to moderate Mask induction if severe Maintain with isoflurane or sevoflurane Maintain blood pressure and fluid balance Use reversible drugs whenever possible	Acepromazine
Cesarean section	Propofol or mask induction Maintain with sevoflurane or isoflurane Epidural analgesia is helpful to reduce the need for other analgesics Minimize anesthetic time If opioids used before delivery, administer one to two drops of naloxone sublingually to neonates If needed to stimulate breathing, administer one drop doxapram sublingually to neonates	α^2-agonists Opioids before delivery
Respiratory disease	Preoxygenate and minimize stress Premedicate with opioids and benzodiazepines Any induction agent that allows rapid control of the airway and ventilation Place endotracheal tube rapidly and be prepared to ventilate if needed Maintain with isoflurane or sevoflurane	α^2-agonists Mask induction
Kidney disease	Premedicate with opioids + or − benzodiazepines Mask, propofol induction Maintain with isoflurane or sevoflurane Maintain blood pressure and fluid balance	α^2-agonists Ketamine in blocked cats

ASA, American Society of Anesthesiologists.

To induce anesthesia, the patient is placed in the chamber, the lid closed, and the breathing tubes attached to the ports of a semi-closed rebreathing system. Oxygen is delivered at 5 L/minute and isoflurane at 3% to 5% or sevoflurane at 4% to 6%. As soon as the patient can no longer stand, the chamber is shaken gently to assess the patient's mobility. When the patient is immobile enough to allow it to be safely handled, the patient is removed from the chamber, a mask is placed, and the procedure continued as with mask induction.

Patients can easily experience problems while inside a chamber because of stress, trauma, vomiting, airway blockage, or other issues. Because it is impossible to accurately assess most monitoring parameters while the patient is inside a chamber, the anesthetist must be vigilant and prepared to act quickly if the patient shows signs of compromise.

TECHNICIAN NOTE

Patients must be restrained and watched *carefully* during both mask and chamber inductions, because the animals can become compromised suddenly and unexpectedly and cannot be monitored closely under these circumstances.

Maintenance of Anesthesia

After anesthetic induction and endotracheal intubation, the patient must be maintained with injectable anesthetics, inhalant anesthetics (isoflurane at a rate of 1.5%–2.5% or sevoflurane at a rate of 2.5%–4%), or a combination of these. The goal during maintenance is to administer enough anesthetic to keep the patient in the desired plane of surgical anesthesia. This requires that the anesthetist frequently evaluate the patient by watching for subtle changes and then adjust the amount of anesthetic administered because of this observation.

Most patients are in light anesthesia immediately after intubation and must be brought to surgical anesthesia. Because inhalant anesthetics are most used to maintain anesthesia, this discussion will focus on maintenance with the use of these agents. During maintenance with inhalant agents, a delayed effect is noted between the time the vaporizer dial setting is changed and the time the anesthetic depth changes, because it takes time for the new concentration to fill the breathing circuit, reach the patient's lungs, and equilibrate with blood and tissues. The time required is influenced by several factors, including the patient's respiratory drive, the agent used, the carrier gas flow rate, and the volume and type of breathing circuit used. For this reason, vaporizer setting adjustments must be anticipated as much as possible through close monitoring. In general, if the patient's anesthetic depth is significantly light or deep, larger dial changes are indicated, whereas if the patient's anesthetic depth is slightly too light or deep, more subtle changes are needed. Familiarity with appropriate dial changes is acquired through experience.

IV maintenance agents, such as propofol or alfaxalone, may be used to maintain general anesthesia by repeat boluses administered every few minutes to effect or by constant infusion via a syringe pump. A syringe pump is a device that automatically delivers the drug through an IV line at a calculated infusion rate.

Patient Positioning, Comfort, and Safety

Some considerations that must be observed throughout the anesthetic induction and maintenance periods are as follows:

- Prevent patient trauma by supporting the patient's body as consciousness is lost.
- When using an IV agent for induction, as soon as the patient is intubated, remove the needle and syringe to prevent accidental overdose.
- After intubation, position the patient in lateral recumbency, and secure and cuff the tube.
- Before surgery begins, check the tube for proper placement and cuff inflation.
- Check the endotracheal tube for kinks or bends. An open airway must be always maintained.
- Temporarily disconnect the endotracheal tube from the breathing circuit while turning the patient to prevent trauma to the trachea caused by torsion of the tube.
- Support the corrugated breathing tubes so that they do not exert traction on the endotracheal tube.
- Place the patient in a position that is as normal as possible during the procedure, without hyperflexion or hyperextension of the neck or limbs.
- Do not compress the chest with restraining devices or instruments.
- Place the patient on a heat-retaining surface, such as a warm-water circulating blanket. Do *not* use an electric heating pad, which can burn the patient.
- Do not restrict blood flow by overtightening limb restraint ropes.
- Place sterile lubricant in the eyes every 90 minutes.
- If one lung is diseased, place the normal side up to maximize oxygen exchange.
- Avoid elevation greater than 15 degrees in the caudal aspect of the body to prevent pressure on the diaphragm.

Recovery From Anesthesia

The recovery period is the time between discontinuation of anesthesia and the time when the patient can walk without assistance. Many factors affect recovery, including length of the procedure, anesthetic protocol, patient condition, body temperature, and patient signalment.

Preparation for Recovery

Upon completion of the procedure, the patient is transferred to a recovery area, where it can be extubated and monitored. The inhalant anesthetic is turned off, but oxygen administration is continued at a rate of 50 to 100 mL/kg per minute (0.5–1 L/10 kg body weight up to a maximum of 5 L/minute) for 5 minutes or until the animal swallows. If the patient is in light anesthesia and must be extubated, oxygen may be administered via a mask, or an oxygen source placed close to the nose for 5 minutes. All ties, catheters, monitoring devices, and other unnecessary equipment are removed. The patient is kept warm and turned at least every 10 to 15 minutes.

Monitoring During Recovery

During recovery, the patient must be watched on a continual basis at close range. The patient must be placed in the cage in a position that allows observation of the mucous membranes and respirations but never left in an open cage or on a table unattended, because a recovering patient may fall and be injured. Monitoring must be performed at least every 5 minutes, paying particular attention to vital signs and watching for and reporting unusual signs, such as vomiting or hemorrhage.

> **TECHNICIAN NOTE**
>
> Many anesthesia-related accidents occur during recovery. Monitor at close range and do not let down your guard. Never leave a patient unattended on a table or in an open cage, because patients may awaken rapidly, chew on the endotracheal tube, fall, or be injured.

Signs of Recovery

During recovery, the patient should be gently comforted and reassured. Recovery may be hastened through gentle stimulation by talking softly to the patient, by rubbing or patting the chest, and by turning the patient. Gentle movement of the endotracheal tube will stimulate breathing.

As the patient recovers, it will progress back through the stages and planes of anesthesia. Passage through stage II during recovery may result in a variety of alarming signs, including excitement, vocalization, hyperventilation, and head thrashing. It is important to be prepared to prevent self-trauma if the recovery is unusually violent or stormy; this may require IV sedation.

Extubation

To prepare the patient for extubation, the cuff is deflated by drawing out all the air until the pilot balloon is empty. Since many patients will regurgitate at the time of recovery, the endotracheal tube cuff should remain inflated until the anesthetist is ready to extubate the patient. The tube is untied to prepare for rapid removal. Both before and after removal, the neck of the patient is kept in a natural but extended position to protect the airway. The endotracheal tube is removed gently when the swallowing reflex returns, using a slow, steady motion. It may also be removed when signs of imminent arousal are evident, such as voluntary movement of the limbs or head, movement of the tongue, or chewing. Extubation should be delayed in brachycephalic dogs until the patient is able to lift its head unassisted. A small mouth speculum can be used to prevent the patient from biting the tube.

The Postanesthetic Period

After recovery, most SA patients should be given nothing by mouth for the first hour or two and no food for at least several hours. At discharge, the client should be instructed to provide water in a gradual manner after arriving home and to feed a small meal after several hours. Exceptions to these rules include small and neonatal patients, which require shorter withholding times. The patient should be monitored for signs of pain, and analgesics should be administered as prescribed.

Equine Anesthesia

All of the basic principles discussed under SA anesthesia apply to anesthesia of the horse. Additional challenges for the equine anesthetist include temperament and physical size of the patient, effects of inhalant anesthetics on cardiorespiratory physiology, and management of recovery. As with SA anesthesia, a successful anesthetic procedure requires careful preparation and a good understanding of the sequence of events involved in taking a horse from consciousness to surgical anesthesia and back to consciousness. Procedure 30.2 summarizes these events when a horse is induced with injectable agents and is maintained with an inhalant agent.

Selecting a Protocol

As for SA anesthesia, protocols are commonly selected by the attending veterinarian. A suitable protocol takes into account patient signalment, pre-existing problems, physical status class, and the procedure to be performed. After the protocol is determined, all drug dosages, oxygen flow rates, and fluid administration rates are calculated and checked *carefully*.

Patients in physical status class ASA III to ASA V require use of modified protocols based on the primary condition (Table 30.11).

Equipment Preparation

It is critical in equine anesthesia to be prepared and to check equipment before use, including any hoists and hydraulic tables that are to be used for lifting and positioning horses. If recovery pads, ropes, and other equipment are used, they should be organized before induction if possible.

The Preanesthetic Period

The preanesthetic procedure in horses differs slightly from that in SAs. After appropriate patient assessment, the first step is placement of an IV catheter, almost always in one of the jugular veins. Some horses object to venipuncture and must be sedated first. Xylazine IV or IM is commonly used for this purpose. Once the horse is cooperative, a small bleb of local anesthetic is administered over the proposed catheterization site to desensitize the skin.

After catheterization, the horse's mouth should be rinsed out with a dose syringe placed between the cheek and the teeth on each side of the mouth to flush out any feed material. This prevents aspiration of the material during intubation or recovery. Feet should be cleaned before sedation, and then shoes should be removed or wrapped. Typically, the patient is premedicated with

---

PROCEDURE 30.2

Sequence of Events for an Equine Anesthetic Procedure[a]

1. Assess, prepare, and weigh the patient (see the section on "Patient Preparation" in this chapter).
2. Prepare equipment and place an intravenous (IV) catheter, which may require IV or intramuscular (IM) sedation in some horses (clippers, local anesthetic, antiseptic scrub, IV catheters, tape, saline flush, suture material, catheter cap, and/or extension line with three-way stopcock).
3. Rinse the horse's mouth, clean the hooves, and remove or wrap shoes when appropriate.
4. Determine the protocol (anesthetic agents, including dosages, routes, and sequence of administration).
5. Calculate the volume of each agent to be given, including fluid administration rates (preanesthesia, induction, maintenance, and analgesic agents).
6. Review oxygen flow rates (see Box 30.3).
7. Prepare equipment required to administer drugs (scales, syringes, needles, agents, reversal agents, emergency cart, controlled substance log).
8. Prepare fluid administration equipment (fluids, administration extension set, syringe pump, tape, saline flush).
9. Prepare equipment for endotracheal intubation (see the section on "Principles of Endotracheal Intubation" in this chapter).
10. Prepare monitoring equipment, including arterial catheterization materials, anesthesia record, monitors, and probes (see the section on "Monitoring the Anesthetized Patient" in this chapter).
11. Assemble and test the anesthetic machine and ventilator (see the section on "Anesthesia Equipment" in this chapter).
12. Administer premedications intramuscularly approximately 20 to 30 minutes before or intravenously approximately 5 to 10 minutes before anesthetic induction.
13. If the horse is adequately sedated, administer the induction agent as a rapid bolus so that the horse will assume recumbency in a rapid and predictable sequence with minimal excitement; otherwise, give additional IV sedation and reassess before induction.
14. Check the patient's readiness for intubation.
15. Place and secure the endotracheal tube (see the section on "Principles of Endotracheal Intubation" in this chapter).
16. Check the patient's vital signs.
17. Hoist, position, and secure the patient for the procedure, with attention to padding of the face and limbs if the horse is in lateral recumbency and for maintenance of an open airway, unrestricted blood flow, and unrestricted chest excursions.
18. Remove the halter.
19. Turn on the oxygen, then connect the endotracheal tube to the breathing circuit.
20. Turn on the inhalant anesthetic to the appropriate level.
21. Determine the patient's anesthetic depth and commence regular monitoring.
22. Attach monitoring devices, including placement of an arterial catheter.
23. Continue to monitor and adjust the anesthetic and oxygen levels as needed until completion of the procedure.
24. Prepare the patient for recovery, including placement of a nasopharyngeal tube and removal of monitoring equipment, and ensure that the recovery area has been prepared. Administration of intranasal phenylephrine spray can help alleviate congestion and reduce obstruction.
25. Discontinue the anesthetic and transfer the horse to the recovery area, paying attention to positioning.
26. Extubate the patient at the appropriate time and ensure that the horse can breathe through its nostrils without obstruction.
27. Assist the horse until it stands as directed by the veterinarian. Be prepared to administer sedatives if needed.
28. Prepare the patient for continued hospitalization or discharge by applying bandages, administering medications, and performing any other procedures ordered by the veterinarian.

[a]Induction with an IV agent and maintenance with an inhalant agent.

TABLE 30.11	Recommendations for Physical Status Class ASA III to ASA V Equine Patients	
Primary Condition	**Example Protocols and Other Considerations**	**Avoid These Agents/ Circumstances**
Colic	Premedicate with xylazine to effect Induce with a ketamine-based protocol Maintain blood pressure in normal range	Acepromazine
Cesarean section	Premedicate with xylazine to effect Induce with ketamine Maintain with isoflurane or sevoflurane Epidural analgesia is helpful to reduce the need for other analgesics Minimize anesthetic time Monitor oxygenation	Opioids before delivery

ASA, American Society of Anesthesiologists.

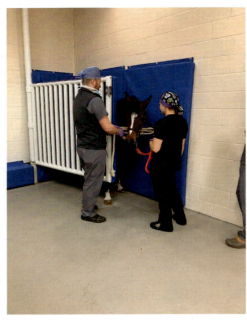

• **Fig. 30.29** A horse is positioned behind a gate, which is secured to the fixed wall with a rope. Note the relatively wide-based stance and the lowered head position. The horse is not particularly interested in its surroundings. This indicates that the horse is adequately sedated before induction.

tranquilizers, α^2-agonists, opioids, or a combination of these by IV injection or, less commonly, IM injection. Just before or immediately after premedication, the horse is positioned in an induction area or is placed adjacent to a tilt table. Some horses startle easily in a strange environment, and some breeds (e.g., Arabians and Thoroughbreds) have a higher drug tolerance. An excited horse should never be induced to anesthesia, because this will increase the drug requirement for anesthetic maintenance. This may cause difficulty keeping the patient anesthetized because of high levels of circulating catecholamines, requiring dangerously deep levels of anesthesia. Sedation is considered adequate when the horse's head (and lower lip) droops, the horse no longer pays attention to its surroundings, and demonstrates a wide-based stance or reluctance to move (Fig. 30.29).

TECHNICIAN NOTE

Never induce anesthesia in a horse that is not adequately sedated.

Induction of Anesthesia

Intravenous Induction

Horses are generally induced to anesthesia by IV administration of drugs. Equine patients are most often induced with ketamine, a combination of ketamine and diazepam or midazolam, or guaifenesin followed by ketamine. Induction typically occurs in a special induction stall that has padded walls and often a padded floor. Induction may be done "free fall" or behind a gate that restrains the horse. The induction stall is sometimes also used for recovery. In contrast to SAs, in which IV induction is given to effect, the goal of induction in horses is to rapidly take the horse from standing (sedated) to lateral recumbency (unconscious) to minimize

excitement; this can cause the horse to injure itself or personnel. All drugs are thus given as a bolus except for the muscle relaxant guaifenesin, which is administered rapidly intravenously to effect by placing it in a pressure bag. Once the horse shows signs of ataxia—typically knuckling of the forelimbs at the fetlocks and carpi—the induction agent is given as a bolus.

Once anesthesia has been induced, vital signs should be briefly checked. The horse is then intubated (see Fig. 30.18A and B).

In some practices, the floor of the induction stall forms part of the surgery table, but in many, the horse must be hoisted onto a table (Fig. 30.30A). It is important to understand how the hoist functions so that the horse can be transported safely and any problems can be resolved rapidly.

It is essential to ensure that muscles and prominent nerves are protected when a horse is placed on a surgical table or surface (see Fig. 30.30B). Many table designs are available, and the anesthetist should make sure that muscle groups are well supported to prevent myopathy ("tying up") and that facial and radial nerves are supported. Horses in lateral recumbency should have the forelimb closest to the table pulled forward if possible to decrease pressure placed on it by the chest and the opposite (i.e., uppermost) limb.

Maintenance of Anesthesia

Of all domestic species, horses present the biggest challenge to the anesthetist. Sudden, unexpected movement can occur with no change in signs of depth of anesthesia. As a result of large breathing circuit volume and patient size, response to changes in inhalant anesthetic and oxygen flow rates occur too slowly to return the patient to surgical anesthesia simply by altering machine settings. A syringe of ketamine is typically drawn up before anesthesia and may be attached to a three-way stopcock in the fluid administration line or kept close to the IV port for this purpose. Approximately one-fifth of the IV induction dose is administered to the horse to return it to surgical anesthesia.

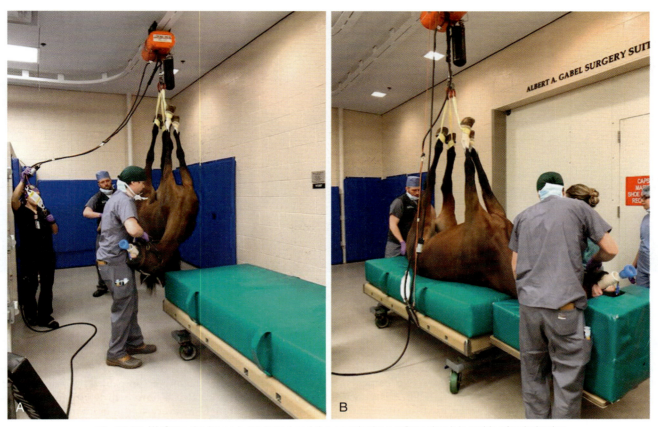

• **Fig. 30.30** (A) Once the horse is intubated and the anesthetist confirms that it is stable after induction, it is hoisted for placement on the surgery table. The anesthetist controls and supports the head while the patient is on the hoist. (B) The horse is positioned on a thick foam pad to prevent muscle damage. Once the horse is positioned, it will be connected to a large-animal (LA) anesthesia machine.

Compared with other species, horses are more likely to develop hypoxemia, hypoventilation, and hypotension during maintenance of anesthesia, particularly when inhalant agents are used. To monitor blood pressure accurately and to obtain arterial blood gas values, it is recommended that horses anesthetized with inhalants for procedures lasting longer than 1 hour have an arterial catheter placed in a peripheral artery (facial, transverse facial, or greater metatarsal) (Fig. 30.31). Blood gas samples should be taken every 30 to 60 minutes or more frequently if the situation warrants.

Hypoventilation is so common in anesthetized horses, particularly those placed in dorsal recumbency, that a ventilator is often used to maintain normal ventilation. Hypotension (mean arterial pressure <70 mm Hg) has been shown to contribute to myopathy, so treatment with drugs is frequently indicated if increased IV fluid rate, decreased depth of anesthesia, and surgical stimulation do not increase blood pressure. The drug most often used to support blood pressure is the positive inotrope dobutamine (typically administered via a syringe pump). Dobutamine and many other positive inotropes may cause arrhythmias, so it is important to monitor the ECG closely when starting an infusion.

Hypoxemia can occur in any horse regardless of the physical status class but is more common in horses that are obese or pregnant or have intestines that have become twisted (e.g., colon torsion), and in those that are placed in dorsal recumbency. Hypoxemia has several possible causes, including hypoventilation, lung disease, and low cardiac output. Wherever possible, the cause should be investigated and corrected.

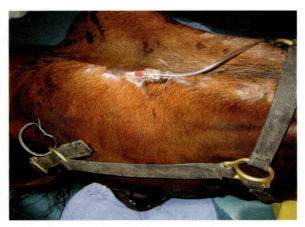

• **Fig. 30.31** Placement of a catheter in the facial artery for monitoring blood pressure and taking blood samples for arterial blood gas analysis.

In horses, anesthesia is usually maintained with isoflurane (at a concentration of 1.5%–2.5%) or sevoflurane (at a concentration of 2.5%–4%). IV maintenance of anesthesia in horses is generally reserved for shorter procedures (<1 hour) in healthy patients and for procedures carried out away from a veterinary practice ("field anesthesia"). Additional doses of xylazine and ketamine are typically administered intravenously to prolong anesthesia at approximately one-fourth the amount of each

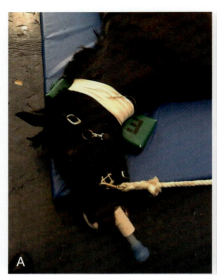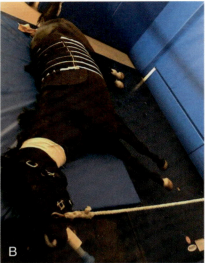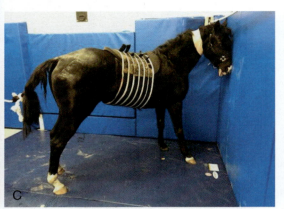

• **Fig. 30.32** Recovery. (A) A horse recovering from anesthesia in a padded stall. Note that the intravenous (IV) catheter is still in place and the neck is supported with additional padding. (B) Placement of head and tail ropes for recovery. (C) Recovered horse standing quietly.

drug used to sedate and induce the horse. Total IV induction and maintenance of anesthesia in horses (known as *total intravenous anesthesia* [TIVA]) is generally characterized by higher blood pressure, better breathing, and more active palpebral reflexes than are seen with inhalant anesthetics. TIVA is associated with recoveries of good quality when used for procedures lasting less than 1 hour.

Recovery From Anesthesia

Horses have an instinctive need to stand shortly after awakening from anesthesia, which makes recovery particularly dangerous. Some steps can be taken to minimize injury to the horse and the anesthetist, but the incidence of complications is high during recovery from anesthesia in horses, and clients should be informed of the risks.

Preparation for Recovery

The following should be done to prepare for recovery: replace the halter and place a nasopharyngeal tube before movement if nasal edema is present (Fig. 30.32A). Upon completion of the procedure, turn off the inhalant anesthetic and transfer the horse to a padded recovery stall, where it can be extubated and monitored. If possible, and particularly if the horse was hypoxemic during anesthesia, provide oxygen support using a demand valve or insufflation (5–10 L/minute delivered nasally or through the endotracheal tube via tubing that is connected to an oxygen flowmeter) until the horse is extubated or is too light to tolerate an insufflation hose. If recovery is assisted by ropes, attach a head rope to the halter and tie another rope to the tail (see Fig. 30.32B and C).

Monitoring During Recovery

During recovery, it is ideal to watch the horse continuously so that it can be assisted or sedated if necessary. While the horse is lying quietly, the anesthetist should watch respirations to make sure that the horse is breathing normally. The anesthetist is positioned at the head of the horse, taking the pulse from the facial artery and assessing the eye for depth of anesthesia.

Signs of Recovery

As the horse recovers, it will go back through the stages and planes of anesthesia. Many horses develop nystagmus during recovery, and rapid nystagmus accompanied by "paddling" of the limbs generally means that a horse will try to get up too soon and will have a "rough" recovery. In this event, it may be prudent to sedate the horse with 50 to 100 mg xylazine IV. Administration of 5 to 10 mg of acepromazine IV is also a useful sedative in recovery, providing it is not contraindicated (i.e., hypotension, hypovolemia, breeding stallions), as it will reduce excitement without producing ataxia. Generally, maintaining control of the head by sitting on the neck or holding the head up off the floor will provide some control over the horse. However, once the horse is strong enough to lift the anesthetist off its neck, the anesthetist should retreat to a safe distance from which to observe the remainder of recovery.

Extubation

The following actions should be taken to prepare the patient for extubation: deflate the cuff by drawing out all of the air until the pilot balloon is empty. Both before and after removal, keep the neck in a natural but extended position to protect the airway. Remove the endotracheal tube gently when the swallowing reflex returns, using a slow, steady motion or when signs of imminent arousal are present, such as voluntary movement of the limbs or head, movement of the tongue, or chewing. Check to make sure that the horse can breathe without obstruction. Horses can breathe only through their noses and will become distressed and compromised if they are unable to do so. If a nasopharyngeal tube has not been placed and the nasal passages are or become obstructed, place one immediately. If a nasopharyngeal tube does not alleviate the obstruction, a tracheostomy must be performed by the veterinarian, so ensure that materials for performing this procedure are always close to the recovery stall.

The Postanesthetic Period

Once the horse is standing and can walk steadily, it can be returned to its stall. This can be assessed by walking the horse in a circle inside the recovery stall. Once back in its own stall, the horse should be muzzled for 1 to 3 hours but should have free access to water.

Ruminant Anesthesia

Ruminants do not pose the same challenges to the anesthetist as those posed by horses; however, an understanding of their unique digestive physiology is important, because it affects the well-being of the patient under general anesthesia. Additionally, ruminants present for general anesthesia less frequently compared with SAs or horses, so it takes longer to gain experience in anesthesia in these animals. There are several reasons for this. Because of their calm nature, ruminants require general anesthesia for relatively few procedures. Many surgical procedures can be performed by using local or regional anesthetic techniques. A discussion of local and regional anesthesia is beyond the scope of this chapter; students may refer to veterinary anesthesia textbooks. Finally, administration of general anesthesia to production animals is often not economically viable.

The general principles discussed for other species also apply to ruminants, and careful preparation and planning are important for a successful outcome. Procedure 30.3 summarizes the sequence of events involved when a ruminant is induced with injectable agents and is maintained with an inhalant agent.

Selecting a Protocol

As with other species, protocols are commonly selected by the attending veterinarian. A suitable protocol considers patient signalment, pre-existing problems, physical status class, and the procedure to be performed. After the protocol is known, all drug dosages, oxygen flow rates, and fluid administration rates are calculated and checked *carefully*.

Patients in physical status class ASA III to ASA V require use of modified protocols based on the primary condition (Table 30.12).

Preanesthetic Fasting

It is essential to ensure that ruminants have been adequately fasted before anesthesia, including water deprivation. Fasting reduces the size of the rumen and decreases microbial activity. This in turn decreases gas production during anesthesia. Normally, ruminants eructate to expel gas from the rumen; however, this does not happen under anesthesia, and bloating may occur. A bloated rumen can put pressure on the diaphragm and large blood vessels (aorta, caudal vena cava) in the abdomen, resulting in respiratory and circulatory compromise. Once an anesthetized ruminant develops severe bloat, it can be difficult to treat and may lead to death if it goes unnoticed or untreated.

Equipment Preparation

Any specialized equipment required for restraining or positioning anesthetized ruminants, such as head gates, transporters, and tilt tables, should be checked. In addition to the standard equipment, it is extremely helpful to have suction available for small ruminants to allow feed material, regurgitus, or saliva to be removed from the pharynx during intubation.

PROCEDURE 30.3

Sequence of Events for a Ruminant Anesthetic Procedure[a]

1. Assess, prepare, and weigh the patient (see the section on "Patient Preparation" in this chapter).
2. Prepare equipment and place an intravenous (IV) catheter, which may require restraint in a chute with a head gate for larger or aggressive cattle (clippers, local anesthetic, antiseptic scrub, IV catheters, tape, saline flush, suture material, catheter cap, and/or extension line with three-way stopcock).
3. Determine the protocol (anesthetic agents, including dosages, routes, and sequence of administration).
4. Calculate the volume of each agent to be given, including fluid administration rates (preanesthesia, induction, maintenance, and analgesic agents).
5. Review the oxygen flow rates (see Box 30.3).
6. Prepare equipment required to administer drugs (scales, syringes, needles, agents, reversal agents, emergency cart, controlled substance log).
7. Prepare fluid administration equipment (fluids, administration extension set, syringe pump, tape, saline flush).
8. Prepare equipment for endotracheal intubation. Have suction equipment assembled and turned on for small ruminants. Remove all jewelry and watches, and ensure that fingernails are trimmed short for digital intubation of adult cattle (see the section on "Principles of Endotracheal Intubation" in this chapter).
9. Prepare monitoring equipment, including arterial catheterization materials, anesthesia record, monitors, and probes (see the section on "Monitoring the Anesthetized Patient" in this chapter).
10. Assemble and test the anesthetic machine and ventilator (see the section on "Anesthesia Equipment" in this chapter).
11. Administer premedications intramuscularly approximately 20 to 30 minutes before or intravenously approximately 5 to 10 minutes before anesthetic induction if this is considered necessary.
12. Administer the induction agent.
13. Check the patient's readiness for intubation.
14. Place and secure the endotracheal tube (see the section on "Principles of Endotracheal Intubation" in this chapter).
15. Check the patient's vital signs.
16. Hoist or lift (as appropriate), position, and secure the patient for the procedure. It is imperative that the pharynx be positioned higher than the head whenever possible.
17. Turn on the oxygen and connect the endotracheal tube to the breathing circuit.
18. Turn on the inhalant anesthetic to the appropriate level.
19. Determine the patient's anesthetic depth and commence regular monitoring.
20. Attach monitoring devices and place an arterial catheter.
21. Continue to monitor and adjust anesthetic and oxygen levels as needed until completion of the procedure.
22. Prepare the patient for recovery, including removal of monitoring equipment, and ensure that the recovery area has been prepared.
23. Discontinue the anesthetic and transfer the patient to the recovery area.
24. Place and support the patient in sternal recumbency so that it can eructate. Extubate the patient at the appropriate time with the cuff partially inflated.
25. Prepare the patient for continued hospitalization or discharge by applying bandages, administering medications, and performing any other procedures ordered by the veterinarian.

[a]Induction with an IV agent and maintenance with an inhalant agent.

TABLE 30.12	Recommendations for Physical Status Class ASA III to ASA V Ruminant Patients	
Primary Condition	**Example Protocols and Other Considerations**	**Avoid These Agents/ Circumstances**
Cesarean section (C-section) requiring general anesthesia (live calf)	No premedication Induce with ketamine-based protocol Maintain with isoflurane or sevoflurane Epidural analgesia is helpful to reduce the need for other analgesics Minimize anesthetic time	α^2-agonists Acepromazine Opioids before delivery
C-section requiring general anesthesia (dead calf, septicemic cow)	No premedication or benzodiazepines Induce with ketamine-based protocol Maintain with isoflurane or sevoflurane Support blood pressure	α^2-agonists Acepromazine
Urethral obstruction	No premedication or premedicate with benzodiazepines (e.g., diazepam) Obtain and evaluate an electrocardiography (ECG) before drug administration Induce with "double drip" or diazepam-ketamine Maintain with isoflurane or sevoflurane Monitor electrolytes preoperatively and intraoperatively Maintain blood pressure and fluid balance	Acepromazine α^2-agonists

ASA, American Society of Anesthesiologists.

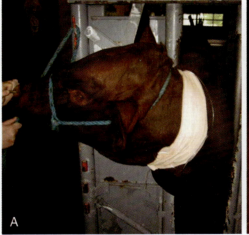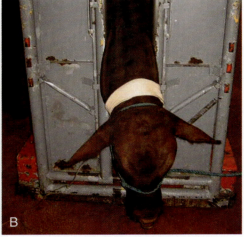

• **Fig. 30.33** (A) A 500-kg bull is restrained for jugular catheterization in a transporter with a head gate. (B) The same bull after sedation with intravenous (IV) 25-mg xylazine.

The Preanesthetic Period

Many ruminants are calm and tractable enough to allow IV catheterization and induction of anesthesia with minimal or no premedication and with mild restraint. Adult cattle are typically restrained using the head gate of a transporter or chute. Premedication is often reserved for patients that are aggressive, excited, or stressed. Typically, IV or IM tranquilizers, α^2-agonists, opioids, or combinations of these are used. Although many ruminants do not require sedation before anesthesia, premedication will provide benefits, such as decreased dose of induction and maintenance drugs and improved muscle relaxation (Fig. 30.33).

TECHNICIAN NOTE

Ruminants are sensitive to xylazine and require, at most, 10% of the dose that horses do.

Induction of Anesthesia

Intravenous Induction

In ruminants, anesthesia is typically induced with a combination of ketamine and diazepam or midazolam, ketamine, and guaifenesin ("double drip"), or Telazol. Induction in large cattle may occur in a special induction stall that has padded walls, in a transporter, or on a tilt table. In smaller ruminants anesthesia can generally be induced next to the surgery table or, if the animal is small or severely compromised, while it is lying on it. Although ruminants do not typically become excited during induction of anesthesia, the goal with larger ruminant patients is similar to that in horses: to rapidly produce unconsciousness while minimizing injury to the patient and to personnel. Drugs are thus given as an IV bolus, except for "double drip," which is administered rapidly IV to effect. Smaller ruminants, particularly those that are compromised, can be given induction drugs intravenously to effect, as for SA patients.

Once the patient is unconscious, it should be kept in sternal recumbency for intubation whenever possible. It is important to be vigilant for regurgitation, which can occur at any point in the anesthetic procedure but occurs most frequently when anesthesia is light or too deep. If regurgitation occurs, the head should immediately be positioned so that it is lower than the body to prevent aspiration. Suction equipment should be available at the time of induction in small ruminants. Once the patient has been induced, vital signs should be briefly checked before intubation (see Fig. 30.19).

All ruminants should be positioned for surgery with the mouth at a level lower than the pharynx to allow drainage of saliva and any regurgitated material from the mouth, preventing buildup in the pharynx, which could lead to aspiration during recovery. Ruminants produce copious amounts of saliva each day, which is normally swallowed. This cannot occur under anesthesia, so it must be allowed to drain. Ruminants, even large cattle, are not as predisposed to developing myopathy or neuropathies as horses are; however, appropriate physical support and padding during anesthesia are prudent and desirable.

Maintenance of Anesthesia

Healthy ruminants typically have relatively few problems during the maintenance phase of anesthesia. Blood pressure is usually well maintained and often is much higher than that seen in SA and equine patients. However, ruminants do tend to hypoventilate and are often observed to breathe rapidly and shallowly, somewhat like a panting dog. This type of breathing pattern tends to lead to hypoxemia and difficulty keeping the patient anesthetized because of inadequate delivery of inhalant anesthetic to the lungs. Patients that demonstrate this breathing pattern should be placed on a ventilator.

Most ruminants have accessible arteries in their ears; these are often catheterized so that blood pressure can be monitored directly and blood samples can be taken for blood gas analysis (Fig. 30.34).

Anesthesia is often maintained with isoflurane (at a concentration of 1.5%–2.5%) or sevoflurane (at a concentration of 2.5%–4%). IV maintenance of anesthesia in ruminants is generally reserved for shorter procedures (<20 minutes) in healthy patients, although if the patient is intubated, the duration of anesthesia can be extended. "Double drip" is commonly used for this purpose.

Recovery From Anesthesia

Unlike horses, ruminants are generally content to lie in sternal recumbency after they wake up from anesthesia. Complications caused by recovery from anesthesia are generally limited to the residual effects of bloat. Ruminants rarely develop nasal edema during anesthesia and usually do not require nasal intubation.

Preparation for Recovery

Upon completion of the procedure, the inhalant anesthetic is turned off and the patient is transferred to a padded recovery stall, where it can be extubated and monitored (large cattle), or to a quiet, clean area on the floor (small ruminant). Ruminants should be supported or propped up in sternal recumbency when recovering from anesthesia to allow eructation to occur.

Monitoring During Recovery

The patient should be monitored for signs of excessive bloating (a visually large abdomen that feels tight to the touch, particularly on the left side).

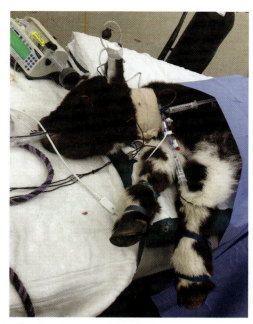

• **Fig. 30.34** A calf under general anesthesia. Note intra-articular (IA) catheterization of an auricular artery.

Signs of Recovery

As the patient recovers, it will go back through the stages and planes of anesthesia. Generally, this is not as dramatic an event in ruminants as it is in horses, even if the patient did not receive premedication. Eructation of rumen gas commonly occurs during the recovery period.

Extubation

In contrast to other species, the endotracheal tube cuff should be kept inflated or only partially deflated to prevent aspiration of any material that may have become lodged in the pharynx during anesthesia. The anesthetist should wait for strong swallowing movements or coughing before extubation. The neck should be kept in a natural but extended position to protect the airway both before and after removal. The endotracheal tube is removed gently by using a slow, steady movement. If removing the tube is difficult, some more air should be removed from the cuff and removal tried again.

The Postanesthetic Period

Once a ruminant is awake and lying in sternal recumbency without support and is no longer in danger of bloating, it can be left unattended for short periods (15–20 minutes). It is prudent to check on the animal periodically, because if a ruminant later assumes lateral recumbency, it will not eructate effectively and may need to be assisted again into sternal recumbency. Many ruminants will lie quietly after anesthesia, standing only after some time has passed unless they are stimulated to rise. It is not necessary to withhold food or water from ruminants postoperatively unless specifically instructed to do so.

Manual and Mechanical Ventilation

Ventilation is a process in which air or anesthetic gases are artificially forced into a patient's lungs. Although ventilatory support is necessary in patients with pre-existing problems, such as lung disease, obesity, abdominal distention, or brain trauma, some ventilatory support is needed even in healthy patients to compensate for the respiratory depression that accompanies general anesthesia. This is especially true in healthy LA patients; therefore many practices ventilate all horses and ruminants under general anesthesia.

Under certain circumstances, such as loss of a normal negative pressure in the chest cavity (e.g., thoracotomy for repair of diaphragmatic hernia, thoracic injury, or pneumothorax) or paralysis of the respiratory muscles when neuromuscular blockers are used as part of the anesthetic protocol, a patient may be unable to breathe. At these times, ventilation is mandatory throughout the procedure to keep the patient alive.

This support can be provided by the anesthetist by applying pressure to the reservoir bag with the pop-off valve fully or partially closed (manual ventilation) or by using a ventilator (mechanical ventilation). For safety reasons, when providing manual or mechanical ventilation pressure in the breathing circuit should never be allowed to exceed 15 to 20 cm H_2O in SAs or 30 to 40 cm H_2O in LAs unless the chest is open, in which case higher pressures may be required. Additional details regarding manual and mechanical ventilation may be found in most anesthesia texts.

Anesthetic Problems and Emergencies

Most general anesthetic procedures are uneventful, but from time to time, problems do develop and have the potential to cause transient or permanent harm to the patient. Most studies show that although as many as 10% of patients have complications of one sort or another, on average only one or two out of 1000 healthy patients die from complications of anesthesia. Horses have the highest mortality rate of commonly anesthetized species (approximately 1 in 100 within 7 days of an anesthetic event). Therefore it is likely that a technician will have experience with many successful anesthetic procedures before a serious complication is ever encountered. This can easily lead to a false sense of security which, unless tempered with increased watchfulness, may impair readiness to handle a crisis.

Although patients with pre-existing conditions, such as major organ disease, are more likely to develop complications, healthy patients may be at greater risk because of species, age, breed, reproductive status, body conformation, or a variety of other factors. For instance, brachycephalic dogs and geriatric, young (<8 weeks old), obese, and pregnant patients are at greater risk. Ruminants may bloat, leading to cardiorespiratory compromise, and recovery from anesthesia in equines has many risks, including myopathy and neuropathy. Therefore the anesthetist must approach any anesthetic procedure prepared for problems that are likely to arise.

Adverse drug reactions, equipment malfunctions, anesthetic overdose, complications of surgery, and human error are other possible causes of anesthetic problems and emergencies. Most can be managed successfully, however, if recognized early and acted upon before they reach a crisis level. Many indicators of developing problems may be detected by careful and frequent observation throughout the procedure. These indicators usually come from the machine (e.g., an overfilled reservoir bag, exhausted CO_2 granules), the patient (e.g., a patient that will not stay anesthetized or that is experiencing a rough recovery), or monitoring devices (e.g., an SpO_2 <95%, a cardiac arrhythmia).

The anesthetist may be able to manage some problems independently and quickly, whereas other problems require rapid and effective communication with the veterinarian in charge in addition to further exploration. For instance, mildly excessive or inadequate depth of anesthesia can, in most cases, be managed by the anesthetist by simply adjusting the vaporizer setting and oxygen flow rate, or by altering the administration of injectable agents. However, some problems, such as hypotension or cardiac arrhythmias, may require more complex action, such as changing the anesthetic protocol, treating blood loss, or interpreting data from a monitoring device. The remainder of this section highlights causes, solutions, and prevention of common anesthetic problems and emergencies.

Inadequate or Excessive Oxygen Flow

A flowmeter or oxygen tank pressure gauge that registers zero indicates that the flowmeter is turned off or that the oxygen tank is empty or turned off. If the primary tank is empty, the reserve tank is opened. If it is impossible to solve the problem right away (if there is no reserve tank on the machine and there is only one machine available) the endotracheal tube should be disconnected from the breathing system until the problem is solved, although there is a risk that the patient may wake up or become hypoxemic in the interim.

Lack of movement of the reservoir bag or of the unidirectional valves when the patient is breathing usually indicates that the endotracheal tube is not in the trachea, is disconnected, or is blocked. A disconnected or misplaced tube will result in difficulty keeping the patient anesthetized. A blocked tube will usually cause dyspnea and cyanosis. To manage this problem, first, the tube is checked to see if it is connected to the breathing circuit and is correctly placed. Next, the tube is disconnected from the breathing circuit, and the anesthetist listens or feels for airflow when the patient breathes to rule out a blockage. If the tube is blocked or is incorrectly placed, the tube is immediately removed and the patient reintubated. If reintubation is not possible (e.g., there is no one to help), oxygen and anesthetic are administered via mask until the tube can be replaced.

An overinflated reservoir bag or a pressure manometer reading greater than 2 cm H_2O while the patient is breathing spontaneously occurs most commonly when the pop-off valve has inadvertently been left too far closed. Occlusions of the scavenging system, high oxygen flow, and overzealous use of the oxygen flush valve are other possible causes. If the pop-off valve is closed, it should be opened immediately. If the pressure is dangerously high (>20 cm H_2O), the endotracheal tube is immediately disconnected from the breathing circuit and the primary problem corrected. If pressure builds again when the tube is reconnected, the scavenging system is checked for a blockage. If high oxygen flow is causing the bag to overfill, the pressure in the circuit should not increase but will remain less than 2 cm H_2O, even though the bag appears to be overinflated. In this case, the bag is gently pressed to empty it as needed and, if safe to do so, the oxygen flow is reduced.

An underinflated reservoir bag indicates inadequate oxygen flow, a leak in the system, a maladjusted scavenging system, or a pop-off valve that is open too far. If it is completely deflated, the oxygen flow is immediately increased, or the oxygen flush valve is used to fill the bag one-half to three-fourths full. Then the pop-off valve, machine assembly, and scavenging system adjustments are checked. If the problem cannot be corrected quickly, it is better to change to another machine.

Saturation of Carbon Dioxide Absorbent Granules

Violet or off-white, brittle absorbent granules indicate saturation of the CO_2 absorbent. The resulting increase in CO_2 in the breathing circuit will cause increased inspired and expired CO_2 levels on a capnograph and may also cause tachypnea or tachycardia. The solution to this problem is to change the granules as soon as the machine is no longer in use. The patient should be changed to another machine for the duration of the procedure. If only one machine is available, high oxygen flow (1 L/5 kg body weight/minute) is used, close monitoring continued, and the patient awakened as soon as possible or, if the patient weighs less than 7 kg, changed to a nonrebreathing system.

A Patient That Will Not Stay Asleep

Difficulty keeping a patient adequately anesthetized is most often related to problems in the machine and associated equipment. It must be ensured that the oxygen is on and flow is adequate, the vaporizer is not empty and is turned on, the machine is correctly assembled, no system leaks are present, and the endotracheal tube is properly placed and cuffed. RR and depth should also be checked. If either one has decreased, the patient's respiratory minute volume may be insufficient to draw enough anesthetic into the lungs. If this is the case, the patient should be manually ventilated every 5 to 10 seconds until in surgical anesthesia. If anesthetic depth is inadequate, it may be necessary to prevent the patient from chewing the tube by applying gentle but firm pressure to the muzzle and to give additional injectable anesthetic until the source of the problem is identified and corrected.

Excessive Depth of Anesthesia

Excessive depth of anesthesia usually results from excessively high vaporizer settings, equipment problems, or pre-existing medical problems. The veterinarian should be immediately informed, administration of all anesthetics stopped, and the flow of oxygen increased; then it is safe to proceed as ordered by the veterinarian. Patients in excessively deep anesthesia may require mechanical ventilation (or squeezing the rebreathing bag), IV fluid support, measures to increase body temperature, reversal agents or other drug therapy, and even resuscitation in extreme situations. If a vaporizer problem (overfilled, tipped over, out of calibration) is suspected, change to another machine until the problem is corrected.

Cardiopulmonary arrest most often follows uncorrected excessive anesthetic depth but can happen at any time during anesthesia. Patients in physical status classes ASA III to ASA V are at especially high risk for cardiopulmonary arrest. A patient that has arrested has no heartbeat, pulse, or respirations and requires prompt initiation of cardiopulmonary resuscitation. The reader is directed to Chapter 25 for a complete discussion on cardiopulmonary resuscitation (CPR).

Apnea and Hypoventilation

Apnea or hypoventilation commonly occurs after any episode of hyperventilation as a result of a decrease in blood CO_2 levels. Apnea or hypoventilation is also common after induction with drugs that depress the respiratory system but can indicate excessive anesthetic depth and, in some cases, even respiratory arrest. To manage apnea, the veterinarian should be immediately informed, other vital signs checked, and anesthetic depth then determined by assessing other monitoring parameters. If the patient is stable and at an appropriate depth of anesthesia, it may be necessary to "bag" the patient two to ten times per minute until normal respirations resume. The low end of this range should be used if apnea is secondary to hyperventilation to allow normalization of CO_2 levels.

Hypotension

Hypotension is a common anesthetic complication caused by pre-existing conditions, blood loss, shock, cardiac arrhythmias, excessive anesthetic depth, and adverse effects of drugs. Hypotension is confirmed by using a Doppler monitor, oscillometer, or direct blood pressure monitoring but may be suspected on the basis of pale mucous membranes, increased CRT, and weak pulses. After the veterinarian has been informed, hypotension should be treated as ordered. Treatment often includes IV fluid therapy, decreased delivery of anesthetic, administration of additional oxygen, warming of the patient, and drug therapy.

Cyanosis or Low Oxygen Saturation

Cyanosis or low oxygen saturation indicates hypoxemia and can be caused by cardiopulmonary disease, ineffective respirations, airway blockage, or machine problems. Cyanosis is a medical emergency that requires immediate action. Dyspnea often accompanies or precedes cyanosis and must also be treated aggressively. Low oxygen saturation is defined as SpO_2 less than 95% on a pulse oximeter. If it is believed that the value is correct and is not caused by a machine or probe problem, first, the veterinarian is informed and then the oxygen flow and machine assembly should be checked, and the endotracheal tube should be checked for blockage. RR and V_T should also be checked to find out if they are adequate.

Vomiting or Regurgitation

Vomiting or regurgitation may occur at any time during an anesthetic procedure and can result in serious complications from pulmonary aspiration if the airway is not protected with a cuffed endotracheal tube. Vomiting is more common during induction and recovery, whereas regurgitation is more common during surgical anesthesia because of relaxation of the lower esophageal sphincter. The tube should always be kept cuffed and the head positioned level with or slightly higher than the rest of the body during surgical anesthesia to decrease the likelihood of regurgitation. If the patient begins to retch or vomit at any time during general anesthesia, the patient's head should be quickly positioned lower than the body so that the vomitus flows out of the oral cavity and away from the pharynx. When the vomiting stops, the oral cavity and the pharynx are carefully cleaned with swabs, gauze, or suction.

Prolonged Recovery

Prolonged recovery may be seen in patients with pre-existing disease or hypothermia, in those that have received dissociatives, or after prolonged procedures. Patients must be supported with IV fluids, good nursing care, measures to treat hypothermia, administration of reversal agents if indicated, and careful monitoring.

Rough Recovery

A rough or stormy recovery is one in which a patient thrashes, vocalizes, paddles, tries to bite, falls over, or exhibits any other uncontrolled behavior that can result in injury of the patient or of personnel during the recovery period. Rough recoveries are more common in nonpremedicated patients and may result from pain, fear, or disorientation. To manage a rough recovery, the patient should be approached with caution and sedatives or analgesics administered as ordered by the veterinarian; the patient is then calmed, and padding, restraint, and bandaging techniques are used to prevent self-trauma.

Acknowledgments

The authors would like to acknowledge the invaluable contribution of our colleague, John A. Thomas, whose original work is foundational to this chapter.

The authors also acknowledge Steven Ahern, AA, AAB, and William Fogarty, MEd, at the Cuyahoga Community College, for photography and art direction for many of the figures in this chapter (Figs. 30.1–30.28, except for Figs. 30.4, 30.5, 30.13, 30.14, 30.17A, 30.18, 30.19, and 30.20).

Bibliography

Recommended Websites

Academy of Veterinary Technicians in Anesthesia and Analgesia (AVTAA): https://www.avtaa-vts.org.

American College of Veterinary Anesthesia and Analgesia (ACVAA): http://www.acvaa.org.

Association of Veterinary Anaesthetists: https://ava.eu.com.

Veterinary Anesthesia and Analgesia Support Group (VAASG): http://www.vasg.org.

Recommended Readings

American College of Veterinary Anesthesia and Analgesia. Guidelines for anesthesia in horses; Small animal monitoring guidelines; and Control of waste anesthetic gases. Available at: http://www.acvaa.org/veterinarians/guidelines.

Grubb T, Sager J, Gaynor JS, et al. 2020 AAHA Anesthesia and monitoring guidelines for dogs and cats. *J Am Anim Hosp Assoc.* 2020;56(2):59–82.

Cooley KG, Johnson RA. *Veterinary Anesthetic and Monitoring Equipment.* Hoboken, NJ: John Wiley & Sons, Inc; 2018.

Duke-Novakovski T, deVries M, Seymour C. *BSAVA Manual of Canine and Feline Anaesthesia and Analgesia.* 3rd ed. Quedgeley, UK: BSAVA; 2016.

Grimm KA, Lamont LA, Tranquilli WJ, et al. *Veterinary Anesthesia and Analgesia.* 5th ed. Ames, IA: Wiley-Blackwell; 2015.

Haskins SC. Anesthesia and analgesia. In: MacIntire D, Drobatz K, Haskins S, et al., eds. *Manual of Small Animal Emergency and Critical Care Medicine.* Ames, IA: Wiley-Blackwell; 2012.

Ko JC. *Small Animal Anesthesia and Pain Management.* 2nd ed. Boca Raton, FL: Taylor & Francis Group, LLC; 2019.

Ko JC, Krimins R. Anesthetic monitoring: devices to use & what the results mean. *Tdy Vet Pract.* 2012;2.

Lin H, Walz P. *Farm Animal Anesthesia: Cattle. Small Ruminants, Camelids, and Pigs.* Ames, IO: John Wiley & Sons, Inc; 2014.

Muir WW, Hubbell JAE. *Equine Anesthesia.* 2nd ed. St. Louis, MO: Saunders; 2010.

Muir WW, Hubbell JA, Bednarski RM, et al. *Handbook of Veterinary Anesthesia.* 5th ed. St. Louis, MO: Mosby; 2013.

Robertson SA, Gogolski SM, Pascoe P, et al. AAFP feline anesthesia guidelines. *J Feline Med Surg.* 2018;20:7.

The Association of Veterinary Anaesthetists. Guidelines for Safer Anaesthesia; Anaesthesia records and checklists. https://ava.eu.com/resources/.

Thomas JA, Lerche P. *Veterinary Anesthesia and Analgesia for Veterinary Technicians.* 6th ed. St. Louis, MO: Elsevier; 2025.

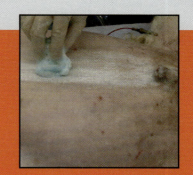

31

Surgical Instruments and Aseptic-like Technique

GEORGE W. MCCOMMON

CHAPTER OUTLINE

LEARNING OBJECTIVES

When you have completed this chapter, you will be able to:

1. Pronounce, define, and spell all key terms in this chapter.
2. Do the following regarding general surgery instruments and stapling equipment:
   - Name and describe commonly used surgical instruments.
   - Know the basic operation and properties of carbon dioxide and diode lasers and develop a basic knowledge of laser safety protocol.
   - State advantages of surgical stapling and list common surgical stapling devices.
3. Discuss vascular sealing devices and list commonly used instruments and equipment for ophthalmic, orthopedic, arthroscopic, and laparoscopic procedures.
4. Do the following regarding surgical instrument packs, instrument care, and the use of surgical drapes and gowns:
   - List surgical instruments and supplies routinely included in general and emergency surgical packs for small and large animals.
   - Describe procedures for cleaning, packing, and sterilizing instruments.
   - Describe procedures for folding and packing cloth surgical drapes and gowns.
5. Do the following regarding the processes of sterilization and disinfection as part of aseptic technique:
   - Differentiate between sterilization and disinfection.
   - List and describe physical and chemical methods of sterilization and methods of quality control of sterilization methods.
   - Know the appropriate sterilization processes for sensitive equipment.
   - State safe storage times and conditions for sterile packs.
   - List and describe common antiseptic and disinfectant compounds.
   - Describe requirements for preparation of the operating room and maintenance of operating room sterility.
6. Describe preparation requirements for both small animal and equine patients, including skin preparation, patient positioning, and draping.
7. Describe preparation requirements for the surgical team and explain the procedures that may be used for hand scrubbing before surgery, the procedure for donning surgical attire, and the procedures for opening sterile items.

KEY TERMS

Antisepsis
Antiseptic
Antiseptic agents
Asepsis
Aseptic technique
Assisted gloving
Autoclave
Box lock
Chemical sterilization
Closed gloving
Coherent light
Cold trays
Collateral thermal damage
Disinfectant
Endogenous route
Ethylene oxide
Exogenous route
External fixation
Filtration
Flash sterilization
Gas sterilization
Incise drape
Ingress port
Insufflate
Joule

Latent thermal damage
Obturator
One-step prep
Open gloving
Osteochondral fragments
Paralumbar fossa
Peritoneal lining
Physical sterilization
Plume
Prosthesis
Quarter drapes
Ratchet
Recumbency
Residual activity
Scrub in
Scrub suit
Sterilization
Sterile field
Sterile technique
Strike-through
Subchondral bone
Towel clamps
Triangulation
Watts (W) per unit time (seconds)

Introduction

To be thoroughly prepared for surgery, it is critical that the veterinary technician be comfortable with all types of equipment and the steps involved in ensuring that **aseptic technique** is maintained. Instrumentation is constantly being changed and improved, and it is often the responsibility of the veterinary technician to prepare, handle, and maintain instruments before, during, and after surgery. Patients need to be appropriately prepared for surgery, and dedication to the proper techniques of surgical preparation is essential to decrease the incidence of surgical site infection. The veterinary technician plays a crucial role in all steps.

Instrumentation

A complete description of all possible surgical instruments is well beyond the scope of this chapter. The goal of this section is to familiarize the technician with the most used instruments and related surgeries to be encountered in general small and large animal practices. Additionally, some of the more advanced items of equipment will be briefly discussed to familiarize the surgical technician with these new devices.

> **TECHNICIAN NOTE**
> Each instrument is designed for a specific purpose, such as cutting, holding, clamping, or retracting, and should only be used for its designated purpose.

General Surgery Instruments

Scalpel

Scalpels (or blades) are the instruments used to make most incisions. Scalpels are available in a variety of different sizes and shapes, with the most common being the disposable versions that are placed onto surgical steel scalpel handles. There are also sterile, plastic-handled scalpels, which may be used once before being disposed of. Although the choice of scalpel blade varies by clinician, certain blades are used for specific tasks. The most used scalpel handles include the Bard-Parker No. 3 (for scalpel blades #10, #11, #12, and #15) and No. 4 (for scalpel blades #20, #21, and #22). Small animal surgeries are generally performed with a No. 3 handle, whereas large animal surgeons usually require a No. 4 handle (Fig. 31.1).

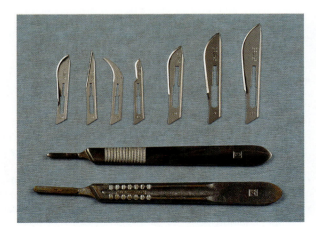

• **Fig. 31.1** Scalpel handles and attachable surgical blades. Surgical blades #10, #11, #12, and #15 fit the Bard-Parker No. 3 scalpel handle, and surgical blades #20 to #22 fit the Bard-Parker No. 4 handle. The No. 3 handle and the #10 blade are commonly used in small animal surgery. The No. 4 handle and the #20 blade are commonly used in large animal surgery.

Electrosurgery

Electrocautery has become common in both general and specialty veterinary practices. The main advantage of this technology is that it allows the clinician to cut while limiting bleeding through electrocoagulation. This is done by passing a high-frequency alternating electrical current through the tissue from the handpiece to the electrical ground plate positioned under the patient. Cutting and/or coagulation can be performed through the same handpiece, and the surgeon can activate it by using a switch on the sterile handpiece or a foot pedal. A nonsterile technician is required to adjust the power level for most units (Fig. 31.2A and B); newer electrosurgery systems also allow this task to be performed by the surgeon on the handpiece (Fig. 31.2C). It is important that adequate contact is made between the patient's skin and the ground plate, or the patient can be burned at the site of the ground plate. Good contact can be made by placing a damp surgical towel between the patient and the ground plate or by using electrocautery gel (Fig. 31.2D). It is not necessary to clip the hair between the patient and the ground plate. In *bipolar electrosurgery*, the current passes between two tips on the handpiece (Fig. 31.2E), which grasp the tissue. The most common application of bipolar cautery is the delicate sealing of small vessels in areas where cauterization of surrounding tissues must be minimized (e.g., neurosurgery, cardiac surgery). No ground plate is needed for bipolar electrosurgery.

Biomedical Lasers and Laser Safety

Laser Properties

"Laser" is an acronym for *l*ight *a*mplification by *s*timulated *e*mission of *r*adiation. Several different types of lasers are used in veterinary medicine. Energized light coming from a laser unit is generated from gas, liquid, or crystal. The beam of light coming from a laser is highly focused and intense, with very little divergence of a laser

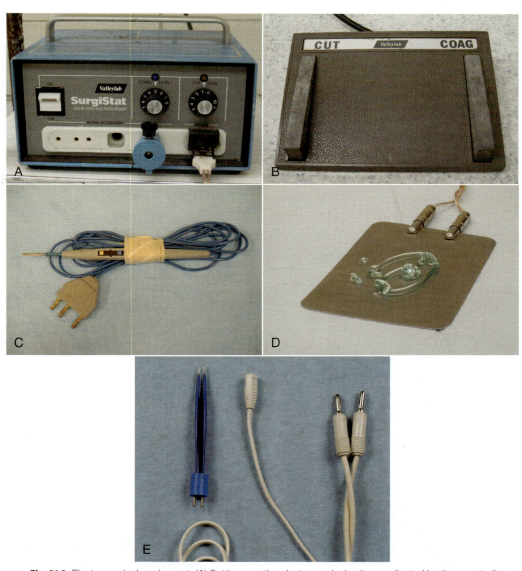

• **Fig. 31.2** Electrosurgical equipment. (A) Settings on the electrosurgical unit are adjusted by the nonsterile technician. (B) The electrosurgical foot switch is placed near the surgeon's foot. (C) Monopolar electrosurgery handpiece. If the handpiece has a cutting coagulation button, a foot switch is not needed. The handpiece is sterilized and is given to the surgeon. The surgeon passes the end of the cord to a nonsterile assistant, who plugs it into the electrosurgical unit. (D) Ground plate on the surgery table with gel to improve skin contact when the animal lies upon it. Good contact is important for proper function. (E) The bipolar handpiece is sterilized for use. A nonsterile foot switch is needed for activation.

beam. Unlike light from a flashlight, the light from a laser is uniform in wavelength and frequency. This is referred to as *coherent light*, and it does not scatter in different directions once emitted from a laser unit.

The effect of a laser on tissue depends on its wavelength within the light spectrum. The resulting interaction depends on the density and makeup of the tissue and may include beam scatter, transmission reflections, or absorptions. For example, bone is more likely than muscle to cause scatter because of lack of absorption. However, most lasers have a thermal effect, resulting in cutting, vaporizing, coagulating, or welding. The amount of laser energy applied to tissue is measured in **joules**, or **watts (W) per unit time (seconds)**. As an example, if a laser is set at 20 watts of power and is applied to tissue for 4 seconds, 80 joules of energy have been applied to the tissue.

An important property of laser surgery is latent and collateral thermal damage. Some lasers cause delayed cellular death, which is referred to as *latent thermal damage*. Lasers can also cause cellular damage or death wider than the actual path of the laser beam; this is referred to as *collateral thermal damage*. The desired effects determine whether a laser can be used for a surgical procedure. Lasers are activated with a foot or hand switch. Most laser beams are invisible, so laser units are built with a helium-neon (He-Ne) visible guide light (Fig. 31.3).

Types of Lasers

The most commonly used lasers in the veterinary field include carbon dioxide (CO_2), neodymium: yttrium-aluminum-garnet (Nd: YAG), and diode lasers. The CO_2 laser is a free beam laser directed by a handpiece, which is held slightly above the tissue surface. Because it does not touch the tissue directly, it is categorized as a noncontact laser (Fig. 31.4). YAG and diode lasers, in contrast, are directed by a hand-held quartz fiber whose tip can be directly applied to tissue; they are therefore regarded as "contact lasers" (Fig. 31.5).

CO_2 Laser. The laser beam is produced from a gas medium (CO_2). The beam is then transmitted down an arm with reflective mirrors, or it can pass through a tube called a *reflective waveguide* (Fig. 31.6).

Nd: YAG and Diode Lasers. YAG and diode lasers are very similar in their properties as their wavelengths are very similar (1064 micrometers [µm] versus 980 µm). The laser beam of the Nd: YAG is produced from a crystal of yttrium, aluminum, and garnet, "doped" with neodymium. The diodes are gallium (indium) aluminum arsenide lasers (Fig. 31.7). Both transmit the laser beam through a quartz fiber (Fig. 31.8).

Laser Safety

Safety when working with lasers cannot be stressed enough as serious injury can occur because of contact with surgical laser beams (Fig. 31.9). All veterinary technicians working with lasers must be trained to follow safety measures when a laser is used in the operating room (Fig. 31.10). Veterinary technicians should know whom to contact immediately if a laser-related issue develops during surgery. The veterinary technician who controls the laser unit

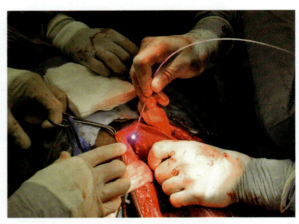

• **Fig. 31.4** A handpiece directs an operating carbon dioxide laser (noncontacting laser), which is held slightly above the surface of the surgical tissue.

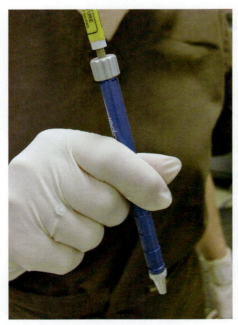

• **Fig. 31.3** The beam from a laser is invisible, but the use of a helium-neon (He-Ne) guide light generates a visible red color that allows the surgeon to see the direction of the laser beam during operations.

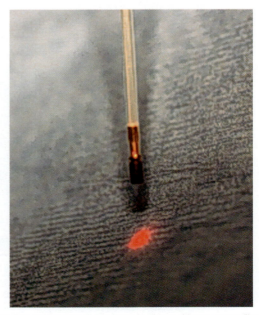

• **Fig. 31.5** The beam of a diode laser is directed by a quartz fiber. The tip of the fiber is applied directly to the surgical tissue.

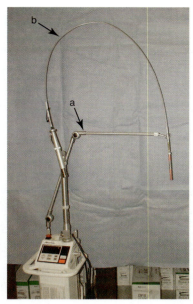

• **Fig. 31.6** A carbon dioxide laser can pass through an arm with reflective mirrors (a) or through a flexible tube called a *reflective wave guide (b)*.

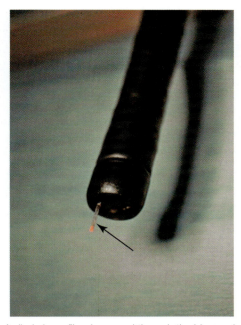

• **Fig. 31.8** A diode laser fiber is passed through the biopsy channel of an endoscope in preparation for transendoscopic laser surgery in a pony.

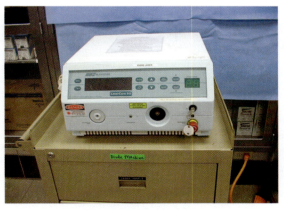

• **Fig. 31.7** Diode laser unit.

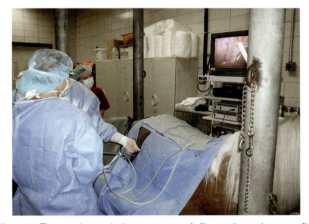

• **Fig. 31.9** Transendoscopic laser surgery. A fiberoptic endoscope fitted with a laser has been introduced into the abdominal cavity of a pony. Note that the tip of the laser is visible on the monitor screen in the background.

during surgery must be skilled in its operation and emergency shutdown. Most lasers are equipped with an emergency shutdown button (Fig. 31.11).

Laser Hazard Classification

Lasers are divided into four classes according to their ability to inflict damage to skin or eyes (Table 31.1). Most medical lasers, which are class IV lasers, can cause skin and eye damage.

Laser Safety Protocol for Personnel

Protocols for the safety of personnel should be developed in each hospital regarding laser use (Box 31.1). These should be tailored to the specifications of each practice, but all must provide a safe

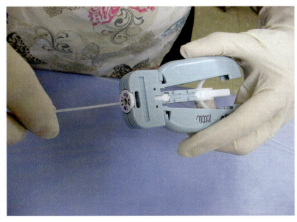

• **Fig. 31.10** The flammable polyethylene coating is stripped off a laser fiber before it is used.

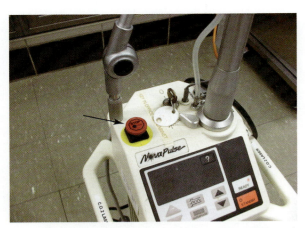

• **Fig. 31.11** Emergency shutdown button on a laser unit *(arrow)*.

TABLE 31.1	Laser Hazard Classification	
Class	**Description**	
I	Not harmful for direct viewing or skin contact	
II	Not harmful for vision, if momentary	
III	Harmful for direct viewing	
IVᵃ	Will cause skin or eye damage Any laser with power greater than 0.5 watts for longer than 0.25 seconds May pose fire hazard	

ᵃIncludes most surgical lasers.

• BOX 31.1   Laser Safety Protocol for Personnel

- Laser surgical procedures are to be performed exclusively in an operating room or in another room specifically designed for the purpose.
- The person at the laser control must be familiar with the operation and shutdown, including emergency shutdown of the laser.
- Laser warning signs are to be posted on the operating room door.
- All personnel must wear wavelength-specific eye protection.
- All windows in the operating room are to be covered with a nonreflective material during laser use.
- The laser is placed on "standby" by the control operator when not being actively used by the surgeon.
- The plume evacuator must be in use during lasing.
- Laser-specific face masks should be worn during laser procedures.

---

working environment by using appropriate safety equipment and gear. Safe use of lasers has been outlined by the American National Standards Institutes (this information is provided at www.ansi.org). The area of risk during laser operation may be defined as the *nominal hazard zone*. The nominal hazard zone is the space within the level of direct, reflected, or scattered radiation during normal operation that exceeds the applicable *maximum permissible exposure* (MPE) level. The MPE is the maximum laser radiation exposure that can occur without causing adverse biologic effects on the eyes or the skin. The eyes are most vulnerable to laser injury; however, using one type of eye protection does not protect staff from all types of lasers. It is important to note that *wavelength-specific eye protection* is available for each laser and must be consistently

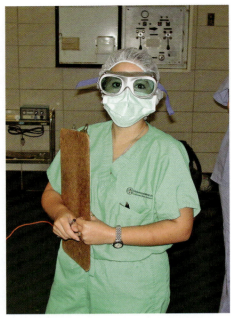

• **Fig. 31.12** Laser eye protection must be worn by all surgical staff whenever a laser is in use. The type of eye protection to be worn varies with the type of laser being used. It is important to wear the *correct eye protection*.

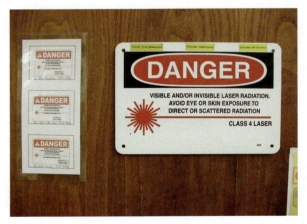

• **Fig. 31.13** A warning sign alerts staff when a laser is in use.

employed during surgeries that involve lasers (Fig. 31.12). It is important that the staff is aware of which type of laser is in use and which eye protection should be worn. *Laser warning signs* should be posted at the door of the operating room, stating that a laser is in use and that proper eye protection is required (Fig. 31.13). Because some lasers, such as the diode laser, can penetrate clear glass, accidental transmission of a laser through a surgery window should be prevented by use of a nonreflective material (i.e., cloth) placed on windows (Fig. 31.14).

Laser Plume Control

Another hazard associated with lasers is the generation of ***plume***, or smoke. Plume generated from lasering tissue may contain toxic substances that can have deleterious effects on veterinary personnel and on the patient. Plume can be controlled with the use of a plume evacuator (Fig. 31.15A), which creates suction to pull the plume through a hand-held sterile tube and into a filtered container (Fig. 31.15B). Filtering face masks specifically made for

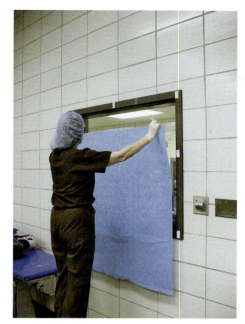

• **Fig. 31.14** All windows in the surgery suite must be covered with nonreflective material to prevent inadvertent laser beam transmission through the glass.

lasering should be worn in lieu of conventional surgical masks when lasers are in use.

Laser Safety Protocol for the Patient

A safety protocol must be established for the patient whenever lasers are to be used (Box 31.2). Sterile saline should be always readily available for the surgeon to protect against the possibility of flash fires in the surgical field. Flammable anesthetic agents, such as pressurized oxygen, should never encounter the laser beam, because this creates an explosive fire hazard. The patient's eyes should be shielded from the beam and shielded endotracheal tubes used if laser penetration of the trachea or upper respiratory tract is possible.

Scissors

Surgical scissors are among the most used surgical instruments in small animal and large animal surgery alike. Each type of scissors has a specific function and is used only for that function (Fig. 31.16). Operating scissors are classified by multiple features, including blade type (straight or curved), the character of their points (blunt-blunt, blunt-sharp, or sharp-sharp), and the design of the cutting edge of the blades (plain or serrated). *Mayo dissecting scissors* are heavy-duty operative scissors used primarily for cutting fascia and other, denser, tissues; their blades may be straight or curved, blunt or sharp, and plain or serrated. Their size and length may also vary. *Metzenbaum dissecting scissors* are fine, straight, or curved scissors used for cutting delicate tissue, such as fat or thin muscle. Metzenbaum scissors are preferred for most soft tissue dissection and come in a wide variety of sizes, with most having rounded points and plain blades. They should never be used for cutting sutures, because this dulls the edges, causing the blades to separate and lose effectiveness. *Stitch scissors* or *Littauer suture removal scissors* are used to cut all sutures except wire sutures, which is what *wire-suture–cutting scissors* are designed for. Suture scissors should not be used for cutting tissues. *Lister bandage scissors* are available to cut bandage material and should not be used for tissue or bone. One blade of the Lister scissors is blunted to facilitate sliding under a bandage without injuring the skin.

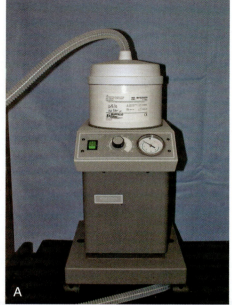

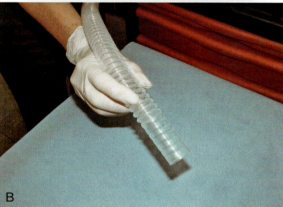

• **Fig. 31.15** (A) Plume evacuator. (B) The plume evacuator hose is sterilized so that it can be used at the surgical site and directed by sterile personnel. The circulating nurse attaches the hose to the evacuator and controls the unit.

• **BOX 31.2** Laser Safety Protocol for Patients

- Areas rinsed in alcohol must be completely dry before laser use to avoid combustion.
- Sterile saline must always be available for the surgeon.
- The patient's eyes are to be shielded during laser use.
- Tissues surrounding the laser surgical field are to be covered with moistened sponges.
- A backstop, such as moistened gauze sponges, is to be used to prevent laser penetration beyond the desired depth. This is especially important when working over hollow organs.
- Flammable anesthetic agents, including pressurized oxygen, must not come in contact with the laser beam.
- Shielded endotracheal tubes must be used if laser penetration of the trachea or the upper respiratory tract is possible.

TECHNICIAN NOTE

Scissors are specifically designed for many purposes, including dissecting tissue and cutting suture or bandage materials. Each pair of scissors should be used only for its intended purpose.

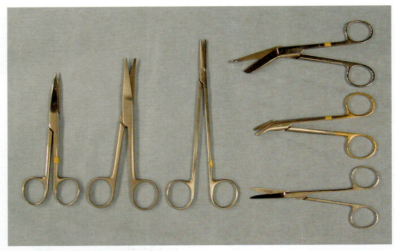

• **Fig. 31.16** Scissors. *Left to right:* sharp-sharp operating scissors. Mayo dissecting scissors, and Metzenbaum dissecting scissors. *Right, from top to bottom:* Lister bandage scissors, wire cutting scissors, Littauer suture removal scissors.

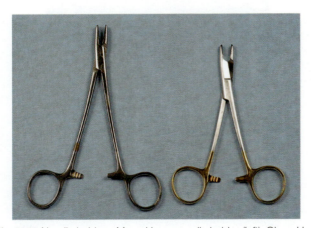

• **Fig. 31.17** Needle holders. Mayo-Hegar needle holder *(left)*, Olsen-Hegar needle holder *(right)*.

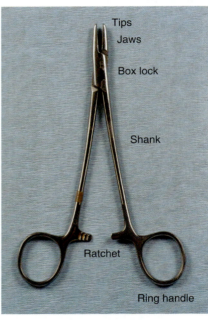

Tips
Jaws
Box lock
Shank
Ratchet
Ring handle

• **Fig. 31.18** Basic components of a surgical instrument.

Needle Holders

Needle holders, also called *needle drivers*, are used to grasp and pass suture needles with suture through tissue; needle holders can also be used to perform tying of suture knots. The two most common needle holders used in veterinary medicine are *Mayo-Hegar and Olsen-Hegar* (Fig. 31.17). The primary difference between Mayo-Hegar and Olsen-Hegar needle holders is the presence of built-in scissors. The Olsen-Hegar needle holder contains built-in scissors, whereas Mayo-Hegar holders do not. Advantages of the Olsen-Hegar needle holder include potential increase in surgical speed and the surgeon being able to work alone without the assistance of another individual to cut the suture. Other scissor designs have been manufactured for specific uses in microsurgery and ophthalmic surgery and should only be used for their intended purposes.

Needle holders have a set of jaws and a **box lock**; furthermore, a ratcheted locking device allows suture needles to be held within the jaws of the needle holder without falling out or twisting (Fig. 31.18). Improper use of needle holders (e.g., using a needle holder that is too small for the size of the needle or using a needle holder to bend or twist wire) may not only damage the jaws but also spring the box lock and *ratchet*, thereby ruining the instrument. High-quality needle holders often contain replaceable tungsten carbide inserts within their jaws. These inserts allow for excellent grip and are resistant to wear. When jaws or inserts become worn down, the jaws of a needle holder may close incorrectly, preventing appropriate grasping of the needles or accidental cutting of suture. It is important to replace worn-down inserts to prevent these potential complications.

TECHNICIAN NOTE
Needle holders are designed for handling the suture needle and performing instrument suture ties.

Thumb Forceps

Thumb forceps have a spring action, and the jaws are opposed by manually compressing the two metal handles together. These forceps are important in the manipulation of tissues and are designed in several different sizes and grasping surfaces to be selected according to the intended use (Fig. 31.19A–C). *Brown-Adson thumb forceps* are commonly used and have multiple intermeshing teeth with a broad tip to provide good tissue and suture needle handling for most routine suturing and wound/incisional closures. *Rat-tooth thumb forceps* have large interdigitating teeth and are used primarily for the skin or fascia. *Adson thumb forceps* have delicate intermeshing teeth that provide a good, atraumatic grasp of delicate tissues. They are commonly used during dissection of muscle and more delicate connective tissues. *Cooley* and *DeBakey thumb forceps*, which have long, narrow jaws with multiple delicate sets of teeth, are relatively atraumatic and are especially well suited for vascular surgery. *Russian thumb forceps* have a broad, curved surface that serves well for needle handling, but they cause trauma when used to hold tissues. Additionally, many thumb forceps intended for skin manipulation (e.g., Brown-Adson thumb forceps) contain replaceable tungsten carbide inserts that facilitate secure needle handling during suture application, like those present on high-quality needle holders.

> ### TECHNICIAN NOTE
>
> Thumb forceps are commonly used to hold tissues while dissecting or suturing.

Tissue Forceps

Tissue forceps are locking instruments that clamp tissues (Fig. 31.20). Like needle holders, they contain a set of jaws, a box lock, and handles with a ratcheted locking device. Various tooth patterns allow different types of tissue forceps to grip tissue with variable strength and secondary tissue trauma. *Allis tissue forceps* securely grasp tissue but cause significant tissue crushing. Allis tissue forceps are therefore considered to be "traumatic forceps" and should be used only on tissues that are being removed from the patient (e.g., tumors, damaged bowel, etc.). These tissue forceps are also commonly used to secure patient drapes and instrument cords (e.g., cautery and suction). *Babcock forceps* are similar in shape to Allis tissue forceps but are considerably less traumatic for tissues, owing to their smoother grasping surface and less stiff design. *Doyen intestinal tissue forceps* are designed with flexible, atraumatic jaws that allow them to safely clamp off viable portions of bowel and other delicate tissues. As has been discussed, generally, the less traumatic the forceps, the less security they afford for tissue holding.

> ### TECHNICIAN NOTE
>
> Tissue forceps use a self-locking mechanism to clamp and hold tissues. They should be chosen according to the damage that may be inflicted to tissue and used accordingly.

Hemostatic Forceps

Hemostatic forceps, also known simply as *hemostats*, are tissue forceps named for their function—to stop bleeding by crushing tissues and associated blood vessels (Fig. 31.21A and B, Fig. 31.22A and B). Types of hemostatic forceps are classified according to their size, the pattern of the grooves on the inside surface of the jaws, and whether they are straight or curved. Most hemostats have transverse grooves

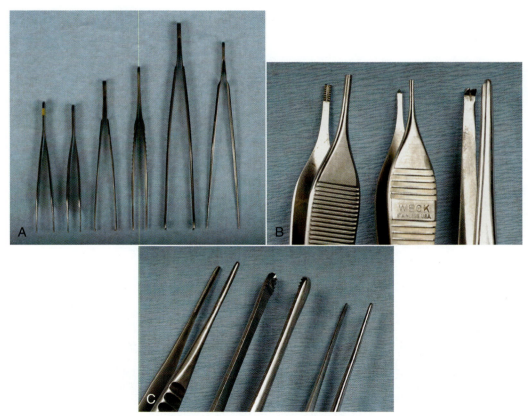

• **Fig. 31.19** Thumb forceps. (A) *Left to right*: Brown-Adson thumb forceps, Adson thumb forceps, rat-tooth thumb forceps, DeBakey vascular thumb forceps, Russian thumb forceps, dressing thumb forceps. (B) Close-up of tips *(left to right)*: Brown-Adson thumb forceps, Adson thumb forceps, rat-tooth thumb forceps. (C) Close-up of tips *(left to right)*: DeBakey vascular thumb forceps, Russian thumb forceps, dressing thumb forceps.

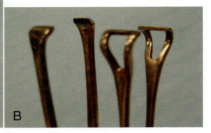

• **Fig. 31.20** Tissue forceps. (A) *Left to right:* Allis tissue forceps, Babcock tissue forceps, Doyen intestinal tissue forceps, Backhaus towel clamps (two sizes). (B) *Close-up of tips:* Allis tissue forceps *(left),* Babcock tissue forceps *(right).*

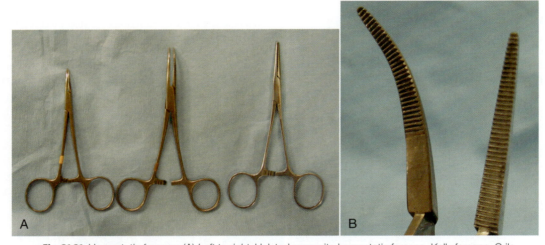

• **Fig. 31.21** Hemostatic forceps. (A) *Left to right:* Halsted mosquito hemostatic forceps, Kelly forceps, Crile forceps. (B) Close-up of jaws: curved Kelly *(left),* straight Crile *(right).*

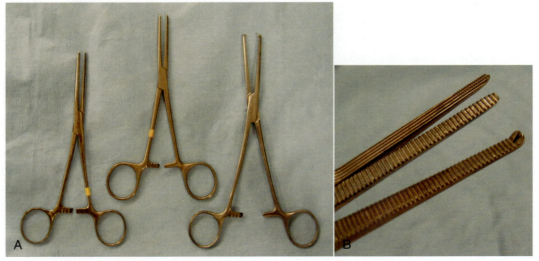

• **Fig. 31.22** Hemostatic forceps. (A) *Left to right:* Rochester-Carmalt forceps, Rochester-Péan forceps, Rochester-Ochsner forceps. (B) Close-up of jaws *(left to right):* Rochester-Carmalt forceps, Rochester-Péan forceps, Rochester-Ochsner forceps.

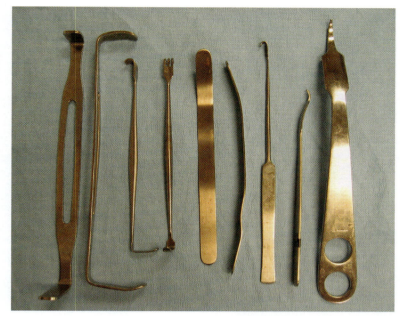

• **Fig. 31.23** Hand-held retractors. *Left to right:* two Army-Navy retractors, two Senn retractors, two small malleable retractors, Snook ovariohysterectomy hook (spay hook), two Hohmann retractors (different sizes).

on the inside surface of the jaws to better grasp the tissue. *Halsted mosquito hemostats* are small and are designed to occlude small vessels. They are similar in design to mosquito hemostats, but Halstead mosquito hemostats are larger for use in crushing larger tissues and vessels. Crile and Kelly forceps differ in their jaw tooth pattern. Crile forceps contain transverse grooves that extend the entire length of the jaws. Kelly forceps contain grooves associated with only the most distal aspect of the jaws. *Rochester-Péan forceps* are large, transversely grooved forceps that are used to clamp tissue bundles and large vessels. *Rochester-Ochsner forceps* are likened to Rochester-Péan forceps, except that they have interdigitating teeth at the tips that aid in grasping the tissue. Rochester-Ochsner forceps are used most in orthopedic or large animal surgery. *Rochester-Carmalt forceps* are large, crushing forceps with longitudinal grooves and cross grooves at the tip to provide greater traction. These forceps are used for clamping across tissue that contains vessels. The most common use of Rochester-Carmalt forceps is to crush and hold the tissues and vessels of the ovaries during routine spaying procedures in small animals.

Retractors

Surgical retractors are commonly used to atraumatically improve the field of visualization in both soft tissue and orthopedic surgical procedures. Properly placed hand-held or self-retaining retractors should not interfere with surgery but rather, should provide more room for the surgeon to work. The most used hand-held retractors are shown in Fig. 31.23. The *Army-Navy retractor* and the *Senn retractor* are double-ended hand-held retractors commonly used to retract skin, fat, or muscle. The Army-Navy retractor has smooth blades, whereas the Senn retractor has one smooth blade and one blade with three sharp or blunt prongs. The *malleable retractor* is made of thin metal that is easily bent to the desired shape and is especially useful for retracting the abdominal and thoracic organs.

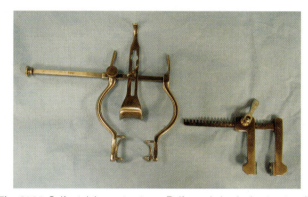

• **Fig. 31.24** Self-retaining retractors. Balfour abdominal retractor *(left)*, Finochietto rib retractor *(right)*.

The *Snook ovariohysterectomy hook*, or "spay hook," is a specialized type of hand-held retractor used to grasp the horn of the uterus during an ovariohysterectomy. The *Hohmann retractor* is used almost exclusively in orthopedic surgery and consists of a single blade and a handle that is used to lever tissues out of the way for better visibility.

In contrast to hand-held tissue retractors, self-retaining retractors (Figs. 31.24 and 31.25) can be locked in place and maintained in an optimal position without the need for a surgical assistant for tissue retraction. The *Balfour retractor* provides increased exposure of the abdominal cavity through the use of wire like blades to distract the abdominal incision and a solid spoon like blade that is hooked onto the sternum to distract it cranially. It is important to ensure that no abdominal contents (e.g., bowel, spleen) are entrapped between the body wall and the retractor during placement. The *Finochietto rib spreader* retracts the ribs to expose the surgical field within the thoracic cavity. The ratcheted part of the retractors is positioned at the dorsal or cranial aspect of the thoracic incision so that it does not interfere with the surgeon. *Gelpi retractors* and *Weitlander retractors* are self-retaining retractors commonly used for muscle retraction, especially in orthopedic and neurologic surgeries.

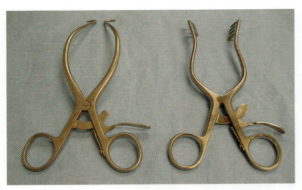

• **Fig. 31.25** Self-retaining retractors. Gelpi retractor *(left)*, Weitlaner retractor *(right)*.

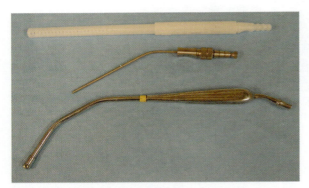

• **Fig. 31.26** Suction tips. *Top to bottom:* Poole, Frazier, Yankauer. The suction tip is attached to a sterile hose. The surgeon hands the other end of the hose to a nonsterile assistant to plug it into the suction unit.

> **TECHNICIAN NOTE**
> Retractors are used to retract tissues and provide good visibility of the surgical site.

Suction Tips

Various suction tip designs are commonly used in both small and large animal surgeries (Fig. 31.26). Many suction tips may be prepackaged, sterile, and disposable. The suction tip is attached to a long, sterile suction tube that is connected to a vacuum source. The *Poole suction tip* is used primarily in the abdominal or thoracic cavity because it has an outer sleeve with small holes to prevent tissue, such as fat, from becoming entrapped in the tip. The *Frazier tip* is used most in orthopedic and neurologic surgery. The *Yankauer tip* is a general purpose suction tip.

Stapling Equipment

Several surgical stapling devices are available (Figs. 31.27 and 31.28) and offer the advantage of fast and easy closure as opposed to suturing. The most used stapling devices include the ligate-divide-separate (LDS), thoracoabdominal (TA), gastrointestinal (GI), and gastrointestinal anastomosis (GIA) staplers, and surgical clips (Ligaclip, Ethicon, Somerville, NJ) and skin staples. Some stapling devices (LDS and GIA) also cut tissue after stapling. The staplers are named by an abbreviation of their designed function (Table 31.2). A number may be used after the name "thoracoabdominal stapler (TA)" or "gastrointestinal stapler (GIA)" to indicate the length of the row of staples (e.g., a TA 30 places rows of staples in a line 30 mm long).

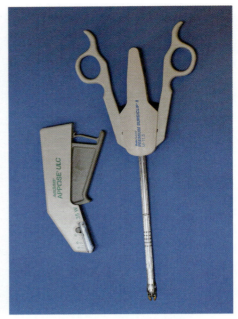

• **Fig. 31.27** Stapler *(left)* and Hemo-clip *(right)*.

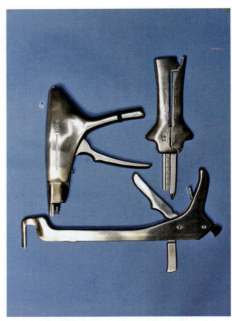

• **Fig. 31.28** Surgical stapling equipment. *Left*: The LDS stapling device applies two staples to tissue and cuts between staples. *Right*: The GIA stapler. A cartridge of staples for one-time use is purchased in a presterilized package. *Bottom*: The TA stapler. Staple cartridges are purchased as for the GIA; shown here without staple cartridges in place.

Vascular Sealing Devices

Various vascular sealing devices allow for ligation of vessels much larger than that afforded by traditional bipolar and monopolar electrocautery units. Such devices use a combination of pressure and energy output to achieve adequate vessel fusion (e.g., sealing of vessels upward of 7 mm in diameter compared with 1 to 2 mm, which is achievable with traditional monopolar and bipolar cautery) (Fig. 31.29A and B). Many of these devices have been designed for both open surgical techniques (e.g., laparotomy, thoracotomy) and minimally invasive surgical techniques (e.g., laparoscopy, thoracoscopy).

Ophthalmic Instruments

Ophthalmic surgery, like many other surgical subspecialties, requires specialized, delicate instruments. Gentle, safe handling and appropriate use of such instruments is necessary to keep them functioning properly for extended periods. Basic ophthalmic operative packs include specialized scalpels (e.g., No. 7 scalpel handle), fine scissors (e.g., iris and strabismus scissors), thumb forceps, needle holders (e.g., Castroviejo ophthalmic needle holders), retractors (e.g., chalazion and Graeffe eyelid retractors), and lacrimal duct cannulas (Fig. 31.30).

TABLE 31.2	Stapling Equipment		
Derivation of Name	**Common Use**	**Comments**	
TA—Thoracoabdominal	Lung and liver lobe resection	Places double or triple row of staples	
GIA—Gastrointestinal anastomosis	Gastrointestinal resection and anastomosis	Places four rows of staples and cuts between the middle two rows	
EEA—End-to-end anastomosis	Gastrointestinal anastomosis	Staples two intestinal segments together in a circular manner with a functional lumen	
Ligaclip stapler	Vessel ligation	Places a single staple	
Skin stapler	Skin and fascia closures	Places a single staple	
LAD—Ligate-and-divide stapler	Blood vessel ligation	Places two staples on a vessel and cuts between them	

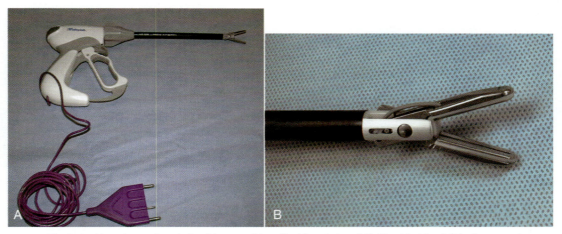

• **Fig. 31.29** Vascular sealing device (Ligasure Atlas, Covidien, Irvine, CA). Hand-held unit (A); close-up of sealing tip (B).

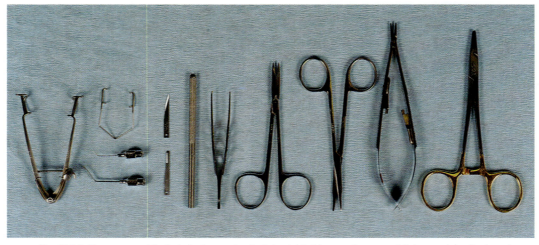

• **Fig. 31.30** Common ophthalmic instruments. *Left to right:* lid speculum, small lid speculum *(top)* and lacrimal cannulas *(bottom),* Beaver blade handle with #64 and #65 surgical blades, Bishop-Harmon thumb forceps, iris scissors, tenotomy scissors, Castroviejo needle holder, and Derf needle holder.

Orthopedic Instruments

Periosteal Elevators

Periosteal elevators are instruments that are used to pry periosteum or muscle from the bone surface. They have a blade like structure at one or both ends of a handle. The blades have sharp or blunt edges and are available in various sizes (Fig. 31.31). The Freer elevator is the most used periosteal elevator in small animal orthopedics.

Rongeurs

Rongeurs are hand-held instruments with sharp, cupped tips that are used to cut small pieces of dense tissue, such as bone, cartilage,

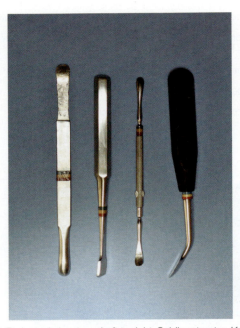

• **Fig. 31.31** Periosteal elevators. *Left to right:* Seldin retractor, Key elevator, Freer elevator, and AO-round edge periosteal elevator.

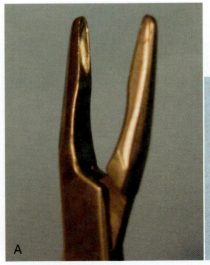

or fibrous tissue (Fig. 31.32A and B). *Bone-cutting forceps* are similar to rongeurs but have paired chisel-like tips. They are used for cutting bone and should not be mistaken or used for wire cutters (Fig. 31.33). Rongeurs have a double or single-action mechanism. *Double-action rongeurs* have a smooth cutting action, are mechanically stronger than single-action rongeurs, and are also larger. Double-action rongeurs are preferred for removing large amounts of dense tissue. *Single-action rongeurs* are more commonly used in confined areas, such as joints and the spinal canal. *Kerrison rongeurs*, which have a gun-shaped appearance, are used specifically in spinal surgery.

Curettes

Curettes are used to scrape hard tissue, such as bone or cartilage. These instruments are often included in both orthopedic and arthroscopic surgical packs. Curettes are designed with a small, sharpened, cup like structure at one or both ends of a handle (like an ice cream scoop) and are available in various sizes (Fig. 31.34). Bone curettes are used to retrieve cancellous bone from

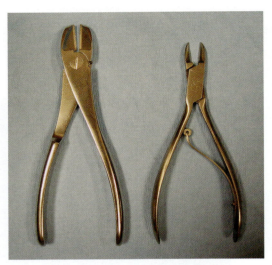

• **Fig. 31.33** Wire cutters *(left)* and bone cutters *(right)*. They look similar but should not be confused—bone cutters have finer jaws.

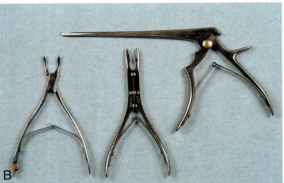

• **Fig. 31.32** Rongeurs. (A) Close-up of tips. (B) *Left to right:* single-action rongeur, double-action rongeur, Kerrison rongeur.

the medullary cavity (tibia, humerus, ilium) for use as a bone graft during fracture repair. Curettes are also commonly used during arthroscopic surgery to debride joint surfaces and dislodge loose, bony fragments within joints for removal.

Bone-Holding Forceps

Bone-holding forceps are designed to hold bone and bone fragments in alignment while orthopedic implants (screws, pins, wires, or plates) are applied. Most bone-holding forceps are self-retaining and are available in a variety of designs and sizes. The

most used types are displayed in Fig. 31.35. *Kern bone-holding forceps* have a ratcheted handle that allows them to be clamped securely onto the bone. Clamshell and point-to-point bone-holding forceps have a locking mechanism like that of needle holders and hemostatic forceps. *Self-retaining bone-holding forceps*, also known as *speed locks*, have a nut that tightens against one handle to squeeze the handles together.

Osteotomes and Chisels

Osteotomes and chisels are used to cut bone by pounding on the flat or flared end of the instrument with a mallet (Fig. 31.36). The cutting edge of the osteotome is tapered on both sides, whereas the chisel is tapered only on one side. Osteotomes and chisels are made of relatively soft metal and should not be used for purposes other than their intended use or they may be ruined.

Gigli Wire

Gigli wire is used to cut bone and horn by placing the wire around the bone and drawing it back and forth in a sawing fashion. T-shaped handles hook onto the wire, allowing the surgeon to firmly grasp the wire.

Trephines and Jamshidi Needles

Trephines and Jamshidi needles are specially designed to remove a core of bone for biopsy. Trephines are T-shaped, reusable stainless steel tubular instruments with a cylindrical cutting blade, similar to a traditional punch biopsy blade (Fig. 31.37). The Jamshidi is a similar instrument but is often for single use and is disposable.

Power Equipment

Power equipment is commonly used in orthopedic and neurologic surgeries. Although some drills are electric or battery powered (Fig. 31.38A and B), many orthopedic drills and saws are powered by nitrogen gas that is supplied via a sterile hose (Fig. 31.38C). The Hall air drill is a specialized high-speed burr that grinds bone (Fig. 31.38D) and is most used for spinal surgery. Many of these instruments cannot tolerate autoclave steam

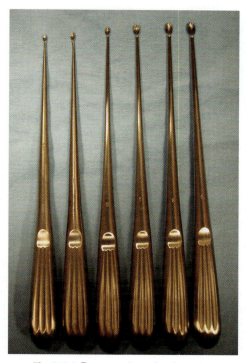

• **Fig. 31.34** Bone curettes of various sizes.

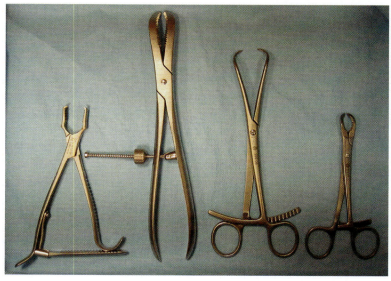

• **Fig. 31.35** Bone-holding forceps. *Left to right:* small Kern forceps, large speed-lock forceps, large point-to-point forceps, small clamshell forceps.

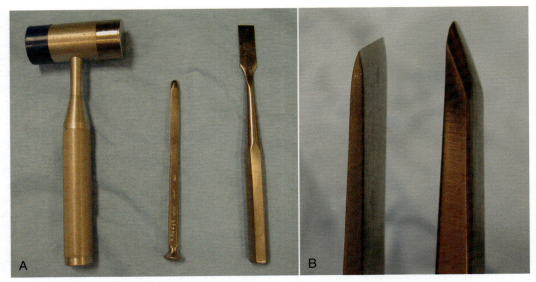

• **Fig. 31.36** (A) Mallet, chisel, and osteotome. (B) Osteotome *(left)* and chisel *(right)*.

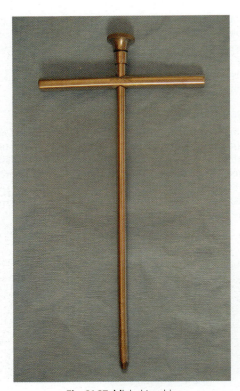

• **Fig. 31.37** Michel trephine.

sterilization or immersion in cold sterilization; therefore *gas sterilization* or covering with sterile coverings is required for their use in sterile procedures.

Orthopedic Implants

Orthopedic surgery may involve the use of various products that are placed into or around the bone and are left in place permanently or for an extended period. Metal implants are usually made of stainless steel alloy, cobalt-chromium alloy, or titanium. Of these three types, titanium is the most resistant to corrosion and has the best fatigue life; it is also the most expensive. Although it is beyond the scope of this chapter to go into detail regarding various orthopedic implants, it is important to be conceptually familiar with general implant types and uses.

Bone Pins

Bone pins vary in diameter, length, and type of point. Three different types of pin point are available—chisel, trocar, or threaded trocar. Steinmann pins are smooth, stainless steel pins ranging in diameter from 1/16 to 1/4 inch. Steinmann pins may also be called *intramedullary (IM) pins*, because they are often placed in the medullary cavity of long bones for fracture fixation. *Kirschner wires (K-wires)* are similar to Steinmann pins, but they are smaller and can be used to pin small bone fragments. Available sizes are 0.035-inch, 0.045-inch, and 0.062-inch diameters. Some pins have threads, like a screw, which are used most for extraskeletal fixator placement (Fig. 31.39). The threads can be located at the end of a pin or in the middle, and they can have a positive or negative profile. A power drill or a Jacobs hand chuck is required to insert the pin into bone, and a pin cutter is necessary to cut it to the proper length (Fig. 31.40).

Interlocking Nails

Interlocking nails are similar to IM pins but have preplaced holes through the pin that allow screw placement. Interlocking nails provide more rigid fixation than is provided by IM pins alone. They provide resistance to compression and rotational forces and require specialized equipment to guide screw placement.

Orthopedic Wire

Stainless steel orthopedic wire or cerclage wire is supplied on spools (Fig. 31.41). The most common sizes used in small animal surgery are 22-, 20-, and 18-gauge (Table 31.3). It is mostly applied in a cerclage fashion by encircling the bone or bone fragments and twisting the ends in a twist-tie fashion using special wire twisters similar in appearance to standard needle holders.

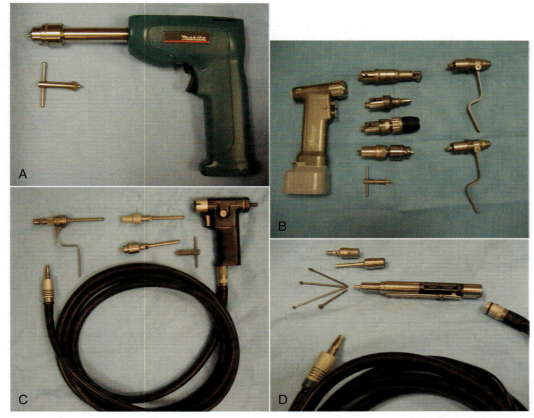

• **Fig. 31.38** Power equipment. (A) The Makita drill is an example of a battery-powered drill. (B) The ConMed Linvatec battery-powered handpiece *(left)*. Attachments shown include *(center, top to bottom)* saw blade attachment, quick release for drill bit, keyless chuck, and Jacobs chuck with key, and *(right)* pin and wire drivers. (C) The 3M minidriver (3M Products, St. Paul, MN) is powered by a tank of pressurized nitrogen gas. It has an attachment for Kirschner wires (K-wires) and quick-release or chuck attachments for drill bits. (D) The Hall air drill has various sizes and shapes of burs and two bur guards of different lengths.

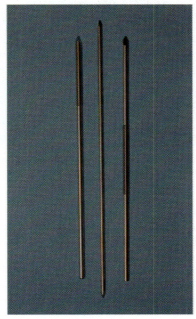

• **Fig. 31.39** Various pin types. *Top to bottom:* positive end-threaded pin, smooth pin, and positive central-threaded pin.

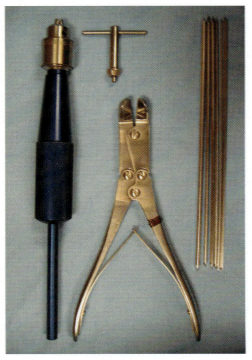

• **Fig. 31.40** Jacobs hand chuck, key, pin cutter, and various sizes of Steinmann pins and Kirschner wires (K-wires).

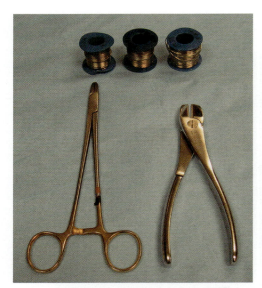

• **Fig. 31.41** Orthopedic wire, wire twisters, wire cutters. Wire twisters look similar to needle holders but are more rugged and are designed to withstand higher forces.

TABLE 31.3	Commonly Used Orthopedic Wire Sizes	
Gauge	Inches	Millimeters
22	0.025	0.64
20	0.032	0.81
18	0.040	1.02

External Fixators

External fixators have gained popularity in recent years because of their ease of placement and as a means of providing fixation without disrupting the fracture site (e.g., closed fracture reduction techniques). External fixation is a means of stabilizing fractures using pins or wire placed through skin and bone. The pins or K-wires are held rigid by metal bars, rings, or acrylic connecting bars attached to the pins at least 1 cm from the skin (Fig. 31.42). If a metal apparatus is used, special clamps are placed to attach a metal connecting bar to each pin.

Bone Screws

Orthopedic screws are available in many different lengths, diameters, and head patterns. Additionally, two basic screw designs are available: cortical and cancellous. Cortical screws are fully threaded screws that are designed for dense (cortical) bone. Cancellous screws may be fully threaded or partially threaded (e.g., lag style) and are made with wider threads to allow for a better grip of softer cancellous bone (Fig. 31.43).

The general steps of screw placement include drilling a hole in the bone, measuring the hole with a depth gauge to determine proper screw length, using a bone tap (a screw like instrument with sharp threads) to cut a screw path in the bone, and inserting the screw with a specialized screwdriver. Newer screw designs include a self-tapping screw (negating the need for a bone tap) and locking screws, in which separate threads engage the bone and the plate. These two newer designs allow for more rapid placement

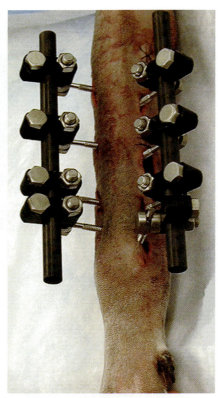

• **Fig. 31.42** An external fixator shown on the radius of a dog. Note the pins that penetrate the skin and bone are fixed to bars with the use of special clamps. (Courtesy Dr. James Toombs.)

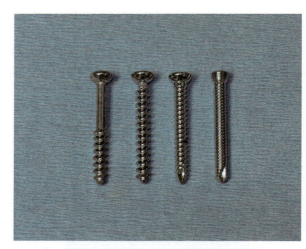

• **Fig. 31.43** Bone screws. *Left to right:* partially threaded 4.0-mm cancellous screw, fully threaded 4.0-mm cancellous screw, fully threaded 3.5-mm nonlocking cortical screw, and fully threaded 3.5-mm locking cortical screw.

and a more stable fixation construct, respectively. Bone screws may be used alone or in conjunction with a bone plate or an interlocking nail.

Bone screws are named by both screw length and thread diameter (in millimeters). Screws commonly used in small animal surgery are 1.5-, 2-, 2.7-, and 3.5-mm diameter cortical screws and 4-mm diameter cancellous screws. Larger (2.7- and 3.5-mm diameter) screws often have hexagonal heads and are driven by the same hexagonal screwdriver; smaller screws (1.5- and 2-mm

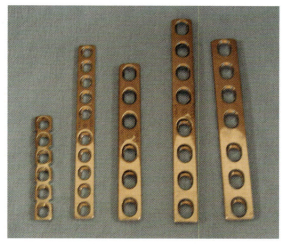

• **Fig. 31.44** Bone plates of various sizes.

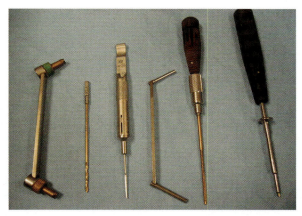

• **Fig. 31.45** Bone plating tools. *Left to right:* drill guide, drill bit, depth gauge, tap sleeve (to prevent soft tissues from being caught on the bone tap), bone tap, and screwdriver.

diameter) have cruciate heads and require a small cruciate screwdriver. Larger screws (4.5-, 5.5, and 6.5-mm diameter) are used in large animal surgery and require a large hexagonal screwdriver.

Bone Plates

Bone plates come in many shapes, sizes, and types (Fig. 31.44) and are named by the number of screw holes and by the screw diameter size that best fits the plate. For example, a seven-hole, 3.5-mm plate would have holes for seven 3.5-mm diameter screws. Additionally, bone plates are classified according to whether they provide compression or not and whether they house locking or nonlocking screws. Bone plates must be bent to match the curve of the bone and fastened with bone screws. Locking plates have specialized inserts that are placed into the threaded screw holes during bending to maintain the correct thread pattern.

Instrumentation required to apply a bone plate is highly specialized and includes drills, drill bits, drill guides, depth gauges, bone taps, tap sleeves, screws, screwdrivers, and plate benders (Fig. 31.45), all of which are included in most general orthopedic plating packs. Although bone plating is more complex than other types of orthopedic fixation and requires an extensive "inventory" of implants, the result is often a more stable construct for healing.

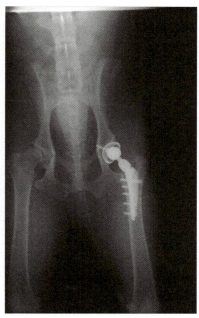

• **Fig. 31.46** Radiograph of a dog with a total hip prosthesis.

Total Hip Prosthesis

The hip joint may be replaced by a *prosthesis* in some dogs with severe arthritis (Fig. 31.46). The femoral prosthesis consists of a long stem placed inside the proximal femur with the use of screws or bone cement, a ball that replaces the femoral head, and a cup replacing the acetabulum.

Arthroscopic Instruments and Equipment

The arthroscope is used as a diagnostic and surgical tool to examine various joints of the horse, including the scapulohumeral, humeroradial, carpal, fetlock, distal interphalangeal, coxofemoral (used in foals only), stifle, and tarsocrural joints. It is also used to examine various joints in the dog. The arthroscope has been used to visualize intra-articular fractures during lag screw fixation, such as third carpal bone slab fractures in the carpus (knee) of horses, and to identify meniscal and cruciate injuries in dogs. Arthroscopy has many uses in both small and large animal surgeries and is used during the removal of osteochondral fragments and osteochondritic lesions on the articular surface in joints of young horses and dogs.

Arthroscope

The arthroscope is a rigid telescope that carries light into a joint cavity and produces a magnified image of the internal structures, which are displayed on a viewing monitor. Different types of arthroscopes with various diameters and viewing angles have been developed, including a 5-mm outer-diameter (OD) arthroscope with a 10-degree, 25-degree, or 70-degree lens viewing angle; a 4-mm OD with a 10-degree, 30-degree, 70-degree, or 110-degree lens angle; a 2.7-mm OD with a 5-degree, 30-degree, or 70-degree lens angle; and a 1.9-mm OD with a 5-degree or 30-degree lens angle. A 4-mm OD, 25-degree or 30-degree angled lens scope is generally used by most equine surgeons (Fig. 31.47), whereas a 2.7-mm OD, 30-degree angled lens scope is commonly used for canine arthroscopy. Most arthroscopes have a small video camera

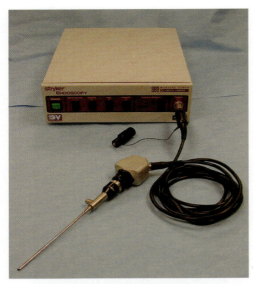

• **Fig. 31.47** A video camera attached to a 4-mm outer-diameter (OD) arthroscope.

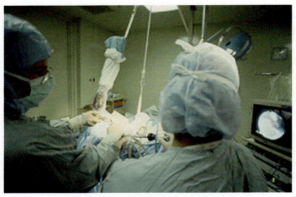

• **Fig. 31.48** Most arthroscopic procedures are viewed on a monitor.

that can be attached, affording the surgeon a larger, crisper image on a video monitor (Fig. 31.48). This greatly improves visualization of the intra-articular space compared with direct viewing through the eyepiece of the arthroscope. This method also allows for better aseptic technique, because the surgeon's face is not near the surgical field, and an assistant can operate the camera-scope unit. A monitor also allows several persons to observe the procedure simultaneously, and a digital record can be made for future replay, both useful functions for academic teaching laboratories and for client education.

Ancillary Arthroscopic Equipment

The arthroscope comes with various instruments used to introduce the scope into the joint and to work inside the joint. Stab incisions are made in the skin over the surgically prepared joint space through which the arthroscope and hand instruments will be inserted.

Sharp Trocar and Sleeve

The *sharp trocar* is a pointed instrument that is inserted into a hollow, cannula-type instrument called the *arthroscope sleeve*

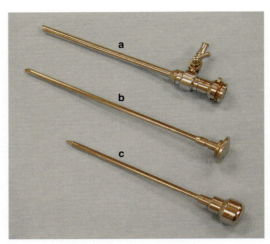

• **Fig. 31.49** The sharp trocar (b) fits inside the arthroscope sleeve (a). The unit is used to penetrate the fibrous joint capsule through a stab incision in the skin. The conical obturator (c) replaces the sharp trocar in the sleeve once the fibrous joint capsule has been penetrated.

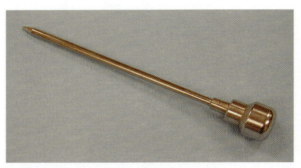

• **Fig. 31.50** The conical obturator replaces the sharp trocar in the sleeve and is used to penetrate the synovial membrane portion of the joint capsule and to advance the sleeve farther into the joint.

(Fig. 31.49). The trocar and the sleeve unit are used to penetrate the fibrous portion of the joint capsule through a stab incision.

Blunt Obturator

Once the sharp trocar has penetrated the fibrous joint capsule, the sharp trocar is replaced by a *conical* (blunt-tipped) *obturator* (Fig. 31.50), which is used to penetrate the synovial membrane of the joint capsule, after which the joint space is distended with a sterile balanced electrolyte solution. The obturator is then used to advance the arthroscope sleeve into the joint space with less risk of damaging the articular cartilage. The obturator is replaced with the *arthroscope* (Fig. 31.51), which is designed to lock onto the sleeve once it is slid into position inside the sleeve.

Light Cable, Light Projector, and Video Camera

Modern arthroscopy is performed with the use of a light source, a video camera, a viewing monitor, and ancillary power equipment. These are collectively stacked on a specially designed cart called the *tower* (Fig. 31.52). A fiberoptic *light cable* (Fig. 31.53) is attached directly to the optical light port on the arthroscope (Fig. 31.54). A high-intensity light generated from a specially designed *light projector* is fed through the fiberoptic cable and arthroscope to illuminate the joint space (Fig. 31.55). It is important to note

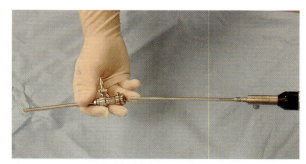

• **Fig. 31.51** Once the sleeve is in position in the joint, the obturator is removed, and the arthroscope is placed into the sleeve.

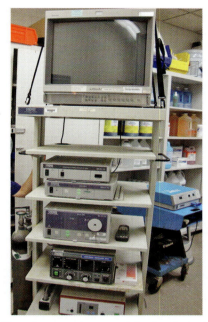

• **Fig. 31.52** The arthroscopy tower contains the stacked power units.

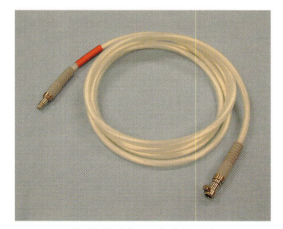

• **Fig. 31.53** A fiberoptic light cable.

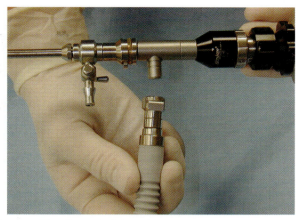

• **Fig. 31.54** The fiberoptic light cable attaches to the light port of the arthroscope.

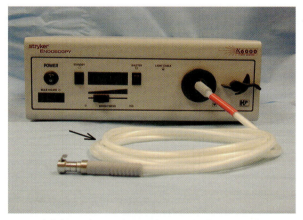

• **Fig. 31.55** A light projector that projects light through a fiberoptic light cable *(arrow)* of the arthroscope.

that fiberoptic cables are easily damaged if excessive bending or kinking occurs and should be handled in a delicate fashion.

Fluid Delivery Systems

Sterile fluid—usually a balanced electrolyte solution—is infused into the joint under pressure to maintain distention of the joint capsule, which is essential for visualization of the intra-articular space. The fluid is infused into the joint space through the sleeve, around the arthroscope. The sleeve has at least one stopcock that is used as an ***ingress port*** to connect a sterile fluid line (Fig. 31.56A and B). Gas insufflation with CO_2 or nitrous oxide has also been used as a method of distending the joint. However, a special system with a pressure-regulating device is required. One disadvantage of gas is that it does not allow for lavage of the joint space if osteochondral fragments become detached within the joint.

Pressurized Bag System

Various systems are available to deliver fluid to the joint. One system has a pressurized bag design, which involves the use of a pneumatic pressure cuff that is slipped around a bag containing sterile fluid. The cuff is inflated with air, which squeezes the fluid bag,

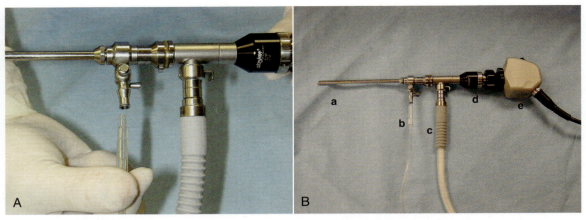

• **Fig. 31.56** (A) The fluid line is connected to the stopcock of the arthroscope. (B) Arthroscopic sleeve *(a)*, fluid line *(b)*, light cable *(c)*, arthroscope *(d)*, and camera *(e)*.

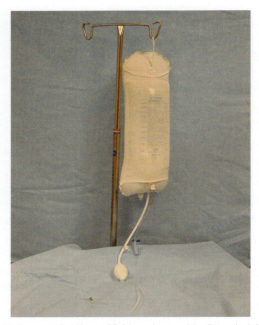

• **Fig. 31.57** A pressurized bag of fluid can be used to distend a joint during arthroscopy.

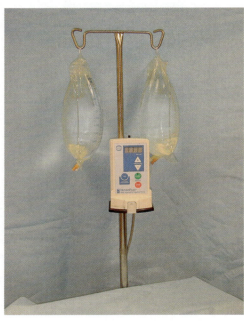

• **Fig. 31.58** An automated fluid pressure pump can be used to infuse sterile fluid into a joint during arthroscopy. Pressure within the joint is automatically regulated by the pump.

thus pressurizing the fluid and regulating the amount of pressure utilized (Fig. 31.57).

Automated Pump System

Another system uses a motorized pump to regulate the fluid rate through fluid lines connected to the arthroscope. One example of this type of system is the Hydroflex (Davol, Inc., Warwick, RI) (Fig. 31.58). Pressure volume and fluid volume going into the joint are automatically regulated within the fluid pump via a pressure feedback control. This allows the pump to maintain a preset pressure within the joint without the need for the surgeon to adjust fluid pressure.

Hand Instruments for Arthroscopic Surgery

Numerous hand instruments of various types are available or have been adapted for arthroscopy. They are used to remove or retrieve osteochondral fragments, to debride articular cartilage

or **subchondral bone**, or to probe cartilage or cartilage lesions. These instruments are inserted into the joint through a separate stab incision, and the arthroscopic operation is performed via a technique called *triangulation*. The hand instruments are often placed in a pack separate from the arthroscope and accessories.

Blunt Probe

The *blunt probe* is used to probe cartilage and subchondral bone in the joint to determine such aspects as cartilage integrity or the extent of a cartilage lesion (Fig. 31.59).

Rongeurs and Grasping Forceps

Various types and sizes of *rongeurs* have been adapted for use in arthroscopy. These instruments have a beveled edge along cupped jaws to cut the attachments of an osteochondral fragment as it is

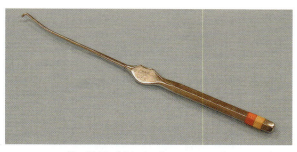

• **Fig. 31.59** A blunt arthroscopy probe.

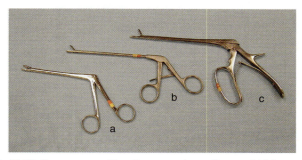

• **Fig. 31.60** Rongeurs used in arthroscopy: Love-Gruenwald *(a)*, grasping forceps *(b)*, and Ferris-Smith *(c)*.

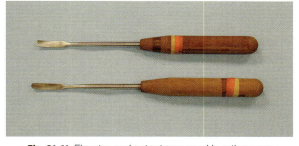

• **Fig. 31.61** Elevator and osteotome used in arthroscopy.

removed (Fig. 31.60). Forceps are used to retrieve loosely attached fragments (see Fig. 31.22).

Elevators and Osteotomes

These instruments have small beveled heads that are designed to cut or break down the attachments of an osteochondral fragment and elevate it from the parent subchondral bone bed (Fig. 31.61).

Curettes

Curettes are inserted into the joint to debride a defect left in the articular cartilage or subchondral bone after removal of an osteochondral fragment or osteochondritic lesion (Fig. 31.62).

Motorized Burrs

Motorized burrs are often collectively referred to as a *motorized arthroplasty system* and consist of a small rounded burr attached to a power-driven shaft. The burr and shaft are enclosed in a sleeve, with a portion of the burr protected to prevent inadvertent damage to surrounding articular cartilage (Fig. 31.63). The burr is also used to debride defects left in the articular cartilage or subchondral bone after removal of an osteochondral fragment or osteochondritic lesion. The speed of rotation of the burr can be

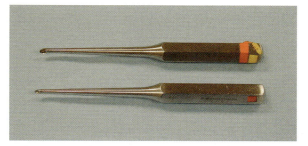

• **Fig. 31.62** Small, cupped bone curettes used in arthroscopy.

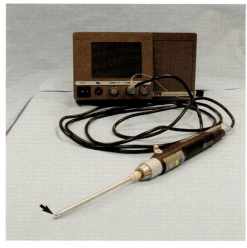

• **Fig. 31.63** A motorized arthroplasty system with burr attachment *(arrow)*.

adjusted and usually operates at several thousand revolutions per minute. Most systems operate with an on-off foot pedal or hand switch controlled by the surgeon.

Radiofrequency Arthroscopic Probes

Intra-articular electrosurgical cutting and coagulation devices are used under arthroscopic guidance to allow for hemostasis of blood vessels and for debridement or resection of damaged soft tissue structures within a joint. Like the aforementioned motorized burrs, most systems operate with an on-off foot pedal or hand switch for the surgeon.

Laparoscopic Instruments and Equipment

Similar to the arthroscope, the laparoscope is a useful diagnostic and surgical tool in veterinary surgery that is used to examine the abdominal and thoracic cavities. The abdominal cavity is accessed via the **paralumbar fossa** (equine) or the ventral abdomen (canine and equine), and gas (CO_2) is used to distend (**insufflate**) the abdomen. Laparoscopy is performed primarily to remove ovaries and retained testicles, to examine/biopsy diseased organs, to repair damaged organs (urinary bladder), and to look for tumors or adhesions. Laparoscopy is performed most often with the patient under general anesthesia; however, it is sometimes performed in horses with the use of sedation and local anesthesia (Fig. 31.64). The laparoscope is coupled with a small video camera that sends the image to a monitor for viewing (Fig. 31.65).

Laparoscope

The laparoscope is, in essence, an oversized arthroscope. Different viewing angles may be selected. Most common are 0-degree and 30-degree viewing angles. A laparoscope with 5-mm OD is

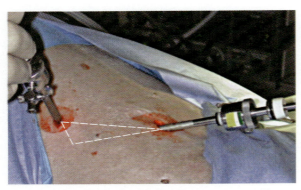

• **Fig. 31.64** Laparoscopic surgery being performed on a pony showing abdominal portals.

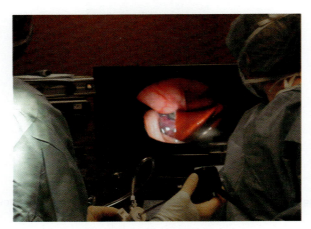

• **Fig. 31.65** Laparoscopic imaging.

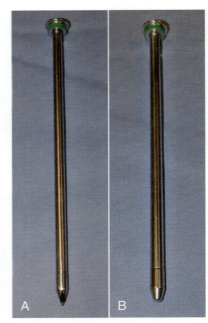

• **Fig. 31.66** (A) Sharp laparoscopic trocar. (B) Blunt laparoscopic trocar.

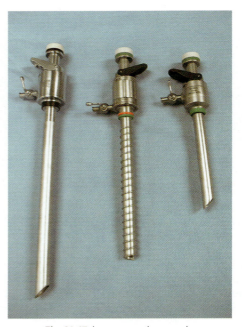

• **Fig. 31.67** Laparoscopic cannulas.

used in small animal patients and one with 10-mm OD in equine patients. The laparoscope measures 33 cm or 57 cm in length.

Laparoscopic Trocars and Cannulas

Sharp Trocars and Cannulas

Various trocars (Fig. 31.66) and cannulas (Fig. 31.67) are used as portals for the laparoscope and for hand instruments. *Sharp trocars* and *cannulas* are used to penetrate subcutaneous tissue and the **peritoneal lining** through a skin incision. Sharp trocars are manufactured with a conical or pyramidal tip. Cannulas are equipped with a valve that prevents escape of gas when a scope or an instrument is not occupying its barrel.

Blunt Trocar

Once the perineum has been entered, the sharp trocar is exchanged for a *blunt trocar* to avoid inadvertent puncture of a visceral organ and ensure safe advancement of the cannula (see Fig. 31.66B).

Light Cable, Light Projector, and Video Camera

As with arthroscopy, it is necessary to have a light source, a video monitor, ancillary power equipment, and a gas insufflator. These electrical units are stacked on a cart called the *tower*. Once the laparoscope has been introduced into the abdomen, a *small video camera* is attached to the eyepiece of the scope. This small camera feeds an image to a *monitor* through a cable for viewing. To illuminate the abdominal cavity, a *light cable* is attached to the light port on the laparoscope and is run to a *light generator*.

Insufflator

Distention of the abdominal cavity is necessary to obtain a safer space for manipulation of the laparoscope and instruments and for better visualization of the viscera. This is accomplished with an *insufflator* (Fig. 31.68). The insufflator creates and automatically maintains the desired degree of abdominal distention during a laparoscopic procedure. CO_2 is the most widely used gas, because it is not combustible. CO_2 is fed into the abdomen through a sterile line (hose) connected to the insufflator and to a port on the cannula. Intra-abdominal pressure generally is maintained at between 10 and 15 mm Hg; higher abdominal pressures decrease ventilation and should be avoided. A flow rate of 9 L/minute is used for insufflation.

Hand Instruments for Laparoscopic Surgery

Numerous hand instruments are available to cut, cauterize, staple, biopsy, and grasp organs and structures (Fig. 31.69A and B). Shafts of most laparoscopic instruments are designed to rotate to attain the most effective angle for use in the abdomen. Because of their length, these instruments are stored in specialized containers (Fig. 31.70).

Instrument Packs

Most veterinary hospitals organize surgical instruments into different surgical packs, depending on the type of practice and surgeries performed. Examples include the following: minor packs (e.g., spay/neuter packs, laceration packs), general packs for more involved soft tissue surgeries, bone packs for orthopedic procedures, specialized packs such as neurologic packs for spinal and brain surgeries, and vascular packs (Tables 31.4 and 31.5). A pack system helps staff members to organize the instruments so that the most used instruments are readily available, and infrequently used instruments are not contaminated and resterilized unnecessarily. For example, all commonly used instruments for spinal surgery are

in one pack, so it is opened, used, cleaned, sterilized, and repacked only when necessary. Infrequently used and large, bulky instruments, such as pin cutters, are typically wrapped individually for use as needed. Commonly used instruments (e.g., scalpel handle, hemostats, thumb forceps, scissors, needle holders, sponges) may be wrapped individually or in plastic self-sealing sleeves to provide access to an additional instrument without the need to open an entire instrument pack. Packs and individually wrapped items should be labeled with the date autoclaved and the initials of the person who prepared the pack.

Packs should be organized in such a way that items are always placed in the same location on the tray (Fig. 31.71A and B). This makes it easier to inventory the instruments and facilitates finding the instruments quickly during surgery. Sponges should be counted at the beginning and at the end of each surgery to ensure that none have been left inside the patient's body. It is

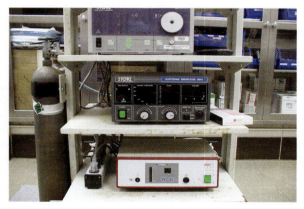

• **Fig. 31.68** The laparoscopic insufflator and air line.

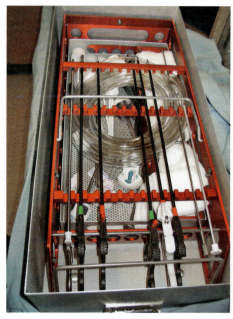

• **Fig. 31.70** A laparoscopic instrument tray.

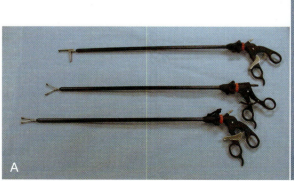
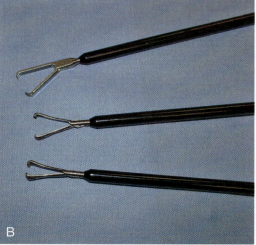

• **Fig. 31.69** (A) Hand-held laparoscopic grasping forceps. (B) Close-up of laparoscopic grasping forceps.

TABLE 31.4	Small Animal Instrument Packs		
Spay/Neuter Pack	**Soft Tissue/General Pack**	**Emergency Pack**	**Orthopedic**
No. 3 scalpel handle	No. 3 scalpel handle	No. 3 scalpel handle	Army-Navy retractors
Brown-Adson thumb forceps	Brown-Adson thumb forceps	Brown-Adson thumb forceps	Senn retractors
Needle holder, Mayo-Hegar	Adson thumb forceps	Needle holder, Olsen-Hegar	Rongeurs
Metzenbaum scissors	Needle holder, Mayo-Hegar	Mayo scissors, curved	Large Kern bone-holding forceps
Sponges (standard count)	Mayo scissors	Mosquito hemostats (3 curved, 3 straight)	Small Kern bone-holding forceps
Sterilization indicator	Metzenbaum scissors	Crile or Kelly forceps (1 curved, 1 straight)	Bone curette
Mosquito hemostats (2 curved, 2 straight)	Wire suture scissors	Allis forceps	Periosteal elevator
Carmalt forceps (2 curved)	Mosquito hemostats (4 curved, 4 straight)	Towel clamps (4)	Steinmann pins (5/64, 3/32, 7/64, 1/8, 9/64, 5/32, 3/16, 1/4)
	Carmalt forceps (2 curved)	Crile forceps (1 curved, 1 straight)	Wire (0.035, 0.045, 0.062)
	Allis forceps (2)	Sponges (standard count)	Jacobs chuck and key
	Towel clamps (8)	Sterilization indicator	Roll 18-gauge stainless
	Towels (6)		Roll 20-gauge stainless
	Stainless steel bowl		Roll 22-gauge stainless
	Sponges (standard count)		Metal ruler
	Lap sponges (2)		Michel clips and applicator
	Sterilization indicator		Sterilization indicator

TABLE 31.5	Large Animal Standard and Emergency Packs	
Standard Pack	**Emergency Pack**	
No. 3 scalpel handle	No. 3 scalpel handle	
No. 4 scalpel handle	No. 4 scalpel handle	
Rat-tooth thumb forceps (3)	Rat-tooth thumb forceps	
Adson thumb forceps (3)	Brown-Adson thumb forceps	
Needle holders (2)	Needle holder	
Mayo scissors (1 curved, 1 straight)	Mayo scissors (1 curved, 1 straight)	
Operating scissors (2 curved, 2 straight)		
Metzenbaum scissors (1 curved, 1 straight)		
Bandage scissors		
Mosquito hemostats (4 straight, 4 curved)	Mosquito hemostats (sharp-sharp)	
Kelly or Crile forceps (2 straight, 2 curved)		
Ochsner forceps, 15 cm (1 curved, 1 straight)		
Allis tissue forceps (2)	Allis tissue forceps (2)	
Towel clamps (16)	Towel clamps (4)	
Towels (4)	Towel (1)	
Saline bowl		
Sponges (standard count)	Sponges (standard count)	
Sterilization indicator		

often recommended to have a list of instruments and ancillary items (towels, sponges, etc.) and a picture of each pack available for review in the preparation area. This may be especially helpful if surgeons have specific preferences or prefer instruments not normally associated with the pack type.

Instrument Care

High-quality surgical instruments are expensive and require specific care and maintenance to keep them functioning properly for their expected lifetime. All instruments should be handled gently; particularly, delicate instruments should be separated from general instruments before being cleaned. Multiple-component instruments should be disassembled before cleaning. Power equipment should be cleaned separately to ensure that water does not get inside the components. Most surgical instruments are made of satin-finished stainless steel. Stainless steel is relatively rust resistant and retains sharp edges when properly sharpened. The satin or dull finish is often favored over the polished finish to minimize glare, although it is less resistant to spotting and discoloration and requires more vigilant cleaning and care.

After each surgical procedure, all instruments that were used or soiled should be rinsed free of blood and organic debris with cold water that is distilled or deionized. Use of tap water can increase staining and rust formation because of the high iron content. Instruments should be soaked in a commercial instrument detergent if a delay is anticipated between completion of a surgical procedure and thorough cleaning of the instruments. After the instruments have been rinsed in cold water or soaked in detergent, each instrument should be inspected and scrubbed with a soft brush in warm water and an instrument detergent of neutral pH (never use abrasive or household cleaning agents). After manual cleaning to remove blood and debris, an ultrasonic (high-frequency sound) cleaner (Fig. 31.72) is used to further remove tightly bound debris and to clean areas that the brush cannot effectively reach. When instruments are placed into the ultrasonic cleaner, box locks should be in the open position. Only

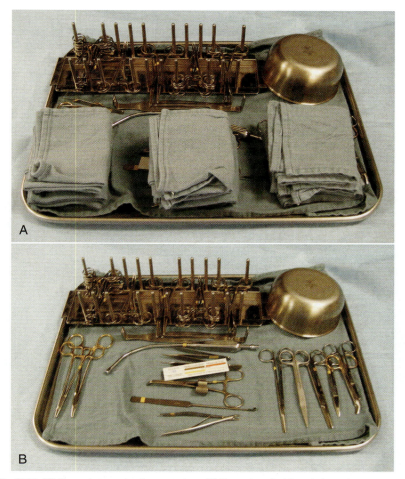

• **Fig. 31.71** (A) Properly organized surgery tray. (B) Same tray, but towels have been removed.

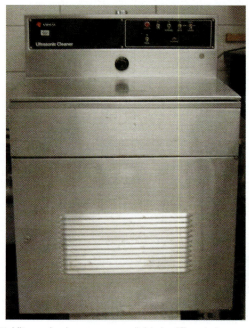

• **Fig. 31.72** Ultrasonic cleaners are available in different sizes and models. Follow the manufacturer's recommendations regarding use.

instruments of similar material should be put together in the ultrasound unit (e.g., stainless steel with stainless steel, chrome with chrome), because intermixing of instruments with different material composition may result in scratching and pitting.

Once properly cleaned, instruments should be thoroughly rinsed with deionized water and allowed to air dry before autoclaving to prevent rust formation. Wiping instruments dry rather than air drying is not recommended as this can leave lint residue. Instruments with a working action, such as a hinge or a box lock, should be treated with a water-soluble instrument lubricant. Milk baths are known to harbor bacteria and must be changed frequently. Instrument lubricants limit rust formation and keep moving parts fluid. Spray lubricants are not oily or sticky and will not interfere with steam sterilization. Working components of power equipment should be lubricated to maximize efficiency and to prolong the working lifetime of the equipment. Before instruments are repacked for sterilization, they should be thoroughly inspected for cleanliness, stiff or "frozen" hinges, improper jaw alignment, rust spots, and worn or broken parts. Defective instruments should be repaired or replaced.

Drapes and Gowns

Surgical drapes and gowns may be made of paper or cloth. Paper drapes and gowns are designed to be disposable and are purchased prepackaged and sterilized for one-time use. Cloth drapes and gowns are designed for repeated use, but they require washing after each use. Immediately soaking the cloth in cold water will prevent blood and other fluid from setting. All cloth drapes and gowns should be washed in a mild detergent and thoroughly dried before sterilization, ideally in a clean, dedicated washer and dryer (clothes and other items should have a dedicated washer and dryer). They should be inspected for holes or other signs of wear and repaired or replaced as needed.

Cloth gowns must always be folded and packed in a correct and consistent manner (Fig. 31.73). This technique allows the sterile gown to be unfolded and put on without contaminating the exterior surface. A cloth or paper towel is often included within the gown pack to facilitate hand drying immediately after scrubbing and before "gowning up."

Cloth drapes must be folded and packed in such a way that sterility can be maintained as they are unfolded and applied to the patient or surgical table. *Accordion folding* allows easy unfolding and placement of the drape (Fig. 31.74). Many specifically designed drapes are available, including adhesive drapes (e.g., povidone-iodine impregnated), transparent drapes, fenestrated drapes, stockinettes, and compressive wraps. After drapes and

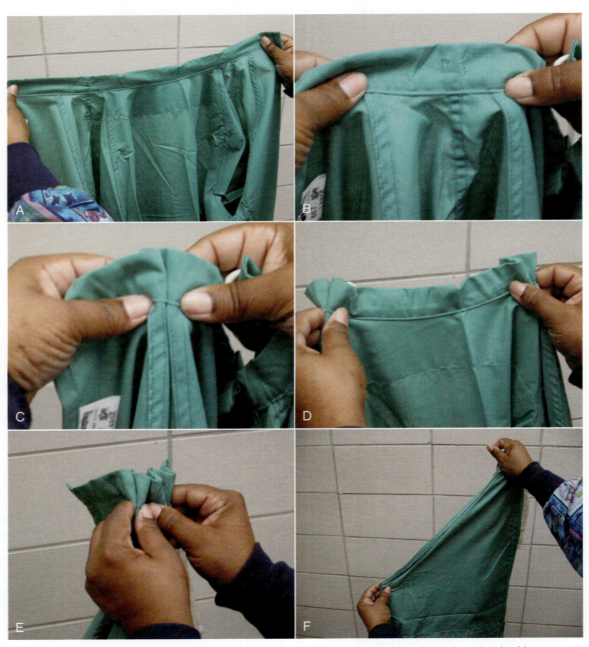

• **Fig. 31.73** Method of folding a cloth surgical gown. (A) The gown is held by the neck so the shoulder seams on the inside of the gown can be seen. (B) Close-up of the three seams of one shoulder. (C) The gown is folded so the outer two seams of one shoulder are touching. (D) The same fold is done with the other shoulder. (E) The gown is folded so the seams of both shoulders are touching. (F) The shoulders are held in one hand while the other hand aligns the armpit seams.

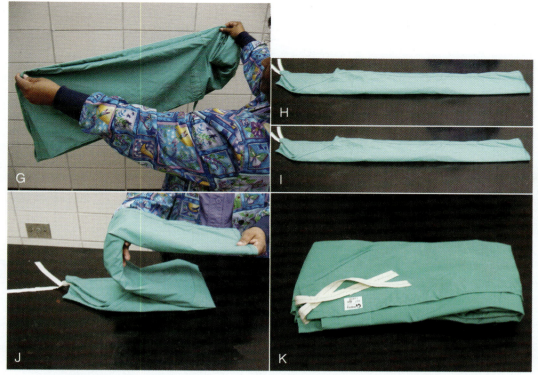

• **Fig. 31.73, cont'd** (G) The shoulders and armpits are held in one hand while the other hand aligns the gown hem. (H) The gown is laid flat on the table. (A tabletop method of folding is to first lay the gown open flat on the countertop with the outside of the gown facing up, sleeves on top. The side edges of the gown are each folded to meet near the middle, and then the gown is folded in half.) Only the inside surfaces of the gown are now exposed. (I) The gown is folded in half lengthwise. (J) The gown is folded in accordion fashion. (K) The gown is laid on the table so the neck ties are uppermost. Proceed to Fig. 31.75, which shows how to wrap the gown.

gowns have been properly folded, they are usually double wrapped in tightly woven muslin fabric or a nonwoven disposable barrier before sterilization (Fig. 31.75).

> **TECHNICIAN NOTE**
>
> Accordion folding of drapes allows for easy unfolding and placement on the patient.

Aseptic Technique

Postoperative infection can have disastrous consequences. **Asepsis** is a condition of sterility wherein no living organisms are present. Aseptic technique includes all steps taken to prevent contamination of the surgical site by infectious agents. A thorough understanding of aseptic technique is required throughout the entire surgical process, from proper sterilization of equipment and cleaning of the operating room to scrubbing and draping of the patient.

The technician may need to act as a circulating nurse by getting the patient into the operating room and opening sterile equipment for the surgeon. Additionally, the technician may be called upon to **scrub in** as a scrub nurse or surgical assistant to organize and pass instruments to the surgeon or to assist with the surgical procedure. A working knowledge of aseptic technique is necessary to perform these tasks correctly and to monitor for inadvertent "breaks" in **sterile technique**.

Microorganisms must be introduced into the surgical site for infection to develop. Sources of microorganisms include *exogenous*

and *endogenous* routes. Exogenous sources of contamination include air, surgical instruments and supplies, the patient's skin, and the surgical team. Endogenous contamination arises from within the patient and reaches the wound through the bloodstream because of bacteremia. Examples of endogenous sources are bacteria from the oral cavity (gingivitis) or the skin (dermatitis).

During every surgery, it is likely that some bacterial contamination will occur at the surgical site, regardless of vigilance to maintain asepsis. The factor most consistently observed to influence the incidence of wound contamination and subsequent infection is the length of time the patient is under general anesthesia. Risk for infection roughly doubles every hour that the patient is under general anesthesia. This fact affirms the importance of an efficient and effective surgical team. Whether contamination progresses to infection depends on many factors, including the general health of the patient, the degree of tissue damage present in the wound, the virulence of the infectious agent, the number of infectious agents, and the use of perioperative antimicrobial agents. The factor over which the surgical team has greatest control is the number of infectious agents that are introduced into the wound by an exogenous route. Strict adherence to the principles of aseptic technique will minimize exogenous wound contamination and will prevent infection.

All procedures do not require the same degree of vigilance regarding aseptic technique. Whether surgery is considered *clean*, *clean-contaminated*, *contaminated*, or *dirty* determines the appropriate degree of asepsis and the need for perioperative antimicrobials. For example, debridement of a cutaneous abscess is a "dirty"

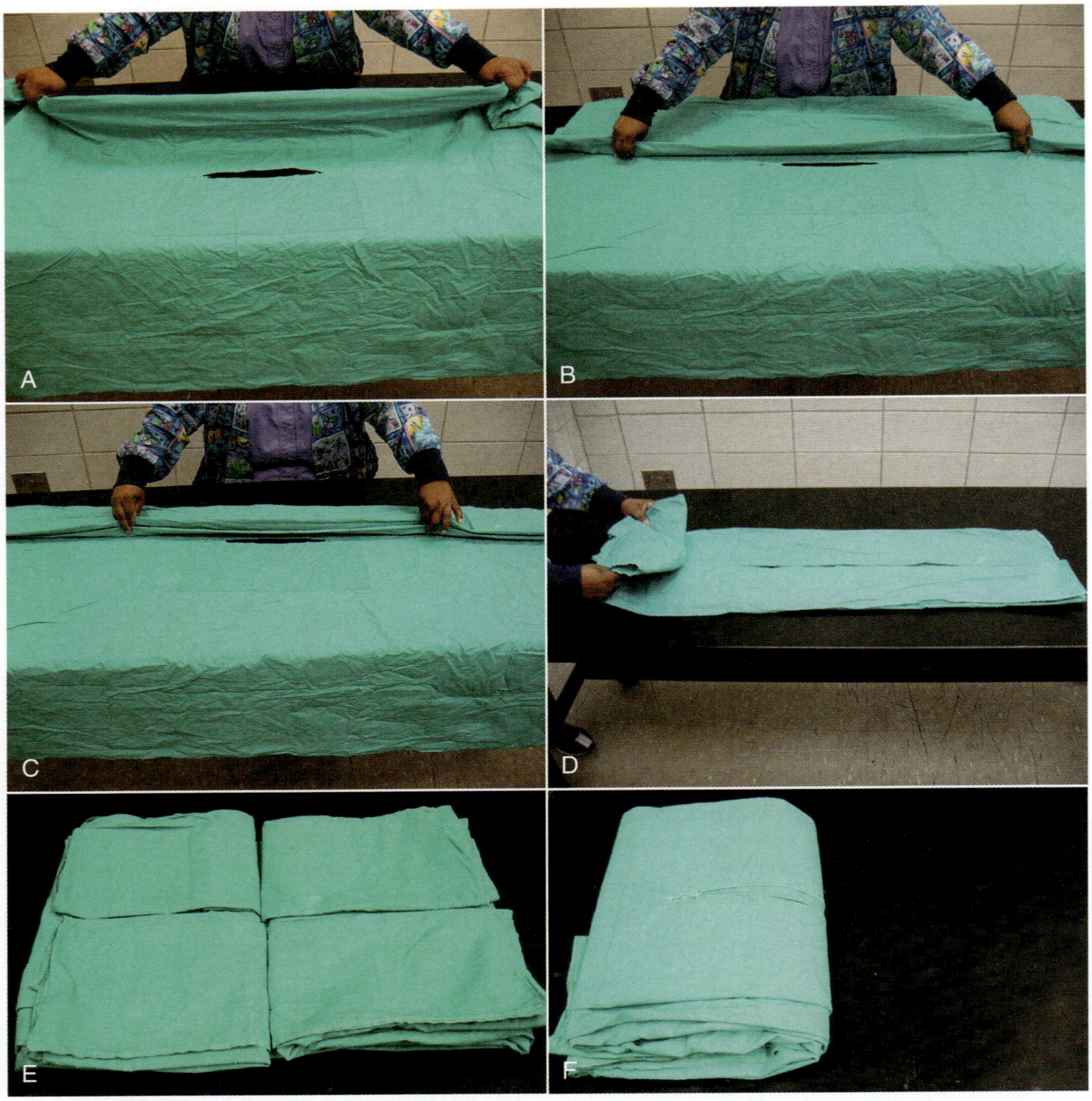

• **Fig. 31.74** Cloth drapes are folded in accordion fashion so that they are easily unfolded onto the patient. (A, B) A lengthwise fold is created in the drape (approximately 30 cm from the middle), and the folded edge is brought to the fenestration at the middle of the drape. (C) This is repeated with a second fold, creating an accordion folding. Each section of folded drape is approximately 15 cm wide. (D) The opposite side is folded in a similar manner. Then one end of the drape is folded to the center in accordion fashion. (E) The opposite end is folded in the same manner. (F) The drape is folded in half (half of the fenestration is visible), and it is ready to be wrapped, as shown in Fig. 31.75.

surgery, so aseptic technique would not be strictly followed. The wound would be scrubbed, but surgical instruments may be disinfected (cold sterilization) rather than sterilized (steam autoclave or gas sterilization), and the surgeon may wear sterile gloves but may forgo complete sterile surgical attire. It may be preferable for such a patient to remain outside the operating room to prevent contamination of an otherwise clean surgical suite and instead put in a treatment or examination room. In stark contrast, for clean surgeries, especially procedures involving placement of permanent implants (e.g., total hip replacement surgery), the surgical team must adhere strictly to aseptic protocol, including limited movement in and out of the surgical suite by personnel during the procedure. Contamination and subsequent infection during these types of procedures can lead to devastating consequences. In each case, the surgeon will determine the degree to which principles of asepsis are to be followed; technicians should clarify this to prepare and stock the appropriate area before the procedure.

Sterilization is defined as the *elimination or destruction* of all living organisms (including viruses) from a material in contrast to *disinfection*, which is the destruction of vegetative forms of bacteria but not spores. Both sterilization and disinfection are used to prepare medical and surgical materials. The process selected, either physical or chemical, depends on the nature of the material and its intended use.

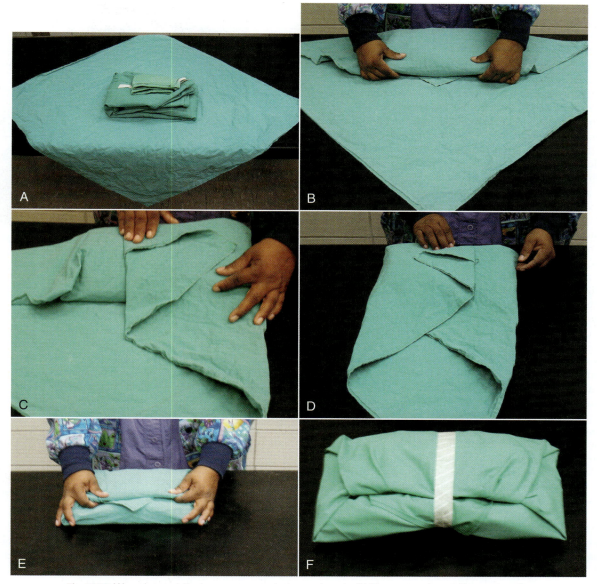

• **Fig. 31.75** Wrapping a cloth drape, gown, or instrument pack. (A) The gown, along with an accordion-folded hand towel and a sterilization indicator, is placed diagonally onto the drapes. (B) One corner is folded over the entire pack and tucked under it, leaving the tip visible. (C) An adjacent corner is folded over the end of the pack and the tip folded back so the drape is flat on top of the pack. (D) The opposite corner is folded the same way. (E) The pack is turned around, and the final corner is folded over the top of the pack and tucked under the folded drape edges, leaving the tip visible. (F) The pack is then wrapped in a second layer in the same manner. The pack is secured with autoclave tape, labeled with the contents, date, and initials of the individual preparing the pack.

PUT INTO PRACTICE

Did you know you control the surgical outcomes based on your skills in maintaining sterile surgical instruments? Make sterility your first priority by following a set protocol that never wavers for cleaning and sterilizing instruments.

Physical Methods of Sterilization

The three general methods of **physical sterilization** include filtration, radiation, and heat. Filtration and radiation are used primarily during the production and packaging of certain surgical products, whereas heat is most often associated with autoclave procedures.

Filtration

The term *filtration* refers to the use of a filter to separate particulate material from liquids or gases. Pharmaceuticals are commonly sterilized by filtration.

Radiation

Some materials that would be damaged by other methods of sterilization can be safely sterilized by radiation, which destroys microorganisms without causing significant temperature elevation.

Gloves and some suture materials are sterilized by radiation during the manufacturing process.

Heat

The method used most for sterilization is heat. There is no single temperature at which all microorganisms are killed instantaneously, because death of bacteria and spores is a function of temperature variance and duration of heat exposure.

The two basic types of heat sterilization are wet and dry heat. Dry heat is used to sterilize materials that cannot tolerate moisture but can withstand high temperatures. Oils, powders, and petroleum products are most effectively sterilized by dry heat, whereas rubber, fabrics, and some metals may be damaged by high temperatures. An advantage of dry heat is that it will not rust or corrode needles or sharp instruments. Dry heat is more difficult to control compared with moist heat, and the sterilization time is longer.

Moist heat sterilization can be accomplished by boiling water or by steam under pressure. Using boiling water at ambient pressures is not a reliable means of sterilization because of its relatively low temperature (100°C); it likely results in disinfection rather than sterilization. The bactericidal effect of boiling water can be enhanced by alkalization with sodium hydroxide (0.1 gram per deciliter [g/dL]) or sodium carbonate (2 g/dL). The addition of these agents reduces instrument corrosion, but they cannot be used with glassware or rubber goods.

The most common method of moist sterilization involves use of saturated steam under pressure; most autoclaves sterilize by this mechanism. Increased pressure causes steam to achieve a higher temperature. Materials to be sterilized in this manner must be penetrable by steam and must not be damaged by heat or moisture.

Dry heat and moist heat destroy bacteria through protein denaturation; more specifically, dry heat kills by protein oxidation, whereas moist heat kills by coagulation of critical cellular proteins. Moisture facilitates the coagulation of protein; thus moist heat kills bacteria and spores at lower temperatures and at shorter exposures than dry heat.

Autoclave Sterilization

Autoclave sterilization is technique sensitive, so operating instructions accompanying the autoclave should be followed. An autoclave load is not sterile unless steam has penetrated the packs completely so that all materials have been exposed to steam at the proper temperature and for the proper duration. This requires that packs be properly prepared and loaded into the autoclave. Most autoclaves used in veterinary practice are *gravity displacement* or downward displacement sterilizers, which means that steam is introduced into the top of the chamber and forces air to the bottom. With *prevacuum sterilizers*, a vacuum pump evacuates the air before steam is introduced. This provides more rapid and even penetration of steam than occurs with gravity displacement, permitting higher temperatures and shorter duration.

Proper pack preparation begins by checking that all materials are thoroughly cleaned and free of grease, oil, or protein residues and are functioning properly. Complex instruments should be disassembled, and any box locks should be open. A sterilization indicator strip should be placed in the middle of pack. The strip will change colors once the correct temperature and pressure are reached inside the middle of the pack. Packs must be properly wrapped with steam-permeable wrappers, such as double-thickness muslin (thread count of 140 threads per 6.45 cm²) or a nonwoven barrier (crepe paper or polypropylene fabric). Muslin wrappers can be washed and reused, but nonwoven barriers are

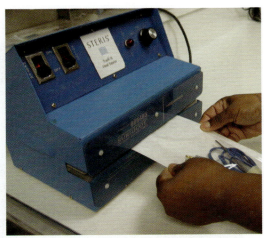

• **Fig. 31.76** Individual instruments may be heat sealed in plastic or paper pouches in preparation for steam or gas sterilization. The instrument should be positioned in the pouch so that the handle will be presented to the surgeon when the pouch is opened.

designed for single use and should not be reused. Packs are usually wrapped in two layers of muslin or nonwoven wrappers. External wraps are folded around a large pack in the same manner as described for drape and gown packs (see Fig. 31.75). Heat-sealable paper or plastic or plastic peel pouches may be used for individual instruments (Fig. 31.76). Each pack must be labeled to identify pack contents, the person who prepared it, and the date it was sterilized. Paper wraps provide longer storage times relative to fabric wraps, regardless of the number of layers. See Table 31.6 for safe storage times for sterile packs.

> **TECHNICIAN NOTE**
> Instruments with hinges or box locks should remain in the unlocked position during autoclaving.

Materials need to be packed as loosely as is practical to ensure good steam penetration. There should be 2.5 to 7.5 cm of space around each pack, and packs should be arranged pyramid-style to allow steam to flow readily from top to bottom. For example, a large pack should not be placed on top of several small ones, because it will block the flow of steam down to the smaller packs. Steam flow may be facilitated by positioning packs vertically (on edge). It is recommended that packs be no larger than 30 × 30 × 50 cm and that they weigh no more than 5.4 kg, depending on the type of material being autoclaved. In many practices, pack size is limited by the size of the autoclave.

Various minimum time–temperature standards have been established for routine sterilization of surgical packs. Exposure to saturated steam at 121°C (250°F) for 20 minutes is a safe minimum standard. Ten to 15 minutes at 121°C (250°F) will destroy most resistant microbes, and an additional 5 minutes provides a margin of safety. When the temperature in the exhaust line reaches the desired level, the entire contents of the sterilizing chamber have been exposed to steam, indicating the beginning of exposure time. The time required to reach the sterilizing temperature is referred to as *heat-up time* and is extremely short (about 1 minute) in prevacuum and pulsing types of sterilizers. Large linen packs require both a longer heat-up time and a longer exposure time. They should be saturated for 30 to 45 minutes at 121°C (250°F)

TABLE 31.6   **Safe Storage Times for Sterile Packs**

Wrapper	Closed Cabinet	Open Cabinet
Single-wrapped muslin	1 week	2 days
Double-wrapped muslin	7 weeks	3 weeks
Single-wrapped crepe paper	At least 8 weeks	3 weeks
Single-wrapped muslin sealed in 3-mL polyethylene		At least 9 months
Heat-sealed paper and transparent plastic pouches		At least 1 year

in gravity displacement sterilizers and for 4 minutes at 131°C (270°F) in prevacuum sterilizers.

TECHNICIAN NOTE

The safe minimum standard for autoclave sterilization is 121°C (250°F) for 20 minutes.

Emergency sterilization, also called *flash sterilization*, is usually performed in prevacuum sterilizers. Recommended exposure time is 3 minutes at 131°C (270°F). Unwrapped instruments are placed in a perforated metal tray, covered with a towel for sterilization, and then carried to the operating room with the use of detachable handles.

After sterilization, it is necessary to allow the packs to cool slowly to reduce condensation formation, which occurs because of too rapid exposure to cool air. This is done by cracking open the autoclave door slightly for a minimum of 20 minutes after the sterilization cycle. If the autoclave door is opened wide, cool outside air will condense steam in the materials, making them soggy and promoting corrosion of metal instruments. Paper-wrapped products should not be left in the autoclave longer than 15 to 20 minutes after the door is cracked. If they are left too long, heat will dry the paper, making it brittle and likely to crack and split when handled.

TECHNICIAN NOTE

Packs should be allowed to cool slowly to reduce condensation formation.

Sterilization Quality Control

Certainty that sterilization has been achieved is attained through use of proper technique and dependable sterilization indicators. Indicators should always be checked before materials are used.

Four types of sterilization indicators are used in autoclaves: (1) autoclave tape, (2) fusible melting pellet glass, (3) culture tests, and (4) **chemical sterilization** indicators. These indicators should be used in combination, because no one test alone can provide quality assurance of sterility.

TECHNICIAN NOTE

The four types of sterilization indicators are (1) autoclave tape, (2) melting pellet glass, (3) culture tests, and (4) chemical sterilization indicators.

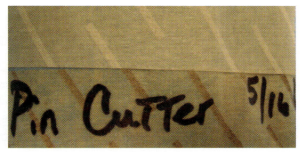

• **Fig. 31.77** Autoclave tape before *(top)* and after *(bottom)* sterilization. Note the darker appearance of the stripes, indicating exposure to steam.

Autoclave tape is useful for identifying packs and articles that have been exposed to steam, but it does not indicate whether proper sterilization requirements (i.e., time, temperature, and steam) have been met (Fig. 31.77). The fusible melting pellet glass indicator indicates that a temperature of approximately 118°C (244°F) was reached but does not show whether proper time or steam saturation was achieved. Culture test indicators are strips that contain a controlled-count spore population of a strain of bacterium (e.g., *Bacillus subtilis* var.). This biological challenge test is useful, because it is the only test that proves microorganisms were killed. Disadvantages of this test include results not being immediately available (results require 1 to 7 days), and does not assess steam penetration. Chemical sterilization indicators are available in many types, which undergo color changes when subjected to saturated steam for adequate periods (Fig. 31.78). Most practices use a combination of autoclave tape on the outside of the pack and a chemical sterilization indicator in the center of the pack to assess sterility.

With prevacuum sterilizers, an air removal test can be run daily to ensure that air is sufficiently removed from the autoclave. With gravity displacement sterilizers, temperature graphs can be kept as a record of autoclave performance. Therefore quality assurance occurs at two levels: to ensure that the pack runs through a sterilization cycle and to ensure that the autoclave system is working properly. Quality control is essential for any surgical practice, because failure to ensure proper sterilization can have far-reaching negative consequences.

Care and Handling of Sterile Packs

Sterile packs should be stored in a dust-free, well-ventilated dry area, away from contaminated equipment. Closed cabinets provide a cleaner storage area than open shelving. Safe pack storage times are listed in Table 31.6. If a pack is dropped, the tape sealing the pack is broken, or the pack wrap becomes wet, punctured, or torn, the pack should be considered contaminated. If there is any doubt as to the sterility of an item, consider it to be nonsterile.

Chemical Methods of Sterilization

Chemical sterilization is performed with certain liquids or gases. Liquid chemicals can be used for instrument sterilization. The agent most used for liquid sterilization is glutaraldehyde. Gas sterilization is used for items that cannot tolerate the high temperatures or steam associated with autoclaving (i.e., power equipment or plastic products). The agents used for gas sterilization are ethylene oxide and hydrogen peroxide gas plasma.

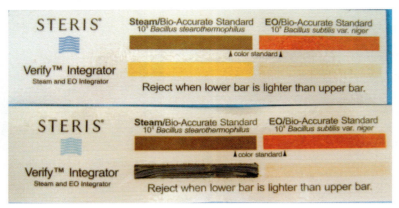

• **Fig. 31.78** Chemical indicator strips to be placed inside packs. This strip can monitor steam (*left*) or gas (*right*) sterilization. The lower strip has been exposed to adequate steam, as indicated by the darkened bar.

Ethylene Oxide

Ethylene oxide is a colorless gas at room temperature. It is flammable, explosive, and toxic. It can cause skin burns, respiratory irritation, vomiting, headaches, and birth defects. Refer to Chapter 4 for a discussion on the occupational hazards associated with ethylene oxide. The manufacturer's guidelines must be followed to prevent injury to hospital personnel and to patients. Ethylene oxide penetrates paper and plastic film packaging. The item to be gas sterilized is wrapped in plastic packaging (polyethylene, poly coated paper, and Mylar) and is sealed with adhesive or heat sealed before sterilization.

Ethylene oxide destroys metabolic pathways within cells by alkylation, and it can kill all microorganisms. Effective sterilization with ethylene oxide is proportionate with the concentration of gas, exposure time, temperature, and relative humidity. Ethylene oxide activity is enhanced by increasing the temperature or the gas concentration. Ethylene oxide sterilizers usually operate at temperatures between 21°C and 60°C (70°F and 140°F). The activity of ethylene oxide approximately doubles with each 10°C increase in temperature. Doubling the ethylene oxide concentration decreases sterilization time by approximately one-half. Moisture is necessary for the lethal action of ethylene oxide, with optimal relative humidity for sterilization with ethylene oxide being 40%, and a minimum of 35% humidity is required for effective sterilization. Exposure time varies from 48 minutes to several hours, but 12 hours of exposure is commonly used for sterilization at room temperature. Specific positioning of packs within the sterilization unit is not as important for ethylene oxide sterilization as it is for steam sterilization. In most ethylene oxide sterilizers, packs are placed inside an air-tight plastic bag, which is then sealed with the vacuum/gas unit in place (Fig. 31.79).

After ethylene oxide sterilization, materials should be quarantined in a well-ventilated area for a minimum of 7 days or in an aerator for 12 to 18 hours. Recommended aeration time varies with the type of material and other factors. Color-coded chemical sterilization indicators are commonly placed within the packs when ethylene oxide sterilization is used. Biological indicators are available for ethylene oxide sterilization and are the only truly reliable test for sterility. Because results are unavailable for several days, biological indicators are most used to evaluate the sterilization system, not individual packs. External tape can be used to indicate exposure to gas sterilization (Fig. 31.80).

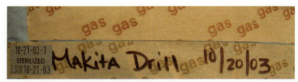

• **Fig. 31.79** Gas tape before (*top*) and after (*bottom*) sterilization. Note the change in color of the word *gas*, indicating exposure.

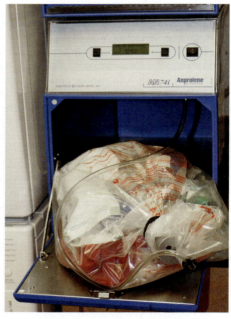

• **Fig. 31.80** An ethylene oxide gas sterilizer.

> **TECHNICIAN NOTE**
>
> Because of the high toxicity of ethylene oxide, it is being replaced by hydrogen peroxide gas plasma sterilization.

Hydrogen Peroxide Gas Plasma

Gas plasma sterilization is often preferred over ethylene oxide because of safety concerns for the environment and personnel. This method inactivates mycobacteria, bacterial spores, fungi, and viruses and can be used to sterilize most items. Items that cannot be sterilized with this method include linen, wood or paper, endoscopes, some plastics, liquids, and tubes or catheters that are long (>12 inches) or of small diameter (<3 mm). Items to be sterilized are wrapped in nonwoven polypropylene fabric or plastic (Tyvek-Mylar) pouches and are placed in the sterilization chamber where a vacuum is drawn, and hydrogen peroxide is injected and vaporized. After 50 minutes, pressure is lowered, and radio waves are applied to the chamber, creating gas plasma, which creates free radicals and kill the microorganisms. The process takes about an hour and requires no aeration. A biological indicator is used to test for sterility, and a chemical indicator is used to show that hydrogen peroxide was present.

Chemical Disinfection

Disinfectants are chemical agents that are applied to inanimate objects to destroy the vegetative form of bacteria but not necessarily the spore forms. Disinfectants classified as "chemical sterilizers" can destroy vegetative bacteria plus spores, tubercle bacilli, and viruses.

Disinfection time is the time required for a particular agent to produce its maximal effect. It is influenced by many factors, including the nature of the material disinfected, the degree of soil and microbial contamination, and the concentration and germicidal potency of the disinfectant.

Antisepsis is prevention of infection by inhibiting the growth of infectious agents and affecting antisepsis in living tissue by antiseptic agents, such as iodine or chlorhexidine.

Antiseptic and Disinfectant Compounds

Chlorhexidine

Chlorhexidine is an **antiseptic** agent that is available in aqueous, tincture, and detergent formulations. It is an effective antimicrobial agent, with activity against bacteria, molds, yeasts, and viruses. Chlorhexidine has a rapid onset and long **residual activity** that is not affected by alcohol, lavage solutions, or organic debris. It has become a popular surgical scrub because of its effectiveness and nonirritating effects on skin. In several human studies, chlorhexidine has been found to be superior to povidone-iodine as a surgical hand scrub. The effectiveness of chlorhexidine and povidone-iodine are similar as choices for surgical scrubs for canine surgery.

> **TECHNICIAN NOTE**
> Chlorhexidine is an effective antimicrobial agent with rapid onset and long residual activity.

As a lavage solution for open wounds, chlorhexidine must be diluted 1:40 with sterile water or saline to produce a 0.05% solution. At this concentration, chlorhexidine has significant antibacterial activity with no cytotoxicity and is superior to povidone-iodine, saline, and other antiseptics. Higher concentrations can cause inflammation and cytotoxicity and are not recommended in open wounds. When chlorhexidine is mixed with electrolyte solutions (e.g., lactated Ringer solution), it will precipitate, but this does not affect antimicrobial activity, and the solution can still be used for wound lavage.

Iodine

Iodine compounds are effective antimicrobial agents with limited activity against bacterial spores. Iodine solutions are used for surgical preparation, topical wound therapy, and joint and body cavity lavage. They are available as aqueous solutions, tinctures, and iodophors. *Aqueous solutions* contain higher levels of free iodine than iodophors and therefore have greater bactericidal activity. However, aqueous solutions are also cytotoxic and cannot be used in living tissue unless they are greatly diluted; they also stain materials and are corrosive to instruments.

Tincture of iodine is a solution of 2% iodine in 50% ethyl alcohol and is intended for use on intact skin. It is not commonly used in veterinary practices.

Iodophors contain iodine complexed with surfactants or polymers so that free iodine is slowly released. Adverse properties of staining and irritation are reduced, and delivery of iodine to tissues is enhanced. *Povidone-iodine*, the most used iodophor, is available in the form of scrubs or solutions. Dilution of stock solutions (common dilutions include 1:10, 1:50, and 1:100) increases bactericidal activity and decreases cytotoxicity. Residual bactericidal activity (i.e., continued action when left on the skin) of povidone-iodine is 4 to 6 hours, but that time is greatly diminished in the presence of organic matter.

Povidone-iodine is one of the most common surgical scrubs and is a relatively safe skin preparation (Table 31.7). It should be noted that alcohol, lavage solutions, or organic debris such as blood will destroy residual bactericidal activity; povidone-iodine can also cause skin irritation or acute contact dermatitis in up to 50% of canine patients, in addition to being a problem for some hospital staff. Rarely, individuals who have repeated contact with iodine scrub solutions may develop systemic iodine toxicity, resulting in metabolic acidosis and thyroid dysfunction.

> **TECHNICIAN NOTE**
> The two most common antiseptic agents used in veterinary medicine are povidone-iodine and chlorhexidine.

Alcohols

Alcohols are used as disinfectant and antiseptic agents and are organic solvents that evaporate rapidly, leaving no residue. Alcohols are bactericidal but ineffective against spores and fungi with no residual effects, but are inhibited by organic debris. Ethyl and isopropyl alcohols are more effective than methyl alcohol as disinfecting agents. Alcohols should never be used in open wounds as they are cytotoxic and can cause pain.

Phenols

Phenols (carbolic acid) have been used historically as both antiseptics and disinfectants but have been routinely replaced by newer, safer, and more effective agents. Hexachlorophene, a skin preparation, was one of the most popular phenols that has been replaced by povidone-iodine and chlorhexidine.

Quaternary Ammonium

Quaternary ammonium compounds are synthetic cationic detergents that act on cell membranes and are effective against bacteria but not against spores and some viruses. These agents are bland and nontoxic, and include benzalkonium chloride, the most commonly used quaternary ammonium compound for disinfection.

Chloride

Antimicrobial chlorine compounds, specifically the hypochlorites, have broad bactericidal and viricidal activity; they can be cytotoxic when improperly used on living tissues. Sodium hypochlorite (bleach) is commonly used as an environmental disinfectant in medical facilities.

TABLE 31.7	Common Antiseptic and Disinfectant Agents			
Examples	**Common Uses**	**Spectrum of Activity**	**Residual Activity**	

Examples	Common Uses	Spectrum of Activity	Residual Activity
Povidone-Iodine Detergent			
Betadine scrub (Purdue Frederick, Stamford, CT) (brown sudsy solution)	Preoperative scrubs	Bacteria, viruses, fungi, protozoa, yeasts	4–6 hours but inactivated by organic debris and alcohol
Povidone-Iodine Solution			
Betadine solution (Purdue Frederick, Stamford, CT) (brown solution)	Preoperative skin preparation; wound lavage when diluted 1:100	Bacteria, viruses, fungi, protozoa, yeasts	4–6 hours but inactivated by organic debris and alcohol
Chlorhexidine Detergent			
Nolvasan scrub (Fort Dodge Laboratories, Madison, NJ) (blue solution), Hibiclens scrub (Stuart Pharmaceuticals, Pasadena, CA) (pink solution)	Preoperative scrubs	Bacteria, viruses, fungi, yeasts	2 days; not inhibited by organic matter or alcohol; less skin irritation
Isopropyl Alcohol-Iodine Povacrylex			
DuraPrep (3M, Maplewood, MN)	Preoperative skin preparation—one step Do not use in open wounds	Bacteria	Rapid onset; at least 1 day residual
Isopropyl Alcohol–Povidone-Iodine			
Prevail-Fx (Cardinal Health, Dublin, OH)	Preoperative skin preparation—one step Do not use in open wounds	Bacteria	Rapid onset; at least 1 day residual
Isopropyl Alcohol–Chlorhexidine Gluconate			
ChloraPrep (Cardinal Health)	Preoperative skin preparation—one step Do not use in open wounds	Bacteria	Rapid onset; 2-day residual; not inhibited by organic matter
Chlorhexidine			
Nolvasan solution (Fort Dodge Laboratories, Madison, NJ) (nonsudsy blue solution)	Preoperative skin preparation; wound lavage when diluted 1:40	Bacteria, viruses, fungi, yeasts	2 days; bactericidal but solution not cytotoxic in open wounds at diluted concentrations
Alcohol, Isopropyl and Ethanol			
Many manufacturers	Surgical preparations; disinfection antisepsis; do not use in open wounds	Bacteria, some fungi	Rapid onset but no residual activity
Ethyl Alcohol–Chlorhexidine Gluconate			
Avagard (3M, Maplewood, MN)	Preoperative hand scrub—waterless	Bacteria	Rapid onset with some residual activity
Phenol, Hexachlorophene			
pHisoHex scrub (Sanofi, Paris, France; Winthrop, Surrey, UK) (white)	Preoperative hand scrub	Bacteria (more effective against gram-positive than gram-negative species)	Up to 2 days
Phenol, Glutaraldehyde			
	Cold sterilization; not intended for living tissues	Bacteria, viruses, fungi, yeasts, spores	None; causes skin irritation

Aldehyde

Formaldehyde and glutaraldehyde are common aldehydes and are both toxic and irritating, restricting them from use on living tissues. They are effective antimicrobial agents but may require several hours of exposure time. Formaldehyde is commonly used in the preservation of tissue specimens. Glutaraldehyde is commonly used for chemical sterilization in cold trays and for endoscopic equipment.

Cold Sterilization

Cold sterilization refers to soaking instruments in disinfecting solutions, such as chlorhexidine or glutaraldehyde. Metal trays used to soak instruments in disinfectant are called *cold trays* (Fig. 31.81). Because sterility cannot be guaranteed, cold-sterilized instruments should be used only for minor procedures (superficial lacerations, dental procedures) or for equipment that cannot tolerate other

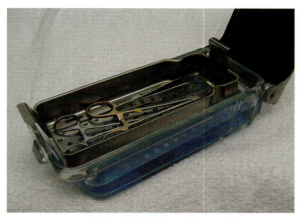

• **Fig. 31.81** A cold sterilization tray. Instruments are kept submerged in disinfectant and are retrieved by lifting the rack.

forms of sterilization, such as endoscopic equipment. Exposure times should exceed 3 hours, with the equipment being rinsed thoroughly before use.

Sterilization of Arthroscopic/Laparoscopic Equipment

All endoscopic cannulas and hand instruments, such as laparoscopic instruments, should be completely disassembled, if possible, before cleaning and disinfecting. Particular attention should be paid to jaws and hinges, because this is where blood and tissue will accumulate. Most hand instruments and ancillary equipment items can be steam sterilized or gas sterilized with ethylene oxide or cold sterilized with a glutaraldehyde-based solution (CidexPlus, Johnson & Johnson Medical Inc., Arlington, TX). Gas sterilization is the preferred method for arthroscopic and laparoscopic equipment, although cold sterilization is an alternative. Cold sterilization, unlike steam and gas sterilization, affords the ability to use equipment more than once in a single day. The arthroscope, laparoscope, light cable, and camera can be gas sterilized or cold sterilized but not steam sterilized.

> **TECHNICIAN NOTE**
>
> The arthroscope or laparoscope, fiberoptic light cable, and the camera should never be steam sterilized.

With cold sterilization, instruments are soaked a minimum of 20 minutes in CidexPlus just before surgery. The electrical plug of the camera cable is not submerged in the cold sterilization solution as this would damage it. The end is draped out over the top of the vessel containing CidexPlus. Use of deep, wide containers will prevent splashes out of the container during transfer of instruments and equipment. The surgeon or assistant double gloves and removes the instruments from the solution. The instruments are then placed in a sterile tray containing sterile water, submerged, gently agitated, individually removed, rinsed with sterile water by a scrub nurse or other assistant, and transferred to the instrument table. The surgeon or assistant removes their outer gloves and dries the instruments. It is important to rinse the instruments thoroughly, because glutaraldehyde, a chemical found in CidexPlus, can cause chemical synovitis and is injurious to chondrocytes.

> **TECHNICIAN NOTE**
>
> Glutaraldehyde is carcinogenic, causes chemical synovitis, and is injurious to chondrocytes.

Operating Room Preparation

Operating room design is important for ease of cleaning. It should be simple and uncluttered, with commonly used equipment and materials readily available. Excess stock should not be stored in the operating room. When additional equipment is needed, it is brought to the operating room by the circulating nurse.

Operating room cleanliness is essential for proper aseptic technique. A routine daily and weekly cleaning schedule should be established to keep the operating room clean and free of contaminants and dust. The surgery table and floor should be cleaned and disinfected immediately after each surgery. A thorough daily cleaning of equipment should be performed at the end of each day, as cleaning creates airborne dust that takes several hours to settle. The operating room is never dry mopped or dusted for this reason as well.

Once a week, the operating room should undergo thorough cleaning from top to bottom (to prevent contamination). Movable equipment is removed and cleaned with a disinfectant solution, sinks and plumbing fixtures should be scrubbed, and buckets and vacuum canisters should be emptied. Permanent structures, such as walls, air vents, window sills, light fixtures, and the surgical table, should be wiped clean. Cabinets should be emptied, wiped, and restocked. All surgical preparation solutions and supplies should be replenished. The operating room floor should be scrubbed and disinfected with a mop, although this may spread dirt and microorganisms throughout the room. To prevent this, the mop head should be laundered daily and not stored in used disinfectant solution. The wet vacuum method, in which the clean floor is flooded with disinfectant solution and then vacuumed, is preferred over mopping.

> **TECHNICIAN NOTE**
>
> Daily and weekly cleaning schedules should be established for the operating room.

Small Animal Patient Preparation

Skin Preparation—Surgical Clip

Generally, small animals are prepared for surgery after being placed under general anesthesia before transport into the operating suite. A #40 clipper blade is used to clip the hair first in the same direction as hair growth and then gently against the direction of hair growth to achieve the closest shave possible. Razors are not recommended, because they have been shown to increase surgical site infections through the creation of microlacerations in the skin. The size of the clip is determined based on the proposed surgical incision. Long hair that is growing near the edge of the clipped area should be trimmed enough that it cannot hang over the site. Larger area preparation may be indicated when large masses are being removed or when skin flaps or grafts are being performed. For abdominal procedures, the clip should extend cranial to the xiphoid, caudal to the pubis, and lateral to the nipples. For orthopedic procedures, the entire circumference of the limb is clipped from the foot up onto the body. In cases where the proposed surgical field includes an open wound and needs to be prepared, sterile,

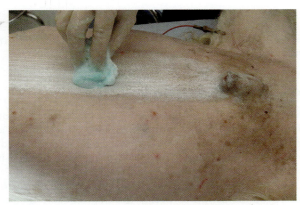

• **Fig. 31.82** Surgical preparation should begin at the proposed incision site and should progress outward, never returning to the proposed incision line with the same gauze sponge. Gloves are worn during the preparation to decrease contamination from the hands.

water-soluble lube should be used to cover the wound before clipping, thereby providing a barrier between exposed tissues and hair clippings. Once the clipping has been performed, the water-soluble lube is rinsed away, and the site is prepared routinely. Particularly contaminated or grossly infected areas should be clipped last. This prevents iatrogenic spread of potentially infectious material across the prepared surgical site. After clipping, a vacuum cleaner may be used to remove loose hairs on the skin prior to the surgical scrub.

Skin Preparation—Surgical Scrub

Initial skin preparation is done in the preparation room to remove gross contamination. Before the abdomen of a male dog is scrubbed, the prepuce should be flushed with an antiseptic solution if it is to be in the surgical field. This is done by using a syringe of preferably 0.05% chlorhexidine gluconate solution to fill the prepuce while sealing the end of the prepuce, allowing the solution to contact the entire area for several seconds. This is done several times before the patient is transferred to the operating room. Examination gloves are worn to decrease contamination from the hands during preparation. The presurgical scrub is performed by alternating an antiseptic scrub (e.g., povidone-iodine or chlorhexidine scrub) with alcohol or sterile saline. (Alcohols or detergents should not be used in open wounds, eyes, or mucous membranes.) Scrubbing should begin over the proposed incision site (Fig. 31.82) and should extend outward in a spiraling pattern, never going back toward the center with the same gauze sponge. The gauze sponge is then replaced with a clean one, and the process is repeated until no dirt is visible on the discarded sponges—often requiring three to five cycles.

The final sterile surgical scrub is performed only after the animal has been properly positioned on the operating table. Sterile gloves should be worn, and sterile gauze sponges are used. If the sterile surgical scrub is performed by alternating povidone-iodine with alcohol, the total contact time of the povidone-iodine should be at least 5 minutes. After the final povidone-iodine scrub, a 10% povidone-iodine solution should be sprayed or painted onto the skin. Alternatively, the sterile surgical scrub may be performed by alternating chlorhexidine gluconate with alcohol or sterile saline. Chlorhexidine or sterile saline may be left on the skin at the end of preparation. Povidone-iodine and chlorhexidine are effective scrub solutions, but the contact time for chlorhexidine is less critical than for povidone-iodine.

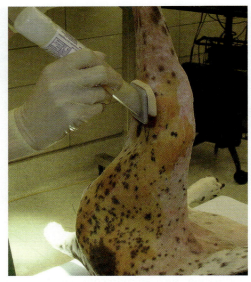

• **Fig. 31.83** Skin preparation using a one-step prep method for sterilization. The applicator sponge is used to paint a single uniform coat of antiseptic solution on the skin, starting at the planned incision site and working outward in a circular pattern. (Photo courtesy Dr. Susanne Lauer.)

> **TECHNICIAN NOTE**
>
> It is recommended that the surgical site be scrubbed and rinsed at least three times. The sterile scrub should provide at least 5 minutes of contact time for povidone-iodine. An antiseptic solution is often applied to the skin after the scrubs.

Several skin preparations are now available that enable a **one-step prep**. The solution is packaged in a small plastic bottle that is directly attached to an applicator sponge. After the bottle is squeezed to activate solution flow, the sponge is used to "paint" a single uniform coat of solution on the skin, starting at the incision site and working outward in a circular motion (Fig. 31.83). The solution requires a 30-second application time and dries within 2 to 3 minutes, so the preparation time is much faster than the traditional alternating scrub described earlier. These one-step solutions contain isopropyl alcohol, which is a broad-spectrum antimicrobial with rapid onset of activity. Other substances in these preparations result in further antimicrobial action and the formation of a film that adheres strongly to the skin and provides long residual activity. These solutions should be applied to clean, dry skin, and the skin should *not* be scrubbed beforehand with povidone-iodine or chlorhexidine gluconate scrub, because residues of these may prevent the one-step preparation from adhering and disinfecting appropriately. These one-step preparations should be applied to intact skin and are not appropriate for use in open wounds or near sensitive eye tissues and other mucous membranes because of the high alcohol content (70%–74%). These preparations enhance the skin adherence to **incise drapes**. The region will be flammable until it dries, so caution should be taken when electrocautery or lasers are used until the scrubbed area is completely dry.

> **TECHNICIAN NOTE**
>
> *One-step preps* are easy to apply, faster than traditional scrubbing techniques, and effective for antimicrobial kill. They have a rapid onset and a long residual effect if used properly.

The surgical preparation technique has many modifications. In preparation for feline orchiectomy (castration), the scrotal hair is plucked, rather than clipped. Feline onychectomy (declawing), tail docking, and dewclaw removal of neonatal puppies are commonly performed without clipping the hair. In these cases, the unclipped surgical site is soaked or gently scrubbed with antiseptic solution and is swabbed with alcohol only before the procedure. When surgery is to be performed on digits or when the entire foot is required to be uncovered in the surgical field, the clipped foot should be soaked in dilute 0.05% chlorhexidine gluconate or 1% povidone-iodine. This can be facilitated by filling an examination glove with the antiseptic of choice and sealing the foot within the glove using surgical tape before the traditional presurgical and sterile scrubs. Bovine and porcine castrations are performed without clipping the hair, and an alcohol or antiseptic wash is used. Equine castrations may be prepared with three thorough washes by using dilute chlorhexidine or povidone-iodine solution.

Small Animal Positioning

Patient positioning for small animal surgical procedures is based on the procedure being performed and surgeon preference. Generally, the position of the animal is described according to the region of the body that contacts the table. For example, right lateral recumbency means the animal is lying on its right side; dorsal recumbency means the animal is on its back; and sternal recumbency means the animal is on its belly. Maintaining patient positioning is facilitated using adjustable surgical tables, portable tabletop V troughs, sand bags, or vacuum-activated "beanbags." It is important to anticipate how the patient should be positioned before patient preparation is begun so that catheters, monitoring equipment, and the like are readily accessible throughout the surgical procedure.

> **TECHNICIAN NOTE**
>
> The dorsal recumbent position is commonly used for abdominal surgical procedures.

In orthopedic surgery, the affected limb is often suspended from an overhead support or intravenous (IV) stand during skin preparation and initial surgical draping. The advantage of hanging the limb is that it allows aseptic preparation of the entire circumference of the limb so that the surgeon can manipulate the entire leg during surgery. To hang the limb, the distal unclipped portion is first covered. Additional strips of tape (stirrups) are extended from the end of the foot. The limb is then suspended by these stirrups, allowing for circumferential scrubbing of the limb (Fig. 31.84A–C) from the foot to the level of the inguinal or axillary region. If the distal aspect of the foot needs to be exposed, the preclipped and soaked foot is hung by using one or two towel clamps affixed to the skin or the cornified portion of the toenail.

Equine Patient Preparation

Patient Positioning

Positioning of the equine patient for surgery can be a highly involved process. It requires more personnel than are needed for small animal patients. In most situations, the minimum number of persons required to position a horse on a surgery table is three. A horse can be transported to the surgical suite and ultimately onto the surgical table in various ways. The method used is determined by the physical setup of the facility. An overhead hoist system greatly facilitates lifting and positioning of the horse onto the surgery table. As an example, the horse is walked into a padded induction room and anesthetized while several persons push the horse against one of the walls (Fig. 31.85A). As the animal becomes anesthetized, supporting personnel aid with its "controlled" collapse to the floor and then roll the animal to lateral recumbency. At some surgical facilities, the horse is positioned in the center of a movable induction room floor that rolls into the surgical suite. Nylon leg bands are strapped to the front and rear feet, and an overhead chain hoist is hooked to the bands (Fig. 31.85B). The horse is raised off the floor and is moved onto the surgical table by way of a rail system on which the chain hoist moves. In other facilities, the horse is lifted off the induction floor with a hoist and is transported into the surgery room. Once the animal is over the surgical table, it is gently lowered onto the table in the desired recumbent position. If the horse is to be in dorsal recumbency, it is maintained in this position with the use of side poles, with pads wedged between the poles and the horse (Fig. 31.85C). Once the horse is positioned on the table, the leg bands are removed, and the limbs may be secured to the positioning poles or table to reduce shifting of the horse during surgery. The chain hoist is rolled away, the rolling floor is pushed back into the padded induction room, and the surgical doors are closed. Large examination gloves or obstetric sleeves are used to cover the feet of the horse to reduce contamination of the surgical suite (Fig. 31.85D). During this preparation time, an anesthesiologist or anesthesiology technician is often placing arterial catheters in the hindlimb or facial artery, attaching the electrocardiography monitor, and attaching fluid lines to the IV catheters.

Skin Preparation

For some equine surgical procedures, particularly *abdominal surgeries*, it is difficult to clip the hair and perform an initial skin preparation before the horse is anesthetized; therefore this must be done in the surgical suite. A wide area of hair at the intended surgical site is removed with electric clippers. The hair is collected with a portable vacuum. The initial skin preparation is performed using chlorhexidine or povidone-iodine scrub with a rinse and wipe-down of alcohol. Next, a sterile skin preparation is performed with sterile gloves and sterile sponges. Three to five surgical scrubs alternating with chlorhexidine and alcohol are performed starting at the center of the surgical site and moving outward in a circular fashion (Fig. 31.85E). Preparation is complete when the sponges no longer visibly collect dirt (Fig. 31.85F). A sterile bowl and gauze sponges are used to complete the final preparation of the surgical site on a horse. The inner sterile wrapping is opened with sterile gloves (Fig. 31.86). After the final preparation has been completed, the surgical area is sprayed with a chlorhexidine solution, which is left on the skin.

Before surgeries are performed on stallions and geldings, the opening of the prepuce sheath is packed with gauze sponges and is sutured closed. This prevents urine and smegma from contaminating the surgical field (Fig. 31.87A and B). With female horses, it is imperative that the mammary area is cleaned thoroughly.

Surgical Team Preparation

Attire

Correct surgical attire and proper scrubbing, gowning, and gloving procedures are important aspects of aseptic technique. Street clothing, especially shoes, are a major source of contamination and should not be worn into the operating room. Ideally, each person should have a pair of shoes designated for use only in the operating

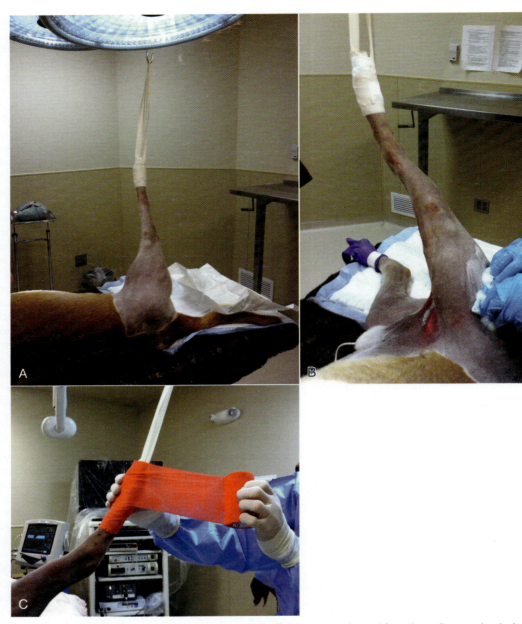

• **Fig. 31.84** Hanging limb surgical preparation. This is commonly used for orthopedic surgeries, including procedures involving the shoulder and hip. (A) Taped stirrups are applied to the distal aspect of a clipped limb. The limb is suspended from the ceiling *(pictured)* or from a fluid stand or pole attached to the surgical table. (B) A surgical scrub is applied to the limb working from the distal aspect of the limb downward in a circular pattern. (C) Using sterile vet wrap, the surgeon covers the distal aspect of the limb before cutting off the taped stirrups. The limb will then be draped and positioned on the surgery table. (Courtesy Veterinary Specialty and Emergency Center, Langhorne, PA.)

room. Disposable shoe covers may be worn in the operating room and discarded upon leaving the room. Lint-free **scrub suits** should be worn in the operating room with the shirt tucked into the pants, reducing the amount of skin debris dispersed into the room.

During surgery, surgical caps, masks, and booties are worn by all persons in the room. The surgical cap covers the hair to reduce airborne contamination. Different types of surgical head covers are available to cover short hair, long hair, or beards (Fig. 31.88A–C). The mask protects the wound from saliva droplets, primarily by redirecting airflow out the sides of the mask and by reducing aerosol contaminants potentially inhaled. It is important for personnel

not to face away from the patient when talking, coughing, or sneezing, because this allows debris to flow from the side of the mask potentially into the surgical field. Plastic face shields are also effective to prevent inhalation of aerosolized particles. Masks are effective for relatively short periods and should be changed between procedures.

TECHNICIAN NOTE

Anyone entering the operating room should wear a cap, mask, booties, and scrub suit.

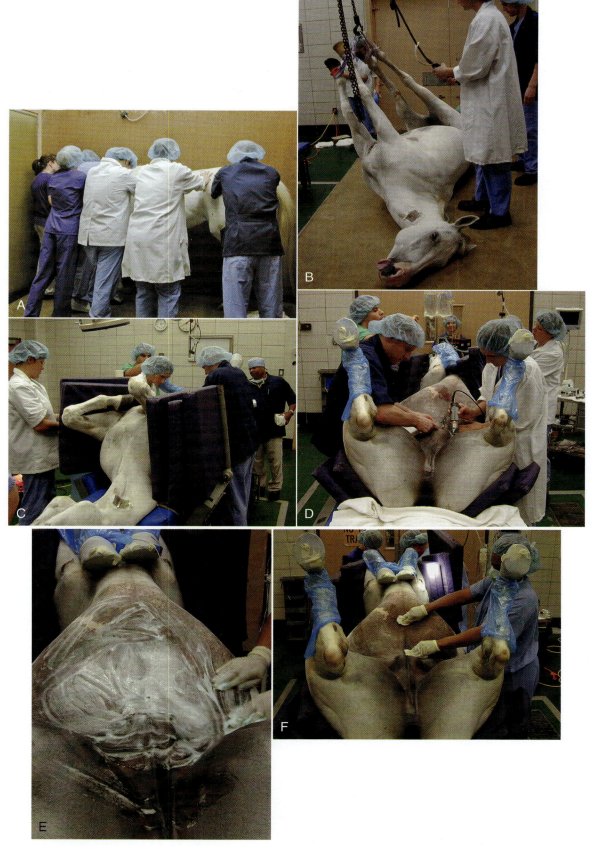

• **Fig. 31.85** (A) During the induction of anesthesia, the horse is positioned against the wall of the induction room by several assistants. As the horse becomes anesthetized, the assistants will keep the horse pressed to the wall as it slides to the floor. (B) Nylon webbing leg bands are strapped to the horse's limbs at the pastern using double half-hitch loops. The leg bands are then attached to a chain hoist to transport the horse to the surgery table. (C) The horse is maintained in dorsal recumbency for surgery using side poles with pads wedged between the poles and the horse. (D) Large examination gloves or obstetric sleeves are used to cover the feet of the horse to reduce contamination of the surgical suite. A wide area of hair is removed with electric clippers, and a surgical scrub of the area is subsequently performed. (E) Three to five surgical scrubs are performed using chlorhexidine. (F) The surgical area is rinsed with alcohol between scrubs.

Hand Scrub

The purpose of the surgical hand scrub is to clean and remove debris and excessive oils from all skin surfaces distal to the surgeon's or surgical assistant's elbows. Scrubbing should be performed before each procedure and followed by gowning and gloving. The surgical scrub provides protection from spreading microorganisms should a breach in sterile technique occur (e.g., torn glove, poor gowning and gloving technique). This scrub is done, because gloves can contain microscopic perforations within the latex and should not be relied upon as the sole mechanism of preventing iatrogenic surgical site contamination from a surgeon's or assistant's hands.

Before the surgical scrub, a surgical cap and mask should be donned, all jewelry removed, and each fingernail cleaned by using a nail pick (included with individually wrapped scrub sponges). The gown pack and gloves should be opened before scrubbing to facilitate gowning and gloving once the surgical scrub has been performed (Fig. 31.89A and B). During and after the surgical scrub, the hands should always be held above the level of the elbows so that any water or soap runs down the arm from "sterile to not sterile." Surgical scrub brushes are commonly purchased as individual, prepackaged, antiseptic-soaked brushes. Reusable scrub brushes, while still available, are somewhat outdated due to the convenience of prepackaged brushes.

The surgical scrub begins distally at the fingers. All four sides of each finger should be scrubbed in a thorough and consistent manner (Fig. 31.90A). The back, both sides, and the palm of the hand are then scrubbed. Next, the wrist and forearm are scrubbed, working toward the elbow to complete the scrub (Fig. 31.90B). After completion of the scrub, the hands are rinsed in water so that the water flows from the fingers to the elbow (e.g., from clean to dirty) (Fig. 31.90C and D).

The two basic methods of surgical scrubs are *counted brush strokes* and *timed*. The counted brush strokes method is performed by counting the number of brush strokes used on each skin surface. Ten to 25 brush strokes are made on each surface of the fingers, hands, and arms before rinsing. This is done four times. The timed method is used more commonly and is done by repeatedly scrubbing and rinsing for a set period.

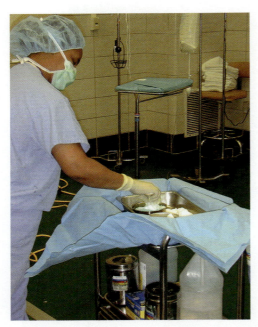

• **Fig. 31.86** A sterile bowl and gauze sponges are used for the final preparation of the surgical site on a horse. The inner sterile wrapping is opened with sterile gloves.

TECHNICIAN NOTE

The surgical hand scrub requires that all surfaces of the fingers, hand, and forearm be scrubbed. Skin-to-soap contact time should last 5 minutes.

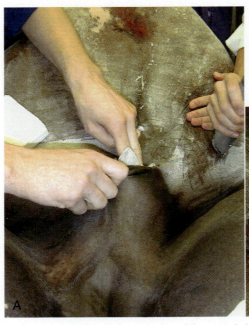
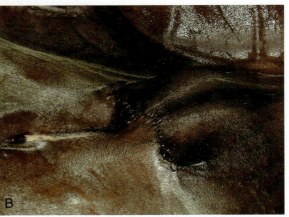

• **Fig. 31.87** Surgical preparation of the ventral abdomen of a horse. (A) During the initial preparation of the ventral abdomen of a horse for surgery, the opening of the male's sheath (gelding or stallion) is packed with gauze sponges. (B) It is sutured closed to prevent urine and smegma from contaminating the surgical field.

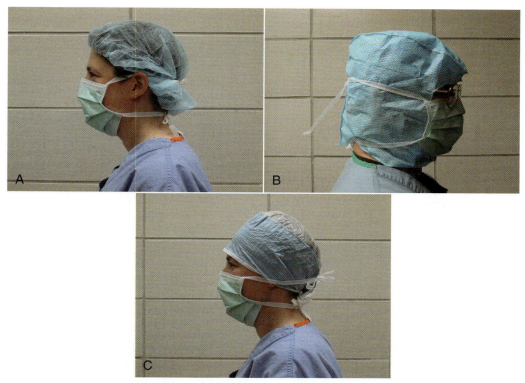

• **Fig. 31.88** Surgical caps and masks. (A) A bouffant head cover is used to cover long or short hair. (B) Hoods are available for individuals with sideburns or beards. (C) A cap may be suitable for covering short hair.

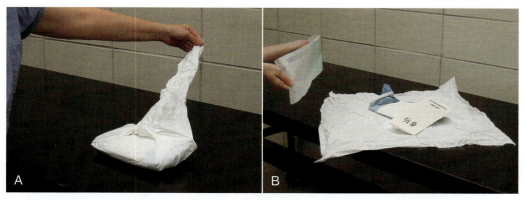

• **Fig. 31.89** An open gown pack. (A) The gown pack may be opened before scrubbing so that the hand towel is available. When opening a pack, always open the flap away from you first. Keep the arm off to the side, not directly over the pack. Open the other three sides, touching only the corners of the wrap on the outside surface. (B) The sterile gloves are opened onto the gown. With the package positioned at the edge of the sterile field, it is opened symmetrically. This gives the contents enough forward momentum to fall onto the sterile field without the need for the clinician to reach over it.

Waterless hand antiseptics can be considered a supplement to traditional scrubbing. These newer alcohol- and chlorhexidine-based antiseptics have been shown to be at least as effective, if not more effective, in reducing skin bacterial numbers. The alcohol solution provides rapid bactericidal and other antimicrobial functions. Similar to traditional surgical scrubbing, hands must be clean and free of debris. In general, it is recommended that a traditional scrub be performed to remove any debris; waterless hand antiseptics can be used as a supplement throughout the day as hands remain clean. The solution is rubbed briskly and evenly over one hand and forearm; a second scrub is applied to the other hand and forearm. A final application is applied to both hands and is allowed to air dry. Waterless antiseptics are fast, effective, easy to apply, and nonirritating.

TECHNICIAN NOTE

Waterless hand antiseptics are easy to apply and are a supplement to traditional hand-scrubbing techniques, effective against microorganisms, and nonirritating to the skin. They should not replace surgical hand scrubbing.

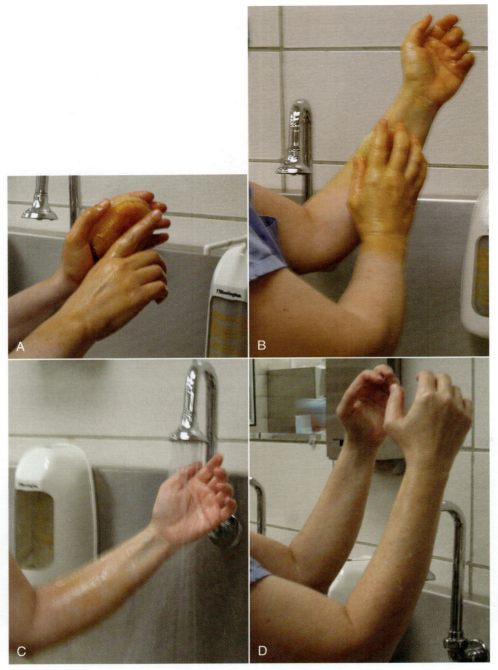

• **Fig. 31.90** Surgical hand scrub. (A) Scrub each surface of each finger, the palm, back, and sides of the hand. (B) Scrub each side of the forearm. (C) Rinse the hands and forearms after scrubbing. The hands are always kept above the elbows. (D) Let the excess water drip off the elbows (running from sterile to nonsterile areas).

Gowning and Gloving

The hands and arms are thoroughly dried with a sterile towel (Fig. 31.91A–D) before gowning and gloving. Gowning is performed first. The folded gown is grasped at the upside surface, and sleeve openings are identified (Fig. 31.92A and B). While the gown is held in this region, it is allowed to unfold without touching any nonsterile surfaces (Fig. 31.92C). The arms are then inserted into each sleeve, and gowning is completed with the help of a nonsterile assistant by tying or fastening the gown around the surgeon's or surgical assistant's neck and waist without touching the front of the gown (Fig. 31.92D–G).

The two methods used for gloving oneself are **closed gloving** and **open gloving**. The risk for contamination is minimized with closed gloving (Fig. 31.93A–E), because the outside of the gloves never contacts the skin. The risk for contamination is much higher during open gloving (Fig. 31.94A–D), and it is generally reserved for minor procedures for which a gown is not worn (e.g., sterile patient scrub, urinary catheterization). If it is necessary to replace

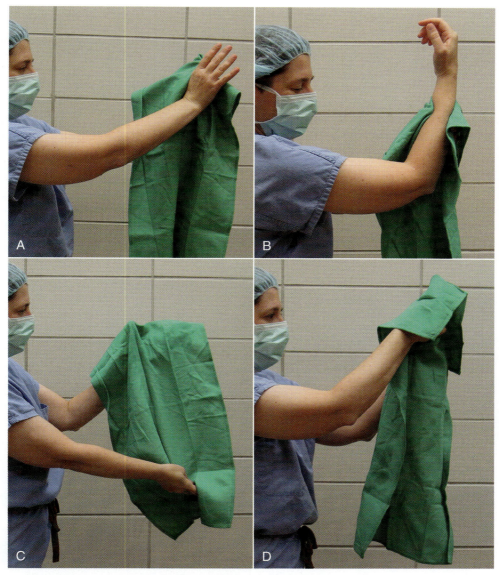

• **Fig. 31.91** Towel drying. (A) One hand is dried first, with the towel held away from the body. (B) Move the towel down to dry the arm, using only the top end of the towel. (C) The dry hand now grasps the dry end of the towel. (D) The other hand and arm are dried. Note that the hands do not switch sides of the towel during the process.

gloves during surgery, the surgeon should allow a nonsterile assistant to grasp the end of the old glove that covers the sleeve and pull both (without touching the sleeve) so that the gown sleeve covers the hands. (Fig. 31.95A and B). The surgeon may then don new gloves using the closed gloving method or by **assisted gloving** (Fig. 31.96A and B).

Maintaining Sterility

It is important for all members of the surgical team to be conscientious about sterility, even if they are not "scrubbed in" (i.e., gowned and gloved). Nonsterile personnel should touch only nonsterile items or areas and should not lean over or reach across sterile fields. Those who are scrubbed in should touch only sterile items or areas and should always face the sterile field, which is limited to the table in front of them. Only sterile items can be placed on a sterile field. If anyone on the surgical team notices a potential source of contamination or "break" in sterile technique, this should be mentioned immediately and steps taken to reduce the risk for further contamination.

Scrubbed-in Personnel

The sterile area on a person is the front of the gown, from just below the shoulders (the neckline is not sterile) to the waist or the level of the table. The gown sleeves are also considered to be sterile. Note that the back of a gowned person is nonsterile, so it should not be turned to face any sterile field, and people attempting to pass one another in the operating room should do so "back-to-back." Gloved hands may be rested on a sterile drape or clasped (prayer like) in front of the body in the zone between the shoulders and the waist. The arms should not be folded across the chest, because the armpit region is nonsterile.

> **TECHNICIAN NOTE**
>
> After gowning and gloving, the sterile region includes the gown sleeves and the front of the gown between the waist and just below the shoulders but not the gown back.

The Patient

Sterile surgical drapes are used to maintain a sterile field around the surgical site. Draping is performed by personnel who have scrubbed in. First, four small towels (cloth or paper) are placed to surround the area where the surgical incision will be made. These drapes, which are called *quarter drapes*, are secured to the skin using towel clamps. *Towel clamps* are forceps used to attach towels and drapes to the patient. These forceps have pointed tips that curve and join like ice tongs and are available in different sizes. *Backhaus towel clamps* and *Roeder towel clamps* are two common designs. The Roeder towel clamp has a metal bead or ball stop attached to the jaws that prevents deep tissue penetration and prevents the towel from slipping toward the box lock of the forceps. Alternatively, a "fenestrated" drape may be placed over the proposed incision site.

During draping procedure, one must avoid brushing the front of the surgical gown against the surgical table. A large drape may be placed over the animal, the surgical table, and the instrument stand to provide one continuous sterile field. Cloth drapes with an opening, or *fenestration*, may be positioned over the surgical site. If a disposable paper drape is used, an appropriately sized

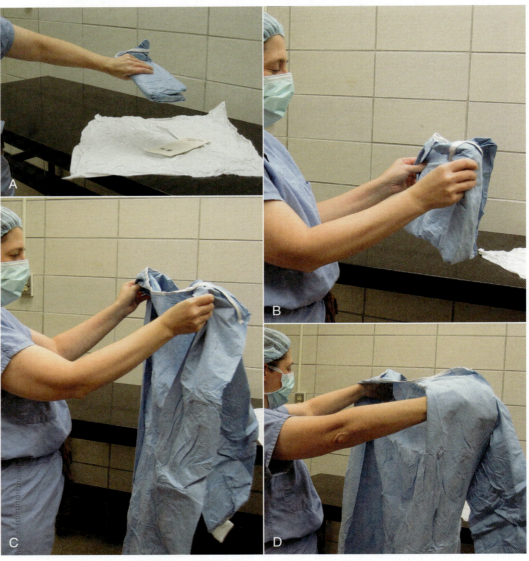

• **Fig. 31.92** Gowning. (A) The gown is picked up in its folded state. This same technique is used when picking up sterile folded towels or drapes. This reduces the risk of accidental contamination. (B) Move to a spacious area to reduce the risk for contamination. (C) The gown is held away from the body by the inside shoulder seams and is allowed to unfold. (D) The arms are slid into the sleeves, but the hands should not extend through the cuff openings.

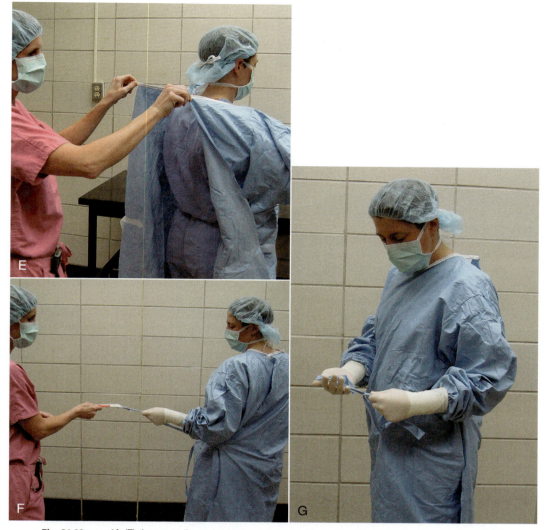

• **Fig. 31.92, cont'd** (E) A nonsterile assistant pulls the gown over the shoulders and ties the back of the gown at the neck and waist. (F) If the gown has a wraparound back, the last tie is performed after the surgeon has gloved. The surgeon hands the sterile tag to a nonsterile assistant. The assistant holds the end of the tag while the surgeon turns around, causing the gown to cover the surgeon's back. The surgeon takes the gown tie and pulls, releasing it from the tag that is still in the assistant's hand. (G) The final tie is done in front by the surgeon.

hole may be cut after the drape has been placed. Because skin preparations do not sterilize but only disinfect the skin, additional incisional drapes or plastic incise drapes may be used to provide a sterile surface at the start of surgery. Incisional drapes are attached at the incision edges using *Michel clips* (Fig. 31.97), scalp clamps, or towel clamps. Such incisional drapes have largely been replaced by translucent, self-adhesive coverings. These newer skin coverings are used to completely cover any visible skin after the barrier drapes have been applied before the skin incision is made. Additionally, incise drapes are often impregnated with an antiseptic (e.g., Ioban; 3M Products, St. Paul, MN). The surgeon can cut through the incise drape when making the skin incision.

If a limb has been suspended in preparation for an orthopedic procedure (as described under "Patient Positioning"), quarter drapes are placed on the body at the base of the limb. The nonscrubbed distal portion of the limb is then covered first with an impermeable sterile material (e.g., aluminum foil), followed by covering with a sterile towel or adhesive material (e.g.,

gas-sterilized Vetrap [3M Products, St. Paul, MN]). During this process, a nonsterile assistant cuts the stirrups, allowing complete covering of the distal limb with the impermeable sterile material and wrap. A sterile cotton stockinette or adhesive incise drape may be used to cover the entire limb. Finally, the limb is passed through a hole in the large sterile drape that covers the entire animal and surgical field.

After draping is completed, sterile instrument packs, light handles, and other sterile equipment may be opened. Draped tables

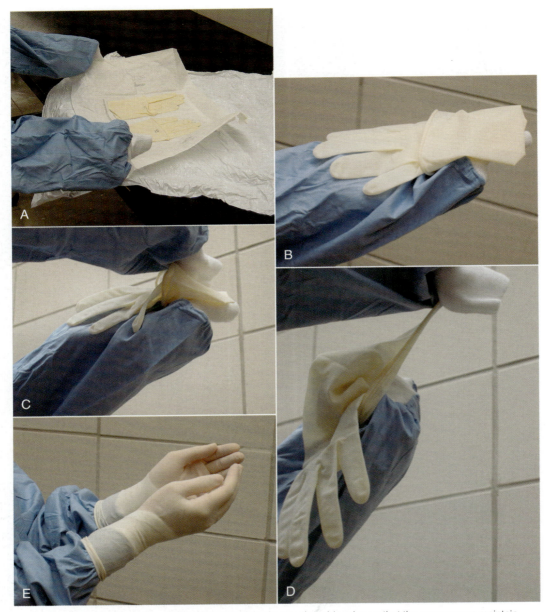

• **Fig. 31.93** Closed gloving. (A) The sterile pack is close to the table edge so that the surgeon can maintain some distance from the table to prevent contaminating the sterile gown. The sterile paper wrap containing the gloves is unfolded, and one glove is picked up. It is easiest for most people to glove their nondominant hand first. The fingers must be kept inside the sleeves at all times during closed gloving. (B) The glove is laid on the hand to be gloved, with the glove fingers pointing toward the elbow and the glove thumb lying against the sleeve. The edge of the glove cuff is grasped through the gown sleeve. (C) The opposite side of the cuff is grasped in the other hand. (D, E) The glove is pulled over the hand. Now the gown and the glove cuff may be grasped together to pull the glove completely onto the hand.

and instrument trays are regarded as "sterile" only on the top of the draped surface, so if part of a sterile item slips below the level of the tabletop, it is considered contaminated and should no longer be touched by the surgeons.

Opening Sterile Items

Nonsterile assistants must open all sterile items for the surgeon. Nonsterile assistants can touch only the outside of sterile packs and should never reach over a sterile field. Large or heavy packs, such as an instrument pack, may be set on a table to be opened.

The four folded edges of the outer wrap are opened one at a time, and the hand and arm are never extended over the top of the pack, in the same fashion that a sterile gown is opened. If the pack can be placed on a *Mayo instrument stand*, this can be accomplished by moving around the stand and pulling each fold away from the center. The inner wrap may be opened by the surgeon or a nonsterile assistant. Once the instrument tray is exposed, the surgeon can pick it up and set it on the draped instrument stand. The outer and inner wraps are discarded as waste by dropping onto the floor for retrieval by nonscrubbed personnel when possible.

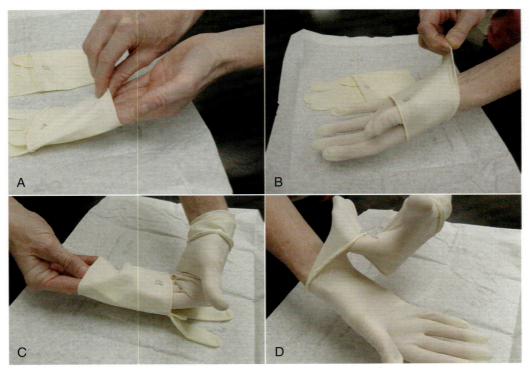

• **Fig. 31.94** Open gloving. (A) The glove pack is opened near the edge of a table. The hand is inserted into the glove opening, taking care not to touch the outside of the glove. The inside of the glove will not be sterile, so the cuff may be touched. (B) The glove is pulled on by grasping the cuff fold with the other hand. The cuff will still be folded, but the glove is on well enough to allow use of the hand. (C) The gloved hand is placed between the cuff and the palm of the glove to assist gloving of the other hand. This protects the gloved hand from accidental contamination on the arm. (D) The cuff can be unfolded. Now adjustments can be made to both gloves, taking care to touch only the sterile areas of the gloves.

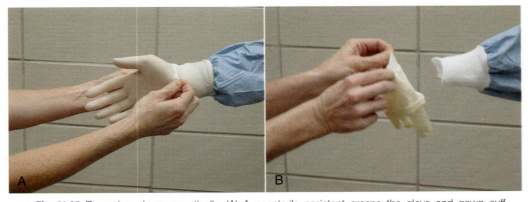

• **Fig. 31.95** Removing gloves aseptically. (A) A nonsterile assistant grasps the glove and gown cuff together, without touching the gown sleeve. (B) As the glove is removed, the gown is pulled over the fingers. The gown cuff is considered contaminated. The surgeon can reglove, taking care not to contaminate anything with the gown cuff. It may be preferable to perform an assisted gloving, as shown in Fig. 31.96.

A smaller wrapped pack may be opened while it is held in one hand (Fig. 31.98A and B). As each corner of the pack is unfolded, it is grasped by the hand that is holding the pack. This prevents the edges of the wrap from contaminating the pack's contents. The exposed item may be grasped by the surgeon or carefully set on the sterile field with wrappings discarded.

To open a plastic or paper pouch, scalpel blade, or suture package, the edges of the wrapper should be peeled back slowly and symmetrically, keeping the package opening directed away from the body.

Some items may be dropped onto the sterile field; care must be taken not to lean or reach across the sterile field. If the item is small or awkward to handle, the surgeon can grasp it with a gloved hand or a sterile instrument. The item should not be allowed to touch the peeled edges of the pouch, because the edges are considered contaminated.

TECHNICIAN NOTE

While opening a pack, make sure that the opening faces away from you.

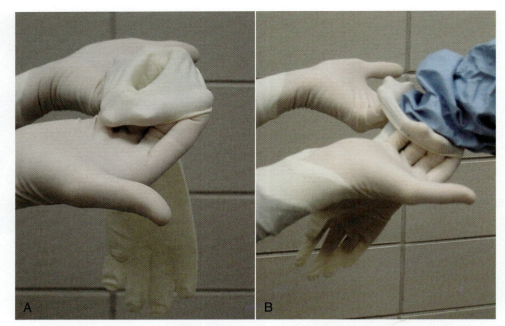

• **Fig. 31.96** Assisted gloving. (A) A sterile assistant picks up the appropriate sterile glove, holding it so the location of the glove thumb is apparent. The assistant hooks their fingers under the glove cuff and pulls to make the glove opening as large as possible. (B) The surgeon slides their hand into the glove while the assistant pulls the glove cuff up to be sure it covers the gown cuff before releasing.

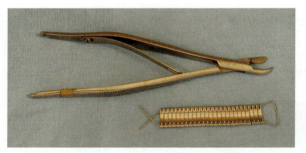

• **Fig. 31.97** Michel skin clips and Michel clip forceps.

Sterile saline may be poured into the sterile saline bowl. To avoid reaching over the sterile field with the saline container or spilling onto the draped surface, the surgeon may hold the bowl away from the instrument tray or position it on the tray at the edge of the sterile field. The lip of the saline container should be a few inches above the rim of the bowl to reduce the risk of touching it but not so high that the saline splashes as it is poured. If drapes or gowns (especially those made of cloth) become wet with saline or blood, they may no longer be impermeable to bacteria and are said to have **strike-through**. If this occurs, the instruments in contact with the region of strike-through should no longer be considered sterile and should be removed from the surgical field and replaced with sterile ones.

TECHNICIAN NOTE

If drapes or gowns (especially those made of cloth) become wet with saline or blood, they may no longer be impermeable to bacteria and are said to have *strike-through*. They should be removed and replaced.

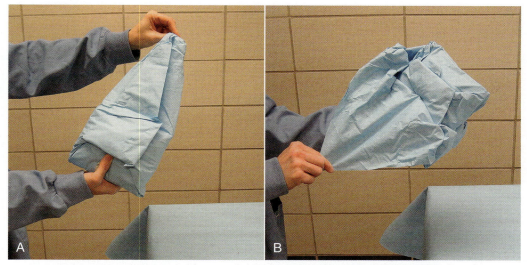

• **Fig. 31.98** Opening a sterile pack that can be held in one hand. (A) Open the first flap away from you. (B) As each flap is opened, it is held together with the hand holding the pack. After the fourth flap is pulled back and secured, the inner package may be grasped by the surgeon. Move the wrap down and toward you as the surgeon lifts the contents up and toward themselves. Alternatively, the package may be set on a sterile field near its edge to avoid reaching over the field.

Acknowledgments

The authors and publisher wish to acknowledge the contribution of James A. Perry, William T. N. Culp, and Daniel J. Burba to previous editions of this chapter.

Recommended Readings

Bartels KE. Lasers in veterinary medicine—where have we gone, and where are we going?. In: Bartels KE, ed. *The Veterinary Clinic of North America, Small Animal Practice*. Philadelphia, PA: Saunders; 2002.

Beale BS, Hulse DA, Schulz KS, et al. *Small Animal Arthroscopy*. St. Louis, MO: Saunders; 2003.

Chamness CJ. Nondisposable instrumentation for equine laparoscopy. In: Fischer JrAT, ed. *Equine Diagnostic Surgical Laparoscopy*. Philadelphia, PA: Saunders; 2002.

Cockshutt J. Principles of surgical asepsis. In: Slatter D, ed. *Textbook of Small Animal Surgery*. 3rd ed. St. Louis, MO: Saunders; 2003.

Fry TR. Laser safety. In: Bartels KE, ed. *The Veterinary Clinic of North America, Small Animal Practice*. Philadelphia, PA: Saunders; 2002.

Hobson HP. Surgical facilities and equipment. In: Slatter D, ed. *Textbook of Small Animal Surgery*. 3rd ed. St. Louis, MO: Saunders; 1993.

Kronberger C. The veterinary technician's role in laser surgery. In: Bartels KE, ed. *The Veterinary Clinic of North America, Small Animal Practice*. Philadelphia, PA: Saunders; 2002.

Lemarie RJ, Hosgood G. Antiseptics and disinfectants in small animal practice. *Compend Cont Educ Pract Vet*. 1996;17:1339.

McIlwraith CW, Nixon AJ, Wright IM, et al. *Diagnostic and Surgical Arthroscopy In The Horse*. 4th ed. Philadelphia, PA: Mosby; 2015.

Mitchell SL, Berg J. Sterilization. In: Slatter D, ed. *Textbook of Small Animal Surgery*. 3rd ed. Philadelphia, PA: Saunders; 2003.

Nieves MA, Wagner SD. Surgical instruments. In: Slatter D, ed. *Textbook of Small Animal Surgery*. 3rd ed. Philadelphia, PA: Saunders; 2003.

Pavletic MM. Surgical stapling. *Vet Clin North Am*. 1994;24:225.

Shmon C. Assessment and preparation of the surgical patient and the operating team. In: Slatter D, ed. *Textbook of Small Animal Surgery*. 3rd ed. Philadelphia, PA: WB Saunders; 2003.

Sonsthagen TF. *Veterinary Instruments and Equipment: A Pocket Guide*. 3rd ed. St. Louis, MO: Mosby; 2014.

Tear M. *Small Animal Surgical Nursing*. 3rd ed. St. Louis, MO: Mosby; 2017.

32

Surgical Assistance and Suture Material

NANETTE WALKER SMITH

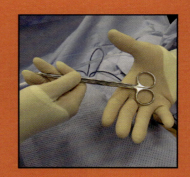

CHAPTER OUTLINE

LEARNING OBJECTIVES

When you have completed this chapter, you will be able to:

1. Pronounce, define, and spell all key terms in this chapter.
2. Describe the role of the veterinary technician in surgical assistance for large and small animal patients.
3. Explain preoperative preparation as it applies to the small animal surgical patient, including review of clipping and surgical scrub techniques with respect to patient positioning, and discuss considerations for operating room (OR) sterility and instrument table organization.
4. Discuss intraoperative duties of the surgical assistant, including surgical lighting, instruments, hemostasis, suture cutting, lavage and suction, camera manipulation, tissue manipulation, retraction, and organ positioning.
5. Describe the most common temporary and permanent forms of surgical implants and their uses.
6. Discuss the considerations involved in choosing a type of suture material, and list and describe commonly used suture materials and needles and their application.
7. Describe the role of the surgical assistant in the postoperative management of patients.
8. Discuss surgical assisting in equine patients, including draping techniques, instrument setup, tissue handling, and common types of suture materials.

KEY TERMS

Fenestrated
Impervious
Ingesta
Laparotomy
Monofilament

Multifilament
Orthopedic
Retroperitoneal
Swaged

Introduction

Small and large animal patients are anesthetized, positioned on the operating table, and prepared for surgery by veterinary technicians who serve as anesthetist, OR technician, and surgical assistant. In some practices, a single veterinary technician may juggle all three of these roles; at other practices, specialized veterinary technicians may individually carry out the various roles.

Surgical outcomes are improved by ensuring that effective sterile techniques and proper OR conduct are carried out before, during, and after each surgical procedure. This chapter focuses on the role of surgical technicians and assistants, and presents surgery-specific techniques and duties, correct instrument handling, and suture material types and characteristics.

Refer to Chapter 31 for information about surgical instrumentation and aseptic preparation of the patient.

General Concepts in Veterinary Surgical Assisting

Role of the Surgical Assistant

Veterinary technicians who serve as surgical assistants must possess a thorough understanding of preoperative patient preparation, positioning, intraoperative techniques, instrumentation, instrument handling, and postoperative wound and patient care. The surgical assistant collaborates with the surgeon for the procedure details specific for the patient. The surgical assistant then ensures that the patient is properly clipped, scrubbed, and positioned, and confirms the presence of equipment needed with the veterinary OR technician. The OR technician prepares the required instruments, tools, and materials on the surgical instrument tables so they are available for quick and easy access throughout the surgical procedure.

Preoperative Preparation

Preparation of the Surgical Patient

Assessment of Clipping and Surgical Scrub

Instructions for clipping hair from the incision site, performing an initial scrub, and transporting the patient to the OR from the prep area are presented in Chapters 31 and 32. The surgical assistant is responsible for assessing the surgical site for proper dimensions and sufficient hair removal to prevent contamination of the surgical site before completion of surgical preparation and moving the patient to the OR. Aseptic preparation of the distal limb is particularly important for hanging limb positioning procedures as the distal limb will be located within the sterile field.

Positioning and Draping

The surgical patient is positioned by the OR technician on the basis of several factors:
1. The particular surgery to be performed
2. The number of surgeries to be performed on the patient
3. The surgical approach
4. The draping technique for that procedure

As the patient is positioned, a warming blanket may be placed along with an electrocautery plate, if required for the procedure. The warming blanket must be located away from the surgical site

and should only be turned on once the patient has been properly draped to prevent contamination of the surgical field. Electrocautery plates should always be in direct contact with the patient. Long and/or thick haircoats can impair the conductivity of the unit and decrease its effectiveness (Fig. 32.1).

> **TECHNICIAN NOTE**
>
> Assess the location of the warming blanket and the electrocautery plate before draping to prevent surgical site contamination.

Patients can be maintained in the desired position by a variety of means. Tape can be passed over the patient and secured to the table, and/or sandbags can be used to prevent movement of the patient. Vacuum bags are an alternative to tape and sandbags (Fig. 32.2). These bags are generally placed inflated under the patient and the patient is held in position by assistants while air is evacuated from the bag. When air has been sufficiently removed from the bag, it maintains rigid positioning of the patient. Care should be taken to minimize abnormal positioning or overdistention of limbs for extended periods during a surgical procedure.

Drapes are typically wrapped and sterilized in a package that can be placed on an instrument table and opened at the onset of surgery (Fig. 32.3). Once surgical site preparation is finished and the surgeon and the surgical assistant are fully gowned and gloved, the patient is draped by the surgeon and the surgical assistant, taking care to establish a sterile surgical field. Because skin cannot be sterilized, it is considered nonsterile, even after surgical scrubbing. Placement of sterile surgical drapes increases asepsis during surgery and diminishes postoperative complications from infection by establishing an **impervious** barrier, decreasing the possibility of contact by sterile instruments and gloved hands with nonsterile skin and hair.

Many types of drapes are available, and their specific purpose and need determination should be understood. Initially, at a minimum, quarter drapes, towel clamps, and a single large surgical drape capable of covering the patient and the entire surgery table should be available to the surgical team (Fig. 32.4).

The quarter drapes are used to create a sterile surgical field. Each drape laid down is secured with a Backhaus towel clamp. The appropriate quarter drape placement technique to prevent contamination is as follows:

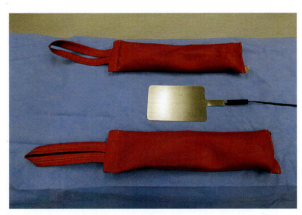

• **Fig. 32.1** The surgery table has been prepared with the cautery plate in the center of the table. Sandbags are used to stabilize the patient in the proper position.

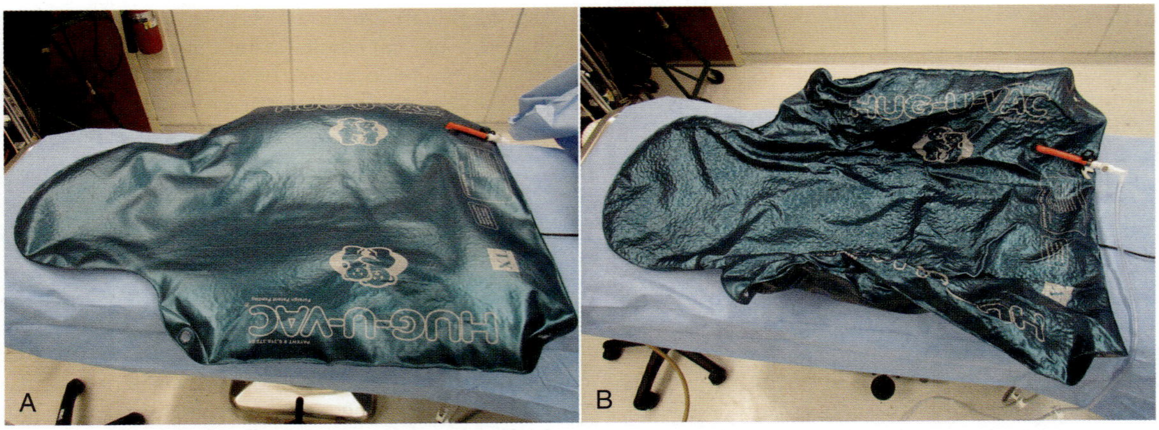

• **Fig. 32.2** (A) A vacuum bag is present on the table. The patient will be placed on the bag and held in position by OR technicians; air will be evacuated from the bag by attaching suction tubing to the bag. (B) This bag was held in position and the air was evacuated. The bag is maintained in position after removal of the air.

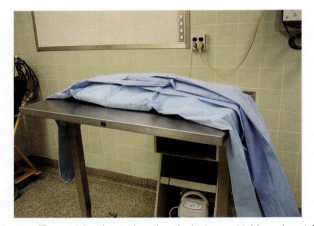

• **Fig. 32.3** The pack has been placed on the instrument table and contains the drapes and instrumentation needed by the surgeon and the surgical assistant to drape at the surgical site.

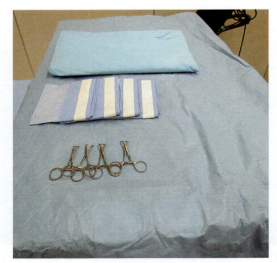

• **Fig. 32.4** The necessary equipment for draping (quarter drapes, towel clamps, and a large surgical drape) is located on the instrument table.

1. The surgical assistant grasps the quarter drape, steps away from the instrument table, and gently opens it to its fullest length and width. The top edge of the drape is folded under and away from the surgical assistant. The corners of the drape are grasped by extended fingers and rolled outward so that the drape wraps around the palms and fingers to protect the drape from contamination (Fig. 32.5A and B). The drape is then floated above the patient before it is placed so that it is not dragged along the contaminated body of the patient. The assistant should maintain a safe distance from the patient to prevent contamination of the assistant's gown.

2. The folded layer of quarter drape is positioned a few centimeters from the proposed incision site. Once placed, the drape should never be advanced toward the proposed incision to avoid dragging contaminants toward the incision site. The double layer of drape provides extra protection in the surgical region, where it can absorb fluids, such as blood and sterile saline lavages.

3. Once positioned, the four quarter drapes are secured to the patient and to each other with Backhaus towel clamps (Fig. 32.6). The towel clamp tips are considered nonsterile once they perforate skin and should not be moved once placed. If they must be removed, they should be handed off to a nonsterile technician and a new, sterile clamp should be used.

4. Once quarter drapes are secured, a large final drape is placed over the patient, the surgical table, and the instrument table; final draping generally requires two people to ensure sterility and coverage (Fig. 32.7A–D). Sterile instrument packs can now be opened and instruments organized on the table. A **fenestrated** surgical drape (see Fig. 32.7D) or disposable nonfenestrated (solid) drape may be chosen; the surgeon will use a scissors to make a fenestration in the solid drape over the surgical site.

Some surgeons elect to attach additional drapes or sterile towels to an incision using Michel clips, which prevent skin from being exposed and provide an additional layer of protection against surgical site infection. Drapes that have a sticky surface, such as Ioban (3M, St. Paul, MN), can also be used after placement of surgical drapes. These sticky drapes allow the entire skin surface to be covered. An incision can be made directly through the translucent Ioban material. A stockinette may be used to cover the distal extremity, allowing the surgical team to maneuver the limb during the procedure without touching the skin (Fig. 32.8A and B).

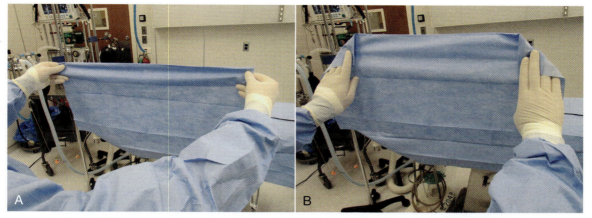

• **Fig. 32.5** The proper technique for grasping and placing the quarter drapes. (A) The quarter drape has been opened to maximum width and a fold has been maintained in the region closest to the incision. (B) The assistant's fingers are wrapped around the end of the drape that is going to be placed down. The palms are now facing the patient, but the hands are protected by the drape from touching the contaminated skin of the patient.

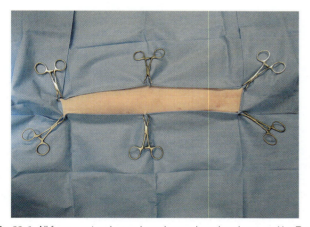

• **Fig. 32.6** All four quarter drapes have been placed and secured by Backhaus towel clamps to isolate the region where the incision will be made.

If penetration of a sterile field is noted, action should be taken to secure the field. Sterile drapes can be added to the now contaminated region and the drapes secured with nonpenetrating clamps. If a surgeon's or surgical assistant's gown or glove comes into contact with a contaminated region, they should step away from the surgical table, the item(s) should be removed, and a sterile replacement should be obtained. Depending on the location and the degree of contamination, postoperative antibiotics may be warranted as ordered by the veterinarian.

Specific examples of patient positioning and draping of each body part are discussed in the following sections.

Abdomen

Most ventral abdominal surgical approaches involve a ventral midline incision for access to the peritoneal cavity and retroperitoneal space. The most common surgeries used for this position are ovariohysterectomy, gastrotomy, and abdominal exploration. Patients are placed in dorsal recumbency. Drapes are placed as previously described and shown in Fig. 32.7. If a vacuum bag positioning device has been used, inflation should not rise above (laterally) or interfere with access to the abdomen.

Extremity

For extremity surgeries in which the surgeon wishes to maintain mobility of the limb, it should be prepared with a hanging limb technique (Fig. 32.9A–D). This technique allows the limb to be held away from the body (generally attached to an intravenous [IV] pole or ceiling hook) so that the limb can be prepared aseptically and draped into the sterile field. Once the limb is aseptically prepared, it should not be touched until it has been properly draped for surgery by the surgeon or assistant. After the foot has been draped, the entire limb can be passed through a fenestrated drape to include it within the surgical field. If surgery is not being performed on the distal limb, the foot should be encompassed with an impervious drape that is secured with sterile bandaging material, such as Vetrap (3M).

Oral Surgery

Positioning for oral surgery depends on the procedure that is to be performed, because patients may be in dorsal, ventral, or lateral recumbency. Draping can be difficult, because the anatomy of the nose, mouth, and orbit prevents easy drape positioning. Most oral surgeries are not considered sterile procedures, but surgeons and surgical assistants should always attempt to perform these surgeries as aseptically as possible.

Perineum

Surgical procedures involving the perineal region, such as anal sacculectomy, episioplasty, or rectal pull-through, may require patients to be placed in ventral recumbency on a perineal stand. The perineal stand allows the patient to be presented in a raised position, preventing the hindlimbs from interfering with the surgery. It is essential that the ventral abdomen be cushioned with padding or several soft towels when using this positioning technique as the hindlimbs often hang freely, causing pressure on the pelvis and the abdomen as a result of the "dead weight" of the hindlimbs. Standard draping technique is used; however, the instrument table cannot be easily draped with the usual drape for a large patient unless it is placed over the patient. Often, a second instrument table drape is used, because the table is positioned off to the side of the surgeon and surgical assistant.

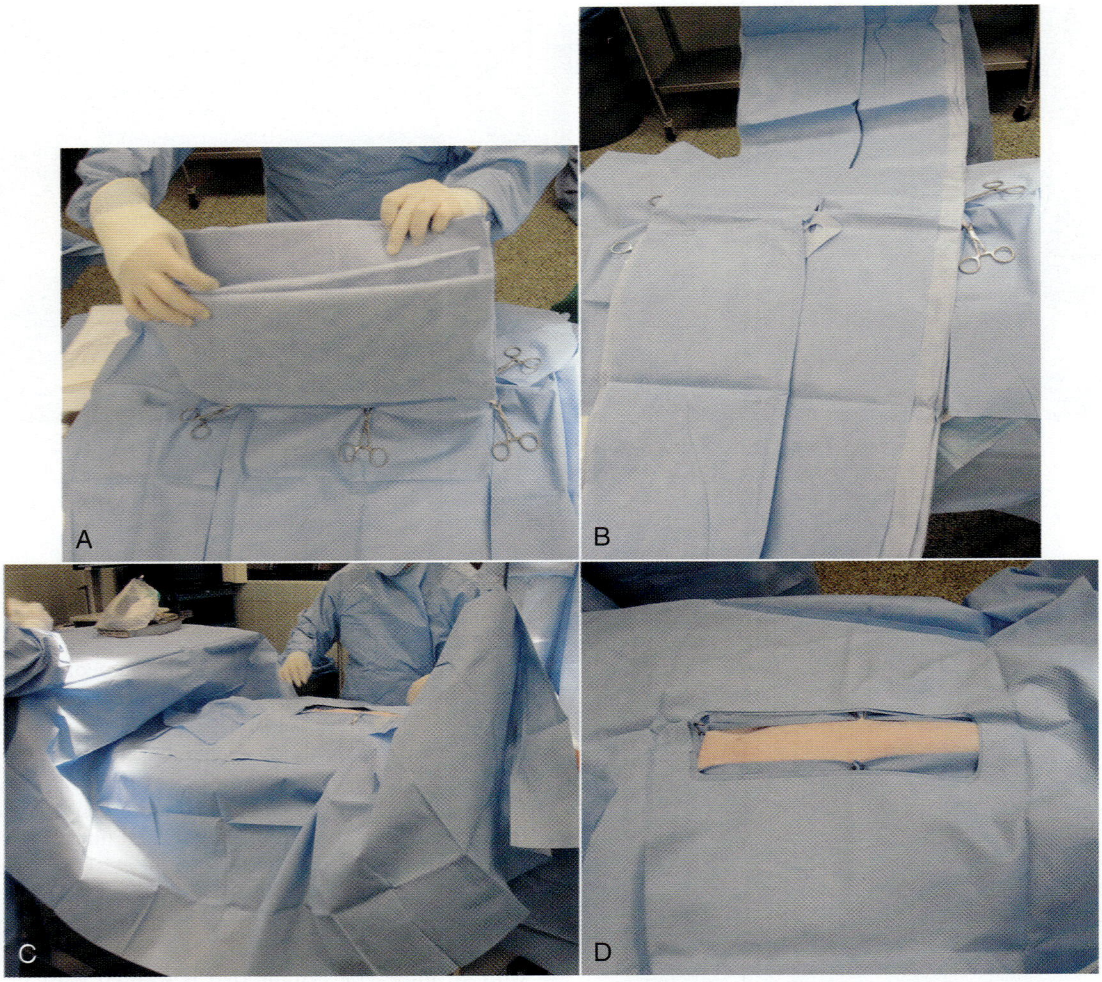

• **Fig. 32.7** (A) The quarter drapes have been placed. A single large drape is positioned so that its fenestration covers the proposed incision site. (B) The surgeon and the surgical assistant have extended the drape out from the patient. (C) The drape has been placed over the patient and instrument table and secured to prevent it from moving. The front part of the drape has been elevated to allow the anesthesia team to have access to the patient. (D) The large drape is covering the quarter drapes and the towel clamps while allowing access to the proposed incision site.

Spine

The spine can be approached both dorsally (for hemilaminectomy or dorsal laminectomy) and ventrally (for a cervical ventral slot). For both approaches, the standard draping technique is used. Many surgeons elect to use an added layer of drapes (attached with Michel clips or Ioban), because the spinal cord is often exposed during neurologic surgery and susceptible to site infection.

Thorax

Most approaches to the thorax are performed with the patient in dorsal (for median sternotomy) or lateral (for intercostal thoracotomy) recumbency. For example, the patient is placed in left lateral recumbency for a right lateral intercostal thoracotomy. The thorax is generally greater in length in the dorsal-to-ventral plane, especially in deep-chested dogs, and therefore requires proper positioning to prevent the patient from shifting during a ventral midline approach. For both thoracic approaches, the patient is draped, as previously described, with four quarter drapes and a large drape to cover the entire patient and the instrument table.

Operating Room Sterility

The surgeon, surgical assistant, and OR technician are responsible for maintaining OR sterility. For the surgeon and the surgical assistant, the focus should be on maintaining the sterility of gowns, gloves, drapes, and instruments. Circulating OR technicians should monitor the surgeon and the surgical assistant, the anesthesia team, and any other observers in the room. The most likely times for breaks in sterility to occur are when the patient is being draped and surgical and instrument tables are being set up.

PUT INTO PRACTICE

Remember to clean "everything" regularly in the surgical suite, including tops of lights, wall fixtures, and the base of the operating table. Such areas can harbor dust and microbial life.

Once scrubbed and gloved in sterile gloves, the hands of OR personnel should always be maintained above the waist and below the shoulders (Fig. 32.10). The only part of the surgery gown

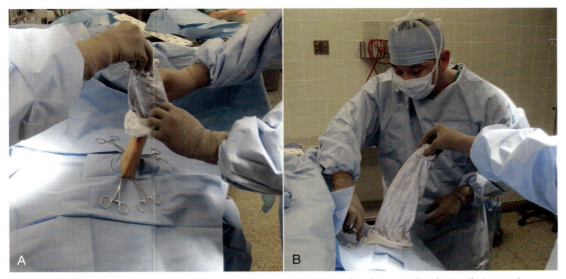

• **Fig. 32.8** (A) A stockinette has been added to cover the limb and to decrease the chance that a surgical site infection may develop. (B) The stockinette is being clamped to the other drapes to prevent it from slipping during the procedure.

considered sterile is the front region from the shoulders to the waist; neither the back of the surgery gown nor any area below the surface of the surgery table is sterile.

Surgical Instruments and Instrument Table Organization

The surgical assistant is often responsible for instrument selection. A "pick sheet" that contains the instruments used or needed for each surgical procedure can help ensure these instruments are available when needed by having them close by in the room or already opened on the instrument table. For example, a pick sheet for a hemilaminectomy (performed to treat intervertebral disk disease) often includes Gelpi retractors, rongeurs, and a surgical drill. Pick sheets may also be used to indicate surgeon preference regarding instruments for a procedure. Commonly used surgical instruments are covered in Chapter 31.

Each surgical team may have slightly different requirements and preferences for setup and instrumentation; however, a few general principles should be considered. The most used instruments should be placed in an easily accessible location by the team. This equipment often includes thumb forceps, scissors, and needle holders that are used on a regular basis (Fig. 32.11). Generally, instruments should be organized as they are returned to the instrument table after use to help prevent delays in accessing them again. Sharp instrumentation (blades and needles, etc.) should be positioned appropriately to minimize possible injury. A magnetic box used to hold sharp instruments is preferable, because this will decrease the likelihood of an accident (Fig. 32.11).

When an instrument is contaminated by a dirty wound or tumor cells, it should be removed from the instrument table (passed off to an OR technician) or placed on an isolated region of the instrument table and not reused. The surgical assistant is responsible for ensuring that contaminated instruments are not used again in a surgical wound, because this may increase the risk of a surgical site infection or seeding of tumor cells. Additionally, any surgical gloves, gowns, gauze, or other materials that have been in contact with a contaminated instrument or wound should be changed and removed from the area.

Surgical sponges and gauze should be counted before surgery begins. Gauze placed into a cavity should be accounted for and tracked closely; the surgical assistant should ensure that all gauze has been removed and accounted for before closure of that cavity. Gauze may contain radiopaque strips (Fig. 32.11) that can be visualized on radiographs if accidentally left inside a patient.

Intraoperative Techniques and Duties

As a surgical team, the critical thinking, communication (verbal or not), proficient ability to predict the surgeon's needs, maintaining the patient's anesthetic comfort and vitals, and being constantly alert for asepsis or other emergent issues are all key to a successful surgery. Immediately after draping the patient, the surgical assistant should work with the surgeon to perform tasks that keep the procedure moving smoothly and improve surgical outcomes. These tasks may include setup of suction and/or electrocautery, placement of light handles, orientation of lighting, placement of scalpel blades on scalpel handles, and assisting with hemostasis and ultimately suturing, in addition to others.

Surgical Lighting

Light handles or sterile light covers should be placed after the patient has been draped (Fig. 32.12A and B). The surgical lights can then be focused and aimed at appropriate sites.

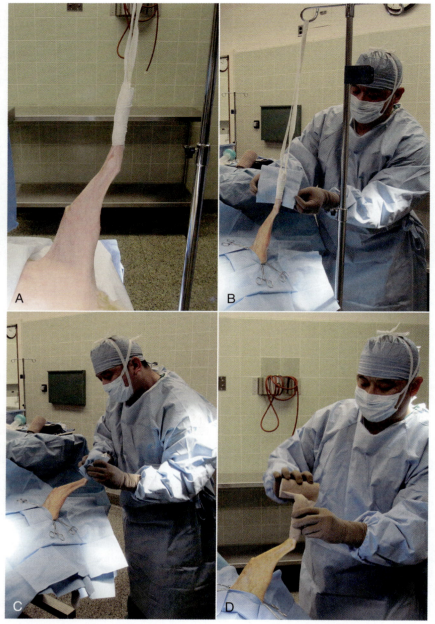

• **Fig. 32.9** "Hanging limb" draping technique. (A) The lower limb has been taped and attached to an IV pole to allow for preparation with aseptic technique and draping. (B and C) After draping-in the limb with quarter drapes, a sterile drape is being placed around the distal limb to allow grasping of the limb and subsequent draping. (D) A sterile outer layer of a self-adherent wrap is then placed over the sterile distal limb drape to maintain the quarter drape in position.

TECHNICIAN NOTE

Light handles or sterile light covers should be placed after the patient has been draped.

In certain procedures, a headlamp may be required to improve lighting at the surgical site, especially deeply positioned surgical fields, such as neurologic and aural surgeries. The surgeon or the surgical assistant may wear the headlamp.

Instrumentation Cords and Tubing

Power units are often best located behind or beside the instrument table, because this minimizes the risk of cords or tubing pulling instruments from the table or contaminating the table by pulling cords over sterile drapes or the patient.

Suction tubing may be secured to the surgical drapes with a nonpenetrating instrument, such as an Allis tissue forceps, which will keep the suction tubing and tip from falling off the table (Fig. 32.13). When an electrocautery handpiece is used, the plug for the device should be passed off the surgical table and attached to the cord, which should be secured to the drape or the table to prevent contamination (see Fig. 32.13).

Additional tools (drills, saws, scopes, fluid delivery, etc.) need to be safely secured to the drapes and/or to the instrument table; placement may need to consider tubing attachment to a tank that is off the instrument table. Tubing should be positioned where it cannot be inadvertently pulled or kinked, resulting in loss of the instrument off the table or, worse, trauma to the patient.

Examples of procedures requiring additional tools include arthroscopy, laparoscopy, and thoracoscopy, which may require carbon dioxide for visualization or fluid delivered to a joint (arthroscopy), where the medium is transported via tubing attached to the port. All "-scopy" procedures require the use of a camera and a light source, both of which have cable attachments to be secured as discussed above and passed off the table to a nearby tower.

Scalpel Use

Numerous scalpel blades are available, and the blade chosen depends on the indication for use. Scalpel blades are placed onto scalpel handles (never by hand) using needle holders to prevent accidental injury (Fig. 32.14). When discarded, scalpel blades should be passed away from the surgery area for disposal in a sharps container. The scalpel blade should never be left in the surgical field.

Three primary grips may be used to hold the scalpel blade: pencil grip, fingertip grip, and palm grip. The pencil grip is employed when the surgeon is attempting to make a very precise cut or when a "stab" incision is necessary to open a structure, such as during a cystotomy or gastrotomy. The fingertip grip is recommended for longer incisions, such as a skin incision for ventral celiotomy. The palm grip is rarely used but allows the surgeon to generate greater force, because the palm is positioned directly over and onto the scalpel handle. Understanding grip positions enables the surgical assistant to be prepared for what may come next.

The scalpel and blade should be passed with care and only when the surgeon is aware and ready to receive them; the blade should be passed with the sharp edge facing away from the surgeon's hand to prevent accidental injury. Scalpels should never be laid on the surgical instrument tray with exposed blades.

Instrument Passing

The surgical assistant is often requested to hand instruments to the surgeon; this responsibility requires knowledge of instruments,

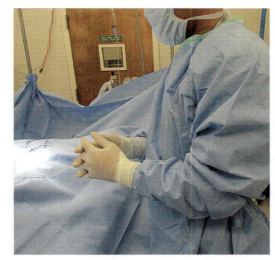

• **Fig. 32.10** The surgical assistant is maintaining proper hand position while facing the operating table. Anything below the waist is considered nonsterile; all sterile personnel should keep their hands above their waist.

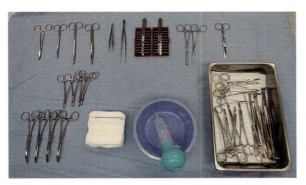

• **Fig. 32.11** An organized instrument table.

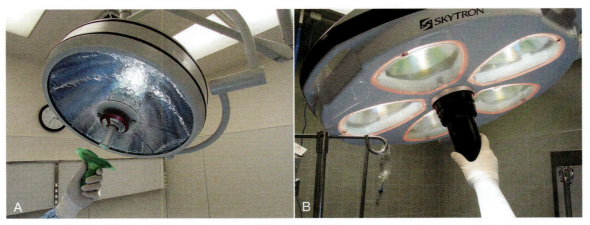

• **Fig. 32.12** Light handle sterile technique. (A) This light maintains a permanent handle, and a temporary collapsible sterile light handle cover is placed during every surgery. (B) A sterile light handle sleeve is placed to control this light. This particular light has a camera incorporated into the design that allows video capture of a procedure.

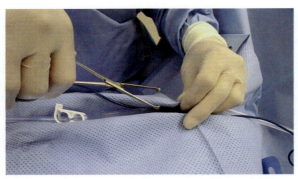

• **Fig. 32.13** Suction tubing and the electrocautery cord are secured to the drape by means of a sterile instrument, such as an Allis tissue forceps.

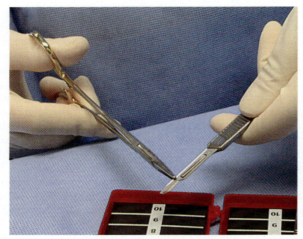

• **Fig. 32.14** Proper placement of a scalpel blade onto a scalpel handle.

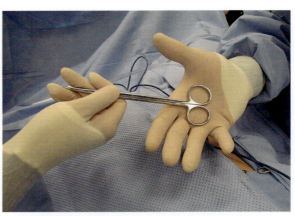

• **Fig. 32.15** The instrument is being passed to the surgeon in the proper orientation. Note that the instrument is being placed into an open hand to allow more immediate use.

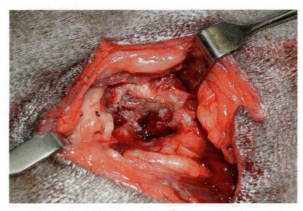

• **Fig. 32.16** Use of hand-held retractors (Senn retractors) to expose a surgical site while a biopsy sample is being obtained.

anticipation, and proper placement of the instrument in the surgeon's hand. Experience with the surgeon and procedures will facilitate readiness and decreases surgical time, ultimately benefiting the patient.

Instruments should be placed in the surgeon's open palm with sufficient forcefulness to allow them to grasp the instrument and prevent it from falling and in a position that allows easy manipulation and usage of the instrument (Fig. 32.15). Any sharp instruments (needles, bladed scalpels, retractors) should be passed with the sharp edge facing away from the surgeon's hand to prevent accidental injury.

Retraction

Retractors, such as Army-Navy retractors, Senn retractors, and malleable retractors, are designated for specific tissue types and methods of retraction (Fig. 32.16). Retraction is a learned skill that requires attention to detail and a focused mind to prevent damage to surrounding tissues while allowing sufficient exposure of the surgical site, often for a significant amount of time.

Hemostasis

Hemostasis can be achieved through a variety of techniques:
• Pressure applied via gauze sponges may be sufficient for small bleeding vessels; pressure and blotting with gauze is preferred over the wiping motion, which removes blood clots that have been established.
• Hemostats contain a ratchet that allows them to be placed onto a larger vessel and maintained in position for a short time to cause hemostasis of a vessel that is not going to be spared.
• Suture ligation, vascular clips, or electrocautery may be warranted when ligating a larger blood vessel. The surgical assistant may gently hold the vessel away from the surrounding tissue using hemostats or other forceps to allow the surgeon to tie off (ligate) the vessel with suture.
• Vascular clips can be placed only on the bleeding vessel using a clip applier. Gentle manipulation of the vessel will prevent tearing of the vessel or release of the vessel back into the surgical wound.
• Electrocautery uses an electrical current that conducts heat through a metal probe to destroy bleeding tissue, thereby controlling blood loss and decreasing surgical time. Electrocautery coagulation devices can be monopolar or bipolar (Fig. 32.17). Monopolar electrocautery passes a current through the target tissue and disperses the current through the patient to a ground pad underneath the patient's body; the patient acts as part of the electrical circuit. Monopolar handpieces are often equipped with both cutting and coagulation modes and are most efficient in a dry surgical site. A gauze blotting technique or gentle suction may be needed initially to decrease blood in the region.

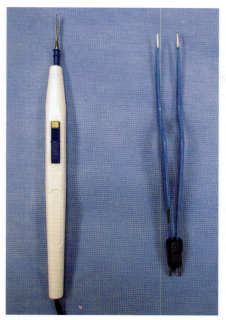

• **Fig. 32.17** Examples of handpieces used for performing cauterization: monopolar *(left)* and bipolar *(right)*.

The monopolar electrocautery probe can also be applied to an instrument (e.g., a DeBakey thumb or hemostatic forceps) that is clamped to a blood vessel for precise cauterization of a blood vessel.

• A bipolar electrocautery unit passes a current between two tips of a forceps; the current is often controlled by a foot switch. Bipolar electrocautery is generally used in surgeries where precisely targeted cauterization is necessary, such as ophthalmic and neurologic procedures.

Several hemostatic agents have been designed to assist with control of intraoperative bleeding. Bone wax is a mixture of beeswax, paraffin, isopropyl palmitate, and a wax-softening agent that can be applied to actively bleeding bone. Bone wax functions by occluding the bleeding channel and effectively controls bleeding that occurs at the site of medullary bone (e.g., during hemilaminectomy) or from within a cut bone (e.g., mandibulectomy). Bone wax is nonabsorbable. Gelatin foams (Gelfoam) can be cut or torn into shapes that can be placed more effectively into a bleeding site and provide a framework for the initiation of clotting; the foam is absorbed over time. Oxidized cellulose (Surgicel) is designed as a sheet that can be cut to specific sizes and placed on organ surfaces. Once bleeding has sufficiently stopped, the cellulose should be removed from the wound.

Suture Cutting

The surgical assistant should cut the suture using the tips of suture scissors to prevent accidental trauma to adjacent normal tissue or cutting previous sutures while the surgeon is suturing.

TECHNICIAN NOTE

Surgical assistants should use only suture scissors and focus on using the tips of suture scissors to cut sutures.

Lavage and Suction

Fluid is routinely used to lavage a wound and should be sterile and iso-osmotic. Examples include lactated Ringer solution and normal strength saline. These fluids may be kept on the instrument table in a sterile bowl and can be transferred to the surgical site via a bulb syringe or by direct pouring of the lavage fluid into a body cavity; liters of fluid may also be used via sterile tubing.

Suction is used to remove lavage fluid or body fluids from a body cavity or wound site. Large suction tips with multiple holes, such as the Poole tip, are used most often in the abdominal or thoracic cavity. Smaller suction tips with a single end-on hole, such as the Frazier tip, may be used for more focal, small amount suctioning, such as that required during neurosurgeries (see Chapter 31). Surgical assistants can suction blood and improve visualization in times of excessive bleeding, enabling the surgeon to identify the source of bleeding.

Camera Manipulation

Minimally invasive procedures, such as arthroscopy, laparoscopy, and thoracoscopy, require a camera be placed into the body cavity or joint that is being evaluated, with an image generated and viewed on a monitor positioned near the surgery table. The surgical assistant is often responsible for pointing the camera in the appropriate direction, because the surgeon typically uses both hands to direct the camera (see Chapter 31).

Tissue Manipulation, Retraction, and Organ Positioning

Skin

Although it is necessary to incise the skin during initiation of surgery, surgeons and assistants should avoid regular contact with the skin during surgery. Once the incision has been made, the skin edges should be handled as gently and atraumatically as possible. Each manipulation of the skin results in trauma or a chance for infection; excessive force should be avoided.

Abdomen

Surgical assistance during abdominal procedures is often warranted, because most procedures begin with abdominal exploration. Anatomic knowledge and organ positioning is important, because each surgeon has their preferred approach to exploration. Surgical gloves or gauze pads should be moistened with iso-osmotic fluid when abdominal organs are touched, particularly the gastrointestinal (GI) tract, to minimize tearing of the serosal layer or damage to the organs.

The liver is a fairly mobile organ consisting of six major lobes in the cat or the dog. The left side of the liver can be gently retracted to the right to view the abdominal esophagus and the stomach (Fig. 32.18). The gallbladder is generally evaluated at this time and can be expressed for assessment of the patency of cystic and common bile ducts.

The pancreas consists of right and left limbs and a central body. The right limb is easily visible and is closely associated with the duodenum. The left limb is located caudal to the stomach and can be viewed by entering the omental bursa. Overmanipulation of the pancreas can result in pancreatitis and should be kept to a minimum.

The spleen is a highly mobile organ and can often be lifted out of the abdomen. During splenectomies, the assistant often

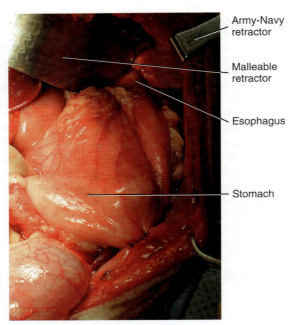

• **Fig. 32.18** During this celiotomy to correct a hiatal hernia, an esophagopexy and a gastropexy have been performed. The malleable retractor is being used to retract the left side of the liver to the right to allow visualization of the abdominal esophagus. The Army-Navy retractor is retracting the left body wall to further increase visualization.

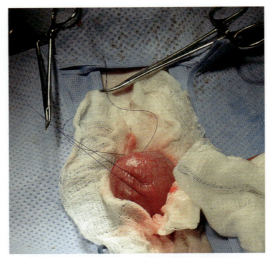

• **Fig. 32.19** Stay sutures attached to hemostats have been placed in the bladder. Stay sutures are commonly used to facilitate manipulation of hollow organs.

handles the spleen, allowing the surgeon to assess the splenic vascular supply. The spleen can vary in size, even within the same animal, because it has the capacity to contract and expand often in the presence of certain medications.

The GI tract can be palpated along its entire length for any abnormalities; overstretching or overmanipulation of the intestines should be avoided. During enterotomies, intestinal resections, and anastomoses, it is important that the surgical team ensure microbe-rich intestinal contents *not* be released into the abdominal cavity to avoid contamination of the peritoneal cavity.

The more ventrally located organs need to be moved aside to view the retroperitoneal structures (kidneys, ureters, adrenal glands, aorta, caudal vena cava). Right-sided retroperitoneal structures can be viewed most easily by retracting the duodenum ventrally and to the left. Left-sided retroperitoneal structures are best viewed by retracting the descending colon and spleen to the right.

The urinary bladder is located in the caudal abdomen and, in some cystotomies, this organ is approached via a minimal caudal celiotomy incision. The ureters enter the urinary bladder on the dorsal surface, so careful attention is necessary when surgery of the dorsal bladder is performed.

The urinary bladder is often manipulated with the use of stay sutures, which allow both the ventral and dorsal aspects of the bladder to be seen. Stay sutures are sutures that are placed into the lumen of a hollow organ, such as the stomach or the bladder, to allow that organ to be manually manipulated (Fig. 32.19). The assistant is responsible for clamping the free ends of the stay sutures together with a hemostat and cutting the suture ends for removal. The surgical assistant often holds the organ in a particular position to allow the surgeon to continue the surgery.

Thorax

Although gentle retraction is always important, within the thorax, overmanipulation of the heart or lungs can result in life-threatening consequences. Large retractors (e.g., flat malleable retractors) are often used in the thorax, particularly when a median sternotomy has been performed to access the heart, cranial mediastinum, or lung lobes. Surrounding the malleable retractor with a moistened laparotomy pad will help decrease the chance of iatrogenic trauma to intrathoracic organs. Retraction may also be necessary when surgery is performed to stabilize fractured ribs (Fig. 32.20).

Musculoskeletal System

Gentle muscle retraction and manipulation by the surgical assistant (see Fig. 32.16) during surgical approaches to bones and joints will decrease trauma and iatrogenic bleeding and facilitate an effective surgery. Tearing and further muscle trauma can be avoided by minimizing excessive force or traction and by keeping the tissues moist.

Although generally more resistant to iatrogenic injury than muscle, bones should be treated with care, and soft tissue attachments to bones should be preserved as much as possible. Bone forceps can be used to hold fractured bones in reduction during repair (see Chapter 31) or to retract bones during certain joint surgeries to improve visualization.

Vascular and Nervous Systems

The surgeon is responsible for manipulation of involved vascular and neurologic structures and placement of retraction devices in the correct location during these delicate surgeries. The surgical assistant may be required to maintain the position of these devices by using extreme focus and care to avoid injury.

Surgical Implants

Implants are devices that are left in the surgical wound to perform a function; they may be permanent or temporary in nature.

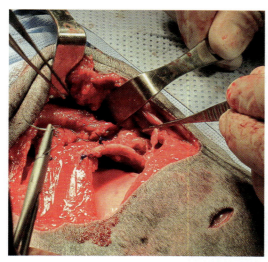

• **Fig. 32.20** Two Army-Navy retractors are being used to improve visualization during repair of a region of thoracic trauma secondary to bite wounds.

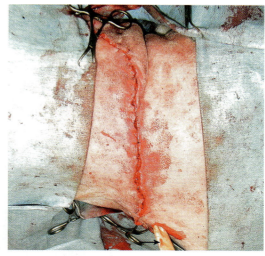

• **Fig. 32.21** A passive drain (Penrose) has been placed to allow drainage of a wound that has been debrided and closed after a traumatic bite wound.

Permanent

Permanent implants are placed with the intention of being left in place for the patient's life; however, if failure or infection occurs, these implants may have to be removed. Each fracture repair or joint stabilization surgery is unique, but having a basic knowledge of the steps involved in the repair process and of **orthopedic** procedure, the instruments, and implants used, such as plates, pins, wires, and screws, will enhance the efficiency of the procedure.

Temporary

Drains are the most common temporary implant used in veterinary medicine. Drains are devices inserted into postsurgical wounds or body cavities to allow for drainage of accumulated fluid and to help eliminate dead space. Drains are generally classified as passive or active, and both must be removed as their presence within tissue stimulates fluid production. Drains are generally removed when fluid production has slowed or ceased.

> **TECHNICIAN NOTE**
>
> Drains, when present in tissue, may stimulate fluid production.

Passive Drains

Passive drains are used most often to drain subcutaneous wounds (Fig. 32.21). These drains are less rigid than active drains and need to be secured in place, with the secured location readily accessible at the time of removal. Passive drains are gravity dependent, requiring the lowest drainage point to be in a dependent location. Passive drains should never be used to drain the abdomen.

Penrose drains made of soft latex are the most common type of passive drain (see Fig. 32.21). Penrose drains generally exit from a single hole in a dependent location; occasionally, a two-hole technique can be used. The drain is secured by placing a suture percutaneously through the nonvisible or upper aspect of the drain. An additional suture can be placed in the visible or lower aspect of the drain; however, this suture should not cause closure of the drain's exit site in the skin.

Active Drains

Active drains use negative pressure to suction fluid and air from a wound. Active drains can be used in medium-to-large subcutaneous wounds and are the drain of choice for abdominal drainage. For smaller wounds, an active drain can be created by placing the tubing from a butterfly catheter into the wound and attaching the needle to a vacutainer to maintain negative suction. Alternatively, the hub from butterfly catheter tubing can be attached to a syringe that is pulled back to negative pressure and secured in place with a needle to prevent the plunger from returning to neutral position.

Larger, commercially available drains consist of a multifenestrated component that is placed within the wound and externally attached to tubing, which is then attached to a suction canister (bulb) that continually generates a negative pressure, causing air and fluid within the wound to be evacuated. Like passive drains, active drains need to be secured to the skin to prevent inadvertent removal (Fig. 32.22A–C).

> **TECHNICIAN NOTE**
>
> Both passive and active drains need to be secured to the skin to prevent premature removal.

Suture Material

Suturing is the act of joining two surfaces together with a stitch or a series of stitches. A suture aims to hold the wound edges in apposition to one another until the tissue has sufficient time to heal. Wound edges may include the obvious integument or body cavities and refer to the edges of incised organs (i.e., biopsy sites); transected or avulsed ligaments or tendons; "-pexy" techniques; elimination of dead space (tacking skin to underlying tissue); and support repairs from wounds, such as hernias. Suturing requires knowledge of multiple available suture material types, sizes, and the suture pattern(s) that may be used. The surgical team must be prepared for the likelihood of multiple considerations, including the preferences of the surgeon(s) involved.

Considerations When Choosing Suture

Wound Type

Just as sutures can enhance wound closure, they can also play a part in the development of wound infections. Wicking action

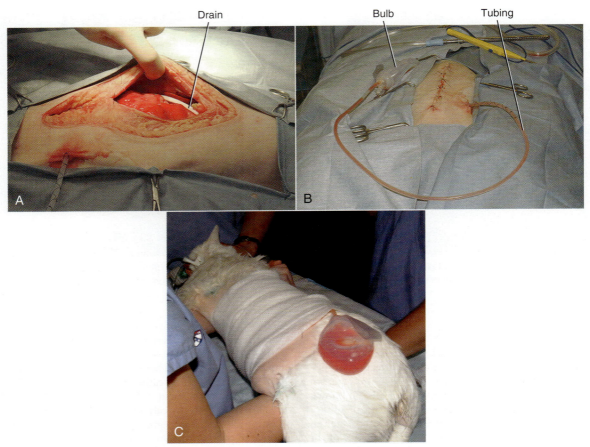

Drain

Bulb   Tubing

A

B

C

• **Fig. 32.22** A Jackson-Pratt drain has been placed intra-abdominally in this feline patient to allow active drainage postoperatively. (A) The drain component can be seen intra-abdominally before closure of the abdomen. (B) The tubing is exiting through a hole lateral to the midline. The tubing is sutured to the skin to prevent inadvertent removal. The suction canister (bulb) is gently squeezed and capped to generate suction. (C) Postoperatively, the patient is bandaged to decrease the likelihood of inadvertent removal and to decrease the chance of infection and pain associated with the drain.

along the suture can draw contaminants into the wound, either during the suturing action or during healing if the suture stability is decreased. If a patient is debilitated with a chronic disease process that affects healing, such as diabetes, or is on long-term medication, such as steroids, metabolic factors can further affect the healing components and suture stability.

The type of organ being sutured is an important factor when choosing the suture material. Sutures placed into hollow organs are often exposed to intraluminal materials that may degrade the suture. Foreign material (suture) placed into contaminated tissue may exacerbate inflammation and lead to infection; some suture types break down more quickly in infected environments. Absorbable sutures are most often used in tissues that heal quickly, such as those of the stomach, intestine, and bladder. Nonabsorbable sutures may be prudent in tissues that heal more slowly, such as fascia and tendons.

Construction

Sutures can be **monofilament** (composed of a single strand) or **multifilament** (several filaments twisted or braided together). Monofilament sutures are generally considered easier to pass through tissue, because they cause less resistance. However, this suture tends to be slippery and knots have a propensity to untie,

so careful attention to knot technique is needed. Multifilament sutures hold knots much more easily but have greater capillary action, making them more susceptible to bacterial colonization than monofilament sutures. Use of multifilament sutures in infected wounds should therefore be avoided.

> **TECHNICIAN NOTE**
>
> Sutures are constructed in monofilament or multifilament forms. Monofilament sutures are more resistant to contamination in infected wounds compared with multifilament sutures.

Size and Strength

The nomenclature of suture sizes has been derived by the United States Pharmacopeia (USP). Most sutures are referred to in terms of their USP size, which correlates with a diameter size (in millimeters) of the suture. Sutures are available in sizes from 11/0 or 11-0 (read as "11 ought"), which is the thinnest suture at 0.02 mm, to 0 (#0 or "ought"), to the thickest suture '7' at 0.9 mm (#7). The greater the number of zeroes, the smaller the diameter of the suture.

The strength of a suture is measured by the force required to break a knotted suture strand. Factors that can weaken a suture include knots; wetness; absorption; placement in an environment that can break the suture down, such as inflamed and/or infected tissue; and inappropriate manipulation of the suture with instruments.

The suture selected should be at least as strong as the normal tissue through which it has been placed and the smallest diameter suture that will adequately hold healing tissues together. The larger the suture and needle, the higher the likelihood of increased trauma, often resulting in wound site compromise or foreign material being pulled into the wound.

TECHNICIAN NOTE

The suture selected to close a wound should be at least as strong as the tissue that it is holding together and the smallest diameter to hold the tissues together.

Handling

A suture material's memory is the capacity of it returning to a previously determined shape after undergoing deformation of the suture. A suture with "lower" memory or no memory is a beneficial characteristic, because these sutures are easier to handle, with improved knot quality. Some suture material can be gently pulled to remove the curl, decreasing its memory and thereby improving handling.

Knot Security

Knots are formed when "throws" or strands of suture are wrapped around each other and pulled together. The knot is the weakest point in a tied suture. The security of a knot is affected by the quality of the knot, knot-tying technique, the coefficient of friction, and the size of the suture material. Knot security can also be affected by tissue fluid.

Suture Classification and Examples

Sutures can be classified by numerous different methods, including type of material (natural or synthetic), biological behavior (absorbable or nonabsorbable), and method of construction (monofilament or multifilament). For purposes of this text, sutures will be classified into broad categories of absorbable and nonabsorbable; specific examples of each will be discussed.

Absorbable

Absorbable sutures are those that lose most of their breaking strength within 60 days of placement. Absorbable suture material can be either natural or synthetic (manufactured); both are available as monofilament-type or multifilament-type threads. Natural suture is absorbed by enzymatic degradation; synthetic suture is absorbed by hydrolysis.

Natural

Natural absorbable sutures consist of catgut or collagen. Catgut is a multifilament suture constructed from the intestines of sheep, goats, or cattle and consists mostly of collagen, packaged in solutions of alcohol. The strength of catgut is maintained for only a short time (plain gut, 7–10 days; chromic gut, 10–14 days); the rate of absorption is variable and unpredictable, but it is essentially gone after 2 weeks. Catgut can also stimulate a severe inflammatory reaction. Because of these qualities, catgut has limited use as an option for securing support layers or structural layers, such as the linea alba. Chromic gut is catgut that has been treated with

a chromium solution that extends its breakdown time, allowing more time for tissue apposition to heal.

Reconstituted collagen made from bovine flexor tendon, a natural absorbable suture, is an alternative to catgut; it has a similar rate of absorption as catgut. This type of suture is generally only used in microsurgeries, such as ophthalmic surgery.

Synthetic

Synthetic absorbable sutures provide predictable degradability in a biological environment; wounds that are infected or inflamed do not significantly affect the degradation of these sutures. The most used synthetic absorbable sutures in veterinary medicine include polyglactin 910, polyglycolic acid, poliglecaprone 25, polydioxanone, and polyglyconate.

Polyglactin 910 (Vicryl) is a braided multifilament suture with good handling characteristics that causes minimal tissue inflammation. It is stable in contaminated wounds; however, because of the nature of the filament, it is less resistant to contamination compared with monofilament suture. Absorption is generally complete at 60 to 70 days. An antibacterial version of polyglactin 910 (Vicryl Plus) is coated with triclosan, an ingredient that assists in preventing bacterial contamination.

Polyglycolic acid (Dexon) is a braided multifilament suture that rapidly loses strength and is weaker than other synthetic absorbable sutures. Its knot security is considered relatively poor and it may cut through friable tissue. Polyglycolic acid loses approximately 35% of its tensile strength by 14 days and is usually completely absorbed between 60 and 120 days. This suture is not recommended for use in the oral cavity or in the presence of infected urine, because the rate of breakdown may be increased by the alkaline pH of the urine or saliva.

Poliglecaprone 25 (Monocryl) is a monofilament suture that is one of the strongest absorbable sutures made; however, by 14 days, approximately 80% of its tensile strength is lost. This suture has good knot security and handling characteristics, and is absorbed by 90 to 120 days.

Polydioxanone (PDS) is a monofilament suture that has greater initial tensile strength compared with the multifilament sutures polyglactin 910 and polyglycolic acid. Although polydioxanone has poor knot security, its approximate strength loss at 14 days is only 14%. This suture is generally completely absorbed at 180 days. Polydioxanone is often used to close the bladder, even in the presence of infected urine.

Polyglyconate (Maxon) is a monofilament suture that is very similar to polydioxanone. Polyglyconate maintains approximately 70% strength at 14 days after placement, and absorption occurs by 180 days after placement.

Nonabsorbable

Natural

Silk is a multifilament suture that consists of braided or twisted strands. Silk has no memory, which makes it the near-perfect suture to handle; however, it has several disadvantages, including poor strength, high capillarity, and the ability to stimulate an intense inflammatory reaction. The tissue reaction that it causes results in loss of tensile strength by 180 days and increases the risk for contamination.

Metallic sutures (stainless steel) are available in monofilament and multifilament forms. Stainless steel has the greatest tensile strength and knot security of all suture materials. Stainless steel sutures result in virtually no inflammatory reaction and can be used in contaminated or infected wounds. Disadvantages include poor handling quality and the tendency of the suture to kink or break when bent repeatedly. Additionally, tissue necrosis can occur from tissue movement over knot ends.

Synthetic

Polyamide (nylon) is available in both monofilament and multifilament forms. Polyamide sutures cause minimal tissue reaction, and the monofilament form has no capillarity. Polyamide has poor handling characteristics and knot security but is suitable for skin sutures. Although polyamide is considered a nonabsorbable suture, 30% of its tensile strength is lost by 2 years after placement.

Polypropylene (Prolene) is a monofilament suture that has the greatest strength of the synthetic nonabsorbable sutures. This suture exhibits minimal tissue reactivity, resists weakening by tissue enzymes, and has low thrombogenic potential. It has high memory and slippery handling characteristics and is suitable for use in the skin.

Polybutester (Novafil) is a monofilament suture that has excellent stretching ability, which makes it an excellent choice for suturing tendons and ligaments. Polybutester stimulates minimal tissue reaction and has good tensile strength, knot security, and handling characteristics.

Polyester (Mersilene) is a braided multifilament suture that retains excellent strength and is suitable for use in slowly healing tissues. Polyester has poor handling and knot security and stimulates a tissue reaction that is greater than that of other synthetic suture materials. Polyester is not recommended in infected wounds, because it can trap bacteria between the fibers, making them impervious to phagocytic cells.

Suture Needles

Suture needles can be preloaded with suture (**swaged**) or can require loading onto an eyed needle (Fig. 32.23A–D). Swaged needles produce minimal tissue damage and are less traumatic than eyed needles. Eyed needles can be closed or French (containing a slit to ease threading). In certain surgeries (e.g., cardiovascular), a double-armed suture may be used, which contains a needle on both ends of the suture.

> **TECHNICIAN NOTE**
>
> Eyed needles require a loop of suture through the needle eye, which causes greater tissue trauma than swaged needles.

Suture needles are classified according to size, shape, and type of needle point. The goal of selection is to decrease needle-induced tissue trauma. The length and diameter of the needle should be considered as should be tissue thickness and depth of the incision so that the smallest needle that can effectively reach both sides of the incision is chosen.

Several needle shapes are available; common shapes include straight, half-curved, and parts of a circle (¼-circle, ⅜-circle, ½-circle, and ⅝-circle), with ⅜ and ½ needles being most commonly used (see Fig. 32.23A–D). Straight needles are generally used only in locations (surface of the body) where the fingers can be used to pass the sutures. Curved needles are manipulated with needle holders.

Needle points are categorized as cutting, tapered, or blunt. Cutting needles are recommended for tough tissue (e.g., skin) and are

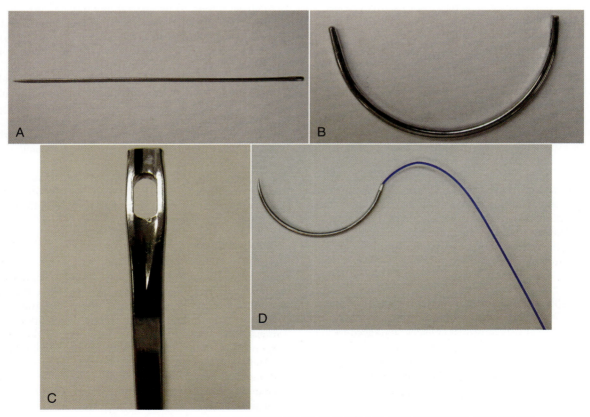

• **Fig. 32.23** Surgical needles. (A) Straight surgical needle. (B and C) A ½-circle eyed needle. Note the hole or eye in part C to allow suture passage. (D) A swaged ½-circle needle.

available in conventional and reverse-cutting forms. Conventional cutting needles have three cutting edges, with the third edge on the inside (concave) curvature. Reverse-cutting needles have three cutting edges; however, the third edge is on the outer (convex) curvature of the needle, and these needles are designed to resist tissue cutout compared with conventional cutting needles. Taper needles contain a sharp tip that is capable of piercing and spreading tissue without cutting surrounding tissues. Locations where taper needles are commonly used include the intestines, subcutaneous tissue, and fascia. Blunt-point needles have a tapered body with a rounded, blunt point able to dissect through friable tissue without cutting/damaging the tissue and are generally recommended for suturing the liver and the kidneys.

Suture Placement and Removal

Suture packages are generally opened by OR staff in a sterile manner and can be passed directly to a surgeon or surgical assistant, or can be dropped onto the instrument table (Fig. 32.24). Suture packages are designed to have their outer packaging peeled back to expose the inner packaging, which houses the suture. The surgical assistant can grasp the inner packaging and position the needle (visible within the package) to be grasped by needle holders perpendicular to the long axis of the needle holder. The position in which the needle is placed within the tips varies per task. The needle should be positioned near the tip when the needle is passed through dense tissue, near the middle for most general purpose suturing, and near the eye for fine suturing of delicate tissues.

The surgical team will consider the wound, closure technique, and the suture types and patterns needed to ensure that the tissue is handled as infrequently as possible. Tissue forceps with teeth should be used to grasp the tissue, and needles should be inserted perpendicular to the tissue. Only the needle holder should be used to grasp the needle for safety.

Basic suture patterns include interrupted and continuous forms; both patterns have advantages. Interrupted suture patterns allow increased control of suture tension and apposition of wounds and avoid potential complications, such as wound dehiscence with subsequent tissue herniation and/or infection, which a single continuous suture strand may allow if it breaks. Continuous suture patterns decrease operative time and form an air-tight and water-tight seal.

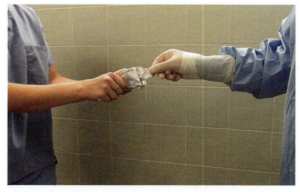

• **Fig. 32.24** The outer layer of a pack of suture material is being opened by the OR technician and offered to the surgeon or the surgical assistant, using proper sterile technique. The inner lining of the suture pack is sterile and can be grasped by sterile personnel.

Postoperative Management

The surgical assistant is often actively involved in the immediate postoperative management of the patient. The wound and surrounding skin should be cleaned immediately after closure with sterile, clean lavage fluid to remove any remaining blood or debris; this minimizes patient discomfort upon awakening.

A sterile wound cover can be placed on the incision after cleaning to prevent the wound from coming into direct contact with the environment. When mid- to distal limb surgery has been performed, the wound is often bandaged postoperatively to decrease swelling and to protect the wound.

Any biopsy samples obtained during surgery should be appropriately identified and submitted by the surgical assistant. If surgical margins are to be evaluated, the assistant can mark the margins with ink or suture material and properly orient the sample for histopathologic evaluation.

The surgical report is an account of all procedures performed during surgery, including use of any implants or sutures. It is part of the patient's medical record and it may be necessary to refer back to the report should a problem arise or if the patient is evaluated at another clinic.

> **TECHNICIAN NOTE**
>
> The surgical assistant can assist in the postoperative care of a surgical patient by cleaning the wound, placing a bandage, submitting a biopsy sample, and/or writing the surgical report.

Surgical Assisting for Equine Patients

Surgeons rely on veterinary technicians to be prepared and to keep things moving in an efficient manner in surgery. Being prepared is most critical to the equine patient in minimizing anesthesia and surgery time, thus lowering the risk of postanesthetic complications, which can occur with large animals under general anesthesia for prolonged periods. Efficient and critical care before and during surgical anesthesia increases the outcome for maximum postoperative comfort and care.

> **TECHNICIAN NOTE**
>
> It is particularly important with large animal surgeries that veterinary technicians, regardless of their roles, anticipate what is needed throughout the procedure to reduce anesthesia time. This will lower the risk of postanesthetic complications, which can occur with large animals under general anesthesia for prolonged periods.

Draping for Abdominal Surgery

The size of the patient and surgery to be performed will dictate the size of the team. As in small animal surgeries, the function of draping is to separate the sterile surgical site from the rest of the contaminated area around the patient. Draping should be performed only by aseptically gowned and gloved members of the surgical team.

Abdominal surgery is one of the most common surgical procedures performed on horses. The animal's abdomen is aseptically prepared, and sterile stockinettes or leg drapes are placed individually over each hindlimb (Fig. 32.25). Next, sterile towels are placed in a four-quarter fashion around the incision site (Fig. 32.26) and secured with several Backhaus towel clamps. With the surgical team positioned on opposite sides of the patient, the large prefenestrated laparotomy drape is carefully unfolded in a coordinated fashion to cover the entire animal (Fig. 32.27) and secured by clamping Backhaus towel clamps to each of the towel clamps underneath the drape (Fig. 32.28A). Each exposed towel clamp is covered with a single 4 × 4-inch gauze sponge (see Fig. 32.28B), and an adhesive, impervious drape is placed directly over the incision site (see Fig. 32.28C). An adhesive spray may be needed for good contact. The gauze sponges prevent the adhesive drape from sticking to the clamps. Care to ensure that all gauze sponges are accounted for before closure is critical.

> **TECHNICIAN NOTE**
>
> It is important that no gauze sponges fall into the abdominal cavity without being retrieved. Account for all gauze sponges prior to abdominal closure by conducting an accurate count as they are used.

Draping for Orthopedic Surgery

The way in which a horse is positioned on the surgery table for an orthopedic procedure depends on which part of the affected limb is to be addressed. Arthroscopic procedures are commonly

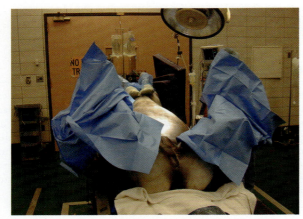

• **Fig. 32.25** Draping of an equine surgery patient. Leg drapes are used to cover the hindlimbs of the patient.

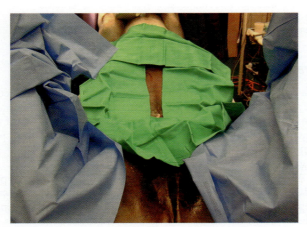

• **Fig. 32.26** Draping the ventral abdomen of an equine surgery patient. Hand towels are placed in a four-quarter fashion around the incision site.

performed with the patient in dorsal recumbency (Fig. 32.29). When the patient is positioned on the surgery table, an electrocautery plate with contact gel is placed underneath the patient, and associated cords are connected to the nearby unit. Impervious plastic drapes are used to reduce strike-through contamination and tearing. An adhesive, impervious type of drape is used directly over the surgical site (Fig. 32.30). If the horse is positioned in lateral recumbency, the affected limb is prepped for surgery by suspending it from an IV fluid pole by using tape placed around the hoof (Fig. 32.31). Once the limb has been aseptically prepared, the area proximal to the surgery site is draped off with sterile hand towels (Fig. 32.32). The circulating OR technician removes the limb from the IV pole by removing the foot from the hanger and grasping a nonprepped area of the limb. The surgeon or the surgical assistant grasps the limb with a sterile hand towel or drape (Fig. 32.33). A sterile surgical glove is placed over the hoof by the surgeon or the surgical assistant. A sterile hand towel is then wrapped around the hoof, or an impervious orthopedic stockinette is placed over the limb. A large drape is fenestrated by cutting a "cross" in the center of the drape to accommodate the limb (Fig. 32.34), which is then fed through the fenestration up to the sterile hand towels, and the entire animal is draped off (Fig. 32.35). The drape is secured at the top of the surgical field with towel clamps. An adhesive, impervious plastic iodine-impregnated drape is then wrapped over the incision site.

Instrument Setup and Handling

If adequate numbers of surgical technicians are present, the surgical instrument packs are opened while the surgeon and the surgical assistant are draping the horse. This reduces anesthesia time. Occasionally, as during some orthopedic surgeries, two tables may be draped, depending on the number of instruments needed for the procedure. The instrument table is draped by a nongloved, gowned OR technician (Fig. 32.36). The surgical instrument packs needed for the surgery are placed on a Mayo instrument stand or a similar type of table and, by using sterile technique, the OR technician opens the outer wrap only (Fig. 32.37). The gloved surgical assistant then opens the sterile inner wrap and removes the sterile instrument tray, placing it onto the draped instrument table. Sterile light handles, suction hose, electrocautery, fluid bowl, gauze sponges, scalpel blade, and suture are arranged on the instrument table. If the horse is draped for abdominal surgery, the surgeon and

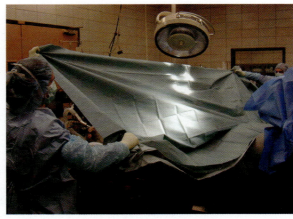

• **Fig. 32.27** Draping of an equine surgery patient. Two individuals are required to drape this patient.

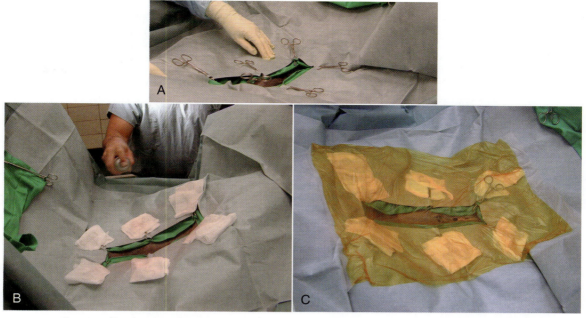

• **Fig. 32.28** Draping the ventral abdomen of an equine surgery patient. (A) Towel clamps are used to secure the laparotomy drape by clamping to the towel clamps underneath the drape. (B) Each exposed towel clamp is covered with a single 4 × 4 inch gauze, and adhesive spray is used to improve the adhesiveness of the adhesive drape. (C) An adhesive, impervious drape is placed directly over the incision site. The gauze pads prevent the adhesive drape from sticking to the clamps.

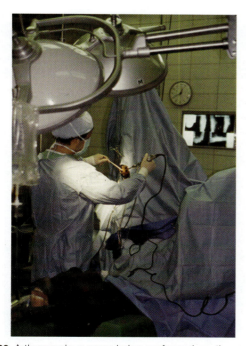

• **Fig. 32.29** Arthroscopic surgery being performed on the carpus of a horse.

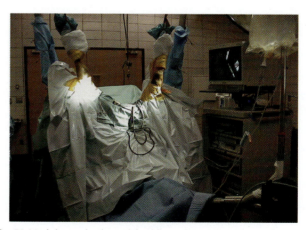

• **Fig. 32.30** A horse is draped for bilateral carpal arthroscopic surgery. Adhesive, impervious drapes are placed around each carpus to reduce surgical wound contamination.

the surgical assistant create a pouch between the back legs of the horse by clamping a hand towel folded to the drape using a nonpenetrating instrument, such as an Allis tissue forceps (Fig. 32.38). The suction hose and the electrocautery line are held in this pouch. The ends of the lines run over the drapes between the limbs of the horse and are connected by the OR technician. A sterile IV fluid line, used to lavage the abdominal organs, may also be set up at this time. The surgical assistant organizes the surgical instruments on the instrument table. The instrument tray is placed on the back of the surgical table, a hand towel is placed in front of the tray, and frequently used instruments are placed on the towel to allow immediate access (Fig. 32.39). Disposable scalpel blades are attached to the scalpel handles. The fluid bowl is positioned on the back edge of the table so that sterile saline can be poured into the bowl by a circulating OR technician. The sterile saline is used to wipe instruments clean during the procedure by taking a wet 4 × 4–inch sponge, gently wiping the blood from the used surgical instrument, placing it back onto the instrument table, and discarding used gauze. Contaminated instruments, gloves, or gowns are removed from the surgical area and replaced.

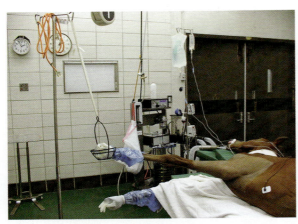

• **Fig. 32.31** An IV fluid pole used to suspend the horse's limb for surgical preparation.

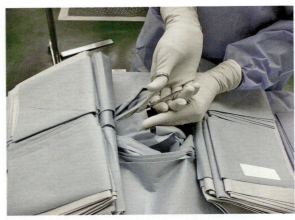

• **Fig. 32.34** A large drape is fenestrated by cutting a cross in the center of the drape to accommodate the limb.

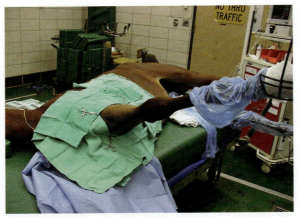

• **Fig. 32.32** The area proximal to the surgery site is draped off with sterile hand towels.

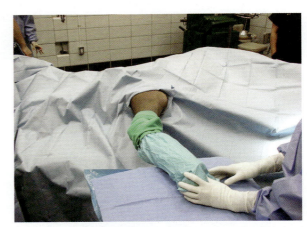

• **Fig. 32.35** To drape a limb for orthopedic surgery, the limb is placed through a fenestrated drape.

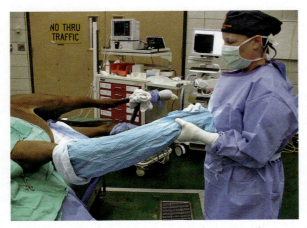

• **Fig. 32.33** During draping of the horse's limb for surgery, the surgeon or assistant grasps the limb with a sterile, impervious orthopedic stockinette.

TECHNICIAN NOTE

Any instrument that becomes contaminated during surgery is immediately removed from the surgical table. Replacements should be at hand in the event of contamination.

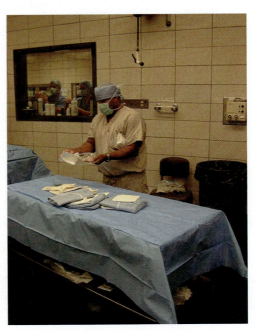

• **Fig. 32.36** An OR technician setting up the instrument table for equine surgery.

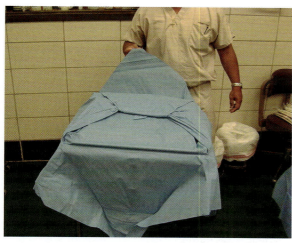

• **Fig. 32.37** Preparing for equine surgery. The OR technician opens the outer wrap of the instrument pack. One member of the surgical team will aseptically open the inner wrap and move the pack onto the instrument table.

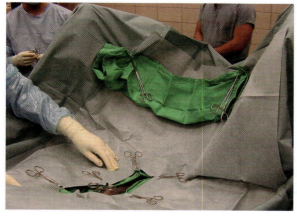

• **Fig. 32.38** A pouch is made from a sterile folded hand towel and is clamped to the surgery drape by nonpenetrating clamps between the horse's hindlimbs to hold the suction hose and cautery line.

Tissue Handling Techniques

Surgical manipulation of tissue in the horse is similar to that in the small animal; the differences are discussed in the section that follows.

Hollow Organ Surgery

Surgical procedures involving hollow organs, especially intestinal structures, are complicated in the horse because of the sheer size, weight, and length of the intestinal tract. The small intestine, for example, is more than 80 feet in length. The large intestine contains many pounds of ingesta, creating a problem during manipulation, and the risk of the intestine tearing and ultimately contaminating the abdominal cavity is high. Thus surgical assistants must be both strong and careful when handling the large intestine (colon) (Fig. 32.40). If the contents from the large colon are to be evacuated, a colon tray is positioned alongside the horse and draped with sterile impervious drapes. The large colon is placed onto the tray away from the abdominal opening, allowing the colon to be

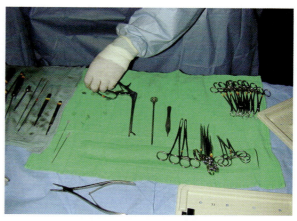

• **Fig. 32.39** The most frequently used instruments are placed closest to the surgeon in front of the instrument pack on a hand towel for easier access.

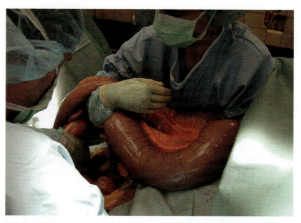

• **Fig. 32.40** During abdominal surgery, the large intestines must be carefully handled during exploration of the abdominal cavity. In this photo, the large colon is being cradled by the surgical assistant.

evacuated without risk of contaminating the abdominal cavity (Fig. 32.41). The surgical assistant must maintain the large colon on the tray during the evacuation process so that it is not unintentionally pulled back into the abdominal cavity. If a small intestinal resection is performed in a horse, the segment intestine is isolated from the rest of the abdominal cavity with laparotomy sponges and impervious drapes. In a coordinated effort between the surgeon and the surgical assistant, the small intestine must be kept properly orientated on the table, and the segments must be kept in check during intestinal resection and anastomosis to maintain their proper positioning for the surgeon during closure and suturing of the enterotomy site. Any instruments that come in contact with the ingesta should be removed from the surgical table and replaced with a sterile replacement. Immediately after closure of the intestine, the surgeon and the surgical assistant must change gloves and gowns for clean, sterile ones before the abdomen is closed.

The intestinal organs can easily become dehydrated and damaged if they are left outside the abdominal cavity for an extended period, creating areas for possible adhesion formation. The surgical assistant should ensure that the exposed intestinal segments be kept moist by applying sterile saline or iso-osmotic fluid via a pressurized fluid bag or bulb syringe (Fig. 32.42).

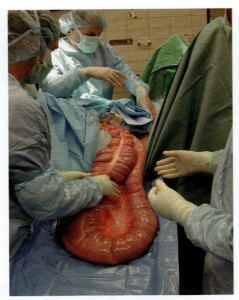

• **Fig. 32.41** The large colon is placed on the colon tray in preparation for an enterotomy and content evacuation. Note that the opening of the abdominal cavity is being draped off.

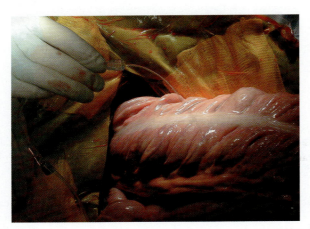

• **Fig. 32.42** A segment of the large colon of a horse. It is imperative that the surface of the intestines be kept moist to prevent drying and subsequent tissue damage.

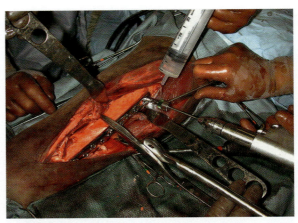

• **Fig. 32.43** Repair of a radial fracture in a foal. Note that the drill bit is bathed with sterile saline to reduce thermal damage to the bone. Surgeons are using transparent sterile gloves (note the powder on the hand to the right).

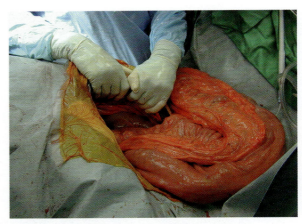

• **Fig. 32.44** Abdominal exploration on a horse. Retraction of the ventral abdominal wall is manually performed by an assistant.

> ### TECHNICIAN NOTE
> It is imperative that a glove that is torn during surgery be replaced immediately.

Bone and Joints

Aseptic technique is an absolute must during orthopedic surgeries because of the severe consequences of infection in bone and joints. Punctured or torn gloves from instruments or sharp ends of fractured bones should be replaced immediately. Surgical assistants will aid in proper tissue retraction and fragment reduction during fracture repair. Frequent irrigation of the tissue is vital during bone drilling (Fig. 32.43), because heat generated from drilling can cause thermal damage to bone, resulting in tissue necrosis. Blood should be actively removed from the surgical field via suction or blotting to allow visualization of affected structures. The surgical assistant is responsible for keeping the surgical table and instruments clean and in order.

> ### TECHNICIAN NOTE
> Constant irrigation of the drill bit is necessary while bone drilling is performed during fracture repair.

Retraction Techniques

Retraction techniques in equine surgery are similar to those in small animal surgery, except during abdominal surgery. Hohmann retractors are effective hand-held retractors for deep tissues surrounding equine bone. Because of the sheer size of the incision sites, it is difficult to maintain self-retaining retractors of any type; therefore the assistant may be called upon to physically retract the abdominal wall with their hands (Fig. 32.44).

Hemostasis

Blood loss in most surgical procedures of horses is not a major concern. Blood loss can become a concern during certain procedures, such as open sinusotomies, nasal septum resections, ovariectomies, castration, uterine trauma repair, and cesarean sections (C-sections). Sponges are avoided in abdominal surgery, because

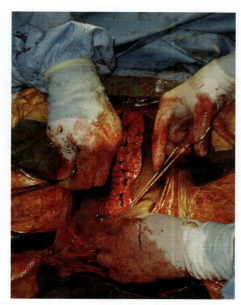

• **Fig. 32.45** Closure of a ventral abdominal incision. Large suture material is needed to maintain closure.

lost sponges cause severe inflammatory reactions, resulting in peritonitis and intra-abdominal adhesions that could impair the normal function of the equine GI tract and be life-threatening to the horse. Therefore suction is used to evacuate fluids from the abdominal surgery field. If large vessel hemorrhage occurs, the vein or the artery is clamped and ligated with suture material. With small vessel abdominal bleeding, it is common to apply hemostats in combination with electrocautery to fuse the vessel walls together.

Suture Materials Used in Horses

Often, the required sutures are discussed before surgery. It is common practice for the surgical assistant to open the suture material and have it ready by arming a needle holder with needle and suture before it is requested by the surgeon. Strong, thick suture material is required during equine surgeries because of the animal's large size. For closure of abdominal organs, a No. 2 to No. 0 absorbable material is commonly used. Closure of the ventral abdominal wall of a horse requires at least a No. 2 or a No. 3 absorbable suture material (Fig. 32.45). PDS and Vicryl are commonly used suture materials. For closure of the subcutaneous space, a No. 0 absorbable suture material often is used. No. 0 or No. 2 to No. 0 nonabsorbable material (nylon or Prolene) is used for apposition of the skin; however, skin staples are also commonly used. In most cases, suture material with swaged needles is used to save time and improve efficiency.

Acknowledgments

The authors and publisher wish to acknowledge the contribution of Susanne K. Lauer to previous editions of this chapter. The authors also wish to acknowledge the veterinary technicians who assisted in the preparation of this chapter.

Recommended Readings

Auer JA, Stick JA. *Equine Surgery*. 4th ed. Philadelphia, PA: Saunders; 2012.

Colville T, Bassert JM. *Clinical Anatomy and Physiology for Veterinary Technicians*. 3rd ed. St. Louis, MO: Mosby; 2016.

Evans HE, Christenson GC. *Miller's Anatomy of the Dog*. 3rd ed. Philadelphia, PA: Saunders; 1993.

Fossum TW. *Small Animal Surgery*. 4th ed. St. Louis, MO: Mosby; 2013.

Sonsthagen TF. *Veterinary Instruments and Equipment, a Pocket Guide*. 3rd ed. St. Louis, MO: Mosby; 2014.

Tracy DL. *Small Animal Surgical Nursing*. 3rd ed. St. Louis, MO: Mosby; 2000.

33

Small Animal Surgical Nursing

NANETTE WALKER SMITH

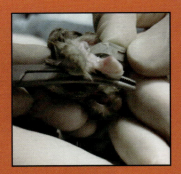

CHAPTER OUTLINE

LEARNING OBJECTIVES

When you have completed this chapter, you will be able to:

1. Pronounce, spell, and define all key terms in the chapter.
2. Regarding surgical preparation and animal positioning:
   - Describe the perioperative responsibilities of the veterinary technician.
   - Describe indications and use of prophylactic antibiotics.
   - Describe signs of blood loss in the postoperative patient.
   - Discuss concerns related to hypothermia in perioperative patients and be able to manage it.
   - Evaluate surgical incisions for complications and be able to remove skin sutures or staples.
3. Understand restraint of the anesthetized patient for surgical procedures.
4. Differentiate between elective and nonelective surgeries.
5. List and describe perioperative considerations for commonly listed surgical procedures.
6. List considerations related to client education for discharged surgical patients.

KEY TERMS

Abdominocentesis
Anastomosis
Arthrodesis
Capillary refill time
Celiotomy
Cellulitis
Cystotomy
Dehiscence
Enterotomy
Evisceration
Gastrotomy
Hydrometra
Ileus

Intussusception
Mucometra
Onychectomy
Orchidectomy
Ostectomy
Osteochondrosis
Ovariohysterectomy
Pseudocyesis
Pyometra
Seroma
Strangulation
Thoracocentesis
Urethrostomy

Introduction

Duties of the veterinary technician include appropriate animal restraint; sample collection and diagnostic evaluation; administration of sedation, anesthesia, and pain medication; instrument preparation; operating room (OR) preparation; appropriate patient preparation and positioning for surgery; aseptic handling of patients and instruments; patient monitoring; direct surgical assistance; patient recovery; and securing of the OR. Many of these topics are covered within this text in more detail; readers should consult the index for specific chapters. This chapter focuses on familiarizing the veterinary technician with specific surgical procedures and relevant anatomy and highlighting technician responsibilities in the preoperative, intraoperative, and postoperative periods. A working knowledge of common surgical procedures will ensure proficiency in surgical assistance, decrease surgery time, enhance the flow of surgery, and improve patient care.

The veterinary technician's role in surgical nursing is an important part of patient management. Preoperative, intraoperative, and postoperative responsibilities should be considered for a successful outcome. The surgical candidate must undergo preoperative assessment, including a physical examination, laboratory evaluation, and appropriate patient preparation and positioning for surgery. The technician's responsibilities during surgery include patient monitoring and surgeon assistance. In the postoperative period, patient monitoring and supportive care are important for postoperative recovery and healing.

Preoperative Patient Assessment

The surgical candidate should undergo a complete preoperative assessment that is based on an understanding of the animal's primary problem so that specific needs can be met. Elective surgical procedures do not have the same demands as urgent surgical procedures. Nevertheless, a good patient history is important in all cases. Eating, drinking, urination, and defecation habits should be ascertained. An animal that has not been eating or drinking will likely require rehydration before anesthesia. Rehydration may necessitate blood or plasma transfusion because of the dilution of red blood cells that occurs with rehydration. However, fluids should not be withheld in an attempt to prevent anemia. Fasting requirements vary in accordance with age and condition of animal. The American Animal Hospital Association (AAHA) recommended in their 2012 *Anesthesia Guideline for Dogs and Cats* that animals up to 16 weeks of age should not be fasted longer than 4 hours before surgery. It has been suggested by other resources that healthy adult animals may be fasted 6 to 12 hours, with special attention paid to diabetic patients, which may or may not be fasted. If the animal has eaten on the day of scheduled surgery, the procedure may need to be delayed to decrease the risk of aspiration of stomach contents. Emergency surgeries will have to be performed whether the animal has eaten or not, but owners should be warned of the increased risk for aspiration. It is also important to know what medications the animal is receiving, including all prescriptions and over-the-counter supplementation that may be given in or with food, water, or other forms, because this may affect perioperative protocols for that patient. A history of previous medical concerns; sedative or anesthetic concerns, complications, or successes; and surgical procedures should be noted and brought to the attention of the surgeon and surgical team. Vaccination status should be ascertained. A young puppy

or kitten is best vaccinated 2 weeks before surgery rather than the day of surgery to minimize the effect of anesthesia on the immune response to immunization. Temperature, pulse rate and quality, respiration rate and character, capillary refill time, mucous membrane color, body weight, and demeanor should be assessed and recorded before surgery. Abnormalities should be brought to the attention of the surgeon.

Preanesthesia screening will depend on the animal's condition and the reason for surgery. Specifics of this are covered in Chapter 30. It is important to discuss with the surgeon what diagnostics are appropriate before surgery and to ensure that they are performed. Diagnostics may be best performed 1 or 2 days before surgery to allow the surgeon to evaluate the patient's status and establish preoperative and surgical protocols. Diagnostics might include blood work (i.e., packed cell volume [PCV], total plasma protein [TP] concentration, blood urea nitrogen [BUN] concentration, blood glucose concentration, complete blood count [CBC], complete biochemical analysis); heartworm test; blood gas analysis; electrocardiography (ECG); radiography; fecal analysis; and/or urinalysis.

Surgical Preparation and Animal Positioning

The veterinary technician should be familiar with the type of surgery to be performed so that patient preparation is adequate and is consistent with the surgeon's preferences, have all necessary equipment readily accessible, and confirm with the surgeon prior to surgery if any changes are needed. The OR should be clean, and anesthesia equipment checked for functionality and made ready for use. A heated circulating water blanket should be placed on the operating table, turned on, and covered with a towel so that it is warm by the time it is needed. Clean, designated, surgical hair clippers and skin cleansing solutions should be used for surgical preparation. Clipper blades and cleansing solutions used on general wounds should not be used to prepare a surgical site. If possible, clipping of hair and initial scrub should be performed in a separate prep room and the final sterile scrub performed in the surgical suite. Appropriate warming blankets should be placed over the patient before surgical draping (Fig. 33.1). The postoperative cage should be set up with appropriate warming equipment

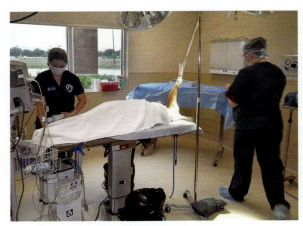

• **Fig. 33.1** This dog is lying on a heated surgical table and has been appropriately covered with a warming air blanket and a towel over the blanket to provide additional warmth during surgery. All areas of the body not involved in the surgical field can be covered.

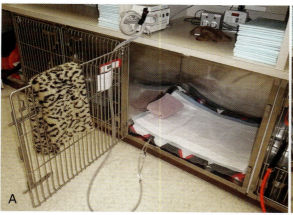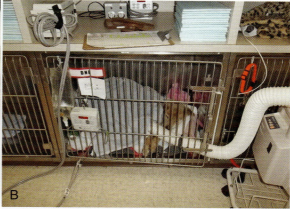

• **Fig. 33.2** (A) This cage has been set up for a postoperative patient. The cage heat is turned on, and adequate bedding is provided. Note the blanket hanging over the door, ready to be placed over the patient at recovery. (B) When this animal was placed in the cage for recovery, a warming air blanket was close by and was immediately placed over the animal for additional heat support.

turned on (Fig. 33.2A and B) and ready to receive the patient postoperatively.

Inadequate animal preparation or inappropriate positioning can hinder surgical technique, increase risk of infection, and result in wasted time spent correcting deficiencies. Aseptic protocol should always be followed with patient preparation, draping, and surgical instrument handling. The hair should be liberally clipped around the surgical site and the skin cleansed appropriately (refer to Chapters 31 and 32).

> **TECHNICIAN NOTE**
>
> Inadequate surgical preparation can hinder surgical technique, increase the risk of infection, and result in prolonged anesthesia.

Perioperative Antibiotics

Prophylactic antibiotics are used to decrease the risk of infection in clean or clean-contaminated surgeries, but they will not eliminate surgical site infections. Use of antibiotics to treat an active infection after surgery is not "prophylactic" use and will not be discussed here. Antibiotics should not be given indiscriminately to animals undergoing surgery, because these agents have potential side effects and their use increases the cost of surgery. More important, indiscriminate use of antibiotics contributes to the development of resistant strains of bacteria that are difficult to treat (hospital "superbugs" such as methicillin-resistant *Staphylococcus aureus* [MRSA]).

> **TECHNICIAN NOTE**
>
> Antibiotics should never be given indiscriminately to animals undergoing surgery, because this contributes to the development of resistant strains of bacteria that are difficult to treat (hospital "superbugs" such as methicillin-resistant *Staphylococcus aureus* [MRSA]).

Indications for Prophylactic Antibiotics

• Operative time is longer than 90 minutes. Open surgical wounds are exposed to bacteria from the animal's skin, operative team, and air. The longer the wound is open, the higher the chance of infection. Prolonged anesthesia also increases the risk for infection, because the lungs are usually not inflating

as they would normally if the patient were awake (unless on a ventilator).
• The patient is immunosuppressed. Factors that suppress the immune system include immunosuppressive drugs (steroids), Cushing disease (hyperadrenocorticism), some cancers, chemotherapy or radiation therapy, and certain infections.
• A hollow viscus is to be entered (e.g., gastrointestinal [GI] tract, urinary bladder).
• Surgery site will be difficult to aseptically prepare (mouth, toe, or ear).
• Orthopedic implants are to be placed or a joint will be entered.
• The consequences of infection could be devastating (joint replacement and neurosurgery).
• Prophylactic antibiotics are not recommended for short, clean surgical procedures, such as simple mass removal or biopsy, ovariohysterectomy, and castration.

Therapeutic drug levels must be present in the wound fluid (serum and interstitial tissues) at the time of surgical incision or the antibiotic will be ineffective. They should be given at least 20 minutes before the surgical incision is made. Antibiotics given 3 or more hours before the procedure select for resistant bacteria and, when given more than 3 to 5 hours after the surgical incision has been made, will likely not be effective in preventing infection. There is no advantage in continuing antibiotics beyond 6 to 24 hours after surgery unless it is necessary to treat an active infection or if a break in sterile technique occurred during surgery. The appropriate antibiotic would be effective against the potential contaminant (usually broad spectrum), achieve good tissue concentrations, and cause minimal side effects. The surgeon is responsible for selecting the appropriate antibiotic.

Monitoring

Intraoperative and postoperative monitoring is critical for proper surgical nursing care. Chapter 30 covers anesthetic monitoring in detail. Some important components of patient monitoring as they pertain to surgery and recovery will be discussed here.

During surgery, maintaining a surgical plane of anesthesia is crucial. Careful monitoring during this time and afterward can alert the observer to potentially fatal complications. Anesthesia and surgery can result in several potential problems, including blood loss, hypothermia, pain, and cardiac and respiratory issues.

The technician must be prepared to address issues as the need arises. Monitoring should involve a series of evaluations. Decisions regarding complications and treatment are based on a group of signs consistent with a problem and abnormal trend in values—not just one abnormality. The postoperative phase is a critical transition period from general anesthesia to consciousness, and monitoring should be continued until the animal is safely extubated, normothermic, and responsive. Complete reporting during anesthetic procedures is also helpful for future patient procedures to avoid complications or repeat of unsuccessful encounters.

Patient monitoring does not stop once the animal has recovered from anesthesia. As long as the animal is hospitalized, evaluation of vital signs, behavior, appetite, and the surgical incision should be performed on a continuous basis. Depending on the status of the animal, daily or more frequent observation is performed and recorded, with abnormalities reported to the surgeon.

> **TECHNICIAN NOTE**
>
> A single abnormal vital sign does not necessarily identify a significant clinical problem. All indicators (temperature, pulse, respiration, capillary refill time [CRT]/mucous membranes) should be evaluated serially to detect a trend in the animal's condition. This trend will determine the severity of the postoperative problem and will likely dictate appropriate treatment.

Blood Loss

Many procedures can result in blood loss as a complication, or blood loss may be caused by the inherent nature of the animal's disease. A baseline PCV and TP should always be assessed for anemia before surgery and values reviewed, along with any additional blood work, with the surgeon. If substantial blood loss occurred during surgery, PCV and TP should also be assessed serially after surgery. It can be difficult to determine whether an animal has lost a substantial amount of blood immediately postoperative, because a recovering animal that is in pain can exhibit similar clinical signs such as continued hypothermia, a drop in body temperature, rapid heart rate with weak peripheral pulses, rapid respiratory rate, and/or pale or white mucous membranes. Other signs include incisional swelling or oozing of blood, abdominal enlargement if intraabdominal hemorrhage occurs, and/or dyspnea with decreased lung sounds if intrathoracic hemorrhage occurs. Abnormalities should be reported to the surgeon immediately. Frequent recording of the patient's clinical signs is important to assess change. Changes in PCV and TP may not occur immediately with blood loss, and these tests may have to be repeated every few hours to document abnormalities or to assess continued blood loss. Note that it is not unusual for PCV and TP to drop up to 10% as a result of anesthesia and surgery, even when no major blood loss has occurred.

> **PUT INTO PRACTICE**
>
> Someone once said, "You can paint a wall with a tablespoon of blood." While not true, you should be attentive to the amount of blood loss experienced by small patients.

Besides PCV and TP determination, abdominocentesis (aspiration of fluid from the abdomen), thoracocentesis (aspiration of fluid from the thoracic cavity), or fine-needle aspiration beneath the incision can be performed when hemorrhage is suspected. If the sampled fluid has a PCV nearly equal to the systemic PCV and clinical signs are consistent with hemorrhage, the index of suspicion should be high. Treatment strategies include crystalloid

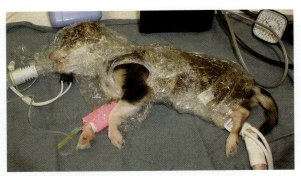

• **Fig. 33.3** One method of heat retention during surgery is wrapping the animal in plastic. This works well for small dogs and cats.

fluid bolus, colloidal fluid administration, blood transfusion, pressure bandage, and reoperation to stop the source of hemorrhage. The treatment of choice depends on the animal's status and ability to maintain a stable condition. Readers should review the clinical signs and treatment strategies for various types of fluid therapy and shock discussed in Chapters 24 and 25.

Hypothermia

Hypothermia is defined as a subnormal body temperature. Once an animal is anesthetized, its body temperature begins to drop. It is important to monitor body temperature throughout general anesthesia and during recovery. All anesthetized animals should be actively warmed to help maintain body temperature. An open body cavity, large clipped area, and application of fluid lavage hastens hypothermia as a result of an increase in exposed surface area and evaporative cooling. Mechanisms of active warming include placing animals on heated circulating water blankets; wrapping paws and the body in plastic wrap to prevent heat loss (Fig. 33.3); wrapping warm water bottles (or gloves filled with warm water) in a towel and placing them next to the animal; covering areas not involved in the surgical procedure with an insulated blanket; using actively warmed cages and surgery tables; and using a warmair blanket (Bair Hugger, Arizant Healthcare, Inc., Eden Prairie, MN) on areas not involved in the surgical procedure. Heat lamps and electric heating pads are not recommended, because they can cause thermal burns caused by the concentration of heat in an anesthetized animal that cannot respond to painful stimuli or move away (Fig. 33.4). Unless a warm air blanket is used, all heat sources should be applied with a towel between the heat source and the animal. If the body temperature rises above normal during the procedure (although rare), the heat source can be turned off.

After surgery, the animal is placed in a warm area to recover, and any necessary heat sources are used. If the patient is severely hypothermic, a warm air blanket and/or a warm water bath can be used to raise the temperature quickly (Fig. 33.5). Body temperature should show a steady rise as the animal recovers. When the animal's temperature approaches 99°F to 100°F, heating sources should be discontinued; however, the animal should be kept covered and body temperature re-evaluated within an hour and then periodically to ensure it returns to and remains normal. Heat should be reapplied if the animal's body temperature begins to drop after heat sources are removed.

Pain

Intraoperative and postoperative pain assessment is important for animal well-being. Pain management is discussed in Chapter 29

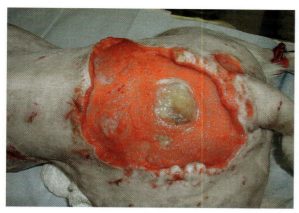

• **Fig. 33.4** The area of denuded skin over the rump of this dog is a result of a thermal burn sustained from an electric heating pad used to maintain body temperature during ovariohysterectomy.

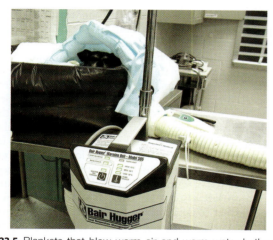

• **Fig. 33.5** Blankets that blow warm air and warm water baths can be used to bring the body temperature up quickly. Note that the dog is placed under the blue hot air blanket in a well-constructed water bath. A large container is filled with warm water and is covered with thick plastic and a towel. The dog or the cat is placed on the towel in the container and is allowed to sink down into the warm water, with the plastic preventing soaking. The animal must be monitored carefully to prevent accidental puncture of the plastic and drowning.

and will be briefly addressed in this chapter. Pain should be assessed preoperatively, perioperatively, and postoperatively. Proper preoperative pain management sets the stage for a smoother anesthetic procedure and recovery and for reduction of preoperative fear, anxiety, and stress that the patient may be experiencing. If an incision is made during surgery, the animal is going to experience pain. It is up to the veterinary technician and the surgeon to decide how much pain a particular procedure might cause. Painful procedures include fracture repair, amputation, declawing, joint surgery, and any major abdominal procedure. Moderately painful procedures include minor abdominal procedures (spaying, cystotomy) and simple body wall hernia repair. Mildly painful procedures might include simple removal of a mass or biopsy. Use of a pain scale that assesses a combination for parameters, such as vital signs, behavior, mobility, and sensitivity to touching the incision, can help the veterinary team determine the need for relief of pain. Pain medication should be administered at dosing intervals appropriate for the medication to keep the animal comfortable,

not on an "as-needed" basis, which implies that medications are not given unless pain is present.

Incision Evaluation

The surgical wound should be inspected visually and palpated daily (see Chapter 27 for detailed information on wounds and healing). The surgical incision may be covered with an adhesive or a wrap bandage for the first few days after surgery to keep it clean, prevent contact with the hospital environment, and absorb seepage; however, bandage care and frequent checks must be conducted to avoid trauma to surgical wound under the bandage, such as excess seepage, infection, dehiscence, and so on. Ointments and creams (even antibiotic topicals) should not be placed on the incision, because they can cause irritation, and components of the ointment can delay wound healing.

Abnormalities that can occur in the early postoperative period (1 to 3 days) include redness, swelling, drainage, and **dehiscence** (wound breakdown). An incision should be evaluated with respect to the type of surgical procedure performed. Elective operations, such as ovariohysterectomy and castration, can be expected to produce mild redness and swelling, with no drainage from the incision site (Fig. 33.6A and B). However, if the wound was contaminated (e.g., laceration, perianal wound) or if surgical exposure was extensive, the incision is expected to be somewhat swollen, reddened, and warm to the touch and may have mild to moderate drainage in the first 24 to 48 hours postoperatively. Swelling secondary to surgical trauma will usually resolve within 3 to 7 days after surgery. However, a **seroma** (serum accumulation under the incision) or a hematoma (blood accumulation under the incision) may persist for weeks.

It is surprising that most animals do not lick or chew at the surgical incision. Animals usually lick or chew at the incision only if the incision is irritating. Contributors to incision irritation include sutures placed too tight, traumatic tissue handling, suture reaction, tension on the suture line, clipper burn, prepping irritation (clipper burn and solution reaction), incision infection, and seroma formation. Only rarely will an animal chew the sutures just because it can. However, if an animal begins to traumatize the incision by licking or scratching, an Elizabethan collar, bandage, neck brace, T-shirt, and/or chemical restraint should be used to protect the incision and the root cause of the irritation addressed.

A seroma can form if extensive surgical dissection occurred beneath the incision, tissue planes could not be or were not adequately closed, or excessive motion occurs at the incision site. A seroma formation is recognized as a localized area of fluctuant swelling that is not usually painful or warm to the touch (Fig. 33.7). Seromas usually resolve without treatment in a few weeks. Warm compresses, hydrotherapy, and bandaging may aid in resolution. Seromas are not typically drained because of the increased chance for infection and decrease in self-resolution; however, if the seroma is very large and/or causing impairment, drainage is warranted. Drainage should be performed aseptically, and an active, closed drain should be placed. It is important to keep animals calm

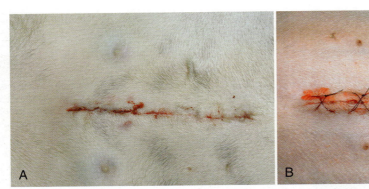

• **Fig. 33.6** These photographs were taken 4 hours after surgery. (A) A celiotomy incision after routine ovariohysterectomy. (B) A celiotomy incision after severe traction on the skin during surgery for exposure. Note the minimal redness, swelling, and drainage from the incision in (A) compared with the incision in (B).

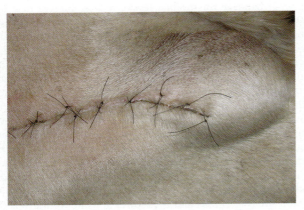

• **Fig. 33.7** Note the swelling on the right beneath the incision; the diagnosis is a seroma. The swelling did not elicit pain on palpation, and the dog's vital signs were normal.

during the postoperative period to decrease the chance of seroma formation. Hematomas are treated similarly; however, because cellular components are present, there is an increased infectious risk. Thus following aseptic techniques is even more important.

If incision swelling occurs 4 to 6 days postoperatively, is warm to the touch, is associated with an elevated body temperature, or is reddened and/or draining, the possibility of infection or **cellulitis** (infection along tissue planes, generally without large pockets of fluid) must be considered (Fig. 33.8). Abscess or infection must be treated with drainage, warm compresses, and systemic antibiotics. Cellulitis is typically treated with warm compresses and systemic antibiotics but is not drained. Aseptic aspiration of fluid or tissues beneath the incision should be performed for cytology and culture before empirical antibiotic therapy is started, where possible. Some infected incisions need to be flushed and managed with an active, closed suction drain or be left open (see Chapter 27 for details on infected and open wound management).

Wound dehiscence is the separation of the layers of an incision or wound. Early recognition is imperative in any wound, especially in abdominal and thoracic incisions, because of their proximity to multiple organs. The most common factors that contribute to wound dehiscence include use of inappropriate suture or suturing technique to close a wound, tension on the incision line, incision infection, seroma formation, and disease and/or drug therapy leading to delayed wound healing. Incision complications and/or the status of the animal may also play a role in surgical wound dehiscence. Rarely, an animal self-mutilates an incision, causing dehiscence. It is important to promptly apply a protective device if licking or chewing at the incision is noted and work with the surgeon to investigate and resolve the reason for the self-mutilation.

Early detection of incision problems is of paramount importance to prevent more serious complications. If dehiscence is suspected, the reason for dehiscence should be ascertained and the surgeon alerted. The technician can clean the area around the wound and provide a sterile covering and an Elizabethan collar to prevent further trauma until it can be assessed by the surgeon. Complete dehiscence of an abdominal wound can result in **evisceration** (exposure) of the abdominal organs, with subsequent contamination and infection. Complete dehiscence of a thoracic wound will result in pneumothorax (air within the chest, causing collapse of the lungs), a problem that may result in sudden death. Animals should be treated immediately if either of these situations is noted.

Suture Removal

Suture removal is commonly performed by the veterinary technician. The procedure is usually performed 10 to 14 days after surgery, because this is the approximate time needed for the wound to begin to strengthen (see Chapter 27 for wound suturing and Chapter 32 for suture types). If internal sutures were placed in the dermis in addition to external sutures, suture removal can be performed in 5 to 7 days, because the internal suture layer will hold the incision closed while healing continues. The incision should be inspected carefully for adequate healing before removal. A healed incision is usually confluent, slightly raised, whitish in color, and has no gaps between skin edges (Fig. 33.9). Incisions

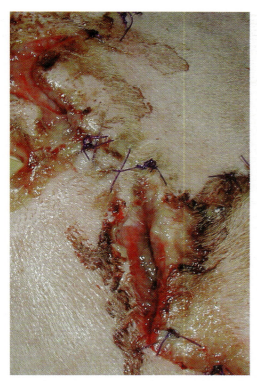

• **Fig. 33.8** Incisional infection is recognized by drainage, redness, swelling, fever, dehiscence, and/or abscess formation. Note the purulent discharge and partial dehiscence of the incision.

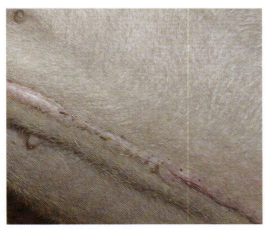

• **Fig. 33.9** Healed incision, 12 days after surgery. Note that the incision is not red, swollen, or draining. The skin edges are apposed, and the scar is slightly raised.

that are swollen, draining, or reddened or display obvious separation should be inspected by the surgeon before suture removal.

Skin sutures are usually easy to remove when the animal is in a calm state. Suture scissors are simple to use and allow removal with minimal discomfort. The suture should be grasped with thumb forceps. Gentle traction is placed on the suture, and the suture is cut near the skin surface (Fig. 33.10). The suture is manually pulled out of the skin after cutting. If metal staples were placed, a skin staple remover should be used to allow removal with minimal discomfort. The staple remover is placed under the staple according to manufacturer instructions (Fig. 33.11A) and squeezed to bend the staple ends up and out of the skin (see Fig. 33.11B).

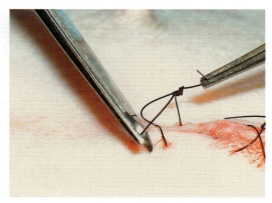

• **Fig. 33.10** Suture removal. The suture is grasped with forceps or fingers and is gently tensioned. It is cut with suture scissors near the skin and then is pulled with slow, steady traction until completely removed.

Bandage Care

If a bandage was placed on a limb, that limb should be monitored carefully. In general, bandages should be kept clean and dry, the bandaged area should be checked twice daily for complications, and the bandage changed at intervals designated by the surgeon. Bandages covering open wounds will need to be changed more frequently than other types of bandages, because wounds can drain excessively, causing serum to seep through the bandage and extend to the external environment. This is called *strike-through* (Fig. 33.12), a condition that must be prevented to circumvent wound infection, because bacteria have better access to a wound or incision when they can migrate through the moisture of a wet bandage. Bandage placement and care are discussed in more detail in Chapter 27.

Drain Care

Drains are placed to collect fluid under a wound or surgical incision. They are often placed when large amounts of tissue are resected (mammary chains, some amputations, large skin masses) or when a large amount of drainage is expected (i.e., contaminated or infected wound). An Elizabethan collar should be fitted on the animal to prevent premature removal of the drain or drain trauma. Active drains (drains that are sealed to the environment and actively collect fluid from the wound into a reservoir) should be emptied as needed (Fig. 33.13A). Passive drains, which are drains providing an exit port for fluid to the external environment, are not ideal because of the risk for ascending bacterial infection and the difficulty in their maintenance; they should be covered and changed frequently to prevent strike-through (see Fig. 33.13B). Drains are removed when the amount of drainage has substantially decreased; some minor drainage because of tissue irritation caused by the drain is to be expected as long as a drain is in place.

> **TECHNICIAN NOTE**
>
> Some minimal drainage because of tissue irritation caused by the drain is to be expected as long as a drain is in place.

Restraint

Animal restraint is important for appropriate surgical technique, patient safety, and patient comfort. The animal's activity should be well controlled after surgery to minimize complications, with

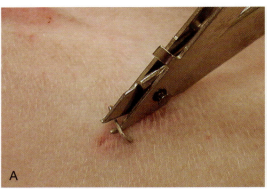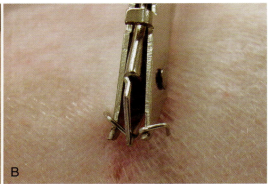

• **Fig. 33.11** Staple removal. Staple remover is used. (A) Staple remover is slipped under the staple. (B) Staple remover is closed, causing the staple to be folded at its midsection and the teeth on either end of the staple to be dislodged from the skin.

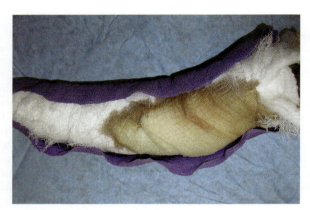

• **Fig. 33.12** Strike-through. Note the red-tinged fluid seeping through the bandage from the wound bed.

the length and degree of confinement depending on the type of procedure performed. Animals undergoing routine sterilization or simple mass removal usually require 10 to 14 days of restricted activity, whereas animals undergoing orthopedic surgery will likely require 6 to 8 weeks of confinement. No animal should be allowed to roam free immediately after surgery to prevent trauma to healing tissues. Elizabethan collars, neck braces, bandages, shirts, and socks can also be used to prevent self-trauma. Cages, crates, fencing, small rooms, leashes, and braces/casts may be appropriate to restrict motion. Refer to Chapters 6, 28, and 30 for more information on restraint devices and drugs used for sedation and restraint.

Noxious-tasting agents are used to prevent animals from licking or chewing on the sutures, but they must be used with discretion. Commonly used substances include Bandguard Cream (Schering-Plough, Kenilworth, NJ), Bitter Apple (Grannick's Bitter Apple Co., Norwalk, CT), Tabasco sauce, and various preparations designed to prevent thumb sucking in children. The agent can be impregnated into the bandage material, and some can be placed directly on the skin around the incision. These agents should never be placed directly on the incision, because they can burn, irritate the incision, and possibly delay wound healing. Caution should be used when any chemical is directly placed on the skin, because a reaction can occur, even if it is labeled for dermatologic usage. If an animal is licking, biting, or chewing at a wound or bandage, a determination should be made as to the source of irritation, rather than just applying a noxious agent. Assessment of the area for irritation, pain management, behavior characteristics, and so on should all be considered regarding self-mutilation.

Common Surgical Procedures

The veterinary technician must have a working knowledge of the common surgical procedures to properly prepare an animal preoperatively, act as an efficient surgical assistant, manage immediate and long-term postoperative care, and be able to clearly converse with pet owners about a performed procedure. The remainder of this chapter reviews common small animal surgical procedures performed in veterinary practice. A brief description of the procedure, with emphasis on the role of the veterinary technician, is given. Details on aseptic technique, surgical site preparation, gowning, and gloving are discussed in other sections of this book and are covered in Chapters 31 and 32.

> **TECHNICIAN NOTE**
>
> The veterinary technician must have a working knowledge of common surgical procedures to properly prepare the animal for surgery, act as an efficient surgical assistant, have discussions with the owner, and manage immediate and long-term postoperative care.

Elective Versus Nonelective Surgery

Surgical procedures are divided into *elective* and *nonelective procedures*. Elective procedures are performed at the veterinarian's and the owner's convenience, usually in healthy animals. Spaying, neutering, and declawing are examples. Some procedures must be done to improve the animal's quality of life but are not necessarily urgent; these include stifle stabilization for cranial cruciate ligament rupture, correction of patellar luxation, and tumor resection in cancers. For these procedures, if animals are not ideal candidates for surgery at the time of presentation, surgery can be delayed. Nonelective surgical procedures must be done urgently. These are usually emergency procedures performed on compromised animals.

Tail Docking and Dewclaw Removal in Puppies

Definition

Tail docking refers to partial amputation (removal) of the tail. *Dewclaw removal* is amputation of the vestigial first digit on the forelimbs and hindlimbs.

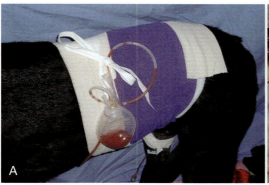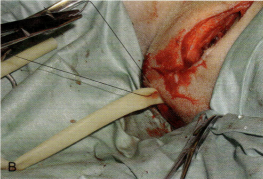

• **Fig. 33.13** Drains. (A) Active drains actively suck fluid from the wound bed into a sealed reservoir and are preferred over passive drains. (B) Passive drains are placed under incisions and just provide surface area for fluid to drain from the wound with gravitational forces. They are more prone to ascending infection and are more difficult to manage. In photo (B), the wound is being closed over a rubber drain *(yellow)*. The incision and the drain will be bandaged afterward.

Indications

Tail docking and dewclaw removal in young puppies are performed primarily for aesthetic reasons and to meet breed standards. Tails are docked and dewclaws removed according to breed standards set forth by the American Kennel Club. For Great Pyrenees and Newfoundland breeds, the presence of dewclaws is necessary for proper show quality. For hunting dogs, dewclaws are removed to prevent trauma during hunting.

> **TECHNICIAN NOTE**
>
> Hunting dogs may have dewclaws removed for practical reasons, such as trauma that can occur when running through thick brush. Other breeds, such as the Great Pyrenees and Newfoundland breeds, will not be of show quality without their dewclaws.

Preoperative Considerations

The dam can get upset as puppies are removed from her presence for these procedures and may even get aggressive. Care must be taken during removal of puppies from the dam and their replacement. If the dam becomes overly upset, it may be necessary to separate her from the puppies during the procedure.

Tail docking and dewclaw removal should be performed during the first week of life (age 3 to 5 days). It must be remembered that puppies of this age are immunogenetically naïve; therefore aseptic technique is paramount to a positive outcome. It is important to perform the procedures in an area where the puppies will not be exposed to high concentrations of infectious agents.

Technique and Intraoperative Considerations

The puppy should be cradled in the palms of both hands and the surgical site prepared by using aseptic technique. The limb or tail is extended toward the surgeon for improved accessibility.

Tail Docking

The desired length of remaining tail is marked, and the skin of the tail is retracted cranially (toward the base of the tail). The tail is amputated with a pair of sharp scissors, bleeding is controlled with electrocautery or pressure, and the skin is released, allowing it to retract over the exposed bone. One simple interrupted absorbable suture is placed to appose the skin edges, or the edges are glued with tissue adhesive.

Dewclaw Removal

The puppy is cradled in the palm of one hand, and the extremity is extended with the other hand. Sharp scissors are used to amputate the claw. Hemorrhage is controlled with electrocautery or pressure. The skin edges may be left to heal by secondary intention or apposed with one absorbable suture.

If a surgical laser is used to remove the tail and the dewclaws, the technician should ensure that appropriate equipment and eye protection are available for the surgical team and that the surgery site is not prepared with alcohol. Plenty of saline-soaked sponges should be available to cover exposed areas close to the laser beam, instruments, and the surgeon's fingers to absorb extraneous laser energy and prevent iatrogenic laser burns. It is best to use instruments approved for laser surgery to prevent reflected laser beams from causing damage. A second technician must be available to vacuum away the emitted plume (smoke) from the laser because it is harmful to humans and animals.

Postoperative Considerations

Puppies should be returned to the dam as soon as hemorrhage is controlled. During the week after surgery, the tail and the feet should be monitored daily for bleeding, drainage, redness, and swelling. The suture remains until it is absorbed or licked out by the mother. Complications are not expected after tail docking or dewclaw removal but might include hemorrhage and infection. If too much skin is removed during amputation of the tail, some animals may have chronic wound healing problems and bone exposure at the amputation site. Revision of the surgical site may be necessary to correct the problem.

Tail Docking and Dewclaw Removal in the Adult Dog

Tail docking and dewclaw removal should ideally be done within the first week of life if performed for aesthetic purposes. Occasionally, these procedures are necessary in adult dogs.

Indications

Indications for tail docking or dewclaw removal in the adult dog include aesthetics, trauma, infection, and neoplasia.

Preoperative Considerations

One must consider the reason for tail or claw amputation before prepping the animal and initiation of the procedure. If the procedure is done to treat cancer, the appropriate amount of skin must be prepared before surgery to obtain acceptable tumor-free margins. Removed tissue will have to be fixed in formalin to submit for biopsy. If trauma is the reason for the procedure, the animal may have to be stabilized before anesthesia can be safely performed. If amputation is performed as treatment for infection, the veterinary technician should have culture swabs available for the surgeon to collect samples for possible identification and sensitivity testing.

Technique and Intraoperative Considerations for Dewclaw Removal in the Adult Dog

The animal must be placed under general anesthesia. The surgical site is clipped and prepared by using aseptic technique. The surgeon makes an elliptical incision at the base of the dewclaw. The dewclaw is dissected free and is transected at the carpometacarpal joint in the front paw or at the tarsometatarsal joint in the hind paw. Hemorrhage is controlled with suture, electrocautery, laser, and/or direct pressure. If a surgical laser is used, one should take the same precautions as those noted under tail docking and dewclaw removal in puppies. The skin edges are apposed with suture. The paw is usually bandaged to control postoperative swelling and bleeding.

Technique and Intraoperative Considerations for Tail Amputation in the Adult Dog

The tail should be clipped and hung from an intravenous (IV) stand or another secure object. The skin should be prepared using aseptic technique. If the tail is to be amputated near the base, the rump adjacent to the tail base must also be clipped and aseptically prepared. If the base of the tail is not to be included in the surgical field, before the animal is draped for surgery, a tourniquet may be placed at the base of the tail to help control hemorrhage. The surgeon can use a sterile tourniquet otherwise. Although a tourniquet should not stay in place longer than 90 minutes in humans, there is no particularly safe time established for animals. The surgeon should be alerted after 30 minutes and then 60 minutes so that the tourniquet can be released for a time and then repositioned to improve the tissue environment.

The tail is amputated at the desired location with a skin incision and disarticulation of the caudal vertebra at the appropriate site. The skin incision is made 1 or 2 cm distal to the expected amputation site to ensure adequate skin coverage of the stump. Blood vessels are identified and ligated. Skin edges are sutured over the remaining vertebrae and the tourniquet removed.

Postoperative Considerations

Surgical sites should be monitored for hemorrhage, swelling, drainage, redness, evidence of self-trauma, and dehiscence. Elizabethan collars should be placed on animals that attempt to traumatize the surgical site. Bandages placed on the foot should be maintained as previously discussed and as directed in Chapters 27 and 32. Skin sutures are removed in 7 to 14 days, depending on how the incision was closed. Pain medication is generally needed for 4 to 5 days after the procedure. Complications are rare for these procedures, even in adult animals.

Feline Onychectomy

Definition

Onychectomy (declawing) is the removal of the claw and its associated distal phalanx on each digit.

Indications

Onychectomy is an elective procedure done to prevent cats from scratching owners and household items. Declawing is generally recommended on the front feet only, because this does not significantly impair the cat's ability to climb trees or defend itself from intruders. Onychectomy is often performed at the same time as castration or ovariohysterectomy.

Preoperative Considerations

Onychectomy is a painful procedure. Preoperative analgesics should be administered.

Technique and Intraoperative Considerations

The cat is placed under general anesthesia. The nails are left long to facilitate nail manipulation during the procedure. The feet are surgically scrubbed but need not be clipped unless the cat is a long-haired breed. A digital nerve block (e.g., bupivacaine) for pain should be administered at this time for effective pain control. If laser is to be used during the procedure, alcohol should not be used to prepare the toes, because it is flammable. A tourniquet should be placed loosely over the foot just distal to the elbow to prevent nerve damage before aseptic preparation and tightened to help control hemorrhage when the surgeon is ready to perform the procedure. The radial nerve is more superficial just proximal to the elbow and can be permanently damaged if the tourniquet is tightened over that area. The tourniquet should be managed as discussed for tail amputation. The surgeon will squeeze the distal limb to help decrease pooling of blood (Fig. 33.14).

Three techniques can be used to remove the claws: (1) use of the Rescoe (nail trimmer), (2) the scalpel blade, and (3) carbon dioxide laser techniques. All are effective means of performing the procedure. In the nail trimmer technique (Rescoe), a guillotine-type nail trimmer is positioned snugly onto the dorsal surface of the toe between the second and third phalanx (Fig. 33.15). During positioning of the nail trimmer, the claw should be pulled cranially. A minimal amount of skin should be excised. The cutting edge of the nail trimmer is positioned at the cranial edge of the footpad. As the cutting edge is advanced, the pad is moved caudally, while the nail is rotated dorsally and caudally. The third phalanx is then excised by the nail trimmer, taking care not to cut the footpad, and the procedure is repeated. A portion of the third phalanx is usually left behind with this technique, but the entire germinal layer is removed to prevent regrowth of the nail. A dedicated pair of Rescoe trimmers should be used, and the blade should be kept clean and sharp to minimize infection and excess trauma.

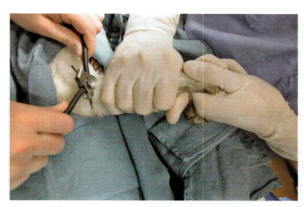

• **Fig. 33.14** Declawing. The surgeon or another assistant is squeezing the distal limb before the tourniquet is tightened to help move blood out of the distal limb. The tourniquet should always be placed distal to the elbow *(as shown)* rather than proximal to the elbow to help prevent permanent radial nerve damage.

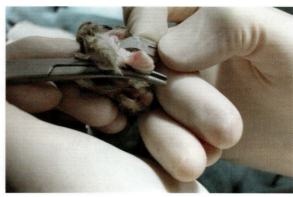

• **Fig. 33.16** Declawing. The scalpel blade was positioned dorsally between the second and third phalanges and the dorsal joint capsule severed, along with the collateral ligaments. The blade is subsequently manipulated dorsally to avoid cutting the digital pad, located ventral to the blade.

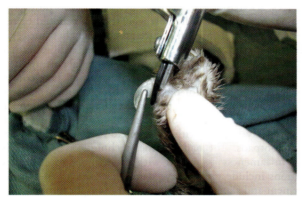

• **Fig. 33.15** Declawing. The nail trimmer has been placed over the claw in such a way that the blade is between the second and third phalanges, and the bottom support is in front of the digital pad. The nail will be pulled forward as the nail trimmer is squeezed to remove the claw.

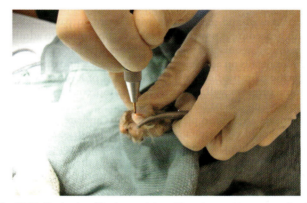

• **Fig. 33.17** Declawing. The laser pictured here is used to remove the third phalanx during declawing. Note the absence of blood. A tourniquet is not required.

The blade technique amputates the entire third phalanx by using a No. 12 scalpel blade. The phalanx is disarticulated dorsolaterally, first by cutting through the joint capsule between the second and third phalanges and then by cutting the collateral ligaments (Fig. 33.16). Next, the nail is cut away from the underlying tissue and digital pad, with as minimal skin trauma as possible. The pad is moved out of the way by positioning the blade more dorsal to prevent inadvertent laceration of the pad.

The laser technique is similar to the blade technique, except that it uses laser energy instead of a blade to dissect the third phalanx free from the second phalanx. The surgical site usually does not bleed with the laser technique, so a tourniquet is not necessary (Fig. 33.17). If a laser is used, the technician should be familiar with safety protocols before the use of a laser, including the avoidance of alcohol prep.

One to two sutures are often placed to appose the skin edges after nail removal, regardless of technique used. Surgical glue (cyanoacrylic tissue adhesive) is used instead of sutures in some instances. If surgical glue is used, it should never be placed on the exposed bone of the second phalanx or dropped inside the void (wound) created by removal of the third phalanx. Instead, the wound should be manually closed and a drop of glue placed only on the skin edges of the closed wound (Fig. 33.18A and B). Dropping glue into the wound can cause chronic lameness and

foreign body reaction. Some veterinarians do not appose the skin edges with anything other than a bandage.

> **TECHNICIAN NOTE**
>
> Do not place tissue glue into the open wound formed after a claw is removed, or chronic lameness and foreign body reaction may result. The wound should be manually apposed and the glue placed only on the skin edges.

After surgery, the paws are bandaged snugly. Two methods are most common: gauze sponge and strips of tape: The sponge is placed over the ends of the digits. Strips of tape are placed longitudinally along the leg and distally around the paw. Tape is then placed circumferentially around the paw up to the elbow. Care is taken to lay tape on the leg and not to pull too tightly. The alternative method uses a gauze sponge over the ends of the digits, strips of tape longitudinally along the leg (stirrups), and vet wrap wrapped distal to cranial, only very slightly taut; then the tape strip is incorporated into the vet wrap and wrapped cranial to distal to finish the bandage. This latter bandage minimizes tape removal from skin/fur. Bandages placed too tightly can result in vascular compromise to the foot, resulting in skin sloughing. The tourniquet is removed as soon as bandaging is complete.

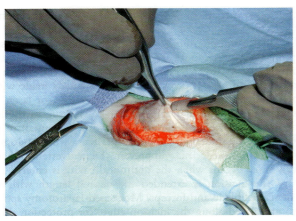

• **Fig. 33.21** This image shows the linea alba tented (raised) with forceps and a scalpel blade in position to penetrate the linea to enter the abdominal cavity.

The abdomen is usually sutured closed in at least three layers. The linea alba is the "layer of strength" and must be securely closed. The subcutaneous tissues are then sutured to decrease the amount of dead space. This helps reduce the frequency of postoperative hematoma or seroma formation. The skin is sutured to complete the celiotomy closure.

> **TECHNICIAN NOTE**
>
> Preoperative and postoperative sponge counts are recommended, and instruments should be assessed to prevent objects from being left in the abdominal cavity.

Postoperative Considerations

During the first 24 hours, the skin incision should be examined carefully for swelling, drainage, excessive redness, dehiscence, and evidence of self-trauma. An Elizabethan collar should be considered if the animal appears to lick or chew the sutured incision. Incision problems should be brought to the attention of the veterinarian; evidence of dehiscence may require emergency closure. Incision monitoring should be continued for 2 weeks after surgery or until suture removal. Animals should be exercise restricted until the abdominal wound has healed.

Some animals may be inappetent or may vomit after celiotomy. Intestinal and pancreatic manipulation can lead to intestinal **ileus** (temporary loss of intestinal motility), nausea, and/or pancreatitis. One or two episodes of vomiting or lack of appetite for the first 24 to 48 hours after celiotomy is usually not a matter of concern in and of itself. However, if the animal appears ill or is vomiting frequently and/or if inappetence continues, further evaluation should be considered. Animals that are not eating or drinking after surgery should be supported with IV fluid therapy until oral alimentation is resumed.

Gastrointestinal Surgery

Definition

Gastrotomy is an incision (opening) into the stomach. **Enterotomy** is an incision into the intestine. These procedures are often done to obtain biopsies, remove damaged tissue or tumors, or to remove foreign material. **Anastomosis** is the suturing of the portions of the GI tract back together to allow ingesta (substances taken into the body as nourishment) to flow normally.

Indications

Abdominal exploration and GI surgery can be indicated for a variety of reasons: GI foreign body, trauma, or obstruction of unknown cause; neoplasia; or biopsy of various tissues for vomiting or diarrhea of unknown origin.

Preoperative Considerations

Preoperative concerns stem from the animal's underlying and current condition. Vomiting and not eating are common clinical signs; thus the patient should be stabilized and dehydration should be addressed before surgery, if possible. The animal should be intubated as soon as possible with a cuffed endotracheal tube to help decrease aspiration of stomach contents should the animal vomit during induction. The veterinary technician should make sure that extra instruments and gloves are available in case the primary pack is contaminated with intestinal contents during the procedure. Prophylactic antibiotics are used if the GI tract is to be entered.

> **TECHNICIAN NOTE**
>
> It is important to remember that GI contents are not sterile and anything that touches the contents is considered contaminated. Contaminated objects should be kept isolated to a single area during surgery. Glove changes and new packs are often required during surgery before closure of the abdomen and should be kept on hand.

Technique and Intraoperative Considerations

When an animal is prepared for a full midline celiotomy, the procedure is initiated with an incision made in the linea alba (see Fig. 33.21), with care taken to avoid damaging underlying structures. An abdominal exploration is performed. The normal GI tract is pink, has visible vasculature on the surface, and has active peristaltic motility (Fig. 33.22A). Abnormalities are noted. Foreign bodies leading to GI obstruction are removed via gastrotomy or enterotomy. In some instances, devitalized tissue must be removed via resection and anastomosis. Devitalized intestine is discolored and lacks blood supply. Purple or red discoloration does not necessarily imply devitalization; blood supply must be evaluated by direct visualization of cut sections, Doppler ultrasonography, or injection of vital stains. If the tissue is questionable, it should be resected (see Fig. 33.22B).

Characteristics of intestinal devitalization include the following:
- Lack of motility
- Gray, green, or black discoloration
- Severe thinning of the visceral wall
- Lack of bleeding on the cut section
- Lack of fluorescein dye uptake
- Lack of Doppler blood flow

For biopsy or foreign body removal, the affected portion of the GI tract is isolated with laparotomy pads (Fig. 33.23). Laparotomy pads are placed to prevent intestinal contents from leaking into the abdomen if accidental spillage occurs. Stay sutures are placed to steady the tissue on either side of the incision. The surgical assistant holds the stay sutures steady during the procedure.

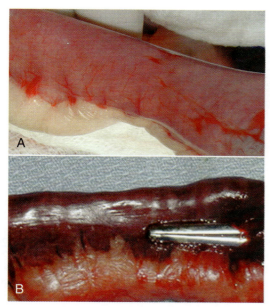

• **Fig. 33.22** The normal intestine is pink with visible vessels and motility. Note the difference in color between the normal intestine (A) and the devitalized segment of bowel (B).

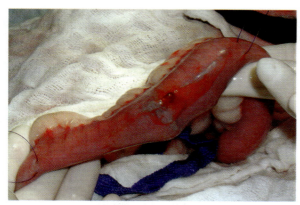

• **Fig. 33.23** If a biopsy is to be performed on the GI tract, the segment is packed with laparotomy (white) pads to prevent leaking ingesta from contaminating the abdominal cavity. Ingesta is prevented from leaking from the cut surface of the intestine by placement of intestinal clamps or by having an assistant gently pinch off the intestinal lumen on either side of the incision with fingers.

Biopsy is performed by making a stab incision into the stomach or intestine between the stay sutures and removing a full-thickness portion of the tissue with a blade or scissors. If the incision is made simply to remove intraluminal material, the stab incision is extended enough to remove the material, and no tissue is removed for biopsy. The incision is closed in an interrupted pattern with absorbable monofilament suture.

If resection and anastomosis are to be performed, the vasculature to the portion of the intestine to be removed is ligated; the intestines are clamped with Doyen forceps, or the surgical assistant supports the intestines with fingers to prevent ingesta from leaking onto the surgical field; the portion of the intestines to be removed is excised; and the viable intestinal ends are sutured together in an interrupted pattern likened to a biopsy site. After completion of the anastomosis, the intestine is evaluated for leakage. This is accomplished by occluding the intestine on either side

of the anastomosis site and filling the enclosed space with sterile saline using a syringe and a small-gauge needle (Fig. 33.24A and B). The surgeon and the surgical assistant check for leaks along the incision. Leaks are sealed with additional suture. The intestine is flushed, and the laparotomy pads are removed from the abdomen and surgical field and counted, with care taken to avoid contaminating the rest of the abdomen or the surgical field with ingesta that might have leaked onto the pads. The technician should ensure that warm isotonic saline is available for flushing the abdominal cavity. The abdomen is flushed and omentum is placed over intestinal incisions. The celiotomy is closed routinely. Many surgeons will ask for a clean surgical pack, gloves, and drape to perform the celiotomy closure to prevent contamination of the celiotomy wound with ingesta from instruments used during the intestinal procedure.

Postoperative Considerations

Careful patient monitoring is important after intestinal surgery. The main consideration is evaluation for intestinal leakage. If intestinal dehiscence or leakage occurs, septic peritonitis will develop. Animals should be monitored for inappetence, vomiting, fever, painful abdomen (tucking), abdominal enlargement, incision drainage, and shock, all of which are potential indicators of peritonitis. Most animals are willing to eat within 24 hours of intestinal surgery. Minor vomiting (one or two times) is to be expected. However, protracted vomiting and inappetence should alert the technician to a potential impending problem with the intestinal surgery site. If intestinal leakage is suspected, abdominal ultrasonography or abdominocentesis is performed. Material collected is evaluated for cell population and bacteria. If material obtained for evaluation from simple abdominocentesis is not sufficient, but leakage is still suspected, a diagnostic peritoneal lavage should be performed. A septic abdominal tap warrants emergency abdominal exploration and correction of the problem.

Feeding animals after intestinal surgery is another consideration. The GI tract requires food for cellular health and proper functioning. Intestinal surgery can result in ileus and may cause inappetence, nausea, and vomiting. However, animals without complications are most often willing to eat within 24 hours. Unless the animal is vomiting, oral alimentation should be initiated as soon as the animal has an appetite. Animals should be introduced to water first. If no vomiting occurs after water intake, then food is introduced. A small amount of highly digestible, bland food should be fed initially. Many diets are available; the choice depends on the surgeon's preference. If no vomiting occurs over 2 to 4 hours, another small amount can be fed. If vomiting does not occur, the amount fed can be gradually increased and frequency decreased. Animals are reintroduced to their normal or another maintenance diet gradually after recovery. Monitoring as discussed for routine celiotomy should also be done.

Gastric Dilatation-Volvulus

Definition

GDV is dilatation of the stomach with ingesta and gas (commonly termed *bloat*), coupled with a signature rotation of the stomach into an abnormal position. This life-threatening condition typically occurs in deep-chested, large, and giant breed dogs but can be seen in other breeds as well. The cause is not specifically known, but genetics and chest/abdomen configuration may

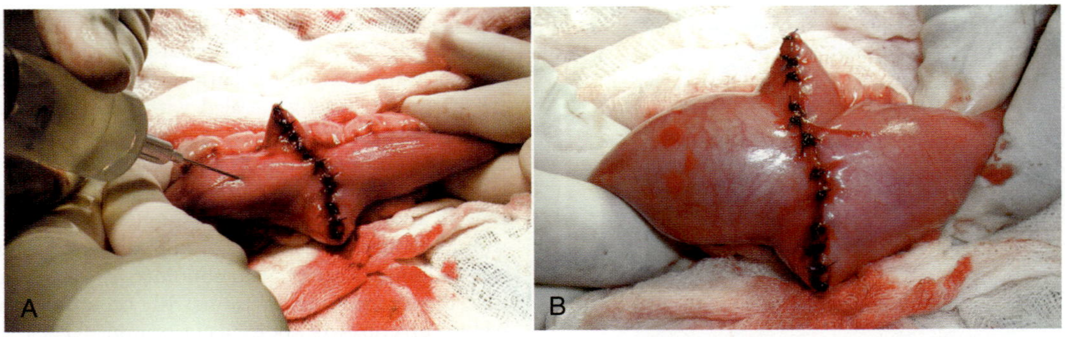

• **Fig. 33.24** (A) To check for leaks after intestinal anastomosis, the intestine is occluded on either side of the incision, and the occluded segment of intestine is filled with sterile saline. (B) The incision is checked for leakage while the segment is filled with saline.

play a role. There are reports of some animals having eaten a large meal, consumed a large portion of water, and/or engaged in heavy exercise after either; however, others have not. Some animals develop the condition during times of stress, such as hospitalization or boarding. Vomiting, retching, and *bloating* (severe distention of the stomach) are classic clinical signs. Surgical correction of GDV is an emergency procedure. The twisting of the torsion of the stomach causes constriction of musculature and blood vessels and may also incorporate other organs such as the spleen, causing tissue decompensation. Gastropexy is surgical attachment of the stomach to the body wall with the goal of creating a permanent adhesion. It is performed to substantially decrease the chance of further stomach rotation, but it does not prevent the stomach from bloating. Partial gastrectomy is removal of part of the stomach, which may be needed if the vasculature was compromised enough to cause tissue decompensation to parts of the stomach. Splenectomy is removal of the spleen, which is often done if any portion of it is incorporated in the volvulus.

Preoperative Considerations

Animals suffering from GDV are usually in shock. If left untreated, these animals will die of cardiovascular collapse. The enlarged stomach compresses the caudal vena cava and affects venous return to the heart, leading to hypovolemic shock. Large-bore catheters should be placed immediately. It is important to place the catheters in the forelimbs or jugular vein, because venous return from the caudal half of the body is impaired by the dilated stomach. These dogs are often large and require a substantial amount of fluid. It is best to place at least two catheters. Baseline blood work, coagulation assessment, ECG, and blood gas are typically obtained shortly after presentation. The veterinary technician should review information about the treatment of hypovolemic shock (see Chapters 24 and 25).

> **TECHNICIAN NOTE**
>
> Large-bore IV catheters should be placed in the front half of an animal suffering from GDV. Venous return from the back half of the dog is compromised because of compression of the vena cava from the dilated stomach.

After fluids are started, the stomach must be decompressed to help stabilize the animal and decrease the chance of gastric wall necrosis secondary to vascular compromise from severe distention

and volvulus. An orogastric tube is placed. (Refer to Chapter 17, "Diagnostic Sampling and Therapeutic Techniques.")

If the tube cannot be passed after sedation, the stomach should be decompressed by trocarization. The disadvantage of trocarization is potential leakage of gastric contents into the abdominal cavity at the stomach puncture site or stomach rupture. For trocarization, the right side of the stomach is aseptically prepared behind the last rib. Decompression is performed by gently passing a large-bore needle or a large-bore IV catheter attached to a 60-mL syringe with a three-way stopcock into the dilated stomach percutaneously. Air is aspirated until the stomach is decompressed enough to stabilize the dog.

After stabilization is under way and vital signs are improving, right lateral abdominal radiographs are obtained. This view is best for evaluating the stomach for bloat with or without rotation present. Thoracic radiography should also be performed because aspiration is a possibility. The dog should also be started on broad-spectrum antibiotics to help prevent septicemia resulting from vascular compromise of the stomach wall leading to bacterial translocation from the GI tract to the bloodstream. The animal is further stabilized and prepared for emergency surgery.

Anesthesia can be challenging in these cases. Respiratory compromise often occurs because of compression of the diaphragm by the gas-distended stomach. Blood pressure is often low and difficult to maintain. If possible, an arterial access port should be established for continuous pressure and blood gas monitoring. Cardiac arrhythmias can occur and may need to be treated. The reader should review Chapter 30.

Technique and Intraoperative Considerations

The dog is prepared for a full ventral midline celiotomy. The abdomen is opened carefully to prevent puncture of the stomach, because gas distention pushes the stomach against the ventral aspect of the abdomen (Fig. 33.25A and B). The veterinary technician should make sure that a stomach tube, bucket, and pump are available in the OR, because if the stomach is substantially distended at the time of surgery, further decompression will be needed to make manipulation easier. The tube should be gently passed down the esophagus after lubrication while the veterinarian manipulates the tube into position within the stomach. The veterinarian can often gently express gas and fluid from the stomach through the tube. If decompression cannot be achieved in this manner, it can be performed with a syringe, three-way stopcock, and needle under direct visualization by the surgeon. The stomach must be handled with care. The stomach wall is often

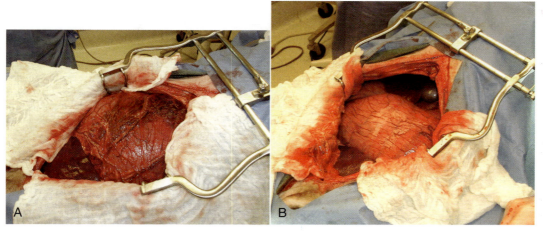

• **Fig. 33.25** (A) Note how the dilated, rotated stomach is pressed against the ventral abdominal wall and protrudes out of the abdomen. Inadvertent stomach puncture can occur if the abdomen is not entered carefully. (B) The normally positioned stomach is still dilated but recesses back away from the ventral incision and lies completely within the abdomen.

friable because of vascular compromise of the tissues. Ingesta and fluid that accumulate in the stomach after GDV are heavy and can contribute to tissue tearing during manipulation of the stomach back into its normal position. Extreme care must be taken to prevent inadvertent damage. Once the stomach is in its normal position, it is evaluated for viability. The stomach is often discolored at the start of the procedure, but this usually improves as blood supply and venous drainage return. A complete abdominal exploratory is performed while circulation is allowed to return to the stomach. The spleen is carefully evaluated. Vascular compromise to the spleen can occur with dilatation and/or rotation of the stomach; the spleen may rotate independently of the stomach or with the stomach, further compromising the vasculature. If the spleen is discolored, the vascular pedicle is relieved of compromise, and the spleen is gently placed out of the abdomen and covered with moistened laparotomy pads. After abdominal exploration, the stomach is re-evaluated for viability. Partial resection (gastropexy) is performed, if needed. A gastropexy is performed on the right ventrolateral aspect of the body wall, near the last rib. Many different techniques may be used to perform gastropexy; a discussion of each technique is beyond the scope of this chapter. The technique used depends on the comfort level and skill of the surgeon performing the procedure. The surgical assistant is responsible for retraction of tissues and suture manipulation to keep the procedure running smoothly. It will often help the veterinary surgeon if the assistant stands on the right side of the dog and holds the body wall up with towel clamps during the gastropexy. This will often expose the entire surgical field for the surgeon.

After gastropexy, the spleen is re-evaluated. In most instances, the normal character of the spleen will return once the blood supply has been reestablished. If all or a portion of the spleen does not appear viable, all or part of the spleen is removed; this is referred to as *splenectomy*. The abdomen is flushed, and the celiotomy incision is closed routinely.

Fixation of the stomach into the celiotomy incision at the time of closure is not recommended, because future abdominal surgery can result in accidental perforation of the stomach when the abdominal cavity is entered.

Postoperative Considerations

Dogs suffering from GDV can have many postoperative complications. Arrhythmias can continue for 2 to 3 days postoperatively. Treatment of arrhythmias should be initiated if vascular compromise is present or is expected on the basis of the type of arrhythmia present and cardiovascular stability. The veterinarian should be alerted about the type of arrhythmia present. Hypotension and hypovolemia can continue postoperatively and should be treated as needed. Urination should be monitored, because prolonged hypotension under anesthesia can affect renal function. A urinary catheter should be placed if urine production is questionable. Some dogs will require a blood transfusion because of hemorrhage associated with tearing of blood vessels during bloating and rotation of the stomach and/or spleen. If a partial gastrectomy was performed, the dog should be monitored for evidence of gastric wall dehiscence. Some dogs continue to develop gastric wall compromise after decompression and surgery. Fever, persistent inappetence, and vomiting may indicate that this is occurring, with signs being similar to intestinal incision dehiscence, as previously discussed. Antibiotics should be continued for at least 7 days postoperatively. Immediately after surgery, IV antibiotics should be given to avoid oral administration. GI protectants, such as histamine type 2 blockers, should be administered for 2 to 4 days postoperatively. Some surgeons prefer to place these animals on a gastric motility modifier to help treat ileus. Finally, gastric dilatation can again occur in the postoperative period, necessitating decompression; however, gastropexy should prevent rotation of the stomach. Extreme caution is needed if passing an orogastric tube soon after the initial surgery.

Oral alimentation should be initiated slowly. Water is given in small amounts at first. If no vomiting occurs, food is gradually introduced. Feeding can start as soon as the animal is willing to eat—often within 24 hours of surgery. Some animals may require antiemetics in the perioperative period to control nausea and vomiting. Long-term dietary management should be considered. Once home, dogs should be on a feeding schedule of smaller meals three to four times a day. If possible, a feeding schedule of two to three times a day should be continued for the rest of the dog's life. Once-a-day feedings are not recommended, both for nutritional reasons and to avoid large amounts of food in the stomach at one time. Water should always be available, but gulping of water should be discouraged. Heavy activity should be avoided after feeding. Owners should be warned that bloating can still occur, even if gastropexy was performed, but the presence of a gastropexy is likely to prevent life-threatening gastric rotation. Stomach decompression may be needed if bloat is severe.

Ovariohysterectomy in Dogs and Cats

Definition

Ovariohysterectomy ("spaying") is surgical removal of the uterus and ovaries.

Indications

The primary indication for ovariohysterectomy is prevention of pregnancy and subsequent production of unwanted puppies and kittens. Other indications for ovariohysterectomy include

endocrine imbalance, infection (see Case Presentation 33.1), injury, cyst, tumor, prevention of unwanted behavior, and congenital abnormalities. Endocrine disturbances are associated with various clinical manifestations, such as sterility, skin lesions, mammary tumors, pseudocyesis (false pregnancy), and nymphomania. Ovariohysterectomy before the first estrus will greatly decrease the chance of mammary neoplasia in dogs. Uterine diseases that may require ovariohysterectomy include metritis, pyometra, uterine prolapse, endometrial hyperplasia, neoplasia, injury, neglected dystocia, and congenital abnormalities.

Preoperative Considerations

Ovariohysterectomy is usually performed between 5 and 6 months of age in most medium to small dogs and all cats. The veterinarian may recommend that large dogs wait to between 6 and 18 months or 18–24 months of age in giant breeds, but the procedure can be performed at almost any age and during any phase of the reproductive cycle. Performing ovariohysterectomy at around 6 months of age decreases the risk of anesthetic complications in younger

---

CASE PRESENTATION 33.1

Signalment: Lady, 6-year-old female Labrador Retriever (Fig. 33.A)

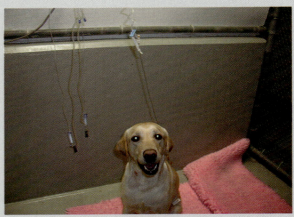

• **Fig. 33.A** Lady, a 6-year-old female Labrador Retriever, brought in for treatment of inappetence and lethargy.

History: Two-week history of increased drinking and urination. Lady showed progressive lethargy and decreased appetite over the 3 days before presentation. For 24 hours before presentation, Lady was inappetent, depressed, and extremely lethargic. The owner noticed some blood-tinged fluid coming from the vulva 4 days ago and that Lady has been licking her vulva regularly. The owner noticed some blood in Lady's urine when she started having accidents in the house about 1.5 weeks before presentation.

Technical considerations: The dog is an intact female; she has not been eating or drinking for 24 hours, has blood in her urine, has a bloody discharge from her vulva, and has been drinking and urinating more frequently than she normally does.
Other questions asked:
1. Is Lady current on vaccinations? *Answer:* Yes, rabies, distemper, and *Bordetella* infection
2. Has Lady ever had puppies? *Answer:* Yes, two litters, all healthy
3. When was her last heat cycle? *Answer:* About 8 weeks ago
4. When was the last time Lady was bred? *Answer:* 3 years ago

5. Are there toxins around your home and can Lady roam freely? *Answer:* No toxins that owners are aware of, and Lady stays indoors or in a fenced yard
6. Has she had any other illnesses? *Answer:* No
7. Did Lady have any dietary items out of the ordinary before this started? *Answer:* No, she eats adult-maintenance dry food (1 cup twice a day) and milk bones only. The owner did try to feed her steak last night because she was not eating, but Lady turned that down.
8. Any coughing, sneezing, runny eyes, vomiting, or diarrhea? *Answer:* No

Examination: Physical examination revealed Lady to be depressed and her abdomen to be tense and painful. Lady had a mucopurulent discharge coming from her vulva. Other findings include fleas, waxy debris in both ears, and moderate dental tartar.
Temperature: 104.5°F
Pulse: 110 beats per minute (bpm), pulses weak and thready
Respiratory rate: 50 breaths per minute
Mucous membranes: Pale and tacky
Capillary refill time: 3 seconds
Technical assessment: Lady is febrile, tachycardic, and tachypneic; has weak and thready pulses; and has pain in the abdomen. Lady appears to be dehydrated and in early shock.

Diagnostic Tests and Findings
- *CBC:* Mild nonregenerative anemia; mildly low total protein (TP); leukocytosis (increased white blood cell count) consisting of neutrophilia (a high neutrophil count) with a left shift (too many immature neutrophils) and toxic changes to the neutrophils; and mild thrombocytopenia (low platelets)
- *Biochemistry panel abnormalities:* Elevated sodium and chloride, mildly low potassium, elevated BUN (i.e., high-protein diet, renal insufficiency, GI bleeding, and/or dehydration), elevated creatinine (kidney value—"high" means renal insufficiency or the animal is dehydrated), mildly low albumin, mildly low TP, and elevated alkaline phosphatase (liver enzyme)
- *Abdominal radiography:* Tissue-dense mass in the caudal abdomen displacing the intestines cranial and dorsal and the intestinal ileus. The mass is consistent with an enlarged uterus (Fig. 33.B).
- *Abdominal ultrasonography:* Enlarged, fluid-filled uterus

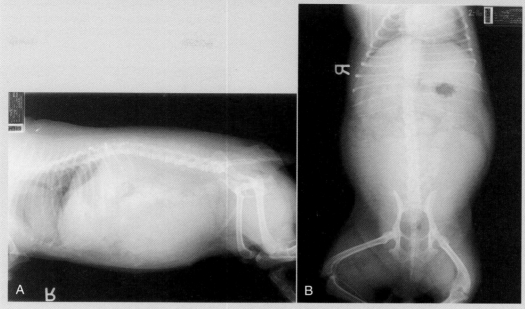

• **Fig. 33.B** Abdominal radiographs of Lady, showing a large tissue-dense mass in the caudal abdomen (large, dense [more white] structure that is irregular and is pushing the intestines cranially and dorsally). (A) Lateral radiograph. (B) Ventrodorsal view.

Urinalysis collected at the time of ultrasonography by cystocentesis: Numerous bacteria, increased white blood cells, hematuria (blood in the urine), urine specific gravity of 1.012 (urine is not concentrated—in a dehydrated dog, this number should be higher. This means that the kidneys may not be functioning normally, or the toxins from the disease are causing diuresis—increased filtration of fluid through the kidneys).

Veterinarian's diagnosis: Pyometra (open), anemia, possible renal insufficiency, possible sepsis.

Technical considerations: Lady has been diagnosed with an open pyometra, because she has purulent drainage from her vulva (e.g., an open wound). She will require emergency surgery to remove the source of infection (her uterus). However, she is azotemic (has an elevated BUN and creatinine), dehydrated, potentially septic, anemic, thrombocytopenic, and in the early stages of shock. This makes her a poor candidate for anesthesia, because she is systemically unstable.

Veterinarian's Treatment Orders

1. Place an IV catheter.
2. Give shock dose of IV crystalloid therapy (may consider adding in a colloid because the protein is low).
3. Begin a cooling process with fans and fluid therapy.
4. Obtain ECG and blood pressure measurements.
5. Obtain a coagulation profile to check for evidence of early *disseminated intravascular coagulopathy* (a disease that involves severe metabolic disruptions that leads to generalized blood clotting throughout the body, followed by hemorrhage).
6. Start Lady on broad-spectrum IV antibiotics.
7. Continue crystalloid and/or colloid therapy until improvements in body temperature, pulses, and respiration are noted.
8. Initiate pain control.
9. Start GI protectants because of GI stasis and inappetence caused by the stress of being in the hospital.
10. Repeat CBC and chemistry panel after Lady's condition begins to stabilize.

What to consider at this point: Lady's systemic condition should begin to stabilize within a few hours of admission to the hospital. She has a life-threatening infection of her uterus and must go to surgery sooner rather than later. As soon as she appears to be out of shock and

rehydrated (it is hoped that BUN and creatinine would come down), she should be prepared for surgery. Lady has bacteria in urine, and a urine sample should be turned in for culture and sensitivity.

Anesthetic considerations: Lady is not a stable patient. *Adequate monitoring:* Blood pressure, temperature, pulse, oxygen saturation, and vitals should be monitored. Only light anesthetics would likely be required and are desired. Instead of using rapid inducing agents that lead to apnea and decreased blood pressure, a muscle relaxant (e.g., midazolam) and a dissociative anesthetic (e.g., ketamine) have the potential to better maintain blood pressure. Because inhalant anesthetics are notorious for dose-dependent effects on the cardiovascular system, a constant rate infusion of pain medication and high epidural should also be considered to keep gas anesthetic administration to a minimum.

Surgical considerations: Lady should be prepped quickly and moved into the OR for surgery. The technician should ensure that the OR is set up with all necessary equipment and suture so that the surgery proceeds quickly. A general abdominal pack would be required. Culture swabs and a bucket for the uterus should be available. The surgeon would likely hand the infected uterus to the technician, and the technician would have to cut into the uterus with sterile technique and obtain a culture—this should be done outside of the OR (Fig. 33.C). The surgical technique would be ovariohysterectomy. However, a wide abdominal preparation will be required, because a large incision will be needed for gentle uterine handling and abdominal exploration (Fig. 33.D). A sponge count should be performed before abdominal incision and before closure of the incision to ensure that none of the sponges are left in the abdomen. The surgical assistant should remember to keep the tissues moist and to avoid pulling on the uterus, because it will be friable and will tear easily, causing septic fluid to leak onto the surgical field and into the sterile abdominal cavity. Tissue and culture samples should be promptly submitted.

Considerations for recovery: Lady will likely be hypothermic, even though she had a fever before surgery, and should be warmed appropriately. Although the infected uterus was removed, she could still experience complications of septicemia to include fever, low blood pressure, anemia, shock, organ failure, and death. All vitals, PCV, TP, ECG, blood

Continued

CASE PRESENTATION 33.1—cont'd

pressure, and mucous membranes should continue to be monitored until Lady is stable.

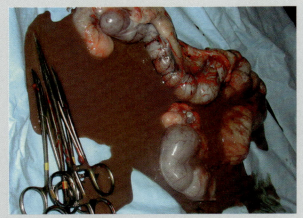

• **Fig. 33.C** This uterus has been cut open with sterile instruments. Note the brown fluid that exudes from the cut uterus. The fluid should be cultured using sterile technique by advancing a culture swab into the uterine lumen through an aseptically made incision.

Other postoperative care: Pain should be controlled with injections rather than with oral medications, and injections should be administered on a routine schedule (do not wait for Lady to exhibit pain). IV fluids should be continued until Lady is eating and drinking. Food and water should be offered 12 hours after surgery. PCV and TP should normalize within a few days, but if they drop too low, colloidal fluid support and/or blood transfusion may be necessary. Coagulation times, CBC, and biochemistry panel should be re-evaluated 24 hours after surgery to ensure improvements. The incision should be monitored for oozing of fluid, which might occur in a dog with low protein and platelets; this should improve in 24–48 hours. A bandage should be placed around the belly if incisional oozing occurs. GI protectants are continued until

Lady's appetite returns to normal. As she improves over 24 to 48 hours and begins to eat and drink, fluid therapy is decreased and then stopped, and oral antibiotic therapy is continued based on culture and sensitivity results.

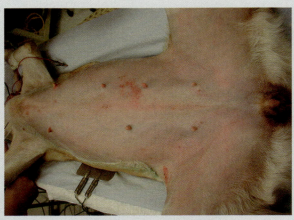

• **Fig. 33.D** This dog's abdomen has been aseptically prepared for pyometra surgery. Note the wide abdominal clip so a full surgical approach to the abdomen can be made.

Postoperative events and client education: Surgery was a success, and Lady recovered without complications. Her blood work abnormalities began to normalize, and her appetite returned within 36 hours. She was discharged from the hospital 3 days after surgery with a prescription for enrofloxacin and tramadol. Initial culture results from urine and uterus revealed *Escherichia coli* sensitive to enrofloxacin. The owners were instructed to monitor the incision daily and to return for suture removal and blood work in 7 days. Lady was back to normal at that time.
Note: Pyometra generally has a good prognosis if diagnosed early and treated appropriately. Recovery is often quick, provided the animal does not have complications, including septicemia.

animals and usually allows the procedure to be performed before the first estrus. If performed during estrus or pregnancy, increased vasculature may be encountered, with the potential for increased hemorrhage. This is more important for dogs than for cats. The most favorable time to spay a mature dog is 3 to 4 months after estrus. After whelping, the operation should be done as soon as the puppies or kittens have been weaned and lactation has ceased, about 6 to 8 weeks after parturition.

Technique and Intraoperative Considerations

The animal is clipped and aseptically prepared for a ventral midline celiotomy. The skin incision extends caudally 3 to 6 cm from the umbilicus in the dog. In the cat, it extends from 2 cm caudad to the umbilicus and 3 to 4 cm caudally. When the abdominal cavity is entered, the uterine horns are located and exteriorized from the abdomen using a spay hook or digital manipulation (Fig. 33.26A). The suspensory ligament holds each ovary tight in the abdominal cavity and must be severed or torn to exteriorize the ovaries, especially on the right, for proper ligation. This is often the most painful part of the procedure, and the animal may begin to wake up. The anesthetist should be prepared for this. The ovarian arteries and veins (pedicles) are ligated with absorbable suture

material of appropriate size (see Fig. 33.26B) and then severed. Usually, two circumferential ligatures are placed. The broad ligament is broken down, and the uterine body is exteriorized and ligated with transfixation and/or circumferential sutures (see Fig. 33.26C and D). The uterus is removed, along with the ovaries. The assistant or surgeon checks to ensure that both ovaries were completely removed (Fig. 33.27). Leaving ovarian tissue behind can lead to recurrent heat cycles and stump pyometra caused by the presence of hormones that can influence any remaining uterine tissue. The abdominal cavity is carefully examined for hemorrhage. The celiotomy incision is closed routinely.

Intraoperative complications include hemorrhage and anesthetic problems. If excessive intra-abdominal blood is seen during surgery, both ovarian pedicles and the uterine stump should be evaluated before celiotomy closure. The abdominal incision will likely have to be extended cranially. This is why adequate preparation before surgery is important. The left ovarian pedicle is evaluated by retraction of the descending colon to the right and viewing of the pedicle just caudal to the left kidney. The right pedicle is evaluated by retraction of the descending duodenum to the left and viewing of the pedicle just caudal to the right kidney. The uterine stump is visualized between the urinary bladder ventrally and the colon dorsally. Bleeding stumps are ligated again before abdominal closure.

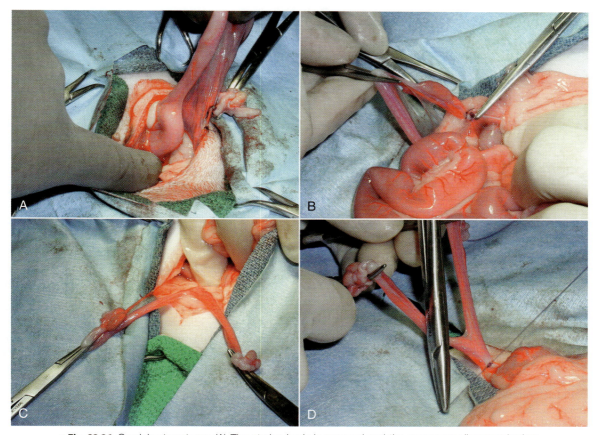

• **Fig. 33.26** Ovariohysterectomy. (A) The uterine body is exposed and the suspensory ligament broken down so the ovarian pedicles can be ligated. Both uterine horns are shown in this figure as digital manipulation is used to bring the uterus out of the abdomen. (B) Once the ovarian pedicle is freed, two circumferential sutures are secured on the portion that will remain in the animal. The ovarian pedicle would be severed proximal to the ovary but distal to the placed ligatures. (C) The uterine body is fully exposed with gentle traction once the ovarian pedicles are ligated and severed and after the broad ligament is broken down. (D) The uterine vessels are ligated with transfixation sutures that individually ligate the vessels on either side of the uterine body and/or as shown with circumferential ligatures that encircle the entire uterine body and the uterine vessels.

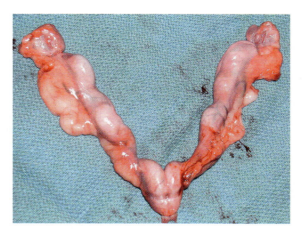

• **Fig. 33.27** Ovariohysterectomy. The uterus is positioned with the ovaries to the top of the picture. Note that the ovaries are not well visualized and look like a continuation of the uterine horns. The ovaries should be exposed from their bursae to ensure that ovarian tissue was not left behind.

Postoperative Considerations

Postoperative intra-abdominal hemorrhage can occur and may be fatal if not treated appropriately. After ovariohysterectomy, the technician should monitor the animal carefully for the first 24 hours. Abnormalities should be promptly reported to the veterinarian in charge.

Incision complications can also occur after ovariohysterectomy. These include irritation, premature suture removal by the animal, seroma formation, infection, suture reaction, and dehiscence. Only rarely are these complications serious. The veterinarian should be alerted to impending incision complications.

Some animals experience renal dysfunction secondary to accidental ureteral ligation during surgery. Ligation typically occurs when overzealous attempts are made to alleviate hemorrhage from a bleeding stump with mass ligation of tissues and poor visualization. It is important to ensure that the ureters are visualized and are not in the mass of tissue to be ligated when hemorrhage from bleeding ovarian or uterine stumps is controlled. Animals are unlikely to show signs of renal failure if only one ureter is ligated, but this may be seen later in

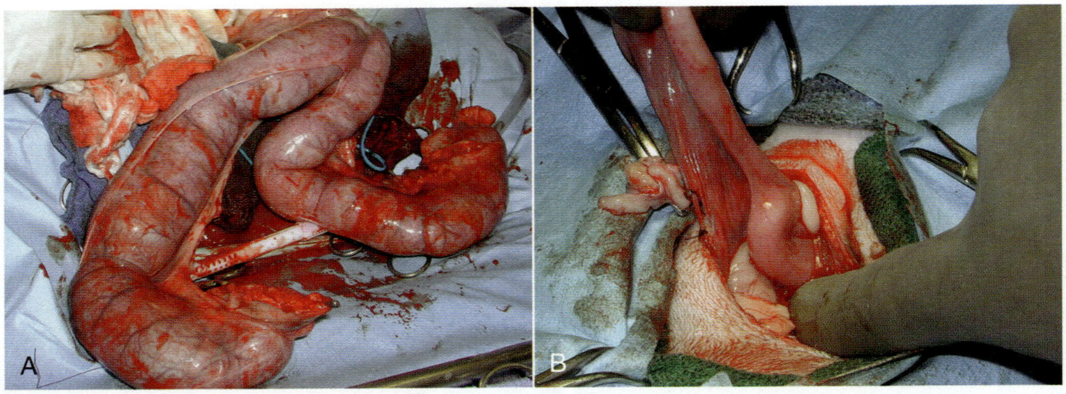

• **Fig. 33.28** Pyometra. The uterus must be carefully handled in cases of pyometra, because it is often large, friable, and heavy. Compare the pyometra uterus (A) with the normal uterus (B).

the form of abdominal enlargement, abdominal pain, or signs consistent with renal infection. If both ureters are inadvertently ligated, the animal will begin to show signs within 24 hours and will die if steps are not taken to alleviate the obstruction of urine flow.

Body weight gain may occur as a late sequela to ovariohysterectomy. Reasons for this excessive weight gain are poorly understood, but it may be caused in part by ovarian endocrine deficiency. Obesity can be controlled by proper diet and exercise. Other late complications include loss of stamina in working dogs (eunuchoid syndrome) and urinary incontinence. Although incompletely understood, urinary incontinence may be related to endocrine alteration after ovariohysterectomy or scar tissue formation around the urinary bladder and proximal urethra. These appear to be rare complications.

Pyometra

Definition

Pyometra is a condition of the uterus in which endometrial hyperplasia has resulted in increased uterine secretions and accumulation of fluid in the uterus with secondary infection. Progesterone production from the ovaries during diestrus contributes to uterine gland hyperplasia and the disease process. The process typically occurs in middle-aged to older intact dogs 4 to 8 weeks after estrus. **Mucometra** or **hydrometra** is enlargement of the uterus with a sterile mucoid or serous fluid, respectively.

Indications

Ovariohysterectomy is the recommended treatment for pyometra. This is especially true for closed (nondraining) pyometra. Some owners will elect conservative management for open (draining) pyometras in valuable breeding dogs, but this should be discouraged because of the risk of septicemia and endotoxemia, and the incidence of recurrence is high. Conservative management of closed pyometra is not recommended because of the risk for uterine rupture, septicemia, endotoxemia, and possibly death.

Preoperative Considerations

An intact female dog with fever, lethargy, polyuria, polydipsia, vaginal discharge, abdominal pain, abdominal enlargement, inappetence, vomiting, and/or diarrhea should be evaluated carefully for pyometra. Animals with closed pyometra are more likely to have severe clinical signs. Baseline biochemical values and blood cell counts should be obtained. Many of these animals are dehydrated or inappetent and have metabolic and/or electrolyte abnormalities at the time of presentation (renal or hepatic dysfunction, glucose imbalance, etc.). They should be started on IV fluids and their metabolic/electrolyte abnormalities corrected, if possible, before surgery. If left untreated, open or closed pyometra can result in septicemia and/or endotoxemia and possible death. Additionally, uterine rupture and peritonitis are possible. Palpation of the abdomen should be done with extreme care, as should any restraint or movement incorporating the abdomen (e.g., lifting), and cystocentesis for urine collection should be avoided in animals suspected of having pyometra. Broad-spectrum IV antibiotic therapy is initiated before surgery.

Technique and Intraoperative Considerations

The animal is prepped for a ventral midline celiotomy. A routine ovariohysterectomy is performed with some exceptions. The uterus is usually large, heavy, and friable (Fig. 33.28A and B). It should be manipulated with extreme care during the procedure to prevent rupture and contamination of the abdomen. This means that the celiotomy incision should extend from the xiphoid to the pubis so that excessive tension is not placed on the uterus during manipulation. Vessels are usually prominent and may be increased in number, so care must be taken to ligate and separate vessels appropriately to prevent hemorrhage. Uterine contents should be cultured for aerobic and anaerobic bacteria and a bacterial sensitivity test performed after the uterus is removed from the surgical field. This is done via aseptic aspiration of the fluid with a needle and syringe before the uterus is contaminated but after removal from the surgical field to prevent contamination of the abdomen with purulent material. Taking care to follow sterile precautions, the uterus can be placed on a surgical drape on a table away from the sterile operating field, and an assistant can take the samples needed by using aseptic technique. The abdomen should be flushed before closure. Abdominal closure is routine.

Postoperative Considerations

Animals should be monitored as for ovariohysterectomy. Special considerations include continued antibiotic therapy in the postoperative period and significant fluid component loss as a result of the removal of the fluid-filled uterus. Septicemia can lead to severe complications, such as shock, disseminated intravascular coagulopathy, and death. IV antibiotics are given until the animal is stable and eating. Antibiotic therapy is continued for 7 to 10 days after surgery according to culture and sensitivity results. Electrolyte and metabolic abnormalities can continue postoperatively, and monitoring for this is important and should be corrected. IV fluids should be given until the animal is stable, eating, and drinking.

Canine Castration

Definition

Orchidectomy (castration or neuter) is the removal of both testicles. Scrotal ablation is removal of the scrotum with the testicles at the time of castration.

Indications

Numerous indications for canine castration are known; the most common is an elective procedure in the young male dog to help prevent roaming, aggressiveness, unwanted breeding, or a combination of these. Several medical problems may also be treated by castration, including prostate disorders, anal and perianal tumors, perineal hernias, and testicular tumors. Older dogs with a well-developed scrotum and animals with scrotal abnormalities should undergo scrotal ablation to prevent severe scrotal swelling, improve postoperative aesthetics, and/or treat disease.

Preoperative Considerations

An optimal age for canine castration is not known, but the procedure is often performed at around age 6 months. Performing castration before the development of unwanted male behavior—before sexual maturity—may help prevent this behavior from occurring. Castration after development of this behavior will often improve behavior but may not eliminate it in all male dogs. In large breed and giant breed dogs, recent orthopedic studies are showing that castration too early can cause significant changes in the maturation of the long bones and appendicular joints of these dogs, adding to arthritic and other joint dysfunctions during adult life. Lengthening the time these larger dogs have to complete their growth phases to 12 months or even 2 years is beneficial. Once the dog stops adding significant weight each month in proportion to height is a good indicator the growth phases are completing and the joints and long bones will be appropriately calcified prior to castration. Before surgery, a careful examination should be performed to ensure that both testicles lie within the scrotum.

Technique and Intraoperative Considerations

The abdomen is clipped from the tip of the prepuce to the margin of abdominal skin and scrotal skin. The clipped area should extend widely into the inguinal region. The scrotum typically is not draped into the surgical field and is not normally clipped during surgical preparation. The scrotum has delicate, thin skin that is easily subject to clipper burn and laceration. If, however, long scrotal hairs are protruding into the surgical field, they should be trimmed without touching the clippers to the scrotal skin. If scrotal ablation is to be performed, the scrotum is clipped and prepared aseptically, along with the rest of the surgical field (Fig. 33.29).

For simple castration, the dog is secured in dorsal recumbency, and standard surgical preparation of the prescrotal skin (cranial to the scrotum) is performed. A testicle is pushed cranial beneath the prescrotal skin. A midline incision is made in the prescrotal skin centrally and over the cranially displaced testicle. With gentle pressure, the testicle is exteriorized through the incision by carefully incising

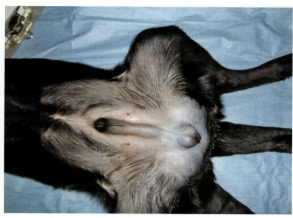

• **Fig. 33.29** Canine castration. Proper positioning and preparation for canine castration via scrotal ablation. Note that the scrotum is clipped. The same positioning is used for routine castrations, but the scrotum does not require clipping.

over the common tunic (tissue that encases the testicle). The testicle is pulled away from the body for ligation as the remaining scrotal ligament is gently dissected from the testicle. Ligation can proceed with an open technique or a closed technique. For the closed technique, two ligatures are placed external to the tunics of the pedicle such that all the vessels and the vas deferens are ligated as a unit. This technique is fast, but if it is not carefully done, the vascular pedicle can slip inside the tunics and into the abdominal cavity, causing uncontrolled hemorrhage. The closed technique is best used on very small patients. The open technique allows individual ligation of the vas deferens and its blood supply and the pampiniform plexus. The testicle is then removed with sharp severance distal to the ligatures. The opposite testicle is handled similarly and is exteriorized through the same incision as the first. The incision is closed with a continuous subcuticular suture pattern. It is best to bury the suture here, because potential irritation might increase the urge to lick.

For scrotal ablation, the incision is made circumferentially around the base of the scrotum (Fig. 33.30A). Care must be taken to avoid removal of too much skin around the scrotum to prevent excessive tension on the closure. The subcutaneous tissue is bluntly dissected to expose the testicles and associated structures. Castration is carried out via ligation of these structures as for simple castration (see Fig. 33.30B). The testicles and scrotum are removed and the incision closed in two to three layers.

Postoperative Considerations

Several postoperative complications can occur. If the preoperative preparation is not done carefully to preclude scrotal dermatitis (clipper burn, excessive scrubbing), the dog will lick aggressively at the scrotum and the incision. This often results in severe inflammation and swelling of scrotal and prescrotal skin. If this problem is not detected early, results can include premature suture removal and wound dehiscence. The best treatment is prevention; if scrotal dermatitis does occur, an Elizabethan collar should be applied on the dog.

Another less common complication is hemorrhage. When the testicles are removed from the scrotal sac, free space remains in the scrotum. If any hemorrhage occurs from the subcutaneous tissue or the common tunic, either from a minor vessel leakage from the surgery or continuous stimulation of the area by the dog because of irritation from licking or nuzzling, the space will fill with a considerable amount of blood before enough pressure is present to create hemostasis, resulting in a large hematoma within the scrotum.

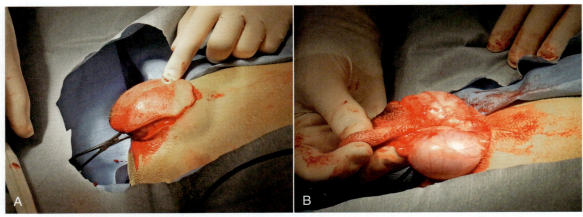

• **Fig. 33.30** Canine scrotal ablation. (A) An incision has been made around the scrotum, ensuring that enough skin would be available for closure post castration. (B) The testicles are exposed through blunt and sharp dissection after the skin incision is made.

If a hematoma is detected early, before the scrotum is full, cold compresses can be applied with slight pressure to the scrotal area to encourage hemostasis. If the scrotum becomes excessively large, not only is it unsightly, but trauma and skin sloughing may occur. At this point, removal of the scrotum may be necessary.

A scrotal seroma is more likely to occur than hemorrhage and can result in scrotal swelling, and can be exacerbated by stimulation of the area by the dog. In older dogs with well-developed scrotal tissue, fluid accumulation after castration can be excessive. Some advocate performing scrotal ablation at the time of castration to prevent this complication in older animals. Treatment is the same as for hematoma. It is important to restrict activity in these dogs to decrease the amount of fluid accumulation.

Feline Castration

Definition

Feline orchidectomy (neutering) is the removal of both testicles.

Indications

Major indications for feline castration are to prevent fighting, roaming, and urine spraying, and to decrease urine odor. Castration in the cat may lead to a rapid response (2 to 4 weeks) to these objectionable characteristics, although complete resolution may not occur owing to age, learned behaviors, or other stressors in the cat's life that were not corrected with castration alone.

Preoperative Considerations

The cat is usually castrated at around age 6 months. Preanesthesia evaluation should include palpation of both testicles to confirm the gender of the cat and to detect retained testicles before surgery.

Technique and Intraoperative Considerations

Several acceptable techniques may be used for feline castration. The patient is generally placed in dorsal recumbency with the legs restrained gently (Fig. 33.31). Unlike in the dog, the scrotum is the site of the primary incision and should be aseptically prepared for surgery. Scrotal dermatitis is not a major concern in the cat, although alcohol is not recommended for use on the scrotum during surgical

preparation. Warmed sterile saline is a good substitute for alcohol. Scrotal hairs are gently plucked from the scrotum with thumb and finger (Fig. 33.32). This is easily accomplished by grasping the base of the scrotum with the thumb and index finger of one hand and gently pushing the testicles into the scrotum. The thumb and finger of the other hand are used to gently strip hair from the scrotal skin. The scrotum is then scrubbed and draped in an aseptic manner.

An incision is made directly through the scrotum, then the testicle is pushed through the incision by gentle pressure with the thumb and index finger (Fig. 33.33A and B). The testicle and its spermatic cord (vessels) are exteriorized with gentle traction and stripping (see Fig. 33.33C). The spermatic cord may be ligated with suture, ligated with metal clips, tied in a knot on itself, or the vessels can be separated from the vas deferens and tied in a square knot. The testicle is then removed by severing the spermatic cord with a blade distal to the ligation site. The scrotum is not sutured, which is why alcohol prep is not recommended (see Fig. 33.33D).

Postoperative Considerations

Scrotal swelling and bleeding are the two most common complications of feline castration. Scrotal swelling is due primarily to traumatic surgical preparation and hair plucking. An Elizabethan collar may be necessary to control licking. If scrotal hemorrhage is noted after surgery, cold compresses on the scrotum for 5 to 7 minutes will help encourage hemostasis (but practically, this is difficult to accomplish). Severe hemorrhage can and may occur intra-abdominally. The veterinary technician should monitor these animals carefully and should bring clinical abnormalities to the attention of the veterinarian (see the section "Blood Loss"). Scrotal infection occurs rarely and should be treated with drainage (if not already draining), scrotal flushing, use of the Elizabethan collar, and appropriate antibiotics.

When the cat is sent home, the owner should be informed to change the litter from a gravel type to shredded paper or pelleted type for the first 5 to 7 days. This will prevent pieces of litter from contaminating the surgical site.

Cesarean Delivery

Definition

The term *cesarean delivery* is derived from the name of Caesar, who allegedly was the first human to be delivered by such a technique.

The procedure involves making an incision into the abdominal cavity and then into the uterus to deliver a neonate. It is usually performed on animals experiencing dystocia. Dystocia (Greek: *dys,* "difficult" + *tokos,* "birth") literally translated means "difficult birth."

Indications

Cesarean delivery is indicated when a bitch or queen cannot deliver puppies or kittens through the birth canal by normal

uterine contractions because of maternal or fetal abnormalities. Some breeders schedule planned cesarean deliveries in dog breeds that might typically have birthing problems, such as Bulldogs. Common causes of dystocia are presented in Table 33.1. Normal stages of parturition are discussed in Chapters 10 and 21.

Preoperative Considerations

The aim of treatment should be the successful delivery of live and undamaged puppies or kittens without harm to the dam. Medical

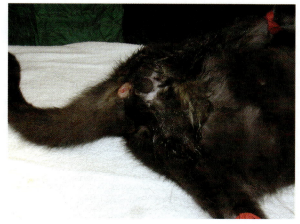

• **Fig. 33.31** Proper positioning for feline castration. The legs are pulled gently forward, and the cat is in dorsal recumbency.

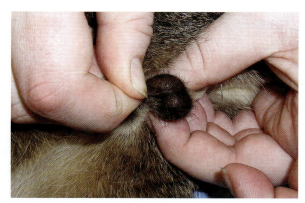

• **Fig. 33.32** Technique for scrotal plucking to remove hair in preparation for surgery.

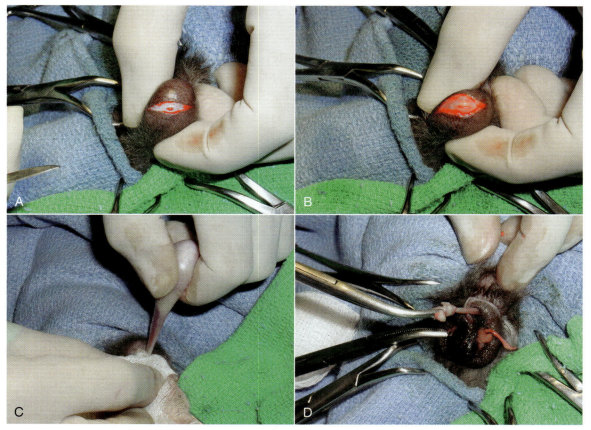

• **Fig. 33.33** Feline castration. (A) A skin incision is made directly over the scrotum, as pictured. (B) Manual pressure is applied to the testicle to exteriorize it through the incision. (C) Traction is then applied to the testicle to pull it out of the scrotal sac for ligation. (D) In this image, the spermatic cord has been knotted on itself and then will be released to go back into the scrotal sac. The scrotal sac will be left unsutured.

TABLE 33.1	Common Causes of Dystocia		
MATERNAL FACTORS			**FETAL FACTORS**
Contraction Forces	**Birth Canal**		**Oversize Fetus**
Uterine inertia (lack of contractions) • First degree (primary) Uterine muscle defect Oxytocin deficiency Premature birth • Second degree	Inadequate pelvis • Immature • Fracture • Breed • Disease		Faulty pelvic presentation • Caudal simultaneous • Head flexion • Limb flexion
Abdominal • Age • Pain • Hernia of uterus • Uterine rupture	Insufficient dilatation • Uterus • Cervix • Vagina • Vulva		

therapy to increase uterine contractures or to treat metabolic abnormalities in the dam should be considered before surgery; however, a diagnosis of the cause of dystocia must be made first. Medical therapy may do more harm than good when used in the wrong type of dystocia (e.g., giving a drug [oxytocin] that would increase uterine muscular contractions to a dam that has a uterine obstruction from a malpositioned or overlarge fetus or uterine torsion). When proper diagnosis of the type of dystocia is made and medical therapy is contraindicated or is not effective, the dam should be prepared for surgery. Dehydration and other metabolic alterations should be addressed before anesthesia, if possible. If not, treatment during and after surgery may be necessary.

The anesthetic regimen is of prime importance when cesarean delivery is considered. The dam that is dehydrated and exhausted and has potential metabolic abnormalities from a prolonged attempted delivery is a poor candidate for anesthesia. Anesthetic complications may be encountered. Selected anesthetic agents should have minimal effects on the newborn and should be safe for the dam.

Technique and Intraoperative Considerations

Clipping is performed before anesthesia. Care should be taken to avoid damaging enlarged mammary glands and nipples. After anesthetic induction and maintenance, the dam is placed in dorsal recumbency. It is important to remember that increased weight of the gravid uterus on the diaphragm may compromise the normal breathing capacity of the dam, and intermittent manual respiration or a ventilator should be considered.

A ventral midline celiotomy is performed in which the uterus is exteriorized and isolated with moistened surgical towels. Uterine isolation helps prevent uterine contents from entering the abdominal cavity. An incision is made into the ventral aspect of the uterine body. Care is taken to avoid cutting a fetus. A neonate and its associated fetal membranes are advanced through the uterine incision by applying gentle manual traction and pressure to the uterine wall. On fetal presentation, the fetal membranes are removed, the umbilicus is clamped or ligated, and the neonate is handed to an assistant. Fetal membranes can be firmly attached to the uterus if the fetus was not full term. Severe hemorrhage can

result if membranes are pulled from the uterus under these circumstances. Each successive neonate is handled similarly until all are delivered. The birth canal (uterine body and vagina) is checked carefully before closure to ensure that a fetus is not wedged there. The uterine incision is closed in two layers. The abdominal cavity is flushed to remove any debris that might have leaked into it from the gravid uterus. The celiotomy incision is closed routinely. The skin should be closed internally with an absorbable suture to prevent premature removal by puppies or kittens during nursing. Puncture of swollen mammary tissue with the needle during closure should be avoided, because puncture can lead to milk leakage and subsequent irritation of tissues.

Some owners prefer that the dam be spayed at the time of cesarean delivery. This can be accomplished in two ways: en bloc removal of the gravid uterus with secondary extraction of the neonates, or cesarean section followed by uterine body closure and ovariohysterectomy. En bloc resection entails clamping both the ovarian pedicles and the uterine body, cutting the gravid uterus out of the dam, then going back and ligating all vasculature in the dam. The gravid uterus is given to an assistant, who then cuts each neonate carefully from the uterus by using sterile instruments and ligates or clamps the umbilicus. The technique chosen by the surgeon depends on preference and assistance available to care for the neonates. No proven benefit or downfall is associated with either technique if performed appropriately. Removal of the uterus and ovaries at the time of delivery does not affect milk production or motherly instincts. Alternatively, the dam can be returned for ovariohysterectomy after the neonates have been weaned.

Postoperative Considerations for the Neonate

The assistant should be ready to grasp the neonate from the surgeon, receiving it in a dry towel. The assistant can then massage the animal gently to stimulate respiration, dry any secretions around the mouth and nose, and dry the remainder of the body to decrease the risk of hypothermia. The mouth should be inspected for evidence of mucus that may be plugging the airway. Gentle suction of the nostrils or mouth may be necessary to remove debris. Weak neonates and those with faint respirations may be stimulated by placing doxapram (a respiratory stimulant) under the tongue. A thorough examination for congenital defects is performed, and the neonate is placed in an incubator or a warm, padded area. Neonates stressed from the prolonged attempted delivery may not survive or may already be dead by the time cesarean delivery is attempted.

Neonates should be returned to the dam as soon as she has recovered from anesthesia. Care should be taken to avoid returning them so early that the dam may unknowingly harm them by stepping or lying on them. The dam should be returned to her home environment as soon as possible so that she can begin caring for the neonates and to prevent transmission of pathogenic organisms to immune-challenged neonates.

Postoperative Considerations for the Dam

The dam should be awakened from anesthesia as soon as possible so that the neonates can begin to nurse. The mother and neonates should be monitored carefully as they are introduced to each other. Most dams accept the young readily, but some may be aggressive. Pain medication should be administered judiciously, because most medications are secreted in the milk and can affect the neonates. Epidural drug administration before surgery can provide pain relief for 4 to 8 hours and will minimize the need for pain medication and transmission of these drugs to the neonate. Other considerations include the development of metritis secondary to retained fetal membranes or infection, excessive uterine hemorrhage from overzealous fetal membrane removal, and all potential complications discussed for routine celiotomy or ovariohysterectomy, if that was performed at the same time. Some dogs may experience infertility after cesarean delivery as a result of scar tissue formation.

Cystotomy

Definition

Cystotomy means incision into the urinary bladder to expose the lumen, or the interior of the urinary bladder.

Indications

The most common indication for cystotomy in small animals is for removal of cystic calculi (i.e., bladder stones). A cystotomy is also indicated to remove tumors, to correct congenital defects, or to repair traumatic rupture of the urinary bladder. A final indication for cystotomy is placement of a cystostomy tube (a tube exiting the urinary bladder and abdominal wall) to provide an alternative outlet of urine in the case of tumor, calculi, or scar tissue causing obstruction of urine flow through the urethra.

Preoperative Considerations

Animals undergo cystotomy for various reasons. If urinary flow was obstructed, the animal should be stabilized before anesthesia, and surgery should be performed. Severe metabolic and/or electrolyte abnormalities might be present. Imaging studies may be necessary to identify the extent of disease and its exact location.

Technique and Intraoperative Considerations

The abdomen is widely clipped from the xiphoid to the pubis. In male dogs, care is taken to clip the hair from the prepuce. The preputial orifice and the penis are then gently flushed with a 1% povidone-iodine (Betadine) solution.

The animal is placed in dorsal recumbency and is prepared for surgery with a standard skin preparation. For male dogs, the abdominal skin incision should curve laterally to avoid the prepuce (see Fig. 33.20D). Care should be taken to thoroughly prepare this area aseptically. The prepuce is draped into the surgical field for urinary calculi removal. This allows placement of a urinary catheter through the urethra for flushing of the urethra to aid in calculi removal. Although it is more common for urinary stones to lodge in the urethra of the male, a urethral catheter should be passed in the female, because urethral calculi have been reported to lodge there occasionally. The urinary catheter in the female dog is usually placed aseptically before surgery. Care should be taken if bladder expression is attempted before celiotomy, because an outflow obstruction from tumor, calculi, or scar tissue may result in inadvertent bladder rupture. Bladder expression should be avoided in those cases or when urinary bladder wall fragility is expected (e.g., urinary flow obstruction or tumor).

In the female, a standard caudal midline celiotomy is performed. In the male, a caudal midline skin incision is made from the umbilicus to the sheath of the penis and is then extended

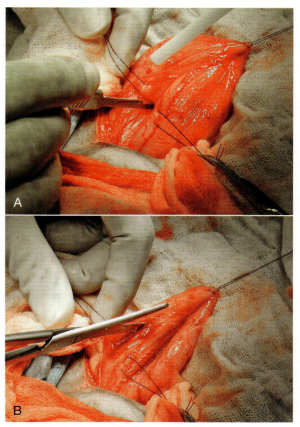

• **Fig. 33.34** Cystotomy. (A) Note the stay sutures in the urinary bladder. Stay sutures are held by the surgical assistant to help stabilize the tissue for the surgeon. This technique can be used for any hollow organ, including the stomach, small intestine, colon, and gallbladder. (B) An incision has been made into the urinary bladder between the two stay sutures and is being extended with scissors.

lateral to the sheath. The caudal superficial epigastric artery and vein lateral to the prepuce are encountered. These are ligated and transected. The sheath is retracted laterally, and a ventral midline celiotomy is performed. The bladder is exteriorized and is packed off with laparotomy pads to preclude urine spillage into the abdominal cavity. If urinalysis and urine culture were not obtained before surgery, a syringe and needle are used to obtain a urine sample before cystotomy. An avascular area on the ventral aspect of the bladder is visualized and two stay sutures placed along the intended incision line (Fig. 33.34A). An incision is made along the proposed incision line between preplaced stay sutures (see Fig. 33.34B). If cystic calculi are present, they are removed and submitted for stone analysis. If biopsy samples are taken for a suspected tumor, samples are placed in formalin and submitted for histologic analysis. Sample collection containers should be readily available; urinary calculi are not typically placed in formalin, and it is best to ask for clarification on appropriate sampling technique from the laboratory to which they will be submitted. Culture of crushed bladder stones, the bladder wall, and urine samples is performed to ascertain pathology.

Because calculi can lodge in the urethra, after removal, the entire lower urinary tract (bladder to urethra) is flushed with sterile physiologic saline solution until all calculi have been removed. The bladder wall is inspected for abnormalities and then closed with a simple interrupted or inverted suture pattern.

Laparotomy pads are removed and counted, lavage of the abdomen is done with sterile physiologic saline solution, and the abdominal incision is closed routinely. A postoperative imaging study may be necessary to determine whether all calculi were removed.

Postoperative Considerations

The animal should be placed on IV fluids after cystotomy to dilute blood clots and flush the urinary bladder. Urine production should be carefully monitored. If the incision was close to or involved with the proximal urethra, postoperative swelling can obstruct urine flow. Also, blood clots can accumulate in the bladder and migrate into the urethra, obstructing urine flow. The veterinarian in charge should be alerted if the animal is straining to urinate and does not produce a urine stream or has not produced urine in 12 hours. Some straining to urinate can be expected after cystotomy because of swelling and bladder irritation, but a urine stream should accompany the straining and the bladder should be nearly empty afterward. During the first postoperative week, mild hematuria (bloody urine), with or without blood clots, and frequent urination can be expected. If this continues or worsens instead of improving, the animal should be re-evaluated.

> **TECHNICIAN NOTE**
>
> During the first week after cystotomy, mild hematuria, with or without blood clots, and frequent urination can be expected.

Treatment ultimately depends on urinalysis, urine culture, and identification of the type of disease present (type of calculi, type of tumor, and type of congenital defect). If cystic calculi were removed, stone analysis must be performed before an appropriate treatment regimen can be initiated. Therapy will likely involve dietary alterations and/or antibiotics. Owners should be informed that recurrence of calculi is a possibility and that dietary recommendations should be followed strictly to decrease that risk.

Postoperative complications are rare after cystotomy. They include urinary outflow obstruction because of swelling or lodging of blood clots in the urethra, celiotomy incision complications, uroabdomen secondary to urine leakage through the cystotomy incision, and recurrence of the primary problem. If the animal is unable to urinate after cystotomy, a temporary urinary catheter may have to be placed to keep the bladder decompressed until surgical swelling decreases. This is not done routinely, because catheter placement can cause further irritation to the healing cystotomy incision and increases the chance of infection. An animal that could not urinate before surgery and had blood work abnormalities should have blood work (renal values, electrolytes, and PCV/TP) reassessed serially to ensure that values are returning to normal postoperatively. If the animal is not producing urine or is producing minimal urine and abdominal distention is detected, a complete biochemistry panel, CBC, and paracentesis should be performed. Fluid taken from the abdomen should be centrifuged for determination of PCV, creatinine, and BUN. Values higher than serum values indicate a problem and should be reported to the veterinarian in charge. Urine leakage through a cystotomy incision is treated with an indwelling urinary catheter or reoperation and appropriate urinary bladder incision closure.

Urethrostomy

Definition

Perineal urethrostomy is the process of making an external opening in the urethra in the area of the perineum that is large enough for passage of urine, mucus, crystals, and small calculi without obstruction. It bypasses the narrow penile urethra, where obstruction often occurs. The procedure is performed in male cats with recurrent urethral obstruction secondary to feline urologic syndrome. Urethrostomy is also performed in other locations, and procedures are named by their location (scrotal urethrostomy, prescrotal urethrostomy, antepubic urethrostomy, etc.). Scrotal urethrostomy, rather than perineal urethrostomy, is performed in male dogs prone to calculi obstruction or in those with penile scar tissue preventing normal urination, because this location provides the best functional outcome. The general technique is the same.

Indications

The primary indication for a perineal urethrostomy is multiple episodes of obstruction in association with feline urologic syndrome. Other less common indications include rupture of the penile urethra secondary to traumatic catheterization or blunt trauma (e.g., hit by a vehicle, kicked in the abdomen), stricture of the penile urethra, and obstruction secondary to cancer.

Preoperative Considerations

A cat with feline urologic syndrome can present with an array of clinical findings, as in the case of dogs with urethral obstruction. The presentation often depends on the duration and completeness of the urinary obstruction. A common factor is straining to urinate. If the animal is brought for examination early, there is little chance that other organ systems are affected. If the animal is brought in 12 to 24 hours after a complete obstruction, severe electrolyte abnormalities, cardiac arrhythmias, kidney dysfunction, and shock can be present. These animals must have the obstruction removed and must be stabilized with establishment of improved or normal renal function before surgery when possible. Catheterization with or without light sedation may be necessary. IV fluid therapy to help remove toxins is also needed. Some animals will require lifesaving measures to protect the heart from severe electrolyte abnormalities (high potassium). Preoperative ECG monitoring and blood work are key diagnostics to determine the state of the patient. Obstruction of urine flow is an emergency in both cats and dogs.

Depending on the suspected cause and location of the obstruction, preoperative imaging studies will be necessary to determine the exact location and extent of the problem.

Technique and Intraoperative Considerations

For perineal urethrostomy, the hair on the perineum and external genitalia is clipped, and the cat is placed in ventral recumbency with the perineum elevated approximately 30 degrees (Fig. 33.35). The tail is extended directly over the dorsal midline and is immobilized with tape. A purse-string suture is placed in the anus to eliminate fecal contamination of the surgical field. Standard skin preparation is performed. For perineal urethrostomy, an elliptical skin incision is made around the scrotum and the prepuce. The testicles are removed if the cat is intact. The penis

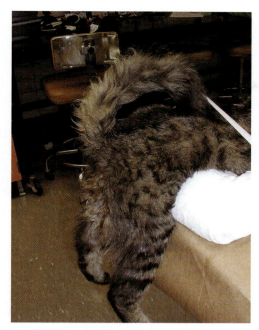

• **Fig. 33.35** The perineal position can be used in the dog or the cat.

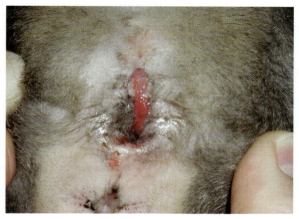

• **Fig. 33.36** This is the appearance of the urethrostomy opening 14 days after surgery.

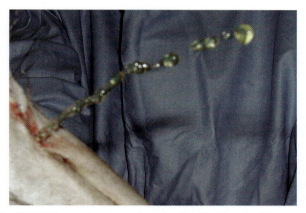

• **Fig. 33.37** After urethrostomy in cats, the bladder should be gently expressed to ensure easy passage of urine.

is dissected free from its pelvic attachments. A catheter is placed in the urethra, and a longitudinal incision is made through the penile urethra, extending cranial to the level of the pelvic urethra. The diameter of the pelvic urethra is approximately two times that of the penile urethra. This allows normal urination in the face of crystalluria (sandlike material in urine) and mucous plugs. The urethral mucosa is sutured to the skin. The remaining portion of the penis is amputated during urethral suturing, and the urinary catheter is removed. The result is a new, permanent opening that will accommodate the excess mucus and crystals (Fig. 33.36). The bladder should be expressed at completion of the procedure to ensure that a good urine stream is obtained (Fig. 33.37).

For scrotal urethrostomy in male dogs, the animal is placed in dorsal recumbency, and the area is prepped as for castration and scrotal ablation. Scrotal urethrostomy in male dogs is performed as in perineal urethrostomy, except that the penis is not amputated. A skin incision is made in the area of the scrotum (castration with scrotal ablation is performed in intact dogs), followed by a urethral incision over a preoperatively placed urethral catheter and then suturing of the urethral mucosa to the skin as for perineal urethrostomy. Gentle urine expression should be done to clear contents and check patency.

Postoperative Considerations

The purse-string suture is removed from the perineum. Immediate postoperative care includes placement of an Elizabethan collar and examination of the surgical site for evidence of hemorrhage. The Elizabethan collar is essential to keep the animal from licking the sutures and should be worn until normal urination has returned without hematuria or straining. Mild hemorrhage during urination is expected for the first 1 to 2 weeks after surgery. Dripping blood is possible, mostly after urination. This usually is of no consequence and will resolve on its own. Rarely is the bleeding severe enough to require additional surgery or transfusion. Animals should be placed on IV fluids for at least 24 hours after surgery, especially if urinary outflow obstruction was encountered,

to maintain normal renal function and flush the urinary bladder and urethra.

The animal should be monitored carefully for normal urination in the early postoperative period. If no urine is produced 12 hours after surgery, the bladder should be manually (firmly but gently) expressed until normal urination is seen. Postoperative catheters are discouraged because of the increased incidence of strictures at the surgery site. Some animals may have a distended and flaccid urinary bladder that will not contract normally after surgery because of overstretching of the bladder and loss of neuromuscular connections, damaged muscle tissue, and formation of scar tissue. The bladder may not function normally for several days in these animals, and manual expression of urine and possible catheterization may be needed. Animals are prone to urinary tract infection and potential overflow incontinence. The urethrostomy site should be manipulated as little as possible. Ointments and warm cleansings are discouraged. These may delay healing or aggravate hemorrhage. For cats, the use of shredded paper or pellets in the litter box is recommended for the first 6 to 10 days. Dietary alterations may be necessary, depending on the composition of the mucous plug, grit, or calculi causing the obstruction, and the presence or absence of a urinary tract infection. Owners should consult with the veterinarian before returning the animal to regular litter, regular exercise/activity, removal of the Elizabethan collar, or modifications in diet.

The most common postoperative complication is stricture, a narrowing of the urethral opening caused by excessive scar tissue formation that requires surgical correction. Self-mutilation of the surgery site by licking can increase the chance of stricture formation and must be prevented. Strictures typically manifest as chronic stranguria (straining to urinate). Complete obstruction of urine flow may also be noted.

Hernias

The strict definition of a *hernia* is the protrusion of tissue from its normal cavity (generally the abdominal cavity) through a congenital or acquired defect in the wall of that cavity. Common hernias in the dog and cat include umbilical, inguinal, and diaphragmatic hernias.

Umbilical Hernia

Definition

An *umbilical hernia* is one in which bowel or, more commonly, omentum and intra-abdominal fat protrude through a defect in the abdominal wall under the skin at the umbilicus. This hernia is most commonly congenital and it is recognized on physical examination by the presence of swelling at the umbilicus (Fig. 33.38).

Preoperative Considerations

Most umbilical hernias are not life-threatening and are surgically repaired at the time of ovariohysterectomy or castration. Small hernias in young dogs (2 to 4 months of age) may be self-limiting. Larger hernias or those in older dogs (6–9 months of age) generally require surgical repair. Large umbilical hernias can result in intestinal entrapment (incarceration) within the confines of the hernia, with resultant **strangulation** (loss of intestinal blood supply with devitalization and possible intestinal perforation). If intestinal strangulation occurs, emergency surgical repair is necessary.

Technique and Intraoperative Considerations

The abdomen is widely clipped from xiphoid to pubis before placing the patient in dorsal recumbency and performing standard skin preparation. A ventral midline incision is made directly over the hernia with care taken to avoid perforating hernia contents. The skin is dissected away from the hernial sac; the contents are then exposed and may be replaced into the abdominal cavity (intestine) after inspection and any surgical resection required, or excised (falciform or omental fat). The edges of the hernial ring are trimmed to ensure healing of the defect. The abdomen is closed with a routine celiotomy incision.

Postoperative Considerations

Postoperative care is like that provided for any celiotomy incision. Recurrence is a rare complication of repair, and reoperation is necessary for correction.

Inguinal Hernia

Definition

An *inguinal hernia* is one in which intestine, uterus, broad ligament, intra-abdominal fat, and/or another abdominal organ protrudes through the inguinal canal because of a defect in the constraints of the canal. This is more common in the bitch than in the male dog. An inguinal hernia is diagnosed on physical examination by the presence of a soft, doughy, nonpainful mass in the inguinal region.

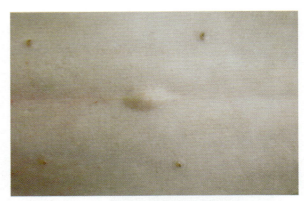

• **Fig. 33.38** Note the raised lesion in the region of the umbilicus (umbilical hernia) on the ventral abdomen.

Inguinal hernias can develop early or late in life; they do not spontaneously regress, and surgical correction is necessary.

Preoperative Considerations

The opposite inguinal ring should be carefully palpated for weakness. Owners should be told that hernias can develop bilaterally, even if a hernia is not present on the opposite side at the time of presentation. Owners should also be told that recurrence is rare but possible.

Technique and Intraoperative Considerations

The abdomen is widely clipped from the umbilicus up to and including the inguinal area. The animal is placed in dorsal recumbency and standard skin preparation is performed. A midline skin incision is made in the caudal abdomen between the inguinal folds. The abdominal cavity is not entered. Lateral dissection is performed carefully to expose the affected inguinal ring with its hernial sac and external pudendal vessels. The hernial sac is emptied of its contents with gentle manipulation and pressure toward the abdominal cavity. The empty sac is then excised and sutured along with the margin of the inguinal ring. Care is taken during closure to avoid the external pudendal vessels that exit from the caudal medial aspect of the ring. The skin incision is closed as for celiotomy.

Postoperative Considerations

The incision is monitored similarly to any abdominal incision. The owner should monitor for recurrence or occurrence on the opposite side.

Diaphragmatic Hernia

Definition

In a *diaphragmatic hernia*, abdominal contents protrude through an opening in the diaphragm into the thoracic cavity. Diaphragmatic hernias may be congenital or caused by trauma.

Preoperative Considerations

Any animal with a history of trauma or suspected trauma should be examined for the presence of a diaphragmatic hernia. Diaphragmatic hernias can be immediately life-threatening or insidious and difficult to identify. Presumptive diagnosis is based on a thorough physical examination. Classic signs of diaphragmatic hernia include a "tucked-up" abdomen (thin, empty abdomen), intestinal sounds in the chest, muffled heart and lung sounds, and dyspnea. However, some animals have only decreased lung sounds over the area of the hernia and mild exercise intolerance, if any. The diagnosis is confirmed by thoracic radiographs.

TECHNICIAN NOTE

Animals with a diaphragmatic hernia should have oxygen and cage confinement to ensure maximal oxygenation, minimal stress, and constant monitoring for respiratory insufficiency before surgery.

An animal with a massive hernia will have a diminished intrathoracic space as a result of the presence of abdominal contents within the thoracic cavity. The resultant space-occupying mass does not allow the lungs to expand normally and compromises delivery of oxygen to blood. These animals can have life-threatening respiratory compromise and should be treated appropriately. Any animal with respiratory compromise should be stabilized by ensuring minimal stress, oxygen cage or nasal oxygen insufflation, confinement, sternal recumbency, and constant monitoring for respiratory insufficiency or arrest. Holding the animal gently and with the head up and the hindlimbs hanging down may allow some abdominal contents to shift back into the abdomen. Along the same lines, the animal can be propped up in such a way that the front half of the chest and shoulders is positioned higher than the hindquarters. IV access should be established in case of an emergency, provided the stress of catheter placement does not cause further respiratory distress. Thoracic radiography will be necessary for diagnosis and to assess for other pathologic conditions. Oxygen therapy should be given to compromised animals during workup and catheter placement. The animal should be stabilized before anesthesia. Rarely is diaphragmatic hernia repair an emergency. Mortality is actually higher in those animals operated on acutely for the problem. Only in cases of severe respiratory distress, gas distention of a herniated viscus (stomach) in the chest, or intestinal strangulation is immediate operation necessary. However, animals with chronic hernias have a greater chance of severe complications that could result in death. In general, operation for a diaphragmatic hernia should occur 1 to 3 days after presentation if the animal is stable. Blood work should be obtained in all traumatized animals to assess overall health and organ function.

TECHNICIAN NOTE

Positioning an animal with a diaphragmatic hernia in sternal recumbency with the shoulders higher than the pelvis or gently raising the animal up from the front end may help reduce abdominal structures back into the abdomen from the thoracic cavity and improve respiration.

Technique and Intraoperative Considerations

One of the most critical times for an animal with a diaphragmatic hernia is anesthetic induction. It is important to be thoroughly familiar with induction procedures and resuscitative techniques in the event of respiratory or cardiac arrest. The animal is placed in dorsal recumbency on an incline, with the head slightly higher than the hindquarters. It is important to remember that severe respiratory compromise may result when the animal is placed in dorsal recumbency, and the technician should be prepared to provide breathing assistance to the animal. Mechanical ventilation or intermittent manual respiration will be necessary throughout the procedure.

The skin is widely clipped from about 3 inches cranial to the xiphoid to the pubis. The lateral thoracic wall on at least one side, preferably the side of the hernia, should be clipped and aseptically prepared for potential chest tube placement or thoracocentesis. A ventral midline celiotomy from xiphoid to near the pubis is performed. The edges of the incision are protected with laparotomy pads, and a Balfour self-retaining abdominal retractor is placed to enhance visualization. The diaphragmatic defect is inspected and any herniated contents are gently reduced into the abdominal cavity. If the herniated contents do not reduce easily, the diaphragmatic defect is enlarged slightly to allow easy reduction. A thorough inspection of abdominal and thoracic viscera is made to rule out organ rupture or vascular compromise.

Repair of diaphragmatic hernia can require working in a deep cavity if the tear is found along the dorsal or lateral components of the diaphragm. Ventral hernias are more easily exposed for repair. Gentle retraction of viscera to expose the defect during repair is necessary to preclude damage to abdominal organs and to allow adequate visualization by the surgeon (Fig. 33.39A and B). The diaphragmatic defect is sutured in a simple continuous suture pattern. This will create an air-tight and water-tight seal.

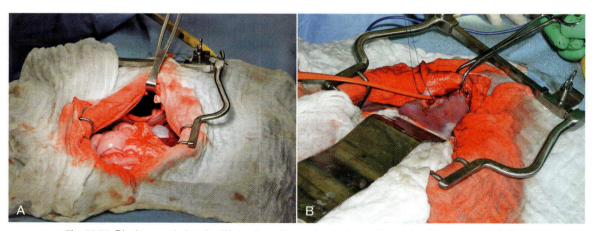

• **Fig. 33.39** Diaphragmatic hernia. (A) An Army-Navy retractor is positioned to show a large hole in the diaphragm at the cranial edge of the incision *(top of picture)*. The abdominal contents have been removed from the chest cavity and have been returned to the abdominal cavity. (B) The defect in the diaphragm has been closed, and a red rubber catheter has been inserted into the right side of the defect near the sternum *(the left side of the picture)* for restoration of normal intrathoracic pressure before the abdominal cavity is closed.

Air is evacuated from the chest by thoracocentesis through the diaphragm or with chest tube placement. The celiotomy is closed routinely. After celiotomy closure, the chest cavity is once again aspirated from the lateral thoracic wall. If a chest tube was placed, evacuation of the thoracic cavity is done through the chest tube.

Postoperative Considerations

The animal should be monitored carefully for signs of respiratory distress. It is best to waken the animal with oxygen supplementation provided through placement in an oxygen cage or through nasal insufflation. If a pulse oximeter is available, oxygen saturation should be checked frequently, especially during attempts made to wean the animal off oxygen. The animal should remain on oxygen until oxygen saturation is maintained at a rate greater than 94% on room air. If dyspnea occurs or if the animal cannot maintain normal oxygen saturation, the chest should be evacuated with a hypodermic needle, a three-way stopcock, and a large syringe, or evacuation can be done through the chest tube. A rapid return to normal negative thoracic pressure and normal lung capacity should be seen with evacuation of air and fluid. In some cases, pulmonary trauma may also be present. This could lead to continued respiratory compromise and/or pneumothorax in the early postoperative period. Therefore thoracic radiography should be considered in the animal that is having respiratory compromise after surgery.

If an indwelling chest tube was placed, periodic aspiration using positional changes (right lateral recumbency, left lateral recumbency, standing on hindlimbs, standing on forelimbs) will afford maximal removal of air and fluid. It is of utmost importance to keep the animal from chewing a hole in the drain or removing it from the chest cavity, and those involved in tube management should be informed on how the tube should be handled. An Elizabethan collar will be necessary, and the chest tube should be covered with a bandage and the animal closely monitored. It is imperative to keep all connections on the chest drain air tight. A security clamp should be placed on the tube to keep air from leaking into the chest if the free end of the tube is inadvertently opened. Premature removal, puncture, or inappropriate management (leaving the three-way stopcock open to the atmosphere) can result in acute animal death secondary to pneumothorax and resultant pulmonary dysfunction. Proper management of a chest tube requires full-time patient monitoring and knowledge of appropriate chest tube emptying. A chart quantitating the amount of air and fluid removed during a given period (12–24 hours) will help determine when the tube should be removed. Most chest tubes are removed immediately after surgery once negative intrathoracic pressure is obtained or within 12 hours of hernia repair. Otherwise, the tube can be removed safely as the amount of air and fluid decreases toward zero.

> **TECHNICIAN NOTE**
>
> An animal with a chest tube should be handled carefully to prevent inadvertent introduction of air around the lungs and death of the animal. Make sure the tube is air tight, that all connections to the environment are closed, and that it is equipped with a protective clamp.

Lumpectomy

Definition

Lumpectomy refers to local surgical resection of a mass, often a cutaneous or subcutaneous mass.

Indications

Indications for lumpectomy include masses of cancerous origin, masses that appear to be changing over time, rapidly growing masses, ulcerative masses, or masses that are impairing function.

Preoperative Considerations

Some masses are related to biochemical or blood cell alterations. Blood work should be performed to evaluate for these abnormalities. Where possible, abnormalities should be corrected before anesthesia. Additionally, many animals undergoing surgery for mass resection are older and may have organ system failure, which should be evaluated before anesthesia. After a mass has been diagnosed, fine-needle aspiration of the mass may be performed. If the mass is considered benign (e.g., lipoma), resection can proceed, or the owner can monitor the mass. If the mass is suspected to be cancerous, or if it is in a location at which future resection may not be possible if growth occurs, resection should be considered. If the mass is suspected of being cancerous, further workup for detection of metastasis should be considered. This would involve blood work, urinalysis, three-view thoracic radiography, abdominal radiography, and possibly, abdominal ultrasonography. Advance imaging or sampling of other areas may also be needed, depending on the location and character of the mass. All surgically resected masses should be submitted for histologic evaluation. Diphenhydramine injection is recommended before surgery or aspiration if the mass is suspected to be a mast cell tumor because of increased risk associated with degranulation of these tumors.

Technique and Intraoperative Considerations

The skin around the area to be resected is prepared for surgery. It should be remembered that a generous clip needs to be performed, because normal margins will have to be removed with the mass. Additionally, large mass resections will require that normal skin around the mass be pulled into the surgical field during closure. If the skin was not prepared aseptically before surgery, this will contaminate the surgical field. Masses should be manipulated as little as possible before surgery. A sterile marker may be used to draw an elliptical pattern around the mass to be removed after the animal is draped for surgery (Fig. 33.40). Include 1 to 3 cm of normal tissue in the resection plane; large margins are reserved for cancerous lesions. The mass is removed and the wound closed in three or more layers, depending on the depth of dissection and resected tissue. Where large amounts of tissue were resected, active drains may have to be placed beneath the wound to prevent fluid accumulation, or advanced surgical techniques may be needed to close the area. Rarely, some excised areas may have to be managed as an open wound. The mass is marked with ink or suture to note cranial and lateral margins for the pathologist evaluating the mass. This will facilitate future surgical planning if the mass was found to be incompletely resected.

Postoperative Considerations

The surgical wound should be monitored as any other surgical procedure. Large resections will result in tension on the incision line, making dehiscence more likely. Animals should be exercise restricted until the wound is healed and sutures have been removed. Owners should be told that additional steps for treatment may be needed once a diagnosis has been obtained (future

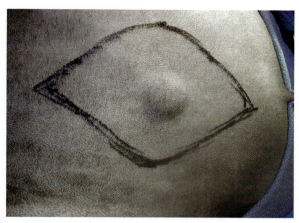

• **Fig. 33.40** Surgical margins have been outlined around this skin mass for removal of the mass and a margin of normal tissue.

surgery if complete resection was not obtained, chemotherapy, radiation therapy, etc.).

Removal of Mammary Neoplasia

Definition

Mammary neoplasia is cancer of the mammary gland. It is the most frequently occurring neoplasm in the female dog and the third most frequently found tumor in the female cat. Mastectomy is removal of a mammary gland. Radical mastectomy is removal of a chain of mammary glands on one or both sides of the animal. Lumpectomy is removal of a mammary tumor with approximately 1 cm of normal marginal tissue—not the entire mammary gland.

General Information and Indications

In dogs, a significantly higher incidence of mammary gland tumor has been noted in intact females and in females that are spayed after their first estrus. Spaying before the first estrous cycle provides a definite protective factor against mammary tumor development.

In the initial stages, the tumor usually appears as a small, firm, pea-shaped mass in one or more of the glands of the mammary chain. Long-standing or fast-growing tumors may present a sizable mass with ulceration and drainage. Early diagnosis and therapy is best.

Before surgery is considered, an examination is done to detect possible metastasis of the tumor. Malignant tumors generally metastasize to the lymph nodes and lungs. Chest radiography may detect pulmonary metastases, and abdominal radiography may show iliac lymph node enlargement suggestive of metastasis. Approximately 50% of mammary tumors in dogs are malignant, and about 80% to 90% of mammary tumors in cats are malignant. Surgery is currently considered the most effective therapy. The primary objectives of surgical treatment are to remove the tumor tissue completely for potential cure and to obtain a histologic diagnosis of tumor type and behavior. Surgical resection of tumors that have already metastasized does not improve the prognosis.

Technique and Intraoperative Considerations

Two techniques are available for tumor resection. In dogs, there appears to be no advantage of radical gland resection versus lumpectomy unless the tumor has been incompletely excised. Lumpectomy affords the same long-term outcome associated with varying forms of mastectomy as long as the tumor is freely movable, small, and on the periphery of the gland. If the tumor is centralized within a gland, multiple tumors are present within a gland or a chain of glands, or the tumor is large and/or fixed, a more radical excision is warranted. In cats, unlike in dogs, recurrence is decreased if a unilateral mastectomy is performed, rather than local excision of the mass. If bilateral radical mastectomy is necessary, the procedure must be staged (removal of one side at a time) to allow less tension on the skin closure. The skin is clipped widely to include all affected mammary glands. The animal is placed in dorsal recumbency, and a standard skin preparation is performed. An elliptical incision is made, attempting to include a 1-cm margin around the tumor. The skin and tumor, with or without the mammary gland, are gently undermined and removed. The skin incision is often gaping if an entire gland is removed, requiring meticulous subcutaneous closure. Subcutaneous tissues are closed with a simple interrupted pattern using absorbable suture material. An active drain may be placed if a large amount of tissue is removed to prevent fluid accumulation under the skin. The skin is closed routinely. The excised mammary masses are placed in formalin for biopsy.

Postoperative Considerations

Major complications that can occur postoperatively are generally related to tension placed on the skin to adequately close the wound when large amounts of tissue are removed. Seroma formation is common, especially if a drain was not placed at the time of surgery and the resection was large. It is best to bandage these animals for 48 to 72 hours postoperatively to prevent large amounts of fluid from accumulating under the incision and to make the animal more comfortable if radical excision was performed. Warm compresses may be needed after seroma development, but cold compresses can be used to decrease swelling and improve pain relief in the first 24 to 48 hours after surgery. Dehiscence is not common, but the incision should be examined daily for evidence of separation, especially if a large amount of tissue is removed. Bruising along the incision edges is common and should be expected. Immediate postoperative hemorrhage can occur. In the event of oozing blood, an abdominal bandage should be applied with gentle pressure. If a drain was placed, a bandage should be placed over the drain, which will be emptied several times a day, and is removed when minimal drainage is noted. If the animal irritates the sutured incision by licking, an Elizabethan collar should be applied until suture removal. An Elizabethan collar should be applied if a drain is in place to prevent self-inflicted pulling or breaking of the drain. The animal should be exercise restricted to help prevent dehiscence and seroma formation, especially if a large incision under tension is present. Radical mastectomy is a painful procedure and pain management should be continued for at least 5 days postoperatively.

Amputation

Definition

Amputation refers to partial or complete removal of a body part, such as a limb or a toe. This section covers limb amputation.

Indications

Indications for amputation include appendicular cancer not amenable to local excision or another treatment modality; severe neurologic dysfunction resulting in repeated trauma to a limb; nonunion fractures that will not result in limb function with orthopedic repair; irresolvable osteomyelitis; vascular disease of the limb, such as thrombosis or arteriovenous fistula; severe trauma to the limb; and congenital deformity resulting in a nonfunctional limb that is not amenable to orthopedic repair. Simple limb fracture is not an indication for amputation, although some veterinarians may perform the procedure to remedy that problem.

Preoperative Considerations

Amputation can involve considerable blood loss. It is important to perform preoperative blood work, including assessment of coagulability, to determine the animal's overall health and to identify any concerns regarding anesthesia. Abnormalities should be corrected, where possible, before anesthesia. Thorough orthopedic and neurologic examinations should be done to assess for concurrent problems. The owner needs to be aware of other orthopedic or neurologic conditions and how they may affect function after amputation. Problems in other limbs can make ambulation after amputation difficult, depending on the severity and the type of problem. When amputation is done because of neoplasia, the animal should be screened appropriately for metastasis before surgery. The amputation must be planned so that adequate margins of normal tissue are obtained if cancer is involved. Amputation is a painful procedure, and analgesics are best initiated before surgery and continued without interruption in the postoperative period.

For hindlimb amputations with disarticulation of the coxofemoral joint in intact male dogs, scrotal swelling is a major concern. Seroma formation after amputation is common and fluid tends to accumulate in the scrotum. Scrotal swelling can become so severe that ablation is necessary. Additionally, the scrotum is more visible after amputation and may not be aesthetically pleasing to some owners. It is best to perform a scrotal ablation and castration at the time of amputation in these dogs.

Technique and Perioperative Considerations

The limb is suspended from an IV fluid stand. The limb is clipped and aseptically prepared for surgery. The clip should be generous and should include the skin around the base of the limb to prevent contamination during closure. In general, a skin incision is made around the limb in the area to be amputated. A surgical assistant is needed to help hold the limb in various positions during surgery while dissection occurs. Vessels are ligated and transected, and nerves may be blocked with local anesthesia and then transected. Subcutaneous and muscle tissues are dissected and transected for removal of the limb. Depending on the site of amputation, the limb may have to be disarticulated or the bone severed to remove the limb. Remaining muscle and subcutaneous tissue are closed over the bone and/or the wound bed. The skin is closed in three layers. If a large amount of dead space is present at the time of closure, a closed active drain may have to be placed.

Thoracic limb amputation can be done by removal of the scapula and the entire forelimb (forequarter amputation), by disarticulation of the scapulohumeral joint, or by ostectomy (excision and removal of all or part of the bone) at the level of the proximal humerus. Forequarter amputation offers the advantages that major vessels and nerves are well visualized, sectioning of the bone is not required, and the prominent scapular spine will not be present as the scapular muscle mass atrophies. It is also indicated in neoplastic diseases of the humerus (especially proximal) or of the scapula. Disarticulation leaves a fuller appearance to the thorax and requires less extensive dissection, but muscle atrophy over the scapula can be unsightly. If disarticulation is performed, the acromion process should be excised to improve appearance. Proximal humeral amputation may be faster for some.

Pelvic limb amputation can be accomplished with disarticulation of the coxofemoral joint or with proximal femoral ostectomy. Proximal femoral ostectomy yields a more cosmetic result, particularly in an intact male dog. It is faster and easier than disarticulation. Neoplastic diseases of the femur will require disarticulation to obtain a normal margin of tissue.

Postoperative Considerations

Postoperative complications are not a major concern but should not be ignored. Analgesics must be given postoperatively in scheduled doses rather than on an as-needed basis for several days to keep the animal comfortable after this painful surgery.

Seroma formation is common. The area can be treated with cold compresses for the first 24 to 48 hours after surgery; if a seroma forms, warm compresses can be initiated. The limb should be bandaged for the first 24 to 48 hours, if possible (Fig. 33.41), to provide some comfort and help minimize seroma formation. The animal should be exercise restricted because motion will increase the size of the seroma. Hematoma formation is also a possibility.

Formation of a seroma or hematoma after surgery can increase the risk of infection. If infection occurs, the incision site may have to be opened and drained and a culture and sensitivity test performed. Anemia can occur in the postoperative period because of blood loss at the time of surgery. Transfusion may be necessary. IV fluids should be administered postoperatively until eating and drinking are resumed. Additionally, the animal should be kept in a well-padded area and supported with a sling when taken out for a walk (until the animal learns to ambulate on three legs). Tension on the incision line, seroma formation, or infection may lead to dehiscence. Depending on the cause and degree of dehiscence, this is managed conservatively or with surgical closure. Animals with neoplasia may develop metastatic disease or may have tumor recurrence at the surgery site.

Amputation is generally a more traumatic experience for the owner than for the pet. Dogs and cats that have had their limbs amputated continue to be excellent pets, and it is important to help the owner understand this. Most animals begin to ambulate within 24 hours of surgery (Fig. 33.42), but some may take a little longer. Almost all are ambulatory within 2 days of surgery. Animals should be kept in the hospital until they are ambulating and their pain is well controlled. Amputees have an excellent prognosis unless the limb was amputated to treat neoplastic disease, in which case the prognosis depends on the type of tumor.

Care of the Neurologic Patient

The most common neurologic disorder in the dog is intervertebral disk rupture. Disks are normally found between the vertebral bodies in the spine and act as shock absorbers during spinal movement and also provide structural support. Over time, disks can undergo degeneration and calcification. When this occurs, the normal shock absorber–like effect is impaired, and extrusion (rupture) of

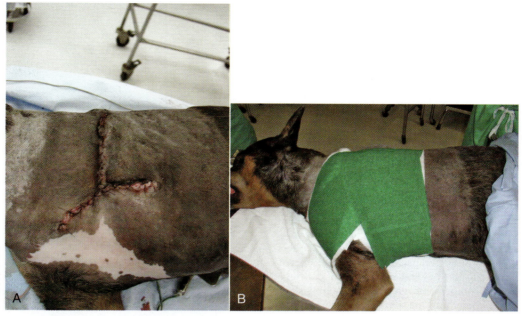

• **Fig. 33.41** (A) Amputation incision immediately postoperatively. (B) A bandage has been applied to the surgical area to provide compression and incisional protection.

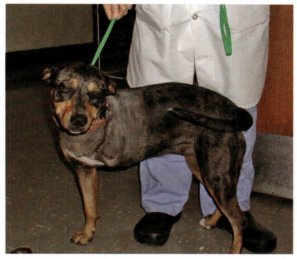

• **Fig. 33.42** This dog's forelimb was amputated the day before this picture was taken. Note how willing the dog is to be up and moving around and how support is not needed, even on postoperative day 1.

disk material into the spinal canal can occur. This puts pressure on the spinal cord and can cause an array of neurologic deficits or pain. Other neurologic disorders that may be encountered include atlantoaxial subluxation (abnormal articulation between the first and second cervical vertebrae); cervical vertebral malarticulation/malformation (wobblers); lumbosacral stenosis/malarticulation or cauda equina (compression of the lumbosacral nerve roots); acute spinal trauma (fracture or luxation); spinal cyst; cancer of the brain, nerves, or spinal cord; malformation of the caudal brain fossa; and hydrocephalus. Many animals with neurologic problems are referred to specialty hospitals for surgery. However, the veterinary technician should be familiar with some of the procedures that might be performed and should understand how to

manage such patients if they return to the veterinary hospital for care after surgery.

One neurosurgical procedure that is occasionally performed in small animal practice is intervertebral disk fenestration. During this procedure, each disk that is calcified or that may become calcified is removed (scraped) from the intervertebral space. This procedure is performed to help deter rupture of the disk material into the spinal canal, although its benefit is unproven. Dogs may develop spontaneous intervertebral disk extrusions in the cervical spine (neck) or the thoracolumbar spine (lower back). If the disk has already ruptured and the animal's ability to ambulate is affected, a decompressive procedure can be performed to alleviate compression on the spinal cord. The most common decompressive procedures are ventral slot (for cervical disk rupture) and hemilaminectomy (for thoracolumbar disk rupture). For acute disk herniation, the most affected breed is the Dachshund, but the Beagle, Pekingese, Poodle, Cocker Spaniel, and Terrier breeds also frequently experience disk herniation.

Surgical Technique and Perioperative Considerations

When an animal with spinal column instability is anesthetized, the normal protective abilities of muscle support and conscious perception of pain are removed, which can lead to additional trauma to the spine during manipulation. Conditions that can result in instability include spinal fracture or luxation and atlantoaxial instability. Animals with such conditions as simple disk herniation or spinal malformation may be worsened by excessive manipulation while under anesthesia. It is the responsibility of the veterinary staff to protect the animal from further neurologic damage by handling the spine with care while the animal is under anesthesia. It is important to keep the neck and the back as straight as possible when moving the animal. To accomplish this, the animal can be taped to a rigid, flat surface; can be carefully cradled in the arm; or can be placed in a stiff blanket sling supported on all sides. The goal is to avoid manipulation of the affected area. The means of transportation is often dictated by the size of the animal, but a rigid, flat surface is the preferred method for transporting animals with severe instability of the thoracolumbar spine. For cervical instability, a neck brace can be placed. Sometimes, however, it is easiest to place the unrestrained animal on blankets or on a firm surface in a basket or a topless carrier so that the blanket or hard surface can just be lifted out with the animal supported. The awake animal will often protect a painful spinal fracture and mostly will lie still without the need to be taped down. Greater concern is evoked about the animal that is thrashing, severely sedated, or anesthetized.

Animals undergoing cervical disk surgery are placed in dorsal recumbency with the head and neck in slight extension (Fig. 33.43). The ventral aspect of the neck is widely clipped from the manubrium sterni to the cranial aspect of the larynx. Standard skin preparation is performed. A ventral midline incision is made through the skin and muscles to expose the intervertebral spaces. For fenestration, a dental tartar scraper, a curved needle, a fenestration hook, or a curette can be used to remove disk material from the interspace. If decompression is needed, an oblong slot is made through vertebral bodies into the spinal canal using a pneumatic or electrically powered bur. The disk material is then carefully removed from the spinal canal. Muscles, subcutaneous tissue, and skin are closed routinely.

Animals undergoing thoracolumbar disk surgery are placed in ventral recumbency. For fenestration, the dorsum over the back is widely clipped from the midthoracic region to the pelvis. Standard skin preparation is performed. A skin incision is made from T11 to L6. Careful dissection between epaxial muscles (muscles of the back) allows palpation and limited visualization of the disk spaces. For fenestration, each space between T10 and L5 is curetted with a technique like that described for cervical disk fenestration. If decompression is needed, a portion of the bony lamina covering the spinal cord is removed with a pneumatic or electrically powered bur. The ruptured disk material is then carefully removed from the spinal canal. Muscles, subcutaneous tissue, and skin are closed routinely.

Postoperative Considerations

Preoperative and postoperative care of neurologic patients depends on their neurologic status and the type of neurologic disease that they have. Management for the nonambulatory animal is demanding as they are subject to decubital ulcers or pressure sores (Fig. 33.44), urinary bladder infections, joint stiffness, muscle atrophy (muscle wasting), pneumonia, and GI ulceration. Preventing these conditions from occurring is the main objective of proper postoperative management, and steps should include the following:

- Passive range of motion exercises, muscle massages, underwater treadmill activity, sling walking, and whirlpool baths encourage joint motion and muscular activity and help decrease the occurrence of pressure sores. Passive range of motion should be performed at least three times a day on all affected limbs until the animal is able to ambulate normally.
- Urinary bladder expression should be performed four or five times per day to keep the urinary bladder empty. This will help keep the animal clean, will prevent detrusor muscle atony (i.e., flaccid bladder) secondary to bladder overdistention (which can lead to permanent bladder dysfunction), and might lower the incidence of infection resulting from urine retention.

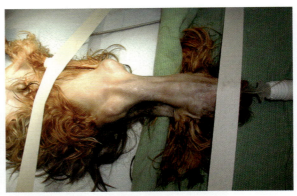

• **Fig. 33.43** Proper positioning for cervical disk surgery.

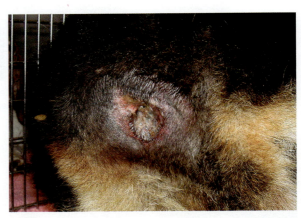

• **Fig. 33.44** Decubital ulcer (pressure sore). The ulcer developed over the greater trochanter of this dog as a result of improper care during recovery from spinal surgery.

TECHNICIAN NOTE

For animals that are unable to urinate, the urinary bladder must be emptied often by urinary catheterization or manual expression to prevent overdistention with permanent urinary bladder dysfunction, keep the animal clean, and help decrease the infection rate.

- Turn (feet under, not over the back) the completely down animal frequently (every 4 hours) to reduce the incidence of pneumonia and to help prevent pressure sore formation. Slings and wheelchairs can be used to get the animal up and off pressure points for a time if the spinal injury is stable.
- Monitor the animal daily for fever, cough, or respiratory distress. The down animal is at risk for pneumonia. Daily coupage and encouraging the animal to stand up and move will help prevent this.
- Keep the animal in a well-padded area to prevent the formation of sores. A waterbed mattress works well for large dogs.
- Keep the animal clean and dry. Soiling will increase the chance of pressure sore formation. This can be challenging when incontinence and immobility play a role.
- Observe the stool daily for evidence of fresh blood (bright red on feces or thermometer) or digested blood (dark, tarry feces), respectively, which may be an indicator of colonic or gastric ulceration, which can occur after spinal cord injury, hospital stress, and/or steroid therapy.

- Observe the vomitus. If it contains coffee ground–like material, it is indicative of gastric bleeding secondary to ulcer formation and should be reported to the veterinarian immediately.
- Observe the animal daily for evidence of pressure sores. Although prevention is the best form of therapy, sores tend to form over bony prominences, especially in large dogs. Prompt treatment should be initiated to prevent severe complications. Treatment consists of frequent turning, whirlpool baths, massages, antibiotics, clipping and cleaning of the area, surgical debridement, and/or bandages placed to alleviate pressure over a prominence, depending on the severity of the lesion.

TECHNICIAN NOTE

It is better to prevent pressure sore formation than to have to treat a pressure sore once it has occurred.

- Animals that have lost pain sensation in one or more limbs should be monitored carefully. These animals may begin to lick or chew the asensory (lack of feeling) portions of their limbs, especially if the area becomes traumatized. Some will even chew off toes or whole limbs. An Elizabethan collar should be placed immediately and the animal closely monitored if chewing or licking is noted.
- Animals that cannot feel their legs may develop ascending or descending myelomalacia. This rare problem is associated with severe spinal cord damage and loss of deep pain sensation, in which progressive loss of spinal cord function occurs as the result of progressive hemorrhage and destruction of normal tissue by inflammatory mediators. Animals that develop this problem may be experiencing great pain and exhibit progression of hindlimb paralysis to forelimb involvement, a change from upper motor neuron myotactic reflexes to lower motor neuron, and gradual loss of panniculus ("fly twitch") response along the back. It is important to alert the surgeon if this is suspected. Most of these animals will eventually suffocate because of loss of function of the diaphragm. Euthanasia before this occurs is recommended.
- Animals that cannot walk should not be allowed to roam free without protection and monitoring. They will traumatize the skin as they drag themselves around and can develop serious abrasions and ulcers.
- Animals with some motor function in the limbs and a stable spinal injury should be assisted/encouraged to get up at least three times a day and encouraged to use their limbs. Ambulatory but ataxic animals should be supported when ambulating to help prevent falls that might lead to further spinal damage. Rehabilitation through specialized centers offering underwater treadmill work and other rehabilitation techniques should be considered.

TECHNICIAN NOTE

To prevent further cervical damage, animals with injuries to the cervical spine should always be placed in a harness rather than in a collar.

All animals with neurologic injuries require cage rest and controlled activity to allow the spinal column to heal. All should be leashed when outdoors, crated when indoors, and restricted according to the surgeon's protocol. Cervical patients should always be placed in a harness, rather than a neck collar, to prevent further cervical damage. Owners should be carefully counseled on the importance of confinement for prevention of further spinal injury.

TECHNICIAN NOTE

All animals with a spinal injury will require cage rest, regardless of if surgery is done. It is important to emphasize to owners that cage rest is important for proper healing, even if the pet is walking and feeling normal.

Orthopedic Surgery

Long Bone Fractures

Preoperative Considerations

When an animal with a fracture is brought to the veterinary hospital, several steps must be taken to prepare the animal for a permanent repair. First, the animal must be stabilized with respect to all other body systems (treated for shock, chest injuries, and abdominal injuries). Second, any open wounds associated with the fracture should be managed. Third, the fracture must be immobilized by means of a bandage, cast, or sling if the fracture is in a location amenable to bandaging (see Chapter 27). Once these three steps have been achieved, fracture repair can be safely considered. Most long bone fractures are not life-threatening and do not require emergency surgery. Stability of the animal determines when the fracture is repaired.

TECHNICIAN NOTE

Most long bone fractures are not life-threatening and do not require emergency surgery.

Intraoperative Considerations

The limb is usually suspended by the foot. An extensive hair clip is required on all limb preparations. The limb will usually undergo extensive manipulation during reduction and repair. For this reason, the limb is clipped from the level of the metacarpus or metatarsus to the scapula or pelvis, respectively, including medial and lateral aspects of the extremity. This may vary slightly, depending on the bone that is fractured, but the general rule should be to perform a wide and thorough clip. The remaining hair at the tip of the paw is covered with a rubber glove or plastic wrap that is taped to the clipped skin. Refer to Chapters 32, 33, and 34 for detailed instructions on preparing limbs for orthopedic surgery.

Positioning

Animal positioning depends on the specific bone that is fractured. Generally, the following positions are recommended for different types of fractures:
- *Femur:* lateral recumbency, affected side up
- *Tibia-fibula:* dorsal recumbency, affected leg hanging
- *Humerus:* lateral recumbency, affected leg up
- *Radius-ulna:* dorsal recumbency, affected leg along the side, or lateral recumbency, affected leg up
- *Pelvis:* lateral recumbency, affected leg up

With so much skin exposed, skin preparation can be time consuming, but it must be meticulous. The surgeon eventually covers the extremity with sterile draping, but this should not preclude aseptic skin preparation.

Surgical Assistance

Orthopedic procedures are often difficult and time consuming and may demand the help of an assistant. Often, the veterinary technician is called on to participate as a surgical assistant and therefore should have a general understanding of orthopedic tissue handling and instrumentation (specifics of intraoperative assistance are covered in Chapters 31 and 32).

Several basic maneuvers commonly required by the surgeon are often performed by the veterinary technician. They include retraction, muscle fatigue, alignment and reduction, and suction of the field. Proper techniques for each are discussed separately.

Retraction

Care should be taken to preserve the soft tissues in the operative field. It will be necessary to have functional muscle groups remaining when the bone is repaired. Retraction should be firm but not so traumatic as to bruise or tear the muscle.

Muscle Fatigue. Fractures in large breed dogs or fractures that are 3 to 5 days old may be difficult to reduce because of heavy muscle mass or severe muscle contraction, respectively. In such cases, constant, steady traction on the muscle groups will cause them to fatigue and relax, thus facilitating reduction. Epidural anesthetics and/or paralytics can be used to aid in muscle reduction (review Chapters 28 and 29).

Alignment and Reduction

For repair of fractured bones, the ends must be reduced and aligned. It is often necessary for an assistant to hold reduction during fixation of the fracture. Pins, wires, screws, and plates of stainless steel may be used to achieve the necessary fixation.

Suction and Tissue Care

Whenever a fracture occurs, bleeding into the fracture site can be massive. Some continuous oozing occurs during fixation. A clean surgical field is of the utmost importance in facilitating early and accurate reduction and fixation. Pay particular attention to ensuring that fracture lines remain visible, because the surgeon needs to see them for reduction and alignment. Also, the tissues should be kept moist. Tissue desiccation can cause tissue death and loss of function. It is imperative that tissue manipulation is performed gently.

Postoperative Considerations

Some postoperative orthopedic patients may require external coaptation. Applied bandages should be managed as discussed in Chapter 27. Animals recovering from orthopedic surgery will likely require a limited time of passive activity but with specific instructions to the owners to ensure a smooth transition back to full use of the limb. Animals should be encouraged to use the operated limb to increase blood supply to the fracture site, to maintain joint and muscle health, and to speed fracture healing. However, limb use should be slow, deliberate, and well controlled. No off-leash activity, running, jumping, or playing with other animals should be allowed. A crate is the best place for animals that are recovering from an orthopedic procedure. The only orthopedic procedure in which activity is strongly encouraged is femoral head and neck excision, for which rehabilitation, building of muscle mass, and encouragement of weight bearing are extremely important for optimal limb function. The relatively unsure gait of a three-legged dog or cat makes it very important to consider the surfaces the animal will be walking on; avoid slippery surfaces (vinyl or wet floors) especially if the animal is unrestrained (e.g., owners putting animal in a bathroom rather than in a crate). Cement, grass, dirt, carpet, or rubber matting provides a much more sure-footed environment.

Rehabilitation is an important part of recovery. Slowly flexing and extending affected joints, along with muscle massage, will improve limb blood flow, maintain joint health, improve joint range of motion, improve muscle tone, and reduce muscle contraction. Range of motion exercises should be repeated two to three times per day with 10 to 15 repetitions of the exercise. A demonstration of proper technique by the technician will help the client understand the therapy. Slow leash walking is performed to encourage limb use initially. The sooner the animal is initially walked in a slow, controlled manner, the more likely it will be able to use the affected limb and work toward strengthening muscle and circulation.

Joints

Preoperative Considerations

Most orthopedic procedures involving a joint are elective, and patients rarely need emergency care. Traumatic fractures and luxation, however, do require urgent treatment. Indications for joint surgery include dislocations, ligament ruptures, infections, fractures, synovial biopsy, arthrodesis (surgical fusion of a joint), and treatment of osteochondrosis (abnormally thickened portion of the articular cartilage). Preoperative management should include limiting the animal's activity and controlling pain. External coaptation is rarely necessary for nonurgent cases but will make the traumatically injured animal (animals with luxation or fracture) more comfortable if the particular area involved is amenable to bandaging.

Intraoperative Considerations

An extensive clip, as for fractures, should be done for joint surgery. Positions will vary, depending on the joint involved. Generally, the following positions are recommended:

- *Hip:* lateral recumbency, affected leg up
- *Stifle:* lateral recumbency, affected leg up, or dorsal recumbency, leg hanging off the end of the table
- *Tarsus:* lateral recumbency, affected leg up for lateral; dorsal recumbency for medial approach
- *Shoulder:* lateral recumbency, affected leg up
- *Elbow:* lateral recumbency, affected leg up; dorsal recumbency for medial approach
- *Carpus:* lateral recumbency, affected leg up; dorsal recumbency for medial approach

Intraoperative assistance in joint surgery is like that necessary in fracture repair. Some special precautions should be taken while the joints are exposed.

Retraction

Care should be taken to avoid placing retractors in direct contact with the articular cartilage. This would damage the cartilage, which has a relatively poor response to trauma. When exposure of the joint is necessary, sharp retraction of the joint capsule will decrease trauma while increasing exposure.

> **TECHNICIAN NOTE**
>
> Care should be taken to avoid placing retractors in direct contact with the articular cartilage, and the cartilage should be kept moist to prevent permanent cartilage damage.

Flush

The cartilage should be frequently flushed with saline to keep it from drying out during the procedure. This is true of all tissues, especially the articular cartilage, because of its poor regenerative ability.

Postoperative Considerations

Postoperative care of animals undergoing joint surgery varies, depending on the surgical procedure, the joint involved, and the surgeon's preference. Early passive range of motion activity with light joint usage is recommended for most animals undergoing joint surgery. Heavy joint use is discouraged in the early postoperative period. Animals should be encouraged to use the affected joint during slow, leash-controlled walks, but are discouraged from running or jumping on the limb. Joint use is increased gradually over the course of recovery, which varies depending on the procedures performed. Joint immobilization is necessary in some cases, such as luxation, but is discouraged in most instances and can result in severe limitations in joint range of motion if care is not taken to rehabilitate the joint carefully.

TECHNICIAN NOTE

It is important to encourage limb use for optimal recovery after long bone or joint surgery. This is best done by slow, controlled leash walking at limited times throughout the day. Running, jumping, and off-leash activity are not allowed.

Client Education

The care an animal receives at home is just as important as the care it received at the veterinary clinic. In a matter of seconds, a surgery can be undone with inappropriate care. Failure to communicate concerns associated with the patient's primary problem and postoperative care can make the clinic liable for some complications.

The surgical patient has special needs. Some of these needs are general for all surgical patients, and others are specific to the surgical procedure performed. The following questions help guide client education and communication with the pet owner at the time of discharge.

1. *What is the intensity of patient care required after discharge?* Veterinary technicians communicate to clients the level of patient care required at home. Simple procedures require minor confinement, few medications, and incision monitoring; other patients may require more intensive home care. If the intensity of care needed is beyond the level that a layperson can be expected to provide, discharge should be reconsidered and delayed until the level of care needed is reduced to a manageable level. Transfer to a specialty clinic for 24-hour care may be another option, although the cost of prolonged care or specialized care may be challenging or prohibitive for the client. More frequent rechecks or progress checks may be needed to assess the patient and continue to update and reinforce home care.
2. *Can the owner provide the needed home care?* Pet owners are capable of providing home care, but it will be dependent on the individual's physical abilities, time constraints, and circumstances. Veterinary technicians should confirm that if the owner is not able to care for the pet, alternative sources of care are provided.
3. *What form of communication is best for helping the client understand the animal's needs at the time of dismissal?* Several methods of client education are available; what works best will depend on the nature of the surgical procedure performed and the personality of the client. Forms of communication include written instructions, handouts, verbal instructions, personal demonstrations, computer-based resources, and videos. In most cases, more than one form of communication may be needed. Showing the owner the surgical site and discussing what is normal/abnormal and when to do something about it should be the minimum communication. If any physical therapy, massage, or special care is needed, that, too, should be covered. Owners should not be dismissed until all questions are answered.
4. *What major concerns should be relayed to the owner for monitoring purposes?* Not only should general care be relayed to the client, but pet owners should also be made aware of potential complications, symptoms of concern, and particular concerns that the surgeon may have relative to the surgical procedure. The owner should be instructed on how to best monitor the patient for these potential complications.
5. *If complications or emergencies arise, what should the client do?* The veterinary clinician should make sure that owners receive clear contact instructions in case of an emergency or complication, depending on the time of day that the emergency occurs. Also, the clinician should educate clients about on-call emergency schedules and let them know that the pet's surgeon may not be available during an emergency. Clients should be given numbers to call for general concerns and questions.
6. *When should the animal return to the clinic for repeat evaluation?* If bandage changes or rechecks will be needed, those visits ideally should be set up on the day of discharge. Veterinary technicians should keep a list of animals that were discharged so that a callback system can be established to check on the client and the pet 1 to 2 days after discharge.

Guidelines for Discharge Instructions

Discharge instructions should be tailored to the procedure performed. A single form should not be used for every procedure, because specialized care may be required for some patients. However, general instructions that can be followed for every procedure should be provided, along with modifications based on need. Basic instructions would include medication administration, incision monitoring, activity restriction, and contact information in the event of a problem. Refer to Chapter 3 and to the Medical Record Forms (Evolve site) for specific examples of discharge instructions. If some form of rehabilitation is required, instructions and methods should be both written and demonstrated for the client. The same holds true for any specialized treatment technique, such as feeding tube management, wound care, drain care, and feeding instructions.

The veterinary technician should include in the medical record all communications and a copy of the discharge instructions. Maintaining appropriate medical record details is important for future reference and is a legal responsibility. Discharge instructions are generally posted as the last entry in the medical record before the patient's return for the follow-up visit. It must be ensured that the record is complete with a surgery report from the surgeon, a list of treatments performed, and signed consent forms. The technician must also remember to place the client on a future communication reminder for a follow-up phone call 1 to 2 days after discharge.

Recommended Readings

Dunning D. Surgical wound infection and the use of antimicrobials. In: Slatter D, ed. *Textbook of Small Animal Surgery. Vol 1*. 3rd ed. St. Louis, MO: Saunders; 2002.

Licroy MD, Bartels KE. Surgical lasers. In: Slatter D, ed. *Textbook of Small Animal Surgery. Vol 1*. 3rd ed. St. Louis, MO: Saunders; 2002.

Quandt JE. Postoperative patient care. In: Slatter D, ed. *Textbook of Small Animal Surgery. Vol 1*. 3rd ed. St. Louis, MO: Saunders; 2002.

Swim IIIHB, Creed JF. Restraint techniques for prevention of self-trauma. In: Bojrab MJ, ed. *Current Techniques In Small Animal Surgery*. 4th ed. Baltimore, MD: Williams & Wilkins; 1998.

Shmon C. Assessment and preparation of the surgical patient and the operating team. In: Slatter D, ed. *Textbook of Small Animal Surgery. Vol 1*. 3rd ed. St. Louis, MO: Saunders; 2002.

Tear M. *Small Animal Surgical Nursing: Skills and Concepts*. St. Louis, MO: Mosby; 2017.

34
Large Animal Surgical Nursing

AMY A. GEEDING AND MARGARET L. TRENTA

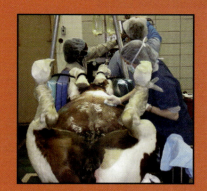

CHAPTER OUTLINE

LEARNING OBJECTIVES

When you have completed this chapter, you will be able to:

1. Pronounce, spell, and define all key terms in this chapter.
2. Describe the preoperative preparation needed for equine patients, as well as the responsibilities of the veterinary technician before, during, and after equine surgery, including postoperative monitoring, medication administration, bandage care, and grooming.
3. List the surgical procedures commonly performed in equine patients and describe indications and preoperative, intraoperative, and postoperative considerations for common surgical procedures in equine patients.
4. List the surgical procedures commonly performed in bovine patients and describe indications and preoperative,

intraoperative, and postoperative considerations for common surgical procedures in bovine patients.
5. Discuss the surgical procedures of young stock, including dehorning, castration, and umbilical hernias and infections.
6. Do the following related to small ruminants:
   - Discuss selected conditions of small ruminants related to the urinary and ophthalmic systems.
   - Describe the surgical procedures commonly performed in small ruminants, including indications and preoperative, intraoperative, and postoperative considerations for common surgical procedures in small ruminants.

KEY TERMS

Anastomosis
Arthroscopy
Celiotomy
Chondritis
Colpotomy
Cryptorchidectomy
Desmotomy
Entropion
Enucleation
Extra-label
Fetotomy
Hemiplegia
Herniorrhaphy

Hyperplasia
Laminitis
Laparotomy
Laparoscopy
Ostectomy
Pneumovagina
Rumenotomy
Sinusitis
Transfaunation
Trephination
Urachus
Urolithiasis

Introduction

The large-animal nursing skills of a veterinary technician are essential to the quality and efficiency of patient care. Veterinary technicians who work with large-animal patients routinely monitor those patients, execute patient treatments, assist the surgeon in the operating room (OR) by performing the roles of both circulating and scrub technician, provide client education, perform general nursing care, and maintain OR conduct. Because of the breadth of responsibility placed on the veterinary technician in a large-animal practice, large-animal surgical nursing requires substantial knowledge of surgical instruments, equipment, and implants, strong observational and communication skills (often helpful when acting as liaison between client and surgeon), clinical knowledge, and technical ability to provide the patient with the best care possible. Expertise in large-animal handling, restraint, and pre-, intra-, and postoperative care are critical to successful outcomes with these surgical patients.

Because of patient size, large-animal patient management can prove to be more intricate when compared with the management of small-animal patients. Despite their size difference, large-animal patients are just as fragile as small animals. A technician familiar with large-animal behavior and physical examination techniques can more quickly recognize signs of change in a patient's status, appearance of infection, and development of neurologic or respiratory clinical signs. Noting these changes and relaying them to the surgeon in a timely manner is invaluable in determining the course of patient treatment and to the overall outcome for the patient.

Surgical Nursing of Horses

Preoperative Preparation

Large-animal technicians are often responsible for appropriate preparation of the equine patient for anesthesia and surgery. Several steps need to be completed before a patient is ready for the OR, often based on the surgeon's specific preferences. It can be helpful, especially in a practice with multiple technicians and surgical staff, to develop checklists, thus ensuring accuracy when prepping equine patients. Communication is crucial; each patient will have individual needs and requirements. Communication between the surgeon, the OR staff, and the anesthesia staff prevents mistakes, ensures the efficiency of the surgical process, and allows for the best possible surgical outcome.

PUT INTO PRACTICE

Preparing for large-animal surgery procedures can be time consuming and intimidating. Break down the steps and learn each one. Preparing for each surgery should become a routine that you can do, no matter what the case. Patient preparation, room preparation, and communicating with your surgeon is the same, no matter what procedure you are set to do.

Because horses generally live outdoors, they may present in quite a dirty state. The surgical preparation process can be expedited by providing the patient with a thorough grooming to ensure a smoother procedure by keeping excess dirt out of the OR. This may not be safely possible with young or fractious equine patients but is a good practice to employ when feasible. A rubber currycomb used in a circular motion will loosen mud, dirt, and dander that has been worked into the patient's coat. A stiff bristle brush is used to remove debris and pick dirt and shavings from the

horse's feet. Dried mud and an animal's natural oils can dull clipper blades quickly. Using water and a mild soap to bathe a patient can help soften the hair and rid the area of dirt and oil, extending the life of the clipper blade. Before clipping the surgery site, if the patient is particularly dirty, it may be beneficial to wash the general area where surgery is to be performed or bathe the entire patient ahead of surgery.

A complete physical examination should be done for all patients going to the OR. This should include TPR (temperature—pulse rate—respiration rate) and auscultation of the heart and lungs. If there is evidence of an abnormal heart rhythm, the surgeon may order electrocardiography (ECG) to gain a better understanding of the patient's cardiac function and to assess anesthetic risk more fully. Preoperative blood work should, at the minimum, include a complete blood count (CBC) and fibrinogen determination, providing a snapshot of the patient's overall health and informing the surgeon of any underlying infection or factors that may adversely affect postsurgical recovery. Depending on the patient's overall health, some surgeons may also elect to perform a blood chemistry panel.

If a horse is wearing shoes, they may need to be removed before surgery. Shoes can be a hazard to a horse recovering from anesthesia and damage certain recovery stall floorings. If the shoes cannot be removed, it is best to cover them with gauze and elastic tape to provide better traction to the patient and protection of the floor.

Depending on the surgeon's preference and the indicated surgery, the site of surgery may be clipped prior to anesthesia to reduce anesthesia time and the amount of debris being introduced to the operating area. The clipping of the surgical site should still occur as close to the time of surgery as possible, as studies have shown an increase in surgical site infection potential with the increase in time between surgical clip and surgery. Communication with the surgeon is imperative before beginning clipping to ensure a wide margin around the surgical site. Should the surgeon need to extend the surgical incision during the surgery, they should not be prevented from doing so by an insufficiently sized clip area. Although clients will never see the surgery itself, they will see the technician's clip job; an untidy clip job is not only detrimental to aseptic technique but also a distraction during the postoperative period. Careless clipping suggests disorderly surgery, despite the two tasks usually being performed by separate individuals.

Hair should be clipped with a No. 40 blade against the grain of the hair, in a symmetrical fashion, and ensuring straight edges. When clipping a thick winter haircoat, it can be helpful to spray the coat liberally with alcohol immediately before clipping to dissolve oils and lubricate hairs for ease of clipping; however, hair soaked in alcohol does not vacuum well. Care should be taken to avoid clipping hair on the horse's mane and tail; those areas should only be clipped when necessary. Before clipping any part of a horse's mane or tail, such plans should be communicated to the clients, because they may need time to process the loss of their horse's mane or tail and should not be surprised by it upon the animal's return.

Once the surgical area has been clipped, it should be thoroughly cleaned with an aseptic scrub solution. Despite prior grooming/bathing, it is highly likely that the patient's skin may still be dirty. When applicable, the mane and/or the tail should be braided out of the way and secured with tape.

Most surgeons and anesthesiologists will want an intravenous (IV) catheter placed in the jugular vein prior to induction, with care taken not to interfere with the surgical site. Venous access for

IV administration during surgery allows for quick drug or fluid administration as needed.

Whenever IV catheterization occurs, care must be given to aseptic techniques to avoid complications, such as phlebitis and septicemia, which can arise from inadequate skin disinfection and trauma caused during catheterization. The catheter site should be clipped and scrubbed before the skin is adequately disinfected. To avoid discomfort, a bleb of local anesthetic is injected subcutaneously over the middle of the jugular vein. Sterile gloves should be donned before inserting the catheter, which must be secured with suture and/or super glue. A variety of different IV catheters are available. Consideration should be given to the length of time a patient is expected to need IV access and how quickly fluids will need to be administered.

For surgeries of a short duration performed in the field (e.g., equine castration), anesthesia may be maintained via IV injections by using only a syringe and needle. For standing surgeries, in which a patient is merely sedated and left standing for the duration of the procedure, placement of an IV catheter is left to the discretion of the surgeon, with the technician often being responsible for maintaining sedation. Other factors influencing the decision to catheterize for a standing procedure include the patient's receptiveness to frequent injections, the handler's ability to administer IV injections quickly and accurately, and the expected duration of the surgery. When in doubt, an IV catheter should be placed prior to the start of a standing surgery; attempting to place one on an uncooperative patient under surgical drapes creates a potentially dangerous scenario for surgeons, technicians, and the patient.

Prior to surgery, equine patients should be fasted for 4 to 6 hours to allow the stomach to empty, thus ensuring better ventilation. In most cases, fasted horses should still have access to drinking water. Foals of nursing age do not need to be fasted; however, if it is desired, they may be denied nursing for only 1 to 2 hours preoperatively. Horses have a strong grazing instinct and, when food is denied during their regular feeding schedule, they often eat things they should not, including stall bedding. Because of this, it is best to muzzle a patient while it is being fasted in preparation for surgery. Fasting as preparation for emergency surgery is usually not feasible.

Approximately 15 to 30 minutes before induction, the patient should receive any desired preoperative medications, such as antibiotics and anti-inflammatories, according to the surgeon's instructions; this allows time to observe for any allergic reaction while maximizing prophylactic benefits. The patient should also receive a tetanus toxoid vaccination if it was not previously administered.

When gas anesthesia is to be used immediately before induction, the patient's mouth should be thoroughly rinsed with a dose syringe or water hose until feed is no longer observed. Despite the patient having been fasted, hay or grass may still be packed in the patient's teeth and cheeks. Rinsing the patient's mouth avoids the risk of feed material being pushed into the airway during intubation. Once the horse has been anesthetized and intubated, the cuff should be inflated to prevent aspiration pneumonia.

Intraoperative Nursing

Efficiency by the team can help reduce the length of time the patient is under anesthesia, thereby reducing anesthesia-related morbidity and mortality. A smooth intraoperative experience depends on attention to detail and effective communication. Consultation with the surgeon should occur prior to anesthetic induction to confirm the instruments, equipment, and supplies expected to be used during the procedure, because these can vary from patient to patient. In larger practices with several surgeons, it is useful to keep a record of the specific preferences of each surgeon.

The most common method of tracking surgeon preferences is by using a "preference card" system, in which an index card is created detailing a specific surgeon's routinely requested instruments, equipment, and supplies for each procedure. Although such a system increases efficiency by ensuring that commonly used items are at hand, it does not preclude the need for a preoperative planning discussion between the OR technician and the surgeon. Patient positioning; the surgical plan, including contingency plans; and anomalies unique to the patient that may impact intraoperative care should be part of the preoperative planning discussion. This will allow for better anticipation of potential surgical complications. Additionally, any preoperative images as required should be available for the surgeon's reference throughout the procedure.

Maintenance of hemostasis during some procedures performed on a patient's limb can be promoted by the placement of a tourniquet. A flat, wide, rubber elastic bandage should be wrapped around the circumference of the limb, beginning distally and moving in a spiral fashion to a point just proximal to the surgical site. This will force blood out of the limb distal to the bandage. A wide bandage is preferred over a narrow bandage to restrict blood flow. The bandage can be secured in place by using adhesive tape at the proximal end, unwound from around the limb distally, and left in place during the procedure to function as a tourniquet.

Alternatively, a pneumatic tourniquet can be applied at the proximal end of the bandage and the bandage can then be removed. The benefit of both methods is to reduce the amount of blood in the surgical field, increasing visibility and thus reducing surgical and anesthetic times. A pressure bandage should be applied after closure of the surgical site and before releasing the tourniquet. Serious side effects can result from leaving a tourniquet in place for longer than 2 hours; therefore this is the maximum recommended length of time for use of a tourniquet.

Patient positioning is important in equine surgery, not only for ease of surgical performance but also because of potential complications related to the patient's size. The pressure created by the patient's body weight makes equine patients prone to myositis (muscle damage) when lying recumbent while under anesthesia. Myositis can increase morbidity and mortality, so the OR technician should ensure that adequate padding is used when placing an equine patient on the surgery table. Patients in lateral recumbency require padding under the face and limbs. Pulling the dependent forelimb forward as far as possible minimizes triceps and radial nerve pressure. Both hind limbs should be extended and parallel to the ground, with ample support.

Patients in dorsal recumbency require padding under their backs (Fig. 34.1). Sufficiently padded restraints should also be used to ensure that the patient does not move from side to side, because such motion will distribute pressure unevenly over the shoulders. All four limbs should be allowed to flex into a relaxed position, except the limb on which surgery is being performed. Hind limb extension should be reserved for aseptic surgical site preparation and the performance of surgery, as leaving a hind limb extended can lead to severe myopathy or neuropathy. Ultimately, the patient should be positioned in a manner which is safe for the patient while allowing the surgeon to access the surgical site easily and comfortably. Positions not providing easy access to the surgical site or that put the surgeon in uncomfortable or awkward positions contribute to prolonged surgical and anesthetic times and increased morbidity and mortality.

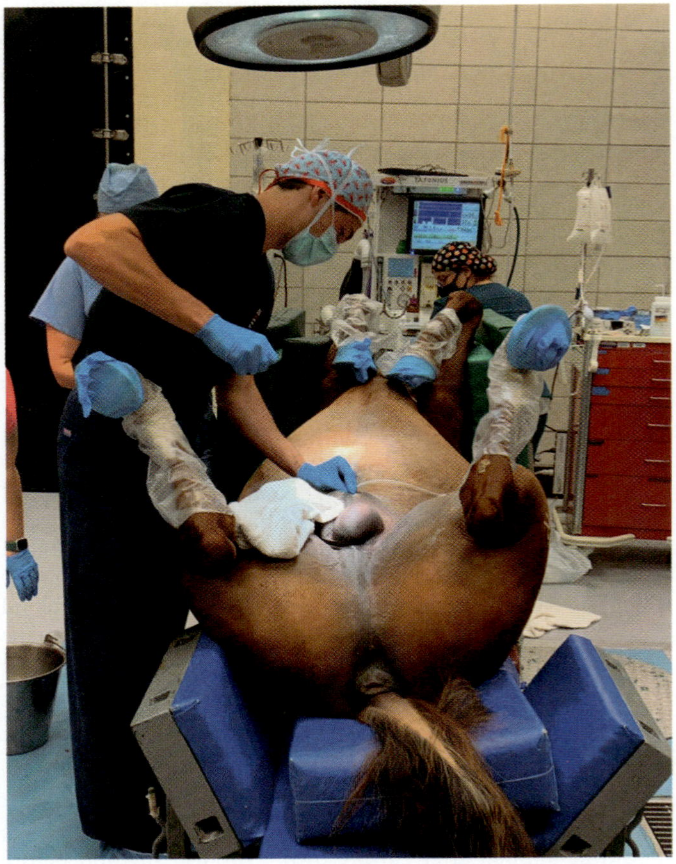

communication among the team members; verify key elements of the procedure, such as patient identity and surgical site location; and serve as a formal beginning to the procedure. A similar pause should occur as the procedure is ending. Although sample checklists are available, each practice should develop its own so that its checklist appropriately addresses its workflow.

Postoperative Nursing

Veterinary technicians are integral to the success of surgery and a surgeon's first line of defense against postoperative complications. Technicians are often responsible for providing the bulk of postoperative monitoring, administering treatments, and watching for subtle changes that could affect the overall outcome of surgery. Paying attention to detail and communicating any changes to the veterinarian quickly and accurately is important. Physical examinations should be performed twice daily at a minimum on all postoperative patients. Examinations and observations should be completed by using a consistent and methodical approach to ensure completeness and accuracy. Each process should be logged into the patient's records. Consistency in the examination process and documentation style across various technicians and work shifts is paramount.

When performing a postoperative physical examination, it is imperative to not only note the quantifiable values of the TPR but also to examine changes in incision site skin integrity, discharge (presence of and changes to), fluctuations in patient attitude and manner, and changes in gait. Some equine patients are very stoic, and an elevated heart rate may be the only early indication of increasing pain.

In equine patients, **laminitis** is an especially concerning postoperative problem. Changes in digital pulse palpation and hoof and coronary band temperature are early indications of laminitis. These should be communicated to the veterinarian immediately. Fever onset, diarrhea, and changes to respiration are all signs of infection and causes for concern in the postoperative equine patient. Early detection is essential in effectively treating postoperative issues. Any changes, both positive and negative, should be appropriately documented in the patient's chart and communicated to the veterinarian.

Veterinary technicians are often responsible for administering treatments as prescribed. These treatments may include providing and monitoring fluid therapy, administering antibiotics and anti-inflammatories, providing pain management therapy, and performing physical therapy.

Care should be taken to carry out orders accurately as ordered by the surgeon. Technicians must monitor prescribed dosages, route of administration, and frequency. Carelessness and inattention can lead to mistakes, some dangerous and potentially fatal to the patient. Furthermore, a technician should be aware of normal postoperative protocol and be able to recognize mistakes in the given orders; such errors should be discussed with the veterinarian before any changes are made. When mistakes are detected, they should immediately be communicated to the surgeon.

Surgical Considerations

Abdominal Surgery

Colic

Colic is many owners' worst fear, because it strikes rapidly with little to no warning, is the leading cause of death in horses, and is an emergency. *Colic* refers to nonspecific abdominal pain. More

• **Fig. 34.1** Stallion under general anesthesia in dorsal recumbency being prepared for a celiotomy to treat colic. A urinary catheter is being placed prior to scrubbing the surgery site. Note obstetric sleeves and exam gloves placed over the horse's limbs and hooves to prevent contamination of the surgical site.

Asepsis is vital to a successful surgical outcome and, as a member of the surgical team, the OR technician plays a key role in its maintenance. When preparing for the procedure the OR technician should ensure that all surgical packs and instruments have been appropriately cleaned, packaged, and sterilized. In preparing the surgical site for the procedure, the OR technician should adhere to the aseptic technique during the sterile or final prep. The scrubbed surgical team should follow the aseptic technique, beginning with applying their surgical scrub and through the gowning process. After opening the surgical packs, instruments, and supplies, both the OR technician and the scrubbed surgical team should visually and verbally confirm that all internal process indicators show adequate changes to denote the sterility of the instruments. Throughout these processes and the surgical procedure, the OR technician should observe the room with an eye toward maintaining asepsis. Should a break in aseptic technique occur, the OR technician should not hesitate to point it out. Breaks in asepsis put the patient's safety and the procedure's success at risk. If there is any indication that the aseptic technique may not have been strictly followed, the surgical team should respond as though a break in asepsis has occurred and act to rectify it as quickly as possible.

To ensure that the entire surgical team is thoroughly prepared and working from the same information, a surgical checklist, time-out, or call-out should be performed before the initial surgical incision is made. This brief pause is meant to facilitate than 70 causes of colic have been identified. Most, although not all, involve the gastrointestinal (GI) system, and the treatment may or may not be surgery. Horses are unable to vomit because of their anatomic features, including the long mesentery of the small intestine, the unfixed position of the left colon, termination of the right dorsal colon into a much narrower transverse colon, and narrowing of lumen at the pelvic flexure. Because of this, they are predisposed to complications of colic. Such factors as diet changes, habitat, weather changes, routine, vices, parasite control, and medical history are all important considerations when examining a patient brought in for colic. Although the causes vary, it is believed that most colic cases in adult horses are caused by impactions of the cecum and large colon, and spasmodic and flatulent colic, more commonly known as "gas colic." Retained meconium and gastric ulcers are the primary causes of clinical signs of colic in foals.

From the perspective of large-animal nursing, treatment for colic, whether surgical or medical, is among the most intense when considering patient care needs. Regardless of the cause of colic, the manifestations of pain include pawing, rolling, lying down, kicking or biting the abdomen, looking at the flanks, and sweating. Even the gentlest horse may quickly become violent, kicking, striking, or throwing itself down, thus putting the client and medical team at risk. Safety for veterinary personnel, the client, and the patient must be paramount during hospital admission and the initial examination.

To both improve safety and relieve some of the initial pain, the patient can be sedated with an alpha$_2$ adrenoceptor agonist such as xylazine, which offers some analgesia by suppressing central nervous system (CNS) neurotransmission and muscle relaxation. At high doses (1.1 mg/kg IV), xylazine is effective for the control of abdominal pain. A lower dose (0.30–0.7 mg/kg IV) is often preferred to provide effective analgesia. Its short duration of action allows for repeated assessment of the patient's condition without long-term masking of clinical signs. The most potentially serious dose-dependent side effects of alpha$_2$ adrenoreceptor agonist drugs are hypertension, decreased cardiac output, ileus, and decreased intestinal blood flow. Other α^2- agonists, such as detomidine, or nonsteroidal anti-inflammatory drugs (NSAIDs), such as flunixin meglumine, may offer better and more long-lasting GI pain management; however, they are not recommended during the initial examination of a horse that may require surgery.

Controlling the patient's pain at the start of the examination allows for safer diagnostic procedures required for a thorough assessment of the patient. Everyone involved in working up a colic case should be hypervigilant and remain aware of the patient's condition while assessing pain.

Several diagnostic aids are used to evaluate a colic patient and determine whether surgery is necessary and warranted. Large-animal technicians should have a good understanding of general physical examination, auscultation, passage of a nasogastric tube, rectal examination, transabdominal ultrasonography, abdominocentesis, and clinical pathology.

For patients in severe pain, nasogastric intubation should be performed at the examination initiation after baseline TPR and auscultation. Because the horse cannot vomit, the passage of a nasogastric tube allows for decompression of the stomach and anterior GI tract by providing an outlet for the reflux of gas and fluid (Fig. 34.2). This reduces pain of distension and aids in the prevention of gastric rupture. During this procedure, never stand directly in front of the horse, and keep a hand on the horse's head. A painful and frustrated horse may swing its head or strike at the handlers. Many patients

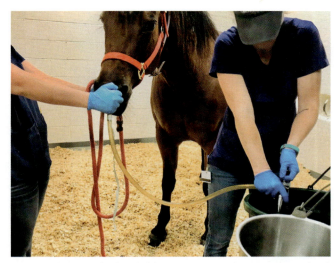

• **Fig. 34.2** A large-animal technician pumps water into a nasogastric tube to decompress the stomach of a horse exhibiting signs of colic. Note that the handler is standing to the side of the horse and supporting the tube in the nose.

may require a nose twitch to insert a nasogastric tube effectively. Regular manipulation of the tube, priming of the tube with water, and suction of the tube are necessary for gastric decompression, and the net amount of the reflux obtained should always be measured and recorded. In cases where reflux persists, an indwelling tube can be left in place by plugging the tube with a syringe, muzzling the patient, and taping the coiled tube to its halter.

Rectal examination is useful in horses to assess intestinal position and size, thickness, evidence of edema, tight mesenteric bands, or distention caused by gas and the presence of fluid or ingesta. Rectal examinations should be performed by a veterinarian using a thin plastic sleeve and ample lubricant to avoid excessive internal irritation, which can lead to rectal rupture. Even a horse being rectally palpated in stocks poses a safety risk, and the technician should communicate immediately if the examiner's safety may be at risk.

Transabdominal ultrasonography is a valuable tool for examining a horse with clinical signs of colic. It provides an image of the GI organs, giving clinicians a better picture of bowel placement, thickness, motility, and abdominal fluid. The composition of the abdominal fluid is determined by the condition of the organs bathed by it. Abdominocentesis is a reliable way to assess the condition of the abdominal contents. The ventral abdomen behind and to the right of the xiphisternum should be clipped and aseptically prepared. A local anesthetic may be used subcutaneously and via injection into the entry site. Depending on the sampling instrument (18-gauge × 3-inch spinal needle, teat cannula, or bitch catheter), the clinician may elect to make a stab incision with a No. 15 scalpel blade. When performing a stab incision, it is important to insert the cannula through a piece of sterile gauze to avoid the sample being contaminated by blood. When fluid is not immediately obtained, rotation of the needle, injection of air with a sterile syringe, or temporary obstruction of the patient's nostrils can be helpful.

Abdominal fluid is graded by gross appearance, cell count, and total protein (TP) concentration. Clinical pathologic examinations provide an invaluable adjunct to diagnosis when defining the cause or severity of GI disease. Routinely, packed cell volume (PCV) and TP will be determined during the initial examination

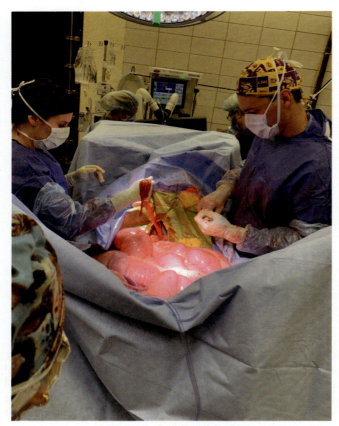

• **Fig. 34.3** Exploratory celiotomy being performed on an equine patient that was presented with clinical signs of colic.

of a patient exhibiting colic clinical signs. Subsequent clinical pathology may also be desired, such as CBC, blood chemistry, and blood gas analysis.

After careful consideration of the initial examination and diagnostics, the decision regarding surgical intervention is made. Decisions regarding surgical management should be made, because the more longstanding the problem, the less likely there will be a successful long-term outcome. There are several reasons to perform a celiotomy; however, GI tract surgery due to colic is the most common in equine patients.

Abdominal surgery can be complex, so a fully prepared surgical team is necessary to ensure an efficient procedure with the best possible outcome. Exploratory abdominal surgery, or celiotomy, is performed for generalized abdominal disease, including colic (Fig. 34.3). Although celiotomy can be performed through a flank incision on a sedated standing patient, it is most frequently performed via a ventral midline incision with the patient fully anesthetized.

The patient is placed into dorsal recumbency, and the hair of the ventral abdomen is clipped from the xiphoid to the pubis, with the lateral margins of the clip extending to both flank folds. If the patient is cooperative and if time permits, the abdomen may be clipped just prior to anesthesia induction. If the patient's hair is clipped on the surgical table, all clipped hair must be removed with a vacuum to avoid contaminating the surgical field, followed by a rough prep and then a sterile prep of the clipped area.

The surgical instrument table should be covered with a sterile drape, and the OR technician opens the necessary supplies for celiotomy; the supplies should include gowns and gloves for the scrubbed surgical team and a surgical pack containing towel clamps and draping materials, scalpel blades and handles, a variety of tissue forceps and clamps, a variety of scissors, and needle drivers. A variety of sutures should also be available. Celiotomy frequently requires sterile bowls, sterile suction supplies that connect to a nonsterile unit, and monopolar cautery.

If monopolar cautery might be used, the OR technician should ensure that a grounding pad is in place before beginning the surgical site prep. An ample stock of sterile lavage and sterile lubricant, which is used to break down adhesions and prevent further formation, should be easily accessible. A stock of sterile needles may also be needed to assist intestinal gas decompression or aspiration of fluids from abdominal organs.

In addition to celiotomy supplies, the OR technician should ensure that extra drapes and duplicate instruments are available if an enterotomy is to be performed (Fig. 34.4A and B). Many practices also use a tray and/or large bucket to strain debris removed during enterotomy to maintain a clean operating environment and to avoid overwhelming the OR drains (Fig. 34.5). GI stapling devices and cartridges may be required if intestinal resection and anastomosis are performed (Fig. 34.6).

Many factors can affect the overall prognosis of a patient recovering from GI surgery for colic. Nursing requirements for care immediately after surgery can often be even more intense. Many patients will require a nasogastric tube, and reflux may continue after surgery. Close attention must be paid to the patient's hydration status, fecal and urine outputs, pain display, and incisional integrity. Any changes should be reported and noted in the records.

The success of a postsurgical colic patient's recovery extends to the quality and detail of the discharge instruction provided to the owners. The return to forced exercise and athletic function is a long, slow process. Postsurgical colic patients should remain on stall rest, with frequent hand walking and grazing for the first 30 days following surgery. Patients may receive small paddock turnout (60' × 60') for the following 30 days. Sixty days postsurgery, patients may be turned out in a large pasture. Postsurgical colic patients should be re-evaluated after 90 days and only then be slowly reintroduced to exercise.

Hernia Repair

Hernias, defined as any abnormal protrusion of viscera through the body wall or other confining structure, are a common congenital condition. Umbilical hernias are the most common hernias seen in equine veterinary practice and may resolve without medical attention. Ligation of the umbilical cord, manual breaking of the cord, and cord infection with abscesses are predisposing causes of umbilical hernias.

To examine an umbilical hernia, the herniating tissue should be manually reduced and the defect in the linea alba accessed. Hernias that admit two or fewer fingers should be allowed time to resolve on their own. Hernias that admit more than two fingers when being manually reduced require elective surgical reduction. A strangulated umbilical hernia, recognized by a hard, painful swelling at the navel that does not reduce with pressure, requires immediate surgical correction.

Inguinal hernias occur when the hernia sac containing fat or a loop of abdominal contents, usually small intestine, enters through the inguinal ring and into the inguinal canal. Inguinal hernias usually occur in foals but can also occur in breeding stallions due to trauma, breeding, or physical exertion (Fig. 34.7A and B). Usually, inguinal hernias can be reduced by pushing the bulge back up through the inguinal ring in the abdomen. Small inguinal hernias tend to correct spontaneously as the foal grows older.

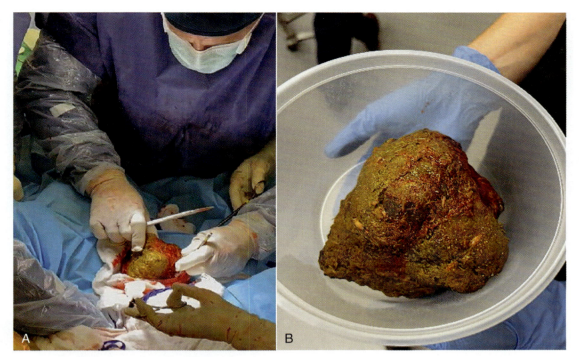

• **Fig. 34.4** Removal of an enterolith *(left)*. An enterolith removed from an equine patient during colic surgery *(right)*. Enteroliths are stones that form when mineralized salts are deposited around a foreign object, such as a pebble, within the intestines of horses. Enteroliths become symptomatic when they grow large enough to obstruct the bowel. Horses suspected of having an impaction but that fail to respond to treatment may have an enterolith. Enteroliths must be removed surgically.

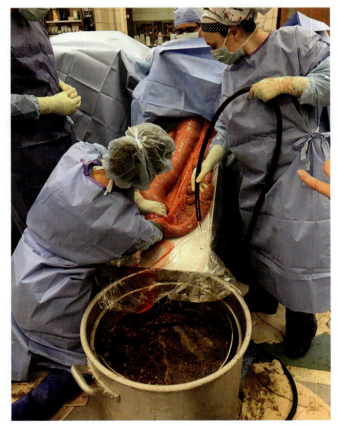

• **Fig. 34.5** Large colon being flushed during colic surgery and the contents strained. Note that the opening of the abdominal cavity is draped to prevent contamination from fecal material splashing into the sterile field.

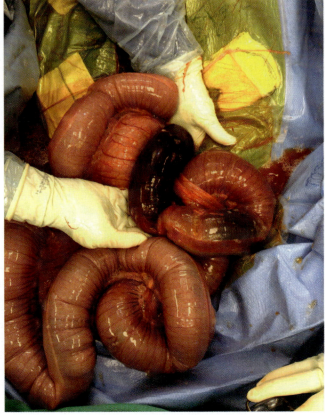

• **Fig. 34.6** Discolored loop of small intestine indicates that the tissue has been compromised and resection and anastomosis should be considered.

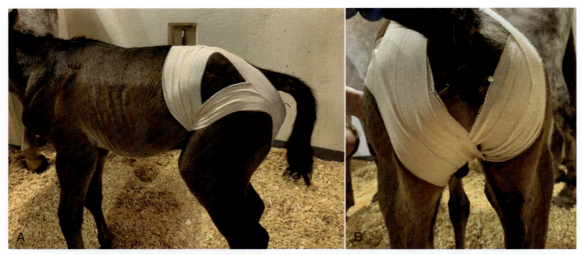

• **Fig. 34.7** One-day-old Thoroughbred foal fitted with support bandage for the treatment of bilateral congenital inguinal hernia. Lateral *(left)* and posterior *(right)* view of a foal shows bandage tied around waist, inguinal region, and hips.

Scrotal hernias are seen exclusively in stallions. These are inguinal hernias that have descended into the scrotum, producing an obvious swelling around the testicle (Fig. 34.8). Both inguinal and scrotal hernias are typically unilateral, with the left side statistically affected more frequently.

Congenital scrotal and inguinal hernias are usually large, reducible, and nonstrangulating, and may be treated with daily manual reduction coupled with a support bandage. Acquired inguinal and scrotal hernias are considered emergencies and can occur in stallions after breeding or jumping, presumably because of increased abdominal pressure. They can also occur spontaneously. This is a very painful condition and often presents with coliclike clinical signs. For differential diagnosis, the spermatic cord, testes, and inguinal rings should be carefully palpated on stallions exhibiting signs of colic. If discovered early, manual rectal reduction may be successful. If reduction cannot be accomplished with gentle traction, surgery is indicated.

Often, the size and location of the incision for a hernia repair are determined by the size and location of the hernia and by patient positioning for surgery. The patient's hair should be clipped with appropriately wide margins around the hernia site to provide the surgeon access to tissues that could be involved in the procedure. A **herniorrhaphy**, or hernia repair, uses the same materials as a general celiotomy, with the potential addition of a mesh implant.

Urogenital Tract Surgery

Umbilical Repair

An umbilical infection, or "navel ill," is a serious and frequently fatal disease in newborn foals. It is caused by a bacterial infection of the umbilical structures, which include the artery, vein, and urachus. Clinical signs of a diseased umbilicus include depression, inappetence, and fever, with the navel area exhibiting swelling, heat, and drainage. It is acquired either during foaling or from subsequent contamination of the healing umbilical stump. Several bacteria may cause infection, but *Streptococcus* is the most common. In the septicemic form, the bacteria enter the bloodstream through the umbilical vessels, spreading to the liver, joints, and elsewhere.

Umbilical infections can be prevented by good management practices, including providing a sanitary environment for foaling,

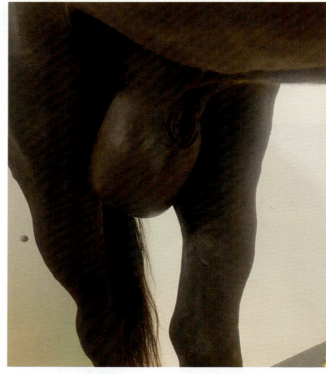

• **Fig. 34.8** Scrotal hernia in an adult stallion.

applying a tincture of dilute chlorhexidine to the umbilical stump after the foal is born and multiple times over the first few days of life, and ensuring that the foal receives enough colostrum within 12 hours of birth.

Ultrasonography is the ideal means of assessment of the internal umbilical structures and can show signs of infection, even with normal findings on palpation. IV antibiotics should be started at the first signs of navel infection to prevent death and the effects of joint ill. All navel abscesses should be opened and drained. The infected umbilical structures should be surgically removed, and the umbilical area kept clean and dry.

Patients undergoing surgery for umbilical remnant resection should be positioned, clipped, and prepped for celiotomy. The OR technician should also be prepared with the same basic supplies used for a celiotomy as well as suction supplies, and Doyen intestinal forceps should be available in case the urachus is still patent.

Castration

Castration is routinely performed on males; only horses intended to be used for breeding are left intact. Intact males (stallions) often have behavioral issues and can pose management challenges. Because of this, castrated males (geldings) are generally preferred by the average horse owner. Medical indications for castration include testicular disease, undescended testicles or cryptorchids, and inguinal hernia. Castration can be performed at any age; however, most horses are "gelded" around 12 to 18 months to allow for physical development before behavioral changes occur.

A complete physical examination should precede castration. Infectious diseases, anemia, and unthriftiness caused by parasites or malnutrition should be corrected prior to surgery and tetanus toxoid booster and antibiotics administered.

Routine castrations are typically performed with the patient in lateral recumbency; however, dorsal recumbency is sometimes preferred (Fig. 34.9). It is common for equine castrations to take place outside of the OR, often in a shaded, grassy paddock (Fig. 34.10). When performing a field castration in lateral recumbency, the "up" hind limb can be restrained by a rope looped around the pastern and either held forward by an assistant or tied with a quick-release knot low around the patient's neck. Occasionally, the veterinarian will choose to perform a castration on a standing patient that is under sedation and local anesthesia. A standing castration is considered safer for the horse, because it eliminates the risks associated with general anesthesia; however, it can present accessibility and safety challenges for the veterinarian.

Little to no clipping is required, but the OR technician should make sure that the area over and around each testicle is free of hair. Basic surgical instruments are used, along with the surgeon's preferred type of emasculator (Fig 34.11A and B). The incisions are typically left open, and the patient should be monitored for excessive hemorrhage, excessive swelling, and herniation of intestines or omentum through the incision site.

Cryptorchidectomy is required if either or both testicles have not completely descended. The incision site for this procedure can vary, depending on the location of the undescended testicle(s). In extreme cases, celiotomy will be required to find a testicle still located in the abdominal cavity. The clipped area for a cryptorchidectomy should be broad enough to allow the surgeon to explore a sufficient area if the testicle is not palpable.

Although castration is a simple procedure with rare complications, the patient needs to be monitored for excessive hemorrhage and local swelling around the penis and prepuce for 24 hours following surgery. Bleeding more significant than countable drops is a cause for concern and should be communicated immediately as it is possible that the patient will need to be reanesthetized for additional ligation. Excessive swelling is generally caused by a scrotal skin incision that is too small, limiting drainage and promoting swelling. Usually, swelling can be remedied through light exercise, although the incision may occasionally need to be extended.

Ovariectomy

Removal of both ovaries is a major operation and therefore not commonly performed for sterilization, as it is in small-animal

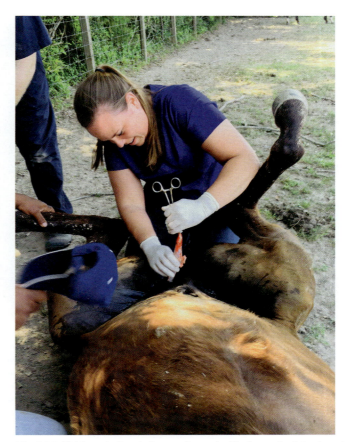

• **Fig. 34.9** Field castration being performed with the patient in dorsal recumbency.

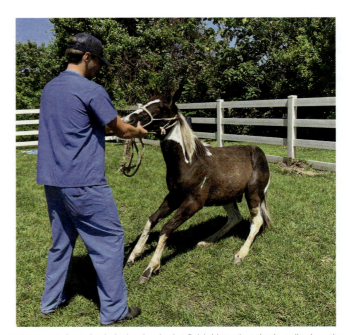

• **Fig. 34.10** Anesthetic induction in the field. Note that the handler has the patient in a flat, open, grassy area with minimal obstacles. The patient's head is being supported and a sitting motion encouraged, aiding with control of the fall to prevent injury.

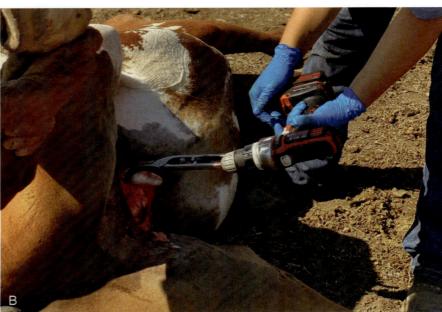

• Fig. 34.11 Serra emasculators *(left)* are a commonly used tool for castration in horses. Emasculators are placed around the spermatic cord so that the nut on the emasculators is located toward the testicle, ensuring that the spermatic cord is crushed toward the body side and that the cord is cut toward the testicle side. The phrase "nut to nut" is often used to ensure proper placement of emasculators during castration. Field castration using a power drill–mounted Henderson castration tool *(right)* on a patient in lateral recumbency. This method uses a twisting action to sever and seal the spermatic cord as opposed to the crushing action of the Serra emasculators. This is thought to minimize the risk of blood loss and other postcastration complications.

patients. The typical reasons for ovariectomy are removal of an ovarian neoplasm, elimination of estrous behavior in a mare that is not going to be bred, or modification of aggressive or nymphomaniac behavior. A unilateral ovariectomy is the recommended treatment for mares diagnosed with a granulosa-theca cell tumor. These mares often display aggressive, stallionlike behaviors due to the large amount of estrogen, inhibin, and testosterone being produced by the tumor. There is a favorable prognosis for returned fertility after unilateral ovariectomy to remove a granulosa cell tumor.

Prior to an ovariectomy, the mare should be fasted for 24 hours, with unlimited access to fresh water. This is to ensure that the colon is free of fecal material, which may impede easy access to the ovaries. Fecal balls remaining in the digestive tract may feel like ovaries during palpation.

Ovariectomies can be performed through a vaginal approach **(colpotomy)**, through the flank, or a ventral midline or paramedian approach. The approach depends on the surgeon's preference, available equipment and assistance, temperament of the mare, size of the ovary, and economic constraints of the client. Routine ovariectomies can be performed by using standard celiotomy equipment. The clip margins for the procedure are predicated by the location of the incision(s) (ventral midline, flank, or lateral). Some equine ovariectomies can be performed laparoscopically through small lateral incisions. Laparoscopic ovariectomies in equine patients are typically performed on sedated standing patients. These procedures carry all the benefits associated with minimally invasive surgery, including not placing the patient under anesthesia. A laparoscope, a camera, a light source and fiberoptic cable, and a carbon dioxide (CO_2) insufflator with sterile tubing are needed, as well as a variety of laparoscopic

instruments. A laparoscopic vessel–sealing device can significantly reduce the amount of time spent sealing/ligating and transecting the ovarian pedicles.

Postoperative care for ovariectomy patients is dependent on the type of approach used. Patients that undergo colpotomy should be placed on stall rest for a week and preferably kept standing to minimize the risk of evisceration. The patient should receive systemic antibacterial and anti-inflammatory therapies for 4 to 5 days, return to light exercise after a week, and return to full athletic function after 2 weeks. Ovariectomies from a flank approach involve similar postoperative care; however, they require a longer lay-up period of 4 to 5 weeks. With a ventral midline or oblique paramedian approach, the time before the patient can return to work is often a minimum of 10 weeks.

Reported complications for ovariectomies include nerve paresis, generalized myositis, hemorrhage from the pedicle, adhesions, wound infection or dehiscence, herniation, postoperative colic, and peritonitis. Mares should be monitored closely for the first 24 hours after surgery, especially for signs of shock suggestive of internal blood loss. Long-term complications are rare.

Perineal Surgery

Caslick Procedure

The Caslick procedure is a very common surgery performed in mares with pneumovagina (i.e. wind sucking). This defect allows air and fecal material to enter and pool in the vagina, resulting in a persistent source of bacterial infections that may contribute to difficulties with breeding management and pregnancy maintenance. Mares with **pnuemovagina** frequently lose the protective value of the vulvovaginal sphincter; this can occur with aging, weight loss, or the presence of vaginal tears associated with prior deliveries.

Ideally, the vulva and the anus are on the same plane. If more than 4 cm of the vulva lies dorsal to the pelvis, a Caslick procedure should be performed with the mare standing and placed under sedation and local anesthesia. The edges of the dorsal vulvar labia are incised and sutured together with a continuous suture pattern (Fig. 34.12). The edges of the vulva will heal together, remaining connected even after the suture is removed. The Caslick suture must be reopened on mares when foaling is imminent and sometimes before the act of breeding. Because this technique is routinely used on broodmares, with each breeding year after year, the vulvar lips become less resilient and more scarred over time. Scarring makes it more difficult for the vulvar lips to heal and align.

Dystocia: Fetotomy and Cesarean Section

Labor in the mare is an explosive event and completed quickly, usually in 15 to 20 minutes. Because of this, there is extremely limited time to correct dystocia. During the first stage of labor, the foal moves into an anterior and dorsosacral presentation. When labor is prolonged or there is a lack of progress in the first or second stage of labor, dystocia should be suspected. Early intervention is essential to ensure a successful delivery. Failure to deliver a foal in 30 minutes of onset of second-stage labor is associated with a dramatically increased rate of foal mortality.

The position of the foal should be carefully examined when there is a lack of progress in delivery. The mare's perineal region should be washed thoroughly with a mild aseptic solution and the vulvar lips dried. The arms of the examiner should be well lubricated and the position of the foal assessed so that decisions can be made for correcting the dystocia. Cesarean section (C-section) should be considered if the foal is alive and cannot be delivered vaginally within 30 minutes. A prolonged attempt at vaginal delivery is the most common cause of mortality in mares and foals and of subsequent impaired fertility in the mare.

C-section is indicated in cases of abnormal presentations, particularly transverse presentation; abnormal fetal size or posture; fetal deformities; abnormalities involving the mare's pelvic canal; uterine torsion; and certain abnormalities of the abdominal wall. Cesarean deliveries are typically performed under general anesthesia either through either a ventral midline or a flank incision (Fig. 34.13). Efficiency is especially critical during C-sections to ensure the best outcome for both mare and foal. General celiotomy instruments are used for C-section, although additional personnel and instruments may be required to help revive the foal.

Postoperative care is similar to any abdominal surgery, except for management relative to the placenta. If the placenta is not expelled soon after the mare recovers from surgery, oxytocin and NSAID therapy may be used in conjunction with uterine lavage. In some cases, icing the mare's feet to prevent laminitis, a complication from retained placenta, may be warranted.

Fetotomy should be performed if the foal is dead and the malposition cannot be corrected manually. This technique involves dissecting a fetus through the mare's vagina to make birth possible and may provide an alternative to a C-section, because it avoids major abdominal surgery and results in a shorter recovery time for the mare. It is best to perform a fetotomy with the mare standing and sedated, although this is not always possible, in which case epidural anesthesia should be provided. It is essential that the fetotome, an instrument used for fetotomies, be placed in the uterus and that the cervix is not cut inadvertently.

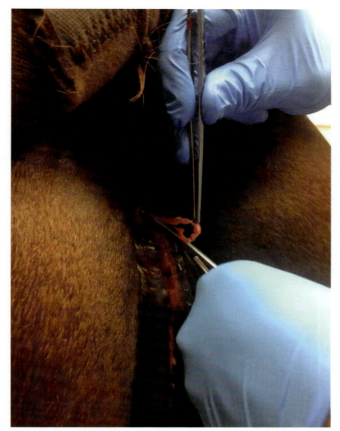

• **Fig. 34.12** Caslick procedure. The edges of the dorsal vulvar labia are incised in preparation for suturing.

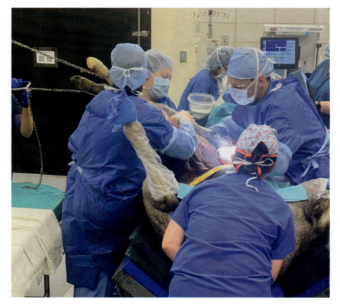

• **Fig. 34.13** Foal being delivered via cesarean section. Note the foal's hind limbs are being hoisted out manually with the use of obstetric chains and the help of the surgical team. An operating room technician is simultaneously pushing the foal backwards through the mare's vagina to aid with the birth.

There must be ample room in the birth canal, and the cervix must be effaced completely for fetotomy to be performed. Fetotomy should be avoided in mares with protracted uterine involution and fetal emphysema, where space is severely compromised, or in cases requiring more than one or two cuts to adequately dismember the fetus. Severe damage to the mare's genital tract is a risk, and C-section is indicated when per vaginal efforts may impair the mare's fertility.

Uterine Torsion and Rupture

Uterine torsion is the rotation of the uterus on its long axis. A rare condition, a hard fall, episode of violent rolling, or an excessively active fetus have been implicated as potential causes. When the uterus rotates 180 degrees, the broad ligament becomes stretched, compromising the blood supply to the uterus and fetus. A 360-degree rotation cuts off the blood supply to the uterus completely and leads to death of the fetus within hours. Torsion nearly always occurs in the last few months of pregnancy, when the uterus is rapidly increasing in size. Mares with uterine torsion will exhibit clinical signs of colic, frequent urination, listlessness, and loss of appetite. Torsion and the direction of the twist can be confirmed by rectal palpation.

Rolling an anesthetized mare with the aid of a wooden plank in the direction of the torsion may correct the rotation; in most cases, it is necessary to make a flank incision and twist the uterus back into its normal position.

Uterine rupture may occur as a sequel to torsion but generally happens during active labor of a large foal, twins, abnormal presentation, or other contributor to prolonged, difficult labor. When the uterus ruptures completely, the foal, along with the placenta, may be extruded from the abdomen, accompanied by sudden vaginal or abdominal bleeding, along with shock during foaling. This indicates the need for a rapid delivery or emergency C-section. A partial tear of the uterus may go unnoticed during foaling and then cause postpartum peritonitis several hours later; these tears can be sutured through the birth canal after delivery. If not possible, repair of the uterus can be done through a midline incision under general anesthesia.

Musculoskeletal Surgery

Lameness

Problems involving the musculoskeletal system are common reasons for veterinary attention and for interruptions in training and performance of the equine athlete. Lameness is defined as any deviation from the normal gait or posture resulting from pain, mechanical dysfunction, or neurologic disease. Lameness can be acute or chronic and can stem from a wide variety of factors, including age, breed, and performance use.

Lameness examinations begin with a precise history to determine whether the onset was acute or insidious, the relationship of the presenting signs to exercise, details of medications received, and shoeing history. Evaluation of conformation and symmetry of the musculoskeletal system should be made, noting any swellings or muscle atrophy. Gait disturbances may be caused by neurological diseases and musculoskeletal conditions. Behavior such as head pressing, staggering, swaying, lack of coordination, extreme head bobbing, or paralysis should receive a neurological examination before or in conjunction with a traditional lameness workup.

PUT INTO PRACTICE

Properly presenting an equine patient for a lameness exam is very important for the veterinarian to obtain a correct diagnosis. This process takes practice and communication with your veterinarian. Learning what your veterinarian wants during these exams will take time but, once you know the process, your help will be invaluable.

A patient being examined for lameness should initially be hand walked on a hard surface to observe limb coordination and any indications of lameness before being viewed in a straight line and a circle at the trot.

In forelimb lameness, as weight is placed on the affected limb, the head will lift; the head will drop when weight is placed on the unaffected forelimb. This drop of the head on the unaffected forelimb is where the phrase "down on sound" originates. The head appears to lower at the same time the sound foot hits the ground, suggesting that the opposite limb is the one exhibiting unsoundness. In hind limb lameness, head movement may be more subtle, requiring the examiner to observe for symmetry in the hips and tail head instead; as the affected hind limb is bearing weight, the tail head will rise.

When the veterinary technician presents a lame horse to be examined by the veterinarian, it is important to work the horse in straight lines, keeping the trot slow and controlled while giving freedom to the patient's head. Too much restraint of the head may inhibit movement that demonstrates lameness, leading to misdiagnosis.

It is helpful for the patient to be viewed while moving in a circle. When working a horse in a circle by using a lunge line, avoid pulling on the horse's head and taking away its natural balance. Instead, forward movement should be promoted by the handler staying behind the horse's shoulder and driving it from the rear. Some clinicians prefer horses be trotted in a circle in hand instead of having them presented at the end of a lunge line. The nonhalter-trained juvenile patient may need to be observed while moving at liberty, either in a small paddock or pen.

Most conditions causing lameness occur in the carpus or distally in the forelimb and in the tarsus or distally in the hind limb, necessitating the examination be concentrated on the distal limb and rule it out before moving proximally. Diagnostics for lameness will include a methodical system of palpation, limb flexion (Fig. 34.14), synovial fluid analysis, intrasynovial and joint blocks, and imaging. Diagnostic imagining traditionally includes radiography and ultrasonography but may also require computed tomography (CT) scan, magnetic resonance imaging (MRI), or nuclear scintigraphy (bone scan). It is important for the technician presenting the patient inbetween flexions and blocks to remain consistent and not add additional variables to the examination. When handling a horse for flexions or blocks, it is important for the technician to stay on the same side of the horse as the examiner and well to the side of the horse, particularly when a forelimb is being addressed. Patients that are experiencing pain because of injuries or musculoskeletal disease may quickly pull their limbs away from the examiner and cause injury to the person restraining the patient. After performance of diagnostics, a treatment plan is determined, which may include surgery.

Fracture Stabilization

Fracture is a loss of the structural continuity in the mineralized connective tissue of a bone and may be either complete or incomplete. A complete fracture is one where there is total loss of function in the bone. An incomplete fracture describes a fracture where only partial structural integrity is lost, with subtle signs of pain and inflammation. Displaced fractures often cause injury to surrounding soft tissue structures. The location, configuration, degree of comminution, and displacement of fracture fragments are of therapeutic and diagnostic importance. Surgical veterinarians must provide clients with a realistic appraisal of the injury, implied costs, and complications that may be encountered with treatment.

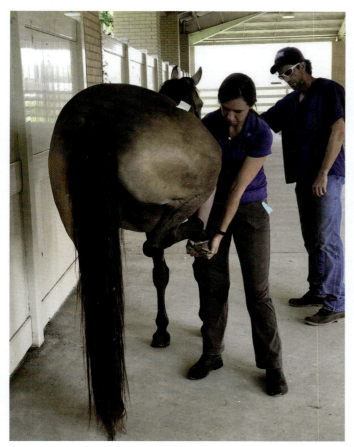

• **Fig. 34.14** Hind limb flexion on a horse being examined for lameness. Note that the handler is on the same side of the horse as the examiner, attentive to the task at hand.

Initial management of a fracture begins with stabilization. An equine patient that is experiencing instability of a limb is often anxious and stressed; therefore restraint should be applied immediately to prevent further injury to surrounding soft tissue. Analgesics should be used to reduce the patient's anxiety along with NSAIDs, such as phenylbutazone, to provide pain relief and help minimize inflammation at the fracture site. Use of analgesic/sedative combinations, such as xylazine or detomidine, should be used conservatively to prevent ataxia.

In an open fracture, the skin should be prepared aseptically before bandaging to prevent further contamination of the fracture site. Some form of immobilization should be used to protect the soft tissues around the fracture, neutralize the forces on bony fragments, and allow the horse limited but protected use of the limb. This will help reduce anxiety and fatigue while decisions about treatment options are being made, during transport, and while waiting for preparation of the OR and induction of anesthesia.

There are several methods of fracture stabilization, and the choice of method is decided by the surgeon and based on fracture type and location. Although once considered unrepairable, significant long bone fractures in equine patients may now be corrected by using advanced techniques and surgical implants (Fig. 34.15A–C). Most of these fractures are best repaired with bone plates and screws, although the OR technician should have at least a basic knowledge of all orthopedic implants and fracture repair methods.

The bone plates most often used in equine surgery are the dynamic compression plate (DCP), the limited contact dynamic compression plate (LC-DCP), and the locking compression plate (LCP). Because LC-DCPs and LCPs carry a higher cost and the size of the equine patient typically requires a larger/longer plate, DCPs are more widely used in equine fracture stabilization. Because of patient size and the weight-bearing load placed on a stabilized fracture, it is common to use more than one plate on a single fracture in an equine patient.

Using plate benders, DCPs and some LC-DCPs will need to be contoured to match the shape of the bone. As with plates, there are several types of screws available for use in fracture stabilization. Equine fracture stabilization relies most heavily on the cancellous, locking, and cortical screws. Cortical screws are available as both self-tapping and non–self-tapping screws. Locking screws can only be used with LCPs and in the threaded section of the "figure-of-eight" holes on an LC-DCP.

The surgeon will determine which variety is most appropriate to the specific fracture and stabilization method. To facilitate the placement of bone screws, the surgical technician should ensure that a drill, appropriately sized drill bits and taps, drill guides, screwdrivers, and a depth gauge are available (Fig. 34.16). Some fractures can be stabilized through the placement of at least one screw but without the use of a bone plate. These screws can be placed in "lag fashion," which requires the use of a countersink in addition to the standard instrumentation used in screw placement.

Countersinking a screw will allow for the top of the screw head to sit flush with the bone. This method of screw placement also requires the use of two different sizes of drill bits, one equal to the diameter of the screw shaft and the other equal to the diameter of the screw threads. Some fractures and their stabilization may also require the use of orthopedic wire placed circumferentially around the bone (cerclage) or through holes drilled into the bone (tension band wiring). The tension band wiring technique may also make use of intramedullary pins in a pin and wire technique. The OR technician should be familiar with basic orthopedic instrumentation. As with any surgical procedure, adherence to aseptic technique is key to the success of orthopedic surgeries, especially those involving implants.

Arthroscopic Surgery

Arthroscopy (Fig. 34.17) is performed on equine patients for a variety of reasons, ranging from diagnosis of joint disease to lavage of septic joints to removal of joint lesions and bone chips. Arthroscopy has specific advantages as a diagnostic and surgical technique. The equine joint can be examined more thoroughly while being relatively noninvasive. Surgical trauma and recovery time are minimal, yielding outstanding cosmetic and functional outcomes.

The type of arthroscopy to be performed and the joint(s) affected will determine the patient's position on the surgical table. Many arthroscopic procedures on equine patients require the use of table-mounted poles or ceiling-mounted chains used to maintain the affected limb in a position that allows access to the necessary joints. The clip margins should extend far enough distally and proximally from the incision site(s) to avoid limiting access to all involved joints. The clip should also extend around the entire circumference of the affected joints except with stifle joints, where a wide enough margin can be clipped without extending to the caudal aspect of the limb.

Arthroscopy is preferred to arthrotomy for joint surgery in equine patients because of its lower morbidity and mortality rates

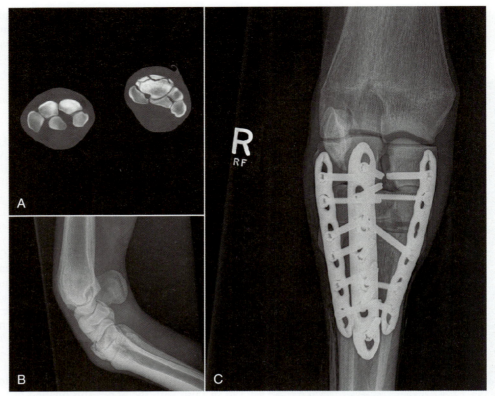

• **Fig. 34.15** (A) Presurgical computed tomography and (B) radiograph images of an equine patient with a right carpal bone fracture. (C) This fracture was repaired under general anesthesia with surgical implants, as seen in the intraoperative radiograph images.

as a result of its minimally invasive nature. Like **laparoscopy**, arthroscopy requires the use of a scope, camera, and light source with a fiberoptic cable; a sterile physiologic solution is used to distend the joint. This solution is typically delivered by an electronic pump to ensure that intra-articular pressure is steadily maintained.

Standard draping materials, scissors, tissue forceps, needle drivers, and scalpel blades and handles are used. The OR technician should ensure that an ample stock of 1.5-inch–long sterile needles are available to the surgeon for pinpointing incision site locations and assisting with fluid egress. Arthroscopic trocars, cannulas, and egress ports will also be used. Additionally, a variety of curettes, arthroscopic rongeurs, and knives may be used to debride the affected areas of the joint or to remove bone chips.

An intra-articular shaver or synovial resector can aid in removal of joint lesions. An intra-articular radiofrequency electrode system (VAPR VUE; DePuy Synthes, Raynham, MA) can be used for ablation of soft tissues within the joint. A variety of tips are available for both the shaver and the VAPR systems; multiple tips should be available for the surgeon to choose the most appropriate one for the situation.

The use of multiple monitors or a centrally located, ceiling-mounted monitor on a boom, if available, can assist in maintaining asepsis during multijoint procedures and in eliminating the need to move scope tower equipment around the patient, risking contamination. If preoperative radiographs have been acquired, they should be displayed in the OR throughout the procedure.

Postoperative complications from arthroscopic procedures include sepsis and swelling. Adherence to the principles of aseptic technique is an extremely important component of avoiding postoperative sepsis. Preoperative antibiotics should be given routinely to arthroscope patients as a preventive against sepsis. Postoperative swelling is a result of subcutaneous extraversion of fluid at the time of surgery and will usually resolve quickly with use of a pressure bandage.

Weak Flexor Tendons and Flexural Deformities

Two types of tendon problems occur in young horses. The first is weak flexor tendons in newborn foals, usually associated with immaturity or septicemia. Weak flexor tendons are exhibited when the foal stands, usually affecting just the hind limbs but occasionally, all four limbs. The plantar aspect of the fetlock will descend toward the ground because of overextension. Most cases of weak flexor tendons self-resolve within 2 to 3 days after birth. Improvement can be encouraged by providing a firm surface to stand on and by keeping stall bedding shallow. Short periods of controlled exercise will help develop muscle tone and tendon strength. Thick supports, such as bandages or casts, are likely to worsen flaccidity and should be avoided. Severe or nonresponsive cases may require heel extension shoes.

The second type of tendon problem seen in young horses is flexure deformity, which is sometimes a congenital condition but may also be acquired in older foals and yearlings. Flexural deformities present as obvious changes in the contour of the limbs. This often results in the foal or weanling standing very upright, usually on the forelimbs. Severe cases exhibit an inability to stand, or knuckling over on the dorsal surface of the hoof wall may be observed.

Flexural deformities are most often seen in the forelimb and are often bilateral, but congenital fetlock deformities can also occur in the hind limbs. Flexural deformity of the coffin joint, sometimes referred to as contracture of the deep digital flexor tendon,

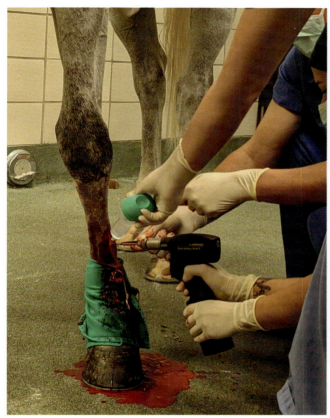

• Fig. 34.16 An osteostixis (or forage) procedure to repair a dorsolateral cortical fracture being performed on an equine patient under standing sedation. Note that an assistant is using a bulb syringe to drip saline solution on the drill bit during drilling to prevent the drill bit and bone from getting hot.

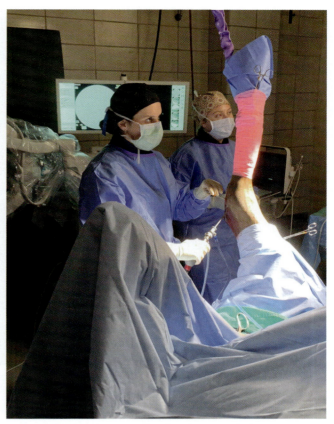

• Fig. 34.17 Hock arthroscopy. The limb is suspended to ensure proper positioning and is fully draped, leaving only the surgery site exposed.

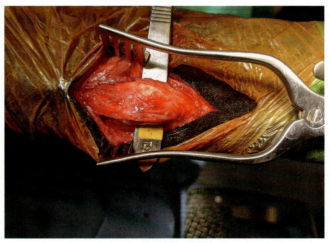

• Fig. 34.18 Ligament desmotomy being performed to correct an angular limb deformity in an equine patient.

or most commonly by horse owners as "club foot," occurs over time. Flexural deformity of the fetlock joint or contracture of the superficial digital flexor tendon might be referred to as "post-leggedness." Foals with flexural deformities of the carpus are likely to be described as "over at the knees."

Flexural deformity of the coffin joint is often managed conservatively, especially when diagnosed early. Nonsurgical treatments include lowering the heels, elevating the toe with a shoe, and decreasing the patient's caloric intake. In newborn foals, oxytetracycline can be used intravenously in conjunction with other treatment modalities; however, this drug can affect renal function, so caution should be exercised when used in foals that are systemically ill. Phenylbutazone may be prescribed to address potential pain stemming from physitis and osteochondrosis, and to promote weight bearing on the affected limb. Controlled exercise in conjunction with corrective trimming and shoeing is usually indicated.

If the deformity is severe at presentation or worsening despite conservative therapies, an inferior check ligament **desmotomy**, or surgical dissection of the ligament, is indicated (Fig. 34.18). This procedure is performed with the animal under general anesthesia and placed in dorsal recumbency with the limb suspended. Desmotomies can typically be performed with basic surgical instrumentation, although special knives may be required. Controlled exercise immediately after surgery is important for correction of the deformity.

Flexural deformities of the fetlock are common in newborns and usually respond to conservative therapy consisting of controlled exercise, physical therapy in the form of manual extension, and support wraps. Some foals may require splints or full-limb wraps but care must be taken to prevent pressure sores. Surgical management via superior check ligament desmotomy or inferior check ligament desmotomy is recommended for severe or nonresponsive cases. Regardless of the technique used, immediate postoperative therapy should include hand walking, backing, and traveling up and down inclines—all therapies that will stretch the flexor tendons and suspensory ligaments.

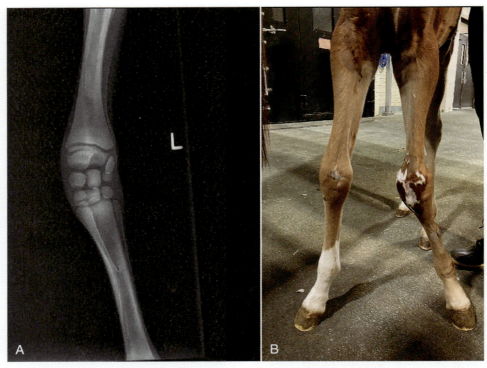

• **Fig. 34.19** (A) Left digital palmar radiographs of a foal with (B) bilateral carpal valgus limb deformities.

Congenital flexural deformity of the carpus or a young horse that is "over at the knee" can initially be treated with support wraps, splints, or casts. Splints and casts can result in pressure sores and so should be well padded and closely monitored. Surgical management for severe, nonresponsive cases is considered a "salvage" effort.

Angular Limb Deformities

Angular limb deformities are characterized by deviation in the forelimbs. Valgus deviation of the carpus is the most common limb deformity in growing foals and results in deviation of the third metacarpal bone medially toward the midline of the limb when viewed from the front of the foal (Fig. 34.19A and B). These foals are more commonly referred to as being "knock-kneed." Various deviations, those that deviate laterally and that are "bow-legged," are less commonly seen in the carpus but often found in the fetlock.

Angular limb deformities are described as either congenital or developmental. Congenital angular limb deformities may be caused by inappropriate intrauterine positions, locoweed ingestion by the mare when pregnant, nutritional imbalances, hypothyroidism, prematurity or dysmaturity, ligamentous laxity, disproportionate osseous development, and general muscular weakness. Developmental angular limb deformities may occur days to months after birth and can be secondary to incomplete ossification or collapse of cuboidal bones, nutritional disorders, excessive exercise, physeal osteochondrosis, or physeal trauma.

Most foals are born with a certain amount of angular deviation, and many of these problems resolve spontaneously without treatment. Lameness is rarely associated with angular limb deformities but, when seen, is suggestive of a grave prognosis that rules out a future athletic career. Early recognition is crucial for the successful management of angular limb deformities. Diagnosis requires observation of the limb in both neutral weight-bearing and non–weight-bearing positions. The ability to correct a deviation manually suggests laxity in the ligaments or incomplete ossification of the cuboidal bones. The inability to correct the deformity manually suggests a developmental deviation secondary to disproportionate growth.

Stall rest in conjunction with controlled exercises multiple times per day can be an effective treatment in newborns with ligament laxity and incomplete ossification. Radiographs should be taken at the start of treatment to establish a baseline. They should be repeated every 2 weeks throughout treatment until the deformity is corrected. Corrective trimming and shoeing may also be included, along with conservative management.

Surgical intervention of angular limb deformities, which involves the manipulation of physeal growth, can be considered when conservative therapies are unsuccessful, the deformity is severe, or the foal is beyond the neonatal period. A periosteal stripping procedure that transects and elevates the periosteum near the affected growth plate will lead to more rapid bone growth on the shorter side of the bone. This typically leads to correction of the disproportionate bone growth; however, if it is not completely corrected, the procedure can be repeated 4 to 6 weeks later. This procedure does not carry the risk of overcorrection or creation of the same deformity on the contralateral side of the limb.

A transphyseal bridging procedure in which at least one screw is placed into the long side of the bone can be used to correct more severe deformities. Depending on the severity of the deformity, the surgeon can either place a single transphyseal screw or two screws with a wire wrapped around them in a "figure-of-eight" pattern. The implants will need to be removed when the initial deformity has been corrected to avoid overcorrection.

For both procedures, affected limbs should be clipped circumferentially to include the joint at the distal and proximal ends of the affected bone and the animal presented in dorsal recumbency. General surgical instrumentation will be used in addition to orthopedic elevators and self-retaining retractors, such as Gelpi or Weitlander retractors. Transphyseal bridging will also require the use of a drill, drill bits, bone taps, a depth gauge, a countersink, screws, a screwdriver, and potentially, orthopedic wire, a wire cutter, and a wire twister.

Postoperatively, the limb should be kept bandaged until the implants are removed to minimize the risk of trauma to the surgical site. Foals should be kept confined to minimize trauma to the physis and the implants. Once implants are removed, the limb only needs to be bandaged until the skin incisions are closed and the sutures removed.

Tendonitis

Because of the structural and functional roles of tendons and ligaments, injuries to them may result in dysfunction due to both pain and mechanical impairment to function. Tendons are a specialized form of dense connective fibrous tissue that transmits the force of muscle contraction to bone. Tendons are surrounded by connective tissue, providing a low-friction gliding environment, blood supply, and structures that influence the line of tendon action. In horses, tendons serve principally as load-bearing structures; therapy is oriented toward restoration of strength.

Injury to the superficial deep digital flexor tendon, is known as a "bowed tendon," is a common injury among performance horses, especially racehorses. Injury occurs when the tendon is strained beyond its normal range. Tendon failure can be acute or result from cumulative episodes of tearing of tendon fibers. Conformational factors, including long, sloping pasterns and low heels, can contribute to a horse's predisposition to tendon injuries. Fatigue, poor/soft surface conditions, and primary degeneration are also common components that contribute to tendon injuries. Horses with superficial deep digital flexor tendon injuries present with local edema and pain upon palpation and, depending on the degree of injury, may present without lameness. Ultrasonography is used to diagnose tendonitis and should be used periodically throughout the treatment process to monitor progress.

Tendons are poorly vascularized and heal very slowly. The primary aim of treatment should be to reduce the acute inflammatory response and promote reorganization of scar tissue into a functional unit. In the acute phase, NSAIDs should be used to reduce the inflammatory reaction in conjunction with complete stall rest, because continued exercise may result in additional tearing of fibers. Bandaging, massage, and cold hose therapy should also be implemented to reduce the initial reaction. Once the tendon is cold and nonpainful, hand walking should be introduced, with subsequent controlled turnout on a firm surface; however, careful attention should be paid to ensure that heat and pain do not return.

Prognosis of superficial digital flexor tendonitis is guarded because of a high incidence of reinjury in either the same limb or the opposite supporting limb. Previously affected horses should be carefully monitored when resuming training and have a long conditioning period, bringing them back to full athletic exertion slowly.

Deep digital flexor tendonitis is less commonly encountered than superficial digital flexor tendonitis, and draft breeds used for pulling heavy loads are most affected. Deep digital flexor tendon injuries are usually the result of an acute traumatic event or strain rather than fatigue injury. Affected horses present with acute lameness proportional to the extent of the injury, edema localized to the injured area, and pain upon palpation.

Treatment of acute deep digital flexor tendonitis and treatment for superficial digital flexor tendonitis are similar: rest, anti-inflammatory drugs, and local therapy. Re-establishment of the correct hoof angle in horses with low, underrun heels may help relieve strain on the tendon. Prognosis varies with the severity of the injury, although horses seem to return to full function better than with superficial digital flexor tendon injuries. Attention to

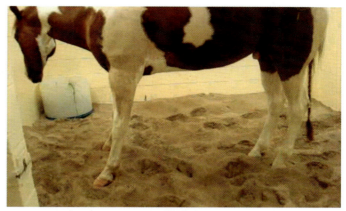

• **Fig. 34.20** Typical posture of a horse with laminitis walking or turning on a hard surface. Note how the horse has extended his forelimbs to shift weight to his hindquarters and off his front toes.

shoeing, proper condition, and monitoring of the affected area when training is resumed can help prevent recurrence.

The most common procedure for the treatment of tendonitis is tendon splitting. Tendon splitting removes the core lesion in the tendon and encourages rapid healing. Superior check ligament desmotomy is another surgical method used to treat superficial digital flexor tendonitis, improving the quality of healing and preventing the recurrence of injury.

Laminitis

Laminitis, commonly referred to as "founder," is a severe and life-threatening disease process that causes reduced blood flow to the horse's foot and subsequent breakdown of the attachments of the hoof. Endotoxins dilate the large arteries leading to the feet, increasing blood flow while causing intense constriction of the small capillary vessels that nourish the laminae. The result is a large volume of blood going down to the feet but being shunted around the laminae. Deprived of blood and oxygen, the laminae swell. Because the hoof is rigid, the swelling compresses the laminae, causing further tissue compromise. If the situation is not relieved, the sensitive inner structures of the feet will die. Several causes, including grain overload, acute endometritis, endotoxemia, infection, walnut shavings toxicosis, chronic obesity, and secondary to Cushing disease, have been identified. Although all four feet can be involved, the forelimbs are commonly affected, with affected horses showing reluctance to move and often taking a "dog-sitting" stance, with the forelimbs well out in front of the body (Fig. 34.20).

Acute laminitis may begin suddenly with fever, chills, sweating, diarrhea, increased pulse, and rapid, heavy breathing. Examination will reveal increased heat in the feet and around the coronary band as well as pain. Most horses will also respond positively to hoof tester evaluation, especially of the toe region of the distal phalanx. Palpation of the palmar arteries over the abaxial surface of the sesamoid bones, otherwise known as the "digital pulse," will reveal an increase in both rate and amplitude of the pulse.

When laminitis becomes chronic, with persistent pain and lameness, there may be permanent damage to the foot. A serious complication of laminitis is rotation of the coffin bone, which may happen as early as 48 hours after an acute episode. Rotation occurs when the coffin bone becomes detached from the hoof wall and, aided by the pull of the digital flexor tendon, rotates away and drops down. All degrees of rotation, from mild to severe, are possible, with severe cases demonstrating the tip of the coffin bone penetrating the sole of the foot.

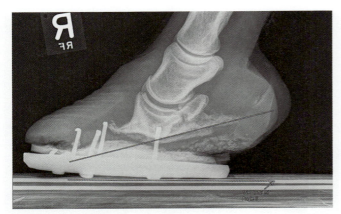

• **Fig. 34.21** Lateral radiograph of the forefoot of a horse with laminitis that has evidence of rotation of the coffin bone.

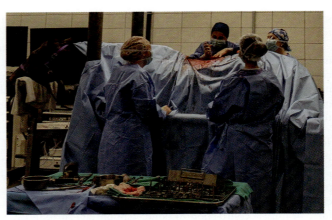

• **Fig. 34.22** A spinous ostectomy being performed on a standing patient to treat impinged dorsal spinous processes. The patient is being restrained in stocks, with the aid of sedation. A technician is supporting the patient's head on a head stand, ensuring that there is no pressure on the airway from the stock door.

Signs of severe rotation will include palpable indentation at the dorsal aspect of the coronary band and protrusion of the sole dorsal to the apex of the frog. Taking radiographs at the onset of disease is important to monitor its progression over time. Lateral radiographs should be taken to determine the degree of rotation of the coffin bone (Fig. 34.21).

There is no cure for laminitis. In acute cases of laminitis, it is important to establish the cause so that treatment can be directed at eliminating the source. Supportive therapy includes controlling pain and inflammation through use of NSAIDs and analgesics, and by promoting blood flow with vasodilator drugs. Icing a horse's feet has also been shown to have therapeutic benefits if done early.

Corrective hoof trimming and shoeing is essential in treating laminitis. It is important to trim back excessively long heels to maintain a normal hoof height and to square the toe to facilitate breakover. Special shoes may also be used to provide necessary support. Egg bar shoes with or without pads can be used on horses with laminitis, providing improved support to the heel region of the horse's foot. Most veterinarians will solicit the help of a skilled farrier when treating patients with laminitis. Hoof wall resection is indicated where there is discernible separation and the dorsal lamina is not providing support to the coffin bone or is applying excess pressure, preventing normal growth.

Nursing care is essential to the management of a patient with chronic laminitis. Laminitis is an extremely painful, crippling disease, and critical patients will spend most of the day recumbent; therefore stalls will need to be kept dry and heavily bedded, preferably with a thick layer of straw. Efforts to prevent pressure necrosis should be ongoing. Patients' feet will require routine hoof soaking and bandaging. A horse wearing ice boots will need to be attended to, at the minimum, every other hour as the ice melts.

Subsolar Abscess

Subsolar abscesses (sole abscesses) are likely the most common cause of acute lameness. Abscesses usually result from injury to the ground contact surface of the hoof, at which time bacteria gain access to the sensitive structure of the foot, usually via cracks in the sole or hoof wall. Horses with chronically poor hoof condition and a hoof wall with poor integrity are prone to bruising and abscesses. Horses with hoof wall separation (seedy toe) or laminitis are particularly at risk. Subsolar abscesses usually present acutely, with severe lameness that is not associated with exercise. Horses with sole abscesses will be reluctant to bear weight on the affected limb. If left untreated, the infection may underrun the hoof wall

and ultimately form a sinus, with a discharging point at the coronary band.

Subsolar abscesses can be identified using hoof testers by demonstrating severe, localized pain over the sole. Paring the sole with a hoof knife may indicate the site of penetration of the sole. The affected foot should be soaked with povidone-iodine and magnesium sulfate. A poultice dressing should then be applied to the foot to encourage drainage. Soaking should be repeated and the poultice bandage changed daily for three to five days, because effective drainage is key to successful treatment.

Impinged Dorsal Spinous Processes

The ridge down the center of the horse's back is composed of 18 thoracic and 6 lumbar vertebrae. Normally, these vertebral spinous processes are separated by interposed muscle. In a horse with impingement of the dorsal spinous process, more commonly known as "kissing spines" disease, the spines impinge on one another or overlap, causing pain and muscle spasms, especially when being ridden or performing athletically. Friction caused by the spines rubbing together results in periostitis with new bone formation, often leading to arthritis of the vertebral column. There is thought that kissing spine may have a genetic component, but it is also common in short-backed horses that have had a history of falling or going over backwards, or that are involved in activities that produce maximum flexion and extension of the spine. Kissing spine is most prevalent with barrel racers as well as hunters and jumpers.

Horses that show signs of back and loin pain, are sensitive to downward pressure on the back, and seem to resent being saddled may be affected by kissing spine. Radiographs can confirm the severity and location of kissing spine lesions, which may be managed with NSAIDs or local injections of corticosteroids and muscle relaxants; however, surgery is the recommended treatment for clients wanting their horses to return to full athletic function.

Subtotal spinous **ostectomy** is an effective method of surgical treatment for impinged dorsal spinous processes. While this surgery has been performed on horses under general anesthesia in lateral recumbency, spinous ostectomies can be performed safely and effectively on the standing patient with IV sedation and analgesia provided (Fig. 34.22). A standing surgery eliminates risks associated with anesthetics and subsequent recovery, and provides the surgeon with easier access to the surgery site and reduces the risk of hemorrhage (Case Presentation 34.1).

CASE PRESENTATION 34.1

A 15-year-old, 1200-lb Thoroughbred gelding was seen for evaluation of chronic back pain. The horse's owners noted that there had been a decrease in ability to perform athletically, reluctance to allow vigorous grooming over the lumbar region, and a new sensitivity to tightening the girth on the saddle. While being ridden, the horse had become less cooperative in performing skills that previously came easily.

A routine physical exam was performed, along with a basic lameness exam, to observe the patient walking and trotting on a hard surface in both a straight line and in a circle on a lunge line. The patient's distal limbs and cervical spine were palpated, with unremarkable findings. The patient responded negatively to palpation along both sides of his back, especially in the thoracic and lumbar regions and over the hips.

Digital radiographs were taken to confirm overriding and impingement of dorsal spinous processes, specifically between T13-L2, most severely affecting T14-T17 (Fig. 34.23). A subtotal dorsal spinous process ostectomy was scheduled for the following morning.

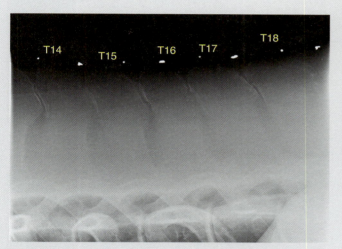

• **Fig. 34.23** Radiographs showing the impingement of multiple dorsal spinous processes. For this patient, a complete wedge ostectomy was created in the dorsal processes of T11, T13, and T15 and a partial ostectomy of T17.

Skin staples were placed under radiographic guidance prior to surgery and left in place to act as surgical markers. The dorsal midline region of the spine from T3-L5 was clipped and aseptically prepared using 2% chlorhexidine scrub and 70% isopropyl alcohol before routine surgical draping was performed. A 22-gauge, 1.5-inch needle was used to administer local anesthetic (lidocaine 2%) subcutaneously over the dorsal midline. The patient was maintained via standing sedation for the duration of the procedure.

A #10 blade was used to incise through skin, subcutaneous tissue, and the supraspinous ligament from the level of T10-T18. A combination of blunt and sharp dissection was performed using a periosteal elevator, Mayo scissors, and Metzenbaum scissors to separate the affected dorsal spinous processes from surrounding tissue and the infraspinous ligament. Lidocaine was deposited locally around the spinous processes using an 18-gauge, 3.5-inch spinal needle. Bleeding was controlled with mosquito hemostats and pressure applied with 4 × 4 gauze and lap sponges.

Using an oscillating bone saw, cranial and caudal complete wedge ostectomies were created in the dorsal processes of T11, T13, and T15

(Fig. 34.24). Continuous saline lavage at an approximate 30-degree angle was used to keep the saw blade and cut bone cool. A cranial wedge partial ostectomy was created in the dorsal process of T17. All fragments were removed with rongeurs, and the surgical sites were thoroughly lavaged with sterile saline. The supraspinous ligament was closed with 0 polyglactin 910 on a taper needle in a simple continuous pattern. Subcutaneous sutures were placed in a simple continuous pattern using 2-0 polyglactin 910 on a taper needle. The skin was apposed with staples, and silver spray was applied over the incision. Recovery from sedation was uneventful.

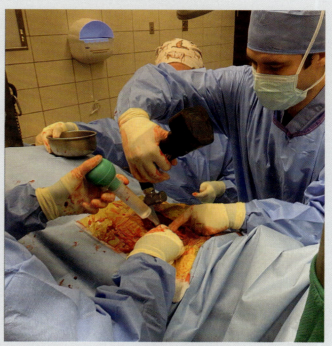

• **Fig. 34.24** An oscillating bone saw is used to create wedge ostectomies of the dorsal spinous processes when surgically treating impinged dorsal spinous processes. A bulb syringe is used to drip saline solution on the saw blade while it is in use to prevent the buildup of heat and to clear saw dust from the site.

The patient was monitored overnight, with no notable issues. Pain and inflammation levels remained within the expected parameters. The patient was discharged from the hospital with a 10-day course of oral trimethoprim-sulfamethoxazole and phenylbutazone paste. It was recommended that the incision site receive cryotherapy with a soft ice pack wrapped in a towel for 10 minutes twice a day, for 5 days to combat inflammation.

Under the care of his owners, per the recommendations of the surgeon the patient received 2 weeks of stall rest with 20- to 30-minute hand walks twice daily. This was followed by another 2 weeks of small paddock turnout. Four weeks following surgery, the patient was turned out in a larger paddock and received aqua treadmill therapy at the owner's discretion up to two to three times weekly. A follow-up exam was scheduled for 14 weeks post surgery. Permission to begin riding was granted at that time. This patient experienced no known complications from surgery.

Poll Evil and Fistulous Withers

Fistulous withers involves the bursal sac overlying the first thoracic vertebral spines. The disease first presents as a swelling on one or both sides of the poll. The initiating event may be pressure at the withers from a badly fitting saddle or harness. Extensive involvement can lead to osteomyelitis of the vertebrae. Poll evil is much like fistulous withers except that it affects the poll of the head, just behind the ears. There may be a history of trauma, such as striking the back of the head against the top of a door. Involvement of the neck ligament causes intense pain when the horse moves its head.

Both fistulous withers and poll evil are often associated with *Brucella abortus*, a bacteria more common to cattle. Horses can pick up the bacteria by ingesting contaminated food or water, or by direct penetration through mucous membranes. However, not all cases of fistulous withers and poll evil are caused by *Brucella abortus*. The bacteria *Streptococcus zooepidemicus* and *Actinomyces bovis* may be found alone or combined with *B. abortus*. Additionally, the hairlike worm parasite *Onchocerca cervicalis* has been implicated in the initial stages of fistulous withers.

Fistulous withers and poll evil are difficult to treat due to their deep-seated nature. Horses that culture positive for *B. abortus* should be quarantined to prevent contact with other horses and humans. Brucellosis causes undulant fever in humans, so the infected tissue and discharge should be handled with caution. Ivermectin should be administered to eliminate potential *Oncocerca cervicalis* involvement. Antibiotic therapy is effective in the early stages but has limited effectiveness once the condition becomes chronic with draining sinuses. Surgical intervention, including wide removal of devitalized and infected tissue, is required for a permanent cure (Fig. 34.25). In the case of fistulous withers, a subtotal spinous ostectomy of the dorsal spinous processes within the affected region is necessary to ensure full debridement of the area.

Cribbing

Cribbing, sometimes referred to as "wind sucking," is a common vice among horses that are kept in stables with minimal enrichment. The act of cribbing involves a horse setting its front teeth on a horizontal object such as the edge of a stall, bucket, or fence post, arching its neck, pulling back, and swallowing huge gulps of air, often accompanied by a grunting sound. The act of cribbing is a coping mechanism for stress or boredom and is thought to release endorphins, causing a sense of pleasure. Cribbing, along with chronic wood chewing, can damage front incisors, occasionally to the extent that a horse can no longer graze. Some horses can become so addicted to the act of cribbing that they fail to consume enough food and begin to lose weight, sometimes causing chronic gastritis. Horses that have not previously been known to crib may learn the behavior from other cribbers housed nearby.

Management techniques to prevent or reduce cribbing may be used such as increased turnout, socialization, and enrichment. Some horses respond well to "toys," such as hanging a milk jug with a few rocks in it from the stall ceilings, or metal mirrors. Commercial devices used to reduce cribbing include cribbing collars that fit tightly around a horse's throat, which increases discomfort when the act of cribbing takes place, or use of a hollow bit, which makes it difficult for a horse to form a seal with its lips on an object.

For young horses, there has been success treating a cribbing habit with surgery. Horses are placed in dorsal recumbency under general anesthesia. Surgical correction of a cribbing habit involves transecting the rostral portion of the sternomandibularis, sternothyroideus, and omohyoideus muscles, as well as the spinal accessory nerve on each side of the neck (Fig. 34.26). A diode laser is used to reduce seroma or hematoma formation. Active drains, typically Jackson-Pratts, are added, with bulb collection reservoirs at both the caudal and cranial ends of the incision. These should remain in place and be monitored until output is minimized (Fig. 34.27).

Enucleation

Enucleation is the removal of the eyeball globe, along with the adjacent connective, muscular, and glandular tissue (Fig. 34.28). Enucleation is warranted in cases of ocular trauma, perforating

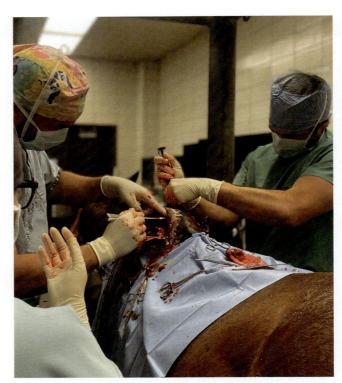

• **Fig. 34.25** Debridement surgery on an equine patient with fistulous withers. Draining tracts were opened bilaterally.

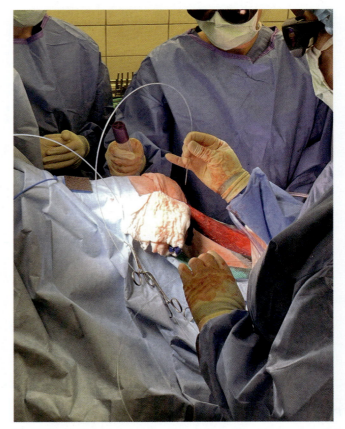

• **Fig. 34.26** Diode laser being used to cut the omohyoideus muscle during cribbing surgery. An assistant is holding a vacuum to capture the laser plume smoke. The entire surgical team is wearing protective goggles while the laser is in use.

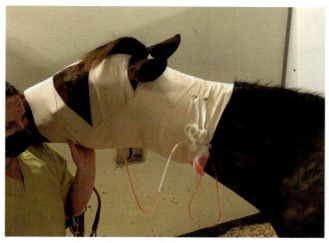

• **Fig. 34.27** An equine patient following cribbing surgery. Note the two bulb collection reservoirs at the end of cranial and caudal Jackson-Pratt drains, accessible outside of the patient's bandage. In the days immediately following surgery, these drains must be frequently monitored and emptied as necessary to help prevent the development of a seroma.

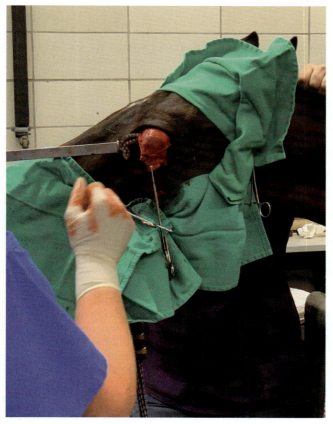

• **Fig. 34.28** An ecraseur being used to perform an enucleation on a sedated standing equine patient.

corneal ulcers, squamous cell carcinoma or other cancerous growths in and around the eye, or end-stage uveitis or glaucoma. Often, enucleating an injured or diseased eye is the best treatment to manage pain and restore quality of life. It is often cost effective when considering the management for chronic ailments and should be considered, especially when prognosis for long-term medical management is poor. Some horse owners may be reluctant to consider enucleation because of cosmetic as well as

management challenges. Most horses adapt extremely well to having only one eye; however, some activities, such as being groomed on the blind side, riding in unfamiliar areas, and loading onto a dark trailer may take some adjustment time. When working around an enucleated or blind horse, one should remain especially cognizant of safety, ensuring that the patient is aware and not startled. There also should be precautions taken to protect the seeing eye to prevent total blindness, which is not often well tolerated in horses.

Enucleations can be performed standing with sedation or under full anesthetization. To prevent discomfort during the procedure, local anesthetic is used. There are two variations of surgical enucleations: transpalpebral and subconjunctival. Transpalpebral enucleations are performed when there is a need to control the spread of infection or cancerous growth. They require the removal of additional surrounding tissue within the eye socket. Subconjunctival enucleations are commonly performed in cases where the eye is injured or perforated. Glandular tissue is always removed during enucleation surgeries, because remnants are likely to cause chronic drainage from the surgery site.

Preparation of the eye and a small area of the surrounding skin should be aseptically performed using a dilute Betadine solution. Eyelashes should be trimmed during the surgical clip. The OR tech should be prepared for the procedure with general surgical instruments and drapes, as well as a sharply curved vascular clamp (such as a Satinsky) and a chain ecraseur or sharply curved Mayo scissors, depending on the surgeon's preference. Some clients may elect to have a prosthetic eye placed during surgery to provide a more esthetic appearance. There is little difference between performing enucleations on equine patients and food-animal patients (Case Presentation 34.2).

Lacerations and Puncture Wounds

Lacerations are the most common type of open wound and commonly include injuries by barbed wire, sharp objects, and animal bites. Irregular edges, extensive damage to the surrounding soft tissues, and heavy contamination is observed. Unless large vessels are severed, hemorrhage is usually not profuse, as the vessels are often stretched, torn, thrombosed, or vasoconstricted. Avulsion refers to a laceration in which tissues have been torn away.

Puncture wounds tend to go together with lacerations, because they are also caused by sharp objects. Punctures usually cause little superficial damage and may initially go unnoticed; however, bacteria and debris carried into deep tissue may result in infection, with wounds involving the thoracic cavity, joints, tendon sheaths, and bursae, causing increased concern. Puncture wounds should be surgically prepared, lavaged, and debrided. Plain and contrast radiography can be helpful to assess the extent of the injury. Unremoved debris and foreign bodies will often result in chronic drain tracts. It is recommended to leave puncture wound injuries open to allow healing by second intention.

The initial goal of wound preparation is to decrease the threat of additional contamination by cleaning the skin surrounding the wound. Subsequently, the wound itself is cleaned and debrided. Often, chemical restraint, combined with regional and local analgesia, will be necessary.

The wound site should be protected from loose hair and debris by applying a water-soluble sterile lubricant while preparing the skin surrounding the injury. Wetting the hair surrounding the wound before clipping can help prevent wound contamination. It is common for blood or fluid running down a horse's chest or limb during wound care to cause the patient to want to move. Draping

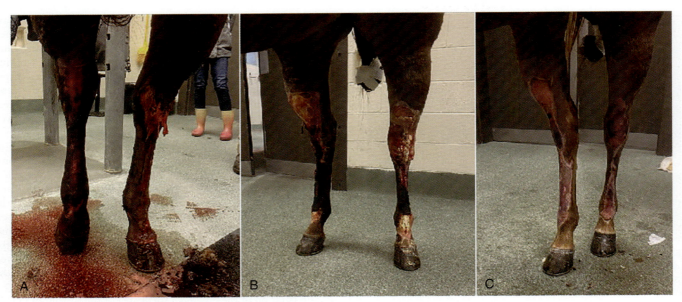

• **Fig. 34.29** Laceration and wound management can be a slow, meticulous process. (A–C) The healing illustrated in these three photos is over 10 weeks, with work yet to be done.

or periodically wiping the fluid can help soothe the patient and discourage movement.

Wounds on the face and upper neck tend to heal faster and more cosmetically than those on the trunk, which tend to heal faster and more cosmetically than those on the extremities. Wounds on the distal extremities are complicated by the lack of soft tissue covering, poor circulation, joint movement, and the greater opportunity for contamination and subsequent infection. Furthermore, persistent exuberant granulation tissue, or proud flesh, is of particular concern on areas below the carpus and tarsus. These factors, in addition to the time that has passed before treatment is initiated, the available facilities, the temperament of the horse, its intended use, and the size and location of the wound, are considerations that help determine the course of treatment, which should be both practical and cost effective (Fig. 34.29).

Upper Respiratory Tract Surgery

Laryngeal Hemiplegia

Laryngeal **hemiplegia** is an upper respiratory disease affecting a horse's upper airway and resulting in paralysis of the arytenoid cartilage. The left recurrent laryngeal nerve is involved in more than 90% of cases. These horses are referred to as "roarers" because of the loud breathing noise they make when being worked due to their inability to abduct the arytenoid during inspiration.

Diagnosis is based on a history of exercise intolerance and endoscopic evidence of hemiplegia or hemiparesis. The slap test can assist in diagnosis of laryngeal functional status and is best used to determine complete laryngeal hemiplegia from other variants of asynchrony. A series of sharp slaps to the lateral aspect of the withers or thorax stimulates adduction of the contralateral arytenoid cartilage to produce glottic closure. Inability to adduct the arytenoid cartilage may indicate a recurrent laryngeal neuropathy.

Treatment options range from conservative management, such as decreasing the level of performance, to surgical treatment involving a tie-back procedure, in which a suture is placed between the appropriate cartilage and muscle to replicate the action of the cricoarytenoideus dorsalis muscle in abducting the cartilage. The

suture placement can be facilitated by using J-shaped cruciate needles. The OR tech may also want to have a selection of deep retractors on hand to aid in maintaining access while the suture is being placed. The surgeon will use an endoscope intraoperatively to visualize the surgical site. This visualization will allow the surgeon to ensure that no additional tissues are affected by the suture placement and that the abduction achieved by the suture is adequate.

Arytenoid Chondritis

In **chondritis**, a condition most commonly affecting young racehorses, one or both arytenoid cartilages undergo dystrophic changes, including enlargement, inflammation, mineralization, and the deposition of granulation tissue, all of which causes a reduction in the laryngeal luminal diameter. Arytenoid chondritis presents with a decreased exercise capacity and inspiratory stridor, specifically during higher-speed exercise, because of restricted airflow at the larynx. Without careful observation, arytenoid chondritis can be confused with laryngeal hemiplegia.

Palpation of the larynx may reveal abnormalities of the affected cartilage. Diagnosis is usually confirmed during endoscopic examination, which will reveal the deformed arytenoid cartilage with little to no abduction. Changes may be mild, consisting of hyperemia, ulceration, and granulation tissue formation at the dorsomedial aspect of the cartilage. Unilateral involvement is most commonly observed but may occur bilaterally.

Arytenoid chondritis can rarely be effectively managed with conservative treatment therapies and nearly always requires surgical intervention. The most common surgical procedure for the treatment of arytenoid chondritis is removal of the affected arytenoid cartilage by way of a ventral laryngotomy. As with a tie-back procedure, the surgeon will use an endoscope to aid with visualization during the procedure. The laryngotomy is most easily performed by passing a diode laser fiber through the channel of the endoscope. While the active end of the laser fiber is nearly always inside the patient's mouth and throat, standard laser safety precautions should still be taken. Esophageal grasping forceps are also important for retraction and gathering of the tissue

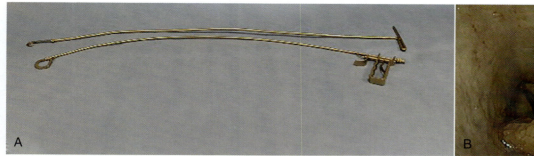
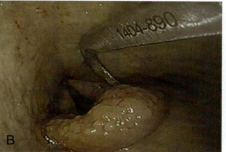

• **Fig. 34.30** (A) An epiglottic knife is used to cut through mucosal folds that (B) form an entrapment over the epiglottis.

being removed. Ventral laryngotomies in equine patients typically require a tracheotomy to be performed for ventilation while the patient is under anesthesia.

The tracheotomy tube is usually left in place for the first few days after surgery to ensure that the patient has an airway of adequate diameter and has unrestricted breathing. Such patients must be monitored closely to ensure that the tube does not become dislodged or obstructed with mucus (which may need to be suctioned away). Laryngotomy and tracheotomy sites require daily cleaning. Application of petrolatum on the skin surrounding the incisions will protect them from drainage during the healing process, which requires approximately 3 weeks.

Epiglottic Entrapment

In a horse with epiglottic entrapment, mucosal folds surrounding the epiglottis become excessively large, creating a mass that envelops the epiglottis and narrows the airway. Due to the narrowed airway, affected horses are exercise intolerant, breathe noisily, and can cough during exercise or after eating. Nasopharyngeal endoscopy reveals redundant folds, often swollen and ulcerated, obscuring the view of the epiglottis. The "hook" procedure, using an epiglottis knife, is performed to free the epiglottis from the redundant mucosal folds (Fig. 34.30A and B). This is a quick surgical procedure performed on the standing patient sedated with a combination of xylazine or detomidine and butorphanol. A nasopharyngeal endoscope provides visual guidance for the surgeon manipulating the epiglottis knife passed through the opposite nostril.

Sinusitis

A horse has six pairs of paranasal sinuses: the frontal, sphenopalatine, and maxillary sinuses, and the dorsal, middle, and ventral conchal sinus. These air-filled cavities accommodate some of the maxillary premolar and molar tooth roots, facilitate passage of facial nerves, and extend around the horse's eyes, ending around the facial crest.

Signs of sinusitis include unilateral facial swelling, purulent ocular and/or nasal discharge, and a dull sound when the sinuses are percussed. Sinusitis refers to any infection or inflammation of one or more sinuses; however, the cause may be either primary or secondary. Primary causes are typically related to upper respiratory infections caused by *Streptococcus* and can be treated with appropriate antibiotic therapy and lavage by way of a catheter placed through a small percutaneous trephine hole into the affected sinus. Secondary sinusitis is an infection from another cause, such as an infected tooth, bone fracture, or sinus cyst. Radiography and endoscopy are helpful in diagnosing the cause of secondary

sinusitis. Whether the sinusitis is primary or secondary, the goal of treatment is to address the underlying cause of the sinusitis and to restore the horse's natural sinus drainage mechanisms.

There are two surgical approaches to the sinus cavity: sinus trephination and sinusotomy. Both trephination and sinusotomy can be performed on a standing patient under sedation and local anesthesia, although some surgeons prefer to perform sinusotomy with the patient under general anesthesia. Sinus trephination involves drilling a hole through the horse's head (face) and into their sinus cavity to allow sinus lavage and for antibiotics to be instilled directly into the sinuses when indicated. The hole will be made using a Galt trephine. Fluid and discharge draining from the nostril during lavage indicates that patency has been established.

Sinusotomy, commonly called "face flap surgery," involves the creation of a bone flap into the affected sinus, allowing for better access (Fig. 34.31). The flap is created using osteotomes and a bone mallet. Periosteal elevators will also be needed to aid in the approach to the bone. For either surgical option, it is a good idea for the OR tech to have bone curettes available to the surgeon. Depending on the need for subsequent lavage or treatment, sinusotomies may be reopened several days in a row.

Postoperative care includes appropriate antibiotics to treat the underlying cause of the sinusitis, anti-inflammatories to reduce inflammation and discomfort, and bandaging. Care should be used when bandaging so as not to occlude the horse's eye. Despite the seemingly grotesque nature of sinus surgery, cosmetic results typically are very good. Horses usually return to full athletic performance after treatment.

Surgical Nursing of Food Animals

Although both food-animal and equine patients tend to be lumped together in large-animal veterinary practice, food animals offer a unique set of challenges. Food animals are just that, animals whose meat is intended for human consumption and that have a limited life span. Although there is a growing number of companion food animals, there generally is a significant economic drive behind clients seeking veterinary care in the food-animal industry. The cost of treatment and the profit potential must align favorably for the client, because herd health management and preventive medicine are paramount.

Food-animal practice facilities must take into consideration functionality and safety. Veterinary practices intending to handle food-animal cases on site must be equipped with appropriate fencing and restraint equipment (nasal tongs) so that these large, sometimes fractious animals can be restrained and examined safely (Fig. 34.32). Tilt tables allow practitioners to perform more surgical and diagnostic procedures with animals under sedation or

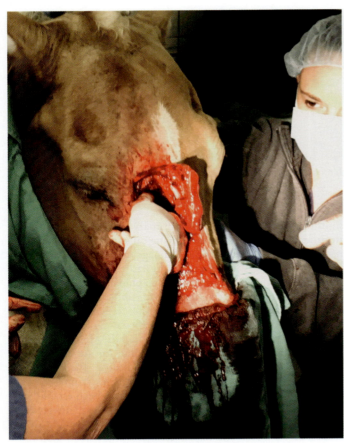

• **Fig. 34.31** A horse with a sinusotomy or "face flap" to treat secondary sinusitis.

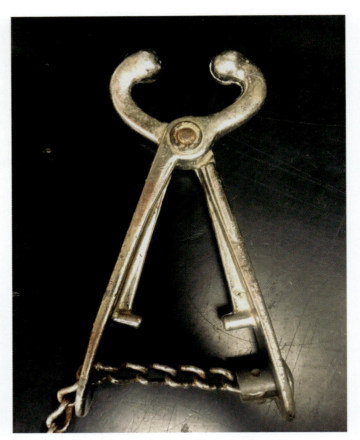

• **Fig. 34.32** Nose tongs used for restraining cattle.

general anesthesia, and are an excellent tool in food-animal practices (Fig. 34.33). Devices for smaller food-animal species are also commercially available and of immense value to the food-animal practitioner.

Preoperative Nursing

Food-animal technicians often are tasked with the initial patient examination. A complete patient history should be obtained from the client or herd manager, including a clear understanding of their interpretation of the clinical signs. More importantly, in internal medicine and surgical cases, the technician should ask questions about overall herd health, environment, how long the presenting issue has been a problem, if it has spread to others, and what action the client has taken to deal with the problem.

Physical examinations on a food-animal patient should start from a distance. Behavior and mentation are most accurately observed when the animal is in its natural environment with minimal human disturbance. Breed and conformation should be considered. With additional restraint, the heart and the lungs should be auscultated, and the body temperature obtained.

Blood work (CBC, chemistry profile) should be done preoperatively; however, economic factors must be considered. Minimally, PCV and TP should be obtained if the patient is to go under general anesthesia or if significant blood loss is of concern.

Intraoperative positioning mandates the need for preoperative fasting. For adult patients in dorsal or lateral recumbency, 36 to 48 hours of fasting is indicated. Because of the capacity of the rumen,

water should be withheld for 12 hours prior to surgery; fasting is not required for patients undergoing standing procedures.

Prior to surgery, an IV catheter should be placed in food-animal patients with appropriate restraint. In most cases, this is best placed in the jugular vein, although for patients with large ears, particularly pigs and Brahman cattle, catheters may be placed in the auricular vein. Restraint of small ruminants may involve holding; cattle should be placed in a squeeze chute or head gate, haltered, and the lead secured with a quick-release knot. Nose tongs can be used to control the animal's head when a halter is not sufficient. The area over the jugular vein should be clipped and aseptically prepared, and the local anesthetic injected subcutaneously. To aid catheter placement on cattle, it is recommended that a stab incision be made using a No. 15 scalpel blade to prevent burring of the ends of the catheter. IV catheters should be secured with either suture or glue.

When allowed, it is recommended that the patient's hair be clipped around the surgical site before moving the animal to the OR. This reduces the debris that is brought into the OR, thus decreasing infection risks. As with horses, this should be done as close as possible to the time of surgery. Once the patient has been anesthetized and positioned for surgery, the surgical site should be aseptically prepared with a scrub solution, ridding the skin of dust, hair, and dander.

Interoperative Nursing

Many food-animal surgeries are performed in the field and are considered "clean" surgeries. When performing surgery in the field, environmental hazards need to be considered. Unlike in a traditional OR setting, insects, dust, and dirt are all significant

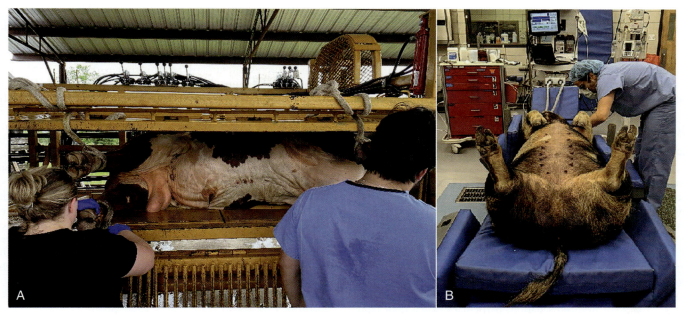

• **Fig. 34.33** (A) Bovine patient being restrained in lateral recumbency using a tilt chute. Limbs are secured for the patient's safety as well as the handler's. (B) A pig under general anesthesia in dorsal recumbency on a surgery table in preparation for a laparoscopy.

factors unique to working outdoors. Restraint techniques are also different when operating in the field. Ropes and halters need to be readily accessible and should be made of a material (preferably thick cotton) that does not burn humans or animals. Having all supplies and equipment ready will ensure efficiency.

Appropriate padding must be used if an animal is to be recumbent during surgery. Attention must be paid to the weight of the animal and the estimated time of recumbency. If the patient is placed in lateral recumbency, the distal forelimb should be pulled cranially, with cushioning placed under the point of the down shoulder. The uppermost hind limb should be elevated off the down hind limb using pads or a bale of shavings or straw, although complications from myositis or radial nerve paralysis can still develop due to restricted blood flow and excess pressure placed on the muscles and nerves. After recovery, these conditions must be addressed. Most patients recover in 1 to 2 days. Because of economic concerns, lack of facilities, and transportation challenges, many surgical procedures are performed with the food-animal patient standing with proper restraint in all scenarios.

Postoperative Nursing

Due to altered gastrointestinal motility associated with the pain, reduced food intake, and anesthesia that accompany surgery, special attention must be paid to ensure that analgesia and nutrition are being considered in the postoperative food-animal patient. Evaluation of the gastrointestinal tracts, especially the forestomach and abomasum, is fundamental to postoperative care of a ruminant patient. The goal of nutritional support following surgery is focused on returning the gastrointestinal tract to its normal function over specific long-term nutritional needs.

Technicians charged with providing care for and observation of postoperative food-animal patients should make note of and communicate any changes in a patient's mentation, appetite, and indication of pain. Frequent TPRs and physical exams will aid in the monitoring of these changes.

Drug Withdrawal and Extra-label Use

In a food-animal practice, drugs that are administered to patients must be labeled for use in that species or be listed as an **extra-label** use drug. If this information is not already listed on the bottle or package insert, it can be found on the Food Animal Residue Avoidance Databank (FARAD) website (www.FARAD.org). If any antibiotics, analgesics, or anesthetics are used, the veterinarian, technician, and owner must follow the recommendations regarding withdrawal times from meat, milk, and eggs. Withdrawal time refers to the period before marketing or slaughter during which the drug cannot be used in an animal. This allows for the drug in the animal's system to be depleted to a below-tolerance concentration.

Extra-label use refers to the use of a new animal drug in a food-producing animal in a manner that is not in accordance with the regular use of the drug as labeled. This should only be considered in extraordinary circumstances and under adherence to strict criteria. To use an extra-label drug in a food animal, a careful medical diagnosis should be made by the veterinarian in the context of a valid veterinary client-patient relationship (VDPR). A determination should be made that there is no marketed drug labeled for the treatment of the condition diagnosed or that drug therapy at the dosage recommended by labeling has been clinically ineffective. There must be a procedure in place to ensure that the treated patient's identity is carefully maintained. Finally, a significantly extended period must be assigned for drug withdrawal before marketing meat, milk, or eggs, and steps should be taken to ensure that the assigned time frames are met so that no illegal residues remain.

Drugs and chemicals play a key role in the production of meat and poultry supply, and consumer concerns are at an all-time high. Residue awareness, prevention, and control has evolved into an intricate pattern of veterinary and nonveterinary involvement; however, veterinary medicine remains at the heart of the discussion. There are intense ethical issues pertaining to residues in meat and poultry for veterinarians in private practice, the food-animal industry, pharmaceutical companies, and regulatory agencies. Veterinary professionals must be diligent regarding client education. It is important to communicate with the owner or producer regarding drug residue in food-producing animals and the required withdrawal time that should be allotted before treatment, because this may not only have an economic effect on the client but may also influence how to appropriately treat the patient.

Surgical Considerations

Laparotomies

Laparotomies are performed in cattle for a variety of reasons; however, rumenotomies, rumenostomy, and C-sections are among the most common. Laparotomies are performed on the standing animal, because this facilitates intra-abdominal exploration and manipulation, and for the standing animal, there is minimal intra-abdominal pressure, which reduces the risk of evisceration. The animal should be restrained in a squeeze chute that provides ample access to the left or right flank, depending on the indication. Ideally, the rumen contents are reduced, although this may not be feasible, especially in cases of impaction.

Most animals need no sedation, particularly when their clinical condition is serious. With fractious animals, xylazine can be administered intravenously. It should be noted that although xylazine is significantly more potent in ruminants than in other species, specific breeds, such as Hereford and Brahman, are especially sensitive to the drug and require only very small doses. Any time sedation is being used on any animal, particularly ruminants, the dose should start small and be worked up to the amount needed for desired effect as the animal's individual response to the drug is better known.

The incision site should be chosen based on the suspected problem. For example, the left paralumbar region is best in a case of traumatic reticuloperitonitis, because the left flank provides access to the reticulum and its associated diaphragmatic area, along with the rumen, spleen, left margin of the liver, left kidney, viscera within the omental bursa, uterus, and bladder. From the right flank, the examiner should be able to palpate the greater omentum and mesoduodenum with the descending duodenum, the abomasum and pyloric area, omasum, visceral surface of the liver, gallbladder, right half of the diaphragm, visceral structures within the omental bursa (small and large intestine and cecum), left and right kidneys, bladder, and uterus. This makes the right paralumbar fossa ideal for conditions such as abomasal volvulus, cecal dilatation and volvulus, intussusception, and intestinal phytobezoar. The rumen will act as a retainer for abdominal contents in many procedures.

Rumenotomy

Rumenotomy is indicated when a ruminant has gorged on feed or ingested a foreign object and, because of rumen stasis or "bloat," the contents of the rumen must be manually evacuated. The position of the rumen against the left body wall makes it an easy portal for other GI structures.

A large area of the left flank is clipped, prepped, and aseptically prepared. Local anesthetic should be provided by using an inverted "L" block behind the last rib and just below the transverse process of the lumbar vertebrae. Lidocaine must be placed under the skin, into the muscle, and to the level of the peritoneum for the block to be successful. When using large amounts of lidocaine, care must be taken to avoid exceeding the toxic dose (lidocaine 6–8 mg/kg). Attention should be paid during surgery to ensure that the patient

remains standing for the entire procedure. General surgical supplies, including towel clamps and draping materials, scalpel blades and handles, a variety of tissue forceps and clamps, a variety of scissors, and needle drivers, should be available.

After successful surgery, healthy rumen contents need to be replaced in the animal by performing a rumen **transfaunation**. In rumen transfaunation, rumen fluid from the rumen of a healthy donor animal is transferred to the compromised recipient animal. The donor fluid contains a broad spectrum of microorganisms, including bacteria, protozoa, fungi, and archaea. This fluid can be obtained from a healthy cow by using a stomach tube and a dose syringe. A cow with a fistulated rumen is invaluable to any food-animal practice for harvesting of rumen fluid (Fig. 34.34).

Few complications are associated with rumenostomy, and the outcome is largely dependent on the presenting complaint. Peritonitis is of concern in cases where rumen contents have spilled into the abdomen. Antibiotics and analgesics will need to be given postoperatively. Daily care of the incision is important, especially keeping the area clear of flies and other insects. Clean and dry the area for 7 to 10 days.

Cesarean Section

C-section is indicated when the calf is too large or has congenital defects, the cow has abnormal pelvic bone conformation, or there is a chance of delivering a live calf during a dystocia malposition. The left flank is the most common approach for this surgery, although the right flank, paramedian, and ventral midline approaches can also be used. The technique is determined by the size, temperament, and physical condition of the cow, in addition to the surgeon's preference.

Surgical preparation in the standing patient involves using an inverted-L nerve block in the left paralumbar fossa and using the rumen to retain the small intestine. Keeping the cow standing during the procedure is often preferred, although surgery can be performed on a cow in right lateral recumbency if she is very sick or if the calf has been confirmed dead. A cow that is straining should receive an epidural to reduce pushing efforts. IV fluid therapy is warranted in cows with severe dehydration.

When performing a C-section, the uterus should be exteriorized unless it is impossible to do so. Exteriorizing the uterus prevents the uterine contents from contaminating the abdominal

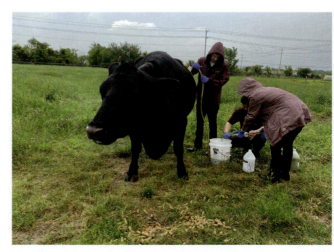

• **Fig. 34.34** Veterinary technicians collecting rumen fluid from a fistulated cow to be transferred into a compromised recipient animal.

cavity and reduces the risk of infection. This is paramount in cases where there is a dead, deteriorating fetus.

Supplies used to receive a live calf should be readily available in cases where viability is unknown. Towels, obstetric chains, Ambu bag, emergency drugs, gloves, and umbilical tape are all necessary for successful delivery. The veterinary technician plays a vital role in caring for the calf (Fig. 34.35).

After surgery, the cow and calf should be left alone to bond (Fig. 34.36). When cleaning the calf, the technician should be sure to leave some of the afterbirth on the calf so that the cow can identify its offspring. The calf should stand within the first 30 minutes and nurse within the first hour to get the colostrum needed for immunity. The calf's navel should be treated with a diluted chlorhexidine solution.

Oxytocin should be given to the cow to aid in expulsion of the placenta and involution of the uterus. During forced fetal extraction, obstetric chains should be looped above the calf's fetlocks and half-hitched below the fetlocks to distribute the pulling forces more evenly on the limbs and prevent physeal (growth plate) fractures.

Abomasal Displacements and Volvulus

Abomasal displacement is a common problem of high-producing dairy cows fed high-concentration and low-roughage diets. Displacements are most likely to occur in the first 6 weeks after calving. Hypocalcemia, along with mastitis, metritis, ketosis, and lack of exercise, can lead to abdominal displacement. Clinically, cows with a displaced abomasum will be reluctant to eat and have reduced manure output and milk production. Cows with volvulus will have an elevated heart rate, be dehydrated, and have large amounts of gas and fluid collected on the right side. Left displaced abomasum (LDA) is much more common than right displaced abomasum (RDA). Because of trapped gas, LDA and RDA can be diagnosed by auscultating a distinct "ping" in the left or right paralumbar fossa.

The Liptak test can be used to diagnose LDA. Percussion of the abomasum on the left side under the last few ribs, an area just below where the gas ping is heard, corresponds to the fluid level in the abomasum. This serves as a landmark that indicates which area should be clipped and surgically prepared. Centesis is performed using an 18-gauge × 1.5-inch needle to collect fluid. If the pH is less than 4.5, it confirms the presence of an LDA. The aspirated gas will have a burnt almond smell.

Conservative treatment involves physically rolling the patient to try to encourage the abomasum to flip back into place. When successful, this tends to be a temporary fix, because the abomasum usually displaces again. Blind tacking or a toggle pin can be used to blindly secure the abomasum to the body wall, but such measures have a high rate of complications, including infection and damage to internal organs.

Surgery is usually necessary to correct abdominal displacements. If the cow has not eaten recently, transfaunation of healthy rumen fluid will speed recovery time. A diet consisting of only roughage should be fed for the initial few days of recovery. If necessary, grain can be gradually introduced back into the patient's diet once full recovery has been made.

Postoperative feeding after a laparotomy should be gradual and occur only after all signs of sedation or general anesthesia have disappeared. A well-bedded, dry stall in a clean, comfortable environment will ensure a speedy recovery. If the incision is kept clean, little else is needed. The surgery site should be monitored

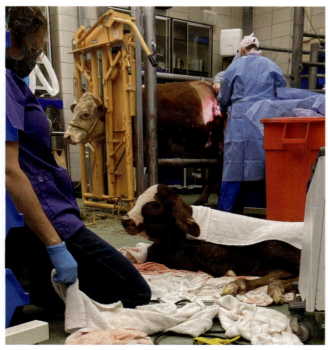

• **Fig. 34.35** A veterinary technician works to warm up a calf recently delivered via cesarean while the surgical team works to complete surgery.

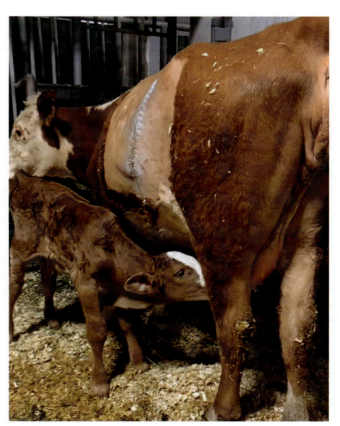

• **Fig. 34.36** New calf born via cesarean section nursing from its mother soon after surgery. The shaved area and incision on the cow are typical of bovine laparotomies.

for swelling, discomfort upon palpation, and discharge of any kind. Antibiotics, analgesics, and tetanus vaccination should be given postoperatively. Stall rest is recommended for 7 to 10 days.

Traumatic Reticuloperitonitis

Traumatic reticuloperitonitis (TRP), more commonly known as "hardware disease," is a medical condition caused by ingestion of foreign material, resulting in a perforation of the reticulum. Patients usually present with acute anorexia and fever, may be reluctant to lie down or move, and display shallow breathing, constipation, and dehydration. Local pain in the region of the xiphoid cartilage manifests as a characteristic grunt upon percussion. Dairy cows will have decreased milk production. Animals that develop peritonitis may have diarrhea. TRP is best diagnosed using radiography.

To treat TRP conservatively, a rumen magnet is administered to immobilize the foreign object in conjunction with systemic antibiotics to control infection. Rumenotomy is effective in cases where the foreign body remains embedded in the wall of the reticulum or the problem is caused by nonferrous foreign material. TRP may lead to peritonitis, liver or reticular abscesses, pericarditis, vagal indigestion, or other secondary problems.

Pericarditis is a common complication of hardware disease. A swollen brisket is a hallmark clinical sign of pericarditis and, although it stems from a secondary issue, it can sometimes be the first sign of TRP noticed by the client. When sharp objects, such as pieces of wire, nails, or barbed wire, are ingested, they can pierce the reticular wall and injure the pericardium. Fluid builds up and compresses the heart, sending the patient into congestive heart failure.

Appropriate animal husbandry should be discussed with clients who have recurrent issues with hardware disease. Farm implements and equipment in disrepair should not be left lying around in the same areas where cattle are housed.

Urogenital Surgery

Umbilical Hernias and Infection

As in other species, the umbilicus in newborn calves consists of the urachus, a tube that connects the fetal bladder to the placental sac, and the remnants of the umbilical vessels that transported blood between the fetus and its mother. These structures normally shrink until only small remnants remain within the abdomen; however, if bacteria gain entry through the umbilicus, those remnants can become infected and require surgical removal (Fig. 34.37). The umbilical body wall is a common site for herniation, with the intestine protruding through the defect, and is common in Holstein dairy calves.

Calves with simple hernias will likely seem normal but have a reducible hernia protruding from the abdomen. Inappetent and febrile calves are likely to have an infected umbilicus. Calves with hernias may be observed urinating more frequently than normal or urinating through the umbilicus itself, suggesting a patent urachus. Calves with suspected umbilical hernias should be closely examined. If possible, it is best to examine the patient on its back in dorsal recumbency. Ultrasonography is a valuable tool for diagnosis of umbilical hernia.

Surgical repair is the treatment of choice and can often be performed in the field by using sedation and nerve blocks; however, general anesthesia is preferred. The umbilicus and all the associated structures will need to be removed. If infection extends to the bladder, a portion of it may also need to be removed. The entire

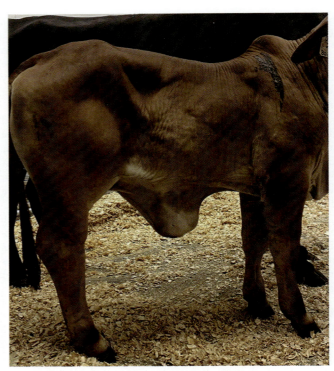

• **Fig. 34.37** A calf with an abscessed umbilicus requiring surgical intervention.

abdomen should be clipped and aseptically prepped. General surgical instrumentation is used, as are Doyen intestinal forceps.

The prognosis for calves with umbilical hernias is very good. Unless the infection is severe, systemic antibiotics need to only be given at the time of surgery. Animals that have received umbilical surgery should be managed in a clean, dry stall for 4 weeks. Too much exercise could lead to incisional complications. Postoperatively, patients should be reintroduced to feed slowly.

Castrations

Castration is a routine practice in large-animal medicine. Castrating male animals offers greater control over breeding programs and reduces management issues associated with aggression. More importantly, castration yields a better product. Postweaning performance tends to be greater, bringing higher market value. Beef, pork, and chevon from castrated males is more consistently of higher quality and palatability compared with those from their intact male counterparts.

There are several techniques for castration that can be used on calves and small ruminants. As with dehorning, castrations are best done early in development, preferably before 2 months of age, to reduce stress in the animal. Calves can be castrated without analgesia while being restrained on the ground or in a chute with the tail pushed straight up over their back. Restraining a calf in this manner is referred to as "tail jacking."

Open castration is the most common castration method used in calves and small ruminants. In open castration, the bottom third to bottom half of the scrotum is excised, exposing the testicles. When incising the scrotum, a horizontal cut can be made with a scalpel blade, or a vertical incision can be made with a Newberry knife to obtain better exposure of the testicles. The testicles are then pulled until the cords break.

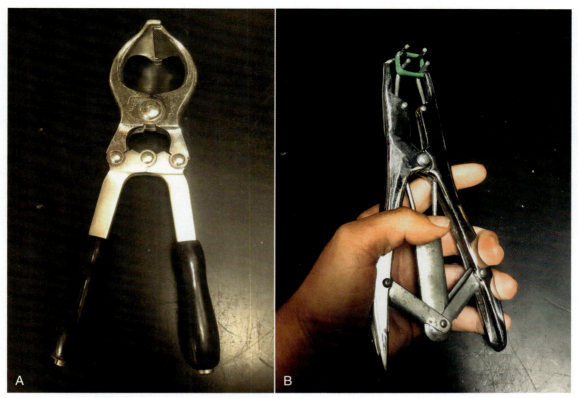

• **Fig. 34.38** (A) Burdizzo clamps used for castration in food animals. (B) Elastrator pliers with band used for castration in food animals.

In older calves, an emasculator may be used to crush and cut the cord, using the same technique of restraint (Fig. 34.38A). This is commonly known as the Burdizzo method. In this method, the blood vessels and spermatic cords are crushed without cutting the scrotal skin itself. Only one spermatic cord is crushed at a time, one higher than the other. If not performed in this staggered manner and the spermatic cords are crushed straight across, blood flow to the scrotum will be compromised. This leads to gangrene in the scrotum, which will eventually rot away. The Burdizzo method is a bloodless procedure and rarely causes infection; however, the urethra can be damaged when it is not performed correctly. Clinical signs that suggest damage done to the urethra include blood in the urine, swelling under the abdomen and around the penis, and severe pain.

Elastration is another bloodless method of castration. In this method, elastrator pliers are used to put a rubber elastrator band around the scrotum above the testicles (Fig. 34.38B). The band will cut off blood flow and cause the testicles to slough off within 2 to 3 weeks. This method should be applied within the first 10 days of life. This is thought to be a more painful method and tends to cause more complications from infection.

In the case of goats, it is recommended that bucks not be castrated until they are 5 to 6 months of age to allow the urethra time to mature and detach itself from the glans penis. When this fails to happen, a condition known as **urolithiasis** can occur. With urolithiasis, stony concretions form in the urinary tract and effectively "block" the urethra. This is a very painful condition that often requires surgery.

Castration in commercial swine should be performed as early as 3 to 4 days after birth. Anesthesia is not required, and the incision is left open to drain. Although they are routinely treated by food-animal veterinarians, pot-bellied pigs are often viewed more as companion animals. Because of this, they are castrated under cover of general anesthesia. A prescrotal incision is made, and both the inguinal rings and the skin are closed. When performing the aseptic prep of the surgical site, sterile saline should be used instead of 70% alcohol as pig skin is more sensitive than the skin of other companion animals. Care should be taken to inhibit activities for 3 to 4 days after surgery to avoid dehiscence of the incision and formation of a seroma or a hematoma. Vaccines and analgesics should be used as appropriate for the species.

Urolithiasis

Urolithiasis refers to the formation of "stones" or concretions of mucus, protein, and minerals in the urinary tract of male small ruminants. These formations can get caught in the urethra and cause obstruction. Most commonly, urethral obstruction is seen in show or pet goats and lambs that are being fed a high-grain, low-roughage diet. Normally, a ruminant will remove phosphorus from its body through its manure; however, diets high in phosphorus and magnesium but low in roughage and calcium force the body to remove excess phosphorus through the kidneys and the urinary tract system. When phosphorus is excessively high, it can consolidate into stonelike pellets too large to pass through the urethra.

Early clinical signs of a small ruminant being "blocked" or having a urethral obstruction are straining to urinate, dribbling urine, decreased urine production, painful urination, and tail flagging. If the condition is left untreated, the patient is likely to lose its appetite, become depressed, have swelling around the prepuce,

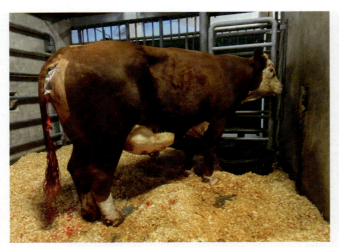

• **Fig. 34.39** An adult steer with a ruptured urethra and free fluid in the abdomen.

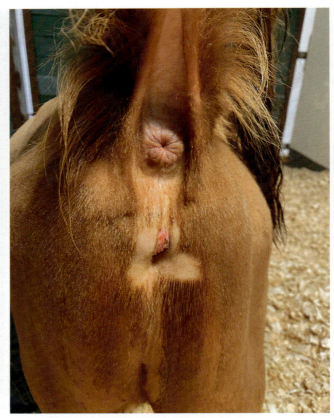

• **Fig. 34.40** Perineal urethrostomy site on a 10-month-old calf that was treated for a ruptured urethra 6 months after surgery.

or experience abdominal swelling caused by a ruptured bladder (Fig. 34.39). Severely affected animals will become recumbent and refuse to get up. They may eventually have a seizure or die suddenly.

Physical examination will often reveal increases in heart rate and respiratory rate, and possibly a distended abdomen caused by an enlarged bladder. Most uroliths in small ruminants lodge at the "urethral process" or "vermiform appendage," a small, tubelike extension of skin and urethra at the tip of the penis. The second most common site is at the "distal sigmoid flexure," an S-shaped curve in the lower half of the penis. Uroliths trapped in the urethral process can often be felt during physical examination.

Surgery is usually required to remove uroliths and to relieve blockages. Farm management practices should be reviewed to prevent the recurrence of urolithiasis. Postoperative care of the patient is dependent on the type of surgery performed.

Urethral process amputation involves removing the urethral process with a scalpel blade. This procedure requires little postoperative care; however, if there are additional uroliths higher in the urinary tract or if management practices are not satisfactorily adjusted, it will not correct the problem permanently.

A perineal urethrostomy, or PU, is a procedure that creates a new opening in the urethra (Fig. 34.40). Animals that have received a perineal urethrostomy appear to urinate like a female as the opening created is closer to the anus. After surgery, the site should be evaluated daily to ensure that the opening does not demonstrate strictures. The animal can no longer be used for breeding purposes after perineal urethrostomy, because it no longer has a functioning penis.

Tubal cystostomy can be used to divert urine from the urethra in a tube to allow time for swelling to subside. This procedure is used in conjunction with urethral process amputation and surgical removal of uroliths from the bladder. The tube is kept in until urine is seen dripping from the prepuce for 48 hours. The tube is then clamped to force the animal to urinate through its urethra. Once the animal can successfully empty its bladder through the urethra, the tube is removed. This may not happen on the first attempt. Many patients require the tube to be left in for 10 or more days.

For animals that have narrowed perineal urethrostomy sites and subsequent obstruction, a permanent opening can be made between the bladder and the belly wall near the prepuce. This procedure, prepubic cystostomy, is also called bladder marsupialization.

This procedure is considered a last resort and poses postoperative complications, such as chronic urine scald and infections.

In male goats with recurrent obstructive urolithiasis, vesicopreputial anastomosis (VPA) has been shown to be a feasible surgical option providing favorable clinical outcomes. During a VPA, the prepuce is incised but left intact to be closed later, the penile shaft is amputated, and a stoma is created between the bladder and the prepuce, combining elements of the previously described surgical treatments for caprine urolithiasis. A Foley catheter is placed into the bladder and the prepuce is closed around it, leaving the tip of the catheter exposed out of the tip of the prepuce. The Foley catheter will then serve as a stent to promote healing of the prepuce. It will also function as a temporary replacement for the urethra until postoperative healing is complete (10–30 days). Care must be taken to avoid contamination of the Foley catheter as it is not connected to a closed collection unit but carries the same infection potential as other urinary catheters. A common aid for maintaining Foley cleanliness in VPAs is a sterile glove perforated and taped over the exposed tip (Fig. 34.41).

Vaginal and Uterine Prolapse

Prolapse of the vagina usually involves prolapse of the floor, the lateral walls, and a portion of the roof of the vagina through the vulva (Fig. 34.42). Occasionally, the entire vagina and the cervix will prolapse through the vulva. This can be seen in all species but is most common in the cow and the ewe. Vaginal and vaginocervical prolapse are most common in the last 2 to 3 months of pregnancy, when large amounts of estrogenic hormone is being secreted by the placenta. This causes the pelvic ligaments, the vulva, and the vulvar sphincter muscles to relax. When the

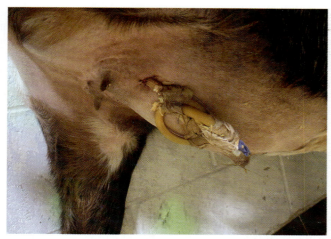

• **Fig. 34.41** The abdomen of a goat with a cystostomy tube placed in the bladder. The fingertip of an exam glove is placed on the end of the tube and punctured to allow urine to drip but prevent debris from getting inside.

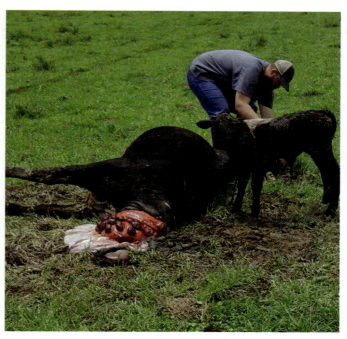

• **Fig. 34.43** Uterine prolapse seen in a cow immediately after calving. Uterine prolapse is a life-threatening emergency and requires prompt veterinary treatment.

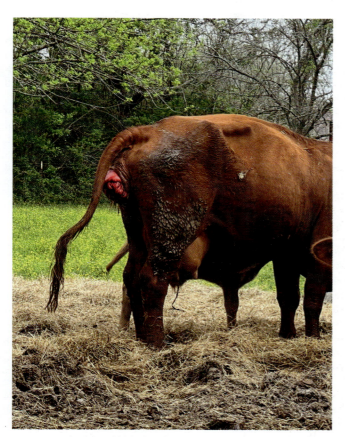

• **Fig. 34.42** Vaginal prolapse in a postpartum cow.

animal lies down, there is an increase in intra-abdominal pressure, particularly in late pregnancy, forcing the vagina and the related structures through the vulva. Once prolapse of the vagina has occurred, the exposed mucous membranes become very edematous, inflamed, and irritated.

Vaginal prolapse can be classified according to the duration and severity of the condition. First-degree prolapse is slight, intermittent protrusion of the floor of the vagina when the animal is lying down. With second-degree vaginal prolapse, the floor of the vagina protrudes through the vulva continuously. In third-degree vaginal prolapse, most of the vaginal floor, including the urinary bladder and the cervix, continuously protrudes from the vulva. Fourth-degree prolapse is a second- or third-degree prolapse that has been exposed for a long enough duration that necrosis and fibrosis have occurred.

The primary objective of treatment is to replace the prolapsed tissues and retain them in place, deliver a live neonate, and salvage the breeding animal. Replacement of the prolapsed tissues is best accomplished with the aid of epidural anesthesia. In small ruminants, an epidural is not usually necessary, because the animal can easily be restrained by being held up by the hind limbs. The prolapsed mass should be cleaned by using a mild aseptic solution. If the urinary bladder is within the prolapsed mass, firmly elevating the prolapse toward the anus will help express the bladder and reduce the size of the mass. Once the prolapsed material has been replaced, a retaining suture is necessary to prevent recurrence.

Uterine prolapse is a life-threating emergency. Prognosis for survival and future reproduction are improved by owner recognition and prompt veterinary treatment. Uterine prolapse usually occurs in the first 24 hours after parturition and happens in a female that continues pushing after giving birth (Fig. 34.43). This continued pushing forces the uterus to evert and pass through the cervix. Hypocalcemia, an abnormal calcium-to-phosphorus ratio, prolonged dystocia, and vaginal injury are all factors that may increase an animal's predisposition for uterine prolapse.

Animals should be handled quietly to avoid possible trauma to the uterus. It is not advisable to transport the affected cow, because it increases the risk for vascular rupture and fatal hemorrhage. Because of their size, smaller ruminants can be transported more safely. Uterine replacement can be performed with the cows in standing or recumbent position and with the animal under epidural anesthesia. Placing recumbent cows on their sternum with their limbs stretched behind them helps tilt the pelvis cranioventrally, facilitating replacement. If it can be done without causing hemorrhage, the placenta should be removed from the uterus.

The uterus should be cleaned with a mild aseptic solution and water to remove contamination and debris. Edema can be reduced through massage and handling of the uterus in early replacement attempts. The cervix is the portion of the uterus nearest the vulva. Replacement begins by pushing this tissue back into the vagina by applying firm and steady pressure, slowly reducing the prolapse. Once the prolapse passes anterior to the vulva, it is important to completely straighten out the uterine horns. Failure to do this step will lead to subsequent prolapse, adhesions, or necrosis. The uterus can be filled with a warm antiseptic solution in water to facilitate this process; however, it also increases the risk for uterine rupture. Once the uterus is back in place, oxytocin should be administered to assist in uterine involution. This may be all that is necessary in an ambulatory female. In a female that is weak and recumbent, it is recommended that vulvar retention sutures be placed. A complication associated with retention sutures for uterine prolapse is that subsequent prolapse will go unnoticed and necrosis will occur within the pelvic canal. Animals that have received retention sutures should be re-evaluated the following day to ensure this has not happened.

Prognosis is dependent on the promptness of placement, external trauma and contamination, and whether the animal is ambulatory. Generally, the uterus recovers very well and animals can be rebred within the same season.

Preputial Prolapse

Preputial prolapse is commonly seen in cattle, specifically breeds with *Bos indicus* influence, such as Santa Gertrudis, Brahman, or Zebu (Fig. 34.44A and B). These breeds tend to characteristically have a pendulous sheath, a large preputial orifice, and a relaxed preputial membrane and penis.

There are four categories of preputial prolapse, as noted below and in Fig. 34.45A and B.

Category	Presentation	Treatment	Prognosis for Return to Service
I	Slight-moderate edema, no lacerations, necrosis, or fibrosis	Conservative	Well
II	Moderate-severe edema, superficial lacerations, slight necrosis, no fibrosis	Surgery	Guarded
III	Severe edema, deep lacerations, moderate necrosis, slight fibrosis	Surgery	Guarded
IV	Severe edema, deep lacerations, necrosis, fibrosis and abscesses	Surgery or salvage by slaughter	Guarded to poor

Regardless of the treatment plan, the prolapsed area should be carefully washed and dried, and an emollient antiseptic ointment applied, with support bandaging to reduce edema and prevent further secondary injury. A sling can be fashioned with a large piece of burlap, heavy netting, or other loosely woven material and held in place with strips of inner tube or bungee cords across the bull's back. Once edema is reduced on bulls with category I or II prolapse, the prepuce should be reduced back into the preputial cavity and held in place by elastic tape. Latex tubing should be positioned in the preputial lumen for urine drainage. These bulls return to service after a series of bandages that aid in reduction of edema and sufficient healing. Bandages should be monitored to ensure that they do not roll or shift, causing increased pressure on sensitive areas.

Hydrotherapy is especially helpful in patients that have lacerations or tissue necrosis. These areas of skin must be covered by healthy granulation tissue and be free of edema before reversion or surgery can take place. Once inflammation and infection are under control, a surgery, commonly referred to as "reefing," to remove scar tissue and to shorten the prepuce, may be considered if the bull is valuable. Without surgery, the recurrence rate for preputial trauma and repeat prolapse is high.

Lacerations

In large-animal practice, lacerations are of greater concern with equine patients than their food-animal counterparts because of a much higher risk of incidence and number of potential accompanying complications. Furthermore, food-animal species tend to heal without the production of exuberant granulation tissue. Regardless, wound management is important with all species of large-animal patients. Emphasis should be placed on wounds of the distal limbs, where wound healing can be the most difficult. Successful treatment of lacerations and wounds relies on thorough debridement, meticulous hemostasis, elimination of dead space, insertion of drains when warranted, and proper suture placement.

Lacerations

Oral Lacerations

Cattle are naturally curious creatures and have indiscriminate eating habits, which make them prone to such conditions as oral lacerations. Injuries can occur on the tongue, the cheeks, or the palate when pieces of wire or other sharp objects are chewed and potentially swallowed. Clinical signs of an oral injury include excess salivation or bloody oral discharge, along with varying degrees of dysphagia and, if debris is packed in the mouth, malodorous breath.

Most oral lacerations heal without surgical intervention by feeding a soft diet, using daily mouth lavage, and use of systemic antibiotics; however, in severe cases that involve the body of the tongue, surgical management is often indicated to promote healing and prevent deformity. Because of the tongue's crucial role in grasping food, as much of the tongue as possible should be preserved. If tissue is devitalized, it may be necessary to perform a partial glossectomy (tongue amputation) as a last resort.

Teat Lacerations

Traumatic teat injuries are common in dairy cows and goats. Due to the size and pendulous nature of a lactating udder, females can step on their own teats, causing lacerations and abrasions. Occasionally, traumatic injury from sharp protrusions in the

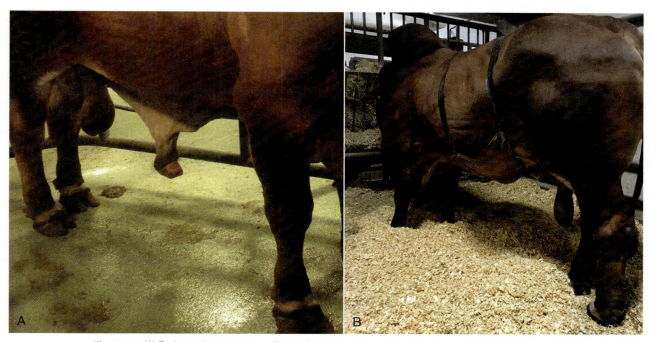

• **Fig. 34.44** (A) Prolapsed prepuce on a *Bos indicus* bull with a pendulous sheath. (B) To protect the prepuce during the healing process and prevent reinjury, the bull has been fitted with a sling made from burlap fabric and a bicycle inner tube.

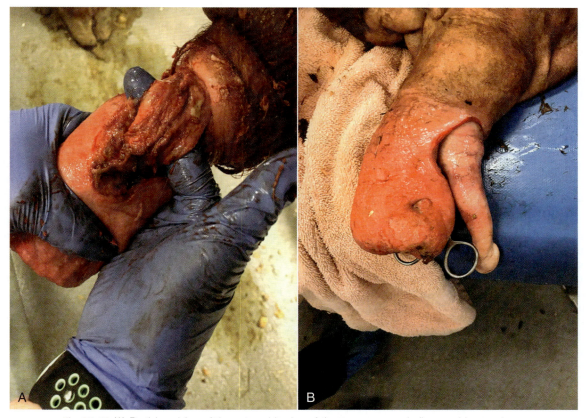

• **Fig. 34.45** (A) Partial avulsion of the external lamina of the prepuce on a bull caused by an abscess sustained during a breeding injury. (B) Complete avulsion of both the external and internal preputial lamina, with the penis exteriorized.

environment are to blame for cuts. Most teat injuries are treated conservatively, but surgical repair is sometimes warranted.

Teat injury that does not involve the teat cistern should be cleaned with mild antiseptic solution and any devitalized skin debrided with a scalpel blade, allowing healing by second intention. A sterile teat cannula can be inserted if the patient will not tolerate being milked. Strict attention to hygiene must be observed when using a teat cannula because of increased risk for mastitis.

Lacerations into the teat cistern require surgical repair; otherwise a leaking fistula will develop. The patient should be sedated and the teat blocked with local anesthetic. The wound must be meticulously cleaned and debrided prior to surgical repair. A teat cannula should be placed and milking avoided until healing is complete.

Perineal Lacerations

Birth-related injuries to the vagina and vulva are common, especially in young stock delivering their first offspring as well as stock that go through a difficult delivery or prolonged labor. Most perineal lacerations are caused by the feet of the fetus making their way through the birth canal. In severe cases, feet can tear through the shelf between the vagina and the rectum and protrude through the anus during birth.

There are three degrees of perineal lacerations. A first-degree tear involves only the mucosa of the vulva, vestibule, and vagina. A second-degree tear involves full thickness of the vulva, vestibule, and vaginal wall but not the rectal wall or anus. A third-degree tear is one in which both the vagina and rectum are torn, creating a rectovaginal fistula.

When perineal injury is anticipated, a dorsal episiotomy can be performed to prevent such severe lacerations. An episiotomy is a surgical incision used to increase vaginal outlet circumference as a fetus is progressing through the pelvis, but the birth is impeded by a small vaginal outlet.

Surgery is essential if the patient is intended to be maintained as a breeding animal following a third-degree perineal laceration. Left untreated, feces will infiltrate the vagina, inspiring an inflammatory process and infection that will spread to the cervix and uterus. Surgery should be delayed up to 4 to 6 weeks until the defect is completely epithelialized and the procedure can be performed with caudal epidural analgesia in the standing patient.

Musculoskeletal System

Lameness

Lameness in production animals is not only a welfare issue but has a fiscal impact. Food animals that are lame tend to be under greater stress and have reduced productivity. Lameness impairs the ability of the animal to move and gain access to food and water, reducing their performance as a producer but also their general well-being. Lame dairy cows are likely to produce less milk and have lower conception rates. If antibiotic therapy is indicated, their milk must be discarded because of the presence of the drugs in it. Meat-producing animals may be reluctant to eat and exhibit a decrease in effort toward obtaining food among other herd members, thus failing to maintain or gain weight.

There are many factors that may contribute to lameness in the food-animal patient. Conformation, age, and genetics play a large part in an animal's resilience. Nutrition, systemic disease, and herd management practices can also contribute to risk factors. Animals

in poor condition tend to be predisposed to lameness and will often be culled from the herd. Livestock kept in intensive housing, especially those with unfavorable hygiene and unforgiving flooring, tend to see a higher incidence of lameness.

Problems in the foot are responsible for most lameness that occurs in cattle, including foot problems originating in the claws, especially the front medial and hind lateral claws, which bear the most weight. Foot problems should be addressed early; if not properly treated, they can progress to osteomyelitis and/or septic arthritis. When cattle need veterinary care for lameness, a few surgical procedures may be warranted.

Regional analgesia (IV retrograde block analgesia) of the distal limb is commonly performed before a claw amputation or corn removal; it can also be used as a diagnostic aid in lameness examinations. A tourniquet is applied in the metacarpal/metatarsal area. A superficial vein—the common dorsal metacarpal (metatarsal) vein or the palmar (plantar) metacarpal (metatarsal) vein—is identified and aseptically prepared. In some larger animals, using anatomic landmarks will aid in venipuncture, because the veins in these animals cannot be easily visualized. An IV injection of 2% lidocaine by using a butterfly catheter will provide analgesia in 5 minutes and will be maintained until the tourniquet is removed.

This same technique can be used to perfuse regional antibiotics to a distal limb. Cephalosporins can be diluted with sodium chloride to a volume of 20 to 30 mL and slowly injected intravenously. The tourniquet can be left on for up to 45 minutes, maximizing antibiotic absorption in the affected area; however, the tourniquet should not stay on any longer than 45 minutes.

Subcutaneous implantation of antibiotic-impregnated polymethyl methacrylate (PMMA) beads near an infected joint offers slow release of antibiotics at the site of infection and can effectively aid in the treatment of septic arthritis, especially in calves. Systemic antibiotics along with joint flushing, regional perfusion, and PMMA beads can be effective in treating septic arthritis.

Ideally, a tilt table is most useful for examining foot problems in cattle; however, one is not always available. There are several methods to restrain the limb of a standing animal in a chute. Proper restraint is extremely important to prevent injury to both humans and animals.

When restraining the limb of a standing animal, its head should be tied in the direction opposite the affected limb. For hind limb restraint, a rope with an eye or quick release should be looped around the cow's pastern. The rope should pass upward over a beam or through a hook over and slightly behind the cow. Passing down from the beam hook, the end is brought around the limb above the hock, going from the medial to the lateral side, to form a half hitch. The cow's foot is lifted off the ground and the slack in the rope taken up.

When restraining a forelimb of a cow, a rope is used to form a loop around the pastern. The other end of the rope passes over the withers, where it should be held by an assistant so that it can be released quickly if the cow starts to go down.

Interdigital Hyperplasia

Interdigital **hyperplasia**, also referred to as *interdigital fibroma* or *corn* by livestock managers, is thickening of the interdigital skin that causes a mass to protrude between the claws (Fig. 34.46). This is most common in the larger of the beef breeds and can involve one or more feet at a time. Chronic irritation between the claws causes this condition to develop, although there is a hereditary component. A large mass can cause pain from the fibroma

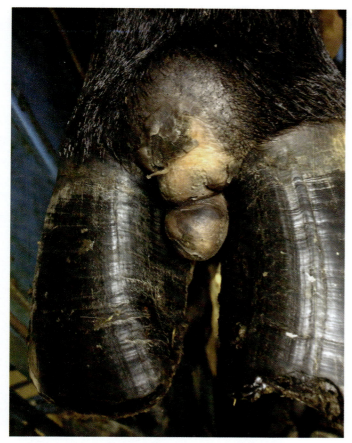

• **Fig. 34.46** Interdigital hyperplasia (fibroma or corn) between the toes of a bull's foot.

becoming eroded, ulcerated, and even infected, leading to swelling and lameness. Removal is determined by the size of the mass and the degree of lameness. After removal, a wire can be used to hold the toes together by drilling holes in the toe region and using cerclage wire or a wire coat hanger to secure the toes.

After the procedure, a bandage will need to be placed to control the bleeding and protect the surgical site. The patient should be kept in a clean, dry area for 3 to 5 days, with one to two bandage changes during that time. Analgesia is also warranted.

Claw Amputation

Unfortunately, the feet of cattle can become infected in the deep tissues of the claw, involving one or more ligaments and tendons and even invading bones, causing a septic joint. This causes severe lameness. Claw amputation may be the best treatment option to provide relief to the patient, but it must not be the weight-bearing claw (front medial or hind lateral) of the animal. Claw amputation should be thoroughly discussed with the producers prior to the procedure. Economically, the value of the animal may not warrant the cost and management challenges posed by postoperative care. Claw removal is usually a salvage procedure used as a short-term solution. Breakdown of the supporting claw happens eventually, the speed of which is dependent on the weight of the animal and the surface it stands and walks on in its everyday environment.

If claw amputation is the agreed-upon treatment plan, radiographs should be obtained prior to surgery to identify how much sepsis is present. Claw amputation is best done on a tilt table with the animal under local anesthesia. A tourniquet is placed above the fetlock and an IV retrograde block is used for anesthesia and analgesia. The claw is removed by using obstetric wire (Gigli wire) just above the area where the infection stops, as shown by the radiographs.

After surgery a pressure bandage should be placed on the foot to aid in hemostasis. Bleeding will increase after the tourniquet is removed and strike-through on the bandage can be expected. The bandage should be changed after 24 hours and then once every 3 days until the exposed bone has granulated over with healthy tissue.

Head and Neck Surgeries

Entropion

Entropion most commonly occurs as a birth defect in which a neonate's eyelid rolls inward, causing the eyelashes to rub against the surface of the eye. This can be seen unilaterally or bilaterally. Entropion can also occur due to severe dehydration, malnutrition, prematurity, or scarring of the eyelid following an injury or infection. Entropion can cause keratitis, or inflammation of the cornea, if not treated promptly. The eyelid is blocked with a local anesthetic and a suture is placed to draw the eyelid back and into the correct position. Usually, the suture can be removed in 48 to 72 hours. The eye should be treated with an antibiotic ointment and ophthalmic lubricant for several days to be proactive against any abrasions.

Dehorning

Dehorning is the act of removing horns on cattle, goats, and sheep with the intention of obtaining overall management benefits. Horns can be sharp and pose a safety risk to anyone, human or animal, interacting with them. Horned animals may require specialized equipment, such as gates, feeders, and chutes, to accommodate the additional space they require. Horned animals are more likely to get caught in fences and vegetation, causing self-injury.

Dehorning is best performed within a chute or head gate for cattle and similar species. It is recommended that cattle be dehorned when they are 8 to 12 weeks of age, before the horn material attaches to the skull. Once horns have attached to the skull, much greater effort is required to remove them. Typically, in mature cattle, calves, and small ruminants older than 6 months of age, the frontal sinus will be exposed when the horns are removed. This leaves the animal at greater risk for sinusitis until the opening closes. Closure can take up to 6 weeks.

Although not required, using a local anesthetic to block the cranial nerve is recommended before dehorning. Injecting lidocaine under the frontal crest halfway between the lateral canthus of the eye and the base of the horn will provide some analgesia for the patient. An electric dehorner or a Barnes dehorner is used to remove the horns (Fig. 34.49A). The Barnes dehorner is a hinged device with a set of sharp scoops (Fig. 34.49B). The scoops are placed over the horn, against the base and the surrounding skin. Opening the handles forces the cutting edges together, slicing through the skin and under the horn.

Large horns on adult cattle, sheep, or goats are generally removed with a dehorning saw or Gigli wire. This method is purely functional. A more cosmetic approach can be used in show cattle and goats. This requires surgical removal of the horns by using local or regional anesthesia and results in a more symmetric

CASE PRESENTATION 34.2

A 7-year-old female Juliana pig presented for an enucleation of the right eye. The patient had been diagnosed with retinal detachment 13 months prior. Subsequent exams revealed cataract development, blindness, and severe anterior uveitis with phthisis of the bulbi. The patient had been medically managed with neo-poly-dex ophthalmic ointment as well as diclofenac to control inflammation and pain, as well as to provide the eye with lubrication. The patient's left eye remained normal, with no intraocular inflammation. A small cataract was present in the left eye, but it was determined not contribute to vision impairment. The left retina was normal, with no signs of partial lifting or detachment. It was felt that the patient's level of discomfort had increased, and enucleation was chosen as the most appropriate treatment option.

The patient was placed under general anesthesia. A retrobulbar block (0.5% bupivacaine) of the right eye was performed prior to surgery. The patient was placed in left lateral recumbency, and the area around the left eye was aseptically prepared for surgery using sterile saline and a sterile dilute Betadine solution (1:20). A transpalpebral approach was used to enucleate the eye. The eyelids were sutured together using 0 poliglecaprone 25 in a simple continuous pattern. An elliptical cutaneous incision was made approximately 3 to 5 mm away from the lid margins with a #10 scalpel blade, and the palpebrae were temporarily clamped rostrally with Backhaus towel clamps within the exposed subcutaneous tissue. Sharp and blunt dissection were employed to extend the incision following the orbit, using a #10 blade and Metzenbaum scissors. The medial and lateral canthal ligaments were transected by traction and sharp incision using a #10 blade. Metzenbaum scissors were used to dissect to the level of the sclera and clear away overlying subcutaneous and periorbital tissue for 360-degree scleral exposure. Extraocular muscle tendons were transected at their scleral insertions when visualized. The optic nerve and retractor bulbi muscle were transected (Fig. 34.47).

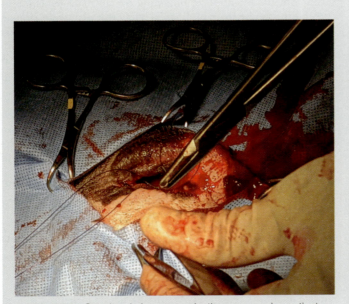

• **Fig. 34.47** Suturing during an enucleation on a porcine patient.

The specimen was collected to be submitted for histopathological assessment. Hemostasis was achieved by packing the orbital space with 4 × 4 gauze and applying digital pressure for a period of 4 minutes; the orbit was then lavaged with sterile saline. The superficial subcutaneous layer was closed in a simple continuous pattern with 2-0 poliglecaprone 25. The skin was closed in a simple cruciate pattern with 0 poliglecaprone 25. Silver spray was then topically applied to the area (Fig. 34.48).

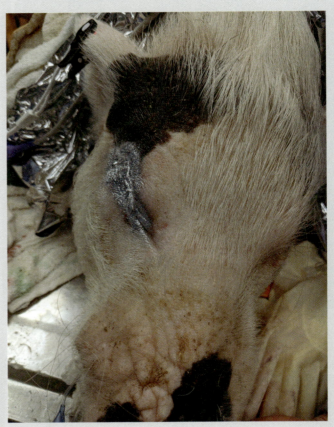

• **Fig. 34.48** Pig following enucleation surgery. The eyeball and surrounding tissues have been removed and the skin sutured closed over the empty orbit. Silver spray has been sprayed topically.

It was noted that the patient became both hypothermic (95.5°F) and bradycardic during surgery; however, recovery was routine and uneventful. The patient's temperature returned to normal within an hour of discontinuing inhalant anesthesia. Heart rate steadily increased to normal over the course of 12 hours following surgery.

The patient was discharged from the hospital 2 days following surgery with a 3-day course of meloxicam to manage inflammation and pain, as well as a 7-day course of omeprazole as a gastric protectant to aid in preventing side effects from the prescribe meloxicam.

The patient continued to recover well at home and experienced no known adverse effects from surgery.

---

appearance of the poll, reducing the chances of hemorrhage and infection.

If the sinuses are opened during surgery, a light bandage must be applied to the patient's head to protect the sinuses from dirt and debris. This area should be kept bandaged until the surgical site has granulated in with healthy tissue. To prevent sinusitis, if bandaging is not an option, the animal should be fed in a manner

that prevents it from placing its head in hay and dust. Furthermore, dehorning should be avoided during heavy fly season as this can contribute to irrigation and infection.

If the patient seems uncomfortable, oral analgesics can be given for 2 to 3 days after dehorning. It is important to know the patient's vaccination history prior to surgery, specifically tetanus vaccination. If the patient's dam was vaccinated for tetanus prior

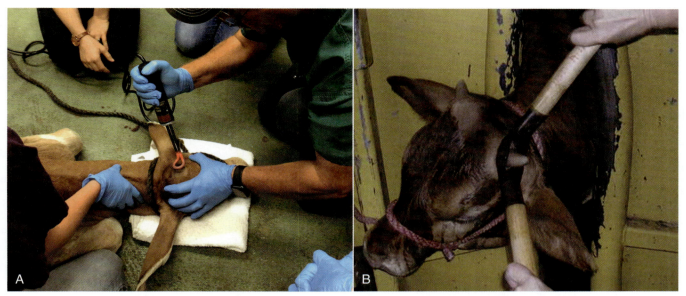

• **Fig. 34.49** (A) Calf being manually restrained and dehorned with an electric dehorner. (B) Use of a Barnes dehorner or scoop for removal of the horns in a young calf being restrained with a head gate and halter.

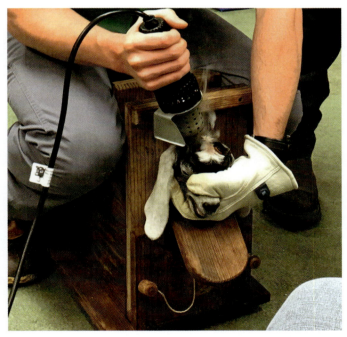

• **Fig. 34.50** Disbudding of a goat less than 2 weeks of age with an electric dehorner. The goat is being restrained by using a bud box.

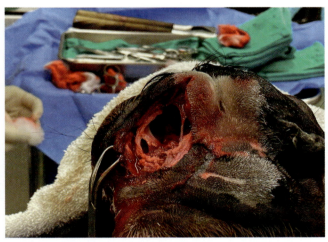

• **Fig. 34.51** Cosmetic dehorning on a juvenile goat that developed scurs following a traditional disbudding.

to giving birth, tetanus toxoid vaccine can be administered to the patient. If the vaccination history is unknown, vaccinating the patient with tetanus antitoxin in conjunction with tetanus toxoid is recommended.

Small ruminants should be dehorned, or disbudded, before the age of 2 to 3 weeks (Fig. 34.50). Waiting until a later age will make the procedure much more painful, and earlier attention reduces the risk for infection. Small ruminants can be held by a confident assistant or placed in a "bud box" for the dehorning procedure. A bud box holds a kid or a lamb in place while their horn buds are being removed. Horn buds can be removed in two ways—using

a bud cauterizer or dehorning paste. Both methods kill horn-producing cells at an early age, thus preventing these structures from developing. Goats should not be dehorned by using a Barnes dehorner because of the risk for skull fracture. In adult goats, horns can be trimmed with Gigli wire. Complete dehorning in adult goats should be avoided, because it has been shown to cause depressed behavior after horn removal. As the animal ages, the risk for complications from dehorning increases. Failure to remove the horn bud completely with inadequate depth of cauterization can result in regrowth or "scurs" (Fig. 34.51).

Tusk Trimming

Dental issues in pigs are rare; however, older stock will develop long and extremely sharp canines. When left untouched, these tusks can become dangerous to both handlers and other pigs. With the increased popularity of companion pigs not intended for consumption, tusk trimming, often done in conjunction with routine hoof trimming, is becoming more routine.

Tusks do not have a pulp cavity above the gingival margin, so they can be cut off without causing pain or infection. Equine molar shears can be used to cut tusks and allow for the task to be achieved quickly. Restraining a boar can be difficult, which is why a hog snare should be utilized. It is suggested that tusks be cut while the boar is mounting a sow.

Recommended Readings

Auer JA, Stick JA, eds. *Equine Surgery*. 5th ed. Philadelphia, PA: Saunders; 2019.

Brink P. Subtotal ostectomy of impinging dorsal spinous processes in 23 standing horses. *Vet Surg*. 2014;43:95–98.

Cypher E. Vesicopreputial anastomosis for the treatment of obstructive urolithiasis in goats. *Vet Surg*. 2017;43:281–288.

Delacalle J, Burba D, Tetens J, Moore, R. Nd: YAG Laser–Assisted Modified Forssell's Procedure for Treatment of Cribbing (Crib–Biting) in Horses. Vet Surg, 31(2), 111–116; 2002.

Divers TJ, Peek SF. In: *Rebhun's Diseases of Dairy Cattle*. St. Louis, MO: Saunders; 2001.

Fackelman GE, Auer JA, Nunamaker DM, eds. *AO Principles of Equine Osteosynthesis*. Davos Platz [Switzerland]: AO Pub; 2000.

Fubini SL, Ducharme NC. *Farm Animal Surgery*. 2nd ed. St. Louis, MO: Saunders; 2017.

Gawande A. *The Checklist Manifesto*. New York, NY: Picador; 2010.

Holtgrew-Bohling K. *Large Animal Clinical Procedures for Veterinary Technicians*. 3rd ed. St. Louis, MO: Mosby; 2001.

Hawkins J, ed. *Advances in Equine Upper Respiratory Surgery*. 1st ed. Ames, IA: Wiley-Blackwell; 2015.

Holzman G, Raffel T. *Surgical Patient Care for Veterinary Technicians and Nurses*. Ames, IA: Wiley-Blackwell; 2015.

Koterba AM, Drummond WH, Kosch PC, eds. *Equine Clinical Neonatology*. Philadelphia, PA: Lea & Febiger; 1990.

Mitchell C, Fugler L, Eades S. The management of equine acute laminitis. *Vet Med Res*. 2014:39–47.

Orsini JA, Divers TJ. *Equine Emergencies: Treatment and Procedures*. 4th ed. St. Louis, MO: Saunders; 2014.

Pugh DG. *Sheep and Goat Medicine*. 2nd ed. St. Louis, MO: Saunders; 2012.

Reed S, Bailey W, Sellon D, eds. *Equine Internal Medicine*. 3rd ed. St. Louis, MO: Saunders; 2009.

Riggs L. How to Perform Non-surgical Correction of Acute Uterine Torsion in the Mare. In: *Proceedings of the AAEP annual convention*. San Antonio; 2006.

Smith BP. *Large Animal Internal Medicine*. 5th ed. St. Louis, MO: Mosby; 2014.

35
Veterinary Dentistry

MARY LYNN BERG

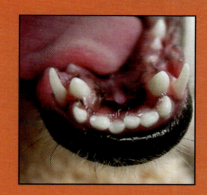

CHAPTER OUTLINE

LEARNING OBJECTIVES

When you have completed this chapter, you will be able to:

1. Pronounce, spell, and define all key terms in this chapter.
2. Explain terminology used in veterinary dentistry to designate location and direction; describe the modified Triadan system for numbering teeth; and describe normal occlusion in dogs and cats, common malocclusions, and orthodontic treatment in small animals.
3. Discuss aspects of the complete medical history as they relate to veterinary dentistry and describe aspects of extraoral and intraoral examinations in dogs and cats.

4. Describe equipment and supplies used for dental radiography and understand the different angles used in dental radiography.
5. Differentiate between the stages of periodontal disease seen in dogs and cats, including gingivitis and periodontitis, and state the goal of periodontal debridement.
6. Describe equipment and procedures for professional dental cleaning with power and hand scalers and explain methods for sharpening dental instruments.
7. Discuss the rationale and procedures for polishing teeth.

8. Compare and contrast regional nerve blocks for oral surgery for dogs and cats.
9. Explain the grading system for periodontal disease and the importance of home care in veterinary dentistry.
10. Discuss indications for restorative dentistry, endodontics, and exodontics.
11. Describe common dental conditions and pathology seen in small animals.
12. List and describe equine dental clinical practices and common problems and treatments.

KEY TERMS

Anisognathism
Apex
Brachycephalic
Brachygnathism
Brachydont
Calculus
Canine
Caries
Carnassial
Cementum
Cingulum
Deciduous
Diastema
Diphyodont
Distal
Distoclusion
Dolichocephalic

Enamel
Endodontics
Exodontics
Furcation
Hypsodont
Incisors
Malocclusion
Mesaticephalic (mesocephalic)
Mesial
Mesioclusion
Modified Triadan system
Molars
Occlusion
Periodontium
Plaque
Prosthodontics
Pulp

Introduction

Veterinary dentistry has been recognized as a specialty for more than 30 years. Historically, few veterinarians and technicians have received formal training in dentistry and oral surgery because of few educational opportunities. However, the number of opportunities for dental training has dramatically increased over the past 10 years. Dental disease is one of the most common diseases in companion animals, with greater than 80% of adult dogs and cats having the condition. The number of animals receiving treatment in veterinary practices is low compared with the number with the disease. When the veterinary team understands the role of a healthy mouth in relationship to the pet's overall health, they are better able to communicate this to the pet owner. Dentistry is performed at varying levels at most small-animal practices. A well-educated veterinary technician can be empowered within the scope of dental practice to (1) educate the clients on the importance of professional dental cleaning to maintain oral health and the relationship to systemic health; (2) execute professional dental cleanings, including periodontal debridement and polishing; (3) obtain diagnostic information through dental charting and dental radiography; (4) provide intraoperative assistance with dental and oral surgeries; and (5) perform discharge appointments that provide client education, including postprocedure care, proper use of appropriate dental home care products, and preventive techniques. Most veterinary practices provide professional dental cleanings and exodontics for their patients. Veterinary dentists provide advanced dental care, such as endodontics, exodontics, orthodontics, prosthodontics, and advanced periodontal therapy. In the process of providing routine care, technicians have an opportunity to identify dental disease in its early stages. Technicians play a vital role in veterinary dentistry and are often on the front line of identifying oral disease. A solid foundation in oral anatomy and associated pathologic conditions is important, along with the knowledge required for disease recognition and treatment principles. In addition, veterinary technicians must be knowledgeable in periodontal disease, including pathophysiology, treatment, follow-up, and prevention.

Scaling and polishing procedures are the most common dental procedures performed in practice, making instrumentation and the techniques of proper periodontal therapy vitally important. These procedures are often mistakenly referred to as *prophylaxis*, *prophy*, or *a dental*. Because of the variation in severity of disease at the time of treatment, the term professional dental cleaning or comprehensive oral health assessment and treatment (COHAT) are replacing these terms. The veterinary technician involved in performing a COHAT should be capable of performing an oral assessment, periodontal debridement (supragingival and subgingival scaling), polishing, home care education, and counseling about proper diet, treats, and toys as they relate to dentistry.

PUT INTO PRACTICE

As a veterinary nurse/technician, performing COHATs and dental radiography can help you become an asset to your practice. Attending labs and lectures to increase your knowledge and skill can be very helpful to increasing your value. It is important to know the laws in your state regulating how much a veterinary nurse/technician can legally do as a part of this process.

Dental radiology is extremely important in veterinary dentistry, because disease is often missed or underestimated when teeth are not examined beneath the gingival margin. Techniques for taking diagnostic dental radiographs and interpretation of normal and abnormal dental anatomy on radiographs are necessary for

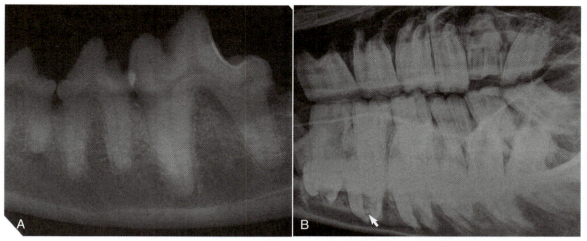

• **Fig. 35.1** Radiograph of brachyodont teeth of the dog (A) and hypsodont teeth of the horse (B).

successful radiographs. There are subspecialties of dentistry, including endodontics, exodontics, orthodontics, and restorative dentistry. Equine dental anatomy and pathologic conditions are also valuable for veterinary technicians' knowledge base, along with preventive and therapeutic treatments for common equine dental problems.

Ethical and Legal Aspects

The level of dental care a veterinary technician may provide varies from state to state, and the laws and regulations for the state of practice must be understood before dental care is provided. The American Veterinary Dental College (AVDC) and the Academy of Veterinary Dental Technician (AVDT) have both published position statements regarding veterinary dental health care providers. These statements provide recommendations for the qualifications of persons who perform veterinary dental procedures. The AVDC considers it appropriate for the veterinarian to delegate certain dental tasks to veterinary technicians. Tasks appropriately performed by veterinary technicians include professional dental cleanings and certain procedures that do not result in alterations in the shape, structure, or positional location of teeth in the dental arch. The American Veterinary Medical Association (AVMA) has created a resource that describes the scope of what veterinary technicians and nonveterinarians can do in each state, which can be seen at: https://www.avma.org/Resources-tools/avma-policies/veterinary-dentistry.

> **TECHNICIAN NOTE**
>
> The level of dental care the technician can legally provide varies from state to state. Become familiar with the laws regulating veterinary dentistry in your state by accessing https://www.avma.org/Resources-tools/avma-policies/veterinary-dentistry.

In addition, the AVDC and the AVDT support advanced training of veterinary technicians to perform additional dental services, such as taking impressions, making models, charting veterinary dental lesions, taking dental radiographs, and performing nonsurgical subgingival root planing.

> **TECHNICIAN NOTE**
>
> The Academy of Veterinary Dental Technicians (AVDT) consists of technicians who have completed a credentialing process and passed a specialty examination demonstrating their enhanced knowledge of veterinary dentistry.

Dental Morphology

Morphology refers to the form and structure of an organism and its parts. Teeth can be classified as **brachydont** or **hypsodont**, based on their crown and root structure (Fig. 35.1). All teeth of humans, carnivores, and pigs are brachyodontic teeth. Brachyodont teeth have relatively small, distinct crowns compared with the size of their well-developed roots. The apices (singular, **apex**) of the roots are open for a limited time during the eruption and development of teeth; therefore teeth do not continually grow or erupt. This contrasts with hypsodont teeth (seen in horses, rodents, and lagomorphs), which have a comparatively large reserve crown beneath the gingival margin and root structure, allowing for continued growth and/or continued eruption during all or most of an animal's lifetime. Hypsodont teeth can be divided further into two categories: *radicular* and *aradicular* hypsodont teeth. Cheek teeth in horses are an example of radicular hypsodont teeth. The apices of these teeth remain open for a significant portion of adult life but eventually close, after which continued growth of the tooth ceases, and occlusal wear is offset only by continued eruption. Cheek teeth and incisors in rabbits and some rodents are aradicular hypsodont (also called *elodont*) teeth, indicating lack of a true root structure and lifelong tooth growth that compensates for occlusal wear.

Dogs and cats have four types of teeth: incisors, canines, premolars, and molars. Incisor teeth are the most rostral teeth and are used for gnawing and grooming. Canine teeth are **distal** to the incisors. They are long and are used for prehending and holding. Premolars and molars (often referred to as "cheek teeth") are used for shearing and grinding.

Most mammals are *diphyodonts*, meaning that they have two sets of teeth. The first set of teeth is referred to as *deciduous* (also referred to as *primary* or *baby teeth*); these are replaced by permanent teeth (also referred to as *secondary* or *adult teeth*). Mammals show great variety in the numbers and types of teeth, depending on the species. Dental formulas used to classify numbers and types of teeth are listed in Box 35.1. Normal eruption times of deciduous and permanent teeth in dogs and cats are provided in Table 35.1, although it should be mentioned that normal variation exists.

It is important to be aware of the number of roots of each tooth. Table 35.2 lists the number of roots of each tooth of cats and dogs. Anatomic variation does occur, so performing preoperative dental radiography is important to confirm the numbers and shapes of tooth roots before extraction or other procedures

• BOX 35.1   Dental Formulas

Dog
Deciduous teeth 2 × (I 3/3, C 1/1, P 3/3) = 28 teeth
Permanent teeth 2 × (I 3/3, C 1/1, P 4/4, M 2/3) = 42 teeth

Cat
Deciduous teeth 2 × (I 3/3, C 1/1, P 3/2) = 26 teeth
Permanent teeth 2 × (I 3/3, C 1/1, P 3/2, M 1/1) = 30 teeth

Horse
Deciduous teeth 2 × (I 3/3, C 0/0, P 3/3) = 24 teeth
Permanent teeth 2 × (I 3/3, C 1/1 or 0/0, P 3 or 4/3 or 4, M 3/3) = 36 to 44 teeth (depending on the presence of canine and wolf teeth)

TABLE 35.1   Approximate Eruption Schedule for Teeth of Dogs and Cats (in Weeks)

	DECIDUOUS TEETH		PERMANENT TEETH	
	Puppy	Kitten	Dog	Cat
Incisors	4–6	3–4	12–16	11–16
Canines	3–5	3–4	12–16	12–20
Premolars	5–6	5–6	16–20	16–20
Molars	—	—	16–20	20–24

involving subgingival pathologic conditions. For example, the maxillary third premolar is usually a two-rooted tooth in dogs and cats, but it is common to see a third root in some of them.

The veterinary dental technician must understand dental anatomic terminology to accurately describe the location of a structure or lesion. Table 35.3 provides a description of the commonly used terms in veterinary dentistry. The concepts of mesial and distal surfaces are difficult to describe without referring to a diagram. Fig. 35.2A and B is a diagram showing these terms.

Referring to teeth by using a numeric system, rather than descriptive terminology, saves time when detailed charting is performed. The most used numbering system is the **modified Triadan system**. Teeth in the maxillary right quadrant comprise the *100 series*, and the left maxillary quadrant is called the *200 series*. The left mandibular quadrant is the 300 series, and the right mandibular quadrant is the 400 series. Each tooth within the quadrant has a two-digit number, starting at the anterior midline and moving along the dental arch in a caudal direction. The right maxillary first incisor is 101, right maxillary second incisor 102, right maxillary third incisor 103, right maxillary canine 104, and so on. The left maxillary canine is 204, left mandibular canine 304, right mandibular canine 404, and so on (Fig. 35.3). Deciduous teeth are designated as the 500 series for the right maxillary quadrant, 600 series for the left maxillary quadrant, 700 series for the left mandibular quadrant, and 800 series for the right mandibular quadrant.

TECHNICIAN NOTE

Remembering the "rule of 4 and 9" helps when using the modified Triadan numbering system. The canines will always be 04 and the first molar is 09.

Cats have fewer teeth compared with dogs, but even when teeth are missing, those that are present will have a predictable number with the modified Triadan system. For example,

TABLE 35.2   Permanent Dentition of the Dog and the Cat

Dog—Permanent Dentition

Mandible	Tooth	Roots
Incisors	1st, 2nd, 3rd	1
Canines	1	1
Premolars	1st	1
Premolars	2nd, 3rd, 4th	2
Molars	1st, 2nd	2
Molars	3rd[a]	1 (or 2)
Maxilla	Tooth	Root
Incisors	1st, 2nd, 3rd	1
Canines	1	1
Premolars	1st	1
Premolars	2nd, 3rd[a]	2
Premolars	(3rd[a]), 4th	3
Molars	1st, 2nd	3

Cat—Permanent Dentition

Mandible	Tooth	Roots
Incisors	1st, 2nd, 3rd	1
Canines	1	1
Premolars	1st, 2nd	Not present
Premolars	3rd, 4th	2
Molars	1st	2
Maxilla	Tooth	Roots
Incisors	1st, 2nd, 3rd	1
Canines	1	1
Premolars	1st	Not present
Premolars	2nd[a]	1 (or 2)
Premolars	3rd[a]	2 (or 3)
Premolars	4th	3
Molars	1st[a]	1 (or 2)

[a]Anatomic variation in root numbers is common. An extra root may be present or may be partially fused to the normal root(s).

tooth 108 always refers to the right maxillary fourth premolar, whether one is discussing the teeth of a dog, a hyena, a cat, or a lion. Because the cat does not have a maxillary first premolar, the premolar closest to the canine tooth is tooth 106 (Fig. 35.4). Cats do not have the mandibular first and second premolars, so the premolars closest to the mandibular canine teeth are numbered 307 and 407, respectively, for the left and right mandible. Keeping these numbers consistent among species allows veterinary professionals to quickly equate a tooth number with an anatomic location. When someone says that tooth 208 is fractured, one should think of the left maxillary fourth premolar, regardless of species.

TABLE 35.3 Common Terminology of Dentistry

Terminology	Definition	Abbreviation
Canine teeth	Also known as *cuspids*; sharp, pointed teeth caudal to the incisors and used to tear food	C
Deciduous teeth	Also known as *primary* or *baby* teeth	D
Dental formula	Indicates the number of teeth found in one side of the mouth	
Dental pad	The padded upper jaw observed in ruminant animal species. The pad acts as a compressor of food and shears forage against lowest incisors	
Incisors	Most forward teeth in mouth; are used for cutting food	I
Molars	Large teeth found caudally to premolars. There are three per side on top and bottom jaws and similar to premolars, are large and flat, and used to grind food	M
Premolars	Also known as *bicuspids*, located caudally to canines. There are four per side on top and bottom jaw and have large, flat surfaces used to grind food	P

Occlusion

Occlusion refers to the spatial relationship of teeth within the mouth. *Malocclusion* refers to the incorrect alignment of teeth or jaws. Although cosmetic issues of misaligned teeth are not typically a concern in dogs and cats, malocclusions can result in discomfort from impingement of teeth on soft tissue structures of the opposing dental arcade. Dogs and cats with a normal occlusion have a "scissors bite," in which the incisors come together to closely overlap like the blades of scissors (Fig. 35.5). When teeth are properly aligned in *scissors occlusion*, there is maximal function of all teeth with no occlusal trauma. Variations of dental occlusion in dogs and cats occur, depending on the breed and the skull type. The relationships of brachydont teeth in normal occlusion are discussed in the sections below.

Incisors

The mandibular incisors should be palatal to (behind) the maxillary incisors, and the coronal third of the mandibular incisors should rest on the cingulum of the maxillary incisors. The cingulum is a smooth, convex bulge located on the palatal side of the gingival third of the incisor teeth.

Canines

When the mouth is closed, the mandibular canine tooth is distal to the maxillary third incisor and **mesial** to the maxillary canine, and it should be centered between these two teeth, without touching either of them.

Premolars

The premolar cusps point to the interdental space of the opposing premolar teeth. The mandibular fourth premolar cusp points in the interdental space between the maxillary third and fourth premolars. When the mouth is closed, the mandibular first premolar is mesial to the maxillary first premolar. The premolars are not in occlusion with the opposing premolar teeth but, when the mouth is closed, the cusp tips should intersect a plane drawn midway between mandibular and maxillary occlusal planes.

Carnassial Teeth

The term *carnassial*, interpreted literally, means "tearing of flesh." This adjective is used to describe the largest shearing teeth of the upper and lower jaws in dogs, cats, and other carnivores. These teeth work together during mastication and contribute most significantly to the masticatory effort. The carnassial teeth of dogs and cats are the maxillary fourth premolar and the mandibular first molar teeth. In most species, the upper jaw is wider than the lower jaw; this is referred to as **anisognathism**. Therefore the maxillary fourth premolar tooth normally occludes lateral (buccal) to the mandibular first molar tooth.

Molars

Humans have many flat occlusal surfaces of the maxillary and mandibular molars that come together during chewing to crush food particles. In contrast, carnivores have sharp, shearing cusps and fewer flat occlusal surfaces. Two maxillary and three mandibular molars of dogs have flat occlusal surfaces that are capable of grinding and crushing hard food particles. Cats, having the dentition of a true carnivore, have molars with few flat occlusal surfaces. Flat occlusal surfaces are often susceptible to the development of **caries** lesions (i.e., *cavities*) in pits and fissures that occur because of incomplete development of **enamel** on the occlusal surface. The relative lack of occlusal surfaces in dogs and cats partly explains their decreased susceptibility to carious lesions compared with humans.

Oral Examination and History

The patient's medical history should be assessed before dental procedures are performed, because dental procedures require elective anesthesia. The veterinary technician should obtain the complete medical history and the history specifically pertinent to dentistry. Clinical symptoms to inquire about include pawing at the mouth, dropping food, walking away from the food bowl after showing initial interest in food, rubbing the face along furniture, and showing uncharacteristic aggression when approached or touched around the facial region (Box 35.2). These signs can indicate oral disease and may manifest earlier in the disease process than would anorexia or oral bleeding. A history of sneezing after drinking water is suggestive of the presence of an oronasal fistula—a common problem in small-breed dogs with severe periodontal disease.

Oral home care history should be obtained by the veterinary technician and include inquiry about any current home care regimen. If no home care regimen is present, the veterinary technician should inquire further to determine whether the client is willing or able to provide oral care at home. If the client has tried home care and has not been successful, the technician should find out what was tried so that alternative methods may be suggested. If the client is currently providing home care, the veterinary technician should ask about the frequency and

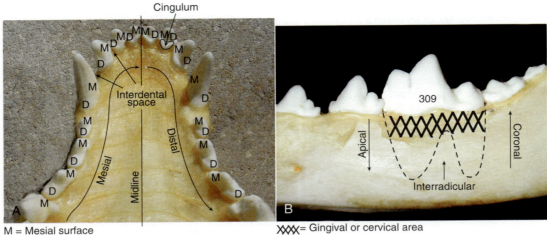

• **Fig. 35.2** Positional terminology commonly used in dentistry. (A) Palatal view of the canine maxilla. (B) Left mandibular first molar. *D,* Distal; *M,* mesial.

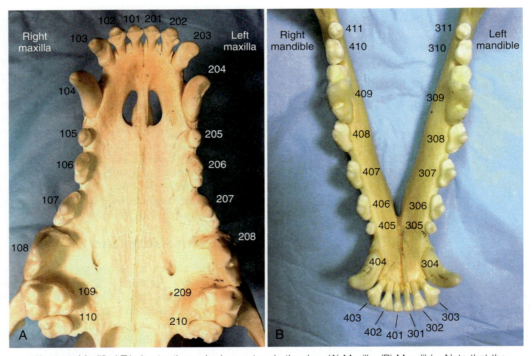

• **Fig. 35.3** Modified Triadan tooth numbering system in the dog. (A) Maxilla. (B) Mandible. Note that the canine tooth always ends with the numbers "04" and the first molar always ends with the numbers "09," regardless of species.

the techniques and products that are being used and history pertaining to diet, treats, and toys. The veterinary technician should ask the client about the following: if the pet is fed dry, canned, or semimoist food; the kind of treats the pet is eating, to determine what role treats are playing in the development or prevention of dental disease; what kinds of toys the pet plays with; and whether it has any inappropriate habits that may increase the risk for dental fracture. Once the dental history has been established, the veterinary technician is in a perfect position to provide counseling on proper home care techniques, diets, and toy products.

The dental or oral surgical procedure, whether routine or emergency, should begin with comprehensive extraoral and intraoral examinations. The mouth can be an indicator of general health, and a thorough oral examination is an integral part of any diagnostic sequence. The veterinary technician plays a crucial role in providing dental care and services, so it is imperative to be familiar with the normal anatomy of the oral cavity and the surrounding structures. By performing examination techniques on a regular basis and by establishing a routine sequence of examination, the clinician and veterinary technician can efficiently and accurately recognize

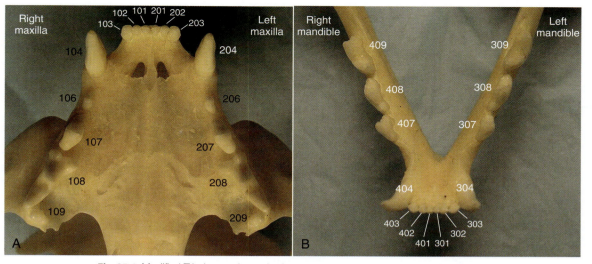

• **Fig. 35.4** Modified Triadan tooth numbering system in the cat. (A) Maxilla. (B) Mandible.

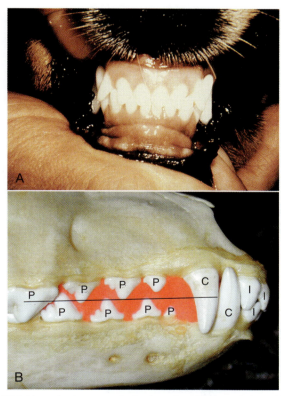

• **Fig. 35.5** Normal scissors occlusion in a dog. (A) Rostral view of incisor and canine teeth in a dog. (B) Lateral view of a dog skull. Premolar cusps interdigitate toward the opposing interdental space. *C*, Canine; *I*, incisor; *M*, molar; *P*, premolar.

abnormalities. All information gathered during the examination should be recorded on a dental record—the legal document of clinical data and dental services that becomes part of the patient's medical record (Figs. 35.6A and B and 35.7A and B). Any abnormalities should be brought to the attention of the veterinarian so that a diagnosis and a proper treatment plan can be established for the patient.

> **• BOX 35.2 Clinical or Behavioral Signs of Oral Disease**
>
> - Pawing at the mouth
> - Facial swelling
> - Dropping food
> - Face rubbing
> - Unusual aggression
> - Sneezing or snorting after eating or drinking
> - Difficulty or pain when opening the mouth
> - Anorexia
> - Jaw opening reflex ("chattering" of the lower jaw)
> - Difficulty swallowing (dysphagia)
> - Excessive drooling (ptyalism)
> - Oral bleeding
> - Resenting touch or manipulation of the head

> **TECHNICIAN NOTE**
>
> Every dental procedure should begin with a comprehensive oral examination to evaluate extraoral structures, including the face, head, neck, and intraoral structures, including the soft tissues of the oral cavity and teeth and their supporting structures.

Extraoral Examination

The examination begins with extraoral assessment of the head, face, eyes, ears, and neck by using direct visual observation, palpation, and smell. The technician performs the following steps: using both hands, palpate each side of the face, head, and neck for symmetric comparison; feel the temporal and masseter muscles for the presence of atrophy, enlargement, or pain; and palpate the ventral, lateral, and medial surfaces of the left and right mandibles for the presence of swelling, which could suggest neoplasia or fracture. Small-breed dogs with advanced periodontal disease are commonly affected by bone loss and pathologic fracture of the mandible, which can be incidental findings in the examination room.

Visual inspection of the ears is performed and evidence of discharge, odor, or pain on palpation is noted, because middle ear disease may be a cause for the presenting complaint of pain on opening

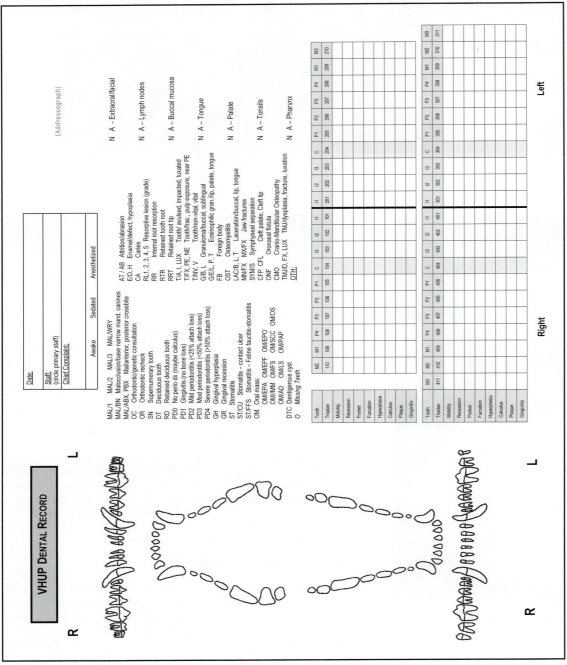

• **Fig. 35.6** Canine dental chart. (A) Front used to document diagnosis.

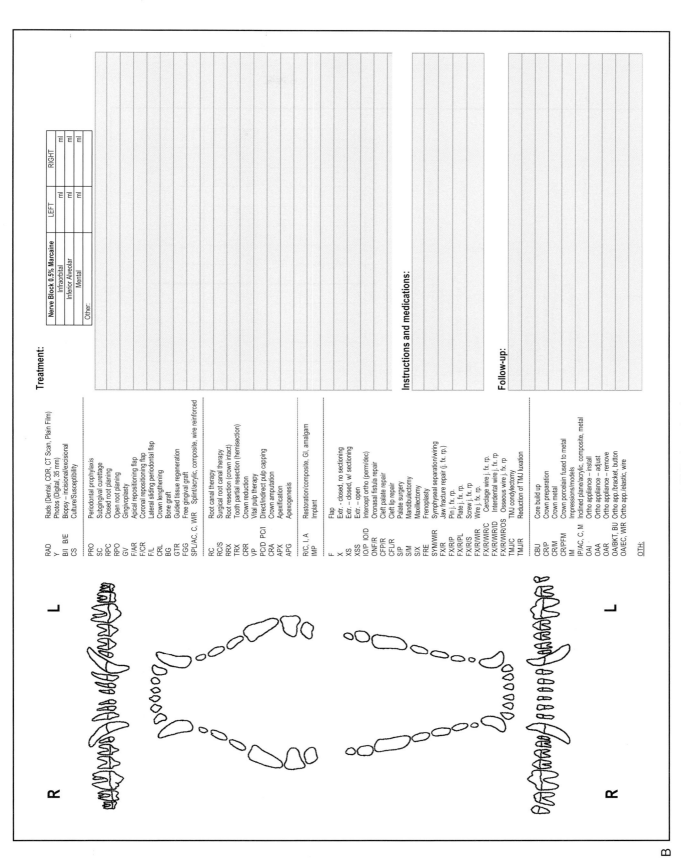

Treatment:

Nerve Block 0.5% Marcaine	LEFT	RIGHT
Infraorbital	ml	ml
Inferior Alveolar	ml	ml
Mental	ml	ml
Other:		

RAD — Rads (Dental, CDR, CT Scan, Plain Film)
Y — Photos (Digital, 35 mm)
B/I B/E — Biopsy – incisional/excisional
CS — Culture/Susceptibility

PRO — Periodontal prophylaxis
SC — Subgingival curettage
RPC — Closed root planing
RPO — Open root planing
GV — Gingivoplasty
F/AR — Apical repositioning flap
F/CR — Coronal repositioning flap
F/L — Lateral sliding periodontal flap
CRL — Crown lengthening
BG — Bone graft
GTR — Guided tissue regeneration
FGG — Free gingival graft
SPL/AC, C, WIR — Splint/acrylic, composite, wire reinforced

RC — Root canal therapy
RC/S — Surgical root canal therapy
RRX — Root resection (crown intact)
TRX — Tooth partial resection (hemisection)
CRR — Crown reduction
VP — Vital pulp therapy
PC/D PC/I — Direct/indirect pulp capping
CRA — Crown amputation
APX — Apexification
APG — Apexogenesis

R/C, I, A — Restoration/composite, GI, amalgam
IMP — Implant

F — Flap
X — Extr. – closed, no sectioning
XS — Extr. – closed, w/ sectioning
XSS — Extr. – open
IO/P IO/D — Intercept ortho (perm/dec)
ONF/R — Oronasal fistula repair
CFP/R — Cleft palate repair
CFL/R — Cleft lip repair
S/P — Palate surgery
S/M — Mandibulectomy
S/X — Maxillectomy
FRE — Frenoplasty
SYM/WIR — Symphyseal separation/wiring
FX/R — Jaw fracture repair (j. fx. rp.)
FX/R/P — Pin j. fx. rp.
FX/R/PL — Plate j. fx. rp.
FX/R/S — Screw j. fx. rp.
FX/R/WIR — Wire j. fx. rp.
FX/R/WIR/C — Cerclage wire j. fx. rp.
FX/R/WIR/ID — Interdental wire j. fx. rp
FX/R/WIR/OS — Osseous wire j. fx. rp
TMJ/C — TMJ condylectomy
TMJ/R — Reduction of TMJ luxation

CBU — Core build up
CR/P — Crown preparation
CR/M — Crown metal
CR/PFM — Crown porcelain fused to metal
IM — Impressions/models
IP/AC, C, M — Inclined plane/acrylic, composite, metal
OAI — Ortho appliance – install
OAA — Ortho appliance – adjust
OAR — Ortho appliance – remove
OA/BKT, BU — Ortho app./bracket, button
OA/EC, WIR — Ortho app./elastic, wire

OTH:

Instructions and medications:

Follow-up:

• **Fig. 35.6, cont'd** (B) Back used to document treatment.

B

VHUP DENTAL RECORD

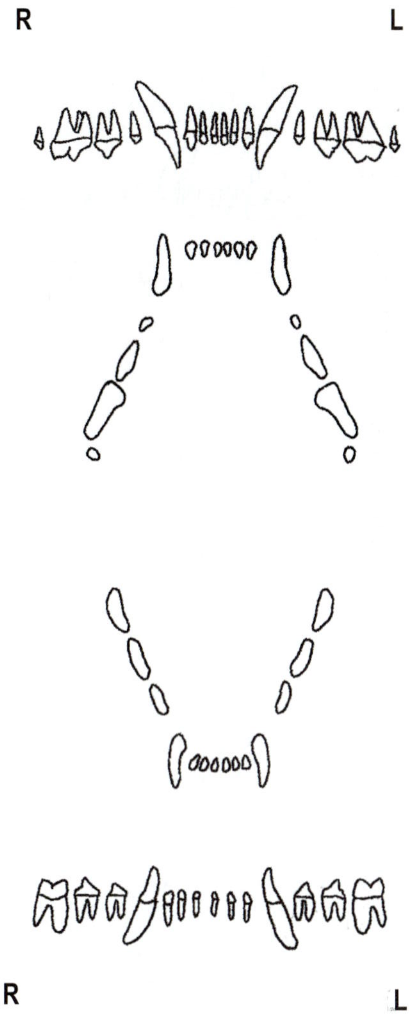

(Addressograph)

Date:

Staff:
(circle primary staff)

Chief Complaint:

	Awake	Sedated	Anesthetized

MAL/1   MAL/2   MAL/3   MAL/WRY
MAL/BN   Malocclusion/base narrow mand. canines
MAL/ABX, PBX   Mal/anterior, posterior crossbite
OC   Orthodontic/genetic consultation
OR   Orthodontic recheck
SN   Supernumerary tooth
DT   Deciduous tooth
RD   Retained deciduous tooth
PD0   No perio dx (maybe calculus)
PD1   Gingivitis (no bone loss)
PD2   Mild periodontitis (<25% attach loss)
PD3   Mod periodontitis (<50% attach loss)
PD4   Severe periodontitis (>50% attach loss)
GH   Gingival hyperplasia
GR   Gingival recession
ST   Stomatitis
ST/CU   Stomatitis – contact ulcer
ST/FFS   Stomatitis – Feline faucitis-stomatitis
OM   Oral mass:
      OM/EPA   OM/EPF   OM/EPO
      OM/MM   OM/FS   OM/SCC   OM/OS
      OM/AD   OM/LS   OM/PAP
DTC   Dentigerous cyst

O   Missing Teeth

AT / AB   Attrition/abrasion
E/D, H   Enamel/defect, hypoplasia
CA   Caries
RL,1, 2, 3, 4, 5   Resorptive lesion (grade)
RR   Internal root resorption
RTR   Retained tooth root
RRT   Retained root tip
T/A, I, LUX   Tooth/ avulsed, impacted, luxated
T/FX, PE, NE   Tooth/frac., pulp exposure, near PE
T/NV, V   Tooth/non-vital, vital
G/B, L   Granuloma/buccal, sublingual
G/E/L, P, T   Eosinophilic gran./lip, palate, tongue
FB   Foreign body
OST   Osteomyelitis
LAC/B, L, T   Laceration/buccal, lip, tongue
MN/FX   MX/FX   Jaw fractures
SYM/S   Symphyseal separation
CFP CFL   Cleft palate, Cleft lip
ONF   Oronasal fistula
CMO   Cranio-Mandibular Osteopathy
TMJ/D, FX, LUX   TMJ/dysplasia, fracture, luxation
OTH:

N A - Extraoral/facial

N A – Lymph nodes

N A – Buccal mucosa

N A – Tongue

N A – Palate

N A – Tonsils

N A – Pharynx

R   L

R   L

Right

Left

Tooth	M1	P4	P3	P2	C	I3	I2	I1	I1	I2	C	P2	P3	P4	M1
Triadan	109	108	107	106	104	103	102	101	201	202	203	204	206	207	208	209
Mobility															
Recession															
Pocket															
Furcation															
Hyperplasia															
Calculus															
Plaque															
Gingivitis															

Tooth	M1	P4	P3	C	I3	I2	I1	I1	I2	I3	C	P3	P4	M1
Triadan	409	408	407	404	403	402	401	301	302	303	304	307	308	309
Mobility														
Recession														
Pocket														
Furcation														
Hyperplasia														
Calculus														
Plaque														
Gingivitis														

• **Fig. 35.7** Feline dental chart. (A) Front used to document diagnosis.

A

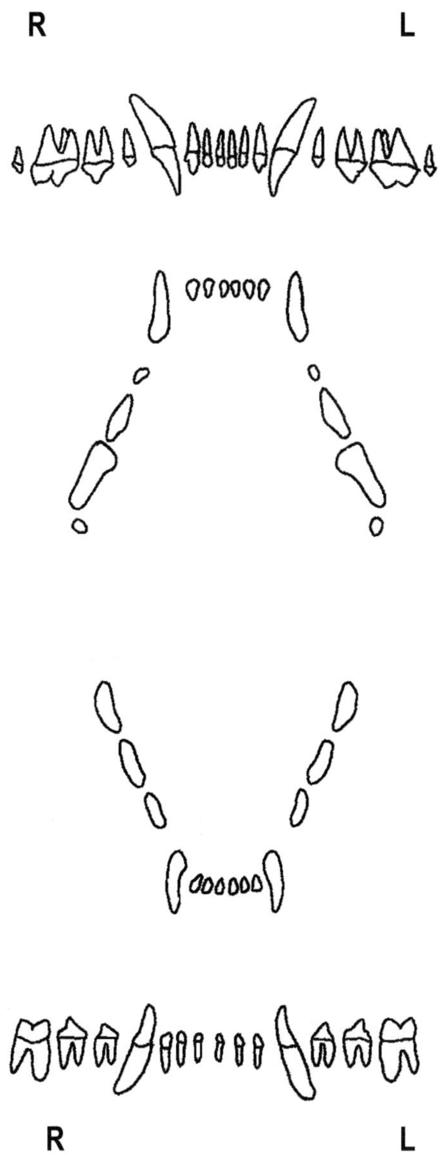

Treatment:

Nerve Block 0.5% Marcaine	LEFT	RIGHT
Infraorbital		
Inferior Alveolar	ml	ml
Mental	ml	ml
Other:	ml	ml

Instructions and medications:

Follow-up:

R L

RAD	Rads (Dental, CDR, CT Scan, Plain Film)
Y	Photos (Digital, 35 mm)
B/I B/E	Biopsy – incisional/excisional
CS	Culture/Susceptibility

PRO	Periodontal prophylaxis
SC	Subgingival curettage
RPC	Closed root planing
RPO	Open root planing
GV	Gingivoplasty
F/AR	Apical repositioning flap
F/CR	Coronal repositioning flap
F/L	Lateral sliding periodontal flap
CRL	Crown lengthening
BG	Bone graft
GTR	Guided tissue regeneration
FGG	Free gingival graft
SPL/AC, C, WIR	Splint/acrylic, composite, wire reinforced

RC	Root canal therapy
RC/S	Surgical root canal therapy
RRX	Root resection (crown intact)
TRX	Tooth partial resection (hemisection)
CRR	Crown reduction
VP	Vital pulp therapy
PC/D PC/I	Direct/indirect pulp capping
CRA	Crown amputation
APX	Apexification
APG	Apexogenesis

| R/C, I, A | Restoration/composite, GI, amalgam |
| IMP | Implant |

F	Flap
X	Extr. – closed, no sectioning
XSS	Extr. – closed, w/ sectioning
XSS	Extr. – open
IO/P IO/D	Intercept ortho (perm/dec)
ONF/R	Oronasal fistula repair
CFP/R	Cleft palate repair
CFL/R	Cleft lip repair
S/P	Palate surgery
S/M	Mandibulectomy
S/X	Maxillectomy
FRE	Frenoplasty
SYM/WIR	Symphyseal separation/wiring
FX/R	Jaw fracture repair (j. fx. rp.)
FX/R/P	Pin j. fx. rp.
FX/R/PL	Plate j. fx. rp.
FX/R/S	Screw j. fx. rp.
FX/R/WIR	Wire j. fx. rp.
FX/R/WIR/C	Cerclage wire j. fx. rp.
FX/R/WIR/ID	Interdental wire j. fx. rp
FX/R/WIR/OS	Osseous wire j. fx. rp
TMJ/C	TMJ condylectomy
TMJ/R	Reduction of TMJ luxation

CBU	Core build up
CR/P	Crown preparation
CRM	Crown metal
CR/PFM	Crown porcelain fused to metal
IM	Impressions/models
IP/AC, C, M	Inclined plane/acrylic, composite, metal
OAI	Ortho appliance – install
OAA	Ortho appliance – adjust
OAR	Ortho appliance – remove
OA/BKT, BU	Ortho app./bracket, button
OA/EC, WIR	Ortho app./elastic, wire

OTH:

R L

• **Fig. 35.7, cont'd** (B) Back used to document treatment.

B

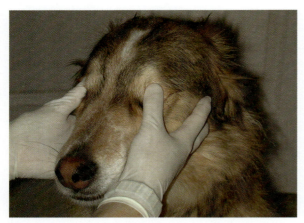

• **Fig. 35.8** Retropulsion of both eyes is an important component of the extraoral examination.

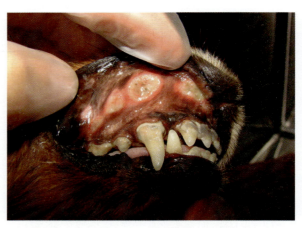

• **Fig. 35.9** Contact ulcerative stomatitis (CUS), also called *contact stomatitis*, in a dog.

the mouth. The eyes are visually inspected and then palpated by using the thumbs on the closed eyelids to gently push (retropulse) both eyes at the same time. Bilateral retropulsion allows for symmetric comparison of depth and firmness (Fig. 35.8). Often, if a space-occupying mass (a result of neoplasia, inflammation, or infection) is present behind or beneath the eye, retropulsion may reveal decreased ability of the globe to move caudally in the orbit on one side compared with the opposite side. Ability to retropulse varies depending on facial conformation. Retropulsion of the eyes in brachycephalic dogs and cats results in less movement of the globe, so comparison of both eyes is important for determining relative differences. The technician should observe for evidence of ocular discharge, which may be caused by blockage of the nasolacrimal duct by a pathologic process, such as a tooth root abscess or neoplasia. The soft tissue in the area ventral to the medial canthus of the eye is then palpated. Swelling in this area may be caused by a tooth root abscess of the maxillary fourth premolar. Evaluation of the neck includes palpation of the right and left mandibular salivary glands beneath the skin of the ventral neck. The mandibular salivary gland is the only easily palpable major salivary gland in dogs and cats. The other three major salivary glands may be too diffuse to palpate easily (parotid, sublingual glands) or not superficial enough to palpate (zygomatic gland). The mandibular gland is easily distinguished from the mandibular lymph nodes because it is softer, larger than, and caudomedial to the mandibular lymph nodes. Once the salivary glands are located, the mandibular lymph nodes can be identified by moving the fingertips cranially. The lymph nodes are palpated bilaterally for symmetry and firmness. In the cat, mandibular lymph nodes are difficult to palpate unless they are enlarged. In the dog, mandibular lymph nodes are almost always palpable, ranging in size from 0.5 to 1.5 cm in diameter, depending on the size of the patient. Although the term *mandibular lymph node* is often used in the singular, the area contains anywhere from one to five nodes. Other nodes that drain the head (retropharyngeal, parotid) are not normally palpable. Nine percent of dogs have another lymph node that is palpable in the subcutaneous tissue dorsal to the maxillary third premolar tooth. This node is referred to as the *facial* or *buccal lymph node* and is often bilateral when present.

> **TECHNICIAN NOTE**
>
> The major salivary glands of the dog and the cat are the paired mandibular, sublingual, zygomatic, and parotid glands.

The occlusion should be evaluated before intubation by noting any teeth that are abnormally positioned. The veterinary technician should pay attention to discrepancies in jaw length, the spatial relationships of teeth as they erupt, and the relationships of erupting teeth to the soft tissues of the opposing jaw. Any deciduous teeth that have not exfoliated by the time their permanent counterparts have erupted should be noted, because persistent deciduous teeth may create situations of periodontal disease and redirection of permanent tooth eruption. Once the deciduous and permanent canines begin to erupt, the relationship of the mandibular canines and the space between the maxillary third incisor and the canine teeth should be routinely monitored. Deviations from normal canine positioning can cause trauma to the palate and require treatment.

Intraoral Examination

A thorough intraoral examination can only be done with the patient under general anesthesia and consists of evaluations of the soft tissues of the oral cavity, the dental structures, and the **periodontium**, a term that describes the supporting structures of teeth. A standard approach to the oral examination allows for efficiency and thoroughness. The veterinary technician should begin by observing the skin and mucosa of the upper and lower lips. Some breeds are prone to lip fold dermatitis caudal to the mandibular canine tooth, which can cause oral malodor unrelated to periodontal disease. *Buccal mucosa* refers to the mucosa that begins at the mucocutaneous junction and lines the cheeks and lips. *Alveolar mucosa* refers to the mucosa that lies against the bone of the upper or lower jaw and meets the gingiva at the mucogingival junction. The normal appearance of the mucosa may be pink or pigmented, and the mucosa should exhibit no lesions, ulcerations, or swellings. Particular attention should be paid to areas of the mucosa that lie adjacent to periodontally diseased teeth, because bacteria in the **plaque** may contribute to painful mucosal ulcerations, often referred to as *contact ulcerative stomatitis* (CUS) or *contact stomatitis* (Fig. 35.9). The caudal cheek lining in the region of the carnassial and molar teeth should be inspected. This mucosa frequently becomes pressed between teeth during chewing, creating a condition known as *cheek-chewing lesions (CLs)* (Fig. 35.10). Similarly, the mucosa beneath the tongue may show signs of CLs referred to as *chewing lesions (lingual/sublingual mucosa/tongue)*, which are usually bilateral (Fig. 35.11). These lesions usually do

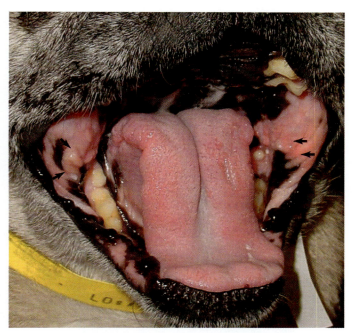

• **Fig. 35.10** Bilateral cheek-chewing lesions (CL) in a dog *(arrows)*. These lesions can be proliferative and sometimes ulcerated.

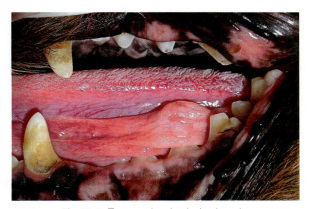

• **Fig. 35.11** Tongue-chewing lesion in a dog.

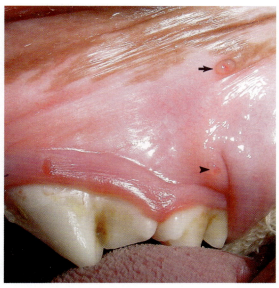

• **Fig. 35.12** Parotid *(arrow)* and zygomatic duct *(arrowhead)* openings in a dog. When the mucosa are not being retracted caudally, the parotid opening is rostral and dorsal to the zygomatic duct opening.

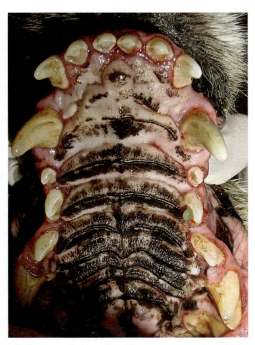

• **Fig. 35.13** Palatal rugae in a dog. The rugae may be widely spaced in dolichocephalic dogs or close together in brachycephalic dogs.

not require treatment unless they are not bilaterally similar or are ulcerated. In these cases, the affected mucosa may be removed and submitted for histopathologic evaluation.

Two raised bumps are found on the alveolar mucosa dorsal to the maxillary fourth premolar and the first molar teeth. Salivary secretions from the parotid and zygomatic salivary glands travel through ducts leading to these duct openings (Fig. 35.12).

The roof of the mouth is composed of a hard palate and a soft palate. The hard palate forms the rostral two-thirds and is covered by palatal mucosa arranged in prominent ridges called *rugae* (Fig. 35.13). These rugae range from eight to 10 in number. In brachycephalic dogs, the rugae are closely positioned, and hair and debris can accumulate in these rugal folds, which should be monitored by owners. The incisive papilla, which is a round, slightly raised structure, is located at the midline of the hard palate just caudal to the incisor teeth (Fig. 35.14). Lateral to the incisive papilla, a small bilateral communication with the incisive duct and the vomeronasal organ can be found. The vomeronasal organ is a

sensory organ involved in detection of pheromones and other chemical compounds. Palpation of the area lateral to the incisive papilla may normally feel as if air is trapped beneath the mucosa because of the communication between the mouth and these nasal structures. The soft palate consists of mucosa and muscle that separate the oropharynx from the nasopharynx. Two prominent bony structures can be palpated just lateral to the midline of the soft palate; these are the hamular processes of the bilateral pterygoid bones. One or both hamular processes may be difficult to palpate in the presence of a nasopharyngeal mass.

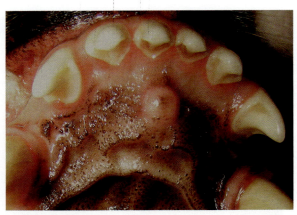

• **Fig. 35.14** Incisive papilla in a dog. The left and right incisive ducts open on the lateral aspects of the papilla.

The pharynx should be evaluated for evidence of inflammation or neoplasia. When the patient's mouth is open, bilateral folds of pharyngeal mucosa will be evident lateral to the tongue. These are referred to as the *palatoglossal folds*, and this area and the mucosa lateral to these folds may be inflamed in cats with lymphocytic–plasmacytic stomatitis (Fig. 35.15). Inflammation of this area of the oral cavity is referred to as *caudal stomatitis (ST/CS)*.

The tip of the tongue is held gently to enable visual examination of the dorsal, ventral, and lateral surfaces. The tongue should be lifted to observe the mucosa of the floor of the mouth and the base of the tongue. In the conscious patient, the examiner's thumb may be used extraorally to push the tongue dorsally for better visualization of the ventral surface of the tongue. The dorsal surface of the tongue is covered by thousands of papillae, some of which contain taste buds. The large, distinctive papillae located at the caudal third of the tongue are the vallate papillae, which are spaced in a curved line separating the body of the tongue from the root. The tongue is depressed to visualize the tonsils, noting any enlargement or change in color or texture. The color of a normal tonsil typically is more hyperemic than the color of adjacent mucosa. Normal tonsils may be fully contained within the tonsillar crypt and may be difficult to visualize.

During examination of the soft tissue, any tissue variations from normal should be described by recording size, shape, color, surface texture, and consistency (e.g., soft, firm, hard, fluctuant). A dedicated area on the dental record may be created to allow for documentation of any abnormalities of oral soft tissue structures (see Figs. 35.6A and B and 35.7A and B).

The next step in the intraoral examination is the evaluation of teeth and their supporting structures. First, the presence or absence of teeth in each quadrant is determined. Missing teeth can be documented on the dental chart by darkening or circling the drawing. Further radiographic evaluation of areas of missing teeth is imperative, because dentigerous cysts can develop as a result of an unerupted tooth. To evaluate the condition of teeth and the periodontium, the technician must use a periodontal probe and a dental explorer. These dental instruments are important clinical tools for obtaining information about the

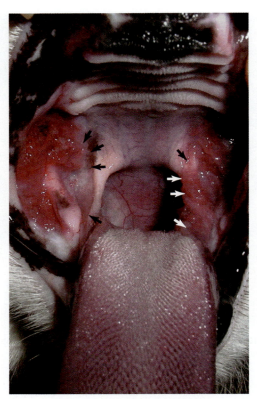

• **Fig. 35.15** Lymphocytic-plasmocytic stomatitis in the area lateral to the palatoglossal folds in a cat *(arrows)*.

health status of each tooth (patient). The canine mouth should be considered as containing 42 patients and the feline mouth as containing 30 patients, with each patient requiring a thorough evaluation. The periodontal probe has a round or flat working end that is marked in millimeter increments, ending in a blunt tip. The probe is used as a miniature intraoral ruler to measure attachment levels, sulcus and pocket depths, loss of bone in **furcation** areas, and size of oral lesions. It is also used to assess the mobility of teeth and the presence of gingival bleeding. Periodontal probes are available in an assortment of design styles, with variations in the thickness of the diameter of the working end and variations in increments of millimeter markings (Fig. 35.16). Probes with Williams markings have millimeter increments at 1, 2, 3, 5, 7, 8, 9, and 10 mm. The University of North Carolina-15 (UNC 15) probe has millimeter markings at 1, 2, 3, 4, 5, 6, 7, 8, 9, 10, 11, 12, 13, 14, and 15 mm; it is useful for evaluating large dogs and patients with deep periodontal pockets. Some probes have a small 0.5-mm ball on the end to minimize tissue trauma; however, these probes typically have markings at 3.5, 5.5, 8.5, and 11.5 mm, resulting in inexact determination of pocket depth. Although many probes are available, a probe with markings beginning at 1 mm is necessary for assessing subtle pocket depths in cats. The Michigan "O" probe with Williams markings is best suited for use in cats, because the diameter of the working end of the probe is narrowest. Some styles have color-coded bands for easier viewing of calibrations.

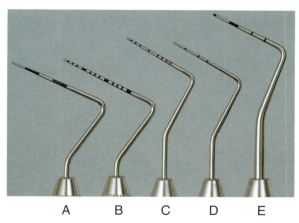

• **Fig. 35.16** Periodontal probes with different calibrations. The blunt-tipped working end is used to measure sulcus or pocket depth, tooth mobility, furcation involvement, gingival recession, and gingival hyperplasia. (From Newman MG, Takei HH, Klokkevold PR, Carranza FA. *Carranza's Clinical Periodontology*. 10th ed. St. Louis, MO: Saunders; 2006.)

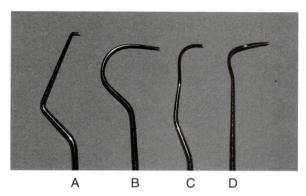

• **Fig. 35.17** Dental explorers with sharp, wirelike tips are used to explore the topography of tooth surfaces. (A) Tufts 17. (B) Shepherd's hook 23. (C) ODU (Old Dominion University) 11/12. (D) 2A Pigtail.

The dental explorer has a slender, wirelike working end that tapers to a sharp point and is used to explore the topography of the tooth surface. When the explorer is held with a light modified pen grasp, the veterinary technician will acquire a tactile sense to locate tooth surface irregularities, such as caries, feline resorption, **calculus** deposits, and **pulp** exposure. Tactile sensitivity is achieved when the flexible working end of the explorer vibrates as it detects surface irregularities. Vibrations are transmitted from the tip to the handle as felt by the veterinary technician. The explorer is also used to determine the completeness of treatment after calculus debridement and to ensure smooth transitions of dental restoratives (fillings). Several designs of explorers are available (Fig. 35.17). Varying degrees of flexibility contribute to the degrees of tactile sensitivity. The "shepherd's hook" is the most common explorer in most veterinary practices and is often paired with a periodontal probe as a double-ended instrument. Although it is convenient to have a shepherd's hook on the opposite end of a probe, it is bulky, inflexible, and less adaptable for subgingival use compared with other explorers. The Tufts #17 explorer has a 2-mm tip that is bent at a 90-degree angle from the shank, allowing it to be used in the subgingival region with little tissue distention (stretching of the gingiva away from the tooth) or trauma to the epithelial lining of the sulcus. The 2-mm tip of the Tufts #17 may have limitations in determining the depth of a dental lesion, such as caries or feline resorption. The curved 11/12 ODU (Old Dominion University) explorer is an ideal choice for veterinary use. The curvature of the long shank and the working ends make it adaptable for use on rostral and caudal teeth supragingivally and subgingivally, and its smaller working end allows for detection of subtle hard tissue defects.

Periodontal instruments, including the probe and the explorer, are held with a modified pen grasp (Fig. 35.18), which is a variation of the grasp used for writing. This recommended grasp facilitates good fingertip tactile sensitivity and precise control of the instrument's working end, decreasing risk of trauma to tissues. The modified pen grasp uses three fingertips placed in a triangular (tripod) position plus a rest finger. The pads of the index finger and the thumb rest on the instrument where the handle and shank meet to hold the instrument. The pad near the fingernail of the middle finger rests on the shank (the portion of the instrument that connects the handle with the working end) (Fig.

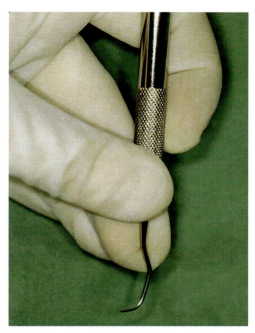

• **Fig. 35.18** Modified pen grasp hand position for periodontal instrumentation: the thumb and index finger hold the instrument handle; the corner of the middle finger rests on the shank. The ring finger is used as a fulcrum and for control.

35.19). Proper placement of the middle fingertip pad against the shank is important for enhancing tactile sensitivity and helping to guide and control the working end. The ring finger should rest on an oral structure, such as a tooth located close to the working area, to provide stability to the hand for added control. Keeping the ring finger in contact with the middle finger will ensure proper wrist motion by limiting the amount of finger motion and will prevent finger fatigue. The little finger should be relaxed and has no specific function in this grasp.

Assessment of the periodontium and teeth should begin at the midline of the mouth; each tooth should be systematically evaluated, one at a time, through visual observation and tactile use of the probe and the explorer. Excessive tooth mobility can be detected by first placing the tip of the probe against the tip of the tooth and gently attempting to move the tooth in the buccolingual direction. Movement is estimated on a scale of 1, 2, or 3, based on the number of millimeters beyond normal physiologic

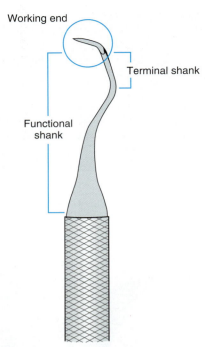

• **Fig. 35.19** Parts of the instrument include the handle, shank, and working end. The functional shank extends from the handle to the working end, and the terminal shank is the part of the shank closest to the working end. (From Daniel SJ, Harfst SA, Wilder R. *Mosby's Dental Hygiene: Concepts, Cases, and Competencies*. 2nd ed. St. Louis, MO: Mosby; 2008.)

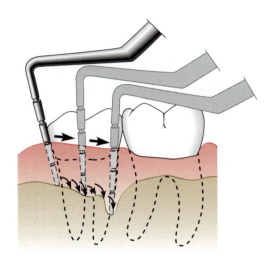

• **Fig. 35.20** While keeping the side of the tip of the probe in contact with the tooth and using a light touch, the probe is "walked" around the circumference of the tooth with short up-and-down strokes every few millimeters. (From Newman MG, Takei H, Klokkevold PR, et al. *Carranza's Clinical Periodontology*. 12th ed. St. Louis, MO: Saunders; 2015.)

mobility that the tooth moves in a single direction (Box 35.3). A slight amount of movement caused by the periodontal ligament that connects the tooth to alveolar bone is normal. The most severe mobility, with a classification of 3, includes any tooth with vertical movement. As each tooth is evaluated for mobility, the characteristics of the gingiva, including color, shape, texture, and consistency, should be noted on visual inspection. Healthy gingival tissues are pink (except where normally pigmented), stippled (orange peel appearance), firm, tapered to a thin margin, and scalloped to follow the contour of the cementoenamel junction (CEJ) and underlying alveolar bone. Any area of the gingiva that deviates from these normal characteristics should be examined more closely with the probe.

TECHNICIAN NOTE

The *periodontium*, that is, the attachment structures of teeth, includes gingival connective tissue, alveolar bone, periodontal ligament, and cementum.

The probe is gently inserted into the sulcus, or pocket, with the probe kept as close to parallel with the long axis of the root as possible and with the side of the probe tip in contact with the tooth. When physical resistance is felt at the base of the sulcus or pocket, the marking level on the probe that is adjacent to the gingival margin is noted. The probe is then "walked" around the tooth with up-and-down bobbing strokes approximately 1 to 2 mm in height (↕) and in 1- to 2-mm horizontal steps (↔) to assess the entire circumference of the tooth (Fig. 35.20). Abnormal measurements (those >3 mm in dogs and >1 mm in cats) should be noted on the dental chart, along with the specific location of the pocket measurement (e.g., MB for mesiobuccal). Probe measurements

between millimeter markings are rounded up to the larger measurement. For accurate readings, it is essential for the technician to develop skill in consistently probing forces (10–20 *g* [gravity] of pressure). This amount of pressure can be attained by pressing the probe tip into the pad of a thumb until the skin is depressed approximately 2 mm.

In areas where the height of the free gingival margin has migrated apically toward or beyond the CEJ, the probe is used to measure gingival recession. Recession is measured in millimeters from the CEJ to the level of the gingival margin. *Attachment loss* (i.e., level) is a term that truly describes the periodontal state of a tooth, because it accounts for both pocket depth and gingival recession (Fig. 35.21). Gingival hyperplasia occurs when the free gingival margin migrates coronally, toward the crown of the tooth. Hyperplasia is measured in millimeters from the CEJ to the gingival margin, which covers a portion of the tooth crown. Increased pocket depth may be caused by hyperplasia or attachment loss, so clinical examination findings are necessary to determine whether the increased probing depth is caused by a true pocket or a pseudopocket.

When multirooted teeth are approached, the probe is used to assess loss of bone in the areas between and around the roots. Bifurcation, which is the furcation between two-rooted teeth, should be assessed from the buccal and lingual-palatal surfaces.

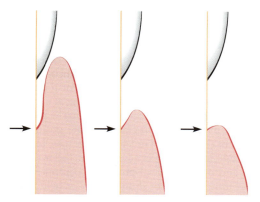

• **Fig. 35.21** Attachment level is measured from the bottom of the pocket *(arrows)* to a fixed point on the tooth, such as the cementoenamel junction (CEJ). Attachment level is a better indicator of periodontal status than is pocket depth, because gingival recession or hyperplasia can greatly affect pocket depth measurement. Note that the three examples have the same level of attachment loss yet different pocket depths as a result of gingival recession. (From Newman MG, Takei H, Klokkevold PR, et al. *Carranza's Clinical Periodontology*. 12th ed. St. Louis, MO: Saunders; 2015.)

Trifurcations of three-rooted teeth should be assessed between each of the three roots. The extent of bone loss determines furcation classification (Box 35.4). The periodontal probe should be placed such that tip can be held as perpendicular as possible to the long axis of the tooth (Fig. 35.22). The tip is gently moved horizontally across a root, dipping into the furcation area and continuing to the adjacent root. The depth of penetration into the furcation area determines the classification. Care must be taken to minimize tissue distention.

During the periodontal evaluation of each tooth, the hard structures of the tooth are also observed, and the dental explorer is used when any chips, fractures, pulp exposure, or abnormal wear pattern of abrasion or attrition is noticed. *Abrasion* (AB) refers to tooth wear associated with aggressive chewing on external objects, such as toys, rocks, and ice cubes. *Attrition (AT)* refers to wear associated with tooth-to-tooth contact over time.

Dental caries (i.e., "cavities") (CA) result from demineralization of enamel and dentin caused by acids produced by certain oral bacteria. These lesions occur most commonly on occlusal (flat) surfaces of the molar teeth. The veterinary technician should gently explore for pits and fissures of the occlusal surfaces of the maxillary first and second molars and the distal half of the mandibular first molar, feeling for areas of demineralization. The explorer should be used to check for clinical signs of feline resorptive lesions by dragging the sharp point horizontally across the cervical portion of each tooth. Sometimes, it is challenging to determine whether a concavity in the area of a furcation is a resorptive lesion or merely mild furcation exposure. If a resorptive lesion is present, the explorer tip will "catch" on the edge of the concavity, while the explorer will freely move out of the concave area as easily as it fell into it when mild furcation exposure is encountered. When tooth fractures are present, the sharp point of the explorer should be gently moved across the tooth surface, feeling for any openings into the pulp. Teeth with significant abrasion may have a brown or black dot in the center of the worn tooth. This can be a sign of chronic pulp exposure or it may be a reparative material produced by the tooth in response to chronic wear (tertiary dentin). Pulp exposure can be distinguished from tertiary dentin with the use of an explorer. If a tooth has pulp exposure, the tip of the explorer

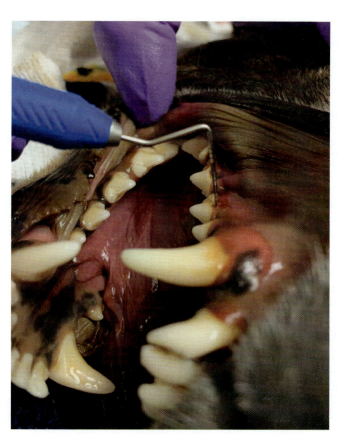

• **Fig. 35.22** The proper probe placement to evaluate furcation exposure. Care must be taken to minimize tissue distention.

will "fall into a hole," while a discolored area caused by tertiary dentin will feel smooth as glass when the explorer is run over this area. This is an important clinical distinction, because treatment of pulp-exposed teeth is necessary, but worn teeth with tertiary dentin usually do not require treatment (Fig. 35.23).

Dental Radiography

Intraoral radiography is essential for planning and assessing outcomes of dental treatment for dogs, cats, horses, and exotic species. Radiography provides the clinician with an important diagnostic tool to detect pathologic conditions that are not clinically visible in the mouth. The types of pathologic findings for which dental

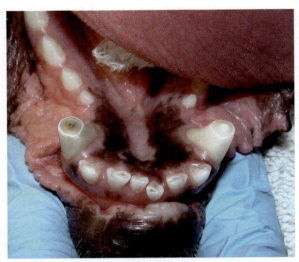

• **Fig. 35.23** Abrasion of the mandibular canine teeth of a dog. Rapid abrasion results in pulp exposure of the dog's right mandibular canine; this is determined by running an explorer over the flat surface and "falling into" the pulp chamber. Slowed abrasion allows the dog's left mandibular canine tooth to respond by producing tertiary (reparative) dentin, which feels smooth as glass when the surface is explored. Both teeth should be radiographed to assess for endodontic pathologic conditions, but the tooth with pulp exposure definitely requires extraction or root canal therapy.

radiography is useful are as follows: root resorption, caries, periapical radiolucency (often seen with tooth root abscesses), periodontal bone loss, retained root tips, unerupted teeth, osteomyelitis, neoplasia, tooth and jaw fractures, foreign bodies, and disease of the temporomandibular joint. The veterinary patient must be sedated or anesthetized to facilitate obtaining quality dental radiographs. Intraoral dental radiography is becoming more routine in general veterinary practice.

Equipment

The dental x-ray machine may be wall mounted, may stand on the floor with wheels that permit storage when not in use, or be a hand-held model. The unit is composed of three primary parts: the control panel, a long (72–86-inch) arm that extends from the control panel, and a tube head that is attached to the end of the arm. The control panel, which is typically mounted on a wall near the dental workstation, contains the power switch, selector buttons for kilovoltage (kV) and milliamperes (mA), a dial or buttons for changing exposure time, and a button that is located at the end of a 6-foot coiled cord. Most dental x-ray units have an internally set level of kilovoltage and milliamperes, and only exposure time may be changed for a darker or lighter technique. The timing selection may be located at the end of the cord of some newer models. An indicator light and an audible sound are emitted from the control panel when exposure is attained.

> **TECHNICIAN NOTE**
>
> The dental radiograph machine should be inspected for leakage. Many US states require regular inspections.

With experience in using the radiograph machine, the technician will be able to determine proper exposure times based on the size of the patient and the density of the tissues through which the x-ray beam must penetrate. The technician needs only to select "dog" or "cat" and patient size.

All veterinary staff members must become familiar with radiation safety guidelines. The timer switch can be remotely wired and mounted outside of the dental treatment room, or at least 6 to 12 feet away from the tube head. Standing at a distance behind a barrier or at a 90- to 130-degree angle that is perpendicular to the beam will place the technician in a safe position away from the direction of the beam. Hand-held units have leaded shields to protect the operator, but it is advised that the technician wear a lead apron and other personal protective equipment when using a hand-held unit. The sensor should never be held in the patient's mouth by the technician while the radiograph is taken; therefore anesthesia is necessary not only to ensure diagnostic-quality images but also to ensure safety. The machine should be inspected regularly for leaks by a competent radiation expert as may be required by state regulations. Development of skills will minimize unnecessary radiation from retakes caused by poor technique or positioning. The ALARA (As Low As Reasonably Achievable) principle, a regulatory safety requirement, should be applied to minimize radiation doses to all patients. As with any radiation exposure, all individuals should wear a dosimeter during the procedure.

Digital Radiography

Traditionally, since the 1920s, intraoral film had been used to obtain dental images. However, with the advent of digital radiography, film is rarely used today. Use of digital radiography in veterinary practice is increasing as practitioners become more aware of its benefits compared with conventional radiographic techniques. The quality of digital imaging has been improving since its first introduction into dentistry; today, the resolution is similar in quality to that of nonscreen dental film radiography. With digital radiography, less time is needed to obtain the image, and no chemicals are used in the process. Direct radiography (DR) technology, which is commonly used today, requires an electronic intraoral sensor, a computer, and an x-ray machine. The sensor, called a *charged coupled device*, may be cordless or may be attached to a cord that connects to the computer. After the sensor is covered with a plastic infection barrier, the sensor is placed into the patient's mouth to capture the image and convert it to the digital format of "pixels"—picture elements in various shades of gray. A remote module transmits the data to the computer so that the image can be immediately viewed, manipulated, and stored. The images can be magnified, and enhancements in contrast or darkness can be made. DR sensors are available in sizes comparable with those used with traditional dental film sizes 0, 1, and 2, limiting application in large-breed dogs, which may take many more views to obtain a full mouth series. A digital option that allows for digital size 4 images is an indirect digital system or computed radiography (CR) that uses phosphor plate technology and a scanner to produce digital images within seconds of processing a reusable plate through a digital scanner. When digital technology is used, caution must be taken to ensure adequate depth of anesthesia, because replacement of a damaged charged coupled device sensor is costly.

Digital technology reduces radiation exposure by 50% to 90% compared with the use of D- and E-speed film. Most modern dental x-ray machines are compatible with digital radiology if they have timers that allow the exposure setting in a $\frac{1}{100}$ of a second time frame. A disadvantage of digital radiography is the high initial cost of the sensor and the software. However, the expense is offset by the savings incurred by not requiring film and processing chemicals.

Exposure and Positioning Errors

Errors in sensor exposure and processing account for unnecessary radiation exposure and additional anesthesia time for the patient. Cone cutting occurs when the beam does not impact portions of the sensor, plate, or film, resulting in areas with no image. Elongation and foreshortening (stretched and shortened images, respectively) are caused by inaccurate vertical angulation during alignment of the beam (Fig. 35.24). To correct elongation or fore-shortening, it helps to think about the position of the sun during the day. When the sun is low in the sky (morning or evening), the shadow is long; at midday, the shadow will be very short. Images that are too dark or too light can result from errors in exposure times. When conventional films are used, variations in processing time can also affect the darkness of the film.

> ### TECHNICIAN NOTE
>
> An image that appears too dark is often the result of greater-than-necessary exposure time. However, digital images may be modified in brightness and degree of contrast. Postprocessing an image will decrease the integrity of the image. It may be better to adjust the exposure time and retake the image.

Techniques

The goal of dental radiology is to obtain a diagnostic image. A diagnostic image must include 2 to 3 mm of bone around the apex of the tooth and the level of the alveolar bone. A radiograph displaying the entire crown is not necessary to ensure a diagnostic image. Two techniques (parallel or bisecting angle) are commonly used to obtain dental radiographs. Each technique varies in the relationship of the beam to the sensor and the teeth to be imaged. The sensor or phosphor plate is placed into the mouth and is held in position with gauze.

The paralleling technique requires the sensor to be placed parallel to the long axis of the tooth (Fig. 35.25A). The beam is directed perpendicular to the sensor and teeth and is positioned to aim for the center of the sensor (Fig. 35.25B). The parallel technique can be used only on the mandibular teeth caudal to the mandibular fourth premolar, where the sensor can easily slide between the jaw and the tongue.

The symphysis at the rostral portion of the mandible and the flat palate of the maxilla prevents use of the paralleling technique. To minimize inherent distortion of dental structures when the paralleling technique is not an option, the bisecting angle technique is used.

The x-ray beam is projected at a right angle to an imaginary line that cuts in half (bisects) the angle formed by the plane of the sensor and the long axis of the tooth (Fig. 35.26A and B). The bisecting angle technique can be intimidating and difficult to understand but is necessary.

Techniques have been developed to obtain nondistorted images by using angles and proper patient and sensor placement. Most dental radiology units have angles on the tube head where it joins with the arm of the unit. The patient should be placed sternal recumbency for maxillary views and dorsal recumbency for mandibular views.

In sternal recumbency, the patent's maxilla should be parallel to the table and not tilted. A square water bottle or tub can be placed under the chin to help maintain this position. The sensor

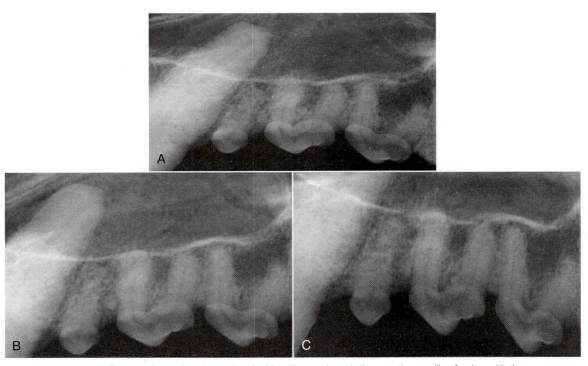

• **Fig. 35.24** Three radiographs taken using the bisecting angle technique on the maxilla of a dog with three different position-indicating device (PID) angles. (A) Foreshortened image from PID positioned too dorsally. (B) Correctly determining the bisecting angle results in an image that most closely represents the size and shape of subgingival structures. (C) Elongated image from PID positioned too ventrally.

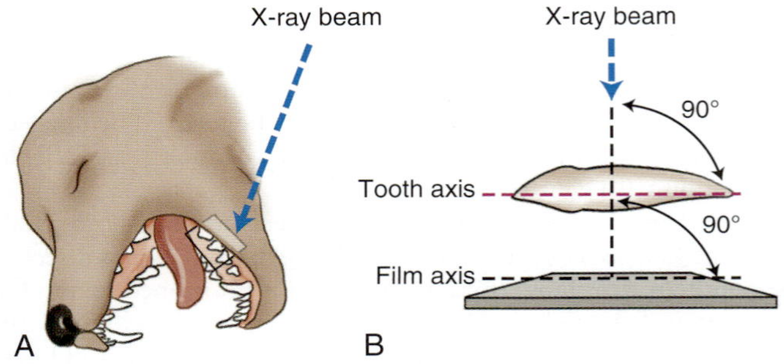

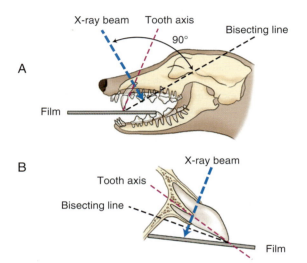

• Fig. 35.25 The paralleling technique is useful for caudal mandibular teeth, for which the sensor is placed parallel to the teeth; the beam is directed at a 90-degree angle to the sensor and teeth.

• Fig. 35.26 The bisecting angle technique is used for the maxilla and the rostral mandible, for which the sensor cannot be placed parallel to the roots. First, determine the angle created by the plane of the tooth and the plane of the sensor. Bisect that angle and direct the beam at a right angle to the bisecting line.

should be flat, with the cord coming out of the front of the mouth for all maxillary views. If the sensor will not remain flat, place a small piece of gauze between the palate and the sensor to help with positioning. Teeth should always be placed on the very edge of the sensor, with the rest of the sensor on the inside of the mouth. It is important to remember that if the desired image has not been obtained, the sensor placement should be checked first before adjusting the tube head. The cone on the dental generator does not have a collimating light or cross hairs to help determine the center point of a radiograph. Most dental radiology tube heads have lines at 90-degree angles, which can be used to obtain the desired radiograph. Hands-on training for dental radiograph positioning is helpful and can be an asset to veterinary practices.

Radiographic Interpretation

To assess the presence of intraoral pathologic conditions on radiographs, it is essential to have knowledge of the appearance of normal radiographic anatomic structures (Fig. 35.27). The radiodensity of the components of teeth and supporting structures varies widely; therefore the terms *radiopaque* and *radiolucent* are used to describe the relative radiographic appearance of oral

and dental structures. Radiodense (radiopaque) structures, such as **cementum**, dentin, and bone, block or absorb radiation, causing that portion of the processed radiograph to appear light or white (Fig. 35.28). The thin layer of enamel covering the crown is the most radiodense structure of the tooth. The lamina dura, which is a cribriform plate of bone lining the tooth socket, appears as a white line adjacent to the periodontal space surrounding a healthy tooth. Beyond the lamina dura, the trabecular pattern of bone may vary in radiodensity. The cortex of the mandible is radiodense.

In contrast, radiolucent structures, such as soft tissue and periodontal ligament space, appear dark or black, because x-ray photons can easily pass through to the sensor. The periodontal ligament fibers are not visible on the sensor; however, the space they occupy can be traced as a black line surrounding the roots. Because pulp is soft tissue, it appears as a dark area (less radiodense) in the center of the tooth.

The radiolucent mandibular canal lies apical to most of the mandibular tooth roots. In small-breed dogs, the apices of the mandibular first molar roots may be seen at a level at or even below the mandibular canal, extending into the ventral cortex. Normal anatomic structures must be distinguished from pathologic structures. For example, the middle mental foramen is located apical to the mandibular second premolar in dogs and can be misinterpreted as a periapical pathologic condition if superimposed over a tooth root. It is helpful to refer to a textbook with images of normal and pathologic radiographic appearances (see "Recommended Readings").

Periodontal Disease

The periodontium is composed of four supporting structures of the tooth: (1) periodontal ligament; (2) gingival connective tissue; (3) alveolar bone forming the tooth socket; and (4) cementum covering the surface of the root. Healthy gingiva has a sharp, tapered edge (margin) that lies closely against the crown of the tooth. The free gingiva forms a moat around the tooth, called the *gingival sulcus*. The epithelial attachment to the tooth crown forms the bottom of the gingival sulcus. The depth of this sulcus varies (up to 3 mm in the healthy mouth of a dog and up to 1 mm in the cat).

Gingivitis refers to inflammation of the gingiva. *Periodontitis* describes inflammation not only of the gingiva but also of other structures of the periodontium. Gingivitis represents the earliest stages of periodontitis and is easily reversible with proper treatment and home care. Once advanced periodontitis occurs, these changes are more difficult to reverse. Periodontitis is the most common disease of animals.

Periodontitis is caused by accumulation of subgingival plaque and the body's response to it. Plaque is a white-tan film that collects around and within the gingival sulcus of the tooth. It is composed of bacteria, food debris, exfoliated cells, and salivary glycoproteins (Fig. 35.29). Plaque begins to form by laying down a biofilm within 20 to 30 minutes after cleaning. If left undisturbed, as quickly as within 24 to 48 hours, plaque will mineralize on the teeth to form dental calculus (sometimes referred to as *tartar*)—a light brown or yellow, raised, irregular deposit adherent to the tooth and root surfaces. This irregular, plaque-retentive surface of calculus allows for further plaque accumulation. As plaque accumulates within the gingival sulcus, it damages the gingival tissues by releasing bacterial by-products that can damage the periodontium. The patient's immune response may also cause tissue damage through the release of inflammatory cytokines from

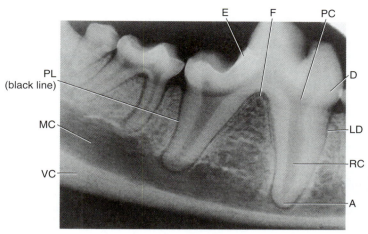

• **Fig. 35.27** Normal radiopaque and radiolucent structures. *A,* Root apex; *D,* dentin; *E,* enamel; *F,* furcation area; *LD,* lamina dura; *MC,* mandibular canal; *PC,* pulp chamber; *PL,* periodontal ligament; *RC,* root canal; *VC,* ventral cortex.

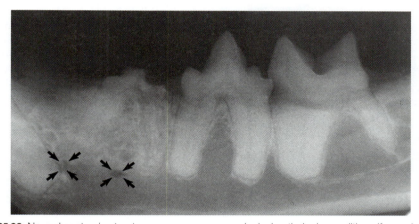

• **Fig. 35.28** Normal anatomic structures may appear as periapical pathologic conditions if superimposed over a root. The middle mental foramen (superimposed over the apex of the canine tooth root) and the caudal mental foramen are labeled with arrows.

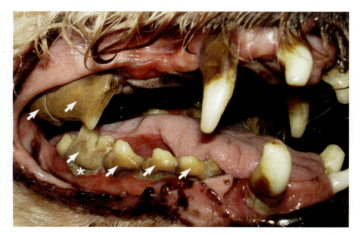

• **Fig. 35.29** Plaque and calculus in a dog. Plaque is white-tan *(asterisk)* and accumulates on the rough surface of calculus. Plaque that is not removed within approximately 24 hours will become mineralized, adherent calculus *(arrows).*

white blood cells as they attempt to destroy bacteria. In the early stages, the gingiva becomes inflamed and bleeds easily. Progression of periodontitis results in loss of attachment. Attachment loss is clinically detectable in its earliest stages by measuring pocket depths with a periodontal probe in the anesthetized patient (Figs. 35.30 and 35.31).

> **TECHNICIAN NOTE**
>
> Plaque begins to form within 20 to 30 minutes after cleaning and, if not removed, it will begin to mineralize into calculus as early as 24 to 48 hours after adhering to the tooth surface. Therefore daily brushing is necessary to minimize calculus formation.

Periodontal disease is difficult to control once it has developed. For this reason, great emphasis must be placed on its prevention. Other diseases can contribute to the severity of periodontal disease, but bacteria in plaque are the primary cause. Early in the formation of plaque, the bacterial population consists mainly of gram-positive aerobic bacteria. Once these bacteria accumulate in substantial numbers, the oxygen gradient of the subgingival environment changes to support

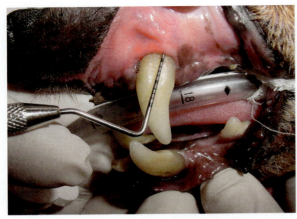

• **Fig. 35.30** A probe is inserted to determine pocket depth.

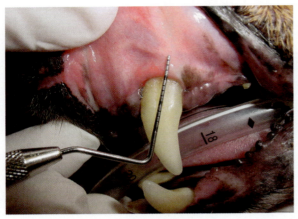

• **Fig. 35.31** A probe is removed to show the degree of attachment loss, which is pocket depth plus gingival recession.

a shift to predominantly gram-negative anaerobic rods and spirochetes. Gram-negative bacteria can produce endotoxins, which have direct adverse effects on the cells of the periodontium, resulting in a more severe immune response. Endotoxins are believed to be attached to the tooth surface, loosely embedded in cementum, and unattached in the sulcular space. When periodontitis is already present, destruction of the junctional epithelium at the base of the gingival sulcus has begun and will continue if not treated. Once the junctional epithelium and the periodontal ligament become destroyed, it is difficult to stimulate regeneration. As the tooth begins to lose its periodontal attachment, it becomes more susceptible to plaque accumulation in the deep periodontal pockets that form around the tooth roots. When the tooth loses a significant portion of its periodontium, it becomes mobile. The infection and inflammation associated with periodontitis are present for months to years before the tooth is eventually lost. Throughout the duration of periodontitis, bacteremia occurs, with the potential for colonization of bacteria at distant sites, including the liver, kidneys, heart, and lungs.

For patients with periodontal disease, the treatment goal is removal of plaque and calculus from the teeth, both supragingivally and subgingivally. General anesthesia is necessary to provide access to subgingival areas, where bacteria can reside and contribute to local and sometimes systemic inflammation. A second and equally important goal is minimization of plaque

reattachment through proper home care and appropriate follow-up treatment.

Periodontal Debridement

Removal of bacterial plaque, endotoxins, and hard calculus deposits is essential to halting the disease process. Home care can be effective in removing supragingival debris when the client is educated to perform the procedures on their pets daily. If oral hygiene is not performed thoroughly, subgingival biofilm will mature and within 48 hours, will contain enough periodontal pathogens to cause gingivitis. Professional clinical care is required to remove pathogens and calculus that harbor bacteria.

Periodontal debridement is the term used to refer to nonsurgical instrumentation that focuses on removal of hard and soft deposits from supragingival and subgingival surfaces of teeth, along with disruption of nonadherent bacteria within the sulcus. The goal of periodontal debridement is to prevent or arrest the infection and restore oral soft tissues to health. Hand and power instruments are used for removing plaque, scaling, root planing, and polishing. The traditional approach to scaling and root planing was based on the belief that bacterial endotoxins were firmly attached to the pitted, irregular surfaces of cementum. Instrumentation with a curette included root planing to remove all damaged layers of cementum, resulting in a glossy, smooth surface that would be less plaque retentive. Current research has shown that endotoxins adhere only lightly to cementum and that removal of the superficial layers of cementum is adequate to achieve the goals of periodontal debridement.

Power Scaling

The use of mechanized instruments for periodontal debridement by using ultrasonic technology was first introduced in the early 1950s to remove foreign material during treatment for caries in human patients. When high-speed air-driven handpieces were introduced shortly thereafter, the ultrasonic application was deemed to be too slow for removal of tooth structure. In 1955, ultrasonic scalers were introduced. The capabilities of the original scalers, with their bulky tip design, were limited to removing supragingival deposits. More definitive scaling was routinely accomplished with hand scalers and curettes. During the 1980s, thinner, probelike tips were developed, and continued advances in technology have expanded their current application to subgingival use. Knowledge of the instrument and of tooth morphology is critical for the safe use of these scalers. No longer considered to be an adjunct to hand instrumentation, ultrasonic scalers are now considered the primary instrument in veterinary practice for use in routine debridement and advanced periodontal therapy.

> ### TECHNICIAN NOTE
>
> When performing periodontal debridement, a cuffed endotracheal tube should be used along with gravity (tipping the nose lower than the rest of the head) to prevent aspiration of fluids and debris.

Power scaling instruments use a water-cooled vibrating tip to remove hard and soft deposits from teeth and periodontal pockets. Vibrations are measured by frequency or the number of times that the tip moves back and forth in 1 second (cycles per second [cps], also called *Hertz* [Hz]). Most units used in veterinary medicine are automatically tuned and have frequencies that are controlled by the unit. Research indicates that when skillfully used, ultrasonic

• BOX 35.5 Benefits of Power Scaling

- Ergonomically superior for reducing hand fatigue and the need for repetitive, intricate hand movements
- Reduces total time patient must remain anesthetized
- Causes less tissue distention than curettes (when slim tips are used subgingivally)
- Causes less root surface damage when used correctly
- Lavage is destructive to bacteria (cavitation, acoustic turbulence, and streaming)

instrumentation is as effective as hand instrumentation. Box 35.5 lists the benefits of power scaling.

Two types of power scalers—sonic and ultrasonic—are categorized by frequency of tip vibrations and the type of power used to create movement at the working end.

Sonic Scaler

The sonic scaler is powered by an air compressor on a dental unit and is attached to the high-speed air line. It operates at a frequency between 2000 and 9000 cps. The tip vibrates in an elliptical pattern, with all surfaces around the diameter of the tip active. The vibrations are audible to the human ear, creating a sound that may be uncomfortable to some operators. Sonic scalers were very popular in the 1990s; however, they have lost favor because of the low frequency. The sonic scaler has less ability to remove heavy, tenacious calculus and is slow to accomplish its task.

Ultrasonic Scaler

Ultrasonic devices use electrical energy that converts the working tip to mechanical energy in the form of rapid vibrations to effectively remove biofilm and calculus deposits. Ranging in frequency from 18,000 to 50,000 cps—above the audible human range—they are more popular and practical for veterinary use compared with the sonic scaler. The ultrasonic scaling unit contains the electronic generator inside a plastic housing. A hose connects the unit to the water supply, which may consist of a portable pressure tank or a quick-disconnect pipe at the sink. A cable attaches the unit to a foot pedal (cordless foot pedals are also now available), and the handpiece is attached by tubing that transports the water to be used as a coolant. A power cord is also attached. Unlike hand scalers that only remove debris with direct contact, ultrasonic scalers provide the additional benefit of a stream of water coming from the tip that acts as a coolant and lavage, flushing debris from the sulcus. The flushing action is destructive to the biofilm by causing acoustic turbulence and cavitation. Acoustic turbulence, also known as *acoustic microstreaming*, is defined as disruption of bacteria in plaque caused by streaming of fluid over the tooth surface or churning of fluid within the confined pocket space. *Cavitation* is defined as the energy that is created from the mist of water. As the water coolant exits the handpiece and strikes the vibrating working end, it creates thousands of water bubbles. These water bubbles implode with enough energy to disrupt bacterial cell walls.

TECHNICIAN NOTE

The transducer converts the electrical energy to mechanical energy. In a magnetostrictive ultrasonic scaler, it may be a metal stack or a ferrite rod. The transducer in a piezoelectric ultrasonic scaler may be a quartz crystal or a ceramic disk.

Safety Precautions

Because water is a necessary part of dental cleaning, appropriate safety precautions must be taken for the safety of the veterinary technician and the patient. To reduce the quantity of aerosolized bacteria, the patient's mouth may be rinsed with chlorhexidine (0.12%) before scaling. This pre emptive rinse may reduce the severity of the bacteremia that invariably occurs during dental cleaning. Another more rapid and efficient option to reduce bacteria and other debris in the oral cavity prior to cleaning would be to use a soft bristled toothbrush and brush all tooth surfaces, followed by a thorough rinsing by using both the air and water buttons on the air/water syringe. This technique will remove most of the plaque and other extraneous material from teeth and give the technician a cleaner area to work with. The veterinary technician and all coworkers in the vicinity of the workstation should wear gloves, masks capable of high bacterial filtration, eye protection such as plastic goggles or disposable face shields, and a gown or scrub top that can be changed after the procedure. The patient's eyes should be lubricated and covered to protect against entry of debris and contaminated fluid. The single most important safety precaution involves intubating the patient and checking to ensure that the endotracheal cuff is fully inflated. The air-tight seal of the cuff should be checked occasionally to prevent the patient from developing aspiration pneumonia. However, care should be taken to avoid excessive inflation of the cuff, which may result in excess pressure on the tracheal lining or a tracheal tear.

Tip Designs

The broad tips are designed for removing medium and heavy deposits, while slim-tip designs allow better access to subgingival pockets and furcation areas. Many practices only use the "universal" tip, which is slower and less effective on supragingival calculus and too large to be effective below the gumline. The use of the board ("beaver tail" or gross removal) tip on the crowns of teeth and the periodontal tips for subgingival cleaning will be more efficient. The "universal" tip can be reserved for use on cats or small dogs with minimal calculus. Approximately 30% to 40% narrower than standard tips, periodontal (slim) tips are approximately 0.5 mm in diameter at the blunt end and are designed to mimic periodontal probes. The slim profile enables easier access to the base of deeper pockets and improves tactility for better detection of calculus. Tips are available in straight and curved designs. Precision tips are available in diameters as narrow as 0.2 mm at the tip for use in advanced periodontal procedures. They are extremely fragile and must be used with a light touch. Another tip option is the diamond-coated tip used with the slow-speed handpiece. If used incorrectly during a nonsurgical procedure, the diamond coating can cause soft tissue damage and excessive loss of tooth substance; therefore this design should be reserved for use during open-flap procedures and should be used only by highly skilled clinicians. Some tips have a built-in light-emitting diode (LED) light (Fig. 35.32). LED technology tends to offer only minimal additional light when used with a good surgical overhead light.

Tips should be checked for possible replacement at least annually or when the metal stacks of the insert become bent or worn down (Fig. 35.33). The tip of piezo scalers wears away with use; it becomes shorter, and the effectiveness of scaling diminishes. Some ultrasonic scaler manufacturers offer a wear indicator card that helps to measure the amount of wearing of the tip (Fig. 35.34). For each millimeter of wear, a 25% decrease in efficiency has been noted. Tips should be discarded when worn down to 2 mm.

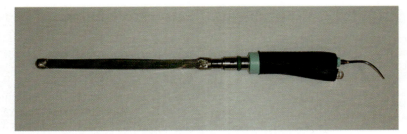

• **Fig. 35.32** Magnetostrictive ultrasonic insert: a metal stack transducer and light-emitting diode (LED) light at the working end.

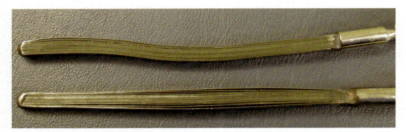

• **Fig. 35.33** Damaged ultrasonic inserts. Magnetostrictive inserts should be discarded when the metal stack becomes bent or splayed.

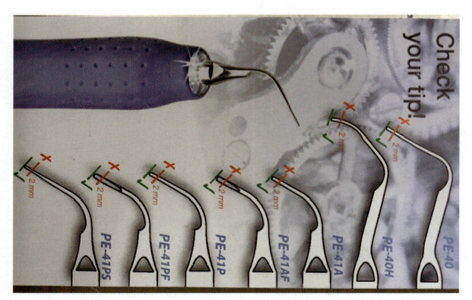

• **Fig. 35.34** The manufacturers of piezoultrasonic scalers have wear indicator cards that helps measure the wearing of the tips. For each millimeter of wear, a 25% decrease in efficiency has occurred. The tips should be replaced when 2 millimeters of wear has taken place.

Energy Dispersion

For hand scalers to be effective, only the sharp cutting edge of the working end must come in contact with the calculus. In contrast, ultrasonic scalers disperse energy over a 360-degree circle around the tip of power instruments. Vibrating activity occurs on the back, face (concave surface), two side (lateral) surfaces, and on the point; however, each surface has varying degrees of vibration, depending on the type of scaler used. Typically, the strongest vibrations are concentrated at the end, 2 to 4 mm from the tip. Veterinary technicians must know the specific type of unit they are working with and must understand the differences in energy dispersal among different tip surfaces to correctly adapt the tip to the tooth for efficient scaling.

Types of Ultrasonic Scalers

Ultrasonic scalers are available in two types—magnetostrictive and piezoelectric. Each type is distinct in its mechanism of action, type of transducer, and direction of tip movement. The transducer is the portion of the handpiece that converts electrical energy into mechanical energy. The magnetostrictive scaler was the most common type of power scaler used in both human and veterinary dentistry but has lost favor to the piezoelectric scalers.

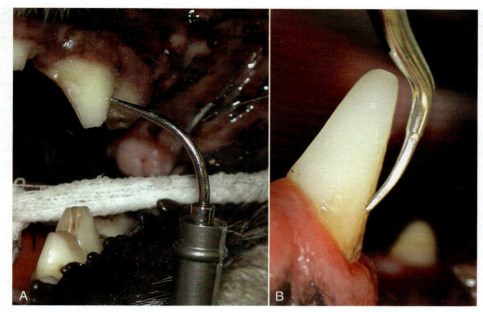

• **Fig. 35.35** (A) The tip of the ultrasonic insert will cause damage if directed at a 90-degree angles to the tooth surface. (B) Correct angulation of the tip. The insert tip should be held at an angle of 0 to 15 degrees from the long axis of the tooth.

The typical magnetostrictive unit has an insert that slides into the handpiece. The insert has two connected parts: the transducer and the working end. The magnetostrictive transducer is a stack of thin nickel alloy metal strips. When a magnetic field is created from the copper coil inside the handpiece, the dimension of the strips is altered by lengthening and shortening, sending vibrations to the tip. Movement of the tip occurs in an elliptical pattern with energy dispersion around the entire diameter of the tip, providing vibrations on all five surfaces. The point of the tip, having the highest power dispersion, can cause damage when directed at a 90-degree angle to the tooth, acting like a jackhammer on hard dental tissue (Fig. 35.35). The face (concave surface) has the next highest powerful vibrations, followed by the back. The two side surfaces have the least powerful vibrations. The back and side surfaces are used most often for scaling, because it is good practice to adapt the surface with the least amount of vibrations that will accomplish the task of debris removal. Magnetostrictive units range in frequency from 18,000 to 42,000 cps (18–42 kHz). Another type of magnetostrictive scaler uses a transducer that is a ferrite rod which produces rotational tip movement. Differences in operation between magnetostrictive units require close attention to manufacturers' recommendations. See Procedure 35.1 for preparation guidelines for a magnetostrictive unit with a metal stack transducer.

TECHNICIAN NOTE

The ultrasonic scaler tip should never be directed at a 90-degree angle toward the tooth surface, because the tip will cause damage to the enamel.

The piezoelectric scaler uses a ceramic disk or quartz crystal as the transducer to produce the straight, linear movement of the tip. Electrical energy causes the disks to alter dimension by expanding and contracting, sending vibrations to the tip at a frequency ranging from 25 to 50 kHz. Because of the back-and-forth motion, the tip is active only on the two lateral surfaces,

forcing the operator to pivot the wrist as the tip is moved around the tooth. If the other surfaces are accidentally adapted to the tooth, the operator will be warned by a different sound and by signs of incomplete removal of debris. Limitations of effective vibrating surfaces cause the piezoelectric scaler to be more technique sensitive compared with other power scalers. The ceramic disk of the transducer is fragile and is easily breakable if the handpiece is accidentally dropped.

Knob Settings and Safety

The power knob adjusts the amplitude—the distance the tip is moving back and forth in one cycle. Greater distance is higher power. Higher power is necessary to remove heavy deposits, while low power is satisfactory for removing plaque. Low power should always be used with thin subgingival tips to prevent the tips from breaking. It is a good principle to use the lowest power setting that will accomplish the task.

The water knob adjusts the flow of water through the handpiece. Because ultrasonic scalers produce heat, fluid must be adequate to prevent pulp damage caused by heat during scaling. Pressure of the water supply line to the unit must measure a minimum of 25 psi (pounds per square inch). A warm or hot handpiece indicates that water pressure is inadequate, and the clinician must immediately stop and adjust by increasing the amount of water and checking the water pressure (if a portable water tank is used). With magnetostrictive units, the water knob should be turned until water exits the tip as a mist, rather than just as a straight stream. Water on the piezoelectric unit should be adjusted to a steady drip when using the periodontal tip below the gumline. The ultrasonic or piezoelectric handpiece should be held using a modified pen grasp. The operator should use a very light touch and let the instrument do the work of removing the calculus from the tooth. Too much pressure on the handpiece can transfer the energy from the instrument to the tooth, resulting in thermal damage and possible death of the tooth.

PROCEDURE 35.1

Techniques for Preparation and Instrumentation When a Magnetostrictive Ultrasonic Scaling Unit Is Used With a Metal Stack Transducer[a]

- Plug the electrical cord into the outlet.
- Run water through the handpiece for a minimum of 2 minutes (each morning) to flush the biofilm from inside the handpiece and cable, draining into the sink.
- Disinfect the handpiece.
- Hold the handpiece upright, perpendicular to the floor, while stepping on the pedal to completely fill the handpiece with water.
- Choose the tip design.
- Remove your foot from the pedal and slide the insert into the handpiece until resistance is met at the rubber "O" ring. Gently twist as the insert is completely seated (if using a metal stack transducer).
- If using a unit with screw-in tip, insert the tip and tighten with the supplied wrench.
- Hold the handpiece parallel to the floor to adjust the power to low-medium and water to a spray. Use the lowest power setting that will accomplish the task.
- Wear gloves, mask, and a face shield or goggles.
- Place gauze or a lap sponge in the back of the patient's throat.
- Protect the patient's eyes (lubricate and cover).
- Check the endotracheal cuff for leakage and make adjustments if necessary.
- Flush the patient's mouth with chlorhexidine (0.12%) or gently brush all surfaces and rinse with the air/water syringe.
- To reduce the pulling weight of the cord, wrap the cord around the forearm or pinky finger or drape over the neck.
- Hold the handpiece lightly with a pen or modified pen grasp.
- Establish a comfortable finger rest.
- Retract the patient's cheeks, tongue, and lips to prevent contact with any portion of the metal tip. A dental mirror is useful for retraction.
- Activate the tip before touching the tooth or calculus.

- Adapt the side of the tip to the tooth in a similar fashion to using a periodontal probe at an angle of 0 to 15 degrees to the tooth.
- With light pressure, move the tip in a sweeping motion as if using a pencil eraser, keeping the end 2 mm of the tip in constant contact with the tooth surface. Use of hard pressure is counterproductive, because this will diminish the vibrations. Vertical, horizontal, or oblique strokes may be used.
- REMEMBER: never hold the point at a 90-degree angle to the tooth, because scratching and gouging of the enamel or cementum may occur.
- Move the tip in a direction beginning on the crown and advancing toward the apex of the tooth to the bottom of the sulcus or pocket. This is opposite to the approach used with hand instrumentation, in which the curette is adapted at the base of the pocket and is moved coronally.
- Assess the surface of the tooth for smoothness by using the tip without activating the vibrations—like using an explorer.
- When encountering stubborn, tenacious pieces of calculus, use light tapping motions against the surface of the calculus or increase the power setting.
- Check for remaining residual calculus by using compressed air from the air or water syringe on the dental unit. Missed calculus will appear chalky white.
- Rinse the mouth with chlorhexidine, flushing any loose debris from tongue, cheek, and lip vestibules.
- If used, remove gauze from the throat, checking for debris before extubation.
- Wipe the unit, handpiece, and cords with a federally approved, nonimmersion type of disinfectant. Follow the manufacturer's instructions for sterilizing the handpiece and tips.

[a]Slight variations may be seen with other types of units; follow the manufacturer's instructions.

Hand Scaling

Periodontal debridement may be accomplished with the use of hand instrumentation. Successful use of hand instruments is dependent on the technician's understanding of instrument design and knowledge of the basic principles of instrumentation.

In general, dental instruments consist of three parts: the handle, the shank, and the working end (see Fig. 35.19). The handle contains the instrument's identification, a description of the instrument with abbreviations that include the name of the designer or the school where it was designed, the manufacturer, the classification type, and the design number. Classifications are determined by the design of the working ends and the intended purpose of the instrument. Examination instruments include probes and explorers. Scaling instruments include curettes, sickles, files, and hoes. Current trends in handles include hollow, lightweight designs that are more efficient in transmitting vibrations detected through tactile sensitivity. Use of wider handle sizes minimizes finger pinching and hand fatigue. Various patterns of surface texture are knurled into the handle to prevent slipping of fingers.

The shank connects the handle to the working end. The curvature of the shank determines the best location within the mouth for use of the instrument. In relation to the long axis of the handle, a straight shank for rostral teeth and an angled shank for caudal teeth (Fig. 35.36). When the shank is bent to form an angle, the terminal shank is the portion below the bend and closest to the working end. The length and diameter of shanks vary; therefore the instrument of choice may depend on the situation for which the instrument is needed. Elongated shanks are useful for accessing deeper pockets and reaching farther caudal in the mouth. A thick, rigid shank is useful for removing heavy, tenacious calculus, because the shank will not flex when pressed against the tooth. Thin, flexible shanks are better suited for removing light calculus deposits or plaque.

The working end of an instrument may be blunt, as in a probe, or pointed, as in an explorer, or it may have sharp cutting edges like those of scaling instruments. An instrument handle may have a single working end or it may be double-ended, with two working ends. The working end of a hand-scaling instrument is called the *blade* and has several parts: the two lateral sides, the face, the back, the heel, and the toe or point (Fig. 35.37A). The face and the lateral surfaces meet to form a cutting edge. The back is formed by the convergence of the two lateral surfaces. Instruments used for supragingival scaling have a pointed tip, while subgingival scalers, known as *curettes*, have a rounded tip. The tip of a curette (known as the *toe*) is designed to minimize trauma to the soft tissue lining the sulcus or the pocket.

The angulation of the face of the blade in relation to the terminal shank classifies the instrument as universal or area specific. To determine this classification, position the instrument handle so the terminal shank is perpendicular to the floor, then identify the face. If the angle between the face and the terminal shank is

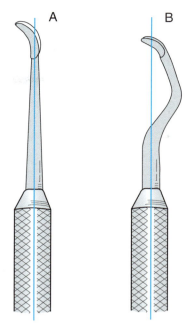

• **Fig. 35.36** (A) A straight shank is best used for scaling teeth in the rostral portion of the mouth. (B) A bent shank is designed for working on premolars and molars. (From Daniel SJ, Harfst SA, Wilder R. *Mosby's Dental Hygiene: Concepts, Cases, and Competencies.* 2nd ed. St. Louis, MO: Mosby; 2008.)

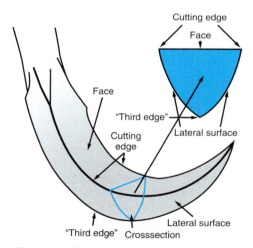

• **Fig. 35.37** The parts of the working end of a hand instrument include the face, cutting edges, lateral sides, back, and toe (tip). (From Darby ML, Walsh MM. *Dental Hygiene Theory and Practice.* 3re ed. St. Louis, MO: Saunders; 2010.)

90 degrees, the instrument is universal—that is, when in use, the handle is placed parallel to the long axis of the tooth and then is slightly tipped left or right to permit either cutting edge to be adapted to the tooth. If the face is offset at an angle of 60 to 70 degrees, as in Gracey curettes, the instrument is considered area specific, and only one of the cutting edges may be adapted to the tooth (Fig. 35.37B).

Supragingival Instruments

Sickle scalers are used to scale the crowns of the teeth. The flat face may be straight or curved lengthwise; the straight lateral surfaces are flat and converge to form a pointed back and tip. When the

cross section of a sickle is envisioned, the instrument is characteristically triangular with 70- to 80-degree internal angles between the face and the lateral surfaces. The sharp tip will cause lacerations if the instrument is used subgingivally; however, it may be used with caution slightly below the gingival margin where the gingiva is spongy and loose enough to permit insertion. Because the sickle is a universal instrument, either cutting edge may be used, depending on how the handle is tipped. Because of the straight side surfaces, the sickle is not conducive to following the curved contours of roots and therefore is reserved for coronal scaling.

> **TECHNICIAN NOTE**
>
> Scalers are designed to be used on the tooth crown, and curettes are designed to be used subgingivally.

When the handle, shank, and blade are on the same plane, the instrument is designed for use toward the front of the mouth. For caudal teeth, the shank will be angled and the instrument will be double-ended to provide mirror images. This style is useful for veterinary patients during scaling of the buccal groove of maxillary carnassial teeth. One working end is contoured for scaling the mesial edge of the groove and the contralateral end contours with the distal edge of the groove.

When the blade is placed against the tooth, the face should be at an angle between 45 degrees and 90 degrees to the tooth surface; however, the ideal scaling angle is between 60 and 70 degrees. The cutting edge is directed to the apical edge of the calculus, lateral pressure is placed against the tooth, and the instrument is used with a short pull stroke to disengage debris.

Subgingival Curettes

Curettes may be used for supragingival scaling, although they are designed for subgingival scaling and root planing. The flat face is curved lengthwise from the heel to the toe, meeting the lateral surfaces to create a cutting edge that extends around the toe. Unlike the flat lateral sides of the sickle scaler that converged to form a pointed back, the sides of the curette are rounded, creating a round back that is easier to insert into a sulcus or pocket. The cross section of the curette is classically shaped like a semicircle, with internal angles of 70 degrees to 80 degrees between the face and the lateral surfaces (see Fig. 35.35).

A universal curette can be adapted for use on all tooth surfaces, while use of an area-specific curette would require several different instruments to scale each tooth in the mouth. Use of area-specific instruments is an advanced concept, and they should be used only by veterinary technicians who understand the inherent design features and possess a thorough knowledge of root anatomy and shape. Incorrect use of an area-specific instrument can cause trauma to hard and soft tissues.

The terms *site specific* and *area specific* are often used interchangeably regarding Gracey instruments, although other area-specific instruments are available. Gracey curettes are designed for use as a set, with each instrument having a complex curvature of the shank for better access to specific teeth. Unlike the universal curette, which is curved only on the plane of the face, the Gracey curette is also curved on the plane of the lateral surface. To help identify the two curved planes, hold the instrument with the terminal shank perpendicular to the floor and view the face at eye level. The face will slope downward, rather than being parallel with the floor and perpendicular to the terminal shank, and the lateral surfaces will be curved to the left or right. This curvature enables adaptation around the contours of roots. As with universal curettes, site-specific curettes have two cutting edges; however, the site-specific curette is unique in that only one edge is designed for use. Before adapting the blade to the tooth, the veterinary technician must confirm that the appropriate edge is chosen. To determine the correct cutting edge, the terminal shank is held perpendicular to the floor to view the honed face from above, enabling the lateral curves to be seen. One cutting edge forms an inner curve; another edge forms an outer curve that appears larger and closer to the floor. The proper cutting edge is always the curve that appears lower and farther from the terminal shank. Unlike universal instruments, which require parallelism of the handle with the tooth, area-specific instruments require parallelism of the terminal shank with the tooth. When in this position against a tooth surface, if the correct edge has been chosen, only the back should be visible. If the face is visible (reflecting light), the instrument is flipped to use the contralateral working end.

> **TECHNICIAN NOTE**
>
> When an area-specific curette is used, the proper cutting edge is the lower edge, as determined by holding the terminal shank perpendicular to the floor. The terminal shank of an area-specific curette is kept parallel to the long axis of the tooth during a vertical scaling stroke. The handle of the universal scaler is kept parallel to the long axis of the tooth during a vertical scaling stroke.

Langer curettes have a combination of universal curette qualities (i.e., they face 90 degrees to shank) with the Gracey curvature of shanks. Langer and Gracey curettes are available with blades that are shorter (mini), which makes them particularly suitable for use on small dogs and cats.

Principles of Scaling

Adaptation of hand-scaling instruments involves the application of the cutting edge against the tooth. Approximately one-third of the cutting edge of the tip should remain in contact with the tooth; constant attention to this detail will prevent damage to the soft tissues as a result of trauma from the tip or the toe (Fig. 35.38). As the curvature of the tooth changes, adjustments must be made to that portion of the cutting edge that is adaptable to the tooth. Use of the thumb against the handle will enable the instrument to be rolled to maintain the contact of the cutting edge around curves.

Angulation refers to the relationship of the face of the instrument to the tooth. When a curette is inserted into a pocket, the angulation of the face should be as close to zero as possible (Fig. 35.39). In this position, the face would be parallel with the root surface, and the back of the blade would be against the soft tissue lining of the pocket. When the blade is positioned at the bottom of the pocket or apical to the intended piece of calculus, the angle should be opened by tilting the handle to the scaling and root planing angle of 45 to 90 degrees—more often between 60 and 80 degrees. Using an angle that is too closed will cause burnishing (smoothing) of the calculus, rather than biting into it for removal. An angle that is too open will place the noncutting edge sharply against the lining of the pocket when a curette is used. This technique is useful if the operator deliberately wants to perform a gingival curettage.

Strokes used when dental procedures are performed will vary depending on the task. With hand scaling, the initial stroke assesses tooth surface topography by lightly feeling for irregularities. This exploratory stroke is also performed with an explorer or with the tip of a power scaler when the power is not activated. When scalers

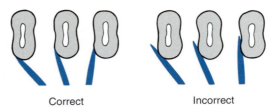

• **Fig. 35.38** Correct adaptation. The lower third of the working end of the instrument must remain in contact with the tooth surface to prevent trauma to soft tissues.

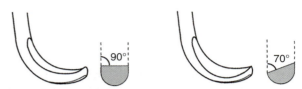

• **Fig. 35.39** Universal versus area-specific (Gracey) curettes. The angle between the face and the terminal shank is 90 degrees on the universal curette and 70 degrees offset on the area-specific curette. Note that one cutting edge is lower when the face is offset. The lower cutting edge is the correct one when an area-specific curette is used. (From Fehrenbach MJ, Weiner J. *Saunders Review of Dental Hygiene*. 2nd ed. Philadelphia, PA: WB Saunders; 2008.)

and curettes are used, once an irregularity is detected, the working stroke is performed by applying lateral pressure against the tooth and pulling the blade vertically, horizontally, or obliquely in a short, controlled stroke. A root planing stroke is longer, and light lateral pressure is used. Apply the minimum number of strokes necessary to accomplish the task.

Sharpening

Thorough periodontal debridement with the use of scalers and curettes can be accomplished only with sharp instruments. Each stroke of a sharp instrument against the tooth will wear away the metal of the cutting edge, causing it to transform from a precise, sharp line at the junction of the face and the lateral surfaces into a dull, rounded surface. Using a dull surface requires heavier lateral pressure against the tooth, reducing tactile sensitivity and creating hand fatigue. The dull surface will burnish the calculus, rather than causing it to be shaved off. Once burnished, this calculus becomes difficult to detect and remove.

Instrument sharpening can be accomplished manually using sharpening stones or with the help of mechanical sharpening devices. Either way, it is critical to have a thorough understanding of the instrument design, including the cross-sectional shape and the line angles between surfaces, to enable a sharp cutting edge to be re-established without creating changes in the instrument's original design.

Sharpening stones typically used for dental instruments include Arkansas, India, and ceramic stones and a synthetic composition, each differing in coarseness. A few drops of lubricant are required on most stones to keep metal particles from embedding into the stone and to reduce heat friction. Lubricate with sharpening oil on the Arkansas and India stones; the ceramic stone can be lubricated with water or used dry; and the composition stone requires water.

Several methods of manual sharpening can be used; however, the technique that requires the instrument to be held stationary while the stone is moved provides an unobstructed view of the blade so that the angle can be precisely controlled. The instrument should be held in a palm grasp, with the blade facing the technician and the face of the blade parallel to the floor. Elbows should be braced against the side of the body for stability, and the procedure should be performed under good lighting that reflects off the face. The stone should be held perpendicular to the face of the blade (Fig. 35.40), beginning at a right angle (90 degrees), and then the stone is tilted against the lateral surface so that the angle opens to 100 to 110 degrees. An angle guide can be purchased or made by using a protractor to aid in visualizing the correct angles.

TECHNICIAN NOTE

When hand instruments are sharpened, the angle between the stone and the face of the blade should be approximately 110 degrees. When sharpening curettes, remember to continue sharpening around the toe.

Using light pressure, the stone is moved in short up-and-down strokes against the lateral surface of the instrument, beginning at the heel of the instrument and working toward the toe, continuing around the toe when sharpening curettes (Fig. 35.41). At the point where sharpening allows the lateral surface to meet sharply with the face of the blade, a black "sludge" will appear on the face of the blade. The step is finished with a few more light strokes, ending with a down stroke of the stone to remove wire particles that have been lifted from the metal.

Sharpening methods that include sharpening of the face should be avoided, because the blade will be weakened and may break during debridement. Instruments that have been oversharpened and are excessively thin should be discarded.

Polishing

Polishing is the final but critical step performed on an anesthetized dental patient as part of routine cleaning or advanced periodontal therapy. During nonroutine dental procedures, such as endodontic therapy or jaw fracture repair, polishing may be the initial procedure performed to remove plaque from the treatment area.

The rationale for polishing teeth in veterinary patients is to smooth the surfaces that have been microscopically scratched during scaling procedures and to remove any extrinsic stains that were not removed with hand or power scalers. Extrinsic stains are discolorations that accumulate on the surfaces from pigments in food, blood, and some antiplaque products, such as chlorhexidine rinses. Intrinsic stains, often seen on the occlusal surface of maxillary molars in dogs, are within the tooth substance and are not removable by polishing procedures. Causes of intrinsic staining include exposure to certain drugs during tooth development (e.g., tetracyclines), trauma, and developmental defects.

The most common method of polishing uses an instrument driven by an electrical motor or an air compressor from a dental unit. A low-speed handpiece is used with a rubber cup. A prophylaxis angle, also called a *prophy angle*, is the attachment that is connected to the handpiece and holds the rubber cup. The cup is available in soft, flexible rubber or firm rubber. Prophy angles may consist of single-use plastic disposable or autoclavable metal. A disposable angle with a soft cup is preferred. The rubber cup can be filled with a polishing paste that contains an abrasive agent available in flour, fine, medium, and coarse grits. Because the act of polishing removes tooth substance, the prophy paste chosen should contain the least abrasive agent that will accomplish the task. Fine or flour pumice is recommended as the grit for a final polish. This grit will ensure the smoothness of the enamel and provide less surface area for plaque to accumulate.

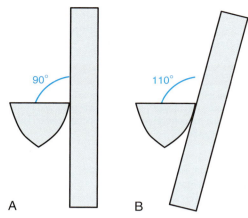

• **Fig. 35.40** (A) Initial setup of a sharpening stone is 90 degrees to the face of the instrument. (B) Open the angle to 110 degrees for sharpening. (From Daniel SJ, Harfst SA, Wilder R. *Mosby's Dental Hygiene: Concepts, Cases, and Competencies*. 2nd ed. St. Louis, MO: Mosby; 2008.)

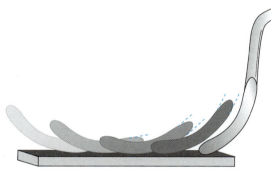

• **Fig. 35.41** To maintain the original design of the instrument, when sharpening curved curettes, begin at the heel, sharpening small sections while working toward the toe. (From Fehrenbach MJ, Weiner J. *Saunders Review of Dental Hygiene*. 2nd ed. Philadelphia, PA: WB Saunders; 2008.)

Friction from the rotating rubber cup creates heat that has the potential to injure the pulp. The handpiece should be used at a low revolutions per minute (rpm) level to minimize adverse effects. Also, adequate paste should be applied, refilling the cup for each tooth, especially when polishing teeth in large dogs. When using a low-speed handpiece without a gauge, the handpiece should be activated to full speed before touching the rubber to the tooth by depressing the foot pedal. The technician should listen for the pitch clues of the rpm level of the low-speed unit and then ease off the pedal to less than one-quarter of the maximum rpm. Light pressure should be used against the tooth—just enough to cause the rim of the cup to flare slightly and polish each tooth surface for only 3 to 5 seconds. The procedure is completed with a gentle rinse with water or chlorhexidine to flush out residual prophy paste from the mouth. Eye protection should be worn by the operator, and the patient's eyes should be protected during the polishing procedure.

Regional Nerve Blocks for Oral Surgery in Dogs and Cats

Regional nerve blocks are essential tools for controlling intraoperative and postoperative pain in dogs and cats during oral surgery. Benefits include pre-emptive analgesia and prevention of "wind-up pain," postoperative analgesia when long-acting anesthetics are used, and decreased concentration of inhalant anesthetic gas needed during the procedure (therefore potentially safer and more cost effective).

Local anesthesia has three basic uses. The term *splash block* refers to wound irrigation directly into an open incision, providing topical anesthesia. *Local anesthesia* refers to infiltration of local anesthetic along planned incision lines or into the periodontal ligament of a tooth of interest. *Regional anesthesia* refers to the delivery of a local anesthetic to specific nerves to block an entire region of the body. Box 35.6 lists materials needed to perform regional nerve blocks for oral surgery. Bupivacaine 0.5% is the most commonly used local anesthetic because of its long duration of action, providing intraoperative and postoperative pain relief. Bupivacaine takes effect in 6 to 10 minutes and lasts from 4 to 8 hours. Lidocaine 2% takes effect in 2 to 5 minutes, and the effect lasts for 30 minutes to 2 hours. The maximum safe dose of bupivacaine is 2.0 mg/kg in dogs and 1.0 mg/kg in cats. Combining lidocaine and bupivacaine is not recommended, because studies have shown reduced efficacy of both drugs when combined. If blocks are required in all four oral quadrants, it is important to keep in mind that the total possible volume should be divided by four to ensure that each quadrant can be effectively blocked. In general, the authors use 0.1 to 0.2 mL of 0.5% bupivacaine for any of the regional blocks described later in cats, and 0.2 to 0.8 mL for a regional oral block in dogs, depending on the size of the patient. Box 35.7 provides an example calculation of four-quadrant nerve blocks in a cat.

Infraorbital Nerve Block

The infraorbital nerve block prevents sensation from the tip of the needle rostrally on the ipsilateral maxilla. The infraorbital foramen is located dorsal to the roots of the maxillary third premolar tooth. The foramen is palpated through the oral mucosa. The needle is inserted through the mucosa into the foramen at the level of the mesial root of the third premolar. The needle is gently redirected if its tip does not advance easily. The needle tip is advanced caudal to the level where the caudalmost extent of oral surgery will be performed, so a 1¼-inch needle is usually necessary in dogs. In cats, the infraorbital canal is shorter and wider; therefore care should be taken to avoid angulation of the needle tip toward the ocular structures. Aspiration should be performed before injecting to ensure that the needle is not in a blood vessel. If blood is aspirated, the technician must reposition and try again or obtain a new needle and syringe. Digital pressure is used over the site after the needle is removed to encourage caudal diffusion and decrease hematoma formation. The foramen is large enough that a 25- or 27-gauge needle can be inserted, with minimal risk of causing damage to the nerve. The extent of the region blocked depends on how far the needle is inserted into the foramen.

Middle Mental Nerve Block

The middle mental nerve block prevents sensation of the ipsilateral rostral lower lip from the labial frenulum rostrally; this block may

also provide decreased sensation of the ipsilateral incisors and canine teeth, although not predictably. The foramen is palpable below the mesial root of the mandibular second premolar in medium- and large-size dogs within the labial frenulum. The foramen is not easily palpable in cats and small dogs. Significant resistance may be felt when the needle is inserted because of the narrowness of the foramen; forceful insertion of the needle should be avoided. Instead, placement of a bleb of anesthetic at the opening of the foramen with a 27-gauge needle is followed by massage of the anesthetic into the foramen. The needle should be inserted into the region of the foramen and infused with the anesthetic. Aspiration should be performed before injecting to prevent intravascular infusion.

Inferior Alveolar Nerve Block

The inferior alveolar nerve block prevents sensation of the soft tissue and bone of the entire ipsilateral mandible. This nerve block has the potential to result in self-trauma to the tongue upon recovery, and patients are not aware of it because they cannot feel self-inflicted trauma when the tongue is numb. This potential complication is rare, but any person who performs nerve blocks should be aware of it. This complication may be avoided by staying close to the medial surface of the mandible and using a small volume of anesthetic to prevent medial diffusion, which results in loss of sensation not only of the inferior alveolar nerve but also of the lingual nerve.

Lidocaine, rather than bupivacaine, may be a good option for this block when the procedure is of short duration and whether the block will be placed in the correct position is a matter of concern. To perform this block, the foramen is palpated intraorally on the medial surface of the caudal mandible. The foramen is caudal and ventral to the mandibular third molar in the dog and caudal and ventral to the mandibular first molar in the cat. In a mid-sized dog, the foramen is approximately 1 cm dorsal to the ventral cortex of the caudal mandible, where the ventral cortex of the mandible curves slightly dorsally. No attempt is made to enter the foramen with the needle; instead, a bleb of anesthetic is placed at the foramen, close to the medial surface of the mandible. Two approaches may be used for placement of this bleb. The intraoral approach involves insertion of a 27-gauge needle along the medial surface of the bone into the region of the foramen. The needle is inserted at a 20-degree angle from the long axis of the mandible approximately 1 cm caudal to the M3 (dog), or 0.5 cm caudal to the M1 (cat). The extraoral approach involves a two-handed technique. Palpate the midpoint of the zygomatic arch between rostral and caudal aspects and move ventrally to the mandible. This should approximate the location of the facial vascular notch on the ventral cortex of the mandible—a dorsal deviation of the ventral cortex of the mandible. A 27- or 25-gauge needle is inserted through the skin at this region (25-gauge may be necessary to penetrate tough skin), staying as close as possible to the medial surface of the mandible. The gloved index finger of the opposite hand is used to feel for the foramen and to assess whether the tip of the needle is in the correct position. The extraoral technique is a good option for beginners, because it allows the operator to feel where the bleb is being deposited.

Maxillary Nerve Block

The maxillary nerve block prevents sensation in the entire maxillary quadrant on buccal and palatal sides of teeth. The same area may be blocked by performing an infraorbital block with a long needle. The approach to the maxillary block is an intraoral

approach using a 27-gauge, 1¼-inch needle on a 3-mL syringe (dog), or a 27-gauge, ½-inch needle on a 1-mL syringe (cat). The needle is bent approximately 1 cm from the tip. The caudalmost aspect of the hard palate is identified just caudal to the maxillary second molar (dog) or the maxillary first molar (cat). The needle is inserted perpendicular to the soft palate just caudal to the molar, approximately ½ cm deep in cats and 1 cm deep in dogs. Care must be taken to avoid inserting the needle too far because of being directly ventral to the eye. Bending the needle 1 cm from the tip provides a reference point as to how far the needle has been inserted. It is important to be careful when bending the needle to avoid creating a rough edge at the tip, which might result in undue trauma when inserted. As with all blocks described here, aspiration should be done on the plunger of the syringe before placement of the bleb to ensure that the needle tip is not in a vessel. Fig. 35.42A–D shows intraoral approaches to the most common regional nerve blocks used in oral surgery.

Periodontal Surgery

A grading system that has been created to categorize periodontal disease helps provide generalizations for appropriate treatment (Box 35.8).
- *Grade I periodontal disease* refers to inflammatory changes confined to the gingiva (gingivitis); this is an easily reversible sign that suggests the need for a routine dental cleaning and increased home care regimens.

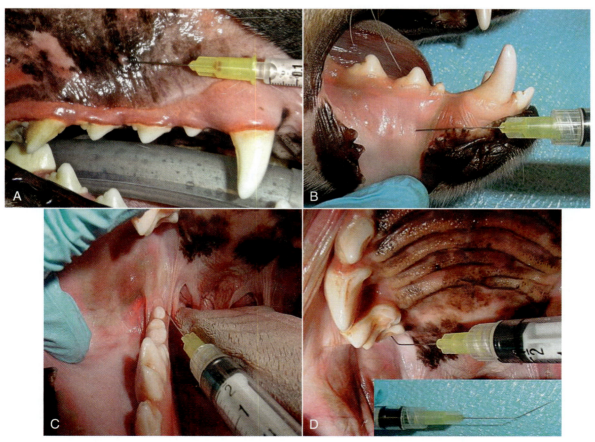

• **Fig. 35.42** Common regional nerve blocks used in dentistry and oral surgery. (A) Infraorbital nerve block. (B) Middle mental nerve block. (C) Inferior alveolar nerve block. (D) Maxillary nerve block (note that the needle is bent 1 cm from the tip).

- *PD 0:* clinically normal
- *PD 1:* gingivitis with no attachment loss
- *PD 2:* less than 25% attachment loss
- *PD 3:* 25% to 50% attachment loss
- *PD 4:* greater than 50% attachment loss

- *Grade II periodontal disease* is an early form of periodontitis in which evidence of loss of attachment is noted, and root debridement or subgingival curettage may be required.
- *Grade III periodontal disease* is considered moderate periodontitis in which 25% to 50% of the attachment structures of the tooth have been lost; root debridement, gingival curettage, and periodontal surgery are often required. Teeth with grade III periodontal disease have a fair to guarded prognosis.
- *Grade IV periodontal disease* is considered severe periodontitis. With attachment loss of 50% or greater, these teeth often require extraction.

Deep periodontal pockets may warrant complex periodontal surgery to be performed by a veterinarian with advanced training. One technique for dealing with unexpected periodontal pocketing in the context of a busy private practice is staging the procedure over two visits. The first visit involves baseline charting, radiography, cleaning, and polishing, along with closed root planing, gingival curettage, and placement of a doxycycline gel, followed by a return visit for more involved periodontal surgery to be scheduled 1 to 2 months later. Doxycycline gel may be placed into a freshly debrided periodontal pocket, provided that the pocket is 4 mm or deeper to allow for retention of the product. Doxirobe (Zoetis, Parsippany-Troy, NJ) is an antibiotic (i.e., doxycycline) mixed with a slowly absorbable polymer that allows delivery of the product in gel form. This treatment provides several beneficial effects. Doxycycline is an antimicrobial with a good spectrum of action against various periodontal pathogens. Doxycycline has anti-inflammatory effects that are beneficial in decreasing damage to periodontal tissues that may be mediated by the response of the immune system to periodontal pathogens. Finally, the space-occupying effect of the polymer prevents the treated pocket from filling with food and debris immediately after the procedure, allowing the site to heal from the most apical aspect coronally. Another product containing clindamycin (Clindoral, Trilogic Pharma, Opelika, AL) is commercially available.

Examination under anesthesia should be performed 2 to 4 months after pocket treatment. Pocket depth should be gently probed once the patient is under general anesthesia. If the pocket depth is normal, no further treatment is necessary, and home care can be continued with routine checkups and periodontal debridement, as necessary. If the abnormal pocket depth is still 5 mm or greater in dogs or 3 mm or greater in cats, periodontal surgery is indicated if the client would like to save the affected tooth. A variety of periodontal surgical procedures have been documented; each technique is appropriate in different situations. Creation of a flap and open root planing usually are necessary with pocket depths of 5 mm or greater. In the past, periodontal disease was considered irreversible; however, with advances in surgical technique and materials, periodontal disease is now considered reversible if dealt with before severe damage to the periodontium occurs. Without proper postoperative home care, the condition will invariably recur. Pets with advanced periodontal disease may require periodontal debridement every 3 to 4 months until evidence suggests that the disease is controlled. A periodontitis treatment decision tree is provided in Fig. 35.43.

Vertical bone loss and horizontal bone loss represent two vastly different challenges in periodontal surgery. Vertical bone loss occurs along the long axis of the tooth root and is easier to deal with than widespread horizontal bone loss, wherein multiple furcations are exposed. After debridement of the vertical infrabony defect, an osteoconductive or osteoinductive material may be placed in the defect. Osteoconductive materials will not induce new bone but rather, will act as scaffolding for new bone cells to traverse the defect. In contrast, osteoinductive materials stimulate progenitor cells of osteoblasts to differentiate and form new bone in an area. In veterinary dentistry, an example of an osteoconductive product is Consil (Nutramax Laboratories, Edgewood, MD). An example of an osteoinductive material is Osteoallograft (Veterinary Transplant Services, Kent, WA). These products generally require a means of retention, which may be an absorbable or nonabsorbable membrane or flap that is repositioned in a coronal location to hold the material once placed. Any foreign material may contribute to continued infection, so the placement site must be adequately debrided before placement of these products is considered. Lavaging the surgical site with 0.12% chlorhexidine, followed by lactated Ringer solution to minimize the cytotoxic effects of chlorhexidine, is appropriate. The flap is closed with 4-0 or 5-0 absorbable monofilament suture material placed interdentally in a simple interrupted pattern, and digital pressure is applied to the gingiva for 60 seconds. Occasionally, a sling suture may be used to provide a purse-string effect to encourage the gingival portion of the flap to reattach. The patient should be placed on a soft food diet with no hard toys or treats for 2 weeks, and antibacterial mouth rinses (0.12% chlorhexidine) may be prescribed. The owner should begin brushing the animal's teeth 1 week postoperatively by using the modified Stillman technique (described in the next section) at the surgery site.

TECHNICIAN NOTE

Attempts to save teeth with advanced periodontal surgery should not be made unless the client is able to perform daily brushing of the animal's teeth.

Home Care

Client communication regarding dental home care is an important veterinary technician skill. The technician will spend time with the client to demonstrate brushing techniques and to provide recommendations for various diets and products that can be used at the patient's home to reduce accumulations of plaque and calculus. Reduction of bacteria in the mouth can be accomplished through brushing, proper diet, and use of toys.

The mechanical cleansing provided by daily tooth brushing provides the most thorough method of plaque control for pets. Several methods may be used; the most widely accepted is the Bass technique, which concentrates the bristles along the gingival margin and in the sulcus (see Fig. 35.44). With a soft toothbrush, the bristles are directed at a 45-degree angle toward the gingival margin so that some of the bristles enter the sulcus while other bristles are resting on the tooth adjacent to the margin. While pressing lightly, short back-and-forth strokes are used and the 45-degree angle maintained for 5 to 10 seconds before repositioning the brush along the next group of teeth.

The modified Stillman technique is sometimes used in areas of periodontal surgery to minimize plaque accumulation while

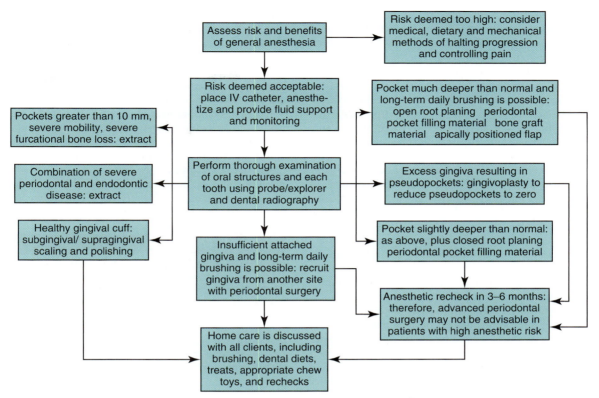

• **Fig. 35.43** Decision tree for patients with periodontal disease.

preventing trauma to the reattaching gingival tissue (see Fig. 35.44). This technique involves placement of the bristles apical to the gingival margin with a gentle sweeping motion in the coronal direction against the gingiva and crown of the tooth, without placing the bristles into the healing sulcus.

Brushing should be initiated at a young age to allow the patient to become accustomed to oral care. Before a toothbrush is introduced, the puppy or the kitten should be given gum massages so that the animal has the experience of the mouth being manipulated. Veterinary patients are reluctant to keep their mouth open, so it is best to brush while the animal's mouth is closed, gaining access to teeth by gently lifting the lips. This brushing technique should be performed with the bristles rinsed in water rather than covered with a veterinary dentifrice (toothpaste), as the animal patients may try to eat the brush if its bristles are covered with dentifrice.

When brushing is completed, the dentifrice can be applied into the mouth as a treat and to confer enzymatic or antiseptic benefits. Many human toothpastes contain xylitol which is toxic to dogs and therefore should not be used. The client should be instructed to prioritize brushing the areas that collect the heaviest debris (usually the buccal surfaces of the caudal teeth) in case the patient becomes uncooperative before the task is completed, and then to move to lingual and palatal surfaces as the patient allows.

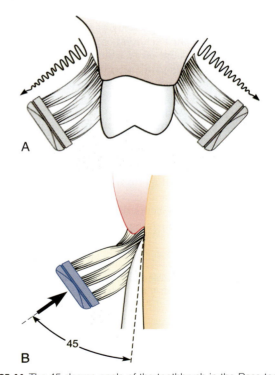

• **Fig. 35.44** The 45-degree angle of the toothbrush in the Bass technique aims the soft bristles toward the gingival margin and into the sulcus. Use short back-and-forth motions without dislodging the bristles from the sulcus. Gentle pressure should elicit blanching of the gingival tissues. In the modified Bass technique, the Bass method is followed by gentle rolling of the bristles over the coronal portion of the teeth. ((A) From Newman MG, Takei H, Klokkevold PR, et al. *Carranza's Clinical Periodontology.* 9th ed. St. Louis, MO: Saunders; 2002. (B) From Newman MG, Takei H, Klokkevold PR, et al. *Carranza's Clinical Periodontology.* 11th ed. St. Louis, MO: Saunders; 2012.)

TECHNICIAN NOTE

The Bass technique of tooth brushing places the bristles of the brush at a 45-degree angle against the tooth along the gingival margin to enable some bristles to slide into the sulcus. The Stillman technique is used in areas of periodontal surgery where bristles apical to the gingival margin are moved with a gentle sweeping motion in the coronal direction against the gingiva, without placement of bristles into the healing sulcus.

Feeding a diet of soft food that adheres to tooth surfaces may contribute to periodontal disease. Plaque control can be augmented by feeding a dental diet that has been manufactured and tested to reduce accumulations. The Veterinary Oral Health Council (VOHC) was established in 1997 by veterinary dentists and researchers to recognize products that have been shown to meet predetermined standards for plaque and calculus retardation. The VOHC seal of acceptance is issued to products that have proven to reduce plaque and/or calculus based on generally accepted protocols. (For a complete list of VOHC-approved products, visit www.VOHC.org.)

Diets reduce accumulation through mechanical or chemical action. The first dental diet was created to take advantage of mechanical cleansing. Long fibers within large pieces of kibble oriented in one direction help keep the biscuit from crumbling readily when a dog or a cat bites into it. This design allows the kibble to mechanically scrape the sides of teeth clean as the teeth penetrate the biscuit. An example of a chemical used to control calculus is hexametaphosphate, which works by sequestering the calcium in plaque fluids to reduce formation of calculus by preventing mineralization of plaque. Use of dental diets alone is generally not as effective as tooth brushing. A regimen that combines special diets with tooth brushing is recommended for optimal plaque control.

Many home care products, including treats, rinses, and water additives, are available. Veterinary technicians should assess each product before offering recommendations to their clients. During home care instructions, the veterinary technician should also offer counseling regarding toys that may be harmful to pets' teeth. Rawhide has an excellent cleansing action; however, the size and shape of the product must be correctly matched with the chewing habits of the dog. Rawhide should be taken away after 20 to 30 minutes of gnawing to decrease the likelihood of gastrointestinal problems caused by ingestion of a large piece. Allowing the partially chewed rawhide to harden overnight will minimize the chance that the pet may encounter gastrointestinal or choking problems associated with ingestion of a large piece of rawhide.

The mandible of a dog does not move side to side, so when a dog chews on a very hard object, there is risk of tooth fracture caused by the shearing action. Many toys found in pet stores, including cow hooves, hard nylon bones, antlers, and natural sterilized bones, are harmful to pets' teeth and can cause dental fractures. Aggressive chewing of tennis balls causes abrasion of teeth, especially when dirt and sand become incorporated within the outer coating of the ball. Clients should be instructed to always monitor their pets when providing chew toys.

TECHNICIAN NOTE

A safe toy or chew should be flexible and be easily bent with one's hands. It should also be soft enough to indent with a fingernail.

Exodontics

The AVDT's position statement states: "Extraction of teeth is considered oral surgery and should not be performed by a veterinary technician; however, it is important that the veterinary technician understand the process to better assist the veterinarian during the surgery." (See www.AVDT.us for the complete statement.)

Although attempts should be made to save teeth whenever possible, extraction (exodontics) or oral surgery is necessary when the prognosis for the affected teeth is grave and when financial constraints or medical conditions prevent multiple anesthetic

episodes that may be necessary to salvage these teeth. Extraction of a tooth with severe periodontal disease may be straightforward if many of the attachment structures of the tooth have been lost; however, because of the large root surface area of canine or feline teeth, their extraction can be challenging. The extraction process begins with placement of a regional nerve block to decrease inhalant anesthesia requirements.

Possible complications should be discussed with the owner before the procedure is begun. Complications include those associated with anesthesia, hemorrhage, ocular trauma, jaw fracture, and displacement of a root into an inaccessible area, such as the nasal passage. Iatrogenic jaw fracture can occur easily when diseased mandibular first molars or mandibular canine teeth are extracted in cats and small-breed dogs, especially when significant periodontal disease already exists.

TECHNICIAN NOTE

Per AVMA and AAHA 2019 Dental Guidelines: "extraction of teeth is oral surgery and should only be performed by a licensed veterinarian…" These positions directly supersede state practice acts as of 2019. The American Veterinary Dental College (AVDC) and the Academy of Veterinary Dental Technicians (AVDT) position statements indicate that dental extractions are oral surgery and should only be performed by a veterinarian. The veterinary technician's role in oral surgery is to have the proper equipment ready, place the regional nerve block, take preoperative and postoperative dental radiographs, retract tissue, and assist in hemostasis.

TECHNICIAN NOTE

A pet's tooth should not be extracted without the direct permission of the client. Always obtain a contact phone number to discuss any unexpected findings.

TECHNICIAN NOTE

Regional nerve blocks used during extractions not only lower inhalant requirements but also provide postoperative pain relief.

Closed Extractions

All oral surgery should be done with a regional block in place, and a pre-extraction radiograph of the tooth should be taken to assess for evidence of root pathologic conditions that may affect the surgical approach. A closed technique is best reserved for single-rooted teeth and for teeth that have severe periodontal disease. Once the regional nerve block has been placed, the gingival attachments around the tooth are separated with a periosteal elevator, a dental luxator, or a scalpel blade. After the soft tissue attachments have been severed, a dental elevator of appropriate size and shape is placed in the periodontal space on the mesial or distal surface of the crown. Once placed in the space, gentle pressure is placed to seat the elevator within the tooth, and the alveolar bone and the handle of the elevator are rotated slightly to stretch the periodontal ligament fibers. If elevation is done correctly, the tooth will be observed to move slightly when the elevator is rotated. Pressure is held for 10 seconds. Then the elevator is advanced apically and rotated against the root in the opposite direction to create pressure, and pressure is held again. The goal is to fatigue the periodontal ligament and prevent tooth root fracture. Larger elevators are used as the periodontal ligament breaks down, which allows more room for placement of a larger instrument. The temptation to wiggle the elevator to obtain a deeper position in the periodontal space should be avoided, because this will often cause breakdown of the alveolar bone and loss of leverage. The elevator may also be placed on the palatal or lingual surface and the vestibular surface within the periodontal space to stretch periodontal ligament fibers around the entire circumference of the tooth. Elevators come in a variety of shapes and sizes, and it is important to have access to assorted sizes for different situations. When a dental elevator is grasped, the handle should rest securely in the palm of the hand. The index finger should be extended so that if the elevator slips, the finger will help stop the advancing of the elevator into deeper structures (Fig. 35.45). Ocular trauma and brain trauma have been documented in cases where dental elevators have slipped during extraction procedures. To prevent this, forces used must be well controlled and should be generated in the lateral, medial, or coronal direction, rather than in the apical direction. The gingival tissue is apposed to close the extraction site with 4-0 or 5-0 monofilament absorbable suture in a simple interrupted pattern. Sterile extraction packs containing the necessary instruments should be prepared for use.

Surgical Extractions

As a result of the large surface area and the multirooted nature of carnivore teeth, surgical extraction is often a less traumatic option than attempts to remove a firmly rooted tooth with closed extraction. As with closed extraction, gingival attachments are separated from the tooth crown with a periosteal elevator, a dental luxator, or a scalpel blade. A flap is created depending on the location and the underlying root structure. The type of flap created should provide optimal access and tension-free tissue closure while inflicting the minimum amount of soft tissue trauma.

Once the flap is raised, a round carbide burr is used in a water-cooled high-speed handpiece to create a window in the buccal bone of roots to be extracted. Multirooted teeth are separated with a tapered fissure burr. Once the window is created

and roots are sectioned, minimal force is necessary to gently pry the roots and attached crown segments from their sockets. Once the roots have been removed in their entirety, rough bone edges are smoothed with a large, round diamond burr. The alveolus of each root is curetted and lavaged with sterile isotonic solution or 0.12% chlorhexidine. The flap is closed with 4-0 or 5-0 absorbable monofilament suture in a simple interrupted pattern.

Occasionally, osteoconductive or osteoinductive products may be placed in the alveolus before closure if it is suspected that the product will not act as a nidus; they will help prevent significant bone loss in the area of the extraction. A postextraction radiograph should be taken to document complete removal of roots in cases where the roots were not retrieved easily.

When a root fractures, additional instruments will be needed to retrieve the retained tooth root. Root tip elevators and root tip forceps are valuable tools in root tip retrieval (Fig. 35.46). Care should be taken to prevent dislodgement of the root tip into the nasal passage or the mandibular canal. Cotton-tipped applicators are helpful for controlling hemorrhage in the alveolar socket to allow visualization of the root tip. Blowing air from an air or water syringe into the socket should be avoided. Although this may facilitate visualization of the root, a fatal air embolism may occur. The pet should be given no hard food or treats for 14 days postoperatively. Postoperative antibiotics generally are not necessary after extraction procedures.

Advanced Dental Procedures

Endodontics

Endodontics is a subspecialty of dentistry that deals with the treatment of the inside of the tooth (pulp) and periapical tissues. This treatment is reserved for veterinary dentists or veterinarians with additional education and experience.

Periapical tissue is located around the tip (apex) of the tooth root. The tooth pulp consists of nerves, blood vessels, lymphatics, and connective tissue. Pulp tissue is found in the pulp chamber

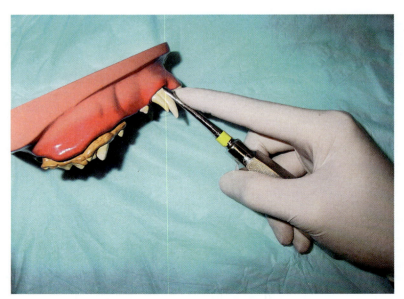

• **Fig. 35.45** Proper grasp of a dental elevator. The index finger is extended to minimize soft tissue trauma if the elevator should slip.

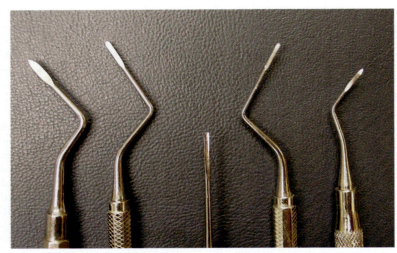

• **Fig. 35.46** Root elevators in various shapes and sizes. These instruments are fragile and should be used with minimal force as they will quickly be damaged.

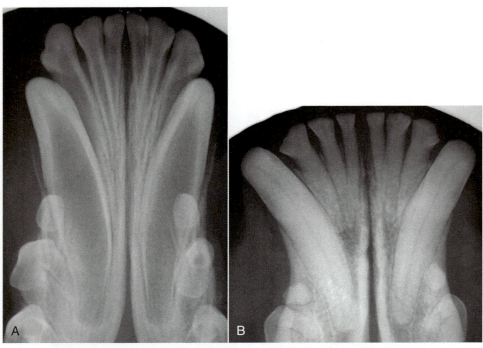

• **Fig. 35.47** Radiographs of the immature permanent teeth of a 6-month-old dog (A) and of the permanent teeth of a 6-year-old dog (B). Note that the secondary dentin produced in the older dog has strengthened the tooth and narrowed the pulp chamber and root canal.

(crown) and root canal (root) of the tooth and enters the tooth through numerous small openings in the apex of the tooth root, called the *apical delta*.

The dental pulp is important for the development of the tooth in a young animal. It supplies nutrients needed by the odontoblasts to deposit secondary dentin. This makes the walls of the root and crown thicker so that the tooth is stronger. The root apex should be closed once the dog or the cat is 10 to 18 months of age. As the animal continues to age, the pulp chamber and canal will become smaller, because odontoblasts will continue to produce secondary dentin, which makes the tooth stronger (Fig. 35.47).

Treatment options for teeth with endodontic disease depend on the age of the animal, the duration of endodontic disease, and the anatomy of the tooth. Conventional root canal therapy is usually performed on dogs and cats 12 months of age and older with endodontic disease. Treatment involves removing dead or dying pulp tissue from the tooth, disinfecting and shaping the root canal, and filling the canal (obturation) with an appropriate material to seal the apex from periapical tissues. Radiography is necessary to ensure that a proper apical seal has been achieved. Teeth that have undergone pulp death become more brittle over time, because they lack the hydration that was originally provided by the pulp tissue. A good history should always be taken to try to determine how the pet fractured the tooth. Inappropriate chew toys in the environment should be removed. A metal crown may be indicated to minimize the likelihood of repeat fracture of the tooth. Endodontically treated teeth should be assessed radiographically at least yearly. There are specific instruments that are associated with endodontic procedures (see Box 35.9).

Restorative Dentistry

Restorative dentistry is the subspecialty of dentistry that restores or maintains the structure and function of a tooth. No restorative material is as strong as the original tooth structure, so an attempt is always made to preserve as much of the original tooth as possible. Indications for restorative dentistry include teeth with dental caries (cavities), fractured teeth, and endodontically treated teeth.

Metal or zirconium crowns are placed on fractured teeth to protect the tooth, especially in working dogs or in cases where repeated tooth trauma is expected. Crowns are most placed in dogs on the canine and maxillary fourth premolar teeth (Fig. 35.48).

Specific Conditions in Dogs and Cats

Tooth Resorption

Tooth resorption is common in cats and becoming a more common finding in dogs. The thought is that with more radiographs

---

• **BOX 35.9** **Endodontic Instrument and Materials Setup**

- Dental radiography
- High-speed handpiece and burrs
- Barbed broaches
- Endodontic files and file organizer
- Rubber stops
- Endodontic ruler
- Canal lubricant, irrigant, and irrigation needles
- Paper points
- College pliers
- Zinc oxide, eugenol
- Glass slab, mixing spatula
- Gutta percha points
- Lentulo, paste fillers
- 10:1 reduction gear contra-angle
- Pluggers and spreaders
- Heating instrument
- Restorative materials and instruments

---

being taken, more pathology is being found. Prevalence studies have found that 20% to 70% of cats are affected by this problem, depending on the population of cats and the investigative methods employed. The lesions are usually appreciated clinically at the cervical portion of the tooth (the junction of where the crown meets the root, sometimes referred to as the "neck" of the tooth), which is often hidden by the gingiva. However, recent histologic studies have found that these lesions begin on the root surface, and radiographic changes can often be seen before a clinical lesion becomes obvious. When a lesion develops at the gingival margin, the adjacent gingiva often covers these lesions with a combination of hyperplastic gingiva and granulation tissue (Fig. 35.49A). There are five stages of tooth resorption, based on the amount of the tooth affected and three types based on the structure of the root. (See https://avdc.org/avdc-nomenclature/ for a complete set of drawings and photos of tooth resorption; search under Teeth Abnormalities and Related Procedures.)

A fine explorer should be used to check for irregularities, as described earlier in this chapter. In the past, restorations have been placed in lesions, but follow-up studies have shown poor long-term results with restoration. Therefore extraction or crown amputation is the treatment of choice. The choice is dependent on dental radiography findings. Dental radiography is necessary to evaluate the severity of resorption and to guide treatment.

Sometimes, it is not possible to perform a complete tooth extraction because of severe root resorption, in which a portion of

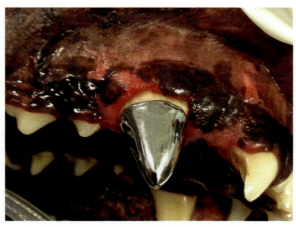

• **Fig. 35.48** A full metal jacket crown has been placed over an endodontically treated maxillary canine tooth.

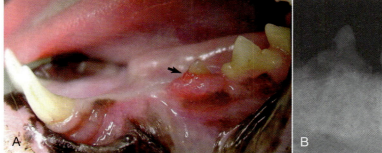
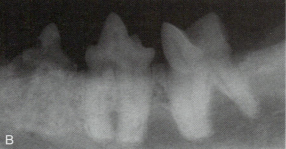

• **Fig. 35.49** (A) Photograph of a mandibular third premolar affected by idiopathic feline tooth resorption *(arrow)*. (B) Radiograph of the left mandible using the paralleling technique. The mandibular left third premolar has undergone significant root replacement resorption, as seen by decreased root density and loss of the normal periodontal space.

the root has been replaced by a reparative bone-cementum material. When this occurs, the tooth root becomes incorporated into the adjacent alveolar bone. Radiographic evidence of this is seen by loss of periodontal ligament space and decreased root density, approximating that of surrounding bone density (see Fig. 35.49B).

When this radiographic appearance is seen in the absence of periodontal or endodontic disease, it is possible to perform a crown amputation, during which hard tissue with characteristics of tooth root is removed, and resorbed root that has been replaced by bone is not removed. The tooth crown and the coronal root segment are removed with a dental burr and a high-speed handpiece. The crestal alveolar bone is smoothed with a dental burr, and the gingiva is closed with absorbable suture over the crown amputation site.

Orthodontic Problems

Malocclusions

Four classes of malocclusions are used. Class I malocclusion occurs when the maxillary and mandibular jaw lengths are normal, but one or more teeth are in an abnormal position. Class I malocclusions are the most common type of malocclusion receiving orthodontic correction in pets. Common examples of class I malocclusions are lingually displaced (base-narrow and/or in-standing) mandibular canines, anterior cross bite, and lance canine teeth. When the mandibular canines are displaced lingually, they often cause occlusal trauma to the palatal mucosa and/or gingiva because of their long crown height. Severe cases can result in complete penetration of the palatine process of the maxillary bone and/or the incisive bone, resulting in an oronasal fistula.

A rostral cross bite occurs when closed-mouth examination reveals that one or more maxillary incisors are positioned lingual to the mandibular incisors. A caudal cross bite occurs when one or more maxillary premolar or molar teeth are positioned lingual to the opposing mandibular premolar or molar (Fig. 35.50). It is important to evaluate the entire dentition and jaw length relationships if proper classification is to be made, because clinical presentations similar to those described earlier can occur as a result of abnormalities in jaw length rather than abnormalities in tooth position. The remaining classes refer to skeletal malocclusions associated with jaw length discrepancies.

A class II malocclusion is also referred to as *distoclusion*, *overjet*, or *overshot*, and sometimes is incorrectly referred to as an *overbite* (Fig. 35.51). In a class II malocclusion, the mandible is relatively shorter than the maxilla; this can be the result of an abnormally long maxilla (maxillary prognathism) or an abnormally short mandible (mandibular **brachygnathism**). The AVDC-accepted term for this occlusion is *mandibular distoclusion*.

A class III malocclusion is also referred to as *mesioclusion*, *underjet*, or *undershot*, and sometimes is incorrectly referred to as an *underbite* (Fig. 35.52). In a class III malocclusion, the maxilla is relatively shorter than the mandible; this can be the result of an abnormally long mandible (mandibular prognathism) or an abnormally short maxilla (maxillary brachygnathism). The AVDC-accepted term for this occlusion is *mandibular mesioclusion*.

Mandibular mesioclusion is an accepted breed standard of some breeds, including Boxers, Boston Terriers, Bulldogs, and Pugs. Therefore malocclusions in brachycephalic breeds are referred to as *normal class III occlusions*.

A general understanding of these terms allows veterinary professionals and personnel to communicate with breeders and pet owners who may use lay or other scientific terms to describe a

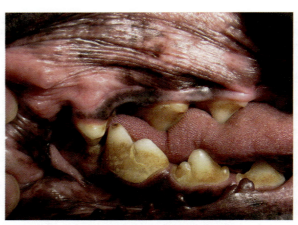

• **Fig. 35.50** Caudal cross bite. The mandibular first molar is buccal, or vestibular, to the maxillary fourth premolar. This may result in abnormal accumulation of plaque and calculus on the buccal surface of the mandibular molars, increasing the need for brushing in this area.

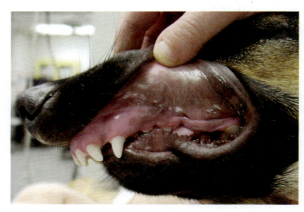

• **Fig. 35.51** Class II malocclusion (mandibular distoclusion). The mandible is relatively shorter than the maxilla, which results in palatal trauma from the mandibular canine and sometimes mandibular incisor teeth.

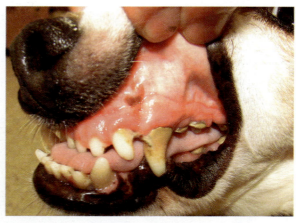

• **Fig. 35.52** Class III malocclusion (mandibular mesioclusion). The maxilla is relatively shorter than the mandible, which may result in attrition of the teeth or trauma to the mandibular mucosa beneath the tongue.

malocclusion. A detailed study of occlusion is necessary before orthodontic treatment for pets or counseling breeders on the role of genetics in malocclusion is considered. Although the genetics of malocclusion in dogs and cats has not been fully elucidated, skeletal malocclusions (class II–IV) are of genetic origin, and some class I malocclusions (e.g., lance canines in Shetland Sheepdogs) are considered to have a genetic component.

The shape of a dog's or a cat's skull must be evaluated when a dental occlusion evaluation is performed. Three types of skulls are recognized: **brachycephalic**, **mesaticephalic** (or **mesocephalic**), and **dolichocephalic**. Brachycephalic breeds have wide skulls with a short maxillae. Examples of these breeds are Boxers, Bulldogs, and Persian cats. Mesaticephalic breeds have well-proportioned skull width and maxillary length. Examples include Beagles, Labrador Retrievers, and German Shepherds. Dolichocephalic breeds have narrow skulls and a long maxillae; examples include sight hounds (Greyhounds, Whippets) and Siamese cats.

Wry bite is a nonspecific term for a form of unilateral maxillary-mandibular asymmetry in which one segment of the jaw is disproportionate to the other segment (e.g., the left mandible is longer than the right mandible). The disproportionate jaw length can occur in the maxilla or the mandible, resulting in what appears to be a curvature of the jaw toward the shorter side.

Impressions and Models

Impressions and models are important in treatment planning of orthodontic disease and in creation of orthodontic devices and restorations. Veterinary technicians and dental assistants can play an important role in obtaining impressions and pouring stone models. Stone dental models also serve as a part of the medical record for documentation of the starting point and of treatment progress.

Alginate is the material that records the imprint of the teeth when full-mouth impressions are taken. Teeth should be cleaned before impressions are taken. A dental impression tray of appropriate size is selected for the patient. Impression trays for dogs and cats can be purchased or fabricated. Once the negative alginate impression is removed from the mouth, dental stone is used to make the positive image of the mouth.

Interceptive Orthodontics

Interceptive orthodontics involves the extraction of persistent deciduous or adult teeth that are causing or will cause problems associated with malocclusion (Fig. 35.53). Interceptive orthodontics can be extremely beneficial, and abnormally erupting permanent teeth sometimes will correct after extraction of retained deciduous teeth. The most important factor determining success with this treatment is early detection of the problem. Many puppies and kittens have completed their vaccination series by the time they reach this mixed dentition stage and will not be seen again before spaying or neutering unless a dental examination can be scheduled to ensure that early orthodontic problems do not go undetected.

Persistent deciduous teeth can occur in any breed of dog or cat, but they are seen most in small-breed dogs, such as Yorkshire Terriers, Poodles, and Dachshunds. Deciduous teeth should have been shed before eruption of their permanent counterparts. When persistent (previously and mistakenly referred to as *retained*) deciduous teeth are identified, they should be extracted before they cause misalignment of their permanent counterparts. Most permanent teeth will erupt lingual or palatal to the retained deciduous teeth, with one exception. Maxillary canine teeth erupt mesial to the persistent deciduous teeth. This is noteworthy, because misalignment will decrease the space between the maxillary canine and the third incisor tooth, where the mandibular canine occludes. When this space is too narrow, one or both maxillary teeth will interfere with the mandibular canine tooth, and tooth wear (attrition) can occur.

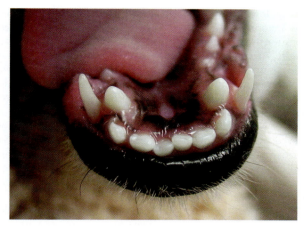

• **Fig. 35.53** Persistent deciduous teeth may contribute to orthodontic (linguoverted or base-narrow permanent canine teeth) and periodontal problems.

Extraction of persistent deciduous teeth is a challenge because of their long, thin roots, which can fracture easily. The goal is to remove the entire tooth root to provide space into which the permanent tooth can move. The immature jaw contains numerous developing permanent tooth buds that can be damaged by dental elevators. Clients should be cautioned about the possibility of permanent tooth damage or discoloration during extraction of deciduous teeth. A skilled veterinary dental surgeon can minimize these complications significantly.

Base-narrow or In-standing Mandibular Canine Teeth

Lingually displaced mandibular canine teeth may result from deciduous teeth that do not exfoliate properly, but other factors may play a role, including the genetics responsible for the development of normal mandibular width. These malocclusions can be corrected by orthodontics in most cases, but clients must be willing to invest the time and expense necessary to clean the oral appliance and return for rechecks as needed. Orthodontic treatment generally is more expensive than tooth extraction and involves additional anesthetic procedures. Orthodontics can be an important treatment option when alternatives to extraction of large teeth, such as canine teeth, are considered.

Crown height reduction, along with partial pulpectomy and direct pulp capping under sterile conditions, may be an option for animals with malocclusions. This combination of procedures entails shortening the tooth to remove the interference it is causing with another tooth or surrounding soft tissue. This method is less invasive than extraction, removes the animal's source of discomfort, and achieves results more rapidly than orthodontic movement. However, it does permanently alter the appearance and, to some degree, the function of the tooth. The pulp chamber is exposed when the crown height is reduced, and a small percentage of these teeth may become nonvital after this procedure.

Dental Trauma

Dogs and cats can generate large quantities of biting, pulling, and grinding forces, and their teeth are often subjected to dental trauma. This trauma can be exhibited as wear (attrition or abrasion), uncomplicated tooth fracture (no pulp exposure), or complicated fracture (pulp exposure).

Many dogs will cause severe abrasion of their teeth by chewing on inappropriate objects, such as rocks or fences. The teeth most often fractured are canines and maxillary fourth premolar teeth. Attrition and abrasion usually occur on incisors and canines but can be seen on premolars and molars. If dental wear occurs slowly, odontoblasts will deposit tertiary (reparative) dentin within exposed dentinal tubules to prevent pulp exposure as enamel and dentin are lost. Tertiary dentin may be seen on the surface of worn teeth as brown or black dots. A dental explorer is moved over the tooth surface to ensure that the pulp tissue is not exposed. When the pulp tissue is exposed, the tip of the dental explorer will fall into the pulp chamber as it crosses the surface of the tooth, while tertiary dentin feels smooth as glass with the explorer.

In acute fractures with pulp exposure, the tooth may bleed from the exposed pulp surface. If the tooth is treated within the first 48 hours, vital pulp therapy may be successful. This procedure involves removing the coronal pulp tissue (the pulp tissue in the tooth root remains), covering the pulp tissue with a medicament, and sealing the coronal exposure site with appropriate dental restorative materials.

All teeth with exposed pulp tissue should be treated with endodontic treatment (conventional root canal, vital pulp therapy) or by extraction. If left untreated, infection from the exposure site will spread to the periapical tissues and over time, a periapical abscess will develop. The client may notice ipsilateral facial swelling (Fig. 35.54) or a draining tract just below the medial canthus of the pet's eye. Most periapical abscesses will not form a fistula through the skin; this means that unless the teeth of these pets are examined for endodontic disease, many abscesses will go untreated. These abscesses can be painful and serve as sources of infection which can spread to other areas of the body.

Discoloration is another sign of endodontic disease; it is commonly seen as a result of prior trauma to the pulp, resulting in pulpitis (Fig. 35.55). Ninety-two percent of discolored teeth show evidence of partial or complete pulp necrosis on exploratory pulpotomy. Because dogs and cats do not articulate their discomfort, evidence of pulpitis warrants endodontic or exodontic therapy to relieve possible pain in a tooth affected by pulpitis.

TECHNICIAN NOTE

A tooth with pulp exposure requires endodontic treatment or extraction. A "wait and see" approach is not appropriate, because dogs and cats hide their level of discomfort.

Oral Neoplasia

Oral tumors account for only 6% of all cases of neoplasia in dogs and 3% to 12% in cats; these tumors are often aggressive, and prognosis depends on early detection. The most common oral tumor in cats is squamous cell carcinoma (SCC), which accounts for approximately 70% of all oral tumors in cats (Fig. 35.56). If a cure for SCC is to be achieved, early detection is particularly important in smaller patients (cats and small dogs) because of the need to obtain clean surgical margins while maintaining adequate function.

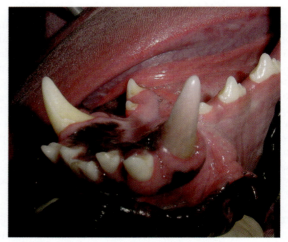

• **Fig. 35.55** Discoloration of the left mandibular canine tooth from pulpitis (inflammation of the tooth, often the result of blunt trauma).

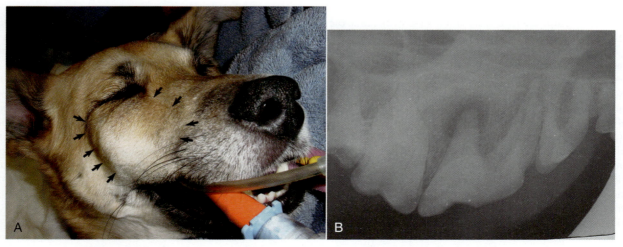

• **Fig. 35.54** (A) Facial swelling associated with a periapical abscess of the right maxillary fourth premolar tooth *(arrows)*. (B) Radiograph shows severe periapical lucencies (bone loss at the root tips as a result of infection).

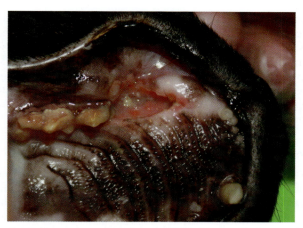

• **Fig. 35.56** Squamous cell carcinoma (SCC) of the maxilla in a cat. Note the lack of a distinct mass but rather, just an area of ulceration and tooth loss. SCC accounts for approximately 70% of oral tumors in cats.

TECHNICIAN NOTE

Squamous cell carcinoma (SCC) accounts for approximately 70% of oral tumors in cats.

In dogs, tumors may be benign or malignant. The most common benign tumor in dogs is a gingival tumor which, in the past, has been referred to as an *epulis* (plural: *epulides*). The epulides were categorized as fibromatous, ossifying, and acanthomatous; the latter is the most locally invasive. Fibromatous and ossifying epulides are also referred to as *peripheral odontogenic fibromas*. Acanthomatous epulis is now referred to as *canine acanthomatous ameloblastoma*. Peripheral odontogenic fibromas do not typically invade bone and usually do not recur if the tooth of origin and its periodontal ligament are removed (Fig. 35.57A). Canine acanthomatous ameloblastoma requires removal of the tumor with a minimum of 1 cm of normal tissue in all directions to prevent recurrence (see Fig. 35.57B). Most oral tumors are not entirely responsive to chemotherapy or radiation, but canine acanthomatous ameloblastoma often responds to radiation. Surgery (mandibulectomy or maxillectomy) is often the treatment of choice as a result of the documentation of the development of malignant tumors at the site of radiation being reported with this tumor type.

The most common malignant oral tumors in dogs are malignant melanoma, SCC, fibrosarcoma, and osteosarcoma. These tumors are locally invasive and have the potential to metastasize to regional lymph nodes or to the lungs. After staging to determine the extent of disease, surgery or radiation is usually recommended to deal with the primary tumor, and metastases are dealt with by chemotherapy, radiation of metastatic nodes, or immunotherapy. Malignant melanoma may be pigmented or amelanotic (lacking in melanin). Dogs and cats that undergo radical maxillectomy and mandibulectomy for removal of an oral tumor generally function well postoperatively, and most clients are pleased with their pets' long-term quality of life and appearance. Cats recover more slowly from maxillectomy and mandibulectomy, and often require placement of a feeding tube (usually an esophagostomy tube) during the recovery period, whereas dogs usually eat and drink within 24 hours after surgery.

Stomatitis

Diffuse inflammation of the entire oral cavity is seen commonly in cats and occasionally in dogs. Inflammation confined to the gingiva

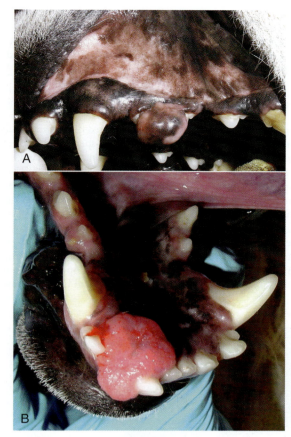

• **Fig. 35.57** (A) Peripheral odontogenic fibroma (also referred to as an *ossifying epulis*) in a dog. (B) Acanthomatous ameloblastoma in a dog (previously referred to as *acanthomatous epulis*). Acanthomatous ameloblastoma is locally invasive but does not metastasize, making these patients good candidates for surgery if margins are attainable.

is referred to as *gingivitis*. Inflammation that extends beyond the mucogingival junction is called *stomatitis* (Fig. 35.58). Stomatitis may result from a variety of causes, including ingestion of a caustic substance, uremia, viral exposure, plant foreign bodies, allergic response to drugs, and, most commonly, immune-mediated causes. Cats are often affected by a type of stomatitis referred to as *gingivostomatitis*, which can involve gingiva, alveolar mucosa, buccal mucosa, sublingual mucosa, and even the mucosa of the caudal oral cavity lateral to the palatoglossal folds. Cats often have decreased appetite or anorexia, halitosis, dehydration, and blood-tinged saliva.

The cause of stomatitis is not clear, but it appears that cats develop inappropriate inflammation in the presence of even small amounts of plaque accumulation. Many cats with stomatitis concurrently shed both herpesvirus and calicivirus. These viruses may influence the immune system, resulting in an overzealous or deficient immune response to bacterial plaque. Therefore plaque control in the form of frequent dental cleaning and home care is important. Unfortunately, many cats with stomatitis are in so much pain that home care is not feasible. Immunosuppressive agents, such as corticosteroids and cyclosporine, help in many cases, but when medical therapy fails or causes unacceptable side effects, full-mouth extractions or nearly full-mouth extractions have been shown to provide resolution of oral discomfort in approximately 80% of cases. In dogs, stomatitis may be caused by autoimmune diseases, such as pemphigus vulgaris or bullous pemphigoid.

Masticatory Myositis

Masticatory myositis is an immune-mediated disease in which the immune system forms antibodies toward a specific component of myosin found only in muscles of mastication. Pets affected by this disease may be seen in the acute phase of the disease, which is painful, or in the chronic phase of the disease, where much scarring has already taken place. Patients in the acute phase often exhibit pain upon mouth opening, decreased appetite, or dropping of food. They often have swelling of the temporal, masseter, and/or pterygoid muscles, which occasionally may also cause exophthalmos. Patients in the chronic phase often have severe temporal and masseter muscle atrophy and inability to open the mouth as a result of severe scar tissue formation. The goal is to diagnose the

disease before these chronic changes occur, because this condition is difficult to deal with in the chronic phase. A diagnosis is made by sending serum and muscle samples to the Comparative Neuromuscular Laboratory at the University of California, San Diego (San Diego, CA). Treatment at the acute phase involves a long, slow taper of oral corticosteroids, beginning dogs at an immunosuppressive dose of 1 mg/kg twice daily. To prevent recurrence, some patients need to take some level of steroids for life.

Jaw Fractures

Jaw fractures are common in dogs and cats that have experienced motor vehicle trauma, high-rise syndrome, or severe periodontal disease resulting in a pathologic fracture. Most jaw fractures benefit from some type of rigid fixation. One of the most common types of jaw trauma is symphyseal separation, in which the right and left mandibles separate at their rostral fibrous union, called the *symphysis*. A cerclage wire placed behind the canine teeth for no longer than 4 weeks provides stability while the symphysis heals (Fig. 35.59A and B).

More involved jaw fractures may be repaired with the use of interdental wire and acrylic composite, transosseous wiring, miniplates, external fixation, or maxillomandibular fixation. Sometimes, teeth along the fracture line can be used as anchor points, but teeth affected by severe periodontal disease should be removed, because the fracture likely will not heal when the diseased tooth acts as a nidus for infection.

Patients that present acutely with a mandibular fracture may benefit from placement of a tape muzzle (Fig. 35.60) to stabilize the fracture until surgical treatment is performed. The tape muzzle is created by using one piece of tape (adhesive side outward) around the muzzle itself, which is attached to a second piece that wraps around the head below the ears. The muzzle should be tight enough to minimize motion but loose enough to prevent irritation of the soft tissue and to allow the tongue to move between the incisor teeth for drinking and eating food of a slurry consistency. Tape muzzles are sometimes considered the definitive treatment of choice in young patients for whom rigid fixation may adversely affect growth of the healing mandible.

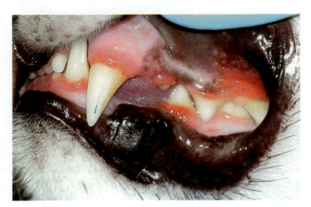

• **Fig. 35.58** Stomatitis in a cat. Inflammation extends beyond the gingiva into the alveolar mucosa; often, the buccal mucosa lateral to the palatoglossal folds is also inflamed.

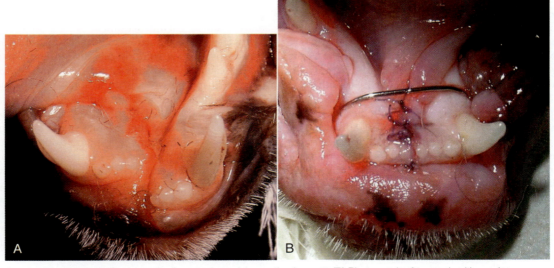

• **Fig. 35.59** (A) Photograph of a symphyseal separation in a cat. (B) Photograph after repair with cerclage wire.

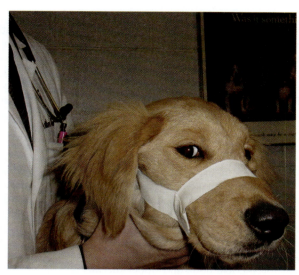

• **Fig. 35.60** Tape muzzle for stabilization of a mandibular fracture in a young dog.

Equine Dentistry

Dental Anatomy and Physiology

Horses have 24 deciduous teeth and 36 to 44 permanent teeth, depending on the presence or absence of canine and first premolar teeth. At eruption, the occlusal surfaces of equine teeth are fully covered by cementum compared with dogs and cats, in which cementum covers only the root. A thin layer of crown enamel is present beneath the crown cementum. Both layers get worn away, exposing an intricate, wavy combination of cementum, dentin, and enamel on the occlusal surface.

Equine mandibular incisor teeth develop features of their occlusal surface that have been traditionally used to estimate age. However, because much variation is seen in the rate of tooth wear based on breed, type of food, and environment, the age of the horse determined via this technique is an estimate at best. Eruption times provide the most accurate method of determining age but can be used only in horses in which their complete permanent dentition has not erupted.

Of all changes on the occlusal surface of the incisors, the appearance of the dental star is one of the more reliable features. The dental star is composed of dentin, and the position of the star moves from the lingual edge of the occlusal surface to the center as the horse ages. The Galvayne groove, a groove that appears on the labial surface of the third incisor in some horses more than 10 years of age, was once considered to be an excellent method of determining the age in horses 10 to 30 years of age. It has since been established that its presence is inconsistent and is of little value in determining the age of a horse.

The canine teeth are usually absent or rudimentary in female horses, but males typically have four permanent canine teeth that erupt at 4 to 6 years of age in the **diastema** between the incisors and cheek teeth. The permanent first premolars, which are referred to as "wolf teeth," are much smaller and located rostral to

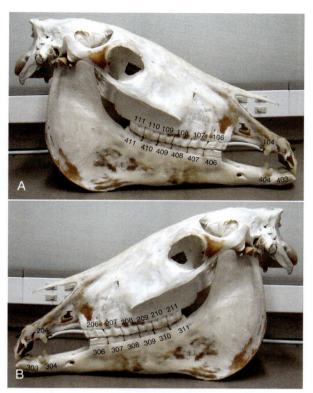

• **Fig. 35.61** Skull of a horse showing the modified Triadan tooth numbering system. (A) Right side. (B) Left side. Wolf teeth, when present, end in the numbers "05."

the other premolars. The first premolar has no deciduous precursor. Wolf teeth are present in 24.4% of female horses and 14.9% of male horses. Wolf teeth occur more commonly on the maxilla. These teeth are often extracted because of concern for causing oral discomfort, especially when the bit contacts the tooth. The premolars and molars are collectively referred to as "cheek teeth." Not including the wolf teeth, each quadrant should contain six cheek teeth (second, third, and fourth premolars, and first, second, and third molars).

A numbering system that is based on the modified Triadan system has been developed for equine teeth (Fig. 35.61). Cheek teeth are closely arranged, with no spaces in between them, so the six teeth in one quadrant function as a single unit. The occlusal surfaces of cheek teeth have many grooves and ridges composed of enamel, cementum, and dentin, which provide varied surfaces for grinding food material. The upper jaw is wider than the lower jaw—a condition referred to as *anisognathism*. The occlusal surface is normally angled at 10 to 15 degrees in a downward slope toward the buccal aspect of the teeth. In horses with painful dental disease or in those fed an inappropriate diet (too little forage), this angle may be increased, resulting in more vertical angulation of the occlusal surface. This condition is termed *shear mouth*.

In horses, the left and right mandibles are not separated by a symphysis, as in dogs and cats. In the horse, the mandibles fuse at the midline at approximately age 3 months. In contrast to carnivores, the temporomandibular joint is designed for horizontal movement, and the muscles necessary to provide this movement are more developed. On the tops of their heads, dogs and cats have large temporal muscles that provide strength in vertical movement of the mandible, whereas horses have well-developed masseter and pterygoid muscles that allow horizontal grinding movement.

Horses have well-developed muscles of the lips that allow them to prehend food, and the commissure of the lips is positioned rostrally, making examination of the caudal cheek teeth challenging.

Common Dental Problems of Horses

Endodontic abnormalities occur because of disease of the inner chamber of the tooth, which is most commonly seen in the form of a tooth root abscess. Tooth root abscesses occur as a result of exposure of the pulp to the oral environment or death of a tooth, with hematogenous spread of bacteria to the compromised site. Pulp exposure may occur due to tooth fracture, excessive wear, or decay. Tooth root abscesses may cause a large swelling of the surrounding bone and soft tissue (Fig. 35.62).

The caudal maxillary tooth roots (fourth premolar and first, second, and third molar) are located just ventral to the maxillary sinus, so infection of any of these teeth may lead to sinusitis and

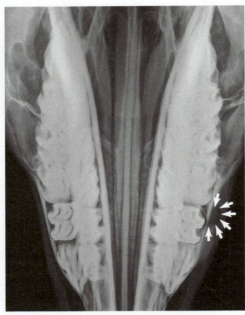

• **Fig. 35.62** Radiograph of a horse with facial swelling caused by a periapical abscess. Arrows point to bone loss associated with an infected maxillary third premolar.

chronic unilateral nasal discharge. Infection caused by a tooth root abscess will not permanently resolve with administration of antibiotics, although antibiotics may provide temporary improvement. Extraction or endodontic therapy is necessary for long-term success. Extraction is often difficult because of limited access and the large amount of subgingival tooth structure. Although incisors, wolf teeth, and canines can usually be extracted via an intraoral technique, cheek teeth most often need to be approached through extraoral techniques such as buccotomy or repulsion.

Orthodontic abnormalities refer to those abnormalities of occlusion (the normal spatial relationship of teeth and jaws) caused by abnormal development, eruption, or wear. Mandibular brachygnathism or mandibular distoclusion (commonly called "parrot mouth") is a developmental disorder in which the lower jaw is relatively shorter than the upper jaw. One goal of treatment is to prevent or minimize the degree of abnormal tooth wear that can occur from malocclusion. Orthodontic procedures can be performed to prevent or correct ventral deviation of the incisive bone and upper incisors and to attempt to overcome the jaw length discrepancy early in life, while growth is still occurring. The opposite of parrot mouth is referred to as "monkey mouth," occurring when the maxilla is relatively shorter than the mandible (resulting from maxillary brachygnathism or mandibular mesioclusion). This condition is seen most in miniature horses.

Horses with jaw length discrepancies require more frequent occlusal adjustments, but any horse should be evaluated at least yearly for abnormal wear patterns. *Floating* is the term used to describe the process of mechanically adjusting the occlusal surfaces of teeth. Flat files or floats (Fig. 35.63) are available in hand and electrically driven versions and are used to remove raised areas, such as hooks, ramps, or points. Removal or loss of a tooth can result in drift of adjacent teeth into the vacancy, leading to abnormal occlusion patterns. Similarly, the tooth from the opposing arcade may overgrow into this void because of lack of normal wear. Patients with these problems will require more frequent examinations and occlusal equilibrations as necessary (Box 35.10).

Another orthodontic problem seen in foals is wry nose. *Wry nose* is a deviation of the incisive bone, maxilla, and nasal septum laterally from the midline. Affected foals may have difficulty suckling or prehending forage, and they display dyspnea resulting from deviation of the nasal septum that can be so severe that a tracheostomy may be necessary. This is believed to be a hereditary condition most seen in Arabians and miniature horses. Orthognathic

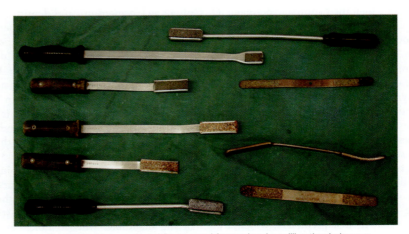

• **Fig. 35.63** Various dental floats used for occlusal equilibration in horses.

• **BOX 35.10** **Suggested Schedule for Routine Dental Examination of Horses**

- *Birth:* examine for malocclusions and congenital defects affecting the tongue, lips, and palate.
- *6–8 months:* examine for eruption of incisors, check occlusion, remove sharp points or hooks if present (float teeth).
- *16–24 months:* examine for presence of wolf teeth, ulcers, points, or hooks; float if necessary.
- *2–3 years:* examine for presence of wolf teeth, bit injuries, deciduous eruption, points, or hooks. Remove wolf teeth; float if necessary.
- *3–4 years:* examine size and shape of jaws; check for retained third premolars, blind wolf teeth, bit injuries, points, or hooks. Remove wolf teeth, caps; float if necessary.
- *4–5 years:* examine all teeth for proper eruption, occlusion, and presence of cysts; remove deciduous teeth and hooks; float if necessary. Remove tissue of cyst structure if present.
- *5+ years:* evaluate jaw excursion; examine mouth for hooks, abnormal wear patterns, periodontal disease, dental decay. Correct uneven wear patterns, float teeth; shorten incisors if necessary.

Adapted from Easley KJ. Equine dental development and anatomy. Proc Am Assoc Equine Pract. 1996;42:1.

surgical correction often requires two separate surgeries and usually is attempted at ages 5 and 7 months.

Periodontal abnormalities refer to loss of or damage to the attachment structures of teeth, which consist of the periodontal ligament, cementum, alveolar bone, and gingival connective tissue. Gingivitis is one of the earliest signs of periodontal disease; gingiva may appear hyperemic, edematous, and bleed more readily than normal. Gingival recession may be seen or loss of periodontal ligament attachment may result in development of a periodontal pocket. Although the cause of periodontal disease in horses is like that described for dogs and cats earlier in this chapter, treatment is challenging because of limited accessibility of cheek teeth in horses. The tooth-cleansing process associated with mastication of abrasive substances is an important part of keeping teeth periodontally sound. Therefore any dental pathologic condition, such as abnormal wear and oral ulceration, should be corrected to prevent preferential use of certain teeth and disuse of others. Depending on their accessibility, deep periodontal pockets may be debrided and lavaged. Off-label use of a canine doxycycline gel (Doxirobe) has been described to deal with periodontally affected teeth that have not lost enough attachment to require extraction; teeth with severe attachment loss and mobility require extraction.

Cemental hypoplasia is a developmental abnormality that can occur in all equine teeth and may predispose the maxillary cheek teeth to endodontic disease, tooth fracture, abnormal occlusal patterns, and caries. Caries are a result of tooth decay caused by bacterial fermentation of food. When a carious lesion occurs within the infundibulum (the infoldings of the occlusal surface of incisors and cheek teeth) of a tooth, this is referred to as *infundibular decay*. Restoration of these lesions with composite filling material has been advocated by some equine dentists, but treatment is controversial.

TECHNICIAN NOTE

Infundibular decay in horses is most likely to affect the maxillary first molar tooth.

Recommended Readings

Baker GJ, Easley J. *Equine Dentistry*. 2nd ed. Philadelphia, PA: Elsevier; 2005.

Beckman B, Legendre L. Regional nerve blocks for oral surgery in companion animals. *Compend Cont Educ Pract Vet.* 2002;24:439.

Bellows J. *Small Animal Dental Equipment, Materials and Techniques: A Primer.* Ames, IA: Blackwell; 2004.

Berg ML. *Companion Animal Dentistry for Veterinary Technicians.* Minneapolis, MN: Bluedoor, LLC; 2020.

DuPont GA, DeBowes LJ. *Atlas of Dental Radiography in Dogs and Cats.* St. Louis, MO: Saunders; 2009.

Gawor J, Niemiec B. *The Veterinary Dental Patient—A Multidisciplinary Approach.* Hoboken, NJ: Wiley Blackwell; 2021.

Harvey CE, Emily PP. *Small Animal Dentistry.* Philadelphia, PA: Mosby; 1993.

Holmstrom SE. *Veterinary Dentistry for the Technician & Office Staff.* Philadelphia, PA: Saunders; 2000.

Holmstrom SE. *Veterinary Dentistry: A Team Approach.* St. Louis, MO: Saunders; 2013.

Lobprise HB, Dodds JR. *Wigg's Veterinary Dentistry: Principles and Practice.* Philadelphia, PA: Lippincott-Raven; 2019.Nield-Gehrig JS. *Fundamentals of Periodontal Instrumentation.* 6th ed. Baltimore, MD: Lippincott Williams & Wilkins; 2008.

Niemiec BA. *A Color Handbook of Small Animal Dental, Oral and Maxillofacial Disease.* London, UK: Manson; 2010.

Niemiec BA. *Veterinary Endodontics. Practical Veterinary.* San Diego, CA: Publishing; 2011.

Reiter AR, Lewis JR, Okuda A. Update on the etiology of tooth resorption in the domestic cat. *Vet Clin North Am Small Anim Pract.* 2005;35:913.

Perrone JR. *Small Animal Dental Procedures for Veterinary Technicians and Nurses.* Hoboken, NJ: Wiley Blackwell; 2021.

Rieter AM, Garcis M. *BASVA Manual of Canine and Feline Dentistry and Oral Surgery.* Gloucester, UK: BSAVA; 2018.

Verstraete FJM. *Self-Assessment Colour Review of Veterinary Dentistry.* London, UK: Manson Publishing; 1999.

36

Geriatric and Hospice Care: Supporting the Aged and Dying Patient

MARY ELLEN GOLDBERG AND KRISTINA L. ROTHERS

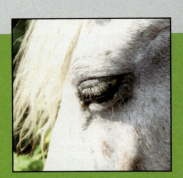

CHAPTER OUTLINE

LEARNING OBJECTIVES

When you have completed this chapter, you will be able to:

1. Pronounce, define, and spell all key terms in the chapter.
2. Discuss the aging process and explain when dogs and cats are geriatric.
3. Identify and explain changes seen in various body systems as dogs and cats age.
4. Identify cognitive impairment and how it might influence geriatric pet behavior.
5. Discuss the management of quality of life as pets age.
6. Discuss what is involved in a geriatric wellness program.

7. Explain hospice and palliative care, including pain management and physical rehabilitation for the geriatric patient.
8. Explain the nursing care of the geriatric patient, including hydration, assisted nutrition, bladder and fecal hygiene, and mobility assistance.
9. Discuss companion animal death and dying.
10. Explain the changing nutritional needs of aging pets.
11. Discuss components of hospice nursing care for geriatric dogs and cats, including identifying the appropriate time to discuss euthanasia with a pet's owner.
12. Discuss components of the physical examination of a geriatric horse.
13. List and describe disorders commonly seen in geriatric horses, including oral/nasal, vision, cardiac, respiratory, gastrointestinal, kidney, skin, neurologic, and orthopedic problems.
14. Identify and explain the chronic conditions that most commonly affect geriatric horses, such as pituitary pars intermedia dysfunction (PPID), equine odontoclastic tooth resorption and hypercementosis (EOTRH), heaves, laminitis, dental problems, sinusitis, equine recurrent uveitis (ERU), and neurologic and musculoskeletal defects.
15. Discuss geriatric horse management, nutrition, and nursing care, including end-of-life issues.

KEY TERMS

Animal hospice
Anosmia
Anterior uveitis
Assistive devices
Cachexia
Cognitive dysfunction
Corneal edema
Decubitus ulcers
Degradation
DISHA
End of life
Enucleation
Frailty
Fungal ulcers
Geriatrics
Gerontology
Heaves

Hirsutism
Hospice
Hypertrichosis
Hyphema
Hypopyon
Hyposmia
Incontinence
Laminitis
Neovascularization
Pain
Palliative care
Quality of life
Sarcopenia
Senescence
Subpalpebral lavage system
Wave mouth

GERIATRIC DOGS AND CATS

Introduction

Gerontology is the study of the aging processes and individuals as they advance from middle age through later life. **Geriatrics** is the study of health and disease in later life.

Hospice care is designed to support individuals in the final phase of a terminal illness, with a focus on comfort and **quality of life** (QOL), rather than cure. Goals include making patients comfortable and pain-free to live each day as fully as possible.

Palliative care is specialized medical care for animals living with serious illnesses. This type of care is focused on relief from the symptoms and stress of a severe illness to improve QOL for both the patient and the family.

Although these are definitions for human patients, they can also be applied to veterinary patients. Advances in veterinary medicine have enabled animal patients to live longer, allowing the veterinary technician to study the care of patients through their different life stages and become familiar with the physical, mental, and emotional changes that occur.

As veterinary patients age, they experience **senescence** (the condition or process of deterioration with age), characterized by decreased function and **degradation** (decreased function and degeneration of organ systems) of their bodies. These changes cause a slow decline and can lead to functional issues, such as reduced fine motor control and weakness. The aging process is not a disease process but is a decline in reserves and strength and other changes in body systems, increasing the likelihood of disease development. Clinical issues that present would be decreased proprioception and muscle atrophy.

Clients with geriatric animals will likely be concerned with QOL issues, such as mobility, **pain** level, fecal and urinary continence, appetite, and maintenance of human-pet interaction within the household. These issues can be further complicated by behavioral changes, or **cognitive dysfunction**. Treatment for the geriatric patient entails addressing such issues as pain while taking care to avoid exacerbation of weakness and cognitive impairment; improving mobility and function; and addressing medical and nursing care issues. Creating a geriatric wellness program is beneficial.

TECHNICIAN NOTE

Medical issues commonly encountered in geriatric patients include obesity, degenerative joint disease (DJD), neoplasia, and endocrine disease. Aging can be compounded by cognitive dysfunction and quality of life (QOL) issues, such as mobility changes, pain, fecal and urinary **incontinence**, appetite changes, and maintenance of human-pet interactions within the household.

The Aging Process

Aging is a term that refers to a complex set of biological changes that result in a progressive reduction in the ability to maintain

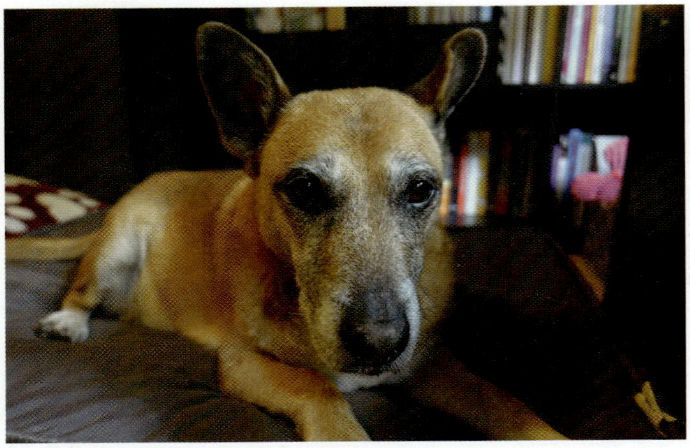

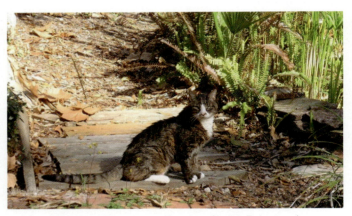

• **Fig. 36.1** Geriatric dog; note gray facial hair and loss of facial muscle mass. (Courtesy Sheilah Robertson.)

• **Fig. 36.2** Geriatric cat. (Courtesy Sheilah Robertson.)

TABLE 36.1	Comparison of Canine Age With Human Age			
Dog's Age (Years)	0–20 lb	21–50 lb	51–90 lb	>90 lb
5	36	37	40	42
6	40	42	45	49
7	44	47	50	56
8	48	51	55	64
9	52	56	61	71
10	56	60	66[a]	78[a]
11	60	65	72[a]	86[a]
12	64	69[a]	77[a]	93[a]
13	68	74[a]	82[a]	101[a]
14	72[a]	78[a]	88[a]	109[a]
15	76[a]	83[a]	93[a]	115[a]
16	80[a]	87[a]	99[a]	123[a]
17	84[a]	92[a]	104[a]	
18	88[a]	96[a]	109[a]	
19	92[a]	101[a]	115[a]	

[a]Geriatric.

Adapted from Tomlinson J. AARP for Our Patients. *Proceedings from STAAR Conference 2016.* Florham Park, NJ, April 14–17, 2016.

homeostasis when exposed to internal physiologic and external environmental stresses. These changes ultimately lead to decreased vitality, increased disease vulnerability, and death. The rate at which an individual cat or dog exhibits signs of aging may be influenced by breed, size, genetic makeup, exposure to injuries and disease, physical environment, stress, and nutritional status (Figs. 36.1 and 36.2).

When Are Dogs and Cats Considered to Be Senior or Geriatric?

Veterinary professionals consider dogs to be senior at an earlier age than pet owners do. Small, medium, and large dogs are considered seniors around the age of 7 years by veterinary professionals. Giant-breed dogs have shorter lifespans and are seniors as early as age 5 years. Most veterinary professionals consider cats senior at age 9 and geriatric at age 13 (Tables 36.1 and 36.2).

Longevity is characterized by a long lifespan during which an individual is generally healthy and free from severe disease. Genetics, breed, disease predisposition, lifestyle (sedentary versus active), socioeconomic factors, and nutrition (overweight versus underweight) all influence an animal's lifespan. Remember:

- Mixed-breed dogs have a longer life expectancy than purebred dogs.
- Obese dogs have shorter lifespans than animals that are not obese.

- Castrated dogs live longer on average than those that are not castrated.
- Pet dogs living inside live longer than dogs that are housed outside.
- All of the above applies to cats, too!

Typical factors for aging processes are progressive and irreversible. All the processes can be accelerated by stress, environment, genetics, side effects of various diseases, premorbid and comorbid conditions, malnutrition, and lack of mobility and exercise.

> **TECHNICIAN NOTE**
>
> Small, medium, and large dogs are in the senior life stage at age 7 years. Small and medium dogs are geriatric at 11 years and large dogs at age 9 years. Giant-breed dogs are senior pets at age 5 years and geriatric at age 7 years. Cats are senior pets at age 9 years and geriatric at age 13 years.

Physiologic Changes Associated With Aging

A study conducted by the American Veterinary Medical Association (AVMA) in 2015 concluded that the significant physical and functional changes that occurred in aging patients fell into the following categories:

1. Behavioral changes: changes in sleep cycle, responses to verbal commands, and interactions with family and other pets

<table>
<tr><th colspan="3">**TABLE 36.2**   Comparison of Feline Age With Human Age</th></tr>
</table>

Life Stage	Age of Cat	Human Equivalent
Kitten Birth to 6 months	0–1 month 2–3 months 4 months 6 months	0–1 year 2–4 years 6–8 years 10 years
Junior 7 months to 2 years	7 months 12 months 18 months 2 years	12 years 15 years 21 years 24 years
Adult 3–6 years	3 years 4 years 5 years 6 years	28 years 32 years 36 years 40 years
Mature 7—10 years	7 years 8 years 9 years 10 years	44 years 48 years 52 years 56 years
Senior 11–14 years	11 years 12 years 13 years 14 years	60 years 64 years 68 years 72 years
Geriatric 15 years+	15 years 16 years 17 years 18 years 19 years 20 years 21 years 22 years 23 years 24 years 25 years	76 years 80 years 84 years 88 years 92 years 96 years 100 years 104 years 108 years 112 years 116 years

Adapted from: http://icatcare.org/sites/default/files/PDF/how-old-is-your-cat-posterweb.pdf.

2. Changes in appearance: gray, dull, dry haircoat; loss of muscle mass; and development of cataracts and nuclear sclerosis
3. Changes in daily function: functional changes in the musculoskeletal system (decreased activity and mobility) and special senses (impaired vision, smell, and hearing)

TECHNICIAN NOTE

Physiologic changes that occur in dogs and cats as they age are categorized as changes in behavior, appearance, and daily function. Physical health changes occur in cats. The three most common physical changes are related to digestive organs (53.39%), cat weight (49.51%), and skin and hair (37.38%).

Effects of Aging on Organ Systems

Cardiopulmonary System

Aging affects the entire body and its functions. Cardiac output starts to decline in midlife, and cardiovascular disease is more common in older dogs and cats. As the heart loses pumping efficiency, cardiovascular endurance decreases. The lungs lose elasticity as the basement membrane thickens ("old dog lungs"), decreasing lung

• BOX 36.1   Cardiopulmonary Changes in Geriatric Dogs

- Declining cardiac output
- Decreased elasticity of pulmonary tissue
- Increased fibrosis of pulmonary tissue
- Decreased cough reflex
  - Pulmonary secretions have low viscosity
  - Increased chance of respiratory disease
- Monitor for pneumonia
- West Highland White Terriers—pulmonary fibrosis
- Chronic bronchitis—older small-breed dogs
- Congestive heart failure, exercise intolerance, and slowly progressive cough
- 75% of dogs over 16 years old have atrioventricular (AV) valve thickening
- Geriatric onset laryngeal paralysis polyneuropathy (GOLPP) can be associated with polyneuropathy, neoplasia, and hypothyroidism
- Of 32 dogs with idiopathic laryngeal paralysis, 100% had esophageal dysfunction; of the 24 dogs evaluated 1 year later, 100% had neurologic signs (ataxia, weakness, conscious proprioceptive [CP] deficits, muscular atrophy)

capacity. The brainstem's control of breathing also changes with age, reducing the ability to respond to increased demand and causing older patients to become less tolerant of exercise. Panting tends to become less efficient, making it harder for older dogs to cool themselves, a factor that must be considered when exercising elderly dogs. The most common cardiac disease in cats older than 6 years is hypertrophic cardiomyopathy (HCM). In dogs, mitral valve degeneration accounts for approximately 75% of heart disease and primarily affects small- to medium-sized breeds. Chronic valvular disease is found in approximately 30% of older dogs (Box 36.1).

TECHNICIAN NOTE

Geriatric dogs and cats become less tolerant of exercise because of a reduced ability of the brainstem to respond to increased oxygen demands. Panting also becomes less efficient, making it more difficult for older dogs to cool themselves.

Integumentary System

The haircoat, skin, and nails can undergo changes as animals age. The skin typically loses elasticity and becomes less pliable. Older dogs are more likely to develop cutaneous neoplasia, with lipomas, adenomas, and mast cell tumors representing the most common types. Callus formation can result in painful weight bearing and altered foot placement.

Aging cats often experience a thinning haircoat, focal alopecia, and increased production of white hairs. Changes in sebum production and reduced self-grooming activity can lead to scaly skin and cause the coat to become dry, oily, and dull. Decreased skin elasticity and brittle claws have also been noted in apparently healthy older cats.

Immune and Endocrine System

Changes in the immune system (Boxes 36.2–36.4) result in reduced ability to combat infection and longer healing times. Endocrine diseases stem from imbalances in hormone levels, as in hypo- and hyperthyroidism. Metabolic systems are likely to be affected with age. For example, aging adrenal glands often increase cortisol production in response to stress and may also affect electrolyte balance. There is also an age-related decrease in basal metabolic rate, so the risk for obesity is higher. There will be reduced absorption, slower drug metabolism and elimination, reduced ability to combat infection, and resistant urinary tract infections. Healing can take longer, and decubital ulcers form over bony prominences when cushioning is not provided.

Gastrointestinal System

Changes that occur in the aging canine gastrointestinal (GI) system include reduced colonic and rectal elasticity, reduced salivary and gastric acid secretion, smaller intestinal villus size, slower rate of cellular turnover, slower colonic motility, and alterations in the intestinal microbiota. Canine maintenance energy requirement decreases by approximately 20%; however, energy digestibility remains constant, so aged dogs should be fed approximately 20% less calories.

Aging cats may experience a reduced appetite because of many factors, including painful dental issues; altered taste or olfaction; compromised prehension, mastication, or swallowing ability; and slowed GI motility.

Hepatobiliary Changes With Age

As animals age, liver size and weight can decrease secondary to decreased hepatocyte number and increased hepatic fibrosis and nodular regeneration. Decreased liver tissue perfusion and regenerative ability make older dogs and cats likely candidates for the development of liver disease. Liver failure occurs when approximately two-thirds of liver function is lost, and this can impair the ability to process and biotransform common medications, making dosage adjustments necessary.

Oral Cavity

Calculus (tartar) accumulation, gingivitis, and periodontal disease can all occur as pets age. Mouth size is a significant risk factor for periodontal disease in dogs. Smaller dogs tend to have greater calculus accumulations, are more likely to develop periodontal disease at an early age, and develop more severe disease than larger dogs.

As cats age, the dentin layer thickens, resulting in greater tooth density, with a yellow, tan, or off-white appearance. Breed type is a significant risk factor for oral disease development in cats. Brachycephalic cats (e.g., Persians, Himalayans) often have crowded teeth, leading to a more significant accumulation of plaque, oropharyngeal inflammation, and periodontal disease.

Renal and Urinary Systems

A gradual decline in renal function is normal in older animals; however, development of chronic renal failure (CRF) is quite common in older cats. The reported prevalence of CRF in older feline populations varies, ranging from 28% in cats older than 12 years of age up to 80.9% in cats of 15 to 20 years. CRF is often advanced when diagnosis is made, as 75% of nephron function is lost before clinical signs are apparent. Other urinary diseases affecting geriatric pets include chronic urinary tract infections, pyelonephritis, and renal neoplasia.

In aging spayed female dogs, urinary incontinence caused by urethral sphincter mechanism incompetence is common. The hallmark sign of urinary incontinence observed by owners is urine leakage while at rest, resulting in a wet spot where a dog sleeps. In intact male dogs, prostatic enlargement can cause straining to urinate or defecate, and this can sometimes lead to the development of a perineal hernia.

Age-related decreased renal glomerular filtration rate (GFR) and tubular function can cause electrolyte imbalances, increased urination, and altered drug excretion.

TECHNICIAN NOTE

Chronic renal failure is common in aging cats, with up to 28% of cats older than 12 years of age affected. Clinical signs are apparent when 75% of nephron function is lost, so most cases are only diagnosed once the disease is advanced.

Nervous System

Special Senses

As the nervous system and associated special senses age, changes are commonly seen (Box 36.5). Age-related hearing loss may occur but is difficult to assess in dogs and cats, as equipment to test hearing is not widely available. Retinal degeneration with night vision loss is common in older dogs; home adaptations using night lighting can help the pet remain active. Cataract formation is also more likely in older pets (Fig. 36.3). It is likely that olfaction decreases with age

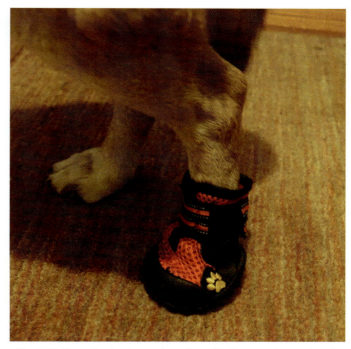

• **Fig. 36.4** Protective boot worn by a dog with degenerative myelopathy. (Courtesy Sheilah Robertson.)

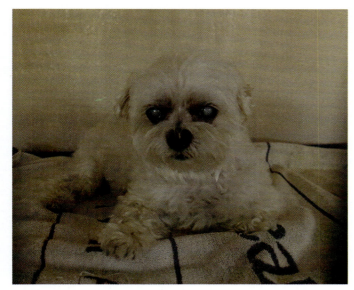

• **Fig. 36.3** Geriatric dog with bilateral cataract formation. (Courtesy Sheilah Robertson.)

in dogs and cats. A decrease in a pet's sense of smell may be partial (**hyposmia**) or complete (**anosmia**) and can lead to decreased appetite, weight loss, or malnutrition, because smell is a critical component of "tasting" food. Changes in flavor perception are often caused by changes within the nose rather than a decrease in the number or function of taste buds.

Central Nervous System

Age-related brain size reduction can cause slower reaction time, loss of fine motor control, and decreased body awareness (proprioception). This may result in difficulty with balance, coordination, and normal gait, although ataxia is never a normal age-related change.

Older pets can develop central nervous system (CNS) neoplasia, with meningiomas being the most common primary brain tumor diagnosed in dogs and cats. Other common primary tumors of dogs are gliomas, astrocytomas, and oligodendrogliomas. Lymphosarcoma is the second most common brain tumor

in cats, occurring either as a primary neoplasm or as part of a multicentric disease.

Two common neurologic diseases of older dogs are degenerative myelopathy (DM) and intervertebral disk disease (IVDD). DM is a slowly progressive degeneration of the white matter of the spinal cord primarily seen in German Shepherds, although other purebred and large mixed-breed dogs may also be affected by this condition. Clinical signs typically consist of a slowly progressive, nonpainful T3-L3 myelopathy. Later in the disease process, urinary and fecal incontinence may develop, and the disease can progress to involve the thoracic limbs and eventually the brainstem. Unfortunately, no treatment has been shown to reverse the signs. Supportive therapy for DM involves physical rehabilitation to maintain muscle mass and nursing care. Protective boots may be worn to prevent injury to the toes and feet resulting from scuffing and dragging (Fig. 36.4).

IVDD causes extrusion or protrusion of intervertebral disk contents into the spinal canal, which places pressure on the spinal cord, causing clinical signs ranging from pain and decreased range of motion to complete paralysis. Two basic types of IVDD disease are seen: type I and type II. Older large-breed dogs, such as German Shepherds, Labrador Retrievers, and Doberman Pinschers, can experience type II IVDD, which is characterized by a slow degeneration and protrusion of the disk into the spinal canal. Conservative management and surgical intervention are available.

Musculoskeletal System

Mobility and strength naturally decline with age (Box 36.6). Age-related loss of muscle mass, or **sarcopenia**, causes a decrease in muscle fiber number and size and slower response to exercise. However, muscles can still respond to strength training (i.e., physical rehabilitation). The first muscles to atrophy are the slow-twitch postural muscles (e.g., spinal epaxial muscles), because these are extremely sensitive to reduced load. With atrophy comes

- Sarcopenia
  - Muscle fibers are replaced with fat first—no loss of muscle circumference
  - Then replaced with fibrous tissue—physical loss of muscle circumference
  - Causes increased stiffness
- Reduced oxygenation of muscle fibers
- Loss of strength of muscles and tendons
- Sarcopenia causes
  - Decreased support of the joints
  - Decreased chondrocytes
  - Reduced ability to respond to growth factors
- With cage rest, significant atrophy of muscles is seen, especially at the insertion of the collateral ligaments
- Aging decreases tensile strength of ligaments secondary to loss of collagen
- Fun bone facts
  - Animals fully change bone content every 5 years
  - Lifetime of weight-bearing exercises decreases bone loss normally seen with aging
  - Weight-bearing training before a bone fracture results in faster healing times
  - Shock wave therapy may aid bone healing, specifically in geriatric dogs
- Water content in the cartilage decreases
  - Thinning of cartilage layer
    - Chondrocytes synthesize smaller, less uniform aggrecan molecules and less functional link proteins
    - Decreased mitotic activities
    - Decreased response to anabolic mechanical stimulants and growth factors
  - Combined with stress on joints secondary to loss of muscle strength, leads to eburnation of subchondral bone and osteoarthritis
- No osteoporosis noted in pets, but bones become more brittle due to infiltration of fat into bone marrow and thinner cortexes
  - Fracture healing is slower
  - More difficult to form a callus
  - Obesity and brittle bones exacerbate progression of osteoarthritis

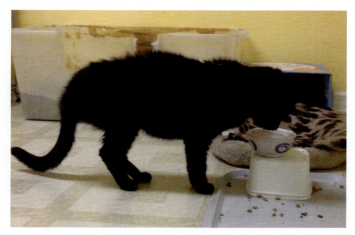

• **Fig. 36.5** Geriatric cat with significant muscle atrophy. (Courtesy Sheilah Robertson.)

decreased ability to maintain normal posture, so the process becomes cyclic (Fig. 36.5). Water content of tendons decreases, muscle fibers are replaced with fat, and the physical loss of muscle mass causes increased stiffness and loss of strength.

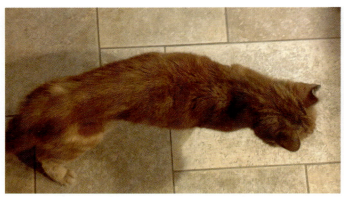

• **Fig. 36.6** This cat displays loss of lean body mass, which is characteristic of cachexia. (Courtesy Sheilah Robertson.)

TECHNICIAN NOTE

Sarcopenia is the aging-related degeneration of muscle mass and is accompanied by a decline in mobility and strength. Frailty is characterized by a decline in the body's functional reserve, lower energy metabolism, smaller muscle cells, and altered nervous, hormonal, and inflammatory functions.

For cats, significant musculoskeletal changes that occur with age include a decrease in lean body mass (muscle, bone, skin, and organs), deterioration of joint components, and functional decline.

The term *frailty* has also been used in relation to age-related musculoskeletal deterioration. **Frailty** is a multisystem impairment associated with increased vulnerability to stressors and describes the condition of individuals that are at increased risk of adverse health outcomes. Frailty is related to but not synonymous with comorbidity and disability. Frailty is characterized by a decline in the body's functional reserve, lower energy metabolism, smaller muscle cells, and altered nervous, hormonal, and inflammatory functions. It is not a disease process, but it leads to increased susceptibility to disease and functional dependency. Frailty is also seen with decreased muscle mass and loss of strength and endurance.

Cachexia is the loss of lean body mass (LBM). It affects a large percentage of dogs and cats with age-related diseases, such as congestive heart failure (CHF), CRF, and cancer (Fig. 36.6). It is characterized by weakness, anorexia, and perceived poor QOL, and is associated with decreased survival. Cachexia literally means "the flesh is consumed and becomes water" (Hippocrates) (Box 36.7).

Cognitive Impairment and Other Behavioral Issues

Cognitive dysfunction (Box 36.8) is a neurodegenerative disorder of senior dogs and cats that is characterized by gradual cognitive decline over an extended period. Diagnosis of cognitive dysfunction syndrome (CDS) is based on recognition of behavioral signs and exclusion of other medical conditions and drug side effects which, in some cases, can mimic or complicate CDS. Clinical manifestations include disorientation; alterations in social interactions, sleep-wake cycle, elimination habits, and activity; increasing anxiety; and learning and memory deficits. The diagnosis of CDS was initially based on clinical signs represented by the acronym **DISHA**, representing Disorientation, altered Interactions with people or other pets, altered Sleep-wake cycles, House soiling, and Activity changes.

• BOX 36.7 Muscle Changes in the Geriatric Dog

- Lactic acid builds faster
  - Glycogen depletes faster
- Decreased creatine phosphate (used first as a fuel in muscle)
- Cannot build muscle strength or endurance as well as younger dogs
- Muscle capillarization decreases with age
- Decreased oxygen supply to muscles
- Decreased endurance
- Type II muscle fibers decreased by ~25%
- Strength
- Type I muscle fibers can increase or stay the same
  - Endurance and postural muscles
- Disuse atrophy—decrease type I muscle, especially those that cross one joint, and postural muscles

• BOX 36.8 Cognitive Dysfunction Changes in the Geriatric Patient

- Cognitive changes
  - Increased oxidative stress
- Deposition of B-amyloid plaques (similar to Alzheimer patients)
- DNA fragmentation or damage
- Changes in intracellular signaling, leading to a loss of neurotrophic factors
- Anatomic changes in the brain
  - Cortical atrophy
  - Increased ventricular volume
  - Reduced neurogenesis in hippocampus
  - Responsible for learning and memory
- Progressive neurodegenerative disorder
- Diagnosis of exclusion
- Clinical signs include
  - Change in sleeping habits
  - Lack of environmental recognition
  - Decreased interaction with human and animal family
  - Restlessness
  - Apathy
  - Anxiety
  - Altered appetite
  - Aggression or irritability
  - Vocalization
  - Incontinence
- Therapy includes
  - Antioxidants—vitamin B, C, and E; fruits and vegetables
  - Fatty acid supplementation
  - Mitochondrial cofactor supplementation—carnitine, alpha lipoic acid (omega-6 fatty acid), coenzyme Q10
  - Phosphatidylserine (phospholipid that improves cognitive deficits and memory)
  - Gingko biloba—a monoamine oxidase inhibitor (MAO-A and MAO-B)
    - Increases dopamine levels and protect neurons from apoptosis induced by B-amyloid
  - Selegiline— a MAO-B inhibitor (Anipryl, L-deprenyl)

Signs of Cognitive Impairment

- Confusion
- Altered relationships and social interactions
- Altered response to stimulation
- Changes in activity—increased anxiety, repetitive behaviors (vocalizing, pacing), apathy, depression
- Altered sleep-wake cycles; reversed day/night schedule, night-time pacing (the most common owner complaint)

TABLE 36.3 Feline Mobility/Cognitive Dysfunction Questionnaire

My Cat	Yes	Maybe	No
Is less willing to jump down			
Will only jump up or down from lower heights			
Sometimes shows signs of being stiff			
Is less agile than previously			
Shows signs of lameness or limping			
Has difficulty going through the cat flap			
Has difficulty going up or down stairs			
Cries when picked up			
Has more accidents outside the litter box			
Spends less time grooming			
Is more reluctant to interact with me			
Plays less with other animals or toys			
Sleeps more and/or is less active			
Cries loudly for no reason/to try to gain my attention			
Appears forgetful			

Note: It is important to ensure there are no environmental reason(s) for these behavior changes.

Adapted from Gunn-Moore DA. Cognitive dysfunction in cats: clinical assessment and management. *Top Companion Anim Med.* 2011;26:17-24; Gunn-Moore DA. Dementia in ageing cats. *Vet Times.* 2014;2014:14-16.

- Learning and memory problems: house soiling; deficits in work, tasks, and commands
- Getting stuck behind doors

TECHNICIAN NOTE

The diagnosis of cognitive dysfunction syndrome (CDS) was initially based on clinical signs represented by the acronym DISHA, representing Disorientation, altered Interactions with people or other pets, altered Sleep-wake cycles, House soiling, and Activity changes.

Behavioral signs are often the first or only indication of pain, illness, or cognitive decline and identifying the contributing factors can be a challenge for the owner and the veterinary team. Senior pets may be less able to cope with stress, making them more susceptible to environmental changes (e.g., a new cat or house). A variety of behavioral problems ranging from avoidance, decreased activity, and inappetence to irritability, restlessness, and aggression could result from underlying pain. It is the job of the veterinary team to discern pain resulting from stress and anxiety, even in a patient with CDS. The veterinarian may treat pain and assess for clinical response when in doubt.

Age-associated cognitive and physiologic assessment should be conducted annually in senior dogs and cats. Clients with elderly animals will not always mention behavior changes during veterinary visits, so veterinary technicians should ask clients direct questions about changes in their pets' behavior (Tables 36.3 and 36.4).

<table>
<tr><td colspan="2">TABLE 36.4   Mobility Questionnaire for Dogs</td></tr>
</table>

Owners should assign a grade to each question based on the rating scale. Rating System: 0 = none; 1 = mild; 2 = moderate; 3 = severe
Difficulty walking
Difficulty moving from lying down to standing position
Difficulty moving from standing to lying down position
Difficulty moving from sitting to standing position
Difficulty moving from standing to sitting position
Difficulty holding posture to defecate
Difficulty to hold posture to urinate
Difficulty ascending stairs
Difficulty descending stairs
Difficulty jumping
Difficulty running
Difficulty climbing inclines
Difficulty losing weight
Difficulty gaining weight
Difficulty with endurance

Adapted from Shearer TS. Managing mobility challenges in palliative and hospice care patients. *Vet Clin Small Anim.* 2011;41(5):609-617.

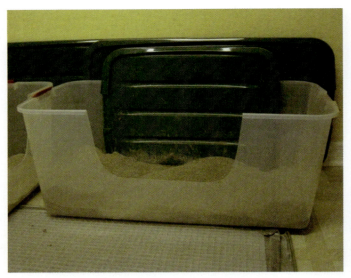

• **Fig. 36.7** A litter box constructed from a plastic storage tub with a lower entry point for easier access for cats with degenerative joint disease. (Courtesy Sheilah Robertson.)

In cats, a thorough medical and behavioral history is required for diagnosis. Cognitive and motor performance appears to decline from approximately age 10 to 11, but age-related brain changes have been seen by age 6 to 7. It can be difficult to differentiate between signs of cognitive dysfunction and those caused by osteoarthritis-related mobility issues. Both conditions often occur concurrently in old cats, and many treatments for one condition will also help the other.

The most common behavioral changes in old cats are grouped under the acronym VISHDAAL and refer to inappropriate behaviors. The three most common behavioral changes in old cats are altered activity (49%), altered learning and memory (21%), and soiling of the house (19%).

The anacronym VISHDALL stands for:

V = vocalization
I = changes in interaction with us and other pets
S = changes in sleep-wake cycle
H = house soiling
D = disorientation
A = changes in activity
A = anxiety
L = learning and memory

TECHNICIAN NOTE

Cognitive dysfunction syndrome (CDS) and age-related impairment can cause behavior changes related to anxiety, reduced mobility, restlessness, reduced interaction with owners, polydipsia/polyuria, and neurologic or circulatory disorders.

Quality of Life

The World Health Organization (2012) defines QOL as "the individual's perception of their position in life in the context of the culture and value systems in which they live and in relation to their goals, expectations, standards, and concerns." QOL in animals has been defined as the affective (emotional) response of an individual animal to their circumstances and the extent to which the circumstances meet their expectations. In the context of animal hospice and palliative care, QOL assessments reflect how an animal's physical, emotional, and social well-being is affected by disease, disability, or changes related to advanced age. There are specific QOL questionnaires for clients to fill out that help assess the pet's QOL. A recent paper by Fulmar et al. is an excellent review article of QOL instruments available (see Recommended Readings, Geriatric Dogs and Cats section).

Management Strategies to Improve Quality of Life

Geriatric animals need to be able to navigate their surroundings easily. This can be particularly challenging for animals with medical problems affecting mobility, including conditions associated with chronic pain, such as DJD and spinal problems. Cats with DJD prefer a litter box with low sides that is easier to get into for toileting needs (Fig. 36.7).

Conditions that reduce sensory abilities, such as vision and hearing loss or cognitive dysfunction, can be associated with impaired spatial awareness and navigational ability. Important resources that need to be accessible include food, water, comfortable resting places, toilet locations, and, for cats, places to withdraw to or hide if they do not wish to interact with people or other animals in the home. Cats like to have food, water, and toilet areas kept separate, and all must be easily accessible from the cat's resting area. If a cat spends time on different floors in the home, it is wise to locate a full set of resources, including a litter box, on each floor.

Once resources have been located appropriately, they should always be kept in the same places so that the animals can find them

TABLE 36.5	Suggestions for Improving the Environment and Increasing Access to Resources for Elderly Cats and Dogs	
Resource	**Dogs**	**Cats**
Food and water	Raising bowls off the ground will help dogs with joint and spinal problems eat and drink more comfortably. Nonslip matting underfoot will prevent a dog from slipping when eating or drinking.	Raise bowls off the ground by a few inches to enable cats with joint and spinal problems to eat and drink more comfortably. Cats used to being fed on raised surfaces (e.g., windowsills or worktops) may need a ramp or steps to enable access, or food and water should be provided in more accessible locations.
Toileting areas	Dogs with mobility problems may need to learn to use a toileting area closer to the house, or even be provided with a toileting area indoors (e.g. by placing puppy pads in a large tray). Owners may need to encourage dogs to go to their toilet area regularly because they may no longer indicate when they need to eliminate.	Needs to be separate from feeding and drinking locations. Cats with mobility problems will prefer large, low-sided litter boxes. Finer-grained litters are easier to stand on and dig in than coarser litters. Cats that have previously eliminated outside may no longer be able to access these locations, and will need to be provided with indoor litter boxes.
Sleeping areas and beds	Beds should be comfortable and supportive (e.g. memory foam), easy for animal to get into and out of, and large enough for them to stretch out in, if they wish. Elderly animals become cold very easily; sleeping areas should be kept warm, especially at night in the winter. Electric heated beds may be welcomed. An Adaptil diffuser plugged in close to the bed may help reduce anxiety and help dogs relax better at night. Items containing the owner's scent may also help some dogs relax better at night.	Beds should be comfortable and padded, easy for the cat to get into and out of, and large enough for them to stretch out in if they wish. Cats prefer to rest in raised places, but animals with mobility problems may need ramps or steps in order to access these locations. Elderly animals become cold very easily; sleeping areas should be kept warm, especially at night in the winter. Electric heated beds may be welcomed. A Feliway diffuser plugged in close to the bed may reduce anxiety and help cats relax better at night.
Moving around inside and outside home	Nonslip matting or carpet in locations of important resources and on the walkways between important areas can improve accessibility for elderly animals with mobility problems. Nonslip ramps can help dogs navigate steep steps outside the home and get into and out of cars. Specially designed harnesses can be helpful for supporting dogs with mobility problems to enable exercise and access to toilet areas.	Nonslip matting or carpet in locations of important resources and on the walkways between important areas can improve accessibility for elderly animals with mobility problems. Most cats prefer raised resting places where they can feel safe and observe household activity from a safe distance. Providing ramps or steps may enable cats with mobility problems to continue to use withdrawal as a way of avoiding things that scare them. Cats with mobility problems may no longer be able to use a cat-flap so owners will need to let them in and out, unless they prefer to stay indoors.

Adapted from Warnes C. Changes in behaviour in elderly cats and dogs. Part 2: management, treatment and Prevention. *Vet Nurse.* 2015;6(10):590-597.

easily. If other animals are in the home, then it is imperative that there is no unnecessary competition for these resources (Table 36.5).

Other Considerations for Geriatric Pets

Introducing a new pet into the household can be extremely stressful for an older animal with mobility problems, especially for one with cognitive dysfunction. Clients may be better advised not to do this, especially with cats and any dog that does not have good social skills or is showing severe cognitive dysfunction.

Play can be associated with a positive emotional response, and an increase in aerobic activity will also boost circulation, enhancing oxygen supply to the brain and muscles. Low-impact games, such as gentle throw-and-fetch or search games, are appropriate for most elderly dogs. For dogs with vision loss, search games to find food or toys are particularly suitable. Short play sessions with fishing rod toys or toys that roll and/or make sounds will suit most cats. Older pets can become bored with toys quickly, so the toys need to be rotated every few days.

Dogs with mobility problems can be taken out in the car and then given a short walk in a new location, or they can accompany their owners on longer walks by riding in a modified baby stroller. Some elderly cats prefer to remain indoors, but if cats do want to go outside, they can do so more safely if they wear a harness or have access to a screened-in area. Screened-in back porches are excellent for environmental stimulation (Fig. 36.8). Animals with severe cognitive dysfunction or anxiety must have an environment that remains stable and unchanged. Highly anxious animals, especially cats, may cope best when restricted to a single room containing food, water, a litter box, and resting and hiding places. It is important to keep furniture and resources in the same places and to avoid big changes in the scent profile of the room; for example, use of strongly scented cleaning products or deodorizers should be avoided. A consistent routine ensures that important events occur in the same order and at approximately the same times every day.

Geriatric Wellness Programs

Geriatric patients often present with several issues (Box 36.9). Experts recommend that dogs and cats in the last 25% of their predicted lifespans have routine health care visits, including updates to a minimum laboratory database, every 6 months. During these visits, a thorough history should be obtained, and a complete physical examination, including evaluation of physical condition, vital signs, skin, coat, lymph nodes, and hydration, should be performed. The examination should also include assessing the cardiopulmonary and

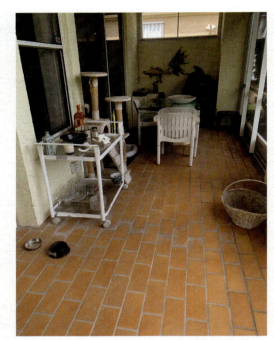

• **Fig. 36.8** Access to a screened back porch can provide environmental stimulation for older cats. (Courtesy Mary Ellen Goldberg.)

• **BOX 36.9** Common Presentation With Geriatric Pets

- Reduced mobility—difficulty with stairs, difficult getting in and out of car (offer some assistance), difficulty rising, shorter walks, cannot jump up on favorite spot to rest
- Pain
- Urinary or fecal incontinence
- Change in appetite
- Decreased alertness
- Change in interaction with the family

---

neurologic systems, abdominal and rectal palpation, and a complete orthopedic examination. The minimum laboratory database should include a complete blood count (CBC); urinalysis; fecal analysis; and serum biochemical panel, including measurement of blood urea nitrogen (BUN), creatinine, glucose, total calcium, total protein (TP), albumin, bilirubin, serum alanine aminotransferase (ALT), and alkaline phosphatase (ALP) (Box 36.10).

TECHNICIAN NOTE

It is recommended that dogs and cats in the last 25% of their predicted lifespans have routine health care visits, including updates to a minimum laboratory database, every 6 months. A geriatric health care program is beneficial to a pet's geriatric lifestyle.

Nutrition

Two major effects of aging include decreased ability to adapt to changes in nutrition and a decrease in the capacity to handle large nutritional excesses or deficiencies. Older patients often have subclinical diseases that further affect their nutritional status and health. Because of this, the role of nutrition becomes an increasingly important consideration not only in the prevention of disease, but also in

---

• **BOX 36.10** Ten Steps to Making a Geriatric Health Care Program Successful

1. The practice decision maker must be convinced that a senior/geriatric health care program will become a significant asset to the practice before investing the time, energy, training, and resources necessary in developing and maintaining the program.
2. Convince the entire staff of the significant health benefits the program offers the senior pet. Critical to the success or failure of a senior/geriatric health care program is the involvement and buy-in of your staff.
3. Create a very specific and detailed program, including age of onset, frequency of visits, scheduling periods, fee structure, educational materials, and marketing strategies. Decide exactly which tests are to be included in the program.
4. Convince the owners of the significant health benefits the program offers their aging pet. A percentage of your practice will readily accept the program, but the rest will need repeated convincing. Increased client knowledge usually equates to increased client acceptance and compliance. Early and continued owner education is a long-term investment in a senior/geriatric health care program.
5. A well-designed market strategy correlates with success. Use newsletters, reminder cards, invoices, telephone directory ads, Web pages, and social media to educate your current and prospective clients on age-related problems and solutions. Client marketing efforts should emphasize all the advances in veterinary medicine, including newer diagnostic testing, improved anesthetics and anesthetic monitoring equipment, behavioral drugs, newer arthritis therapy options, leading-edge cancer chemotherapy, more effective cardiac medications, dental care, and available nutritional advancements.
6. Bundle the fee structure to include a senior pet discount. Discount the fee for all the services and consider a cost reduction in the senior diets for any patients already on the program.
7. Start slow and be patient, and the program will grow. A senior/geriatric health care program is a long-term hospital investment. It is much easier to add a test and expand the program than take one away, because the cost was considered excessive for the average owner. Unfortunately, an overzealous program coupled with underdelivery of value is commonplace. The seeds of program success and client subscription begin when outlining a lifelong preventive health care program the first time a new owner visits the practice, even for puppies or kittens.
8. Because a comprehensive health examination will require more time in the exam room, try to schedule these appointments during slow days or during periods of the day when you can devote the time necessary for a complete evaluation.
9. An attractive three-color trifold brochure for your practice's program is an easy and time-saving marketing tool. The brochure should be uniquely branded to your practice. Highlight the specifics of your program (age of onset, visits per year, etc.), but keep the piece simple for an easy read. Emphasize the advantages of the health program to older pets and the early warning disease signs to watch for.
10. Periodic program review by your clients and staff is essential in maintaining the consistently high standard of care you have established for your senior patients. Do not be afraid to modify the program to meet the emerging minimum database protocols.

---

helping maintain the aging pet's QOL. Body weight, body condition score (BCS), and muscle condition score (MCS) should be regularly assessed in dogs and cats.

Obesity is currently the most common nutritional disorder of pet dogs and cats (Fig. 36.9). Several health problems, including chronic inflammation, osteoarthritis, pulmonary and cardiovascular diseases, pancreatitis, hypertension, insulin resistance, glomerular hyperfiltration, and increased anesthesia-related morbidity and

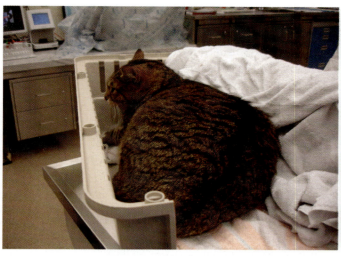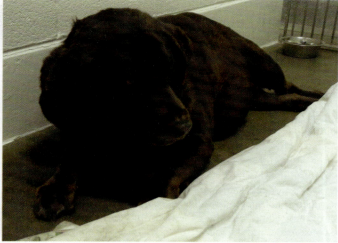

• **Fig. 36.9** Obesity is a concern in older dogs and cats, and can exacerbate other health conditions. (Courtesy Sheilah Robertson.)

mortality rates, are caused or complicated by obesity in dogs. In addition, excess body weight decreases both QOL, as indicated by an increased incidence and severity of osteoarthritis, and life expectancy, and adversely affects immune function. Obesity in cats is associated with increased risk for reduced mobility and diabetes mellitus.

Wellness examinations that include BCS and MCS evaluations can be an effective method for early detection of weight gain or muscle loss and allow for appropriate invention to slow progression and minimize potential adverse effects. Older dogs and middle-aged cats tend to have reduced energy needs and, if calorie intake is not adjusted accordingly, weight gain will result. The primary indicator of energy requirement in normal pets is LBM, which tends to decrease with age. This, in addition to a decrease in activity, can contribute to the reduction in maintenance energy requirement (MER) seen in aging dogs and middle-aged cats. However, a nutritional assessment should be completed on each patient to determine its individual needs, rather than assuming all older pets need a reduced calorie intake. For more information regarding nutrition, refer to Chapter 9.

> **TECHNICIAN NOTE**
>
> Obesity is currently the most common nutritional disorder of pet dogs and cats. Dogs that weigh 10% to 20% more than their ideal body weight are generally classified as "overweight," whereas those that weigh 20% more than their ideal body weight are classified as "obese."

Anesthesia

The topics of anesthesia and analgesia are covered in detail in Chapters 29 and 30; however, anesthesia for dogs and cats at either end of the age spectrum deserves special attention. One of the most common mistakes made when anesthetizing older patients is depending primarily on inhalant agents and avoiding preanesthetic agents because of the misunderstanding that inhalant agents are somehow safer. Presedation is recommended to decrease anxiety and fear that lead to increased catecholamine release, which predisposes patients to cardiac arrhythmias, peripheral vasoconstriction, increased cardiac work, and decreased tissue perfusion. Good outcomes are related to appropriate drug choice and administration. Therefore it is prudent to choose drugs that are reversible, can be given to effect, and have a short duration of action.

> • **BOX 36.11** **Medical Conditions Appropriate for Hospice or Palliative Care**
>
> - Terminal diagnosis
> - Chronic, progressive disease
> - Progressive, undiagnosed disease
> - Chronic disability
> - Terminal geriatric status

Hospice and Palliative Care

Animal hospice is a program of care that addresses the physical, emotional, and social needs of animals in the advanced stages of a progressive, life-limiting illness or disability. Palliative care is treatment that supports or improves QOL for patients and caregivers by relieving suffering; this applies to treating curable or chronic conditions and **end-of-life** (EOL) care (Box 36.11).

Developing an effective, patient-specific EOL care treatment plan is a collaborative effort involving the veterinary team and the client. Treatment goals described by the client should be as specific as possible and recorded in detail in the patient's medical record. The veterinarian should discuss the client's ability and willingness to provide the increased level of caregiving generally required for a terminally ill patient. The plan should be presented in words the client can understand without overreliance on medical terminology. When the health care team collaborates with the pet owner to successfully address the patient's physical, social, and emotional needs, you are best able to maximize comfort and minimize suffering (Table 36.6).

> **TECHNICIAN NOTE**
>
> The client's capacity to care for their pet is an important consideration in developing a treatment plan, because it relies on their active involvement.

Special Nursing Considerations

The most important goal of palliative care and hospice is to help patients achieve a good QOL. Suffering occurs if clinical signs of disease become uncontrolled or overwhelming, so medically managing symptoms forms the foundation of comfort care for such patients.

Pain Management

Many practitioners are hesitant to treat geriatric animals with analgesic agents, sedatives, and anesthetics. Unfortunately, this means that many older patients needlessly suffer from pain associated with chronic conditions or are denied the benefit of procedures that require sedation or anesthesia. Pain is a complex multidimensional experience with sensory and emotional components, and it can have a significant and negative impact on an animal's QOL and the human-animal bond. Age- and disease-related changes in organ function and body composition can impact drug pharmacokinetics. Dose and dosing intervals may require adjustment in geriatric patients, with renal, hepatic, and cardiac disease all being of concern.

Clinical metrology instruments (CMIs) for dogs and cats measure activity, mobility, and function. CMIs help clients identify pain and functional limitations, and objectively measure response to treatment. They require that the same client fill out the form each time for consistency, and are repeated every 2–4 weeks after starting the treatment plan. They can be extremely helpful with EOL decisions.

Examples of CMIs for dogs are:
- Helsinki Chronic Pain Index (HCPI)
- Canine Brief Pain Inventory (CBPI)
- Cincinnati Orthopedic Disability Index (CODI)
- Health-Related Quality of Life (HRQL)
- Liverpool Osteoarthritis in Dogs (LOAD)

- Canine OsteoArthritis Staging Tool (COAST)

Examples of CMIs for cats are:
- Feline Musculoskeletal Pain Index (FMPI)
- Feline Physical Function Formula (FPFF)
- Owner Behaviour Watch (OBW)
- Zamprogno Question Bank (ZQB)

TECHNICIAN NOTE

Pain is a complex multidimensional experience with both sensory and emotional components, and it can have a significant and negative impact on an animal's quality of life (QOL) and the human-animal bond.

When managing pain, a pre-emptive, multimodal approach should be implemented. With this approach, pharmacologic and nonpharmacologic therapies complement one another, working better together than any single therapy. Integrative veterinary medicine (IVM) combines complementary and alternative therapies with conventional care to allow for intervention at multiple places along the nociceptive pathway, increased effectiveness of analgesic drugs, and use of lower drug doses. A multimodal pain management approach can include the use of anti-inflammatories, opioids, tricyclic antidepressants, anticonvulsants, N-methyl-D-aspartate (NMDA) receptor antagonists, nutraceuticals, and

TABLE 36.6 Components of an Integrated Approach to End-of-Life (EOL) Care

Component	Objective	Intervention
Physical care	Pain management Management of clinical signs Hygiene Nutrition Mobility Safety Environmental needs	Anticipate, prevent, control, and regularly monitor acute and chronic pain; provide multimodal pain relief through: • Pharmacologic management • Environmental modifications • Dietary management • Gentle handling techniques Examine patient to diagnose and treat dyspnea, gastrointestinal (GI) abnormalities, cognitive dysfunction, anxiety, pruritus and skin problems (e.g., local infections, pressure sores), dental health, respiratory conditions Maintain urine and feces sanitation, access to elimination sites Perform dietary and body condition assessment; monitor dietary habits and changes; maintain balanced nutrition, adequate food intake, and hydration to the extent possible, keeping in mind that decreased food and water intake are normal in the dying process Provide nonskid flooring in pet's living area, accessible litter box location and design, physical assistance devices (harnesses, slings, carts, and wheelchairs), range-of-motion exercises Restrict access to environmental hazards (e.g., swimming pools); protect from aggressive pets, observe for self-trauma Provide comfortable bedding, temperature and ventilation control, adequate space, peaceful environment
Social well-being	Engagement with family Isolation avoidance Interaction with other pets Mental stimulation	Involve pet in family activities as illness allows; maintain regular owner-pet interaction Avoid or minimize extended periods of isolation or nonsocialization Maintain appropriate interaction with other pets; monitor pet-to-pet hierarchal changes and adverse socialization behaviors Offer regular play opportunities and environmental enrichment
Emotional well-being	Preservation of dignity Stress reduction Preserve pet's household role Maintain the will to live	Minimize house soiling, manage incontinence, maintain good hygiene and grooming Minimize exposure to stress and changes in routine; assess pet's willingness to receive needed treatments Continue expectations for companionship, surveillance, or other household roles; adhere to daily routines Monitor behavior; ensure regular interaction with family members; observe for signs of withdrawal, depression, or resignation

Adapted from Epstein M, Griffenhagen G, Kadrlik J, et al. 2015 AAHA/AAFP Pain Management Guidelines for Dogs and Cats. *J Am Anim Hosp Assoc.* 2015;51(2):67-84.

TABLE 36.7 Examples of Pain Severity Based on Common Diseases Seen in Hospice Patients

Pain Severity	Disease
Mild	Dental disease, mild cystitis, osteoarthritis
Moderate	Cystitis, osteoarthritis
Moderate to severe	Osteoarthritis, capsular pain caused by organomegaly, intervertebral disk disease, oral cancer, corneal abrasion/ulceration, pleuritis, hollow organ distension, trauma, peritonitis, hemoabdomen, pancreatitis
Severe to excruciating	Thrombosis/ischemia, inflammation (cellulitis), neuropathic pain (nerve entrapment, inflammation, disk herniation), bone cancer/pathologic fracture, central nervous system infarction/tumors, necrotizing pancreatitis, aortic saddle thrombus

From Cox S. Chapter 18. Pharmacology interventions for symptom management. In: Shanan A, Pierce J, Shearer T, eds. *Hospice and Palliative Care for Companion Animals: Principles and Practice.* Ames, IA: John Wiley & Sons; 2017:165-180,

adjunct physical modalities. (See Chapter 29, "Pain Management," for details about pain scoring, pain assessment, and use of pain medications; and Table 36.7.)

Physical Modalities for Pain Management in Geriatric Patients. Nonpharmaceutical treatments are significant in effectively treating pain in geriatric patients. Loss of muscle mass can result in the animal's inability to perform basic body functions, including eating, drinking, and posturing to urinate and defecate. Rehabilitation is useful in halting or reversing these changes and may be used to alleviate pain via several methods, including increasing joint mobility, stimulating neuromuscular input, and reducing inflammation. A slow pace of conditioning should be considered, including balance exercises, neuromuscular stimulation, and core strengthening. The core of animal rehabilitation involves positive interactions between the animal and the therapist.

Additionally, some exercises can be safely taught to animal caregivers, allowing for frequent therapy in the home setting and reduced clinic visits. There are many other tools at the therapist's disposal, including laser therapy, pulsed electromagnetic field therapy, shock wave therapy, and acupuncture. Alternative therapies can often be used in the presence of organ dysfunction and in conjunction with pharmaceutical agents, including chemotherapy and analgesic drugs. (See Chapter 23, "Rehabilitation and Alternative Medical Nursing," for information about alternative therapies that may benefit geriatric patients.)

Nursing Care

The veterinary hospice nurse's role can be divided into three core competencies:

1. *Medical caregiver:* This role requires the veterinary hospice nurse to be able to assess the level of pain and discomfort, to intervene to keep the patient comfortable, and to know when and how to use other health care resources.
2. *Educator:* In this role, the veterinary hospice nurse delivers information from the medical team to the animal's caregivers to ensure the best care for the patient.

3. *Advocate:* The veterinary hospice nurse can be the bridge between patient, family, and the hospice team by intervening on the patient's and caregiver's behalf, taking on the role of communicator and translator of information and feelings. The veterinary hospice nurse advocates, providing guidance and support to the human members of the family during the final journey with their pet by using knowledge, communication skills, intuition, and empathy.

> **TECHNICIAN NOTE**
>
> The veterinary hospice nurse's role can be divided into three core competencies: medical caregiver, educator, and advocate.

Geriatric animals may respond poorly to changes in their environment, and many have clinical signs of cognitive dysfunction. Faced with a hospitalization or extensive inpatient treatments, some of these animals seem to "give up" within moments of being in a strange environment. This may include refusal to eat, drink, or interact with caretakers. Owners should be encouraged to leave familiar toys or blankets to comfort these patients. Keeping the hospital stay as short as possible will be beneficial; scheduling appointments first thing in the morning may allow patients to be discharged on the same day.

Nursing care is especially important in aging animals. Special attention should be paid to food and water intake; hand-feeding may help. Padded bedding should be used for all geriatric animals, as most suffer from some degree of DJD. Time should be taken to socialize with hospitalized animals (at times separate from visits to perform medical procedures, such as administering medications or taking rectal temperature) to make them feel more relaxed, prevent anticipation of what they may perceive as "something bad," and provide opportunities to look for signs of pain that might not be immediately evident from distant observation or during treatments.

> **PUT INTO PRACTICE**
>
> Conversations with clients about their aging pets can be a challenge, but, as a veterinary nurse/technician, you will be building relationships over time. You can assist your clients in recognizing changes in their pets that will help the pets live their best lives. While these conversations can be challenging, your knowledge of their lives and their pets will assist with nutrition, cognitive issues, and other issues that occur as their pet ages.

Fluid Therapy

Dehydration assessment is challenging in emaciated and geriatric patients, because they have poor skin elasticity, which can mimic dehydration. In these patients, when compatible history and physical examination findings are present, it is reasonable to assume 7% dehydration and treat accordingly. Once a patient has been stabilized by volume replacement, maintenance fluid administration should be considered to maintain hydration, which can significantly improve QOL. Subcutaneous administration can be equally efficacious to intravenous fluid administration and is more suitable for home and outpatient care. Caregivers can easily be taught to administer subcutaneous fluids at home after observing them performing this task to ensure it is being done properly. (Refer to Chapter 24, "Fluid Therapy and Transfusion Medicine," for more information regarding fluid administration.)

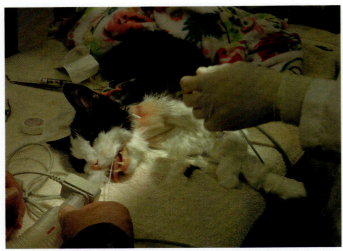

• **Fig. 36.10** Placement of a feeding tube in a cat under anesthesia. (Courtesy Sheilah Robertson.)

Feeding Tubes

If a feeding tube is placed, fluid therapy can be administered enterally. Indications for feeding tube use include older animals with no obvious physical problems other than an unwillingness to eat and pets with inappetence associated with advanced chronic disease, untreated pain, fear, or anxiety. An honest discussion about the realities of artificial nutrition should precede any decision to place a feeding tube. The most common types of feeding tubes inserted in dogs and cats are nasoesophageal, esophageal, and gastrostomy and jejunostomy tubes. All of these, except the nasoesophageal tube, require anesthesia for surgical placement (Fig. 36.10). Nasoesophageal and jejunostomy tubes are used only in hospitalized animals, whereas esophageal and gastrostomy tubes can be managed by owners at home.

Because many owners are unfamiliar with the use of syringes and the procedure for administering food through feeding tubes, it is often necessary to spend a significant amount of time with them when the animal is being discharged from the hospital. Detailed instructions should be given regarding tube maintenance, administration technique, and feeding amounts. It is helpful to supply the owners with well-written, concise instructions and video links to help them establish reasonable expectations. Although feeding tubes require routine daily care, owners are usually happy with the results when they see how much better their pet feels. (For more information about feeding tubes, see Chapter 9, "Animal Nutrition.")

Hygiene, Bladder, and Fecal Maintenance

Pets approaching the end of life may develop fecal and/or urinary incontinence, so caregivers must often be trained to provide hygienic care to prevent urine and fecal scald and transmission and spread of infections. It is commonly presumed that there is also a psychological benefit to hygiene maintenance, through prevention of the loss of dignity associated with the loss of lifelong

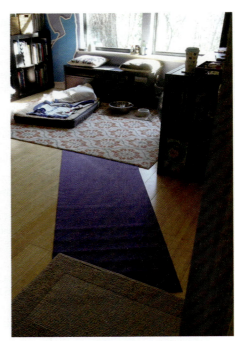

• **Fig. 36.11** Rugs and yoga mats can be used to create a path on slippery floors for pets to access common areas. (Courtesy Sheilah Robertson.)

toileting habits and the unpleasant effect associated with the sensations and odors of uncleanliness. Hair around the anus and genitals can be trimmed to more easily clean and dry the skin, and the pet owner should be taught to use baby wipes or mild soap and water to clean around the genitals and the anus, taking care to remove all urine and feces from the haircoat and skin. The owner should rinse the area well and make sure it is completely dry. A moisture-barrier ointment and cornstarch baby powder should be applied after each cleansing.

Some pets may require diapers to contain urine and stool. Pet diapers with replaceable liners are commercially available, or human diapers may be used. Any time diapers are required for containment, it is important to do regular checks to quickly change them when they become soiled to avoid tissue breakdown.

Cats may become too weak or uncomfortable to climb over the side and into the litter box. In this case, the client should replace the litter box with a low-sided one.

Care of the Recumbent Patient

Recumbent patients require soft bedding to avoid **decubitus ulcers** ("bedsores"), impeccable hygiene, and frequent turning to avoid complications, such as limb edema, joint and muscle stiffness, hypostatic pneumonia, or atelectasis. Bedding changes must occur as often as needed. If the patient is unable to hold itself up sternally, foam rolls, pads, wedges, or rolled-up towels can be used to help them maintain a sternal position and prevent them from falling over. If assisted to get up, patients require a nonslippery floor surface for traction. The use of yoga mats and rugs can allow better traction on slick flooring (Fig. 36.11).

Decubitus ulcers usually occur over bony prominences, such as the hips, elbows, stifles, shoulders, and cheeks, and result from loss of blood supply, with necrosis of subdermal tissue. The skin becomes red and alopecic and then progresses to black and necrotic. Decubitus ulcers can be avoided in recumbent animals if adequate padding is used. Tegaderm Gel over decubitus ulcers,

1. With your pet lying on its side, place hands in a prayerlike fashion over the area where you imagine the bladder is located. If your pet is strong enough to support its weight, then this procedure can be done while standing. You may find this procedure works better for you if your hands are facing toward the front of the animal as opposed to the rear.
2. Slowly apply equal and progressively increasing pressure to the body wall and, by extension, the urinary bladder. Slow, steady, and progressive pressure is the key. This is a skill that your pet likely requires, so be patient, keep trying, and DO NOT BECOME DISCOURAGED.
Watch for male dog: https://www.youtube.com/watch?v=G8kuOD2Iup4
Watch for female dog: https://www.youtube.com/watch?v=Qyc181o-g0A
Watch for cat: https://www.youtube.com/watch?v=9KH_eMDJBC8

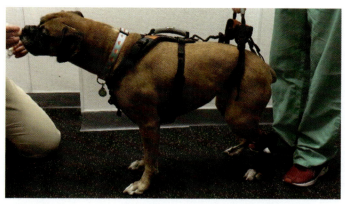

• **Fig. 36.12** The Help 'Em Up harness is an example of a lifting device that can be used to aid mobility in geriatric dogs. (Courtesy Sheilah Robertson.)

covered with Tegaderm Pads (3M, St. Paul, MN), is very helpful for ulcer management. Additionally, the Assisi Loop and laser therapy can be beneficial in treating decubitus ulcers. (For more information regarding wound management, refer to Chapter 27, "Wound Management and Bandaging.")

Recumbent patients may require manual bladder expression to urinate. It is important to teach those caring for the patient how to palpate the bladder and assess bladder function (Box 36.12). Bladder management can involve frequent trips to places where your dog or cat typically urinates—the smell and familiarity of a safe environment may allow them to relax and eliminate.

Bladder expression is tailored to the individual patient. Cats and small dogs have easily palpable bladders that can be held in one hand. Grasping the bladder in one hand and providing gentle but firm compression may help achieve the desired results. For larger patients, a two-handed technique is required. The patient may be lying in lateral recumbency or standing with support. Using the flat surfaces of the hand, not the tips of the fingers, palpate the bladder. While isolating the urinary bladder, the hands are pushed together, simultaneously pushing toward the animal's back. This traps the bladder between the hands and the back, thus allowing urine to flow out through the urethra.

Mobility Assistance with Slings and Carts

Assistive devices such as harnesses or wheelchairs may be necessary for an aging pet, especially if neurologic or musculoskeletal disease is present. Mobility slings and harnesses can be used to move pets more comfortably while minimizing injury to the pet and the owner. Slings and harnesses are designed to accommodate forelimbs, hind limbs, or all four legs. When choosing a sling, patient comfort and ease of use should be considered. Homemade slings, such as a cloth log carrier for larger dogs, may work well; however, technical advancements have made commercial products more comfortable for the pet and the owner. Some homemade slings, or towels used as slings, may apply added pressure to the bladder and cause the pet to urinate inappropriately, whereas most commercial slings are designed to prevent this problem. Slings should have a soft lining against the animal's skin to avoid causing irritation and sores, and should be washable. Observing the pet for pain, discomfort, and respiratory distress is critical, as slings can place pressure on the chest wall, and debilitated pets may have trouble breathing if the sling does not fit correctly.

Harnesses are often a more useful aid to mobility. They can be worn for several hours a day and provide easy access to a handle to lift the dog up (Fig. 36.12). There are also harnesses available with long straps that are useful to prevent back strain for owners of small dogs.

Carts can allow functional independence for impaired animals. They aid in ambulation and can be used to provide therapeutic exercise. They are normally suggested for paretic or paralyzed patients, patients with severe osteoarthritis, and obese patients, and may be used with other devices. When determining the most appropriate cart, the size and weight of the dog or the cat, the amount of support needed, the patient's residual strength and mobility, and the caretaker's physical abilities should be considered. Getting a patient into and out of a cart can be difficult and may require lifting.

Companion Animal Death and Dying

Caring for animals facing imminent death is guided by the same principles that guide caring for all hospice patients: maximizing patient physical and emotional comfort so the death experience is as peaceful, dignified, pain-free, and surrounded by loving care as much as possible; and supporting the animal's caregivers so they experience peace and confidence in their own decisions. Emotional support, guidance, and education are provided by the hospice team to maximize a caregiver's sense of having made the right choice and to minimize guilt, internal conflict, and complicated grief. It is imperative that both euthanasia and natural (unassisted) death be discussed as soon as a caregiver-hospice provider relationship has been established. Educating clients about the euthanasia procedure itself and encouraging them to ask questions is an important and sensitive task. Information should be provided about the drugs that will be given, how they will be administered, and how long it will take for sedation and death to occur. It is best practice to provide families with available resources for support prior to euthanasia, because anticipatory grief can be as debilitating as grief resulting from the actual loss.

GERIATRIC HORSES

Horses are living longer than ever before; it is not uncommon for many horses in their 20s to still be ridden and even shown. As a result, owners are becoming more interested in preserving health and QOL for their equine partners throughout their retirement years. Despite a deep emotional attachment to their aging equine, the stress to both the horse and the owner when transporting a horse that may not have been off the farm for many years and the financial burden may prevent an owner from taking the horse to a veterinary hospital for treatment when a problem or

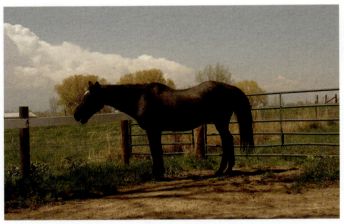

• **Fig. 36.13** A 34-year-old geriatric Thoroughbred horse in good body condition and with a shiny haircoat. (Courtesy Mike Thero.)

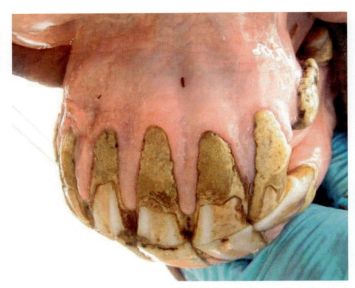

• **Fig. 36.14** External appearance of the maxillary and mandibular incisors in a horse with equine odontoclastic tooth resorption and hypercementosis prior to tooth extraction. (Courtesy Jennifer Rawlinson.)

emergency arises. Therefore many equine veterinarians in private practice manage geriatric horses on the farm. Keeping the geriatric horse healthy and comfortable at home should be paramount in the decision process used by both the veterinarian and the owner.

Aged horses are often defined as those older than 20 years of age. Age itself is not a disease and, with proper care, it is possible for a horse to live out its later years comfortably and happily (Fig. 36.13).

Physical Examination

An annual physical examination is important to identify signs of disease conditions in the aged horse. The general physical examination of a geriatric horse follows the same guidelines as an examination performed on a younger one. (Refer to Chapter 7 for a detailed description of physical examination of the equine patient.) An annual (ideally biannual or even quarterly) BCS is helpful to determine whether the aged horse is maintaining an adequate body condition. (Refer to Chapter 9 for the equine BCS scale.) A score of 1 indicates that a horse is emaciated, and a score of 5 indicates obesity. Acute or chronic weight loss indicates an underlying problem, such as tooth loss, inability of the GI tract to absorb nutrients, or neoplasia.

The horse's attitude is assessed as bright and alert or lethargic. The horse's haircoat should be short and smooth. Older horses suffer from a myriad of health problems, including pituitary pars intermedia dysfunction (PPID), dental problems (particularly equine odontoclastic tooth resorption and hypercementosis, or EOTRH), DJD, equine recurrent uveitis (ERU), heaves, laminitis, neurologic deficits, parasitism, and sinusitis.

Common Problems in Aging Horses

Oral and Nasal Health

Performing an oral examination is important as many older horses are missing teeth or have sharp points (hooks) on their teeth, preventing normal chewing. A severe change that can occur over time is called a *wave mouth*, which occurs when the horse's teeth are of different lengths, preventing normal chewing action. Another condition that is being recognized more often in the aging equine population is EOTRH, which is a syndrome in horses that results from resorptive lesions of the incisors and sometimes canine teeth (Fig. 36.14). Geriatric horses are also more prone to chronic sinus infections, and the presence of nasal discharge and a dull sound when the sinuses are percussed indicate that the sinus cavity contains fluid.

Vision

An ophthalmic examination is performed to check the horse's eyes for certain diseases, such as ERU and cataracts. It is not uncommon for an older horse to have significant visual impairment that is only apparent during an ophthalmic examination. Many older horses are housed on the same farm for years and can learn to compensate for vision loss. If they are moved to a new location, the owner will discover that the horse has difficulty maneuvering in the new environment because of decreased vision.

Cardiac Disease

Cardiac auscultation is important for assessing resting heart rate and the presence of murmurs or arrhythmias. It is helpful to feel the pulse while heart rate is assessed to ensure that they are synchronous and to ensure the pulse is strong and has a normal rhythm. Mitral regurgitation is the most common valvular lesion in horses older than 15 years of age, causing a systolic murmur on the left side of the thorax. Aortic regurgitation occurs in older horses and is clinically associated with a diastolic murmur on the left side. The most common arrhythmia in older horses is atrial fibrillation and is often an incidental finding on physical examination. The rhythm is irregularly irregular and is accompanied by an elevated resting heart rate (>44 beats/minute). Many horses can tolerate this arrhythmia for years and appear healthy but may exhibit exercise intolerance at high levels of exercise.

Respiratory Disease

A respiratory examination evaluates respiratory rate, respiratory effort, and the presence of nasal discharge or coughing. Older horses often have heaves (moderate to severe equine asthma or recurrent airway obstruction) and will have an increased respiratory rate and effort. Chronic cases develop a heave line (hypertrophy of abdominal muscles) resulting from increased expiratory effort.

Gastrointestinal Disease

The GI tract is assessed initially by evaluating the consistency and amount of manure, which should have a normal consistency and should not contain large pieces of hay or grain. If large pieces are present, the horse is not chewing its food properly, and an oral examination is warranted. The presence of diarrhea may indicate chronic colitis or malabsorptive disease.

Kidney Disease

The horse's renal system can be assessed initially by evaluating the amount of water consumed daily and the frequency of urination. Annual urinalysis is important to assess the concentrating ability of the kidneys and to ensure the urine does not contain abnormal amounts of certain substances, such as protein or glucose.

Skin Disorders

The horse's integument is examined for dermatitis and abrasions, especially around bony areas, such as the pelvis. Reproductive organs are visually examined. Elderly male horses may develop tumors on their sheath (prepuce) or penis that are often squamous cell carcinomas and require treatment. The rectal area is evaluated for the presence of melanomas (generally a problem for gray horses) and normal anal tone. Melanomas are often left alone unless they are large enough to interfere with defecation, at which point they may require surgical excision; however, regrowth is common.

Neurologic Abnormalities

On general neurologic examination, older horses may be found to drag their hind limbs and may have blunted toes owing to neurologic deficits or musculoskeletal pain (e.g., DJD in the hocks). The horse's neck should be examined for evidence of pain. This can be done by offering the horse a carrot or a handful of grain to encourage it to touch its nose to its shoulder. If the horse is reluctant or is unable to perform this action, this may indicate the presence of neck pain. Neck pain is sometimes the result of a fractured cervical vertebra, which can be diagnosed with cervical radiographs. DJD of the cervical vertebrae is also common in older horses and may be treated with steroid injections.

Orthopedic Disease

The musculoskeletal examination is an important part of a general physical examination. Older horses are prone to laminitis and may have changes such as rings on the hoof wall that indicate chronic inflammation (Fig. 36.15). They also often have DJD in multiple joints (e.g., carpus, hock) and become stiff without regular pasture turnout. Muscle atrophy is common, especially on the dorsum and around the gluteal area.

> **TECHNICIAN NOTE**
>
> Geriatric horses are likely to have general health problems. At a minimum, an annual (preferably a biannual) physical examination is important to identify and treat problems early.

Chronic Diseases of the Geriatric Horse

Geriatric horses often have multiple problems that require close attention to minimize complications. Common problems in older

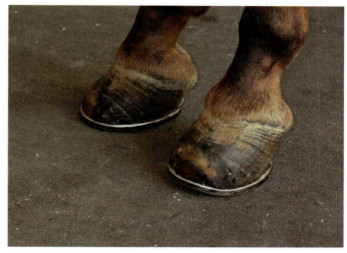

• **Fig. 36.15** A horse with rings on its hoof wall, indicating chronic laminitis. (Courtesy Britta Leise.)

horses include PPID, heaves, laminitis, dental problems, sinusitis, ERU, neurologic deficits, DJD, and parasitism.

Pituitary Pars Intermedia Dysfunction

PPID was originally termed equine Cushing disease (ECD) because of features that resembled Cushing disease in humans; however, there are several differences between the diseases. PPID is a common disease of older horses, especially those over 15 years of age. All breeds of horses can develop PPID; however, it has been suggested that it is more common in ponies and Morgan horses. PPID causes a collection of clinical signs that result from chronic high blood cortisol levels. In most cases, the pituitary gland, which stimulates cortisol production via adrenocorticotropic hormone (ACTH), is enlarged and overactive. As many horses affected by PPID may have concurrent insulin dysregulation, the veterinarian may recommend checking their insulin levels in addition to endogenous ACTH.

Clinical signs of PPID vary among patients. Earlier in the disease process, the horse may exhibit decreased athletic performance, lethargy, delayed shedding, loss of epaxial muscle mass (topline), regional adiposity (crest, tail head), and laminitis, which is also associated with insulin dysregulation. As the disease advances, additional signs (Fig. 36.16) include lack of seasonal shedding or **hypertrichosis** (overly long haircoat), skeletal muscle atrophy, "hay belly," abnormal sweating, polyuria/polydipsia, recurrent infections, bulging supraorbital fat, infertility, persistent lactation, seizurelike activity, blindness, parasitism, and tendon laxity. Supportive findings on blood work (CBC and chemistry profile) include hyperglycemia (blood glucose level >180 mg/dL), hyperinsulinemia, hypertriglyceridemia, neutrophilia, and lymphopenia.

Diagnosis of PPID is made based on the horse's history, signalment, physical examination, and ancillary diagnostic blood tests. Testing is not recommended in the absence of clinical signs. Of the tests available, no single test is 100% accurate.

Three tests that are typically used include the dexamethasone suppression test (DST) to assess cortisol response, measurement of endogenous ACTH, and the thyrotropin-releasing hormone (TRH) stimulation test. In early PPID, the recommended testing is a TRH stimulation test with ACTH measured, or a baseline ACTH if TRH is not readily available. For moderate to advanced PPID, the recommended testing is a baseline ACTH concentration or TRH stimulation test with ACTH measured. Often, these

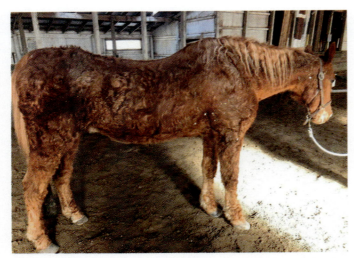

• **Fig. 36.16** Horse with untreated pituitary pars intermedia dysfunction (PPID). Note the hypertrichosis, loss of muscle mass, regional adiposity (tail head), and hoof rings, indicating chronic laminitis. (Courtesy Luke Bass.)

aged horses are in some type of chronic pain. Low to moderate pain of at least 24 hours' duration does not appear to impact diagnostic testing with baseline ACTH or TRH stimulation testing. In aged horses with generalized hypertrichosis, initiation of treatment without further testing is also appropriate.

The primary treatment for PPID is the dopamine agonist pergolide, which is administered once daily and comes as a small tablet that most horses will readily eat in a small handful of grain, making owner/patient compliance more likely. Many clinical signs will significantly improve with treatment. Horses with PPID often appear quiet and depressed, but after treatment is initiated, they become much more alert and act youthful. Rechecking blood tests after starting medication will aid in determining the optimal pergolide dose. Some horses show a transient reduction in appetite. To address this problem, stop treatment until appetite returns and/or decrease the dose by half for 3 to 5 days, then titrate back up in 0.5–1 μg/kg increments every 2 weeks until the desired dose is achieved.

> **TECHNICIAN NOTE**
>
> Pituitary pars intermedia dysfunction (PPID) is common in older horses. Clinical signs vary, but horses often have hypertrichosis (excessive long hair growth throughout the body) and depression. PPID can cause immunosuppression, so diagnosis and treatment are imperative to maintain the health of the geriatric horse.

Heaves (Recurrent Airway Obstruction or Equine Asthma)

Most evidence suggests that **heaves** is the result of the lung's hypersensitivity to inhaled antigens, although multiple theories exist regarding exactly why it occurs. Heaves is similar to asthma in people and has allergic and inflammatory components. The most common allergic triggers are mold, organic dust, and endotoxins present in hay and straw. Horses living in a dusty stable with minimal pasture turnout and that are exposed to cobwebs, straw, and hay are more prone to heaves, as exposure to these allergens leads to airway inflammation and bronchoconstriction. Some horses are affected only a few weeks each year, whereas others are affected year-round. Clinical signs of heaves include increased respiratory rate (tachypnea) and increased effort (dyspnea), nostril flare, dry cough, and fever (unless a secondary infection is present), and they may have a clear nasal discharge. Horses with chronic heaves are often in poor body condition, with a heave line (extreme development of the external abdominal oblique muscles owing to increased effort on exhalation). The horse may extend its head on exhalation to improve airflow; upon thoracic auscultation, wheezes will be heard.

Diagnostic tests to confirm and characterize the lower airway inflammation include upper airway and tracheal endoscopy, bronchoalveolar lavage (BAL), lung function testing, thoracic radiography (x-ray), and ultrasound examination. BAL is indicated in horses with poor performance and coughing but is not necessary in horses with severe disease and suggestive clinical signs. Excess white blood cells (WBCs; neutrophils) seen on cytology confirm the presence of lower airway inflammation and are suggestive of heaves. Radiographs are recommended for horses that fail to respond to standard therapy or to further characterize airway inflammation. Usually, if a horse acutely develops signs of heaves, careful management can minimize clinical signs. Changing the horse's environment to minimize allergens is an important component of treatment. Increasing pasture turnout, soaking or steaming hay before feeding, and eliminating dusty bedding are excellent ways to minimize clinical signs. Medications, including steroids and bronchodilators to control inflammation and bronchoconstriction, are administered systemically or locally (e.g., by using an inhaler). Horses with heaves require management changes, close monitoring, and early treatment at the onset of clinical signs but can live comfortably for a long time if treated properly.

Laminitis (Founder)

Laminitis is a devastating, sometimes fatal, disease of horses. Laminitis results from the disruption of blood flow to the laminae, which secure the coffin bone (P3) to the hoof wall. Inflammation often permanently weakens the laminae and interferes with the wall/bone bond. In severe cases, the bone and hoof wall can separate, and the bone may rotate, sink, and penetrate the bottom of the foot (sole), necessitating euthanasia. Laminitis can affect one or all feet, but it is most often seen in the forefeet concurrently, which likely results from horses bearing more weight on their forelimbs (about 60%).

Although extensive research has been conducted, the exact pathophysiology is still poorly understood. Laminitis may be secondary to a primary problem (e.g., endotoxemia, fracture repair) or may develop acutely with no apparent cause; however, it most commonly occurs in the geriatric horse because of PPID or insulin dysregulation. This could be attributed in part to elevated insulin levels that cause decreased blood flow to the foot via vasoconstriction, which results in damage to the laminae. Some breeds (e.g., Quarter Horses, ponies, and draft horses) are more prone to developing laminitis. Acute laminitis is characterized by pain, inflammation, enzymatic activation, vascular derangements, and lamellar destabilization. The severity of the initial insult often determines the outcome, regardless of treatment.

Treatment strategies should be directed at halting disease progression during the development and acute phases. It is therefore critical that owners are well informed of the early signs of laminitis so they can be on the lookout for such symptoms and can contact their veterinarian early in the disease process, which will hopefully lead to a better outcome.

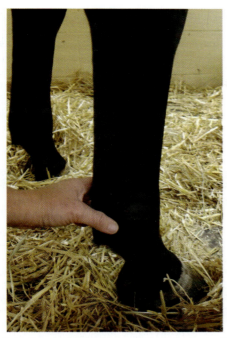

• **Fig. 36.17** Palpation of digital pulses over the fetlock near the sesamoid bones, both laterally and medially. (Courtesy Kristina Rothers.)

Laminitis is a painful condition, because the horse is standing on the affected foot/feet and often cannot find relief from pain. Clinical signs of acute laminitis include reluctance to walk and turn, shifting weight when standing, feet that are warm to the touch, bounding digital arterial pulses palpated over the fetlock near the sesamoid bones (Fig. 36.17), pain in the toe region when pressure is applied with hoof testers, and a "sawhorse stance" in which the forefeet are stretched out in front of the horse to try to take pressure off their heels. Chronic laminitis signs include rings on the hoof wall, bruised soles, frequent abscesses, and dished hooves resulting from unequal rates of hoof growth. Diagnostic tests include radiography of the feet, along with additional tests to diagnose the inciting cause.

Treatment for laminitis itself is often symptomatic, with a primary focus on pain control, and includes regular trimming or possibly therapeutic shoeing, foot pads (e.g., Soft Rides [Soft-Ride Inc., Bacliff, TX]), deep bedding in the stall (e.g., 6–8 inches of shavings or sand), and use of nonsteroidal anti-inflammatory drugs (NSAIDs; e.g., phenylbutazone, firocoxib). If the patient is obese, it is also important to implement a safe weight loss strategy, limiting their diet to only good-quality grass hay and eliminating sources of sugar, such as certain grains and treats. If the owner insists on giving the horse treats, low-sugar, commercially available treats or celery can be offered sparingly. Laminitis may be acute or chronic; geriatric horses often develop chronic laminitis and require regular foot care every 4 to 5 weeks to minimize clinical signs. Recovery can be complete or permanent damage to the laminae may occur, so long-term care is provided individually.

TECHNICIAN NOTE

Laminitis is a painful and sometimes fatal disease that can affect all horses but is of special concern in the older horse. Early diagnosis is critical to a successful outcome, and owner education is a critical role of the veterinary technician.

Dental Problems and Sinusitis

Geriatric horses often develop dental disease as they age. As their teeth wear down or fall out, the opposing tooth will become too long or will develop points (sharp areas on the tooth). This causes abnormal occlusion and interferes with chewing. *Wave mouth* is a severe malocclusion of all teeth; it commonly affects geriatric horses and causes extreme difficulty chewing food.

Clinical signs of dental abnormalities include poor body condition, slow chewing, dropping grain or hay from the mouth, discomfort when chewing, and whole (unchewed) grain in the manure. A thorough dental examination should be performed at least annually (preferably biannually) on horses 20 years of age or older to detect and treat abnormalities. When proper dental care is provided, many older horses can chew their food well and maintain their body condition.

EOTRH is a common inflammatory disease syndrome in aging horses that results in resorptive lesions of the incisors and sometimes canine teeth. As the disease progresses, the roots of the incisors start to resorb. Some horses also develop hypercementosis, which is an excessive buildup of cementum (calcified tissue) on the roots of one or more teeth that can give the appearance of bulblike swellings around the roots of the affected teeth. Affected teeth start to loosen and become painful, and weakened teeth may even fracture in some horses.

EOTRH is a painful disease, and the most common initial sign reported by owners is the horse's reduced ability to grasp apples and carrots. Over time, many horses will eventually stop taking these treats entirely. Some horses become incredibly adept at grasping feed with their lips, sliding it past the incisors and moving it into the mouth through the bar region.

Oral examination can be quite challenging as horses with dental pain are resistant to manipulation of the lips and pressure on the affected teeth. Placement and opening of an oral speculum can elicit possibly dangerous behavior, even under heavy sedation. EOTRH diagnosis necessitates intraoral radiography of both the incisors and the canines. Radiographic findings may include loss of the periodontal ligament space, disruption of alveolar and regional cancellous bone, osteomyelitis, and tooth fracture. Moderate to severe cases require staged or complete extraction of the affected incisors and canines. This is generally achieved with the animal under heavy standing sedation, because there are additional risks, not to mention cost, with placing a geriatric horse under general anesthesia. It is important to let the owner know that after complete extraction of the incisors, the horse's tongue may stick out, at least initially, as the horse learns to hold it differently without the incisors to keep it in the mouth. See Case Presentation 36.1 diagnosis and treatment example of a horse with EOTRH.

Chronic sinusitis of one or both sinuses is also common in older horses and is often caused by tooth root abscessation. Clinical signs include purulent unilateral nasal discharge. Percussing the sinuses in the middle of the horse's head will elicit a dull sound, indicating fluid accumulation. Diagnostic tests include an oral examination to look for tooth root abscessation, upper airway endoscopy, and skull radiography. Treatment options include administering long-term antimicrobials, flushing the sinuses, and/or removing an infected tooth root.

Equine Recurrent Uveitis (Moon Blindness)

Geriatric horses often develop eye problems, with the leading cause of blindness in horses being ERU. ERU is a progressive disease that causes frequent episodes of inflammation and degeneration in one or both eyes. Some breeds, such as Appaloosas, are more commonly affected. Clinical signs include a swollen and painful eye, blepharospasm, *corneal edema* (bluish-white tint to the cornea); iris color change; *neovascularization* (blood vessel growth on cornea); *anterior uveitis* (inflammation in the front chamber of the eye); *hypopyon* (cellular debris in the eye); and *hyphema* (hemorrhage in the eye). A horse with a swollen, painful eye is treated as an emergency, because the cornea is thin (1.5 mm thick) and has no blood supply, so the eye can rupture if not treated quickly. Both eyes should be evaluated, because

many geriatric horses also have cataracts and degenerative retinal changes.

Horses live in a contaminated environment and may develop bacterial and fungal ulcers that can be resistant to therapy. Fungal ulcers can be particularly difficult to treat, often requiring medication(s) to be applied several times per day. Diagnostic evaluation includes performing a thorough ophthalmologic examination, applying fluorescein stain to evaluate the cornea for ulceration, and taking samples for cytology and culture. Treatment depends on whether the cornea

CASE PRESENTATION 36.1

Equine Odontoclastic Tooth Resorption and Hypercementosis (EOTRH) in an Arabian Gelding

A 23-year-old Arabian gelding was presented for weight loss of several months' duration and lack of interest in treats, which he had always enjoyed. The gelding was evaluated by his equine veterinarian and veterinary technician. On physical examination, the horse was in poor body condition (body condition score [BCS] 3/9), and a mild heart murmur (grade 1/5) was noted. The remainder of the physical examination was unremarkable. Routine blood work was performed (complete blood count [CBC], diagnostic panel) and no abnormalities were noted. The patient was sedated (with 5 mg detomidine and 5 mg butorphanol intravenously), and an oral speculum was placed to perform oral examination and dental floatation. Despite sedation, he was very resistant to having the oral speculum placed. Intraoral radiography was performed and revealed moderate to severe hypercementosis of the upper (maxillary) incisors, with multifocal punctate lysis of the incisor roots and bulbous enlargement of some of the tooth roots (Fig. 36.A). The radiographic findings, in conjunction with physical and oral examination findings, were consistent with EOTRH.

The radiographic abnormalities involving the maxillary incisors were more severe than those of the mandibular incisors, and they were suspected to be the cause of most of the pain in the horse. Given the progressive and painful nature of EOTRH, staged extraction of all maxillary incisors with standing sedation was recommended after discussion of the findings with the owner.

After removal of the maxillary incisors and complete healing, the gelding would be re-evaluated for comfort level and weight loss to determine whether removal of the lower incisors was further indicated at that time.

To perform the extraction, a 14-gauge Mila Quick Cath was aseptically placed in the left jugular vein, and the horse was maintained under sedation by using a detomidine continuous infusion for the procedure. The incisors were extracted in a routine fashion. As is typical with EOTRH, the teeth were found to be weakened and misshapen (Fig. 36.B). The sites were then sutured closed (Fig. 36.C). The sutures usually fail within a few days after extraction; however, primary closure still allows for initial healing. In this case, if suture dehiscence did occur, the owner was instructed to rinse the tooth sockets with saline solution twice daily for 7 days. The horse recovered well from the standing sedation, and the catheter was removed. The owner was given instructions to monitor the sutures, and the horse was placed on oral antibiotics for 7 days postoperatively.

At a recheck evaluation 3 months postoperatively, the horse was found to be in improved body condition (BCS 5/9). The owner reported that the animal was brighter and more interactive and that he was once again eager to receive treats. The owner was grateful to be able to enjoy her relationship more fully with her long-time equine partner once more.

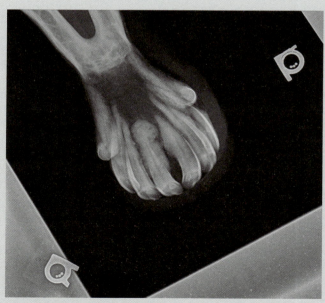

• **Fig. 36.A** Radiograph of maxillary incisors of a horse with equine odontoclastic tooth resorption and hypercementosis (EOTRH). Note the moderate to severe hypercementosis with multifocal punctate lysis of the incisor roots and bulbous enlargement of some of the tooth roots.

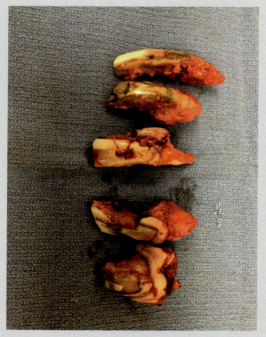

• **Fig. 36.B** The affected teeth after extraction. Note the varying degrees of resorption. (Courtesy Luke Bass.)

CASE PRESENTATION 36.1—CONT'D

Equine Odontoclastic Tooth Resorption and Hypercementosis (EOTRH) in an Arabian Gelding

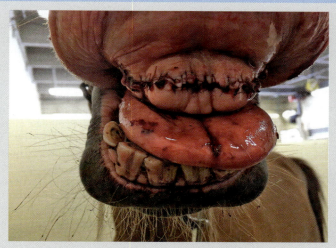

• **Fig. 36.C** The mouth after extraction of incisors. Sutures will often fail after a few days; however, primary closure still allows for initial healing. Also note the tongue sticking out slightly. (Courtesy Luke Bass.)

has only inflammatory changes or if a corneal ulcer is present. If no ulcer is present, medications (topical steroids, atropine, serum, and systemic NSAIDs, such as flunixin meglumine) are used to eliminate inflammation and dilate the pupil. If an ulcer is present, steroid use is contraindicated. In this case, topical antimicrobials (+/−fungicides) and other medications are given until the ulcer resolves, and then steroids can be used to manage inflammation. It is important to get a sample from the ulcerated area and examine it under a microscope so that an appropriate treatment plan can be formulated. An ulcer may not respond to treatment if the underlying cause (e.g., fungal) has not been appropriately identified. In fact, the ulcer may progress and can quickly lead to an emergency, so it is important to implement an appropriate treatment plan as soon as possible.

It is often difficult to treat a horse with a painful eye, so a subpalpebral lavage (SPL) system can be placed for ease of treatment. When the system is being placed, it is important to ensure the foot plate that anchors the system to the eyelid is far enough from the cornea so as not to be another source of trauma.

When a horse has an SPL system in place, it is also important to ensure that the owner watches for excessive tearing or squinting, because it could be a sign that the SPL has shifted and is rubbing the cornea. Surgery may also be required to treat an ulcer. Once the episode has resolved, preventive treatment, such as using a fly mask and anti-inflammatory medications, is often needed to minimize additional episodes. Enucleation (removal of the affected eye) is the last resort in older horses, because both eyes are often affected. Without treatment, the horse will be in pain, and the affected eye will become smaller over time.

TECHNICIAN NOTE

A swollen, painful eye in a horse is considered an emergency, because the eye can rupture if this is not treated quickly.

Neurologic Deficits

Older horses can develop mild or progressive neurologic deficits owing to trauma or chronic changes, such as cervical fractures or osteoarthritis compressing the spinal cord. Clinical signs in an affected horse may include depression, dragging of the toes, ataxia, difficulty standing, and reluctance to turn the neck. Diagnostic tests include thorough physical and neurologic examinations, blood work, cervical radiography, and, possibly, cerebrospinal fluid aspiration (to rule out an infectious cause). Treatment includes anti-inflammatory medications and small paddock turnout/stall confinement, if needed. These horses are often weak and may lose their position in the hierarchy. Therefore, it is important to place them with other horses in similar condition and to feed them individually to ensure that they are receiving adequate nutrition.

Musculoskeletal Conditions

Geriatric horses often have multiple sites of DJD or osteoarthritis and can be lame at the walk and trot. Lower limbs, hocks, carpi, and cervical vertebrae are most affected. Soft tissue problems include suspensory ligament degeneration (noted more often in older broodmares). Diagnostic tests include lameness examination, nerve blocks, and ultrasonography and radiography to identify affected areas. Treatment includes local joint injection of steroids and/or chondroprotective agents (e.g., hyaluronic acid) to relieve clinical signs; however, extreme caution should be used if the horse has PPID, because steroid administration has been linked with potentially causing laminitis in these cases. If the horse has PPID, it may be prudent to discuss alternative therapies, such as platelet-rich plasma (PRP) or stem cell therapy instead of steroid administration. Many of these horses require long-term NSAID administration to have a good QOL. Monitoring with diagnostic tests, such as a chemistry profile, packed cell volume (PCV), TP, and urinalysis, is important with long-term NSAID use. Although side effects such as renal insufficiency or right dorsal colitis may be noted with long-term NSAID use, it is paramount to keep a geriatric horses comfortable at the end of its life. Pasture turnout as much as possible is important, because older horses become stiff when standing in a stall for too long. Nontraditional therapies, such as chiropractic and acupuncture, have also been shown to be effective in some cases.

> **TECHNICIAN NOTE**
> Geriatric horses often have multiple problems that require careful monitoring and treatment to ensure optimal health and longevity.

Management, Nutrition, and Nursing Care of the Geriatric Horse

Geriatric horses can have a good QOL with proper care, but they require close monitoring. Many are turned out in pasture and are not monitored well. They may have poor body condition hidden by a thick haircoat, so it is best to train the owner to assess the horse's body condition. Clipping older horses and placing a blanket in the winter can keep them comfortable. Frequent hoof trimming every 4 to 5 weeks is important to maintain the horse's comfort, especially if the animal has DJD and lameness. If the horse's hoof grows too long, the angle of the foot changes and makes walking more difficult. Routine dental floating every 6 months will keep the horse comfortable and eating well, and will prevent problems such as wave mouth.

It is notoriously difficult to maintain weight and body condition in older horses. It is especially difficult to improve a horse's condition if it has lost weight or is already thin. Frequent pasture turnout can be helpful for maintaining body condition and GI tract health and for minimizing stiffness. If the older horse is in poor body condition, feeding the animal individually is important to ensure that the horse is receiving enough food and to assess appetite. Feeding free-choice high-quality hay with supplementation of alfalfa (hay or soaked alfalfa cubes or pellets) will aid in maintaining weight.

Feeding an equine senior feed or a calorie-dense diet can also help maintain weight if a horse has lost teeth. There are several high-quality commercial feeds available that are high in fat so the horse does not need to eat a large quantity to help maintain condition (e.g., Purina Amplify; Purina Animal Nutrition, LLC, Gray Summit, MO). Corn oil (¼ to 1 cup per day) added to the feed provides additional calories and is inexpensive; however, sometimes horses do not find corn oil palatable, so monitoring to make sure the horse is consuming the feed and that the feed does not sit and turn rancid is important. Additionally, sometimes corn oil can cause loose feces, so the horse's fecal output needs to be monitored to make sure it is tolerating the oil.

General management recommendations include regular deworming, frequent manure removal, and low stocking density (e.g., a few horses in a large pasture) to minimize parasite burden in a pasture. Periodic fecal egg counts should be performed to assess whether the deworming schedule is adequate. Regular vaccination, with use of the recommended vaccine protocol for the area, is recommended. The American Association of Equine Practitioners has guidelines for core and risk-based vaccination of horses posted on its website (www.aaep.org). If the horse has a history of vaccine reactions, it may develop more severe reactions over time, so geriatric horses with a history of vaccine reaction are at higher risk. Pretreatment with an antihistamine or an NSAID may help, but if the horse still has a reaction despite pretreatment, only core vaccines should be administered to minimize complications. It is also helpful to spread vaccinations out so as not to overwhelm the immune system. Splitting the vaccines between the spring and fall can also be a good strategy to ensure biannual evaluation. At a minimum, annual physical examinations and annual blood tests (e.g., CBC, chemistry profile) are important for early detection of problems such as renal and liver insufficiency.

Additional considerations must be noted in treating geriatric horses, because they may be more sensitive to certain medications, such as sedatives and NSAIDs. This sensitivity may be a result of a combination of decreased muscle mass and renal and/or liver insufficiency. Many aged horses receive long-term daily NSAID treatment for chronic DJD (osteoarthritis), so it is important to provide them with the appropriate dose. It is also important to monitor the horse's attitude, appetite, manure production, renal values (creatinine, BUN), urinalysis, PCV, and TP. If any changes in these values are observed, the patient and the treatment protocol should be reassessed.

End-of-Life Issues

When a geriatric horse is no longer enjoying a good QOL, euthanasia may be considered by the owner and/or recommended by the veterinarian. Considerations for euthanasia are often multifactorial but are usually based on GI or orthopedic concerns. GI-related concerns can include poor body condition that is not responding to increased caloric intake, rapid weight loss, or declining appetite. Orthopedic concerns can include refractory pain (e.g., acute, severe laminitis) or severe DJD, leading to chronic, severe lameness.

Additional considerations include episodes of frequent falling and impending cold weather. Cold weather and snow are difficult for older horses to manage. Even with blanketing, it can be hard for an older horse to maintain decent body condition in the winter months. If the horse slips on the snow and ice, it may be impossible for it to get back up again, necessitating emergency euthanasia. These geriatric horses have often been a part of the family for years, and usually the entire family wants to be present during the horse's final moments. Scheduled euthanasia can allow the family to say goodbye and can offer a peaceful end to a beloved horse.

Recommended Readings

Geriatric Dogs and Cats

Bellows J, Center S, Daristotle L, et al. Aging in cats common physical and functional changes. *J Feline Med Surg.* 2016;18:533–550.

Bellows J, Center S, Daristotle L, et al. Evaluating aging in cats: How to determine what is healthy and what is disease. *J Feline Med Surg.* 2016;18(7):551–570.

Bellows J, Colitz CMH, Daristotle L, et al. Common physical and functional changes associated with aging in dogs. *J Am Vet Med Assoc.* 2015;246(1):67–75.

Bishop G, Cooney K, Cox S, et al. 2016 AAHA/IAAHPC End-of-Life care guidelines. *J Am Anim Hosp Assoc.* 2016;52:341–356.

Brooks D, Churchill J, Fein K, et al. AAHA weight management guidelines for dogs and cats. *J Am Animal Hospital Assoc.* 2014;50:1–11.

Epstein M, Kuehn NF, Landsberg G, et al. AAHA senior care guidelines for dogs and cats. *J Am Anim Hosp Assoc.* 2005;41(2):81–91.

Epstein M, Griffenhagen G, Kadrlik J, et al. 2015 AAHA/AAFP pain management guidelines for dogs and cats. *J Am Anim Hosp Assoc.* 2015;51(2):67–84.

Fulmer AE, Laven LJ, Hill KE. Quality of life measurement in dogs and cats: a scoping review of generic tools. *Animals (Basel).* 2022;12(3):400.

Hammerle M, Horst C, Levine E, et al. 2015 AAHA canine and feline behavior management guidelines. *J Am Anim Hosp Assoc.* 2015;51:205–221.

Vogt AH, Rodan I, Brown S, et al. AAFP–AAHA: feline life stage guidelines. *J Feline Med Surg.* 2010;12:43–54.

World Health Organization. 2012. https://www.who.int/tools/whoqol#:~:text=WHO%20defines%20Quality%20of%20Life,%2C%20expectations%2C%20standards%20and%20concerns. Accessed 8/7/2024.

Geriatric Horses

Beech J, Boston RC, McFarlane D, et al. Evaluation of plasma ACTH, α-melanocyte-stimulating hormone, and insulin concentrations during various photoperiods in clinically normal horses and ponies and those with pituitary pars intermedia dysfunction. *J Am Vet Med Assoc.* 2009;237:715.

Bentz AI. Fare thee well: how to help owners (and yourself) deal with the death of a horse. *Compend Cont Educ Vet.* 2009;31:514.

Bertone J, ed. *Equine Geriatric Medicine and Surgery.* Philadelphia, PA: Elsevier; 2006.

Donaldson MT, Jorgensen AJ, Beech J. Evaluation of suspected pituitary pars intermedia dysfunction in horses with laminitis. *J Am Vet Med Assoc.* 2004;224:1123.

Donaldson MT, McDonnell SM, Schanbacher BJ, et al. Variation in plasma ACTH concentration and dexamethasone suppression test results with season, age, and sex in healthy ponies and horses. *J Vet Int Med.* 2005;19(2):217–222.

Endocrine and metabolic diseases. In: Smith BP, ed. *Large Animal Internal Medicine.* 5th ed. St. Louis, MO: Mosby; 2015.

Hart, K, Durham, A, et al. Recommendations for the Diagnosis and Treatment of Pituitary Pars Intermedia Dysfunction (PPID) Revised October 2021 by the PPID Working Group. https://sites.tufts.edu/equineendogroup/files/2021/12/2021-PPID-Recommendations-V11-wo-insert.pdf. Accessed on May 16, 2023.

McGowan C. Welfare of aged horses. *Animals.* 2011;1(4):366–376.

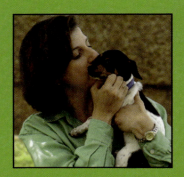

CHAPTER OUTLINE

LEARNING OBJECTIVES

When you have completed this chapter, you will be able to:

1. Pronounce, define, and spell each of the key terms in this chapter.
2. Discuss aspects of the human-animal bond.
3. List and describe the elements of grief and the role of veterinary professionals in grief counseling.
4. Do the following regarding euthanasia:
   - Discuss the impact of euthanasia and client grief on members of the veterinary health care team.
   - Discuss the legal and ethical issues related to euthanasia.
   - Discuss the role of the veterinary health care team in counseling owners facing the death of their pet and factors

that owners need to consider when making decisions regarding euthanasia, natural death, and aftercare.
   - Describe the considerations in training staff and preparing for unexpected events during euthanasia.
   - List the signs and symptoms of staff burnout.
   - List and describe the common methods of euthanasia in large and small animals.
   - Discuss the special considerations related to euthanasia of large animals.

KEY TERMS

Anticipatory grief	Human-animal bond
Bond-centered care	Moral injury
Burnout	Mourning
Compassion fatigue	Natural death
Complicated grief	Normalizing
Disenfranchised grief	Opisthotonos
Dysthanasia	Paradigm
Empathy	Partnering
Euthanasia	Trauma exposure
Extravasation	

Introduction: The Human-animal Bond

In the first quarter of the 21st century, domestic animals of a wide variety of species have continued to experience an ongoing transformation of status in human society from property, livestock, and commodities to companions, family members, and children. Research and observation along several lines have illustrated and explained this transformation. Recent discoveries in animal cognition and ethology have established animals as sentient beings, with complex emotional and social makeups. On the human side, it has become widely established that animals provide psychosocial benefits to people in a myriad of ways. Even the terminology used has changed from *pet owner* to *pet parent* and from *pet* to *fur baby*. Many studies have documented *mutual* benefits enjoyed by both the animal *and* the human in the relationship, down to the physiologic level.

One of the results of the human-animal bond transformation is that people now devote an increasing amount of time, energy, and resources, both financial and emotional, to the care of their animals. It follows that the most important stage of the animal's life in which to ensure that ideal care is given is the end-of-life stage. On that basis, many veterinary professionals are devoting a greater portion of their time, energy, and resources into supporting the patient, client, and family through the final stage of an animal's life in many more ways than just medical.

The findings of present and ongoing research can only be expected to reinforce the current consensus that animals are essentially family members. The physiological, emotional, cognitive, spiritual, and social effects of humans living and interacting with animals of all species are more deeply understood than ever before. Therefore when a beloved animal dies, the human brain makes no distinction between the loss of a pet and the loss of a human family member, requiring veterinary professionals, especially veterinary technicians, to face all types and degrees of grief and help clients experiencing them. When faced with losing a beloved pet, clients also face the danger of stigmatization by those in their social sphere who may unintentionally underestimate or underappreciate the true depth and length of pain that is very likely to be present. These clients feel misunderstood and isolated. This reality presents an opportunity for technicians to support, validate, and partner with the client experiencing loss within their unique bond with animals (Box 37.1).

At the end of life, the "unit of care" must expand to include the pet's family and any other stakeholders in the animal's life. The needs, hopes, fears, and concerns of all members of the unit require the attention of the entire end-of-life care team to deliver what is now known as *bond-centered care* (Fig. 37.1).

> **TECHNICIAN NOTE**
>
> The reality of the human-animal bond requires veterinary professionals to include the human client as part of the unit of care, especially at the end of the animal patient's life.

Bond-centered Care

The most important shift in the approach to caring for the veterinary patient nearing the end of life is the shift from keeping a body alive to supporting the bond between two or more beings as the beloved animal approaches the end of its life. In supporting the relationship between clients and veterinary professionals at this stage of the animal's life, the veterinary technician can become an anchor of trust by listening to anything the clients may wish to talk about, helping clients understand the dying process and euthanasia, assuring clients that their emotions surrounding the death of their pets are normal, and much more. As will be described, clients enter the grieving process well before the actual death of their pets, and often, the client feels safest with the veterinary technician in sharing their true thoughts, hopes, fears, and wishes.

The Interdisciplinary Team

The hallmark of bond-centered end-of-life care is that it is delivered by a team of diverse professionals uniquely trained and equipped to support the unit of care (pet *and* human caregivers) through the final stage of an animal's life. Core members of the team are the attending veterinarian, the veterinary technician/nurse, and the human mental health professional, the last most often a licensed social worker. Depending on the needs of the client and the family, the team may expand to include clinical psychologists, members of the clergy, integrative medicine practitioners, energy workers, and animal communicators. In recent years, many organizations have been formed, with the mission to provide pet loss support in the form of literature, in-person counseling, and support groups.

For some veterinary technicians, the desire to help clients through grieving the loss of their pets expresses itself in the pursuit of education in social work and clinical counseling. Indeed, some veterinary schools have begun offering credentials in *veterinary social work* to qualified individuals, establishing a formal

- Terminology is changing from *owner* to *pet parent* and from *pet* to *fur baby.*
- Pet loss can be traumatic, regardless of outward appearances.
- Animals and humans derive mutual benefits from the bond.
- Anthropomorphism is increasingly accepted and even encouraged.
- Animals of many species have acquired the status of family member.

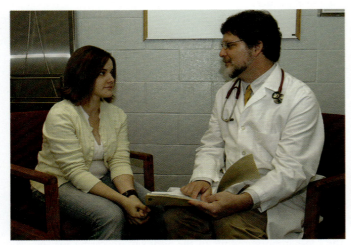

• **Fig. 37.1** The status of animals as family members has become commonplace as an outward expression of the human-animal bond. The human-animal bond becomes the focus of care at the end of life between clients and veterinary personnel.

link between veterinary care and human emotional support. This link also extends in a critical way to veterinary professionals themselves: mental health support as an integral part of the culture of veterinary medicine itself addresses the very real dangers of exposure to suffering and death in the normal course of one's duties. Paradoxically, pursuing excellence in euthanasia may be a mechanism for improving one's own professional quality of life.

Paradigm Shifts

A **paradigm** is any kind of philosophic or theoretical framework that underlies and guides a school of thought. In both human and veterinary medicine, the dominant paradigm is typified by the mandate to diagnose, treat, and prevent disease. This paradigm is responsible for great scientific advancements, improvements in overall health and longevity, and the eradication of some diseases altogether. At the end of life, this paradigm can become a reason for unnecessary suffering for the patient, client, and veterinary medical professional.

When faced with the fact that every single human or animal is going to die someday, one very quickly encounters profound and dangerous limitations in the disease/medical paradigm. In the desire to fight against disease, pain, and suffering, other factors, such as comfort, joy, love, and family, get left out. Worse still, patients' own feelings about their quality of life (QOL) are often ignored or misinterpreted. In veterinary medicine, these problems are compounded because of the nature of the human-animal bond, the mystery surrounding animals' ability to communicate

their desires, and the reluctance of many veterinary professionals to trust or even acknowledge the client's knowledge and intuition about what their pet needs and wants in life.

In all too many cases, euthanasia or even natural death is viewed as a failure or "giving up." This is an example of a flawed paradigm at the heart of veterinary medicine, which fails to acknowledge that not every pet will get this or that disease but that all pets will die, that death is a natural part of life, and that death has meaning. The end of life cannot be approached with the same philosophy as that which underlies annual vaccinations, emergency surgery, differential diagnosis, or any other approach that seeks to fight disease and put off the inevitable. A major source of client stress and emotional trauma is bringing the so-called "medical" model into end-of-life situations. At some point, one must realize that the patient is not sick but is dying and needs an entirely different kind of care.

Ultimately, end-of-life care requires a paradigm shift that touches every aspect of the relationship between the animal's family and the veterinary professional. The medical model no longer applies. Comfort, meaning, and support are now the priorities. Death is no longer the enemy, but a stage of life to be approached with dignity, compassion, and highly refined skill.

> **TECHNICIAN NOTE**
>
> In bond-centered end-of-life care, priorities shift from fighting disease to promoting comfort in recognition of the inevitability of death.

The Veterinary Technician's Roles Before, During, and After Euthanasia

Euthanasia is one of the most performed procedures in veterinary medicine. Paradoxically, perhaps tragically, euthanasia is the one aspect of veterinary practice in which veterinary students receive little to no formal training. Several resources that seek to remedy this discrepancy are available (see the Recommended Reading section at the end of the chapter), and veterinary technicians are offered rich opportunities to obtain deeper education and skills in helping clients and patients through the death experience. In exploring the different roles of the veterinary technician in end-of-life cases, many new discoveries will emerge and will deepen and enhance the care of clients and patients to higher standards than have been traditionally accepted. The main roles to be understood and mastered are education, medical care, and advocacy. These are known as the *core competencies*, which were first delineated by the International Association for Animal Hospice and Palliative Care.

Education and Communication

The veterinary technician is often the best-equipped and best-positioned member of the care team to talk with and listen to clients as they learn to navigate the last months, weeks, days, and moments of their pets' lives. In general, technicians spend more time with clients compared with the veterinarian and, in many cases, clients feel a more significant connection with and a sense of trust in their technician, and are therefore more likely to voice their deepest desires regarding the care of their pets. For this reason, it is critical that the technician be equipped with communication skills that are most likely to honor the bond. These skills include open-ended questions; generous, judgment-free listening; healthy empathy; and appropriate body language.

Open-ended questions are constructed to avoid soliciting a "yes" or "no" response. The goal in asking this type of question is to invite clients to engage and share their knowledge and understanding of their pet's condition or diagnosis; their feelings about different care options, including the decision to end their pet's life; and any other information considered important in managing the case. In this way, a deliberative partnership, rather than a paternalistic one, is created between client and veterinary professional—another example of the paradigm shift required when approaching the end of a pet's life.

The client's greatest need currently is a human being who listens without judgment and without the need to understand, agree with, or even like what the client is saying. Technicians must feel no need to impart knowledge or even reassurance when listening. The only skill requirement is the ability, developed through daily attentive practice, to accept both what the client is saying and allow the situation to be what it is. The only priorities are trusting the client's intuition and being open to a sense of awe as one listens.

Empathy is the ability to identify with the emotions and feelings of others. Although empathy is revered as a virtue in the veterinary profession, it is not without its dangers. Empathy has been observed to take at least two forms. First is the experience of actually feeling what the other person is going through as if it were happening to the listener. This triggers the involuntary stress response and ends up reducing helpful behavior. On the other hand, simply cognitively appreciating what the client is experiencing and feeling bypasses the stress response and increases helpful behavior.

Of all the communication skills discussed, nonverbal communication and body language are the most important. Within the context of a deliberative partnership, technicians should pay attention to the flow of nonverbal communication when conversing with clients who are navigating the end-of-life process with their pets. Open and inviting postures, judicious use of eye contact, and positioning oneself at the same level will help clients feel safe to share difficult feelings and grapple with important questions.

Advance Directives

In human medicine, the advance directive is an indispensable tool for ensuring that the dying person's wishes are honored, especially if the person becomes unable to communicate. Because animals cannot speak, it is even more essential to discuss clients' wishes and desires as early as possible if their pet receives a life-limiting diagnosis or even while the pet is still in good health. There is no evidence that such discussions create or increase clients' fear or depression; on the contrary, they serve as an important touchpoint in the client–veterinary professional relationship and as a safeguard against procedures and measures to which the client may not wish to subject their pet, much less what the pet may choose for itself if it could.

Clients' wishes regarding the aftercare and memorialization of their pets should be an essential part of early end-of-life conversations. These decisions are best made before a potential crisis occurs and before the planned euthanasia or natural death experience begins, when the client's decisions are less governed by the emotion of the end-of-life experience. Technicians may feel reluctant to bring up these questions for fear of upsetting the client. It is important to remember that although it may be difficult for the client to consider questions of aftercare while their pet is still alive and while euthanasia may not yet be a necessary consideration,

studies have shown that these discussions do not compound or intensify the client's grief but, in fact, can liberate them to enjoy and appreciate their pet's last days of life, knowing that a plan is in place when the time comes.

Some clients may not wish to think about or make these decisions because of anticipatory grief. The veterinary staff should never insist that a decision be made immediately. Clients should be reassured that they need not decide right away and encourage them to take comfort in the fact that there is plenty of time to find the option that feels most appropriate and meaningful to them. Once determined, the client's wishes should be entered into the patient's medical record and communicated to all who are involved in the case.

Discussing Euthanasia

In the early stages of end-of-life conversations, technicians can perform quality-of-life assessments, which include discovering "lines in the sand" that would trigger the client to arrange a euthanasia appointment. As discussions progress, clients' wishes can be identified and put together to form the advance directive for their pet. Box 37.2 contains some essential questions to ask during these discussions.

Some clients may wish to be present for the entire experience, some for the presedation period only, and others may not wish to be present at all, instead choosing to say their farewells before the procedure begins. It is important to assure the client that no matter what they choose, their feelings and wishes are normal and their choice is supported.

The veterinary technician may also educate the client about the euthanasia experience itself. In early end-of-life conversations, the process can be outlined in general terms, and the technician may even ask clients how much information and detail they feel comfortable hearing. Clients' feelings may range from their desire to ensure a quick, painless procedure for their pets to their need to understand what their pets may be experiencing as the drugs for sedation, anesthesia, and euthanasia are administered.

Discussing Natural Death

During end-of-life discussions, clients almost always express the wish that their pets would die naturally and peacefully in their sleep. Other clients may have a firm, definite desire that their pet experience a natural death without euthanasia because of ethical, religious, or spiritual beliefs. In the emerging field of animal hospice and palliative care, there are many groups and practitioners who dedicate their work to providing *hospice-supported natural death*. In this type of end-of-life care, the patient and family are supported around the clock while allowing the natural dying process to unfold. For the patient, pain control, hygiene, comfort,

> **• BOX 37.2 Essential Questions to Ask in Early End-of-Life Conversations**
>
> - What is your understanding of your pet's condition and prognosis?
> - What are your greatest hopes and fears?
> - What is most important to you as time grows short?
> - What are your wishes and desires for your pet's end-of-life-transition?
> - Who will be present and for how much of the euthanasia appointment?
> - What are your wishes for aftercare?

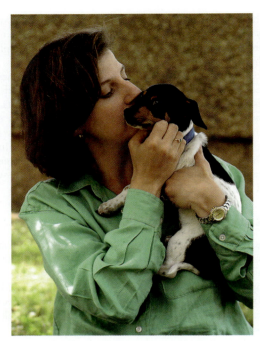

• **Fig. 37.2** The technician often plays a central role in assisting in a good death.

and environment are all addressed. If any of these elements become impossible to provide for at any point during the process, euthanasia remains an option should it become the most humane course of action. The technician can describe the pros and cons of both euthanasia and hospice-supported natural death, and help the client better interpret their desires and make decisions based on a solid understanding of both.

TECHNICIAN NOTE

The technician's role as educator in end-of-life cases requires a deeper knowledge of the dying process, whether via euthanasia or natural death, and the ability to listen without judgment.

Medical Care

In recent years, well-educated and trained veterinary technicians have been entrusted with an increasing percentage of animal medical care tasks. Depending on state guidelines, many care tasks can legally be performed in the home by the veterinary technician, saving the attending veterinarian time, the client money, and the patient potential stress and anxiety. This leveraging of the technician's abilities can only benefit the quality of care provided, preserve and strengthen the bond between patient and client, and infuse the technician's work with more meaning and significance. The paragraphs below touch on some aspects of medical care that are specific to end of life and can be performed by the veterinary technician (Fig. 37.2).

Preparation for Euthanasia

When euthanasia has been chosen, the veterinary technician plays a crucial role in preparing the patient, the space, and the client for the death experience. The top priority is comfort for all involved. The client must be allowed and encouraged to maintain as much close and loving contact with their pet as desired. Blankets, beds,

---

• BOX 37.3   **Preparing a "Sacred Space" for Euthanasia**

- Choose and dedicate a comfortable space, away from normal clinic activities.
- Provide comfortable arrangements for human family members to gather.
- Consider soft music, lighting, and aromatherapy options to minimize fear and stress
- Eliminate any aspects that denote a "medical" feel.
- Provide blankets and beds for patient comfort.
- Include absorbent pads in case of bladder/bowel release, without distracting from the overall purpose of the euthanasia space.

---

and absorbent pads should be used to provide the patient and the client maximum comfort before and after administration of sedation and/or anesthesia drugs. All necessary supplies should be within reach without intruding on the overall setting of a "sacred space."

The well-established practice of in-home euthanasia is a compelling option for many pet owners. Offering this option to clients very often dramatically reduces the stress of the euthanasia experience for both client and patient. All of the skills and roles of the technician during euthanasia apply to the in-home service setting. For many technicians, this practice has given greater meaning to their work.

In the clinic setting, it is advisable to designate a space or spaces dedicated to the euthanasia experience. "Comfort rooms" are common and are often simply examination rooms that have been appointed with comfortable sofas, carpet, art on the walls, colors chosen for their calming effect, and even music and aromatherapy diffusers. Other options include an outdoor "memory garden," or other type of secluded, quiet space away from the main events in the clinic. Whatever the arrangement, it is important that the space allows families maximum opportunity to be comfortable and free of distraction, and that any sort of "medical" feel is minimized or avoided (Box 37.3).

Assisting With and Performing Euthanasia

Whether the euthanasia experience occurs in the clinic or in the home, the veterinary technician can and should serve as an essential member of the care team at the time of the death of the pet. In keeping with the concept of bond-centered care, the most obvious place for a technician's abilities is in preparing the sedated or anesthetized patient for euthanasia by placing the intravenous catheter. A high level of confidence and skill is required in this situation. All too often, the patient is taken from the client to the treatment area to place the catheter. This practice needs to be eliminated from veterinary practice, because it threatens the human-animal bond at precisely the time when it should be most strongly supported. The technician can narrate the process and usually perform the task without help, provided the patient is adequately sedated or anesthetized. Furthermore, because the patient is asleep, if a vein is not accessed within a few seconds, an alternative route of administration of the euthanasia solution can be selected.

If the attending veterinarian is to administer the euthanasia solution, the technician can play an important role in skillfully and gracefully holding off a vessel, passing supplies to and from the veterinarian, and managing the patient during the euthanasia. Ideally, the technician is an essential partner in the "dance" of the euthanasia experience, imparting the practiced skill of purposeful

• BOX 37.4 **Essential Tasks for the Euthanasia Appointment**

- Consider scheduling the appointment outside of busy times in the clinic.
- Arrange for and receive payment prior to the appointment whenever possible.
- Verify consent and aftercare wishes.
- Keep the space stocked with essential supplies, such as syringes, needles, gauze, intravenous catheters, facial tissues, grief support materials, etc.
- Eliminate any need for removing the pet from the client.
- Allow time alone for the client at any stage and remain available at all times.
- Deliver proper techniques and methods, whether or not in tandem with the attending veterinarian.
- Establish and follow protocols for confirming death.
- Be mindful of exits and clients' need for privacy.

yet highly sensitive care, which powerfully supports clients as they say farewell to their beloved pets.

TECHNICIAN NOTE

Never remove an animal from a client to place an intravenous (IV) catheter in preparation for euthanasia unless the client requests it.

PUT INTO PRACTICE

Do you feel you are too emotional during euthanasia? It is okay to feel sad or tearful. It shows your true caring and empathetic self, which is something that clients will appreciate. It's okay to excuse yourself if you are overwhelmed.

Preparing the Pet's Body for Aftercare

The preparation and care of a pet's body for either burial, transport to a cremation facility, or other form of care is a task that is practiced with alarming inconsistency in veterinary medicine. It may be highly unlikely that the average veterinary practice would allow a client to witness the handling of their deceased pet after euthanasia. Recognizing that veterinary practices may be ill equipped or underequipped to raise the level of dignity in the care of recently deceased pet above that of trash bags and freezers, a few simple additions to the euthanasia process may be beneficial.

First, allowing clients the opportunity to view or be with the body after death can fulfill wishes that clients were unaware that they had; this opportunity can manifest itself in a variety of ways. Second, technicians and even clients can wash the pet's body in a final gesture of love before the body is removed. Additionally, the time between death and aftercare can be used for making paw- or hoofprints, trimming hair, and any other meaningful task of memorialization requested by the client (Box 37.4; Fig. 37.3A–C).

Advocacy

Underlying all of the roles for veterinary technicians to play on the care team is the central role of advocate—for the patient, the client, and the standards of care held by the practice overall. In no other situation is advocacy more necessary than end-of-life situations. Pet parents often feel too overwhelmed or distracted by their normal emotions to insist or even voice their wishes after the death of their pet. Being the team members who spend the

greatest amount of time with clients and patients, technicians are in an ideal position to ensure that clients' and patients' wishes and needs are known and followed to the best of the team's ability (Case Presentation 37.1).

Another area of advocacy in which technicians can be effective is in maintaining the overall standards and protocols practiced by the veterinary care team. An essential element of high-quality end-of-life care is the consistency of the euthanasia experience offered by the practice. Technicians can spearhead meetings and training sessions to codify the agreed-upon standards of end-of-life care that will form the basis of the practice's services. Advocating for high, consistently practiced standards of care will increase clients' trust and comfort, especially if they are faced with more than one pet's death over the years. Ultimately, clients will often forgive almost any medical or surgical error, misdiagnosis, or unintended consequence of treatment. If, however, they have a traumatic experience during euthanasia, they are likely to feel unable to return to the practice.

TECHNICIAN NOTE

Advocating for a high standard of end-of-life care *is* advocating for the human-animal bond.

Decisions: Goals of Care, Euthanasia, and Natural Death

Although it is *not* the technician's role to recommend for or against euthanasia, within the conversations described in the previous paragraphs, the technician is still an essential resource for clients who may be struggling with questions of suffering, QOL, and the fear of making the decision to end their pet's life too soon or too late. At this stage, the client is experiencing anticipatory grief and the fear of the unknown that appears as the client contemplates the inevitable death of the pet. It is important to reassure the client at every step of the process that their feelings are normal.

Quality of Life and the Will to Live

QOL is composed of objective and subjective factors that exist within the personalities of the pet, the client, and all who care for the bond. In making the decision to end a pet's life, it is essential to consider the pet's own opinion of its life, and the client is the most reliable resource for this information. The pet's physical appearance is perhaps the least significant parameter in determining quality of life, let alone whether life should be terminated. The technician can help the client to weigh the various parameters that make up the pet's QOL. Two parameters commonly and erroneously cited in negatively assessing an animal's QOL are appetite and weight loss (Fig. 37.4).

Appetite is sometimes a reliable barometer for QOL, but it is important to consider that some animals (especially horses) may retain a good appetite well past the point where euthanasia was the best option. Conversely, the loss of appetite does not necessarily mean that the animal is suffering; it may be that the animal's body simply no longer requires nutrition as it moves on through the natural dying process. It should never be assumed that if an animal stops eating at some point in its dying process that it will starve to death. The important question is, how much does eating and the pleasure of eating *matter* to the animal? Furthermore, many clients may inadvertently prolong (or be inappropriately encouraged to

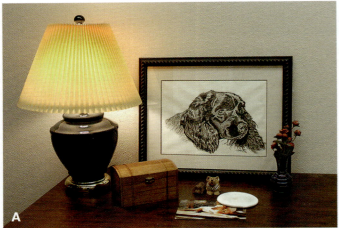

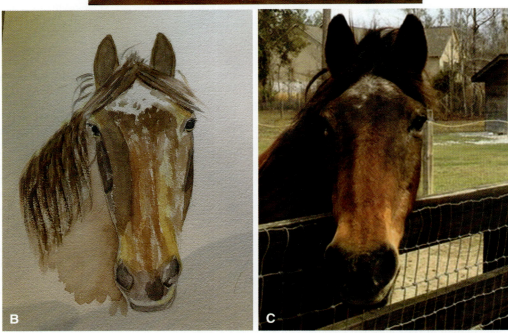

• **Fig. 37.3** Memorialization is the process of learning to love the absent pet and adjust to the transformed bond.

prolong) their pet's life because "she's still eating," even though the pet's pain and discomfort can no longer be controlled, and the rest of the pet's daily life is characterized by restlessness, lack of engagement, and inertia. In these situations, question what the pet would lose if their life were to end today. If the answer is, for example, "5 minutes of eating," the picture becomes clearer and the road to an informed decision better defined.

Weight loss often brings up questions regarding euthanasia. Clients often worry when their pet's body condition deteriorates near the end of life. Provided there is no physical danger, weight loss does not matter to the animal. Pets do not look at themselves in a mirror and worry that their ribs are showing. This perspective often comes as a relief to clients who may have been feeling pressured to euthanize their underweight pet when so many other parameters that mean more to the animal were still intact. With large animals, loss of body condition is more of a concern, because it relates to the animal's ability to get up and down.

Overriding all questions of QOL is the animal's own desire to live. Again, the client is uniquely positioned to assess this question and, notwithstanding the animal's QOL "score," the decision to end life depends on subjective parameters that lie at the heart of the human-animal bond. At this point in the end-of-life process, it is critical to assure the client that *they are the world's expert on their pet*. This assurance is the counterbalance to the overwhelming burden associated with making the decision to end their pet's life at some point in time. The technician and the client together can develop a plan for monitoring the patient's QOL, with "lines in the sand," established based on the individual patient and the client's own goals of care, which ultimately guide and support the client's informed decision regarding the patient's final days.

Suffering

The most common statement made by clients regarding a dying pet is, "I don't want them to suffer." This statement reveals one of the greatest fears and potential grief triggers that exist within the human-animal bond. It also reveals the need and the opportunity to help the client interpret signs their pet may be showing and

CASE PRESENTATION 37.1

Advocacy

You are called upon to accompany your attending veterinarian to a farm call. Petunia, a 16-year-old Paint Horse, took a bad fall while running in the pasture and has likely fractured her right foreleg. The owner, a former event rider who is now in her 60s and has owned and trained Petunia from when she was a foal, is heartbroken and shows no signs of being willing to leave Petunia's side. The owner is aware that Petunia's condition is terminal and that her limbs are very unstable but refuses to leave her beloved horse, stating her firm desire to be present through every step of the euthanasia procedure.

You assure her that you and the veterinarian will sedate and anesthetize Petunia to lay her down in the most relaxed way possible and that there is no need to step away during a potentially disturbing event. After explaining that the safest vantage point for Petunia's transition to recumbency is 20 feet away, the veterinarian administers 6 mL of 100 mg/mL xylazine intravenously and, over the next few minutes, Petunia's head drops between her knees. You hold Petunia's head as the veterinarian administers the anesthetic induction syringe. Within seconds, Petunia sinks onto her hindquarters, and you and the veterinarian gently guide her into lateral recumbency, placing her head gently on the ground with smooth, easy movements.

Petunia's owner is then invited to sit at Petunia's head and given the chance to say her farewells over the 12 to 20 minutes of anesthesia time. The veterinarian informs Petunia's owner that Petunia is ready for the injection that will help her to pass, and Petunia dies peacefully, with her head held in her owner's arms.

At the conclusion of the appointment, Petunia's owner embraces you and thanks you for advocating her wish to be present for Petunia's last moments. She states that watching her beloved horse lie down under anesthesia was the most peaceful way she could imagine to say goodbye to her beloved partner.

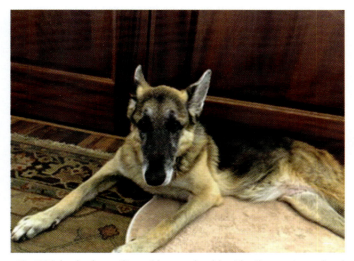

• **Fig. 37.4** Lack of appetite or thinness should not be the most prominent factors in the decision for end-of-life measures.

understand what their pet is experiencing in the weeks and days leading up to the time of death.

Suffering is nothing more than a spectrum of painful experiences capable of being experienced by a sentient being. In discussing suffering with clients, several important points can help dispel the emotional and fear-based responses to the idea of suffering in pets. First is the idea that death is not painful, but disease is. Second, harmful effects of suffering depend on the individual's ability

• BOX 37.5   Ethical Factors Affecting Euthanasia

1. Prolonging life versus doing harm
2. Objective and subjective perceptions of animal welfare
3. Behavior as a terminal disease
4. Animal use in research
5. Convenience versus practical/financial barriers to care

CASE PRESENTATION 37.2

Ethical Challenge

The owner of two 6-year-old Chow Chow littermates brings both dogs to your practice for their yearly checkups. A concerning mass is found on one of the dogs, and additional diagnostics reveal an aggressive cancer that has already metastasized to her chest. Several weeks later, after numerous conversations about humane endpoints and weighing treatment options (the owner decided against oncologic therapy), the owner decides that euthanasia is the best choice for her dog. While making the euthanasia appointment, the owner states her wish to euthanize the dog's littermate at the same time. The littermate has no health problems, but the client expresses a deeply held belief that the littermate would be irretrievably traumatized by the loss of its sibling and that she prefers to "send them to Heaven" together.

Upset by this request, you confer with your supervisor and attending veterinarian. Rather than trying to argue and convince the client out of her beliefs, the team decides to refer the client to another provider, citing the practice's commitment to its core value and policy of only performing euthanasia for the relief of intractable suffering and to spare the terminal patient from the worst that the disease has in store. The client understands and respects the practice's stance.

to cope or adapt. Third, suffering must be weighed against that capacity for pleasant, positive affective experiences. Approaching suffering in this way offers an opportunity for the technician to build further trust with the client, by framing the discussion in a thoroughly individualized way. Suffering thus loses its domination over human perception and interpretation of animals' experience. New priorities of comfort, happiness, and meaning emerge. This change of perspective empowers the client as the world's expert on their pet and may help avoid premature euthanasia.

> **TECHNICIAN NOTE**
> Questions of quality of life (QOL) and suffering are subjective and individual. The answers that inform end-of-life decisions lie in those aspects of life that matter to the animal and depend on the intuition and insight of the client.

Ethical Considerations

Every euthanasia event carries an ethical dimension. Inevitably, technicians will encounter cases that either challenge or run counter to deeply held values and beliefs about how animals should be cared for. The veterinary care team should establish self-governing guidelines on how to deal with cases that may present ethical challenges, including the option to refuse wishes deemed unethical (Box 37.5 and Case Presentation 37.2).

Convenience

The decision to euthanize an animal in the absence of terminal disease, intractable suffering, or any other of the commonly cited indications may be termed "convenience" euthanasia. Technicians may encounter clients who, for whatever reason, are unwilling or unable to properly care for an animal and request that the animal be euthanized. Clients in these situations must never be made to feel judged. At the same time, they should be educated and offered options for rehoming the animal or seeking some other arrangement that would allow the animal to receive the treatment it requires.

As with most other aspects of end-of-life care, these issues are matters of opinion. It is important that the practice establish policies for handling cases of convenience that minimize ethical conflicts and preserve staff morale. It is always appropriate to refuse to euthanize for the sake of convenience and refer the client to another practitioner if one's own deeply held values would be compromised.

Shelter and Research Situations

Technicians working in shelter and research environments are subject to the unique stresses of euthanizing otherwise healthy animals when no other viable options exist or in the normal course of the facility's operations. It is critical that technicians in these situations have every opportunity for self-care and receive emotional support as an essential part of their terms of employment. These professionals are particularly susceptible to burnout and compassion fatigue, which often manifests in bitterness and anger toward real or imagined abuse and neglect on the part of persons who may have been responsible for placing animals in these situations. Regular meetings with staff to share their feelings and unburden themselves from the challenges of their work can help ensure the awareness and minimization of dangerous mental health hazards.

Whatever the circumstances faced by the technician involved in depopulation, research-associated, and shelter-based euthanasia, encouragement and meaning may be derived from implementing similar standards of care to those of a veterinary practice or euthanasia service. All the essentials of the "good death" can be incorporated into the euthanasia practice of the shelter or research facility. Presedation, anesthesia, skillful application of techniques, and dignified body care can all contribute to minimizing the effects of the increased exposure to death faced by technicians working in shelters and research (Fig. 37.5).

Welfare

Euthanasia for welfare reasons in otherwise treatable cases is another complex and highly emotionally charged issue. Technicians whose work brings them into contact with neglected animals for whom euthanasia is deemed the best option carry a very heavy emotional burden. Welfare also becomes an issue when an owner is no longer financially able to care for an animal with special physical needs. Although the animal may still have excellent QOL (from its own point of view), the lack of any other future prospect other than being surrendered to a shelter or turned out to pasture (in the case of many large-animal species) precludes the animal's right to a good death. Rescue organizations can only do so much. Most rescues, although well intentioned, often fail to consistently apply the principles of animal welfare, especially to address the individual social, emotional, and psychological needs of the animals.

Behavior

A particular type of case that challenges technicians' deepest values is that of a patient with intractable and dangerous behavior that has not responded to treatment. This type of euthanasia case

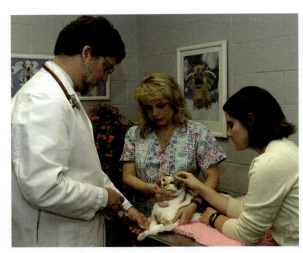

• **Fig. 37.5** Letting the pet decide. When comfort measures are effective, the pet's physical appearance is of little concern in assessing quality of life and making end-of-life decisions.

requires the technician to hang on tightly to the paradigm of comfort versus cure. The proper approach is to assume that behavior problems are indeed a type of disease and that animals with such behavior problems are indeed suffering. Behavior problems should be discussed in the same way as any other life-limiting diagnosis, and with the same bond-centered orientation.

Euthanasia: An Experience, Not a Procedure

However well informed the decision may be, it is ultimately based on the belief that death is preferable to the present condition, that comfort is no longer sustainable or achievable, and that the human-animal bond would be best served with a dignified, peaceful death via medical intervention. There is no definitive or objective "code" that bestows upon any decision to euthanize the description "this is absolutely the right time." The layers of "unknowns" that surround euthanasia are the major causes of grief in veterinary clients, and it is at this point that the technician can support the client in the fact that there is no "bull's eye" to be aimed for, but that all who were involved in the animal's care had done the best they could with the information available, and that the animal had been allowed to express its own desires and provided with all the comforts that veterinary medicine and nursing can provide, even unto the end of life.

> **TECHNICIAN NOTE**
>
> Ultimately, the decision to euthanize an animal is based on the belief that death is the most humane course of action given the available information.

Euthanasia: The Art of Providing a Good Death

The term *euthanasia* derives from the Greek roots *eu-* (good) and *thanatos* (death). The American Veterinary Medical Association (AVMA) lists 12 criteria for evaluating euthanasia methods (Box 37.6). This section will explore the methods that meet the criteria most completely, especially because they can be adjusted to enhance and support the human-animal bond.

From *AVMA Guidelines for the Euthanasia of Animals*, 2020. https://www.avma.org.

BOX 37.6 Criteria for Humane Euthanasia

- Ability to induce loss of consciousness and death without causing pain, fear, or distress
- Reasonable time to induce loss of consciousness
- Reliability
- Safety for personnel
- Irreversibility
- Compatibility with requirement and purpose
- Emotional effect on observers or providers
- Compatibility with future examination (i.e., necropsy)
- Drug availability and potential for human abuse
- Compatibility with species, age, and health status
- Ability to maintain equipment
- Safety for predators/scavengers in case of carcass consumption

Common Methods

The most common category of method for the euthanasia of most small and large domestic species is the noninhalant pharmaceutical category. The most common vehicle for noninhalant pharmaceutical euthanasia is a barbiturate overdose. Barbiturates have historically been used for induction and maintenance of general anesthesia and to control seizures. When given as a lethal dose, barbiturates directly depress the neurons in the brainstem that are responsible for sustaining life. This overdose can be given as the sole agent or after sedating and/or anesthetizing the animal. After the initial brain death, respiration ceases, followed by cardiac arrest. The pharmacodynamics of the euthanasia drugs can provide an important touchpoint with clients who may worry about what their pets may be experiencing during the process. It can be a great relief for some clients to know that the drug works in the brain first and that as breathing and heartbeat fade and disappear, the animal is not aware of the body shutting down. It is always appropriate to ask clients how much detail they prefer to receive before beginning early end-of-life conversations.

Sodium pentobarbital is the most common injectable barbiturate used for euthanasia. Depending on the manufacturer's composition, the drug may hold a Drug Enforcement Administration (DEA) Schedule II or III Controlled Substance designation. Practices should ensure compliance with documentation regulations and determine who is authorized to handle controlled drugs.

Other AVMA–accepted noninhalant pharmaceutical methods include the use of intravenous or intracardiac potassium chloride or magnesium chloride. A relatively new method involves the use of intrathecal lidocaine, which directly blocks the brainstem, causing eventual respiratory and cardiac arrest. Each of these methods require the animal to be in a deep surgical plane of anesthesia in order to be effective.

TECHNICIAN NOTE

Explaining how the various drugs work can help calm clients' fears surrounding their pets' experience of euthanasia. Clients should be asked for the level of detail that they prefer before beginning the conversation.

Small-animal Protocols

All euthanasia protocols will feature varying uses of the following steps: presedation, anesthesia, and euthanasia. Practitioners are increasingly implementing the anesthesia step into their protocols because of the greater control, ease, and safety of presedation and anesthesia and the bond enhancement and support that they can provide. For the person performing the euthanasia procedure, having the pet heavily sedated or in a deep plane of anesthesia eliminates the need for restraint, allows for many other options than intravenous injection of the euthanasia solution, and most importantly, allows the client to remain in close contact with the pet throughout the procedure.

Steps

Presedation With or Without Anesthesia

In small-animal patients, particularly dogs and cats, presedation options will include an α_2-agonist sedative, such as dexmedetomidine, plus an opioid, such as butorphanol, combined in one syringe and administered either subcutaneously or intramuscularly. When dosed appropriately, this drug combination can provide profound sedation sufficient to proceed with euthanasia with use of minimal restraint, thus promoting closeness between pet and client. It should be explained to clients that the alpha$_2$ drugs decrease cardiac output and may slow the action of the euthanasia solution somewhat, but that death will be peaceful and the patient will be unaware. Acepromazine is often added to the presedation cocktail, especially in larger, nervous, or anxious dogs. Caution should be used when administering α_2-agonists to cats because of the risk of vomiting. In aggressive or dangerous-to-handle dogs, oral formulations (i.e., dormosedan gel) can be administered without directly touching the animal. Onset of action is longer, but the dramatically reduced stress and risk both to patient and professional are well worth the extra time to achieve adequate sedation safely. Even with heavy sedation, animals can be unpredictably aroused by visual, auditory, or tactile stimuli, so the veterinary professionals should still be on their guard as they proceed with the euthanasia.

Anesthesia may be combined with presedation to produce sleep that can allow for a variety of options for euthanasia, ease the sense of urgency, and thereby remain bond centered. Clients almost always express the wish that their pets would die peacefully in their sleep. Technicians can explain that the anesthesia step *gives* the animal that sleep, which can be a profound relief to clients. Pre-euthanasia anesthetic protocols involve a dissociative agent, such as ketamine, often combined with a benzodiazepine, such as midazolam, which is added to the presedation syringe. Alternatively, many providers reconstitute a vial of Telazol (tiletamine + zolazepam) with other combination agents, such as acepromazine and butorphanol or ketamine and xylazine, and use that combination as the sole presedation/anesthesia injection. Many variations exist and are preferred in different situations (Table 37.1). When anesthesia is chosen, clients should be reassured that their pets can still hear their voices and feel their presence but will not react to anything the veterinarian or technician does, such as placing an intravenous catheter or administering the euthanasia injection. It can often be a great comfort for the client to know that this is the most comfortable their pet has been in a long time. Anecdotal evidence suggests that a chief benefit of anesthesia is that it allows injection of the euthanasia solution very slowly, which is thought to reduce or even eliminate involuntary side effects, such as agonal breaths, limb stretching or paddling, and release of bladder and bowel contents.

TECHNICIAN NOTE

A euthanasia protocol involving presedation and anesthesia allows many benefits for the patient and comfort for the client, in addition to smoothly facilitating the provider's task.

TABLE 37.1 Common Presedation, Anesthesia, and Euthanasia Drugs and Their Uses

Drug/Class	Dose	Purpose	Route	Caution
α²-agonists: xylazine, detomidine, dexmedetomidine	0.005 to 0.015 mg/kg 1 to 1.1 mg/kg, depending on agent and concentration	Pre-euthanasia sedation, enhance/deepen anesthesia	SQ, IM, PO, IV	Reduces cardiac output; evaluate safety in heart patients, consider avoiding in cats
Opioids: butorphanol, morphine, hydromorphone, nalbuphine	Depending on concentration, 0.1–0.2 mg/kg	Enhance/deepen sedation, analgesia	SQ, IM, IV, PO	Pure mu-agonists may cause vomiting
Dissociative: ketamine, tiletamine	Ketamine = 2.2–5 mg/kg in dogs and horses, generally 0.5 mL per 10#	Anesthesia	SQ, IM, IV	Combine with a benzodiazepine to counteract muscle rigidity and stage-2 excitement
Benzodiazepines: diazepam, midazolam	0.2–0.4 mg/kg 5.0 mg/kg	Paired with dissociative for anesthesia/muscle relaxation	*Diazepam IV only; all others SQ, IM, IV; midazolam also rectally or intranasal	None; wide dose range; can control concurrent seizure/neurologic disease
Phenothiazines: acepromazine	0.01–0.02 mg/kg	Tranquilization; synergistic with other sedation/anesthesia drugs	SQ, IM, IV, PO	Avoid in heart patients or when vasodilation would compromise euthanasia efficacy
Barbiturates: pentobarbital	85-255 mg/kg based on route	Euthanasia	IV, IH, IC, IR, IP, PO	Anesthetize patients for all routes other than IV
Combinations: tiletamine/zolazepam	13.6 mg/kg	Anesthesia	SQ, IM	Patients may exhibit agitation associated with stage 2 of anesthesia

IC, Intracardiac; *IH*, intrahepatic; *IM*, intramuscular; *IP*, intraperitoneal; *IR*, intrarectal; *PO*, oral; *SQ*, subcutaneous.
Adapted from Companion Animal Euthanasia Training Academy certificate course, attended 4/2018, Loveland, CO.

Euthanasia

Sodium pentobarbital is the most common injectable agent for achieving a quick, painless death in small and large domestic species and is said to be the one drug that fulfills the AVMA's criteria by itself. If used as the sole agent in a one-step protocol, it is only appropriately administered intravenously or orally in awake or sedated patients. Barbituric acid derivatives have a high pH and cause severely painful irritation and tissue necrosis if the agent is inadvertently administered outside a vessel, causing unnecessary pain and discomfort in the awake or sedated patient. A well-placed intravenous catheter can minimize the risks of extravasation, but not all patients have ideal veins, and patients deserve to be spared the discomfort caused by the struggle to locate and access a vessel.

Instead, in the anesthetized patient, the full potential of sodium pentobarbital is realized because of the availability of alternative routes of administration if a vein is not quickly and easily accessed. In cats, the intrarenal, intrahepatic, intracardiac, and intraperitoneal routes are all possible when the animal is under anesthesia. In small dogs, intrahepatic and intracardiac routes are often chosen. In large dogs, the intracardiac route is the most common alternative. For all intraorgan injections except intracardiac ones, the normal dose of euthanasia solution is doubled or tripled, and the solution is still injected slowly. The skilled provider will shield their hands under blankets while administering the injection, all the while explaining to the client that the dying process may take longer but that their pet is in no distress whatsoever. Many clients worry about the idea of an intracardiac injection. The best explanation to reassure them is that the heart is just a big vessel and is the quickest and most efficient way to get the drug where it needs to go (the brain) to produce its intended effect.

TECHNICIAN NOTE

Training in the performance of intraorgan injections frees the provider from the potential stress of locating a vessel to inject the euthanasia solution.

Large-animal Considerations and Protocols

The human-animal bond, with all its attributes, emotional content, and history, is, in many ways, deeper and more intense with large animals, particularly horses. Evidence indicates that the grieving/mourning process among horse owners often lasts longer and is more deeply felt than among dog and cat owners. For this reason, even more care and effort should be undertaken to support the bond in end-of-life situations with large animals (Fig. 37.6A and B)

Safety

With euthanasia of large animals, safety is the top priority for all involved. Whenever possible, a setting that causes minimal fear, anxiety, and stress for the animal and, at the same time, provides handlers, providers, and onlookers with a safe place to participate

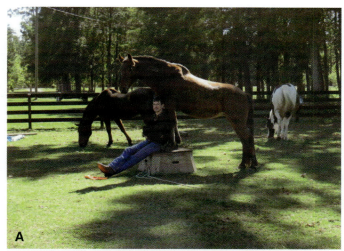

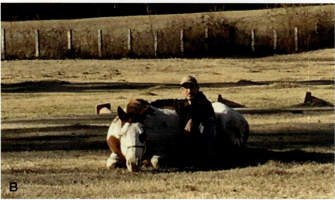

• **Fig. 37.6** (A, B) Pet parents of large animals, particularly horses, have been reported often to have a stronger bond with their animals compared with parents of smaller companion animals.

or be present should be chosen. The steps and protocols in large-animal euthanasia are fairly similar to those for small animals; however, there are added risks involved in positioning the animal into recumbency. Very rarely is a horse already down (although this is one of the main reasons for choosing euthanasia) when the team arrives to perform the euthanasia. Historically, clients have been discouraged from being present for the euthanasia of their beloved horse, which can have a profoundly traumatic effect on the bond and can complicate the grieving process. Through training and the use of a two-step anesthesia protocol, the unpredictability of laying the horse down is drastically diminished, and owners can maintain a greater closeness throughout the procedure.

Steps

Presedation With or Without Anesthesia

The most common presedation protocol in horses is anchored around α²-agonist sedatives, such as xylazine, romifidine, or detomidine. These can be combined with a tranquilizer, such as acepromazine, and an opioid, such as butorphanol, to deepen the sedation effect, and administered intravenously, almost always in a jugular vein. When the level of sedation is adequate (head lowered to the level of the carpi), the provider can proceed with either anesthesia or euthanasia.

It is at this point that the human-animal bond is at the most vulnerable state—when the time comes to lay the horse down, either through anesthesia or euthanasia. Inducing anesthesia to

lay the horse down has anecdotally been reported to result in a much smoother "fall," with none of the undesirable and disturbing esthetic effects that are often associated with the one-step or two-step (without anesthesia) protocols. A simple induction dose of ketamine plus diazepam, given as a rapid intravenous bolus, provides the greatest means for a smooth transition to the ground and up to 20 minutes of anesthesia time for the horse's loved ones to gather and say their farewells. In this and previous descriptions of the two-step protocol, it may be inferred that the final injection is almost an afterthought, woven into a larger process with much greater meaning.

Euthanasia

When used in a one-step protocol, the euthanasia solution is most often administered in the jugular vein and as a rapid bolus to avoid the excitement and agitation of Stage 2 of anesthesia. As with small animals, presedation and anesthesia may slow the effects of the euthanasia solution because of decreased cardiac output but, again, clients can easily be reassured and supported while their beloved animal passes away. In all cases, death is confirmed via cardiothoracic auscultation to confirm absence of heartbeats and the absence of corneal reflex.

Physical Methods

In some cases, physical methods of euthanasia are indicated, preferred, or required, depending on the species and situation. Physical methods most commonly consist of gunshot or captive bolt, both of which disrupt the brainstem tissue, causing respiratory and cardiac arrest. Highly trained personnel and perfectly functioning equipment are required for the proper delivery of physical euthanasia methods. Although these methods may be visually upsetting to the layperson, unconsciousness is immediate and, in many situations, this is the most humane option.

TECHNICIAN NOTE

Large animals and their human families deserve the same standard of end-of-life care as that given to small animals.

Dysthanasia

The side of euthanasia feared by all veterinary professionals is its opposite, **dysthanasia**. Dysthanasia occurs when the patient or client suffers during the dying process because of unexpected occurrences. Many practitioners have described the distress and emotional trauma of a euthanasia procedure that did not go according to plan. Some common situations include a malfunctioning intravenous catheter; extravascular administration of the euthanasia solution; adverse patient reactions, such as vocalizing and exhibiting signs of pain or distress to administration of either presedation or euthanasia; and complicated emotional states in the clients. Perception is an important issue to consider. Some involuntary signs the patient shows during the death process, such as agonal (labored) breathing and **opisthotonos** (stretched limbs and a backward-arched head) are not indicative of distress, but the client may interpret these as adverse events. It is essential to educate and inform the client ahead of time that certain signs may occur, but the pet is not aware of the body's dying process and these signs in no way mean that something is going wrong. Some practitioners describe these signs to the client as "energy leaving the body," which can be reassuring. Still, many adverse signs, whether real or perceived, are avoidable through careful selection and efficient execution of protocols, which often include presedation and anesthesia as described earlier.

Client suffering can occur surrounding the death of a pet when communication and attention are lacking or when full understanding of either euthanasia or natural death has not been achieved. Profound feelings of guilt, fear, and anger are very common when the client feels inadequately supported or perceives that their pet has not died well or has suffered at the end. Dysthanasia is a major reason for the loss of a client; therefore it deserves intense attention and requires rigorous, ongoing staff training to ensure that the risk of a bad death is minimized and that processes are in place to ensure that clients are properly cared for when unexpected situations occur (Table 37.2).

Handling the Unexpected

Even when every precaution has been taken, every skill has been practiced correctly, and every step has been taken with the greatest

TABLE 37.2	Summary of Agents and Methods of Euthanasia: Characteristics and Modes of Action				
Acceptability	Mode of Action	Ease of Performance	Safety for Personnel	Species Suitability	Efficacy and Comments
Barbiturates					
Acceptable	Direct depression of cerebral cortex, subcortical structures, and vital centers; direct depression of heart muscle	Animal must be restrained unless sedated or anesthetized; personnel must be skilled to perform intravenous injection	Safe except human abuse potential; DEA-controlled substance	Most species	Highly effective when appropriately administered; acceptable by intravenous and in small animals
Benzocaine					
Acceptable	Depression of CNS	Easily used	Safe	Fish and amphibians	Effective but expensive
Carbon Dioxide					
Acceptable	Respiratory acidosis and decrease in intracellular pH	Used in closed container	Minimal hazard	Small laboratory animals, birds, cats, small dogs, mink (high concentrations), zoo animals, amphibians, fish, some reptiles, swine; conditionally acceptable for nonhuman primates and free-ranging wildlife	Effective, but time required may be prolonged in immature and neonatal animals
Carbon Monoxide (Bottled Gas Only)					
Acceptable	Combines with hemoglobin, blocks oxygen uptake by erythrocyte	Requires appropriately maintained equipment	Extremely hazardous, toxic, and difficult to detect	Most small species, including dogs, cats, rodents, mink, chinchillas, birds, reptiles, amphibians, zoo animals, rabbits; conditionally acceptable for nonhuman primates and free-ranging wildlife	Effective; acceptable only when equipment is properly designed and operated
Cervical Dislocation					
Conditionally acceptable	Disruption of electrical activity of brain	Requires training and skill	Safe	Poultry, birds, laboratory mice, and rats weighing less than 200 g or rabbits less than 1 kg	Irreversible, violent muscle contractions can occur after cervical dislocation
Clove Oil, Isoeugenol, and Eugenol					
Acceptable	Inhibits voltage-sensitive sodium channels in the CNS	Easily used	Safe	Finfish, both freshwater and marine	Effective

Continued

TABLE 37.2   Summary of Agents and Methods of Euthanasia: Characteristics and Modes of Action—cont'd

Acceptability	Mode of Action	Ease of Performance	Safety for Personnel	Species Suitability	Efficacy and Comments
Decapitation					
Conditionally acceptable	Direct depression of brain activity	Requires training and skill	Guillotine poses potential employee injury hazard	Laboratory rodents, small rabbits, birds, fish, amphibians, reptiles	Irreversible, violent muscle contractions can occur after decapitation
Electrocution					
Conditionally acceptable	Causes cerebral hypoxia	Not easily performed in all instances; animal should be unconscious before procedure being performed	Hazardous to personnel	Used primarily in foxes, sheep, swine, mink (with cervical dislocation), ruminants	Violent muscle contractions can occur at same time as loss of consciousness
Gunshot					
Conditionally acceptable	Direct concussion of brain tissue	Requires skill and appropriate firearm	May be dangerous	Large domestic and zoo animals, reptiles, wildlife	Instant unconsciousness, but motor activity may continue
Inhalant Anesthetics					
Acceptable (isoflurane, enflurane, sevoflurane, desflurane are clinically available in the United States)	Direct depression of cerebral cortex, subcortical structures, and vital centers	Easily performed with closed container; can be administered to large animals by mask	Must be properly scavenged or vented to minimize exposure to personnel	Small animals weighing less than 7 kg	Highly effective, provided subject is sufficiently exposed
Microwave Irradiation					
Acceptable	Direct inactivation of brain enzymes by rapid heating of brain	Requires training and highly specialized equipment	Safe	Mice and rats	Highly effective for special needs
Nitrogen, Argon					
Acceptable	Displaces oxygen, causing anoxia	Use closed chamber with rapid filling	Safe if used with ventilation; is nonflammable and nonexplosive with minimal hazards to humans	Turkeys, chickens, and pigs	Effective except in young and neonates; an effective agent but other methods preferable; not acceptable in most animals younger than 4 months of age
Penetrating Captive Bolt					
Acceptable	Direct concussion of brain tissue	Requires skill, adequate restraint, and proper placement of captive bolt	Safe	Ruminants, horses, swine	Instant unconsciousness, but motor activity may continue
2-phenoxyethanol					
Acceptable	Depression of the CNS	Easily used	Safe	Finfish not to be consumed	Effective but expensive
Pithing					
Conditionally acceptable	Trauma of brain and spinal cord tissue	Easily performed but requires skill	Safe	Ruminants and frogs that have been rendered unconscious	Effective, but death not immediate unless brain and spinal cord are pithed

Continued

TABLE 37.2	Summary of Agents and Methods of Euthanasia: Characteristics and Modes of Action—cont'd				
Acceptability	Mode of Action	Ease of Performance	Safety for Personnel	Species Suitability	Efficacy and Comments
Potassium Chloride					
Acceptable in unconscious animals (when combined with magnesium chloride OR magnesium sulfate)	Direct depression of cerebral cortex, subcortical structures, and vital centers secondary to cardiac arrest	Requires training and specialized equipment for remote injection with the ability to give intravenous injection of potassium chloride	Anesthetics may be hazardous with accidental human exposure	Most species	Highly effective; some clonic muscle spasms may be observed
Thoracic Compression					
Conditionally acceptable	Physical interference with cardiac and respiratory function	Requires training	Safe	Small to medium-sized free-ranging birds	Apparently effective
Tricane Methane Sulfonate					
Acceptable	Alters nerve conduction and decreases cardiovascular function	Easily used	Safe	Fish and amphibians, other aquatic cold-blooded animals	Effective but expensive

CNS, Central nervous system; *DEA*, Drug Enforcement Administration.

Modified from *AVMA Guidelines for the Euthanasia of Animals*, 2020. https://www.avma.org/sites/default/files/2020-02/Guidelines-on-Euthanasia-2020.pdf.

attention to all details, things can still go wrong with euthanasia. The intravenous catheter can malfunction, a vein can "blow," or a patient can unexpectedly vocalize during euthanasia, even when an appropriate dose of anesthesia was given. It is at times like these when one's interpersonal and technical skills are tested to their limits. If unexpected events are discussed well in advance in accordance with the bond-centered paradigm, the practitioner is free to be in the moment with the client and patient. By including the unexpected in the range of allowable situations during euthanasia, the technician and veterinarian can strengthen to relationship with the client and preserve as much meaning in the experience as possible.

Establishing Protocols and Training Staff

To minimize the chances of dysthanasia and promote a consistent client experience, a detailed, principled, agreed-upon body of training and protocol must be established for the practice to provide good euthanasia (Box 37.7). Every staff member should be familiar with how euthanasia appointments are handled and be able to explain the hospital's protocol to inquiring clients. All departments should be well versed in the proper conduct when euthanasia cases arrive and the procedure is in progress to minimize trauma to grieving clients.

Furthermore, all veterinary practices should build into the structure of their time the opportunity to debrief, process, and share with one another about difficult or challenging cases. Regular times to connect with coworkers in this way improves the health of any practice. If painful feelings brought on by work are safe to mention, they are also subject to change through establishing healthy workplace cultural norms.

> **• BOX 37.7   Staff Training Essentials to Ensure a Good Euthanasia Experience**
>
> - Discover and discuss staff beliefs about euthanasia.
> - Discuss and agree on roles of different personnel.
> - Establish consistent protocols and procedures.
> - Establish protocols for sending sympathy cards and offering grief support.

> **TECHNICIAN NOTE**
>
> Acceptance of the unexpected, gained through training and experience, will carry clients and providers through difficult situations.

Hospice-supported Natural Death

Over the course of their careers, technicians will encounter some clients who, for ethical, spiritual, religious, philosophical, or other reasons, are firmly opposed to euthanasia or wish for their pet to die naturally in its own time. It is well within the grasp of modern veterinary medicine to support patients and clients through the natural dying process. Pain and symptom control, hygiene, environmental enhancement for the patient, and emotional support and respite care for the client, usually around the clock near the end of the animal's life, are the hallmarks of hospice-supported natural death. If all requirements for patient comfort are met, allowing the pet to die naturally in the loving presence of its human companion can be a powerfully moving and deeply meaningful event.

Deep Questions

Part of the reason for the growing interest in hospice-supported natural death is our own growing understanding of animal cognition. Recalling the previous discussion of QOL and what it means to the individual animal, several important questions emerge: Do animals have a sense of past or future? Can they hope for things? If an animal has an incurable disease or devastating injury or cannot function in a way that is considered "normal," does that mean that the animal would prefer to die? Can animals choose pain and suffering for some unknown purpose? Is death via euthanasia the only answer to suffering?

As we can see, hospice-supported natural death challenges virtually all the most deeply held assumptions about the inner life of animals or at least exposes them as assumptions. Just as there are humans who respond very differently to life-limiting diagnoses, it stands to reason that some animals may prefer to endure pain and suffering rather than choosing to die. At the very least, it is recommended that those clients who wish for a natural death for their pets should be educated about euthanasia and those who opt for euthanasia be educated about natural death, so that both options can be demystified and any fears or worries discussed and alleviated. There are several organizations dedicated to supporting pets and people through the natural dying process. Recalling the technician's role as educator, the act of helping clients understand the signs of active dying, from weeks to days to hours before death, is essential in supporting the bond through the process.

Signs of Active Dying and Caring for the Dying Patient

The most important component of supporting the natural death of a pet is informing the client about what to expect in the last weeks, days, and hours of their pet's life. Understanding the various signs is extremely helpful to the client who may be worried about the animal's physical appearance or that certain signs might mean that the pet is in pain or distress. Learning to interpret the signs of approaching death even weeks away empowers clients and caregivers to address comfort-related needs and to allow normal signs of dying to come and go.

In the last month to 3 months before death, pets exhibit behavioral changes, ranging from withdrawal to increased attention seeking. Appetite begins to decrease, along with weight and muscle mass. Signs of dehydration can also appear. Although the body is still able to absorb subcutaneous fluids, they can be offered if administration does not cause undue stress or fear. When fluids begin accumulating in the distal limbs and axial regions, the body no longer requires them and administration should stop. As dehydration continues, endorphins are released to relieve the discomfort associated with cessation of nourishment.

One to two weeks before death, clients may notice disorientation, confusion, and agitation, which can be signs of cognitive dysfunction, but these have been described as the animal drifting back and forth between consciousness and unconsciousness. Appetite and water intake continue to wane. Body temperature may decrease, along with blood pressure.

Days to hours before death, pets may exhibit a "swan song" period of resurging energy before the final decline. Incontinence and irregular breathing occur. Extremities continue to become cooler as blood pressure drops. As the kidneys fail, the pet may smell "like death." Heart rate and rhythm become slower and irregular.

Minutes before death, agonal breaths may appear. Limbs will stretch, and the head may arch backward. Bladder and bowels will empty. Terminal gasps will give way to respiratory arrest and eventual cardiac arrest. Pupils will become fixed and dilated with brain death.

Throughout this process, clients must be supported in caring for any of the pet's physical or mental/emotional needs until the final moment and beyond and, above all, they must be reassured that death does not cause pain, but disease does, and that the point of hospice-supported natural death is to minimize or eliminate the unpleasant effects of disease so that death can be welcomed in its own time.

> **TECHNICIAN NOTE**
>
> Clients who desire and are prepared to ensure a natural death for their pets without euthanasia need intensive, often around-the-clock support during their pet's dying process.

Aftercare and Memorialization

In early end-of-life conversations, client's wishes for the care of their pet after death is an essential part of the information needed to ensure the best care and support of the bond. Decisions made before a potential crisis are always less stressful, even if they are sad to contemplate.

Burial

Burial is a very common form of aftercare. Many clients even preselect a special area on their home property where they wish to lay their pets to rest. As tactfully as possible, it is important to educate the client about the potential for euthanasia drugs to leach into the soil and aquifers and for the body to be exposed to scavengers. If the burial is not completed in a timely fashion (as is sometimes an issue with large animals) or if the animal is not buried deep enough (generally, 4 feet of earth on top of the body is required), and an endangered or protected scavenger is harmed by ingesting contaminated flesh, the veterinarian can face severe consequences from fish and wildlife authorities.

Cremation

Increasingly, clients are opting to have their pets cremated. There may be concerns about the possibility of relocating and the emotional ramifications of leaving a buried pet behind. Clients need to know the difference between individual and communal cremation, especially if they wish to have their pet's ashes returned to them. The veterinary practice must maintain a close relationship with a trusted cremation service and be able to articulate the different options clearly.

Water-based Cremation

In some areas, veterinarians who dedicate their practice to providing euthanasia and end-of-life care exclusively also operate their own aftercare facilities to provide their clients with an all-inclusive, consistent experience. One of the most recent advances in nonburial aftercare is water-based cremation, also called "aquamation." An environmentally friendly alternative to burial or flame-based cremation, aquamation is based on the chemical process of *alkaline hydrolysis*, where the use of potassium hydroxide and sodium hydroxide in water act to speed up the natural decomposition process. At the end of the 20-hour process, only bones remain, which are dried, pulverized, and returned to the client. The nonsolid remains are inert and nontoxic and can be used to irrigate gardens or fields.

Return to the Elements

Seen most often in large animals, a patient euthanized without drugs (i.e., by physical methods) may simply be left for scavengers and for the natural decomposition process to return the body to simpler forms of matter that will support new plant and animal life. Whatever the clients' wishes may be for aftercare, each option can be made as dignified and meaningful as possible, and the technician is the main contact in facilitating early discussion and decision making.

> **TECHNICIAN NOTE**
>
> Clients' wishes for aftercare should be an integral part of early end-of-life conversations.

Honoring the Death and Nurturing the Memory

Just as grief and mourning are unique to every individual, so are the nearly infinite ways in which clients may wish to memorialize their pets. In practice, technicians can offer to create paw- or hoofprints, and to trim and save fur or the hair of a mane and tail. Dozens, if not hundreds, of services exist around the world to help facilitate the client's memorial wishes for their pets to find full expression (Fig. 37.7).

Grief and Loss: Human and Animal Perspectives

The human-animal bond does not end with the death of the animal. In this section, we will explore some of the most profound, intangible, mysterious yet crucial aspects of the veterinary profession. Within the capacity of a veterinary technician, understanding the elements of the effects of loss on pet owners and the care team as well as the animals themselves can help add meaning to the reality of death and the feelings that come with experiencing loss as part of one's job. Technicians can do this by partnering with the grieving client in the immediate aftermath of euthanasia and maintain that contact at different intervals such as anniversaries by sending sympathy cards or otherwise communicating the acknowledgement of a pet's memory.

The first and most important idea to understand is that grief is associated with any kind of loss. The human brain does not make any distinction between the loss of a pet and the loss of a human loved one. Grieving pet owners often feel stigmatized by the rest of society and made to feel as though their emotions are out of proportion, unnecessary, or inappropriate simply because they have experienced the loss of an animal as opposed to that of a human. When veterinary technicians encounter pet owners facing or dealing with the death of a pet, they meet someone who is experiencing fear of the unknown. In this situation, a deep understanding of all the elements of the pet owner's grief equips the technician to provide a uniquely profound and powerful kind of help.

Grief is the natural response to loss. All sentient beings experience grief, and every individual grieves and mourns differently. Grief is an internal process, consisting of thoughts and emotions surrounding the loss. *Mourning* is the *act* of grieving, the outward manifestation of the internal landscape of the bereaved.

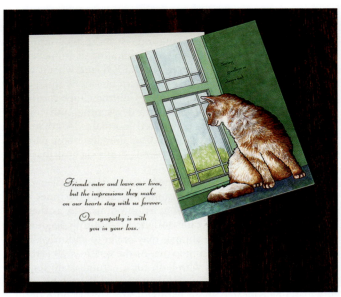

• **Fig. 37.7** A card thoughtfully signed and sent by members of the veterinary health team may be of comfort to grieving pet parents.

Anticipatory Grief

Clients experience **anticipatory grief** any time they contemplate the death of their pet. The feeling intensifies when faced with a terminal diagnosis or other life-limiting condition. In early conversations, the technician should reassure clients that their feelings are normal. Many clients fear the initial questions or subjects that may be brought up in discussing their pet's condition and prognosis and may not wish to talk about them. It is important to never force the client to engage in end-of-life discussions. By remaining open and nonjudgmental, the technician creates a safe space where the client will eventually arrive at the willingness to talk about the end of their pet's life. Recognizing and acknowledging anticipatory grief keeps the channels of communication open.

"Normal" Grief

Grief is universal and unique at the same time. As various theories that characterize stages or phases of grief have accumulated, it has been recognized that grief is nonlinear, dynamic, and has no timeline. In the context of the human-animal bond, a subtler and more universally applicable approach is needed, an approach that recognizes grief as a range of thoughts and feelings that operate uniquely within each individual's consciousness. The technician learns to normalize whatever the client is expressing, and the client feels safer having shared their pain.

Emotional Responses to Loss

Sadness and *loneliness* are the most deeply felt emotions in the grieving client. They often elicit intense physical expressions. Reassurance that it is all right to cry and long for the pet helps the client feel safe and minimizes the loneliness and isolation that accompanies sadness and depression. Almost everyone experiencing a profound loss feels *numbness* at the same time. In the early aftermath of euthanasia, numbness should be normalized, as it is the brain's way of protecting a person from feeling too much at once.

Anger is another normal emotional response to loss. Sometimes, anger finds a target in the veterinary professional. This is only because the source of the client's frustration (the circumstance of loss) is irreversible. Patient, respectful listening as the anger is fully vented and dissipates is the way to help clients who feel like this. Also, anger can be turned on oneself, not only in clients but also in veterinary professionals, and can lead to depression.

Guilt and *shame* are often woven together with anger at the feeling that others may not understand or appreciate the depth of grief felt with the loss of the pet. The speculation and the fear that the client expresses through questioning what they did wrong or what they could have done or should not have done can only be supported with understanding, not by trying to talk them out of their feelings of guilt (Case Presentation 37.3).

Relief is an unexpected but essential emotional response which, again, the client may wrongly self-interpret as selfishness. This sense of relief is caused by release from sometimes years-long worry, stress, and energy spent managing or treating the pet's disease process. In the same way that death can end the suffering of the animal, it can also end a measure of the client's suffering (Case Presentation 37.4).

TECHNICIAN NOTE

Grief contains a vast range of emotions that, when acknowledged by the technician, can help normalize one's experience.

Complicated Grief

Complicated grief is an extremely intense, prolonged, and mentally and physically debilitating permutation of normal grief. Complicated grief is a risk factor in clients who have not experienced major losses in their lives or have experienced multiple losses within a short period or under sudden, traumatic circumstances.

In addition, clients without a reliable support system may experience complicated grief. Complicated grief is a major risk factor for major depression, posttraumatic stress disorder, and even self-harm or suicidal ideation. Any sign of complicated grief should be an automatic trigger for referral to a human mental health professional (Box 37.8).

Disenfranchised Grief

Perhaps the most dangerous form of grief experienced by the client is that which is met with ignorance or lack of understanding or minimization by those in the client's social circle. **Disenfranchised grief** isolates the bereaved pet owner through exposure to the all-too-common sentiments: "She was just a dog; you'll get over it; there are so many other dogs/cats/horses that need homes; she's in a better place," and so on. Although these statements are not meant maliciously, the pain of grieving pet parents is compounded and prolonged when they feel that they are misunderstood and isolated and that their pain is underappreciated because the object of their grief was not a human. This type of grief especially needs the support of the veterinary team and particularly of the human mental health professional.

Partnering With the Grieving Client

Much earlier in this chapter, the necessity for a paradigm shift in veterinary medicine from a disease model to a comfort model was explained as a necessary philosophic anchor in the practice

---

CASE PRESENTATION 37.3

Guilt

Polonius, a 15-year-old Labrador Retriever, is presented to your practice for decreased mobility, occasional urinary and fecal incontinence, and intermittent inappetence. No definitive diagnosis has been made, but Polonius's parents are afraid that his quality of life and ability to perform his normal daily activities are rapidly deteriorating. As the technician, you listen to their hopes and fears. In this type of case, it is most important that clients be encouraged to identify clear "lines in the sand" that would trigger a euthanasia appointment. Polonius's owners note that he seems to show signs of distress and potential loss of dignity when unable to rise to take care of his elimination needs. To maximize Polonius's comfort, the attending veterinarian places him on nonsteroidal anti-inflammatory drug (NSAID) therapy combined with gabapentin for musculoskeletal discomfort, and Polonius enjoys several weeks of increased mobility and his surroundings.

One day, you receive a call from Polonius's owner, stating that she believes that he has taken a permanent turn for the worse and needs advice on arranging a euthanasia appointment. She asks if it is appropriate to arrange a preplanned appointment or just to wake up one morning and decide that "today is the day." You explain that both thoughts are valid and normal and that there is nothing wrong with setting a date for the near future, then observing that the day may not be *the* day when the time arrives, or to decide before the appointment that today *is* the day and know that all considerations have been addressed. Conversely, if specific "lines in the sand" have been established in early end-of-life conversations and the client feels that the next decision to make is when to euthanize, the technician can offer the idea that Polonius and his owner have been given a "window" to make the decision, free from the demands of a crisis or emergency.

As it happens, Polonius's owner schedules the euthanasia appointment and brings him to your clinic. She expresses profound guilt as the main theme of her anticipatory grief. This guilt stems from Polonius's owner's unwillingness to subject him to advanced diagnostics and treatments, knowing as she does his fragile and easily upset emotional nature. You assure her that opting not to avail oneself of every possible treatment available through advanced veterinary medicine in no way means that one is robbing Polonius of the chance for a longer life. You also assure her that feelings of guilt in this context are normal and that you are available to listen whenever she needs a professional ear. The euthanasia goes perfectly, and Polonius's owner expresses her profound appreciation for your acknowledging her concerns and for allowing her to navigate the final stage of her beloved dog's life in the best way she knew how.

---

of veterinary palliative, hospice, and end-of-life care. Before the death of the pet, priorities shifted toward symptom control and physical, mental, emotional, and social stimulation. The goal was not to "fix" the patient. After the death of the pet, the client should be approached in much the same way. It is no one's job to "fix" the client. The healthiest way to help grieving clients is by **partnering** with them and **normalizing** their feelings (Boxes 37.9 and 37.10). Partnering with a grieving client does not require an expert. A helping attitude, willingness to listen, and the unique relationship between client and technician are the only requirements. Through the course of partnering with the grieving client, technicians may be surprised to find moments of humor and laughter in their interactions with the client. "Gallows humor" is a normal and healthy response to an otherwise traumatic situation and should not be discouraged. The human psyche has evolved many mechanisms, as described earlier, to protect itself from excessive exposure to the effects of trauma, and humor is one of them. The author of this chapter has shared many moments of laughter with clients during the euthanasia appointment, even during the actual

CASE PRESENTATION 37.4

Relief

The owner of Skeezix, a 19-year-old cat in chronic kidney failure, comes in for a quality-of-life consultation after observing 2 weeks of almost total inappetence in his pet. Skeezix's owner has not considered that his cat may be facing an end-of-life situation and is very reluctant to consider euthanasia because of previous experience. He has been giving Skeezix subcutaneous fluids twice a day for the past 4 months, and both Skeezix and the client have been agreeably participating in the procedure. Nevertheless, Skeezix's inappetence is threatening to overshadow all the home care that his owner has been providing through the last several months.

Upon conferring with the attending veterinarian, it is determined that Skeezix's condition is terminal and neither reversible nor realistically treatable. At the euthanasia appointment, you notice the owner smiling as he holds his beloved cat for the final injection. Seeing your acknowledgment, the owner remarks that his life had been dominated by caring for and worrying about Skeezix for most of the past year. Now, he says, he feels released from a great burden of responsibility and investment of time and energy, and that Skeezix certainly must feel a similar sense of release. You agree with his assessment and reinforce his feeling that sometimes the death of a beloved pet can bring with it the sense of profound relief: from worry, lost sleep, energy and money spent, and the fear surrounding the uncertainty of the disease process and prognosis. Paradoxically, in this case, death provides relief for both human and animal.

• BOX 37.8   When to Contact a Human Mental Health Professional

Clients:

- Are fearful and anxious about the care plans and decisions for the pet yet unclear about their wishes.
- Express intense confusion or avoidance about the pet's disease process and necessary decisions.
- Are intrusive upon the time and energy of the hospice team beyond agreed-upon boundaries.
- Ask a hospice team member to distort the facts of the case to children or other family members.
- Express disagreement among family members about the best course of action for the pet's care.

• BOX 37.9   Principles of Partnering With the Grieving Client

- Allow the situation to be exactly what it is.
- All feelings are acceptable and mentionable.
- Be a companion, not an expert.
- Grief is not a problem to be solved.
- Things do not happen "for a reason," or follow any kind of order or plan embedded in Nature.

• BOX 37.10   Talking With Children About Death

- Be honest and accurate; avoid euphemistic language, such as "put to sleep." Children may become afraid that when they go to sleep, they will not wake up.
- Do not be afraid to use such words as *die* and *death*. It is important that children understand the uniqueness of the situation.
- Explain that in euthanasia appointments, the medications given to the pet are not medications that people take.
- Allow children to be present at the euthanasia appointment and to come and go as they wish, and to sit with and touch the pet's body.
- Respect family wishes and beliefs.
- Provide children with books on the subject of pet loss.

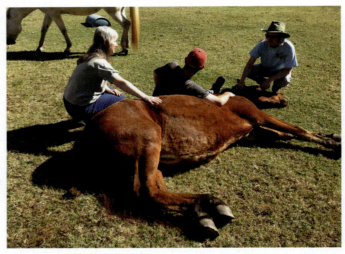

• **Fig. 37.8** The ideal in bond-centered care is for a meaningful death welcomed by those in the animal's circle of care. This deceased horse is surrounded by human caregivers.

TECHNICIAN NOTE

The act of partnering with the grieving client results in profound levels of connection, which may have unintentional humorous aspects.

Animals' Understanding of and Responses to Death

All species have some form of social structure. Attachments with a herd, pack, or flock can run very deep (Fig. 37.9). It is natural and inevitable to observe changes in the behavior of animals in the time leading up to and sometimes long after the death of a friend. Clients with several pets in the household almost always ask whether the other pets should be allowed to witness the death or to view the body, whether they experience the same types of emotions as people, and what the clients can do to help. In keeping with the concept that animals have a rich cognitive and affective life, clients can be assured that it is normal and even advisable to allow the other pets to interact with or observe the death as they feel the need. It is often surprising to see animals take on a serious, thoughtful demeanor when encountering the body of their deceased friend or to observe a normally aloof pet refuse to leave the side of a dying housemate.

administration of the euthanasia solution. These moments in no way detracted from the significance of the experience, but rather, added to the close bond of support between client and provider.

Bond-centered care contains a vast body of knowledge and skills to learn to do well. When practiced with a team approach with safe, open lines of communication, euthanasia increases its capacity for meaning and can sometimes approach beauty (Fig. 37.8).

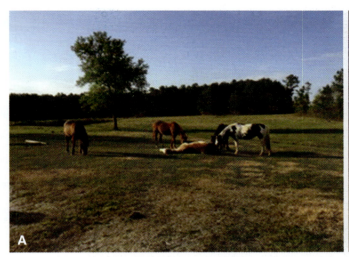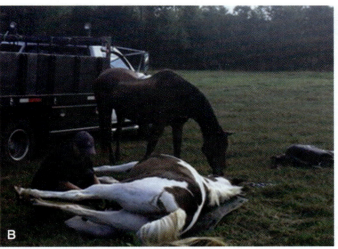

• **Fig. 37.9** (A, B) Allowing other animals to view the body and process what has happened is an important part of the period immediately after the death of a pet and provides a profound insight into the inner lives of animals.

After the death, animals may continue to look for their friend who has passed, checking areas with lingering scents, or simply wait as if expecting their friend to return. These and other related behaviors can last for weeks until finally the new reality is integrated into the surviving animals' lives and their behavior returns to a "new normal." During this time, it is always appropriate to give extra attention and affection to the remaining animals as they process the change in their lives and allow the emotional and behavioral changes to follow their natural course (Fig. 37.9A and B).

> **TECHNICIAN NOTE**
>
> Animals have their own processes of grieving and mourning. Technicians should encourage clients to treat their other pets as companions in bereavement.

The Critical Need for Self-care and Mental Health Support

For technicians who choose to pursue work in end-of-life care, those working in general practice and, indeed, in any capacity that involves patient care, the reality of death is almost a daily occurrence. The accumulation of experience brings with it the danger of mental and emotional occupational hazards, which occupy two main categories, *trauma exposure* and *moral injury*. These two categories originate in the work environment and should be understood as the mechanisms for such commonly mentioned problems as *burnout* and *compassion fatigue*.

Moral Injury and Burnout

Moral injury occurs when one is tasked with doing anything that violates one's deeply held values. Recalling the experience of the shelter and research environments, the prevalence of behavioral euthanasia, and the financial barriers to care experienced by pet owners, technicians are particularly vulnerable to moral injury. Moral injury is also often experienced by technicians tasked with

performing extensive and intensive care to patients with obviously terminal diagnoses and intractable suffering. Futility makes caring feel like torture. All these emotional stressors accumulate and drive *burnout*, which is often blamed on a lack of resilience or emotional stamina on the part of the sufferer. Burnout is therefore simply a group of symptoms of emotional exhaustion, protective cynicism, and loss of personal accomplishment caused by sustained exposure to morally hazardous situations in the workplace.

Trauma Exposure and Compassion Fatigue

Compassion fatigue, also referred to as vicarious trauma or secondary traumatization, is the gradual loss of the ability to respond with helpful empathy as a result of the frequency and number of demands for such responses. From an environmental and physiological perspective, the best term for the technician's experience of these stressors is *trauma exposure*. The body systems involved in the stress response are activated, whether one is experiencing or only hearing about the actual trauma. Technicians become containers for the pain of others and cannot escape its effects. These hazards are among many major causes for technicians leaving the profession and can even be early precursors to suicide, which occurs with alarming frequency in veterinary medicine (Box 37.11). The two main areas of potential change, self-care and workplace culture, are how technicians can mitigate and detach from the mental and emotional stressors of their work.

Ways to combat moral injury and trauma exposure begin with the right culture of the workplace. Discussions of burnout and compassion fatigue must never be off limits in communications among coworkers. No one should ever feel isolated or weak for experiencing either problem. Regular meetings should be held to allow staff to share their feelings, talk about emotionally exhausting cases, and to strengthen practice policies on supporting staff members.

Along with the practice's responsibility to care for its employees, coworkers also have a responsibility to care for each other. Offering a sympathetic ear or a shoulder to cry on, relieving a teammate who needs a break, and handing over a case to a fresh coworker are all examples of a team supporting itself.

- Ongoing physical and mental exhaustion
- Irritability
- Self-contempt
- Sleeplessness/excessive sleep
- Weight loss
- Emotional detachment from clients and coworkers
- Headache
- Job dissatisfaction
- Addiction
- Crying spells
- Physical fatigue
- Withdrawal from family and friends
- Increased alcohol intake
- Eating disturbance (overeating/inability to eat)
- Loss of interest in things usually enjoyed
- Persistent thoughts and images related to the problems of others
- Distraction
- Aggressive behavior

Ultimately, every technician is also responsible for their own self-care—the first line of defense against the emotional hazards of the work. When needed, technicians should feel justified in taking all their allowed vacation days, rotating away from the most emotionally intense areas of the job and, above all, feeling all right about refusing to sacrifice one's own well-being. Technicians who care well for themselves are therefore able to care for clients and patients, especially in supporting the human-animal bond in the most delicate specialty in veterinary medicine, end-of-life care (Box 37.12).

TECHNICIAN NOTE

Do not wait for signs of burnout or compassion fatigue to appear. Caring for oneself is easier when done in health and not when having to repair mental and emotional damage.

Summary: Key Points

Euthanasia is an experience, not a procedure. The human-animal bond is at its most vulnerable at the end of life. Every aspect of the technician's job, from caregiver to educator to advocate, must function at a high level to provide the best care.

The end of life is a stage of life. All pets will die. This fact requires a high level of training in the care of the pet's physical, mental/emotional, and social needs and the client's well-being. The human-animal bond continues after death, and the client needs support, even when the pet is no longer physically present.

Death is natural, inevitable, and meaningful to both the dying and the bereaved. The reality of death requires veterinary medicine to shift from a paradigm of fighting disease to one of improving life, where comfort, not longevity, is the priority.

Technicians are essential members of the interdisciplinary team.

Owners have the right to mourn the loss of their pets and to the support of the veterinary team and human mental health professionals.

Self-care and mental health support are essentials of veterinary practice.

• **BOX 37.12** **Strategies for Self-Care**

- Eat, exercise, and sleep well and enough.
- Take all the vacation and paid sick days every year.
- When away from work, do not remain available or "on call."
- Find and nourish creative pursuits.
- Meditate or engage in other meaningful spiritual activity.

Recommended Readings

Argus Institute. Making Decisions. https://www.argusinstitute.colostate.edu. Accessed 5/2017.

Ariadne Labs. *Serious Illness Conversation Guide*. Patient-tested Language; 2023. https://www.ariadnelabs.org/wp-content/uploads/2023/05/Serious-Illness-Conversation-Guide.2023-05-18.pdf.

Bishop G, Cooney K, Cox S, et al. 2016 AAHA/IAAHPC End-of-Life Care Guidelines. *J Am Anim Hosp Assoc*. 2016;52(6):341–356.

Buffone AEK, Poulin M, DeLury S, Ministero L, Morrisson C, Scalco M. Don't walk in her shoes! Different forms of perspective taking affect stress physiology. *J Exp Soc Psychol*. 2017;72(2017):161–168.

Butler C, Lagoni L. Euthanasia and grief support in an equine bond-centered practice. In: Bertone JJ, ed. *Equine Geriatric Medicine and Surgery*. Elsevier; 2006:231–243.

Cooney KA, Kogan LR, Brooks SL, Ellis CA. Pet owners' expectations for pet end-of-life support and after-death body care: Exploration and practical applications. *Top Companion Anim Med*. 2021;43(2020):2–7.

Coyle N. Palliative care, hospice, and bioethics: A natural fit. *J Hosp Palliat Nurs*. 2014;16(1):6–12.

Dean W, Talbot S, Dean A. Reframing clinician distress: Moral injury not burnout. *Fed Pract*. 2019;36(9):400–402.

Gawande A. *Being Mortal: Medicine and What Matters in the End*. New York, NY: Metropolitan Books; 2014.

Ireland J. Demographics, management, preventive health care and disease in aged horses. *Vet Clin North Am Equine Pract*. 2016;32(2):195–214.

Lagoni L, Butler C. *The Human-Animal Bond and Grief*. Philadelphia, PA: WB Saunders; 1994.

Leary S, Underwood W, Anthony R, et al. AVMA Guidelines for the Euthanasia of Animals: 2020 Edition. www.avma.org/resources-tools/avma-policies/human-animal-interaction-and-human-animal-bond.

Matte AR, Khosa DK, Meehan MP, Coe JB, Niel L. An exploratory study of veterinary professionals' self-reported support of bereaved clients before, during, and after companion animal euthanasia in Southwestern Ontario, Canada. *Omega (Westport)*. 2021;83(3):352–370.

McGowan CM, Ireland JL. Welfare, quality of life, and euthanasia of aged horses. *Vet Clin North Am Equine Pract*. 2016;32(2):355–367.

McMillan FD. *Mental Health and Wellbeing in Animals*. Oxford, UK: Blackwell; 2007.

Peereboom K, Coyle N. Facilitating goals-of-care discussions for patients with life-limiting disease-communication strategies for nurses. *J Hosp Palliat Nurs*. 2012;14(4):251–258.

Pope G Soar. *My Butterfly: The Animal Dying Experience*. Sebastapol, CA: Brighthaven; 2015.

Shanan A, Shearer T, Pierce J. *Hospice and Palliative Care for Companion Animals: Principles and Practice*. Hoboken, NJ: John Wiley; 2017.

Spitznagel MB, Marchitelli B, Gardner M, Carlson MD. Euthanasia from the veterinary client's perspective: Psychosocial contributors to euthanasia decision making. *Vet Clin North Am Small Anim Pract*. 2020;50(3):591–605.

Stull C. Death and euthanasia as contemporary topics in equine curricula. *J Equine Vet Sci*. 2013;33(5):309–314.

Temel JS, Greer JA, Muzikhanski A, et al. Early palliative care for patients with metastatic non-small-cell lung cancer. *N Engl J Med*. 2010;365(8):733–742.

Glossary

Abdominal pinging Technique of identifying abdominal gas accumulations by simultaneous percussion and auscultation of the abdominal wall.

Abdominocentesis Sampling of free fluid within the peritoneal space.

Aberrant/erratic parasite Parasite that has wandered into an organ or location where it is not normally found.

Abomasum The "true stomach" of the ruminant; secretes acids, mixes and contracts ingesta, and moves liquid chyme into the small intestine.

Abrasion An area of skin that has been superficially scraped, creating a wound. Also, tooth wear associated with chewing on objects, such as rocks, ice cubes, toys, and bones.

Abscess Localized collection of pus (composed of dead neutrophils) in any part of the body, usually associated with bacterial infection, inflammation, and swelling around the site.

Absorption Uptake of substances into or across tissue.

Acanthocephalans Also known as spiny-headed or thorny-headed worms, the necrotrophic worms live as adults in the small intestine; common parasites of wildlife and some domestic animal species but rarely found in humans.

Acariasis Any infestation/infection with acarines—mites or ticks. For example, infestation with *Demodex canis,* the follicular mite of dogs, is referred to as *demodectic acariasis.*

Accounts receivable Money that is due to the practice from the sale of goods or services.

Acid-fast staining Procedure that uses the acid-fast stain to distinguish bacteria that have mycolic acid incorporated into their cell walls.

Acidosis Elevated levels of metabolic acids within blood or tissue.

Acids Compounds whose water-based solutions have a sour taste, turn blue litmus paper red, and can combine with metals to form salts and yield hydrogen ions or protons when dissolved in water.

Aciduric Capable of growing well in extremely acid media, pH below 7. Associated with aciduria.

Activated clotting time (activated coagulation time, ACT) Inexpensive but relatively insensitive test to evaluate the intrinsic and common pathways of coagulation. The test uses a special ACT Vacutainer tube containing a diatomaceous earth activator that must be prewarmed before use. The test should not be performed in animals that are severely thrombocytopenic.

Activated partial thromboplastin time (APTT) Test used to evaluate the intrinsic and common pathways of coagulation. The test requires citrated plasma and careful adherence to collection and processing requirements.

Active drain Commonly referred to as closed-suction drains, they create a vacuum within the wound and allow wound fluid to be removed via a rigid fenestrated drain into an external collection container.

Active immunity Production of substances in the body (e.g., antibodies and interferon) that render the animal immune from disease. Active immunity can occur via immunization, as an immune response caused by natural exposure to the antigen, or as a sequela of the disease.

Acupuncture Use of needles (or injection of fluid, laser, ultrasound, surgically implanted material, or electrical stimulation) to stimulate specific predetermined "acupuncture" points in the body to produce chemical or physiologic changes in the body. It is combined with herbs and massage to make up traditional Chinese medicine (TCM).

Acute radiation toxicity Side effects caused by radiotherapy that occur between day 1 (the start of radiotherapy) and day 90. Side effects are characterized by toxicity to rapidly proliferating normal tissues such as skin, mucous membranes, intestinal tract, and bone marrow, and often resolve within days to weeks.

Adjuvant Substance, such as aluminum phosphate, that increases the efficacy of a vaccine without having any immunologic property of its own.

Adjuvant therapy Cancer treatment that is given in addition to the primary or initial treatment. The most common examples are radiotherapy that is given to treat residual cancer remaining after an incomplete surgical resection and postoperative chemotherapy that is administered to prevent or treat systemic metastasis. The overall purpose of adjuvant therapy is to decrease the likelihood of cancer recurrence.

Adsorbent Solid substance that attracts and holds a substance to its surface.

Agammaglobulinemic Description of a pathologic condition in which the body forms few or no gammaglobulins or antibodies.

Agglutination Visible or microscopic irregular, variably sized clumping of red blood cells (RBCs) that form because of excess antibodies bound to the surface of RBCs.

Aggression Behavior that is angry, destructive, and intended to be injurious; behaviors that result in harm to the opponent. Threats and aggression exist along a continuum. An inhibited bite that leaves a red mark or indentation on the skin or that only pulls hair from another animal usually reflects intent to warn (threat) rather than to harm (aggression).

Agonist Substance, such as a drug, that produces a physiologic or pharmacologic effect characteristic of the receptor to which it binds.

Alkali Alkaline substances produce hydroxide ions on contact with water; alkaline or basic chemicals found in numerous bathroom and household cleaners, alkaline batteries, and cement.

Alkaluric Of alkaline condition, pH above 7 and decreased H+.

Allantois Innermost portion of the fused chorioallantoic membrane, which assists in the transfer of nutrients, oxygen, and waste products to and from the fetus.

Allodynia Recruitment of nonpainful nerve fibers that transmit information as pain, resulting in previously pleasant or neutral sensations experienced as unpleasant.

Allogrooming Grooming performed by one animal on another animal of the same species.

Alopecia The partial or complete absence of hair from regions of the body where it normally grows.

Amino acids Nitrogen-containing compounds that constitute the "building blocks" or units from which more complex protein is formed. They contain both an amino (NH_2) group and a carboxyl (COOH) group. Approximately 11 essential amino acids must be provided in the diet, along with approximately 10 nonessential amino acids, which can be synthesized in the body.

Amnion Membrane that separates the amniotic lubricating fluid surrounding the fetus from the urine like fluid within the allantois membrane.

Anaerobe Bacterial organism that is unable to grow in the presence of oxygen.

Analgesia Pain relief.

Anaphylaxis Allergy or hypersensitivity (to foreign proteins or drugs) resulting from sensitization after prior contact with the causative agent. Severe anaphylaxis can be fatal if untreated because of hypoxia.

Anastomosis Reconnecting (suturing) of bowel after resection of a portion of bowel.

Anechoic Structure in an ultrasound image that does not produce echoes and appears black.

Anemia Condition in which the blood is deficient in red blood cells or hemoglobin.

Anestrus Period of no or least reproductive activity.

Anger Stage of grief during which anger is the primary emotion, expressed directly, indirectly, and specifically or generally.

Animal hospice A program of care that addresses the physical, emotional, and social needs of animals in the advanced stages of a progressive, life-limiting illness or disability.

Animal Medicinal Drug Use Clarification Act (AMDUCA) Amendment to the Federal Food, Drug, and Cosmetic (FFD&C) Act that regulates extra-label drug use for the treatment of veterinary species, provided specific conditions are met.

Anisocoria Unequal pupil sizes

Anisocytosis Variation in red blood cell (RBC) size that can be detected by examining a blood smear or by measuring an increase in the RBC distribution width (RDW). Anisocytosis is often increased in animals with regenerative anemia but may occur in other conditions, such as iron deficiency.

Anisognathism Condition in which the maxilla and the mandible are not equally wide.

Anode Positively charged side of the x-ray tube that receives oncoming electrons from the cathode. Both heat and x-rays are produced as a result of interactions between electrons and the metal anode.

Anorexia Loss of appetite or absence of food, especially when prolonged.

Anosmia Complete loss or impairment in sense of smell.

Antagonist Drug that blocks activation of a receptor by its agonists (including the receptor's endogenous substrate).

Antecedent The first step of the applied behavior analysis (ABC) model for determining an animal's motivation for performing a behavior. Antecedents are stimuli that precede the unwanted behavior.

Anticipatory grief Feelings of grief experienced when contemplating the future death of a pet; this feeling intensifies when faced with an animal's terminal diagnosis or other life-limiting condition.

Anticoagulants Additives used in blood collection bags for blood banking to keep blood from clotting; a substance that hinders the clotting of blood.

Antiemetic Drug used to treat or prevent vomiting.

Antimicrobial susceptibility test Test to determine whether an antimicrobial agent will kill or inhibit the growth of a bacterial organism.

Antiseptic Antimicrobial agent that kills or inhibits the growth of microorganisms on external surfaces of the body. Antiseptics generally should be distinguished from drugs, such as antibiotics, which destroy microorganisms internally, and from disinfectants, which destroy microorganisms found on nonliving objects.

Antitoxin Antibody produced in response to a toxin, such as tetanus, that is capable of neutralizing the toxin.

Anxiety Anticipation of future or potential danger that may be unknown, imagined, or real. Leads to a physiologic response similar to that of fear.

Aortic stenosis Congenital cardiac anomaly resulting in resistance to flow of blood from the left ventricle into the aorta.

Apex Tip of the root of a tooth.

Apnea Temporary absence of spontaneous breathing.

Appendicular skeleton Bones of the limbs (appendages).

Appointment system System by which clients call ahead and are given a specific time and date to come into the practice.

Apteric Normal area of skin of birds where feathers do not grow, including the face, abdomen, and feet.

Arrhythmia Abnormal heartbeat rhythm detected during palpation of the chest or pulse during auscultation or recorded on an electrocardiogram (ECG).

Arthrocentesis Aspiration of fluid from a joint.

Arthrodesis Surgical fusing of a joint together such that all motion at the joint is lost.

Arthropod Any member of the phylum Arthropoda. Most of the members of this phylum have jointed appendages in the adult stage. Relative to veterinary parasitology, arthropods include a wide variety of creatures with "jointed feet," such as centipedes, millipedes, crustaceans, insects, and mites and ticks.

Arthroscopy A medical procedure that allows for examination of the interior of a joint via endoscope which is inserted into the joint area through a small incision.

Artificial insemination (AI) Placement of semen within the uterus or oviduct by other than natural means so that fertilization of oocytes can occur.

Ascariasis A roundworm infection of the intestine with ascarids.

Asepsis Condition of sterility wherein no living organisms are present.

Aseptic technique Methods used to prevent contamination of a surgical site or wound by disease-producing organisms.

Assisted feeding Providing energy and nutrients when animals are not eating adequate amounts. Enteral feeding uses the gastrointestinal tract, and parenteral feeding uses the venous (blood circulatory) system.

Assisted gloving Method of putting on sterile gloves in which a sterile gloved assistant holds the glove open to allow the surgeon to advance their hand into the glove without touching the outside.

Assistive devices Resources such as harnesses, wheelchairs, mobility slings, carts, and other devices may be necessary to assist with mobility for the aging pet, especially if neurologic or musculoskeletal disease is present.

Asystole Type of arrhythmia characterized by a "flat line," or the absence of heartbeats.

Ataxia Uncoordinated muscle movements when walking, usually associated with neurologic dysfunction.

Atelectasis Collapse of a portion of or all of one or both lungs.

Atlas First cervical vertebra, which forms the atlanto-occipital joint with the occipital bone of the skull and the atlantoaxial joint with the axis (second cervical vertebra).

Atrial fibrillation Very rapid, uncoordinated contractions of the atria of the heart, resulting in lack of synchronism between heartbeat and pulse beat.

Atrial premature complexes Premature contractions of the atria initiated by one of the atria from a location other than the normal sinus heartbeat, which originates in the sinoatrial node.

Atrioventricular (AV) valve Heart valve located between an atrium and a ventricle. The right AV valve is the tricuspid valve, and the left AV valve is the mitral valve.

Atwater factors Average energy content of macronutrients. For human foods, the Atwater factors are as follows: 4.0 kcal for 1 g protein or 1 g carbohydrate, and 9.0 kcal for 1 g fat. For commercial pet foods, modified Atwater factors are used, including 3.5 kcal for 1 g protein or 1 g carbohydrate, and 8.5 kcal for 1 g fat.

Aural In or of the ear.

Autoclave Machine that uses pressurized steam to sterilize objects.

Autolysis Self-digestion of tissues or cells by enzymes that are released by their own lysosomes.

Average daily gain The average amount of weight an animal will gain each day.

Axillary Under the armpit.

Axis Second cervical vertebra that forms the atlantoaxial joint with the first cervical vertebra (the atlas).

Ayre T-piece Nonrebreathing circuit with corrugated tubing but no reservoir bag or pressure relief valve, in which the fresh gas inlet is located near the patient, and the waste gas exits away from the patient; Mapleson E circuit.

Azotemia Condition in which blood has increased concentrations of nitrogenous wastes, such as blood urea nitrogen (BUN). Azotemia may be further characterized as prerenal azotemia caused by dehydration, as renal azotemia caused by impaired kidney function, or as postrenal azotemia caused by obstruction of the urinary tract.

Backward conditioning One of the four different timing options for pairing stimuli during classical conditional or counterconditioning; involves distraction, such as offering food before attempting to touch the animal.

Bactericidal Describes an agent that kills bacteria such as antiseptics.

Bacteriostatic Describes an agent that inhibits bacterial multiplication.

Bain coaxial circuit Nonrebreathing circuit with a reservoir bag and corrugated tubing in which the fresh gas inlet is located near the patient and the pressure relief valve is located away from the patient; Mapleson D circuit.

Band neutrophil Immature neutrophil characterized by a U- or S-shaped nucleus with generally parallel sides. The number of band neutrophils increases in some animals with inflammation.

Barbering Behavioral problem in which the animal obsessively grooms to the point of damaging the hair and skin.

Barbiturates Nervous system depressants used to induce sleep and, in high doses, as anesthetics and euthanasia agents.

Barrier nursing Nursing of patients using stringent and enhanced infection control practices to prevent and discourage infections or spread to other patients.

Basophil Type of granulocyte with a segmented nucleus and granules that stain blue to purple with Wright stain or quick stains. Marked species variation in the appearance of the granules has been noted. Basophils from dogs have a few darkly purple-staining granules, basophils from cats have numerous gray to lavender granules, and basophils from horses and cows have numerous darkly purple-staining granules.

Behavior The second step of the applied behavior analysis (ABC) model for determining an animal's motivation for performing a behavior. Behavior is what the animal actual does. There may be many behaviors happening close together and in rapid succession.

Bereavement State of sadness, grief, and mourning after the loss of a loved one.

Binocular vision Vision in which both eyes are used synchronously to produce a single image.

Bioavailability (F) Fraction of a drug dose that reaches the bloodstream.

Biological value Percentage of protein of a feed that is usable as a protein by the animal. A protein that has a high biological value is said to be of good quality.

Biosecurity Series of steps implemented to prevent or reduce the spread of infectious disease. Veterinary personnel who travel between production farms are required to implement

biosecurity practices, such as changing or sanitizing boots, changing coveralls, and, on some farms, driving through an antiseptic tire bath when entering a farm.

Biotransformation Chemical modification of a drug to an active, inactive, or toxic metabolite.

Blind spot Area directly behind, directly in front of the nose, or between the eyes of a horse, where the field of vision is extremely limited and the horse is unable to see a person.

Blood smears Thin films of anticoagulated blood prepared on glass slides that are air dried, stained, and evaluated for cell morphology and differential leukocyte counts.

Blood type Reflects the presence of specific erythrocyte antigens that have the potential to cause immune stimulation.

B-mode Brightness mode ultrasound image display. It forms the basis of two-dimensional ultrasound images so that anatomic structures can be assessed in real time on a monitor.

Body condition score (BCS) Estimate of body fat composition, with higher scores indicating overweight or obese animals and lower scores indicating thin or emaciated animals.

Body language The primary language used by animals to communicate with one another and with humans.

Bond-centered care A part of end-of-life care in which the focus of care becomes the bond between the veterinary patient and client; end-of-life care that considers how the human-animal bond might be affected.

Borborygmi Rumbling noises caused by propulsion of gas and ingesta through the intestines (sing. borborygmus).

Box lock Hinged part of a needle holder, tissue forceps, or hemostatic forceps.

Brachycephalic Head shape that is shortened in the rostrocaudal dimension, as seen with such breeds as Pugs, Boston Terriers, and Boxers.

Brachydont Tooth type with a small, distinct crown compared with large, well-developed roots.

Brachygnathism The uneven alignment of the upper and lower teeth in animals, such as when the mandible is relatively shorter than the maxilla because of abnormally short mandible (mandibular brachygnathism).

Bradyzoite Literally, "a slow-growing, tiny organism." This is a term for a tissue stage, for example, a slow-growing developmental stage that occurs in cysts in the life cycle of *Toxoplasma gondii.*

Burnout Exhaustion caused by sustained exposure to highly emotional situations in the workplace.

Cachexia Weight loss, loss of muscle mass, and general debilitation that may accompany chronic disease.

Calculus Plaque that has become calcified and is firmly adhered to teeth.

Calibrator Standardized material with known quantitative or qualitative characteristics (e.g., concentration, activity, reactivity, intensity, size) that is used to adjust (or calibrate) an instrument or a measurement procedure. The instrument or procedure is adjusted to yield results that match the calibrator.

Calorie Also called a kilocalorie (kcal), the amount of heat required to raise the temperature of 1 kg of water 1°C. In nutrition, calories are the basic unit of energy used when discussing food or exercise.

Capillary refill time Time required for blood to refill the small capillary beds of the mucous membranes after digital blanching.

Carcinogen Substance or agent that causes cancer in animals or people.

Cardiopulmonary resuscitation Emergency procedure performed in an effort to manually preserve intact brain function until further measures are taken to restore spontaneous blood circulation and breathing.

Caries Tooth decay caused by bacterial acid production and demineralization of tooth substance.

Carpal flexion sling Forelimb sling used in small animals that flexes the wrist joint and is used to protect flexor tendon repair and prevent weight bearing while allowing movement of the elbow and the shoulder.

Cash flow Measurement of a practice's inflow and outflow of cash over a period.

Cassette A rectangular or square container designed to hold radiographic film.

Catalase Enzyme required to convert hydrogen peroxide to hydrogen gas and water.

Cathartics Medications that through their chemical effects serve to promote the clearing of intestinal contents.

Cathode Negatively charged side of the x-ray tube that produces electrons from a metal filament when it is heated.

Cationic detergents Nonsoap surfactants that are in a positive state; can be found in fabric softeners, germicides, disinfectants, and sanitizers, and are rapidly absorbed and may produce severe local and systemic toxicity.

Celiotomy Surgical opening of a coelomic cavity (e.g., the abdominal cavity).

Cellulitis Sterile or nonsterile inflammation of the interstitial tissues.

Cementum Hard tissue that covers the root of brachyodont teeth and portions of the crown of some hypsodont teeth.

Center for Veterinary Medicine (CVM) Governing body that regulates the manufacture and distribution of drugs, food additives, and medical devices used in veterinary species under the Federal Food, Drug, and Cosmetic (FFD&C) Act.

Cestode Adult stage of a tapeworm. Usually found in the intestinal tract of the definitive host. Tapeworms are long and flattened parasites. The three basic parts of a tapeworm are the scolex, the neck, and the strobila. The strobila is composed of proglottids. Three types of proglottids are known: immature, mature, and gravid.

Chelonian Turtles and tortoises.

Chemical restraint A type of restraint that uses specific drugs to achieve an appropriate level of patient compliance for successful completion of specific veterinary procedures and to ensure the safety of both the veterinary medical team and the patient.

Chemical sterilization Use of liquid or gas to sterilize surgical materials. Glutaraldehyde is a liquid that is commonly used to sterilize surgical instruments. Ethylene oxide and hydrogen peroxide are vaporized to sterilize delicate equipment, instruments, and plastic items that cannot tolerate the high temperatures, pressures, and steam associated with autoclaving.

Chemotherapy Use of chemical substances to treat disease, primarily with cytotoxic drugs used to treat cancer. Chemotherapy is usually systemic therapy and is given intravenously or by mouth.

Chest tube Flexible tube inserted through the intercostal muscles into the pleural space.

Choke Obstruction of the esophagus.

Chondritis Inflammation of the cartilage that connects the ribs to the breastbone. The cause is often not clearly known or understood.

Chorioallantois membrane Membrane formed by the fusion of the chorionic and allantoic membranes.

Classical conditioning Also known as *respondent conditioning*. The animal learns the association between events—one event (the conditioned stimulus) predicts another (the unconditioned stimulus). Emotional behaviors are easily classically conditioned.

Clinic A veterinary or animal clinic is a facility in which the practice is conducted typically and may include inpatient and outpatient diagnostics and treatment.

Cloaca In birds and reptiles, a single terminus of the urinary, intestinal, and reproductive tracts.

Closed gloving Method of putting on sterile gloves whereby the hands are kept hidden within the sleeves of a sterile gown during gloving.

Coagulase Enzyme required to convert fibrinogen to fibrin.

Coagulation cascade The interaction of multiple activated proenzymes (clotting factors) involved in secondary hemostasis, resulting in cross-linked fibrin strands that stabilize the primary platelet plug.

Coagulopathy Disease or condition that affects the ability of blood to coagulate.

Coccidia Microscopic, single-celled parasites that spread from one animal to another (including humans) by contact with infected feces.

Cognitive dysfunction A neurodegenerative disorder of senior dogs and cats that is characterized by gradual cognitive decline over a long period.

Colic Severe abdominal pain of sudden onset caused by a variety of conditions, including obstruction, twisting, and spasm of the intestine.

Colitis Inflammation of the colon.

Collagen Proteins that make up most of the skin, bone, cartilage, tendons, and other connective tissue.

Colloid Substance that consists of particles that are dispersed throughout a solution and are too small for resolution with an ordinary light microscope but are incapable of passing through a semipermeable membrane.

Colostrometer Tool that measures colostrum quality.

Colostrum The first milk, which contains the antibodies.

Colpotomy Incision through the wall of the vagina.

Committee on Veterinary Technician Specialties (CVTS) Committee that helps guide and structure the development of specialties for veterinary technicians and provides a standardized list of criteria and assistance for societies interested in attaining academy status.

Compassion The quality of understanding the suffering of others and wanting to do something about it.

Compassion fatigue The gradual loss of the ability to respond with empathy as a result of the frequency and number of demands for such responses.

Compendium of Veterinary Products (CVP) A comprehensive reference of approved pharmaceuticals and biologics.

Complementary medicine A group of preventive, diagnostic, and therapeutic philosophies and practices which, at the time they are performed, may differ from current scientific knowledge, or whose theoretical basis and techniques may diverge from veterinary medicine routinely taught in accredited veterinary medical colleges, or both.

Complete blood count (CBC) Test used to evaluate peripheral blood that typically includes packed cell volume (or hematocrit), a red blood cell (RBC) count, hemoglobin concentration, RBC indices, a platelet count, a white blood cell (WBC) count, and a WBC differential.

Complete feeds A type of feed for horses typically made of a mixture of roughage and concentrate (usually 80% roughage and 20% concentrate) manufactured by grinding the food and formulating it into pellets.

Complicated grief An extremely intense, prolonged, and mentally and physically debilitating permutation of normal grief.

Computed radiography (CR) Similar to digital radiography except that an x-ray receiver similar to a film cassette is used and must be processed in a special machine. The special cassette contains a photostimulable phosphor that changes x-ray photons into a latent electronic image when read by a laser.

Computed tomography (CT) An x-ray imaging technique that creates detailed pictures, or scans, of areas inside the body. It is also known as *computerized axial tomography* (CAT).

Concentrates Broad classification of feedstuffs that are high in energy and low in fiber.

Conflict-related aggression Aggression toward people, often over resources and in similar contexts as dominance aggression but with the dog showing ambivalent visual cues. These dogs are often submissive or fearful in other contexts and are likely to be submissive or fearful immediately after an attack. Many clients will say that the dog acted like it "was sorry for what it did."

Congenital Born with a specific condition. Can be genetic or environmentally induced.

Conjunctivitis Inflammation of the tissue under the lid margins and surrounding the visible globe.

Consequence The third step of the applied behavior analysis (ABC) model for determining an animal's motivation for performing a behavior. Consequences follow behavior and drive future behavioral decisions.

Considerate Approach A concept that encompasses the interaction between the veterinary team and the patients and inputs from the environment while veterinary care is being administered; setting up the environment and each interaction to be sensitive to the needs of patient.

Conspecific Describing animals of the same species.

Constipation A difficulty in passing stool from the body, often coupled with straining to defecate.

Consultation Specific period of time that the veterinarian meets with the client and the patient for the purpose of diagnosis/treatment.

Contamination The presence of disease-producing bacteria or other microorganisms on the surface of a wound or surgical field.

Contralateral The opposite side.

Control Standardized material that is used to monitor an assay to ensure that it is working correctly, consistently, and within desired limits. Controls are used to determine whether the instrument or the measurement procedure is yielding expected results for a sample with known characteristics. Controls are usually within the range of what you might expect to see in your patients. At least two control levels (normal and abnormal) are run. Low, normal, and high controls may be run if

both high and low values of the analyte are clinically important. Control materials should be different from calibrator materials to ensure independent assessment of performance of the procedure.

Controlled substances Controlled substances that are regulated by federal law with regard to their manufacture, distribution, and dispensing.

Corpus hemorrhagicum (CH) Structure formed within the ruptured follicle immediately after ovulation.

Corpus luteum (CL) Structure that replaces the corpus hemorrhagicum and is capable of production of progesterone.

Corrosive Highly reactive substance that causes obvious damage to living tissue.

Counterconditioning An interventional technique to replace an existing conditioned response.

Coupage The act of striking the chest wall rhythmically with cupped hands. Cupping the hands creates an air cushion on impact so that tenacious mucus is dislodged.

Cow kick A kick from a hind limb directly to the side and the back.

Cradle A barred restraint device. The bars are tied together like a nonridged fence. It is tied around the neck of a horse like a loose splint and prevents the horse from biting or licking itself.

Crepuscular An adjective referring to animals that are active at dawn and dusk (twilight).

Crop Dilatation of the esophagus of birds at the base of the neck where food is stored, is softened with fluids, and is passed to the stomach in small amounts.

Cross match Testing of compatibility of the blood of a transfusion donor and the blood of a recipient by mixing the serum of each with the red cells of the other, and examining the samples for the presence or absence of agglutination reactions.

Cross-ties Common method of restraining a horse for simple procedures, such as grooming. The horse is tied to a pillar on either side by the square metal pieces on either side of the halter.

Cryotherapy Application of cold to the body to decrease pain and inflammation; therapeutic techniques used to decrease tissue temperature; cold therapy.

Cryptorchidectomy The excision and removal of an undescended testicle which may be done through an open or minimal (laparoscopic) surgical procedure.

Cryptorchidism Refers to males with one or both testes not in the scrotum.

Crystalloid fluid Solution composed of electrolytes and water.

Crystalluria The presence of crystals in the urine.

Cutaneous larval migrans Zoonotic skin condition caused when an infective third-stage larval of a hookworm (usually *Ancylostoma braziliense*) penetrates the skin of a human being and travels within the superficial layers of the epidermis, producing highly pruritic, serpentine (twisting) tracts in the skin. Common names for this skin condition include sandworms, creeping eruption, and plumber's itch.

Cyanosis Bluish discoloration of the mucous membranes or skin caused by severe reduction of hemoglobin in blood.

Cylindruria The presence of casts in urine.

Cysticercoid Type of metacestode stage found in the intermediate host in the life cycle of a tapeworm. The cysticercoid is usually found within an invertebrate intermediate host, such as a flea or a grain mite. A cysticercoid

is a single, noninvaginated scolex within a small, fluid-filled vesicle, cavity, or bladder. In its life cycle, *Dipylidium caninum* uses the cysticercoid stage, which may be found within the intermediate host, an adult flea. See **Metacestode**.

Cystocentesis Method of obtaining a urine sample by inserting a needle through the abdominal wall and into the urinary bladder and withdrawing urine from the bladder into a syringe. The bladder may be located by palpation or under ultrasound guidance.

Cystotomy Incision into the urinary bladder.

Cytochrome oxidase Respiratory enzyme found in bacteria that conserves energy released when oxygen is reduced.

Cytology Microscopic evaluation of cell morphology in samples collected by fine-needle aspiration or impression smears of tissue or fluid accumulations. Cytology is often used as a screening test to determine whether inflammation or neoplasia is present, although definitive diagnosis of specific causative agents or neoplasms can sometimes be made.

Cytotoxic Agent or process that kills cells. Chemotherapy and radiotherapy are forms of cytotoxic therapy.

D-dimers Specific proteolytic fragments that result from plasmin digestion of cross-linked fibrin and contain two D domains and one E domain of the original fibrinogen molecule. D-dimers are sometimes measured in animals with suspected disseminated intravascular coagulation (DIC) or other diseases associated with increased fibrinolysis.

Dead space Space between tissues created by a wound, allowing accumulation of fluid.

Debridement Removal of foreign matter and dead tissue from a wound.

Decontamination Removal or neutralization of injurious agents.

Decubitus ulcers Pressure sores (bed sores) that develop when an animal lies on a bony prominence for too long.

Defibrillation Process of converting a fibrillation arrhythmia to a normal heartbeat (usually via electrical shock with a defibrillator).

Definitive host Within the life cycle of a parasite, the host that harbors the adult, sexual, or mature stage of a parasite is the definitive host. For example, the definitive host for *Dirofilaria immitis*, the canine heartworm, is the dog. Adult male and female heartworms are found within the right ventricle and pulmonary arteries of the canine definitive host.

Definitive treatment Treatment intended to cure or permanently control a cancer. One or a combination of anticancer therapies may be used, including surgery, radiotherapy, and chemotherapy.

Degloving injury Injury—typically to the distal limb—in which a large section of skin is torn off the underlying tissue in a glove like fashion.

Degradation The act or process of degrading.

Dehiscence Loss of integrity of the sutured layers of an incision.

Dehydration Abnormal depletion of body fluids.

Delay conditioning One of the four different timing options for pairing stimuli during classical conditional or counterconditioning; method in which the conditioned stimulus is presented and remains present for a fixed period (the delay) before the unconditioned stimulus is introduced.

Dermatophyte Fungus that infects the skin and nails.

Dermis The vascular, thick layer of the skin lying below the epidermis.

Desensitization Gradually introducing a stimulus to a learner such that the learner does not respond to it; involves identifying a nonstressful starting point, providing gradual planned exposures that do not elicit a visible response from the learner, and very gradually increasing the stimulus intensity over repeated exposures.

Desmotomy The surgical cutting of a ligament that removes or frees the tensile strength.

Diagnosis The act of identifying a disease, illness, or problem by examining a human or animal.

Diagnostic peritoneal lavage Insertion of fluid into the peritoneal cavity; fluid is allowed to dwell for a short time and then is drained. Gross, microscopic, and chemical analyses are performed on the returned fluid.

Diagnostic ultrasonography (DUS) An imaging technique that uses high-frequency sound waves to produce images of internal structures in the body; also known as *sonography* or *diagnostic medical imaging*.

Diaphragm Thin, dome-shaped sheet of muscle that forms the boundary between thoracic and abdominal cavities; it helps to produce inspiration when it contracts. The diaphragm is dome-shaped at rest, with its convex surface directed cranially. When it contracts, the dome of the diaphragm flattens out; this increases the volume of the thoracic cavity and causes air to be drawn into the lungs.

Diarrhea The abnormally frequent discharge of soft or liquid feces, if unchecked can cause dehydration.

Diastema Gap between teeth, as seen between incisors and the cheek teeth of a rabbit.

Differential media Media that detects differences between two organisms on the basis of a biochemical test, for example, MacConkey agar differentiates between lactose-fermenting bacteria and lactose nonfermenters on the basis of color (positive organisms are pink on this medium, and negative organisms are white).

Digenetic fluke Digenetic trematode that has two intermediate hosts—a first intermediate host and a second intermediate host—in addition to the definitive host.

Digestible energy (DE) Energy that remains after the energy lost in feces is subtracted from gross energy.

Digestion Process of protein, carbohydrate, and fat breakdown into absorbable nutrients.

Digital fluoroscopy (DF) An imaging technique that projects a radiographic image on an image-intensifying fluorescent screen, which is coupled to a digital video recorder. The video images are digitized and stored.

Digital imaging and communication in medicine (DICOM) DICOM 3.0 is the current standard format for digital images in veterinary and medical fields.

Digital radiography (DR) A digital imaging technique in which the x-ray tube is coupled to a specialized receiver that changes x-rays into electrical signals. The analog image is digitalized and is displayed on the integrated computer screen.

Diplomate of the American College of Veterinary Behaviorists (DACVB) Veterinary designation for completing a formal residency, taking advanced continuing education classes in the field of animal behavior, and passing a rigorous examination process. These veterinarians are qualified to diagnose and treat behavior disorders in animals.

Disenfranchised grief When someone experiencing grief is met with ignorance, lack of understanding, or minimization, such as when animal owners feel that they are misunderstood and isolated and that their pain is underappreciated because the object of their grief was not a human.

DISHA Acronym for **d**isorientation, altered **i**nteractions with people or other pets, altered **s**leep–wake cycles, **h**ouse soiling, and **a**ctivity changes. The diagnosis of cognitive dysfunction syndrome was initially based on the clinical signs of this term.

Disinfectant Chemical agents that are applied to inanimate objects to destroy the vegetative form of bacteria, but not necessarily the spore forms.

Disk diffusion Also known as the Kirby-Bauer method, test in which paper disks infused with a particular concentration of an antimicrobial agent are applied to mature cultures of microbes. Effectiveness in killing or retarding the growth of microbes is noted and directs a specific treatment protocol. The test is used to provide effective antimicrobial therapy for treatment of susceptible microbial infections. Effective testing increases the likelihood of providing effective treatment and reduces the risk of microbial resistance.

Displacement behaviors Behaviors observed in dogs and cats that serve as a coping mechanism intended to help the pet reduce its anxiety level. Displacement behaviors include grooming (in cats), yawning, scratching, and licking lips (in dogs).

Disseminated intravascular coagulation (DIC) Pattern of generalized concurrent intravascular thrombosis and bleeding. This is among the most serious complications of shock.

Distal In dentistry, a positional term that refers to the surface of the tooth farthest from the rostral midline of the dental arch.

Distocclusion A malocclusion in which the upper teeth are mesial to the lower teeth. It is also known as an *overbite*.

Distribution Dispersion of a drug that is systemically available from the intravascular space and of extravascular fluids and tissues to target receptor sites.

Diversionary restraint Type of restraint in which varying techniques or devices are used to distract the horse.

DNA sequencing Determining the order of nucleotides in deoxyribonucleic acid (DNA) from which amino acids in a polypeptide chain can be predicted and used to identify pathogens and rapidly identify bacteria, fungi, and viruses.

Dolichocephalic Head shape that is longer than average in the rostrocaudal dimension, as is seen in Greyhounds and Collies.

Dolichocephalic breeds Breeds of animals with a relatively long skull (typically with a breadth of less than 80 [or 75] percent of the length. These may be confused with brachiocephalic breeds.

Doppler ultrasonography A noninvasive test used to measure the blood flow through blood vessels by bouncing high-frequency sound waves off erythrocytes.

Dosage The expression of the amount of drug per body weight (e.g., milligrams per kilogram [mg/kg]).

Dose-dependent drug reactions An adverse drug reaction (ADR) that occurs based on a particular volume of drug that is given. Non-dose-dependent drug reactions may occur regardless of the amount of drug administered.

Dosimetry The calculation of a dose of radiation. Based on the severity of side effects, if any, the dose may be adjusted.

Down animals Animals that are not able to stand.

Drug Any chemical agent that affects living processes.

Drug clearance (Cl) The rate at which a drug is removed from an organ or from the body, expressed as the volume of plasma cleared of drug per unit time (milliliters per minute [mL/minute]). This value is used to measure the efficiency of drug elimination.

Drug compounding Any manipulation of a drug (combining, mixing, or altering) other than that provided for on the approved drug label.

Drug Enforcement Agency (DEA) Agency in the US Department of Justice that is responsible for enforcement of laws governing the uses of controlled substances.

Duodenum The first segment of the small intestine after the stomach. Chyme enters the duodenum from the stomach.

Dysbiosis Imbalance in intestinal bacteria that precipitates changes in the normal activities of the gastrointestinal tract.

Dysphoria An emotional state characterized by anxiety, depression, or unease.

Dyspnea Difficult or labored breathing.

Dysthanasia Pertaining to suffering during the dying process as a result of unexpected occurrences, such as prolonging the life of animals that are seriously or even terminally ill and that are potentially experiencing suffering.

Dystocia Difficult birth. This term can be applied to difficult birth in any species, which can result from a number of causes such as large fetus, small dam, or malpositioning.

Ecdysis Shedding of the outer integument (layer of skin).

Ectoparasite Parasite that is found on the exterior of the definitive host. Ectoparasites infest the host; they produce an infestation or ectoparasitism. For example, *Ctenocephalides felis*, the cat flea, is an ectoparasite found within the pelage (hair coat) of the cat.

Efficacy A drug's capacity, once bound to its receptor, to produce an effect.

Egg packet The typical reproductive "offspring" produced by adult *Dipylidium caninum*. Egg packets are discharged through either of the lateral genital pores of this tapeworm.

Ehmer sling Pelvic limb sling used in small animals that prevents weight bearing and helps force the femoral head into the acetabulum by abduction and internal rotation of the femur.

Electrocardiography Measurement of the electrical conductance of the heart; ECG rhythm strips.

Electronic medical record (EMR) An electronic record in chronological order of a patient's medical data, which include the primary purposes such as diagnostic procedures, diagnoses, prognoses, and treatment, and secondary purposes such as evaluations of medical information for business, legal, and research purposes.

Elimination The act of urination and/or defecation.

ELISA **E**nzyme-linked **i**mmunosorbent **a**ssay is a method used to measure a substance (antigen or antibody) by linking formation of an antigen-antibody complex to a detection method, typically a color change mediated by an enzymatic reaction (see Fig. 12.4).

Elongation The act of lengthening.

Embryo Structure formed by fertilization of the oocyte by sperm.

Emergency facility A veterinary emergency facility is one with the primary function of receiving, treating, and monitoring emergency patients during its specified hours of operation.

A veterinarian is in attendance at all hours of operation, and sufficient staff is always available to provide timely and appropriate care. Veterinarians, support staff, instrumentation, medications, and supplies must be sufficient to provide an appropriate level of emergency care. A veterinary emergency service may be an independent, after-hours service; an independent 24-hour service; or part of a full-service hospital or a large teaching institution.

Emetics Agents used to induce vomiting.

Emotional medical record Record of behavior that the veterinary team can refer to before handling the animal; includes what the animal prefers for distractions, the best location to work with this animal, if there is a provider preference, and specific handling notes and responses for each visit.

Empathy The ability to identify with the emotions and feelings of others.

Enamel Hard tissue of high mineral content that covers the crown of a tooth.

End of life Period at the end of a patient's life.

Endodontics Branch of dentistry dealing with disease of the pulp.

Endometrial Belonging to the mucous membrane lining the uterus.

Endoparasite Parasite that is found on the interior of the definitive host. Endoparasites infect the host; they produce an infection or endoparasitism. For example, *Dirofilaria immitis*, the canine heartworm, is an endoparasite found within the right ventricle and pulmonary arteries of the dog.

Endoscopy Instrument for visualizing the interior of a hollow organ or part (such as the bladder or esophagus) for diagnostic or therapeutic purposes and that typically has one or more channels to enable passage of instruments.

Endotoxemia The presence of poisonous substances in bacteria; separable from the cell body only upon its disintegration.

Energy density The number of calories provided in foods. For pet diets, energy density is expressed as kcal/g.

Enrichment media Culture media used to enhance the growth of specific bacteria.

Enterohepatic recirculation Occurs with some compounds that are metabolized in the liver. The metabolites are emptied in the bile and are reabsorbed in the small intestines.

Enteropathy Disease of the intestinal tract.

Enterotomy Incision into a small intestinal lumen.

Entropion A condition in which the eyelid is turned inward which can lead to irritation of the eyeball from contact with eyelashes.

Enucleation Scientifically refers to the removal of the nucleus of a cell, medically refers to the removal of a tumor, gland or the eyeball itself.

Environmental Protection Agency (EPA) Government agency charged with protecting human health and the environment. The Pesticide Regulation Division, under the Federal Insecticide, Fungicide, and Rodenticide Act, oversees pesticides.

Eosinophil Type of granulocyte with a segmented nucleus and granules that stain pink to red with Wright stain or quick stains. Marked species variation in the appearance of the granules has been noted. Eosinophils from dogs have numerous round, reddish granules; eosinophils from cats have numerous rod-shaped, reddish granules; eosinophils from horses have numerous large, round reddish granules; and eosinophils from cows have numerous small, round, reddish granules.

Epidermis Outermost layer of the skin.

Epithelialization Process of wound coverage by epithelial cells during the final stage of the proliferative phase of wound healing.

Eructation Act or instance of belching.

Eschar A thick, leathery, black layer of dead tissue; a scab, especially after a burn.

Esophagostomy tube Tube placed into an artificial opening in the esophagus when oral feeding is impossible because of injury or surgery.

Estrogen Hormone found in both males and females that primarily encourages female characteristics and aids in the signs of estrus.

Estrus Period of sexual activity in nonhuman female mammals that includes proliferation of uterine mucosa, swelling of the vulva, ovulation, and acceptance of coitus.

Ethylene oxide Gaseous substance used as a sterilant for instruments and articles that would be damaged by steam sterilization. Ethylene oxide is suspected to cause cancer in some animals in cases involving very large or long exposures. It is a colorless gas at room temperature; is flammable, explosive, and toxic; and can cause skin burns, respiratory irritation, vomiting, headaches, and birth defects.

Etiology Study of the cause of disease.

Euthanasia Greek for "good sleep." Method of intentionally ending a life to relieve suffering.

Evisceration Uncontrolled exposure of organs through an incision as a result of dehiscence or trauma.

Excoriation Skin lesions caused by the self-trauma of scratching.

Exodontics Extraction of teeth via closed or surgical techniques.

Exposure time In radiology, this is the amount of time that the x-ray beam has contact with the patient, and simultaneously with the digital collector or radiographic film.

External coaptation Use of a rigid external device such as a bandage, splint, or cast to align fractures.

Extracellular matrix Meshwork like substance attached to the outer cell surface that provides support and anchorage.

Extracorporeal shockwave A high-energy, focused sound wave that delivers energy to a specific focal point in the body; these sound waves dissipate mechanical energy into tissues, which initiates biological responses at the cellular level to decrease inflammation and speed healing.

Extra-label The usage of a pharmaceutical or chemical in a manner that is not recommended by the manufacturer such as treating a species or condition with a drug not specifically designed/approved for that species or condition.

Extra-label drug use Actual use or intended use of a drug in an animal in a manner that is not in accordance with approved labeling.

Extravasation Leakage of something out of its container or normal location, such as a drug out of a vein.

Exuberant granulation tissue Excessive formation of vascularized fibrous tissue (granulation tissue) in an open wound. Granulation tissue is considered exuberant when it grows above the level of the skin. Also referred to as *proud flesh*.

Failure of passive transfer (FPT) Deficient levels of antibodies absorbed by the gut in animals dependent on colostrum for immunologic protection. Failure can occur because colostrum contains inadequate levels of antibodies, or because the animal is not able to absorb adequate quantities of antibodies.

Farrowing The act of a sow giving birth to piglets.

Fastidious Describes bacteria that have specific growth requirements.

Fatty acid Building block of animal or vegetable fats and oils with varying carbon chain lengths. Several essential fatty acids must be provided in the diet.

Fear Feeling of apprehension experienced when an animal perceives that some nearby place, thing, or event may be dangerous. This emotion usually leads to avoidance of fear-inducing stimuli. Physiologic changes (increased heart rate, respiratory rate, blood pressure, and dilated pupils) involve autonomic arousal, stimulation of the hypothalamic–pituitary–adrenal axis (HPA), and release of stress hormones.

Fear, anxiety, and stress (FAS) An animal's changing emotional state marked by fear, anxiety, and stress demonstrated by signs of distress, including fear-induced defensive aggression. Fear Free uses the FAS score as a numeric value assigned to the patient's level of fear, anxiety, and stress.

Fear Free A certification program for members of the veterinary profession and other pet care professionals (e.g., trainers, groomers, walkers) that provides in-depth instruction on how to interact with animals and strives to provide the highest quality veterinary medical care by protecting the emotional welfare of the patient.

Fear-related aggression Aggression displayed when the dog perceives a threat. Most dogs demonstrate fearful body postures and possibly physiologic signs. Over time, as the dog learns that these behaviors are effective, it can begin to demonstrate more offensive body postures.

Fecal transfaunation Repopulation of the gut of a horse with healthy flora from another horse.

Federal Food, Drug, and Cosmetic (FFD&C) Act Federal law regulating drug approval, use, safety, and efficacy.

Fenestrated Having a window or one created in a surgical drape.

Fetal membranes Membranes that support fetal development by providing nutrition and enabling respiration and excretion. Fetal membranes include yolk sac, allantois, amnion, and chorion.

Fetatome Device used to cut a dead fetus into smaller parts that can be more easily extracted vaginally when a fetotomy is performed.

Fetotomy Procedure in which a dead fetus is cut into smaller pieces so that it can be extracted vaginally.

Fever Elevation of body temperature caused by a temporary increase in the body's thermoregulatory set point, usually caused by infection, inflammation, or neoplasia.

Fibrin(ogen) degradation products (FDPs) Small-molecular-weight polymers that result from plasmin cleavage of fibrinogen and fibrin. FDPs are sometimes measured in animals suspected of having disseminated intravascular coagulation (DIC) or other disorders of fibrinolysis.

Fibrinolysis Enzymatic breakdown of fibrin, usually by plasmin. Fibrinolysis is the part of normal coagulation that results in dissolution of clots as part of the healing process. Some diseases are associated with increased fibrinolysis.

Fibroblasts Cells that are recruited into a wound during the proliferative phase of wound healing that help form granulation tissue.

Fight-or-flight response A state of alert experienced when a threat to survival is perceived. A series of physical responses, including stimulation of the sympathetic nervous system, increased heart rate, and increased blood flow to muscles, to prepare the animal to avoid the threat (flight) or confront the threat (fight).

First-degree burn Superficial burn on the outermost layer of the skin (epidermis). Affected skin is reddened and painful but re-epithelializes within 1 week with topical wound management.

First-pass effect The portion of a drug that is lost during the process of absorption, which occurs typically in the intestinal wall and liver. Large amounts of a drug may be readily metabolized before entering general circulation, and this necessitates a higher initial dose to be effective.

Flash sterilization Emergency sterilization in which the instrument is placed unwrapped in an autoclave and is taken directly to surgery after sterilization. It is not recommended as a routine sterilization procedure.

Flight zone Area surrounding a livestock animal that, when entered by a predator, will cause the animal to move.

Fluid resuscitation Use of fluid therapy to treat low blood pressure or severe dehydration.

Fluoroscopy Presentation of a continuous x-ray image, which involves directing the x-ray beam through the patient and onto an image intensifier.

Foal Juvenile horse nursing from its mother.

Focal–film distance Distance between the target in the x-ray tube and the surface of the x-ray cassette.

Foley catheter Catheter threaded through the urethra to the bladder, where it is held in place with a tiny inflated balloon.

Follicle Structure on the ovary within which the oocyte develops.

Follicle-stimulating hormone (FSH) Hormone produced in the anterior pituitary that when released encourages follicular development and spermatogenesis.

Fomite An object that in itself is harmless, such as clothing or instruments, but is able to harbor pathogenic or infectious agents and serve as an agent of transmission of infection.

Forage Vegetative portion of plants in a fresh, dried, or ensiled state; it is fed to livestock (as pasture, hay, or silage).

Foramen magnum Large hole in the occipital bone through which the spinal cord exits the skull.

Foreshortening The visual effect of an object appearing to look shorter than it is because it is angled toward the viewer.

Forestomach Prestomach chambers in a ruminant animal. Includes reticulum, rumen, and omasum.

Fourth-degree burn Involves tissue extending beyond the dermis, including muscle, tendon, and bone. Surgical intervention is required to prevent scarring that restricts movement. Animals with fourth-degree burns are critically ill and require intensive care to survive.

Frailty A multisystem impairment associated with increased vulnerability to stressors; the condition of individuals that are at increased risk of adverse health outcomes. Frailty is related to but not synonymous with comorbidity and disability and is characterized by a decline in the body's functional reserve; lower energy metabolism; smaller muscle cells; and altered nervous, hormonal, and inflammatory functions.

Frustration Experienced when an animal is in a situation in which it is prevented from performing a behavior that it is highly motivated to perform.

Furcation Region of a multirooted tooth where the roots diverge from the crown.

Gangrenous mastitis Necrosis of a large area of a mammary gland or glands secondary to infection. One or more anaerobic bacteria are often attributed to the infection. It is known as "blue bag" because of the dark blue color of the necrotic mammary tissue.

Gas sterilization Use of chemical vapors to sterilize surgical materials and instruments that cannot withstand the high temperatures associated with stream sterilization in autoclaves. The most commonly used chemical gas is ethylene oxide.

Gastric lavage Irrigation of the stomach, the contents of which are gently pumped out; usually done to remove ingested poisons.

Gastrointestinal parasite A parasite of the intestinal tract.

Gastrostomy Method of enteral feeding in which a tube is surgically introduced through the abdominal wall.

Gastrotomy Incision into the stomach.

Generic name The chemical name of a drug rather than the brand name under which the drug is sold.

Genetic Inherited. In general, one parent or both parents transmit disease-causing genes to the offspring, unless it is a new mutation in the patient. The disease may not show up until much later in life.

Gentle control A concept of animal care that uses the following: distractions when possible; stabilization rather than forcible restraint to encourage stillness; gentle support so the animal feels secure; animal gently kept in place with attention paid to all six directions of possible movement (up, down, right, left, forward, back); safe prevention of harm to the pet and the veterinary team; and a plan for ways to stop the procedure and safely move away if the fear, anxiety, and stress score (FAS) increases rapidly.

Geriatrics Branch of medicine that deals with the problems and diseases of old age and aging people.

Gerontology The study of the aging processes and individuals as they advance from middle age through later life.

Giardia Flagellated protozoal parasite of the small intestine. Animals with giardiasis may have watery diarrhea. *Giardia* can be spread to humans via contaminated water.

Glucose absorption test A test used to determine whether a horse is properly absorbing nutrients.

Glycosuria The presence of glucose in the urine.

Gonadotropin-releasing hormone (GnRH) Hormone produced in the hypothalamus that when released can initiate the release of follicle-stimulating hormone or luteinizing hormone in the male or female.

Goniometer Tool used to measure joint range of motion.

Gram stain Commonly used stain named after its developer Hans Christian Gram that is used to differentiate bacteria on the basis of the composition of their cell walls. Gram-positive organisms have peptidoglycan in their cell walls and lack an outer cell membrane. Gram-negative bacteria have an outer cell wall that comprises a lipid bilayer with lipopolysaccharide. ram-positive bacteria retain crystal violet in the Gram stain reaction and stain blue, whereas gram-negative bacteria do not and stain red.

Granulation tissue Vascularized fibrous tissue that covers a full-thickness skin wound if the wound is left to heal by secondary intention.

Gray (Gy) A unit of ionizing radiation in the International System of Units (SI). It is the absorption of one joule.

Gregarious Animals that tend to live in groups.

Grid A thin sheet of lead strips with radiolucent spacers encased in an aluminum cover, giving the appearance of a thin, flat rectangular tray. A grid is placed between the patient and the film cassette to absorb scatter radiation so it does not reach the cassette and affect image quality.

Gross energy (GE) Total potential energy of a foodstuff determined by measuring the total heat produced when the food is burned in a bomb calorimeter.

Gross pathology Refers to pathologic changes in tissue that are visible with the unaided eye.

Gross revenue Money generated by a business through the sale of goods or services before any expenses are deducted.

Gulick A calibrated tape measure used to accurately measure body circumference.

Habituation A type of conditioning in which the learner's response to the same stimulus decreases in intensity over time.

Half-life Time required for the amount of a drug in the body to decrease by one-half, or 50%. Used to estimate the dosing interval.

Halitosis A foul odor to the breath.

Haul-in facility Large-animal facility to which animals are brought to the practice for examination or treatment.

Hazardous chemical (also known as *hazardous material* or *hazmat*) Any chemical or chemical product that may present a physical or health hazard, including, but not limited to, carcinogens, irritants, sensitizers, toxins, flammable materials, and products that may be reactive with other common chemicals.

Heaves Recurrent airway obstruction (or equine asthma). Clinical signs include increased respiratory rate (tachypnea) and increased effort (dyspnea), nostril flare, and dry cough.

Heel effect The x-ray beam produced through interactions with the anode has a spectrum of x-ray energies. The x-ray beam is more intense at the side of the cathode than in the center of the beam or on the anode side.

Hematemesis Vomiting blood.

Hematochezia Presence of blood in feces.

Hematocrit (HCT) The percentage of a specific volume of blood that consists of packed red blood cells (RBCs). Although hematocrit often is used synonymously with packed cell volume, it is used most correctly to refer to a value measured by an automated hematology analyzer and calculated from the mean cell volume multiplied by the RBC count.

Hemiplegia One-sided weakness or paralysis or weakness of the face, arm, or leg; this may be a sign of stroke or other neurological injury/deficit.

Hemocytometer Specialized counting chamber with a surface that contains a pair of etched counting grids and a special weighted coverglass used for manual determination of cell counts. Detailed manufacturer instructions must be followed carefully for accurate results.

Hemoglobin Specialized, iron-containing protein in red blood cells (RBCs) that binds oxygen in the lungs for transport to tissues. Hemoglobin concentration is measured by most automated hematology analyzers as an index of RBC mass.

Hemolysis Destruction of red blood cells with liberation of hemoglobin. In microbiology, hemolysis refers to the clearing of media around a bacterial colony.

Hemoptysis Coughing up blood, or blood in sputum.

Hemostasis Process of vasoconstriction, platelet plug formation, and blood coagulation resulting in clot formation in response to vascular injury.

Hepatic encephalopathy Altered cognitive and neurologic function as a result of buildup of toxins in the bloodstream that are normally removed by the liver.

Hermaphroditic Refers to the condition in which a single adult organism has the reproductive organs of both the male and the female of the species. Cross fertilization and self-fertilization are possible with hermaphrodites. Most digenetic flukes of domesticated animals are hermaphroditic.

Herniorrhaphy The surgical repair of a hernia.

Hertz (Hz) Unit of measurement used to quantify the frequency of ultrasound waves; 1 cycle per second.

Heterogonic life cycle One of two pathways in the life cycle of *Strongyloide stercoralis.* The heterogonic cycle takes place when environmental temperatures are fair (not extremely cold or hot).

Heterophil Type of granulocyte in birds, guinea pigs, and rabbits. Heterophils have bilobed or segmented nuclei and numerous red-staining, seed-shaped or rod-shaped granules. Heterophils function similarly to neutrophils, but there are differences in the granule content.

Hirsutism Abnormally excessive hair growth associated with Cushing disease in horses and ponies.

Histopathology Refers to pathologic changes in tissue that are microscopic and can be seen only with the use of a microscope.

Hobbles Leather straps fastened around the pasterns of horses; can be placed on all four limbs and tied together with a rope, or just on forelimbs or hind limbs to keep a horse from kicking.

Homogonic life cycle One of two pathways in the life cycle of *Strongyloides stercoralis.* The homogonic cycle takes place when environmental temperatures are adverse (harsh weather).

Hospice Facility or program designed to provide a caring environment to meet the physical and emotional needs of the terminally ill.

Hospital A veterinary or animal hospital is a facility in which the practice conducted typically or may include inpatient and outpatient diagnostics and treatment.

Hospital Safety Manual A collection of written safety-related policies unique to a specific workplace.

Human-animal bond The recognized emotional relationship that exists between humans and companion animals.

Humane twitch Mechanical restraint device with a metal hinge that is placed over the upper lip of the horse, squeezed, and clipped to the halter.

Hydrocarbons Any of a large class of organic compounds that contain only carbon and hydrogen. Examples include natural gas, propane, butane, kerosene, gasoline, and motor oil.

Hydrometra A condition in which the uterus fills with sterile fluid that causes mild to moderate distention.

Hydronephrosis Dilatation and distention of the renal pelvis and calices, usually caused by obstruction of the flow of urine from the kidney.

Hydrophilic Having an affinity for water; soluble in water. Hydrophilic drugs often are poorly absorbed and distributed and therefore require administration by injection (parenteral administration) to achieve effective therapeutic levels.

Hydrotherapy Use of water to promote physical activity for therapeutic effects.

Hyoid bone Bone in the neck region that supports the base of the tongue, the pharynx, and the larynx and aids the process of swallowing. The hyoid is usually referred to as a single bone, but it is composed of several portions. The hyoid bone is attached to the temporal bone by two small rods of cartilage.

Hyperalgesia Lowering of the pain threshold, resulting in less stimulation required to produce pain.

Hypercarbia Elevated carbon dioxide levels in blood.

Hyperechoic Structure in the ultrasound image that appears bright or white compared with adjacent structures.

Hyperplasia The abnormal increase in the number of cells in an organ or tissue that leads to abnormal enlargement. A benign example is a callus formation where there is constant friction of pressure.

Hypersensitivity Exaggerated immune response to some source of stimulation.

Hyperthermia Elevation of body temperature caused by inadequate heat-dissipating mechanisms to overcome excessive ambient heat without a change in the body's thermoregulatory set point.

Hypertonic Having an osmolality higher than that of blood and providing electrolytes in greater proportion than water.

Hypertrichosis An abnormal growth of hair over the body, it is classified into two types: localized or generalized.

Hyperventilation Increased ventilation; a respiratory pattern that results in lower carbon dioxide blood levels.

Hypnotic Drug that induces sleep.

Hypobiosis A life cycle term that means "being in suspended animation" or "undergoing arrested development."

Hypoechoic Structure in the ultrasound image that appears darker than adjacent structures.

Hypoglycemia Lower than normal levels of blood glucose resulting in lack of fuel to the brain and other organ systems.

Hyposmia Partial decrease in sense of smell.

Hypotension Abnormally low blood pressure.

Hypothermia Abnormally low body temperature. The measured body temperature must be compared with what is normal for the age group because neonates have lower body temperatures than adults.

Hypoxic ischemic encephalopathy (HIE) A medical emergency believed to result from oxygen deprivation during the birthing process that can vary in severity, depending on the age of the fetus, length of oxygen deprivation, and severity of hypoxia. Foals often seem normal after birth but develop progressive symptoms, including failure to recognize the mare; inability to stand, walk, or nurse; vocalization; and seizures. Commonly referred to as "dummy foal" or "equine maladjustment syndrome."

Hypotonic Having an osmolality lower than that of blood and providing water in greater proportion than electrolytes.

Hypoventilation Decreased ventilation; a respiratory problem that results in higher blood levels of carbon dioxide.

Hypovolemia Decreased circulating blood volume.

Hypoxemia Low blood oxygen levels.

Hypoxia Low tissue oxygen levels.

Hypsodont Tooth type with a long reserve crown and roots that allow for continued growth and/or continued eruption.

Icterus Yellow discoloration of tissues, serum, or plasma caused by the presence of bilirubin. Icterus, also referred to as *jaundice,* may develop as a result of hemolytic disease (prehepatic), liver disease (hepatic), or cholestasis (posthepatic or obstruction of bile flow).

Idiopathic Arising spontaneously or from an obscure or unknown cause.

Idiosyncratic drug reaction An unpredictable reaction to a drug that does not occur immediately but occurs after several days of treatment; often associated with an immune system response.

Ileus Functional loss of intestinal motility.

Impervious Waterproof. Does not allow water to penetrate.

In situ In its normal place; confined to the site of origin.

Incise drape A sterile, adherent, plastic surgical drape. It is often impregnated with an antiseptic. The drape is incised along with the skin.

Incontinence Involuntary urination or defecation.

Indigenous flora Bacteria that normally inhabit an anatomical site. Also called *normal flora* or *microflora.*

Inflammatory phase The first phase of wound healing. Characterized by formation of a blood clot within the wound, release of growth factors, and recruitment of macrophages and neutrophils to clean up the wound and to modulate healing.

Ingesta Food material in the intestinal tract.

Ingress port Port on a tubular instrument used to infuse a solution into a cavity, such as a joint.

Inguinal Pertaining to the groin area.

Insufflate To pump a gas or medicinal substance into a body cavity.

Integrative medicine An approach to treatment that uses complementary, holistic, and conventional treatments in a rational, evidence-based way.

Intensifying screen A fluorescent screen that lines a radiographic cassette so that it has close contact with the radiographic film placed in the cassette. The screen produces photons when exposed to x-rays, which intensifies the effect of the x-ray beam. This dual exposure reduces the patient's exposure to radiation.

Intermediate host Within the life cycle of a parasite, the host that harbors the immature, asexual, or larval stage of a parasite.

Intervertebral disk disease A condition in which disks between the vertebrae of the spine herniate into the space occupied by the spinal cord. The herniated material compresses portions of the spinal cord, causing pain and possible paralysis or paresis.

Intraosseous Administration of a drug or fluid into the bone.

Intussusception Telescoping of a portion of the bowel into another.

Ionizing radiation Any radiation that is capable of displacing electrons from atoms or molecules, thereby producing ions. Examples include alpha particles, beta particles, gamma rays or x-rays, and cosmic rays. In medicine, ionizing radiation arises from radiotherapy, x-ray machines, and radioactive substances. Ionizing radiation also enters the atmosphere of the earth from outer space. At high doses, ionizing radiation increases specific types of chemical activity inside cells.

This effect can be used to treat cancer, but it also leads to health risks, such as induction of cancer.

Irritant Agent that causes pain or inflammation at the site of injection.

Ischemia Deficient supply of blood to a body part, such as the heart or brain, caused by obstruction of the inflow of arterial blood.

Isoechoic Structure in the ultrasound image that is of equal echogenicity to another structure.

Isotonic Having the same osmolality as that of blood.

Joule Unit of energy or work. The amount of work required or energy needed to produce 1 watt of power per 1 second.

Jugular vein Consists of paired veins running in the neck that drain the brain, face, and neck.

Keratoconjunctivitis Combined inflammation of the cornea and the conjunctiva.

Ketosis Nutritional disease of cattle and sometimes sheep, goats, or swine that is marked by reduction of blood glucose and the presence of ketone bodies in blood, tissues, milk, and urine; it is associated with digestive and nervous disturbances.

Kilojoule Amount of mechanical energy needed for a force of 1 newton to move a weight of 1 kg a distance of 1 m. Used as a measure of food energy in Europe, with conversions of 1 kcal = 4.184 kJ and 1 kJ = 0.239 kcal.

Kilovolt peak (kVp) Quality factor that regulates the energy of the x-ray beam. The higher the kVp (kilovoltage), the higher the energy of the x-ray photons. Regulates contrast in the radiographic image. The higher the kVp, the lower the contrast.

Laceration Sharp cut or tear through the skin and possibly deeper tissues.

Lag phase A period in the life cycle of bacteria in which the population remains constant while adjusting to the environmental conditions in which it is attempting to grow. This is often measured in laboratory experiments surrounding bacterial cell cultures.

Laminae Interdigitations between the corium and the hoof that serve as attachment sites between the hoof and the coffin bone; bony plates that form the roof of each arch of each spinal vertebra.

Laminitis A serious and sometimes fatal disease in horses in which the hooves become inflamed (can affect one or all feet, but it is most often seen in the forefeet concurrently). Laminitis results from the disruption of blood flow to the laminae, which secure the coffin bone (P3) to the hoof wall. Inflammation often permanently weakens the laminae and interferes with the wall-bone bond.

Laparoscopy A surgical examination of organs or internal structures of the body which is done under general or local anesthesia.

Laparotomy Surgical incision into the abdominal wall.

Left shift An increased number of immature granulocytes, typically used to refer to an increased number of band neutrophils. The presence of a left shift often indicates inflammation.

Lesions Alterations or abnormalities in a tissue (pathologic changes); for example, wounds, sores, ulcers, tumors, cataracts, and any other tissue damage.

Leukocytosis Condition characterized by an abnormally high total number of circulating leukocytes. Neutrophilia indicates increased numbers of circulating neutrophils.

Levey-Jennings chart Graph on which quality control data are sequentially plotted for rapid visual inspection (see Figure 12.3). The x-axis may show the date or control run number, whereas the y-axis depicts the concentration of the control. The mean and ±1, 2, or 3 standard deviations from the expected mean of the control material are indicated on the graph.

Lipemia Turbidity of serum or plasma due to the presence of lipids that contain a high concentration of triglycerides. Lipemia may occur after a meal or in association with various metabolic diseases.

Lipid Any fat, oil, or related compound that is insoluble in water but soluble in nonpolar solvents.

Lipophilic Soluble in lipids. Drug absorption across cell membranes is most effective for drugs that are lipophilic.

Low-level laser therapy (LLLT) A treatment using low-level or "cold" lasers to stimulate healing in body tissues. The laser is applied to the surface of the body or inserted in an orifice. Treatment is intended to speed the rate of healing and is used on wounds, tendon injuries, and painful muscles; also known as *laser therapy* and/ or *photobiomodulation.*

Luteinizing hormone (LH) Hormone produced in the anterior pituitary that when released can initiate follicular maturation, ovulation, and spermatogenesis.

Lyme disease Also called *borreliosis*; an infectious disease caused by bacteria from the genus *Borrelia*. The bacteria typically are spread through the bite of an infected deer tick.

Lymphocyte Variably sized, round leukocyte with a round nucleus, condensed chromatin, and minimal pale cytoplasm, resulting in a relatively high nuclear-to-cytoplasmic ratio. Most lymphocytes normally present in the circulation are small. B and T lymphocytes mediate humoral and cell-mediated immunity, respectively.

Lymphosarcoma Also known as *lymphoma*; cancer of lymphocytes and lymphoid tissues and the third-most commonly diagnosed cancer in dogs.

Magnetic resonance imaging (MRI) A noninvasive imaging system that uses powerful magnets to generate images of internal structures in the body. The images produced by MRI reflect information about the chemical makeup of tissues and can distinguish between normal and abnormal tissues and those that have been traumatized or are cancerous.

Magnification The process of making an image appear larger. In light microscopy, the power of the ocular multiplied by the power of the objective equals the total magnification of the image.

Maintenance rate The amount of fluid needed to fulfill the physiologic requirement for water.

Malocclusion Incorrect alignment of jaws or specific teeth within the jaws.

Many-host tick An individual tick that is capable of feeding on many different hosts. Many-host ticks make frequent visits to different hosts.

Mare Adult female horse.

Massage Systematic and scientific manipulation of the soft tissues of the body for the purpose of obtaining or maintaining health, to promote relaxation, to decrease pain, or to promote circulation to surrounding tissues.

Master problem list Complete list of diagnoses given to a patient during its lifetime.

Mastitis Inflammation of the mammary gland. Typically occurs during lactation. If endotoxins are absorbed from septic secretions within the udder, endotoxemia can result, and the condition is termed *toxic mastitis.*

Maternal aggression Aggression typical of a female that is attempting to prevent access to her offspring (usually neonates). May also occur during pseudopregnancy (pseudocyesis), when females nest and guard items as if they are neonates, in the absence of actual pregnancy.

Maturation phase The third and final phase of wound healing. During this phase, collagen fibers remodel and align, and there is a final gain in wound strength.

Maximum permissible dose (MPD) The total dose of ionizing radiation that is considered safe for a patient.

Mean corpuscular hemoglobin concentration (MCHC) The average concentration of hemoglobin in a volume of blood. MCHC is calculated from the hemoglobin concentration divided by the packed cell volume (hematocrit) and is used to characterize red blood cells (RBCs) in anemic patients.

Mean corpuscular volume (MCV) Average volume of red blood cells (RBCs). MCV is measured by most automated hematology analyzers and is used to characterize the RBCs in patients with anemia. It also may be calculated by dividing the packed cell volume by RBC count obtained through manual methods.

Mediastinum Space in the thorax between the lungs that contains the trachea, esophagus, heart, nerves, lymphatic vessels, and major blood vessels.

Medication administration/order records (MAOR) Records used by the entire veterinary health care team to help organize the management and care of hospitalized patients.

Melena Passage of dark tarry stools that contain decomposing blood; usually an indication of bleeding in the upper part of the alimentary tract, especially the esophagus, stomach, and duodenum.

Meninges Connective tissue layers that cover the brain and the spinal cord.

Mentation Mental activity or acuity of a patient.

Mesaticephalic (mesocephalic) Refers to a head shape of moderate length in the rostrocaudal dimension, as is seen in Beagles.

Mesial Positional term in dentistry that refers to the surface of the tooth along the dental arch that is closest to the rostral midline of the dental arch.

Mesioclusion Also known as *prognathism*; a malocclusion in which the mandibular arch is mesial to the maxillary arch. It is colloquially known as an *underbite.*

Metabolic acidosis Acidosis resulting from excess acid in the blood caused by abnormal metabolism, excessive acid intake, renal retention, or excessive loss of bicarbonate (as in diarrhea).

Metabolism The ability of a living organism to modify the chemical structure of drugs so that they are no longer active.

Metabolizable energy (ME) Energy available to the animal after energy from feces, urine, and combustible gases has been subtracted from gross energy. Used to express the energy content of foods and commercial diets.

Metabolizable (maintenance) energy requirement (MER) Average amount of energy used by an animal with normal activity, exercise, and growth, or other energy demands beyond resting.

Metacestode A larval tapeworm. Stage of the tapeworm found within the vertebrate or invertebrate intermediate host. Examples of metacestode stages include cysticercoid, cysticercus, coenurus, and the hydatid cyst (both unilocular and multilocular).

Metastasis Process by which a malignant cancer spreads from the primary or original site to a distant location in the body.

Metritis Inflammation of the uterus. This condition can be associated with buildup of septic fluid within the uterus. If endotoxins are absorbed from the septic uterine fluid, endotoxemia can result, and the condition is termed *toxic metritis*.

Metronomic therapy Treatment including continuous or frequent administration of low doses of chemotherapy drugs.

Microfilaria (pl. microfilariae) This "prelarval" developmental stage is often associated with *Dirofilaria immitis*, the canine heartworm.

Milliamperage (mA) The milliamperage setting controls the quantity of electrons boiled off the filament in the x-ray tube.

Minimum inhibitory concentration (MIC) Lowest concentration of an antimicrobial agent that will inhibit the visible growth of a microorganism after overnight incubation.

Miosis Constriction of the pupil of the eye.

Miracidium A ciliated, motile stage that emerges from the operculated egg of a digenetic fluke. The miracidium is covered with tiny moving hairs that allow it to swim in the water and to come in contact with the first intermediate host of the fluke, which is usually a snail.

M-mode Motion mode image display in ultrasound imaging wherein motion of the body, usually the heart, is observed by scanning a thin slice of it over time.

Mobile facility A mobile practice is a veterinary practice conducted from a vehicle with special medical or surgical facilities, or from a vehicle suitable for making house or farm calls. Regardless of mode of transportation, such practices have a permanent base of operations with a published address and telecommunication capabilities for making appointments or responding to emergency situations.

Modified Robert Jones bandage Bandage that is similar to a Robert Jones bandage but with a much thinner secondary layer.

Modified Thomas splint Traction splint constructed of rods; used to stabilize long bone fractures in large animals.

Modified Triadan system A current detailed nomenclature scheme/diagram that is used by veterinary medicine in which a three-digit number is assigned to each tooth with the first digit representing the quadrant of the mouth, and the second and third number indicating the location of the tooth in the quadrant.

Modulation Process of amplifying or dampening incoming pain signals after arrival to the spinal cord.

Moist wound healing Maintaining a moist wound environment by using an occlusive or semi occlusive primary bandage layer.

Molting A normal process that is seen in birds and some reptiles in which feathers or skin or shed and replaced with new. In reptiles this is also referred to as ecdysis.

Monocyte Largest circulating leukocyte in health; monocytes are characterized by abundant basophilic cytoplasm that often contains clear vacuoles and/or small pink granules. Nuclei are oval, indented, or ameboid in shape and have chromatin that is less condensed than in lymphocytes.

Monofilament A type of suture material consisting of a single synthetic strand rather than a cluster of twisted fibers. The relatively smooth outer surface of a monofilament suture decreases the likelihood of its harboring microbes.

Moral injury A distressing aftermath that may be expressed psychologically, behaviorally, socially, or spiritually as a result of exposure to events that contradict one's beliefs, morals, or expectations.

Mourning The act of grieving; the outward manifestation of the internal bereavement.

Mucometra Sterile mucus within the uterus causing mild to moderate distention.

Multifilament A suture material composed of two or more threads twisted around one another.

Multilocular hydatid cyst A type of metacestode/larval tapeworm that is closely associated with *Echinococcus multilocularis*. The multilocular hydatid cyst consists of many tiny, spherical, fluid-filled vesicles or cysts; however, these cysts are not enclosed by a thick, fibrous cyst wall of host origin, as in the case of *Echinococcus granulosus*.

Multimodal analgesia Use of two or more drugs to affect different phases of nociception simultaneously.

Multiple organ dysfunction syndrome (MODS) A complication of shock in which generalized microvascular clotting causes sufficient organ damage to result in failure of multiple organs.

Mutagen Chemical or physical agent that causes permanent deoxyribonucleic acid (DNA) injury and alteration within a cell. These changes are separate and distinct from those that normally occur during genetic recombination.

Mydriasis Dilatation of the pupil of the eye.

Myelosuppression Condition in which normal bone marrow activity is decreased, resulting in fewer white blood cells (WBCs; especially neutrophils), platelets, and red blood cells (RBCs) in the circulation. Myelosuppression is a potential side effect of some cancer therapies (e.g., radiotherapy, chemotherapy).

Myiasis Infection of fly larva in tissue.

Myocardium Middle layer of the heart and the main muscle layer responsible for contraction during systole.

Myofibroblast Type of fibroblast with contractile properties similar to those of smooth muscle cells, which are responsible for wound contraction.

Myositis Inflammation of muscle.

Myotherapy (or *trigger point therapy*) Form of massage that uses ischemic compression to relieve pain and muscle spasms.

Nadir Lowest circulating neutrophil count after administration of a chemotherapy drug. The nadir occurs at a predictable time point after therapy that varies depending on exactly what drug has been given.

Nares Nostrils.

National Association of Veterinary Technicians in America (NAVTA) An association dedicated to representing and promoting veterinary technology.

Natural death Death occurring in the course of nature and from natural causes (as age or disease).

Necropsy Examination of an animal after it has died to determine abnormal and disease-related changes that occurred during its life. The term *necropsy* originates from the Greek language and means "viewing the dead." Necropsy is also known as *autopsy*, which is Greek for "seeing with one's own eyes."

Needle (canine) teeth Deciduous third incisors and canines of piglets. These "baby teeth" are very sharp and should be nipped to protect the sow during suckling.

Negative punishment Decreases the frequency of a behavior because something pleasant is taken away (subtracted) after that behavior.

Negative reinforcement Increases the frequency of a behavior because something unpleasant is taken away or avoided (subtracted) after that behavior.

Negative-pressure wound therapy (NPWT) The controlled application of a vacuum to a wound; can be used in situations where normal drains cannot be used, such as distal limb wounds, wounds with extensive dead space and a large amount of expected fluid production, or before the use of skin flaps and grafts.

Nematode A roundworm.

Neonatal period In puppies and kittens, the first 2 to 4 weeks of life are characterized by complete dependence on the mother for nutrition, warmth, care, and overall survival because of incomplete neurologic functions, such as audio and visual abilities and proper spinal reflexes.

Neoplasm Abnormal growth of tissue that may be benign or malignant.

Net energy (NE) Energy available to the animal after energy from feces, urine, combustible gases, and loss of body heat has been subtracted from gross energy.

Net income Total income after the expenses are subtracted from the revenue.

Neurologic larva migrans A zoonotic condition caused by ingestion of an egg that contains an infective second-stage larva of the roundworm *Baylisascaris procyonis*, which is commonly referred to as the *raccoon ascarid*.

Neuromuscular electrical stimulation (NMES) A modality of physical therapy in which small electrical impulses are sent through the skin to underlying nerves and muscles, creating an involuntary muscle contraction. NMES is helpful in maintaining muscle tone in patients with muscle atrophy caused by disuse and incapacitation.

Neurotransmitter Chemical substance released from the axon terminal of a presynaptic neuron; diffuses across the synaptic cleft to excite or inhibit the target cell.

Neutropenia Abnormal decrease in the number of neutrophils (the most common type of white blood cells [WBCs]) in the blood.

Nociception Term used to describe three neuralgic phases of the pain pathway: transduction, transmission, and modulation. The perception of a painful or injurious stimulus both while conscious or unconscious; included in three of the four neuralgic phases of the pain pathway: transduction, transmission, and modulation.

Nonadherent dressing Primary layer that does not adhere firmly to the wound surface.

Nonocclusive Permeable to moisture and air; used in reference to bandage materials.

Nonparenteral A route for the administration of medication that is not intravascular. Nonparenteral routes include oral, sublingual, topical, transdermal, ophthalmic, otic, nasal, rectal, and vaginal routes.

Nonprotein nitrogen (NPN) In animal nutrition, refers to components such as urea, ammonia salts, ammoniated by-products, or free amino acids that are not proteins but can be converted into proteins by microbes in the ruminant stomach; should be used cautiously to prevent potential excess or deficiency, which may result in toxicity.

Nonrebreathing system Breathing circuit in which exhaled gases are carried away from the patient into a scavenging system.

Nonsteroidal anti-inflammatory drugs (NSAIDs) Large group of anti-inflammatory agents that work by inhibiting the production of prostaglandins. Examples include ibuprofen, ketoprofen, naproxen, and aspirin. These compounds also possess analgesic, antipyretic, and anti-inflammatory effects; they reduce pain, fever, and inflammation but can cause vomiting, stomach ulcers, and acute renal failure in animals.

Normalizing Allowing or encouraging something to be viewed as normal, as in encouraging feelings of grief after a pet's death.

Nosocomial infection Infection that hospitalized patients acquire from the hospital environment, another patient, or a health care provider.

Nuclear medicine The branch of medicine that makes use of radioactive substances.

Nutraceutical Naturally occurring and biologically active products (nondrug substances) administered orally to provide substances required for normal body structure and function with the intent of improving the health of animals.

Nutrients Substances that provide nourishment for growth and maintenance of life.

Obturator Stylus or removable plug used during insertion of a tubular instrument.

Occlusive Impermeable to moisture. Used in reference to bandage materials. An occlusive primary layer is used for moist wound healing.

Occupational Safety and Health Act Law in the United States that established the Occupational Safety and Health Administration. It gives every American worker protections and responsibilities in the area of safety. The Act applies to all workplaces in the United States and its territories that have at least one employee.

Occupational Safety and Health Administration (OSHA) Agency of the US government that is charged with enforcing the Occupational Safety and Health Act, which enforces federal laws that help ensure a safe workplace for American workers. Twenty-one states and territories have OSHA programs administered by the state; the remainder fall under federal OSHA jurisdiction.

Ocular larval migrans (OLM) Zoonotic condition caused by the migration of nematode larvae (usually *Toxocara canis*) through the eyes of children. Children become infected with these larvae by ingestion of eggs containing the infective second-stage larvae of *T. canis*.

Office A veterinary office is a veterinary practice in which a limited or consultative practice is conducted and that typically provides no facilities for housing or for inpatient diagnostics or treatment.

Omentopexy Surgical fixation of the omentum to the body wall.

Omentum Supportive mesenteries, which arise from the greater and lesser curvatures of the stomach.

Omphalophlebitis Umbilical infection or inflammation.

Oncotic pressure The portion of total osmotic pressure contributed by colloids.

One-host tick An individual tick that will feed on a single animal or on a single species of animal.

One-step prep Alcohol-based solutions containing other antiseptics that form a film when painted on the skin. Provide rapid onset of antiseptic effect and a long residual effect.

Onychectomy Removal of a claw.

Oocyst The "egg like offspring" produced by coccidial parasites such as *Cystoisospora (Isospora)*.

Oocyte Female component of the embryo that originates from the follicle of the ovary.

Open gloving Method of putting on sterile gloves when the person is not wearing a sterile gown or when the hands are protruding through the ends of the gown sleeves.

Operant conditioning Also known as *instrumental conditioning*; based on the principle that the consequences of a behavior will influence its frequency; known as the *Thorndike law of effect*. Behaviors that result in pleasant outcomes will increase in frequency, whereas those that result in unpleasant outcomes will decrease.

Operculated egg An egg that possesses a "tiny, cap like door" at one pole. Operculated eggs are produced by digenetic trematodes and pseudotapeworms.

Opportunistic infection Infection caused by an organism that is usually harmless but that causes disease under certain circumstances, such as failure of host defenses.

Orchidectomy Removal of the testicles.

Orthopedic Related to surgery on the skeleton.

Orthopnea Shortness of breath when lying down. Animals in congestive heart failure will stand and resist lying down to facilitate respiration.

Osmolality Concentration of osmotically active particles in solution expressed in osmoles or milliosmoles per kilogram.

Ostectomy Removal of a portion of bone.

Osteochondral fragments Fracture involving the articular cartilage and underlying bone.

Osteochondrosis Defect in cartilage maturation that causes lack of ossification of maturing cartilage.

Otoacariasis Infestation of the external ear canal with mites or ticks. *Otobius megnini*, the spinose ear tick, and *Otodectes cynotis*, the ear mite of dogs and cats, produce otoacariasis.

Outpatient Patient that comes into a practice for treatment and is discharged without being admitted for an overnight hospital stay.

Ovariohysterectomy Spay; removal of the uterus.

Over-the-counter (OTC) drug A nonprescription drug, as opposed to a legend drug.

Oxidase An enzyme, such as cytochrome oxidase, that catalyzes an oxidation-reduction reaction using oxygen as the electron acceptor.

Oxygen saturation The amount of hemoglobin bound to oxygen at any given moment. This value is measured in percent and reflects the degree of blood oxygenation.

Oxytocin Hormone produced in the hypothalamus and stored in the posterior pituitary which, when released, enhances milk "letdown" into the teat canal and uterine contractility.

Packed cell volume (PCV) The percentage (%) of red blood cells (RBCs) in a specific volume of blood; determined by centrifugation of a microhematocrit tube filled with anticoagulated blood. PCV is commonly used in veterinary medicine as an index of RBC mass.

Pain A complex multidimensional experience with both sensory and emotional components; it can have a significant and negative impact on an animal's quality of life and the human-animal bond.

Palatability Description of the taste, texture, aroma, and other characteristics of pet food. Highly palatable foods tend to be rich in fat and have added flavor enhancers.

Palliative care Specialized medical care for animals living with serious illnesses. This type of care is focused on relief from the symptoms and stress of a serious illness, with the goal of improving quality of life for both the patient and the family.

Palpebral edema Swelling of the eyelids.

Pancytopenia A decrease to below normal in the concentration of the three major blood cell types: red cells, white cells, and platelets.

Panleukopenia Viral infection of cats that is not considered zoonotic but is highly contagious from cat to cat.

Paradigm Any kind of philosophic or theoretical framework that underlies and guides a school of thought.

Paralumbar fossa Depression in the dorsocaudal abdominal body wall of quadrupeds bordered by the costal processes of the lumbar vertebrae, the last thoracic rib, and the tuber coxae.

Paraneoplastic syndrome Symptoms that result from effects on organs or tissues distant from the site of a primary tumor or its metastases. The underlying cause is usually a substance that is produced by the tumor and then is released into the systemic circulation. Almost any organ or tissue can be affected.

Paratenic host/transport host A host in which a parasite does not undergo further development but in which it remains encysted or in "suspended animation," serving as a source of the definitive host when the definitive host ingests the paratenic host.

Parenteral Administration by injection.

Parthenogenesis Modified form of sexual reproduction characterized by the formation of an ovum without the fertilization of a male's spermatozoan.

Partnering Participating in an activity or working with another individual, such as a provider showing a helping attitude and a willingness to listen to a client experiencing grief over the loss of a pet.

Parturition Process by which delivery of mammalian offspring occurs.

Parvoviral enteritis Viral infection of dogs that is not considered zoonotic but is highly contagious from dog to dog.

Passerine Of or related to the largest order (Passeriformes) of birds, which includes more than half of all living birds and consists chiefly of altricial songbirds.

Passive drain A drain that functions by allowing fluid to flow along the drain surface as the result of capillary action (e.g., the Penrose drain).

Passive immunity Type of immunity incurred via one of the following ways: (1) in utero when antibodies pass through the placenta from the dam to the fetus; (2) in newborns from the consumption of antibody-rich colostrum (first milk); or (3) by intravenous infusion of antibody-rich plasma (usually given to neonates that failed to gain adequate levels of antibodies in steps 1 and 2 here).

Passive range of motion (PROM) Joint movement caused by a therapist who moves a limb with no assistance from the patient; the use of stretching to prevent loss of normal range of motion, return normal range of motion if absent, increase cartilage nutrition in the joint, and stimulate cartilage regeneration.

Patent ductus arteriosus Congenital cardiac anomaly that results in persistent vascular communication between the aorta and the pulmonary artery.

Pathogenesis Sequence of events that leads to or underlies a disease.

Pathology The science and study of disease, especially the causes and development of abnormal conditions.

Penetrating wounds Injuries that often cause extensive injury to deeper tissues not apparent on inspection of the skin, making them challenging to assess; these wounds can be caused by factors such as bites, bullets, arrows, sticks, and antlers.

Percutaneously Term that refers to administering something through the skin.

Pericarditis Inflammation of the pericardium.

Perineal The area between the anus and the dorsal part of the external genitalia, especially in the female.

Perineal hernia Herniation of abdominal contents through the pelvic diaphragm, resulting in swelling on either side of the anus.

Periodontium Supporting structures of the tooth, including the periodontal ligament, gingival connective tissue, alveolar bone, and cementum.

Peritoneal lining A thin, transparent membrane (serosa) that lines the peritoneal cavity. It is also called the *parietal peritoneum.*

Persistent infection (PI) Chronic infection that does not resolve despite use of antimicrobials.

Personal protective equipment (PPE) Any piece of clothing or article worn by the user that is designed to prevent injury. PPE places a physical barrier between the wearer and the hazard; examples include gloves, glasses or goggles, aprons, boots, smocks, and masks.

Petechiation Small, visible pinpoint hemorrhage lesions less than 1 mm in diameter.

pH Measurement of the concentration of hydrogen ions in a solution. pH indicates whether a solution is acidic (pH < 7.0), neutral (pH = 7.0), or basic (pH > 7.0).

Pharmacodynamics (PD) Study of the biochemical and physiologic effects of drugs.

Pharmacokinetics (PK) Study of the movement of drugs in the body (i.e., absorption, distribution, metabolism, and excretion).

Pheromone Chemical substance that is usually produced by an animal and serves especially as a stimulus to other individuals of the same species for one or more behavioral responses.

Phlebitis Inflammation of a vein.

Phobia Fear of a specific stimulus that is excessive and persistent. The response usually seems out of proportion to the threat.

Physical restraint A type of restraint that uses physical measures such as stocks, halters, and lead ropes to control an animal for the purpose of examination or treatment.

Physical sterilization Use of filtration, radiation, and heat applied to medical products to eliminate or destroy all living organisms (including disease-producing organisms such as viruses) from a material.

Picture archival computing systems (PACS) A remote hard drive used to store data permanently and to move images around to different computer workstations within a single hospital or between hospitals; required to store, send, receive, print, and view images from all imaging modalities.

Pineal gland The endocrine structure within the brain that acts to correlate the length of daylight to reproduction.

Pituitary gland The "master endocrine gland." A pea-sized endocrine gland located at the base of the brain, made up of the anterior pituitary gland, which produces seven known hormones, and the posterior pituitary gland, which stores and releases two hormones from the hypothalamus; also called the *hypophysis.*

Placenta Structure that consists of the yolk sac, the amnion, the allantois, and the chorion; responsible for the passage of oxygen, nutrients, and waste products between fetus and dam.

Plaque An accumulation of food particles, saliva, minerals, and bacteria that appears as a white-tan, easily removable film on the teeth.

Plasmin Proteolytic enzyme formed from plasminogen in blood. Plasmin cleaves fibrin to dissolve clots and reestablish blood flow in areas of vascular injury.

Platelets (thrombocytes) Non nucleated fragments of megakaryocyte cytoplasm that circulate in blood and are involved in primary hemostasis. Platelets usually are smaller than red blood cells (RBCs), and the cytoplasm contains numerous small blue to purple granules, the contents of which are important in hemostasis.

Play-related aggression Behavior typical of play, usually nonaffective, and often simply referred to as inappropriate play behavior when directed toward humans.

Pleural effusion Fluid buildup in the space surrounding the lungs within the thorax.

Plerocercoid (sparganum) The infective developmental stage that parasitizes the second intermediate host in the life cycle of a pseudotapeworm.

Pleural effusion The accumulation of excess fluid in the pleural cavity (i.e., the space between the lungs and the chest wall).

Plume Smoke created from laser application on tissue.

Pneumovagina Seen primarily in horses, a condition in which there is poor vulvar conformation in mares which can lead to ascending infections, lack of establishment in breeding or survival of fetus.

Pneumothorax Abnormal accumulation of air in the space between the rib cage and the lung. This abnormal air pocket compresses the lung, resulting in respiratory distress. The lung may collapse. This condition may be caused by injury to lung tissue, rupture of air-filled pulmonary cysts, or puncture of the chest wall.

Poikilothermic Describes organisms, such as fish or reptiles, whose body temperature varies with the ambient temperature. Poikilotherms are commonly known as "cold-blooded" animals.

Point of balance The point on a livestock animal where if one takes a step in either direction, the animal moves in the opposite direction.

Polioencephalomalacia Also known as *cerebrocortical necrosis,* is characterized by altered function of the central nervous system. Brain swelling and inflammation lead to necrosis of brain tissue and death. Diagnosis is confirmed postmortem. Causes may include ingestion of grain diets and plants high in thiaminases, which inactivate vitamin B_1.

Polydipsia A condition evidenced by increased levels of thirst and excessive drinking (adj., polydipsic).

Polymerase chain reaction (PCR) An in vitro technique that is used to rapidly synthesize large quantities of a given deoxyribonucleic acid (DNA) segment. This involves separating the DNA into its two complementary strands, binding a primer to each single strand at the end of the given DNA segment where synthesis will start, using DNA polymerase to synthesize two-stranded DNA from each single strand, and repeating the process.

Polyuria Excessive production of urine.

Positive punishment Decreases the frequency of behavior because something unpleasant is added after a behavior.

Positive reinforcement Increases the frequency of behavior because something pleasant is added after a behavior.

Positron Emission Tomography (PET) An imaging test that uses radioactive drugs to examine metabolic activity within tissue or organs.

Practice acts Primary laws or statutes written and passed by the legislature to govern the practice of a profession. Typically, each state has its own practice act for each licensed profession.

Precocious Relatively developed, mature, and mobile at birth, such as animals born with full haircoats, open eyes, and teeth.

Pre-emptive analgesia Pain management administered before any trauma occurs to prevent expected pain.

Preferred optimal temperature zone (POTZ) Proper temperature at which enclosures should be kept to care for species such as fish, reptiles, and amphibians.

Pregnancy toxemia Sudden demand for energy by fast-growing fetuses that can occur in the last few weeks of pregnancy. Occurs more commonly in ewes with twins than with a single fetus. Rapid breakdown of body stores releases ketones, leading to ketoacidosis.

Preoxygenation Providing oxygen by mask or cannula for 5 to 10 minutes prior to a medical procedure to allow the lungs to fill with an increased percentage of oxygen.

Prescription drug A pharmaceutical drug that requires a prescription for it to be legally dispensed.

Previous history Medical history preceding the events surrounding the current problem, including the patient's origins, behavior, previous conditions, and treatments.

Primary closure Surgical closure of a fresh, clean wound, leading to primary-intention healing.

Primary-intention wound healing Healing of a wound across a surgically closed incision.

Primiparous Describes an animal that has given birth once.

Problem-oriented veterinary medical record (POVMR) A record keeping system in which clinical data are organized by medical problem. This approach is more labor intensive and generates more voluminous records than the source-oriented veterinary medical record (SOVMR), but it offers a comprehensive written evaluation of the patient.

Procercoid The developmental stage that parasitizes the first intermediate host in the life cycle of a pseudotapeworm. This host is usually an aquatic crustacean.

Profits The amount left over after all normal and necessary operating expenses of a business are subtracted from the gross revenue.

Progesterone Hormone present primarily in the female that is related to the presence of a corpus luteum and to pregnancy.

Proglottid One of the individual units of the tapeworm that make up the strobila. Proglottids are arrayed in a chain like manner (much like boxcars in a freight train).

Progress notes Chronologically ordered notations made in the medical record that describe the events of each patient's examination, diagnosis, and treatment.

Prolactin Hormone secreted by the pituitary gland that, in concert with progesterone, estrogen, and other hormones, stimulates milk formation.

Proliferative phase The second phase of wound healing, characterized by invasion of fibroblasts, formation of granulation tissue, deposition of collagen, epithelialization across healthy granulation tissue, and wound contraction by myofibroblasts.

Proprioceptive Activated by, or related to, stimuli that arise within an animal.

Prosector The person performing the necropsy.

Prosthesis Synthetic material used to replace some tissue or part of the body.

Prosthodontics A dental specialty that creates artificial teeth to replace missing or damaged teeth.

Prothrombin time (PT) Test used to evaluate extrinsic and common pathways of coagulation. This test requires citrated plasma and careful adherence to collection and processing requirements.

Protozoan (pl. protozoa) A unicellular (one-cell) organism.

Pruritic Itchy.

Pseudocyesis False pregnancy.

Pseudoparasite Object that is mistaken for a parasite.

Pseudopregnancy Anestrous state resembling pregnancy that occurs in various mammals, usually after an infertile copulation; pseudocyesis, false pregnancy.

Pulmonary artery Artery arising from the right ventricle that delivers blood into the pulmonary circulation.

Pulmonary edema Fluid buildup within the alveoli or interstitial spaces of the lung.

Pulp Soft tissue within the center of a tooth, consisting of cells, vessels, and nerves.

Pulse deficit As detected by simultaneous cardiac auscultation and pulse palpation, a condition wherein each audible heartbeat is not accompanied by a palpable pulse wave.

Pulse oximeter Instrument used to noninvasively measure the oxygen saturation of hemoglobin. This value serves as an indirect assessment of the animal's oxygenation status.

Pulse pressure The difference between systolic and diastolic pressures. This determines the intensity of the sensation when peripheral pulses are palpated.

Punishment Anything that decreases the future frequency, intensity, or duration of a behavior.

Pyometra Bacterial infection of the uterus with purulent fluid accumulation.

Pyrethrin A natural insecticide derived from plants that is used to control various ectoparasites.

Pyuria Refers to the presence of inflammatory cells (neutrophils) in urine.

Quality control (QC) Method or program that uses specific decision criteria or rules to determine whether an analytical test is producing accurate, consistent, and reliable results. QC uses control materials to determine whether a procedure is in control (performing acceptably) or out of control (failing to perform within acceptable control limits). A QC system is designed to detect problems before test results are transmitted to the clinician, thus avoiding implementation of treatment based on erroneous test results.

Quality of life Overall enjoyment of life and general well-being.

Rabies Viral disease spread by the saliva of infected animals, primarily through bite wounds. Human and animal vaccines are available and effective, but once symptoms of the disease appear in a patient, mortality is nearly 100%.

Radiographic contrast The difference in the density of two separate areas in a radiograph. Increased contrast between adjacent anatomical parts facilitates interpretation of the radiograph.

Radiographic density The level of darkening in various areas of the radiograph. Air density, for example, gives rise to the darkest parts of the radiograph. In contrast, a metal density gives rise to white regions in the film.

Radiographic detail The combined effect of radiographic contrast and definition.

Radiology information systems (RIS) The electronic management system of radiology departments; may include a variety of features such as patient scheduling, storage and retrieval of imaging files, veterinarian's interpretive findings, results distribution, and billing.

Raptorial species Of, related to, or being a bird of prey.

Ratchet Part of an instrument—usually located near the rings or handles—that allows the instrument to be maintained in one position after it has grasped or retracted the tissue.

RBC indices Measurements or calculations that are part of the complete blood count (CBC). Mean corpuscular volume (MCV) and mean corpuscular hemoglobin concentration (MCHC) are used to describe the average RBC volume and hemoglobin concentration, respectively. RBC indices may be useful in the classification of anemia.

Rebreathing system Breathing circuit in which exhaled gases are recirculated to the patient after carbon dioxide is removed.

Recent history Information about the current medical problem, including the presenting complaint and circumstances, date and location, and treatment.

Recumbency Lying down. This adjective indicates which part of the body is on the ground or table. For example, *lateral recumbency* means that the animal is lying on its side; *dorsal recumbency* means that the animal is lying on its back; and *sternal recumbency* means the animal is on its belly.

Red blood cells (RBCs) (also called erythrocytes) Circulating cells that contain hemoglobin to carry oxygen from lungs to tissues. In most mammals, RBCs are round and anucleate, although in camelids, RBCs are oval. In nonmammalian species, RBCs are oval and have nuclei.

Re-epithelialization Regrowth of epithelial cells over a wound. Cells advance in a single layer across the wound until they meet in the middle, when migration stops as the result of contact inhibition.

Referral facility Provides services by veterinarians with a special interest in certain species or a particular area of veterinary medicine.

Refractometer Instrument that measures the bending of light (angle of refraction) as it passes between liquid and air. Because the angle of refraction and the concentration of solutes are relatively linear, refractometry can be used to approximate total protein concentration in serum or plasma.

Regional nerve block Procedure whereby a relatively small amount of local anesthetic is injected near a nerve, causing desensitization to a larger area on the body. Proximal and distal paravertebral nerve blocks are examples of regional nerve blocks used to anesthetize the flank area.

Registered Veterinary Technologists and Technicians of Canada/Technologues et Techniciens Vétérinaires en Registrés du Canada (RVTTC) The national association of registered veterinary technician and technologists in Canada.

Regurgitation Flow of stomach contents into the esophagus and mouth unaccompanied by retching, as distinguished from vomiting, which occurs as forceful expulsion of stomach contents into the esophagus and mouth, preceded by retching.

Rehabilitation Restoration of health.

Reinforcement Anything that increases the future frequency, intensity, or duration of a behavior.

Relaxin Hormone secreted by the corpus luteum in the ovaries of pregnant animals. It relaxes the pubic symphysis, softens the cervix, and inhibits uterine contractions.

Renomegaly Enlargement of one or both kidneys.

Reperfusion injury Tissue injury resulting from the re-establishment of blood flow after a period of oxygen deprivation.

Repetitive behavior A repeated action or behavior in an animal, often an unwanted behavior, such as cribbing, wood sucking or chewing, stall walking and weaving, kicking stalls, and frequent pawing (also called stable vices). Some of these behaviors are true stereotypies: repetitive behaviors with no discernible, immediate function.

Replacement fluid rate Volume and rate of fluids needed to replenish fluid deficit and replace ongoing losses. Replacement fluid rate is equal to dehydration plus ongoing losses plus maintenance.

Residual activity Continued bactericidal activity that persists after antiseptic or disinfectant has been applied.

Resolution Stage during which there is no longer anger or depression but acceptance.

Respiratory minute volume (RMV) The amount of air that moves into and out of the lungs in a minute; tidal volume multiplied by respiratory rate.

Resting energy requirement (RER) Average amount of energy used by an animal while resting in a thermoneutral environment. The formula used to estimate RER for dogs and cats is $RER = 70 \times BW_{kg}^{0.75}$ kcal/day.

Reticulocyte Red blood cells (RBCs) stained with new methylene blue or other vital stains that form visible aggregates of ribosomal ribonucleic acid (RNA; reticulum). RBCs that contain reticulum are immature and are counted as an index of a bone marrow regenerative response to anemia.

Retroperitoneal Of or pertaining to the body cavity located behind the peritoneum, including structures such as the kidneys, which are found between the peritoneum and the body wall.

"Right to know" law A common name for the hazard communication standard of the Occupational Safety and Health Administration (OSHA). This standard requires an employer to inform employees when they may be exposed to hazardous chemicals while performing their duties and requires workers to wear prescribed safety equipment when using any product containing a hazardous chemical.

Ringworm Contagious fungal infection of the skin. Fungal spores of the genera *Trichophyton* and *Microsporum* are the most common causative agents.

Robert Jones bandage Distal limb bandage for which a large amount of rolled cotton is used; aids in immobilization of fractures. Rigid material can be incorporated into this bandage.

Rotating anode Anode plate in an x-ray tube that rotates around a stem made of molybdenum to aid in heat dissipation.

Roughage Coarse, bulky feeds, essential to the diets of ruminants and horses but largely indigestible if fed to species other than ruminants and horses. High in fiber, low in digestible carbohydrates and proteins.

Rouleaux formations Rouleaux formation refers to red blood cells (RBCs) in chains that resemble a stack of coins. In horses and cats, rouleaux formation is common, whereas in dogs, rouleaux formation may be an indication of inflammation or an artifact of smear preparation.

Rounds Scheduled one-on-one visit, at least once daily within the hospital setting with each patient to assess their progress and adjust treatment as needed for a positive outcome.

Rules and regulations Secondary mandates written by the state board.

Rule of Twos Method of determining whether some treatments may be given at another time, less frequently, or only as needed in an effort to keep patients calm. If a procedure requires more than 2 attempts, causes more than 2 seconds of intense struggling, or requires more than 2 arms on the animal to stabilize it, a different plan is preferable.

Rumen The first chamber of the ruminant digestive tract; used for storage of ingested food and initial digestion of protein and simple carbohydrates.

Rumen tympany Rumen distention with air, commonly referred to as *bloat*.

Rumenostomy Surgical procedure whereby a permanent hole is created from the skin into the rumen.

Rumenotomy Surgical incision into the rumen.

Safety data sheet (SDS) A system for cataloging important safety information regarding hazardous chemicals in the workplace. SDSs should be available to workers in the area where the chemicals are stored and should include product information regarding spill-safety procedures, toxicology information, and emergency procedures. SDS formats can vary from state to state.

Sarcopenia Age-related loss of muscle mass.

Sarcoptic mange Also called *scabies*, sarcoptic mange is a parasitic infestation of the skin of animals with the mite *Sarcoptes scabiei canis*. Common symptoms include hair loss, itching, and inflammation.

Scatter radiation Lower-energy x-ray photons that have undergone a change in direction after interacting with structures in the patient's body.

Schistosome A "blood fluke" that inhabits the blood vasculature of its definitive host.

Sciatic nerve Nerve that runs along the caudal aspect of the femur beneath the biceps. It is important to avoid this nerve when giving intramuscular injections.

Scrub in Disinfecting the hands and donning sterile gown and gloves to participate in a sterile procedure.

Scrub suit Shirt and pants worn into the operating room. Usually made of a lint-free cotton or polyester material.

Scutes The external scales covered with horn found on the feet of crocodilians and birds and on the shell of turtles.

Seasonally polyestrous Having repeated estrous cycles that occur during the breeding season of a species.

Second-degree burn The result of full-thickness epidermal and partial-thickness dermal injury. The epidermis can appear yellow-white, black, or charred and may slough and leak plasma; will usually heal by epithelialization with minimal scarring in 10 to 21 days, although some may require surgical intervention.

Second intention wound healing Healing of a wound by granulation tissue formation, epithelialization, and contraction.

Secondary closure Wound that has formed healthy granulation tissue and is then closed by apposing the skin over the granulation tissue.

Seed ticks The six-legged larval stages of ticks.

Segmented neutrophil A mature neutrophil with a segmented nucleus.

Selective medium Culture medium that reduces the growth of unwanted bacteria to allow the growth of other bacteria. MacConkey agar is selective because it inhibits the growth of gram-positive organisms.

Semi occlusive Allowing air and moisture to move through. Used in reference to bandage materials. A semi occlusive primary layer is used for moist wound healing.

Senescence The condition or process of deterioration with age.

Sensitization Occurs when the animal develops a stronger response over time to the same stimulus.

Sepsis A state of systemic inflammation characterized by deteriorating vital signs and the presence of infection.

Septicemia Invasion of the bloodstream by microorganisms (usually bacteria) from a focus of infection. It is accompanied by fever, chills, prostration, pain, nausea, and diarrhea.

Seroma Sterile fluid accumulation beneath an incision after surgery.

Serous Of, related to, producing, or resembling serum.

Shock A condition of decreased perfusion and decreased oxygen delivery to vital organs.

Spica splint A splint that maintains the forelimb or the pelvic limb in extension through application of a soft, padded bandage and a strong lateral support splint that curves over the shoulder or pelvis.

Sievert (Sv) A measure of the health effect of low levels of ionizing radiation on the human body. The Sievert has the same units as the Gray and is equal to the absorbed dose times the quality factor, which compares the health consequences of that type of radiation with those of x-rays.

Signalment Information about a veterinary patient, including its name, age, sex, breed, species, electronic ID, reproductive status, color, and distinctive markings.

Simultaneous conditioning One of the four different timing options for pairing stimuli during classical conditional or counterconditioning; method in which the conditioned and unconditioned stimulus are presented at the same time.

Sinusitis An infection of the sinuses of the head.

SOAP Acronym for **s**ubjective, **o**bjective, **a**ssessment, and **p**lan (SOAP); the format for recording each visit or examination used to evaluate hospitalized or sick patients.

Social hierarchy Social structure that allows for division of resources, rights, and privileges. Animals in higher social positions tend to have priority access to resources. However, social hierarchies are flexible, not absolute. Hierarchies can change over time and can be different in different contexts; they vary according to the specific individuals that make up the hierarchy.

Socialization Process by which an animal develops appropriate social behaviors toward members of its own and other species. The process of socialization requires providing to the young animal pleasant experiences with people, situations, inanimate elements of the environment, and other animals.

Societies Organizations formed by veterinary technicians who share a common interest in a particular aspect of veterinary technology.

Source image distance The distance between the beam of the x-ray and the spot where the image is formed. Distortion and magnification may be controlled or enhanced by managing the distance while taking images.

Source-oriented veterinary medical record (SOVMR) Record keeping system that enters medical information from multiple sources in chronologic order and is organized by subject matter.

Sparganosis A zoonotic condition resulting from a second intermediate host (sometimes a human) becoming infected with the plerocercoid or sparganum in the life cycle of a pseudotapeworm. Sparganosis is a condition that is commonly associated with the pseudotapeworm, *Spirometra mansonoides*.

Sparganum See **Plerocercoid**.

Specialty facility A veterinary or animal facility that provides services by board-certified veterinarians/specialists.

Specific gravity (SG) The ratio of the density of a fluid to the density of pure water. SG depends on both the number and the molecular weight of solutes found in the solution. SG is used as an indicator of solute concentration in the urine and, by extension, the concentrating ability of the kidney.

Spectrophotometry Measurement of the amount of light that a substance absorbs. Spectrophotometers are instruments that pass a beam of light of a specific wavelength through a substance, such as serum or plasma. The amount of light that passes through the sample is then measured by a photodetector. Typically, an analyte will absorb some of the photons from the light beam, thus reducing the light that reaches the detector in proportion to the quantity of analyte present in the sample.

Spherocytes Red blood cells (RBCs) that lack a central zone of pallor and appear slightly smaller and denser than normal RBCs. Spherocytes result from binding of antibody to the RBC surface and removal of a portion of cell membrane by macrophages in the spleen. This occurs most commonly in immune-mediated hemolytic anemia.

Spica splint Full-limb bandage, including a lateral splint that reaches over the shoulder or hip, that is used to aid in immobilization.

Stationary anode Anode block in an x-ray tube that does not move and is embedded in copper to aid in heat dissipation. Found exclusively in portable equipment used in field work.

Steady state After repeated drug dosing, a drug's plasma concentration reaches steady state (or stable concentration in the blood) when the amount of drug administered equals the amount of drug eliminated.

Stenotic nares A constriction or narrowing of one or both nares, may or may not be due to an obstruction.

Sterile field An area that has been prepared for the use of sterile equipment. This includes the area around the wound, incision site, or body orifice into which an instrument or catheter will be passed. It also includes the area covered by sterile drapes and the sterile region of properly attired personnel.

Sterile technique Creating a sterile field and working within it by not contaminating it with nonsterile objects.

Sterilization The elimination or destruction of all living organisms (including disease-producing organisms such as viruses) from a material.

Sternum The breastbone. The series of rod like bones called *sternebrae* that form the floor of the thorax.

Stertor Inspiratory noise similar to snoring, usually caused by obstruction to airflow at the pharynx or larynx.

Stocks Vertical metal or wooden pillars, arranged in a rectangular shape and connected by horizontal bars, designed to restrain horses or cattle standing within.

Strangulation Encircling of a tissue with suture or internal structures (e.g., slipping of bowel into a hernia or through scar tissue) such that blood supply to the tissue is lost and death of the tissues ensues unless the tissue is released and blood flow can resume.

Stranguria The act of straining to urinate.

Strategic planning An organization's process for defining or updating its vision, mission, and strategy, and allocating resources toward achievement of these goals.

Stress Any pressure or strain placed on a system. If pressure is great enough or persistent enough, for example, an animal that is unable to escape from a fear-inducing stimulus, constant stimulation of the hypothalamic-pituitary-adrenal axis (HPA) can lead to immune suppression and increased susceptibility to disease. Animals that experience frequent frustration or conflict are likely to be stressed.

Stridor A harsh, high-pitched respiratory sound, usually caused by obstruction of airflow at the pharynx or larynx.

Strike-through When fluid penetrates a surgical drape or gown, it creates a pathway by which organisms can invade the sterile field.

Subchondral bone The bone that lies just beneath joint cartilage.

Superfecundation Successive fertilization of ova involving multiple episodes of coitus during the same heat. Fertilization is provided by different males.

Superfetation Fertilization of two or more ova in the same female during different heats. In this way, a pregnant dam may ovulate and become pregnant a second time.

Swaged Squeezed on, as with a suture needle onto suture.

Syncope Fainting.

Systemic inflammatory response syndrome (SIRS) Widespread inflammation caused by an underlying disease process. Often causes generalized tissue damage and can be a complication of shock.

Tachycardia Rapid heart rate; the opposite of bradycardia.

Tachypnea Fast, shallow breathing.

Tachyzoite Literally "a fast-growing, tiny organism." This is a term for a tissue stage, for example, a fast-growing developmental stage that occurs in cysts in the life cycle of *Toxoplasma gondii.*

Tail tie Restraint of an equine or bovine tail by tying a quick-release knot in the switch and tying the free end to the animal, often around its neck.

Technician assessment Clinical judgment that the veterinary technician makes regarding the physiologic and psychological problems and needs of a patient. The technician assessment comprises the "A" portion of the veterinary technician SOAP—the list of technician evaluations arranged in order of priority with reference to the psychological and physiologic needs of the patient.

Technician evaluation The second phase of the veterinary technician practice model. Conclusions drawn from patient assessment and analysis of the database related to the animal's (or the owner's) physical and psychological response to a veterinary medical condition.

Technician intervention The third phase of the veterinary technician practice model. An action planned and implemented by the veterinary technician using independent critical thinking to address a patient's reaction to illness and risk for future problems, as well as owner knowledge deficits. Typically, a technician intervention is carried out to address each of the technician evaluations.

Teleradiology Transmission of digital images from one hospital to the next via computer cable connections. Teleradiology allows rapid turnaround in assessment of images and improves access to expert opinions on patient findings.

Tenesmus Distressing but ineffectual urge to evacuate the rectum or urinary bladder.

Teratogen Agent or substance that may cause physical defects in a developing embryo when a pregnant female is exposed to that substance.

Therapeutic blood level Range of concentrations of a drug in the bloodstream at which the drug is expected to have the desired effect.

Therapeutic drug monitoring Periodic measurement of the amount of a drug in blood.

Therapeutic ultrasonography Penetrating tissue through high-frequency sound waves to decrease pain and improve healing of tissues.

Thermotherapy The use of heat for rehabilitation purposes such as pain relief, decreasing inflammation, calming muscle spasms, and increasing blood flow. Thermotherapy may include the application of hot cloths or water bottles, ultrasound, heating pads, hot baths, whirlpool therapy, and heat wraps to the body to reduce pain.

Third-degree burn Full-thickness injuries of the epidermis and deep-layer dermis, characterized by a thick, leathery, black layer of dead tissue called eschar, that are insensitive to the touch. Treatment may require surgical interventions, wound debridement, and skin grafts; can be life-threatening.

Third-intention wound healing Healing of a wound that has already formed granulation tissue and undergone secondary closure.

Thoracocentesis A procedure in which air or fluid is removed from the chest (pleural space), using a syringe and needle aseptically.

Three-host tick An individual tick that will feed on three individual animals or three different species of animal.

Thrombocytopenia Occurs as a decrease in the number of platelets in the blood.

Thromboembolism Formation of a blood clot that lodges in or obstructs a blood vessel.

Thrombophlebitis Inflammation of the vein associated with a thrombus.

Thrombosis Clotting of blood within a vessel that results in obstruction of blood flow.

Tidal volume The volume of a normal breath (≈10–15 mL/kg body weight).

Tortoise A land turtle.

Total digestible nutrients (TDNs) Term that indicates the energy value of a feedstuff. TDN is calculated by using the following formula % TDN = % DCP + % DCF + % DNFE + (%DEE × 2.25), where DCP = digestible crude protein, DCF = digestible crude fiber, DNFE = digestible nitrogen-free extract, and DEE = digestible ether extract.

Touch Gradient A method of touching animals in a systematic and sensitive way to decrease fear, anxiety, and stress during handling. Consists of two main components: maintaining continuous hands-on contact with the patient throughout the entire procedure or examination, and acclimating the patient to increasing levels of touch intensity while continuously measuring the patient's acceptance and comfort.

Toxic change Occurs when several morphologic abnormalities indicate intense stimulation of neutrophil production and shortened maturation time. Toxic changes include Döhle bodies, cytoplasmic basophilia and vacuolation, toxic granules and nuclear vacuolation, hyposegmentation, ring formation, and fragmentation. Rarely, formation of giant neutrophils occurs.

Toxicosis (pl. toxicoses) Any disease of toxic origin; a pathological condition caused by the action of a poison or toxin.

Toxin A poisonous substance that is a specific product of the metabolic activities of a living organism and is usually very unstable.

Toxoid A toxin that has been altered so that it does not cause disease but is able to induce the production of protective antibodies. The immunogenicity, however, remains intact and makes toxoids suitable for use as vaccines. Immunizations against tetanus and botulism are examples of toxoids.

Toxoplasmosis Infestation with a single-celled parasite called *Toxoplasma gondii.* Toxoplasmosis is a disease of concern primarily for pregnant women and for people with compromised immune systems.

Trace conditioning One of the four different timing options for pairing stimuli during classical conditional or counterconditioning; method in which a conditioned stimulus and an unconditioned stimulus are presented following each other, but separated by a gap.

Tracheostomy Surgical creation of a hole from the skin to the trachea.

Tracheotomy Surgical act of making an incision on the ventral aspect of the neck and opening a direct airway through an incision in the trachea.

Trade name The name of a drug or pharmaceutical used by a particular manufacturer. For example, atorvastatin is the generic name for the same drug called Lipitor by Viatris.

Traffic flow Pattern of movement of patients through the practice (e.g., reception to examination room, ward to reception).

Transcutaneous electrical nerve stimulation (TENS) The therapeutic use of electric currents to stimulate nerves. It typically involves the use of a hand-held, battery-operated unit that can modulate pulse width, frequency, and intensity. The unit is usually connected to the skin using two or more electrodes.

Transduction Conversion of unpleasant stimuli into nerve signals at the point of injury.

Transfaunation Transfer of beneficial microorganisms from the rumen of one individual to that of another.

Transfusion reaction Adverse events that occur as a result of receiving a transfusion.

Transmission The sending of pain signals via nerve fibers to the spinal cord.

Transport media Media that maintains bacteria in original concentrations without encouraging growth or causing death of the bacteria.

Trauma exposure The exposure to an event that is considered traumatic such as death, threatened death, actual or threatened injury or sexual or other violence.

Trematode Digenetic fluke. See **Digenetic fluke.**

Trephination A historical ancient surgical procedure in which holes are created in the skull often to relieve pressure; also referred to as "burr holing", it is commonly used for the release of pressure in fingernails and toenails in human medicine.

Triadan system Tooth numbering system applicable to multiple veterinary species.

Triage The act of sorting patients quickly into groups on the basis of a rapid initial assessment of disease or injury severity.

Triangulation Technique used in laparoscopic and arthroscopic surgery that establishes two reference points—one using the scope and the other the surgical hand instrument—to target a third point, the surgical site. This enables the surgeon to visualize the site of interest while at the same time manipulating surgical instruments inside a body cavity to make surgical corrections.

Trombicula species Chiggers. The six-legged larval chigger is the only stage of this mite that is parasitic. Chiggers are periodic parasites that attach to the skin of their hosts. Their salivary secretions liquefy the host tissue, which is sucked up by the feeding larval mite.

Trophozoite Literally, "a tiny, moving organism"; defined as fast-growing organisms in developmental stages occurring as cysts in the life cycle of *Toxoplasma gondii* and other similar apicomplexan parasites.

Tube cystostomy Surgical procedure in which a Foley catheter is placed through the abdominal wall and into the bladder. The catheter allows urine to drain passively from the bladder while urolithiasis is managed.

Tumor grade Microscopic assessment of the degree to which particular cancer cells are similar in appearance and function to normal cells of the same tissue type. In general, cancer cells that differ markedly from normal cells or are poorly differentiated (high grade) have a more malignant clinical behavior.

Tumor stage Clinical assessment of how much cancer a patient has (volume of disease) and how much it has spread. Tumor stage is determined by the results of diagnostic tests, such as blood work, radiography, and tissue biopsy. The tumor stage considers the size and degree of invasion of the primary tumor, whether it has metastasized to any lymph nodes, and whether it has spread to distant organs. In general, the higher or more advanced the tumor stage, the worse the patient's prognosis.

Turtles Any of an order (Testudinata) of land, freshwater, and marine reptiles that have a toothless, horny beak and a shell of bony dermal plates, usually covered with horny shields, enclosing the trunk and into which the head, limbs, and tail usually may be withdrawn.

Twitch Device used in restraining horses; consists of a wooden handle and a chain loop or rope loop that is twisted around a horse's nose; it is believed that the nose is a pressure point and, once it is squeezed by the twitch, endorphins are released, relaxing the horse.

Two-host tick An individual tick that will feed on two individual animals or two different species of animal during its life cycle.

Tympany Hollow sound produced when a body cavity containing air is sharply tapped.

US Department of Agriculture (USDA) Government agency that regulates veterinary biologics (vaccines, antitoxins, and diagnostics that are used to prevent, treat, or diagnose animal diseases).

US Food and Drug Administration (FDA) Government agency charged with ensuring the safety and efficacy of human and animal drugs and the safety of cosmetics, foods, and other consumer items.

US Pharmacopoeia (USP)–National Formulary (NF) The official legal drug compendium for the United States. A compilation of all drug substances and products focused on providing active ingredients.

Unilocular hydatid cyst A single hydatid cyst formed by an *Echinococcosis*-type tapeworm.

Unwanted behavior Action or behavior by an animal that is undesirable to humans and that can damage or sever the human-animal bond. Many unwanted behaviors are normal for the species but may be objectionable to humans.

Unwanted elimination An unwanted behavior involving the act of urination and/or defecation at inappropriate locations and times.

Urachus A remnant of the fetal allantois that drains the fetal urinary bladder and exits the fetal abdomen via the umbilical cord.

Urethral process The portion of the urethra that extends beyond the end of the glans penis in the male goat, sheep, and horse.

Urethrostomy A surgical procedure that creates a permanent opening in the urethra. The procedure is most commonly performed in male cats that have a history of multiple urethral blockages. In this species, a urethrostomy is made in the perineum.

Urine specific gravity Laboratory test showing the number and molecular weight of particles in urine used as an indicator of the concentrating ability of the kidney; measured with a refractometer.

Urolithiasis The process of forming stones in the urinary tract.

Uterine prolapse Condition that occurs when the uterus folds inside out through an open cervix and protrudes through the vulvar lips.

Uterine torsion Condition in which the uterus twists, preventing delivery of the fetus. Uterine torsion occurs in cattle and in camelids and can be a cause of dystocia.

Validation Process of understanding and expressing acceptance of another person's emotional state.

Vasodilatation Dilatation of the blood vessels; the opposite of vasoconstriction.

Velpeau sling Nonweight-bearing forelimb sling that flexes the entire limb; primarily used for medial shoulder luxation.

Ventricular premature complexes Premature contraction of the ventricles, initiated by one of the ventricles from a location other than the normal cardiac conduction system.

Ventricular tachycardia An abnormally high heart rate initiated and sustained by one of the ventricles outside the normal cardiac conduction system.

Vesicant Agent that causes tissue destruction or necrosis on extravasation.

Veterinarian A graduate of an accredited school of veterinary medicine. Veterinarians typically complete 4 years of undergraduate study and acquire a bachelor's degree before completing an additional 4 years of postgraduate study in veterinary medicine.

Veterinarian-client-patient relationship (VCPR) Set of requirements that must be met for a veterinarian to use a prescription or a veterinary feed directive drug.

Veterinary assistant The adjectives "animal," "veterinary," "ward," and "hospital," combined with the nouns "attendant," "caretaker," and "assistant," are titles sometimes used for individuals involved in the care of animals whose training, knowledge, and skills are less than those required for a veterinary technician, laboratory animal technician, or veterinarian. They are responsible for assisting the veterinary technician and the veterinarian and are trained on the job or complete 4 to 6 months of training.

Veterinary medical databases National data banks that include medical data supplied by veterinary medical schools to assist in conducting retrospective studies and in predicting clinical outcomes. They are often used to teach veterinary students.

Veterinary nurse A paraprofessional providing supportive care to animals treated within a veterinary facility, clinic, or institution. Often this term is synonymous with the term veterinary technologist or veterinary technician.

Veterinary physical rehabilitation Physical therapy and rehabilitation for animals, particularly dogs. Veterinary physical rehabilitation is adapted from human physical therapy and is used to increase the rate of healing and functionality postoperatively, following injury, or during disease processes that adversely affect mobility.

Veterinary practice Modern veterinary practices are often owned by corporations or teams of veterinarians and often employ many veterinarians and a staff of veterinary technicians, assistants, receptionists, and kennel workers. Practices can also be privately owned or be specialty or referral practices that employ veterinarians who have completed advanced, specialized training in a particular aspect of veterinary medicine or surgery.

Veterinary spinal manipulative therapy The practice of chiropractic medicine on animals. It involves manipulation and alignment of the spinal column to remove vertebral subluxations that may hamper optimal neural transmission through the spinal cord and peripheral nerves. Pain caused by muscle spasms and decreased function of organs are thought to be caused by subluxations of the spine. Veterinary spinal manipulative therapy is performed primarily on horses, dogs, and cats.

Veterinary teaching hospital A facility at which consultative, clinical, and hospital services are rendered and in which a large staff of basic and applied veterinary scientists perform significant research and teach professional veterinary students (DVM or equivalent degree) and house officers.

Veterinary technician Carries out the veterinary technician practice model and completes all patient care duties except those exclusive to the practice of veterinary medicine. Veterinary technicians are graduates of American Veterinary Medical Association (AVMA)-accredited programs of veterinary technology and have successfully completed the Veterinary Technician National Examination.

Veterinary technician evaluation The assessment portion of SOAP where a veterinary technician lists the patient's physical, psychological, social, and environmental conditions, with the patient's most important needs listed first, followed by the less critical needs in decreasing order of importance.

Veterinary Technician National Examination (VTNE) A national examination for veterinary technicians required in most US states and Canadian provinces.

Veterinary technician practice model Serves as the foundation for the practice of veterinary technology and includes a series of prescribed steps taken by veterinary technicians engaged in patient care. These include the following:

1. Gather data about the patient.
2. Identify and prioritize patient evaluations.
3. Develop and implement a plan for patient care by establishing a series of veterinary nursing interventions.

4. Evaluate the patient's response to the plan of care.
5. Gather additional data (go back to step 1 and re-evaluate the patient).

Veterinary technician specialist (VTS) Credentialed veterinary technician who has completed the requirements established by the Committee on Veterinary Technician Specialties (CVTS), such as graduating from an AVMA-accredited program and completing the education and training required by the respective academy of specialists.

Veterinary technologist A graduate of a 4-year baccalaureate American Veterinary Medical Association (AVMA)-accredited program in veterinary technology.

Veterinary technology The science and art of providing professional support to veterinarians. The American Veterinary Medical Association (AVMA) accredits programs in veterinary technology that graduate veterinary technicians and/or veterinary technologists.

Visceral larval migrans (VLM) Zoonotic condition caused by ingesting an egg containing an infective, second-stage larva of a roundworm (usually *Toxocara canis*). These larvae migrate from the host's intestine and travel throughout the visceral organs, usually the liver and/or the lungs.

Vomiting The act of expelling the contents (often undigested) from the stomach through the mouth.

Walk-in system A approach for veterinary or medical care that does not involve pre-arranged appointments and is often associated with clinics or emergency facilities.

Waste anesthetic gas (WAG) Gas used in inhalation anesthetic machines that is not metabolized by the patient and is given off in respiration.

Watts (W) per unit time (seconds) A unit of power in the International System of Units that is defined as 1 joule per second. The watt (symbol: W) is named after the Scottish engineer James Watt (1736–1819).

White blood cells (also called *leukocytes*) A series of cells that lack hemoglobin and therefore appear to be clear under the microscope. Though fewer in number than red blood cells, they are larger and play a vital role in protecting the body from microinvaders.

Wind-up phenomenon Alterations in the nervous system (hyperalgesia and allodynia) that occur when the central nervous system is bombarded by persistent pain impulses, altering pain processing and causing untreated or inadequately treated pain, leading to untreatable pain states (nonresponsive or chronic intractable pain); also known as *central sensitization*.

Withdrawal time The time required for a drug and its residue to be cleared from the meat or milk of an animal used for human consumption.

Working problem list List of a patient's problems pertinent to the current hospital stay that is often used to assist the veterinary health care team to work through current problems.

X-ray Form of electromagnetic radiation that can be used in diagnostic imaging to produce radiographs or computed tomographic images.

Yeasts Unicellular fungal organisms that reproduce by budding.

Zone of inhibition In agar plates, the clear region around the paper disk saturated with an antimicrobial agent. The region indicates that the antimicrobial agent contained in the disk was successful in inhibiting microbial growth.

Zoonosis Any disease that is transmissible from lower animals to humans (e.g., rabies, plague, trichinosis). *Visceral larva migrans* caused by *Toxocara canis* is a zoonotic condition that may be transmitted from dogs to humans.

Zoonotic disease Disease that is common to both animals and humans; often describes a disease that is easily transmissible between animals and humans.

Index

A

Abdomen, acute, 788, 789b
Abdominal aorta, necropsy examination, 483
Abdominal auscultation, in horses, 231–232, 231f, 232b
Abdominal cavity
    fluid evaluation, 623
    necropsy examination, 481
Abdominal exploration, emergency, 804, 804b
Abdominal palpation, 218–219
    per rectum, in horses, 803, 803b
Abdominal pinging, 235
Abdominal surgery, 1094–1098
    draping for, 1043–1044, 1044f–1045f
    incision, 1037–1038, 1038f
    preoperative preparation for, 1031, 1032f–1033f
Abdominocentesis, 1054
    emergency, 779, 779f, 803, 804t
    in large animals, 561–565, 561b, 562f
      horses, 803, 804t
    in small animals, 515
Abducens nerve, 222–223, 223t
Abomasal displacements and volvulus, in cattle, 1117–1118
Abomasum, 485
Abrasions, 845
Abscesses
    skin, 408t–409t
    subsolar, 1108
    swabs, 407
Absorbable sutures, 1041
Absorbed dose, 449–450
Absorption, drug, 894–895, 894f
Abuse, animal, 25
Academy of Veterinary Behavior Technicians (AVBT), 119t
Acanthocephalans, 373
Acanthocytes, 347
Acariasis, 374–375
Accelerated idioventricular rhythm (AIVR), 797–798, 798f
Accessory nerve, 222–223, 223t
Accounts receivable, 35, 37, 60, 66
Accreditation Policies and Procedures Handbook, 5
ACE inhibitors, 891t

Acepromazine, 145t–146t, 934
Acetaminophen, 836–837, 837b, 913
Acid-fast bacteria, 421, 421b
Acid-fast staining, 412–414, 413b–414b
Acidosis, 774
Acids, in cleaning agents, 828–829, 829b
Aciduric urine, 367
Acoustic enhancement, ultrasound, 461
Acoustic nerve, 223t
Acquired chronic kidney disease, 589
Acquired myasthenia gravis, 595
Actinobacillus spp., 421
Actinomyces spp., 420
Activated charcoal, 825–826
Activated clotting time (ACT), 353–354
Activated partial thromboplastin time (APTT), 354
Active drains, 844–845, 1039, 1039b, 1040f
Active immunity, 240, 240b
Active prevention, and intervention, 139
Acupressure, 743–744, 744f
Acupuncture, 673, 742–745
    cautions and contraindications, 745, 745b
    clinical indications, 744–745
    definition and mechanisms of action, 742–743
    methods of stimulation, 743–744, 744f–745f
    points, 743
Acute abdomen, 788, 789b
Acute enteritis, 586t
Acute gastritis, 586t
Acute radiation toxicity, 662, 662f
Acute renal failure, 616
Acute tumor lysis syndrome (ATLS), 671
Ad lib (free) feeding, 272, 272b
Adamantanes, 898t
Addison disease, 594, 887
Additives
    fluid therapy, 760–761
    pet food, 278, 285
Adenoma, 657
Adjuvant therapy, 661
    to vaccines, 240
Adrenal disease, drugs for, 887, 887b
Adriamycin. *See* Doxorubicin
Adrucil. *See* Fluorouracil

Adsorbent, 825
Advance directives, 1201
Advanced life support, 784–785, 785b
Adverse drug reactions, 896, 896b
Advertising, 55
Advocacy, 1203, 1203b, 1205b
Aelurostrongylus abstrusus, 391–392, 392f, 392b
Aerobic and anaerobic swabs, 407
Aeromonas, 421
Afoxolaner, 886t
Agar gel immunodiffusion (AGID), 364
Age/sex terminology
    for horses, 225t
    for ruminants, 225t
Agglutination, 344, 345f, 764
Aggression. *See also* Restraint
    animal behavior problems and, 118
    in cats, 142–143, 143b
      fear-related, 144
      during play, 144
      preventable aggressive behavior, 142–143
    in dogs
      fear-related, 144
      play-related, 144
    in horses, 149–150
      toward humans, 150
AGID. *See* Agar gel immunodiffusion
Aging
    drug pharmacokinetics and, 897
    effects on organ systems, 1177–1180
    physiologic changes associated with, 1176–1177, 1177b
    process, 1175–1176, 1176f, 1176b
Agonists, 896, 915, 933
Alanine aminotransferase (ALT), 360
Alcohols, as disinfectants, 1011
Aldehyde, 1012
Alfaxalone, 937, 963
Alignment and reduction, long bone fractures, 1088
Alkalis, 829, 829b
Alkaluric urine, 367
Alkeran. *See* Melphalan
Allantois, 331
Allergies
    food, 283
    history, 209

Page numbers followed by "f" indicate figures, "t" indicate tables, and "b" indicate boxes.